Don't Go

TO THE

Cosmetics Counter Without Me

8th Edition

A unique, professionally sourced guide to thousands
of skin-care and makeup products from today's
hottest brands. Shop smarter, look beautiful, and
discover which products really work!

PAULA BEGOUN
The Cosmetics Cop
with Bryan Barron

Contributing Author: Bryan Barron
Editors: John Hopper, Stephanie Parsons, Jill Irwin
Art Direction, Cover Design, and Typography: Erin Smith Bloom,
    Beginning Press
Printing: RR Donnelley
Research Director: Daynah Burnett
Research Assistant: Brooke Young

Copyright © 2010, Paula Begoun
Publisher: Beginning Press
            1030 SW 34th Street, Suite A
            Renton, Washington 98057

Eighth Edition Printing: January 2010

ISBN: 978-1-877988-34-9
10 9 8 7 6 5 4 3 2 1

This book is distributed to the United States book trade by:

Publishers Group West
1700 Fourth Street
Berkeley, California 94710
(800) 788-3123

And to the Canadian book trade by:

Raincoast Books Limited
9050 Shaughnessy Street
Vancouver, British Columbia, V6P 6E5 CANADA
(604) 633-5714

And in Australia and New Zealand by:

Peribo Pty Limited
58 Beaumont Road
Mount Kuring-gai NSW 2080 AUSTRALIA
Tel: (02) 9457 0011

BEAUTYPEDIA.COM
YOUR ULTIMATE SOURCE FOR
COSMETIC PRODUCT REVIEWS

Free Content
A selection of free reviews and free access to Paula's extensive Cosmetic Ingredient Dictionary

Searchable Database
Search reviews from over 260 cosmetic lines.

Subscribe Today
Subscribers have complete access to over 45,000 product reviews, full ingredient lists for all skin-care products, plus concise information that lets you shop for only the best products!

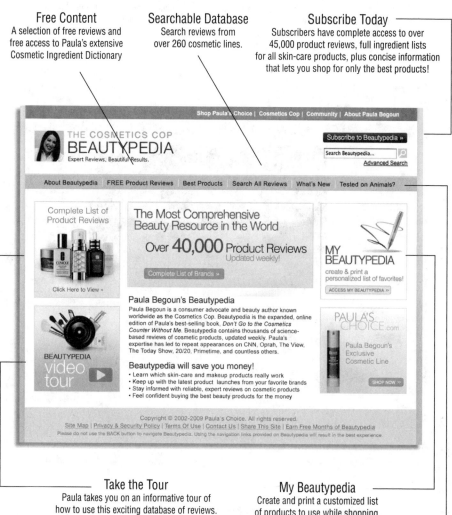

Take the Tour
Paula takes you on an informative tour of how to use this exciting database of reviews.

My Beautypedia
Create and print a customized list of products to use while shopping.

Hundreds of Brands Reviewed
Find out if the brand you're interested in has been reviewed.

Animal Testing Report Card
Find out if your favorite brands are tested on animals.

COSMETICSCOP.COM
SUPERIOR SKIN-CARE & EXPERT INFORMATION

Shop
Learn about Paula's state-of-the-art skin-care products. Whether your concern is acne, wrinkles, dry skin, or anything in-between, we have the best products to choose from.

FREE email Beauty Bulletins
Sign up for Paula's Beauty Bulletins and enjoy free product reviews, informative articles, and more.

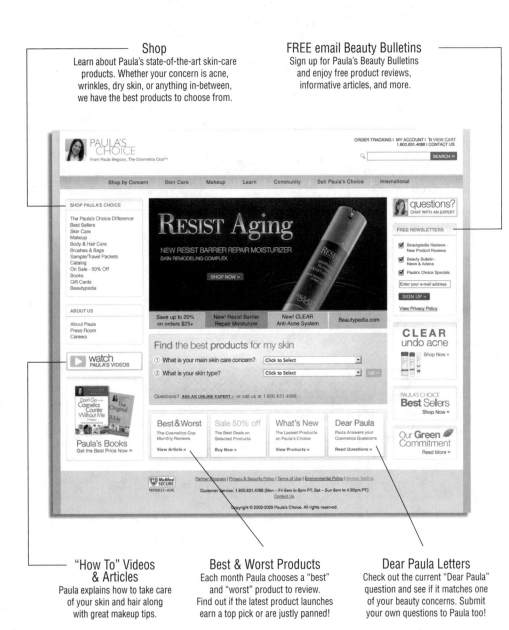

"How To" Videos & Articles
Paula explains how to take care of your skin and hair along with great makeup tips.

Best & Worst Products
Each month Paula chooses a "best" and "worst" product to review. Find out if the latest product launches earn a top pick or are justly panned!

Dear Paula Letters
Check out the current "Dear Paula" question and see if it matches one of your beauty concerns. Submit your own questions to Paula too!

FROM THE PUBLISHER

Paula Begoun is the best-selling author of *Don't Go to the Cosmetics Counter Without Me*, *The Original Beauty Bible*, *Don't Go Shopping for Hair Care Products Without Me*, and *Blue Eyeshadow Should Be Illegal*. She has sold millions of books, educating women about the facts and secrets the beauty industry doesn't want them to know. Paula also spearheaded the creation of the world's most extensive database of product reviews at www.Beautypedia.com.

Paula is nationally recognized as a consumer advocate, covering the cosmetics industry. She is called upon regularly by reporters and producers from television, newspapers, magazines, and radio as a cosmetics industry expert. She has appeared on hundreds of talk shows over the years, including *The View*, *Dateline NBC*, *Good Morning America*, *20/20*, *Today*, *Later Today*, *CBS Morning News*, *Hard Copy*, *Canada AM*, and National Public Radio, and has made more than a dozen appearances on *Oprah*. Today, with the success of Paula's Web sites, www.CosmeticsCop.com and www.Beautypedia.com, women all over the world consider Paula the most reliable source for straightforward information about all their beauty questions.

In 1996 Ms. Begoun launched her own line of skin-care products, called Paula's Choice. This distinctive line of products, available online at www.paulaschoice.com, is renowned for its effectiveness and ease of use. While Paula is proud of her line, she realizes that there are vast numbers of product options for women to consider. As a result, she continues to provide her readers with substantiated and documented studies and analysis about skin-care and makeup products from other lines based on her extensive research and years of experience. In her reviews and critiques, it is clear that Paula continues to maintain her evenhanded approach to offering readers an unprecedented assortment of smart choices for their cosmetic purchases.

PUBLISHER'S DISCLAIMER

The intent of this book is to present the author's ideas and perceptions about the marketing, selling, and use of cosmetics. The author's sole purpose is to present consumer information and advice regarding the purchase of makeup and skin-care products. The information and recommendations presented strictly reflect the author's opinions, perceptions, and knowledge about the subject and products mentioned. Some women may find success with a particular product that is not recommended or even mentioned in this book, or they may be partial to a skin-care routine Paula has reviewed negatively. It is everyone's unalienable right to judge products by their own criteria and to disagree with the author.

More important, because everyone's skin can, and probably will, react to an external stimulus at some time, any product can cause a negative reaction on skin at one time or another. If you develop skin sensitivity to a cosmetic, stop using it immediately and consult your physician. If you need medical advice about your skin, it is best to consult a dermatologist.

ACKNOWLEDGMENTS

There are no words that can adequately express the challenge and commitment required for writing a book of this scope and nature. The energy and resourcefulness needed to research, compile, review, write, and edit a 1,000+ page book is an almost endless undertaking. If it were not for my team of Bryan Barron, Daynah Burnett, and Brooke Young, this book would not have been possible. Their perseverance and devotion to completing the project go beyond anything I could have hoped for. Not only did they meet deadline after deadline, they did it with an accuracy and exactness that exceeded my every expectation. Without their feedback, patience, and contributions, this book would have been a very good idea but an absolutely unconquerable task.

DEDICATION FROM CO-AUTHOR BRYAN BARRON

This book is dedicated to my partner, Benjamin Coles. In the three years he has been a part of my life, I have not only discovered the type of relationship I've always wanted but a stronger sense of self and purpose. Our relationship has truly made me a better person. The happiness and contentment he adds to my life translates to every part of it, including my work on this book. Ben is a constant source of love, support, enthusiasm, and understanding—qualities I hope everyone who reads this book has the privilege to experience in their own lives.

CHAPTER SIX—THE BEST PRODUCTS

CHAPTER SEVEN—
COSMETIC INGREDIENT DICTIONARY ONLINE

CHAPTER ONE

Why You Need a Cosmetics Cop!

The cosmetics industry is a jungle of products and you need someone with experience to help you get through it. As was true for all previous editions of this book, this one covers many of the new lines that have appeared, while many of the previously included lines have been entirely re-reviewed, critiqued, and balanced against current studies to make sure that our analysis reflects the most current research about ingredient efficacy, performance, and product integrity.

If you've ever felt uncertain about a product, or are too short of time or energy to figure out for yourself which foundations are too pink or too orange, which eyeshadows are too shiny or too difficult to use, which powders go on too chalky, which cleansers are too greasy, which toners are too harsh, what makes one moisturizer different from another, or how wrinkle creams differ, then, yes, you need (and will benefit from) this book. As you read the various skin-care and makeup reviews, you will start to get a better understanding of how the cosmetics industry really works. I've also included a summary chapter of best finds and best buys, but don't jump to that one first. It is important to read the individual product assessments and criteria so you understand exactly what standards we used to evaluate each particular category.

Skin-care products were evaluated almost entirely by analyzing the ingredient list (as regulated by regulatory boards around the world) and comparing the ingredients listed to the claims made about the product. For example, if a toner asserts that it is designed for sensitive skin, it should not contain ingredients that irritate skin. If a moisturizer claims it can hydrate the skin, it should contain ingredients that can do just that. If an antiwrinkle product claims it contains a special ingredient that can eliminate wrinkles, we searched medical and biomedical journals to find support, or a lack thereof, for those claims. In addition, I make a point of challenging the inflated claims made about myriad ingredients. I also explain why seemingly impressive-sounding ingredients might indeed benefit the skin or might hurt the skin, and I often elaborate on the validity or usefulness of a specific ingredient or combination of ingredients. In short, the skin-care reviews separate the state-of-the-art products from the so-so and the "Oh, no!" products found in line after line after line, often citing the published research used to make the assessment.

For the makeup reviews, each product is described in terms of its performance, value, texture, application, and effect. Within every category of product—foundations, mascaras, blushes, eyeshadows, concealers, powders, lipsticks, brushes, and pencils—my team and I established specific criteria, and we evaluated the products based on those criteria. For example, according to my criteria, a foundation meant for someone with oily skin should be matte; contain minimal to no greasy or emollient ingredients; blend easily; leave a smooth, even finish; and have no blatant breakout-triggering ingredients. All foundations must match skin tones exactly—they should not be any noticeable shade of orange, peach, rose, pink, or ash—because people are not orange, peach, rose, pink, or ash. I established similar criteria for mascaras, blushes, eyeshadows, concealers, pressed powders, lipsticks, and pencils. I relied on my more than 20 years as a professional makeup artist to help establish guidelines for the quality of a product and its application, and I compared and contrasted hundreds of similar makeup products from different lines throughout the review process.

HOW I BECAME A COSMETICS COP

I often marvel at how I happened into this unusual occupation. It's not as if you can answer an ad for this kind of job, and clearly the cosmetics industry and beauty magazines aren't interested in hiring someone to do what I do. Yet, from the beginning, when I wrote my first book, *Blue Eyeshadow Should Be Illegal* in 1984, it was clear there was a demand from consumers for this kind of information. With more than 3 million books sold, I have never once regretted the day I got fired working at cosmetics counters in Washington, D.C., where I was living at the time, and eventually began writing my books.

For me the cosmetics industry was always a love-hate relationship. From a very young age I struggled with debilitating, painful eczema over most of my body. Then at puberty I developed acne, which lingers even now (although it's under control thanks to products I've formulated to manage this often chronic condition). I spent a good deal of my childhood and teen years in dermatologists' offices and at cosmetics counters or drugstores, trying every possible treatment or product that promised to give me normal skin. It never happened. I still had acne; if anything, my skin was more inflamed, irritated, and oily than it had been before. Little did I know then that the very products I was using were making my skin worse, not better.

Trying to find answers for my own skin has been a lifelong quest. Then, in 1977, I took my first job at a department-store makeup counter to supplement my income as a freelance makeup artist (I always had a knack for doing makeup). As a young makeup artist I had built up a list of political and celebrity clients and was doing quite well, both financially and professionally. I found the artistry of creating beautiful makeup styles for women intriguing, and the world of fashion and glamour thoroughly exciting. At the age of 24, I was thrilled with my career. My clients wanted only me, and they were some of the most powerful and formidable women in Washington. But, as with any business, it had its ups and downs.

A store at a mall in Silver Spring, Maryland, had an opening for a cosmetics salesperson. They hired me on the spot because, as I was told, I looked the part, wearing nice makeup and dressing well. Amazingly (to me anyway) they weren't interested in my makeup or skin-care experience; I had to be trained to sell products, especially skin-care products.

Even back then, I knew something wasn't quite right with a lot of the cosmetics and with the advertising for them, particularly in the skin-care arena. Having struggled for years with oily skin and blemishes, I knew from personal experience that astringents didn't close pores, products claiming not to cause breakouts made me break out, and most products that promised to clear up acne only made my skin more red and irritated. I didn't yet know all the technical details of why skin-care products failed abysmally at doing what they claimed they could do, but it was blatantly obvious that plenty of mascaras with claims of being flakeproof weren't, that foundations claiming to keep oil at bay didn't, and on and on. More often than not, the claims made about what the products would do rarely matched their performance. However, while it seemed certain to me that much of the cosmetics industry was grossly misrepresenting its products, at the time I had no way to confirm my suspicions.

On my first day at the department-store cosmetics counter, I was assigned to work behind the Calvin Klein and the Elizabeth Arden counters. With no previous training or information about these lines, I was told to sell the products. I did the best I could. Unfortunately, my ideas of how to help customers was completely different from that of the other salespeople and, more important, different from that of the line manager. My first mistake was telling several customers not to bother using an astringent because alcohol-based products wouldn't stop oil production and would only create more skin problems, causing skin to become dry, red, flaky, and irritated. By the end of the second day, the woman working next to me was mortified. She called in the line representative, who made it clear that I should keep my personal opinions to myself and just sell the products. I said I would do my best. This was only my second day! Things had to get better, I thought. They didn't.

After I complained that the two lines I was assigned to sell didn't always have the best makeup colors or skin-care products for every woman I talked to, the cosmetics manager told me, "All the customer wants to know is what you tell her; the customers never ask questions, because they trust our products." Several disagreements later, I was out of a job.

Shortly after that brief stint in the department store, I read *The Great American Skin Game* by Toni Stabille. It changed my life. This landmark book conveyed in clear, concise terms the processes and techniques the cosmetics industry uses to sell hope to gullible and uninformed consumers. In fact, Stabille was largely responsible for proposing many present-day Food and Drug Administration (FDA) regulations, including advertising guidelines, safety regulations, and mandatory ingredient lists. Her work confirmed what I had already reasoned must be true, and significantly changed the way I approached cosmetics.

Although it sounds a bit melodramatic, I knew then that I couldn't continue to sell something I knew to be a waste of money or just plain bad for the skin. Consumers (including myself) deserved better. I wasn't anti-makeup—just the opposite—but I was (and am) anti-hype and against misleading information. Thus, I took my first steps along what has turned out to be a long career path—longer and more consistent in some ways than I could ever have imagined—that went from owning my own cosmetics stores in 1980 to working as a TV news reporter at a local Seattle TV station, to owning my own publishing company in 1985, and back to creating and owning my own skin-care and makeup company in 1995, Paula's Choice.

With every step, my goal has been to do whatever it takes to find out and expose the truth behind the ads and the literally unbelievable claims thrown about by the cosmetics world. After all, one good sales pitch about an "exclusive formula" or a revolutionary new ingredient, and your pocketbook could easily be lighter—by $100 to $500—for a 1-ounce jar of standard cosmetic ingredients, or for ingredients that can't possibly live up to the claims made for them.

I know that I can't stop the cosmetics industry from force-feeding consumers an endless stream of expensive products and misleading or erroneous claims and information, but I also know there are enough women who are interested in seeing the other side of the picture to motivate me to continue to do what I do. Knowing the "rest of the story" can only help you feel and look more beautiful in the long run.

I WISH WE WEREN'T SO SUSCEPTIBLE

What is difficult for me to comprehend is why so many women believe what the cosmetics industry tells them, and why—even when they don't fully buy into the whole idea—they believe enough to fall into the same traps everyone else does. It doesn't seem to cause any doubts or raise any skepticism for women when cosmetics lines repeatedly bring out new miracle products, like a parade that never ends, particularly when they never tell us what was wrong or not as revolutionary with the earlier products they once claimed were so spectacular for skin, and yet they almost always continue to sell them, too!

Lots of women can't wait to buy the products a celebrity is selling or claims to use because it seems to be accepted as fact that being beautiful or famous means you must know about product quality or what is best for skin care and makeup. After the incessant hype and marketing distortion that accompany all of this, and despite the inevitable disappointments, we still buy whatever the next impressive ad or celebrity is selling. Yet if we weren't disappointed, the same lines wouldn't have to keep creating new antiwrinkle, acne, or myriad other skin-care items, and new lines wouldn't be introduced every year. This pattern repeats, season after season, year after year.

There is a part of me that struggles with what I do. Women would much rather hear that a product can turn back the clock or lift skin or get rid of wrinkles (I would love to hear that, too, if it were true!). I wish I could offer that fantasy, but if it's not true—and it isn't—I can't do it. My fantasy would be to let every woman hear what dermatologists, cosmetics chemists, and those in the industry really say about the products they make and sell. Lots of them are laughing behind your backs and you will never be privy to it.

HOW DO THEY GET AWAY WITH IT?

I'm sure you've heard the remark that if you repeat a lie often enough it can become fact for many people; that is exactly how it is in the cosmetics industry. For example, the need for an eye cream is ludicrous (I will explain why later in this book), but such products are accepted as standard by most women. Many women believe a skin-care product can actually work as well as Botox, dermal fillers, lasers, or other medical cosmetic corrective procedures, after all, that's what the ads say, isn't it? Nothing could be further from the truth.

I am often asked, "How do they get away with it?" How do cosmetics companies get away with what is either misleading information or out-and-out lying to the public? The answer: They get away with it because getting around cosmetics regulations worldwide has become an art, an art that leaves the consumer between a rock and a hard place. Even when the claims are out and out lies, by the time the regulatory boards get around to challenging a cosmetics company's advertising claims the ads have long since been replaced with ads for a new product launch.

The only part of the cosmetics industry that is clearly regulated for the consumer's protection worldwide is the ingredient list, but even there I see lots of problems. Since 1978, in the United States (far later in the rest of the world), cosmetics companies have been required to divulge all the contents in their products, and to list them in the order of concentration from most to least. Unfortunately, the vast majority of consumers don't know how to read a cosmetic's ingredient list because they can be phenomenally technical and extensive (there are thousands and thousands of cosmetic ingredients). That complexity means that most of us must rely on the unregulated claims and assertions that appear in the marketing copy. But taking the time to decipher the ingredient lists is the only way you'll be able to make a rational decision when it comes time to purchase skin-care products. But, then again, that's job security for me and my team!

YOU WOULD BE SHOCKED

I wish there were some way I could teach every cosmetics consumer how to read an ingredient list. Once you became familiar with the chemical names and Latin names of the ingredients and how they function, you would be stunned at how similar the products in a particular category truly are. It's not that there aren't differences among products, there indeed are, but it's astounding how similar many products are. And I mean astounding! It is truly a marketing phenomenon when the cosmetics industry can convince women that there is a qualitative difference between a $10 cleanser and a $50 cleanser, or that a $60 sunscreen is far more advanced than one selling for $25, and so on for each product type. Even Dr. N.V. Perricone, author of *The Wrinkle Cure* (a book describing Perricone's own unsubstantiated, nonscientific data regarding the treatment of wrinkles) and owner of the product line bearing his name, was quoted in the *New York Times* (November 18, 2001, "The Skin Game with New Wrinkles") as saying "Promise them an unlined face, and you can sell them anything." This is exactly what he and hundreds of other companies (including many fronted by dermatologists) are doing, selling empty promises that women fall for every time an ad proclaims the next answer for wrinkles. Add the medical credibility of a doctor endorsing or creating a line, and that's all the convincing many consumers need before handing over their credit cards.

What I hope my book brings to light by the time you are done reading through the various lines and the introductory chapters is that there is an absolutely amazing number of brilliant skin-care products being sold. However, if you are going to take truly beautiful care of your skin, you must also be aware that there are an alarming number of products being promoted by misleading, overrated, and erroneous claims, which are tossed out there by companies because there are no legal restrictions to encourage them to do otherwise. If you are seduced by price and advertising rhetoric, both your skin and your budget run the risk of being damaged, or, at the very least, being poorly taken care of. If you're not seduced by the rhetoric, you can gain some real benefits.

THE BUSINESS OF CLAIM SUBSTANTIATION: "OUR STUDY SHOWS…"

Very few consumers, or reporters for that matter, are aware of the large number of skin-care "research" laboratories, including universities and doctors' offices, whose only clients are cosmetics companies that want to "buy" faux studies so they can cite enticing statistics to "validate" incredible claims that they can use as a marketing strategy.

These research labs exist solely to provide pseudoscientific material for the cosmetics industry, and their "studies" are rarely, if ever, published. That way, if the marketing copy claims that a moisturizer provides an 82% increase in moisturization or a 90% increase in the skin's water content, the company may very well be able to point to a "study" that says this is true. Quoting these inconclusive, vague studies in a news story or ad can make them sound significant and meaningful, but in truth they are more often than not just hype and exaggeration generated exclusively to sell products. One of these claim-substantiation companies actually advertises its ability to deliver "creative claim generation/substantiation."

Here's a perfect example of how these feigned studies are performed. Let's take a typical claim about a moisturizer providing a large increase in the skin's moisture content. Without some basic information about how the study was conducted, that increase is meaningless. You can take almost anyone's skin, rub some alcohol on it or even just wash it with plain soap, then put on any moisturizer in the world, and the skin will reflect anywhere from an 82% to a 200% increase in moisture content. (In fact, you can soak in the bathtub for 30 minutes and come out with your skin well saturated with water and have a 500% increase in its moisture content.) Furthermore, perhaps the test included only five or ten women and compared only two products, one with an unknown formula. It may indicate that for this small group, brand A worked better than brand X—but what about how it worked compared with the 5,000 other moisturizers on the market? Maybe lots of those work just as well as or better than brand A.

According to an article in *Cosmetics & Toiletries* magazine (December 1999, pages 52-53):

> *Skin moisturization studies using bioengineering methods are commonplace today. If data generated for a new test product demonstrate a statistically significant difference between the test product and untreated skin in favor of increased hydration, then claims indicating this to the consumer would be substantiated.… For example, [the claim] "moisturizes your skin for up to 8 hours" would be substantiated by a study where a statistical difference was observed between the test product and untreated skin for up to 8 hours following application of the test product.*

In essence, in examples like this, what the words "our studies show" are telling you is that when compared with plain, unmoisturized, washed skin, the moisturizer made skin moist! That isn't exactly shocking. The use of any moisturizer would show the same results.

Another glaring example is that lots of companies assert they have studies proving their products don't cause irritation, but the testing done to evaluate that reaction looks only at the surface of the skin, not what is taking place underneath. Yet a huge amount of damage to skin from irritation never shows up on the surface. For example, sun damage occurs within the first seconds of skin seeing daylight through a window, but you neither feel it nor see it because the inflammation from the impact of the UV rays is not happening on the surface, but rather underneath, where it is not detectable. The test for a product's potential irritancy is only one very small part of the picture.

I've seen this process at work firsthand, and it is disturbing. Ads for substantiation companies in cosmetic industry magazines state quite clearly that if you need a claim they can get you a test to fit. Whoever is paying the bill hires the research lab. The lab is handed the products and told what to look for and what kind of results are needed—for example, proof of moisturization, exfoliation, increased firmness, reduction of wrinkles, or some other parameter. Then the lab goes about setting up a study to prove that position. Rarely are these studies done double blind, rarely do they use a large group of women or show long-term results, and rarely are these studies ever published—most are never made available to anyone. Yet consumers are led to believe this unverified information is factual when they read about it in editorials in magazines or newspapers.

I could go on and on about this kind of inadequate claim-substantiation business that takes place in the world of skin care, and I do so numerous times throughout this book. What's important to remember is that phrases like "our studies show" or "our research establishes" or "our test results demonstrate" aren't worth the paper they are printed on unless you can see the entire study and can judge for yourself exactly how the research was carried out and whether or not the results are significant or senseless.

(Sources for the above: *Cosmetic Claims Substantiation*, Cosmetic Science and Technology Series, vol. 18, ed. Louise Aust, New York: Marcel Dekker, 1998; and *Cosmetics and Toiletries* article: "The European Group on Efficacy Measurement of Cosmetics and Other Topical Products is considering new cosmetic legislation to regulate claims of efficacy," by G. E. Pierard, Ph.D., Allured Publishing, Boca Raton, FL, 2000.)

BUZZWORDS

The following are a few of the more popular terms you may have seen or heard in marketing jargon for cosmetic products that get hyped and overhyped by the cosmetics industry. Although you might have heard them, you may not be aware that they have little to no meaning when it comes to what you will actually be putting on your skin or to what is effective or a waste of your money. Here's what's behind the buzz.

All Natural or Organic: While this implication of "natural" or "organic" ingredients resonates with consumers, it doesn't assure you that you are getting an accurate picture of safety or effectiveness, much less reliable facts. Further, many companies claim their products are all natural when in fact they contain a preponderance of unnatural ingredients. But even more important, there is no research anywhere showing that natural or organic ingredients are better for skin than synthetic ingredients. In fact, there are lots of natural ingredients that show up in skin-care products that are either toxic (Source: *Toxicology In Vitro*, June 2006, pages 480-489) or carcinogenic, or irritating to skin—and irritation causes all kinds of havoc for skin (Source: *Skin Research and Technology*, August 2004, pages 144-148). And finally, when a plant of any kind is added to a cosmetic, and is preserved, stabilized, and mixed with other ingredients, it loses most, if not all, of its natural orientation (Source: FDA *Consumer* magazine, May-June 1998, revised May 1998 and August 2000).

Hypoallergenic or Good for Sensitive Skin: These terms suggest to the consumer that the product is less likely to cause allergic reactions or skin sensitivities. However, there are no standard testing restrictions or regulations for determining whether a product qualifies as meeting this claim. A company can label their product "hypoallergenic" or "good for sensitive skin" without providing any substantiation for the claim. This is also true for terms such as "dermatologist-tested," "sensitivity tested," "allergy tested," or "nonirritating." None of these terms are required to be backed up by any proof that they are better for your skin than products without these claims, because there are no standardized guidelines (Source: www. FDA.gov). You also will be surprised at the number of products in this edition that get rated with an unhappy face because the product is labeled for sensitive skin, but then contains a preponderance of irritating or sensitizing ingredients.

Fragrance-Free: This is supposed to indicate to the consumer that a product contains no perfume or fragrant ingredients, but it ends up having little meaning. Despite this labeling, many products use fragrant plant extracts that can cause skin irritation, allergic reactions, or a phototoxic response on skin (meaning they enhance the negative effects of the sun on your skin). Fragrances, natural or otherwise, are not benign ingredients (Source: *Acta Dermato-Venereology*, July 2007, pages 312-316). Plus "fragrance-free" is not a term regulated by the FDA; it ends up being useless information on a product label unless you know what to watch out for on the ingredient list (Source: www.FDA.gov).

Noncomedogenic and Nonacnegenic: These terms are not regulated by the FDA or any other regulatory board anywhere in the world, and as such have no legal meaning. Again, any product can spotlight these terms. In real life, the search for products that won't cause breakouts remains a struggle. Given there are millions of combinations of ingredients used in cosmetics, there is no way to determine exactly which combination is a problem (Source: www.FDA.gov).

Dermatologist Tested: No matter how impressive this wording sounds, and as long as there are no reliable published data stating otherwise, this term can mean simply that a doctor applied the product to his or her skin or watched someone else do that and then said they liked the product. It doesn't tell you anything about efficacy or how one product compares with any other product. I've seen lots of products, even with a doctor's name on the label, that make the same absurd, misleading claims as the rest of the industry. I've also seen products that are terribly formulated or contain ingredients that can hurt skin make the same claims.

Essential Oils: There is nothing essential about essential oils. It is a term attributed to fragrant oils to bestow an aura of effective skin care upon them, where, in almost every case, none exists. It is well established in scientific and dermatological journals that fragrance, whether natural or synthetic, is problematic for skin (Sources: *Acta Dermato-Venereology*, 2007 volume 87, issue 4, pages 312-316; *Dermatology*, 2002, volume 205, number 1, pages 98-102; *Contact Dermatitis*, December 2001, pages 333-340; and *Toxicology and Applied Pharmacology*, May 2001, pages 172-178). For any company to suggest that products containing volatile ingredients such as rose, orange oil, pine oil, and lavender, to name a few, are gentle, helpful, or hypoallergenic is not just misleading—it's harmful for skin.

Cosmeceutical: Despite all the medical pedigrees of doctors who love using this word, the term "cosmeceutical" is not in any way regulated or controlled, and anyone can slap that label on their products to promote them as being more "medical." Cosmeceutical is nothing more than a marketing term with illusions of grandeur. Even the FDA and other regulatory boards around the world say cosmeceuticals don't exist, and they consider these products merely cosmetics, albeit with clever marketing language attached (Sources: *U.S. Markets for Physician-Dispensed Cosmeceuticals 2009*, www.the-infoshop.com; *SKINmed*, July-August 2008, pages 214-220; *Archives of Dermatological Research*, April 2005, pages 473-481).

Miracle ingredients: Contrary to what the cosmetics industry at large would like you to believe, skin care does not rely on a single star ingredient to enhance skin's appearance or function or to improve the appearance of wrinkles or any other skin condition. Month after month, consumers are faced with new ingredients, each claiming superiority over any number of predecessors. Everything from vitamin C and collagen to some exotic plant from a distant forest or exotic location, or perhaps a newly derived molecule, is advertised as being the answer for your skin. Yet the vast majority of these have no substantiated, independently funded (i.e., funded by an organization other than the company selling the product or ingredient) research to prove these assertions. Even when there is research showing the ingredient can be effective for skin, that doesn't make it better or more essential than other ingredients. This constant yet ever-changing list of "best" ingredients may keep things interesting for cosmetics marketing departments and the media, but it rarely helps the consumer determine what is needed to maintain healthy, radiant skin. Think about it like your diet—broccoli and grapes may be incredibly healthy to eat, but if you ate only broccoli and grapes you would soon become malnourished and your body would suffer. Skin is the same way—it's a complex structural organ that requires many substances to function in a younger and healthier manner.

Mature Skin: Many products on the market are supposedly designed specifically for women who are in their 30s, or their 40s, or who are 50 or older, but age is NOT a skin type. An "older" person can have the same skin-care concerns as a younger person. Acne, blackheads, eczema, rosacea, sensitive skin, or oily skin can plague women over 50 or in their 30s, and a woman well under 50 can have dry, freckled, wrinkled, or obviously sun-damaged skin. Not everyone in their 40s has the same skin-care needs, or in their 50s or 60s or 70s. In a way it's simple: You need to pay attention to what is taking place on your skin, and that varies from person to person.

YOUR BEAUTY MANTRA: EXPENSIVE DOESN'T MEAN BETTER

The amount of money you spend on skin-care products has nothing to do with how your skin looks. In other words, spending more money does not affect the status of your skin. What does affect the status of your skin are the products you use. An expensive soap by Erno Laszlo is no better for your skin than an inexpensive bar soap such as Dove; in fact, both are bad for skin. On the other hand, an irritant-free toner by Neutrogena can be just as good as, or maybe even better than, an irritant-free toner by Guerlain or La Prairie (depending on the formulation), and any irritant-free toner is infinitely better than a toner that contains alcohol, peppermint, menthol, essential oils, eucalyptus, lemon, or other irritants, no matter how natural-sounding the ingredients are and regardless of the price or claim. Spending less doesn't hurt your skin, and spending more doesn't necessarily help it. Simple, but true!

DON'T LOVE YOUR PRODUCTS OR ANY COSMETICS COMPANY (AFTER ALL, THEY'RE CHEATING ON YOU)

I listen to women say it all the time. It doesn't matter if it is reporters, beauty editors, or women I encounter every day. They exclaim how much they love a product. And other women listen (or overhear) and wonder if they should love it, too. After all, love is a pretty powerful sentiment. Why would someone love a bad product or one that didn't work as claimed? Because we all "love" things that are bad for us. We love that guy who won't call us back or is rude and demeaning. Or we love chocolate cake and french fries. Or we love skin-care products with bad formulas (useless or harmful ingredients), jar packaging, low SPF ratings, and on and on. There are brilliant products available, but without knowing what is best for your skin, you can't possibly know what to love and what to dislike from a rational perspective.

And don't be line loyal. Ask yourself: Why should you be loyal to any cosmetics company when the cosmetics company isn't even loyal to itself? For example:

- **Estee Lauder owns:** Aramis, Aveda, Clinique, Bobbi Brown, M.A.C., Origins, Jo Malone, La Mer, Tommy Hilfiger fragrances, Bumble + bumble, American Beauty, Flirt, Good Skin, Grassroots, Michael Kors Beauty, Darphin, Ojon, and Donna Karan Cosmetics.
- **L'Oreal owns:** Maybelline New York, Garnier, Lancome, Helena Rubinstein, Bio-Medic, Vichy, Biotherm, Shu Uemura, Kiehl's, Soft Sheen-Carson, Redken, Matrix, Kerastase, Giorgio Armani, Inneov, Sanoflore, CCB Paris, Dermablend, The Body Shop, Skinceuticals, Ralph Lauren, and La Roche-Posay.
- **Procter & Gamble owns:** Cover Girl, Max Factor, Anna Sui, Olay, DDF, Aussie, Camay, Clairol, Gillette, Head & Shoulders, Ivory, Infusium-23, Pantene, Gillette, Fredric Fekkai, Noxzema, Pantene, SK-II, Old Spice, and Zest.

- **Johnson & Johnson owns:** Neutrogena, Aveeno, Clean & Clear, RoC, Rogaine, Lubriderm, Purpose, and Ambi.
- **Beiersdorf owns:** Nivea, La Prairie, Eucerin, and Juvena.
- **Unilever owns:** Dove, Pond's, Vaseline, and Sunsilk.
- **Louis Vuitton-Moet Hennessy (LVMH) owns:** Dior, Guerlain, Givenchy, Benefit, Fresh, Make Up For Ever, and Sephora's namesake line.

The truth is we really don't love the product we are using because we are all too ready to toss it when the next new miracle product starts being advertised. My message is that it's a good idea to stop loving your products until you know what you are buying and whether or not the product (or, if you prefer, object of your potential affection) is beneficial. Once you have that information, then you can decide whether or not you "love" the way it feels on your skin.

INGREDIENTS

To make it easier for you to become familiar with what you'll find on ingredient lists, I created and continually update an extensive online *Cosmetic Ingredient Dictionary*. You can access this free dictionary by visiting either www.CosmeticscCop.com or www.Beautypedia. com. Please refer to it when you don't know what an ingredient is or does, or when you hear a claim that a particular ingredient has some miraculous properties for skin. You will be amazed at how legitimate research rarely matches what a cosmetics company wants you to believe.

CHAPTER TWO

How to Take the Best Care of Your Skin

CAN YOU HAVE GREAT SKIN?

The answer is a resounding yes. My book, *The Original Beauty Bible*, 3rd Edition, has extensive information about how to understand what works and what doesn't work for skin. It also has easy-to-follow, skin-care regimens for every skin type, including those with sensitive skin, rosacea, acne, dry skin, sun damage, wrinkles, and on and on. This book, *Don't Go to the Cosmetics Counter Without Me*, is primarily a product review guide. It is meant as a source that tells you specifically what products live up to their claims, what products don't, and what products waste your money.

The Original Beauty Bible teaches you how to understand what types of products you should look for. Over the past several years, the amount of documented and peer-reviewed research on skin-care and cosmetic ingredients has grown tremendously. Serious investigation has increased exponentially on all fronts—from antioxidants, anti-irritants, skin-identical ingredients, and cell-communicating ingredients, to how skin ages, why skin wrinkles, how skin heals, what the effects of hormones are on skin function, and how to treat blackheads and acne—not to mention giving us a better understanding of how sun and oxygen destroy skin and why irritation is harmful for skin. Cosmetic dermatology, cosmetic corrective procedures, and plastic surgery procedures have greatly improved, but the array of options has become more extensive and the risks more difficult to quantify and evaluate. Answers and explanations about all that and more is what you will find in *The Original Beauty Bible*.

The following is a summary of the basics that you need to know if you are going to choose the best products for your skin, and of the overarching standards I use to review all the products in this book.

WHY IRRITATION IS SO BAD FOR SKIN

Throughout this book you will repeatedly read cautions and warnings encouraging you to avoid products or skin-care routines that can cause irritation and inflammation. I cannot stress enough (as you undoubtedly will be able to tell after reading only a few paragraphs of this book) how bad it is to irritate or inflame skin—I mean really, really bad! The research about this issue is overwhelming, yet on an ongoing basis we subject our skin to elements that can cause a long list of unwanted problems.

Irritation and inflammation, whether from unprotected sun exposure, free-radical damage from the very air we breathe, eating unhealthy foods, smoking, or pollution is a terrible problem. Yet equally as problematic are skin-care products that contain irritating ingredients, involve using very hot water, or result in overscrubbing skin. Our skin can barely keep up with the assault. In the long run it doesn't, and it suffers irreparable damage.

There is a litany of negative effects that occur when skin is irritated or inflamed, but fundamentally this results in the skin's immune system becoming impaired, collagen breaking down, and the skin being stripped of its outer protective barrier. What is perhaps most shocking is that all of these damaging responses can be taking place underneath the skin's surface; you won't even notice it, not until many years later. The clearest example of this is the significant and carcinogenic effect of the sun's silent UVA rays. You don't feel the penetration of these mutagenic rays, but they are taking a toll on the skin nonetheless.

Chronic and even acute irritation and inflammation can destroy the skin's integrity by breaking down the skin's protective barrier, and that, over time, damages the skin's collagen and elastin components. Inside the skin, inflammation impairs the skin's immune and healing responses. In addition, breaking down the skin's protective barrier can allow the introduction of bacteria, thus increasing the risk of more breakouts. Any way you look at it, irritating the skin in any manner is almost always not a good idea, and especially not when it happens every day with sun exposure or the skin-care products we use.

THE MOST COMMON IRRITATING INGREDIENTS TO AVOID

(These are of greater concern when they appear at the beginning of an ingredient list.)

- Alcohol or SD-alcohol followed by a number (Exceptions: Ingredients like cetyl alcohol or stearyl alcohol are standard, benign, waxlike cosmetic thickening agents and are completely nonirritating and safe to use.)
  - Camphor
  - Citrus juices and oils
  - Eucalyptus
  - Excessive fragrance
  - Menthol
  - Menthyl lactate
  - Menthoxypropanediol
  - Mint
- Peppermint
- Sodium lauryl sulfate
- Arnica
- Bergamot
- Cinnamon
- Clove
- Eugenol
- Grapefruit
- Lavender
- Linalool
- Wintergreen
- Witch hazel
- Ylang-ylang

(Sources *Inflammation Research*, December 2008, pages 558-563; *Skin Pharmacology and Physiology*, June 2008, pages 124-135, and November-December 2000, pages 358-371; *Journal of Investigative Dermatology*, April 2008, pages 15-19; *Journal of Cosmetic Dermatology*, March 2008, pages 78-82; *Mechanisms of Ageing and Development*, January 2007, pages 92-105; and *British Journal of Dermatology*, December 2005, pages S13-S22)

FORGET THE TERM "MOISTURIZER"

Regardless of the name or claim, "moisturizers" (or antiwrinkle, antigravity, serum, or whatever the industry calls them in terms of their antiwrinkle benefit, whether they are in cream, lotion, serum, or even liquid form) must supply the skin with ingredients that maintain its structure, reduce free-radical damage (environmental assaults on the skin from sun, pollution, and air), and help cells function more normally. When moisturizers contain the well-researched, effective groups of ingredients that can do these things, they are as close to "anti-aging," or "anti-wrinkling," or "repairing" as any skin-care product can get.

All skin types will benefit from daily, topical application of cell-communicating antioxidants, anti-irritants, skin-identical ingredients, and water-binding agents that together work to improve and re-create the structure and function of healthy skin. Those are the ingredients that make the most difference and have the most impact on the function of the skin, making it looking younger, smoother, and potentially blemish-free (and the research, as you'll see, is abundant and overflowing on this topic).

Should You Use a Lotion, Cream, Gel, Serum, Liquid, Mousse, or Balm?

Now that you have learned to ignore the marketing terms cosmetics companies attribute to their potions for skin under the guise of antiwrinkle, the single most important aspect is that they all contain a generous, well-researched, and potent assortment of antioxidants, cell-communicating ingredients, and ingredients that mimic skin structure. With few exceptions, all of the products listed in this book under the ubiquitous "moisturizer" or antiwrinkle or whatever category that gets a happy face meets these fundamental criteria.

The next question is what kind of product has those qualities and what does it look like. In other words, what should the consistency and texture of this product be regardless of the name on the label? The answer: it all depends on your skin type and personal preference. As long as the product contains state-of-the-art ingredients, the ingredients that make the product a gel, cream, lotion, serum, liquid, or mousse are inconsequential except as they relate to your skin type.

Think of it like a chocolate dessert. You might prefer a torte, pudding, bonbon, cake, ice cream, or some other form, but the chocolate is what counts; the other ingredients are there simply to carry the important taste of chocolate to your mouth.

As a general rule, those with oily or combination skin will prefer lighter-weight lotions, gels, serums, or liquids. Those with dry skin usually prefer creams or more emollient formulations to make up for what their oil glands don't provide or what dry, arid climates make worse. And those with blemish-prone skin generally do better with moisturizers that have a thinner consistency.

Daytime versus Nighttime Moisturizers

Putting aside the claims, hype, and misleading information you may have heard, the only real difference between a daytime and nighttime moisturizer is that the daytime version should contain a well-formulated sunscreen. For daytime wear, unless your foundation contains an effective sunscreen, it is essential that your moisturizer feature a well-formulated, broad-spectrum sunscreen rated SPF 15 or higher. Well-formulated means that it contains UVA-protecting ingredients, specifically titanium dioxide, zinc oxide, avobenzone (also called butyl methoxy-dibenzoylmethane or Parsol 1789), Tinosorb, or Mexoryl SX (ecamsule). Regardless of the time of day, your skin needs all the current state-of-the-art ingredients I describe in the following paragraphs. Your skin doesn't do special healing at night nor is it more "receptive" to nutrients, despite what you might hear from a cosmetics salesperson. Diet is the best way to think about this, just like your body needs a healthy diet in the morning as well as at night, skin needs the same: healthy ingredients morning and night.

Skin-Identical Ingredients

Ingredients that mimic skin structure are referred to in different ways. They often are called skin-identical ingredients or intercellular matrix substances, but they also can be termed natural moisturizing factors (NMF), and I often refer to them in my books as water-binding agents. By any name these are brilliant ingredients for all skin types because they improve the function of skin and provide the barrier protection that is critical to having and maintaining healthy skin.

The term "skin-identical ingredients" refers to the substances between skin cells that keep them connected and help maintain the skin's fundamental external structure. Many ingredients have these functions. Humectants, of which glycerin is a classic example, draw water to skin and are one vital component of a moisturizer. But what good is attracting water to the skin if the structure isn't there to keep the water from leaving?

This intercellular structure is made up of many different components, ranging from ceramides to lecithin, glycerin, polysaccharides, hyaluronic acid, sodium hyaluronate, sodium PCA, collagen, elastin, proteins, amino acids, cholesterol, glucose, sucrose, fructose, glycogen, phospholipids, glycosphingolipids, glycosaminoglycans, and many more. All of these give the skin what it needs to keep its cells intact. Just adding water is meaningless if the intercellular matrix is damaged.

Antioxidants

Antioxidants are an essential part of any state-of-the-art moisturizer. An immense body of research continues to show that antioxidants are a potential panacea for skin's ills, and ignoring their benefit while shopping for moisturizers (or any products with names like anti-aging or antiwrinkle or treatment) means you'll be shortchanging your skin. What makes antioxidants so intriguing is that they seem to have the ability not only to reduce or prevent some amount of the oxidative damage that destroys and depletes the skin's function and structure, but also to prevent some of the degenerative effects in skin caused by sun exposure.

The number of antioxidants that can show up in a skin-care product is almost limitless. Yet despite endless cosmetics companies launching new miracle ingredients on a constant, unrelenting basis, there is no single best one. In fact, many work well together and thus a cocktail approach to using antioxidants is preferred. These vital elements for skin can range from alpha lipoic acid, beta-glucan, coenzyme Q10, grape seed extract, green tea, soybean sterols, superoxide dismutase, vitamin C (ascorbyl palmitate and magnesium ascorbyl palmitate), and vitamin E (alpha tocopherol, tocotrienols) to pomegranate, curcumin, turmeric, and on and on and on.

(Sources for the above: *Clinics in Dermatology*, November-December 2008, pages 614-626; *Skin Therapy Letter*, September 2008, pages 5-9; *Journal of Drugs in Dermatology*, July 2008, pages S7-S12; *Dermatologic Therapy*, September-October 2007, pages 322-329; *Dermatologic Surgery*, "The Antioxidant Network of the Stratum Corneum," July 2005, pages 814-817; *Journal of Pharmaceutical and Biomedical Analysis*, February 2005, pages 287-295; and *Cosmetic Dermatology*, December 2001, pages 37-40.)

Cell-Communicating Ingredients

Every cell has a vast series of receptor sites for different substances. These receptor sites are the cell's communication hookup. When the right ingredient for a specific site shows up, it has the ability to attach itself to the cell and transmit information. In the case of skin, this means telling the cell to start doing the things that a healthy skin cell should be doing. If the cell accepts the message, it then shares the same healthy message with other nearby cells in a continuing process.

(Sources for the above: *Microscopy Research and Technique*, January 2003, pages 107-114; *Nature Medicine*, February 2003, pages 225-229; *Journal of Investigative Dermatology*, March 2002, pages 402-408; *International Journal of Biochemistry and Cell Biology*, July 2004, pages 1141-1146; *Experimental Cell Research*, March 2002, pages 130-137; *Skin Pharmacology and Applied Skin Physiology*, September-October 2002, pages 316-320; and www.signaling-gateway.org.)

Anti-Irritants

Anti-irritants are another element vital for good skin-care formulations. Regardless of the source, irritation is a problem for all skin types, causing collagen breakdown, increasing oil production, generating free-radical damage, and hurting the skin's immune response. Many elements are responsible for irritating skin, including hot water, cold water, sun exposure, pollution, irritating skin-care ingredients, soaps, drying cleansers, and overscrubbing the skin. You may think that none of those things bother your skin, but they absolutely are causing an immense amount of damage. Even if your skin doesn't feel or appear irritated after exposure to those things, it is still being irritated. The breakdown of skin under the surface is taking place whether you see it or not. That means if you are out in the sun, sitting in a sauna, or using a skin-care product that contains irritating or sensitizing ingredients, the irritation damage is still taking place even though the skin doesn't show it (Sources: *Journal of Biochemical and Molecular Toxicology*, April 2003, pages 92-94; *Skin Research and Technology*, January 2003, pages 50-58; and *Dermatotoxicology*, edited by Hongbo Zhai and Howard I. Maibach, Seventh Edition, CRC Press, Boca Raton, FL, 2007).

Anti-irritants are incredibly helpful because they allow skin extra healing time and can reduce the problems caused by oxidative and other sources of external damage.

Emollients

For those with truly dry skin—that is, where the dryness is not caused by irritating or drying skin-care products—emollients are the lubricating ingredients critical for making skin feel hydrated. Emollients provide dry skin with the one thing it's missing—moisture—in the form of substances that resemble those the skin should produce for itself. Emollients are ingredients like most nonfragrant plant oils, mineral oil, shea butter, cocoa butter, petrolatum, fatty alcohols, and animal oils. All of these and many more are exceptionally beneficial for dry skin.

For Those with Normal to Oily Skin or Minimal Dryness

Emollients are the last thing someone with any amount of oily skin needs. While any skin type needs the same essential ingredients of antioxidants, skin-identical ingredients, and cell-communicating ingredients, the texture of the product is what makes the difference. Avoid any moisturizer that comes in a thick lotion, cream, balm, or ointment form because it can clog pores and make skin feel oilier than it already is. Use only products that come in a gel, liquid, or extremely lightweight lotion or serum form.

(Other sources for this section: *Current Molecular Medicine*, March 2005, pages 171-177; *Applied Spectroscopy*, July 1998, pages 1001-1007; *Skin Research and Technology*, November 2003, pages 306-311; *Journal of the American Academy of Dermatology*, March 2003, pages 352-358; *Skin Pharmacology and Applied Skin Physiology*, November-December 1999, pages 344-351; and *Dermatology*, February 2005, pages 128-134.)

YOU DON'T NEED EYE CREAMS

Most women believe that eye creams are specially formulated for skin around the eye area. There is no evidence, research, or documentation to validate the claim that eye creams have special formulations that set them apart from or make them superior to other facial moisturizers. I have never found a dermatologist or cosmetics chemist who can tell me what special ingredients the eye area needs that the face doesn't—or vice versa. It only takes a quick look at the ingredient labels of any moisturizer or eye moisturizer to see that they don't differ except for the price and the tiny containers used for the eye creams. Eye creams are a whim of the cosmetics industry designed to evoke the sale of two products when only one is needed.

The only time you might want to use a different product around the eyes is if the skin there happens to indeed be different from the skin on the rest of your face. For example, if your face is normal to oily and doesn't require a moisturizer except occasionally on the cheeks or around the eyes, then an emollient, well-formulated moisturizer of any kind will work beautifully. You don't have to purchase a product labeled "eye cream."

Ironically, one of the real drawbacks of many so-called eye creams is that they rarely contain sunscreen. For daytime, that makes most eye creams a serious problem for the health of your skin. Although you might believe, as the company wants you to, that you are doing something special for your eye-area skin, you actually are putting it at risk of sun damage and wrinkling by using an eye cream without sunscreen. This is another example of the way cosmetics marketing and misleading information can waste your money and hurt your skin.

AVOID JAR PACKAGING!

Packaging plays a significant role in the stability and effectiveness of the products you use. Because many state-of-the-art ingredients, from cell-communicating ingredients, antioxidants, and plant extracts to skin-identical ingredients, are unstable in the presence of air, jar packaging, once opened, permits air to enter freely, which causes these important ingredients, the very ingredients that make a product most beneficial for skin, to break down and deteriorate. Jars also mean that you probably are sticking your fingers into the product, which can transfer bacteria and further cause the great ingredients to break down. Think about how long an unprotected head of lettuce lasts in your refrigerator. Or, after opening a can or jar of food, how long does it take before it's a moldy mess? Airtight packaging, or any packaging that reduces the product's exposure to air, is essential when you are buying the best products for your skin. You should also avoid clear packaging that lets light reach the product. Light of any kind is a problem because it causes sensitive ingredients to break down.

If that isn't enough to make you reconsider jar packaging, it's worth noting that *The Guidelines on Stability of Cosmetic Products*, March 2004, by the CTFA and COLIPA (respectively, the American and European cosmetic governing associations to which most cosmetics companies in Europe and North America belong) states, "Packaging can directly affect finished product stability because of interactions which can occur between the product, the package, and the external environment. Such interactions may include ... barrier properties of the container [and] its effectiveness in protecting the contents from the adverse effects of atmospheric oxygen...."

(Other sources for the above information: *Free Radical Biology and Medicine*, September 2007, pages 818-829; *Ageing Research Reviews*, December 2007, pages 271-288; *Dermatologic Therapy*, September-October 2007, pages 314-321; *International Journal of Pharmaceutics*, June 12, 2005, pages 197-203; *Pharmaceutical Development and Technology*, January 2002, pages 1-32; *International Society for Horticultural Science*, www.actahort.org/members/showpdf?booknrarnr=778_5; and Beautypackaging.com, www.beautypackaging.com/articles/2007/03/airless-packaging.php.)

GENTLE CLEANSING—ANYTHING ELSE HURTS YOUR SKIN

Research proving that you should clean the skin gently is now well established. This is the basic first step for all skin types, from normal to oily, dry, blemish-prone, or sun-damaged.

Expensive water-soluble cleansers will not make your face any cleaner, nor are they necessarily any gentler than the less expensive water-soluble cleansers. In fact, the handful of standard cleansing agents used in cleansers is the same all across the cosmetics spectrum, regardless of price.

One more point: The wrong cleanser can cause problems for your skin. For example, a cleanser that is too greasy can create blemishes and make skin feel greasy or oily. A cleanser that is too drying can create combination skin, because drying up skin doesn't stop or change the amount of oil your oil glands produce.

Bar soaps and bar cleansers are typically far more drying than water-soluble cleansers that use gentle cleansing agents. I do not recommend anyone wash with this type of cleanser.

(Other sources for the above: *International Journal of Dermatology*, August 2002, pages 494-499; *Cosmetic Dermatology*, August 2000, pages 58-62; *Cutis*, December 2001, volume 68, number 5, Supplemental; *Skin Research and Technology*, February 2001, pages 49-55; *Dermatology*, 1997, volume 195, number 3, pages 258-262; and *Journal of the American Medical Association*, April 1980, pages 1640-1643.)

Avoid wiping off your makeup. Pulling at your face tears the elastic support tissue in skin, causing it to sag. Think about women you've seen wearing heavy earrings and how far that pulls the lobe, eventually making it sag even when the earrings aren't there!

Use a gentle makeup remover without fragrance or coloring agents to take off the last traces of your makeup. One way to reduce puffy eyes or irritated skin around the eyes is to be sure you get all your makeup off, remembering to pull and tug at your skin as little as possible.

USE A SUNSCREEN 365 DAYS A YEAR

If you are exposed to the sun, even for as little as a few minutes every day—and that includes walking to your car, walking to the bus, or sitting next to a window during the day (the sun's damaging UVA rays come through window glass)—regardless of the season, that exposure adds up over the years, and it will wrinkle your skin, cause skin discolorations, and potentially result in skin cancer. If exposure that minimal can wrinkle the skin, imagine how much worse the impact of being in the sun for a long period of time can be and how ultimately detrimental sunbathing can be. No skin-care product except a sunscreen with an SPF of 15 or greater that includes the appropriate UVA-protecting ingredients of titanium dioxide, zinc oxide, avobenzone (butyl methoxydibenzoylmethane), Mexoryl SX (ecamsule), or Tinosorb can help prevent that excessive and relentless damage from taking place.

You must apply sunscreen liberally! That means that using an expensive sunscreen can be dangerous if it discourages you from applying it generously. For more specifics about sun protection, including SPF ratings and UVA versus UVB protection, refer to the Sun Facts section of my Web site, www.CosmeticsCop.com.

EXFOLIATE REGULARLY

Exfoliation is the natural process that all skin goes through—the outermost layers of skin are sloughed off and replaced by the new cells that move to the surface. This endless inside-to-outside movement is the hallmark of healthy skin. For many reasons this healthy cell turnover process can be impaired, causing problems for many skin types. An excess of surface skin cells that don't shed normally can be the result of sun damage (sun damage causes the surface layer of skin to become thick and scaly, while it thins and depletes the support structures in the layers below the surface). It also can be caused by oily skin preventing natural exfoliation because the excess oil makes skin cells stick to the surface. Overly emollient skin-care products that basically hold skin cells down can do the same thing. For some skin disorders, and as a result of sun damage, abnormally generated skin cells adhere unevenly and tenaciously to the surface of skin, another problem that slows healthy exfoliation.

What happens when we help the outer layer of skin function more normally? Your face can truly look younger! The best analogy I can think of is to compare it to the heels of your feet. Before you get a pedicure, the built-up, dead layers of skin on your heels look dry, rough, discolored, and scaly, and there are pronounced lines. Once that layer is removed, and it can be removed fairly aggressively without damaging anything, your heels look much better. Moreover, once you apply moisturizer, which can now be absorbed better because it isn't being blocked by the presence of overproduced skin cells, Voilá! You have "younger"-looking feet. The wrinkles are gone, the thick scaly appearance is gone, the dryness is gone, and your heels look beautiful. I'm not suggesting we should be that aggressive from the neck up or on most parts of the body, but the same benefits you gain when exfoliating skin on your feet hold true for the face. You just have to be more gentle than you are with your heels!

Topical scrubs are one way to exfoliate, which can be as simple as using a washcloth, or a cosmetic cleanser that contains a gentle (not gritty or skin damaging) abrasive material. However, research has solidly established that salicylic acid (BHA), for normal to oily or blemish-prone skin, and alpha hydroxy acids (AHAs) or polyhydroxy acid (PHA), for normal to dry skin, are not only effective exfoliants but also increase collagen production, improve the overall health of the skin, increase cell turnover, and reduce the appearance of skin discolorations. Therefore, those types of exfoliants are preferred to scrubs because they deliver greater, multi-faceted results.

(Sources for the above information: *Archives of Dermatologic Research,* April 2008, pages Supplemental S31-S38; *Journal of Cosmetic Dermatology,* March 2007, pages 59-65; *Skin Pharmacology and Physiology,* May 2006, pages 283-289; *Journal of Cosmetic Science,* March-April 2006, pages 203-204; *European Journal of Dermatology,* March-April 2002, pages 154-156; *Food and Chemical Toxicology,* November 1999, pages 1105-1111; and *Journal of the American Academy of Dermatology,* September 1996, pages 388-391.)

SOLUTIONS FOR SKIN LIGHTENING

Skin-lightening products abound in the cosmetics industry. Their promise—making skin lighter or lightening and removing brown skin discolorations—shows up worldwide, but most notably in Asian and Middle Eastern countries where the beautiful darker skin colors are apparently considered less aesthetically appealing than lighter skin tones. The names of the products in this arena are compelling, and of course the all-natural versions boast of plant extracts that claim to do the job and claim to do it better than prescription formulas. As you probably have come to expect from the cosmetics industry, when it comes to what the products and ingredients can actually do, the claims are misleading and often downright deceptive. Almost all of the skin-lightening products offered are enclosed in far prettier packaging and adorned with far more beguiling names than most other cosmetic products, but these gorgeous packages are filled with formulations that barely live up to even a fraction of the illusion they present.

The primary options for skin lightening are reviewed at length in my book *The Original Beauty Bible*, but here is a brief overview.

Use sunscreen. No other aspect of skin care can prevent, reduce, and potentially eliminate sun-induced and hormonal skin discolorations than the diligent use of a well-formulated sunscreen of at least SPF 15 or greater with the UVA-protecting ingredients avobenzone (butyl methoxydibenzoylmethane), ecamsule, Tinosorb, titanium dioxide, or zinc oxide. Using any other product or medical treatment without also using a sunscreen is a waste of time and money.

(Sources: *Journal of the European Academy of Dermatology and Venereology*, July 2007, pages 738-742; *Journal of the American Academy of Dermatology*, December 2006, pages 1048-1065; *Skin Therapy Letter*, November 2006, pages 1-6; and *British Journal of Dermatology*, December 1996, pages 867-875.)

Consider using a product containing hydroquinone. Hydroquinone is a strong inhibitor of melanin production that has long been established as the most effective ingredient for reducing and potentially eliminating melasma (Source: *Journal of Dermatological Science*, August, 2001, Supplemental, pages 68–75). In different concentrations it inhibits or prevents skin from making the substance responsible for skin color. Over-the-counter hydroquinone products can contain 0.5% to 2% concentrations, while 4% concentrations of hydroquinone (and sometimes higher) are available only from physicians.

Though controversial, there is abundant research showing hydroquinone to be safe and extremely effective (Sources: *Cutis*, April 2008, pages 356-371, August 2006, pages S6-S19; *Journal of Cosmetic Laser Therapy*, September 2006, pages 121-127; *American Journal of Clinical Dermatology*, July 2006, pages 223-230; and *Journal of the American Academy of Dermatology*, May 2006, pages S272-S281).

Vitamin A and vitamin A derivatives. A great deal of research shows that vitamin A (retinol) or prescription derivatives found in products such as Renova or Tazorac are extremely effective in treating skin discolorations (Sources: *Journal of the Academy of Dermatology*, December 2006, pages 1048-1065; *Skin Therapy Letter*, November 2006, pages 1-6; and *Bioscience, Biotechnology, and Biochemistry*, October 2008, pages 2589-2597).

AHA and BHA products. AHA concentrations between 4% and 10% and BHA concentrations between 1% and 2% can be effective not only because they accelerate cell turnover of the top layers of skin, but also because they directly inhibit melanin formation. That makes them a formidable asset in reducing or eliminating the appearance of brown discolorations (Source: *Experimental Dermatology*, January 2003, pages S43-S50).

Azelaic acid. Azelaic acid is considered very effective when applied topically in a cream formulation at a 15% to 20% concentration, and should be considered for a number of skin conditions. For the most part, azelaic acid is recommended as an option for acne or rosacea, but there is also some research showing it to be effective for the treatment of skin discolorations. Azelaic acid concentrations of 15% to 20% are available by prescription only. Twenty percent azelaic acid is available by prescription only in Azelex and 15% azelaic acid is found in the prescription-only Finacea (Sources: *Journal of Dermatology*, January 2007, pages 25-30; *Cutis*, February 2006, pages 22-24; and *Medical Hypotheses*, March 1999, pages 221-226). Concentrations less than 15% (usually less than 1%) show up in cosmetic skin-care products.

When combined with other "actives," ranging from retinol to AHAs and vitamin C, it can be another option when you begin experimenting to find what works for you.

Arbutin. Arbutin is a hydroquinone derivative isolated from the leaves of the bearberry shrub, cranberry, blueberry, and most types of pears, and serves a similar purpose. Because of arbutin's hydroquinone content, it can have melanin-inhibiting properties (Source: *Journal of Pharmacology and Experimental Therapeutics*, February 1996, pages 765-769). Although the research describing arbutin's effectiveness is persuasive (even if most of the research has been done on animals, in vitro, or by companies selling products using the ingredient), concentration protocols have not been established. That means we just don't know how much arbutin it takes to have an effect in lightening the skin.

The ingredients listed in this paragraph, along with their Latin or technical name, might show up in a skin-care product claiming to inhibit melanin production, but all have only minimal or no research showing them to be as effective as the options listed above: Paper mulberry (*Broussonetia kazinoke*); Mitracarpe (*Mitracarpus scaber*, an extract of bearberry); Bearberry (*Arctostaphylos uva ursi*); Yellow dock (*Rumex crispus* or *R. occidentalis*); glutathione; leukocyte extract (form of peptide); *Aspergillus orizae* (fungus); Licorice root (*Glycyrrhiza glabra*); and the following Chinese plant extracts: Yohimbe (*Pausinystalia yohimbe*); Cang Zhu (*Atractylodes lancea*), Bai Xian Pi (*Dictamnus dasycarpus* root-bark); Hu Zhang (*Polygonum cuspidatum* or giant knotweed rhizome), Gao Ben (*Ligusticum rhizome* or Chinese lovage root); Chuanxiong (*Rhizoma ligustici*); and Fangfeng (*Radix sileris* also *R. ledebouriella*).

(Sources for the above: *Journal of Investigate Dermatology*, Symposium Proceedings, April 2008, pages 20-24; *Chinese Journal of Integrated Medicine*, September 2007, pages 219-223; *Phytotherapy Research*, November 2006, pages 921-934; and *Household and Personal Products Industry Magazine*, April 2001.)

Vitamin C. Vitamin C is considered a stable and effective antioxidant for skin. For skin lightening, several studies have shown it can have benefit for inhibiting melanin production. What complicates the issue of vitamin C is that the vitamin has many forms, and these are used in skin-care products in a wide variety of concentrations. Options include magnesium ascorbyl phosphate, L-ascorbic acid, ascorbyl glucosamine, and ascorbic acid. While the amount of research isn't definitive, the vitamin offers other benefits along with its skin-lightening ability. Still, there are very few studies showing any of these have any effect on inhibiting melanin production, and the tests that do exist used concentrations far greater than the concentrations in most skin-care products. Generally, the amount of vitamin C in these studies ranged from 5% to 10%; most skin-care products that contain vitamin C usually have less than a 1% concentration (Source: *International Journal of Dermatology*, August 2004, pages 604-607).

When it comes to improving skin discolorations it is essential to use a combination approach. Diligent and consistent use of a well-formulated sunscreen is the first line of defense when tackling skin discolorations. Many researchers feel that 2% to 4% hydroquinone lotions can be more effective when combined with Retin-A or Renova, and exfoliating with AHAs or BHA is optimal. It is also extremely helpful to consider chemical peels or laser treatments to remove or lighten skin discolorations; and then to use the topicals mentioned above to maintain the improvement. Tackling discolorations via a single product approach most likely won't result in significant improvements.

SOLUTIONS FOR BLEMISHES

At the heart of the matter, acne is an inflammatory disorder. Interaction among a whole series of physical triggers creates redness and swelling that ends in the eruption of a blemish. Understanding how to stop this sequence of events from taking place, along with reducing inflammation, will let you begin to create a successful skin-care routine (Source: *Expert Opinions in Pharmacotherapy*, April 2008, pages 955-971).

The five major factors (and one minor one) that contribute to the formation of blemishes are:

1. Hormonal activity (primarily androgens, male hormones)
2. Overproduction of oil by the sebaceous (oil) gland (the oil gland is an important formation site of active androgens, which control oil production)
3. Irregular or excessive shedding of dead skin cells, both on the surface of skin and inside the pore
4. Buildup of bacteria in the pore
5. Irritation
6. Sensitizing reactions to cosmetics, specific foods (rarely), or medicines.

For optimal results when fighting blemishes and acne, what you can do is:

*   Reduce oil to eliminate the environment in which acne-causing bacteria thrive.
*   Exfoliate the skin's surface and within the pore to improve the shape and function of the pore.
*   Disinfect the skin to eliminate acne-causing bacteria.

Over-the-counter and prescription options abound for fighting blemishes, and that makes it a confusing battle to fight. It's confusing because there isn't one routine or medication (or combination of therapies) that works for everyone. Finding the combination that works for you is the goal, and that requires experimentation.

Clearing Blemishes, Step by Step:

Cleansing the Face: Use a gentle, water-soluble cleanser. One of the most common myths in the world of skin care is that a cooling or tingling sensation means that a product is "working," which couldn't be further from the truth. That tingling is just your skin responding to irritation, and products that produce that sensation actually can damage the skin's healing process, make scarring worse, trigger excess oil production, and encourage the bacteria that cause pimples. Using cleansers that contain pore-clogging ingredients (like soaps or bar cleansers) also can make matters worse (Source: *Dermatologic Therapy*, February, 2004, Supplement, pages 16-25 and 26-34).

I repeat: The essential first step is to find a gentle, water-soluble cleanser. If you are removing stubborn or waterproof makeup, you may need to use a washcloth to be sure you really remove all of your makeup. To prevent bacterial growth on that washcloth, use a clean one every time you wash your face.

Exfoliating: Use a 1% to 2% beta hydroxy acid (BHA) product or an 8% alpha hydroxy acid (AHA) product to exfoliate the skin. As a general rule, for all forms of breakouts, including blackheads, BHA is preferred over AHAs because BHA is better at cutting through the oil inside the pore (Source: *Cosmetic Dermatology*, October 2001, pages 65-72). Penetrating the pore is necessary to exfoliate the pore lining. However, some people (including those allergic to aspirin) can't use BHA, so an AHA is the next option to consider.

A topical scrub or a washcloth can be used as a mechanical exfoliant to remove dead skin cells. This is helpful for some people—but it does not in any way take the place of an effective BHA, AHA, or topical prescription treatment. Be careful never to overscrub when using a mechanical scrub because too much abrasion can disrupt the skin's ability to heal. And remember, acne cannot be scrubbed away!

Topical Disinfecting: Benzoyl peroxide is considered the most effective over-the-counter choice as a topical disinfectant to fight blemishes (Source: *Skin Pharmacology and Applied Skin Physiology*, September-October 2000, pages 292-296). The amount of research demonstrating the effectiveness of benzoyl peroxide is exhaustive and conclusive (Sources: *American Journal of Clinical Dermatology*, April 2004, pages 261-265; and *Journal of the American Academy of Dermatology*, November 1999, pages 710-716). Among benzoyl peroxide's attributes is its ability to penetrate into the hair follicle (pore) to reach the problem-causing bacteria and kill them—with a low risk of irritation. Furthermore, it doesn't pose the problem of bacterial resistance that occurs with some prescription topical antibacterials (antibiotics) (Source: *Dermatology*, 1998, pages 119-125).

There aren't many other options for disinfecting the skin. Alcohol and sulfur are good disinfectants, but they are also too drying and irritating, and they can make matters worse for skin by damaging the skin's ability to heal (Sources: *American Journal of Clinical Dermatology*, April 2004, pages 217-223; *Cosmetics & Toiletries Magazine*, March 2004, page 6; and *Infection*, March-April 1995, pages 89-93).

Absorbing Excess Oil: This is perhaps one of the most difficult skin-care problems to control. Because oil production is triggered only by hormones, there is nothing you can apply topically to stop your skin's oil glands from making more oil. What you can do to make sure you don't make matters worse is avoid products that contain oils or emollient ingredients. To absorb surface oil, forms of clay masks can help a lot, although avoid masks that contain irritating ingredients. As strange as it sounds, Phillip's Milk of Magnesia can be used as a facial mask. It is nothing more than liquid magnesium hydroxide, which does a very good job of absorbing oil. How often to use a mask depends on your skin type; some people use it every day, others once a week. A well-formulated absorbent mask may be used after cleansing, left on for 10 to 15 minutes, and then rinsed with tepid water.

Medical Options:

Retinoids: Aside from exfoliation, there are prescription options for improving the shape of the pore, including Retin-A (tretinoin), Differin (adapalene), and Tazorac (tazarotene). There is an immense amount of research showing that these are effective in treating acne (Source: *Journal of the American Medical Association*, August 11, 2004, pages 726-735). Depending on your skin type, you can use them up to twice a day. You also can try using them only at night, and then using a BHA or AHA during the day. As an alternative, some dermatologists recommend applying the BHA or AHA first, then applying Retin-A, Differin, or Tazorac. The theory is that the BHA or AHA boosts the effectiveness of the prescription products by helping them penetrate the skin better. Again, talk to your doctor and experiment to see which frequency, combination, and sequence of application works best for your skin.

Oral Antibiotics: If topical exfoliants, retinoids, and antibacterial agents don't provide satisfactory results, an oral antibiotic prescribed by a doctor may be an option to kill stubborn, blemish-causing bacteria. Several studies have shown that oral antibiotics, used in conjunction with topical tretinoins or topical exfoliants, can control or reduce many acne conditions

(Sources: *Cutis*, August 2008, pages S5-S12; and *International Journal of Dermatology*, January 2000, pages 45-50).

As effective as oral antibiotics can be, however, they should be a near-last resort, not a first line of attack. Oral antibiotics can produce some unacceptable long-term health problems.

For more detailed information on solutions for blemishes, please refer to my book *The Original Beauty Bible*, 3rd Edition, or visit my Web site at www.cosmeticscop.com.

SOLUTIONS FOR WRINKLES AND DRY SKIN

The plan presented in this section is designed to improve the overall appearance of your skin by supplying it with gentle, effective, and protective ingredients that have a proven track record for helping wrinkled skin look and feel better. Providing such benefits to skin on a daily basis will enhance its health and appearance, encourage collagen production, and help generate normalized skin cells, which altogether means greatly reducing wrinkles! Notice that I did *not* write that wrinkles can be "eliminated"! Regrettably, there is no magic potion or combination of products in any price range that can make wrinkles truly disappear. The wrinkles you see and agonize over (not to be confused with fine lines caused by dryness, which are easily remedied with a good moisturizer) are the result of cumulative sun damage and the inevitable breakdown of the skin's natural support structure. Skin-care ingredients, no matter who is selling them or what claims they assert, cannot replace what plastic surgeons or cosmetic dermatologists can do.

With those factors in mind, the basic place to start is to follow a step-by-step plan that provides what the skin needs to repair itself and to function optimally.

Use a state-of-the-art sunscreen, SPF 15 or greater whose formula goes beyond basic (and critical) sun protection and includes antioxidants, anti-irritants, cell-communicating ingredients, and ingredients that mimic the structure and function of healthy skin. An abundant and ever-expanding amount of scientific research is proving how antioxidants not only boost a sunscreen's efficacy, but also play a role in mitigating sun damage by reducing the free radicals and skin inflammation that sun exposure generates (Sources: *Experimental Dermatology*, January 2009, pages 522-526; *Journal of the American Academy of Dermatology*, June 2005, pages 937-958; *Photodermatology, Photoimmunology, and Photomedicine*, August 2004, pages 200-204; and *Cutis*, September 2003, pages 11-15).

Exfoliate with an effective AHA or BHA product. One significant consequence of sun damage is that the outer layer of skin becomes thickened, discolored, rough, and uneven. The best way to help skin shed abnormally built-up layers of dead, unhealthy skin is to use a well-formulated alpha hydroxy acid (AHA) or beta hydroxy acid (BHA) product. Such exfoliation not only will even out skin tone, but also will significantly improve the texture of skin. Another benefit is that exfoliating accumulated layers of dead skin cells helps other products you use, particularly moisturizers, penetrate your skin and be far more effective. The most researched forms of AHAs are glycolic or lactic acids; salicylic acid is the sole BHA option. For AHAs, look for products that contain at least 5% AHA, but preferably 8% to 10%. If the percentage isn't listed on the label, then the ingredient should be at the top of the ingredient list. For BHA products, 0.5% to 2% concentrations are available.

The difference in concentrations between the AHAs and BHA is not a qualitative one. Rather, it's just that leave-on, daily-use AHAs are effective at 5% to 10% and BHA is effective at 1% to 2% (Sources: *Women's Health in Primary Care*, July 2003, pages 333-339; *Journal of*

Dermatological Treatment, April 2004, pages 88-93; *Dermatology*, January 1999, pages 50-53; and *Journal of the American Academy of Dermatology*, April 1997, pages 589-593).

A well-formulated, state-of-the-art moisturizer is basic. Choose a product, regardless of the name on the label, appropriate for your skin type and loaded with antioxidants, skin-identical ingredients, and cell-communicating ingredients. If you have normal to oily or blemish-prone skin it should have a liquid, gel, or thin serum consistency. For normal to dry skin, use a lotion or lightweight cream, and for dry to very dry skin, use a very emollient or balm-like cream.

Explanation of Reviews

HOW PRODUCTS ARE RATED

Rating a wide variety of cosmetic products is a rigorous, complex process. Establishing criteria that will let someone distinguish and differentiate a terrible product from a great one, or a good product from one that's just mediocre, requires exact and consistently applied guidelines, and, moreover, guidelines that must be substantiated with published research that used clear criteria and rigorous scientific methods. These are exactly the criteria I've created for each product type that I review in this book.

First—and above all—**you need to know that my team and I do not base any rating decision on our personal experience with a product.** In other words, just because I like the way a cleanser or a moisturizer feels on my skin, I know it doesn't mean that thousands of others will feel the same way about it. Personal feelings won't help you evaluate whether a product may hurt your skin or live up to any part of the claims showcased on the label. There are lots of online beauty chat rooms and blogs, fashion magazines, and friends who love to share their personal experiences about the products they use (many of them post reviews). That might be interesting and entertaining, but it's important to recognize that lots of people also like things that aren't good for them. Some people may like sun tanning; others may use products that contain irritating ingredients because they believe the tingling feeling means it's "working." Most people have no idea what kinds of ingredients can damage skin.

Think about it like diet. If you based what you eat on what you liked, you might be eating only ice cream or pizza or chocolate cake. If you had to choose between broccoli and chocolate cake, the choice would be chocolate cake. The only reason you consider eating broccoli or spinach is because the research clearly indicates that they are healthy for your body. The same is true for skin. There is abundant, thorough research showing what is good for skin, which cannot be determined by common sense or feelings.

If you're going to spend money on a product, why not find out first whether or not it can live up to its claims—based on formulary or comparison performance issues—and then see how you can expect it to perform on you? That is what you will find out from the reviews in this book.

All of the ratings for the skin-care products in this book are based primarily on the formula of the individual product. I have consulted countless published, peer-reviewed studies about the ingredients in the product, and have considered the possible resulting interactions, with each other and with your skin. I also evaluate these formulas based on published cosmetics chemistry data about ingredient performance and consistency. From that I can assess a product's potential for irritation, dryness, breakouts, sensitivities, greasiness, and other issues of texture and performance.

Makeup products are evaluated more subjectively than skin-care products with regard to their application, color selection, texture, and how they and their performance compare with similar products from myriad other lines. Formulation is also a consideration in reviewing makeup products, but predominantly for claims made in regard to skin care and for any makeup product that includes an SPF rating.

This rating process is more challenging than I can describe because even if I think a company is absurdly overcharging for its products or is exceedingly dishonest in its claims and advertising, and no matter how unethical it seems to me, it does not prevent me from saying that a product is good for a particular skin type. As you will see, I often say, "This is a good product, but what a shame the price is so absurd and the claims so ridiculous!"

Overall, the evaluation process for this 8th Edition of *Don't Go to the Cosmetics Counter Without Me* is the same as for the most recent previous editions. However, you will find one major difference that has had a direct impact on the product ratings. In this edition, I use a far more stringent standard for excellence for every category of product. Happy faces are no longer awarded to ordinary, perfunctory products with mediocre, standard, or even good formulations. For example, if a product makes claims about containing antioxidants or anti-irritants, then it better contain a convincing amount of these ingredients. Thus, you will notice that many more products receive neutral ratings in this edition than in previous editions, and many of those neutral ratings are because of inadequate packaging.

In this book, I make the final and fundamental determination for each individual product rating based on specific criteria established for each product category. For every category, from lipsticks, blushes, mascaras, and eyeshadows, to concealers, foundations, cleansers, toners, scrubs, moisturizers, facial masks, AHA products, wrinkle creams, and brushes, I've created specific standards that the products in each category must meet to garner a happy, unhappy, or neutral (meaning unimpressive but not bad) face.

Makeup products are assessed primarily on texture and application using professional tools (brushes). For example, was it silky-smooth or grainy and overly dry? Also important are color, ease of use, and price. Color: Was a wide range of colors available? Was there an adequate selection for women of color? Ease of Use: Was the container poorly designed? Were colors placed too close together in an eyeshadow set? Was foundation put in a pump container that squirted too much product or didn't reach to the bottom of the component? And, finally, Price. More specific criteria for each makeup category are discussed further in this chapter.

Skin-care products are evaluated almost exclusively on the basis of content versus claim. For example, if a product claims to be good for sensitive skin, it cannot contain irritants, skin sensitizers, drying ingredients, and so on.

I also asked the following questions to see if a product measures up to its claims, based on established and published research:

1. Given the ingredient list, and based on published research—not just on what the cosmetics company wants you to believe—can the product really do what it promises?

2. How does the product differ from similar types of products?

3. If a special ingredient (or ingredients) are showcased, how much of it is actually in the product, and is there independent research verifying the claims for it?

4. Does the product contain problematic fragrances (including volatile fragrance chemicals), plants, topical irritants, or other questionable ingredients that could cause problems for skin?

5. How farfetched are the product's claims?

6. Based on what's known about the ingredients it contains, is the product safe? Are there risks such as allergic reactions, increased sun sensitivity, insufficient sunscreen formulations, or potentially toxic ingredients?

I wish I had the space to challenge and explain every single exaggerated claim and lofty explanation that accompanies the products listed in this book, but there is just not enough room (or time) to tackle that prodigious task. I cover most of the distortions and some of the hyperbole about products and ingredients in the reviews and in the *Cosmetic Ingredient Dictionary* section of my Web site, www.Beautypedia.com.

DUE DILIGENCE

I can't stress enough how much time and effort my staff and I put into gathering our information. We are diligent about making sure we incorporate accurate and precise information or research for all of the products we review. To accomplish this, the first order of business with every edition is to contact every cosmetics company whose products I'm reviewing and ask them to please send whatever they can about their data or facts regarding their products and claims. Unlike the 7th edition of this book, only a handful of companies were forthcoming with information this time, including ingredient and product lists. Most cosmetic brands we contacted weren't willing to send us anything about their company or their products, let alone details about the "research" or the "studies" they use to "substantiate" their claims.

Let me state clearly that I am more than willing to present any documented research and substantiating information that contradicts or disproves something I've previously written. I am more than willing to revise my previously stated opinions and positions as new research comes to light, showing that earlier information is no longer correct. As an example, over the years I have changed my opinion on sunscreens with regard to the new research on UVA protection. I have modified my attitude toward antioxidants, salicylic acid (BHA), and cell-communicating ingredients, too, given the growing body of literature establishing the positive effects of these ingredients on skin. I also am now more open to layering products when different active ingredients are needed, ranging from skin-lightening products to sunscreens and acne products. I could go on, but I want to be explicit about my desire to present the most up-to-date, currently published research that exists when it comes to skin-care formulations and makeup products.

I also want to thank the companies that did send me their information. While I may not agree with them on the quality of all their products or their advertising claims, their willingness to be forthcoming about their formulations and claims is appreciated.

The following companies were extremely helpful in providing information for the compilation of this book: Alpha Hydrox, BeautiControl, Boots, Cetaphil, DHC, GloMinerals, Laura Geller, Lorac, NeoStrata, Nivea, Olay, ProActiv, Sheer Cover, Stridex, and Trish McEvoy.

IS IT NECESSARY TO TRY A PRODUCT BEFORE REVIEWING IT?

Many people wonder how I can judge the value of a skin-care product by its label. You may be thinking, "Wouldn't that be like judging the taste of a food just by the ingredients in it? What about tasting it for yourself?" Taste is necessary information, but nowadays it is also prudent to judge a food by its ingredient list before you even put it in your mouth. It would be foolish for any of us to consume anything without a clear understanding of how much fat, cholesterol, sodium, preservatives, coloring agents, fiber, vitamins, carbohydrates, or calories it contains, along with myriad other things that are pertinent to our health, both general knowledge of healthy eating habits and personal dietary needs. Without that information, regardless of the taste (and everyone has their own bias when it comes to taste), you would never know what you were putting in your body.

As you are well aware, you can cause yourself harm by eating what isn't good for you. You may love the taste, but eating too much fat, calories, or salt can lead to weight gain, cancer, high blood pressure, and so on. If you aren't getting appropriate nutrition, you can become malnourished. If you have food allergies or sensitivities, you might eat something that is dangerous for you. How would you ever know what you were doing to yourself? The labels on food are every consumer's best friend, whether you're shopping at a discount grocery store or the fanciest gourmet market.

Just as food labels are incredibly important, so are skin-care and makeup ingredient labels. But, cosmetic ingredient labels are much more difficult for consumers to understand, not only because the ingredients have complicated technical names but also because an ingredient may have several names. In addition, there are thousands of cosmetic ingredients that can show up in a product and the combinations of ingredients have significance for different skin types and the overall health of the skin. That's what I can provide. I translate the information on the skin-care ingredient label into what it can really provide for your skin according to published research about that formulary. If a skin-care product says it is good for sensitive skin and won't cause breakouts, but then contains ingredients known to cause irritation and breakouts, that is essential information. If a skin-care product sells for $100, but contains the same ingredients as a product that costs $20, that is, to say the least, very important information. Perhaps even more significant, if a $100 product contains fewer or less effective ingredients than a $20 product, that is crucial consumer information. If a product claims to protect skin from the sun, but doesn't have an SPF 15 or greater and doesn't contain UVA-protecting ingredients, that is vital information, regardless of price. A person may love how the product is packaged, how it feels on their skin, or even the results they see, but that doesn't guarantee they're using an outstanding (or even average) product.

The bottom line is that the ingredient list helps you sort through the jungle of choices. It's a far better starting point than basing decisions strictly on advertising mumbo jumbo or on promises that are never delivered.

EVALUATING SKIN-CARE PRODUCTS

My reviews of skin-care products in each line are, with some exceptions, organized in the following categories: cleansers, eye-makeup removers, scrubs, toners, alpha hydroxy acid or beta hydroxy acid exfoliants, moisturizers and serums (all kinds, regardless of the claim or type, such as eye or neck creams), specialty products, sunscreens for use from the neck down, anti-acne products, facial masks, and lip products. The criteria I used to evaluate the quality of the products in each of the different categories of skin-care products are explained below.

CLEANSERS: In reviewing facial cleansers, the primary criteria are how genuinely water-soluble they are, and how gentle. Facial cleansers should rinse off easily, with or without the aid of a washcloth, and remove all traces of makeup, including eye makeup. Once a water-soluble cleanser is rinsed off, it should not leave the skin feeling dry, greasy, or filmy. And it should never burn the eyes, irritate the skin, or taste bad. Cleansers that meet these criteria and that also are fragrance-free receive my top rating (Paula's Pick).

EYE-MAKEUP REMOVERS: Eye-makeup removers must efficiently and easily take off makeup and they must not contain irritating ingredients of any kind. Makeup removers are one of the few categories in which the products are nearly indistinguishable from one another. They are formulated so similarly that there are no surprises or real cautions needed. Eye-makeup removers rated Paula's Picks are assigned that distinction because of their exceptionally gentle, fragrance-free formulas and because they are effective for their intended purpose.

SCRUBS: Mechanical exfoliation is a fancy name for scrubs, brushes, or washcloths that remove skin cells as you massage them over the skin. Many scrubs are unnecessarily irritating and should be avoided; as a result they get a bad rating. It is also important for scrubs to rinse off easily without leaving any residue or greasy feel on the skin. Some women prefer the feeling of a scrub on their skin, but there aren't many scrubs that are any better than just a clean, soft washcloth with a gentle, water-soluble cleanser, and I often state that in the review. Scrubs rated Paula's Picks meet the criteria of being gentle and easy to rinse and have additional positive traits such as being fragrance-free or containing buffering agents that do not impede rinsing or hinder effectiveness.

ALPHA HYDROXY ACID (AHA) AND BETA HYDROXY ACID (BHA) EXFOLI-ANTS: Without question AHAs and BHA are the most effective exfoliants you can use when they are well-formulated. I apply very specific criteria to determine if an AHA or BHA product will be an effective exfoliant. When it comes to AHAs and BHA, the crucial information comes in two parts. One is the type of ingredient and its concentration in the product; the other is the pH of the product. AHAs work best at concentrations of 5% to 8% in a base with a pH of 3 to 4 (this is more acid than neutral), and their effectiveness diminishes as the pH rises above 4.5. BHA works best at concentrations of between 1% and 2% at an optimal pH of 3, its effectiveness diminishing as the pH increases beyond 4. Generally, the effectiveness of both AHAs and BHA decreases as a product's pH increases and as the concentration of the ingredient decreases. This relationship is so central to the entire subject of exfoliation and cell turnover that it bears repeating: AHAs work best in a 5% to 8% concentration in a product with a pH of 3 to 4; BHA works best in a 1% to 2% concentration, in a product with a pH of 3 to 4 (Source: *Cosmetic Dermatology*, October 2001, pages 15-18).

Salicylic acid (BHA), although it provides more penetrating exfoliation into the pore, can be less irritating than AHAs because of its close chemical relation to aspirin. Salicylic acid is derived from acetylsalicylic acid, which is the technical name for aspirin, and aspirin has anti-inflammatory properties. When applied topically on the skin, the salicylic acid in BHA products retains many of these anti-inflammatory properties. AHAs, on the other hand, have some irritating properties, so AHA products that contain special anti-irritant or antioxidant ingredients receive better ratings than AHA products that do not contain such ingredients.

AHA and BHA products definitely can smooth the skin, improve texture, unclog pores, and give the appearance of plumper, firmer skin because more healthy skin cells are now on the surface. But that change is not permanent; when you stop using the AHA or BHA, the skin goes back to the condition it was in before you started.

Products that contain AHA sound-alikes, including sugarcane extract, mixed fruit acids, fruit extracts, milk extract, and citrus extract, or BHA derivatives, such as wintergreen extract or willow bark extract, cannot exfoliate skin, or do much of anything else, although willow bark does have anti-inflammatory properties. Therefore, I rate products that contain these ingredients not effective. You might think these are better because they appear to be a more natural form of AHA or BHA when you see the less technical, more familiar plant names on the label, but that perception is not reality.

FACIAL MASKS: Many facial masks contain claylike ingredients that absorb oil and, to some degree, exfoliate the skin, which can be beneficial for someone with oily skin. The problem with many masks is that they often contain additional ingredients that are irritating or that can clog pores. Although your face may feel smooth right after you rinse the mask off, after a short period of time you may experience problems created by the mask's drying effect. Even the few clay masks that contain emollients and moisturizing ingredients can still be too drying for dry skin, and they can cause oily skin to break out. There are also a range of masks that contain plasticizing (hairspray-like) ingredients that you apply and then peel off your face like a layer of plastic. Such masks take a layer of skin off when removed, and that can make skin feel temporarily smoother, but there is no long-term benefit to be gained and this amount of film-forming agent isn't the best for skin, so these always receive a poor rating.

The claims that clay from one part of the world or another, or from some part of the ocean or from a volcanic region is best for skin aren't supported by research of any kind showing that to be true. In essence, there isn't any research anywhere showing that clay can do anything beneficial for skin other than absorb oil, and there is not a shred of research showing that plasticizing masks have any benefit whatsoever. Moreover, any skin-care step used only occasionally simply can't have as much value as a better routine used daily.

Another type of facial mask that shows up is the kind with strictly moisturizing ingredients. Basically, these don't differ from moisturizers except that they are thicker formulations. Calling the product a mask seems to make women feel like they are doing something special for their skin, when, with very few exceptions, they aren't. Despite all these shortcomings, which I point out in the individual reviews, there are masks in this book that do get happy face and Paula's Pick ratings, either because they have potential benefit for dry skin (i.e., if they contain ingredients that can address this condition) or because they have absorbent value for oily skin.

Masks are rated based on their compatibility for each skin type and on whether or not they contain irritants. For dry skin the mask must have emollient properties and for oily skin it must have absorbent ingredients. Masks rated Paula's Pick exceed those criteria and go above and beyond by offering either fragrance-free formulas or unique extras with genuine benefit for skin.

TONERS: Toners, astringents, fresheners, tonics, and other liquids meant to refresh the skin or remove the last traces of makeup after a cleanser is rinsed off should not contain any irritants whatsoever. That is the basic standard, but a superior product also should deliver state-of-the-art ingredients to skin, including antioxidants, skin-identical ingredients, and cell-communicating ingredients. Regrettably, this entire category is one where the industry overall offers some of the most ordinary, banal formulas imaginable with very little benefit for skin beyond the basics. Unfortunately, it is still true that many toners (particularly those aimed at people with acne) contain irritants, making them unacceptable for any skin type. Those always receive an unacceptable rating.

When toners are well formulated they can be a great start to any skin-care regimen, adding an extra helping of brilliant, healthy ingredients to skin.

MOISTURIZERS: Despite all the fuss, assertions, and price differences among antiwrinkle, firming, anti-aging, and renewing products that claim to restore youth to skin, in truth these products are nothing more than "moisturizers." A plethora of these products are being marketed to women, but I can tell you that there is not one plastic surgeon or dermatologist going out of business because of them.

As a general category, "moisturizers" are quite easy to review because what constitutes a state-of-the-art product in this category is well established in the scientific literature. They must contain ingredients that can smooth and soothe dry skin, keep moisture in the skin cell, help maintain or reinforce the skin's protective barrier, protect skin from free-radical damage, reduce inflammation or irritation, protect skin cell integrity, and contain cell-communicating ingredients to optimize healthy cell production, all in an elegant, silky emollient base for dry skin or an ultralight gel, serum, or liquid base. Almost all other claims for this immense group of products are exaggerated and misleading, not to mention never-ending!

A recurring myth espoused at cosmetics counters and routinely in fashion magazines is that oily skin needs a moisturizer. In other words, you may be told that oily skin makes more oil because it is combating some form of underlying dryness. No part of that is true. Oil production is controlled and regulated by hormones (Sources: *Clinical and Experimental Dermatology*, October 2001, pages 600-607; and *Seminars in Cutaneous Medicine and Surgery*, September 2001, pages 144-153). If dry skin could induce oil production, then everyone with dry skin would be oozing oil, but they aren't, because physiologically that isn't how skin works (and the insanity of that hurts my brain). All skin types need healthy state-of-the-art ingredients, but they do not have to come in a lotion, balm, or cream form; gels, liquids, and serums serve that purpose perfectly for those with normal to oily or blemish-prone skin.

While multitudes of ingredients are potentially helpful for skin, there are also a number that are a waste of time, or worse. These range from bee pollen to gold to animal extracts from a thymus, a spleen, or a placenta, as well as plant extracts that can be potential skin irritants and actually damage skin—I point out as many of these as I can in my reviews. If there is no research showing these ingredients are helpful for skin, then they are there for marketing purposes only, and that doesn't help your skin.

There are also moisturizers that companies promote as being great for combination skin because they claim they can release moisturizing ingredients over dry areas and oil-absorbing ingredients over oily areas. That is categorically impossible. A product cannot hold certain ingredients back from the skin—where would they go? Imagine a lotion touching your skin and separating so the ingredients for the oily parts get up and run over here and the ones for the dry area get up and head over there. It just isn't feasible in any way, shape, or form. If you have combination skin (meaning slightly dry to dry areas accompanied by oily areas), you need to apply a moisturizer only over the dry parts of your face, including around the eyes, if applicable. If you have combination skin and wish to use something all over your face, shop for water- or silicone-based gel or serum-type moisturizers so you don't make the oily areas worse.

MOISTURIZERS FOR OILY SKIN: Even when skin is oily it can still (and does) benefit from the application of products that contain antioxidants, anti-irritants, skin-identical ingredients, and cell-communicating ingredients.

When a product, particularly a moisturizer, claims to be oil-free, noncomedogenic, or non-acnegenic, it often misleads consumers into thinking they are buying a product that won't clog pores. But those terms are not regulated by the FDA and have no legal meaning. A cosmetics company can use any or all of those terms without any qualifying ingredient listing or substantiation. Legally, you could label bacon grease noncomedogenic, as you could any substance or product, even those that clog pores.

The term "oil-free" is probably the most misleading, because there are plenty of ingredients that don't sound like oils, but that absolutely will aggravate breakouts. Many cosmetics contain waxlike thickening agents that can clog pores. These ingredients are included in moisturizers because they duplicate the natural lipids (sebum or oil) in our skin, or prevent dehydration, and that's great. But if you have problems already with the oil being created in your pores, adding more of the same kind of substance will only make things worse. Despite the problems these ingredients can cause, they show up in lots and lots of so-called oil-free products.

While there is evidence that some specific ingredients can trigger breakouts, there are no absolutes. I wish there were, but there aren't.

There are no easy answers for this one, but you can understand that trying to research, categorize, classify, and make absolute conclusions about thousands of ingredients with an infinite number of possible combinations is just not humanly possible.

However, here are a few ideas to at least point you in the right direction. Because a thicker formulation is more likely to contain problematic ingredients, just as a highly emollient product can, it is far better for those with normal to oily skin to use gel or "serum"-type products that leave out most, if not all, thickening agents. Moisturizers for oily skin are rated as preferred for that skin type if they are lightweight and have minimal to no waxy or emollient ingredients listed near the beginning of the ingredient list (because emollients theoretically can clog pores).

DAY MOISTURIZER VERSUS NIGHT MOISTURIZER: There is no difference between what the skin needs during the day and what it needs at night in terms of state-of-the-art ingredients such as antioxidants, skin-identical ingredients, and cell-communicating ingredients, except for sunscreen. The same way the body needs healthy foods any time of the day or night, so does the skin. Moisturizers labeled daytime moisturizers should absolutely contain sunscreen; if they don't, then the rating is based at least in part on the need to wear another product over it that does provide appropriate sun protection. If the daytime product does contain sunscreen, it is rated higher if it also has a generous blend of state-of-the-art ingredients. Other than that, moisturizers labeled as being for daytime are judged on their formula, the same as so-called nighttime products.

EYE, THROAT, CHEST, NECK, AND OTHER SPECIALTY CREAMS, SERUMS, OR GELS: There is no research showing that skin in the eye area, on the neck or chest, or any other specific area requires different ingredients than skin on the face. Buying a separate product for a special area of the face or body, whether a cream, gel, lotion, or serum, is altogether unnecessary. Almost without exception, the ingredient lists and formulations for such products are identical to the formulas of other creams, gels, lotions, or serums identified as being only for the face. That doesn't mean there aren't some beautifully formulated products labeled for different parts of the body, but their formulas are not special or unique for that area, so why buy a second moisturizer for the eye or neck area when the one you are already using on the rest of your face is brilliantly formulated as well.

The cosmetics industry makes a lot of money selling women extra products they don't need by dividing the body into different segments, each with purportedly different skin-care needs. Because of the relentless advertising pushing this erroneous concept, women stay tied to the belief that the eye area, throat, chest, legs, and hands all have different skin-care needs. Even more bothersome is the fact that most cosmetics companies give you only a tiny amount of the so-called specialty product, and then charge you a lot more for that tiny tube of product than they do for a large container of face cream, despite the similar formulations. Moreover, many eye-area products don't contain sunscreen. If your well-formulated face moisturizer contains sunscreen, but the product for your eye area doesn't, then you are actually allowing damage to occur on the skin around your eye by not using your face moisturizer with sunscreen in this area.

SUNSCREENS: Valid scientific research abounds demonstrating that wrinkles, skin damage, many skin discolorations, and many skin cancers result primarily from unprotected sun exposure (Sources: *British Journal of Dermatology*, July 2007, pages 26-32; *Journal of Cutaneous Pathology*, May 2007, pages 376-380; *Radiation and Environmental Biophysics*, March 2007, pages 61-68; and *Mechanisms of Ageing and Development*, April 2002, pages 801-810). Clearly this subject has to do not only with cosmetics, but also with serious health issues. It is well established that the only true, first-line-of-defense, antiwrinkle product is a well-formulated and carefully applied sunscreen. My Web site, www.cosmeticscop.com, has extensive information on the wide variety of concerns, problems, and cautions regarding sunscreen formulations and application.

The main criterion for a well-formulated sunscreen is the SPF rating, with SPF 15 being the standard considered basic by most dermatology and cancer organizations around the world. However, the SPF number only tells you how long you can stay in the sun without getting sunburned, which is caused by the sun's UVB rays. While that is helpful, it is only part of the protection you need. It is now known that most wrinkling, and possibly skin cancer, results from unprotected exposure to the sun's UVA rays. Because of the difference between UVA damage and UVB damage, and because there is still no UVA rating system, to ensure you are getting adequate UVA protection, your sunscreen must contain one of the five UVA-protecting ingredients and they must be listed as an active ingredient on the label. These active ingredients are avobenzone (also called Parsol 1789 or butyl methoxydibenzoylmethane), titanium dioxide, zinc oxide, Tinosorb, and Mexoryl SX (ecamsule) (Sources: *Free Radical Research*, April 2007, pages 461-468; *Mutation Research*, April 2007, pages 71-78; *International Journal of Radiation Biology*, November 2006, pages 781-792; *Photodermatology, Photoimmunology, & Photomedicine*, December 2000, pages 250-255; and *Photochemistry and Photobiology*, March 2000, pages 314–320).

No sunscreen receives a happy face rating unless one of those UVA-protecting ingredients is listed on the active ingredient part of the ingredient list and it has an SPF of 15 or greater.

Sunscreens rated a Paula's Pick not only provide sufficient UVA protection but also contain several beneficial extras for sun-exposed skin, including potent antioxidants that help boost skin's defenses in the presence of sunlight.

Synthetic sunscreen ingredients can be irritating to skin no matter what the product's label says. (Only titanium dioxide and zinc oxide are considered mineral or "natural" sunscreen ingredients.) You have to experiment to find the one that works best for you. The sunscreens that contain only mineral ingredients are considered almost completely nonirritating; however, they can still pose problems for someone with oily or acne-prone skin because their occlusive composition means they can clog pores and aggravate breakouts. This is not to say that someone with blemish-prone skin should avoid these active ingredients. It is not a given that they will make you break out, just something to be aware of as you're experimenting with various sunscreens.

Applying sunscreen liberally is indispensable for the health of skin, which means that all expensive sunscreens are potentially dangerous for skin, not because they don't provide the proper protection, but because their high cost might discourage you from applying it liberally. Think about it: How liberally will you apply a $50-for-1-ounce sunscreen to your face or body versus a product that costs only $20 for 2, 4, or 6 ounces?

SUNSCREENS FOR OILY OR COMBINATION SKIN: Sunscreens are a very tricky category for someone with oily or combination skin. It takes experimentation to find the one that works best for you. The problem is that the ingredients used to suspend the active ingredients are not necessarily the best for oily skin. What I generally recommend is that someone with oily or combination skin select a foundation or pressed powder that contains well-formulated sunscreens. Before applying your makeup with sunscreen, apply an appropriate lightweight gel moisturizer over dry areas or just use a well-formulated toner all over, which can be enough "moisturizing" for that skin type. Be sure to use a regular sunscreen on all exposed skin from the neck down.

SUNSCREENS FOR SENSITIVE SKIN (INCLUDING ROSACEA): The nonirritating nature of titanium dioxide and zinc oxide, when they are the only actives listed on the ingredient label, assures you that you are getting an optimal product for sensitive skin. Neither ingredient is known for causing an irritant response or a sensitizing reaction on skin (Sources: *Cosmetics & Toiletries*, October 2003, pages 73-78; and *Cutis*, September 2004, pages 13-16 and 32-34).

WATER-RESISTANT SUNSCREENS: In truth, no sunscreen is really "waterproof." You must reapply if you have been sweating or immersed in water for a period of time. The only terms approved for use on sunscreens are "water-resistant" and "very water-resistant." The FDA's ruling on this matter reflects research data from studies that prove these products have only a limited ability to stay in place when people are in water or sweating. To determine a product's water resistance, the SPF value is measured directly after application and then again after a period of immersion in water. A "water-resistant" product means that its labeled SPF value measured directly after application and then again after 40 minutes of immersion is the same; that is, it maintains its SPF value over the entire 40 minutes of immersion. A "very water-resistant" product means that the SPF value on the label remained the same after 80 minutes of water immersion (Source: www.fda.gov).

If you are swimming or sweating outdoors, you absolutely should use a sunscreen that's labeled water-resistant or very water-resistant, and reapply it frequently. These sunscreens are formulated differently from regular sunscreens, using acrylate and silicone polymer technology in their formulations, which helps them hold up remarkably well in water. Acrylate-type ingredients are, like hairspray, holding agents. These plasticizing ingredients form a film over the skin and can take a great deal of wear and tear in contact with water and friction before the sunscreen protection is diluted and rinsed away.

SELF-TANNERS: All self-tanning products, whether you choose one made by Coppertone, Clarins, Decleor Paris, or Estee Lauder, are created equal. The active ingredient in almost every single one of these products is dihydroxyacetone, which is what turns the surface layer of skin brown. This ingredient acts on the skin cells and their amino acid content, causing a chemical reaction that temporarily gives the skin a darker color. These products are considered completely safe for skin (Source: *American Journal of Clinical Dermatology*, 2002, volume 3, number 5, pages 317-318). Rarely, some self-tanners contain erythrulose in addition to dihydroxyacetone. Erythrulose acts similarly to, but more slowly than, dihydroxyacetone, which means it takes longer (usually 2 to 3 days) for it to have an effect on skin color.

Your personal preference as to how self-tanners make your skin appear actually has less to do with the product itself than with the nature of your own skin cells. The interaction between the active ingredient and your skin is controlled more by your body's chemistry than anything else. That's why your friend or sister may have brilliant results with a self-tanner that made your skin look rust-colored or unnaturally orange.

ACNE PRODUCTS: Dermatological journals from around the world make it clear that acne products must deliver four categories of performance to deal with breakouts: (1) gentle cleansing (to remove excess oil and reduce inflammation), (2) effective exfoliation to unblock pores and reshape the pore lining, (3) disinfection, and (4) absorption of excess oil (Source: *American Journal of Clinical Dermatology*, 2001, volume 2, number 3, pages 135-141). I base my reviews for these types of products on how they measure up to these four important skin-care needs. Anti-acne products that contain needless irritants (e.g., alcohol, witch hazel, and menthol) always receive a bad rating because they are damaging to skin and can increase oil production.

CLEANSERS FOR ACNE PRONE SKIN: Using a gentle, water-soluble cleanser is standard for any skin-care routine, and it is equally necessary for those with blemish-prone skin. Often, skin-care routines aimed at those with oily skin or acne recommend cleansers that are exceptionally drying or irritating, which can increase inflammation. Yet, as I've mentioned several times throughout this introduction, inflammation damages the skin's healing process and increases oil production, which only makes matters worse.

I also never recommend bar soap for acne or breakouts. Bar soaps of any kind are kept in their bar form by ingredients that potentially can clog pores. Research also shows that high-pH cleansers (soaps usually have a pH greater than 8) can increase the presence of bacteria in the skin (Source: *Cutis*, December 2001, Supplemental, pages 12-19). To that end, I rate gentle, water-soluble cleansers highly if they do not contain irritating or excessively drying ingredients.

EXFOLIANTS FOR ACNE PRONE SKIN: See the sections above on "Scrubs" and on "Alpha Hydroxy Acid (AHA) and Beta Hydroxy Acid (BHA) Products."

DISINFECTANTS FOR ACNE PRONE SKIN: To kill the bacteria in the skin that cause blemishes (*Propionibacterium acnes*), you need a reliable topical disinfectant (available over the counter) or topical antibiotic (available by prescription). There aren't many options when it comes to disinfecting the skin with over-the-counter products. The best over-the-counter topical disinfectant is either a 2.5%, 5%, or 10% benzoyl peroxide product—but only if no irritating ingredients are added. In fact, research has established benzoyl peroxide as one of the most effective treatments for mild to moderate acne (Sources: *Drugs in Dermatology*, June 2007, pages 616-622; *Cutis*, June 2007, Supplemental, pages 9-25; and *Lancet*, December 2004, pages 2188-2195). As a general rule, it is better to begin with a 2.5% benzoyl peroxide solution to see if it is effective, rather than starting with the more potent, and somewhat more irritating, 5% or 10% concentrations. If one of those doesn't work for you, the next step is to see a dermatologist to investigate the options of a topical antibiotic in association with a topical retinoid such as Retin-A, Differin, Tazorac, or Avita. For more information on topical antibiotics and retinoids along with other treatments for acne, please refer to my Web site www.cosmeticscop.com.

ABSORBING EXCESS OIL: There are many types of skin-care and makeup products designed to create a matte finish or place an oil-absorbing layer of ingredients on the skin. Although these products often work well to absorb excess oil and keep shine under control, none of them can stop oil production because oil production is controlled primarily by your hormones, and that cannot be affected from the outside with cosmetics.

I often point out that oil-absorbing ingredients like rice starch, cornstarch, and other food products typically are considered problematic for those who have breakouts. Food substances can get into pores and encourage bacteria production (after all, bacteria thrive on organic substances), which is not the best when your goal is to fight off the bacteria.

Clay masks are popular options for absorbing excess oil on the skin. While they can help, they often contain other ingredients that are skin irritants, can clog pores, or are too emollient for oily skin. I rate clay masks and other masks primarily on whether or not they contain irritating or emollient ingredients that are not be appropriate for blemish-prone skin.

SKIN-LIGHTENING PRODUCTS: Regardless of whether they come in cream, lotion, gel, or liquid form, all skin-lightening products should contain at least 2% hydroquinone and/ or an impressive amount of alternative ingredients (such as arbutin, niacinamide, or a form of vitamin C) that have research demonstrating their ability to affect melanin production as a means of lightening sun- or hormone-induced skin discolorations. Although there are no formulary protocols for alternative skin-lightening agents, the research that does exist involved higher concentrations than are present in most products. Therefore, products with only minute amounts of alternative ingredients generally are rated poorly.

WHAT WORKS VERSUS MARKETING CLAIMS

While I want to emphasize how extensive the misleading portrayals of skin-care products and their supposed effects and benefits are within the cosmetics industry, I also want to underscore that there are hundreds of great products for all skin types. When I describe my elation or enthusiasm about any product, I am also careful to let you know what you can really expect and, where applicable, how out-of-line the price often is for what you are getting. So, just because I think a formula is amazing for dry skin, that doesn't mean I concur with its claims about firming, lifting, undoing or preventing wrinkling, reducing lines, fighting stress, erasing cellulite, and on and on and on....

INGREDIENT HIGHLIGHTS

When reading ingredient lists, remember, the ingredients are listed in order of their concentration, from most to least. The closer an ingredient is to the end of the ingredient list or the closer it is to a preservative (e.g., phenoxyethanol, methylparaben, propylparaben, ethylparaben, imidazolidinyl urea, or methylisothiazolinone) or to a fragrance (e.g., fragrance, parfum, or often an individual essential oil such as lavender oil or bergamot oil), the less likely it is that there is a significant amount of that ingredient in the product. That means its impact, for better or for worse, is negligible.

When I use the term "thickeners" to describe ingredients, I'm referring to components that add texture, thickness, viscosity, spreadability, and stability to a product. Thickeners that function as emulsifiers are also vital for keeping other ingredients mixed together. Thickening agents often have a waxlike texture or a creamy, emollient feel, and can be great lubricants. There are literally thousands of ingredients in this category, and they are the staples of every skin-care product out there, regardless of the product's price or claims about "natural" ingredients.

Slip agents help other ingredients spread over or penetrate the skin and they also have humectant properties. Slip agents include propylene glycol, butylene glycol, and hexylene glycol, among many others. The misleading information you read about these being bad for skin is related only to the amount. At 100% concentrations, they are definitely too strong and irritating; however, at 100% concentration, lots of things are too strong and irritating, including plants, water, and minerals.

Abrasive or scrub ingredients are found in cleansing scrubs or in some facial masks meant to remove dead skin cells. The most typical scrub particles are polyethylene, almond meal, cornmeal, ground apricot kernels, jojoba beads, and almond pits. Polyethylene is the most common form of plastic used in the world and the most popular scrub agent. It is flexible and has a smooth, waxy feel. When ground up, the small particles appear in scrubs as a fairly gentle abrasive. Seashells (listed as diatomaceous earth on the ingredient label) also are used as abrasives in scrubs, but they can be extremely rough on skin due to their uneven shape and rough edges.

Aluminum oxide (also listed as alumina), the same substance used in microdermabrasion treatments, also shows up in some scrub products. This substance can be extremely gritty and irritating for skin and may be too harsh for regular use, and I mention that in the reviews.

Absorbents in skin-care and makeup products are designed to create a matte finish or oil-absorbing film layer on the skin. These absorbent materials are typically talc, silicates (e.g., magnesium aluminum silicate), clays, dry-finish silicones or silicone polymers (usually cyclopentasiloxane or phenyl trimethicone), nylon-12, and film-forming agents (hairspray-like ingredients), and all of these can absorb oil effectively. Some have drier finishes than others, but that depends on the specific formulation and the amount of the ingredient. As I often point out, my concern about ingredients like rice starch, cornstarch, and other food products is that they are typically problematic for breakouts. Food substances can get into pores and encourage bacteria production, which is not the best when fighting off bacteria is the goal.

Film-forming agents are ingredients such as polyvinyl pyrrolidone (PVP), methylacrylate, and the polyglycerylacrylates presently being used in a vast number of moisturizers, wrinkle creams, and eye gels to help the skin look smoother. Film-forming agents usually are found in hairsprays and hairstyling products like gels and mousses because they place a thin, transparent, plastic-like layer over the hair (and skin). In the past, the kinds of film-forming agents used were problematic for some skin types; today, with the advent of new polymers, these ingredients do a good job of keeping moisture in the skin and generally are present in such tiny amounts that they are unlikely to be a problem for most skin types. Some film-forming agents have oil-absorbing properties. When these film-forming agents are listed relatively higher up on a product's ingredient list, they might be present at an amount that can leave a slightly tacky feeling on the skin.

Most skin cleansers include ingredients known as surfactants. Surfactant is a technical term that refers to a large number of ingredients that can cleanse as well as degrease. When cleansers contain surfactants as the primary cleansing agent, I use the phrases detergent-based, detergent cleansing agent, or standard detergent cleanser. The most common ingredients in this category include cocoamidopropyl betaine, sodium laureth sulfate, TEA-lauryl sulfate, cocamide DEA, ammonium laureth sulfate, and ammonium lauryl sulfate, to name a few. Because sodium lauryl sulfate, TEA-lauryl sulfate, and sodium C14-16 olefin sulfate are very strong detergent cleansing agents and are known for their irritation potential (Sources: *British Journal of Dermatology*, May 2002, pages 792-800; and *Toxicology in Vitro*, August-October 2001, pages 597-600), I warn against using a product that contains them when they appear in the first part of the ingredient list.

A profusion of plant extracts are used in cosmetics, so many that it's impossible to list them all individually and explain their purpose or lack of purpose. As far as the world of cosmetics hype is concerned, if it grows, it can change skin for the better, especially if it is an exotic plant from the Amazon or the Himalayas. You're never going to see a cosmetics company extol the value of any plant extract from Chicago or Seattle. Regardless of the silliness of the marketing angles, there is no consensus on which plant (or plants) is the most beneficial. According to each cosmetics company, it's the plants they include in their products that have the most astonishing merits.

When plants are an issue in a skin-care product, I point out the known benefits of those plants, such as antioxidant, anti-irritant, or antibacterial properties. I also explain when plants are a problem in cosmetics due to their potential for causing irritation or a sensitizing reaction. When a plant has irritation potential and antioxidant properties (e.g., horsetail extract), I generally cite the irritation potential because there are so many other plant extracts that have antioxidant properties without the irritation. Why include plant extracts with a risk to skin?

Nonfragrant plant oils or nonvolatile oils are almost always beneficial as emollients and lubricants and often have potent antioxidant and skin-identical properties.

I often list the exact name of a vitamin included in a product. Regardless of the individual vitamin—whether it is vitamin A, C, or E—vitamins in skin-care products can't feed the skin or provide nutrition from the outside in. However, many of them can work as antioxidants and that can benefit the skin.

Even plain water gets overhyped in skin-care products. Many products use an assortment of exclusive-sounding adjectives—deionized, declustered, purified, triple-purified, demineralized, fossilized—to describe what is nothing more than plain water. These terms indicate that the water has gone through some kind of purification process or was taken from a specific water source, but that is standard for cosmetics. You also will find phrases such as "infusions of" or "aqueous extracts of" followed by the name of one or more plants. That means you're getting what is merely "plant tea," essentially plant juice and water. Although descriptions like this indicate that you are getting mostly water and a hint of plant extract, they sound so pure and natural that they create the impression that they must be better for the skin. It turns out, as you might expect, that water is water. The kind of water does not affect the skin or the final product. After the water is combined with other ingredients, its original status is unimportant.

Silicones are a remarkable, diverse, and ubiquitous group of ingredients that show up in over 80% of all cosmetic products being sold. Silicones may look, act, and have a feel reminiscent of oil, but they are not oils. Technically speaking, silicone as a chemical compound is often discussed in relation to fluid technology. Either way, regardless of the precise name, silicone is an elegant skin-care ingredient that has an exquisite, silky, somewhat slippery feel; it also has an affinity for skin and "dries" to an almost imperceptible finish. Its popularity in formulations reflects its versatility and the finish it gives products. For someone with oily or acne-prone skin, silicone is not necessarily a problem, because there are new silicone polymers that have oil-absorbing properties and can leave a soft, almost powder-like matte finish on skin.

PLANTS: A GROWING ISSUE

Not all plants that show up in cosmetics are beneficial for skin. There are many plant extracts that sound harmless, but the research indicates otherwise. For example, St. John's wort contains several components that are toxic on skin in the presence of sunlight (Sources:

Planta Medica, February 2002, pages 171-173; and *International Journal of Biochemistry and Cell Biology*, March 2002, pages 221-241). *Ephedra sinica*, an extract from a Chinese herb and also known as *ma huang*, has a high tannin and volatile oil content and has been shown to have toxic properties (Source: *Toxicological Sciences*, August 2000, pages 424-430). Or take camphor, an aromatic substance obtained from the wood of a southeast Asian tree *Cinnamomum camphora*. When applied to the skin, this produces a cooling effect and dilates blood vessels, which in turn can cause skin irritation and, with repeated use, dermatitis (Sources: *British Journal of Dermatology*, November 2000, pages 923-929; and *Clinical Toxicology*, December 1981, pages 1485-1498).

The list of problematic plant extracts is long, and their irritant potential will shock you as you read through the reviews in this book. So much for all plants being harmless and good for skin! There are literally hundreds and hundreds of plant extracts included in cosmetics, and most consumers blindly assume that all of these must hold some special benefit for their skin, when in truth that is not always the case.

The issue of natural versus synthetic is one I've written about extensively over the years. To sum it up succinctly, "natural" does not mean good and "synthetic" does not mean bad. Each group has its shortcomings and strengths, but I would no sooner accept any plant as automatically being good for my skin than I would walk naked through a patch of poison ivy assuming that because it's a plant, it must be OK.

"Natural" simply defines the source of the ingredient; it tells you nothing about the ingredient's effectiveness or risks. Menthol and peppermint may have a natural source, but both are serious skin irritants and a problem for skin. Ingredients like silicone and stearyl alcohol are synthetic, but they are remarkably silky-soft ingredients, vital to a vast array of cosmetic formulations. Sodium lauryl sulfate is a detergent cleansing agent derived from coconut, but that doesn't make it good for skin.

"Synthetic" merely tells you that the ingredient was created in a laboratory, and although that kind of origin may sound unhealthy, just as with plants, healthy versus unhealthy can be based only on an ingredient-by-ingredient evaluation.

PARABENS AND PRESERVATIVES

You may not think of preservatives as an essential part of your skin care and cosmetics products, but without question skin-care and cosmetics products need preservatives. This is especially true for products that contain plant extracts—just think about how long a bunch of broccoli lasts in your refrigerator before it becomes a mushy, discolored mess. Whether it is a cleanser, lotion, toner, blush, foundation, or mascara, without preservatives these everyday items will become overloaded with bacteria, mold, and fungus, making them harmful to skin, eyes, and mucous membranes.

Even as necessary as preservatives are to the safety of cosmetics, they've had their share of woes over the years. For example, back in the early 1990s, it was discovered that combining formaldehyde-releasing preservatives (e.g., 2-bromo-2-nitropane 1-3 diol, or dmdm hydantoin) are combined with amines (e.g., triethanolamine), something called nitrosamine forms, and nitrosamine (in its various forms) is, in fact, carcinogenic. This problem was viewed as inconsequential for cosmetics because the amount of preservatives used in cosmetics is minute, and no test has shown it to cause problems for people applying makeup or using skin-care products. Studies related to carcinogenic properties of nitrosamine were done by feeding it orally to laboratory rats. Still, it is not a pleasant thought to associate a "carcinogen" with your cosmetics in any way, shape, or form. As a result, and despite their effectiveness, formaldehyde-based preservatives are not as popular as they once were.

Another group of preservatives, called parabens, is now in a predicament similar to that of formaldehyde-releasing preservatives, and this has become a common subject for questions from my readers. Parabens may come in the form of butylparaben, ethylparaben, isobutylparaben, methylparaben, or propylparaben, and they have been linked distantly (meaning in limited studies and with only a handful of subjects or animal studies) to breast cancer due to their weak estrogenic activity and their presence in breast cancer tumors, as well as to low sperm count rates in men. But even from a distance, that has some people worried, especially considering that, by some estimates, more than 90% of all cosmetics products contain one or more parabens. In fact, parabens are the most widely used group of cosmetic preservatives in the world because of their efficacy, low risk of irritation, and stability. What started the concern about parabens was a study published in the *Journal of Steroid Biochemistry and Molecular Biology* (January 2002, pages 49-60), which evaluated the estrogenic activity of parabens in human breast cancer cells.

The very technical findings of the study, which involved both oral administration and injection into rat skin, did show evidence of a weak estrogenic effect on cells in a way that could be problematic for binding to receptor sites that may cause proliferation of MCF-7 breast cancer cells. A single study identified parabens in human breast tumor samples supplied by 20 patients. This study was concerned primarily with the use of deodorants that contain parabens rather than with cosmetics in general, but it has been extrapolated to the cosmetics industry as a whole, prompting many consumers to check the ingredient lists of the products they're using.

More to the point, however, the presence of parabens in human breast tumors doesn't mean they caused the tumors. Pervasive fear was generated by these well-circulated facts. What didn't make the e-mail spam rounds is that all the researchers who are studying this issue, as well as health organizations around the world, agree that the information to date is hardly conclusive and at best vague, and that parabens require more study (Sources: *Journal of Applied Toxicology*, January-February 2004, pages 1-4, September-October 2003, pages 285-288; and *Journal of the National Cancer Institute*, August 2003, pages 1106-1118).

What is surprising to some is that parabens actually have a "natural" origin. Parabens are formed from an acid (p-hydroxy-benzoic acid) found in raspberries and blackberries (Source: *Cosmetics & Toiletries*, January 2005, page 22). So much for the widely held belief that natural ingredients are the only answer for skin-care products! As yet, no one has any idea (or has evaluated) whether it is the consumption of parabens or their application to the skin that is responsible for their presence in human tissue. And no one knows what the presence of parabens in human tissue means. In terms of the low sperm count in relation to parabens, research published in *Birth Defects Research, Part B, Developmental and Reproductive Toxicology* (April 2008, pages 123-133) concluded that parabens had no effect on sperm count in an in vivo experiment (meaning it was done on real guys). Does this mean you should stop buying products that contain parabens? I mean, who wants this stuff being absorbed through their skin whether there is conclusive research or not? That's a good question, but the answer isn't simple and the studies are hardly conclusive on any front.

Clearly it is a potentially serious issue, and the FDA is conducting its own research to determine what this means for human health (Source: The Endocrine Disruptor Knowledge Base [EDKB], http://edkb.fda.gov/index.html). A definitive answer, however, is far from close. As a point of reference, and just to keep the concern over parabens in perspective, it is important to realize that parabens are hardly the only substances that have estrogenic effects on the body. The issue is that any source of estrogen, including the estrogen our bodies produce or the types associated with plant extracts, may bind to receptor sites on cells, either strongly or weakly. This can either stimulate the receptor to imitate the effect of our own estrogen in a positive way, or it can generate an abnormal estrogen response. It is possible that a weak plant estrogen can help the body, but it is also possible that a strong plant estrogen can make matters worse. For example, there is research showing that coffee is a problem for fibrocystic breast disease, possibly because coffee exerts estrogenic effects on breast cells (Sources: *Journal of the American Medical Women's Association*, Spring 2002, pages 85-90; *Annals of the New York Academy of Science*, March 2002, pages 11-22; and *American Journal of Epidemiology*, October 1996, pages 642-644).

To quote some studies directly: "Although parabens can act similarly to estrogen, they have been shown to have much less estrogenic activity than the body's naturally occurring estrogen." For example, a 1998 study (Routledge et al., in *Toxicology and Applied Pharmacology*, November 1998, pages 12-19) found that the most potent parabens tested in the study, butylparaben, showed from 10,000- to 100,000-fold less activity than naturally occurring estradiol (a form of estrogen) [found in our water systems]. Further, parabens are used at very low levels in cosmetics. In a review of the estrogenic activity of parabens (Golden et al., in *Critical Reviews in Toxicology*, June 2005, pages 435-458), the author concluded that based on maximum daily exposure estimates, "it was implausible that parabens could increase the risk associated with exposure to estrogenic chemicals" (Source: www.fda.gov). Ironically, the endocrine-disrupting potencies of ingredients like parabens or phthalates (a type of plasticizer) "are several orders of magnitude lower than that of the natural estrogens" (Source: *Environment International*, July 2007, pages 654-669). Human endocrine-disrupting sources have their origin in plants, such as marijuana (Source: *Toxicology*, January 2005, pages 471-488), or in medicines such as acetaminophen (Tylenol) (Source: *Water Research*, November 2008, pages 4578-4588).

A study conducted at the Department of Obstetrics and Gynecology at Baylor College of Medicine in Houston, Texas, investigated the estrogenic effects of licorice root, black cohosh, dong quai, and ginseng "on cell proliferation of MCF-7 cells, a human breast cancer cell line...." The results showed that "Dong quai and ginseng both significantly induced the growth of MCF-7 cells by 16- and 27-fold, respectively, over that of untreated control cells, while black cohosh and licorice root did not" (Source: *Menopause*, March-April, 2002, pages 145-150).

Another study concluded that "Commercially available products containing soy, red clover, and herbal combinations induced an increase in the MCF-7 [breast cancer] proliferation rates, indicating an estrogen-antagonistic activity...." (Source: *Menopause*, May-June 2004, pages 281-289). Despite this evidence, when was the last time you read a media report or received a forwarded e-mail about the breast cancer risk from soy or ginseng?

EVALUATION OF MAKEUP PRODUCTS

I developed a list of specific criteria and guidelines that I use for each makeup category, along with other factors, to determine a product's performance, reliability, or value to skin. The following describes the criteria and guidelines I use to evaluate each category of makeup product.

FOUNDATIONS: My fundamental expectation for any foundation, regardless of type (liquid, pressed powder, loose powder, stick, cream-to-powder, or any of the various mineral makeups), is that it not be any shade or tone of orange, peach, pink, rose, green, or ash—because there are no people with skin that color. Consistency, coverage, and feel are vital. All foundations, regardless of texture, must go on smoothly and evenly, not separate or turn color, and be easy to blend. Foundations that claim to be matte must be truly matte, meaning no shine or dewy finish, and they must have the potential to last most of the day. Foundations that claim to moisturize must contain ingredients that can do that, but without being so slick that blending is difficult and coverage spotty.

The very good news is that foundations have improved considerably, in some cases dramatically so. It is easier than ever before to find not only a broad selection of neutral shades encompassing many skin tones, but also superb textures and finishes. Today's best foundations make skin look beautifully smooth and even rather than heavy or mask-like. I am consistently amazed at how many foundations today can make skin look incredible without seeming obvious. Even cream-to-powder foundations have come a long way and have some of the smoothest textures and most natural-looking results around. Ironically, despite the inexplicable popularity of mineral makeup, many of those in loose-powder form don't look nearly as natural on skin as today's best liquid foundations.

FOUNDATIONS WITH SUNSCREENS: Foundations with sunscreens are held to the same standards as all other sunscreens, which means they must have at least an SPF 15 and must list a UVA-protecting ingredient as one of the active ingredients on the label. The only acceptable UVA-protecting ingredients are titanium dioxide, zinc oxide, avobenzone (also called Parsol 1789 or its technical name butyl methoxydibenzoylmethane), Tinosorb (technical name bis-ethylhexyloxyphenol methoxyphenyl triazine), and Mexoryl SX (technical name terephthalylidene dicamphor sulfonic acid; also known as ecamsule). In the reviews, you will notice that foundations with poor or inadequate sunscreens are criticized severely, and do not receive better than a neutral face rating. In some situations, the performance of the foundations was considered excellent, but the foundation could not be relied on for sun protection and would require a well-formulated sunscreen to be worn underneath. For more details, see the information on sunscreens presented in the "Evaluating Skin-Care Products" section.

Beauty Note: The makeup products we used to make color suggestions were purchased, were tested at the tester units available at the cosmetics counter, or were received as samples from the company. The color, shade, or tone of a particular product can fluctuate for a number of reasons. If I refer to a particular foundation as being "too peach" and you find that it's just right for you, it may be that we simply disagree or it may be that the product I tested or bought was different from the one you ended up buying. Whenever possible, every foundation has its entire shade range reviewed in person, with detailed notes about the good and poor shades.

CONCEALERS: Concealers should never be any shade of orange, peach, pink, rose, green, or ash. My team and I look for smooth textures that go on easily without pulling the skin, don't look dry and pasty, provide sufficient coverage, and, perhaps most important, do not crease into lines. I generally do not recommend using thick or creamy concealers over blemishes (liquid concealers with a matte finish are preferred), but there is rarely a problem with using such concealers on other parts of the face if they match your skin. And many women prefer to use a creamy concealer under the eyes.

I don't recommend medicated concealers because they are rarely, if ever, "medicated" with ingredients or formulations that can affect breakouts. For medicated concealers to work, they would need to contain an effective exfoliant or an effective disinfectant, and I have yet to test one that meets those criteria and also has a color that anyone would dare put on their face, although the colors have been getting better.

Despite the claims that a product should be for oily skin versus dry skin, please keep in mind that companies can make these claims regardless of what ingredients the product contains. In general, the thicker and greasier the product, the more likely it is to be problematic for oily, acne-prone skin. However, anything you apply over skin can cause problems. Just because a product does or doesn't contain oil is no guarantee one way or the other that it won't cause problems. There also are lots of ingredients that don't sound like oil but that can cause problems for skin. Generally, a matte-finish product is best for oily skin, but that still won't ensure a lack or reduction of breakouts.

COLOR CORRECTORS: There is no reason to use color correctors in any form. Color correctors usually are applied before you blend your foundation color and they generally come in shades of yellow, mauve, pink, peach, or mint green. Color correctors are marketed as a way to change skin color, so that if your skin has pink undertones, a yellow color corrector is supposed to even that out. The only thing these products do is give the skin a strange hue. Does anyone think the colored layer isn't noticeable? That yellow or mauve layer then mixes with your foundation, giving it a strange color as well. Another problem with this kind of product is that it adds another layer on the skin, and the buildup of cosmetic ingredients on the face can be pore-clogging. A well-chosen foundation color and blush can easily provide the color balance you are looking for without adding another layer of strange makeup colors to your skin. As a result of these limitations, these products are, thankfully, harder to find, but when they appear they are rated accordingly unless their effect is nearly imperceptible on skin.

FACE POWDERS: Face powders come in two basic forms: pressed and loose. I evaluate them on the basis of whether they go on sheer, shiny, chalky, or heavy, and whether they are too pink, peach, ash, or rose. I consistently give higher marks to powders that go on sheer and have a silky-soft texture and a natural beige, tan, or rich brown finish with no overtones of red, peach, orange, yellow, or green. It is getting more and more difficult to find a bad powder in any format. Thanks to improved milling processes and pigment technology, today's best powders are capable of making all skin types look polished while helping to set makeup and prolong its wear.

Talc is the most frequently used ingredient in powders in all price ranges, and it is one of the best for absorbing oil and giving a smooth finish to the face. Some companies make claims about their grade of talc being better than another company's. The issue of a grade difference cannot be proven and is irrelevant unless the product's feel and performance are affected.

Other minerals are used for the same purpose as talc, and though they may sound more exotic, they are not any better for the skin. Including cornstarch or rice starch in powders can help create a beautiful texture and these are interesting substitutes for talc, but they also can be a concern because there is evidence that they can clog pores and cause breakouts. I try to screen for these ingredients in that regard. Mineral makeup is discussed separately in this chapter.

Numerous shiny powders are being sold today in loose and pressed forms, and I rate these products on ease of use, how well they last, how much they flake, and how sheer and easy they are to blend. Shiny powder as an oil-absorbent is never deemed a good idea because if the intent is to powder down shine, then applying more shine doesn't make sense. These products are an option for those who want to add sparkle to their allover makeup appearance.

Powders often are designated by the cosmetics companies as being specifically for dry skin or for oily skin. Those designations are often bogus, however, with little difference between the formulations. I rate a face powder as being good for oily skin if it contains minimal waxy or oily ingredients and has good absorbency without being heavy or thick on the skin. Powders recommended for dry skin are those that contain moisturizing agents or that have a finish that is satin-like rather than blatantly matte. Powders for dry skin should also have an almost creamy texture, despite the absorbent nature of the main ingredients.

MINERAL MAKEUP: As a category, mineral makeup is a caprice of the cosmetics industry. In reality, it is nothing more than a powder makeup and we review it just as we do any other powder: how does it feel on skin, how natural does it look, and how well does it hold up during the day. In terms of marketing, what is maddening from an ingredient standpoint is that there is nothing uniform or consistent about products bearing the "mineral" makeup label. For example, some mineral makeups contain talc, others an ingredient called bismuth oxychloride. Talc is found in most powders with or without the "mineral" label. Bismuth oxychloride isn't even found in nature and isn't preferred in any way, except personal preference. In fact, talc is a far more natural, unadulterated, pure ingredient than bismuth oxychloride. Bismuth oxychloride is manufactured by combining bismuth, a by-product of lead and copper metal refining (the dregs of smelting, if you will), with chloride (a chlorine compound) and water. It's used in cosmetics for its distinct shimmery, pearlescent appearance and its fine white powder texture that adheres well to skin. On the downside, bismuth oxychloride is heavier than talc and can look cakey on skin. Also, for some people, bismuth oxychloride can be irritating due to the manner in which its crystalline particles tend to "poke" at pores.

Actually, bismuth is chemically similar to arsenic. That is more shocking than it is significant, but it's that kind of comparison that mineral makeup companies make to try to scare you about the ingredients in other powders not deemed "mineral makeup." Just as cosmetic-grade mineral oil is not related to the crude petroleum from which it originates, neither is bismuth oxychloride identical to bismuth; therefore, the arsenic association is irrelevant. This is just a good example of how companies can skew the definition of "natural," and how they twist factual information to make other cosmetics brands' ingredients sound harmful.

Beauty Note: Talc often is criticized as an awful cosmetic ingredient that should be avoided. The concern about talc is not about how it is used in makeup, but, rather, its use in large amounts in pure concentrations, in the form of talcum powder. Part of the story dates back to several studies published in the 1990s that found a significant increase in the risk of ovarian cancer from vaginal (perineal) application of talcum powder (Sources: *American Journal of Epidemiology*, March 1997, pages 459-465; *International Journal of Cancer*, May 1999, pages 351-356; *Seminars in Oncology*, June 1998, pages 255-264; and *Cancer*, June 1997, pages 2396-2401). However, subsequent and concurrent studies cast doubt on the way these studies were conducted and on the conclusions they reached (Sources: *Journal of the National Cancer Institute*, February 2000, pages 249-252; *American Journal of Obstetrics and Gynecology*, March 2000, pages 720-724; and *Obstetrics and Gynecology*, March 1999, pages 372–376).

While more research in this area is being carried out to clear up the confusion, none of the research about the use of talc is related to the way women use makeup. There is no indication anywhere that there is any risk from using makeup products that contain talc.

FACE POWDERS WITH SUNSCREEN: There are a few pressed powders available that have a reliable SPF 15 or greater and that contain UVA-protecting ingredients. That is great news. However, I am concerned about this because of the way women often use these products. While I don't doubt the validity of the SPF number, I worry that most women won't apply pressed powders with sunscreen liberally enough to get the amount of protection indicated on the label. If you lightly dust the powder over your skin, you will not get the SPF protection indicated. You must be sure you apply the pressed powder in a manner that liberally, completely, and evenly covers your face. I feel that pressed powders with sunscreen are an iffy choice if they are the only product used for sun protection, although they are a great way to touch up your makeup during the day and to reapply sunscreen at the same time.

BLUSHES: It is essential for blushes to have a smooth texture, to blend on easily, and to have a silky feel on the skin. Overall, I don't recommend obviously shiny blushes. Although they don't make cheeks look as crepey or wrinkly as shiny eyeshadows do the eyes, sparkling cheeks look out of place during the day. There are many blushes whose finish casts an attractive, non-sparkly glow on skin. These are rated highly, provided other attributes remain strong. I also comment when a powder blush's pigmentation is strong, which means less is needed per application (and you may in fact prefer a sheer blush instead).

Cream blushes, cream-to-powder blushes, and liquid or gel blushes are rated on their blend-ability, whether they streak, how greasy or dry they feel, how fast they set, and how well they last. I also describe which cream blushes tend to work better over foundation and which ones perform better if applied directly on the skin. As a general rule, liquid blushes are best used on bare skin and are not recommended for anyone with large pores in the cheek area.

EYESHADOWS: Regardless of color or shine, I evaluate all eyeshadows on the basis of texture and ease of application. I point out which colors have heavy or grainy textures because they can be hard to blend and can easily crease or flake. Eyeshadows that are too sheer or too powdery are also a problem because the color tends to fade as the day wears on; plus they can be difficult to apply, flaking all over the place. I also am leery of eyeshadow sets that include difficult-to-use color combinations. Many lines offer duo, trio, and quad sets of eyeshadows with the most bizarre color combinations imaginable. Sets of colors must be usable as a set and coordinated in complementary colors; they should never paint a rainbow or kaleidoscope of color across the eye. However, if you are looking for a kaleidoscope effect, I've pointed them out; they just have an unhappy face rating next to them.

Generally, it is best to buy eyeshadow colors singly, not in sets. That way you can be as-sured of liking all the colors you buy, not just two out of three or four. Powder eyeshadows are by far the most prevalent format, and as such most of our attention was focused on this type of eyeshadow. Regarding shine, you will notice in this edition that I am more lenient based on the fact that many of the best eyeshadows have a subtle shine that can light up the eye area without looking obvious. Such eyeshadows are a tricky proposition for someone with pronounced wrinkles, but can still be used on the brow bone as a highlighter.

Specialty eyeshadow products such as liquids, creams, powdery or creamy pencils, and loose-powder eyeshadows are evaluated on ease of use, blendability, staying power, and how well they work over and with other products. My reviews indicate a clear bias toward matte eyeshadow powders as opposed to any other type of eyeshadow. I find liquids and creams hard to control, and even more difficult to blend with other colors, though there are some exceptions. Most of them also tend to crease easily, and they almost always lose intensity throughout the day. But again, some products in these formats surprised me, and the positive reviews indicate as much.

EYE AND BROW SHAPERS: Basically, all pencils, regardless of brand, have more similarities than differences. Most eye pencils, lip pencils, and eyebrow pencils are manufactured by the same companies (meaning the same manufacturing plants) and then sold to hundreds of different cosmetics lines. Whether they cost $30 from Chanel or $7 from Almay, they are likely to be exactly the same product. Some pencils are greasier or drier than others, but for the most part there are few marked differences among them. Eye pencils that smudge and smear and eyebrow pencils that go on like a crayon—meaning thick and greasy—are always rated ineffective, because they tend to look artificial and can get very messy as the day goes by. Keep in mind that whether an eye pencil smears along the lower eyelashes depends to a large extent on the number of lines around your eye, how much moisturizer you use around the eye area, the type of under-eye concealer you use, and how greasy the pencil is. The greasier the moisturizer or under-eye concealer, the more likely any pencil will smear, and you can't blame that on the pencil.

Liquid eyeliners are rated on how easy they are to apply, the type of brush, how quickly they dry, and their potential to last all day. The way these types of liners last throughout the day is a consideration because many liquid liners tend to flake and peel. Another bothersome issue with several liquid liners is that the color fades as you apply it along the lash line, meaning you must add successive coats, which increases the chance of smearing.

The long-wearing gel eyeliners were reviewed based on their formula (they must contain ingredients that contribute to long wear), ease of application, drying time, color intensity, and wearability. For the most part, this type of eyeliner from every brand performs well, and is worth strong consideration if you like the look of liquid liner but aren't fond of applying it or if you have oily eyelids and cannot get pencil or powder to last.

Eyebrow pencils were reviewed for ease of application and whether or not they look natural as opposed to greasy or thick when applied. Powder or tinted brow gels needed to have the same attributes.

LIPSTICKS, LIP GLOSS, AND LIPLINER: Every woman has her own needs and preferences when it comes to lipstick. Some women like sheer applications; others prefer glossy or matte finishes. Colors are also difficult to recommend because of the wide variation in taste. Given those limitations, I review the range of colors and textures available, commenting only on texture rather than critiquing it, because personal preference is vital to a final decision. The general groupings are glossy or sheer, creamy, creamy with shine or iridescence, matte, and semi-matte. As a matter of preference, because of staying power and coverage, I give the highest marks to creamy or semi-matte lipsticks that go on evenly and aren't glossy, sticky, thick, or drying.

Several companies offer their versions of the two-step lip paint and top coat, first introduced with Max Factor's Lipfinity. Step 1 involves painting the lips with color, waiting a couple of minutes for it to dry (which becomes increasingly uncomfortable because these paints are not moist in the least), and then finishing with a glossy top coat. The top coat provides moisture, a shiny finish, and doesn't disrupt the color coat applied beneath it. With few exceptions, the lip paints were rated highly, with some clear favorites emerging, from both inexpensive and expensive lines.

I evaluate lip pencils according to whether they go on smoothly without being greasy or dry and how well they stay in place once paired with a lipstick. I also comment on the shade range relative to the number of lipstick shades a company offers. You'd be surprised how many companies offer dozens of lipstick shades and only four or five color options for lip pencil.

Lip glosses were evaluated primarily on their texture, application, finish (particularly degree of stickiness), and longevity. Those that went on smoothly, provided a suitably glossy finish, and came in a beautiful range of colors of varying intensity were rated highest. When a lip gloss has greater pigmentation (some go on as intensely as a lipstick), I mention it in the review. I also screened for irritants often seen in "plumping" lip glosses. Such irritants include peppermint, pepper extracts, ginger, and menthol. For sanitary reasons, lip glosses that come in a tube or wand are preferred to those that come in a pot.

MASCARAS: Mascaras should go on easily and quickly while building length and at least some thickness. Mascara brush shapes have improved phenomenally over the years, although there still are some that are awkward to use because they are too big or too small. When applicable, I comment on a mascara's brush and how it helps or hinders application. Mascara should never smear or flake, regardless of price.

Waterproof mascaras are rated strictly on how well they hold up when splashed with water and how long and thick they make lashes. Keep in mind that, although waterproof mascaras stay on when in contact with water, they break down just as easily when in contact with emollients from moisturizers, sunscreens, eye creams, foundations, creamy under-eye concealers, and other specialty products applied around the eye. Waterproof does not guarantee smudge-proof, all-day wear.

In general, I include information on how quickly a mascara can produce great (or not so great) results, how well it wears, whether or not it makes lashes feel soft and conditioned or brittle and dry, and how easy it is to remove with a water-soluble cleanser.

FACE AND BODY ILLUMINATING/SHIMMER PRODUCTS: Given the ever-expanding number of choices within this group, it was time to separate them when a line offered such products (and clearly, many women want some element of shine to be part of their makeup wardrobe). Whether in liquid, cream, or powder format, shimmer products are rated on texture, application, finish (was it greasy or silky), level of shine, and the ability of the shine to cling to skin rather than flake off onto you and your clothing. I also comment on shade ranges where applicable and mention when certain shimmer products would actually be better mixed with other makeup items, such as foundation. Special attention was paid to whether the amount of shine is a sophisticated, radiant glow or an all-out Las Vegas glitter. The latter types is not rated as highly because, almost without exception, there are performance and aesthetic issues.

BRUSHES: Brushes are essential for applying makeup correctly and beautifully. Blush and eyeshadow brushes are offered by some of the major cosmetics lines, and all of the makeup artistry lines offer at least the essentials for a complete makeup application. Brushes are rated on overall shape and function as well as on the softness and density of the bristles. Eyeshadow or blush brushes with scratchy, stiff, or loose bristles are not recommended. As a rule, be cautious about buying brush sets because many include brushes you don't need or won't use often. Brush cases and other accessories are rated on their functionality, construction, ease of use, and, in some instances, portability. All closures were tested to ensure ease of use, and special care was taken to note the level of craftsmanship, especially for such items sold in department stores.

UNDERSTANDING THE RATING SYSTEM

The rating symbols I use to rate the products reviewed in this book are described below. These simple, but succinct (and cute), symbols denote approval or disapproval of a specific product and provide an at-a-glance comparison of expensive and inexpensive choices.

For those who are familiar with my reviews and ratings from previous editions of my books, this edition, like the seventh, has incorporated a major shift in what constitutes an expensive and reasonably priced product and what constitutes a well-formulated and state-of-the-art product. Products containing antioxidants, plant extracts, vitamins, or any other light- or air-sensitive ingredients are evaluated based on their packaging as well as on their ingredients. A superior formula loaded with these kinds of ingredients is useless for your skin if it is packaged in a container that isn't airtight, or that allows light in, such as a jar or a clear container. Such packaging quickly renders antioxidants and other air- and light-sensitive ingredients ineffective. Consequently, if a product's packaging is inappropriate and allows unstable ingredients to break down, even a brilliantly formulated product is rated with only a neutral face.

✓ ☺ **Excellent (Paula's Pick!) and** ✓ ☺ **$$$ Excellent (Paula's Pick but overpriced).** This rating indicates the products I found to be the best of the best. It is judiciously assigned whenever a product exceeds expectations, meets or exceeds the criteria for a product in its category with minimal to no concerns (except for price, which is indicated by the dollar signs), and surpasses expectations of any comparable product. For this edition of *Don't Go to the Cosmetics Counter Without Me*, you will find that my "Best Products" list now includes only products that receive a Paula's Pick rating, separated according to retail location. This reduces the number of best products in each category (which makes shopping easier) and assures my readers that they are getting what my and my team's experience and substantiated research indicates are truly state-of-the-art products, regardless of how much they choose to spend.

☺ **Very Good.** This smiling face indicates a great product that meets and/or surpasses the criteria set for that category of product, and that I recommend it highly because of its performance or its impressive formulary characteristics. The smiling face means the product is definitely worth checking into and potentially worth buying, especially considering that it is so reasonably priced. Products receiving this symbol have prices that are eminently more affordable on an ounce-per-ounce basis than other similar and equally well-formulated products.

☺ **$$$ Very Good (but overpriced).** This symbol indicates a great product that meets and/ or surpasses the criteria set for that category of product. However, just because the product is well-formulated doesn't mean it is worth the money. Almost without exception there are always reasonably priced versions of a product that meet or exceed the same quality standards as the more expensive versions. Whether or not a product received the "$$$" designation depends on a pricing versus size threshold my team and I set based on industrywide averages per category. For example, if a cleanser costs more than $15 for 4 ounces or less of product, it is considered expensive and has the "$$$" symbol. Same thing for moisturizers priced greater than $30 for 1 ounce, and so on.

☹ **Average.** This neutral face indicates an OK, but unimpressive, product that can cause problems for certain skin types, or a well-formulated product with packaging that compromises the effectiveness and stability of its ingredients. I often use this face to portray a dated or old-fashioned formulation. That doesn't mean it's a bad product, just that it isn't very interesting or it lacks some of the newer cell-communicating ingredients, antioxidants, anti-irritants, emollients, or nonirritating ingredients for its intended skin type. I also use the neutral face to reflect a makeup product that isn't really bad, but that is completely unnecessary or is unnecessarily overpriced for such an ordinary product, which easily could be replaced with a far less expensive version from the drugstore. Depending on your personal preferences, products rated with the neutral face may be worth checking out, but they're nothing to get excited about and, in the case of skin-care items, should be avoided if the neutral face rating is due to poor packaging.

☺ **$$$ Average (but overpriced, so why bother?).** This symbol indicates an ordinary, boring product whose excessive price makes it ludicrous to consider, especially if it is an otherwise great formula with inappropriate packaging. For skin-care products, this rating may reflect a lack of unique or interesting water-binding agents, anti-irritants, emollients, antioxidants, effective exfoliants, gentle cleansing agents, or combinations of those in a given formulation. For makeup, it reflects a performance that pales in comparison to other, far better formulations, but that still can look OK when applied, or an acceptable product for those who want a no-frills product for minimal accentuation.

☹ **Poor (don't buy!).** For many reasons, this frowning face indicates a product that is truly a poor choice for skin from almost every standpoint, including price, dated formulation, performance, application, and texture, as well as potential for irritation, skin reactions, and breakouts. Because any unhappy face rating indicates a product that I would never recommend, you will not find such products rated with the "$$$" designation. After all, who wants to pay extra for a truly inferior product destined to disappoint?

WHY REVIEWS CHANGE

Over the years, in each edition of my books, my reviews and comments change from those in previous editions. There are three major reasons why: (1) I have acquired new research that supports a different evaluation, (2) other products in a category are significantly better and, therefore, the original evaluation of superior performance may be downgraded due to a comparison to superior formulations being sold now, and (3) the company changed the product since I last reviewed it, which happens more often than most consumers know, and, yes, it's just as frustrating for me.

CHAPTER FOUR

This Book is Only the Beginning!

DON'T GO TO THE COSMETICS COUNTER WITHOUT BEAUTYPEDIA.COM!

All of the reviews in this edition of *Don't Go to the Cosmetics Counter Without Me* are also available online at www.Beautypedia.com. This exclusive Web site serves as an extension of the very book you're holding. Beautypedia debuted in January 2008, shortly after the seventh edition of this book was published. Since then, my team and I have provided reviews of more than 260 cosmetics lines and have added several features that make it easier than ever to zero in on the best products the cosmetics industry has to offer. The site has thousands upon thousands of subscribers, and in many ways has succeeded beyond my expectations.

Joining Beautypedia gives you access to more reviews than my team and I could reasonably fit into a book (at least a book that someone could actually carry without causing muscle strain). We update the site weekly and send out e-mail alerts announcing what's new every two weeks. You'll find new reviews are posted in real time, existing reviews are edited as new information (or better products) comes to light, discontinued products are removed, and price changes are made where applicable. Beautypedia is an invaluable online tool that will help you stay informed about all of the latest skin-care and makeup products. I encourage you to visit and see for yourself all that it has to offer! Visitors have access to lots of free content, including my exhaustive *Cosmetic Ingredient Dictionary*, insightful summaries of every brand reviewed on the site (including all of the brands in this book), and a selection of free reviews.

A yearly subscription to Beautypedia will save you money and enable you to take better care of your skin than you ever could have imagined! Take advantage of the special discount show-cased on the postcard in this book, and enjoy 50% off your first year of Beautypedia today!

Stay Beautifully Informed with Beautypedia.com!

The brands on the list below are reviewed exclusively on www.Beautypedia.com and are not in this book:

Alba Botanica	Avage
Aloette	Avalon Organics
Amatokin	Avita
AmorePacific	B. Kamins, Chemist
Arcona	Babor
Artistry by Amway	Beauty Without Cruelty

Becca
Billion Dollar Brows
Bioelements
Bio-Oil
Biotherm
Black Opal
Blinc
Blisslabs
Blistex
Borba Cosmeceutical
Boscia
Botox Cosmetic
Bumble + bumble
Canyon Ranch
Care Skin Care by Stella McCartney
Cellex-C
Chantecaille
Clarisonic
Cosmedicine
CosMedix
Derma E
Dermablend
DERMAdoctor
Differin
Dove Hair Care
Dr. Hauschka
Dr. LeWinn's Private Formula
Dr. Perry
DuWop
Earthscience
Eau Thermale Avene
Elemis
Elizabeth Grant
Eminence Organics Skin Care
Erno Laszlo
Eve Lom
Fashion Fair
Frederic Fekkai
Freeze 24-7
G.M. Collin
Glymed Plus
Green Cream
Green People
Guerlain
Guinot

Hard Candy
Hydroderm
Hylexin
Illuminare
Iman
IsaDora
Jane
Janson Beckett Cosmeceuticals
Jason Natural
JK Jemma Kidd
Joico
Jonathan Product
Juice Beauty
Kate Somerville
Kiss My Face
Lab Series Skincare for Men
Lac-Hydrin
LactiCare
Lauren Hutton's Good Stuff
Lise Watier Skin Care
Lumedia
Lumene
M LAB
M.D. Forte
Mario Badescu
Max Factor
Meaningful Beauty by Cindy Crawford
Mederma
MetroGel, MetroCream & MetroLotion
Mineral Makeup
N.Y.C.
Natura Bisse
Natural Advantage by Jane Seymour
Neways
Nia24
Nicole Miller
Noevir
Nonscents Hair Care
NP Set
Nude Skincare
Obagi
OC Eight
Ojon
Ole Henriksen
Osmotics

PanOxyl
Perricone MD Cosmeceuticals
Pevonia Botanica
pHisoderm
Phytomer
Pixi
Pond's
Prestige Cosmetics
Principal Secret
Pürminerals
Purpose
Quo Cosmetics
Refissa
Remergent
Remede
Ren
Renova
Retin-A
Retin-A Micro
RevaleSkin
ReVive
Rodan + Fields
Sea Breeze
Sense Skin Care by Usana
Shaklee Enfuselle
Sisley Paris
Skin Effects by Dr. Jeffrey Dover
SkinMedica
Skyn Iceland
Sovage Dermatologic Laboratories
Spectro
St. Ives
Studio Gear
Tarte Cosmetics
Tazorac
Tend Skin
Three Custom Color Specialists
Too Faced
Tracie Martyn
TRESemme
Tri-Luma
Ultraceuticals
Vaniqa
Vaseline
Vichy

Victoria's Secret Cosmetics
Vincent Longo
Wei East
Weleda
Wen by Chaz Dean
Yes To
Yon-Ka Paris
Youthful Essence by Susan Lucci
Yves Rocher
Z. Bigatti
Zapzyt
ZO Skin Health

CHAPTER FIVE

Product-by-Product Reviews

AHAVA (SKIN CARE ONLY)

AHAVA AT-A-GLANCE

Strengths: Most of the cleansers are good; all of the sun-care products with sunscreen include avobenzone for UVA protection.

Weaknesses: Expensive; several of the daytime moisturizers with sunscreen do not list active ingredients; Dead Sea mud is not the cure-all for anyone's aging skin; lackluster moisturizers and serums; jar packaging; no AHA or BHA products; no products to manage acne; no products to lighten skin discolorations; average masks.

For more information about Ahava, call (800) 366-7254 or visit www.ahavaus.com or www.Beautypedia.com.

AHAVA DERMUD PRODUCTS

☺ **$$$ Dermud Gentle Soothing Facial Cleanser** *($20 for 4.2 ounces)* is a very standard but good water-soluble cleanser for normal to oily skin. It removes makeup easily and rinses without leaving a residue, though it doesn't have any edge in terms of alleviating the effects of inflammation from external influences. Your skin won't notice the tiny amount of Dead Sea water, but it will be clean!

☹ **Dermud Facial Calming Moisturizer SPF 15** *($30 for 1.7 ounces)* does not list active sunscreen ingredients, but it does contain octinoxate and zinc oxide. Still, this isn't worth considering over many other sunscreens that provide reliable (and FDA-required) labeling. Even with the actives listed, this lightweight sunscreen would not be recommended for any skin type because it contains irritating grapefruit peel oil.

☹ **Dermud Intense Soothing Nourishing Cream** *($30 for 1.7 ounces)* isn't what I or anyone familiar with moisturizer formulations would consider intense or soothing. Anti-irritants are nearly absent, and the grapefruit peel oil can be irritating and possibly cause a negative skin reaction in the presence of sunlight. Beyond these problems lies a very boring moisturizer for normal to dry skin.

AHAVA TIME LINE PRODUCTS

☺ **$$$ 3D Essence Ampoules** *($90 for 0.5 ounce)*. This Ahava serum arrives in packaging that is far more impressive than what you will find inside the capsules. They contain water, silicones, plant extracts, more silicones, more plant extracts, and slip agents. Silicones feel good on your skin, but the other ingredients aren't at all unusual and certainly not "age-defying." The plant extracts are a mix of anti-irritants and irritants, so their effects, in essence, negate each other.

☺ **$$$ Age Defying Continual Eye Treat** *($42 for 0.5 ounce)* consists mostly of water, several silicones, glycerin, and Dead Sea water. The silicones will help smooth and slightly fill in superficial lines around the eye, but this "treat" is missing several key elements to improve your skin's appearance and health. As such, although it's an option for normal to slightly dry skin anywhere on the face, it isn't worth the money and there are far superior options available from a range of product lines.

☺ **$$$ Age Defying Optimizer Serum** *($70 for 1 ounce)* is a light-textured, water-based moisturizer that claims to provide eight hours of continuous hydration. The numerous plant extracts (some helpful, some irritating) aren't moisturizing, and other than these additives you're relying on the water and slip agent (butylene glycol) to do the hydrating. This is a barely OK option for normal to oily skin, and the antiwrinkle claims are sheer fantasy.

☺ **$$$ All Night Nourishment** *($56 for 1.7 ounces)* isn't worth using all night, at least not if you want to treat your skin to the "nourishment" it deserves. Although the main plant extract in this moisturizer for normal to slightly dry skin has possible anti-inflammatory properties, there is not enough evidence to deem it safe or effective for continual use. There isn't really anything else to say about this product, given its ordinary formulation, which is hardly nourishing or helpful for skin. This falls below the median line for a worthwhile moisturizer. Also worth noting, this product contains fragrances known to cause irritation.

☹ **All Day Moisturizer + SPF 15** *($52 for 1 ounce)* does not list its active ingredients, which means it does not comply with FDA regulations. If you don't know what active ingredients you are putting on your skin, you have no way of knowing if you are getting full UVA protection. In addition, the main plant extract in this product (*Zizyphus jujuba*) has a questionable safety profile for skin (Source: www.naturaldatabase.com). Also worth noting, this product contains fragrances known to cause irritation.

OTHER AHAVA PRODUCTS

☺ **$$$ Cleansing Cream** *($20 for 3.4 ounces)* shares a formula that is nearly identical to Ahava's Dermud Gentle Soothing Facial Cleanser, which costs the same but offers almost an ounce more product. Like the Dermud version, this is a good water-soluble cleanser for normal to oily skin (it is not creamy as the name states).

☺ **$$$ Cleansing Milk** *($24 for 8.5 ounces)* is just an overpriced cold cream-style cleanser. It is an option for someone with dry skin, but there are many far less expensive versions that would work as well if not better.

☺ **$$$ Purifying Gel** *($24 for 4.2 ounces)* is an exceptionally standard cleansing gel for normal to oily skin. The basic formula is overpriced for what you get, and Dead Sea water is hardly essential to the cleansing process, but this is nevertheless an option.

☺ **Gentle Eye Makeup Remover** *($18 for 8.5 ounces)*. This uses gentle detergent cleansing agents to remove makeup, and as such must be rinsed from skin to avoid irritation. It works well on most types of eye makeup, but a water-in-silicone makeup remover is preferred for long-wearing or waterproof formulas. This contains rose flower water for fragrance.

☺ **$$$ Mud Exfoliator** *($24 for 3.4 ounces)* is more a water-soluble cleanser than a scrub, but it does contain synthetic scrub particles and sea mud. If you assumed that Dead Sea mud had some special benefits for everyone's skin, then you'd want to leave this on longer than it says to in the directions; however, Dead Sea mud doesn't have any such special effects, so you might as well just rinse it away.

☹ **Matifying Toner** *($21 for 8.5 ounces)*. Because irritating witch hazel distillate (which is mostly alcohol) is listed as the second ingredient, this a poor choice as a "gentle treatment" for oily, acne-prone skin. Alcohol causes cell death and free-radical damage, plus it stimulates oil production in the pore. Otherwise, this is just a very boring toner that has little hope of making blemished skin look better (though the minerals it contains can give a temporary matte finish to your skin).

☹ **Mineral Toning Water** *($21 for 8.50 ounces)* lists the solvent methylal (also called dimethoxymethane, methylene dimethyl ether, among others) as its second ingredient, which is a compound related to formaldehyde. This ingredient is a volatile compound that can be irritating to skin, as can the citrus extracts in this poorly formulated toner.

☺ **Matifying Moisturizer** *($32 for 1.7 ounces)* is a basic blend of water, thickener, absorbent, more thickener, silicone, witch hazel, and preservatives. Its formula makes it barely passable as a moisturizer, and it does contain fragrance. It's such a banal formula it doesn't warrant your attention.

☺ **$$$ Mineral Beauty Serum** *($60 for 1 ounce)* pretends it's an AHA product by listing sugar cane, sugar maple, and various citrus extracts (their "Mineral Osmoter" blend—What a corny marketing name! Who came up with that one?!). None of these ingredients work in the same manner as the AHAs glycolic or lactic acids; even if they did, this lackluster serum's pH is too high for them to function in that manner. The only thing beautiful about this serum is the ridiculous price tag, which is beautiful only to Ahava; the product is not beautiful for your skin.

☺ **$$$ Mineral Eye Cream** *($40 for 1 ounce)* is very similar to Ahava's Continual Eye Treat, but the plant extracts this one contains, which have only minimal antioxidant properties to start with, will quickly lose any possibility of providing a benefit to your skin because the jar packaging won't keep them stable. Why the Continual Eye Treat costs more for half as much product is a mystery, but neither product is even close to being state-of-the-art. This is merely an average option for normal to slightly dry skin. It does contain fragrance.

☺ **$$$ Protective Moisturizer with SPF 15, Normal to Dry Skin** *($35 for 1.7 ounces)*. Although this product claims to offer SPF 15 protection, the sunscreen agents it contains (including zinc oxide for UVA protection) are not listed as active, which is mandatory in the United States and several other countries. Therefore, you cannot rely on this for daytime care. The base formula is light and silky, but lacks state-of-the-art ingredients. For the money, any of the daytime moisturizers with sunscreen we've recommended from Neutrogena, Olay, or Boots are far better choices. If you opt to take your chances with this product, it is best for normal to slightly dry skin.

☺ **Skin Replenisher (Night), for Normal to Dry Skin** *($40 for 1.7 ounces)* is actually one of the few intriguing moisturizers from Ahava because it contains some truly beneficial ingredients for reinforcing a healthy barrier function, such as glycoproteins and jojoba seed oil. Unfortunately, the antioxidants it contains won't last long once this jar-packaged moisturizer is opened. It is, however, formulated for its intended skin type. Ahava's claim that skin can absorb the benefits of minerals only "in the delicate calm of night" is false. More to the point, there are no minerals of note in this product, unless you consider a sprinkling of sea salt noteworthy. Though worth noting, this product contains fragrances known to cause irritation.

☺ **$$$ Skin Replenisher (Night), for Very Dry Skin** *($48 for 1.7 ounces)* offers normal to slightly dry skin a silky finish, but those with very dry skin will want something more emollient.

Overall, all skin types need more than this bland moisturizer can provide; most of the interesting ingredients are present in teeny-tiny amounts, and the product is packaged in a jar.

☺ **Smoothing Moisturizer (Day), for Normal to Dry Skin** *($32 for 1.7 ounces)* is a basic moisturizer for its intended skin type, yet is inappropriate for daytime use because it does not offer sun protection. Water-binding agents are plentiful, but antioxidants are in short supply (and what's here won't hold up for long because of the jar packaging).

☺ **Smoothing Moisturizer (Day), for Very Dry Skin** *($42 for 1.7 ounces)* offers little of substance to those with normal to very dry skin, though its long list of thickeners can provide a smooth, moist feel. All skin types, but especially dry skin, need much more than this average, jar-packaged formula provides. Also worth noting, this product contains fragrances known to cause irritation.

☹ **$$$ Intensive Hydration Mask** *($28 for 3.4 ounces)* is a basic, 1960s style moisturizing mask for normal to dry skin that is mostly waxes and glycerin. It's about as intensive and beneficial as sitting in traffic. All you get is a moisturizer to make dry skin feel less dry, but you can do that for less than $10 at the drugstore, and get a larger container. Ahava sells this as a unique leave-on mask, but the truth is you can leave almost any moisturizing mask on your skin if you want to. The amount of Dead Sea water is almost undetectable, which is fine because this sulfur-laden water doesn't bestow any unique benefits on dry skin.

☺ **Purifying Mud Mask, for Normal to Dry Skin** *($28 for 5.3 ounces)* is primarily a mud and clay mask. For someone with very oily skin this may be helpful, but for someone with dry skin this would be an overly drying experience. There just aren't enough emollients to compensate for the absorbency of the clay and mud.

☺ **Purifying Mud Mask, for Oily Skin** *($28 for 5.3 ounces)* is a very standard clay and mud mask for its intended skin type. The amount of witch hazel distillate is likely too small to be cause for concern (you would typically want to avoid the alcohol it contains), while the plant extracts are a mix of soothing and irritating ingredients, so they cancel each other out.

AHAVA SUN PRODUCTS

☺ **Sun Protection Anti-Aging Facial Moisturizer SPF 50** *($25 for 2.1 ounces)* provides an in-part avobenzone sunscreen and is water resistant, but otherwise this sunscreen lotion for normal to slightly dry skin is downright boring. Neutrogena, Coppertone, and Clinique offer better sunscreens with avobenzone, and they include more than the measly 1% this Ahava product contains.

☺ **Sun Protection Anti-Aging Moisturizer SPF 15** *($22 for 8.5 ounces)* is a water-resistant sunscreen that's suitable for normal to slightly dry or slightly oily skin, but it would have been a lot better if Ahava had included more than a token amount of vitamin E for an antioxidant boost. The Dead Sea minerals are barely present, but that's fine, as they offer no hope of protecting skin from sun exposure.

☺ **Sun Protection Anti-Aging Moisturizer SPF 30** *($22 for 8.5 ounces)* covers the basics in terms of providing UVA protection with avobenzone and of being a water-resistant formula for use during swimming and exercising. However, the lotion formula is really bare bones, and doesn't offer normal to slightly dry skin much beyond sun protection. For the money, that's disappointing.

☺ **Sun Protection Anti-Aging Moisturizer SPF 50** *($25 for 8.5 ounces)* is nearly identical to Ahava's Sun Protection Anti-Aging Facial Moisturizer SPF 50, and the same review applies.

☺ **Sun Protection Anti-Aging Moisturizing Spray SPF 15** *($22 for 8.5 ounces)* is a spray-on lotion version of Ahava's Sun Protection Anti-Aging Moisturizer SPF 15. The formulas are nearly identical, and both include avobenzone for UVA protection. This is an OK option for normal to slightly oily or slightly dry skin.

☺ **Sun Protection Anti-Aging Moisturizing Spray SPF 30** *($22 for 8.5 ounces)* is an alcohol-free, spray-on sunscreen with silicones for a silky application and smooth finish. The water-resistant formula is suitable for all skin types except sensitive. I am concerned that only 1% avobenzone (listed as butyl methoxydibenzoylmethane) is included, because that may not be enough to ensure sufficient UVA protection, especially over a period of hours outdoors. Most broad-spectrum sunscreens with avobenzone rated SPF 30 or higher contain 3% of this active.

☹ **After Sun Rehydrating Balm** *($25 for 8.5 ounces)* offers skin a frustrating combination of beneficial (urea, glycerin) and irritating (menthyl lactate, witch hazel) ingredients, and as such this is hardly a soothing product to use on sun-exposed skin. This also contains lots of preservatives (much more than a typical moisturizer) and volatile fragrant components that can be irritating, especially on sunburned skin. There is nothing "rehydrating" about this balm.

ALMAY

ALMAY AT-A-GLANCE

Strengths: An excellent assortment of foundations with sunscreen; very good powders, liquid eyeliner, lip pencil, and mascaras; inviting and well-organized in-store displays.

Weaknesses: Company discontinued all of their skin-care products; despite their hypoallergenic claims they still included potentially irritating and sensitizing ingredients; mediocre blush and eyeshadows; lipsticks with sunscreen that do not provide sufficient UVA protection; the Pure Blends line is disappointing.

For more information about Almay, call (800) 992-5629 or visit www.almay.com or www. Beautypedia.com.

ALMAY PURE BLENDS

☹ **Pure Blends Makeup** *($13.99).* Almay claims this lightweight tinted moisturizer is 97.4% natural, which appears to be the case, although the process the ingredients go through—getting it out of the ground or off the tree, cleaning it up (you don't want dirt or insects or bacteria in your skin-care or makeup products), creating the extract, preserving it so it doesn't get moldy or become bacteria-laden—isn't such a natural process. But, natural or not, this sheer makeup misses the mark by including a host of skin-irritating fragrant plant extracts and oils that are a problem for skin. This is a great example of how natural doesn't necessarily mean better or safer for skin. Taken on its own as a tinted moisturizer, this isn't bad, but there are better ones that omit irritants and include sunscreen so you get two benefits for the price of one.

☺ **Pure Blends Mineral Makeup SPF 15** *($13.99)* includes 20% zinc oxide, which not only provides excellent broad-spectrum sun protection but also lends an opacity and dry finish to this well-packaged loose powder makeup. The powder is housed in a central chamber and is shot onto an attached (and surprisingly soft) brush, allowing you to dust it over your face. The result is a sheer application whose initial light coverage can be built to medium with successive coats. However, adding more powder tends to make this look and feel too dry, not only because of the amount of zinc oxide but also because the other main ingredient is aluminum starch octenylsuccinate, which has an absorbent finish. Almay wisely recommends using this as secondary rather than primary sun protection because you'd have to pile this on to ensure your skin is sufficiently shielded. The finish feels very matte but tends to look a bit shiny on skin. That helps it not appear too dull, but it won't make someone with very oily skin happy, unless they don't want to downplay the shine. As is typical of Almay, all six shades (including options for fair to medium skin tones) are soft and neutral. This product is recommended as an adjunct to your sun protection, whether it's in addition to your foundation or daytime moisturizer. It doesn't have the best feel or performance when worn alone.

☹ **Pure Blends Loose Finishing Powder - Translucent Shimmer** *($13.99)*. Almay claims this powder is 98.2% natural and the ingredients on the label back up that claim. But, natural or not, the glitter flecks in this powder make it impossible to recommend. The sparkly pieces are messy and flake easily off the skin. The first ingredient, mica, also adds to the pearlescent finish of this pinkish powder, making it appear anything but "98.2% natural" on the skin.

☺ **Pure Blends Loose Finishing Powder - Translucent Matte** *($13.99)*. Almay claims this powder is 98.2% natural and the ingredients on the label back up that claim. The first ingredient is mica, a common shiny mineral found in lots of cosmetic powders to give the skin a glow. While this sheer powder does a decent job of absorbing oil (something any powder can do), it isn't any better or worse for your skin than other loose powders. The mica also keeps it from being matte; so even though the oil that your pores produce will be held back for a while, your face will still look shiny. The one available shade is slightly pink and will work only for fair skin tones. The cardboard packaging is small and convenient for travel, but the included powder puff is a bad option for application; powders of any kind should be applied only with a powder brush.

☺ **Pure Blends Blush** *($11.49)*. The first ingredient in these powder blushes is mica, which is why each of the available shades has shimmer. The sheerness of the powder keeps the shimmer from being overwhelming, and the color goes on much lighter than it appears in the compact. Only Sunkissed (which is designed for bronzing skin) should be avoided altogether, because it's too orange to be flattering. The included brush is too small for proper application and you should toss it. By the way, the formula for Pure Blends Blush is nearly identical to Almay's Pure Blends Eyeshadow, and it contains the same plant extracts that can irritate skin.

☺ **Pure Blends Eyeshadow** *($7.49)*. These soft powder shadows blend and wear well, lasting for hours without creasing. Each of the mostly neutral shades has some shimmer, but the sheerness of these shadows keeps the shimmer from being overwhelming. If you've been waiting for a 98.2% natural eyeshadow, look no further—this fits the bill; however, I am concerned that many of the irritating plant extracts this contains may cause contact dermatitis on the eyelids, which is why this eyeshadow is not rated with a happy face.

☺ **Pure Blends Lipgloss** *($7.99)*. Pure Blends Lipgloss is 95.8% natural (according to Almay) and the ingredient list supports the claim, but natural doesn't add up to a great product; in this case it is 100% ordinary. The fact that this lipgloss is touted as being more natural than those of its competitors doesn't mean it wears any better or longer. In fact, this gloss is thinner and oilier than most glosses, wears off quickly, and needs to be reapplied much more frequently than is the norm. All of the shades are sheer and neutral, but this product is just not worth the trouble.

☺ **Pure Blends Volumizing Mascara** *($6.99)*. The attention-getting claim for this mascara is that it's 97.5% natural. Based on the ingredient list, there's no reason to dispute the claim, but here's the kicker: the core ingredients in this mascara are seen in almost every non-waterproof mascara sold today, which means those are mostly natural, too. Almay's claim may be valid, but it doesn't distinguish this mascara as much as consumers may think. What does distinguish this mascara (and not in a good way) is its uneven, clumpy application and the fact that it requires considerable effort to look decent. It tends to flake shortly after application but the flaking doesn't continue. Still, this is one of Almay's most disappointing mascaras.

ALMAY MAKEUP

MAKEUP REMOVERS: ☺ **Makeup Remover Towelettes, Oil-Free** *($5.99 for 25 towelettes)* are essentially a gentle, water-soluble cleanser in premoistened cloth form. This basic formula will remove a light makeup application but is not capable of removing mascara, long-wearing foundation, or lip color. It is best for normal to slightly dry or slightly oily skin.

☺ **Moisturizing Eye Makeup Remover Liquid** *($5.99 for 4 ounces)* is a standard, mineral oil-based liquid that efficiently removes eye makeup, though not without leaving a greasy residue. The gentle, fragrance-free formula is best used before cleansing.

☺ **Moisturizing Eye Makeup Remover Pads** *($5.81 for 80 pads)*. Moisturizing Eye Makeup Remover Pads are nearly identical to the Moisturizing Eye Makeup Remover Liquid, except for the pad format, which some consumers may prefer.

☺ **Oil Free Eye Makeup Remover Liquid** *($6.29 for 4 ounces)* works well to remove most eye makeup. The lack of silicone or oils makes it a poor choice to remove waterproof mascara.

☺ **Oil Free Eye Makeup Remover Pads** *($5.99 for 80 pads)* are nearly identical to the Oil Free Eye Makeup Remover Liquid, only in pad form, so the same review applies.

FOUNDATION: ✓☺ **Clear Complexion Liquid Makeup** *($12.49)* is a foundation that promises to "heal blemishes." It contains salicylic acid as the anti-acne active, but in an amount that's too low (0.6%) and at a pH that's too high (pH 6) to be helpful for skin. Even though the salicylic acid in this makeup won't help with blemishes, this still offers an enviably smooth, liquid texture that blends onto skin with ease, providing light to medium coverage and a natural matte finish. It is a great example of how beautiful a foundation can look on the skin. Eight shades are available, and almost all of them are exquisite. Only Warm and Honey should be viewed with caution; these may be too peach for some medium to tan skin tones. There are no options for very light or dark skin tones. One caution: Because of the salicylic acid, this product should not be used around the eyes or on the eyelids. This foundation is one to try if you have normal to very oily skin, though it would need to be paired with an effective sunscreen rated SPF 15 or higher for daytime use.

✓☺ **Nearly Naked Liquid Makeup SPF 15** *($12.99)* is easily one of Almay's best liquid foundations. Its lightweight cream texture blends superbly, setting to a smooth matte finish that enhances skin without looking flat, fake, or the least bit unnatural. Well-suited for someone with normal to oily skin, it offers sheer to light coverage and excellent sun protection from its in-part titanium dioxide and zinc oxide sunscreen. More good news: The nine shades are beautifully neutral, with options for fair to tan skin tones.

✓☺ **Smart Shade Smart Balance Skin Balancing Makeup SPF 15** *($11.99)*. This liquid foundation with titanium dioxide and zinc oxide as the only sunscreen ingredients is Almay's latest version of their Smart Shade makeup. The original formula, with the same name, is still available, at least for now; the only differences are the price (this one is $5 more) and the claims Almay makes. This improved version not only carries on the skin-matching pigment technology claim of its predecessor, but also adds the claim of being able to sense where skin is oily or dry and to act accordingly. We've seen this claim before, and it never works. Simply put, there's no way a makeup can know where skin is dry or oily and then be able to deposit the right ingredients to improve these disparate conditions. Where would the moisturizing ingredients go when the oil-absorbing ingredients are "activated," and vice versa? In terms of moisturizing, this silky foundation provides little moisture; the ingredients are primarily about absorbing oil and moisture. It goes on smoothly, blends readily, and sets to a soft matte finish that becomes powdery a short time later. The finish is incredibly skin-like, making this one of the most natural-looking foundations available. Coverage goes from sheer to light. Only three shades are available, and they're said to self-adjust to each level (light, medium, and dark), depending on your skin tone. They can't really do that, of course, but the shades are versatile enough to work for most people with light to slightly tan skin. Note: this foundation dispenses white with small colored specks. The specks "burst" as you blend, and the whiteness disappears, so there's no ghostly look to be concerned about. This foundation is best for normal to oily skin.

✓ ☺ **TLC Truly Lasting Color 16 Hour Makeup SPF 15** *($12.99)* will not remain looking "just-applied" for the full 16 hours (and definitely not over your oily areas), but don't let the exaggerated claim keep you from trying this fantastic foundation. The silky texture is a pleasure to blend, and provides medium coverage that layers well over trouble spots. Gentle, effective sun protection is assured from the blend of titanium dioxide and zinc oxide, while the smooth matte finish helps keep excess oil in check (just not all day) without looking chalky. The eight mostly neutral shades are indicative of what Almay usually produces, which is good. There are no options for dark skin tones, and the lightest shades may present some trouble for fair skin due to overtones of pink and yellow, but they're still worth considering. Avoid the too-peach Warm. By the way, Almay did include vitamins and antioxidants in this foundation, but the clear glass packaging won't keep them stable unless you're diligent about protecting it from exposure to light. In foundations these impressive ingredients are almost always window dressing and should not be construed as turning your foundation into a form of skin care.

☺ **Smart Shade Makeup SPF 15** *($13.99)* is available in only three shades, and the logic from Almay is that this colorless makeup (I'll explain that in a moment) transforms to complement your skin tone, thus taking the guesswork out of choosing a foundation shade. If only it were that simple! Addressing the preliminaries, this liquid foundation has a titanium dioxide and zinc oxide sunscreen, which is great, and it also lends some opacity and coverage. Unfortunately, it also creates a somewhat flat finish. Coverage is sheer to medium (if you're up for layering), and for those with oily skin or oily areas, it does a great job of keeping shine to a minimum. As you dispense each shade, it appears grayish white. As you blend, it turns into a flesh tone and feels surprisingly light. Each shade blends well and does not streak or look "dotted" on skin, though its initial appearance is admittedly startling. Almay has divided the shades by depth of skin color. The Light shade fares best because it is the most neutral, and is a versatile option for fair to light skin, but may be too yellow for some fair skin tones. Light/Medium is OK for medium skin tones, but is too peach for lighter skin, while Medium has a rosy tone that makes it unsuitable for most skin colors. Unlike Cover Girl's TruBlend or Max Factor's Colour Adapt foundations, you won't be able to wear more than one shade and have it look convincing. In fact, given the limitations of the shades Almay created, consumers may end up more frustrated than satisfied by this attempt to streamline foundation shade choices. If one of these shades works for you, this is an impressive, long-wearing foundation for normal to very oily skin. Note, however, that it will take more than a water-soluble cleanser to remove it. (I used a silicone-based makeup remover with a washcloth to get it off.)

☺ **Line Smoothing Compact Makeup SPF 15** *($14.99)* has a creamy texture that blends well and achieves a smooth texture with medium coverage, though it can be blended to have a sheer appearance if desired. It sets to a natural-looking finish that will only slip and fade if you have oily areas. Best for normal to dry skin, Line Smoothing Compact Makeup comes in eight shades, suitable for fair to medium skin, and all of them are outstanding.

☺ **Line Smoothing Makeup SPF 15** *($14.99)* offers excellent UVA protection thanks to its titanium dioxide and zinc oxide sunscreen. It has a slightly thick, initially creamy texture that blends smoothly, provides light to medium coverage, and has a satin matte finish. I disagree with Almay's claim that this formula "hydrates all day" because it contains minimal ingredients with substantial moisturizing properties for skin. The nine shades are mostly neutral and include options for fair to tan skin. Beige and Warm suffer from a noticeable peach cast, and are the only shades to avoid. This foundation is best for normal to slightly dry skin and, contrary to its name, doesn't do much to smooth the appearance of lines.

☺ **Touchpad Nearly Naked Makeup SPF 12** *($12.49)* is a sheer, nonaqueous, silicone-based foundation that has a foundation-soaked sponge firmly attached to the base of a compact. You touch the damp sponge and apply the makeup with your fingers. It's a bit inelegant but nevertheless is a method of application many women won't mind. The good news is double, because this has a titanium dioxide and zinc oxide sunscreen (even if SPF 12 is a bit disappointing, when SPF 15 is the standard set by all medical associations), and it also blends so well, drying to a natural satin-matte finish that feels smooth and weightless. Nearly Naked is aptly named, because this formula isn't much for coverage, though if you prefer sheer to light coverage this won't be an issue. The six shades (though ever-so-slightly peach) are all excellent, but because of the way this foundation is packaged, it is impossible to see the real color, which makes choosing the best shade a guessing game.

CONCEALER: ☺ **Bright Eyes Eye Base + Concealer** *($8.99)*. This sheer liquid concealer is dispensed from a squeeze tube that has a synthetic brush affixed to the opening. Dispensing takes some getting used to; it is easy to squeeze out too much and waste product. It is sold as an eye-area brightener that claims to deflate puffy eyes. The first claim is realistic but the second is just standard cosmetic puffery. Each of the two shades provides a subtle brightening effect thanks to the soft shimmer finish they have, though they do end up with a matte-feeling finish. The silicone-enhanced formula contains several water-binding agents and antioxidant plant extracts, but none of these will reduce puffy eyes. Despite that letdown, artfully applied, a concealer with soft shine can make the eye area look better. As an eye base, the formula helps eyeshadows apply and adhere better versus application over bare skin—but any matte or powder finish foundation or concealer applied to the eyelid can do the same thing. This is best for those who want sheer coverage with a hint of shine.

☺ **Clear Complexion Concealer** *($7.99)* contains, like all of Almay's Clear Complexion products, salicylic acid. It's present here at 1%, but the pH is over 4, so it won't exfoliate skin and can't help to reduce blemishes and blackheads. This is still a worthwhile liquid concealer that provides medium coverage and a soft, somewhat dry matte finish. It's an option for concealing blemishes or red spots, but be aware of the salicylic acid and keep it away from the eyelid area. All three shades are recommended.

☺ **Smart Shade Concealer SPF 15** *($8.99)*. This concealer gets its "smart" name from the claim that it "transforms into your ideal shade." But if that were really true, wouldn't just one master shade suffice because it would "transform" for everyone? Almay offers three shades, so they don't seem to believe their own claim! Aside from the hokey name, this concealer has a slightly liquid texture that provides more slip than necessary, so it's somewhat tricky to get it placed just where you want it because it tends to spread too easily. I add to this precaution the fact that the formula takes longer to set than it should. It ends up having a soft matte finish capable of medium coverage, but you may notice minor creasing under the eyes and fading by the end of the day. Two of the three shades are good and well-suited for light skin tones; avoid Medium, which is quite peachy. The smartest part of this concealer is its titanium dioxide and zinc oxide sunscreen, which is why this is worth considering despite the other shortcomings. It is an excellent choice for use around the eye area, especially if your foundation or daytime moisturizer with sunscreen proves irritating when applied to that area.

☺ **Line Smoothing Concealer SPF 10** *($10.49)* works beautifully as an under-eye concealer thanks to its fluid, smooth application, just the right amount of slip, and soft matte finish. The sole sunscreen active is titanium dioxide, a gentle choice for a product meant to be used around the eyes, but it's disappointing the SPF rating is not 15. Three shades are available, all excellent.

☺ **Nearly Naked Cover-Up Stick** *($7.79)* pales in comparison to Almay's other concealers, but still has merit for someone with dry skin. The coverage this lipstick-style concealer provides is not "Nearly Naked" and it tends to crease into lines under the eye, though that can be reduced by setting it with powder. The wax content of this concealer makes it completely inappropriate for use over blemishes. Three shades are available, each suitably neutral.

POWDER: ✓ ☺ **Nearly Naked Loose Powder** *($12.49)* promises a "flawless, natural-looking finish" and delivers! This talc-based powder has an ultra-silky texture that feels weightless and sets makeup without looking flat or dry. All three shades are suitable for most skin tones since they are so translucent. Someone with very oily skin will likely want a more absorbent powder, but all other skin types will appreciate what this has to offer.

✓ ☺ **Line Smoothing Pressed Powder** *($13.99)* feels silky, goes on sheer and exceptionally smooth, and makes normal to dry skin look polished, not powdered. The slight satin finish of this powder won't exaggerate wrinkles, but powders (this one included) don't do much to smooth their appearance, either. That doesn't mean this outstanding option isn't worth considering, and if you have light to medium skin, the three shades are geared for you.

☺ **TLC Truly Lasting Color Pressed Powder SPF 12** *($12.99)*. In an unusual move for Almay, this talc-based pressed powder with sunscreen lacks sufficient UVA-protecting ingredients (titanium dioxide, zinc oxide, avobenzone [also called butyl methoxydibenzoylmethane], Tinosorb, Mexoryl SX [also known as ecamsule]). Although it's not a pressed powder to consider if you want broad-spectrum sun protection, it has a beautiful, creamy feel that slips over skin and blends to a natural yet polished finish. You may be tempted by Almay's claim of 16-hour wear for this product, but anyone with oily skin will find they need a touch-up before lunch. In terms of wearability, however, this powder does hold up well throughout the day as far as not pooling into pores or looking streaked is concerned, but that's true of many top-rated powders (some with great SPF protection). Among the three shades (suitable for light to medium skin) you'll find Medium and Light/Medium appear a bit peach in the compact, but both look softer and more neutral on skin. The happy face rating for this pressed powder does not apply to its deficient sunscreen.

☺ **Clear Complexion Pressed Powder** *($12.63)* claims to clear blemishes with salicylic acid (present at 0.6%), but since a pH value cannot be obtained from a powder, it won't work for that purpose. The formula is talc-based and the texture is unusually dry, though it doesn't look chalky on skin. It contains cornstarch, not the best ingredient to use on blemish-prone skin, but it is absorbent. Three sheer shades are available, and all have merit.

BLUSH AND BRONZER: ☺ **Smart Shade Blush** *($8.99)* is said to be so smart, it blushes for you—thanks to shade-sensing "smart beads" that transform to your ideal blush color. Available in Pink, Berry, or Natural tones, each offers very soft, sheer color that requires several layers to really register as blush. The liquid texture is surprisingly easy to blend and sets quickly to a soft matte finish. You may be wondering if this blush can really self-adjust to each individual's skin tone, and the simple answer is: it cannot. However, like any color cosmetic, the way it looks on your skin will be (to varying degrees) different from how the same shade looks on someone else's skin. Almay is taking the obvious and trying to make it sound customized, but all they've really created is a good liquid blush for normal to oily skin (Note to those with large pores: This does not magnify them or make them look "dotted with color").

☺ **Touchpad Blush** *($10.29)* takes the concept of sheer blush almost all the way to invisible! An attached "touchpad" sponge is infused with liquid silicone blush and the result is a very soft wash of translucent color. Unfortunately, the slick nature of silicone makes this tricky to blend. It meshes well with skin, but controlling where the blush goes is difficult because of the product's slip. Still, for those willing to be patient and adapt to a unique application, this is a way to (barely) blush and leave skin with a subtle glow, courtesy of each shade's low level of shimmer. The available shades are so sheer, only those with porcelain to medium skin should use them. Darker or tan skin tones will be left wondering why no color is showing up after repeated applications!

☺ **Powder Blush** *($10.29)* is a below-standard pressed-powder blush that comes in an attractive range of shades and has a reasonably smooth application. The problem is the sparkly particles woven into each shade. They don't do this blush any favors, are distracting in daylight, and tend to flake. Powder blush is one area where Almay never seems to pull ahead.

☺ **Powder Bronzer** *($10.29)* is pressed and has a dry texture; the two believable tan shades go on sheer, though each leaves sparkles on skin that tend to flake off and land where you don't want them.

☺ **Smart Shade Bronzer** *($8.99)* is nearly identical to the Smart Shade Blush, except the color saturation is stronger, so you need less per application to produce noticeable results. The blending qualities and soft matte finish remain the same, as does the fact that this liquid bronzer is best for normal to oily skin. The main drawback is the color itself, which tends toward orange regardless of your skin tone. That limits the appeal and doesn't make this preferred to other bronzing options.

EYESHADOW: ☺ **Intense i-Color Eye Shadow Extension Play Up Trio** *($7.49)* has the same texture and application traits as the Intense i-Color Powder Shadow, but most of the trios offer suitable, contrasting shadow shades that really do enhance one's eye color. For example, the Play Up Trio for Browns features a pale peach, medium brown, and muted plum shade, while the Play Up Trio for Hazels features pale pink and taupes, all of which work for, not against, those eye colors. Avoid the Play Up Trios for Green and Blue eyes because each contains at least one inappropriate color.

☺ **Bright Eyes Eye Shadow** *($8.49)* has two eyeshadows in one package, one a softer shade than the other, and each with a cream-to-powder finish. Combining these or using them separately is supposed to create the intensity or brightening you need, but those traits can be attributed to most eyeshadow formulas, depending on the colors you choose. The cream-to-barely-powder finish helps create a sheer application but these eyeshadows remain creamy even after blending and are prone to creasing and fading. Try going for the same effect these provide with a sheer powder eyeshadow that has a soft shine finish, such as those from M.A.C.'s Satin collection.

☺ **Intense i-Color Powder Shadow** *($7.49)* presents a collection of four eyeshadow trios, each with shades meant to complement your eye color (a misguided notion, but I'll get to that in a moment). The texture of these shadows is smooth yet powdery, so unless you're careful some flaking is imminent and application can be messy. These go on quite soft, and every shade in each trio has an obvious shine that borders on overpowering the underlying color of the eyeshadow itself. The trios for green eyes and blue eyes should be avoided because eyeshadow is not about matching your eye color, it's about shading and shaping the eye area. Even if your goal is to enhance your eye color, to do that effectively you would choose contrasting, not matching, shades. For example, if you want to make white look whiter, you don't put another shade of white next to it, you pair it with a dark shade, like slate or black. Applying blue eyeshadow (actually, don't apply it, ever, but just for example …) when you have blue eyes means that you're adding color that will visually compete with your eyes, whereas brown shades, or pale peach, caramel, or taupe colors will enhance them. It really is that simple. These trios from Almay are intended to make eyeshadow shopping easier but end up not helping in the least. They just point women back to a makeup theory that hasn't made it into the fashion magazines since the '70s. I'm sorry to report that, according to the Almay representative I spoke with, these trios have been exceedingly popular.

EYE AND BROW SHAPER: ✓ ☺ **Liquid Eyeliner** *($7.49)* remains one of the very best liquid liners at any price. It goes on smoothly and easily, creating a dramatic line—thin or thick—without flaking, chipping, or looking crinkled. Two shades (classic brown and black) are available, both with all-day longevity.

☺ **Eye Liner** *($8.19)* is a very good, automatic, retractable pencil with a smooth application that is only slightly prone to smudging. It won't outlast the gel-based eyeliners from Stila, Bobbi Brown, and Paula's Choice, but is a worthy contender if you prefer pencils. As claimed, this pencil is waterproof. In fact, it requires an oil- or silicone-based makeup remover to get it to come off completely.

☺ **Intense i-Color Liquid Liner for Eyes** *($7.49)* has a brush and application that are nearly identical to Almay's Liquid Eyeliner, except that each of the four shades are loaded with iridescence. The cool factor of this eyeliner is that the shades alter in changing light (for example, Raisin Quartz is a metallic purple but in certain light takes on a brownish cast). The negative is that this much shine so close to the lashes is distracting, and not flattering if wrinkles are noticeable. Still, teens and twenty-somethings will find this a fun departure, and it does last.

☺ **Brow Defining Pencil** *($7.49)* is ultra-thin and does not require sharpening. It has a suitably dry texture that demands a soft touch while applying, but that's precisely what it takes to get the best results from this long-lasting brow enhancer. The three shades are terrific, including a great option for blonde (but not white-blonde) eyebrows.

☺ **Blendable Eye Pencil** *($7.49)* is a standard pencil with a creamy yet slightly stiff texture that is meant to be smudged (the opposite end of the pencil has a rubber-tip for smudging). If you're looking for long wear, this won't do, but does work to create dramatic, smoky eyes.

☺ **Bright Eyes Liner/Highlighter Duo** *($8.49)*. This dual-sided, needs-sharpening pencil provides an eyeliner shade on one end and a shimmer-infused highlighting shade on the other. The eyeliner applies smoothly and sets to a nearly smudgeproof finish; the highlighter goes on sheer, imparting noticeably more shine than color. Adding shine to drooping eyelids isn't going to have a lifting effect; instead, it will draw attention to the problem. Applying shine to a smooth, taut brow bone is preferred, but with this product, the shine isn't what would be considered subtle. Although the eyeliner portion is good, there are better pencils available that last longer and don't require routine sharpening.

☹ **Intense i-Color Liner** *($6.99)* is an automatic, retractable eye pencil with a stiff texture that makes smooth application difficult. The plus side is that once you apply it, it does indeed last, without smudging or smearing. Each shade is shiny, so this will make wrinkles on the eyelid or under-eye area look more noticeable (and I suspect enhancing those lines is not your intention).

LIPSTICK, LIP GLOSS, AND LIPLINER: ✓ ☺ **Ideal Lipliner Pencil** *($7.49)* is an automatic, retractable lipliner that includes a built-in sharpener. That's a nice touch (the sharpener is concealed in the base of the pencil component), but unless you like a fine, pointed tip you won't need to use it—that's the beauty of an automatic pencil! Although Almay created shades to coordinate with their lipsticks, the lipsticks are not recommended (though the lipliner colors are great). By itself, this lipliner has a smooth, easy-glide application that stays put and does a good job of preventing lipstick from feathering into lines around the mouth.

☺ **Truly Lasting Color** *($10.59)* is another contender in the category of paint-on, Lipfinity-like liquid lipsticks. This option has the same concept as its predecessors from Cover Girl and Max Factor, meaning that you apply it in a two-step process. The lip color goes on first. Allow it to dry for a minute or so, and then apply the glossy top coat for comfortable wear without disrupting the longevity of the color beneath. In most respects, Almay's option is at least comparable to its competitors. However, it doesn't improve on the wear time of Max Factor's Lipfinity or the smooth feel of M.A.C.'s Pro Longwear Lipcolor. Almay's shade selection is a nice assortment of nudes and bright hues, all of which go on sheerer than you'd expect. Layering doesn't build color intensity—what you see from the first coat is pretty much what you'll get, and it's a softer look that lots of women prefer. Almay's glossy top coat is stickier than most, but for gloss lovers this feel probably won't be objectionable. Truly Lasting Color does not stay on for the 12 hours touted on the packaging, but, like others in this category, it lasts much longer than standard matte or cream lipsticks, although you will need to reapply the top coat regularly to maintain a creamy, lipstick-like feel.

☺ **Hydracolor Lipstick SPF 15** *($8.99)* claims to refresh lips with 100 times more water than regular lipsticks, yet that's easy for this water-based lipstick to do because most lipsticks do not contain any water! Water itself isn't enough to keep lips hydrated (it would just evaporate and leave lips feeling even drier), so it's a good thing Almay included emollients and moisturizing agents, too. Regrettably, the sunscreen does not include the UVA-protecting ingredients of titanium dioxide, zinc oxide, avobenzone, Tinosorb, or Mexoryl SX. That's disappointing because Almay has had lipsticks in the past that deliver sufficient UVA protection. Independent of the sunscreen, this lipstick feels water-light and, true to claim, refreshing upon application.

The water content means this doesn't feel as creamy as standard lipsticks, so expect fairly frequent touch-ups to maintain a smooth, moist finish.

☹ **Ideal Lip Gloss** *($7.99)* has a smooth, non-sticky texture and high-shine finish, but the peppermint oil it contains will irritate and burn lips.

☹ **Ideal Lipcolor Lipstick SPF 17** *($7.49)* does not contain the UVA-protecting ingredients of titanium dioxide, zinc oxide, avobenzone, Tinosorb, or Mexoryl SX. That's shocking considering this essential element of sun protection is something Almay clearly knows about. Making matters worse, the creamy formula contains peppermint oil, and for that reason is not recommended.

MASCARA: ✓☺ **Intense i-Color Mascara Volumizing Lash Color** *($7.49)* is an excellent mascara for length with appreciable thickness, but you can ignore the claims that the slight tint of each shade will somehow noticeably enhance your natural eye color. The aubergine tone of Raisin Quartz does little to make green eyes stand out, while Emerald Green will compete with, rather than enhance, green eyes. The Brown Topaz and Black Pearl shades are by far the winners. Best of all, this mascara goes on clump-free while offering long wear without flakes or smudges.

✓☺ **One Coat Nourishing Mascara Lengthening** *($7.01)* has a misleading name because not only does it take more than one coat to achieve results, but this superior mascara thickens as well as it lengthens! It applies cleanly, wears and removes well, and I for one am glad that, aside from the packaging graphics, Almay didn't choose to alter this long-standing great mascara.

✓☺ **One Coat Nourishing Mascara Triple Effect** *($8.19)* is marvelous. It has a dual-sided brush that maximizes length, curl, and thickness, although if you get too enthusiastic while applying, it can go on somewhat heavy and uneven. The brush side with the longer bristles quickly lengthens and separates lashes, while the opposite side has short, closely packed bristles to add thickness and drama. The formula keeps lashes soft and makes it easy to remove with a water-soluble cleanser, making this a top choice and one that rivals the best mascaras from L'Oreal. Of course, there is nothing in it that is nourishing for your lashes.

✓☺ **One Coat Nourishing Mascara Triple Effect Waterproof** *($7.99)* has the same dual-sided brush as the non-waterproof version, but due to the formula changes necessary to create a waterproof mascara (which this is), the application is thinner. That means less drama, but otherwise there's no question that for a waterproof mascara this maximizes lashes quickly and beautifully, and it wears without a hitch.

☺ **One Coat Nourishing Mascara Thickening Waterproof** *($6.99)* applies beautifully and makes lashes noticeably longer and thicker, though I disagree with Almay's claim of "100% thicker lashes." Still, it wears well, is waterproof, and doesn't make lashes feel stiff or brittle.

☺ **One Coat Nourishing Mascara Thickening** *($6.99)* isn't as impressive as the One Coat Nourishing Mascara Lengthening, but is still recommended. Again, the name is not accurate because this mascara lengthens better than it thickens. Slight clumping is apparent, but it brushes through easily, and this isn't a stubborn formula to remove.

☺ **Intense i-Color Lengthening Mascara** *($7.49)* builds OK length with minor clumps that can be combed through with successive coats. Thickness is minor, and in terms of overall performance this stops short of being genuinely impressive, but it's fine if you just want defined, longer lashes. By the way, this is not a gel-based formula as claimed. The main ingredients in this mascara are the same waxes and thickeners that show up in thousands of others.

☺ **Intense i-Color Thickening Mascara** *($5.99)* promises that lashes will look up to 300% fuller, but the results don't turn out that way, at least not the kind of percentage increase most women would want to achieve. Application is on the heavy side, and it requires several comb-through coats to create neatened, defined lashes, with less then desirable thickness. In contrast, this elongates lashes well and wears without smearing or flaking. This mascara teeters between a happy face and neutral face rating, but because there are so many stellar mascaras available in the inexpensive category it really ends up being one that can stay on the shelf.

ALPHA HYDROX (SKIN CARE ONLY)

ALPHA HYDROX AT-A-GLANCE

Strengths: A good selection of well-priced, effective AHA products using glycolic acid; also excels with skin-lightening and retinol products; a small but commendable selection of cleansers.

Weaknesses: Problematic sunscreens and a couple of moisturizers with oxygenating ingredients; reliance on jar packaging for some products with antioxidants.

For more information about Alpha Hydrox, call (800) 552-5742 or visit www.alphahydrox. com or www.Beautypedia.com.

ALPHA HYDROX WHITE PRODUCTS

✓ ☺ **Face Wash** *($5.99 for 6 ounces)* is an excellent, foaming cleanser that produces a soft, creamy lather. The fragrance-free formula removes makeup and rinses clean, so skin is perfectly prepped for the next step, be it toner, AHA/BHA product, or moisturizer. Face Wash is suitable for all skin types.

☺ **AHA Exfoliating Cream** *($8.20 for 2 ounces)* is a very good, though basic, AHA moisturizer that contains 8% glycolic acid at a pH of 3.6. (Alpha Hydrox states that the pH is 4, but our testing revealed otherwise.) There really is nothing about this exfoliant that makes it different from the other Alpha Hydrox AHAs; clearly the marketing is different, but the performance is the same. You do get a smaller amount in this case, however. This fragrance-free formula is ideal for normal to dry skin and it contains a tiny amount of antioxidants. Keep in mind that although the company recommends this for sensitive skin, an 8% concentration of glycolic acid can be too much for those struggling with sensitivities, so tread carefully.

☺ **Swipes 14% AHA** *($16.99 for 24 pads)*. If you prefer to use an effective AHA product in pad form rather than a cream, gel, or lotion, then this is a product worth considering. The AHA content is higher than usual, but this is still an option if your skin can tolerate this amount; however, this percentage of AHA is definitely not for everyone and the FDA has a preferred limit of 8%. If you're one of those people who believes that if a little is good then a lot is better, or if you have very advanced sun damage, then this is a very good option. It is good that Alpha Hydrox included anti-irritants, but not so good that they formulated with methylchloroisothiazolinone as the preservative in the formula, because it's contraindicated for use in leave-on products. Still, you can swipe a pad over your face, let the solution sit for several minutes, and then rinse with water to remove.

☺ **Daily Moisturizer, Extra Hydration for Normal to Dry Skin** *($8.29 for 3 ounces)* is essentially a drugstore version of Clinique's bland Dramatically Different Moisturizing Lotion, which was an antiquated formula 15 years ago. The price for this fragrance-free moisturizer is its most enticing feature.

☹ **Daily Sunscreen, SPF 15 UVA/UVB** *($7.99 for 4 ounces)*. I am generally complimentary about Alpha Hydrox's AHA products. Sadly, I cannot muster even a half-smile for this disappointing daytime moisturizer. The sunscreen actives do not provide sufficient UVA protection and the base formula barely creeps past mediocre. What a sad day for a product line that had cutting-edge products in the early '90s.

☹ **Vanishing Blemish Solution** *($8.20 for 0.5 ounce)*. What a shame this anti-acne product is loaded with alcohol (listed as ethanol). The 2% concentration of salicylic acid and pH of 3.2 guarantee exfoliation and blackhead reduction, but it comes at the cost of irritating already inflamed skin, not to mention that the irritation will trigger more oil production in the pore. The anti-irritants included aren't enough to counteract the damaging effects of the alcohol.

OTHER ALPHA HYDROX PRODUCTS

✓ ☺ **Foaming Face Wash** *($7.49 for 6 ounces)* is water-soluble with a slight foaming action. Expect this to do a sufficient job removing makeup and consider it recommended for all skin types except very oily. Foaming Face Wash is also fragrance-free.

☺ **Nourishing Cleanser** *($7.99 for 4.5 ounces)* contains a couple of vitamins and skin-conditioning agents that aren't all that helpful in a cleanser because they are rinsed from skin so quickly. This is otherwise a standard but good water-soluble cleanser suitable for all skin types except very oily. The tiny amount of corn and soybean oil should not pose a problem for those with blemish-prone skin.

☹ **Toner Astringent for Normal to Oily Skin** *($5.99 for 8 ounces)* lists alcohol as the second ingredient and that is followed by witch hazel and, shortly thereafter, menthol. This toner is not recommended (and, if you're curious, the pH is too high for the glycolic acid to function as an exfoliant). Alcohol in this amount makes oily skin worse because it triggers more oil production within the pore lining.

☺ **AHA Souffle** *($15.99 for 1.6 ounces)*. AHA Souffle includes 12% glycolic acid formulated at a pH of 4, which makes this effective for exfoliation. The lightweight but substantial-feeling cream base is basic, but although a few antioxidants are included, the jar packaging will quickly render them ineffective. This is still an effective AHA option for normal to dry skin.

☺ **Enhanced Creme** *($12.99 for 2 ounces)* is nearly identical to the AHA Souffle, minus the antioxidants (which is fine considering this product is also packaged in a jar) and with a slightly thinner texture. The other difference is the amount of glycolic acid, which is 10% in this product.

☺ **Enhanced Lotion 10% Glycolic AHA** *($11.99 for 6 ounces)* remains the best AHA bargain Alpha Hydrox offers. The standard lotion formula contains 10% glycolic acid at a pH of 4, making it an effective option for exfoliating normal to dry skin. There isn't much else of note to discuss, but if you're looking for a good AHA product with a lotion texture, this is one to try.

☺ **Oil-Free Formula** *($11.99 for 1.7 ounces)* features 10% glycolic acid at a pH of 4 in a lightweight gel base that is indeed oil-free. This is an excellent option for those with oily to very oily skin seeking an AHA product. Keep in mind that if your oily skin is accompanied by blackheads and blemishes, BHA (salicylic acid) offers a greater benefit.

☹ **Eye and Upper Lip Cream** *($9.99 for 0.65 ounce)*. The eye area and upper lip area are definitely two of the most age-prone places on the face, but this product isn't the antiwrinkle answer. It's a basic emollient moisturizer that contains a decent amount of vitamin E, a basic antioxidant addition to most cosmetic formulations. The amount of lactic acid is too low for it to function as an exfoliant, though it does have some benefit as a water-binding agent. This product contains comfrey extract, which isn't something to use near the eye, or anywhere else for that matter. Topical application of comfrey has anti-inflammatory properties, but it is recommended only for short-term use and only then if you can be sure the amount of pyrrolizidine alkaloids (a toxic component of the plant) is less than 100 micrograms per application—something that would be impossible to determine without sophisticated testing equipment, making comfrey an ingredient to avoid. The alkaloid content makes it a potential skin irritant (Sources: *Chemical Research in Toxicology*, November 2001, pages 1546-1551; and *Public Health Nutrition*, December 2000, pages 501-508).

☺ **Night Replenishing Cream** *($9.99 for 2 ounces)* is a very basic, emollient, fragrance-free moisturizer for dry to very dry skin. Alpha Hydrox recommends this for use around the eyes, and it is suitable for that purpose.

☹ **Oxygenated Moisturizer** *($14.99 for 2 ounces)* claims to oxygenate skin while stimulating collagen production, but providing oxygen to intact, otherwise healthy skin is detrimental because it causes free-radical damage (Source: *Aging Cell*, June 2007, pages 361-370; *Journal of Pharmaceutical Sciences*, September 2007, pages 2181-2196; and *Human and Experimental Toxicology*, February 2002, pages 61-62). Alpha Hydrox used peroxidized corn oil in the form of TriOxygen-C, a patented ingredient that is also used in the Neoteric line for treating diabetic skin ulcers (Neoteric is the parent company of Alpha Hydrox). Although this ingredient's function is beneficial for supplying oxygen and promoting healing of ulcers, the physiological process that skin enacts to heal wounds is vastly different from treating wrinkles or supplying oxygen to non-wounded skin. Both repeated use of any peroxidized substance and delivering extra oxygen to skin are damaging (Sources: *Journal of Reconstructive Microsurgery*, May 2007, pages 225-230; *Plastic and Reconstructive Surgery*, May 2007, pages 1980-1981; and *Cell Tissue Bank*, 2000, volume 1, issue 4, pages 261-269).

✓☺ **Retinol Night ResQ** *($14.99 for 1.05 ounces)* ranks as one of the top retinol products available in any price range. Alpha Hydrox uses packaging that keeps the retinol stable and they also included antioxidant vitamins E and C along with an anti-irritant. The fragrance-free base formula is quite thick and preferred for normal to very dry skin not prone to blemishes. Overall, well done! By the way, retinol products from Natural Advantage by Jane Seymour (an infomercial brand reviewed on Beautypedia) and philosophy have nearly identical formulas to this less expensive option!

☹ **Sheer Silk Moisturizer SPF 15** *($15.99 for 1 ounce)* contains an in-part zinc oxide sunscreen, which is excellent. However, the peroxidized corn oil is cause for concern because oxidizing oil can lead to free-radical damage when applied over intact skin.

✓☺ **Spot Light Targeted Skin Lightener** *($9.99 for 0.85 ounce)* is a well-formulated, skin-lightening product that combines 2% hydroquinone with 10% glycolic acid in a base with a pH of 3.3, all in packaging that will keep the hydroquinone stable. The lightweight lotion base is suitable for normal to slightly dry or dry skin, and the only thing missing is a selection of state-of-the-art skin-identical ingredients and more antioxidants (vitamin E is included). Still, this remains one of the better options for those who want to lighten sun- or hormone-induced brown skin discolorations, and the glycolic acid works in tandem with the hydroquinone to improve skin's appearance and texture.

AMERICAN BEAUTY

AMERICAN BEAUTY AT-A-GLANCE

Strengths: Many state-of-the-art moisturizers, though they're not without their issues; Lauder's formulary expertise in the moisturizer category at a lower price point than most other Lauder-owned lines; good foundations without sunscreen; good powders; excellent powder blush; several lip-enhancing options, including a remarkable long-wearing lip paint.

Weaknesses: Problematic toners, lackluster scrub, sunscreens whose UVA-protecting ingredients are present but at questionable amounts. No skin-lightening, AHA, BHA, or effective anti-acne products; foundations and lipsticks with sunscreen that lacks sufficient UVA protection; poor concealer.

For more information about American Beauty, owned by Estee Lauder and sold exclusively at Kohl's, call (866) 352-8337 or visit www.americanbeautycosmetics.com or www.Beautypedia.com.

AMERICAN BEAUTY SKIN CARE

☹ **Fabulous Froth Gel Cleanser** *($12.50 for 5 ounces)* is a standard, detergent-based, water-soluble cleanser that would work for someone with normal to oily skin. The drawback is that it might be too drying for most skin types and the inclusion of irritant menthyl lactate makes it a tough sell.

☺ **Luxurious Lather Creamy Cleanser** *($12.50 for 5 ounces)* is a very good, though very standard, water-soluble cleanser for normal to slightly dry or combination skin. The cleansing agents make it too drying for dry to very dry skin.

☺ **Barefaced Beauty Makeup Remover for Eyes and Lips** *($12.50 for 4.20 ounces)* is a decent, silicone-based makeup remover, but the inclusion of rose extract (relatively high up on the ingredient list) in a product for use around the eyes is not a good idea, especially when there are other similar versions that are fragrance free.

☹ **Extra Clean Balancing Tonic** *($11 for 6.70 ounces)* is mostly water and rose extract, and—strangely enough—it also contains menthol, which is irritating for skin, and not balancing or cleansing in any way. How disappointing, because it does contain some good ingredients for skin, too.

☹ **Extra Clean Soothing Tonic** *($11 for 6.70 ounces)* has several skin-helpful ingredients and would have been a slam-dunk recommendation for a toner, but the menthol is irritating for skin, not soothing in the least.

☺ **Soft Glow Gentle Face Polisher** *($14 for 3.40 ounces)* is a mildly abrasive scrub that uses a mixture of clays to exfoliate the skin. It has a rather thick, pasty feel on the skin, and is a bit tricky to rinse, but for someone with normal to oily skin, it's an interesting change from the typical scrubs you find at cosmetic counters.

☺ **$$$ All Is Forgiven Skin Repair Concentrate** *($35 for 1 ounce)* contains many of the beneficial antioxidants and skin-identical ingredients the Estee Lauder Companies (of which American Beauty is one) use in their lotion-style serums. The difference here is the lack of silicone and the prominent use of the fragrant American Beauty plant extract. It coincides with the name of this line, but has no benefit for skin. That fact keeps this product from earning a higher rating, but it's still a good option for normal to slightly dry skin. It does contain fragrance and the mica/titanium dioxide blend lends a glow to skin.

☺ **Beauty Boost Overnight Radiance Cream** *($28 for 1.7 ounces)* is an emollient moisturizer with a silky texture and a nice blend of antioxidants, ingredients that mimic the structure of skin, and anti-irritants. What a shame the jar packaging renders this all for naught.

☺ **Beauty Boost Overnight Radiance Eye Cream** *($26 for 0.5 ounce)*. The unfortunate choice of jar packaging means that the light- and air-sensitive ingredients (all of the really beneficial ingredients) won't retain their potency once you begin using it. Even in better packaging, however, this eye cream for dry skin would be tough to recommend because it contains fragrant plants that aren't the best for skin, especially in the eye area.

☺ **Moisture-Wise Continuous Hydrating Cream** *($23.50 for 1.7 ounce)* is similar to the Moisture-Wise Continuous Hydrating Lotion below, but the jar package means that the longevity of the impressive ingredients will be too fleeting. What a shame, because the silky-smooth texture and bevy of beneficial ingredients is a bona-fide boon for dry skin.

☺ **Moisture-Wise Continuous Hydrating Eye Cream** *($22.50 for 0.5 ounce)* is almost identical to the Moisture-Wise Continuous Hydrating Cream above, save for a slightly less silky texture. Otherwise, the same basic comments apply: it's a very good, silky-smooth moisturizer for dry skin, with a smattering of ingredients that mimic the structure of skin, plus some anti-irritants and antioxidants.

☺ **Moisture-Wise Continuous Hydrating Lotion** *($23.50 for 1.70 ounces)* is a very good, silky-smooth moisturizer for dry skin, with a smattering of ingredients that mimic the structure of skin, plus some anti-irritants and antioxidants. Someone with dry skin would not be disappointed by this product.

☹ **$$$ Ultimate Diamond Restorative Anti-Aging Cream** *($49.50 for 1.7 ounces)*. There is nothing antiaging or restorative about this cream, at least not any more so than any other ordinary moisturizer. The only unique things about this moisturizer are the claims. It doesn't contain ingredients that can lighten skin discolorations, as in inhibiting melanin production. The diamond powder is commercial grade leftover diamond residue, but it does not add any more glow to skin than any other shine-enhancing ingredients. While shine does make skin look brighter, that is easily accomplished with dozens of products costing a fraction of this amount. Adding diamond dust is nothing more than a marketing angle, a way for a cosmetics company to make a product seem more prestigious than it really is. This is a good moisturizer for normal to dry skin, but the antioxidant plant ingredients, which have the potential to help skin, won't remain stable due to the jar packaging.

☺ **Uplifting Firming Eye Cream** *($23.50 for 0.5 ounce)* contains more rose extract than it does some of the more exciting ingredients that appear toward the end of the ingredient list. Still, it does have all the usual bells and whistles, even if (as with most eye creams) none of them are special for the eye area. In the final analysis, it's the jar packaging that reduces the rating, not the formulation.

☺ **Uplifting Firming Face Lotion SPF 15** *($27 for 1.7 ounces)*. With less than 1% titanium dioxide (you should expect at least 2% or greater when another active is listed, as is the case here), this is not the most uplifting lotion for sun protection, as that small amount limits its ability to defend your skin against the sun's UVA damage. Thankfully, the rest of the formulation is a standout, with an excellent variety of antioxidants, ingredients that mimic the structure of skin, and a cell-communicating ingredient. The firming claim is dubious, but for healthier skin, add this one to your list.

☺ **Uplifting Firming Face Cream SPF 15** *($27 for 1.7 ounces)* is similar to the Uplifting Firming Face Lotion SPF 15, but this cream version comes in a jar and the ingredients can't stand up to the kind of exposure to the air that type of packaging allows.

☹ **Youth-Full Anti-Aging Face Cream SPF 15** *($27 for 1.7 ounces)* covers the UVA spectrum with avobenzone, which is a good start for any sunscreen regardless of the claim on the label. It also has an enviable blend of antioxidants, ingredients that mimic the structure of skin, and a cell-communicating ingredient. All in all, that could have added up to a great rating, but the jar packaging won't keep these ingredients stable. It works as a sunscreen, but everything else is more empty than full.

☺ **Youth-Full Anti-Aging Lotion SPF 15** *($27 for 1.7 ounces).* Youth-Full Anti-Aging Lotion SPF 15, unlike its cream counterpart, comes in packaging that gives the state-of-the-art ingredients it contains (and there are a lot of them) a fighting chance to stick around and actually help your skin. A disappointment, but not a disaster, is the small amount (only 0.98%) of titanium dioxide present. This falls a little short in the UVA-protecting department, but not enough to reduce the rating.

AMERICAN BEAUTY MAKEUP

FOUNDATION: ☺ **Perfect Mineral Powder Makeup** *($25)* is American Beauty's most expensive foundation, and unless you're convinced that mineral makeup is the ultimate option, the cost isn't justified. The mica-based loose powder has no sunscreen, something inherent to many other mineral makeups. It has a silky, weightless texture and soft, dry matte finish that imparts a subtle sparkling shine to skin. Coverage is lighter than similar mineral makeups, but can be built to medium if needed. Among the seven shades, be aware that Bronzer (a sheer tan color) is very shiny, while Medium is too orange to look convincing on anyone. The best shades are for those with fair to light skin.

☺ **Perfectly Even Natural Finish Foundation** *($16.50)* goes on evenly and the coverage is light to medium, so it does look fairly natural on the skin. The silicone-based formula, best for someone with normal to dry skin, does separate, so you must shake it before you apply it. Of the 14 shades, Medium/Warm and Medium/Cool can appear too peach, and Light/Cool can look too pink on the skin.

☺ **Super Plush Powder Foundation** *($17.50)* is a standard, talc-based pressed powder that deposits enough color to be considered a foundation. There are 14 decent shades (Light/Cool may be too pink for some skin tones) worth a test run, but be careful; powder foundation can make dry skin look drier, and can look too thick on oily skin.

☹ **Perfect Lighting Line Smoothing Foundation SPF 15** *($17.50).* Regrettably, the SPF 15 part of this foundation lacks the UVA-protecting ingredients of titanium dioxide, zinc oxide, avobenzone, Tinosorb, or Mexoryl SX, and so this is not recommended, despite the noteworthy color selection and smooth, even application and finish.

CONCEALER: ☹ **Perfecting Concealer** *($12.50)* goes on too sticky, is difficult to blend or smooth out (so it looks uneven and obvious), and, finally, creases endlessly during the day. The only thing perfect about this concealer is the name.

POWDER: ☺ **$$$ Perfect Lighting Line Smoothing Pressed Powder** *($16)* is a traditional talc-based powder with an excellent silky-sheer application. Your lines won't disappear, but the shades are great and definitely natural-looking when applied.

☺ **Perfectly Even Natural Finish Pressed Powder** *($16)* provides slightly more coverage than the Perfect Lighting pressed-powder version, but other than that, these two powders have more in common than they do differences. Both are worthwhile choices, but this won't absorb oil any better than lots of other pressed powders. Only Deep can be too orange on skin; all the other colors are very good.

BLUSH AND BRONZER: ✓ ☺ $$$ **Beloved Rose Powder Blush** *($18)*. This pressed-powder blush promises a true color payoff and it delivers just that from each of its attractive shades. The suede-smooth texture promotes even application while the lovely satin finish adds a shimmering glow to cheeks. Mocha Bloom and Rose Shimmer are the most workable shades, but all of the colors are recommended for those of you who want a very good blush with some shimmer.

✓ ☺ **Blush Perfect Cheek Color** *($15.50)* is a pretty darn near perfect powder blush. There are more than 20 attractive shades with a mix of matte and subtle shine versions. The application is sheer and even.

☹ $$$ **Pretty Bronze Bronzing Powder** *($17.50)* has a dry, powdery texture that applies very sheer and leaves sparkles on skin, which isn't the way to fake a tanned appearance. Both shades are attractive and soft—you just need to apply a lot of it to achieve a bronzed look. Taking a cue from the name, this bronzer is pretty average—and that's not good enough considering its cost.

EYESHADOW: ☺ **Luxury for Lids Eyeshadow Duo** *($15.50)*. Duo eyeshadows usually pose a problem because you almost always end up using one faster than the other, or you use only one because you don't really like the color it's paired with. Luxury for Lids has that basic problem too, although some of the duos, particularly some of the attractive matte duos, do work nicely together. You will also be impressed with the smooth, even application. Still, if you have wrinkled eyelids watch out for some of the shiny shades; they will make your wrinkles more noticeable.

☹ $$$ **Perfect Mineral Loose Powder Eyeshadow** *($15.50)*. When it comes to applying eyeshadow neatly, loose is not the preferred way to go; even if it's in a pressed form, eyeshadow can get sloppy when applied and sprinkled all over the eye area, not to mention your countertop. It's great that American Beauty took steps with packaging to make sure things don't get too messy, and that they included an acceptable brush. What's not so great is that despite a gossamer texture, these sheer, loose eyeshadows impart sparkling shine that clings poorly. You have to apply a lot of any shade to get a reasonable color payoff that lasts, but doing so only makes the flaking more of an issue. This works best for adding a touch of shine to the browbone, but not for application all over the eye area.

EYE AND BROW SHAPER: ☺ **Ultra-Easy Automatic Eyeliner** *($11.50)* lives up to its name. It comes in a twist-up container (no sharpening) and has a soft, smooth application. You get a choice of eight basic colors. For a basic eye pencil, this is very, very good.

☺ **Perfect Brows Automatic Pencil** *($11.50)*. This is a standard, automatic brow pencil that comes in four very good colors. Each applies smoothly and has a soft powder finish. Although perfect brows depend more on your application than on a specific pencil, this is definitely a step in the right direction to help the process!

LIPSTICK, LIP GLOSS, AND LIPLINER: ✓ ☺ $$$ **Super Plush 10-Hour Lipcolor** *($16.50)* is American Beauty's version of Estee Lauder's Double Wear Stay-in-Place Lip Duo and M.A.C.'s Pro Longwear Lipcolour. All of these include a lip color "paint" and glossy top coat packaged in a dual-sided slim component. You apply the lip color, allow one minute for it to dry, then apply the glossy top coat, which ensures comfortable wear. As with the Lauder and M.A.C. versions, the lip color applies smoothly (many of the shades go on opaque and most have some degree of shimmer) and feels drier as it sets. The silicone-based top coat adds a beautiful sheen without feeling slick, sticky, or greasy and the duo wears beautifully. Mine stayed on through coffee, lunch, and a late afternoon snack. As expected, the eventual color fading began at the inner portion of the lips and moved outward. The only drawback to American Beauty's option is that you may find yourself applying the top coat more often than others due to its thinner texture.

☺ **Fabulous Feel Liquid Lipcolor** *($12.50)* is a unique lip color that is neither lipstick, nor lip gloss, nor lip stain. It is a sweep of somewhat sheer color that is more matte than glossy, but it doesn't feel dry on the lips. I was impressed by the uniqueness of this product and suggest you give it a test run because it is not your run-of-the-mill lip product. There are 8 shades waiting for you to experiment with.

☺ **Luxury for Lips Moisture Rich Lipcolor** *($12.50)* is a fairly standard, extremely emollient lipstick with an impressive color selection. Just watch out: This is greasy enough to easily move into lines around the lips if you are prone to that.

☺ **Pretty Glossy Luscious Lipshine** *($12.50)* is a basic, but good, lip gloss with several attractive shades.

☺ **Ultra-Easy Automatic Lipliner** *($11.50)* is no easier than a bevy of standard, twist-up Lipliners, but this is still an excellent one to consider. There are eight beautiful, albeit tame, colors on display.

☹ **Enduring Beauty Longwear Lipcolor** *($12.50)* is about as long-lasting as an ice cube in hot water. This is merely an extremely emollient, standard lipstick that isn't much different from the Luxury for Lips Moisture Rich Lipcolor above.

MASCARA: ✓ ☺ **Perfectly Waterproof Mascara** *($12.00)*. Wow! That was the first word that came to mind as I applied this outstanding waterproof mascara. Just a few sweeps of the wand defined lashes with equal amounts of length and thickness. There was some minor clumping, but that was easily remedied with a few more brush strokes. As with most waterproof formulas, this stays on very well when lashes get wet, and requires an oil- or silicone-based eye makeup remover.

☺ **Double Lush Mascara Plus Primer** *($12.50)* is a two-sided mascara. One side is a white gel mascara meant to prime your lashes, and the other is regular mascara. With or without the two-step process you can get long, thick lashes with just a few strokes. My only concern is that the primer tends to make the lashes look spiky after you're done applying the mascara. Without the primer, you just get long, thick lashes, with only a slight amount of clumping. You get long lashes either way, so I guess you can decide which look you like best.

☹ **Softly Shaping Mascara** *($11.50)* produces decent, attractive, long lashes, but you have to be patient while applying enough layers to get there. It can flake slightly during the day, but not enough to warrant a poor rating.

FACE AND BODY ILLUMINATING/SHIMMER PRODUCTS: ☺ **Luminous Liquid All Over Face Glow** *($15.00)* is a sheer liquid that can be applied over or under foundation to add an extremely subtle glow to the skin. It comes in two shades, and can be a bit tricky to apply without disturbing your foundation, but with practice this can create a nice effect.

ARBONNE

ARBONNE AT-A-GLANCE

Strengths: Most of the NutriMinC RE9 products have merit and contain an exciting blend of antioxidants and ingredients that mimic the structure and function of healthy skin; a small selection of basic but effective cleansers and masks; good powder, eyeshadow, and blush; brush and color sets are worth a look.

Weaknesses: Consistent and pervasive use of volatile fragrant oils that are irritating, allergenic, and/or photosensitizing for skin; no effective AHA or BHA products; no skin-lightening or effective anti-acne products; only one sun-care product that does not contain problematic ingredients; average foundations and eye pencils; unimpressive concealer and mascara.

For more information about Arbonne, call (800) 272-6663 or visit www.arbonne.com or www.Beautypedia.com.

ARBONNE SKIN CARE

ARBONNE CLEAR ADVANTAGE PRODUCTS

☹ **Clear Advantage Acne Wash** *($15.50 for 4 ounces)* uses salicylic acid as its active ingredient, but in a cleanser its benefit for blemish-prone skin is wasted. Even if the salicylic acid may have an impact on skin before rinsing, this water-soluble cleanser is not recommended due to the peppermint it contains.

☹ **Clear Advantage Refining Toner** *($15.50 for 4 ounces)* lists witch hazel as its second ingredient and that, coupled with the peppermint and other plant extracts known for their allergenic potential (dandelion, anyone?), makes this a clear problem, not an advantage, for all skin types.

☹ **Clear Advantage Acne Lotion** *($16.50 for 2 ounces)* proved frustrating because it came so close to being a slam-dunk option. This lightweight lotion contains 1% salicylic acid and has a pH low enough to allow it to work as an exfoliant. However, because Arbonne insists on portraying a natural image, several plant extracts were included, too. The problem? Most of them are either irritating or allergenic for skin (Source: www.naturaldatabase.com). What a shame! Some soothing plant extracts are included, too, but their benefit is canceled out by the problematic extracts.

ARBONNE FC5 PRODUCTS

☹ **FC5 Exfoliating New Cell Scrub** *($28 for 4 ounces)*. The claims for this clay-enriched scrub are quite disconcerting and almost blatantly misleading exaggerations, bordering on lies. You're told to expect a tingling/heating sensation and a reddening effect that may last up to two hours after use. Of course, they claim that this is proof the product is working, but irritation that persists at this level is damaging your skin. This is not akin to getting a peel from an aesthetician or dermatologist, and even if it were, this is not something you should do on a regular basis. This scrub is chock-full of problematic plant extracts and also contains a host of irritating fragrant oils. Bamboo extract is the abrasive agent, while benzyl nicotinate is a stimulant-type ingredient that causes increased circulation, which plays a part in the lingering redness after using this scrub. For the health of your skin, please don't subject it to this damaging scrub; the irritation kills cells and breaks down collagen, counter to what anyone should be doing to their face.

☹ **FC5 Hydrating Eye Creme** *($30 for 0.5 ounce).* Ignore all of the eye-area improvement claims for this product; they're silly and have nothing to do with the formula or with reality, they were merely dreamed up by a clever marketing department. Not only are the claims bogus, Arbonne loaded this product with fragrant oils, which is a problem, especially in the eye area. Some of the citrus oils are known to cause a phototoxic reaction when skin is exposed to sunlight, and that's not the way to make delicate skin around the eyes stronger or more resistant to signs of aging! Even without the irritants, this is as boring a moisturizer as you can get.

☹ **FC5 Oil-Absorbing Day Lotion SPF 20** *($39.50 for 1.7 ounces).* The tiny amount of cornstarch in this daytime moisturizer with an in-part avobenzone sunscreen isn't enough to absorb much oil. This is even truer when you consider the emollient thickening agents that precede it on the list. You may think this would be better for normal to dry skin, but it isn't recommended for any skin type because it contains several fragrant oils known to cause skin irritation. Some of the citrus oils in this product are capable of causing a phototoxic reaction when skin is exposed to sunlight. Knowing this, who cares if this contains fresh kiwi cell extracts, which is the big selling point for the product? You'd be better off running pure kiwi on your skin, though that will make it sticky, so you'd have to rinse afterward.

Arbonne Intelligence Products

☹ **Intelligence Daily Cleanser** *($22.50 for 4.3 ounces)* doesn't even make it to average intelligence thanks to its inclusion of a grocery list of irritating plant extracts (including comfrey), along with menthol and volatile citrus oils. It may smell divine, but what's creating the aroma isn't doing your skin any favors.

☹ **Intelligence Daily Balancer** *($22.50 for 6 ounces)* contains enough comfrey to be problematic (this is a leave-on toner), and the inclusion of irritating citrus oils makes matters worse by compromising skin's barrier properties.

☹ **Intelligence Daily Eye Cream** *($28 for 0.52 ounce)* likely contains too small an amount of comfrey to make it a problem for routine application, but it also contains the preservative methylisothiazolinone, which is contraindicated for use in leave-on products due to its potential to cause allergic contact dermatitis (Source: *Contact Dermatitis*, June 2006, pages 322-324).

☹ **Intelligence Daily Moisturizing Cream, Day & Night** *($38.50 for 4.3 ounces)* contains the problematic preservative methylisothiazolinone as well as irritating citrus oils and cardamom oil. These inclusions are as intelligent as brushing your teeth with a cotton swab.

☹ **Intelligence Rejuvenating Cream** *($35 for 2.2 ounces)* would have been an excellent, ultra-emollient moisturizer for someone with dry to very dry skin if it did not contain irritating citrus oils along with clary and cardamom oils.

☹ **Intelligence Exfoliating Masque with Thermal Fusion** *($32 for 4.6 ounces)* may very well get its thermal qualities from the irritation incited by the volatile citrus oils contained in this exfoliating clay mask. It also contains benzyl nicotinate, which is most often seen in lip-plumping products because it is a vasodilator (an ingredient that increases circulation to the area of skin it is applied to), which can cause capillaries to surge and potentially break within the skin.

Arbonne NutriMinc RE9 Products

☺ **$$$ NutriMinC RE9 REnewing Gelee Creme Hydrating Wash** *($39 for 3.15 ounces)* is a very good, water-soluble cleanser but one whose price should give you serious pause. Of course, the cost supposedly has to do with the bevy of antioxidants and other high-tech ingredients in this cleanser, but your money is better spent on leave-on products that contain these ingredients. The tiny amount of orange oil adds fragrance and may prove problematic for use around the eye area. Otherwise, this is best for those with large budgets and normal to slightly dry or slightly oily skin.

☹ **NutriMinC RE9 REstoring Mist Balancing Toner** *($33 for 3.15 ounces)* lists witch hazel as its second ingredient and also contains a significant amount of comfrey extract *(Symphytum officinale)*, which is a problem in products meant to be left on skin.

☺ **$$$ NutriMinC RE9 REveal Facial Scrub** *($31 for 4 ounces)* is an OK but very overpriced topical scrub that uses walnut shell powder as the abrasive agent. Walnut shells are an option, but one that is not preferred to synthetic exfoliating beads because the shell pieces are uneven and may cause micro-tears in the skin. The oil in this scrub should offset this possibility, and also makes it preferred for those with normal to dry skin.

☺ **$$$ NutriMinC RE9 REgain Illuminating Enzyme Peel** *($40 for 1 ounce)* brings us another product claiming to exfoliate via the power of enzymes. Once again, papaya and pineapple are the fruits said to have enzymatic activity that leads to exfoliation. Well, let me tell you: Any exfoliation your skin gets from this product will be minor, as enzymes are weak exfoliants at best and tend to be unstable in cosmetic formulations. The various fruit extracts are meant to stand in for "chemical" AHAs, but they don't function the same way, and there's no research proving otherwise. The main plant extract in this is bilberry, and although it won't exfoliate (peel) skin, it has potent anti-inflammatory action when ingested (Source: www.naturaldatabase. com), although the anti-inflammatory action has not been confirmed for topical application. Although the citrus extracts in this product can be irritating, this is still an OK product for normal to dry skin. It would be rated higher if the antioxidant vitamins and peptides comprised more of the total formula.

☺ **$$$ NutriMinC RE9 REactivating Facial Serum, Day & Night** *($49 for 1 ounce)* lists several fruit extracts in the hopes that you'll think they exfoliate skin, but they don't. Arbonne also included lactic acid at about 2%, an amount that's below ideal for exfoliation although the pH of this product is in the correct range. The tiny amount of salicylic acid has no exfoliating action on skin. Although not worthy as an exfoliant, this stably packaged serum is packed with helpful ingredients for skin, from antioxidants to nonirritating plant oils and (mostly) soothing plant extracts. Although the tiny amount of comfrey extract is not likely cause for concern, it keeps this product from earning a Paula's Pick rating. This product is best for normal to slightly dry or slightly oily skin.

☹ **NutriMinC RE9 REality SPF 8 Day Creme** *($49.50 for 1.5 ounces)* costs way too much for a product that offers skin an inadequate SPF rating and lacks sufficient UVA-protecting ingredients. It also contains a high amount of comfrey extract, making it even more problematic. This is a hugely embarrassing formula!

☹ **NutriMinC RE9 REpair Corrective Eye Creme** *($49 for 0.6 ounce)* lists comfrey extract as its second ingredient and contains significant amounts of other potentially problematic plant extracts, making it a non-contender.

☺ **$$$ NutriMinC RE9 REversing Gelee Transforming Lift** *($45.50 for 1.5 ounces)* is made to sound like a face-lift in a bottle, and claims to promote the production of collagen, elastin, and ground substance. The latter refers to the intercellular material in which the cells and fibers of connective tissue are embedded, and is part of the lowest layer of the dermis. This product isn't likely to make your skin's ground substance stronger, but it contains many beneficial ingredients that help restore a healthy barrier and allow skin to make collagen, something it does quite well on its own when not impeded by sun damage and topical irritants. This water-based, silicone-free serum is best for normal to oily skin. It does not rank a Paula's Pick due to the inclusion of a small amount of comfrey extract.

☺ **$$$ NutriMinC RE9 REcover Night Creme** *($79 for 1 ounce)* is a marvelously formulated moisturizer that is loaded with antioxidants and contains the cell-communicating ingredient lecithin as well as nonvolatile plant oils and emollients to make dry skin look and feel healthy. What a shame the potency of over a dozen ingredients in this product is hindered by the choice of jar packaging!

☺ **$$$ NutriMinC RE9 REtaliate Wrinkle Filler** *($45 for 0.05 ounce)* consists mostly of water and film-forming agent along with standard emollients. The amount of film-former can help make skin feel tighter temporarily, but if you want a cosmetic wrinkle filler (i.e., those that function like a soft spackle for lines) there are better products from Good Skin (Tri-Aktiline), and Estee Lauder (Perfectionist). However, if you're set on Arbonne, this product contains an impressive assortment of peptides, which theoretically have cell-communicating ability. However, none of the peptides in this wrinkle filler can diminish wrinkles, so please don't invest in this thinking you can go from lined to lineless with a quick swipe of the pen-style applicator.

☺ **$$$ NutriMinC RE9 RElease Deep Pore Cleansing Masque** *($31 for 5 ounces)* is a standard clay mask that is overpriced for what you get, and the amount of comfrey extract is a cause for concern (though less so in a product such as this that would be used infrequently and only left on skin briefly). It's an OK option for normal to oily skin, but calling this "super strength" is stretching things to the point of snapping.

OTHER ARBONNE PRODUCTS

☺ **$$$ Cleansing Cream** *($16 for 2 ounces)* is a standard, cold cream-style cleanser that uses safflower oil to dissolve and help remove makeup. It's an option for dry to very dry skin but will require a washcloth for complete removal.

☺ **About Face Wipe Out Eye Makeup Remover** *($19.50 for 3.7 ounces)* is a water- and glycerin-based eye-makeup remover whose cleansing agents are very mild. As such, this isn't effective for removing waterproof mascara or long-wearing eyeliner, but if that doesn't apply to you, using this is an option.

☺ **$$$ Prolief Natural Balancing Cream** *($34 for 2.5 ounces)* is similar to Arbonne's Phy-toProlief and the same review applies.

☹ **Damage Control Water Resistant SPF 30** *($28 for 6 ounces)* has the ability to protect skin from UVA and UVB rays while remaining water-resistant (though even water-resistant sunscreens require reapplying after swimming or perspiring). It's also loaded with a selection of skin-friendly ingredients, which is why it's so disheartening to find that this otherwise stellar sunscreen also includes so many irritating fragrant oils. In addition to their irritating properties, bergamot and lime oils can cause a phototoxic reaction (Source: www.naturaldatabase.com) and topical application of lavender oil causes skin cell death while increasing free-radical damage (Sources: *Contact Dermatitis*, September 2008, pages 143-150; and *Cell Proliferation*, June 2004, pages 221-229).

☺ **Lip Saver SPF 30** *($8 for 0.17 ounce)* is the only product in Arbonne's sun line worth trying. This oil-based lip balm protects with an in-part avobenzone sunscreen and also contains two forms of antioxidant vitamin C. The amount of arnica extract is likely too low to be a concern for irritation, but it keeps this product from earning a Paula's Pick rating.

☹ **Liquid Sunshine Tan Enhancer SPF 15** *($28 for 6.3 ounces)* features an in-part zinc oxide sunscreen but has troublesome claims (such as increasing the duration of your tan) while assaulting skin with irritants including bergamot, lime, lavender, cedarwood, and geranium oils.

☹ **Made In The Shade Self-Tanner SPF 15** *($28 for 6 ounces)* lacks sufficient UVA-protecting ingredients and contains a litany of irritating fragrant oils, none of which are helpful for skin. Countless self-tanners exist that turn skin brown without this risk of irritation.

☹ **Save Face & Body SPF 15** *($26 for 6 ounces)* wins points for its in-part avobenzone sunscreen, but then its score drops to zero due to the inclusion of the same volatile fragrant oils that all of the Arbonne sun products include. Save your face and body by not purchasing this product!

☹ **Glow With It After Sun Lotion** *($32 for 8 ounces)* contains several fragrant, volatile oils that are irritating to skin and problematic when applied to skin that may be exposed to sunlight. Whether pre- or after-sun, this product is not recommended.

ARBONNE MAKEUP

FOUNDATION: ☺ **$$$ About Face Line Defiance Liquid Foundation SPF 15** *($36)* comes in sleek packaging with a pump applicator, but be careful because it's easy to dispense more product than you need. Texture-wise, this is good, but because the satin matte finish tends to sit on top of skin rather than mesh with it, things like large pores and wrinkles are magnified in an unflattering way almost immediately. What a shame, because this does have an undeniably silky feel and remains so while blending, but the end result is what counts and this just can't compare to myriad other options that are far less pricey. The other downfall is the number of shades that are a far cry from being soft and neutral. You'd think Arbonne would have taken a cue from the countless lines that get skin color right, but they seem to think that a woman's skin should look an unnatural shade of pink or peach. Shades to consider with caution are: 1C, 11C (slightly pink), 5C, 6N, and 7N (slightly peach). The following shades are exceedingly peach, orange, or rose and are a must avoid: 2W, 3N, 4C, 10N, 12C, 13W, and 14N. The only shades that are truly worthwhile are 8W, 9W, and 15C (an excellent dark shade).

☺ **$$$ Mineral Powder Foundation SPF 15** *($34)*. Without question, Arbonne has the sun protection portion of this makeup down pat, but that's where most of the benefits start and stop. This mineral foundation has a thick yet smooth texture and dry finish that feels matte, but looks shiny (matte and shiny is an odd combination). The titanium dioxide and zinc oxide not only provide sun protection, but also lend this makeup its drier finish and medium coverage. As mineral makeup goes, this isn't a bad one; if only the colors were better! Several shades are overtly peach or rose, while many of the more neutral shades (for medium skin tones) have an ashen cast that's hard to ignore, and the ashen cast is more apparent here than in several other mineral makeups my team and I have tested. If you're willing to tolerate the drawbacks and don't mind a shiny finish, the only acceptable shades are 3N, 4C, 6N, 9W, 11C, and 14N. The included Kabuki-style brush is OK; it could be softer, but the fullness enables swift application of this powder foundation. Despite the dry-feeling finish, this mineral makeup is not recommended for those with oily skin or oily areas because the powder tends to pool. It is best for normal skin with minimal to no signs of dryness.

POWDER: ☺ $$$ **About Face Translucent Loose Powder** *($24)* comes in a standard jar with a sifter and enclosed powder puff (though loose powder looks best when applied with a brush). The talc-free formula has a silky, light texture and slightly dry finish, suitable for normal to oily skin. The two shades available appear too pink and peach, but apply so sheer the color becomes inconsequential.

BLUSH: ☺ **About Face Blushers** *($14)*. About Face Blushers have an exquisite texture that applies evenly and imparts soft color that layers well. However, every shade is shiny and sparkling cheeks don't communicate sophisticated daytime makeup. For evening glamour, these are contenders, and there are some good choices for women of color.

EYESHADOW: ☺ **About Face Eye Shadows** *($12)* have an enviable texture that is identical to the About Face Blushers. These cling well, blend smoothly, and build color with ease. Again, the shine speaks louder than the wonderful texture, and most of these shades are shiny enough to emphasize wrinkles or crepey skin, making most of the shades best for younger eyes. The almost-matte options include Shy, Subtle, Suede, Diva, Reckless, Linen, and Sugar Beet.

EYE AND BROW SHAPER: ☺ $$$ **Virtual Illusion Eye Definer** *($16)* is a standard, but very good, automatic pencil that glides on and tends not to smudge or smear. If only the colors weren't so iridescent or, in some cases, just plain tacky. On older skin the iridescence will only exaggerate an imperfect lash line, and the odd colors will serve to detract, rather than enhance. Eclipse, Urban, and Hepburn are the most workable shades.

☺ **About Face Brow Wax** *($18)* contains the same basic ingredients used to create a brow pencil, but this is a hard wax, poured into a compact. It's an OK option to fill in and define brows, but not nearly as efficient or elegant as the best brow pencils and powders because it tends to go on heavy and the finish isn't as long-lasting. The enclosed brush is uncomfortably stiff and scratchy, and best discarded in favor of a softer option. All three shades are good, including Auburn.

☹ **Virtual Illusion Eye Definer** *($16)*. The only illusion you'll see from using this automatic, retractable eye pencil is one of fleeting results. Application is silky-smooth, but you really need to layer it to get defining impact. Whether you layer or not, however, the formula tends to fade and smear in short order. It isn't worth considering over numerous automatic pencils from the drugstore.

LIPSTICK, LIP GLOSS, AND LIPLINER: ☺ $$$ **About Face Lipstick** *($16.50)* features a gorgeous selection of shades (those who prefer a bevy of coral or peach-toned colors will be delighted), each with a creamy texture and slight glossy finish.

☺ $$$ **About Face Sheer Shine** *($16)* is a typical lip gloss that comes with a wand applicator and has a smooth texture and glossy finish that's minimally sticky. There are some great shades to consider.

☺ $$$ **Virtual Illusion Lip Definer** *($16)* is an automatic, nonretractable lip pencil with a very smooth application that doesn't impart strong color but that can be layered for greater definition. Once set, it tends to last about as long as most lipliners, so all told it really doesn't have any edge making it worth the cost when there are great pencils for far less at the drugstore.

☹ **About Face Prep & Plump** *($28)* is a two-step product that involves applying a water- and silicone-based solution to lips along with a gloss that's applied once the base coat has dried. The base coat contains the irritant benzyl nicotinate, which causes lips to feel warm because it increases the blood flow to them. The plumping gloss makes lips temporarily larger by continuing this irritation with the potent menthol derivative menthone glycerin acetal. Be aware that this "burning" sensation can last for several minutes and you may find it too much to bear—I know I did. The irritation this product causes won't be pretty in the long run because irritation makes wrinkles and chapped lips worse. There is nothing in this product that has anything to do with the dermal lip injections that a doctor performs.

MASCARA: ☹ **$$$ About Face Lash Color Mascara** *($19.50)*. This expensive mascara has a sloppy, wet application that does no better than average when it comes to making lashes longer and more defined. Thickness is scant to nonexistent. (I'm not even quite sure how a mascara can actually make lashes look somehow less noticeable, but this one comes close to proving the impossible.) What's more, this tends to flake slightly during wear. An all-around "why bother?" unless you're willing to settle for a lot less while at the same time paying way too much for a bad mascara when there are brilliant mascaras at the drugstore way ahead of this one. By the way, the ingredients in this mascara are present in almost all mascaras; Arbonne's claims that their formula is somehow superior or natural is marketing nonsense.

☺ **$$$ Virtual Illusion Dual Volume Mascara** *($28.50)*. This dual-sided mascara includes a mascara on one end and a special "top coat" on the other, supposedly designed to add shine, lift, and curl. The mascara itself applies heavier and wetter than usual, which leads to some messy clumps that must be neatened. With patience, you can build considerable length and definition with this mascara, but it isn't easy, and clumping is hard to avoid. The clear top coat is applied with a rubber-bristle brush and this lightweight gel makes a slight difference in terms of lashes being able to hold an upswept curl. It isn't enough to make this worth the splurge, but at least the gimmicky top coat isn't a bust in the results department. On the other hand, a great mascara can net you better results without the two-step procedure.

BRUSHES: ☺ **$$$ 10-Piece Precision Brush Set** *($35)* is a jaw-dropping value when you consider that most other lines charge two to three times more for similar makeup brush sets. The essential brushes that make up the bulk of this collection are all soft and well-shaped, though the Powder and Blush brushes could be a bit softer and more dense. The nonessential brushes serve as extras you likely will not use, but these can be removed so you can store preferred additional brushes in the attractive non-leather pouch.

SPECIALTY PRODUCTS: ☺ **$$$ Virtual Illusion Makeup Primer** *($32.50)*. This wonderfully silky, gel-textured primer works beautifully to smooth skin and prep it for makeup. It is similar to a well-formulated serum because it contains some bells and whistles (i.e., antioxidants) not seen in most primers. I'm not a big advocate of primers because they're essentially underwhelming moisturizers or serums, and why add another product when you don't have to? Why not just start out with a well-formulated moisturizer or serum that does it all? My only concern about this product is the presence of the irritant horsetail extract (listed by its Latin name *Equisetum arvense*). The amount is small enough that it isn't likely to be troublesome, but without it, this primer would rate a Paula's Pick. Virtual Illusion Makeup Primer is best for normal to oily skin. Its texture is such that it can, to a limited extent, temporarily fill in large pores and superficial lines around the eye. Don't expect to look years younger, but you will see some improvement

☺ **$$$ Virtual Illusion Lash Enhancer** *($35 for 0.25 ounce)* is Arbonne's contribution to the growing trend of lash growth products. The difference is that Arbonne's version doesn't contain any ingredients known to impact lash length, thickness, or color. Their claims are carefully worded to remain strictly in the cosmetic realm, but there's no reason to believe this brush-on lash product (you apply it like eyeliner) will do a thing for your lashes beyond provide mild conditioning. There are several plant extracts, flavonoids, and minerals, including ingredients such as ginseng root that may stimulate circulation, but none of these substances has ever been shown to make lashes stronger or to cause lost lashes to re-grow (or hair to grow on any part of the body). The tripeptide that's included has no documented evidence that it does anything reliable for skin, let alone for eyelashes.

☺ **Custom Colour Palette** *($18)* is a faux leather tri-fold makeup carrier that has room for every single Arbonne blush and eyeshadow. If the holders could be adapted to fit different sized colors from other lines, this would make sense. As is, you'd have to be completely devoted to Arbonne makeup to make this a useful purchase.

AUBREY ORGANICS

AUBREY ORGANICS AT-A-GLANCE

Strengths: A few decent moisturizer options; one good makeup brush.

Weaknesses: Too numerous to list, but major issues include a lack of sunscreens without a problematic active ingredient; consistent use of ingredients proven to be irritating to skin while offering no substantiated benefit; a complete lack of products to address common skin-care concerns, from acne to pigmentation problems; the makeup is abysmal.

For more information about Aubrey Organics, call (800) 282-7394 or visit www.aubrey-organics.com or www.Beautypedia.com.

AUBREY ORGANICS SKIN CARE

AUBREY ORGANICS COMBINATION/DRY SKIN 2 PRODUCTS

☹ **Sea Buckthorn & Cucumber with Ester-C Facial Cleansing Cream, for Combination/Dry Skin** *($12.98 for 8 ounces)* is similar to the company's Seaware with Rosa Mosqueta Facial Cleansing Cream, for Dry Skin, but with less alcohol. If you think that makes this a gentler cleansing option, think again: the geranium and lavender oils in this product are troublesome for skin and for use around the eyes.

☹ **Sea Buckthorn & Cucumber with Ester-C Facial Toner, for Combination/Dry Skin** *($9.28 for 8 ounces)* lists alcohol and witch hazel as part of this toner's herbal base and contains several other ingredients that, while natural, are also very irritating to skin.

☺ **Sea Buckthorn & Cucumber with Ester-C Moisturizing Cream, for Combination/Dry Skin** *($16.28 for 4 ounces)* appears to be a good moisturizer for normal to dry skin, though the way some of the ingredients are listed leaves you to wonder exactly what is being used. The good news is this product does not contain irritants. Instead, it uses beneficial, nonvolatile plant oils that have antioxidant activity, and plant extracts with proven soothing properties.

☺ **Sea Buckthorn & Cucumber with Ester-C Moisturizing Mask, for Combination/Dry Skin** *($8.98 for 4 ounces)* works better as a topical scrub for normal to dry skin than a mask, and it contains some good anti-irritants, including chamomile oil. The questionable aspects include the mysterious "coconut fatty acid cream base" and the nut meals used as abrasive agents (these tend to be unevenly shaped particles that can be damaging to skin if used too aggressively).

AUBREY ORGANICS COMBINATION/OILY SKIN 4 PRODUCTS

☹ **Blue Green Algae with Grape Seed Extract Facial Cleansing Lotion, for Combination/Oily Skin** *($15.48 for 8 ounces)* has a cleansing base consisting of castile soap, and although this version uses olive oil instead of animal fat, it can still be drying for skin. The lavender oil also contributes to making this cleanser problematic for any skin type.

☹ **Blue Green Algae with Grape Seed Extract Facial Toner, for Combination/Oily Skin** *($9.28 for 8 ounces)* lists alcohol and witch hazel as its main ingredients, making this not recommended for any skin type. This is as soothing for stressed skin as walking barefoot on a hot sidewalk.

☹ **Blue Green Algae with Grape Seed Extract Moisturizer SPF 15, for Combination/Oily Skin** *($16.28 for 4 ounces)* is nearly identical to the company's Green Tea & Ginkgo Moisturizer SPF 15, for Normal Skin, and the same review applies.

☹ **Blue Green Algae with Grape Seed Extract Soothing Mask, for Combination/Oily Skin** *($8.98 for 4 ounces)* contains lavender oil, which makes it too irritating for all skin types.

AUBREY ORGANICS DRY SKIN 1 PRODUCTS

☹ **Jojoba Meal & Oatmeal with Rosa Mosqueta Mask & Scrub, for Dry Skin** *($8.98 for 4 ounces)* lists alcohol as its second ingredient and an unknown detergent cleansing agent as its first. This cleanser/scrub hybrid is too irritating for all skin types. If you want a natural scrub for dry skin, try mixing some cornmeal with a teaspoon or so of plain jojoba oil.

☹ **Rosa Mosqueta & English Lavender Facial Toner, for Dry Skin** *($9.28 for 8 ounces)* lists alcohol as the second ingredient, followed by witch hazel. All the plants in the world can't change how irritating that is for skin. However, several of the plant extracts in this product are either skin irritants or have potential photosensitizing or toxic reactions on skin, including peppermint, coltsfoot, nettle leaf, St. John's wort, watercress, horsetail, arnica, and lemon (Source: www.naturaldatabase.com).

☺ **Rosa Mosqueta Night Creme with Alpha Lipoic Acid** *($21.50 for 1 ounce)* contains a tiny amount of alpha lipoic acid (listed as such, though it should be listed as thioctic acid). But even if it was brimming with it, or other antioxidants, the translucent glass bottle won't hold them stable. This is a decent moisturizer for dry to very dry skin and, thankfully, lacks any of the problematic plant extracts found in most of Aubrey Organics' moisturizers. The amount of alcohol is too small to cause irritation.

☹ **Rosa Mosqueta Rose Hip Moisturizing Cream, for Dry Skin** *($16.28 for 4 ounces)* contains problematic plant extracts and an incomplete ingredient listing that doesn't follow FDA or CTFA regulations.

☺ **Rosa Mosqueta Rose Hip Seed Oil** *($12.98 for 0.36 ounce)* contains nothing more than organic rose hip seed oil. It is a soothing, nonvolatile plant oil that is often touted for its vitamin C content. Although fresh rose hip seed oil is rich in this vitamin, most of this nutrient is destroyed during the drying and processing necessary to create products like this. Still, this product can be a good spot treatment for patches of very dry skin.

☹ **Seaware with Rosa Mosqueta Facial Cleansing Cream, for Dry Skin** *($15.48 for 8 ounces)* lists the second ingredient as alcohol, and that can be drying and irritating for all skin types. The typical detergent-based cleanser in this product is standard in the industry, only here it has a less technical (and mislabeled) name, "coconut fatty acid." Coconut fatty acid goes by many less-friendly names, from tridecyl cocoate to cocamidopropylamine oxide, but if they were on the label, then it would start sounding like everyone else's products and it would be so much harder to convince people that you were all natural. This cleanser can be drying for most skin types.

AUBREY ORGANICS NORMAL SKIN 3 PRODUCTS

☹ **Green Tea & Ginkgo Facial Cleansing Lotion, for Normal Skin** *($15.48 for 8 ounces)* is almost identical to the company's Seaware with Rosa Mosqueta Facial Cleansing Cream, for Dry Skin, only this one is in lotion form. The same concerns apply.

☹ **Green Tea & Ginkgo Facial Toner, for Normal Skin** *($9.28 for 8 ounces)* follows the pattern set by all of the toners in this line: it's an alcohol and witch hazel base coupled with several irritating plant extracts. The anti-irritant plant extracts in this product don't have a flower's chance in a blizzard of helping skin.

☹ **Green Tea & Ginkgo Moisturizer SPF 15, for Normal Skin** *($16.28 for 4 ounces)* lists padimate O (PABA) as its active ingredient, which is too irritating for skin and leaves it vulnerable to UVA damage. Several of the plant extracts are a problem, too, making this a sunscreen that won't keep normal skin in that state for long.

☺ **Green Tea & Green Clay Rejuvenating Mask, for Normal Skin** *($8.98 for 4 ounces)* is a standard clay mask that includes glycerin, plant extracts, and thickeners. It's an OK option for normal to slightly oily skin, but its oil content isn't encouraging for anyone battling blemishes.

AUBREY ORGANICS OILY SKIN 5 PRODUCTS

☹ **Natural Herbal Facial Astringent, for Oily Skin** *($9.28 for 8 ounces)* is similar to all of the toners from Aubrey Organics, and harms skin more than it could possibly help. This is a classic example of why natural ingredients aren't inherently better for skin.

☹ **Natural Herbal Facial Cleanser, for Oily Skin** *($12.98 for 8 ounces)* is painful to even write about! This very irritating cleanser exposes skin to soap, witch hazel, alcohol, eucalyptus, camphor, and menthol, among other problematic ingredients. Ouch!

☹ **Natural Herbal Maintenance Oil Balancing Moisturizer, for Oily Skin** *($13.48 for 2 ounces)* cannot balance oil in the least but does subject skin to many irritating ingredients, including witch hazel, balsam oil, horsetail, balm mint, and coltsfoot, with the latter containing compounds that are carcinogenic (Source: *Toxicology and Industrial Health*, September 2006, pages 321-327).

☹ **Natural Herbal Seaclay with Goa Herb Oil Balancing Mask, for Oily Skin** *($8.98 for 4 ounces)* contains peppermint oil, which sabotages an otherwise effective but average clay mask. Goa herb oil (also known as ringworm oil) is very irritating to skin and mucous membranes, and is also easily absorbed, where it can cause systemic problems (Source: www.naturaldatabase.com).

AUBREY ORGANICS SENSITIVE SKIN 6 PRODUCTS

☹ **Vegecol Facial Cleansing Lotion, for Sensitive Skin** *($15.48 for 8 ounces)* contains several ingredients that are completely inappropriate for sensitive skin, or any skin type for that matter, including St. John's wort, coltsfoot, and lemon peel oil.

☹ **Vegecol with Aloe & Oatmeal Soothing Mask, for Sensitive Skin** *($8.98 for 4 ounces)* contains several ingredients that are completely inappropriate for sensitive skin, or any skin type for that matter, including alcohol, St. John's wort, coltsfoot, and lemon peel oil.

☹ **Vegecol with Aloe Alcohol-Free Facial Toner, for Sensitive Skin** *($9.28 for 8 ounces)* is preferred for sensitive skin compared to Aubrey Organics' other toners, but the witch hazel and lavender water still make it a poor choice for most skin types, particularly sensitive skin.

☹ **Vegecol with Aloe Moisturizing Cream, for Sensitive Skin** *($13.48 for 2 ounces)* contains several ingredients that are completely inappropriate for sensitive skin, or any skin type for that matter, including St. John's wort, coltsfoot, and lemon peel oil.

OTHER AUBREY ORGANICS PRODUCTS

☹ **Sparkling Mineral Water Herbal Complexion Mist** *($7.48 for 4 ounces)* isn't akin to San Pellegrino in a bottle, though misting that on your face would be a far gentler option. This product is not recommended due to a list of irritants that includes balm mint, mistletoe, yarrow, and fragrant oak musk oil.

☹ **Herbessence Makeup Remover** *($6.95 for 2 ounces)* is mostly nonvolatile plant and nut oils, but there's enough lavender oil in here to make it potentially problematic, especially if used to remove makeup around the eyes. Any of the non-volatile oils in this product will help break down makeup without risking irritation, so stick with that approach if you have dry skin and prefer an oil cleanser.

☹ **Natural AHA Fruit Acids with Apricot Exfoliating Mask** *($19.95 for 4 ounces)* lists alcohol as the second ingredient and also contains lemon and jasmine oils to further complicate matters for your skin.

☹ **Natural AHA Fruit Acids with Apricot Toning Moisturizer** *($19.95 for 4 ounces)* does not contain AHAs in any form but instead uses several plant extracts that are irritating for skin, including whole extracts of lavender, peppermint, and coltsfoot. Fragrant oils of jasmine and lavender only make matters worse.

☹ **Amino Derm Gel Clear Skin Complex** *($7.95 for 2 ounces)* is said to help keep skin clear, but what's reliable about this product is how efficiently it causes irritation from the witch hazel, alcohol, and several problematic plant extracts.

☹ **Collagen TCM Therapeutic Cream Moisturizer** *($13.48 for 2 ounces)* claims to deliver 100% pure, soluble collagen and elastin onto the skin, rather than into it. That's an accurate statement because the molecular structure of these ingredients is too large to penetrate into skin, so they do not act to replenish your skin's supply. It's interesting that a company that is so gung-ho to let its customers know it doesn't test on animals resorts to using animal-derived ingredients (at least they're being true to their natural roots). All told, the grain alcohol as the second ingredient and the lackluster formula make this a moisturizer to ignore.

☹ **Lumessence Lift Firming Renewal Cream with CoQ10 Liposomes** *($32.50 for 1 ounce)* contains denatured alcohol mixed with lavender as the third ingredient. Both are damaging to skin cells because both alcohol and lavender cause free-radical damage and kill skin cells, which is not renewing at all for skin of any age. This also contains fragrant rose oil, which only makes matters worse. Plus, the effectiveness of the handful of exciting ingredients in this moisturizer will be compromised because of the jar packaging.

☹ **Lumessence Rejuvenating Eye Creme with Liposomes** *($23.50 for 0.5 ounce)* contains many ingredients that are beneficial for dry skin, though few of them are listed correctly (there's no such ingredient as "humectant liposomes," though at least they indicate what the complex consists of). Unfortunately, lavender is present in an amount significant enough to make it a problem for skin.

☺ **Pure Aloe Vera** (*$7.78 for 4 ounces*) consists of organic aloe vera and natural preservative. Aloe can be soothing to sun-exposed or reddened skin, but I disagree with the company's claim that it is the best ingredient for skin that has endured too much sun exposure.

☺ **Sea Buckthorn with Ester-C Antioxidant Serum** (*$15.98 for 0.36 ounce*). Assuming that the ingredient list is somewhat accurate, this is mostly jojoba oil and some form of vitamin C. That can be helpful for dry skin. Sea buckthorn oil has antioxidant capability, but not in the type of packaging this product has.

☹ **Ultimate Moist Green Tea/Rosemary/Mint Hand & Body Lotion** (*$9.95 for 8 ounces*). I wonder when Aubrey Organics is finally going to get on board when it comes to accurate ingredient lists. There is no such ingredient as "coconut fatty acid cream base" as far as any regulatory board in the world is concerned, so it could be any number of thickening agents or emollients, which could be natural or not. Regardless of the base, this problematic lotion won't do much good for anyone because it contains several known irritants such as eucalyptus, mint, and spearmint, all of which hurt skin.

☹ **Ultimate Moist Morning Meadow Hand & Body Lotion SPF 15** (*$9.95 for 8 ounces*) conjures up images of a peaceful dawn when the grass is still wet with dew, but don't let that cloud your judgment of this sunscreen, whose problems are identical to the Saving Face SPF 10 Sunscreen Protection Spray reviewed below.

☹ **Vegecell Nighttime Hydrator with Green Tea** (*$18.75 for 1 ounce*) is similar to many of the products Aubrey sells, with no mention of skin type. The alcohol, lavender, peppermint, coltsfoot, nettle, sage, St. John's wort, watercress, lemon, ivy, sage, and lemon are all serious problems for skin.

☺ **White Camellia Oil** (*$15.98 for 0.36 ounce*) contains exactly what the name indicates, and nothing more. Aubrey claims this is "a superb complexion oil" but that's either just his opinion or based on anecdotal evidence; there is no substantiated proof. Moreover, white camellia oil is primarily used for fragrance, not skin care, so this product is best dabbed on the wrist, if used at all.

☹ **Natural Lips** (*$7.50*) are simply sheer lip tints. The colors are very soft and pretty, but they all contain enough peppermint oil to sound the irritation alarm for lips.

☺ **Treat 'Em Right Lip Balm** (*$2.95 for 0.15 ounce*) is available in several flavors, and not all of them are recommended. Each flavor has the same wax and plant oil base, and as such they do a good job of protecting lips from chapping and moisture loss, though they aren't the most elegant-feeling balms around. The Raspberry and Vanilla & Honey flavors are an option, while the Peppermint & Tea Tree, Spearmint, and Tangerine each contain potent irritants that don't help dry, chapped lips get better; rather they can make matters worse.

AUBREY ORGANICS SUN PRODUCTS

☹ **Gone! Safe and Natural Outdoor Spray SPF 10** (*$6.58 for 4 ounces*) uses only padimate O (PABA) as its active ingredient, which leaves skin vulnerable to UVA damage, not to mention the substandard SPF rating. This actually qualifies as one of the most irritating skin-care products I've ever reviewed due to the litany of irritants it contains, from eucalyptus oil and alcohol to menthol and lavender oil. The essential oils may naturally repel insects, but I'd save your skin by donning protective clothing instead.

☹ **Natural Sun SPF 12 Protective Tanning Butter** (*$7.25 for 4 ounces*) does contain an in-part titanium dioxide sunscreen, but an SPF 15 is critical and basic to good skin care, and the padimate O (PABA) can still be a problem for most skin types.

☺ **Natural Sun SPF 20 Tinted Sunscreen, for Face & Body** *($8.50 for 4 ounces)* is similar to but has a lighter texture than the Natural Sun SPF 12 Protective Tanning Butter. Although the SPF rating is ideal, the inclusion of padimate O (PABA) still makes this not worth considering over the many effective sunscreens without it. Iron oxides give this lotion a sheer tint, but that's more to offset the whitening effect of the titanium dioxide than to add color to skin.

☺ **Natural Sun SPF 20 Unscented Sunscreen, for Face & Body** *($7.75 for 4 ounces)* is nearly identical to the Natural Sun SPF 20 Tinted Sunscreen, for Face & Body, minus the iron oxides that give the previous sunscreen its "tint."

☺ **Natural Sun SPF 25 Green Tea Protective Sunscreen, Ideal for Children** *($8.50 for 4 ounces)* isn't ideal for children (or adults) because one of the active ingredients is padimate O (PABA), though it is joined by titanium dioxide to provide broad-spectrum sun protection. This ends up being a decent, oil-rich sunscreen for dry to very dry skin. The jasmine oil is present in a tiny amount, but may still cause problems for those with sensitive skin (if the PABA doesn't stir things up first).

☺ **Natural Sun SPF 25 Sunscreen, Ideal for Active Lifestyles** *($8.50 for 4 ounces)* is a repackaged and renamed version of the Natural Sun SPF 25 Green Tea Protective Sunscreen, Ideal for Children, and the same review applies.

☹ **Natural Sun SPF 8 Deep Tanning Sunscreen** *($7.25 for 4 ounces)* has an SPF rating that's too low, an active ingredient that is severely outdated and provides insufficient UVA protection, and still encourages users to get a deep tan. Talk about the fast track to wrinkles and, potentially, skin cancer!

☹ **Saving Face SPF 10 Sunscreen Protection Spray** *($8.00 for 4 ounces)* won't save your face from anything but will encourage wrinkles due to its lack of UVA-protecting ingredients and possibly a phototoxic reaction from the St. John's wort oil it contains.

☹ **After Sun Body & Face Maintenance Moisturizer** *($10.75 for 8 ounces)* contains too many problematic ingredients to make it worthwhile, whether skin is dealing with sun-induced dryness or not.

AUBREY ORGANICS MAKEUP

☹ **Natural Translucent Base** *($23.95)*. The Natural Translucent Base and Silken Earth powders are designed to be used as foundation, highlighter, contour, and blush, but the gritty texture of each and the incredibly dry finish make them all poor candidates—not to mention that each one contains cinnamon powder. That certainly is natural and may smell nice, but it's nevertheless problematic for skin.

☹ **Silken Earth** *($11.95)* is nearly identical to Aubrey Organics' Natural Translucent Base and the same review applies.

☹ **Silken Earth Powder Blush** *($11.95)*. Although silk powder is the main ingredient in this loose-powder blush, its feel and finish on skin is unusually dry. The application is sheer and, yes, silky, but quickly gives way to a parched, chalky feeling finish. This blush made my face sting seconds after applying it, and checking the ingredient list I saw that radish powder is one of the natural colorants. This is an all-natural blush, but that's no guarantee it's going to be a good one because irritation is bad for skin no matter what form it comes in!

☺ **$$$ Silken Earth Body Shimmer** *($23.95)*. This loose-powder shimmer comes in a generously sized tub complete with sifter and a tiny brush that's better than usual, but still impractical if you intend to dust this powder over a larger area. It feels silky and weightless at first, but has a drier finish with sparkles that don't cling well, so flaking is apparent right from the very beginning. Considering the cost and average performance, this isn't worth choosing over shimmer powders from Jane or Wet n' Wild at the drugstore.

☺ **Makeup Brush** *($21.95)* is an OK powder brush if you don't prefer the type that has a full head and soft, domed shape. Aubrey's brush is cut so it is more rounded and flat than domed, but it works to dust on powder or powder blush and the natural hair bristles are appropriately soft.

☹ **Natural Cosmetic Brush** *($3.95)* is inferior to almost any other powder brush you'll find for sale, and although it comes in two sizes (one for powder application and a smaller version for contouring) you're better off ignoring both. If you're intent on supporting a cosmetics company espousing natural ingredients, consider the vastly superior brushes from Aveda or The Body Shop.

AVEDA

AVEDA AT-A-GLANCE

Strengths: Effective use of beneficial plant oils and extracts in some products; one of the few lines that offers a lip balm and sheer lip tint whose sunscreen includes adequate UVA protection; superior tinted moisturizer with sunscreen; good concealer; terrific brushes and refillable compacts.

Weaknesses: Several products contain irritating essential oils or fragrance components known to cause sun sensitivity or skin cell death; substandard cleansers and irritating toners; so-called treatment products that can irritate skin; foundations whose SPF rating falls below the minimum of 15; average to poor blush options; several lip color products contains irritating fragrant oils.

For more information about Aveda, call (866) 823-1425 or visit www.aveda.com or www.Beautypedia.com.

AVEDA SKIN CARE

AVEDA BOTANICAL KINETICS PRODUCTS

☺ **$$$ Botanical Kinetics Purifying Creme Cleanser** *($20 for 5 ounces)* would be a much better lotion-style cleanser without the witch hazel extract, but the emollient ingredients keep it from being a significant problem for the normal to dry skin types this cleanser is best for.

☹ **Botanical Kinetics Purifying Gel Cleanser** *($20 for 5 ounces)* has a considerable amount of lavender and rosemary, two irritants that tarnish this otherwise standard and effective water-soluble cleanser. Several fragrant components (including eugenol and geraniol) are a problem when used around eyes or mucous membranes.

☺ **Botanical Kinetics Skin Firming/Toning Agent** *($19 for 5 ounce)* is a simple rose water toner with a couple of good skin-identical ingredients and a tiny amount of alcohol. It's more akin to misting skin with fragrance rather than with helpful ingredients.

☹ **Botanical Kinetics Toning Mist** *($19 for 5 ounces)* lists peppermint as the second ingredient and also contains witch hazel and alcohol, along with fragrant plant extracts with no established benefit for skin. This toner is not recommended.

☹ **Botanical Kinetics Exfoliant** *($19 for 5 ounces)* has a workable pH of 3, but the amount of salicylic acid it contains is too small for it to function as an exfoliant. This liquid contains several irritating plant extracts, including lavender, witch hazel, and balm mint.

☹ **Botanical Kinetics Hydrating Lotion** *($32 for 5 ounces)* is a basic moisturizer fraught with problematic ingredients, including significant amounts of lavender, rosemary, and comfrey, along with lesser amounts of fragrance components (such as eugenol) that are skin irritants. Eugenol is particularly egregious. It is a major component of clove oil, and research has shown the eugenol content of clove causes skin cell death, even when low concentrations of clove (0.33%) were applied to cultured skin cells (Source: *Cell Proliferation*, August 2006, pages 241-248).

AVEDA ENBRIGHTENMENT PRODUCTS

☺ **$$$ Enbrightenment Brightening Cleanser** *($38 for 4.2 ounces)* is a very basic water-soluble cleanser whose main cleansing agent is combined with a fatty alcohol to produce copious foam. As for the claims, any well-formulated cleanser will do exactly what this one says it will do. The difference is that many other cleansers do it without causing irritation to skin from fragrance and fragrance chemicals, and without the exorbitant price. The amount of salicylic acid this contains is too low for it to affect a single skin cell, plus it's rinsed away before it can initiate any kind of cell turnover. This cleanser is best for normal to oily skin and is capable of removing makeup, but for the price and formulation, it is just too ordinary to give your hard-earned (or even easily earned) dollars for.

☹ **Enbrightenment Brightening Treatment Toner** *($42 for 5 ounces)* is a surprisingly well-formulated toner for all skin types because it contains a potentially efficacious amount of vitamin C, along with plant extracts that research (although limited) has shown do have an effect on improving skin tone and discolorations. The amount of salicylic acid is too low for it to be effective, plus this toner's pH is above 4, so exfoliation won't occur, but that could have been overlooked to some extent if everything else were up to par. So, why is it rated with an unhappy face? The amount of rosemary extract is too large to ignore; the smell is unmistakable—you could spread this on bread with some olive oil and salt and have a tasty snack—OK, not really, please don't try this at home. In addition, this contains potentially irritating fragrance chemicals that all skin types are better off without. What a shame—this could have been a really good skin-care product.

☹ **Enbrightenment Brightening Correcting Cream** *($55 for 1.7 ounces).* The brightening components touted in this facial moisturizer have the potential to lighten skin discolorations, but they end up falling under a dark cloud due to the jar packaging. Continual exposure to light and air will cause the active constituents in most of these ingredients to break down, and that leaves you with an expensive, ordinary moisturizer that isn't worth a fraction of the cost, even in a huge jar. Further trouble comes from the amount of irritating rosemary leaf extract, a plant that has potent antioxidant properties, but its unmistakable fragrance also contains irritating chemicals. This has a lush, emollient texture, but so do many other moisturizers that contain more intriguing ingredients and that omit the irritants, omit the fragrance, and are available in better packaging. There is little hope that daily use of this product will lighten skin discolorations.

☹ **Enbrightenment Brightening Correcting Lotion** *($50 for 1.7 ounces).* Now this is the kind of packaging I'm talking about: unlike Aveda's Enbrightenment Brightening Correcting Cream, Aveda chose an airless pump bottle to preserve the integrity of the light- and air-sensitive plant ingredients they've added to this moisturizer for normal to dry skin. Unfortunately, Aveda also included a skin-irritating amount of fragrant rosemary leaf extract—the smell is potent and you'll feel a tingle as soon as you apply this—and that makes it too irritating for all skin types. Add to that several fragrant chemicals and things go from bad to worse. There is no reason to consider this product over several other skin-lightening products, even if you're looking for all-natural, because this product certainly doesn't qualify unless you define the term "skin-lightening" to mean no results at all other than what moisturized skin can produce.

☹ **Enbrightenment Brightening Correcting Serum** ($50 for 1 ounce) is a water-based serum containing a form of vitamin C that limited research has shown to be effective against hyperpigmentation when combined with niacinamide, which is absent from this product. What this does contain that makes it a poor contender if you're looking to help your skin is irritating rosemary leaf extract and several volatile fragrance chemicals. Rosemary has potent antioxidant properties, but the chemicals responsible for its unique scent are not what anyone's skin needs—not when the goal is to reduce inflammation. Normally I'd look past the rosemary extract because most companies don't include much of it, but in this case, the smell is potent and that spells trouble for your skin (though it would be great emanating from your oven on whatever you were roasting). One more comment: the amount of salicylic acid is too low for it to benefit skin, plus the pH is over 4, so exfoliation is unlikely to occur.

☹ **Enbrightenment Brightening Intensive Massage Mask** ($45 for 4.2 ounces). There are reasons to consider this thick, creamy mask, especially if you have dry skin and want an overnight treatment. Despite that, there are more reasons to leave this pricey mask on the shelf, chief among them being the amount of fragrant (really fragrant, as in hard to miss) rosemary leaf extract. The irritant potential of this plant far exceeds the positive potential of any of the beneficial ingredients in this mask, all of which are present in lesser amounts. If you want to spend in this range for a facial mask and get a better formulated product, look to those from Estee Lauder or Jan Marini Skin Research instead.

AVEDA GREEN SCIENCE PRODUCTS

All of the Green Science products from Aveda carry on about the argan oil they contain. This oil comes from tree nuts native to Morocco, and is said to be rich in vitamin E and linoleic acid. Of course, Aveda also mentions the native Moroccan Berbers, natives who've supposedly used this oil for centuries for medicinal and cosmetic purposes. That must mean it's something special (though keep in mind other natural ingredients, such as lead, were also used for cosmetic purposes until we learned how harmful it can be) but what does published research have to say about argan oil? Not much. The only study concerning topical application of argan oil has shown its oil-controlling, not moisturizing, properties. The remaining body of research has to do with the oil's benefits when consumed orally, and includes studies related to prostate cancer, the circulatory system, and cancer. We do know that argan oil contains beneficial components, including essential fatty acids and the antioxidants vitamin E and ferulic acid. In that sense, argan oil can be considered a reliable antioxidant, though not necessarily any better than other plant oils such as olive or pomegranate (Sources: *Journal of Cosmetic Dermatology*, June 2007, pages 113-118; *Cancer Investigation*, October 2006, pages 588-592; *Clinical Nutrition*, October 2004, pages 1,159-1,166; and *European Journal of Cancer Prevention*, February 2003, pages 67-75).

☹ **Green Science Firming Eye Creme** *($45 for 0.5 ounce)*. In the case of this eye cream, jar packaging will not keep the argan oil and other antioxidant ingredients stable once it is opened. In addition, the amount of rosemary extract in this eye cream and the inclusion of Thai ginger oil (also known as plai oil) makes this too irritating for skin. The science may be green, but that doesn't guarantee smart skin care (Source: *Biotechnology and Applied Biochemsitry*, May 2008, pages 61-69)!

☹ **Green Science Firming Face Creme** *($55 for 1.7 ounces)*. Jar packaging will quickly render the antioxidant capability of argan oil unstable, and will also negatively affect the other antioxidants in this product. The amount of rosemary extract is cause for concern, while the plai oil (also known as Thai ginger oil) retains many of the volatile components that make common ginger so irritating to skin (Source*: Biotechnology and Applied Biochemsitry*, May 2008, pages 61-69). This also contains synthetic fragrance ingredients that can contribute to skin's irritation response and aren't all that "green." What a shame; several ingredients in this moisturizer are a boon for dry to very dry skin.

☹ **Green Science Lifting Serum** *($50 for 1 ounce)* contains several beneficial ingredients, but the amount of rosemary extract is cause for concern, while the plai oil (also known as Thai ginger oil) is a significant irritant. The synthetic fragrances don't help matters either, and aren't in the least "green" ingredients. Lastly, there is no research anywhere showing that the peptides in here will help increase skin cell turnover rate, especially not on the surface of skin—that's what a well-formulated AHA or BHA product does, something Aveda's skin-care range is missing. Estee Lauder, Clinique, and Bobbi Brown offer much more sophisticated serum formulas without irritants (and by the way, it's ironic that Estee Lauder owns Aveda).

☹ **Green Science Line Minimizer** *($85 for 1 ounce)*. The amount of rosemary extract in this water-based serum is cause for concern, as is the plai oil. Also known as Thai ginger oil, plai oil is similar to common ginger, which means it retains this plant's volatile components that can cause skin irritation. This serum also contains several irritating synthetic fragrance ingredients (not exactly green by anyone's standards) and is really unimpressive compared to the best "wrinkle-filling" products available. For example, Good Skin Tri-Aktiline Instant Deep Wrinkle Filler is superior to this product, not only because of its formula but also because its spackle-like texture really does fill in superficial lines (though the effect is temporary). And the Good Skin product costs less than half of what Aveda is charging for this product. Estee Lauder owns Aveda and Good Skin.

AVEDA OUTER PEACE PRODUCTS

☺ **$$$ Outer Peace Foaming Cleanser** *($25 for 4.2 ounces)* is a liquid-to-foam, water-soluble cleanser that contains gentle detergent cleansing agents along with several anti-irritant plant extracts. Salicylic acid is also present, but only a tiny amount, which is rinsed off before it has a chance to work. The amount of alcohol is insignificant, but the salicylic acid means this should not be used around the eyes. This cleanser contains tamanu seed oil, which is reputed to contain a fatty acid (calophyllic acid) said to have an antimicrobial action on skin. There is no substantial information about tamanu oil's effect on acne, although there is some research showing it has wound-healing effects (Source: *International Journal of Cosmetic Science*, December 2002, pages 341-348), but fighting blemishes is completely different from healing wounds. All other claims about tamanu oil's benefit for skin are anecdotal, but its polyphenol content makes it a suitable antioxidant—just not in a cleanser where it is rinsed down the drain, along with the salicylic acid, before it has a chance to work.

☺ $$$ **Outer Peace Acne Relief Lotion** *($40 for 1.7 ounces)* is a lightweight, matte-finish BHA lotion that contains 0.5% salicylic acid and has a pH of 3.9, meaning that exfoliation will occur, but not very much. With the 0.5% concentration, this product is only marginally effective. It would be better for blemish-prone skin if the salicylic acid were present in at least a 1% concentration, and for more stubborn acne, 2% would be preferred. This also contains cornstarch (which contributes to this lotion's matte finish), but as a food-based ingredient, that isn't the best for dealing with the bacterium that triggers blemishes.

☹ **Outer Peace Acne Relief Pads** *($31.50 for 50 pads)* contains 1.5% salicylic acid, but the pH of the base is too high for it to exfoliate skin. Also, the amount of alcohol in this solution is too irritating for all skin types, not to mention that the alcohol cancels out the anti-irritant effect of the much smaller amounts of plant extracts.

☺ $$$ **Outer Peace Acne Spot Relief** *($29.50 for 0.5 ounce)* ranks as an effective, but needlessly expensive, BHA lotion that comes with a frustrating balance of positives and negatives. It's great that the 2% salicylic acid is in a base with a pH of 3.7, which will allow exfoliation to occur. It's not so great that Aveda included alcohol and cornstarch, both of which can exacerbate problems for those battling acne. The amounts of the offending ingredients aren't large, but this product would have earned a Paula's Pick rating without them (even though I still have reservations about the price tag for the tiny amount of product provided).

☺ $$$ **Outer Peace Cooling Masque** *($37 for 4.2 ounces)* is a needlessly expensive clay mask, which doesn't contain anything that brings peace to acne-prone skin. Like all clay masks, this can absorb excess oil and leave skin feeling smooth and looking, at least for the short term, matte. There is more alcohol and preservative in this formula than potentially beneficial plants, and the fragrance is potentially irritating due to the volatile components it is composed of.

AVEDA TOURMALINE PRODUCTS

☺ $$$ **Tourmaline Charged Exfoliating Cleanser** *($29 for 5 ounces)* is a rich, foaming cleanser that uses jojoba beads to gently polish the skin as you wash. This cleanser contains a skin-friendly assortment of nonirritating plant and nut oils, making it a great choice for parched, flaky skin during the winter months. It does contain fragrance and fragrant components along with salicylic acid, but those ingredients would be more of a problem if this product was used around the eyes, and a scrub-type cleanser shouldn't be used in that area anyway. By the way, the antioxidants included are a nice touch, but are needless in a rinse-off product as they end up down the drain instead of being absorbed into your skin where they are needed.

✓ ☺ $$$ **Tourmaline Charged Eye Creme** *($32 for 0.5 ounce)* is a brilliantly formulated moisturizer for the eye area or any other place where skin is slightly dry. It contains mostly silicone, water, glycerin, thickeners, tourmaline, skin-identical ingredients, antioxidants, cell-communicating ingredient, slip agents, fragrance, and preservatives. Tourmaline is a crystalline mineral that Aveda maintains increases the energy (and, therefore, the potency) of the ingredients it is blended with. Although there is research proving tourmaline's worth for removing heavy-metal ions from water (Source: *Journal of Environmental Sciences*, 2006, pages 1221-1225), it has no established benefit for skin, so it's a good thing several other ingredients in this eye cream do!

☺ $$$ **Tourmaline Charged Hydrating Creme** *($35 for 1.7 ounces)* has a frustrating blend of beneficial and problematic ingredients, and the most helpful ingredients (the many antioxidants in this moisturizer) are hindered by jar packaging. This is an OK moisturizer for normal to dry skin, but the tiny amount of eugenol is potentially problematic. By the way, there's only a dusting of tourmaline in this product, though that's just fine since it has no effect on skin.

☺ $$$ **Tourmaline Charged Protecting Lotion SPF 15** ($40 for 2.5 ounces) would rate a Paula's Pick if only the amount of titanium dioxide wasn't so low. As is, the amount (less than 1%), even coupled with octinoxate, is sketchy in terms of reliable UVA protection, especially if you don't apply this product liberally. That said, this moisturizing lotion has an excellent assortment of antioxidants, skin-identical ingredients, and cell-communicating ingredients. It is also free of problematic plant extracts and fragrance components.

☻ **Tourmaline Charged Radiance Fluid** ($40 for 1 ounce) would have been a worthwhile serum-type moisturizer for all skin types were it not for the inclusion of alcohol (it's the second ingredient) and clary extract, along with a list of unnecessary irritants—oils of peppermint, lavender, geranium, marjoram, orange, and lemon peel. When you combine all of these it's quite an assault on the skin, and not what comes to mind when Aveda states that this product "energizes skin with new, visible life." This does contain tourmaline, which has no proven benefit for skin. If Aveda's statements that tourmaline increases the efficacy of the other ingredients combined with it were true, that would mean the many problematic ingredients in this product would be even more irritating.

✓ ☺ $$$ **Tourmaline Charged Radiance Masque** ($29 for 4.2 ounces) is a very good moisturizing mask for normal to dry skin. It contains mostly water, glycerin, thickener, plant oil, emollients, slip agents, nonirritating plant extracts, tourmaline, lycopene (an antioxidant), more emollients, skin-identical ingredients, preservatives, and titanium dioxide (for opacity). Although this mask's claims of boosting skin's radiance due to the tourmaline it contains are unproven, it isn't a problem for skin. As with all moisturizing masks, the longer it is left on the skin the better your results will be, especially if your skin is dry.

OTHER AVEDA PRODUCTS

☺ **Pure Comfort Eye Makeup Remover** ($16 for 4.2 ounces) is a water-based, gentle makeup remover that's essentially a modified version of a water-soluble cleanser. This isn't too effective for removing long-wearing makeup, but it's good news that all the plant extracts used have soothing rather than irritating qualities.

☻ **Dual Nature Face Protection SPF 15** ($26 for 1.7 ounces) combines titanium dioxide and zinc oxide for outstanding broad-spectrum sun protection in a lotion base that has a substantially matte finish, something normal to oily skin not prone to breakouts will appreciate. It's a shame that these positive traits are mixed with fragrant plant oils, including geranium, jasmine, and orange, all of which are potential irritants. In addition, orange oil is phototoxic, which means it can cause adverse reactions on skin that is exposed to sunlight (Source: www.naturaldatabase.com), although there is debate about how much orange oil is needed to cause such a reaction. Many aromatherapy Web sites recommend not using orange oil if skin will be exposed to sun, while others recommend using less than 1.4%, though I could not find research documenting why this specific amount or less is deemed acceptable, so I advise playing it safe and avoiding orange oil altogether.

☺ $$$ **Pure Vital Moisture Eye Creme** ($25 for 0.5 ounce) doesn't hold a candle to the myriad eye creams other Lauder-owned lines offer, though many of those products (like this one) still suffer from reliance on jar packaging. This is an average moisturizer for the eye area or elsewhere, and it's unfortunate that the really intriguing ingredients show up too late in the game to be significant players.

☹ **Brightening Moisture Treatment** *($40 for 2.5 ounces)* is the lotion version of the Brightening Essence, and although this product omits the alcohol present in the Essence, it contains the same group of irritating essential oils. What a shame, because without the irritants this would have been a good anti-inflammatory moisturizer for normal to slightly dry skin. It cannot, however, work to diminish the appearance of sun-induced skin discolorations.

☺ **$$$ Balancing Infusion for Dry Skin** *($21 for 0.34 ounce)* is mostly meadowfoam seed oil and fragrance, along with tiny amounts of vitamins and other plant oils. The fragrance can be a problem for all skin types; you're better off moisturizing with plain olive or jojoba oil than this chancy product.

☹ **Balancing Infusion for Sensitive Skin** *($21 for 0.34 ounce)* contains some plant oils and extracts with established soothing properties, but fragrance is the second ingredient, and the fragrant components in this serum (including linolool and limonene) are an unnecessary pitfall for anyone with sensitive skin.

☹ **Balancing Infusion Oily Skin/Acne Treatment** *($21 for 0.34 ounce)* is completely inappropriate for someone dealing with acne or blackheads, not only because the concentration of salicylic acid (0.5%) is too low, but also because of the plant oils this product contains. Jojoba, sunflower, and soybean oils are great for dry skin, but readily cause problems for someone with oily or blemish-prone skin. Last but not least, the fragrant plant extracts in this product (centered on rosemary) are potent irritants.

☺ **$$$ Deep Cleansing Herbal Clay Masque** *($20 for 4.4 ounces)* is as standard a clay mask as it gets. Although this masque has enough emollients to make it more "comfortable" than many other clay masks, the emollients are more suited to normal to dry skin than oily skin. Clay is not cleansing in the least, though it can absorb oil from skin.

☹ **Intensive Hydrating Masque** *($20 for 5 ounces)* brings the skin a mixed bag of helpful and potentially harmful ingredients and, despite the name, isn't all that hydrating (you won't think so if your skin is dry to very dry). The amount of lavender extract is likely too problematic to make this worthwhile for even occasional use, especially given the selection of moisturizing masks whose formulas best this one without troublesome ingredients.

☺ **Lip Saver SPF 15** *($8.50 for 0.15 ounce)* includes an in-part avobenzone sunscreen and is an outstanding emollient lip balm that's packaged ChapStick-style. The ratio of plant oil and jojoba esters to wax produces a softer-texture lip balm that leaves an attractive sheen on lips. The only drawback is the flavor, which is composed of cinnamon and clove. The amounts of these ingredients aren't enough to warrant avoiding the product, but it would have received a Paula's Pick rating without them. One more point: Aveda claims this is waterproof, but a more accurate term is "water-resistant." This balm will need to be reapplied after swimming or perspiring.

☺ **Sun Source** *($17.50 for 5 ounces)* contains dihydroxyacetone, the ingredient used in most self-tanners to turn skin brown. Although it would be easy to dismiss this self-tanner on its similarity to so many others, Aveda has concocted a thoughtful, irritant-free product that features an elegant moisturizing base that includes antioxidants (and in stable packaging, too). The tiny amount of balsam won't be a problem for skin and likely just contributes to this product's fragrance.

AVEDA MAKEUP

FOUNDATION: ✓ ☺ **$$$ Inner Light Tinted Moisture SPF 15** *($26)* is an outstanding tinted moisturizer that uses titanium dioxide as its sole sunscreen active. It has a smooth, creamy texture that hydrates skin while leaving a satin finish, and is suitable for normal to dry skin, offering sheer coverage and a hint of color. Five shades are available and they are all excellent. Aspen is a real find for someone with fair skin.

☺ **Inner Light Dual Foundation SPF 12** *($21.50)* is a pressed-powder foundation that contains a titanium dioxide–based sunscreen. Although SPF 15 would have been better—and would comply with the American Academy of Dermatology recommendations—this is still a consideration, as long as you understand that (as for any sunscreen product) it must be applied liberally to achieve the stated SPF. And since this is only SPF 12, to truly protect your skin you also need another sunscreen product, such as a moisturizer, to get sufficient protection. In contrast to its predecessor (Dual Base Minus Oil), this powder foundation is talc-free and instead contains mica, which creates a slightly drier texture and imparts noticeable shine, something that's not the best for a natural look in daylight. It maintains a smooth finish and is easy to blend, providing sheer to light coverage when used dry. Aveda claims it can be used wet, too, but as with most powder foundations, this method of application can promote streaks and look uneven. Seven mostly beautiful soft, neutral shades are offered, with options for light (but not very light) to dark skin tones.

☺ **$$$ Inner Light Liquid Foundation SPF 12** *($21.50)* doesn't have a liquid texture, and in fact is so thick that it can be difficult to dispense from the bottle (if any foundation could benefit from a pump applicator, it's this one!). Out of the bottle, this does blend on smoothly and thins out before setting to a soft matte (in feel) finish. A slight amount of shine is apparent, but not enough to make this a problem for daytime wear. The all titanium dioxide sunscreen is great, though SPF 15 is preferred; the lower number keeps this foundation from earning a happy face rating. Twelve mostly exemplary shades are available, with some great neutrals for fair to light skin and non-ashy shades for African-American skin tones. The only shades to approach with caution are Sesame and Cinnamon, as both have a tendency to turn slightly peach. This foundation is best for normal to slightly oily skin.

CONCEALER: ☺ **Inner Light Concealer** *($16)* is a liquid concealer with an initially moist texture that quickly sets to a matte finish, so it must be blended quickly. But if you try to apply this in a sweep of color, it goes on somewhat choppy, providing spotty, rather than smooth, even coverage. It works far better if you apply it in dots over the areas where you need it, and then buff it out so you can get natural-looking coverage capable of concealing dark circles (without creasing) and minor redness. Among the six shades, only Bamboo is questionable because it has a slight orange cast. The others are winning neutrals, with Mahogany a standout for dark skin. Although this concealer has a matte finish, a slight amount of shine is evident. It's a minor issue, but one you should be aware of if you want to avoid shine.

POWDER: ☺ **$$$ Inner Light Pressed Powder** *($20)* is a talc-free pressed powder with a silky texture that feels creamier than most yet remains sheer on skin. Three very good shades are available; however, there are no options for dark skin tones. Keep in mind that because the minerals that comprise this powder have shine, their effect on skin is quite prominent—not really what you want if you're using powder to control or minimize shine.

☺ **$$$ Inner Light Loose Powder** *($22)* comes in only one shade, which is extremely limiting given Aveda's multicultural foundation and concealer colors. Compared to the top loose powders, this talc-free option, while decidedly light, is drier and has way too much shine to look convincing in daylight. It's an option for evening shimmer powder, but given the shine it imparts—just what someone with oily skin is trying to avoid—anyone considering this powder to keep oily areas in check won't be thrilled with the result.

BLUSH: ☺ **Petal Essence Cheek Color** *($15)* has a decently smooth texture but its application imparts almost as much shine as color, and tends to be somewhat uneven. The palette of mostly warm-toned (copper, peach) colors is limiting and, considering the price, this blush isn't in the same league as many others.

☹ **Petal Essence Cheek Tint** *($22)* is blush in stick form, and its stiff, waxy texture must be warmed on the skin prior to applying, which is inconvenient. The vivid yet sheer colors (all have shimmer) blend well and leave a moist finish appropriate for dry skin. The unhappy face rating is due to the inclusion of lavender oil, which is an irritant and a problem for the health of skin cells.

EYESHADOW: ☺ **Petal Essence Single Eye Color** *($12)* retains its silky texture and smooth, flake-free application (quite a feat considering every shade has some amount of shine). The range of colors has been reduced, likely so Aveda can launch seasonal eyeshadow colors, but most of the mainstays are workable, depending on how much shine you want. Only Vinca is too purple to work for anything other than pulling focus from what eyeshadow is meant to enhance: the eyes.

☺ **Petal Essence Eye Color Duo** *($16)* shares the same texture and smooth, even application as the Petal Essence Single Eye Color. Each Duo has some degree of shine, with most having an obvious shimmer. The main problem is that all but one pairing is either too blue, green, purple, or contrasting to consider, unless your intent with eyeshadow is to color (rather than shape and shade) the lid and under-brow area. Gobi Sand/Haze is the least shiny and most workable Duo.

☺ **Petal Essence Triple Accent** *($18)* is a dual-sided pencil meant for use on eyes, cheeks, and lips. One side is more pigmented and works for creamy cheek or lip color, while the opposite side works best as a shimmery highlighter. If you don't mind regular sharpening and like the shade pairings, this is an option, but not one that's easy to blend or long-lasting.

EYE AND BROW SHAPER: ☺ **Petal Essence Eye Definer** *($12.50)* is nothing special, just a nice selection of standard, needs-sharpening pencils with an appropriate dry finish that is minimally prone to smudging. Avoid Indigo (blue).

☺ **Uruku Eye-Lip Color Liner** *($12.50)* is a standard pencil with three colors that work much better for lips than eyes. The uruku pigment lends an orange cast that just isn't that attractive for eye lining.

☹ **Uruku Eye Accent** *($16)* has a creamy, slick texture that glides over the eye area but doesn't set, so it remains movable and will definitely crease. There is no reason to put up with these drawbacks when companies such as Benefit and Revlon offer superior cream eyeshadows that have a powder finish to enhance wear. In case you're wondering, uruku is a natural reddish-orange pigment derived from the urukum palm tree, and although Aveda plays up its presence as a natural colorant in this product, other unnatural cosmetic pigments are used as well, such as manganese violet, which is derived from an inorganic source.

LIPSTICK, LIP GLOSS, AND LIPLINER: ✓☺ **Lip Tint SPF 15** *($12)*. Lip Tint SPF 15, in contrast to many of Aveda's lip products, is free of irritants and contains an in-part titanium dioxide sunscreen! The formula is wholly impressive, containing an excellent array of soothing, nonvolatile plant oils, antioxidants, and ingredients that mimic the structure and function of healthy skin. Each sheer shade is wearable and contains a touch of shimmer for an attractive, slightly creamy finish.

☺ **$$$ Nourish-Mint Sheer Mineral Lip Color** *($14)* only has "mineral" in the name to capitalize on the refuses-to-die trend of mineral makeup. Formula-wise, this sheer lipstick differs little from most others. It has a slightly firmer texture (due to less oil) than Aveda's Nourish-Mint Smoothing Lip Color, and all of the shades have a slight shimmer. Like the original Nourish-Mint, this contains some good antioxidants, but the fragrance components, including eugenol, may cause irritation.

☺ **$$$ Nourish-Mint Smoothing Lip Color** *($14)* is a creamy lipstick that almost crosses the line to greasy, but its lack of slickness helps it stay anchored to lips (for about as long as most creamy lipsticks last). The soft gloss finish and range of shades are attractive, though only the burgundy-to-red shades leave any sign of a stain. Surprisingly, no mint oils or extracts are listed, and this doesn't make your lips tingle upon application. However, this does contain small amounts of fragrance components (including eugenol), which may cause irritation, and that keeps this from earning the top rating. Kudos to Aveda for including several notable antioxidants in this formula.

☺ **$$$ Nourish-Mint Renewing Lip Treatment** *($15)* is a glossy lip balm in lipstick form. The colorless formula feels great over chapped lips and helps prevent moisture loss, just like most well-formulated lip balms. There are no ingredients in this product that plump lips over time; the only reason to consider it over less expensive balms is if you want a noticeably glossy finish and a spearmint flavor (which may prove irritating).

☺ **Lipliner** *($12)* is a standard, needs-sharpening pencil that is nicely creamy and available in mostly workable colors. Nice, but not extraordinary.

☹ **Lip Glaze** *($16)* is a standard tube-type lip gloss with a moderately thick texture and a slightly sticky feel on the lips. Although the shades are gorgeous, this product contains peppermint and ginger oils, which combine to produce a warm, tingling sensation that you should read as a signal that your lips are being seriously irritated. There are so many other excellent choices for lip gloss that share the same positive traits as this one but don't assault your lips with irritants.

☹ **Lip Replenishment** *($14)* is just a colorless lip balm in lipstick packaging. It feels very greasy and, although the emollients included will definitely make dry, chapped lips feel better, the peppermint tends to make chapped lips worse due to its irritating properties.

☹ **Uruku Cheek-Lip Creme** *($16)* presents an all-in-one option for quick lip and cheek color, but the creamy texture and slightly moist finish of this product mean it will fare best as a faint wash of color on the lips. Due to the inclusion of the irritants peppermint and cinnamon (along with fragrant components such as eugenol), this product is not recommended for cheeks or lips.

☹ **Lip Shine** *($14.50)* is a tube-type lip gloss with a light, slick texture. It leaves a smooth, glossy sheen and offers some great colors, but the inclusion of peppermint, anise, cinnamon, and basil oils add up to lip irritation, which dims this gloss' otherwise polished prospects.

MASCARA: ☺ **Mascara Plus Rose** *($12)* produces copious length and decent thickness without clumping or smearing. It still goes on wetter than most mascaras and is not recommended for those prone to watery eyes, but if you're careful not to blink too much this is definitely worth considering as an all-purpose mascara.

☺ **Mosscara** *($15)* claims its conditioning formula is helped by the inclusion of Iceland moss, yet there is not enough moss in it to cover a twig, let alone condition lashes. This is an ordinary mascara formula that produces average length and minimal thickness, but it's hardly exciting or worth considering over the best Maybelline or L'Oreal mascaras.

BRUSHES: ✓ ☺ **Flax Sticks** *($12-$34)*. Aveda's latest brushes are splendid. Each is made with unbelievably soft and functional synthetic hair. Ever the environmentally conscious company, Aveda has provided brush handles that are composed of recycled wood and flax. I found the handles to be a bit awkward due to their squared edges, but that's a minor quibble for an overall superior brush collection. In the Flax Sticks collection, the best brushes include the #5 Eye Smudger ($14), and #8 Complexion Brush ($21) (which is best for eyeshadow application).

FACE AND BODY ILLUMINATING/SHIMMER PRODUCTS: ☺ **$$$ Inner Light Shimmer Accents** *($21.50)* are a great way for those with normal to dry skin not prone to blemishes to highlight and add noticeable, non-sparkling shine to skin. All of the flesh-tone to tan shades are workable and versatile, and each blends well. Aveda claims this is non-acnegenic, but the mango butter and triglycerides in here can definitely pose problems for those battling acne. The other issue is the fragrance, which is quite strong, although it does dissipate. I wouldn't apply this near the eyes (and definitely not on eyelids), but it should be fine if mixed with a moisturizer and applied elsewhere on the face or body.

☺ **$$$ Petal Essence Face Accents** *($20)* is a pressed shimmer powder combining three stripes of shimmer powder in one pressed-powder pan. The various color combinations are all workable whether applied separately or blended together, and each goes on sheer, imparting more shimmer than pigment. This product is remarkably similar to Bobbi Brown's Shimmer Brick Compact ($35), which is also a Lauder-owned company, but Brown's costs twice as much.

SPECIALTY PRODUCTS: ☺ **Essentials Environmetal Compact** *($19)* is a sleek metal compact that can hold two Aveda eyeshadows and one powder blush, or it can house a single pressed powder or powder foundation. The hinge element extends out a bit and can house an Aveda lipstick, making this a clever, portable way to carry your (Aveda) makeup.

☺ **$$$ Professional Environmetal Compact** *($26)* is a large compact that can house up to 16 Aveda eyeshadows or numerous, other combinations of any Aveda makeup product sold in a pan. It's best for someone who uses several colors or who routinely alternates between various blush and eyeshadow combinations.

☺ **Total Face Environmetal Compact** *($14)* is a happy medium between the smaller and larger Environmetal Compacts. This midsize option houses just the essentials: powder, blush, and eyeshadow. If you're sold on Aveda makeup and like the idea of customizing a palette, this is recommended.

AVEENO (SKIN CARE ONLY)

AVEENO AT-A-GLANCE

Strengths: Very good range of sunscreens that include avobenzone for UVA protection, and one outstanding sunscreen with retinol.

Weaknesses: Well-intentioned but ineffective anti-acne products; reliance on a single showcased ingredient (typically soy) that makes their antiaging products less enticing than the competition; no products to address hyperpigmentation; no toners.

For more information about Aveeno, call (866) 428-3366 or visit www.aveeno.com or www.Beautypedia.com.

AVEENO CLEAR COMPLEXION PRODUCTS

☺ **Clear Complexion Cleansing Bar** *($3.39 for 3.5 ounces)* contains 1% BHA in a soap-free bar cleanser, but the pH is too high for the BHA to be effective as an exfoliant and it would be rinsed down the drain before it could have an effect on skin anyway. Bar cleansers can be drying, though this one is gentler than most; it could work for someone with normal to oily skin who doesn't have blemish-prone skin.

☹ **Clear Complexion Cream Cleanser** *($7.49 for 5 ounces)* is medicated with 2% salicylic acid, but it will be rinsed down the drain before it can penetrate pores and help with blemishes. There is a lot of fragrance in this cleanser, and it contains the irritating menthol derivative menthyl lactate, making it not recommended.

☹ **Clear Complexion Daily Cleansing Pads** *($7.49 for 28 pads)* contain a mere 0.5% salicylic acid (BHA), which isn't enough to combat blemishes or stubborn blackheads, plus the pH of the solution is too high for the BHA to exfoliate. These pads are best for cleansing oily to very oily skin because of their detergent cleansing agent, sodium C14-16 olefin sulfonate, which is more drying than most and generally should be avoided. Although it's present here with milder detergent cleansing agents, it is still too potentially drying for most skin types.

☺ **Clear Complexion Foaming Cleanser** *($7.49 for 6 ounces)* is a standard, detergent-based, water-soluble cleanser that contains 0.5% salicylic acid. Such a small amount of salicylic acid (BHA) is only somewhat effective against breakouts, though even if it could have an effect, it would be rinsed down the drain before it had a chance to do anything. This cleanser contains enough of the drying cleansing agent sodium C14-16 olefin sulfonate to make it a problem for almost all skin types. It also contains fragrance.

☺ **Clear Complexion Daily Moisturizer** *($16.99 for 4 ounces)* has enough enticing claims to fulfill the wish list of anyone suffering from bouts of dryness and breakouts. However, this 0.5% BHA lotion shortchanges blemish-prone skin with too little salicylic acid despite an effective pH of 3.7. That's discouraging, and things don't perk up since this is also an extremely ordinary lightweight moisturizer with nary an antioxidant or state-of-the-art water-binding agent to be found. This fragranced product won't do a thing to keep skin clear or help with blemishes you may already have.

☺ **Clear Complexion Correcting Treatment** *($15.99 for 1 ounce)* is a 1% salicylic acid (BHA) treatment, but it has a pH of 5, which means it is ineffective for exfoliating skin or dislodging stubborn blackheads. Its only redeeming quality is the inclusion of retinol, backed up by opaque, airless packaging that will keep it stable. As a retinol product for normal to slightly oily or slightly dry skin, this is recommended.

AVEENO CONTINUOUS PROTECTION PRODUCTS

☺ **Continuous Protection Sunblock Lotion SPF 30** *($10.99 for 4 ounces)* is an effective sunscreen. The standard base formula is suitable for normal to dry skin, and avobenzone is on hand to provide UVA protection. Just don't take the "continuous protection" part of the name seriously. Although an SPF 30 product provides longer protection than an SPF 15 product, you still need to reapply this after swimming, perspiring, or exercising if you want to maintain protection or plan for a full day out in the sun. Aveeno knows this or they wouldn't mention that this product maintains its SPF rating for only 40 minutes in water. After that you should reapply it rather than rely on the misleading name that implies longer protection than competing sunscreens rated at SPF 30.

☺ **Continuous Protection Sunblock Lotion SPF 30, for Face** *($10.49 for 3 ounces)* is similar to the Continuous Protection Sunblock Lotion SPF 30 above. Although it does have a few more bells and whistles than the "body" version, it doesn't contain any ingredients that make it better suited for use on the face.

☺ **Continuous Protection Sunblock Lotion SPF 45** *($9.99 for 4 ounces)* is nearly identical to the Continuous Protection Sunblock Lotion SPF 30 above, and the same review applies. The only difference of note is the slightly higher amount of active ingredients required to net an SPF 45 rating.

☺ **Continuous Protection Sunblock Lotion SPF 55** *($9.99 for 3 ounces)* is similar to the Continuous Protection Sunblock Lotion SPF 30 above, except this product contains a higher amount of active ingredients necessary to achieve its SPF rating. This provides excellent broad-spectrum protection, and it includes antioxidants.

☺ **Continuous Protection Sunblock Lotion SPF 55, for Baby** *($9.99 for 4 ounces)* distinguishes itself from the Continuous Protection Sunblock Lotion SPF 55 in name and with the inclusion of anti-irritant oat flour. A sunscreen with this many active ingredients is ill-advised for babies, whose skin is not developed enough to tolerate them. Babies under six months of age should be shielded from sunlight rather than treated with sunscreens of any kind; beyond six months, the best sunscreen actives for a baby's skin are titanium dioxide and/or zinc oxide (Source: www.cancercare.ns.ca/media/documents/sunexposurebrochurefinal.pdf). This is worth considering by adults.

☹ **Continuous Protection Sunblock Lotion SPF 70, for Face** *($10.99 for 3 ounces)* contains avobenzone for sufficient UVA protection, but it has an SPF rating that, while accurate, may make you think that you can apply this once and be outdoors all day without a care (of course, the "continuous protection" name doesn't help, either). Although this sunscreen contains some good antioxidants and an anti-irritant, it also contains a preservative (methylisothiazolinone) that is not recommended for use in leave-on products due to its sensitizing potential (Source: *Contact Dermatitis*, October 2006, pages 227-229). Without this problematic preservative, this could have been a good sunscreen for normal to oily skin. One more point: Aveeno should not be labeling this "waterproof," because no sunscreen is impervious to water; you'll still need to reapply such sunscreens after swimming or toweling off. "Water-resistant" is the way to describe how a sunscreen like this functions on skin.

☹ **Continuous Protection Sunblock Spray SPF 45** *($10.49 for 5 ounces)* includes avobenzone for sufficient UVA protection, as well as the antioxidant vitamin A and soy extract. Despite those positives, the alcohol content of this spray-on sunscreen, coupled with the high percentage of active ingredients, makes it too irritating for all skin types.

☹ **Continuous Protection Sunblock Spray SPF 70** *($10.99 for 5 ounces)* provides broad-spectrum protection and includes the maximum amount of avobenzone for impressive UVA protection (stabilized by the same ingredient Neutrogena advertises as their Helioplex complex; both Neutrogena and Aveeno are owned by Johnson & Johnson), all in a convenient spray that works from any angle (mothers trying to apply sunscreen to squirming children will love that feature). However, the amount of alcohol is significant, and makes this a tough sunscreen to recommend due to its drying, irritating potential. The alcohol-free spray-on sunscreens from Kinesys (not reviewed in this book), Coppertone Water Babies, or Paula's Choice provide ample sun protection and include ingredients that help rather than harm skin.

AVEENO POSITIVELY AGELESS PRODUCTS

☺ **Positively Ageless Daily Cleansing Pads** *($8.99 for 28 pads)* are an interesting way to cleanse skin and exfoliate immediately after. You use the smooth side of the pad to cleanse and remove makeup, then turn the pad over and use the textured side for a mild, scrub-like effect. The solution these pads are steeped in is gentle and capable of removing most types of makeup, but silicone-based and waterproof formulas won't come off with these pads unless you use a lot of pressure, which isn't the best for your skin. Aveeno recommends these pads for sensitive skin, but the fragrance they've added diminishes the assurance that those with sensitive skin should use them. Other than that, they are suitable for all skin types.

☺ **Positively Ageless Daily Exfoliating Cleanser** *($9.99 for 5 ounces)* is a standard, detergent-based cleanser that also contains polyethylene (plastic beads) for a topical scrub action. That's about all there is to this product, and it's an option for all but very dry skin—as long you don't expect to look ageless after using it.

☺ **Positively Ageless Warming Scrub** *($8.99 for 4 ounces)*. The warming sensation you experience with this scrub occurs when the magnesium sulfate it contains mixes with water (you're directed to apply this to damp skin), causing what's known as an exothermic reaction. It's a neat high school science experiment, but it offers no special benefit to your skin beyond the fleeting feeling of warmth. Otherwise, it's a thick-textured yet rinsable scrub that's preferred for normal to oily skin. It's nice that this is fragrance free, but adding magnesium sulfate raises questions of dryness due to its alkaline nature. This ingredient provides no benefit, so the only thing positive about this product is that it is a good scrub, not bad, but not ageless!

☺ **Positively Ageless Daily Moisturizer SPF 30** *($19.99 for 2.5 ounces)* is a well-formulated daily moisturizer whose sunscreen features avobenzone. It is difficult to assess the relative quantities of the interesting ingredients in this sunscreen because Aveeno chose to list the inactive ingredients alphabetically. This is permitted by the FDA for over-the-counter drug products, but isn't as helpful for the consumer as listing ingredients in descending order would be. The mushroom extracts in this product won't take the years off, but, assuming they're present in sufficient quantities, they can have an anti-inflammatory effect.

☺ **Positively Ageless Eye Serum** *($19.99 for 0.5 ounce)* is a very basic, boring light-weight serum for slightly dry skin anywhere on the face. All the intriguing ingredients add up to less than a dusting, making this pale in comparison to the superior serums from Olay and Aveeno's sister brand Neutrogena.

☹ **Positively Ageless Lifting & Firming Daily Moisturizer SPF 30** *($20.49 for 2.5 ounces)* is a good lightweight daytime moisturizer with sunscreen for normal to slightly dry or slightly oily skin. Avobenzone is on hand for UVA protection accompanied by silicones and absorbent thickening agents to promote a soft matte finish that works well under makeup. Nothing in this formula will lift or firm skin unless you believe that all it takes for that is mushroom extract and a tiny amount of wheat protein. Although sun protection is assured, this product could have been a much stronger contender for your "antiaging" arsenal if it contained more antioxidants and skin-identical ingredients.

☹ **Positively Ageless Lifting & Firming Eye Cream** *($19.99 for 0.5 ounce)* is an incredibly average moisturizer for slightly dry skin anywhere on the face. As far as extraordinary goes, it's extraordinary only if you believe Aveeno's claims about an ingredient it uses known as tetra-hydroxypropyl ethylenediamine. According to Aveeno's sister company RoC (both owned by Johnson & Johnson), this ingredient has been clinically proven (of course, the results of these clinical studies are not available for public scrutiny and they were done by J&J) to tighten epidermal cells, resulting in a lifted, firmed appearance. Technical information about tetrahydroxypropyl ethylenediamine indicates it functions as a neutralizing agent and helps adjust the pH of water-based products. There is no independent, peer-reviewed research demonstrating it to be effective for sagging skin, as RoC claims (unless by tightening they mean constricting due to irritation). Even if there were, once the skin begins to sag due to bone loss and fat pad shifting (something that happens to all of us as we age), no amount of any topically applied ingredient will help. This type of sagging can be remedied only by cosmetic surgery. Any tightening effect this ingredient has on skin cells would be due to the inflammation that occurs if a product is too alkaline or too acidic. But that would be a temporary effect, not even related to the results possible from surgical procedures or a particularly healthy impact on the skin.

☺ **Positively Ageless Lifting & Firming Night Cream** *($19.99 for 1.7 ounces)* sounds like a wonder product, given that Aveeno reports that their clinical studies showed 97% of women saw "significant improvement" in skin firmness after just 4 weeks of use. Since this study is not published, we don't know the number of participants, their age range, whether or not this cream was compared to other products, or how the product was applied. For example, if the skin was first stripped with alcohol, as is often the case in these kinds of so-called studies, then the results would be impressive for any product, which is why so many companies make this claim that their studies show almost everyone was thrilled with the product. Also, what does "significant improvement" mean? Did these women reconsider having cosmetic surgery because this product made their skin so firm, or are we talking a subjective improvement because of how the skin felt after it was placed over irritated skin? It may well be just that, because not a single ingredient in this rather bland, jar-packaged moisturizer can legitimately, noticeably firm skin. Aveeno's sister company RoC claims the ingredient tetrahydroxypropyl ethylenediamine can tighten and lift epidermal skin cells, but their alleged research on this ingredient has never been reproduced—and if this ingredient is the key to firmer skin, why doesn't it show up in products from other J&J company brands such as Neutrogena? Neutrogena has more antiaging products than Aveeno and RoC combined, but uses tetrahydroxypropyl ethylenediamine in only one antiwrinkle product. You have to wonder why.

☺ **Positively Ageless Night Cream** *($19.99 for 1.7 ounces)* makes the tired claim of going beyond being "just" a moisturizer to visibly reduce the signs of aging. It's a basic but effective moisturizer suitable for normal to slightly dry skin, and Aveeno is banking on the mushroom extracts to produce ageless results. Both species used, reishi *(Ganoderma lucidum)* and *Lentinula edodes*, better known as shiitake, have research concerning their benefits when consumed as food, but there is no research showing them to be effective when used topically on skin (Source: www.naturaldatabase.com). Both mushrooms have antioxidant properties (Source: *Journal of Agricultural and Food Chemistry*, October 2002, pages 6072-6077), but their benefits will be short-lived because of this product's jar packaging.

☺ **Positively Ageless Rejuvenating Serum** *($19.99 for 1.7 ounces)* cannot self-adjust to an individual's skin and does not contain ingredients that stimulate exfoliation (Aveeno uses the term "cell renewal"). This is a water- and silicone-based serum that contains a tiny amount of water-binding agent and thickener along with mushroom extracts and the mold *Mucor miehei*. This mold is said to have enzymatic action that causes exfoliation, but there is absolutely no research to support the claim. At best, expect this serum to make skin feel silky and regain its softness.

☹ **Positively Ageless Sunblock Lotion SPF 70 Face** *($10.99 for 3 ounces)* is a basic sunscreen that contains stabilized avobenzone for UVA protection. I am concerned that the percentage of active ingredients required to net an SPF 70 rating may be needlessly sensitizing for many skin types, especially on the face, so you should test this at home before you slather it on and head outside. Remember, an SPF 70 doesn't give you better protection, just longer protection, and there aren't that many hours of daylight anywhere in the world. Adding to this potential irritation is the inclusion of the sensitizing preservative methylisothiazolinone. This isn't a sunscreen I feel comfortable recommending.

☹ **Positively Ageless Sunblock Spray SPF 50** *($10.99 for 5 ounces)*. This spray-on sunscreen mist contains stabilized avobenzone for sufficient UVA protection. That's excellent, but the base formula is mostly alcohol, which makes it too drying and irritating for all skin types. If you're wondering about the sd-alcohol being at the bottom of the ingredient list, it's in that position because Aveeno decided to list the inactive ingredients in alphabetical order instead of descending order. This is permissible because sunscreens are regulated as over-the-counter (OTC) drugs, not as cosmetics, and OTC products can legally play this game with their ingredient lists. As a result, you need to err on the side of caution and assume that alcohol could easily be the first ingredient.

AVEENO POSITIVELY RADIANT PRODUCTS

☺ **Positively Radiant Cleanser** *($7.49 for 6.7 ounces)* is a very good, water-soluble cleanser for all skin types except very dry. The soy sterol and soy protein look good on the label, and they do have water-binding properties, but their benefit is negligible in a product that is quickly rinsed from skin.

☺ **Positively Radiant Daily Cleansing Pads** *($7.49 for 28 pads)* are a convenient way to cleanse skin gently. Aveeno boasts about the soy in these dual-textured pads, but there isn't enough of it to amount to a single bean. The water-based formula is composed of mild detergent cleansing agents. However, the cleansing agents' mildness means they won't do a thorough job of dissolving makeup and removing excess surface oil. Unlike several other cleansing cloths/ wipes, this product does need to be rinsed. Left on the skin, it leaves a slightly sticky finish, and the strong fragrance from these pads isn't what you'd want to leave on your skin all day or night. The textured side of the pads allows for exfoliation during cleansing, and I am pleased to report this aspect of the pads is also gentle and fairly nonabrasive. These pads are best for someone with normal to dry skin who does not wear much makeup, or who is prepared to use these pads with a separate makeup remover.

☹ **Positively Radiant Anti-Wrinkle Cream** *($16.99 for 1.7 ounces)*. This relatively standard moisturizer is only capable of (temporarily) reducing the appearance of wrinkles, and that's about all you can expect from any moisturizer making anti-wrinkle claims. Aveeno is convinced that their "Soy Vitamin Complex" is chiefly responsible for this product's alleged age-diminishing ability. I keep searching for substantiated, independent research pertaining to soy (specifically, soybean seed extract) as an effective topical agent for warding off the signs of aging, but it still doesn't exist. What we do know is that soybean seed extract, which is prominent in this product, is a good antioxidant and anti-inflammatory agent for skin. That's positive, but it's also true of myriad ingredients in skin-care products, and in this one it just won't significantly get rid of wrinkles. This moisturizer would be a much better formulation had Aveeno not stuck with soy as the center-stage antioxidant, because the meager amount of vitamin E it contains is not of any consequence for skin. Moreover, their choice of jar packaging renders both ineffective, making this a nearly do-nothing moisturizer not worth considering over many others.

☺ **Positively Radiant Daily Moisturizer** *($16.99 for 4 ounces)* carries the claim that it is clinically proven to even-out skin tone, though the results of this study aren't available and an even skin tone often comes down to subjective assessment, which isn't saying much. Besides, it would also be nice to know what this product was being compared to in the clinical test, and whether or not skin was irritated before the product was applied. Regardless of the relatively meaningless statement "clinically proven," this is another one-note moisturizer whose only noteworthy ingredient is soy extract. As mentioned, soy has antioxidant and anti-inflammatory benefits for skin, but it would be better if Aveeno's products included more than soy because it is not the be-all and end-all antioxidant. The mica and titanium dioxide add a soft shine to skin (for radiance) and this lotion is best for normal to slightly dry or slightly oily skin. This is only recommended for daytime use if your foundation contains UVA-protecting ingredients and is rated SPF 15 or greater.

☺ **Positively Radiant Daily Moisturizer SPF 15** *($16.79 for 4 ounces)* shares the same claims and general formulary traits as the Positively Radiant Daily Moisturizer above, except this one is preferred for daytime because of its in-part avobenzone sunscreen.

☺ **Positively Radiant Daily Moisturizer SPF 30** *($16.99 for 2.5 ounces)* has a lighter-weight, drier-finish formula than either of the other Positively Radiant Daily Moisturizers, as well as offering longer sun protection, still with an in-part avobenzone sunscreen. It's an OK option for normal to slightly oily skin, assuming you don't mind the soft shine it leaves on skin.

☺ **Positively Radiant Eye Brightening Cream** *($16.99 for 0.5 ounce)* is one of the best products Aveeno offers, though not because it reduces dark circles and puffiness around the eyes, as claimed. Praise is warranted because of its excellent combination of silicones, glycerin, emollients, soy-based antioxidants, vitamins, and skin-identical ingredients, all in packaging that keeps the vulnerable ingredients stable during use. The mineral pigments in this cream produce a slightly reflective (what Aveeno refers to as "brightening") effect on skin, which can cosmetically blur dark circles—but the effect is gone if you stop using the product. This works best when paired with a good concealer.

☹ **Positively Radiant Tinted Moisturizer SPF 30** *($16.59 for 2.5 ounces)*. Although this tinted moisturizer is available in workable colors for fair to medium skin tones, it does not contain the UVA-protecting ingredients of titanium dioxide, zinc oxide, avobenzone (also known as butyl methoxydibenzoylmethane), Mexoryl SX, or Tinosorb and is not recommended. It is also doubtful that this contains enough soy to discourage skin discolorations, but without question the insufficient UVA protection will encourage more of what you don't want to see in the mirror.

☺ **Positively Radiant Triple Boosting Serum** *($15.79 for 1.7 ounces)* has a texture that is more like a lotion than a serum, but the prominence of silicones lends it a silky-smooth finish. Aveeno claims that this fragranced product has their highest concentration of Total Soy Complex, listed as soybean seed extract. They maintain soy will even skin tone, diminish discolorations, and shield skin against further wrinkles. It would be great if soybean extract could accomplish all of that, but it isn't possible. The good news is that research has shown that soy and its components, when taken orally in supplement form (particularly the antioxidants genistein and other isoflavones), have protective properties, such as shielding skin from UV light-induced damage and reducing inflammation (Sources: *Carcinogenesis*, March 7, 2006; and *Archiv der*

Pharmazie, December 2005, pages 598-601). In addition, limited in vitro and in vivo studies have shown that topically applied soybean seed extract increases collagen and hyaluronic acid synthesis in aging skin (Sources: *Photochemistry and Photobiology*, May-June 2005, pages 581-587; and *Journal of Cosmetic Science*, September-October 2004, pages 473-479), but that is true of lots of antioxidants, not just soy. Plus, none of that means soy will forestall wrinkles; you'll still need to wear an effective sunscreen every day and practice smart sun behavior, eat lots of antioxidants, and use skin-care products that are loaded with lots of antioxidants. This product would have been rated higher if Aveeno had included additional antioxidants and perhaps a cell-communicating ingredient or two.

AVEENO ULTRA-CALMING PRODUCTS

☺ **Ultra-Calming Foaming Cleanser** *($7.49 for 6 ounces)* contains feverfew extract, which Aveeno maintains will reduce facial redness and calm skin. However, according to published research, feverfew is a problem for skin because it causes contact dermatitis (Sources: www. naturaldatabase.com; *Medicinski Pregled*, January-February 2003, pages 43-49; and *Contact Dermatitis*, October 2001, pages 197-204). Feverfew is a plant producing pollen and also a must to avoid if you suffer from pollen-related allergies (Source: *Journal of the British Society for Allergy and Clinical Immunology*, January 1991, pages 55-62). This cleanser contains only a tiny amount of feverfew extract and so poses less of a problem, especially because it isn't left on the skin. With a gentle base and an array of skin-identical ingredients (though these are not particularly helpful for skin in a cleanser), this is a good option for normal to slightly dry skin. When complete makeup removal is an issue, a stronger cleanser would be needed. This cleanser is fragrance-free.

☺ **Ultra-Calming Daily Moisturizer SPF 15** *($16.99 for 4 ounces)* is recommended for its in-part avobenzone sunscreen, though I wouldn't call that or the other active ingredients in this moisturizer "ultra-calming." Many people tolerate the sunscreen agents in this product well, but a product positioned as "calming" would be better with just titanium dioxide and/or zinc oxide for sun protection. These mineral sunscreens have almost zero risk of causing irritation, which is what someone dealing with facial redness or rosacea should be considering. Because this sunscreen's base formula is listed in alphabetical order (which is within FDA regulations because it is an over-the-counter drug, not a cosmetic), the relative amounts of the different ingredients are not as clear as when ingredients are listed in descending order. However, it does contain fragrance—another faux pas for an "ultra-calming" product—and lacks antioxidants. If calming isn't your expectation, this sunscreen is an option, just not an exciting one.

☹ **Ultra-Calming Moisturizing Cream** *($16.79 for 1.7 ounces)* contains a significant amount of feverfew extract, which is irritating, not calming, to skin. In addition, it is an exceedingly basic formula that lacks significant amounts of state-of-the-art ingredients.

☹ **Ultra-Calming Night Cream** *($15.79 for 1.7 ounces)*. A moisturizer designed to soothe sensitive skin and reduce redness shouldn't contain fragrance or several of the other ingredients found in this product, such as alcohol and ethylene/acrylic acid copolymer. Aveeno also includes feverfew extract, a plant which has compounds that can cause irritation, rather than prevent it. Feverfew has been shown to have anti-inflammatory properties when consumed orally, and it sounds logical that that benefit should translate to skin if topically applied. However, there are at least 39 chemical components in this plant, and some of them are, in fact, irritating (Source: www.naturaldatabase.com). There are many better anti-irritants to consider, such as oat-derived beta-glucan, willow herb, and licorice extracts to name a few. Even if feverfew were a miracle anti-irritant, this moisturizer for normal to dry skin has an exceptionally bland formula that is void of any state-of-the-art ingredients. In many ways this formula is as out of date as the computer you bought in 1985. Lastly, the jar packaging won't help keep the feverfew stable, although that may actually lessen its irritation potential!

OTHER AVEENO PRODUCTS

☺ **Moisturizing Bar** *($3.39 for 3.5 ounces)* is an oat flour–based bar cleanser that is certainly less troublesome for skin than traditional bar soap. However, because the ingredients that keep this in bar form can leave a residue on skin, this isn't preferred to a well-formulated water soluble cleanser.

☺ **Skin Brightening Daily Scrub** *($7.49 for 5 ounces)* doesn't entice with lots of needless frills. Instead, this standard, effective scrub goes about its business of allowing you to polish your skin while also providing a cleansing action. It is suitable for all skin types except very dry.

☺ **Advanced Care Moisturizing Cream** *($9.49 for 6 ounces)* is a glycerin-rich lightweight cream for those struggling with eczema (also known as atopic dermatitis) or any degree of dry skin. The fragrance-free formula isn't too exciting, but it covers the basics in terms of providing ingredients that help restore a healthy skin barrier and prevent moisture loss. The amount of glycerin is very helpful for those with eczema (Source: *Acta-dermato Venereologica*, 2002, pages 45-47), but aesthetically it tends to leave a slightly tacky finish on skin. Don't let that stop you from trying this gentle moisturizer if eczema is a concern; the finish can be made to feel silkier by adding a couple drops of a nonfragrant plant oil such as jojoba or evening primrose.

☺ **Daily Moisturizing Lotion SPF 15** *($8.79 for 8 ounces)*. Labeling this a "breakthrough body lotion" is a joke because the only breakthrough component is the name. The in-part avobenzone sunscreen is great (and it's stabilized by the same ingredient Neutrogena uses in their Helioplex technology—remember Johnson & Johnson owns Aveeno and Neutrogena), but the base formula is a snoozer and completely devoid of antioxidants. The happy face is strictly about the sun protection; other than that, the formula isn't even a tiny bit interesting for mildly dry skin.

☹ **Essential Moisture Lip Conditioner SPF 15** *($3.69 for 0.15 ounce)* does not contain the UVA-protecting ingredients of titanium dioxide, zinc oxide, avobenzone, Tinosorb, or Mexoryl SX. Aveeno clearly recognizes the importance of UVA protection or they wouldn't be using avobenzone in their Continuous Protection sunscreens.

☺ **Continuous Radiance Moisturizing Lotion, for All Skin Tones** *($15.99 for 7.5 ounces)* is a moisturizer for body or face that contains the self-tanning ingredient dihydroxyacetone. The point of difference here is the dial-type dispensing system, which allows you to control how much self-tanning ingredient is dispensed into the lotion (half the product is self-tanner, the other half an ordinary lotion moisturizer). So you can control the amount of self-tanner that gets mixed into the lotion. It's a clever concept, but has its pros and cons. If you want a faster, darker tan, you would use this product up pretty quickly and be left with just the lotion portion, which has no special benefit. For subtle differences in lighter shades this is an option. The key point is that all self-tanners, regardless of how they are dispensed (lotion, gel, spray, mousse, and others) are more about application technique than anything else.

☺ **Continuous Radiance Moisturizing Lotion** *($8.99 for 8 ounces)* is nearly identical to the Continuous Radiance Moisturizing Lotion, for All Skin Tones, except without the separate dial-dispensing mechanism. Aveeno has an option for fair or medium skin tones, both with the same basic formula but with differing amounts of the self-tanning ingredient dihydroxyacetone. For facial use, this is best for normal to slightly dry skin.

☹ **Intense Relief Medicated Therapy** *($3.69)* comes in two formulas: The stick version uses 1% menthol as one of the active ingredients; the balm portion contains 1% camphor. Both serve their purpose as counter-irritants. What that means is the menthol and camphor in these products cause greater irritation on their own than the irritation or itching you may be feeling on your lips or skin. That's not healthy for skin, and this product is not recommended.

AVON

AVON AT-A-GLANCE

Strengths: Consistent UVA protection from almost all of the products with sunscreen; a few state-of-the-art moisturizers (some with sunscreen) at near-bargain prices; Avon Solutions cleansers; a selection of formidable concealers, powders, blushes, and lipsticks; the company provides complete ingredient lists on its Web site and offers some of the most helpful Customer Service associates in the industry.

Weaknesses: The Clearskin products are mostly irritating and poor choices for anyone battling blemishes; the Anew Clinical lineup won't make you cancel that upcoming appointment for whatever cosmetic corrective procedure you've booked; an overreliance on jar packaging diminishes the antioxidants found in many Avon moisturizers; the marriage of insect repellent with sunscreen is an imperfect union; endless, unnecessarily repetitive moisturizers with exaggerated, outlandish claims; several of the foundations look decidedly unnatural or have SPF ratings that are too low; average eyeshadows and pencils; mostly average to disappointing mascaras.

For more information about Avon, call (800) 500-2866 or visit www.avon.com or www.Beautypedia.com.

AVON SKIN CARE

AVON AGELESS RESULTS PRODUCTS

☺ **Ageless Results Renewing Eye Cream** *($13 for 0.5 ounce)* suffers from jar packaging, which is a shame because it contains several antioxidants. It is otherwise an emollient moisturizer for dry skin anywhere on the face. The mineral pigments titanium dioxide and mica are what's making the eye area appear "brighter."

☺ **Ageless Results Intensive Line Filler SPF 15** *($13 for 0.06 ounce)* includes titanium dioxide and zinc oxide for sun protection, and these mineral ingredients plus mica are what help "blur the look of fine lines." Avon claims this product reduces the look of deep wrinkles in two weeks, but that isn't possible. The base of this product is mostly heavy-duty thickeners and waxes. An intriguing ingredient in this product is retinoxytrimethylsilane. Also known by its trade name of SilCare 1M75, it's an Avon-patented blend of retinol, silicone, and soybean oil that is supposed to be as effective as "straight" retinol without the potential for irritation (Source: www.freepatentsonline.com/7074420.html). There is no published research substantiating the claims for this ingredient, so you're left to take Avon's word for it. However, in theory it should work similarly to retinol, though neither ingredient is capable of making deep, etched lines look significantly better. Avon wisely uses packaging that keeps this retinol derivative stable. This is worth trying for its value as a sunscreen and temporary line-filling effect—but don't expect results that turn back the clock to your pre-wrinkle days.

✓ ☺ **Ageless Results Renewing Day Cream SPF 15** *($15 for 1.7 ounces)* is an outstanding daytime moisturizer for normal to slightly oily skin. It contains an in-part avobenzone sunscreen and covers every base in terms of what skin needs to look and feel healthy, all in stable, hygienic packaging. Well done, and this is noticeably less expensive than some of Avon's pricier but less impressive moisturizers.

☺ **Ageless Results Overnight Renewing Cream** *($15 for 1.7 ounces)* contains mostly water, glycerin, silicone, thickeners, film-forming agent, absorbent, skin-identical ingredients, vitamins, ingredients that mimic the structure and function of healthy skin, more silicone, fragrance, and preservatives. The jar packaging hinders the stability of the vitamins (antioxidants), but this is still a good moisturizer for normal to dry skin.

AVON ANEW PRODUCTS

☺ $$$ **Anew Daily Resurfacing Cleanser** *($15 for 5 ounces)* is a good, basic, though fairly abrasive cleansing scrub for normal to very oily skin. It exfoliates skin and rinses cleanly. Be sure to scrub gently because the alumina crystals are more aggressive then you might think and you can easily over-scrub skin, hurting the skin's protective outer barrier.

☺ $$$ **Anew Luminosity Ultra Advanced Skin Brightener SPF 15** *($22 for 1 ounce)* is an in-part avobenzone-based sunscreen in a decent moisturizing base that contains mostly water, thickeners, slip agent, water-resistant agent, a long list of plant extracts, antioxidants (unfortunately, unstable due to the jar packaging), preservatives, and fragrance. This is a good option for someone with normal to slightly dry skin. Contrary to Avon's claims, Anew Luminosity does not contain any reliable amounts of ingredients known to inhibit melanin production or to lighten skin discolorations, other than the sunscreen itself. This does contain a tiny amount of uva-ursi leaf extract, although how much of this arbutin-containing plant is needed to produce satisfactory results, if any, is undetermined.

AVON ANEW ADVANCED PRODUCTS

☺ **Anew Advanced All-in-One Max SPF 15 Cream** *($16.50 for 1.7 ounces)* is an intriguing way to combine broad-spectrum sunscreen (including avobenzone for UVA protection) along with approximately 2% glycolic acid and the AHA ammonium glycolate. That amount is barely enough for sufficient exfoliation, though the product's pH is low enough for some to occur. The product is also loaded with antioxidants and contains retinol, but the jar packaging means they will be ineffective shortly after the product is opened. This is worth a look if you're curious to try a low-level AHA with sunscreen, and the formula is best for normal to slightly dry skin.

✓ ☺ **Anew Advanced All-in-One Max SPF 15 Lotion** *($16.50 for 1.7 ounces)* is similar to the Anew Advanced All-in-One Max SPF 15 Cream, except for two important differences: packaging that keeps the retinol and antioxidants stable, and larger amounts of glycolic acid and ammonium glycolate. It is an excellent daytime moisturizer for normal to slightly oily skin. The inclusion of enzymes is interesting, but the exfoliation and smoothing benefits this product provides are from the AHAs; the enzymes are too unstable to function in that capacity.

AVON ANEW ALTERNATIVE PRODUCTS

☹ **Anew Alternative Intensive Eye Cream** *($25 for 0.5 ounce).* Claiming to "attack the major signs of dark circles," this won't work beyond making them look less apparent if eye-area skin is dry (something any moisturizer applied to this area will do). Although Avon included over a dozen state-of-the-art ingredients, most are rendered ineffective once this jar-packaged product is opened. Further, Avon's idea of herbaceuticals for this product included a host of irritating fragrant oils, including peppermint, geranium, frankincense, and West Indian sandalwood. Lastly, this contains a high amount of neem extract (listed as *Melia azadirachta* flower extract) from a plant whose profile is a mix of positive and negative effects, and it has no research showing it is a panacea for dark circles (Source: www.naturaldatabase.com).

☹ **Anew Alternative Clearly C 10% Vitamin C Serum** *($20 for 1 ounce)* is a poorly formulated serum for two reasons: the vitamin C will not remain stable due to clear packaging that exposes it to light, and the first ingredient is alcohol, which causes dryness, irritation, and free-radical damage and increases oil production in the pore.

☺ **$$$ Anew Alternative Intensive Age Treatment** *($32 for 1.7 ounces).* Avon's use of words such as "herbaceutical" and phrases like "let the healing age begin" inspired much curiosity in this product, but, as is often the case in the cosmetics industry, the ad slogans and hype don't equal fact. What Avon has produced is a good AHA product, using ammonium glycolate and glycolic acid (at a pH of 3.7) for exfoliation. The AHAs are in a decent moisturizing base of glycerin, thickeners, film-forming agent, and silicone. Plenty of antioxidants are included, but Avon's choice of a jar container means they'll be ineffective shortly after the product is opened. One other ingredient of note in this product is 2-amino-4,5 dimethylthiazole HBR. In order to use this ingredient in their product, Avon signed a nonexclusive licensing agreement with Alteon, a biotech company. It is one of several ingredients Alteon has developed that they claim has an effect on advanced glycation end-products (AGEs). AGEs are abnormal, cross-linked, oxidized proteins that might play a role in the aging process. Here's how AGE affects skin. Sugars, particularly in the form of glucose, are one of the primary ways the body gets its fuel for producing energy and get up and go. Yet glucose, through an enzymatic trigger, can also attach itself to proteins anywhere in the body and form "glycated" substances (advanced glycation end-products or AGEs) that damage tissue by making it stiff and inflexible. AGEs directly affect the surface layers of skin, as well as structures beneath the surface such as collagen and elastin. At this point, we don't know whether AGEs can be stopped, or even inhibited, and there is no published research pertaining to 2-amino-4,5-dimethylthiazole HBR (also known as alagebrium or ALT-711) and its effect on wrinkles or skin. The research that does exist, from Johns Hopkins University, involved 13 elderly men and women with systolic hypertension. The study participants took either daily doses of alagebrium for eight weeks or a placebo. The results showed an improvement in the stiffness of the arteries. At best, this was a small study, and whether that result relates to skin is an even bigger leap of faith. But it does at least show that Avon is making attempts to be more cutting-edge than many of its high-priced competitors. The plant extracts in this product lend an intense fragrance that tends to linger on skin, so if you're considering purchasing this item, ask your Avon lady for a sample first! (Sources: *Journal of Investigative Dermatology*, December 2005; *Annals of the New York Academy of Science*, June 2006, pages 529-532; *Journal of Biological Chemistry*, April 2005, pages 12087-12095; and *Archives of Biochemistry and Biophysics*, November 2003, pages 89-96.)

☺ **$$$ Anew Alternative Intensive Age Treatment SPF 25 Day** *($32 for 1.7 ounces)* makes much ado about the fusion of Eastern and Western technology to create a product that reactivates the skin's healing process, but the big—legitimate—news is that this is an exceptionally well-formulated daytime moisturizer with UVA protection (it contains avobenzone). Although somewhat thick, it has the feel of a lightweight lotion and a soft finish appropriate for someone with normal to slightly oily or slightly dry skin. Housed in stable packaging featuring an airless pump applicator, the formula is loaded with antioxidants, anti-irritants (including several forms of curcumin—an Avon specialty), and ingredients that mimic the structure of healthy skin. The only drawback is the pervasive fragrance. I generally don't comment on a skin-care product's specific scent (it would be best for skin if there weren't any fragrance), but this one is perfume-like to the max, and definitely something to take into consideration before you purchase this otherwise outstanding product.

✓ ☺ **Anew Alternative Photo-Radiance Treatment SPF 15** *($25 for 1 ounce)* is a well-formulated daytime moisturizer for normal to dry skin. It contains an in-part avobenzone sunscreen, several antioxidants, cell-communicating peptides, and Avon's AHA blend of thio-dipropionic acid and ammonium glycolate at a pH of 3.6. In terms of exfoliation, I wouldn't expect too much despite the effective pH value. That's because the amount of AHAs is likely no more than 2%, an amount that provides more water-binding than exfoliating ability. Still, the other attributes of this product make it well worth considering. The mica and titanium dioxide combine to cast a soft, illuminated glow to skin.

AVON ANEW CLINICAL PRODUCTS

☹ **$$$ Anew Clinical Advanced Dermabrasion System** *($28 for 2.5 ounces)* is a new twist on topical scrubs that use alumina particles to try to mimic the kind of exfoliation that occurs with a microdermabrasion treatment. Avon's dual-sided, connected tubes house a lotion-based scrub on one side and what they refer to as an "advanced skin conditioner" on the other. The component's cap allows you to adjust the amount of product dispensed from each tube. Although clever, this is really just another topical scrub whose abrasiveness can be controlled by the user (but it can also be overdone). Most people will want to dispense more scrub than conditioner, because using too much conditioner won't prompt much exfoliation (which is OK if you want a really mild scrub). Regardless of the ratio of product you use, this is not the must-have solution for those with wrinkles, discolorations, or large pores. You cannot scrub away these skin conditions, and no scrub, no matter how it's packaged or dispensed, can make pores smaller. What this will do is smooth a rough skin texture and minimize dry, flaky skin. Keep in mind that a well-formulated AHA or BHA product is preferred over any scrub because it offers a greater range of benefits, including the diminishment of discolorations, improvement in blemishes, and stimulation of collagen production, with studies proving their efficacy.

☹ **$$$ Anew Clinical Advanced Retexturizing Peel** *($25 for 30 pads)* used to be sold as a part of a two-step system involving glycolic acid-steeped disposable pads followed by neutralizing pads (formulated at a higher pH to stop the exfoliating action of the AHA). Clearly consumers didn't like the two steps or Avon wouldn't have changed it. Besides, the neutralizing step was a waste of time anyway, since just splashing skin with tap water will stop the acidic action of chemical exfoliants. These pads are supposed to be akin to a 35% AHA peel, but don't count on it. The water-based pads contain about 10% ammonium glycolate with glycolic acid, at a pH of 4, so exfoliation will occur. However, alcohol is the fourth ingredient listed, and that increases the potential for irritation. Although effective (just not to the extent of a physician-administered AHA peel), there are better, less expensive AHA products available.

☺ **$$$ Anew Clinical Advanced Wrinkle Corrector** *($32 for 1.7 ounces)*. This is sold as the at-home answer to wrinkle-filling injections, but choosing this product over in-office cosmetic corrective procedures is like the difference between looking at pictures of Paris at night and actually being there. The amount of silicone in this product has a minor, spackle-like filling effect on superficial lines, and it does leave your skin feeling very silky. This also exfoliates skin, with a blend of AHAs (approximately 4%) in a pH of 3.6. Using this moisturizer for normal to slightly dry skin around the eye may cause irritation, not only from the AHAs and low pH, but also from the inclusion of a high amount of the sunscreen ingredient ethylhexyl methoxycinnamate, plus fragrance. There is research proving that AHAs stimulate collagen production, but none of the ingredients in this product can regenerate "hydroproteins" (unless that's a fancy way of referring to collagen again). The neutral face rating is due to the jar packaging, which won't keep the numerous plant extracts (antioxidants) in this "Wrinkle Corrector" stable during use. This contains mineral pigments that leave a slight shine on skin.

☺ **$$$ Anew Clinical Crow's Feet Corrector** *($29 for 0.66 ounce)* is another Avon product proclaiming that it can save you from the pain, time, and expense of cosmetic corrective procedures. There is nothing in this product that can remotely duplicate what a cosmetic dermatologist or plastic surgeon can do. The notion is as ludicrous as it is seductive, but it's all flash and dash, and that's bad for your skin and budget. This product involves two steps and is packaged in a sleek, dual-sided pen-like component. Before I discuss each product's formula, you need to know that in no way is this even vaguely akin to having skin (and wrinkles) resurfaced with lasers. Even Avon doesn't believe that, or why would they continue to sell dozens and dozens of other serums and eye creams claiming to get rid of wrinkles? If this product worked as claimed, anyone concerned with wrinkles around the eye could use it for a short time and need nothing else, but that's not the case. Step 1 is the Gentle Resurfacer. This water-based fluid dispenses from an angled tip. You're directed to massage eye-area wrinkles for one minute three times per week. It contains mostly water, slip agents, film-forming agents (think hairspray), mushroom extract, thickeners, preservatives, and cosmetic pigments. It is an ordinary, almost silly formula given the claims, and it doesn't resurface skin. Rubbing the skin is far more exfoliating in itself than anything this product provides. The coloring agents do provide a brightening effect, but that's a cosmetic effect, it isn't skin care. By the way, massaging wrinkles won't improve their appearance. If anything, manipulating the thin skin around the eyes can lead to sagging because it stretches the elastin in skin and makes wrinkles more pronounced. Step 2 is the Crease Filler. This is what Avon claims will reduce the length, depth, and number of crow's feet around the eyes. It contains mostly water, slip agent, a silicone polymer that has a soft spackle effect on wrinkles, emollient thickeners, and plant extracts. Not a single ingredient in this product can mimic the results of laser treatments; it isn't even a very interesting formula in terms of stimulating collagen production, repairing skin's barrier, or protecting from free-radical damage, three critical elements of great skin care. At best, this can temporarily fill in superficial lines around the eyes. Deep lines (the kind that you can still see even when your face is expressionless) will see no improvement. This gimmicky product is a waste of time and money.

☺ **$$$ Anew Clinical Derma-Full Facial Filling Cream** *($34 for 1 ounce)*. Reading the claims for Avon's latest wonder cream (and they launch these at breakneck speed) you just may be tempted to throw out every other Avon product you own—don't do that, because Avon isn't going to discontinue those. Clearly they don't quite trust that this one is the answer in comparison to all the other ones they sell. And the notion that this in any way is akin to injectable fillers is like suggesting a tricycle has a lot in common with a BMW. Give me a break! There is no way this moisturizer with glycolic acid (AHA) can even slightly approximate the results possible from dermal fillers or other cosmetic corrective procedures a dermatologist performs. This isn't even as well formulated as other Avon products. Other than the plumping effect, which you'll get from any moisturizer, you won't see your face restored to its full, lifted, youthful look; it simply isn't possible. But, of course, that doesn't stop companies like Avon from continuing to tempt gullible consumers who are desperate for a solution to an aging face. We've got to get a grip here. Nothing we apply topically can take the place of what happens when a dermal filler is injected into the lower layer (dermis) of skin in a precise, concentrated manner. There are no topical solutions to address the underlying causes of skin sagging. Like many companies making this claim, Avon included sodium hyaluronate, which is the salt form of a popular dermal filler material—hyaluronic acid—that is found in Restylane, Perlane, and Juvederm. As impressive as that sounds, lots of cosmetics companies include the same ingredient (sodium hyaluronate), so the claims would apply to just about any moisturizer with this ingredient. However, even if Avon included hyaluronic acid (the actual ingredient found in the real fillers) in a cosmetic it wouldn't penetrate through the skin, which is a good thing; you should see what happens to skin when a dermal filler is injected into the wrong area of the face—it isn't a pretty picture. What this moisturizer will do is make skin feel silky-smooth, help promote cell turnover, and provide a more even skin tone because it contains an effective amount of glycolic acid (most likely 5%) at a pH that permits exfoliation to occur. The peptides are a nice touch in terms of enhancing skin's ability to hold moisture, but the antioxidants will degrade due to the jar packaging. This is an OK option for normal to slightly dry skin, but in no way, shape, or form should you consider it "injectable-grade facial filler, now in a cream."

☺ $$$ **Anew Clinical Derma-Full X3 Facial Filling Serum** *($54 for 1 ounce)* is a less emollient version of the Anew cream version of this product. The misleading, flawed claims are the same for both products in terms of positioning them as a topical alternative to medical dermal fillers, most notably those that contain hyaluronic acid. The promise of dramatic firming and plumping isn't going to happen, nor will you see deep facial folds and hollowed cheeks diminish beyond the plumping action that occurs when you use any well-formulated moisturizer. As you might expect (at least by now I hope you would), the minimal amount of plumping you'll see is not even remotely akin to the results achievable from dermal fillers or other cosmetic corrective procedures. Such procedures are essential if you truly want to impact the age-related changes of deep wrinkles and sagging skin. Regardless of claims, no skin-care product can address the multiple causes of "aging" skin, such as loss of elasticity, shifting and decreasing fat pads, and loss of the muscle and structure that contributes to a youthful facial structure (to name just a few of the causes of an "aging" face). Although this is not an alternative (I mean really, what a joke!) to actually having dermal filler injected into your wrinkles, this is worth considering if you're looking for a lightweight AHA serum. It contains approximately 5% glycolic acid at a pH that allows exfoliation to occur, and includes a few good water-binding agents and cell-communicating peptides. The mica lends a shimmer finish to this serum, but it's subtle. Despite the claims, this doesn't contain pure hyaluronic acid like you'd get with a dermal filler used by a dermatologist, and even if it did contain the same material, it could not be absorbed into your skin or have any effect on any structures in the dermis.

☺ **$$$ Anew Clinical Expression Line Filler** *($35 for 0.5 ounce)*. You're supposed to believe that this product will regenerate the substances in your skin that naturally plump out any lines. The tacit message is that you'll save money, avoid painful injections, and see your wrinkles disappear just as though you had been to a professional. But, make no mistake about it: that is absolutely not going to be the case with this or any product claiming to replace cosmetic corrective medical procedures. Despite the fact that there are some outstanding skin-care ingredients in this product that can help generate new collagen, improve barrier function, and allow skin to produce healthier cells, there are no skin-care ingredients that function in the same manner as a dermal filler. Injecting substances such as hyaluronic acid or collagen into lines is vastly different in procedure and physiological response then from slathering those ingredients on your skin. When you apply ingredients used in dermal fillers (such as collagen or hyaluronic acid) to skin, they penetrate a few layers of the epidermis. Due to their ability to draw and hold moisture to the surface layers of skin, they have a slight plumping effect on wrinkles. When these same substances are injected into skin in a controlled manner, they work to lift the skin depression (such as a wrinkle) from the inside out, sort of like replacing worn springs in a mattress. The dermal filler plumps the wrinkle from underneath, giving (temporary) new spring to skin. Similar ingredients in a skin-care product can't do this regardless of the particle size (nanometer or otherwise). The main ingredients in this allegedly "concentrated" product are water, slip agents, algae protein, and mushroom extract, none of which can effectively fill in deep lines, although they can have a temporary minor smoothing effect on superficial lines, just like most moisturizers and serums. Avon includes several plant extracts in this product, and most of them function as antioxidants and/or soothing agents. Lesser amounts of cell-communicating peptides are also present, so this certainly isn't a throwaway formula; it's just one whose claims are misguided. You will notice that this product also contains hyaluronic acid, the same substance used in some dermal fillers. Although hyaluronic acid is a very good skin-identical ingredient, topical application isn't going to restore lost volume to skin or fill in wrinkles. All you have in this fairly expensive Avon product is a lightweight hydrating serum for all skin types except sensitive.

☹ **$$$ Anew Clinical Eye Lift** *($28 for 0.66 ounce)* is a two-part product packaged in one jar, and it's made out to be nothing short of an eye-area miracle. If you need to give your eyes a lift or get rid of puffiness, dark circles, or a loss of firmness, Avon insists you should look no further than this product, and they have impressive-looking statistics to back their assertions. However, there are no details of how they came to their conclusions or how many women were involved in their tests. ("Dermatologist-supervised" may sound official, but that doesn't mean that even one iota of their claims is true—since without the study in hand the claims are all embellishment with no substance.) The product consists of an Upper Eye Gel and an Under Eye Cream. The Gel is supposedly responsible for the lifting and tightening actions, yet it doesn't contain ingredients that have that effect. Along with water, glycerin, and slip agents are numerous plant extracts (including several antioxidants, but the jar packaging will make these air-sensitive ingredients ineffective shortly after opening), skin-identical ingredients, film-forming agents, preservatives, and coloring agent. It's a good, lightweight moisturizer with a gel texture, but sagging or drooping skin won't do an about-face. The Cream part is marketed as being able to "accelerate cellular metabolism" and alleviate under-eye darkness and puffiness. In contrast to the Gel, the Cream has a truly emollient texture with many beneficial ingredients for skin. None of them, however, will make dark circles or puffiness things of the past, and it's a shame that the many antioxidants are stalled by the product's jar packaging, though the Cream will unquestionably make dry skin around the eyes look and feel better. In addition, as with all well-formulated moisturizers, it will temporarily reduce the appearance of wrinkles. Cosmetically, the mica and titanium dioxide in the Under Eye Cream will help reflect light, diminishing the appearance of dark circles. Again, the effect is temporary and not as convincing as camouflaging dark circles with a good, neutral-toned concealer. The Cream does not list fragrance on the label, but it does contain fragrance components, so be careful about getting it too close to the lash line.

☹ **Anew Clinical Instant Face Lift** *($28 for 1 ounce)* lists alcohol as the third ingredient, which makes this too potentially irritating for all skin types. The lifting portion comes from the amount of PVP (a film-forming agent commonly used in hairstyling gels) in this water-based serum. When it sets on skin, you may notice a tightening effect, but no actual "lifting" is taking place. This contains tiny amounts of water-binding agents and antioxidants, but the alcohol's presence and the inclusion of menthol derivative menthoxypropanediol makes this a no-go.

☺ **$$$ Anew Clinical Plump & Smooth Lip System** *($25 for 2 ounces)* mentions fuller lips in its description but really plays up the "youthful" results this two-step system provides. Housed in a dual-sided, pen-style component, both steps provide a silicone-enhanced texture coupled with lip-smoothing emollients and some good antioxidants plus retinol. The plumping action doesn't come from those ingredients. Rather, just like most lip plumpers, this version uses irritants (peppermint oil and menthoxypropanediol) to incite fullness and increase circulation to lips, resulting in a rosier color. It's a temporary effect, but too irritating for routine use, so consider this only for special occasions.

☺ **$$$ Anew Clinical Professional Stretch Mark Smoother** *($25 for 5 ounces)*. Avon states that 9 out of 10 women have stretch marks, and that's fairly close to the statistics I've seen in research and literature about this skin complaint. That means there are a lot of women out there who would love to have a product that could do what this product claims to. Sadly, this product is neither clinical nor professional and cannot change the stretch marks on anyone's body. Ignoring the exaggerated claims, what this product ends up being is an alpha hydroxy acid (AHA) body lotion containing approximately 4% AHAs in a base with an effective pH of 3.5. The moisturizing base contains several ingredients that have benefit for skin in terms of supplying antioxidants, but that won't change a single stretch mark. Avon also included a small amount of menthol, probably to make your skin tingle when you apply it, so you'll think it is actually doing something. The menthol is indeed doing something, but what it's doing is called irritation, and that isn't helpful for any skin type. If it weren't for the menthol this would be a decent exfoliating moisturizer for sensitive skin. The one unique ingredient in this product is butea, a plant extract Avon claims can boost elastin production to prevent new stretch marks from forming. There isn't a shred of published research about this ingredient. Plus, stretch marks are damaged elastin fibers—they are permanently damaged, and cannot be repaired—so how could producing more elastin help? There's no proof that stimulating elastin production will repair stretch marks or prevent new ones from forming. So, you ask, what can improve the appearance of stretch marks? Various laser treatments have proven effective, as well as topical use of tretinoin (prescription-only ingredient found in Retin-A, Renova, Tazorac, and other products). While lasers and tretinoin can be effective, neither will completely eliminate stretch marks, and the results vary greatly, depending on the patient's skin tone and individual response to the treatments (Sources: *Dermatologic Surgery*, May 2008, pages 686-691; *Dermatologic*

Clinics, January 2002, pages 67-76; and *Archives of Dermatology*, May 1996, pages 519-526). Although the laser treatments and tretinoin are more expensive than this Avon product, at least there is research indicating that there is the potential for a positive outcome; all you get with Avon's product is a good but fairly ordinary AHA moisturizer.

☺ **$$$ Anew Clinical ThermaFirm Face Lifting Cream** *($32 for 1 ounce)*. Does Avon's alternative even come close to mimicking the effect of Thermage? Not in the least. This is a surprisingly lackluster formula for a cream advertised as having "potent ingredients." It consists primarily of water, slip agents, triglyceride, several thickeners, shea butter, film-forming agent, preservatives, a menthol derivative, several plant extracts, minerals, and a tiny amount of vitamin E. Avon refers to this as their "most advanced and powerful facial lifting product ever." Well, it isn't, at least not from any published research, or any research Avon is willing to part with, and not in comparison to other products Avon sells. At best, this is a decent moisturizer for someone with normal to slightly dry skin, but the menthol derivative (used in a small amount to create the impression that the product is doing something) isn't the best for any skin type.

AVON ANEW FORCE EXTRA PRODUCTS

☺ **Anew Force Extra Eye Cream** *($16 for 0.5 ounce)* contains Avon's patented ingredient trioxaundecanedioic acid (also known as oxa acid). It is said to be an effective exfoliant able to perform better than AHAs, without causing irritation. Yet examination of Avon's patent for this ingredient reveals that oxa acid, like AHAs, requires a pH range of 3 to 4 to be effective. With either of these ingredients, the trade-off for effective results is some amount of irritation from the acidic pH—so Avon's claim that this is a gentler alternative to traditional AHAs doesn't hold up, not even in their own patent! Further, the pH of this product is above 4, which is borderline for accomplishing any exfoliation, based on their own research. There isn't much else of note in this product; the antioxidants would be beneficial if this product did not use jar packaging.

☺ **Anew Force Extra Triple Lifting Day Cream SPF 15** *($22 for 1.7 ounces)* comes with claims that your face "will see a 60% improvement in fine lines and wrinkles in one week." If that happens in just a week, in two to three weeks you should be wrinkle-free, and that's not possible! Aside from the hype, this ends up being a decent moisturizer with a good SPF that includes avobenzone as one of the active ingredients. What makes this product unique, along with a few other Anew products, is Avon's trademark ingredient trioxaundecanedioic acid (also known as oxa acid). A patented ingredient, oxa acid is supposed to be effective as an exfoliant and to perform better than AHAs, without irritation. The only research supporting this notion is a very long, rambling patent held by Avon. What makes it confusing is that while one complaint about AHAs is that the low pH required to make them effective for skin can cause irritation, it seems that oxa acid, according to the patent, has the same problem: "in treating skin conditions [oxa acid] has been found to be affected by the pH of the composition … preferably in the pH range between 3.5 and 4.0." That's the same range that makes for effective use of AHAs. Nonetheless, if you wanted to give another exfoliant a try, this is one to consider, though the pH is definitely higher than the patent for this ingredient suggests. The lightweight lotion contains some good antioxidants, but the jar packaging is a problem.

☺ **Anew Force Extra Triple Lifting Night Cream** *($22 for 1.7 ounces)* won't lift anything and this isn't the best product in the Anew lineup, but it is a good basic moisturizer for normal to dry skin. It contains mostly water, silicone, thickeners, glycerin, Vaseline, more thickeners, Avon's patented oxa acid (see the review for Anew Force Extra Triple Lifting Day Cream SPF

15 above), preservatives, skin-identical ingredients, antioxidant vitamins, and fragrance. The jar packaging won't help keep the antioxidants stable, so they cannot be relied on.

AVON ANEW REJUVENATE PRODUCTS

☺ **$$$ Anew Rejuvenate 24 Hour Eye Moisturizer SPF 25 Day/Night Cream** *($30 for 0.66 ounce).* This two-part product provides an eye-area moisturizer with sunscreen for daytime, A.M. Eye Cream, and a no-sunscreen eye cream for nighttime use, P.M. Eye Cream. Sounds convenient, and the dual-sided jar packaging is clever, but cleverness and convenience don't always add up to good skin care, which is the case with this product. Aside from the jar packaging (Can you believe that?!), the main problem is that the directions for the A.M. Eye Cream, which contains synthetic sunscreen active ingredients, state that you should apply this to your eyelid. Doing that is not a good idea, because it's very likely that the sunscreen ingredients will migrate into your eye and cause irritation (and if you perspire while wearing this as directed, eye contact is guaranteed). For the eye area, titanium dioxide and zinc oxide are the only two active sunscreen ingredients you should use because they won't cause burning or irritation. If the eye area weren't the issue (though given the name and price that is how most women will use it), it does include avobenzone for UVA protection and is formulated in a lightly emollient, silky base. The main plant extract, *Tinospora cordifolia*, has research showing it has immune-stimulating effects when taken orally, and it also is an antioxidant (Sources: *Journal of Ethnopharmacology*, June 1999, pages 277-281; and *International Immunopharmacology*, December 2004, pages 1645-1659). However, there is no research demonstrating the effectiveness of this plant when applied topically. Plus, stimulating the immune system can't affect dark circles or reduce puffiness, which is what this eye cream claims to do. The P.M. Eye Cream is similar to but silkier than the A.M. Eye Cream and, as mentioned, does not contain sunscreen. Both products contain several antioxidants and retinol, but these ingredients are wasted due to the jar packaging, which allows them to degrade and reduces their potency over time. This duo can help make slightly dry skin anywhere on the face look better, but the sunscreen portion should not be applied as close to the eye as Avon recommends.

☹ **Anew Rejuvenate Flash Facial** *($48).* I can't imagine anyone struggling with oily skin, with large pores, and with worries about wrinkles not being tempted by the claims for this serum. Despite the exceedingly high price for an Avon product, I'm betting this will find its way into lots of women's skin-care routines. Unfortunately, that will be a regrettable waste of money. What you are supposed to believe is that this product is similar to an aesthetician cleaning your pores by doing thousands of micro-extractions. That exaggerated claim is just stunning, because this is not a new way to resurface skin or reduce pore size; it doesn't have any positive impact on pores whatsoever. There are products that can temporarily make pores appear smaller, and anything with a matte finish will create this illusion, but nothing permanent is taking place (which you'll see as soon as you wash your face—everything is back to normal). This serum from Avon contains some good absorbent ingredients and silicone for a silky texture, but the combination of slip agents and thickeners won't make for a long-wearing matte finish capable of keeping excess shine in check for long, and I can assure you that the illusion of smaller pores vanishes quickly. Speaking of shine, Avon added it to this serum by including mica. What a bad ingredient choice if what you wanted to do was maintain a matte look and keep oily skin looking refined instead of greasy! Actually, aside from the inane claims, this would have been a well-formulated serum-style moisturizer if it weren't for the menthyl lactate it contains. This menthol derivative is responsible for the serum's cooling sensation, but that's not a benefit, it's an irritant response. For the same amount of money, those with normal to oily skin would be better off using Estee Lauder Idealist Pore Minimizing Skin Refinisher, and for half the price, any of the Olay Regenerist serums are also worth considering. One more comment: Anyone who has ever had professional extractions done knows that the process does not make pores look smaller. If anything, extracting a blackhead often leaves the pore looking larger because once the plug is removed the space within the pore where it was is then exposed (the blackhead fills in some depth that is exposed once the plug is removed). Simply removing a blackhead, whether via manual extraction or with a well-formulated BHA product, is not going to change pore size (though it will improve pore function and likely result in fewer breakouts).

☺ **Anew Rejuvenate Night Revitalizing Cream** *($32 for 1.7 ounces).* Here's one more Avon product promising to help you fight the appearance of aging skin. This time the results are supposed to be similar to a "professional antiaging facial." What a ridiculous claim. First, what exactly is an antiaging facial? To me, it's a vague description that defies comparison, but it does sound impressive. What is certain is that it doesn't work anything like peels or micro-dermabrasion, and when it comes to traditional facials, well, they don't work to prevent aging either. This product ends up being a lightweight moisturizing cream containing Avon's AHA alternative (thiodipropionic acid) along with salicylic acid. Although this blend has the potential to be effective for exfoliation (hardly unique to this product), the cream's pH of 4.4 is too high to ensure exfoliation will occur. Unlike the serum version of this product (Anew Rejuvenate Flash Facial) this cream version omits the irritating menthyl lactate, which is good news. Mica is still included for a shiny finish, but this product is ultimately too emollient to make pores look smaller for long, despite the claim. It does contain some great ingredients for normal to dry skin, but many of them will begin to deteriorate once the jar packaging is opened. Whether you choose to waste your money on an antiaging facial (whatever that means) or this product, either way you won't end up with younger-looking, refined skin.

☹ **Anew Rejuvenate Dial-A-Glow Anti-Aging Moisturizer SPF 15** *($32 for 1.7 ounces).* This self-tanner with built-in sunscreen leaves skin vulnerable to UVA damage because it does not contain the UVA-protecting ingredients of titanium dioxide, zinc oxide, avobenzone, Tinosorb, or Mexoryl SX. As such, it is not recommended.

AVON ANEW ULTIMATE PRODUCTS

☺ **$$$ Anew Ultimate Contouring Eye System** *($30 for 0.59 ounce).* As you may well suspect, nothing about this two-part product has the power to "reshape, repair, and recontour" your eye area—this isn't an eye-lift in a jar, and neither formula should be packaged in a jar in the first place! One part of the dual-sided jar contains **Concentrated Elixir**. This nonaqueous moisturizer has an emollient silkiness and contains enough silicone and wax to serve as a temporary spackle for lines around the eyes. How long the effect lasts depends on how expressive you are and on what else you apply to the eye area (e.g., foundation, concealer). Concentrated Elixir contains the plant oil from *Perilla ocymoides*. Although this oil is a great source of fatty acids for skin and has been shown to have an anti-inflammatory effect when consumed, it is also known to cause contact dermatitis. This is attributed to two constituents present in the oil: 1-perillaldehyde and perillalcohol (Source: www.naturaldatabase.com). Avon would've done better to include a nonproblematic oil, such as evening primrose or borage. The Elixir also contains several ingredients that will quickly lose their potency thanks to the jar packaging.

This includes a form of retinol mixed with liquid silicone (retinoxytrimethylsilane), which is really disappointing. The second part of the product is labeled **Intensive Repair Cream**. It is neither intensive nor reparative in the least because it contains nothing more than water, slip agents, gel-based thickener, preservatives, and iron oxides for color, all-in-all a formula that would have been considered antiquated even 20 years ago. Taken together, Anew Ultimate Contouring Eye System is a mediocre system with the additional misfortune of being stuck in a jar. None of the antioxidants, retinol, or peptides can reduce under-eye bags or sagging skin, nor can they restore elasticity.

☺ **$$$ Anew Ultimate Night Age Repair Cream** *($34 for 1.7 ounces)* is a good AHA moisturizer for those with normal to slightly dry skin who prefer a creamy texture. The blend of ammonium glycolate and glycolic acid seems to be present in an efficacious amount, and the pH of 3.6 permits exfoliation. Avon also includes a smaller amount of antioxidants and plant-based water-binding agents, but the jar packaging won't keep them stable once this product is in use. Still, this has merit if you're looking for a well-formulated AHA product.

☺ **$$$ Anew Ultimate Day Age Repair Cream SPF 25 UVA/UVB** *($34 for 1.7 ounces).* This daytime moisturizer with AHAs has a lot going for it and is definitely a product to consider if you want to combine an in-part avobenzone sunscreen with the exfoliating power of AHAs. This silky, slightly thick cream for normal to dry skin contains a blend of glycolic acid and ammonium glycolate at approximately a 3% concentration and has a pH of 3.6. It is light enough to work well under makeup, too. The downside is the jar packaging, which won't keep the antioxidants and peptides this contains stable during use. You can ignore Avon's claims that this product stimulates youth proteins and restores natural volume to aging skin—this isn't surgery in a jar and there is no such thing as "youth proteins" (there aren't old proteins either). Natural volume in the face is about muscle tone and fat deposits; this product will not do anything to increase or change those aspects of your face. What this will do is provide broad-spectrum sun protection and exfoliation, a combination that is traditionally difficult to pull off because sunscreens require a higher pH to remain stable in emulsions, while AHAs work best at lower pH levels. Somehow Avon has succeeded (NeoStrata also sells sunscreens with AHAs), and that, plus how silky-smooth this feels on skin, are compelling reasons to give this daytime moisturizer an audition.

☹ **$$$ Anew Ultimate Age Repair Elixir** *($54 for 1 ounce)* is disappointing and doesn't match some far better offerings from Avon. It contains mostly water, thickener, slip agents, alcohol, more slip agent, film-forming agent, silicones, more film-forming agent, and a handful of exotic plant extracts. The two promoted peptides are present in tiny amounts, and neither has the ability to lift or firm skin, nor can they restore lost elasticity. And another thing: What is this much alcohol doing in a product designated as skin-repairing? All told, the story behind this product is far more fascinating than the results, and it isn't worth considering over serums from Olay, Neutrogena, Clinique, or Paula's Choice.

☹ **$$$ Anew Ultimate Elixir Premium** *($68 for 1 ounce)* is supposed to retighten and lift skin's structure on the face and neck, all thanks to Avon's Pro-Sirtuin technology. Sirtuins are proteins that help regulate certain biological processes by controlling the chain of events that cause these processes to happen, which is why they're often referred to as information regulators. The antiaging connection has to do with their potential to regulate the cellular processes responsible for aging. It is believed that if certain sirtuins can be modified to work against the mechanisms of aging then the results may be visible on skin (think fewer wrinkles, less sagging, and greater resiliency). However, it's much more likely that any research into sirtuin manipulation will be carried out primarily in an effort to reduce or control age-related degenerative diseases. At best this research is in its infancy and there is no evidence that it is possible or even safe. Of course, those annoying facts don't stop some cosmetics companies from jumping on the youthful skin connection and parlaying the research about sirtuins into skin-care products. What seems promising is that topical application of specific sirtuins derived from yeast and the red grape component of resveratrol (Avon doesn't use either source) seem to have a protective effect on skin in the presence of oxidative and ultraviolet light stress. However, far more research is needed before I'd suggest anyone run out and look for products that increase sirtuin activity in their skin. Not only is there limited research showing how much and what type of sirtuin is needed topically to cause desirable (as opposed to the potential for undesirable) cellular changes leading to younger skin; but also the bioavailability of a topically applied source of sirtuins is questionable given that we don't know how efficiently they penetrate intact skin. (Testing skin cells in a lab setting with concentrated doses of ingredients that stimulate sirtuins often doesn't translate into how it works in skin-care products.) An even bigger concern is that whenever normal cellular processes are manipulated, you run the risk of causing a potential overproliferation of cells, which is the blueprint for cancer. In other words, how would the sirtuin-influenced cells know when too much of a good thing becomes a health-threatening problem? (Sources for the above: *Current Medicinal Chemistry*, 2008, pages 1887-1899; *Journal of Drugs in Dermatology*, June 2007, pages 14-19; and *Nature Reviews: Drug Discovery*, June 2006, pages 493-506). Getting beyond the sirtuin story (and there's no reason to believe any ingredient in this serum will have the claimed effect), it is very disappointing that there's alcohol in this product. The amount likely is too low to cause much harm, but it's listed before several state-of-the-art ingredients, which doesn't make this a serum to contact your Avon salesperson about. When you really examine the formula, the name for this product is downright embarrassing. It isn't "ultimate" or "premium" in any way, save for the deluxe packaging! The only way it can possibly defy the effects of gravity on your face is if you apply it while hanging upside down from a trapeze.

☺ **Anew Ultimate Night Gold Emulsion** (*$34 for 1.7 ounces*). Another Anew Ultimate product. It's funny how there are so many ultimates in the Avon product line, yet if any of them ultimately worked, why would they be launching new ones with such regularity? At least this one is an effective AHA gel-textured moisturizer. It contains approximately 5% glycolic acid and Avon's own AHA ingredient—thiodipropionic acid and trioxaundecanedioic acid. The very fragrant formula is infused with particles of gold shine, no doubt in an effort to reinforce the product's name, not really to provide a precious benefit to skin. Despite the gel texture, this can leave oily skin feeling too slick and greasy. It is best for normal to dry skin.

Pay no mind to Avon's claims that their Pro-Sirtuin TX technology stimulates this special class of proteins. (Sirtuins are types of proteins involved in metabolism, cell growth cycle, and DNA repair.) Lauder also claims to have a special ingredient that does this, reseveratrol, a component of red wine, which of course is completely different from Avon's ingredients. Resveratrol does have research showing it is a very potent topical antioxidant, but neither Lauder nor Avon has research proving they can now reverse aging. As far as Avon's formula goes, there is no research proving any of the peptides or other ingredients in this product, or in any product, have an effect on sirtuins in your skin. Even if they could, Avon's choice of clear jar packaging won't keep the ingredients stable once the product is opened.

AVON CLEARSKIN PRODUCTS

☹ **Clearskin Cleansing Pads for Normal to Oily Skin** *($4.29 for 42 pads)* lists alcohol as the second ingredient, followed by witch hazel and, further down, menthol. Alcohol causes dryness, irritation, and can trigger oil production in the pore lining, which is exactly what those struggling with acne don't need.

☹ **Clearskin Immediate Response Acne Cleanser** *($5.29 for 5.1 ounces)* contains 2% salicylic acid, but it's just wasted because it is rinsed from skin before it has a chance to get into the pore and work. This gel cleanser also contains a drying detergent cleansing agent and the irritant menthyl lactate, which has no effect on reducing redness and swelling from acne. Your skin's immediate response to this cleanser won't be positive, that's for certain!

☹ **Clearskin Purifying Astringent Blackhead Clearing Formula** *($4.29 for 8 ounces)* lists alcohol as the main ingredient, which makes this astringent too irritating for all skin types, plus alcohol stimulates oil production in the pore. The 2% salicylic acid is coupled with a pH above 4, so exfoliation will not occur.

☹ **Clearskin Immediate Response Spot Treatment** *($4.99 for 0.5 ounce)* contains 2% salicylic acid and is formulated at an effective pH of 3.8. What a shame the base for this spot treatment contains enough alcohol to make it an irritating prospect for all skin types. Alcohol increases oil production in the pore, too.

☹ **Clearskin Professional Acne Treatment System** *($34)*. Avon heavily promotes this trio of anti-acne products as an even better version of the popular infomercial brand ProActiv. You can go ahead and read this entire review for the details if you like, or you can stop right now, because I can assure you that this system is not as effective as ProActiv. The reasons, you ask? (1) the formulas include needless irritants and (2) they do not include a topical disinfectant to fight the bacteria that contribute to acne. Avon claims their exclusive zinc hexapeptide-11 ingredient warrants their superior difference because it helps control surface oil. That's not much of a claim when you consider how many other cosmetic ingredients have the same action, such as kaolin, certain silicone polymers, talc, and aluminum starch to name a few. If it can work in some other manner, there is no published research proving that to be true, so consumers just have to take Avon's word for it and the ingredient manufacturer's (and we all know how trustworthy cosmetics companies can be about their claims—not to mention, this isn't the first product Avon has claimed would clear up your acne, clearly the ones that came before didn't work so well). Avon makes a great fuss of the fact that this ingredient is exclusive to their formula but exclusivity doesn't equate to exclusive results. Their oil claim is not unique and their ingredient not the only apple in the barrel. Interestingly, however, there is a growing body of research demonstrating zinc's second-tier role in minimizing acne. The research deals primarily with the oral consumption of zinc, but there have been some intriguing in vitro studies as well that show zinc's role as an anti-inflammatory agent when applied to cultured skin cells. One study compared the effects of topical application of zinc acetate with the effects of common disinfectants such as benzoyl peroxide and topical antibiotics. The zinc acetate didn't win out as the superior choice, but it reasonably held its own by comparison (Sources: *Seminars in Cutaneous Medicine and Surgery*, September 2008, pages 170-176; *European Journal of Dermatology*, November-December 2007, pages 492-496; *Journal of the European Academy of Dermatology and Venereology*, March 2007, pages 311-319; and *The Journal of Dermatological Treatment*, 2006, pages 205-210). However, none of these studies examined what role zinc hexapeptide-11 may have in mitigating acne, reducing inflammation, or affecting oil production. There are three products in this kit: a cleanser/scrub, pre-soaked medicated pads, and a salicylic acid (BHA) lotion. The **Deep Pore Cleansing Scrub** contains a tiny amount of the abrasive agent polyethylene mixed with water, clay, detergent cleansing agent, and alcohol. It features 0.5% salicylic acid as an active ingredient, but this small amount and the fact that the product is rinsed from the skin before it can have a benefit assures minimal to no efficacy. In addition, the scrub also contains menthol, which is irritating, and the formula isn't the easiest to rinse from skin, so we're not off to a good start. Step 2 involves swabbing your skin with **Clarifying Toner Pads**. Avon again disappoints with an alcohol-laden formula and irritating cinnamon bark extract. Alcohol causes free radical damage, inflammation, encourages oil production in the pore lining, and hurts the skin's healing process. What a shame, because there are some state-of-the-art ingredients in this product. The last step is to apply the **Daily Correcting Lotion**, which contains 0.5% salicylic acid, just like the pads in step 2. As a leave-on BHA product this almost has merit for skin. The small amount of salicylic acid isn't necessarily ideal, but the serious cause for concern is the amount of alcohol in this lotion. All told, there is little reason to try this kit. What Avon claims makes it unique isn't proven, and even if it worked as claimed, at best you'd enjoy less oily skin at the expense of causing lots of irritation and doing little to kill acne-causing bacteria. ProActiv and any other cosmetics company making effective yet gentle anti-acne products have nothing to worry about with this problematic trio from Avon. Actually, the dermatologist being profiled in ads for this kit should be ashamed to be fronting for such poorly formulated products.

AVON SOLUTIONS PRODUCTS

☹ **A.M./P.M. Solutions Maximum Moisture Refreshing Day Cleanser/Makeup Removing Night Cleanser** *($12.50 for 6.8 ounces total).* Packaged in one jar are two cleanser formulas: one for daytime and one for evening. The idea is to use a lighter, gel-based cleanser in the morning and a heavier, lotion-like cleanser at night when makeup removal is what you need. There is no logic in using different cleansers in the morning versus the evening. The **Refreshing Day Cleanser** is a gentle option for normal to oily skin, though it isn't great at removing makeup. The **Makeup Removing Night Cleanser** is far too emollient for anyone whose skin is other than normal to dry. It does dissolve makeup, but it isn't easy to rinse without a washcloth and would be problematic for someone with normal to oily skin or skin prone to blemishes. So, to recap, this product contains two different products with two different formulas, one good for normal to oily skin, and the other good for normal to dry skin—they are not both suitable for the same skin type. One well-formulated, gentle water-soluble cleanser for your skin type is all anyone needs. Not to mention that the jar packaging makes the cleansers tricky to use.

☺ **A.M./P.M. Solutions Total Radiance Day Cream SPF 15/Night Cream** *($17.50 for 2.6 ounces total).* Housed in one jar component with a divider between compartments is a daytime moisturizer and a nighttime moisturizer. The daytime moisturizer sensibly contains an in-part avobenzone sunscreen and has a lightweight base suitable for normal to slightly dry skin. The formula contains several intriguing ingredients, but most of them will degrade after opening the jar package. The Night Cream has a richer, silkier texture that's best for dry skin. However, one of its main plant ingredients (Aframomum melegueta) is a type of pepper that contains a volatile oil and other chemical constituents that can be irritating, while imparting no benefit to skin (Source: www.naturaldatabase.com). This plant likely won't retain much of its irritation potential after the product is opened, but inclusion of this amount is still concerning. Note that both products in this duo also are sold separately.

☹ **A.M./P.M. Solutions Total Radiance Refreshing Day Cleanser/Makeup Removing Night Cleanser** *($12.50 for 6.8 ounces total)* is a problematic cleansing duo because both cleansers, which are quite similar, contain the drying detergent cleansing agent sodium C14-16 olefin sulfonate as a main ingredient. The A.M. Formula contains the menthol derivative menthyl lactate, which only makes matters worse.

☺ **Solutions Plus Total Radiance Micro-Exfoliating Cleansing Cushions** *($12.50 for 28 pads)* are textured pads soaked in a standard water soluble cleanser. The pads work well to cleanse skin and remove makeup, but must be used gently to avoid irritating skin. The fact that these contain fragrance doesn't make them suitable for sensitive skin as claimed.

☹ **Solutions Plus Total Radiance Thermal Cleanser** *($12.50 for 3.4 ounces).* This cleanser contains a high amount of magnesium sulfate, an ingredient that, when mixed with water, causes a chemical reaction that generates heat. The sensation may feel nice, but it does nothing to open pores or allow for a deeper cleansing. If anything, exposing skin to this much warmth can be irritating and put skin at risk for broken capillaries. This also contains polyethylene scrub beads to polish skin. It's an OK option as a scrub and the vitamins and other intriguing ingredients are there more for show than effect.

☹ **A.M./P.M. Solutions Maximum Moisture Day Cream SPF 15/Night Cream** *($17.50 for 2.6 ounces total).* This "solution" for your skin includes a day cream with sunscreen and a nighttime moisturizer—two products packaged in one jar component. This may seem handy in terms of saving space, but the Day Cream doesn't provide sufficient UVA protection because it doesn't contain the UVA-protecting ingredients of titanium dioxide, zinc oxide, avobenzone (may be listed as butyl methoxydibenzylmethane), Tinosorb, or Mexoryl SX and is not recommended. The Night Cream has a lush emollient texture suitable for dry skin, but it contains irritating eucalyptus. Plus, the jar packaging won't keep the teeny amount of beneficial ingredients stable after opening. Overall, this is a problem product all around!

☹ **$$$ Solutions Plus Maximum Moisture Eye Cream** *($12.50 for 0.5 ounce)* is a very standard moisturizer that contains a tiny amount of antioxidants whose effectiveness won't last long thanks to the jar packaging. What matters more is that this eye cream contains irritating eucalyptus. Irritation of any kind isn't good for skin, especially on the face, and it definitely isn't good for the eye area.

☹ **Solutions Plus Total Radiance Eye Gel** *($12.50 for 0.5 ounce).* This water-based eye gel isn't a solution for anyone's skin, at least not if the goal is improvement. Irritating witch hazel is a major ingredient, and it is closely followed by aluminum starch, which does little to moisturize skin. This contains an impressive assortment of antioxidants and cell-communicating ingredients, but the jar packaging won't keep them stable. Even in better packaging, the witch hazel base is a mistake.

AVON SKIN SO SOFT PRODUCTS

☹ **Skin So Soft Bug Guard Plus IR3535 Expedition Gentle Breeze SPF 15 Pump Spray** *($12 for 4 ounces)* is a combination insect repellent and sunscreen, but it is not recommended due to the absence of UVA-protecting ingredients and the presence of a high amount of alcohol (which doesn't create "skin so soft").

☹ **Skin So Soft Bug Guard Plus IR3535 Insect Repellent Unscented SPF 15 Sunscreen Spray** *($10 for 4 ounces)* may work to keep mosquitoes and flies away, but fails to provide sufficient UVA protection, while the amount of alcohol is irritating to skin, especially when paired with the chemical insect repellent.

☹ **Skin So Soft Bug Guard Plus IR3535 SPF 15 Sunscreen Cooling Gel** *($12 for 4 ounces)* is similar to the other Skin So Soft Bug Guard products, only in gel form. The same concerns about the lack of UVA-protecting ingredients and high amount of alcohol apply here, too.

☹ **Skin So Soft Bug Guard Plus IR3535 SPF 15 Sunscreen Spray** *($10 for 4 ounces)* contains a different blend of active ingredient to repel insects, but its sunscreen actives and the presence of alcohol match those of the other Skin So Soft Bug Guard products, and it is not recommended.

OTHER AVON PRODUCTS

☺ **Moisture Effective Eye Makeup Remover Lotion** *($4 for 2 ounces)* is a very basic, but effective, water- and oil-based makeup remover. It is fragrance-free and gentle enough to use around the eyes, though it is best used prior to washing with your regular cleanser.

☺ **Dramatic Firming Cream** *($8.50 for 1.7 ounces)* is a lush, emollient moisturizer that provides basic care for dry to very dry skin. It contains a smattering of antioxidants, including potent pomegranate. However, Avon's choice of jar packaging won't keep them stable once you begin using it.

☹ **Hydra-Radiance Intensive Nutrient Night Serum** *($12.50 for 1 ounce)*. Composed primarily of water, film-forming agent (think hairspray-hold ingredient), and alcohol, this serum isn't intensive in a good way regardless of whether it's used at night or not. It contains lesser amounts of some notable ingredients for skin, but the amount of alcohol is too irritating and no one needs this much hair spray. The visible glow you'll get from applying this serum comes from cosmetic pigments, not from any of the vitamins or minerals in this poorly formulated serum. Avon is completely capable of making better formulas than this, but they usually cost more; perhaps this is the bargain offering? Still, even at a bargain, they could have done a better job.

☺ **Lighten Up Plus Undereye Treatment** *($15 for 0.5 ounce)* won't lighten under-eye circles, but is a well-formulated lightweight moisturizer for slightly dry skin. Its silicone content promises a silky finish (great for prepping the eye area for concealer) and it contains vitamin-based antioxidants and some good skin-identical ingredients.

☺ **Moisture Therapy Intensive Extra Strength Cream** *($5.99 for 5.3 ounces)* is a very basic and rather boring moisturizer for dry skin that contains mostly water, mineral oil, Vaseline, thickeners, plant oils, silicone, preservatives, and fragrance.

☺ **Nurtura Replenishing Cream** *($8 for 1.7 ounces)* contains mostly water, thickener, antioxidant plant oils, sunscreen agent, glycerin, more thickeners, preservatives, fragrance, and coloring agents. The jar packaging will keep the plant oils from exerting an antioxidant benefit, but this still addresses the basic needs of dry skin.

☺ **Rich Moisture Face Cream** *($4.99 for 3.4 ounces)* is hardly rich, not with alcohol as its third ingredient. This is a very dated, very basic moisturizer that is barely passable for normal skin.

☺ **Banishing Cream Skin Discoloration Improver** *($8.50 for 2.5 ounces)* used to contain hydroquinone as its active ingredient, but Avon opted to remove this controversial, yet effective skin-lightening agent. Unfortunately, they did not replace the hydroquinone with anything that can produce the same results, so any lightening effect from this product is purely coincidental! Without the hydroquinone, this is a ho-hum moisturizer whose tiny amount of antioxidants is rendered insignificant thanks to jar packaging.

☺ **Care Deeply with Aloe Lip Balm** *($0.99 for 0.15 ounce)* is a standard, effective petrolatum-based lip balm that does its job of making dry, chapped lips feel better. For under one dollar, that's not such a bad deal!

⊗ **Moisture Therapy Intensive Moisturizing Lip Treatment SPF 15** *($1.99 for 0.15 ounce)* lacks sufficient UVA protection, so it is not a good choice for daytime wear if your goal is sun protection for the lips. This is otherwise a fairly standard, emollient lip balm that also contains some good antioxidants and emollient oils, which makes the lack of UVA protection that much more disappointing.

AVON MAKEUP

FOUNDATION: ✓ ☺ **Beyond Color Line Softening Mousse Foundation** *($12)* makes a big deal about the vitamins it contains, but they're barely present in this silicone-based foundation—plus the jar packaging won't keep them potent once the product is opened. Despite that bit of bad news, this foundation has an amazing, almost otherworldly texture that, true to claim, is "light as air" and blends flawlessly. It provides sheer to medium coverage with a silky-soft matte finish, which makes this appropriate for normal to very oily skin. Someone with any degree of dry skin won't appreciate this foundation's finish, though it is far from being a flat, dulling matte. The nonaqueous formula is long-lasting and will require more than a standard water-soluble cleanser for complete removal. Among the 12 mostly beautiful shades, only Warmest Beige suffers from being too peach. The remaining shades include excellent options for fair to dark (but not very dark) skin.

☺ **Anew Age-Transforming Compact Makeup SPF 15** *($15)*. The only skin-looks-younger claim you can count on with this silicone-based compact foundation is the sun protection it provides, and that does count for something. However, the other specialty ingredients are there for show and little more. The sunscreen is in-part titanium dioxide and provides reliable UVA protection. This cream foundation has an initially greasy feel that smooths over skin evenly and sets to a satin finish that feels slightly powdery, but your skin doesn't look the least bit powdered. You'll get sheer to light coverage and this does a fairly good job of not sinking into large pores or wrinkles on the face. It contains some intriguing ingredients, including a retinol blend, but the way this is packaged means it will routinely be exposed to light and air; the compact is larger than most cell phones. Taken on its merits as a foundation with sunscreen, this is a very good option for those with normal to dry skin not prone to blemishes. The range of shades is uniformly excellent. Although several shades look off-putting in the compact, they soften considerably when blended on skin.

☺ **Beyond Color Skin Smoothing Cream Foundation SPF 15** *($12)*. This cream foundation is also called Beyond Color Skin Smoothing Compact Foundation. For our review, we used the name that appears on the product package; the latter is how it is listed on Avon's Web site. It promises to make skin look firmer instantly, but in the words of Mary Poppins, that's a "piecrust promise: easily made, easily broken." Although this foundation contains some notable antioxidants and a retinol complex, those aren't going to firm your skin as instantly as claimed (or even in the distant future), especially when you consider that the packaging will allow the air-sensitive ingredients to be routinely exposed to light and air. What about the foundation itself? It has a silky-smooth, slick texture that slides easily over skin and sets to a soft powder (in feel) finish. Its appearance on skin is satin-like, and as such this is best for normal to dry skin not prone to blemishes. Sun protection is assured with titanium dioxide, though it contributes little to coverage because this foundation goes on quite sheer. Among the dozen shades, there are some great options for fair to tan skin tones. The following shades are too orange or peach to recommend: Buff, Toffee (also known as Caramel), and Porcelain (this would look terribly peach on most fair skin tones).

☺ **Anew Beauty Age-Transforming Foundation SPF 15** *($16)* is a beauty first! This silky liquid foundation not only provides an in-part titanium dioxide sunscreen, but contains approximately 3% glycolic acid at a pH of 3.4, which permits exfoliation. It blends smoothly and offers light to medium coverage with a satin finish that feels moist. So why didn't this innovative foundation receive a Paula's Pick rating? Because, for all its positive traits, it looks very much like a layer of makeup sitting on top of your skin. The formula settles easily into lines, large pores, and facial crevices, and trying to soften this effect noticeably diminishes the coverage it provides. If you decide the benefit of sun protection and AHA exfoliation is worth the trade-off, there are some suitably neutral colors among the 14 shades. The following shades are best avoided due to peachy overtones: Porcelain, Natural, Warmest Beige, and Toffee.

☺ **Ideal Shade Cream-to-Powder Foundation SPF 15** *($10)* claims to contain essential true-tone pigments to match any skin tone, but that doesn't explain why several shades of this cream-to-powder makeup don't resemble real skin tones in the least. Cover Girl and L'Oreal did much better with their foundations for which they make similar claims. More creamy than powdery, this compact foundation with an in-part titanium dioxide sunscreen applies smoothly and blends easily—you can quickly achieve sheer, uniform coverage. The finish hints at being powdery, but any oily areas will be showing shine before you know it. This is a potential winner for those with normal to dry skin. Many of the 18 shades are impressive and blend on softer than those from Avon's Ideal Shade Liquid Foundation SPF 10, reviewed below. The ones to avoid due to overtones of pink, peach, or orange include Light Ivory, Cream Beige, Medium Beige, Soft Honey, and Nutmeg. The darkest shade, Earth, is not that dark and isn't suitable for most African-American skin tones.

☺ **Ideal Shade Liquid Foundation SPF 10** *($10)*. This silky-smooth liquid foundation applies and blends superbly and sets to a radiant, lightweight satin finish that enhances skin while providing light to medium coverage. This feels and looks natural (though make no mistake, it's still makeup), but many of the 16 shades are too peach, pink, orange, or copper. Avoid Light Ivory, Medium Beige, Amber, Nutmeg, and Spice, and consider Pure Beige and Creamy Natural carefully. There's also the issue of the SPF rating. No matter that the sunscreen ingredient is solely titanium dioxide, the SPF is too low for daytime protection. If you decide to try this otherwise very good foundation and are willing to pair it with a product rated SPF 15 or greater, it's best for normal to slightly dry or slightly oily skin. This does contain a rather strong fragrance.

☺ **Ideal Shade Mousse Foundation Stick SPF 10** *($10)* is a stick foundation that should have a higher SPF rating than it does. Given the active ingredients, I wouldn't be surprised if this passed the SPF 15 level during testing, but for whatever reason Avon opted to label it as SPF 10. Because of that, this is not a great all-in-one option for a foundation with sunscreen. The slick, slightly greasy texture is easy to blend and sets to a soft satin finish best for normal to dry skin that's not prone to blemishes. It feels surprisingly light, provides moderate coverage, and looks more natural than stick foundations from several years ago. I wish the colors were better, though. As is, only a handful resemble real skin tones. Avoid Natural Beige, Creamy Beige, Medium Beige, Pure Beige, Earth, and Nutmeg.

CONCEALER: ☺ **Anew Beauty Age-Transforming Concealer SPF 15** *($10)* provides the benefits of an illuminating concealer, an in-part titanium dioxide sunscreen, and glycolic acid in one concealer. The pH of 3.6 allows the glycolic acid (present at about 3%) to exfoliate, but such exfoliation isn't needed for the under-eye area, which is precisely where this concealer is likely to be applied. The click-pen applicator dispenses the product onto a brush, and although initially too slippery, it sets quickly to a matte (in feel) finish that has a soft shimmer. Coverage is moderate; this hides minor redness and dark circles, but requires layering for more pronounced flaws. Six shades are available: Natural Golden is slightly peach but may work for some medium skin tones; Natural Deep turns slightly ash due to the amount of titanium dioxide it contains; Natural Medium is too pinky-peach and best avoided. Based on the formula, this will make skin smoother and protect it from sun damage—just be cautious about using it too close to the eye due to the acidic pH.

☺ **Beyond Color Radiant Lifting Concealer** *($7)* cannot lift skin anywhere, anymore than any cosmetic can. This liquid concealer is outfitted with a precision brush applicator to facilitate application. It does indeed make application convenient, but this product provides such sheer coverage it doesn't do a respectable cover-up job on even minor flaws. If your camouflaging needs include dark circles, broken capillaries, or blemishes, this won't make you happy. For those with near-perfect skin and barely noticeable imperfections who need only minor coverage, this product is worth checking out. It takes longer than usual to set, but once it does, the satin-matte finish lasts well. Five mostly excellent shades are available—watch out for the too-peach Medium, and use caution with Deep, which women of color may find too dark for most African-American skin tones (though it's a great, non-ashy shade).

☺ **Ideal Shade Concealer** *($6)*. This twist-up stick concealer has a thick texture with minimal slip, so initial application is tricky. It is best applied in small dots that you blend together with a concealer brush or clean fingertip. The fact that this concealer has minimal movement impedes blending a bit, but ends up being advantageous because it stays in place and is prone to only minor creasing into lines. Ideal Shade Concealer provides excellent coverage, so unless you have a very dark spot or extreme redness you'll be pleased with the results. Almost all of the shades are recommended. Be careful with the slightly peach Light Medium and avoid the orange-y Dark shade. Fair, Light, and Neutral are the best of the bunch. Two more comments: The waxes and thickening agents make this concealer a poor choice for use on blemishes. Also, this contains ethylhexyl methoxycinnamate, a sunscreen ingredient that may cause irritation when used around the eye. If you notice any stinging or burning when you use this concealer, it may very well be due to this ingredient.

POWDER: ✓ ☺ **Anew Beauty Age-Transforming Pressed Powder SPF 15** *($12)*. This mica-based powder (it also contains a small amount of talc) provides great sun protection with its in-part titanium dioxide and zinc oxide sunscreen. It has a silky, dry texture yet a very smooth application that blends well and provides more coverage than a standard pressed powder. Given the amount of titanium dioxide and zinc oxide, the finish feels matte, but the mica lends a soft sheen so your skin isn't left looking flat or dull. This doesn't soften the look of lines and wrinkles any better than other highly rated powders, but it doesn't exaggerate them either. Most of the six shades are commendable and will work for fair to tan skin tones. Nude Beige is slightly peach, while Dark Beige tends to go on a bit orange and looks slightly ash once blended. This pressed powder with sunscreen is best for normal to dry skin, and it is fragrance-free.

✓ ☺ **Ideal Shade Loose Powder** *($9)*. This talc- and mica-based powder is said to contain light-adjusting pigments so your skin looks its best in any light. The goal is to "glow without the glare," but I've never seen any powder look glaring on anyone's skin, although they can look shiny. Just to be clear, cosmetic pigments used in powders (such as iron oxides) have nothing to do with shine—that's where the mica (a pearlescent mineral pigment) comes into play.

The good news is that this loose powder does add a glow without adding noticeable "glaring" shine. You won't see an adjustment taking place as you go from indoor to outdoor lighting as claimed (other than what light does to shiny particles on the face normally); rather, this powder looks fantastic on skin regardless of the lighting. It has a beautifully silky texture and seamless application; its overall effect and formula are best for those with normal to dry skin. With the exception of Tawny (which is too peach for most medium skin tones), all of the shades are great, including the two offered for darker skin tones.

✓ ☺ **Ideal Shade Pressed Powder** *($9)*. Just like the loose-powder version of Ideal Shade, Avon's pressed powder claims to contain light-adjusting pigments so your skin looks its best in any light. There is much less mica in Ideal Shade Pressed Powder than in the Ideal Shade Loose Powder, but its finish on skin is every bit as glowing (and, yes, not glaring). This smooth, dry pressed powder makes skin look finished without appearing over-powdered. It has a lovely sheer application and absorbent matte finish, making it best for normal to oily skin. All of the shades are soft and neutral, with options for fair to dark (but not very dark) skin tones. Forget the light-adjusting claims—you won't see that happening on your skin as you move from one light source to the next. Instead, this pressed powder looks great regardless of where you are.

BLUSH AND BRONZER: ✓ ☺ **True Color Bronzer** *($10)* is an excellent talc- and silicone-based pressed bronzing powder. The texture is supremely smooth, application is even, and the color payoff is impressive. What a find for those looking for a matte finish bronzer! Only one shade is available, but it's versatile enough to work for most medium skin tones (light skin tones can use it too, but should apply it sheer). This bronzing powder contains some emollient ingredients that make it potentially problematic for blemish-prone skin.

☺ **Smooth Mineral Blush** *($9)*. Using loose powder is not the best way to apply blush, even if you're a fan of mineral makeup. Avon's version has a smooth yet noticeably dry texture that must be applied very sheer or it tends to deposit unevenly, making skin look blotchy instead of softly blushed with color. The shine is of the sparkling variety and it clings decently. Although I suspect most women who want powder blush will prefer pressed instead of loose, this is a viable option for shiny cheeks.

☺ **True Color Blush** *($8)* has a smooth, dry texture and soft, non-powdery application. The palette offers enough enticing options to make this a worthwhile option, but bear in mind that every shade has at least a slight shine. Rose Lustre and Golden Glow Light/Medium have the most shine, though the latter is an acceptable shimmer powder for evening. Earthen Rose is a great tan color for contouring.

☺ **Be Blushed Cheek Color** *($8)*. It's always upsetting when an inferior product replaces a superior option, and that's what we have here. Gone is Avon's brilliant Split Second Blush Stick, whose silky texture and translucent powder finish were benchmarks in the cream-to-powder blush category. Now we have Be Blushed Cheek Color, and it pales by comparison. The powder finish of Split Second Blush Stick has been replaced by the moist, sheer finish of Be Blushed, although both blend on quite well. Be Blushed comes in an array of soft, shimmer-infused colors that gives normal to dry skin an attractive sheen, but it doesn't wear as well as a cream-to-powder formula would. If you were not a fan of Split Second Blush Stick and want a creamier, sheer blush this is worth considering—although it is not recommended for anyone prone to breakouts in the cheek area because the ingredients that create the moist finish and keep this in stick form can exacerbate blemishes.

☺ **Smooth Mineral Blush Duo** *($10)* offers a loose-powder blush or bronzer along with a loose-powder highlighter in one jar. The two products have their own half of one component, and a dual sifter mechanism with a closure is included to keep things tidy. Though the formula is technically mineral-based because it contains mica (a mineral that makes powders shine), the majority of the ingredients in this duo have nothing to do with minerals. That's not a problem at all, just an observation that this product isn't as natural as it's made out to be. Both the blush/bronzer and highlighting powder have smooth, almost creamy textures and apply smoothly (though not as easily as a pressed-powder blush or bronzer). The highlighting powder has a strong iridescent finish that looks more glaring than beguiling. In particular, the Barbie® doll-pink shade of the Warm Ice duo is the fast track to 1980s overdone pastel blush. The other Duos fare better and work best for light to medium skin tones. If you opt to use both products, keep in mind that this much shine is best reserved for evening makeup, and the shine does cling well.

EYESHADOW: ☺ **Heavenly Soft Eyeshadow Trio** *($7)* has a silky softness that's almost creamy and an application that's smooth, even, and nearly flake-free. The question of whether to purchase this comes down to sheerness: every trio deposits minimal color that is too soft for a classic eye design. That is, none of the colors are dark enough for use as liner and the potential crease colors need lots of layering to show up. You'll get sparkling shine that's not too distracting, but that's the most impact these shadows make. If you desire very sheer color for eye makeup, the best sets to consider are Brown Trio, Nude Trio, and Plum Trio.

☺ **Smooth Mineral Eyeshadow** *($8)* is certainly a messier way to apply powder eyeshadow, mineral or not. Pressed powder eyeshadows are simpler and easier to apply. For the record the main minerals in Avon's formula are the same as those used in most eyeshadows, even though they're not marketed or labeled as mineral makeup. On a positive note, compared to other loose mineral powders, Avon took care to choose packaging that minimizes the mess, so if you're extra careful, this works well as a silky-smooth powder eyeshadow with a finish that is either a sparkling shine (Bronzestone, Pixie Dust, Russet, and Pink Sapphire) or a soft shimmer (all the other shades). The shine stays in place reasonably well, though some flaking is inevitable. The gray-blue Breeze shade is the only one to consider avoiding, unless you intend to apply it sheer.

☺ **True Color Eyeshadow Single** *($4)* has a silky, dry texture and sheer application that goes on smoother for the lighter shades than it does for the deeper hues. The shade range is divided into mattes, metallics, and shimmers. Only a few matte shades are available, but they're all genuinely matte. The shiny shades are best for unwrinkled eyes or for judicious use on the brow bone. Whether or not these wear for 12 hours as claimed is debatable. The sheer colors don't go the distance and although the deeper shades hold up better, how long any eyeshadow lasts depends on what you use with it and how you apply it.

☺ **Anew Beauty Eye Lifting Serum Shadow** *($10)* is a liquid eyeshadow that's elegantly packaged and outfitted with a brush applicator that fans out to cover large areas (such as the entire eyelid) or it can be used to define small areas. The water-based formula has nice slip and as such is easy to blend, while the color applies sheer. The downside is the somewhat tacky finish and the iridescent/metallic finish of the shades. Another issue is that the formula contains fragrance and fragrant plant extracts, neither of which are wise to apply to the eyelid or near the tear duct. Needless to say, this won't lift skin anywhere, and the shine can draw attention to wrinkles, not visibly reduce them as claimed.

☺ **Color Trend Dreamy Cream to Powder Eyeshadow** *($2.99)* is an OK cream-to-powder eyeshadow that's packaged in a lip gloss-like squeeze tube with an angled applicator. It is best to apply this to the back of your hand and then dab with a brush to apply to the eyelid area. Application is somewhat uneven, but it can be blended to a sheer powder finish that is minimally prone to creasing and fading. The main issue has to do with the colors, almost all of which are pastel and more garish than attractive. Pink Opal is decent, and Mochachino is preferred, but that's about it. The Shadow Paints from L'Oreal's HIP line are better and easier to work with, and the slightly higher price for the L'Oreal product is worth it.

☺ **Glazewear Diamonds Eye Color** *($7)*. This liquid eyeshadow applies easily without having problematic slip, so you can blend it fairly easily, and it sets to a matte finish (in feel only) that does a decent job of staying put. Those with oily eyelids will get some creasing from this product, and everyone will notice some amount of flaking from the shine particles, which are present in each shade. The color range is limited and on the sheer side, but there are some good options. Avoid Turquoise Dream unless you're dreaming of vividly colored eyelids. If you want to try a superior version of this product, check out L'Oreal's HIP Cream Shadow Paint at your local drugstore.

☹ **Jillian Dempsey for Avon Professional Eyeshadow** *($9)*. Jillian Dempsey is a makeup artist Avon hired to spruce up their makeup line with some "professional" products. I wondered if this would mean an improvement in their makeup collection or did Avon mean that the existing products in the line were unprofessional? Either way, this isn't an improvement. This set includes one cream and two powder eyeshadows. The cream eyeshadow is a good option if you prefer this type of shadow (because it sets to a semi-powder finish), but the powder shadows are sheer and although they apply smoothly, flaking occurs even if you're careful to tap the brush before applying. The fact that 2/3 of this eyeshadow set are merely average not only makes it a tough sell, but also undermines the professional designation Avon was going for. Revlon and L'Oreal have better cream and powder eyeshadows at this same price point.

☹ **Perfect Wear Extralasting Powder Eyeshadow** *($8)* is a loose-powder eyeshadow that comes with a pointed sponge-tip applicator. Why these products keep showing up is anyone's guess—a pressed-powder eyeshadow is so much easier to work with. Although this isn't all that messy to use and the formula sets almost immediately and then doesn't move, you're still left with a stripe of intense shine that may temporarily blind anyone who catches your gaze (OK, I'm exaggerating, but you get the idea). The sponge-tip applicator hurts more than it helps; however, even if you shake some powder out and attempt to apply it with an eyeshadow brush, it grabs on skin right away and won't move, which you might at first think is a good thing, but only if a stripe of glitter is what you are looking for. With all of these drawbacks, does it really matter how long this lasts?

☹ **Smooth Mineral Eyeshadow Duo** *($9)* offers two shades of loose-powder blush packaged in one jar each, side by side and controlled by a dual sifter mechanism with a closure that keeps everything nice and tidy. Despite the name, the majority of the ingredients in this duo have nothing to do with minerals; that's not a problem, it's just an observation that this product isn't as natural as it's made out to be. The lighter shade in each duo is sheer and laced with sparkles that have poor cling, so expect consistent flaking as the day, or night, goes by. The darker shade is suitable for contour or, when used wet, eyelining. It is richly pigmented and applies smoothly (a little goes a long way). Because of the loose format, some flaking is inevitable during application, which doesn't make this preferred over pressed-powder eyeshadows. If you decide to try this anyway, the only duo to avoid is Earthly Blues—earthy blue shades should stay where they originate, on the earth, not on your eyes.

☺ **True Color Eyeshadow Quad** *($8)* has a smooth texture but not the best application. Every shade in these quads is shiny (and the shine tends to flake), making for an overall eye design that's shine overload, not to mention that most of the color combinations are unworkable or predominantly blue, green, or purple.

☹ **Eye Artist Eyeshadow Trio** *($8)*. This trio of powder eyeshadows is housed in a large compact with a large black and white illustration of an eye. The three shades are striped in a wave pattern over this image, meant to resemble how they should be applied on the eye area—but, please, don't follow this pattern, it is too extreme and contrasting. Even the application leaves much to be desired; it is sheer, powdery, and barely shows up on skin no matter how much you apply. Although well-intentioned in terms of showing color placement, the imagery used doesn't help, and poor application is a problem.

☹ **Beyond Color Radiant Lifting Eyeshadow** *($7)* doesn't just add color to eyes, it also claims to reduce lines, wrinkles, and crepey skin while providing a "lifted appearance." Should you cancel your cosmetic surgery appointment? No way! The antiaging ingredients include a selection of B-vitamin polypeptides along with antioxidant vitamins A, C, and E—all listed after the preservative, meaning their presence is insignificant. As an eyeshadow, this product has a thick texture that applies unevenly; it tends to get chunky and then thinner as it is blended. The mostly pastel and pale neutral colors have shimmer, and enough of it to make less-than-smooth eyelids look wrinkled, plus the formula creases slightly. None of this is great news, and makes this difficult to recommend.

☹ **In a Wink Instant Eyeshadow Sheets** *($9)*. Now this is something I haven't seen before and that says a lot, given how many thousands of products I've reviewed over the years! Avon has crafted press-on sheets of eyeshadow meant to simplify eyeshadow application. You simply peel away the plastic cover, position it over your eyelid and under-brow area, press and rub to transfer the shadow, and remove. Avon then advises you to blend with your fingertips, which isn't a smart way to achieve a beautiful eye design; any professional makeup artist worldwide will tell you it's best to blend shadows with brushes, not fingers. But Avon assumes you're in a hurry, so why not? Unfortunately, if time is of the essence, this isn't the eyeshadow solution you may be hoping for; it isn't practical, reasonable, or attractive in the least. The main problems are that these pre-cut sheets won't fit every woman's eye shape—those with small eyes are out of luck, as are those who don't have a prominent eyelid area. As you press and rub this over the eye area, the color transfers readily, but depending on how much you rub the result can look decent to muddy, like a paint-by-numbers project gone horribly wrong. The powder shadow is easy to blend with your fingers, but again, that's not the tool to use (brushes are preferred). Besides, these shadows don't cling very well so they will fade, flake, and crease during the day. Nice try, Avon, but this is a time-waster, not a time-saver, wink-wink!

EYE AND BROW SHAPER: ✓ ☺ **Perfectly Portable Liquid Eye Liner** *($7.50)*. This tiny, slightly stout container of liquid eyeliner includes a felt-tip pen-style brush that applies color evenly. The richly pigmented formula dries quickly and stays put without flaking or smearing. For the money and ease of precise application, it is an outstanding liquid eyeliner. Warm Brown is the only shade available, but it's wearable.

☺ **Color Trend Mini Eye Liner** *($0.99)* is a standard eye pencil except that it's small, roughly half the size of a normal eye pencil. It applies smoothly though sheer, and building color for more intensity leads to some smearing and fading during wear. If you don't mind sharpening and are going for a smoky eye (where you'll smudge the eyeliner for a diffused effect), this is an inexpensive pencil to consider. Avoid the Midnight Blue shade, which isn't dark blue, but actually an aquamarine shade that isn't flattering.

☺ **Feeling Fine Ultra Thin Eye Liner** *($6)* is an ultra-thin, automatic, nonretractable eye pencil that applies effortlessly and sets to a long-wearing finish. It's easy to create a thin or thick line with this pencil, but note that every shade is shiny, and will leave either a shimmer or metallic finish. That won't make a less-than-taut or wrinkled eyelid look any better, but if that doesn't apply to you, this remains a terrific pencil to consider.

☺ **Glimmersticks Waterproof Eye Liner** *($6)* applies easily and the retractable pencil doesn't require sharpening, which is always a plus. These glide so well you'll need to be extra careful to not over-apply, and each slightly to moderately shiny shade sets to a fairly immovable finish. True to the name, this is a waterproof formula, though it does come off with a water-soluble cleanser.

☺ **Glimmersticks Brow Definer** *($6)* has been improved and now this automatic, retractable brow pencil is a strong contender for enhancing brows. Its four colors (including a good option for blonde brows) go on smoothly and evenly, each with a soft powder finish that lasts.

☹ **Anew Beauty Smoothing Eye Liner** *($8)*. "Smoothing" is a good word to describe the effect this eye pencil has on making skin along the lash line look better. Application is also smooth, and despite the fact that the formula remains creamy to the touch, it is only minimally prone to smudging or fading. The shade selection presents mostly classic options. The Emerald shade is worth considering because it is a deep green with black undertones that doesn't look even a little outlandish. If you don't mind routine sharpening, this is a good, inexpensive pencil to consider (it would rate a happy face if sharpening weren't required).

☹ **Big Color Eye Pencil** *($6)* is a standard chunky pencil with a smooth, silicone-enhanced application and a soft, slightly creamy finish. Every color is quite shiny and most are pastel, but if that's your thing these do hold up reasonably well.

☹ **Satin Gel Eye Liner** *($7)* is the least expensive gel eyeliner available, but it ends up disappointing regardless of your budget. They have less intense color and a drier consistency upon application than others in this category. Application with a liner brush is recommended but challenging due to the dry nature of this eyeliner, and you'll need to layer it if you are looking for a darker, more defined line. This gel liner wears well through the day, but the color is disappointingly sheer. Be warned, if you're still committed to giving this liner a try, the Pearl colors are filled with glitter flakes that lack any sort of subtlety.

☹ **Smooth Minerals Eye Liner** *($6)*. This slightly creamy pencil has a smooth application that sets to a soft powder finish. It is slightly prone to smearing and fading; this isn't the pencil to choose if you expect perfect wear all day. It requires routine sharpening. As for the minerals, they're a minor part of the formula so consider them marketing more than functional or even remotely necessary.

☹ **Smooth Over Eye Definer** *($6)* is an eye pencil that needs routine sharpening, yet it holds up better than most, meaning that you won't eat up most of the pencil sharpening it because you need a new point, which wastes a lot of product. Application is undeniably smooth and even—getting a perfect line is a cinch—and although this remains slightly creamy it sets to a long-wearing finish. This pencil isn't advised if you have oily eyelids or watery eyes, but fans of traditional eye pencil should check it out.

☺ **Ultra Luxury Brow Liner** *($5)* is an ordinary brow pencil that has a typical dry texture, but it is easier to apply than most. The price is right, and this is one to consider if you prefer brow pencil to powder and don't mind routine sharpening.

☺ **Ultra Luxury Eye Liner** *($5)* has an attractive price for a standard pencil that applies easily and offers a smooth, dry finish. This is still prone to mild smearing as the day wears on.

☹ **Jillian Dempsey for Avon Professional Kohl Eyeliner** *($6)* has a smooth, powdery texture, but application leaves much to be desired. As you apply the color it goes on heavy in one place along the lash line and becomes weak and choppy in others, so the result is spotty and inconsistent unless you layer it carefully. The problem? Layering helps even things out, but then causes the dry-finish formula to flake. Oddly, using the sponge tip on the opposite end to soften/smudge the line doesn't help matters.

☹ **Glimmersticks Eye Liner** *($6)* is an automatic, retractable pencil with a texture that's too creamy to last for long, particularly as eyeliner. If you prefer pencils, there are better ones available in this price range from Revlon, L'Oreal, and others.

LIPSTICK, LIP GLOSS, AND LIPLINER: ✓☺ **Glazewear Diamonds Lipstick** *($8)* is positioned as a high-performance gloss and luxury lip color in one, and it is. Essentially it's a lip gloss in lipstick form; what sets it apart (aside from some riveting sheer colors) is its smooth, moisturizing yet non-slippery texture and a glossy finish that's free of stickiness. Another plus: These last longer than a standard lip gloss, so frequent touch-ups aren't necessary. This isn't a foolproof product for anyone prone to lip color bleeding into lines around the mouth, but it is a must-try if you love the high shine and shimmer that many lip glosses provide but dislike their brevity.

✓☺ **Glazewear Liquid Lip Color/Glazewear Metallics Lip Gloss** *($6)* is a very good, medium-coverage lip gloss that has a slick application and a non-sticky, glossy finish. The color range is extensive and gorgeous, owing to this product's deserved popularity. Avon occasionally rotates in Glazewear Metallics Lip Gloss, which differs little from original Glazewear save for its metallic finish.

✓☺ **Hollywood Lights Lip Gloss** *($7.99)*. Get this: When you cap the gloss and go to apply it, the underside of the cap lights up to—you guessed it—put your lips in the spotlight! Although clever, it's an unnecessary addition that ties in with Avon's "shine a light on your lips" claim. The gloss itself is marvelous! It's lightweight, applies smoothly, has a non-sticky finish and illuminates lips with an attractive (not the least bit overbearing) glossy sheen. As the Hollywood saying goes, "you gotta' have a gimmick." Lip gloss doesn't need gimmicks, but in this case it's fine because the gloss itself is such a great, inexpensive find.

☺ **Perfect Wear Extralasting Lipstick** *($8)*. This silky, lightweight lipstick is supposed to be transfer-resistant, but it isn't. Even once it sets to a slight matte finish it comes off easily—on cups, significant others, napkins, forks, spoons, and anything else your lips touch. The good news is that the color intensity is so strong that it takes several hours for the color to fade to the point where a touch-up is necessary (though all bets are off if you try to get through an entire meal with this intact). The only other point worth mentioning (other than Avon's impressive, versatile shade selection) is that this isn't the most comfortable lipstick unless you're used to the somewhat dry feel of matte and other transfer-resistant lipsticks. That's not a deal-breaker, but know beforehand that this isn't going to feel lush and creamy for long.

☺ **Pro 3-in-1 Lip Wand** *($9.50)*. There isn't anything particularly professional about this product, but it is a clever, convenient way to combine lipstick, lipliner, and lip gloss in one product. Slightly longer than a standard ballpoint pen, this Lip Wand contains a standard creamy mini lip pencil on one end, a sheer, non-sticky lip gloss in the center, and a mini cream lipstick on the other end. As Avon states, all of the shades are coordinated. You'll go through the pencil and lipliner quickly if you use this daily; it's best for travel, when it's convenient to have all of your lip products together in one component.

☺ **Ultra Color Rich 24-Karat Gold Lipstick** *($8)* is a good, lightweight cream lipstick whose creamy, slightly slick finish isn't for anyone who has problems with lipstick bleeding into lines around the mouth. The "24-karat gold" in the name is because each shade is infused with particles of gold glitter. Although the effect isn't as garish as it sounds, I must say that as this lipstick wears off the glitter begins to feel a bit grainy. Otherwise, most of the shades are attractive and this certainly has a gleaming finish that puts the spotlight on your lips.

☺ **Ultra Color Rich Lipstick** *($6.50)* is a traditional creamy lipstick with a large selection of full-coverage colors, most with a satin finish. The Sheer SPF 15 colors are not recommended due to their lack of sufficient UVA protection.

☺ **Color Trend Mini Lip Liner** *($0.99)*. Although it's one of the least expensive lipliners around, you get only about half as much product as you do with others. The oil-based formula applies well, and there is enough talc to promote a soft matte finish that stays in place reasonably well. You have to tolerate routine sharpening, but at this price that's not such a bad trade-off. The color selection is small, but all are pigment-rich, which aids in longevity.

☺ **Glimmersticks Lipliner** *($6)*. If it weren't for this automatic, retractable lipliner's somewhat tacky finish, it would be among the best for smooth application and ability to keep lipstick from feathering into lines around the mouth. As is, it's recommended for those willing to tolerate the finish, though that becomes less of an issue when paired with a lipstick.

☹ **Anew Beauty Youth-Awakening Lipstick SPF 15** *($10)*. The "youth-awakening" part of this lipstick is based on the claims about its ability to fight the five signs of lip aging, which include loss of rosy color, severity of lip lines, decreased fullness, loss of elasticity, and skin discoloration. What you end up getting is eons from this lofty promise, rather it is merely a very emollient lipstick based on squalane which has no special benefit any more then other oils used in lipsticks. It feels light yet lush and leans toward the greasy side of creamy. Anyone prone to lipstick bleeding into lines around the mouth will find this formula makes a beeline into them due to its slickness. Several ingredients in this lipstick work to smooth and condition lips, but for all the antiaging claims, it is inexcusable that the sunscreen does not provide sufficient UVA protection. All the other claims can also be attributed to any creamy lipstick—apply it and your lips will be better defined, have deeper color, and look smoother. Avon deserves points for at least coming up with a different lipstick formula to support its claims, but simply swapping some ingredients for others in the same category (such as emollients) isn't going to make lips look even one day younger with continued use. Someone at Avon should have awakened to the fact that UVA damage plays an important role in aging lips, and then formulated accordingly.

☹ **Beyond Color Plumping Lipcolor SPF 15** *($8)* lacks the UVA-protecting ingredients of titanium dioxide, zinc oxide, avobenzone, Tinosorb, or Mexoryl SX, but its opacity does provide some element of sun protection. This creamy, full-coverage lipstick feels moist but not too slick, and comes in a color range with something to please everyone. As for the lip-plumping claim, don't count on it—there is nothing in the formula that has this effect.

☹ **Big Color Glossy Lip Pencil** *($6)* is a thick lip pencil that needs inconvenient routine sharpening every time you use it. If you don't mind the sharpening, this applies smoothly and is a cross between a sheer lipstick and a lip gloss. It is minimally sticky and tends to stay in place better than standard lip glosses, so you get more mileage per application. The shade selection is small, but all are attractive and work with a variety of lipstick shades. If not for the sharpening element, this would rate a happy face.

☺ **Pro-To-Go Lipstick** *($9)*. Aside from the clever one-piece, slide-and-glide packaging and the ads featuring actress Reese Witherspoon (remember, she is paid to promote Avon, just like any who celebrity represents a cosmetics line), there isn't much to extol about this lipstick. Its emollient formula feels slippery on your lips and imparts a glossy finish that tends to fade quickly. Anyone prone to lipstick bleeding into lines around the mouth will find this formula moves there in seconds. Otherwise, this is about as no-big-deal as it gets. Unless you're hyped about the novel packaging, there are better cream lipsticks at the drugstore.

☺ **SpectraColor Lipstick** *($9.50)*. Although this is packaged to resemble a lipstick, the product has the texture, slip, and finish of a lip gloss. The selling point with SpectraColor is that you can "dial in" the color you want. The bottom of the tube has a dial at the bottom that goes from 1 (lightest color) to 7 (darkest color). Looking inside the clear center portion of the component reveals two compartments, one housing a light shade and the other a dark shade. Where you set the dial determines the proportion of each shade that's dispensed. The concept is intriguing, and the dial mechanism works to fine tune the color, but dialing back and forth can get messy and potentially lead to streaky, uneven results. It doesn't help that the product itself is so slippery. With a texture of light meringue, it produces a glossy finish, but quickly travels outside the lip's borders, even if lines aren't present. An intriguing concept, but it didn't translate into a useful product.

☺ **Ultra Luxury Lipliner** *($5)* has a great price for a standard pencil that isn't too dry or too creamy for precise application. The fact that it needs sharpening prevents it from earning a happy face rating.

☹ **Plump Pout Lip Gloss** *($7)*. This shimmer-infused, ultra-smooth gloss has a gorgeous finish on lips and is absolutely non-sticky. Why the unhappy face rating, then? From the moment this touches your lips, you'll feel a tingling, burning sensation that just doesn't let up. In almost no time this gloss becomes almost painful to wear—it actually made my lips throb, and that's not good! The fragrance and flavor ingredient in this gloss causes your lips to swell by virtue of strong irritation, and that isn't the way to get fuller lips, especially on a daily basis; plus the minor improvement isn't worth the perpetual irritation, which dries out the lips and cause collagen to breakdown.

☹ **Slick Tint for Lips** *($0.99)*. Sometimes, every so often, with cosmetics you really do get what you pay for. That's certainly true for this ultra-cheap tinted lip balm packaged like a tube of Chapstick. It imparts sheer color and has a soft gloss finish, but feels unusually thick, almost gloppy, and has an off, nearly rancid, waxy odor. The lanolin oil–based formula will quickly travel into any lines around the mouth. For a few dollars more, any of the lip glosses or balms from Wet 'n' Wild beat this hands-down.

☹ **Ultra Color Rich Ultra Plumping Lipstick** *($8)* is supposed to provide rich color while plumping lips. It has a slightly creamy, lightweight texture that glides over lips, but because the center portion of the lipstick is uncolored (the center core is what's said to provide the "plumping power"), application is uneven. You get more color for the edges of your mouth than you do for the center, so some fine-tuning is needed. The plumping comes from this lipstick's minty flavor, while a pepper resin causes a warm tingling that increases circulation to lips. The result is subtle plumping, but it's done by irritating your lips, which isn't a wise thing to do on a daily basis. Avon included retinol, too, but the tiny amount isn't going to enlarge lips or stimulate collagen production, especially not when the mint is causing collagen to break down. This isn't one of Avon's better lipsticks.

MASCARA: ☺ **Daring Curves Waterproof Mascara** *($7.50)* allows you to quickly create long, curvaceous lashes that are defined and separated and that just keep getting longer the more you apply, all without clumping. Thickness is minor, even with successive coats, but the formula is waterproof and recommended if you prefer a lengthening mascara and don't need much volume. This requires an oil- or silicone-based makeup remover.

☺ **Superfull Mascara** *($8.50)* takes some time to build, but with effort lashes end up full, thick, and appreciably long. Clumping is minimal, and the only issue involves the manner in which the rubber bristles deposit mascara—they tend to leave the tips of your lashes with little balls of mascara. These require a lash comb to eliminate, and doing so is a must or you run the risk of flaking during wear. Aside from that caveat, this mascara is enthusiastically recommended.

☺ **Supershock Mascara** *($8.50)* is an impressive mascara, but building lashes to "larger than life proportions" is not in its bag of tricks (and unless you have a measuring tape adaptable to lashes, you can't prove their claim). The large applicator has a brush that contains many tiny, thin bristles that stand up straight. A few coats produces lots of length, but building thickness (volume) is difficult. This is worth considering if you're looking for clump-free length and reliable wear with easy removal. But if you want to spend less and get more bang for your buck, Cover Girl's Lash Blast Mascara trounces this because it allows you to build on the results without messing up a careful application.

☺ **Uplifting Mascara** *($8.50)* brings us yet another mascara with a rubber-bristled brush. The supposedly unique twist here is that the brush is the world's first bendable one, but that claim's not factual. Almost any mascara brush will bend if you want it to, and then there's the issue that simply having a brush that bends doesn't necessarily provide greater results. This is just a fairly good lengthening mascara that applies cleanly and coats lashes evenly and without clumps. You can build some thickness with successive coats, but nothing too prodigious. One caution: The variegated rubber bristles feel scratchy if you're not careful when applying this to lash roots.

☺ **Wash-Off Waterproof Mascara** *($6.50)* provides some length without clumps or smears, but no thickness. That's not terrible, but far better waterproof mascaras are available for the same amount of money from L'Oreal, Rimmel, and Maybelline New York.

☺ **Daring Curves Mascara** *($7.50)* creates softly curled lashes that last all day, but its lengthening prowess is moderate and thickness is scant. It's a good choice if you don't need much lash enhancement beyond a bit of length and curl, but is otherwise unremarkable.

☺ **Daring Definition Mousse Mascara** *($7.50)* has a lightweight, mousse-like texture, but that doesn't make for a better mascara. If anything, the texture of this mascara makes it more prone to clumping during application. It produces impressive length quickly, but loses points for making lashes feel dry and flaking throughout the day.

☺ **Jillian Dempsey for Avon Professional Mascara** *($9.50)* is a dual-sided mascara of which only half has any chance of making your lashes happy, the other half isn't worth anything. One end has a bigger brush that separates and lengthens beautifully without a bit of clumping. But, the other end has a baby brush end, which is meant to be used on smaller lashes, but it is a complete dud. The waterproof formulation and short stumpy brush make getting an even, clump-free application to smaller lashes nearly impossible. The combination of the poorly shaped small brush and the poorly formulated waterproof mascara make for a clumpy mess that smears and requires additional time and effort to clean up. You'll have much better results using the big brush side for all your lashes. However, taken altogether, that means you're getting only half as much mascara as you normally would, so it isn't as much of a bargain as it may seem.

☺ **Mistake Proof Mascara** *($9.50)*. The claim is that you can "be perfect ... every time" when applying this mascara because one end of this two-sided product contains a liquid makeup remover. The idea is that if it smears or if you inadvertently get some on your skin during application, you simply flip the tube around and use the angled applicator to correct the mistake. It works, but the problem with the remover's formula is that it leaves a greasy film on your skin that needs to be touched up. If you neglect to touch up, it can smear the mascara or any other makeup you're wearing. In the end, you're making more work for yourself; most mascara boo-boos can be cleaned up quickly with a cotton swab and a little water. The mascara itself is fantastic; it lengthens and thickens lashes quickly and without clumps or flaking. You won't get super-dramatic lashes, but the enhanced, separated look is perfectly suitable for most, and it wears well throughout the day. But there are lots of other mascaras that do the same or better without taking up space with an unnecessary product.

☺ **Spectralash Mascara** *($9.50)*. Remember Maybelline's Dial-a-Lash Mascara, which allowed users to dial in their preferred amount of mascara prior to application? It was more gimmicky than a true advantage, but Avon has streamlined the concept for Spectralash. Instead of being able to dial from 1 (minimal mascara) to 10 (lots of mascara), you get three levels. Level 1 provides good length and thickness and barely clumps. Even after several coats, it wears evenly. Level 2 offers a slightly heavier application than Level 1, and actually clumps less. You'll get great lash separation and a beautifully long, fringed look for lashes. Going to Level 3 prompts the heaviest, wettest application as well as the most troublesome clumps. The clumps are manageable if you have a lash comb handy, and the payoff with Level 3 is impressively dramatic lashes. There's a big difference between Levels 1 and 3; as expected, Level 2 is the happy medium. This is a mascara to consider if you like the variety it offers, but keep in mind that routinely going from Level 1 to Level 3 will eventually blur the results, because with each switch back and forth you're dealing with excess mascara from Level 3, so your Level 1 results will gradually become closer to the results you get from Level 2. Confusing? Absolutely, that's why this is best left in the Avon catalog.

☹ **Astonishing Lengths Mascara** *($7.50)* produces copious length and does so quickly! What's not so astonishing about this mascara is its tendency to flake and not make it through the day without some smearing.

BRUSHES: ☺ **All Over Kabuki Face Brush** *($4.99)* is impressively dense for the money, so it holds powder well (though it could be softer). The problem is not with the brush itself, but rather using it with the previously mentioned Mineral Makeup. Unless you tap every bit of excess off the brush prior to application, the effect looks very dry and heavy on all skin types. However, using this brush with a better mineral makeup is an option.

FACE AND BODY SHIMMER/ILLUMINATING PRODUCTS: ☺ **Look Alert Eye Brightener** *($3.99)* is a fluid highlighter that's housed in a click-pen applicator with a built-in synthetic brush. It is meant to blur fine lines and "optically airbrush imperfections," but that's a tall order for what amounts to a lightweight, very sheer highlighter with a soft shine finish. It's amazing what shine can allegedly do for skin, isn't it? On the one hand it creates a soft glow (a nighttime prismatic glitter effect), but for those with wrinkles almost any amount of shine is going to draw attention to wrinkles or other imperfections. As a result, this product works well to create a subtle highlight under the eye or on the brow bone, but because it provides almost no coverage, you'll want to brush it on (carefully) after applying concealer. This is recommended as long as you don't expect any of Avon's airbrushed-to-perfection claims to come true.

SPECIALTY PRODUCTS: ☺ **MagiX Face Perfector SPF 20** *($10)* does not contain active ingredients capable of protecting skin from the full range of UVA light, so its use as a sunscreen is not recommended. As a primer for those with oily skin, it is capable of creating a very smooth, matte surface for makeup while keeping excess oil in check for a period of time (the length of time depends on how oily your skin is and what skin-care products you use). The silicone-heavy formula has a silky, dry finish, but cannot "perfect" skin better than many other primers or, better yet, silicone-enhanced serums loaded with antioxidants.

AVON MARK

AVON MARK AT-A-GLANCE

Strengths: Mostly good foundations; incredible powders; great inexpensive eyeshadow; one outstanding mascara; good shimmer products; good cleansers; outstanding daytime moisturizer with SPF 30; some worthwhile moisturizers; good lip balm.

Weaknesses: The lash top coat and some of the makeup brushes fail to impress even a little bit; the products for oily and acne-prone skin are mostly unimpressive and needlessly irritating.

For more information about Avon Mark, call (866) 633-8627 or visit www.meetmark.com or www.Beautypedia.com.

AVON MARK SKIN CARE

☺ **Calming Effect Comforting Milk Cleanser** *($7 for 6.7 ounces)* is a very good, inexpensive water soluble cleanser for all skin types except for very oily. It contains some notable soothing agents, though their effect in a cleanser won't add up to much given how quickly it is either removed or rinsed from skin. A strong point is this takes off makeup without drying skin; and it contains fragrance in the form of vanilla and banana fruit extracts, but those have little to no risk of causing irritation.

☺ **That's Deep Purifying Gel Cleanser** *($7 for 6.7 ounces)*. Although this doesn't clean deeper than any other water soluble cleanser, it is a good option for normal to oily skin. Makeup comes off easily and skin is left soft and refreshed. This contains fragrance in the form of black currant and orange flower.

☺ **Mist Opportunity Multi-Tasking Refresher** *($8 for 6.7 ounces)* is an average spray-on toner for all skin types that would be much better without the fragrant plant extracts, which provide no benefit for skin (eau de cologne is not skin care). It does contain apple fruit extract, which is a good cell-communicating ingredient but not enough to warrant a happy face.

✓ ☺ **For Goodness Face Antioxidant Skin Moisturizing Lotion SPF 30** *($15 for 1.7 ounces)*. What a great name and, thankfully, it is also a great sunscreen with the actives including in-part avobenzone (for UVA protection) in a lightweight moisturizing base. All in all it is a very good daytime moisturizer for normal to oily skin. The airless jar packaging helps keep the many antioxidants and plant extracts in here stable during use, and it also contains a cell-communicating ingredient. Some of the plant extracts are fragrant, but their antioxidant ability offsets this minor setback.

☺ **Light Bright Lighten & Depuff Eye Gel** *($8 for 0.17 ounce)* contains over a dozen plant extracts, none of which are capable of reducing puffy eyes or dark circles. The main plant extract is lotus, and Avon maintains this reduces the look of tired eyes. Don't count on it: the research on lotus doing anything of the sort is conspicuously absent. Some of the plant extracts are there for fragrance, while others have anti-irritant ability or function as antioxidants. All told, this is a good lightweight moisturizer for slightly dry skin anywhere on the face—just don't count on any of the eye-area claims to actually come true.

☹ **Matte Chance Mattifying Lotion** *($15 for 1.7 ounces)* lists alcohol as the second ingredient, which negates the worthwhile ingredients in this serum-type product and makes it too irritating and drying for all skin types. In addition, alcohol triggers oil production in the pore lining, which won't keep skin matte. Clinique and Smashbox offer much better products to mattify skin without the "chance" of irritation.

☺ **Need a Shrink? Pore Minimizer Lotion** *($8 for 0.17 ounce)*. The clever name doesn't reflect a clever product. While it would be nice if this could make pores smaller, at best the absorbent ingredients that comprise the bulk of the formula will help keep excess oil in check for a short period of time. Keeping skin matte can help pores look smaller (pores look larger and more apparent when they're engorged with oil), but that in and of itself doesn't actually reduce their size. Like it or not, pore size is genetically determined and no skin-care product has a permanent effect on reducing their size. This is merely an OK lightweight moisturizer for oily skin, but several of the plant extracts are potentially irritating.

☺ **See Things Clearly Brightening Moisturizer** *($15 for 1.7 ounces)* is a very good shimmery finish moisturizer (the shimmer provides the brightening effect) for normal to slightly dry or slightly oily skin. It contains an impressive amount of antioxidants and cell-communicating ingredients along with a tiny amount of water-binding agents. Some of the plant extracts are potentially irritating, but this is likely offset by the non-irritating plant extracts that precede them. The airless jar packaging will help keep the antioxidant ingredients stable during use.

☹ **Get Clearance Anti-Acne Blemish Treatment Gel** *($8 for 0.17 ounce)*. Despite containing 2% salicylic acid, this ends up being another irritating anti-acne product due to the excessive and unnecessary amount of alcohol it contains. It is not recommended due to the irritation alcohol causes, including increasing oil production in the pore.

☺ **Calm Yourself Hydrating Mask** *($7 for 3.4 ounces)*. Although this gel mask contains some hydrating ingredients, the preponderance of citrus extracts it contains isn't good news for anyone's skin. It's disappointing that the potentially irritating citrus is more prominent in the formula than anti-irritants and non-irritating antioxidants. At best, this is an OK lightweight mask for areas of slightly dry skin. The claim of increasing skin's moisture content by 168% sounds impressive, but remember, when skin swells with water (over 30%), that damages the skin's protective barrier, depleting the healthy substances in skin that maintain its balance, resiliency, and moisture content.

☺ **Shine Fighter Oil-Control Mask** *($7 for 3.4 ounces)*. The combination of absorbent ingredients in this mask for oily skin can help reduce shine and make skin matte, but only for a short time. However, the inclusion of alcohol along with clay and silica can make this an unnecessarily drying experience, even for those troubled by very oily areas. The clay and silica are good, but the alcohol is damaging, causing irritation, free-radical damage, and ironically, triggering more oil to be produced.

☺ **Kiss Dry Goodbye Lip Smoother** *($8 for 0.17 ounce)* takes brilliant care of dry, chapped lips. Unlike many lip balms, this contains antioxidants and omits irritants such as camphor and menthol (though some of the plant extracts are fragrant, but none of these are as much a problem for the lips as menthol and camphor). Note: this is flavored with the artificial sweetener saccharin, a bit shocking given how out-of-date an ingredient that is, but you shouldn't be licking your lips anyway, so if you can avoid doing that, the saccharin isn't much of a problem.

☺ **Kiss Therapy Super Soothing Lip Balm** *($4)* is a glossy, emollient, rose-scented lip balm available in a colorless option or Sheer Red—which is actually fuchsia. It does the trick for dry lips, but the fragrance is intense, and, due to where your lips are located on the face, it's right under your nose.

AVON MARK MAKEUP

FOUNDATION: ✓☺ **Powder Buff Natural Skin Foundation** *($8)*. Avon, the master brand behind the Mark line, has an excellent track record with pressed-powder foundations. Powder Buff Natural Skin Foundation continues their winning streak with its suede-smooth, talc-free formula. This is a top powder foundation that blends beautifully and sets to a satin matte finish that never makes skin look dull or too powdered. Coverage goes from light to barely medium and this also works great dusted on as a pressed powder to set foundation. The formula is geared toward those with normal to dry skin; those with oily areas will want more absorbency than this powder foundation provides. The shade range is excellent across the board, offering neutral colors for light to tan skin tones.

☺ **C-Thru-U Beautifying Sheer Tint SPF 15** *($8)* is indeed a sheer tint for skin, one with a creamy texture that blends well and leaves a slightly moist finish and soft, translucent color. Eight shades are available, and although the four lightest shades are on the peachy side, they're too sheer for that to really matter. Shades 4 and 6 are considered "glow" shades, and impart a soft shimmer. Avon has updated the formula so the active ingredients now include titanium dioxide for sufficient UVA protection. I am pleased to recommend this tinted moisturizer as a very good option for all skin types except very oily.

☺ **Dab Action Face Clearing Foundation** *($8)* is designed as a blemish-fighting foundation, and contains 2% salicylic acid as its active ingredient. Unfortunately, the pH is over 4, so it won't work to exfoliate skin or minimize blemishes and blackheads. The unique part of this foundation is its dab-on applicator. A runny liquid housed in a tube is dispensed onto a thin, sponge-like applicator, which is dabbed onto skin. The foundation blends well (though the thin consistency takes some getting used to) and sets to a somewhat dry, very matte finish. Those looking to conceal blemishes or redness will be disappointed by this foundation's sheer coverage. However, if you have very oily skin without blemishes, this is an original matte foundation to consider. Among the eight shades, only Face 5 and Face 7 are too peachy to recommend. Face 1 is great for fair skin, while Face 8 is a non-ashy option for women of color.

☺ **Face Xpert Flawless Touch Makeup** *($8)* has unique packaging that dispenses a liquid foundation onto a rounded sponge applicator tip. You dab the foundation where needed and blend, either with the attached sponge or your fingers. I recommend blending with a regular-size flat makeup sponge because the sponge that's part of this foundation is too small for an efficient application, plus it tends to apply product unevenly. The foundation has a slightly thick but lightweight texture with enough slip to make blending pleasant. It sets to a silky matte finish that provides light to medium coverage and is ideal for normal to oily skin. The overriding problem with this makeup is the shades, many of which are overtly peach to orange. Among the seven choices, avoid Medium, Honey, and Extra Deep. Medium Tan is borderline peach, but is neutral enough to work for some skin tones. This foundation isn't "perfection in action," but if you can find a shade that works, it's worth auditioning.

☺ **Get A Tint Tinted Moisturizer Lotion SPF 15** *($8)* has a lotion-like consistency and provides titanium dioxide for sufficient UVA protection. Best for normal to slightly dry or slightly oily skin, it slips on evenly and blends readily to a sheer, moist finish. The colors tend toward being peach, with the most obvious being Honey/Golden. Avoid that shade; the others are acceptable but do not include options for fair or very dark skin tones.

☺ **Speedway Do Everything Makeup** *($8)* is a stick foundation whose "Do Everything" name refers to the fact that it functions as foundation, concealer, and powder in one, similar to most stick foundations. This has a very creamy application that spreads easily and feels light on the skin. It provides sheer to medium (if you layer it) coverage and dries to a satin matte finish. If your skin is oily (or if you have noticeably oily areas) you will need to use this with a separate powder for shine control. Those with normal to slightly dry skin would fare best with this product, especially if the goal is an all-in-one makeup. Eleven mostly excellent shades are available, including options for darker skin tones. Shades 5, 7, and 8 tend to be a bit peach, but may work for some medium skin tones. Shades 10 and 11 are beautiful non-ashy shades for African-American skin tones.

CONCEALER: ☺ **Tru-Lie Hook Up Concealer** *($5)* is a liquid concealer with a thinner than usual consistency that provides sheer to light coverage. This is not the concealer to select if you have pronounced dark circles or broken blood vessels to camouflage, but it nicely diffuses other imperfections and dries to a soft matte finish that poses no risk of creasing. The six shades are excellent, though note that Deep may be too peach for some darker skin tones.

☹ **Good Riddance Hook Up Concealer** *($6)*. This is a mini pencil concealer that needs routine sharpening, so expect its lifespan to be brief and usage more time-consuming than any other type of concealer. Actually, you can expect brief results, too, thanks to this concealer's thick, oil-based texture. It covers well and the shades are workable (Light/Medium is slightly peach), but it tends to crease mercilessly and fade within an hour. This simply isn't worth considering over several other concealers from Avon.

☹ **Invisible Touch Perfecting Concealer** *($5)*. Invisible Touch Perfecting Concealer claims "Poof! Perfect skin." However, using this slick, slightly greasy concealer isn't the route to skin perfection. A more accurate description would have been "Poof! Peachy skin" because three of the four shades leave a noticeable peach cast (Deep is the only acceptable shade). In addition, this creases and provides such sheer, fleeting coverage you'll wonder why you bothered.

POWDER: ✓☺ **Matte-Nificent Oil-Absorbing Facial Powder** *($8)* has an adorably clever name and a formula that makes this among the best pressed powders available today for normal to oily skin. This talc-based, fragrance-free powder feels supremely light and looks great on skin, never thick or cakey. It has a smooth, dry finish that nicely controls shine (though not all day—you will need to reapply this occasionally). The four shades are stellar examples of neutral colors, and best for light to medium/tan skin tones.

✓☺ **Powder-matic Go Anywhere Loose Powder** *($8)* is not only a spectacular talc-based loose powder, thanks to its silky, weightless texture and natural, nondrying finish, but is also ingeniously packaged. I'm not a fan of loose powder because it's just too messy compared to pressed powder. However, many women prefer this type of powder and Mark makes it easier than ever to use. Packaged in a deep compact, the powder has a sifter that can be opened and closed, allowing you to control how much powder comes out, and the sifter can be "locked" for traveling or toting in your makeup bag. It works very well and nearly eliminates the messy element of using loose powder. Three shades are available, all sheer and neutral.

BLUSH: ✓ ☺ **Good Glowing Mosaic Blush** *($7)*. This pressed-powder blush has an almost creamy feel and a very smooth, even application that enlivens skin with soft to moderate shimmer (depending on how much you brush on). The mosaic pattern unites a range of complementary colors that come off as one shade on skin, so consider the design more of an aesthetic feature rather than a practical advantage. This inexpensive blush is recommended for anyone looking for glow-y cheeks and soft color. It's advisable for daytime makeup only if you apply it lightly as a finishing/highlighting touch over a matte powder blush. The shimmer doesn't flake.

✓ ☺ **Just Pinched Instant Blush Tint** *($6)*. Fans of sheer cream blush, take note: This is an excellent option. The creamy formula isn't too slick, so blending can be more precise, yet the finish maintains a satin-like creaminess that makes this blush best for dry skin. It is not recommended for those prone to blemishes (powder blush is preferred). All of the shades are attractive but their sheerness makes them preferred for fair to medium skin tones. Just Pinched Instant Blush Tint works well to create that soft, translucent color, but don't expect it to last all day without a touch-up.

☺ **Cheekblossom Cheek Color Tint** *($6)* is supposed to react with your skin's chemistry to change color, but it ends up turning the same soft pink shade on anyone (think of mood lipsticks from the 60s, exact same concept). Those with darker skin will find the silicone-based gel color barely registers even if you apply a lot of it. It has a silky, nearly weightless finish laced with subtle sparkles and is ultimately best for those with fair to light skin.

☺ **Shimmer Cheekblossom Cheek Color Tint** *($6)* is nearly identical to Mark's regular Cheekblossom Color Tint, meaning it is supposed to reflect your body's chemistry and change the appropriate color after you apply it (don't believe it for one second). This version contains more sparkles and they're noticeably gold (these don't change color), so the finish is much more obvious on cheeks. Daytime makeup doesn't call for the kind of sparkling cheeks this provides, even if you're a teen in the mood to experiment with makeup. Just like the regular Cheekblossom product, this turns the same sheer pink color on everyone (think of mood lipsticks from the 60s, exact same concept). It is best reserved for evening makeup and recommended only for those with fair to light skin.

☺ **Good Glowing Custom Pick Powder Blush** *($6)* is a silky, pressed-powder blush whose colors are quite sheer, even on fair skin. The "glowing" part is from the noticeable shine of all the shades, though the shiny particles tend to flake off easily, leaving you with patchy sparkles and barely there color.

EYESHADOW: ☺ **I-Mark Custom Pick Eyeshadow** *($4)* wins points for its ultra-smooth texture that feels almost creamy and applies evenly without flaking. Since this makeup collection was designed to appeal to teens, I understand the fact that almost half of the 19 shades are blue, green, purple, or bright pink—but that doesn't mean I won't encourage teens and young adults to avoid these colors if their goal is to shape and shade the eye rather than color it. Still, there are some worthwhile, easy-to-work-with shades, plus the blue, purple, and green options go on sheerer than they look. Every shade has some amount of shine, but that shouldn't be a problem for teens and most young women prefer it anyway.

☺ **I-Sheer Creamy Hook Up Eye Shadow** *($5.50)* is a sheer liquid eyeshadow that applies smoothly and isn't the least bit creamy, so the name is misleading. It imparts minimal color and moderate shimmer, and the dry finish holds up better than expected. (It definitely lasts longer than true cream eyeshadows.) This is best used over powder eyeshadows to highlight the brow bone; allover use should be reserved for women whose eye area hasn't begun to show signs of aging, because the shine will magnify wrinkles.

☺ **Mini Mark It Stick for Eyes** *($6)*. This tiny, chunky pencil eyeshadow has a beautifully smooth texture; an even application that imparts sheer, shiny color; and a soft powder finish to ensure respectable wear. It's an option if you want sheer, shimmery eyeliner, or you can use any of the lighter shades to highlight the brow bone. The only issue is that this pencil needs routine sharpening, which shortens its lifespan (you lose a lot of the pencil every time you have to sharpen), especially when compared with powder eyeshadows.

☺ **Winkstick Hook Up Eye Shadow Stick** *($5.50)* is a twist-up, creamy eyeshadow stick imbued with sparkles. The sheer colors are easy to work with, though not all of them are reliable if you want an eye design that flatters your eyes rather than competes with them. The biggest issue is that this eyeshadow stick tends to stay creamy after application and is prone to endless creasing and fading during the day. It's a novel way to apply eyeshadow, but no match for the artistry you can create and the longevity you can get from powder eyeshadows.

EYE AND BROW SHAPER: ☺ **Get in Line Hook Up Waterproof Eyeliner** *($5.50)*. This liquid eyeliner must be shaken before use to distribute the cosmetic pigments. Once that's done, the thin, appropriately firm brush makes it easy to draw an even line of soft color. This sets quickly to a subtle metallic finish, and is waterproof as claimed. Whether it wears for 10 hours depends on what else you've applied around your eyes and if you have oily eyelids. This doesn't hold up nearly as well as the numerous gel eyeliners available. Avoid the Deep Aqua shade, which is really a soft teal that competes with, rather than complements, your eye color.

☺ **On the Edge Hook Up Liquid Eyeliner** *($5.50)* has a lot going for it! The long, thin brush isn't as precise as others that are shorter and have a pointed tip, but it works well to apply an even line of color (and the color doesn't peter out before you cover the entire lash line). The formula dries quickly and, once set, is generally impervious to smudging or flaking. Avoid the peacock-blue Calisto shade.

☺ **Metalliner Eye Glam Hook Up** *($5)* works well as a liquid liner under two conditions: you have to adapt to a somewhat flimsy brush that makes application trickier than usual, and you have to want a metallic finish. The blue, bronze, and silver shades are striking but really best for fantasy or nightclub makeup rather than day-to-day colors. The formula dries quickly and wears well, but the shades make this tough to recommend over other liquid liners that perform just as well and come in standard, workable colors.

☹ **Eyemarker Color On Line** *($5.50)*. I always prefer automatic pencils to those that require routine sharpening mostly for convenience, but this automatic, nonretractable option is no better than average. It applies smoothly, though the effect is almost too soft for eyelining unless you layer it, and that isn't convenient. If you do take the time to layer this on, after you apply several layers to build intensity, the line tends to smudge easily and you're left with a too-soft, imprecise, sloppy look. Stick with the automatic eye pencils from major drugstore lines instead.

LIPSTICK, LIP GLOSS, AND LIPLINER: ☺ **Dew Drenched Moisturlicious Lip Color** *($6)* is a good, lightweight cream lipstick that applies smoothly and leaves a soft gloss finish that doesn't feel too slippery on lips. Color impact is minor, so this is definitely a lipstick for those seeking a sheer veil of color. It would be better if the shade selection was larger, but what's available is versatile. Note that this lipstick is flavored with the artificial sweetener sucralose (also known as Splenda®).

☺ **Fresh Kiss Cool Burst Lipcolor** *($6)* is a full-size creamy lipstick in a miniature case. The 15 semi-opaque shades are mostly soft pastel and nude tones, and over half include shimmer. The minty scent and flavor do not translate into lip tingling, which is a good thing, because tingling would mean your lips are being irritated—probably not what you had in mind from a lipstick.

☺ **Glossblossom Ripening Lip Tint** *($6)* gets its "ripening" from the fact that this lip gloss goes on clear and then deepens to a soft pink color. Its supposedly customizes itself to each person's lips, but it isn't some magical formulary trick. Rather, it's simply reminding us that the same color looks different on each person's lips. We've all experienced this, and it isn't unique. With this particular product, the effect is subtle and it remains a fluid, non-sticky, wet-shine lip gloss.

☺ **Glow Baby Glow Luxe Hook Up Lip Gloss/Glow Baby Glow Hook Up Lip Gloss** *($5)* works fine as a lightweight, shimmery lip gloss. It comes in a tube with a brush applicator, and can be "hooked up" with other Mark products (concealer, mascara, nail polish) if desired. This gloss has a slick, non-sticky feel and imparts subtle color and lots of shine. A similar version called Glow Baby Glow Hook Up Lip Gloss is also available. These shades have minimal to no shimmer and feature a sponge-tip applicator.

☺ **Candy Kisses Lip Gloss** *($10)* provides three shades of lip gloss, each individually packaged to resemble pieces of cellophane-wrapped candy. Clearly designed to appeal to pre-teens, the glosses are scented and flavored to be reminiscent of candy. Of course, wearing gloss with the intention of licking your lips to ingest it isn't the goal, but the fact remains that this gloss has a frosting-like smooth texture and completely non-sticky finish. It's comfortable to wear and provides a soft gloss finish and a hint of color.

☺ **Electro-Lights Lip Vitagleam** *($7.50)* has a name that sounds more like a dance club from the 1970s than a simple lip gloss! This wand-style gloss has a syrupy texture that can feel a bit goopy on the lips if you apply too much. Electro-Lights Lip Vitagleam has the wettest-looking finish of all the Mark glosses, and the colors, though neon-like in the tube, go on invisibly.

☺ **Lip Mark-It Color On Line** *($5.50)*. As far as automatic, creamy lip pencils go, this is as good an option as any. The only drawback is the limited color selection.

☺ **Lip Vanitease Glossy Lip Lacquer** *($6)* provides more color and coverage than traditional lip gloss, but feels and finishes glossy. It's neither sticky nor too slippery, and makes its mark as an all-around good lip gloss.

☺ **Metalluscious Lip Cream Hook Up** *($5)* promises "hypnotic color" and although your admirers won't be in a trance, there is no question this liquid lipstick's metallic, shimmer-infused opaque colors are striking. Even better, the formula glides on and feels lightweight and not the least bit sticky. This product may be too much for teens because its sophisticated palette speaks more to adult makeup.

☺ **Tattoo Kiss Superfaithful/Kissink Lip Tintmarkers** *($7)* are long-lasting lip stains that are packaged to resemble Magic Markers. The color is applied from a pointed (but not sharp) tip and darkens as it dries. Because the second ingredient in this simple formula is alcohol, which is necessary for the staining effect and for the product to dry quickly, you'll want to pair it with a lip gloss or balm for comfort. All the shades lean toward being brighter than they appear, and they do last. You'll need an oil- or silicone-based remover, and even it won't remove every trace of color.

☺ **Gleamstick Hook Up Lip Color** *($5.50)* is a basic cream lipstick that leaves lips feeling tingly. The mint scent is likely responsible for the tingling, though no mint extracts or menthol appears on the ingredient list. The colors provide moderate coverage and pigmentation that's stronger than what most teen-appeal lines typically offer. This isn't as moisturizing as the reviews on Avon's Web site claim, and the tingling can cause dry lips and irritation that might temporarily make the lips look bigger but ends up being more of a negative with regular use.

☺ **Juice Gems Squeeze On Lip Gloss with Real Fruit** *($6)* contains fruit extracts, which aren't the same as real fruit. That's a good thing, because real fruit wouldn't last long in a cosmetic. This is a standard, sheer, sticky lip gloss that has a potent fragrance (and, strangely, it isn't the least bit reminiscent of fruit).

☺ **Mini Mark It Stick for Lips** *($6)* is a thick, chunky mini pencil that needs routine sharpening (and that isn't convenient or easy). It has a slightly greasy texture that imparts sheer, sparkle-infused color with a metallic tinge. It isn't as slick and greasy as similar lip pencils of this ilk, but the sparkling effect is dazzling in a pre-teen style rather then an elegant shine. That was likely Avon Mark's goal given the market for their brand, but what is worth keeping in mind if you're considering this product for yourself is exactly what image are you going after. Note that this will be gone in no time due to the constant need for sharpening to maintain the point.

☺ **Pro Glimmer Hook Up Lip Powder** *($5.50)*. Truly an unusual product, this oil-based loose powder is meant to be applied over lipstick or lip gloss to enhance color and staying power. To test how this worked, I first applied Avon Mark's Pro Gloss Plumping Lip Shine and the result was interesting. The Lip Powder is surprisingly easy to apply over a gloss, though you have to use moderate pressure to ensure the powder smooths on evenly and doesn't get clumpy and imbedded in the gloss. The Hook Up Lip Powder turned the gloss into a satin matte finish complete with a metallic shimmer and intense pigmentation. That may or may not be to your liking, but the problem to consider is the slightly rancid, stale wax odor this product has. You're better off choosing a creamy lipstick with a metallic finish rather than dealing with this two-step, potentially messy process.

☹ **Pro Gloss Hook Up Plumping Lip Shine** *($5.50)*. This thick, slightly sticky lip gloss plumps lips temporarily by irritating them with cinnamon bark extract. You'll feel the tingly, warming sensation almost instantly, but that's not the best experience to put your lips through, especially on a daily basis. Although this is not nearly as irritating as many "plumping" glosses, it is still best reserved for only occasional use. The range of shades is great and all impart translucent color via the handy brush applicator.

MASCARA: ✓ ☺ **Comb Out Lash Lifting Mascara** *($6)* uses a comb applicator rather than a standard mascara brush, and the results are exceptional. Lengthening is a breeze and you will also notice perfectly separated, lifted, and curled lashes, all without clumps or smearing. This is a fantastic find for the money!

☺ **Lash Splash Hook Up Waterproof Mascara** *($5.50)*. This standard waterproof mascara stays on quite well if lashes get wet. It requires an oil- or silicone-based remover and tends to make lashes feel more brittle than other waterproof mascaras. Still, for the money, this produces respectable length, minor thickness, and doesn't clump. Several coats are required for best results.

☺ **Tattoo Lash** *($6)* is Mark's volumizing mascara, and it does make good on that promise. Creating long, thick lashes is easy, though not without some minor clumping and a heavy application that may not be to everyone's (especially teens) taste. It wears without flaking or smudging, and is definitely a consideration for dramatic thickening.

☺ **Lashtensions Lash Magnifying Hook Up** *($5)* is a base coat for lashes, meant to "fiber-optically thicken" lashes with panthenol and silk protein. Neither of these ingredients can have an impact on lashes, especially not in the minuscule amounts used in this product. As with almost all lash primers, using it makes little difference compared with what two coats of a good mascara can do. You won't see a difference with this product unless you're using an underachieving mascara, and if that's the case, why not step up to a superior one?

☹ **Make It Big Lash Plumping Mascara** *($6.50)*. This mascara's large, cumbersome brush makes it tricky to apply evenly without getting mascara on the surrounding skin. Given a lot of patience you can do a better job, but the result is still an uneven application that tends to clump and that requires significant comb-through. In the end, the effort it takes just isn't worth its attractive price—not when there are superior mascaras at the drugstore for the same amount of money.

☹ **Scanda-Lash Hook Up Mascara** *($5)* has a great name but doesn't exactly perform scandalously. Its strength is that it doesn't clump and with some effort it does go the distance, but for thickening and impressive length you'll have to turn to other mascaras.

☹ **Dream Gleam Lash Topcoat** *($6)* is a translucent, sea-blue mascara infused with silvery-blue glitter. The idea is to apply it over or under mascara for a gleaming, glossy effect. The comb applicator makes it easy to apply and it leaves lashes looking wet and clustered rather than fringed and separated. The drawback? Removal! This is an incredibly tenacious formula that just won't budge, even after several attempts. Given the so-so results and frustration at getting it all off, it's not recommended.

BRUSHES: ☺ **Concealer Brush** *($5)*. Of the makeup brushes Mark sells, the synthetic hair Concealer Brush fares best and also makes a great eyeshadow brush.

☺ **Go with the Pro Brush Kit** *($15)*. These tiny brushes aren't what any professional makeup artist would turn to, but it's not a bad set to have on hand for secondary, on-the- go use. None of the brushes are that soft, but they work OK for touch-ups. You get a brush for powder, concealer, lipstick/gloss, eyeliner, and one for eyeshadow. The lip brush works better to apply eyeliner, while the eyeliner brush works best to apply lipstick, at least by practical standards. As mentioned, this isn't a professional-caliber set, but it is an option to keep in your office drawer or weekend travel bag where space is limited.

☺ **Powder Brush** *($8)*. Given the price, the Powder Brush is a respectable option, though it could be softer and a bit more tapered

☹ **Blending Brush** *($5)* is a great example of what to avoid when shopping for brushes.

☹ **Blush + Bronzer Brush** *($6)* is a great example of what to avoid when shopping for brushes.

☹ **Eye Shadow Brush** *($5)* is scratchy and too small for all but detail work.

☹ **Eyeliner Brush** *($5)* is too scratchy and full to draw a precise line.

FACE AND BODY SHIMMER/ILLUMINATING PRODUCTS: ✓ ☺ **All Lit Up Face Brightening Wand** *($8)* is a sheer liquid shimmer that comes in a click-pen package with a synthetic brush applicator. Considering Mark's teen appeal, it's surprising this product's shine is so subtle. It's an excellent highlighter for all skin types (and all ages) looking to add a touch of soft radiance to the skin. The amount of shine is barely distracting for daytime wear, but a product like this still works best for evening glamour. Perhaps most impressive is that the shine stays put, so you can highlight small areas (like the brow bone or bridge of the nose) without worrying that sparkles will end up where you didn't want them.

✓ ☺ **Get Bright Hook Up Highlighter** *($6)*. Accurately described as a pearly liquid highlighter, this lightweight fluid is easy to blend and adds just the right amount of subtle glow to skin. It is ideal for highlighting under the eyes, on the brow bone, or on top of cheekbones. The flesh-toned shades correspond to various skin tones, from fair to tan. All of these are sheer and can be used with or without foundation. Consider this inexpensive shine done right!

☺ **Crystal Shimmer Hook Up Shimmer Powder** *($6)* is a decent loose shimmer powder packaged in a glass vial. It can be "hooked up" with other Mark makeup items, such as mascara or liquid eyeliner. The six shades produce a more striking (read: noticeable) shine than the All Lit Up Face Brightening Wand, though it's still on the softer side. Since this is a powder, the shine does not cling to the skin as well. However, it works as well as almost every other shimmer powder if your goal is high shine.

☺ **Glow Xpert Face Shimmer** *($8)*. I'll say up front that I don't care for the packaging and mode of application Mark chose for this fluid shimmer lotion. The lotion is housed in the bottom of a component that's affixed with a tiny plastic sifter. When you unscrew the top, there's a wand attached to it outfitted with a round sponge. The sponge is in direct contact with the sifter, and that's how the shimmer lotion is transferred. You use the round sponge to dab and blend Glow Xpert Face Shimmer wherever you want intense shine. As you can imagine, it's really easy to overdo it with this application method because the sponge tends to pick up a lot of product at once. If you apply carefully, you can achieve a flattering (though still very shiny) effect from any of the workable colors. Once dry, the shine tends to stay in place, which is always a plus. This deserves a happy face for its long-wearing finish, but the application the company devised is definitely tricky (more gimmicky then helpful).

☺ **Shimmer Bars All-Over Face Color** *($6)* is a good shimmer powder for those looking to highlight or add a touch of shine to certain areas of the face. The shine clings well and, if applied sheer, is even suitable for daytime wear.

☺ **Shimmer Cubes All-Over Face Color** *($5)*. These individual cubes of pressed powder come in a small but workable range of shades for use on cheeks and eyes, and it's readily apparent which shades work best on each area—there are colors here that shouldn't go anywhere near your eyes unless you want to look like your allergies are in overdrive. The soft "baked" texture is prone to crumbling, so be sure to purchase this with one of the refillable compacts Mark offers. Color payoff is good and application with a brush is smooth. Indeed, these practically blend themselves. The shine is a subtle to moderate glow depending on how liberally you apply, and it stays in place well.

☹ **Twinklebelle Shimmering Powder Brush** *($9)*. Housed in a cylindrical component with a built-in brush applicator is this chalk-textured, loose shimmer powder. Its finish on skin makes you look ultra-sparkly in no time, but trying to get it on evenly is a chore. If shimmer powder is what you're after, there are much better, neater-to-use options available from Jane or Wet n' Wild. Cute product name, though!

SPECIALTY PRODUCTS: ☺ **Hook Up Connector** *($0.50)* is a small piece of molded plastic with openings on each end. You use it to connect two Mark makeup products, such as concealer and mascara, or lip gloss and liquid lip color. It's not essential, but is convenient if more than one hook-up-able Mark product appeals to you.

☺ **Make Your Own Face Case** *($6)* is a sleek compact that can hold up to four eyeshadows. The tablets are held in place by a magnet, and the compact includes a slim mirror (which isn't very useful) and a dual-ended brush/eyeshadow sponge that doesn't facilitate a smooth makeup application and should be discarded and replaced with something better.

BANANA BOAT (SUN CARE ONLY)

BANANA BOAT AT-A-GLANCE

Strengths: Inexpensive and widely distributed; various textures to please a wide variety of skin types and preferences; great selection of self-tanning products; some good sunscreen options with avobenzone or titanium dioxide (check labels carefully).

Weaknesses: Several sunscreens lack sufficient UVA-protecting ingredients; several sunscreens carry SPF ratings that are miserably low; a selection of products that promote tanning; no sunscreens with formulas suitable for sensitive skin; problematic sunscreens for kids and babies (due to their mild-as-water and gentleness claims).

For more information about Banana Boat, call (800) 723-3786 or visit www.bananaboat.com or www.Beautypedia.com.

BANANA BOAT BABY PRODUCTS

☺ **Baby SPF 50 Sunscreen Stick** *($4.99 for 0.55 ounce)* is a very good sunscreen stick that includes stabilized avobenzone for reliable UVA protection. Although it is too waxy for allover use, it can be spot-applied to areas more prone to sunburn (e.g., bridge of the nose, tops of the feet and ears) after you've applied another sunscreen evenly. This contains some good antioxidants as well as a selection of exotic fragrant plant extracts. It is best for dry to very dry skin and not recommended for use on breakout-prone areas. However, the active ingredients in this shouldn't be used on babies. For babies I strongly recommend using sunscreens that contain only zinc oxide and/or titanium dioxide as the active ingredients. For adults this is a great option, but the baby label is really a problem.

☺ **Baby Tear-Free SPF 50 Continuous Lotion Spray** *($9.99 for 6 ounces)* is a good spray-on sunscreen with avobenzone for sufficient UVA protection, but the tear-free claim is incredibly misleading. All of the actives in this sunscreen can cause eye stinging and tearing if this is not sprayed very carefully (and never sprayed directly on face; apply to hands first, then spread on facial skin). It is good that fragrance was omitted and a couple of vitamin-based antioxidants were included; however, this is not an ideal sunscreen for use on baby's skin. A gentle mineral sunscreen with titanium dioxide or zinc oxide is preferred.

☺ **Baby Tear-Free SPF 50 Lotion** *($10.49 for 8 ounces).* Although it's great that this sunscreen lotion contains an in-part titanium dioxide sunscreen, the claim that this formula is "mild as water" is completely wrong. Several of the sunscreen actives have the potential to cause irritation on baby's skin, whereas plain water has no such concerns. Your child will get broad-spectrum sun protection if this is applied liberally, but the risk of skin stinging and problems with eye contact are real.

BANANA BOAT KIDS PRODUCTS

☺ **Kids Dri-Blok SPF 30 Lotion** *($8.19 for 6 ounces)* is a lightweight, dry-finish lotion with nearly 3% avobenzone for UVA protection. The powdery finish is said to keep sand from sticking to skin and for the most part that's true (sand sticks much more readily to a moist finish, which this sunscreen lacks). This is a good sunscreen option for kids (or adults) who find most high-SPF products feel too thick or goopy on skin.

☹ **Kids SPF 50 Continuous Clear Spray** *($9.99 for 6 ounces).* Yes, sufficient UVA protection is assured with this in-part avobenzone sunscreen but the amount of alcohol makes it too drying and irritating for anyone's skin, including kids.

✓ ☺ **Kids Tear-Free SPF 30 Continuous Lotion Spray** *($9.99 for 6 ounces).* UVA protection is assured thanks to the maximum permitted amount of avobenzone, and this alcohol-free spray-on sunscreen has a light, silky feel. Antioxidants are plentiful and the formula is fragrance-free, which is a benefit for everyone. Although the tear-free, won't-sting-skin, and waterproof claims are without basis (the active ingredients in this sunscreen can definitely irritate the eyes if contact occurs, and some people's skin cannot tolerate these sunscreens without a stinging sensation), that doesn't change the fact that formula-wise, this sunscreen is one of Banana Boat's very best.

☺ **Kids Tear-Free SPF 30 Lotion** *($8.99 for 8 ounces)* is absolutely not "as mild as water" (that's like saying soda pop is as good for you as a glass of milk), but this in-part titanium dioxide lotion has a silky texture and smooth finish that is water-resistant. The tiny amount of antioxidants included here is better than nothing, but they likely convey minimal benefit to skin.

☺ **Kids Tear-Free SPF 50 Continuous Lotion Spray** *($9.99 for 6 ounces).* Labeling this as "gentle" is inaccurate because the actives used in this in-part avobenzone sunscreen have the potential to cause skin reactions, especially on children's skin. And if it gets in the eyes, you'll quickly find out how laughable the gentleness claims are. However, this remains a good option for kids who know how to apply sunscreen correctly or adults with normal to slightly dry skin who want a convenient, spray-on sunscreen that's alcohol-free.

☺ **Kids Tear-Free SPF 50 Lotion** *($10.49 for 8 ounces)* contains an in-part titanium dioxide sunscreen but is not "mild as water"! Several of the sunscreen actives may cause irritation on a child's skin. This is a good sunscreen, just not a gentle one that's special for kids.

BANANA BOAT SPORT PERFORMANCE PRODUCTS

☺ **Kids SPF 50 Sunscreen Stick** *($5.99 for 0.55 ounce)* is a very good sunscreen stick that includes stabilized avobenzone for reliable UVA protection. Although too waxy for allover use, it can be spot-applied to areas more prone to sunburn (e.g., bridge of nose, tops of the feet and ears) after you've applied another sunscreen evenly. This contains some good antioxidants as well as a selection of exotic fragrant plant extracts. It is best for dry to very dry skin and not recommended for use on breakout-prone areas. The active ingredients aren't the best for kids, but most adults will tolerate them just fine.

☺ **Sport Performance Dri-Blok SPF 30 Continuous Lotion Spray** *($9.99 for 6 ounces)* is a very good, in-part avobenzone sunscreen for active people with normal to oily skin. The amount of film-forming agent ensures water- and sweat-resistance, but does not change the fact that, as with all sunscreens, this needs to be reapplied after excessive perspiration or water immersion. It is good news that Banana Boat is offering a spray-on sunscreen that doesn't contain drying alcohol.

☺ **Sport Performance Dri-Blok SPF 30 Lotion** *($8.99 for 6 ounces)* is a very good in-part avobenzone sunscreen for normal to oily skin. It has a smooth texture and soft matte finish plus treats skin to a couple of vitamin-based antioxidants.

✓ ☺ **Sport Performance Lip Balm SPF 50** *($2.99 for 0.02 ounce).* More lips balms with reliable broad-spectrum sun protection are needed, and here's an excellent one to add to your list. UVA protection is assured from avobenzone, and the emollient, balm-like base is ideal for keeping lips protected from chapping and moisture loss. It is fragrance-free and flavored with the artificial sweetener saccharin.

☹ **Sport Performance SPF 15 Continuous Clear Spray** *($9.99 for 6 ounces)* deserves credit for its broad-spectrum blend of sunscreen actives that includes avobenzone, but the amount of alcohol it contains will prove too irritating and drying to skin.

☹ **Sport Performance SPF 15 Lotion** *($8.99 for 8 ounces)* features an in-part avobenzone sunscreen in a lightweight lotion base that is short on frills. However, it is not recommended because it contains the preservatives methylchloroisothiazolinone and methylisothiazolinone. Also known as Kathon CG, this preservative blend is not advised for use in leave-on products. As such, this sunscreen is not recommended. Even if the amount used is lower than what's permissible for use in leave-on products, why take chances with a preservative blend known to be sensitizing?

☹ **Sport Performance SPF 30 Continuous Clear Spray** *($9.99 for 6 ounces)*. There's nothing sporty about needlessly irritating skin with alcohol, and that's what will happen when this in-part avobenzone sunscreen is sprayed on skin. The amount of antioxidant vitamins is too small to counter the damage this much alcohol can cause.

☹ **Sport Performance SPF 30 Faces Oil-Free Sunscreen** *($8.49 for 3 ounces)*. What a shame this in-part avobenzone sunscreen contains the sensitizing preservatives methylisothiazolinone and methylcholorisothiazolinone. Without these problem ingredients, this would be one of Banana Boat's better sunscreens for normal to oily skin.

☹ **Sport Performance SPF 30 Lotion** *($8.99 for 8 ounces)* features an in-part avobenzone sunscreen in a lightweight lotion base that is short on frills. However, it is not recommended because it contains the preservatives methylchloroisothiazolinone and methylisothiazolinone. Also known as Kathon CG, this preservative blend is not advised for use in leave-on products.

☹ **Sport Performance SPF 50 Continuous Clear Spray** *($9.99 for 6 ounces)* is, save for a higher percentage of active ingredient, similar to the Sport Performance Sunblock SPF 15 Continuous Clear Spray reviewed above, and the same review applies.

☹ **Sport Performance SPF 50 Lotion** *($8.99 for 8 ounces)* features an in-part avobenzone sunscreen in a lightweight lotion base that is short on frills (though the amount of avobenzone isn't likely to provide UVA protection worthy of the SPF 50 rating). However, it is not recommended because it contains the preservatives methylchloroisothiazolinone and methylisothiazolinone. Also known as Kathon CG, this preservative blend is not advised for use in leave-on products.

☹ **Sport Performance SPF 85 Continuous Clear Spray** *($11.99 for 6 ounces)* contains avobenzone for sufficient UVA protection, yet once again Banana Boat includes denatured alcohol as the main ingredient in the base formula, which causes free-radical damage and kills skin cells. Alcohol, coupled with the high percentage of active ingredients necessary to get an SPF 85 rating, make this sunscreen too drying and irritating for all skin types. Increasing the amount of synthetic sunscreen agents to obtain an SPF rating this high increases the risk of a sensitizing skin reaction. Besides, there's no need to go for SPF 85 if you have a well-formulated SPF 30 or SPF 45 sunscreen that you apply liberally and reapply as needed.

BANANA BOAT SUN WEAR PRODUCTS

☹ **Sun Wear SPF 30 Faces Oil-Free Daily Sunscreen Lotion** *($9.49 for 3 ounces)* contains the preservatives methylisothiazolinone and methylchlorothiazolinone (Kathon CG), which are contraindicated for use in leave-on products.

The Reviews B

☹ **Sun Wear SPF 50 Daily Sunscreen Lotion** *($9.99 for 6 ounces)* is a good, in-part avobenzone sunscreen in a silky, matte-finish base that contains some very good antioxidants and skin-identical ingredients. What a shame the Kathon CG preservative system makes an otherwise fine sunscreen ill-advised due to its potential for causing a sensitized reaction.

☹ **Sun Wear SPF 50 Daily Sunscreen Lotion Mist** *($9.99 for 5 ounces)*. What a shame this in-part avobenzone sunscreen contains the sensitizing preservatives methylisothiazolinone and methylcholorisothiazolinone. Without these problem ingredients, this would be one of Banana Boat's better sunscreens for normal to oily skin. By the way, the botanical extracts this formula contains have dubious benefit for skin.

BANANA BOAT ULTRA DEFENSE PRODUCTS

☹ **Ultra Defense SPF 15 Sunscreen Lotion** *($8.99 for 8 ounces)* deserves credit for its in-part avobenzone sunscreen, but loses points for including the sensitizing preservatives methylcholorisothiazolinone and methylisothiazolinone. Plenty of broad-spectrum sunscreens use less problematic preservatives, so there's no need to set your sights on this one.

☹ **Ultra Defense SPF 30 Continuous Clear Spray** *($9.99 for 6 ounces)* contains too much drying, irritating alcohol to make it worth considering over several other spray-on options, including those from Banana Boat. Moreover, 1% avobenzone isn't the ideal amount for UVA protection in a sunscreen rated SPF 30.

☹ **Ultra Defense SPF 30 Sunscreen Lotion** *($8.99 for 8 ounces)* deserves credit for its in-part avobenzone sunscreen (though 1% avobenzone isn't what you want to see in a sunscreen rated SPF 30), but loses points for including the sensitizing preservatives methylcholorisothiazolinone and methylisothiazolinone.

☹ **Ultra Defense SPF 50 Continuous Clear Spray** *($9.99 for 6 ounces)*. Although this is a much better formula in terms of UVA protection than Banana Boat's Ultra Defense Continuous Spray Sunblock SPF 30, the amount of alcohol makes it impossible to recommend.

☹ **Ultra Defense SPF 50 Sunscreen Lotion** *($10.49 for 8 ounces)* deserves credit for its in-part avobenzone sunscreen, but loses points for including the sensitizing preservatives methylchloroisothiazolinone and methylisothiazolinone.

☺ **Ultra Defense SPF 80 Sunscreen Lotion** *($9.99 for 3 ounces)*. This Banana Boat Ultra Defense sunscreen fortunately does not contain the same sensitizing preservative system as a few of their other products, and that's good news. It also contains the maximum amount of avobenzone for excellent UVA protection—but SPF 80? It is highly doubtful that anyone's skin sees that much daylight. Even someone whose skin turns pink in 10 minutes would be protected for 800 minutes (over 13 hours), which is overkill to say the least. There's also an issue with the amount of active ingredients required to claim SPF 80—that high a concentration poses a risk of irritating skin—and over 30% of the ingredients in this sunscreen are actives, so a sensitized reaction is much more likely. Still, this will provide longer broad-spectrum protection than several other sunscreens—it's just that the trade-off may not be worth it.

☹ **Ultra Defense SPF 85 Continuous Clear Spray** *($12.99 for 6 ounces)*. Although this sunscreen contains a hefty amount of active ingredients, including avobenzone for sufficient UVA protection and octocrylene to keep it stable, its base formula is mostly alcohol. That means it is too drying and irritating for all skin types.

☺ **Ultra Defense Sunscreen Faces SPF 30 Lotion** *($7.99)* is a well-formulated sunscreen that includes avobenzone for sufficient UVA protection. It has a silky, lightweight texture and matte finish that those with oily skin will appreciate. The inclusion of several antioxidants is impressive, but becomes less so when you realize that all of them are listed after the preservative, so they don't add up to much. Still, given the typical sunscreen formula, you're getting a fairly decent cocktail of antioxidants and this is fragrance-free.

BANANA BOAT AFTER SUN PRODUCTS

☹ **Aloe After Sun Cleansing Wipes** *($3.29 for 16 cloths)* contain witch hazel as the second ingredient, which negates the soothing agents that follow. Your skin deserves better than this after a long day in the sun and heat! Plain, pure aloe vera gel would be preferred.

☹ **Aloe After Sun Gel** *($5.89 for 8 ounces)* lists alcohol as the second ingredient and contains a mere token amount of aloe, making this a bad choice for after sun or any other time.

☺ **Aloe After Sun Lotion** *($6.99 for 16 ounces)* is an OK option for use any time skin is dry. But for after sun, when skin may have suffered some amount of damage (even with the application of a well-formulated sunscreen) there are better formulas to consider from Olay Quench, Curel, and CeraVe.

☹ **Aloe After Sun Spray Gel** *($7.49 for 8 ounces)* cools skin with a fine mist of alcohol, but the overall effect is more irritating than soothing, and truly beneficial ingredients are a foreign concept for this poorly formulated product.

OTHER BANANA BOAT PRODUCTS

☹ **Aloe Vera with Vitamin E Sunscreen Lip Balm SPF 30** *($1.99 for 0.15 ounce)* lacks the UVA-protecting ingredients of titanium dioxide, zinc oxide, avobenzone (also known as butyl methoxydibenzoylmethane), Tinosorb, or Mexoryl SX and is not recommended.

☹ **Dark Tanning Oil SPF 4** *($7.69 for 8 ounces)* has a woefully low SPF rating and its ability to provide UVA protection is inadequate. Moreover, any product that encourages tanning (and dark tanning, no less) isn't one that should be considered by anyone looking to keep their skin young, vibrant, and healthy.

☹ **Dark Tanning Oil, No Sunscreen** *($7.69 for 8 ounces)* is merely a blend of mineral oil with tiny amounts of aloe, various plant extracts, and vitamins. The antioxidant properties of the vitamins won't shield skin from sun damage. If anything, consumers should question the ethics of a company promoting sun protection and tan-attaining products. Disingenuous is one way to put it, but I can think of harsher words! This is only recommended if you long to return to the days when slathering baby oil on skin and baking in the sun was seen as a healthy summer activity. By all medical standards today, this practice is viewed as the fast track to skin damage and, potentially, skin cancer.

☹ **Deep Tanning Dry Oil SPF 4 Continuous Clear Spray** *($9.99 for 6 ounces).* The amount of active ingredients and the SPF rating of this sunscreen make it just pathetic. Add to that the drying, irritating alcohol base and the fact that this product encourages tanning, and Banana Boat has taken pathetic to a new low!

☹ **Deep Tanning Dry Oil SPF 8 Continuous Clear Spray** *($9.79 for 6 ounces)* is very similar to Banana Boat's Deep Tanning Dry Oil SPF 4 Continuous Clear Spray, which isn't encouraging. SPF 8 is better than SPF 4, but still falls below the minimum SPF rating recommended by countless medical organizations. Moreover, this product encourages tanning and its alcohol-based formula causes dryness, irritation, and free-radical damage.

☹ **Deep Tanning SPF 4 Lotion with Green Tea** *($9.49 for 8 ounces).* This unethical sunscreen encourages tanning, which not only causes wrinkles and skin discolorations but also puts your skin at serious risk of skin cancer. Deep tanning? Why doesn't Banana Boat just hand out cigarettes with this product? That would seal up the damage inside and out. An SPF 4 should not be allowed to be sold without a warning, similar to what cigarette companies must include on their tobacco products. This emollient lotion is suitable for dry skin, but the amount of green tea is tiny, clearly an afterthought and for marketing purposes only. Besides, if you're going to encourage tanning, why bother including antioxidants? They can't change or reduce the damage that getting a tan will cause. Clearly, the goal here is to encourage damage instead of protecting skin.

☹ **Deep Tanning SPF 8 Lotion with Green Tea** *($9.99 for 8 ounces)* is similar to Banana Boat's Deep Tanning SPF 4 Lotion with Green Tea and the same comments apply here, too.

☺ **EveryDay Glow SunDial Self-Tanning Moisturizer, For Lighter Skin Tones** *($11.99 for 6.7 ounces)* combines a self-tanning lotion and "primer" in one cleverly packaged product. The user controls how much of each product is distributed by dialing in the desired amount. It's intriguing and the formulas are just fine, but the end result is a sunless tan, just like you achieve from countless products without the packaging gimmick this one has. The only reason to go with this type of product is for times when you only want a little color or need to deepen a previously applied self-tan. However, you can also do that with numerous other self-tanners. This is best for normal to dry skin.

☺ **EveryDay Glow SunDial Self-Tanning Lotion, For Darker Skin Tones** *($11.99 for 6.7 ounces)* has the same packaging and application methods (and caveats) as the EveryDay Glow SunDial Self-Tanning Moisturizer, For Lighter Skin Tones, but the self-tanner portion contains a greater amount of dihydroxyacetone for darker color. Otherwise, the same comments apply.

☹ **Faces Plus UVA & UVB Sunblock Stick SPF 30** *($5.49 for 0.55 ounce)* lacks the UVA-protecting ingredients of titanium dioxide, zinc oxide, avobenzone (also known as butyl methoxydibenzoylmethane), Tinosorb, or Mexoryl SX and is not recommended.

☹ **Protective Tanning Dry Oil SPF 15 Continuous Clear Spray** *($9.79 for 6 ounces).* The SPF rating and in-part avobenzone sunscreen is great, but it's hard to overlook the packaging, which explicitly sells this product as a way to get a tan. Also, the main ingredient in the base formula is skin-damaging denatured alcohol. There are plenty of lightweight sunscreens that provide broad-spectrum protection but that don't expose skin to alcohol and that don't make claims that promote getting "the color you want." You should never get "the color you want" from the sun, at least not if you want to reduce your risk of skin cancer, wrinkles, and skin discolorations.

☹ **Protective Tanning Dry Oil SPF 25 Continuous Clear Spray** *($10.99 for 6 ounces)* is very similar to Banana Boat's Protective Tanning Dry Oil SPF 15 Continuous Clear Spray. It contains a higher amount of active ingredients to achieve its SPF rating, but otherwise suffers from too much skin-damaging alcohol.

☹ **Protective Tanning Oil SPF 15** *($7.79 for 8 ounces)* may make you think this is the safe way to tan, but there's no such thing. Any amount of color skin gets from the sun is a sign of dam-age. This sunscreen does not provide sufficient UVA protection and is little more than fragranced baby oil disguised as a protective product for skin when it's really all about getting a tan.

☹ **Protective Tanning Oil SPF 8** *($7.79 for 8 ounces).* The blend of active ingredients in this tanning oil won't protect skin from the sun very well, especially as far as UVA screening is concerned. The SPF rating is too low for sufficient protection, and the product is designed to encourage tanning.

☹ **Sooth-A-Caine Aloe Vera Spray Gel with Lidocaine** *($6.19 for 8 ounces).* The lidocaine in this spray-on product serves as a good topical anesthetic, but the menthol is a problem. There are other lidocaine products at the drugstore that don't subject skin to further irritation. Plain aloe vera gel would be preferred as a lightweight soothing option for sunburned skin.

☹ **Sport Quik-Dri SPF 30 Body & Scalp Sunblock Spray** *($8.59 for 6 ounces)* dries quickly because of the amount of alcohol it contains, yet that—coupled with the active sunscreen ingredients that include avobenzone—can prove too irritating for all skin types.

☺ **Summer Color Self-Tanning Lotion, Deep Dark Color** *($7.69 for 6 ounces).* Because this lightweight yet moisturizing self-tanning lotion contains dihydroxyacetone as the second ingredient, dark color is assured. This is recommended for those with medium to dark skin tones and/or those who have experience with applying self-tanner (the darker the results, the more one risks a streaked or blotchy appearance). Based on the emollients and thickening agents in this self-tanner, I am doubtful of the company's claim that it "dries in minutes." A gel formula is best if quick drying is what you're after.

☺ **Summer Color Self-Tanning Lotion, Light/Medium Color** *($7.69 for 6 ounces)* is similar to the Summer Color Self-Tanning Lotion, Deep Dark Color, except this lotion has slightly less dihydroxyacetone for a less intense tan.

☺ **Summer Color Self-Tanning Mist, For All Skin Tones** *($10.49 for 5 ounces)* is an alcohol-free, fine-mist self-tanning spray. It uses dihydroxyacetone (DHA), the same ingredient found in most self-tanners to turn skin dark. This option is well-suited for those with oily or breakout-prone skin.

BARE ESCENTUALS

BARE ESCENTUALS AT-A-GLANCE

Strengths: Good makeup removers (unless you wear waterproof formulas); a good loose powder and some impressive mascaras; several elegant brush options; not too expensive.

Weaknesses: The mineral makeup has its share of pros and cons and isn't for everyone; poorly formulated BHA product; several of the loose powder products with shine have a grainy feel and cling poorly; Self-tanner with unidentified essential oils; greasy lipstick.

For more information about Bare Escentuals, call (800) 227-3990 or visit www.bareescentuals.com or www.Beautypedia.com

BARE ESCENTUALS SKIN CARE

BARE ESCENTUALS RAREMINERALS PRODUCTS

☹ **RareMinerals Renew & Reveal Facial Cleanser** *($26 for 2.5 ounces)* is a nonaqueous, clay-based powder cleanser that you mix with water before use. It contains a detergent cleansing agent along with baking soda and other absorbents, including the company's "soil mineral concentrate," which is said to release its benefits (still undocumented and at best completely dubious) when water is added. What I particularly object to is the statement that this cleanser contains no skin-irritating chemicals, because what it does contain are skin-irritating "natural" ingredients, and whether synthetic or natural, irritation is bad for skin. The absorbents and soil mineral concentrate (dirt) can be too drying, which leads to irritated skin, and the several fragrant oils (clove, rosemary, lavender, lime, jasmine, and clary) are absolutely irritating.

☹ **RareMinerals Moisture Burst Facial Mist** *($18 for 3.4 ounces).* The RareMinerals original treatment product (which is nothing more than a loose powder with soil concentrates; in other words, it's powdery dirt) was supposed to be a does-it-all product regardless of one's skin-care concern. Obviously it wasn't capable of that because the company didn't believe their own proclamations; why else would this toner be needed? It turns out this isn't a spray-on toner anyone should use because the sage and rosemary leaf waters pose a risk of irritation. That's made worse by witch hazel water, an ingredient whose alcohol component can be troublesome for skin (though the amount of witch hazel in this toner is smaller than in many other toners that have this ingredient). Don't be swayed by the intriguing claims for this toner—it goes over the top in claiming to provide protection against environmental stressors that lead to premature aging. That claim is better suited to sunscreen, nonirritating plant extracts, and antioxidants, which this toner doesn't provide. As for the soil minerals being able to feed skin? You're better off obtaining "essential nutrients" from a healthy diet and treating your skin to products loaded with researched antioxidants and cell-communicating ingredients.

☹ **RareMinerals Purely Nourishing Facial Moisturizer** *($32 for 1.7 ounces)* isn't a moisturizer anyone should consider. The "soil minerals" (which should be identified but aren't, so who knows what you're actually putting on your skin) aren't essential for anyone's skin. Although this moisturizer contains a roster of impressive nonmineral ingredients, it loses a favorable review because it contains grapefruit and lavender oils, two fragrant additives that are present in amounts very likely to be irritating. And bitter-orange oil, although present in a smaller amount, doesn't improve matters. In fact, the trio of fragrant additives doesn't make this worth considering over any Paula's Pick–rated moisturizer, regardless of price.

☺ **$$$ RareMinerals Skin Revival Treatment** *($60).* The list of claims for this product makes it sound like Nirvana for the skin. For all intents and purposes the showcased ingredient in this product is, well, dirt. (Dirt is my term, Bare Escentuals uses the term "Jurassic, virgin soil," but by any name, soil is just another term for dirt, although I have to agree soil does sounds less, well, dirty). I have to admit that seeing dirt advertised as skin care is a first! RareMinerals Skin Revival Treatment is supposed to contain 72 organic "macro" and "micro" minerals. However, you won't find 72 minerals listed on the ingredients label, just Organic Soil Mineral Concentrate—so you have to take their word that these 72 minerals are present in the "virgin" dirt. According to the company, this mixture, along with the other ingredients, will produce firmer, smoother, and brighter skin while at the same time prompting exfoliation and reducing pore size. Essentially, this is being sold as a one-size-fits-all "skin-care" product "feeding" skin with everything it needs to look its best and function optimally. That part is definitely a stretch because, first and foremost, this powder-based product isn't moisturizing in the least (minerals aren't moisturizing; if anything, they absorb oil), nor does it provide sun protection. Its mica base is there for the shine, and while other absorbent minerals are included they also prevent the skin-identical ingredients in the product from having much, if any, benefit for skin. Actually, the formula isn't too far removed from the original bareMinerals Foundation SPF 15. Both are loose powders that go on smoothly and impart a radiant glow to skin that comes from those shiny particles of mica. RareMinerals Skin Revival Treatment comes in four shades, including a Clear option that still imparts some color, and most of them provide enough coverage to camouflage minor flaws and redness, so you will perceive that your skin looks better. The recommendation to wear this at night is just shocking to me. Be forewarned that sleeping with this product on your face will result in makeup stains on your pillowcase, and that leaving this stuff on overnight would most likely be drying and irritating. Minerals on the skin, even plain talc or chalk or soil of any kind, aren't soothing in the least. They need to be washed off, not worn to bed, and this product is no exception. Getting back to the mineral claims, is there anything to them? Does this "pure mineral concentrate" hold the secret to revitalized, youthful skin? Regardless of the purity of the soil, minerals cannot be absorbed by skin (their molecules are just too big), so any effect would be entirely superficial. Moreover, while there hasn't been much research on topical application of minerals, we do know that whether they are applied topically or ingested, minerals depend on other factors (most notably coenzymes) to work, and even when that happens the benefits aren't all that exciting (Sources: *Cosmeceuticals*, Elsner & Maiback, 2000, pages 29-30; and *International Journal of Cosmetic Science*, 1997, page 105). There is no substantiated research proving that minerals, whether concentrated or not, exfoliate skin or have any effect on pore size. Any perceived reduction in pore size from using this product is solely from its reflective quality and natural opacity, the same as any other powder foundation. It can work to temporarily fill in large pores, but when it's washed off, any potential benefit is washed away at the same time. You may be wondering about the vitamin C (ascorbic acid) in this product. According to the chemists I spoke with, ascorbic acid tends to remain stable in an anhydrous (waterless) product, which this powder certainly qualifies as. How much of the vitamin C reaches the skin is a question, however, along with whether RareMinerals uses an effective amount. The bottom line is that although RareMinerals may be unique in terms of its extraction process and its use of virgin soil, those elements won't translate into skin care. It's just another form of powder, and a rather expensive one at that.

☹ **RareMinerals Blemish Therapy** (*$28 for 0.07 ounce*) is not recommended for several reasons: its active ingredient of 3% sulfur, while it is antibacterial, is way too drying and irritating for skin; the absorbent minerals will only exacerbate the dryness from the sulfur; and the retinol and niacinamide will be useless because of the unfortunate choice of jar packaging and the high pH of the sulfur. It is also interesting to note that high pH products over 8pH can increase the amount of acne-causing bacteria in skin.

OTHER BARE ESCENTUALS SKIN-CARE PRODUCTS

☺ **i.d. bareEyes Eye Makeup Remover** (*$14 for 4 ounces*) is a standard, fragrance-free, detergent-based eye-makeup remover that does the job, but is best used prior to cleansing the face since the ingredients are best rinsed from the skin.

☺ **i.d. On The Spot Eye Makeup Remover** (*$5 for 24 swabs*) provides a very gentle eye-makeup remover inside the hollow center of a cotton swab. Snapping the swab at the indicated point feeds the fluid onto the cotton tip, making for quick, convenient application. This isn't the most economical way to remove makeup, and the formula is too mild for stubborn or waterproof makeup, but it's an option.

☹ **bareVitamins Skin Rev-er Upper** (*$21 for 2.3 ounces*) used to rate as a very good 1% BHA (salicylic acid) product with a pH of 3.5 to ensure that exfoliation will occur. It seems the company changed the formula somewhat (or finally listed all of the ingredients) and not for the better. This contains several plant extracts that are a distinct problem for skin, with the biggest offender being arnica. This also contains St. John's Wort, listed by its Latin name of *Hypericum* *perforatum.* Applied topically, this plant contains several components that are toxic in the presence of sunlight (Sources: *Planta Medica*, February 2002, pages 171-173; and *International Journal of Biochemistry and Cell Biology*, March 2002, pages 221-241). What a shame, because this is no longer a BHA product I can recommend, and there are so few options!

☺ **$$$ bareVitamins Eye Rev-er Upper** *($21 for 0.45 ounce)* claims to make you look like you got 12 hours of sleep, but this rather basic moisturizer doesn't adequately substitute for a good night's rest, or for a better formulated product. It contains mostly water, slip agent, occlusive agent, emollient, thickeners, silicone, antioxidant vitamins, plant extracts, skin-identical ingredients, preservatives, and mineral pigments (that's what creates the cosmetic brightening effect). This is a decent choice for those with normal to slightly dry skin.

☺ **Faux Tan** *($22 for 4.5 ounces)* contains dihydroxyacetone, the same ingredient found in most self-tanning products. This works as well as any, but gets a cautious recommendation because of the fragrance in its blend of essential oils. Without knowing which oils comprise this fragrance, you could be applying irritants to skin whose only benefit is smelling pleasant.

☺ **$$$ bareVitamins Lip Rev-er Upper** *($16 for 0.06 ounce)* is a stick lip balm based on macadamia nut oil. It applies smoothly and the amount of film-forming agent (it's the second ingredient) has some ability to keep lipstick in place, though it's not foolproof. This isn't the best for very dry or chapped lips, but is worth testing if you want something lighter to wear under lipstick.

☺ **Buzz Latte Lip Balm** *($8 for 0.25 ounce)* is a good emollient lip balm in stick form. It contains helpful emollients and waxes along with token amounts of antioxidants.

BARE ESCENTUALS MAKEUP

FOUNDATION: ☹ **bareMinerals Foundation SPF 15** *($25)* is the loose-powder foundation that put Bare Escentuals on the map and it is the backbone of this makeup line. This talc-free, mica-based powder has a soft, almost creamy texture and an undeniably shiny finish (not a good look for someone with oily skin). The titanium dioxide and bismuth oxychloride lend this powder its opacity, medium to full coverage, and slightly thick finish. In addition, with 25% titanium dioxide listed as an active ingredient, broad-spectrum sun protection is assured. This foundation can be tricky to blend, and is best applied with a powder brush. Several shades are available, with the best options being for fair to light skin. There are plenty of shades for women of color, but the high amount of titanium dioxide causes them to look or turn ashy on darker skin. The Tan shade is an excellent choice for loose bronzing powder.

☺ **$$$ bareMinerals SPF 15 Matte Foundation** *($28)*. Now that a matte-finish makeup look is making a comeback (again)—in contrast to the luminescent, nearly glittery appearance of foundation over the past few years—Bare Escentuals decided to put their option out there, but they just didn't pull it off, although it would have been a welcome change of pace from their shiny options. This loose-powder mineral foundation has a very soft texture and smooth application. The sunscreen is a blend of titanium dioxide and zinc oxide, and makes up 20% of the formula. Provided you apply this evenly, sun protection is assured. These minerals also provide opacity and contribute to the matte finish and medium to almost full coverage.

Despite the name, however, this foundation doesn't have a truly matte finish; you still get a soft, non-sparkling glow that someone with very oily skin won't appreciate. The silica base coupled with calcium silicate and the mineral sunscreen agents can make this feel quite dry, which makes it not the best for dry skin. What Bare Escentuals did well is the closure for this loose-powder makeup. The sifter can be completely sealed so powder doesn't spill out all over the place, although you'll still get some residual powder in the cap and on the sifter with each use, but the mess is minor when compared with the mess of many other loose powders.

Where this foundation takes a sharp nosedive is in its shades. Most of the light colors are fine, but all of the darker shades have a strong ashen finish that can make dark skin tones look drab and gray. The following shades are not recommended, either because they are very ash or because they are too peachy, pink, or just plain chalky: Medium, Warm Tan, Dark, Medium Dark, Golden Dark, Medium Deep, Golden Deep, and Deepest Deep. The Golden Medium shade is acceptable, but is too yellow for many medium skin tones, so consider it carefully.

☺ $$$ **bareMinerals Multi-Tasking Minerals** *($18)* are sold as colors to use as an eyeshadow base or as a concealer to be used with the bareMinerals Foundation SPF 15. These loose powders have less shine than the foundation, but are far from matte. A small but good selection of neutral shades (best for fair to light skin) is available, including Well Rested. The Summer Bisque and Honey Bisque shades have 20% zinc oxide as an active ingredient, rating an SPF 20.

POWDER: ☺ $$$ **bareMinerals SPF30 Natural Sunscreen** *($28)* is a loose powder with a sunscreen that's pure titanium dioxide. Housed in a cylindrical component affixed with a soft, decently shaped applicator brush, you shake powder from the base so it feeds through the bottom of the brush, and then apply to your face. The powder has a soft, sheer texture and minimal shine (much less shine than other powders from Bare Escentuals). This is a great way to add to the sun protection you're already getting from your daytime moisturizer or foundation with sunscreen, plus it helps blot excess shine. Three shades are available, and while all are workable, the Tan shade works best as bronzing powder (strategically applied to cheeks and temples) rather than as allover face powder. The titanium dioxide is micronized so it doesn't leave a thick, pasty appearance on skin.

☺ $$$ **Mineral Veil** *($19)* is a talc-free loose powder with a softer and much lighter consistency than the bareMinerals Foundation SPF 15, and it applies matte. The two sheer colors have a dry finish that's best for someone with normal to oily skin. This is cornstarch-based, so avoid it if you're prone to or are battling blemishes.

☹ $$$ **Hydrating Mineral Veil** *($29)*. Don't be misled by the name of this loose powder. Although it is water-based, it contains plenty of absorbent cornstarch, which doesn't make it the least bit hydrating, and cornstarch is not a mineral. Claims for mineral powders are as devious and misleading as it gets in the cosmetics industry, but apparently they're incredibly convincing. This powder has a somewhat heavier feel upon application than most loose powders, but it does quickly lighten, leaving skin feeling very dry and looking very matte. On skin the application looks iridescent, with an almost metallic shade of pink—so this isn't something you want to swirl all over your face during the day or even at night, unless you want a very shiny, somewhat other-worldly complexion. Because of its absorbency and finish this powder is best for normal to very oily skin; however, as mentioned, you must be willing to tolerate a lot of iridescence, which almost always makes oily skin look oilier. Plus, the hydrating claims are ludicrous; this is a drying powder—there is nothing moisturizing about it.

☹ **Mineral Veil On the Go** *($28)*. What a mess this cornstarch-based loose powder is! The packaging features powder with a built-in brush, but the twist-up brush part is way below average quality, the powder dispenses too heavily and unevenly, and what you end up with is a lot of product on yourself and/or your counter. There is no reason to prefer this to a compact pressed powder that is also portable. Fans of Mineral Veil, please test this in the store before buying; you'll save yourself a great deal of at-home frustration by doing so. And just in case you were wondering, cornstarch is not a mineral, so the name is meaningless, just as it always has been with any of these mineral makeup products.

BLUSH: ☺ **$$$ All Over Face Color** *($13)* is in this category because most of the shades are suitable as blush, not colors you'd want to dust all over the face. This is another loose powder with a shiny finish comparable to the bareMinerals Foundation SPF 15. Even the least shiny shade, Soft Focus True, has enough shine to make someone with oily skin nervous.

☺ **$$$ bareMinerals Blush** *($18)* has the same basic texture as the loose foundation, and the comments about its being messy and hard to control apply here, too. There are some matte shades of this product, and the application is soft and relatively even once you've mastered how much loose color to pick up on your brush for best results. Although it's hard for me to encourage this option, I'm sure some women will love it.

☺ **$$$ bareMinerals Blush Compatibles** *($22)* provides two loose powder blushes in one jar, with the colors separated by a divider. The sifter twists so you can more easily control how much powder is dispensed, but this still remains a messy way to apply blush. One shade is almost matte while the other is sparkling, and both have a dry texture that can go on somewhat thick but will blend better than you'd expect. Among the duos, use caution with the odd pairing of Pink Ice and Ginger Spice.

EYESHADOW: ☺ **bareMinerals Eye Shadow** *($13)* has a much silkier, lighter texture than the bareMinerals Foundation SPF 15. It applies and blends well, with most of the shades going on softer than they look. Some of the shades appear matte in the container, but their noticeable shine is revealed on application. Speaking of shine, it runs the gamut here, from a "you're glowing" to a "you're blinding me" finish. This is still a messy way to apply eyeshadow, and the shiniest shades don't cling as well as they should.

☺ **bareMinerals Glimpse** *($13)* is a small collection of loose-powder eyeshadows with more emphasis on sparkling shine than pigment. They're for "whisper soft" eye effects, but the amount of shine these leave isn't more than a whisper amount, and it doesn't stay in place.

EYE AND BROW SHAPER: ☺ **bareMinerals Brow Powder** *($11)* is loose powder for the brows that comes in six suitable colors, though this is an incredibly untidy way to shape and define your brows. Why anyone would choose this over a pressed matte brow powder (or eyeshadow) or even a good, standard brow pencil is a mystery. In addition, all of the colors have a subtle shine.

☺ **bareMinerals Liner Shadow** *($13)* would indeed work as eyeliner, and these intensely pigmented loose powders function wet or dry. They're not as grainy as they used to be, though every shade is imbued with shine, some featuring a metallic or glittery finish (and yes, the glitter flakes). Just as with the Brow Powder, this is a messy way to line your eyes, but if you're willing to tolerate that and have a smooth, wrinkle-free eyelid and lower lash line, go for it—with one caveat: avoid the obvious blue and green shades, which have nothing to do with shaping and defining the eye.

☺ **$$$ Buxom Insider Eyeliner** *($14)* is an automatic retractable pencil available in six shades ranging from purple to pearl. It claims to be gentle enough to line even the inner rim of eyes, but the formula doesn't bear that out. Besides, using any pencil to line the inner rim of the eye isn't a good idea due to the risk of the product getting into the eye. Even if eye health and safety weren't an issue, lining the inner rim of the eye with this pencil is a problem due to the formula's extreme creaminess. You could wait for hours for this to set and you'd still be waiting. All things considered, there are many far better eyeliner options to consider over this one.

LIPSTICK, LIP GLOSS, AND LIPLINER: ☺ **bareMinerals 100% Natural Lipgloss** *($15)*. The name of this lip gloss is enticing, and while it does come close to being 100% natural, it isn't, at least not in terms of ingredients. Perhaps they were referring to the way this will look on your lips, but most consumers think "100% natural" means they are getting a "better-for-you formula." You aren't. Still, you may want to consider this moderately thick, oil-based gloss. It has a stickier finish than glosses rated Paula's Pick, but the colors are sheer and versatile enough to work with most lipsticks. The brush applicator works well and isn't prone to splaying.

☺ **bareMinerals 100% Natural Lipliner** *($11)*. This automatic, retractable lip pencil has a smooth but greasy application due to its plant oil–based formula. Application is swift, but the line doesn't last long and it will bleed into any lines around the mouth. If that's not a concern for you and you want a lipliner whose ingredients are truly 100% natural, give this an audition. The shade range is small, but it's filled with can't-go-wrong colors.

☺ **Buxom Lips** *($18)* pledges to naturally create the look of fuller lips, something most lip glosses with light-reflecting shimmer can do. These sheer, sparkling glosses contain menthone glycerin acetal, which can be irritating, but the amount used doesn't even cause a tingling sensation, which means it's not doing much., and that's not such a bad thing. As is, this is an OK lip gloss whose stickiness doesn't make it preferred to many others, and the plumping effect just doesn't happen.

☺ **Lip Gloss** *($14)* is a standard non-sticky wand lip gloss with some attractive sheer colors. The same type of gloss can be found for less, and the minty fragrance this has makes me nervous.

☺ **Lip Liner** *($11)* does not need sharpening and is retractable, but the texture is too creamy to draw a defined line, not to mention the short wear time.

☹ **Lipstick** *($15)*. The Lipstick offerings have some nice colors, but the formula is very greasy and won't last long, not to mention it will quickly migrate into lines around the mouth. How disappointing!

☺ **Quick Stick** *($14)* is an automatic, retractable lipstick/lip pencil combination. Almost as greasy as the Lipstick, this isn't for anyone prone to lip color bleeding into lines around the mouth. It's an OK option if this type of product appeals to you.

☹ **bareMinerals 100% Natural Lipcolor** *($15)* contains nothing but natural ingredients. But don't take that to mean this emollient cream lipstick is better than others. If anything, quite the opposite is true: the third ingredient in this lipstick is barium sulfate, a natural mineral compound that can be poisonous if ingested and that is noted for the way it frequently causes skin reactions. This same ingredient is consumed orally before having certain types of X-rays taken; it is believed that barium sulfate's low solubility and the body's ability to excrete it both help promote its negligible bioavailability. Still, it's not the best ingredient to see so prominently in a lipstick. Each opaque, highly pigmented shade also contains lavender oil, which can cause skin-cell death even when used in low amounts. This lipstick is a great example of a natural product not being as advantageous as a product with a mix of natural and synthetic ingredients.

☹ **Buxom Big & Healthy Lip Stick** *($18)*. This cleverly named product is merely an automatic, nonretractable lip crayon claiming to be a 3-in-1 product (lipliner, lipstick and lip plumper), but it barely does even one of these right. Used as a lipliner, it sufficiently prevents feathering, but it needs to be manually sharpened into a tip that's fine enough to do so. As a lipstick, it has a lovely semi-matte finish and real staying power, but the formula is so dry that it drags across lips, preventing smooth application. To top it all off, Bare Escentuals opted to include the irritant menthone glycerin acetal to trigger some lip plumping (meaning it causes irritation, which is never good for lips), but it only causes a telltale tingle and a minimal, temporary plumping effect. Although the short list of colors is deep and versatile, this multi-tasking formula simply fails to deliver.

MASCARA: ☺ **Magic Wand Brushless Mascara** *($15)* doesn't have a brush, so the name is accurate. Instead, you get a stick with grooves that grab and coat the lashes, providing dramatic length in the process. It can go on heavy and wetter than usual, which sticks lashes together rather than creating a separated, fringed look. Still, the results are impressive if you're looking for a lengthening mascara.

☺ **Weather Everything Waterproof Mascara** *($15)* stays on no matter how wet lashes get, and manages to make lashes look decently longer with a soft fullness and clean separation. Unlike several waterproof formulas, this one doesn't make lashes feel dry or brittle, though it takes some effort to remove completely.

☹ **$$$ bareMinerals Flawless Definition Mascara** *($18)* has a rubber-bristle brush that you'd think would perform better than it does. As is, application is wetter than usual and can lead to smearing. This darkens lashes considerably and provides ample length, while allowing you to build slight thickness. You'll notice slight clumping, but it's easy to smooth out because this formula doesn't dry quickly. After it sets, minor flaking during wear is apparent, which doesn't bode well considering the number of mascaras that don't flake.

☹ **Big Tease Mascara** *($15)* really is a tease because this is not a mascara that will "get even the most timid lashes noticed." After considerable effort, this builds merely average length and minimal thickness. The dual-sided brush appears useful, but neither the long, thin bristles nor short, thick bristles produce anything resembling big, flirtatious lashes.

☹ **$$$ Buxom Lash Mascara** *($18)*. "Reveals every single lash" is the promise this mascara makes, and it comes through, but there are drawbacks, especially when compared with really great mascaras, many of which cost half the amount of Buxom Lash. For starters, the rubber-bristle brush is enormous. That makes it difficult not only to reach the lashes at the inner corner of the eye but also to avoid getting mascara on your skin during application, although it is possible with patience and practice. Wielding the brush carefully, you can make lashes impressively long, moderately thick, and perfectly separated. Clumping is a minor issue, and this glitch is easily fixed with nimble comb-through. With all of these positives, why the neutral face rating? This mascara tends to flake and can make lashes feel drier than most. The flaking isn't terrible, but at this price, mascara should at the very least provide worry-free wear. Because this mascara doesn't do that, it isn't recommended over many less expensive mascaras at the drugstore, such as Cover Girl Lash Blast or Maybelline New York The Colossal.

☹ **$$$ Double-Ended Mascara & Lash Builder** *($26)* is a dual-sided mascara that includes a colorless lash primer and the same (original) Bare Escentuals Mascara reviewed below. As usual, the Lash Builder (primer) does little to impress. Actually, two coats of the mascara alone produced longer-looking lashes. If you're curious to try this type of product, L'Oreal and Maybelline New York have much better, less expensive options.

☹ **Mascara** *($15)* produces respectable length and some thickness, but not enough to distinguish itself from many less expensive mascaras at the drugstore. It's an OK mascara, but for the money, OK isn't enough.

BRUSHES: ☺ **Bare Escentuals Brushes** *($10-$28)*. The Brushes in this line are impressive, with almost as many options as makeup artist–driven lines such as M.A.C. Unfortunately, many of them use hair that isn't as soft as it could be, or they aren't shaped as well as others. Among the best options are the **Precision Liner Brush** *($12)*; the retractable, synthetic hair **Soft Focus Face** *($30)*, **Soft Focus Liner**, and **Soft Focus Eyeshadow** *($22)*; and the **Covered Lip Brush** *($14)*, **Double Ended Precision Brush** *($28)*, **Blending Brush** *($16)*, **Flawless Application Face Brush** *($22)*, **Eye Defining Brush** *($16)*, **Tapered Shadow Brush** *($14)*, **Wet/Dry Shadow Brush** *($18)*, **Eyeliner Brush** *($12)*, **Heavenly Eyeshadow Buffing Brush** *($16)*, and **Crease Defining Brush** *($18)*.

☺ **Angled Shadow Brush** *($12)*. Angled Shadow Brush is too small for all but the tiniest amount of shading, but other brushes allow you to get the same effect while having other advantages. ☺ **Flathead Shadow Brush** *($15)* is cut straight across, which doesn't really have an advantage other than for applying a thick line of powder eyeshadow, a feat other, more versatile brushes can accomplish. ☺ **Heavenly Eyeliner Blending Brush** *($14)* has enough firmness for eyeliner application, but tends to only draw a thick line and plenty of other tools can be used to soften or smudge eyeliner if smoky eyes are the goal. ☺ **Maximum Coverage Concealer Brush** *($20)* is synthetic and works well to apply liquid products, but is too large for applying concealer to small areas, such as the inner corner of the eye.

I'd advise against the too-stiff, scratchy ☹ **Brow Brush** *($12)*. The ☹ **Full Coverage Kabuki Brush** *($28)* is hard to hold and, for the manner in which it is used, not soft enough. ☹ **Lash Comb** *($10)* features metal teeth that can be severely damaging if you inadvertently scratch your eye. If you prefer using a lash comb, stick with the safer versions that have plastic teeth.

FACE AND BODY SHIMMER/ILLUMINATING PRODUCTS: ☹ **bareMinerals Glimmer** *($13)* is an ultra-shiny loose shimmer powder with a grainier texture than the other bareMinerals powders due to the high amount of mica. Any flaking (and this powder does flake) will be extremely obvious. With almost 30 shades, this is clearly a star attraction of the line, but there are less messy, longer-lasting ways to add intense shine to your routine.

☹ **Foiling Glimmers** *($46)* offer four bareMinerals Glimmer shades in one kit and include a wet/dry eyeshadow brush. This is a lot of money for a lot of flaky shine, but it is eye-catching, and the teens I observed in the Bare Escentuals store were all abuzz over this kit.

SPECIALTY PRODUCTS: ☺ **bareVitamins Prime Time** *($21)* is a standard, silicone-based, waterless primer. Like others cut from the same cloth, it makes skin feel very silky and can improve foundation application. However, many lightweight moisturizers do this too, and also supply skin with more of what it needs to look and feel its best. This product contains vitamin-based antioxidants in stable packaging, and that makes it a step above some other primers, though it's not a must-have if you're already using a silicone-enhanced moisturizer pre-makeup.

☺ **$$$ Quick Change** *($18 for 3.7 ounces)* has its place as a spray-on brush cleanser, especially if you're using the same brushes on multiple people or using one brush to apply very different colors. Those scenarios don't apply to most women, but the fact remains that this product works, albeit the dry time is a bit slow due to the glycerin it contains. For cleaning and sanitizing makeup brushes quickly and easily, I prefer Brush Off, available from www.brushoff. com. Keep in mind that such products are alcohol-based, and consistent use can make natural brush hairs feel dry and brittle, and so are best for occasional use.

☺ **$$$ bareVitamins Prime Time Eyelid Primer** *($16)* is sold as a product to extend the wear of the loose-powder eyeshadows bareMinerals offers. Oddly enough, a product like this wouldn't be needed if bareMinerals offered pressed eyeshadows that adhered to skin better than their loose version (which flakes all over the place as you apply it and as it wears during the day). Other than the shortcomings of loose-powder eyeshadows, is this a worthwhile product to try? Perhaps. Housed in a pen-style applicator with an angled sponge tip, this product is little more than an exceptionally sheer concealer with a matte finish. It feels light, sets quickly, and can help absorb excess oil, which will increase the longevity of your eye makeup. The drawback is the lack of coverage. Why would you use this over the eyelid area when there are many excellent matte-finish concealers that have the same characteristics as this product? Most people will find that eye makeup looks a lot better when they first camouflage and even out the thin skin on the eyelid. Prime Time Eyelid Primer doesn't provide that benefit, but I suppose it's an option for those who either don't mind using two products when one will do or whose eyelids don't need much coverage prior to applying eye makeup.

☹ **Weather Everything Liner Sealer** *($18)* is a tiny bottle of a liquid solution meant to make any bareMinerals powder last through all manner of wet weather or swimming. The formula contains mostly water, alcohol, and film-forming agent (the same type used in hairsprays). It smells medicinal, feels sticky, and although it does work to keep the powder colors in place when wet, the textural (and irritation) trade-offs aren't worth it.

BEAUTICONTROL

BEAUTICONTROL AT-A-GLANCE

Strengths: The Cell Block-C products; several well-formulated moisturizers; decent AHA and scrub products; excellent retinol products; several good cleansers; Lip Apeel; very good lip balm with sunscreen; good self-tanner; some great foundations (including one with full coverage); superior loose powder; very good powder blush and eyeshadow trios; the liquid eyeliner and lip gloss are excellent; some innovative products that make this line deserve a second look.

Weaknesses: Most of the body-care products contain irritating ingredients, as do several others throughout the line; the jar packaging is really disappointing; most of the toners contain problematic ingredients that can hurt skin; limited options for sunscreens, although what's available provides sufficient UVA protection; the Skinlogics Sensitive skin-care line contains ingredients that are problematic for those with sensitive skin; mostly problematic concealers; average eye pencil; limited to poor foundation, concealer, and powder shades for women of color.

For more information about BeautiControl, call (800) 232-8841 or visit www.beauticontrol.com or www.Beautypedia.com.

Note: I would like to acknowledge and extol how exceptionally helpful the staff at Beauti-Control's main office has been in allowing my team and me to compile the information necessary to complete this review. Very few cosmetics companies extend such a high level of service and reliable information to us, and we truly appreciate it.

BEAUTICONTROL SKIN CARE

BEAUTICONTROL BC SPA PRODUCTS

☺ **$$$ BC Spa Resurface Microderm Abrasion for Face** *($50 for 2.5 ounces)*. This absurdly overpriced scrub is a decent option for all skin types except oily or blemish prone because the oils and thickeners it contains aren't good for that skin type. It includes alumina as the abrasive agent, similar to what's used in microdermabrasion treatments. However, massaging this over the skin with your hands isn't the same thing as an in-office microdermabrasion session. To that end, BeautiControl sells the BC Spa Microderm Abrasion Facial Buffer, a battery-powered hand-held device that is equipped with a rotating facial brush that does help to create an impact similar to that of the real deal. The device has two speeds and the brush head is composed of synthetic bristles. Used with this scrub, it produces more thorough results than just using your fingers. However, it's easy to get carried away with this device, and coupled with the scrub particles (which are overly abrasive) you may get more irritation than benefit. For that reason, it's best to use this scrub without the device (you can try the Facial Buffer with your favorite cleanser). Plus the jar packaging isn't the best—dipping wet fingers time and time again into any skin-care product is ill-advised. Resurface Microderm Abrasion for Face is a consideration if used with a gentle touch.

☺ **BC Spa Microderm Abrasion Facial Buffer** *($11.50 for 3 piece system)*. This battery-powered device is meant to be used with BeautiControl's BC Spa Resurface Microderm Abrasion for Face. It includes two detachable brush heads with synthetic bristles, and the device has two speeds (Normal and Gentle). Used with the company's Microderm scrub, it can quickly become an overly aggressive way to exfoliate skin. However, this is a consideration to try with your favorite (gentle) facial cleanser. If you opt to try that, be sure to use only gentle pressure and to keep the brush head away from the eye area. In addition, you must clean it thoroughly after each use or you will be scrubbing bacteria into your face every time you use it.

☺ **$$$ BC Spa Resurface Multi-Acid Resurfacing Peel** *($50 for 30 pads)* contains approximately 10% glycolic acid (AHA) at a pH of 4.1. For an AHA product a slightly lower pH value around 3.5 would have been a lot better. Although this also contains other AHA ingredients—lactic acid, lactobionic acid, and gluconolactone—they don't make up much of the total content, which further reduces the possibility of exfoliation (i.e., "resurfacing"). The pads are meant to be swiped over skin, you leave the residue on for 10-20 minutes, and then you rinse. You'll definitely want to rinse because these pads leave a sticky film on skin that interferes with the application of other products. This doesn't come close to having anything to do with a professional peel from a doctor or aesthetician. And the jar packaging isn't helpful for keeping these ingredients stable. Note that for a lot less money you can purchase well-formulated AHA products from Alpha Hydrox, Neutrogena, or Paula's Choice.

☹ **BC Spa Sculpt Body Sculpting Gel** *($42 for 5 ounces)* is incapable of improving one centimeter of skin on your body. The second listed ingredient is alcohol, which has no positive effect on cellulite or on skin. The alcohol not only generates free-radical damage, but also causes dryness, irritation, and inflammation, thus hurting the skin's healing process. This formula also contains a slew of irritating plant extracts and oils, all of which make this one unhappy product for skin.

☹ **BC Spa Sculpt Firming Body Creme** *($35 for 0.5 ounce)* claims to firm and tone pretty much any part of your body that's begun to sag or lose elasticity. The formula is said to create "the optimal environment for your skin to produce collagen." While it is generally easy to help skin make more collagen, this product gets in the way of helping skin do that because it contains more than a dozen irritating ingredients, which produce inflammation that causes collagen and other healthy elements of the skin to break down. The amount of caffeine may seem impressive, but there is no research showing that caffeine firms skin or improves cellulite the way the claim asserts on the label. If you wanted to check that fact out definitively for yourself, simply use the leftover coffee from a strong pot (after it has cooled) as a toner on your legs or body and see if you get benefit. At least that way you would be delivering far more caffeine to your skin than you would by applying the teeny amount in this product.

BEAUTICONTROL CELL BLOCK-C PRODUCTS

☺ $$$ **Cell Block-C Intensive Multivitamin Face Serum** *($37 for 30 capsules)* comes packaged in single-use capsules, which is a good way to preserve the efficacy of the antioxidant vitamins it contains. The nonaqueous, silicone-based formula feels incredibly silky and is suitable for all skin types except sensitive (due to the ascorbic acid). This is best for those who want a vitamin C–laden serum. Overall, although the formula is good, it's not as impressive as Elizabeth Arden's Ceramide Gold capsules.

✓ ☺ **Cell Block-C Intensive Brightening Elixir** *($26 for 1 ounce)* is a lightweight moisturizer that claims to reduce hyperpigmentation. The various forms of vitamin C in this product may have some impact on discolorations, but the amount is likely not enough to fade discolorations with the same proficiency as hydroquinone or arbutin (Sources: *Dermatologic Therapy*, September-October 2007, pages 308-313; and *International Journal of Dermatology*, August 2004, pages 604-607). Still, even if only minimal fading of discolorations occurs (or if discolorations are not a concern), this moisturizer has a lot going for it in terms of providing an antioxidant boost to normal to slightly dry skin. Moreover, the opaque tube packaging helps keep the vitamin C and other antioxidants in this elixir stable during use. This contains fragrance in the form of citronellyl methylcrotonate.

✓ ☺ **Cell Block-C New Cell Protection SPF 20** *($30.50 for 1 ounce)* is a remarkable mineral sunscreen (titanium dioxide is the sole active ingredient) for normal to dry or sensitive skin. It is fragrance-free and loaded with antioxidants and cell-communicating ingredients, and the packaging will keep these sensitive ingredients stable during use. There are very few sunscreens/daytime moisturizers available that supply skin with such an impressive cocktail of beneficial ingredients, and it has a lovely texture, too. As such, this deserves strong consideration. The only sour note is the price, which may discourage liberal application, which is essential for achieving the sun protection your skin needs daily (though this is still less expensive than many department store offerings).

✓ ☺ $$$ **Cell Block-C P.M. Cell Protection** *($36.50 for 1 ounce)* is an impressive, silky-textured moisturizer for normal to dry skin, and for once the claims of strengthening skin and enhancing its repair process are accurate. That's because the numerous antioxidants, lightweight emollients, and cell-communicating peptides are capable of helping skin help itself when it's exposed to damaging elements (except sunlight, so you'll still need sunscreen). This contains fragrance in the form of citronellyl methylcrotonate (Source: *International Cosmetic Ingredient Dictionary and Handbook*, 11th Edition, 2006, page 516).

BEAUTICONTROL PLATINUM REGENERATION PRODUCTS

☹ **Platinum Regeneration Advanced Eye Repair Creme** *($31 for 0.5 ounce)*. This emollient eye cream contains almost every substance that cosmetic ingredient manufacturers tout as being able to banish all sorts of under-eye problems, from dark circles to wrinkles and puffiness. The bad news is that none of these ingredients work as claimed, and the only "research" to support the claims comes from the companies that sell the ingredients to brands like BeautiControl.

This formula does have merit for dry skin and contains some peptides, antioxidants, and skin-identical ingredients that would have rated it a very good facial product (not just for use around the eyes), but their benefit won't last long due to the jar packaging. If that weren't enough of a letdown, this eye cream contains the menthol derivative menthyl lactate, which makes it too irritating for any part of the face, but especially problematic for the eye area.

☹ **Platinum Regeneration Rejuvenating Eye Treatment** *($42 for 6 pairs)*. These pre-treated eye patches are sold with the promise of giving you younger-looking eyes in 30 minutes. The mundane formula is mostly water, glycerin, film-forming agent (think hairspray), and a small amount of red algae and peony extract, although the latter two have no research showing they are beneficial for the eye area or for skin anywhere else on the body. Glycerin is a good skin-care ingredient, but it's about as basic as you can get. You'll find these patches make the skin around the eyes look smoother and feel a bit tighter, but the effect is temporary (and I mean really temporary) and potentially irritating, because a product with a film-forming agent listed second on the ingredient list is not skin care. This also contains alcoxa, an ingredient that has constricting effects on skin and can be irritating, which is harmful to skin, not helpful.

☺ **$$$ Platinum Regeneration Skin Renewing Serum** *($62 for 1.8 ounces)*. With the exception of the two polyhydroxy acids (PHA)—lactobionic acid and gluconolactone—all of the intriguing ingredients in this serum are listed after the preservative, meaning they are barely present. The formula has a slightly tacky texture, but the amount of PHA may help facilitate exfoliation. It's a good option for normal to dry skin, but not nearly as effective as any of several other well-formulated AHA products from other lines. There is nothing about this product specially formulated for 40+ skin as claimed or for any other age group either, and the price is silly for what you're getting.

✓ ☺ **$$$ Platinum Regeneration Age Defying Lip Treatment** *($23.50 for 0.09 ounce)* is a very well-formulated lip balm. The oil-based formula comes in stick form, and its slim component is great for traveling and on-the-go use. It contains ingredients capable of preventing moisture loss and chapped lips, and includes more bells and whistles than what's seen in the majority of emollient lip balms available today. The extras don't necessarily justify this product's cost, but at least you're getting more than a standard lip balm for your money. This lip product has a slightly sweet scent and flavor.

BEAUTICONTROL REGENERATION PRODUCTS

☺ **$$$ Regeneration Gold Eye Repair** *($28 for 0.5 ounce)* is an OK moisturizer for normal to slightly dry skin anywhere on the face. It contains a small amount of peptides, and although these theoretically could have cell-communicating ability, their stability is fragile even in the best formulation and packaging, so this jar container ensures the ingredients won't remain stable.

☺ **$$$ Regeneration Gold Rejuvenation Face and Neck Lotion** *($58 for 1.8 ounces)*. If you're curious to see what polyhydroxy acids (PHAs), an alternative to AHAs such as glycolic acid, can do for your skin, then this moisturizer is a good option. The pH-correct formula allows exfoliation to occur and is formulated in a base suitable for normal to dry skin. There isn't a strong reason to consider PHAs over AHAs (or BHA), but products that contain them are worth a try if your skin cannot tolerate other forms of exfoliation ingredients.

✓ ☺ **$$$ Regeneration Overnight Retinol Recovery Eye Capsules** *($39.50 for 30 capsules)*. These silicone-based fragrance-free capsules are an excellent way to treat skin to the benefits of stabilized retinol. Each capsule contains enough serum to cover skin around both eyes with little excess, so you're not wasting product. However, you also can apply the contents of these capsules all over the face if desired. Further praise is warranted because the formula contains antioxidant green tea and the anti-irritant bisabolol. This product is suitable for all skin types.

✓ ☺ **$$$ Regeneration Overnight Retinol Recovery Serum** *($45 for 1 ounce)* is a silky, lightweight serum with retinol, an ingredient that helps improve skin by changing the way new skin cells are produced (so in that sense, the core claims made for this serum are accurate). The packaging will keep the light- and air-sensitive retinol stable, though it's worth noting that the component is oversized for what's necessary to hold 1 ounce of product. Not only does this fragrance-free serum contain retinol, it also treats skin to a host of other beneficial ingredients, including antioxidants and several water-binding agents. It is recommended for all skin types, although those with sensitive skin may find the retinol too irritating.

☹ **$$$ Regeneration Platinum Plus Eye Cream** *($35 for 0.5 ounce)* contains several ingredients that are helpful for normal to dry skin, so it's a shame that jar packaging was chosen. Because of that, many of the intriguing ingredients in this product won't remain stable once the product is opened. The last three ingredients in this eye cream are forms of fragrance, so it is not a fragrance-free product as claimed.

✓ ☺ **$$$ Regeneration Platinum Plus Face Serum** *($65 for 1 ounce)* doesn't hold any special secrets to address the needs of women aged 50+ or any age for that matter, and it won't reduce sagging skin—no skin-care product can do that. What it does have going for it is a lightweight lotion texture that's loaded with several beneficial ingredients for skin of any age, and that's why it earns a Paula's Pick rating. This is best for normal to slightly dry skin; it contains fragrance in the form of citronellyl methylcrotonate.

☹ **$$$ Regeneration Skin Renewing Lotion** *($36 for 1.8 ounces)* contains glycolic and lactic acids, but even combined the amount isn't high enough to help exfoliation. Plus the third ingredient is triethanolamine and that high-pH ingredient shouldn't be a primary element of the formula because it is irritating in higher amounts and offers no benefit for skin. Ignore the claims that this product is targeted toward the skin-care needs of women in their 20s, it isn't. There are some great ingredients present, but the amounts are too small to be of help for skin of any age.

✓ ☺ **$$$ Regeneration Tight, Firm & Fill Eye Firming Serum** *($42.50 for 0.46 ounce)* is a lightweight, water-based eye gel that helps smooth and plump skin, including superficial wrinkles, thanks to its blend of hydrating glycerin, peptides, and some good water-binding agents, including hyaluronic acid. It is fragrance-free and also contains some lesser-known antioxidants. This is suitable for all skin types, but please keep your expectations realistic because this won't tighten or fill in wrinkles; it's not even remotely equivalent to the results you get from dermal fillers. BeautiControl doesn't directly make that claim, but the term they use, HylaSponges, makes it sound like the dermal filler Hyaluron, and it isn't.

☹ **$$$ Regeneration Tight, Firm & Fill Face Cream** *($48.50 for 1 ounce)* purports to make skin tighter immediately, but doesn't contain any ingredients capable of doing that. Even if it did, the effect would likely be irritating, and assuredly only temporary (think minutes, not hours). Although this moisturizer for normal to dry skin contains several peptides, the jar packaging BeautiControl chose isn't likely to keep them stable during use. As for the "hyaluronic filling spheres" they claim are in this product—don't count on them performing in any way like the dermal filler products that contain hyaluronic acid. BeautiControl uses the salt form of this ingredient (sodium hyaluronate) and while that's fine, it isn't the same thing as the hylauronic acid you're getting injected via dermal fillers. Therefore, and because this product is applied topically and not injected under the wrinkle, the plumping/line-filling effect isn't even a close comparison (though water-binding agents like sodium hyaluronate can temporarily plump dry skin).

☺ **$$$ Regeneration Extreme Repair Hand Therapy** *($13.50 for 3 ounces)*. The tiny amount of AHAs in this mundane, simple hand cream cannot exfoliate skin. Even if they were present in a larger amount, the pH of 4.7 is too high for exfoliation to occur. Still, this is a decent, slightly emollient hand cream that's among the few fragrance-free options available. It is not recommended for daytime unless you follow with a sunscreen rated SPF 15 or greater.

BEAUTICONTROL SKINLOGICS PRODUCTS

☹ **Skinlogics Cleansing Gel** *($16.50 for 6.7 ounces)* contains several fragrant citrus and other plant extracts (plus jasmine oil) that can be irritating. It would definitely be a problem for use around the eyes, and as a cleanser you'll probably use this around the eyes to help remove makeup.

☺ **$$$ Skinlogics Clear Deep Cleansing Gel** *($16 for 6.7 ounces)* is an OK water-soluble option for normal to oily skin. It would be better without the fragrant plant extracts, but they're not present in the same amount as they are in BeautiControl's Skinlogics Cleansing Gel, and they didn't include the problematic jasmine oil in this formula. This works well to remove makeup and rinses cleanly.

☺ **$$$ Skinlogics Gold Cleansing Foam** *($16.50 for 5 ounces)*. This liquid-to-foam water-soluble cleanser is suitable for all skin types except sensitive. It contains a small amount of fragrant plant extracts, but likely not enough to cause irritation. Gold Cleansing Foam removes makeup and doesn't leave even a trace of residue. The claims are beyond what the formula can actually do, but this is just fine as a cleanser.

☺ **$$$ Skinlogics Platinum Cleansing Lotion** *($17.50 for 6.7 ounces)* is a basic but effective cleansing lotion for normal to dry skin. BeautiControl positions this as a cleanser for women in their 40s, but there's nothing in the formula that's unique to 40-something skin. Women in their 40s can and do have many different skin types—normal, oily, acne prone, blackheads, and rosacea—and this cleanser definitely isn't suitable for any of those skin types. It removes makeup well, but requires use of a washcloth to avoid leaving a residue. This does contain plant extracts that pose a slight risk of irritation.

☺ **$$$ Skinlogics Platinum Plus Nourishing Creme Cleanser** *($20.50 for 6.7 ounces)* is a gentle, water-soluble foaming cleanser that contains emollients helpful for normal to dry skin. This cleanser also contains several antioxidants and skin-identical substances, most of which won't remain on skin after rinsing. It's a nice idea to think that Beauticontrol's Pink Nutrispheres burst open during cleansing to deposit vitamins on skin, but it's doubtful they'll stand up to rinsing and, thus, they shouldn't be relied on for antioxidant benefit. This contains fragrance in the form of methyl dihydrojasmonate.

☺ **$$$ Skinlogics Sensitive Gentle Cleansing Lotion** *($18 for 6.7 ounces)* contains too many ingredients that are ill-advised for all skin types, but especially for sensitive skin. Geranium, lavender, lime, and orange may smell delicious, but all of them spell trouble for skin in a delicate state. Beyond the problematic plants (none of which have even a small benefit for sensitive skin), this is a standard cleanser that would be best for normal to oily skin.

✓☺ **Skinlogics Lash and Lid Bath** *($9.75 for 4 ounces)* is a very good, exceptionally gentle cleanser that BeautiControl positions as an eye-makeup remover. It works well for that purpose, and it's fragrance-free. This is similar to removing your eye makeup with Johnson & Johnson's Baby Shampoo, which means you can expect it to perform gently, but it is incapable of removing long-wearing eyeliner or waterproof mascara. If you don't routinely wear that type of eye makeup, this is worth purchasing.

☹ **Skinlogics Makeup Remover** *($20.50 for 6.7 ounces)* is not recommended because it contains irritating rosemary oil. If you prefer lotion-style makeup removers, those from Avon and Clinique are much better, and less expensive.

☹ **Skinlogics Clear Blemish Control Tonic** *($18 for 6.7 ounces)* is irritating in several ways: its pH of 2 is extremely acidic, which negates the benefits of the salicylic acid. Coupled with the low pH, it is an alcohol-based formula that also contains witch hazel, which adds more fuel to the fire. Alcohol not only causes free-radical damage, but also irritates the skin, which actually can increase oil production directly in the pore.

☹ **Skinlogics Gold Tonic** *($17.50 for 6.7 ounces).* With grapefruit extract high up on the ingredient list, the potential for irritation makes this a tonic to overlook, particularly for sensitive skin. It can't reduce the appearance of puffiness as claimed.

☹ **Skinlogics Herbal Hydrating Mist** *($9.50 for 6.7 ounces)* is a basic toner that contains a problematic amount of irritating ivy and arnica extracts. In addition, the tiny amount of non-irritating plant extracts present offers minimal benefit to skin, making this a toner to ignore.

☺ **$$$ Skinlogics Platinum Tonic** *($17.50 for 6.7 ounces)* is similar to BeautiControl's Skinlogics Gold Tonic but contains a different blend of plants. Most of the plant extracts are helpful for skin, which makes the few problematic ones less of a concern. The antioxidant-rich formula should be kept away from light due to the translucent bottle packaging.

✓ ☺ **$$$ Skinlogics Platinum Plus Relaxing Tonic** *($22.50 for 6.7 ounces)* sells itself as more than just a toner, and it is! Although this has a lingering floral scent some may find unappealing, there's no denying this milky toner is a state-of-the-art formulation for normal to very dry skin. It is loaded with water-binding agents, antioxidants (including nonfragrant plant oils), and ingredients that help reinforce skin's protective barrier. The label does not list fragrance, but the product does contain fragrance chemicals, which it would be better off without.

☹ **Skinlogics Sensitive Rinse & Restore Tonic** *($19 for 6.7 ounces)* contains a significant amount of mugwort extract (listed by its Latin name *Artemisia vulgaris*), a plant whose volatile components, including camphor, are too irritating for all skin types (Source: www.naturaldatabase.com). Mugwort has no known benefit for skin, either—nor do the other problematic plants in this toner.

☺ **$$$ Skinlogics Tonic** *($16.50 for 6.7 ounces)* contains mostly water and slip agents that make skin feel silky, but it isn't as impressive as it could've been. Plus, it's not good news that so many problematic plant extracts are included at higher concentrations than the helpful ingredients. BeautiControl offers better toner formulas than this.

☺ **$$$ Skinlogics Facial Scrub** *($16.50 for 2.6 ounces).* This scrub with cleansing ability would be much more logical for all skin types if it did not contain several fragrant essences. They're not present in great amounts, but including them at all is unnecessary, and keeps this gel-based scrub from earning a Paula's Pick rating. Use this scrub gently because it's more abrasive than many others.

☹ **Skinlogics Clear Purifying Scrub/Masque** *($18 for 5 ounces)* is well-intentioned, but the company made a major misstep by including drying, irritating sulfur. It also contains some plant extracts with irritant potential, but they're less of a concern relative to the amount of sulfur.

☺ **$$$ Skinlogics Thermal Facial Scrub** *($20 for 2.6 ounces)*. Here's another scrub whose novelty is that it warms when mixed with water. This is a simple chemical reaction that's also present in less expensive scrubs from drugstore lines, but the bottom line is that it's not necessary for good skin care. The warming reaction, which begins quite intensely and then subsides, may feel good, but it has zero impact on clogged pores or cleansing skin. If anything, the initial high heat actually can encourage the presence of surfaced capillaries. This type of product can be a problem for anyone with sensitive skin, especially those with rosacea. However, it's a good scrub for someone with normal to oily skin, whether or not you think the warming (thermal) effect is neat.

☹ **Skinlogics Clear Oil Control Moisturizer** *($18 for 3.4 ounces)*. Forget about the claims of controlling oil production or detoxifying the skin because there are no botanicals that can do that, and toxins have nothing to do with acne. This moisturizer goes on silky, but has a slightly tacky finish that doesn't do much to keep skin matte. The amount of citrus extracts is a concern and has no benefit for any skin type; some of the other plant extracts aren't the best, either. It's a shame that there are more potentially troublesome ingredients than beneficial ones.

☺ **Skinlogics Gold Moisturizer** *($19 for 3.5 ounces)*. With the exception of a tiny amount of potentially troublesome plant extracts, this is a very good moisturizer for normal to dry skin. It contains an impressive mix of lightweight emollients, cell-communicating ingredients, soothing agents, and antioxidants. Considering the overall formula, the price is a bona fide bargain.

☹ **Skinlogics Moisturizer** *($19 for 3.5 ounces)* contains a skin-confusing blend of beneficial and problematic ingredients. Overall, the skin-helpful ingredients outweigh the skin-detrimental ones, but really why bother with a product that is fighting itself instead of just focusing on helping your skin?

☺ **Skinlogics Platinum Moisturizer** *($20 for 3.5 ounces)* is a good moisturizer for normal to dry skin. The claim of exfoliation is dubious because this doesn't contain much in the way of exfoliating ingredients; a tiny amount of urea is present but the citrus extracts don't function like AHAs. Formula-wise, this isn't as impressive as BeautiControl's Skinlogics Gold Moisturizer.

✓☺ **Skinlogics Platinum Plus Brightening Day Creme** *($26 for 3.5 ounces)*. Although the claim is that it can lighten age spots (which are really sun-damage spots that can occur at any age), this product is better positioned as a well-formulated moisturizer for normal to dry skin. It contains a very good mix of emollients, cell-communicating ingredients, several antioxidants, and beneficial plant extracts. The alpha-arbutin in this product may have some impact on brown skin discolorations, but I suspect the amount isn't enough to net what most consumers would consider significant improvement. Still, this is definitely worth a try if you need a great moisturizer and want to see if an alternative to hydroquinone may help lighten sun-induced discolorations. Of course, this is recommended for daytime use only if your foundation contains a sunscreen rated SPF 15 or greater, and you'll be applying the foundation evenly and liberally. This does contain fragrance in the form of various fragrance chemicals, though the amounts are likely too small to cause irritation.

☺ **$$$ Skinlogics Platinum Plus Renewing Night Creme** *($31 for 1.4 ounces)* ends up being one of the disappointing BeautiControl moisturizers, but not because the formula is lacking. What separates this from their outstanding options is the choice of jar packaging, which won't keep the antioxidants in it stable during use. Without the boost these ingredients provide, this is relegated to the status of a standard emollient moisturizer for normal to dry skin. Although the label does not list fragrance, the product does contain fragrant chemicals. One more comment: absolutely nothing about this formula is unique to skin over the age of 50.

☹ **Skinlogics Sensitive Hydra-Calm Moisturizer** *($20 for 3.5 ounces).* According to the claims, the arnica extract in this lightweight moisturizer can reduce the appearance of redness. I don't know where the proof is for that, because arnica is a known irritant and the amount of it in this product is bound to be troublesome for all skin types. The arnica's negative impact is intensified with the inclusion of other plant irritants as well, while the anti-irritants are unfortunately a lot less prominent (so their effectiveness is negligible). Whoever was in charge of formulating this moisturizer seemingly has no idea what sensitive skin needs to provide barrier protection and reduce inflammation.

☺ **Skinlogics Sensitive Protective Services Calming Fluid** *($25 for 1.6 ounces)* is an expensive way to get the benefits of topical hydrocortisone, and would be a better option without the irritating plant extracts that Beauticontrol adds to all of their Skinlogics Sensitive products. What's frustrating is that without the problematic plant extracts this would be a very good option for sensitive skin that needs the additional benefit of hydrocortisone. As a reminder: hydrocortisone is recommended only for intermittent or short-term (no more than three consecutive months) use due to the detrimental effect it has on collagen.

☺ **Skinlogics Skin Hydrator Anti-Ash Creme** *($17 for 4.5 ounces).* This thick, somewhat greasy moisturizer is capable of reducing the appearance of ashen skin (caused by a buildup of dead skin cells) but for only a brief period of time. It simply places a layer of emollients over the dry patches, but it does nothing to address the underlying cause, which requires exfoliation. If ashen areas are a concern, you'll get much better results using an AHA or BHA exfoliant formulated in a moisturizing base than you will with this ordinary Vaseline-based moisturizer. The price is actually over the top for what you get, given that most moisturizers in far larger containers are formulated nearly identically, if not better.

☺ **Skinlogics SPF Booster SPF 30+** *($21 for 4.5 ounces)* is a good sunscreen for normal to oily skin. It provides avobenzone for sufficient UVA protection and is formulated in a lightweight lotion base. This would be rated a Paula's Pick if it contained more than a tiny amount of vitamin E for an antioxidant boost.

☹ **Skinlogics Clear Spot Treatment Duo** *($16 for 0.5 ounce)* is a clever two-sided product that combines a topical disinfectant with benzoyl peroxide on one end and a BHA (salicylic acid) gel on the other. Although the pH of the 2% BHA Gel is low enough for exfoliation to occur, it's lower than usual (pH 2.6), which makes it too irritating for skin. That, coupled with the alcohol base, makes this portion of the product too irritating to recommend for blemishes or oily skin. Remember, irritation increases oil production in the pore and alcohol causes free-radical damage. The Clearing Lotion with Benzoyl Peroxide portion is fine, but there are several less expensive products that contain the same amount of this active ingredient.

✓ ☺ **Skinlogics Lip Balm SPF 20** *($10.50 for 0.6 ounce)* is a very good lip balm with an in-part avobenzone sunscreen. It contains effective emollients and leaves a soft gloss finish. The only misstep is the inclusion of orange oil, but the amount is so small as to be inconsequential.

✓ ☺ **$$$ Lip Apeel** *($19.50 for 1.25 ounces)* is a two-part product (peel and balm) that helps the user manually peel dry skin off the lips and then places a thick, glossy balm on them afterward. The peel is a mix of waxes and silicates that can indeed rub off dead skin as you massage the lips. The balm is well formulated, but would be even better without the orange oil. Still, this cleverly packaged product is a very good way to keep lips smooth, flake-free, and moisturized.

OTHER BEAUTICONTROL PRODUCTS

☺ **Microderm Eye-X-Cel Eye Cream** *($20 for 0.5 ounce)* is a standard emollient eye cream that's an OK option for normal to dry skin, at least if you're willing to settle for less than your skin deserves. The small amount of antioxidants won't remain potent for long due to the jar packaging. The "brightness" this eye cream provides is from its mix of cosmetic pigments that leave a slight white cast on skin; that isn't a skin-care benefit, it's merely a cosmetic effect.

☺ **$$$ Leg Apeel Self-Tanner for Legs** *($20 for 4.4 ounces)*. Although lots of women bemoan their white legs during shorts season, BeautiControl didn't need to create a legs-only self-tanner. Although the formula is fine, there's no reason any self-tanner cannot be used on the legs, face, arms—wherever you want color. This product is tinted with caramel so you can see where it has been applied. It contains the same tanning ingredient—dihydroxyacetone—present in almost every self-tanner being sold. Leg Apeel also contains cosmetic pigments for a bit of coverage and shimmer. You'll find less expensive versions of this product from Jergens' Natural Glow line at the drugstore.

BEAUTICONTROL MAKEUP

FOUNDATION: ✓ ☺ **Secret AGEnt Undercover Makeup** *($15)*. Those needing a full coverage foundation, take note: this is an excellent option. Although it doesn't look natural on skin, no foundation with this amount of coverage does; that's the trade-off for the amount of camouflage you get. This isn't as opaque (or nearly as obvious) as Dermablend but it covers quite well and is much easier to apply. It feels silky and sets to a long-wearing matte finish that doesn't look too powdery or flat. Perhaps the best news is that the shades are mostly exemplary. The only ones to avoid due to obvious overtones of peach or pink are Y-4, P-2, P-3, and P-4. Shade P-5 is also not recommended due to a strong copper tone. There are plenty of neutral options for those with fair to medium skin tones, and P-6 is great for dark skin tones.

☺ **$$$ Perfecting Creme to Powder Finish** *($15)* looks beautiful on skin but is very difficult to pick up with a sponge or your fingers. Just swiping your finger across the top barely picks up any product, and with a sponge you almost have to dig in to pick up enough makeup for what amounts to light coverage with a natural satin finish that is best for normal to dry skin that's not prone to breakouts. Almost all of the shades are very good, and provide options for fair to dark skin tones. The ones to avoid due to overtones of peach or orange include P-3, N-4, and P-5. Although this missed being rated a Paula's Pick, it is definitely worth exploring if you prefer this type of foundation (and will apply it over a daytime moisturizer rated SPF 15 or greater).

☺ **$$$ Perfecting Wet/Dry Finish Foundation** *($21)*. This talc-based pressed powder foundation has a smooth texture that's drier than it is silky. Used wet or dry, it provides light to medium coverage and a soft matte finish that is best for normal to slightly dry skin. The formula isn't absorbent enough to handle combination skin with oily areas and definitely not skin that's oily all over. This looks better on skin when used with a damp sponge rather than applying it dry. As usual with wet application, you have to be careful of streaks during blending, but if you opt to try this foundation I suspect you'll prefer how it looks applied wet versus dry. The shades are mostly excellent, particularly those in the Y and N range. BeautiControl only falters with the peach-tinged P-3 and ash P-5 and Y-5.

☺ **$$$ Platinum Regeneration Age Defying Makeup SPF 12** *($25)* is sold as a treatment and liquid makeup in one. The claims made aren't really impressive, but the formula does contain some antioxidants, anti-irritants, and peptides that aren't typically seen in makeup. Does that make this foundation better for your skin? I suppose so, but the edge isn't tremendous when you consider the tiny amounts of the atypical ingredients. What counts most in terms of antiaging is the sunscreen, and this foundation disappoints with an SPF rating that's below standard. The amount of titanium dioxide included belies the low SPF rating, so it's curious why BeautiControl didn't list this as being greater than SPF 12. As for the foundation itself, it has a silky, elegant texture that takes more time than usual to blend. Once set, you get light to medium coverage and a satin finish best for normal to dry skin. The shade range is quite extensive and most of them are workable for light to medium skin tones. N3 is slightly peach, N5 is slightly ash, and P3 is very peach. The oddest shade is P5, which has a copper rose cast that finishes slightly ash. This foundation would earn a happy face rating if its sunscreen was rated SPF 15 or greater.

☺ **$$$ Secret AGEnt Mineral Makeup SPF 15** *($25)* has a different base formula than most mineral makeup, but retains the mineral sun protection seen in most mineral foundations with sunscreen. This loose-powder foundation has a dry texture but smooth application that sets to a matte finish laced with sparkles. It appears slightly waxen on skin and provides medium to nearly full coverage if you brush on several coats. The shade range is mostly impressive, though keep in mind that the high amounts of titanium dioxide and zinc oxide contribute to this foundation's ashen finish on skin. This is less apparent in the lighter shades (Neutral Light and Pin Light are great for fair skin) but the darker shades suffer. These shades are not recommended: Neutral Dark, Pink Dark, and Yellow Dark. This fragrance-free foundation is best for normal to oily skin.

☹ **Creme Sheer Protection** *($14)* is BeautiControl's most dated foundation and the one I recommend you avoid unless you're already using it and cannot fathom changing to something better. It's a greasy cream makeup packaged in a compact that doesn't include an applicator. The colors are average to poor, while the finish is heavy and puts an unbecoming mask on skin rather than enhancing it as today's best foundations do.

CONCEALER: ☺ **Secret AGEnt Coverup** *($5.50)* is too liquidy for its own good! Although the colors are great and the finish is natural while providing coverage for minor imperfections, this takes too long to blend and has an excessive amount of slip. If you have the patience to tolerate this concealer's shortcomings, it may be worth a try. If not, consider L'Oreal True Match Concealer instead.

☺ **Secret AGEnt Maximum Coverage Concealer** *($10.50)*. This mineral oil- and wax-based cream concealer comes in three fairly good colors and provides nearly full coverage. The problem is the texture, which is greasy, and the finish, which readily creases into lines under the eyes, even if set with powder. There are better concealers to consider, even if you need full coverage, such as those from Make Up For Ever or Laura Mercier.

☹ **Platinum Regeneration Age-Defying Concealer** *($17.50)* is a creamy stick concealer that's oil-based and contains a colorless moisture core that, while visually appealing in the package, actually leads to an uneven application that requires more blending than usual. Once blended, this provides spotty coverage. The finish remains greasy, so this fades and settles into lines around the eyes (or mouth) quickly. It contains an impressive amount of peptide (that's where the antiaging claims come into play, even though peptides alone aren't the answer to youthful skin).

☹ **Extra Help Concealer** *($5.50)* provides significant coverage, but that's all it does well. You'll need "extra help" figuring out how to blend this surprisingly lightweight yet greasy concealer, not to mention lots of patience waiting for it to set, which never happens to a satisfying degree. Skin looks greasy wherever this is placed, and it easily creases into lines and sinks into large pores. You've been warned!

POWDER: ☺ **Loose Perfecting Powder** *($14)* is an outstanding loose powder in terms of its gossamer-smooth texture and silky matte finish. The colors tend toward pink, but each goes on soft and sheer, leaving minimal trace of the pink undertone. The sifter is covered with an adhesive seal that's extremely difficult to remove. I stopped trying after several attempts and just pulled the whole sifter cover off to examine the product.

BLUSH AND BRONZER: ✓ ☺ **$$$ BC Color Mineral Blush** *($16)* is terrific! You get two complementary colors in one pan without a divider, so it's best to swirl your brush over both and apply the blush as one color. Application is smooth and even while color payoff is impressive. All of the shades are matte except Tawny, which has a moderate shimmer most will find too much for professional daytime makeup. We have a winner! Buy this blush for its excellent texture and finish, not for the mineral angle. The mineral pigments in this powder blush are used in blushes throughout the cosmetics industry.

☺ **$$$ Secret AGEnt Tri-color Bronzing Powder** *($15.50)* includes a striped design of tan, a mid-tone color, and a pale shade for highlighting. The colors all go on as one when this is applied with a standard powder or blush brush, so the design is more for visual appeal in the container than expert results on your face. The powder has a smooth but flyaway, dusty texture and slightly grainy finish with sparkles that cling poorly. For the money, this isn't one of the better bronzing powders available.

EYESHADOW: ☺ **$$$ BC Color Mineral Shadow Trio** *($18)*. BeautiControl's sole powder eyeshadow option comes in trio form, and I'm pleased to report almost all of the color sets are well coordinated. Each set includes a light, medium, and dark shade, with the darkest shade in each being deep enough to double as eyeliner. The texture is smooth and dry (be sure to knock excess shadow from your brush to prevent fallout) and application is soft and even. Every trio has at least one shiny shade, but the shine isn't glaring and most users will likely appreciate the effect. The best trios are Sedona, Au Natural, Wisteria Lane, and Sandstone. Rainforest favors olive green tones but is workable, especially when blended with a tan or taupe shadow. The minerals in this eyeshadow formula are the same ones used industry-wide in powder eyeshadows.

☺ **Shadow Control Creme** *($8)* does help to keep your eyeshadow on, without creasing, for the entire day. There are four colors, but, like the eyeshadows, they are all shiny. The main ingredient in this product is petroleum distillates, and it forms a waterproof finish that necessitates an oil- or silicone-based makeup remover.

EYE AND BROW SHAPER: ✓ ☺ **Liquid Eye Liner** *($9.50)* is one of the sleeper products in BeautiControl's makeup line and one of the best liquid eyeliners out there. The felt tip–style applicator allows for a precise, thin line and the formula dispenses evenly and dries quickly. Once set, this won't budge until you take it off, so you're in for a day of worry-free wear. Classic black and dark brown shades are available, along with a navy hue that's an attractive alternative to black.

☺ **$$$ Brow Kit** *($18)* provides two matte, pressed brow powders in a thin compact, plus a clear brow wax for a non-sticky finishing touch. The powders apply well and enhance the brows nicely, but toss the included brush, which is too stiff and scratchy. Having two colors to work with isn't a must, but for those who want to customize, these tone-on-tone shades work well together.

☺ **Eye Defining Pencil** *($8)* is a very standard eye pencil that needs routine sharpening. Application is smooth, but the finish remains slightly creamy and is prone to smearing. It isn't worth the trouble unless you smudge the line (and set it with a powder eyeshadow to get it to last) before it does so on its own.

☺ **Eyebrow Pencil** *($12.50)* is a standard, sharpening-required brow pencil with a slightly waxy texture that applies softly without skipping or making brows appear matted. Some seldom-seen colors are included, including Taupe (which can work for some ash blonde brows) and Auburn. Oddly, there are no colors for dark brown or black brows.

LIPSTICK, LIP GLOSS, AND LIP PENCIL: ✓ ☺ **Lip Gloss** *($14)*. BeautiControl hit a home run with this fabulous lip gloss. The texture is light yet moisturizing, and the finish is completely non-sticky. Almost all of the shades are infused with some degree of shimmer, and each goes on softer than it looks. This is highly recommended unless you prefer tenacious, syrupy glosses.

☺ **BC Color Mineral Lip Color** *($14)*. Minerals count for only a small portion of this cream lipstick's formula and if you're thinking the minerals make this a more natural lipstick, think again: one of the main ingredients is (the very synthetic) polyester! Not to worry though, because it contributes to this lipstick's smooth texture and cling. This provides a soft gloss finish and comes in an attractive range of shades that includes bright and softer tones. All of the colors leave enough of a stain to help this lipstick last until lunch.

☺ **Clear Lip Gloss** *($9.50)* is a basic, but good, clear lip gloss whose only drawback is its too-thin texture. The shiny effect doesn't last long, though this isn't the least bit sticky and, being colorless, is compatible with any lip color.

☹ **Platinum Regeneration Age-Defying Lip Color** *($18)* gets its antiaging chops from a tiny amount of peptide it contains plus claims that after several weeks lips are softer and smoother, which would be true after using any lipstick that's as slick and oily as this one. This will quickly travel into lines around the mouth and the glossy, slippery finish is fleeting. A true age-defying lipstick would contain sunscreen, something this formula lacks.

☹ **Lip Shaping Pencil** *($8)* requires routine sharpening but if it weren't for that inconvenience, it would earn a Paula's Pick rating. The texture is smooth and creamy without being overly slick and, once set, this really lasts. It is a very good option for those prone to lipstick bleeding into lines around the mouth. The colors favor bright and dark tones, but there are a few versatile shades, too.

MASCARA: ✓ ☺ **SpectacuLash Mascara** *($10)*. The most spectacular part of this mascara is how well it lengthens lashes without a single clump, smear, or flake to impede the results. You won't get much thickness (the law of diminishing returns applies here) but lashes are left beautifully long and softly fringed. This earns a Paula's Pick rating for those looking to lengthen, not thicken, lashes.

✓ ☺ **$$$ SpectacuLash Thickening Primer and Maximum Length Mascara** *($18.50)*. This dual-sided mascara includes a colorless lash primer and regular mascara. With the **Thickening Primer** applied first, noticeable bulk is added to lashes. When followed with the **SpectacuLash Maximum Length Mascara**, the result is impressive, at least compared to applying the Maximum Length Mascara (which goes on a bit too wet) alone. With the primer, you get more thickness and greater oomph, and the results look great. Although this is recommended, you should know that Maybelline and L'Oreal sell similar (in some instances better) versions of this product for less money.

☺ **SpectacuLash Maximum Volume Mascara** *($10)* isn't as wondrous as the name implies. It's essentially a more dramatic version of BeautiControl's original SpectacuLash Mascara. That means you'll get more noticeable thickness and reasonably long lashes with greater depth. This still doesn't wow in the thickness department, but it's still a good mascara to consider.

☹ **SpectacuLash Waterproof Mascara** *($9)* is waterproof, but that's its only redeeming quality. Considering the wealth of excellent waterproof mascaras, there's no reason to consider this one. It goes on too wet, smears in a blink, and clumps after only a few strokes with the brush. The result is spiky, uneven lashes and it's not a look to covet.

SPECIALTY PRODUCTS: ☺ **Secret AGEnt Color Primer** *($8).* This clear silicone-based primer makes skin feel supremely silky. It is fragrance-free and compatible with most liquid or powder foundations. The texture allows for smoothing and minor "filling" of superficial wrinkles or large pores, but as with most products like this, the effect is fleeting. This contains two good antioxidants, but the clear tube packaging won't keep them stable during use. Although this works well, you can get the same results from a silicone-based serum that's loaded with beneficial ingredients for skin, such as those from Paula's Choice, Olay, or Cosmedicine.

☺ **Secret AGEnt Licensed to Fill Lip Primer** *($12).* This waxy, colorless lip primer is meant to fill in lines around and on the lips for a smoother result and a reduced chance of lip color bleeding into lines. It works respectably, at least to stop feathering. Filling in lines on the lips doesn't work as well because this doesn't have the spackle-like texture that's needed for this cosmetic effect. For less money and a precise tip which allows better application, check out the colorless lip pencil options from The Body Shop and Paula's Choice.

☺ **Makeup Erase Pencil** *($12.50).* This colorless pencil (which for some inexplicable reason is fragranced) is meant to remove minor makeup mistakes such as overdone or less-than-perfect eyeliner. Simply swipe or dab the pencil over the affected area and wipe the mistake away and you're done, right? Not quite. Although this pencil's waxes and silicones remove makeup easily, they leave a film behind that makes reapplication tricky. In essence, you have to wipe away the pencil residue, too, so the question becomes why not just use a cotton swab dipped in makeup remover instead of bothering with this pencil? Still, if the concept of this pencil appeals to you, it works as claimed.

☺ **$$$ Replenishing Conditioner for Lash and Brows** *($28.50 for 0.21 ounce)* purports to make lashes longer and fuller, yet all it contains are thickeners, conditioning agents, and several peptides. This concoction will make lashes and brow hair soft and shiny, sort of like putting a leave-in conditioner in your hair does, but none of this product's ingredients has been shown to stimulate lash growth or increase thickness. The neutral face rating for this product pertains to its lack of impressive results, especially if you were hoping for longer, thicker lashes.

BENEFIT

BENEFIT AT-A-GLANCE

Strengths: One of the few cosmetics lines that try to bring fun back to skin care, but succeed more with their makeup; a good BHA product; Lipscription deserves an audition if you're prone to chapped lips; all of the foundations are good; two of the concealers are exceptional; well-deserved reputation for liquid blush and bronzer; Dallas, Hoola, Dandelion, and Georgia are all great; good brow-enhancing options; several good lip glosses; excellent shimmer products.

Weaknesses: No sunscreens in the skin-care lineup; mostly irritating anti-acne products; clever names and product descriptions are much more interesting than product contents; mostly unimpressive eyeshadows; the chunky pencils; lip-plumping products disappoint; mostly average mascaras.

For more information about Benefit, call (800) 781-2336 or visit www.benefitcosmetics. com or www.Beautypedia.com.

BENEFIT SKIN CARE

☺ **You Clean Up Nice Face Wash** *($25 for 8 ounces)* is a fairly standard water-soluble cleanser for normal to oily skin, but would be better without the peppermint extract. Still, there is very little of it in here and it's not likely to be a problem because this is a product that's rinsed from skin (and the peppermint is the extract rather than the more potent oil form).

☹ **Woman Seeking Toner** *($32 for 6 ounces)* is an abysmal, overpriced formula that includes far too much alcohol (it's the second ingredient) and the preservative is the sixth ingredient.

☺ **Gee... That Was Quick! Oil-Free Makeup Remover for Eyes & Face** *($21 for 8 ounces)* is a basic, gentle, fragrance-free makeup remover that makes quick work of most types of makeup. It's not the best for waterproof or long-wearing formulas, but is otherwise great to use before cleansing.

☺ **$$$ Honey Snap Out of it Scrub** *($28 for 5 ounces)* is marketed as a dual-purpose scrub and mask, but is really just a thick-textured scrub that uses polyethylene (plastic beads) as the main abrasive agent. The plant oil and thickeners make this preferred for normal to dry skin, and the tiny amount of honey won't make skin snap to attention.

☹ **$$$ Dear John** *($32 for 2 ounces)* is described as having "brains and beauty," but in truth this product doesn't have an intelligent formulation. An impressive moisturizer would include recognized, state-of-the-art skin-care ingredients and technology. Instead, this is a paltry mix of water, castor oil, thickeners, a tiny amount of vitamin E, and preservative. Everything else is present in amounts too small to matter, so you have to ask: How beneficial is that? Not in the least. This moisturizer isn't terrible, just really disappointing.

☺ **$$$ Depuffing Action Eye Gel** *($28 for 0.5 ounce)* attempts to send under-eye bags packing, and is accompanied by a very cute description that makes it seem like a cure-all for puffy eyes. Not to burst anyone's bubble, but your puffiness won't recede one bit with this simple formulation that contains nothing unique or special. Given that the primary sources of puffiness and bags around the eye have to do with fat pads, muscles, and edema (swelling), there just isn't a cosmetic that can affect those biological causes. This lightweight, water- and silicone-based gel feels soothing and contains good antioxidants and anti-irritants, and it comes in opaque tube packaging that will keep them stable during use. The hydrolyzed soy flour, which Benefit claims will firm and lift skin, is chiefly used as a thickening agent, and won't lift skin anywhere. This is an option as a lightweight gel moisturizer for around the eyes (it can be used on the rest of the face, too). It does contain fragrance.

☹ **$$$ Eyecon** *($30 for 0.5 ounce)* promises to fade dark circles—a phrase that is a surefire clue that you're reading a science fiction story designed to make you fall for the hope that dark circles can actually be alleviated with skin-care products. You should know that there is nothing in this basic, ordinary moisturizer that can fade dark circles—or even be any real benefit for skin. The hyped ingredients in this product—sweet almond and apple fruit extract—are barely present, but even if they were there in greater amounts, they come up short in comparison to countless other skin-care ingredients. So what you're left with is a moisturizer whose high concentration of film-forming agents may make eye-area skin look smoother and perhaps feel a bit firmer. But the effect is merely temporary, and it should be noted that at these levels the acrylate-based film-forming agents may pose a risk of irritation (Source: *International Journal of Toxicology*, November 15, 2002, Supplement 3, pages 1-50).

☺ **$$$ Firmology** *($32 for 1.7 ounces)* is a standard, water- and silicone-based serum that contains light-reflecting pigments for a nice glow. The silicone makes skin feel silky, but you can find it in lots of other products—including many body lotions at the drugstore—so there's no reason to consider this sounds-exciting-but-is-really-underwhelming product. By the way, the fragrance components in this product may cause a skin reaction if you're not using it with an effective sunscreen.

☹ **Do It Daily! Oil-Free Moisturizing Lotion SPF 10** *($28 for 2 ounces)* isn't worth doing daily or even once a week! In the first place, the SPF rating is too low to provide sun protection that meets the standards recommended by the American Academy of Dermatology (and almost every other medical board concerned about skin or skin cancer), and second, the active ingredients do not provide adequate UVA protection. Even as a moisturizer, this product offers little beyond the mundane for any skin type, and you should consider it a must-avoid product if you're serious about taking the best possible care of your skin.

☹ **Boo-Boo Zap** *($20 for 0.2 ounce)* contains an unknown amount of salicylic acid and has a pH of 2. The pH encourages exfoliation, but coupling the salicylic acid with the alcohol and camphor in this product makes this exceedingly irritating to skin. Benefit's directive to apply this "several times a day" is akin to repeated slaps in the face.

☺ **$$$ Ka-Pow** *($20 for 0.08 ounce)* contains 2% salicylic acid formulated in a surprisingly nonirritating base, but it includes plant oils, which don't belong in an anti-acne product. It would be great if dabbing this solution on blemishes was all it took to eliminate them, but that's not the case. Specifically, this product's pH of 4 is borderline for the salicylic acid to have value as an exfoliant, though it's not a throwaway product.

✓ ☺ **$$$ Lipscription** *($32)* features a tube of **Buffing Lip Beads** that are a gentle, effective way to remove dry, flaky skin from lips. The plant oils provide some moisture, but the **Silky Lip Balm** is the real savior for dry lips. This Vaseline-based balm contains a film-forming agent to help it stay around longer, and enough silicones to warrant the silky portion of the name. Although pricey, this duo will keep your lips smooth, soft, and flake-free.

☺ **$$$ Smoooch** *($20 for 0.25 ounce)* makes mention that the vitamin E in this water-based lip balm will "cure, comfort and heal your lips while you sleep." Vitamin E alone isn't a star ingredient for lips—and pure vitamin E can be sensitizing for them—but more to the point, the amount of it in this product is next to nothing. The emollients, mineral oil, and waxes are what's working to keep lips smooth and soft, though this is a very expensive way to supply lips with those commonplace ingredients.

BENEFIT MAKEUP

FOUNDATION: ☺ **$$$ "Hello, Flawless!" SPF 15** *($34)*. This pressed-powder foundation includes an in-part titanium dioxide sunscreen, so it does double duty and makes an excellent adjunct to your liquid foundation with sunscreen. It has a smooth, dry texture that's more powdery than I was expecting given the product's formula. Applied with a brush (but don't use the one included in the compact; it's awkward and applies powder unevenly) you get sheer coverage; applied with a sponge you get medium coverage and a soft matte finish that looks quite natural. If you're using this to beef up the sun protection your foundation or moisturizer provides, it's best applied with a sponge, and you can use a brush to dust off any excess powder. The shade range includes options for light to medium skin tones. "It's About Me, Me, Me!" Toffee is slightly pink and "Why Walk When You Can Strut?" Hazelnut is slightly peach, but workable. The synthetic sunscreen actives may be a problem for use around the eyes, so use caution and don't apply to the eye area if there are signs of irritation.

☺ $$$ **PlaySticks** *($32)*. PlaySticks is one of the few foundation sticks left and it remains a very good choice. It must be blended quickly because it dries to a powder finish almost immediately, and the finish does have longevity. Coverage can go from light to medium and the drier finish makes this suitable for normal to slightly oily skin only; it won't hold up as the day goes by for those with very oily skin. Each of the ten colors is soft and neutral, and options for fair and dark skin are included.

☺ $$$ **Some Kind-A-Gorgeous** *($28)* is meant to be one-shade-fits-all sheer foundation that "evens skin tone without the look or feel of makeup." Although this is indeed lightweight thanks to its silicone-enhanced cream-to-powder texture, it isn't translucent enough to work on any skin tone. Some Kind-A-Gorgeous is best for fair to almost medium skin tones, and provides minimal coverage with a satin matte finish.

☺ $$$ **You Rebel SPF 15** *($30)* comes up short. Although the sunscreen is in-part avobenzone, only one sheer shade is available. This qualifies more as tinted moisturizer than foundation, and its creamy texture leaves a slightly moist sheen, making it suitable for normal to dry skin.

☹ **You Rebel Lite SPF 15** *($30)* does not improve on Benefit's original You Rebel SPF 15, mostly because this version's sunscreen does not provide sufficient UVA protection. The creamy-smooth texture is great for those with normal to dry skin who prefer sheer coverage and a moist finish, but the sunscreen issue is a big one, and doesn't make this a practical three-in-one product to consider.

CONCEALER: ✓ ☺ $$$ **Lyin' Eyes** *($18)* is the clever name for this click-pen concealer that you apply with a built-in synthetic brush. Each of the three skin-like shades applies with ease and provides medium coverage while setting to a smooth matte finish. It does a great job of convincingly concealing minor flaws without looking like you're hiding something—and that's the truth!

☺ $$$ **Boi-ing** *($18)* is billed as "the world's best concealer," which makes me wonder why Benefit sells several other concealers. If this is the best, then wouldn't everything else pale in comparison? Regardless, this cream-to-powder concealer (which leans toward being creamier) provides almost complete coverage and blends easily. It layers well if you need to camouflage very dark circles, but won't last through the day unless it's set with powder, which can make the under-eye area look dry and cakey. Among the three shades, only Medium is too peach to strongly consider.

☺ $$$ **Erase Paste** *($26)*. This creamy concealer in a pot is almost too creamy for its own good! You'll certainly achieve considerable coverage that can be layered for more camouflage, but doing so requires careful blending and makes this already crease-prone formula more apt to do so. Benefit offers three shades, all of which have potential, though they're not the most neutral around. The selling point is how well this concealer brightens your skin, either under your eyes or elsewhere, but that's hardly a unique trait, and the brightening is from the moist finish (which should be set with powder to minimize creasing and fading).

☹ **$$$ Powderflage Powder Concealer** *($28)*. This product's name is a big-time misrepresentation because it does not provide any camouflage and it doesn't work like a concealer. It's a pale pink loose powder infused with small particles of pearlescent shimmer. Used on its own, it's way too sheer to provide meaningful coverage and it can make the under-eye area look too white. The Sephora salesperson explained that it's best to use it over a regular concealer (such as a creamy concealer) to set it and to add a highlighted finish. This product is expensive, and given how messy it is to use a loose powder around the eyes, plus the fact that doing so can enhance rather than minimize the appearance of wrinkles, you'd be wise to stick with a traditional concealer instead, such as Maybelline Instant Age Rewind Double Face Perfector (at about one-quarter the price and a far better product).

☹ **It-Stick** *($20)* is a thick pencil concealer intended to "cease the crease" and fade expression lines. There is only one color, a fleshy peach, which won't work on most skin tones, and the creamy texture dries to an unflattering finish that looks heavy and tends to crease in your creases.

☹ **You're Bluffing** *($22)* is a twist-up cream concealer meant to camouflage redness, but its single yellow shade would add a strange, obvious hue to most skin tones unless it is blended on very sheerly. Of course, doing so means that blotchy or ruddy spots would receive minimal coverage, so the result is almost no effect at all. You're Bluffing is too slick and creamy to use over blemishes.

POWDER: ☹ **Bluff Dust** *($22* just doesn't look convincing on skin, no matter how sheerly you apply it (or how good your bluffing skills are). This is yet another yellow-toned product meant to conceal redness, but it is so intense that skin ends up looking more yellow. None of this is attractive, and you will find that a natural-looking, skin-tone foundation does a much better job of evening out your own skin tone.

BLUSH AND BRONZER: ✓ ☺ **$$$ BeneTint** *($28)* has become a beauty classic, though it's not for everyone. This simple, rose-tinted, liquid cheek color only looks good on flawless, smooth skin. It can be used as a lip stain, and is relatively long-lasting in that capacity. If you prefer liquid blush, this is deservedly one of the best.

✓ ☺ **$$$ Glamazon** *($26)* is virtually identical to BeneTint, but this is a sheer, believable bronze tint. If your skin is perfectly smooth and even, it will work well. Note: this product and BeneTint dry quickly, so blending must be fast and precise.

☺ **$$$ CORALista** *($28)*. Benefit knows how to make good blushes and bronzers and CORALista is another great option in their lineup. This shimmery, coral pink powder will add a healthy glow to your cheeks. The shimmer is subtle and CORALista will look great on many skin tones. Brushing on a sheer layer wakes up and adds a soft color to your skin. Lighter skin tones can use this as a blush, whereas darker skin tones will find it works best as a highlighter. The moderately sheer color wears well through the day with no flaking or fading. The included brush is too small for proper application and the powder does have a faint peach scent to it, but neither of these factors should keep you from giving CORALista a try.

☺ **$$$ Dallas** *($28)* promises an "outdoor glow for the indoor gal" and it delivers this via shine that leaves skin with a healthy glow. The nude pink shade has a soft tan undertone and is bound to become a Benefit favorite because this color is foolproof for many skin tones.

☺ **$$$ Dandelion** *($28)* is positioned as a highlighting powder but works best as a pale pink blush. It has a very soft gold undertone and a sheer amount of shine. This has a nice, smooth texture and the pressed powder is finely milled, so application is even, if a bit sheer. Color-wise, Dandelion is best for those with fair to light skin tones who want a touch of shine. Although it's pricey, the good news is that the shine is muted enough to not be distracting when worn for daytime makeup.

☺ **$$$ Georgia** *($28)* is a lovely pressed-powder blush that comes in one shade, a soft pink-peach. It goes on smoothly and offers more shine than Dallas or Dandelion, making it trickier (but still an option) for daytime wear.

☺ **$$$ Hoola** *($28)* is a pricey, but excellent, bronzing powder. If you don't mind parting with this much moola, you'll find that Hoola has a smooth texture, minimally shiny finish, and a believable tan color that is very flattering on fair to medium skin.

☺ **$$$ Posietint** *($28)* imparts a translucent flush of warm pink that stays put. The trouble (and major drawback) is with application: this liquid blush sets to a stain almost immediately, so blending must be lightning-fast because it doesn't budge easily once set. For that reason, using this as a sheer cheek tint is difficult. However, using it as a long-wearing lip stain is an option, assuming you like the color. The brush applicator works well on lips, but its size means extra caution if lips are small.

☺ **$$$ Thrrrob** *($28)* has a reasonably smooth yet dry texture and sheer application, imparting a pale, cotton candy–pink shade with a touch of silvery shine. It doesn't impart the rush of color the description mentions; actually, it takes a lot of product to build noticeable color, a point that isn't true for many other powder blushes, including the better options from NARS and Lorac (two companies that offer sexier hot-pink blushes).

☹ **Powder Blush** *($22)* is pricier than ever but doesn't have an outstanding formula to support it. This is a disappointing blush due to its dry texture and uneven, spotty application. Almost all department store lines (and many at the drugstore) have powder blushes whose texture and application best this product.

☹ **Talk to the Tan** *($26)* is not only a needlessly expensive bronzing gel for the face, but also, with alcohol as the second ingredient, is too drying and irritating for all skin types. There are better, irritant-free bronzing gels available from Wet 'n' Wild for less than five dollars.

EYESHADOW: ☺ **Powder Eyeshadow** *($16)* sports an enviably silky texture that glides onto skin and blends easily. All of the shades go on sheer and have at least a slight amount of shine, with the almost-matte options being Pass the Potatoes and Don't Rock the Boat. Those names are a kick, and by far the most entertaining aspect of this product. By the way, Benefit describes their eyeshadow palette as "trendy neutrals," but there are far too many green and blue hues to qualify the collection as neutral!

☺ **$$$ Velvet Eyeshadow** *($18)* is a powder eyeshadow with a very smooth texture and sheer application that imparts proportionately more shimmer than color. Even the darker shades apply quite sheer, and building intensity takes more effort than it's worth. As usual, the shade names are a combination of cute and clever. This eyeshadow blends readily and the shine clings well, but it's only for those who want minimal color and moderate shimmer, not exactly a classic look, but one that can work on some women.

☺ **Creme Eyeshadow** *($19)* has a creamy, slick feel and a minimal powder finish. The formula now creases, which explains why Benefit dropped an earlier portion of the name. The shades are all very shiny and since most are pastel to soft colors these are best for highlighting the brow bone, assuming yours is smooth and firm.

☺ **F.Y...eye!** *($22)* is an overpriced, peach-toned eyeshadow base that adds a subtle, strange tone to the eye area. This stays slick on the skin but has a powdery finish. Your foundation or matte-finish concealer will work better.

☺ **$$$ Lemon Aid** *($20)* is an unnecessary pale yellow eyeshadow base that has a thick, creamy texture; it does not work as well as a neutral foundation for minimizing discoloration.

☺ **$$$ Smokin' Eyes** *($36)*. This is sold as an all-inclusive kit to give your eyes and brows a makeover. Included in one sleek compact are three powder eyeshadows, a powder eyeliner, Benefit's Brow Zings product (in Light, a shade that won't work for everyone), the Eye Bright highlighter (normally sold in pencil form, presented in this compact as a pressed cream), a teeny-tiny pair of tweezers, and a mini dual-sided eye/brow brush. It sounds like quite a deal, but half the products in this kit are merely average and the tools are too small for practical use, although as far as brushes and tweezers go, these are good. The powder eyeshadows are the best part, though each is shiny. They apply evenly and sheer, so you can build to the intensity necessary for smoky eyes. All told, for less money, you can select individual products to create the classic smoky eye look and apply them with full-size brushes rather than miniature versions of the real deal.

EYE AND BROW SHAPER: ☺ **$$$ Badgal Liner Waterproof** *($20)*. This dark black pencil is thinner than the original chunky Badgal that Benefit sells. Badgal Liner Waterproof applies smoothly and wears well through the day. The smudger tip on the opposite end of the pencil is useful for softening and blending the liner once applied. The color will begin to fade after 12 hours or a sweaty workout, but it won't wear off completely. In fact, you'll definitely need an eye-makeup remover to take this off completely at the end of the day!

☺ **$$$ Brow Zings** *($30)* includes two coordinated brow colors (in a creamy wax and powder cake) along with two tiny but functional brushes and a mini pair of tweezers, all in one compact. The nongreasy, wax-based color is good for tinting and grooming unruly brows, while the powder is for softer accenting or less dramatic shading. It's true that brushes this size are no match for those of standard length, but for travel or purse, what's included here is workable and not scratchy or flimsy.

☺ **$$$ Speed Brow** *($16)* works well as a sheer brow tint while helping to groom and keep stray hairs in place. A Clear Speed Brow option is available, as are shades for dark blonde to light brown and medium to dark brows. Speed Brow dries quickly and the brush is small enough to allow for precision grooming of thin or sparse brows. If you're considering the Clear version, keep in mind that a container of Maybelline New York's Great Lash Clear Mascara costs one-third the price and has four times as much product.

☺ **$$$ Babe Cakes** *($22)* is a standard cake eyeliner that is applied wet and then dries to a liquid liner–like finish, though not as intense. One pairing of brown and deep black is available, and is an OK option if you prefer this method for eyelining.

☺ **$$$ Brows A-Go-Go** *($38)* brings together several of Benefit's brow-enhancing products into one cardboard compact. Included are two shades of their Brow Zings powder, a sheer brown brow wax, a pressed yet creamy version of their Eye Bright pencil, a very tiny black eye pencil, mini tweezers, and a mini dual-sided synthetic-bristle brush. Benefit also included simple step-by-step instructions for shading and shaping the eyebrow area, a nice touch. If only all of the products were as helpful as the paper instruction guide! The Brow Zings powder and wax are great, but only if you have light to medium brown brows. The pencil is utterly standard and almost too small to use (sharpen it once and you'll be shocked at how much smaller it gets), as are the tools. The Eye Bright product is OK but its slightly greasy texture doesn't last long; the Brow Highlighter Powder is pale pink with a strong iridescent finish that can look too contrasting next to dark brows (subdued shine is preferred).

The Reviews B

☺ **$$$ High Brow** *($20)* is meant to highlight the brow bone for an "instant brow lift." Applying any lighter eyeshadow to this area will have the same effect and you won't have to deal with the downsides this pencil has: it needs routine sharpening, the creamy texture drags slightly, and unless you apply sparingly and blend very well, it can look opaque and heavy (sort of approaching drag queen makeup). Unless you've been utterly disappointed with trying to highlight your brow bone with powder or cream eyeshadows and want something different, there is no reason to waste money on this pencil.

☺ **$$$ Instant Eyebrow Pencil** *($20)*. Quick, smooth application and two excellent colors (best for light brown to blonde brows) are strong points for this needs-sharpening brow pencil. The pencil has a soft tip, so it requires light pressure or short, feathering strokes through brow hairs for best results. I wish the finish didn't remain tacky on brows because it can feel and look a bit gummy, which may be why Benefit included a spoolie brush at the opposite end of this pencil to smooth out the problem application. All in all this pencil is below many other superior options from dozens of other cosmetic companies.

☺ **$$$ Sketching Pencils Eyes** *($18)* are standard pencils that have a soft, creamy, ready-to-smudge texture. Application is easy, but you might as well use the included smudger before the pencil does so on its own.

☻ **Eye Bright** *($20)* is a pale pink, slightly greasy pencil meant to be used on the dark inner corners of the eyes. It is completely unnecessary because any neutral-shade concealer can do the same without the unflattering pink tint.

☻ **Gilded** *($20)* is a standard chunky pencil that is creamy enough to consistently smear and fade. It may seem impressive that it is heralded by major fashion magazines, but remember, such publications applaud many products that are mediocre to poor, or just plain irritating.

☻ **Bad Gal** *($20)* is a standard chunky pencil that is creamy enough to consistently smear and fade. It may seem impressive that it is heralded by major fashion magazines, but remember, such publications applaud many products that are mediocre to poor, or just plain irritating.

☻ **Mr. Frosty** *($20)* is a standard chunky pencil that is creamy enough to consistently smear and fade. It may seem impressive that it is heralded by major fashion magazines, but remember, such publications applaud many products that are mediocre to poor, or just plain irritating.

LIPSTICK, LIP GLOSS, AND LIPLINER: ☺ **$$$ BeneTint Lip Balm** is a standard, but good, castor oil-based lip gloss with a texture that is not too sticky and a sheer, cherry-red color that would work well on a variety of skin tones.

☺ **$$$ BeneTint Pocket Pal** *($20)* is a dual-sided wand that features a vial of BeneTint liquid on one end and a clear lip gloss on the other. You brush the BeneTint on lips, allow it to dry, and then top it with the lip gloss (which is necessary because BeneTint on its own does not moisturize lips). If you like the way BeneTint colors your lips and want a glossy finish, this is recommended!

☺ **$$$ Full Finish Lipstick** *($18)*. With a name like Full Finish, you might expect full coverage, but that's not what you get with this creamy-smooth lipstick. The shade range is attractive and each leaves a decent, doesn't-fade stain as it wears, but layering any color only adds up to moderate coverage and a soft gloss finish. This is a good cream lipstick to consider; it just has a misleading name.

☺ **$$$ Rush Hour** *($22)* is sold as an instant makeover for lips and cheeks, promising to refresh your look in ten seconds or less. Packaged like a standard slim lipstick, this has a creamy but light texture that's closer to a lipstick than a cream-to-powder blush. The single shade was designed to be so versatile that anyone can use it, and for the most part that's true. It's a medium rosy pink with a hint of mauve that complements many skin tones—just don't expect it to show up well on very dark skin. Rush Hour is comfortable to wear on lips and has a nearly opaque, creamy finish. On cheeks, the shade definitely works for blush and can be sheered out to create a soft flush of color.

☺ **$$$ Lipstick** *($16)* is all about the playful to humorous shade names. Favorites (for names) include "But Officer," "One Hit Wonder," and "Luck Be a Lady." The lipstick itself is rather ordinary, with a texture that's more waxy than creamy and that supplies medium coverage. Despite the fun names, these feel old-fashioned compared to the ultra-smooth, often lightweight lipsticks from lines such as Estee Lauder and Lancome.

☺ **$$$ California Kissin'** *($18)* is a sheer, blue-tinted lip gloss that's also mint-flavored and said to brighten your smile. The blue tint is soft enough to not interfere with whatever lipstick it is paired with, but that also means it won't make teeth look any whiter. It is otherwise a standard emollient lip gloss that's pricey for what you get.

☺ **$$$ Color Plump Plumping Lip Color** *($22)* has a smooth, easy-to-apply texture that feels creamy without being slippery. As for Benefit's claim that their tripeptide complex enhances lip volume, don't bet on it. The amount of peptides in this pencil is minimal (it's the very last ingredient listed) and there is no substantiated proof that peptides in minor amounts, or for that matter even in large amounts, prompt fuller lips—and they are in no way comparable to the results you get from collagen injections. What's making lips look fuller is the soft, reflective shimmer each light-coverage shade has, and that's a benefit you can get from many lipsticks.

☺ **$$$ Cupid's Bow Set** *($28)*. Cute names are one thing Benefit has in spades, but the concept behind this dual-ended, needs-sharpening lip pencil isn't likely to make you fall in love or pucker your lips. One side of the pencil is a creamy lip color, and the sole shade is a largely unappealing drab mauve brown. The other side is a thin-tipped lipliner that is a pale opalescent pink. The idea is to shade the outer portion of your lower lip with the lip color, then highlight the Cupid's bow (central part of the upper lip) and middle of your lower lip. You can do the same thing with a regular lipstick or lip gloss, and in that sense your range of shades is wide open (not to mention the variety of lipsticks and glosses available).

☺ **$$$ D'finer D'liner Clear Lipliner** *($20)* beckons you to "conquer the feather factor," meaning that this needs-sharpening pencil, meant to be applied on the border of your lips, will keep lipstick locked in place for hours. It works marginally well, but the oil-based formula doesn't hold up as long as similar products whose base is made up of stay-put silicones. Although described as clear, this product has a faint pink color and leaves a subtle shimmer finish, so it sort of looks like you missed your lips a bit. Those with a consistent problem of lipstick feathering into lines around the mouth will likely be disappointed by this product's brief staying time.

☺ **$$$ Sketching Pencils Lips** *($18)* has a less creamy texture than most standard lip pencils and glides on easily without smearing. If only it didn't need sharpening—a part of the picture that keeps it from earning a happy face rating.

MASCARA: ☺ **$$$ Get Bent Wonder Lifting Mascara** *($19)* does have a bent brush, and if you like the concept, you can manipulate any mascara brush head in this manner. This "whole new angle" on mascara is more gimmicky than anything else, but that's forgivable because this quickly produces long, lifted, beautifully separated lashes without clumps or smearing. The mascara formula keeps lashes softer than most, and allows you to apply multiple coats without incident—though this does eventually reach the point of diminishing returns.

☺ **$$$ Bad Gal Lash Mascara** *($19)* is not, in the words of Benefit, "like wearing a set of false eyelashes without the glue." From the box to the oversized brush, everything about this mascara is big except the results. It does apply cleanly and evenly, with no clumps in sight, but after much effort for moderate length and minimal thickness, I wasn't ready to put on a black leather jacket and ride off into the night on the back of a motorcycle. I was ready for a nap!

☹ **$$$ Badgal Waterproof Mascara** *($19)*. "Bad" mascara would be a more appropriate name for this lackluster mascara that does little more than add some pigment to the lashes. It doesn't lengthen, thicken, or curl lashes at all. The only good thing to say is it doesn't smudge and it is waterproof, as the name indicates. All in all, it's an expensive mascara with bad performance.

BRUSHES: ☺ **Bluff Puff** *($20)* is a powder brush with a stubby handle that fits easily into the palm of your hand for dusting the face with powder. The brush head is firm but soft, and the densely packed bristles hold powder well and distribute it evenly. I wouldn't use this with Benefit's too-yellow Bluff Dust, but it is a suitable alternative to traditional brushes for applying loose or pressed powders that come in true skin-tone shades.

☺ **$$$ Hard Angle Brush** *($16)* is surprisingly soft for how firm it is! This synthetic brush does a great job of applying wet or cream cake liners in an even, thin line, but performs merely OK with dry shadows since its thin wedge doesn't allow for much grab. The angled cut affords easy lining at the lash line, and could also work well for shaping brows.

☺ **$$$ The Talent Brush** *($18)* is one of Benefit's best brushes. It's a soft, synthetic brush, with a small, rounded tip. The brush's density allows for superior grab that deposits powder shadow evenly (this is especially effective if you use a dabbing motion rather than a sweeping one), and the angled cut makes blending around the eye nearly effortless. Its shape and size make it an option for shading and contouring, too.

☹ **$$$ Concealer Brush** *($20)* is larger than you might expect for a concealer brush, which is problematic if you need to get into tight corners or small spaces around the nose or eyes. It does a superior job at grabbing and blending cream-based products, but is not dense enough to hold its shape and is prone to splaying at the sides.

☹ **$$$ Get Bent Brush** *($16)* features a pointed tip atop an angled head, which seems like a good idea, but actually makes it too awkward to hold the brush steady for precise eye-lining. That issue becomes moot, however, since the soft synthetic hairs are not dense enough at the tip to create precise lines. This brush is workable for creating a thicker, smoky effect around the eye, but nevertheless the novel crooked tip is hard to master.

☻ **Foundation Brush** *($20)* has a flat, sculpted cut that does make blending easy, but still leaves a lot to be desired. With a large surface area that lacks density, it picks up and deposits product unevenly, which can throw a wrench in foundation application, no matter how much you blend. Every single tester (and even a few in the packaging) showed signs of splaying.

FACE AND BODY ILLUMINATING/SHIMMER PRODUCTS: ✓ ☺ **$$$ 10** *($28)* tempts you to "be a perfect 10," and although it takes more than this cosmetic to go from bland to glam, without question you'll be pleased with the wonderfully silky texture and smooth application. This pressed shimmer powder is housed in a large cardboard box and includes a pale pink and sheer bronze shade with no divider in between. The concept is to bronze and highlight, but this is best for highlighting by adding soft touches of shine because the bronze shade is so sheer. The shine clings well and is glow-y without being too show-y, making for an attractive, though pricey, evening look.

☺ **$$$ High Beam** *($24)* comes in a nail polish bottle and is applied to the face with a brush (or you can use a sponge or your fingers). It is a silvery-pink shimmer lotion that dries to a matte finish, leaving the shine behind.

☺ **$$$ Moon Beam** *($24)* is identical to High Beam except for its golden pink color. Both products tend to stay put and are much easier to control than shimmer powders with their minimal ability to cling.

☺ **$$$ Lust Duster** *($18).* This loose powder with the seductively suggestive name is simply meant to highlight the brow bone and tops of the cheekbones. They really play up the mineral angle, but in fact the mineral pigments in this powder are also found in countless other powders. More to the point, although this has a silky, weightless texture that provides a smooth finish and soft shine, lots of pressed shimmer powders can produce the same degree of highlighting, but without the mess of loose powder. The packaging Benefit chose for Lust Duster doesn't minimize the potential for mess, so if you opt to try this, be careful when you're applying it or even transporting it. The pastel-themed shades are indeed suitable for highlighting the afore-mentioned areas, and the shine clings reasonably well, but almost every line at the drugstore offers similar if not better options for far less money.

☺ **$$$ That Gal** *($28)* is a highlighting lotion whose pale pink shimmer adds a soft glow and moist feel to skin. Benefit is selling this as a primer, which means they intend for it to be applied all over the face. That's an option, but only if you have normal to dry skin and want forehead-to-chin shimmer. The click dispenser on top of the glue stick–like package takes some getting used to and can dispense too much product if you're not careful.

☹ **$$$ Miss Popularity** *($24)* is billed as a "precision highlighter for eyes and face," and the pointed sponge-tip applicator makes being precise quite easy, although ultimately this is a very expensive way to add shine to skin. The white-gold loose powder adheres well to skin, so flaking isn't a problem. This doesn't glide over skin with grace, so it's not the best if you're look-ing to apply it to, say, your entire eyelid. Using this to highlight key areas is fine, because you are left with strong shine; just be aware that many of today's better shine-enhancing powders play it soft.

☹ **$$$ Ooo La Lift** *($22)* feels like an "instant eye lift!"—or so Benefit would like you to believe. This is just a pale pink liquid highlighter with a smooth texture and a slight shine. There is absolutely nothing in it to support the "depuffing and firming" claims, though using this under the eyes to banish dark areas will make puffiness less apparent.

SPECIALTY PRODUCTS: ☹ **$$$ Dr. Feelgood** *($28 for 0.85 ounce)* is supposed to be worn either alone or over makeup to smooth skin and fill in fine lines and noticeable pores. I guess you could also call this product spackle, because that is exactly how it works. The waxlike formula melts over the skin and then fills in the flaws (at least somewhat). You won't notice much difference in wrinkles or pore size, but long-term use may lead to clogged pores because of the waxlike thickening agents in this product. The first ingredient is cornstarch, and while this offers a dry finish, it isn't optimum for use over blemish-prone skin because food-based ingredients can feed the bacteria that promote acne. By the way, the tiny amounts of vitamins A, C, and E won't nourish skin and the packaging chosen for this product won't keep them stable.

☹ **$$$ She-Laq** *($30)* is meant as a sealant for lipstick, eyeliner, or brow color. It's a thick, alcohol-based liquid with hairspray ingredients that should not go anywhere near the eye, as the irritation potential is just too high. Otherwise, it's just an expensive variation on brow gel, and the supplied applicators and tools are inferior to professional brushes.

☹ **Lip Plump** *($22)* has been around for too long when you consider its lackluster performance, inconvenient application, and price. It supposedly smooths and builds the contour of the lips, but is really just a lightweight, flesh-toned concealer that minimally fills in lip lines and takes too long to set. Even the Benefit counter personnel agreed this is a product that is difficult to work with, messy to apply, and, perhaps most importantly, doesn't really work. It's not that often I get such candid comments from a line's representatives, but I think they sum up this product exactly!

BIORE (SKIN CARE ONLY)

BIORE AT-A-GLANCE

Strengths: Provides complete ingredient lists for every product on the company Web site; improved cleansers.

Weaknesses: Known for their pore strips, which aren't as helpful as they seem; lots of products that contain alcohol and/or menthol, neither of which improve the look or function of pores; the sole sunscreen option lacks the proper UVA-protecting ingredients.

For more information about Biore, call (888) BIORE-11 or visit www.biore.com or www.Beautypedia.com.

BIORE COMPLEXION CLEARING PRODUCTS

☺ **Blemish Fighting Ice Cleanser** *($7.99 for 6.7 ounces)* gets its icy feeling from menthol, the sole ingredient that sabotages this otherwise very good, water-soluble cleanser. The 2% salicylic acid is useless against blemishes in this product, not only because of a too-high pH but also because of its brief contact with skin.

☺ **Warming Anti-Blackhead Cream Cleanser** *($7.99 for 6.25 ounces)* contains the mineral zeolite, which causes an exothermic (heat-generating) reaction when mixed with water. That may feel interesting but it has no benefit for the skin, so this ends up being more gimmicky than anything else and isn't preferred to other cleansers in the Biore line. The 2% salicylic acid is rinsed down the drain before it can impact skin, and the lack of cleansing agents makes this a poor choice to remove makeup. It's a mediocre cleanser for normal to dry skin.

☹ **Triple Action Astringent** *($7.99 for 8.5 ounces)* contains two types of drying alcohols along with witch hazel and menthol, making this a problem product for all skin types. The amount of alcohol in this toner increases oil production in the pore.

☹ **Pore Unclogging Scrub** *($7.99 for 5 ounces)* is a cleanser, not a scrub, and its wax content impedes rinsing. More of an issue than the name and wax is the menthol, which makes this product too irritating for all skin types.

BIORE DAILY RECHARGING PRODUCTS

☺ **Refresh Daily Cleansing Cloths** *($6.99 for 30 cloths).* These textured cloths help exfoliate and cleanse normal to dry skin not prone to breakouts. The grapefruit extract has irritation potential, so ideally you'll want to rinse your skin after using the cleansing cloth. Otherwise, these work fairly well to remove most types of makeup, an effect that's similar to what you'd get using a washcloth with a cleansing lotion.

☹ **Revitalize 4-in-1 Self-Foaming Cleanser** *($7.99 for 6.7 ounces)* would be a much better cleanser for normal to oily skin if it did not contain the irritating combination of eucalyptus and menthol. They do feel cooling on your skin, but that cooling sensation is an indication of irritation, not revitalizing.

☺ **Detoxify Daily Scrub** *($7.99 for 5 ounces)* is an OK scrub for normal to dry skin. It contains cleansing agents as well, but the amount of wax prevents complete rinsing and so it may leave a film on your skin (which has the potential to clog pores). By the way, a scrub or any other type of exfoliant doesn't detoxify skin—that simply isn't possible. Your pores aren't producing toxic sludge that's waiting to be expunged; simple cleansing twice daily does a good job of removing dirt, debris, excess oil, and perspiration from the skin's surface, and for exfoliation a washcloth is far preferred to this formula.

☺ **Enliven Cooling Eye Gel** *($9.49 for 0.5 ounce)*. If you are looking for an inexpensive, very light gel moisturizer for slightly dry skin anywhere on the face, then this is an acceptable, though completely unexciting, option. Some of the plant extracts have irritation potential, but they are present in amounts so small they are likely not a cause for concern. Biore also includes a preservative (dmdm hydantoin) that is known to be sensitizing, as well as fragrance, but again, in amounts likely too small to be cause for concern; however, for the eye area they should have been left out altogether.

☹ **Nourish Moisture Lotion SPF 15** *($9.99 for 3.4 ounces)* lacks the UVA-protecting ingredients of titanium dioxide, zinc oxide, avobenzone (also known as butyl methoxydibenzoylmethane), Tinosorb, or Mexoryl SX and is not recommended. Although it does contain titanium dioxide, it is not listed as an active ingredient, and therefore this should not be relied on for daytime protection.

☹ **Restore Skin-Boosting Night Serum** *($9.99 for 1.4 ounces)*. Although this water- and silicone-based serum will make your skin feel unbelievably silky and it contains a hefty amount of antioxidant green tea leaf, it also contains plant irritants such as rosemary and sage. The plant *Chelidonium majus*, commonly known as greater celandine, is capable of causing contact dermatitis (Source: *Contact Dermatitis*, July 2000, pages 43-47). The price is attractive, but this serum has too many problems to make it worth considering over far better serum formulas from Olay, Neutrogena, or Clinique to name a few.

☺ **Purify Self Heating Mask** *($7.99 for 2.08 ounces)* claims to open pores and provide "an intensive deep clean," but this relatively standard clay mask does no such thing. Pores cannot be opened (and if they closed we would lose the ability to sweat, which would cause us to overheat), and a mask like this cannot go deeper than the superficial surface layer of skin. This is a good option for oily skin, and the heating effect is primarily a tactile sensation, not a unique benefit. Heat is a problem for blemished or inflamed skin too, so avoid this mask if that describes your skin's condition.

BIORE PORE STRIPS PRODUCTS

☹ **Deep Cleansing Pore Strips** *($10.49 for 14 strips)* is the gimmicky product that put Biore on the map several years ago. Now available in a single package that includes removable strips for the nose and face, the concept remains the same: you place a piece of cloth with an incredibly sticky substance on it over your nose or elsewhere on the face, as you might do with a Band-Aid, wait 15 minutes for it to dry, and then rip it off. Along with some amount of skin, blackheads are supposed to stick to it and come right out of the skin. The main ingredient on the strips is polyquaternium-37, a film-forming, hairspray-type ingredient—so it's basically a piece of gauze with a form of hairspray on it. You may at first be impressed with what comes off your nose. (Well, there is no question: you will be impressed.) Most people do have some oil sitting at the top of their oil glands, and most of the face's oil glands are located on the nose. So whether you use these strips or a piece of tape, black dots and some skin will be removed. Is that helpful? Only momentarily, although if you use the Biore product, the plastic-forming agent can get into the pores and possibly cause breakouts and irritation. The way these strips adhere, they can absolutely injure or tear skin and cause spider veins to surface. They are especially unsafe if you've been having facial peels; using Retin-A, Renova, AHAs, or BHA; or are taking Accutane; or if you have naturally thin skin or any skin disorder such as rosacea, psoriasis, or seborrhea. Biore claims this product can pull an entire blackhead plug out of the skin. It can't. If you could grab a blackhead out of the skin, your skin would be left with an empty hole (and there is nothing in this product that will close it up), but that's not what happens. Instead, just the top layer of the blackhead is removed, and then the blackhead returns because the source of the problem was never corrected. Nothing was done to reduce irritation, exfoliate skin cells, help keep oil flow normal, or close the pore. Without question, this product is not preferred to a well-formulated BHA product, which, in most cases, effectively dissolves and controls blackheads (in addition to its other positive traits).

☹ **Ultra Deep Cleansing Pore Strips** *($7.99 for 6 strips)* are nearly identical to the Deep Cleansing Pore Strips, but here tea tree oil and irritating menthol have been added, too. These are designed for the nose only, and the act of tearing off the strip is irritating enough without adding troublesome ingredients to the mix.

BIORE SKIN PRESERVATION PRODUCTS

☺ **Clean Things Up Nourishing Gel Cleanser** *($7.99 for 6.7 ounces)* is a standard, well-formulated water-soluble cleanser that's suitable for normal to oily skin. It is capable of removing makeup and, unlike many of Biore's cleansers, doesn't contain menthol. This does contain a small amount of *Melissa officinalis* extract, but its potential for irritation is minimal. I don't care for their choice of preservatives, and I don't really like any amount of coloring agents, but in a rinse-off product it is minimally problematic.

☺ **Dual Fusion Moisturizer + SPF 30** *($14.99 for 1.7 ounces)*. The fact that this product is packaged in a component with separate "chambers" for its moisturizing and sunscreen components is of no special benefit for skin. The sunscreen portion needs (and contains) some of the same ingredients found in the moisturizer side, so the separation is a gimmick. Moreover, the concept of dispensing a sunscreen and moisturizer at the same time isn't helpful for skin. That's because you're diluting the sunscreen as you mix it with the moisturizer, so you will not be getting the SPF stated on the label. You're better off using a daytime moisturizer or foundation with sunscreen where everything is blended together and the blended combination was tested to ensure the sun protection stated. The sunscreen part is OK on its own, but the moisturizer portion is a mediocre option for normal to oily skin. If you use this product as directed, its sun protection is most likely hindered by the hokey dual-fusion dilution concept. This product also contains a potentially irritating amount of *Melissa officinalis* extract.

☺ **Even Smoother Microderm Exfoliator** *($14.99 for 3 ounces)*. This scrub can be needlessly abrasive unless used very gently. The base formula helps cushion skin, but not to the extent where caution isn't advised. This rinses quite well and is best for normal to slightly dry or oily skin. Because it's present in only a tiny amount, *Melissa officinalis* extract is not cause for concern as an irritant.

☺ **Hard Day's Night Overnight Moisturizer** *($14.99 for 1.7 ounces)*. A moisturizer claiming to rebuild skin while you rest should contain more ingredients capable of doing that than this product does. The glycerin, vitamin E, and green tea are helpful, as are the thickening agents that give this product its texture, but where are the ceramides, cholesterol, skin-identical and water-binding agents, anti-irritants, and additional potent antioxidants? What about cell-communicating ingredients? The ingredients in this product are like the appetizer that leaves you still hungry for the main course; where's the meat? All of the state-of-the-art ingredients essential to help skin rebuild a strong barrier and gain a healthy appearance are in short supply. Instead of being a hard-working moisturizer, this Biore product is basically a part-time employee who takes too many breaks. As such, you'll get minimal benefit, and why settle for that when there are other moisturizers that provide so much more (and without the couple of questionable plant extracts this one contains)? If you're OK with settling for less than your skin deserves, this is an option for normal to dry skin.

☺ **See the Future Fortifying Eye Cream** *($14.99 for 0.5 ounce)* is an OK lightweight eye moisturizer that can be used anywhere on the face where skin is slightly dry. There are a couple of plant extracts that pose a risk of irritation, especially when used near the eyes. This would be better if it did not contain fragrance (many eye creams omit this type of ingredient because of the potential for irritation).

BOBBI BROWN

BOBBI BROWN AT-A-GLANCE

Strengths: Some good cleansers; a few stably packaged products loaded with advanced ingredients to keep skin in top shape; an easy-to-use, lightweight self-tanner; one of the best neutral shade ranges for foundation; foundation options for all skin types and preferences; very good blush and eyeshadows (powder and cream), including several matte shades; the Gel Eyeliner; Shimmer Brick; mostly excellent brushes; several refillable compact options and other useful accessories.

Weaknesses: As with most Lauder-owned companies, the well-formulated moisturizers are hindered by jar packaging, which compromises the effectiveness of light- and air-sensitive ingredients; several otherwise effective products are marred by irritating fragrant oils or fragrance components; some of the foundations without sunscreen lack sufficient UVA-protecting ingredients; concealers are a mixed bag; are mostly unappealing lip glosses, and none of those with sunscreen provide sufficient UVA protection.

For more information about Bobbi Brown, owned by Estee Lauder, call (877) 310-9222 or visit www.bobbibrowncosmetics.com or www.Beautypedia.com.

BOBBI BROWN SKIN CARE

BOBBI BROWN EXTRA PRODUCTS

☹ **Extra Balm Rinse** *($20 for 1.7 ounces)* is a very rich, luxurious cleansing balm for dry to very dry skin, but the olive oil prevents it from rinsing well without the aid of a washcloth. That's not a big deal, but the amount of the fragrant component limonene in this product is. Limonene is a volatile compound found in most citrus fruits, and its topical application causes contact dermatitis (Source: www.naturaldatabase.com).

☹ **Extra Eye Balm** *($60 for 0.5 ounce)* is an extremely emollient, rich moisturizer that would have been a slam-dunk for those with dry skin (and an imposing skin-care budget) if it did not include appreciable levels of potent irritants like mint oil, orange oil, and galbanum oil, among others. None of these ingredients should go anywhere near the eye. What a shame, because aside from those irritants this is an exceptionally well-formulated product.

☹ **Extra Face Oil** *($60 for 1 ounce)* contains some highly effective oils for dry to very dry skin, including olive, sesame, and jojoba. Not willing to leave well enough alone, this product also contains the irritants neroli, patchouli, lavender, and sandalwood, along with problematic fragrance components such as geraniol and linalool. Using plain olive oil would be preferred to this well-intentioned but faulty product.

☹ **Extra Moisturizing Balm** *($85 for 1.7 ounces)* ends up being a very expensive way to supply skin with Vaseline and silicone, the main ingredients (next to water) in this rich balm. The antioxidant plant oils are rendered ineffective by this product's jar packaging, and the geranium oil, while smelling nice, can cause skin irritation (Sources: *Contact Dermatitis*, June 2001, pages 344-346; and *Journal of Applied Microbiology*, February 2000, pages 308-316). Choosing plain Vaseline not only costs considerably less but spares your skin an irritant response.

☹ **Extra Moisturizing Balm SPF 25** *($85 for 1.7 ounces)* has avobenzone for UVA protection, but contains irritating bitter-orange oil and angelica oil, which is photosensitizing (Source: www.naturaldatabase.com). What's that type of ingredient doing in a product whose intention is to protect skin while outdoors? And even if it didn't include these problem ingredients, how liberally are you going to apply a sunscreen with a price like this?

☹ **Extra SPF 25 Tinted Moisturizing Balm** *($50 for 1 ounce)* includes an in-part avobenzone sunscreen. But in this greasy tinted moisturizer, that benefit is negated by the many fragrant oils, all of which are irritating to skin and counteract the anti-irritants present in the formula. Without them, this would have been a good option for those with very dry skin, and all the shades are impeccably neutral.

☹ **Extra Soothing Balm** *($55 for 0.5 ounce)* contains triglycerides, waxes, emollients, and plant oils that can protect and restore dry skin to a healthier-looking and smoother-feeling state. What's not the least bit soothing is the inclusion of ginger root and bitter-orange oils. Both can be irritating to skin and they keep this product from being a worthwhile purchase (Source: www.naturaldatabase.com).

OTHER BOBBI BROWN SKIN-CARE PRODUCTS

☺ **$$$ Lathering Tube Soap** *($24 for 4.2 ounces)* isn't a true soap, but the name is apropos for the apothecary-style packaging chosen for this product. This is a standard foaming cleanser that uses the soap derivative potassium myristate as the main cleansing agent, one that can be drying and sensitizing for some skin types. However, this cleanser also contains a battery of nonirritating plant oils for extra cushioning while cleansing. There are minute amounts of lavender, jasmine, and grapefruit for fragrance, but likely not enough to be problematic. Though pricey, this is still a decent cleansing option for normal to slightly dry skin.

☺ **$$$ Eye Makeup Remover** *($22 for 3.4 ounces)* is a very standard, detergent-based eye-makeup remover that contains fragrant rose water and soothing cornflower extract. It works well, but so do many similar removers that cost much less than this one and skip the fragrance.

✓☺ **$$$ Instant Long-Wear Makeup Remover** *($22 for 3.4 ounces)* is a standard, but very good, dual-phase makeup remover. The blend of solvent and silicones quickly removes all types of makeup, including waterproof mascara and lip stains. What makes this product a cut above many similar options is its lack of fragrance and any other ingredients problematic for use around the eyes. It is indeed extra gentle, and recommended for all skin types.

☺ **$$$ Buffing Grains for Face** *($40 for 0.99 ounce)* are made to sound special because you can add these loose grains to any cleanser to create a custom scrub. The novelty may be fun, but this concoction is simply polyethylene beads (plastic beads) with adzuki bean powder and tiny amounts of plant oils, plus a detergent cleansing agent that is activated by water. Polyethylene is used in most topical scrub products; you don't need to spend this much money for its benefit. For the money-is-no-object among us, this is a viable option. Still, for many reasons, a soft washcloth works just as well if not better than a scrub.

☺ **$$$ Soothing Face Tonic** *($26 for 6.7 ounces)* is a very good toner for all skin types, though its clear glass packaging hinders the effectiveness of the antioxidants present. Still, this supplies skin with some excellent water-binding and soothing agents, and the tiny amount of lavender is unlikely to be a problem.

☹ **$$$ Hydrating Eye Cream** *($45 for 0.5 ounce)* definitely contains ingredients that can hydrate skin around the eyes or elsewhere on the face, but it's an overall lackluster formula whose antioxidant vitamins are compromised by jar packaging. This eye cream is fragrance-free.

☹ **$$$ Hydrating Face Cream** *($50 for 1.7 ounces)* contains mostly water, silicone, slip agent, thickeners, plant oil, algae, vitamins, fragrant plant extracts, film-forming agent, a cell-communicating ingredient, and preservatives. It's a good option for normal to dry skin but would be much better in packaging that keeps the antioxidant vitamins stable once it's opened.

✓☺ **$$$ Intensive Skin Supplement** *($65 for 1 ounce)* has some impressive ingredients and a lightweight, water-based serum texture built around slip agents and silicones. The amounts of vitamin C and mulberry root extract are probably not enough to have an effect on melanin production, but between them, the other antioxidants, and a cell-communicating ingredient, this is a well-formulated product that can be used by all skin types.

☹ **$$$ Oil Control Lotion SPF 15** *($45 for 1.7 ounces).* Other than having a soft matte finish that someone with oily skin will appreciate, this daytime moisturizer with an in-part avobenzone sunscreen cannot control oil. Oil production is controlled by hormones, and as such is not affected by what you apply topically to your skin (although certain ingredients can absorb excess oil, but that's not the same as controlling oil production). So, with its matte finish and reliable sunscreen, why isn't this a slam dunk for normal to oily skin? Because the amounts of lavender extract and irritating geranium oil surpass the amounts of several state-of-the-art ingredients, including linoleic acid and the antioxidant nordihydroguaiaretic acid. For what this product costs, you should expect more of the good stuff and little to none of the bad.

☹ **$$$ Overnight Cream** *($65 for 1.7 ounces)* is sold as a "technologically advanced repair product for nighttime use," and although it does use ingredients that can repair skin's barrier and improve its appearance, the choice of jar packaging renders the many antioxidants in this product unstable shortly after you open it. This still has merit for dry to very dry skin; it does contain fragrant plant extracts.

☹ **Protective Face Lotion SPF 15** *($45 for 1.7 ounces)* wins points for its in-part titanium dioxide sunscreen and a silky lotion base laced with soothing chamomile, several antioxidants, and cell-communicating ingredients. The problem is the inclusion of fragrance components of linalool, limonene, and cinnamyl alcohol, the latter of which is a known skin sensitizer and inappropriate for use in a product meant to protect skin from sun damage (Source: *Chemical*

Research in Toxicology, March 2004, pages 301-310). It's interesting that cinnamyl alcohol and its aldehyde form are part of a standard fragrance mix used by dermatologists to determine whether a patient is suffering allergic contact dermatitis from fragrance (Source: www.dermatologytimes. com/dermatologytimes/article/articleDetail.jsp?id=396332).

☺ **$$$ Vitamin Enriched Face Base** *($50 for 1.7 ounces)* lists many antioxidant vitamins but what's not explained is the choice of jar packaging, which won't hold them stable once this moisturizer is opened. It contains some good anti-irritants, but these are countered by fragrant geranium oil and lesser amounts of potentially sensitizing fragrance components, further making this product a tough sell, especially given its price.

☹ **Lip Balm SPF 15** *($17 for 0.5 ounce)*. Lip Balm SPF 15 lacks the UVA-protecting ingredients of titanium dioxide, zinc oxide, avobenzone, Tinosorb, or Mexoryl SX, and is not recommended.

☺ **$$$ Sunless Tanning Gel for Face and Body** *($30 for 4.2 ounces)* is a water- and silicone-based self-tanner that uses the same ingredient (dihydroxyacetone) found in almost all self-tanning products. Brown offers two versions, based on whether you have a light to medium or medium to dark skin tone. This does contain volatile fragrance components, and is best used in the evening and rinsed in the morning to avoid the potential for irritation when skin is exposed to sunlight.

BOBBI BROWN MAKEUP

FOUNDATION: ✓ ☺ **$$$ Moisturizing Cream Compact Foundation** *($40)* is a great foundation for the winter season because its formula is helpful for dry skin when cold temperatures take a toll. This foundation is creamy without being greasy and ideal for normal to dry skin. It moisturizes without feeling heavy or looking greasy, and once blended sets to a satin-smooth finish. This can be blended on sheer or built to medium coverage. The range of shades is mostly remarkable, as is typical for Brown's foundations. The only tricky colors are Warm Natural (will be too peach for some medium skin tones), Golden (too orange), and Walnut (may be too red for some dark skin tones). Chestnut and Espresso are beautiful for some African-American skin tones, and there are shades for those with fair skin, too. The tiny amount of lavender is unlikely to cause problems, and the only other caution is that the emollients in this makeup make it not recommended for blemish-prone skin.

✓ ☺ **$$$ Oil-Free Even Finish Compact Foundation** *($40)* is a silicone-based creamy compact makeup that applies and blends beautifully. Along with Clarins' Soft Touch Rich Compact Foundation, it raises the bar for next-generation cream-to-powder makeups. Brown's version has a natural, slightly moist finish that isn't really powdery—it actually leaves skin with a soft glow that only those with oily skin will want to avoid. It provides light to medium coverage but if you layer it you can get nearly full coverage, a feature that also makes it an option for use as concealer. Several shades are available, and the only ones to consider carefully are Golden, Chestnut, and Honey. Brown's lightest shade (Alabaster) is not offered in this foundation, which leaves those with very fair skin at a bit of a loss, but Porcelain may work for some.

✓ ☺ **$$$ SPF 15 Tinted Moisturizer** *($40)* has an in-part titanium dioxide–based sunscreen, and the silicone-based formula has a light but noticeably moist feel on the skin. The colors are exceptional, making this an outstanding tinted moisturizer for normal to dry skin. As expected, coverage is sheer and even.

☺ **$$$ Foundation Stick** *($40)* was the debut foundation from Bobbi Brown, and it's interesting (and worthwhile) to note that the shade range has improved considerably over the years. Initially, the small lineup was very yellow, though it was clear Brown was heading in the right direction—there wasn't a pink or rose-toned shade to be found. Today's assembly of 17 mostly neutral shades runs the gamut from fair to very dark, with just a few missteps along the way. Warm Natural and Honey are slightly peach, but may work for some skin tones, while Chestnut has enough red so it may be problematic for some dark skin tones. Golden is still too yellow, and not recommended. Espresso is a brilliant shade for very dark African-American skin tones, while Alabaster should please those who feel no foundation is light enough for their skin. Texture-wise, this remains creamy, is surprisingly easy to blend, and provides medium coverage that can be sheered if desired. I disagree with the company's "for all skin types except very oily" claim, because this is not the type of foundation someone with blemishes should use, nor does it have a matte quality to please someone with an oily T-zone. It is best for normal to dry skin.

☺ **$$$ Luminous Moisturizing Foundation** *($45)* has an elegant, fluid texture with just enough slip to make blending over normal to dry skin a pleasure. This does indeed have a luminous, satin-like finish, casting a healthy glow (rather than obvious shine) on skin. Coverage goes from light to medium and, as usual, almost all of the shades are flawlessly neutral. I wouldn't label this foundation "super-moisturizing" as the company does, but it will hydrate. Just don't expect it to firm or lift the skin, as the showcase ingredient with that alleged benefit (acetyl hexapeptide-3) is barely present and doesn't work in that manner anyway. The only thing keeping this from earning a Paula's Pick rating is the inclusion of lavender extract, which lends a noticeable lavender fragrance to this otherwise top-notch foundation.

☺ **$$$ Skin Foundation SPF 15** *($45)* is a very good option for fans of tinted moisturizer looking for a bit more coverage and who still want the convenience of an all-in-one product. Skin Foundation SPF 15 provides sheer to medium coverage and broad-spectrum sun protection, though at 1% titanium dioxide the UVA protection is not as impressive as many others with a higher concentration. The creamy texture blends easily, drying down to a satin finish that leaves the skin with a natural-looking yet polished finish. As is the case with most Bobbi Brown foundations, the shades tend to be golden in tone, and while there are some very good options for light to dark skin tones, there are also some shades to avoid. Warm Almond, Almond, Warm Walnut, Walnut, and Chestnut are all likely too orange for anyone. This foundation will work for all skin types.

☺ **$$$ Smooth Skin Foundation** *($40)* has a creamy-smooth, slightly thick texture with a nice amount of slip, so application is easy, though this takes longer to set than similar foundations. It leaves skin with a dewy finish and provides medium coverage. A major selling point of this foundation is that it can supposedly control oily areas while moisturizing dry areas. As I have written several times in the past, it is not possible for the same ingredient to keep oil at bay in one place while intuitively sensing where skin is dry and releasing moisturizing agents only over those areas. Moisturizing and oil-absorbing ingredients can (and often do) coexist in the same product, but once everything is uniformly mixed together, the moisturizing agents and oil absorbers cancel each other out, since neither is able to exert its full benefit on skin. Don't believe the disparate claims, but do consider this foundation if you have normal to dry skin. The shades are mostly gorgeous, but they're not all aces. Avoid Golden (too yellow) and Almond (slightly red; Warm Almond is much better). Walnut is slightly red, but may be an option for some darker skin tones.

☺ **$$$ Moisture Rich Foundation SPF 15** *($42)* has a wonderfully soft, fluid-but-creamy texture that blends beautifully and dries to a natural, soft glow finish. Coverage is in the light to medium range and the shades are almost impeccable—the only ones to watch out for are Golden, which is quite yellow, and Walnut and Almond, both being slightly red. Warm Natural is borderline peach and has a brightness to it that's not exactly skin-true, but it may work for some Asian skin tones. African-American skin tones are well served here, as are those with skin in the very fair range. Lamentably, the sunscreen is without sufficient UVA-protecting ingredients, which means this must be paired with another product that provides that critical protection. How shortsighted—because this is otherwise a formidable foundation for someone with normal to dry skin.

☺ **$$$ Oil-Free Even Finish Foundation SPF 15** *($42)* does not contain the UVA-protecting ingredients of titanium dioxide, zinc oxide, avobenzone, Tinosorb, or Mexoryl SX. That's a shame (and a near-insult at this price level) because this liquid foundation has a smooth, fluid texture that blends beautifully and sets to a soft, natural matte finish. Coverage runs from light to medium, and the formula is best for those with normal to slightly oily skin. Sixteen shades are available, including options for darker skin tones, and almost all of them are praiseworthy. The only ones to consider avoiding are Golden (the lone shade that suffers from being too yellow) and the slightly peach but still passable Almond.

CONCEALER: ☺ **$$$ Creamy Concealer Kit** *($32)* is a two-part product, with a creamy, thick, crease-prone concealer nestled on top of a small jar of loose powder. I suppose this will seem handy for some, but it adds little to the appeal of this product. The pros for the concealer are excellent coverage, reasonably smooth application, and reliable colors—only Beige and Almond are too pink and peach to pass muster. The lightest shade, Porcelain, is a great color for very fair skin, but it is coupled with a Pure White powder that can look ghostly. The rest of the ten shades come paired with Brown's Pale Yellow powder, which isn't as yellow as it used to be, but it's not a one-shade-fits-all deal either. The Creamy Concealer is also available alone, though it offers one less shade than the Creamy Concealer Kit. Powder is absolutely needed with this concealer; without it, expect to see creasing into lines and fading by the end of the day.

☺ **$$$ Face Touch Up Stick** *($22)*. There really isn't anything new, better, or different enough about this stick concealer to justify the price. The creamy texture and medium coverage make Face Touch Up Stick easy to use, blend, and layer, but those are attributes that several less expensive concealers also have. If you're still keen to try this, shop carefully because the following shades are very orange or copper: Warm Almond, Almond, Warm Walnut, Walnut, and Chestnut.

☹ **Corrector** *($22)* has the same texture, application, and level of coverage as Brown's Creamy Concealer, but this version is meant for those with very dark circles. The shades are almost all strongly peach or pink, but the logic from Brown is that such hues cancel the purple tinge dark circles have. They do cancel it, but the effect is not nearly as flattering or neutral as it is from a neutral- to yellow-toned concealer. If anything, using a noticeably pink or peach-toned concealer over purple skin discolorations just replaces one discoloration with another. Regardless of what you need to conceal, no one's skin is this pink or peach. If you're intent on trying this product, the least problematic shades are Deep Bisque and Very Deep Bisque.

POWDER: ✓ ☺ **$$$ Sheer Finish Loose Powder** *($34)* is a talc-based powder that has a light, silky texture and smooth, slightly dry finish thanks to the cornstarch it contains. It feels weightless and looks very natural, yet makes skin look polished. Among the seven shades, avoid

White (which really is pure white) and Golden Orange. Sunny Beige is slightly peach, but may work for some medium skin tones.

✓ ☺ **$$$ Sheer Finish Pressed Powder** *($32)* is also talc-based and shares the silky, light-weight texture and beautiful finish of the Sheer Finish Loose Powder. The same shade cautions apply here too, but there are good choices for fair to dark skin.

☺ **$$$ Face Powder** *($34)*. Bobbi Brown's loose Face Powder is a standard, talc-based powder that has an airy, silky texture and a dry finish. It's not quite as silky as the Sheer Finish Loose Powder, but you get more product for your money (1 ounce versus 0.25 ounce). The colors have been improved, and are not as yellow and orange as they once were, though Golden Orange is still one to check in natural light and carefully consider to make sure it doesn't look too bright.

☺ **$$$ Pressed Powder** *($32)* is virtually identical to the loose Face Powder, with the same colors and same caution about the Golden Orange shade, and, in this case, avoid Sunny Beige, which is too orange.

BLUSH AND BRONZER: ✓ ☺ **$$$ All Over Bronzing Gel SPF 15** *($28)* is a brilliant, easy-to-blend option for bronzing skin, and contains an in-part avobenzone sunscreen for additional sun protection wherever it is applied. More a lotion than a gel, this single shade is a gorgeous, sheer golden tan color without overtones of copper, orange, or peach. The shade works best on fair to medium skin tones, and offers a soft, moist finish without any shine (an all-too-common trait of bronzing products). If you're looking for this type of product, All Over Bronzing Gel SPF 15 should be on your short list of contenders.

✓ ☺ **$$$ Pot Rouge for Lips and Cheeks** *($22)* is an above-average sheer cream blush for dry to very dry skin. Pot Rouge looks greasier than it is. You may be surprised how easily it applies because there's no heavy feel and it's free of excess slip. Its semi-moist finish makes it great for dry skin, but not the best for solo use on the lips or if you have an uneven skin texture or breakouts. If you opt to use this as timesaving lip-and-cheek makeup, you may want to follow up with a lip gloss, particularly if your lips are routinely dry or chapped. This is recommended over Stila's similar, but slightly too greasy, Convertible Color.

☺ **$$$ Blush** *($22)*. The pressed-powder Blush features gorgeous colors that apply and blend evenly with a smooth matte finish (a few shades have a negligible amount of shine). This blush has a good color payoff on the skin, so if you want a sheer look, apply sparingly.

☺ **$$$ Bronzing Powder** *($33)* shows Brown knows what she's doing when it comes to creating believable tan shades for fair to medium skin tones. All of the shades are attractive and convincing, each possessing a smooth application and soft finish with a tiny amount of visible shine. Those with fair skin should apply this sparingly and build as needed—a little goes a long way.

☺ **$$$ Shimmer Blush** *($22)*. If you're looking for a beautiful shiny powder blush, this is a very good one. The color selection is small but what's available is good, especially if you prefer vibrant pastel tones. As for the shine, it's a blend of low-glow shimmer with crystalline sparkles, which tend to flake slightly. The silky, suede-like texture is wonderful and what you should expect from a powder blush at this price point. L'Oreal, Revlon, and Maybelline offer blushes with shine that cost less, but except for the L'Oreal True Match Blush, Brown's has a stronger color payoff.

☹ **$$$ Illuminating Bronzing Powder** *($33)* has a smooth, dry texture that applies softly, but the colors are a mixed bag and the shiny finish tends to look uneven. Shades Maui and

Antigua are not bronze tones but they do work as blush. Fans of Brown's makeup should stick with her original bronzing powder and, if you desire shine, add that separately.

EYESHADOW: ✓☺ **$$$ Long-Wear Cream Shadow** *($22)* takes a cue from Brown's successful Long Wear Gel Eyeliner and merges that technology into a silky, cream-to-powder eyeshadow collection. Application is surprisingly easy, but you better be fast because the formula sets quickly. It also doesn't have as much initial movement as powder eyeshadows, which can make blending difficult to nearly impossible. In terms of long wear, this passes with flying colors and absolutely refuses to crease—though you may notice slight fading at the end of the day. All but two of the shades have shimmer, but the shine level is mostly subtle to moderate. Bone and Suede are completely matte, with the former being a great all-over shade and the latter good for softly defining the crease. All told, this is a very good option if you're looking for a departure from powder eyeshadows, or something novel to use with a powder eyeshadow. And because the two formulas go together easily, you can apply powder eyeshadow over or under Long-Wear Cream Shadow, if you are careful not to rub too hard.

☺ **$$$ Eye Shadows** *($20)* have a silky, smooth-blending texture and most of the colors are beautifully matte (those that aren't true matte have a very soft, nonintrusive shine). There are some great choices for darker skin tones, and many of these shades would work well for lining the eyes or defining the eyebrows. The lighter shades apply sheerer than the medium to deep shades, which isn't necessarily advantageous but can make blending colors a bit easier.

☺ **$$$ Metallic Eye Shadow** *($20)* has a smooth, almost creamy texture that is a pleasure to apply. Considering the amount of metallic shine, the effect is still flattering and it doesn't overwhelm the face, though it must be said that Brown's Shimmer Wash shadows do mesh better with skin. The shine is a mix of finely milled shimmer with large particles of shine; the larger particles exhibit average cling, so expect some flaking unless you apply this sheer. Brown offers many attractive shades, and the pigmentation in each is strong. You can also use these wet for an intensified effect or for eyelining.

☺ **$$$ Shimmer Wash Eye Shadow** *($20)* is how Brown chose to separate her matte eyeshadows from the obviously shiny powder ones. These have the same smooth texture and even application, except every shade has a non-flaky shimmer finish. There are shine-enhancing options for all skin tones.

☺ **Cream Shadow Stick** *($20)* is a creamy eyeshadow in a roll-up stick form. There is only one color left (Vanilla, a soft nude) but it goes on choppy and can be difficult to blend out evenly. Plus, the texture of this starts smooth yet remains sticky once it has set! I'm a bit surprised this hasn't improved.

EYE AND BROW SHAPER: ✓☺ **$$$ Long-Wear Gel Eyeliner** *($21)* is a cream-gel eyeliner that is applied with a brush. It goes on like a liquid liner, and quickly sets to a long-wearing, budge-proof finish. It's truly an extraordinary product for lining the eyes, especially for anyone who finds powders or pencils fade or smear by the end of the day (or sooner). Brown's selection of shades often sees high-shine options rotated in seasonally, but the core assortment of blacks, charcoal brown, and steely grays is perfect.

✓☺ **$$$ Natural Brow Shaper** *($19)* is essentially a lightweight mascara for brows. You can groom and shade your eyebrows with natural-looking color and a soft, natural-looking finish. This is truly best for the brows only; it applies well and dries quickly, yet the bristles on the brush aren't long enough to reach down to the roots of any gray hair you may wish to conceal. The colors aren't the best for very dark brown or black hair, but there is a nice range for lighter hair shades, while the Auburn shade is a neutral tan that is best for someone with light brown or dark blonde brows. A Clear version is also available. One caution: overapplying this can cause flaking, so use it sparingly until you adjust to how much is needed to achieve the desired effect.

LIPSTICK, LIP GLOSS, AND LIPLINER: ☺ **$$$ Creamy Lip Color** *($22)* feels more greasy than creamy, but some women may indeed prefer this super-emollient lipstick with a glossy finish. The texture isn't slick or overtly slippery, but the oils will definitely cause color to migrate into lines around the mouth. This is not as pigmented as Brown's regular Lip Color, and as such doesn't last as long. Still, there are some gorgeous colors to consider, and if the price doesn't bother you and lines around the mouth aren't an issue, you may want to give this a test run.

☺ **$$$ Lip Color** *($22)* is a traditional cream lipstick with nice opaque coverage and great colors, including less conventional but still attractive options. Regardless of depth, the shades have minimal stain, so don't expect long wear.

☹ **$$$ Metallic Lip Color** *($22)*. Many of Bobbi Brown's lipsticks suffer from being too greasy, and this is another one to add to the list. Some women don't mind this because the emollient feel is great, but there are lots of creamy lipsticks that feel moist and smooth without being greasy and slick. Given that, plus the price and the tendency of these metallic-finish colors not to stay on for very long, it's a tough sell. Note that Brown's latest tester units don't separate the various lipsticks by type, so you either need a sharp eye to spot the metallic-finish shades or you need to ask a salesperson for assistance.

☹ **$$$ Lip Gloss** *($20)* is an extremely overpriced, standard thick, sticky gloss with a poor brush that tends to splay after a few uses.

☹ **$$$ Lip Liner** *($20)* is a standard creamy lip pencil that features a smooth application and beautiful shade range, but the pencil has limited longevity compared to many others, including those that need sharpening, as this does.

☹ **$$$ Crystal Lip Gloss** *($17)* is a very thick, sticky and syrupy gloss that comes in a squeeze tube. This will provide a high shine to the lips, but the thick feel is less than pleasant.

☹ **$$$ Brightening Lip Gloss** *($20)* has a thick, syrupy texture that ends up being quite sticky and also tenacious. The brightening part comes from the noticeable shimmer in each shade of this sheer gloss. The brush applicator is a nice touch, but with repeated use it can splay (when is Brown going to change this inelegant feature?), which makes for a messy application if you're not careful.

☹ **$$$ Shimmer Lip Gloss** *($20)* is an extremely overpriced, standard thick, sticky gloss with a poor brush that tends to splay after a few uses; the Shimmer version just adds sparkle.

☺ **$$$ Tinted Lip Balm** *($18)* comes in a glossy black ChapStick-style component and imparts translucent, moisturizing color to lips. This petrolatum-based balm doesn't feel overly thick or greasy and leaves a soft sheen. Although pricey, the colors are versatile and wear is comfortable. You may find this is worth the splurge, although it works best worn alone rather than applied over lipstick.

MASCARA: ✓ ☺ **$$$ No Smudge Mascara** *($22)* really doesn't smudge but its performance goes beyond that. You'll enjoy how quickly this mascara lengthens lashes without clumping, and it provides more thickness than most waterproof mascaras. It stays on all day whether you're swimming or getting caught in the rain, and doesn't make lashes feel dry or brittle. Removing it requires more than a water-soluble cleanser, but that's par for the course. This is one to try if you prefer shopping for mascara at the department store.

☺ **$$$ Everything Mascara** *($22)* is a great all-purpose mascara, but it doesn't excel in any particular area. Moderate length and thickness are both present in equal proportion, so if you're looking to build amazingly long or dramatically thick lashes, this mascara won't bring you "everything." However, it does nicely separate lashes, doesn't clump or smear, and leaves lashes feeling soft rather than stiff or brittle.

☺ **$$$ Lash Glamour Lengthening Mascara** *($22)* is only glamorous if your definition of the word as it pertains to mascara is "minimal length and no thickness after much effort." This mascara is best for a natural look, and it applies cleanly without flaking.

☹ **$$$ Perfectly Defined Mascara** *($22)* is supposed to make the most of every lash yet it goes on too wet and has a tendency to flake throughout the day. On the plus side, the rubber-bristle brush makes lashes considerably long and much thicker. However, when you know you can achieve that from mascaras that cost less, are easier to apply, and don't flake, why pay more for annoyances?

FACE AND BODY SHIMMER/ILLUMINATING PRODUCTS: ☺ **$$$ Shimmer Brick Compact** *($38)* provides five individual shades of powder (which resemble stacked bricks, hence the name), and all of them are viable options for adding a soft shine to the skin. The powder applies well, despite the fact that it feels drier than most, but the shine tends to migrate and dissipate after a few hours of wear. If the colors appeal to you, go for it—just don't expect the shimmer effect to go the distance.

BRUSHES: ☺ **$$$ Bobbi Brown Brushes** *($22-$60)*. Brown's Brushes are quite nice, with well-tapered edges and dense bristles, though the prices are on the high side. Many of the brushes are available in either a travel (4-inch) or professional (6-inch) length. There are some to carefully consider, and some to ignore altogether. The best, most useful brushes are the Ultra Fine Eyeliner Brush, Eye Shadow Brush, Eye Contour Brush, the fabulous Eye Smudge Brush, Foundation Brush, Concealer Brush, Touch Up Brush, and Retractable Lip Brush.

☺ **$$$ Brush Case** *($30-$35)* is available in sizes to fit Brown's short or professional-length brushes, but the cases themselves aren't anything special, especially for the money.

SPECIALTY PRODUCTS: ☺ **$$$ 3-Pan Palette** *($10)* doesn't involve slicing pieces of your makeup up for travel. Instead, this clever, well-designed palette holds three powder-based products in their original containers. It's quick and easy to slip products in and out, and is worth considering if you use several shades of Bobbi Brown eyeshadow or powder blush. The palette includes a built-in mirror but does not have extra room to stow brushes.

☺ **$$$ 6-Pan Palette** *($10)* doesn't involve slicing pieces of your makeup up for travel. Instead, this clever, well-designed palette holds six powder-based products in their original containers. It's quick and easy to slip products in and out, and is worth considering if you use several shades of Bobbi Brown eyeshadow or powder blush. The palette includes a built-in mirror but does not have extra room to stow brushes.

☺ **$$$ Blotting Papers** *($20 for 100 sheets)* are powder-free, tissue paper–style blotting papers that work well to absorb excess oil before you touch up with powder. The only issue is cost; you definitely don't have to spend this much to get an identical product. However, the cost includes an attractive, sturdy case. If you wish to spend less, Brown sells refill packs for these papers for $5.

☺ **$$$ Conditioning Brush Cleanser** *($16.50 for 3.4 ounces)* is nothing more than stan-dard shampoo that will nicely clean your brushes, but it can easily be replaced with much less expensive options from L'Oreal, Johnson & Johnson, or Neutrogena. The formula contains peppermint, which is a strange addition, and not an ingredient you'd want to remain on your brushes, especially those used near the eyes.

☺ **$$$ Face Palette** *($15)* has six compartments in a portable compact. It comes empty, and you fill it with chunks of cream-based products, such as lipsticks or Brown's Foundation Stick (a spatula is included to smush things down). This isn't the best way to travel with makeup, but if you're up for slicing and dicing your full-size cosmetics for on-the-go use, check this out.

THE BODY SHOP

THE BODY SHOP AT-A-GLANCE

Strengths: One of the few cosmetic companies that lists complete product ingredients on its Web site; affordable; the Aloe Products for Sensitive Skin are appropriate for that skin condition; good selection of eye makeup removers; one of the best pressed-powder foundations around; great pressed powder; liquid eyeliner; lip gloss; nice selection of affordable makeup brushes and specialty products.

Weaknesses: The Tea Tree Oil and Kinetin collections; subcategories that focus on one beneficial ingredient (grape seed, vitamin C, etc.) to the exclusion of others, making for several collections of one-note products; no effective routine to address blemishes; poor skin-lightening products; surprisingly lackluster to poor foundations and concealers; poor long-wearing lip product.

For more information about The Body Shop, owned by L'Oreal, call (800) 263-9746 or visit www.thebodyshop.com or www.Beautypedia.com.

THE BODY SHOP SKIN CARE

THE BODY SHOP ALOE PRODUCTS

✓ ☺ **Aloe Calming Facial Cleanser, for Sensitive Skin** *($14 for 6.75 ounces)* is a good, gentle cleansing lotion for normal to dry or sensitive skin. It is fragrance-free and does not contain detergent cleansing agents. The oil content may require the use of a washcloth for complete removal.

✓ ☺ **Aloe Gentle Facial Wash, for Sensitive Skin** *($16 for 4.2 ounces)* is a very good, fragrance-free, gentle water-soluble cleanser for its intended skin type. In fact, this is great for all but very oily skin and rinses cleanly while removing makeup easily.

☺ **Aloe Calming Toner, for Sensitive Skin** *($12 for 6.75 ounces)* doesn't contain any skin irritants, including fragrance, but it's also a really boring concoction of just water, aloe, slip agents, and glycerin. It doesn't provide much benefit to skin other than slight moisture and helping to remove last traces of makeup.

☺ **Aloe Gentle Exfoliator, for Sensitive Skin** *($14.50 for 2.5 ounces)* exfoliates skin with a small amount of mildly abrasive diatomaceous earth derived from tiny sea creatures. This ingredient is cushioned in a slightly creamy base of water, aloe, slip agents, and thickeners. It is a workable option for dry skin and is fragrance-free.

☺ **Aloe Eye Defense** *($17 for 0.5 ounce)* is a good, though relatively unexciting, lightweight moisturizer for slightly dry skin anywhere on the face. Aloe has anti-inflammatory properties, but a product intended to soothe signs of sensitivity should contain more than just aloe as its anti-irritant backbone. This contains a tiny amount of soothing allantoin and some respectable water-binding agents, so it's certainly not a waste-of-time product. For the money, it's not bad if you need a touch of moisture over mild dry spots, including around the eyes. This contains fragrance in the form of p-anisic acid.

☺ **Aloe Protective Serum, for Sensitive Skin** *($20 for 1 ounce)* has some intriguing ingredients for sensitive skin that is slightly dry, though many of them are present in amounts too small for skin to notice. Still, this aloe-based, gel-like serum is fragrance-free and provides antioxidant benefit via its soybean oil content. Although not a true state-of-the-art serum, it is a worthy choice for those with sensitive skin.

☺ **Aloe Soothing Day Cream, for Sensitive Skin** *($16 for 1.7 ounces)* isn't the most soothing moisturizer around, and the tiny amount of oat flour in this fragrance-free moisturizer will barely register on skin. It's just a basic moisturizer for normal to slightly dry skin.

☺ **Aloe Soothing Moisture Lotion SPF 15, for Sensitive Skin** *($18 for 1.7 ounces)* is worth considering as a fragrance-free daytime moisturizer for normal to slightly dry skin. It includes an in-part avobenzone sunscreen and lightweight moisturizing ingredients plus a tiny amount of anti-irritants.

☺ **Aloe Soothing Night Cream, for Sensitive Skin** *($20 for 1.7 ounces)* is a more emollient version of the Aloe Soothing Day Cream, for Sensitive Skin, and contains an additional soothing agent, though not in an amount great enough for irritated skin to notice.

☺ **Vitamin E Everyday Summer Face Lotion** *($20 for 1.7 ounces)* is a mediocre lightweight moisturizer for normal to slightly dry or dry skin. It contains a small amount of the self-tanning ingredient dihydroxyacetone, so can provide a hint of sun-kissed color. That's the only interesting element of this otherwise lackluster formula; the vitamin E isn't present in an amount great enough to warrant it being part of the product name.

☺ **Aloe Protective Restoring Mask, for Sensitive Skin** *($18.50 for 3.3 ounces).* Other than containing one substantial emollient and a small amount of nonfragrant plant oil, this is a boring mask for those with normal to dry or sensitive skin. Aloe isn't a protective ingredient, at least not when it comes to shielding skin from further irritation or helping to improve its barrier function (though that's not to say it doesn't have benefit for skin). A greater concentration of soothing agents and non-jar packaging would have made this mask a much better product.

☺ **Aloe Lip Treatment** *($9.50 for 0.5 ounce)* is a good lip balm packaged in a tube for convenient, take-along use. The simple blend of castor oil and coconut oil does a great job of preventing chapped lips, and The Body Shop was wise to not include any extraneous irritants like mint or menthol as so many other companies do. As for the aloe, its presence is so meager your lips won't notice—but that's OK, because everything that precedes it on the list is helpful.

THE BODY SHOP GRAPESEED PRODUCTS

☺ **Grapeseed Facial Wash, for Normal/Dry Skin** *($12 for 3.4 ounces)* is a slightly water-soluble cleanser due to its plant oil content. Although this is a fine option for normal to dry skin not prone to blemishes, you will need to use a washcloth for complete removal.

☺ **Grapeseed Hydrating Toner, for Normal/Dry Skin** *($12 for 6.75 ounces)* contains more alcohol and fragrance than its namesake grape seed oil and extract, but there's not enough alcohol to make this toner an irritating experience for skin. It's a standard formula that provides an extra cleansing step and softening benefit, but that's about it.

☺ **Grapeseed Daily Hydrating Moisture Cream, for Normal/Dry Skin** *($15 for 1.7 ounces)* contains appreciable amounts of antioxidant grape seed and sesame seed oils, but the jar packaging hinders their effectiveness. This is otherwise a standard moisturizer whose few other bells and whistles are present in token amounts.

☺ **Grapeseed Extra Rich Night Cream, for Normal/Dry Skin** *($17 for 1.7 ounces)* is a more emollient version of the Grapeseed Daily Hydrating Moisture Cream, for Normal/Dry Skin, and although it's preferred for dry skin, the same basic comments apply.

THE BODY SHOP KINETIN PRODUCTS

☹ **24 Hour Treatment Lotion with Kinetin** *($28 for 1 ounce)* contains kinetin and the antioxidant vitamin E, but also has a lot of spearmint and orange oils, both of which are irritating to skin and would offset any potential benefit from kinetin.

☹ **Daily Eye Treatment with Kinetin** *($22 for 0.4 ounce)* isn't that much of a treatment. It's a relatively standard moisturizer that contains a significant amount of Paullinia cupana extract. Also known as guarana, this ingredient's caffeine content has constricting effects on skin and can be an irritant. If you were hoping to get your money's worth from the kinetin in this product, you're out of luck because it is barely present.

☹ **Facial Day Treatment SPF 15 with Kinetin** *($26 for 2 ounces)* covers the UVA spectrum with its in-part titanium dioxide sunscreen and contains a lot of kinetin (though exactly how much is needed in topical products has not been established), but it irritates skin with an appreciable concentration of spearmint and orange oils.

☹ **Illuminating Face Treatment with Kinetin** *($28 for 1.4 ounces)* is a boring, jar-packaged moisturizer that spells trouble for skin in the form of irritating spearmint and orange oils.

THE BODY SHOP MOISTURE WHITE PRODUCTS

☺ **$$$ Moisture White Cleansing Powder** *($24 for 1.67 ounces)* is a nonaqueous, talc-based foaming cleanser that has no whitening effect on skin whatsoever. It's basically a novel way to cleanse skin, and talc has a very mild exfoliating effect. For the money, this doesn't compare favorably to most water-soluble cleansers.

☹ **Moisture White Toning Essence** *($24 for 5 ounces)* lists alcohol as the second ingredient, making this toner too drying and irritating for all skin types.

☺ **Moisture White Brightening Serum** *($38 for 1.5 ounces)* contains mostly water, glycerin, emollients, silicone, slip agents, vitamin C, plant oils, thickeners, preservatives, and fragrance. It's a good lightweight moisturizer for normal to slightly dry skin types curious to try a vitamin C product.

☹ **Moisture White Moisture Cream Plus** *($30 for 1.3 ounces)* is a below-standard moisturizer that contains irritating clove leaf oil and is not recommended. The tiny amounts of vitamin C and licorice extract have no ability to lighten skin.

☹ **Moisture White Night Treatment Cream** *($38 for 1.3 ounces)*. The form of vitamin C in this product is magnesium ascorbyl phosphate, which research has shown to be an effective skin-lightening agent in concentrations of 3% and above (Source: *Skin Research and Technology*, May 2002, pages 73-77). Although this product appears to meet that percentage, the jar packaging won't keep the vitamin C stable once it's exposed to air and light and it contains the fragrant components of linalool, geraniol, limonene, and eugenol, all of which are problematic for skin.

THE BODY SHOP SEAWEED PRODUCTS

☹ **Seaweed Deep Cleansing Facial Wash, for Combination/Oily Skin** *($12 for 3.3 ounces)* has merit as a water-soluble cleanser for its intended skin type but doesn't make it across the finish line because it contains irritating menthol.

☺ **Seaweed Purifying Facial Cleanser, for Combination/Oily Skin** *($14 for 6.76 ounces)* is a good cleansing lotion that omits detergent cleansing agents in favor of silicone and emollients. It is best for normal to slightly dry skin and rinses surprisingly well without the aid of a washcloth. This cleanser isn't more purifying than any other, so ignore that claim.

☹ **Seaweed Clarifying Toner, for Combination/Oily Skin** *($12 for 6.76 ounces)* contains menthol and that additive is made more irritating by the presence of fragrant components such as linalool and citronellol.

☺ **Seaweed Pore-Cleansing Facial Exfoliator, for Combination/Oily Skin** *($14.50 for 2.5 ounces)* is a cleanser and topical scrub in one that uses olive seed powder as the abrasive agent. The jojoba oil is inappropriate for oily areas, but this is an acceptable scrub for normal to slightly dry skin.

☹ **Seaweed Clarifying Night Treatment, for Combination/Oily Skin** *($20 for 1 ounce)* is a boring moisturizer. Despite enticing claims, this product is primarily water, thickener, and preservative. Lots of ingredients follow these basics, but none of them are intriguing for skin and leave it shortchanged yet highly fragranced.

☺ **Seaweed Mattifying Day Cream, for Combination/Oily Skin** *($16 for 1.7 ounces)* offers skin slightly more than the Seaweed Clarifying Night Treatment, for Combination/Oily Skin, but that's not saying much. This is an average water- and silicone-based moisturizer for its intended skin type.

☺ **Seaweed Mattifying Moisture Lotion SPF 15, for Combination/Oily Skin** *($18 for 1.69 ounces)* provides an in-part avobenzone sunscreen in a lightweight lotion base suitable for its intended skin type. What's missing are several essential elements necessary to create a great moisturizer, making this an effective, though average, sunscreen.

☺ **Seaweed Pore Perfector, for Combination/Oily Skin** *($20 for 0.5 ounce)* is a far-from-perfect-for-pores product that contains mostly water, silicone, and alcohol. It's doubtful the alcohol will have a detrimental effect on skin given that the amount is likely less than 5%, but its prominence is definitely a red flag. Plus, this contains lots of fragrance ingredients that have no positive effect on blemishes, and that may cause irritation.

THE BODY SHOP TEA TREE OIL PRODUCTS

☹ **Tea Tree Cleansing Wipes** *($12 for 25 wipes)* are below-standard wipes that have minimal cleansing ability and don't remove excess oil and makeup as well as most water-soluble cleansers. They're pricey for what you get too: these work out to be $0.48 per wipe and you'll be replacing them in less than a month! The amount of tea tree oil is too low to function as a disinfectant, while this contains fragrant oils and fragrance chemicals that cause irritation and are definitely not for use around the eyes.

☹ **Tea Tree Skin Clearing Facial Wash** *($11 for 8.4 ounces)* has the makings of a very good water-soluble option for normal to oily skin, but things get problematic due to the inclusion of menthol and Calophyllum inophyllum seed oil, which is derived from a species of evergreen tree. Research has shown this ingredient is cytotoxic (kills cells) and although it may have antibacterial properties for acne, there are better ingredients to use for this purpose (Sources:

Journal of Photochemistry and Photobiology, September 2009, pages 216-222; and *Phytochemistry*, October 2004, pages 2,789-2,795). The tea tree oil adds a medicinal scent, but the amount in this cleanser isn't great enough to combat acne-causing bacteria, not to mention it's rinsed from skin before it can be of much benefit.

☹ **Tea Tree Skin Clearing Foaming Cleanser** *($13 for 5 ounces)* is a liquid-to-foam cleanser that contains a hefty amount of tea tree oil but also includes menthol, making it too irritating for any skin type. The seed oil from the Calophyllum inophyllum plant is also a problem for skin due to its irritating chemical constituents.

☹ **Tea Tree Skin Clearing Toner** *($11 for 8.4 ounces)* lists alcohol as the second ingredient and also contains a host of other problematic ingredients that won't improve matters for blemish-prone skin. Alcohol in this amount causes dryness, free-radical damage, and irritation that can stimulate more oil production in the pore lining. Actually, this formula is bound to confuse blemish-prone skin because the cornstarch can feed the bacteria that causes acne while the anti-irritants won't be of much help due to the irritating ingredients that dull their impact.

☹ **Tea Tree Blackhead Exfoliating Wash** *($13 for 3.3 ounces)* is a slightly creamy scrub that essentially claims you can scrub blackheads away, which absolutely isn't true. A facial scrub can help remove the top portion of the blackhead, but since you're not doing anything about the underlying cause, the blackhead is back before you know it. Moreover, because this uses apricot seed powder as one of the abrasive agents, it can be rougher on skin than a well-formulated scrub should be. The amount of tea tree oil is too low to have an antibacterial effect against acne, and blackheads have nothing to do with bacteria. This contains the seed oil from the Calophyllum inophyllum plant is also a problem for skin due to its irritating chemical constituents.

☹ **Tea Tree Skin Clearing Lotion** *($13 for 1.69 ounces)* has a silicone-enriched, silky texture but the amount of tea tree oil in this lightweight moisturizer is too low to function as a topical disinfectant for acne. Moreover, this contains some problematic fragrance chemicals and fragrant oils, including Calophyllum inophyllum seed oil, which is derived from a species of evergreen tree. Research has shown this ingredient is cytotoxic (kills cells) and although it may have antibacterial properties for acne, there are better ingredients to use for this purpose (Sources: *Journal of Photochemistry and Photobiology*, September 2009, pages 216-222; and *Phytochemistry*, October 2004, pages 2,789-2,795). Examples are benzoyl peroxide and triclosan.

☹ **Tea Tree Blemish Fade Night Lotion** *($18 for 1 ounce)* contains barely any tea tree oil, instead this lightweight moisturizer relies on laurelwood oil (listed as Calophyllum inophyllum and also known as tamanu oil) for its alleged anti-blemish properties. I wrote "alleged" because there is insufficient evidence available to gauge the effectiveness of this oil for blemishes and it is an irritant (Source: www.naturaldatabase.com). It might work to some extent against blemishes due to its potential antibacterial action and fatty acid composition, but wouldn't you rather spend your money experimenting with proven anti-acne ingredients?

☹ **Tea Tree Oil** *($9 for 0.33 ounce)* lists alcohol as the second ingredient and, despite the name, doesn't appear to contain the requisite amount of tea tree oil to have an anti-blemish effect.

☹ **Tea Tree Blemish Gel Stick** *($9 for 0.08 ounce)* is a poorly formulated product that lists alcohol as the second ingredient and also contains a host of other problematic ingredients, none of which will improve matters for blemish-prone skin. Alcohol in this amount causes dryness, free-radical damage, and irritation that can stimulate more oil production in the pore lining.

☹ **Tea Tree Concealer** *($9 for 0.14 ounce)* has an emollient texture that is a problem for use over blemishes. The ingredients that keep this concealer in stick form can easily clog pores, while the amount of tea tree oil is too low to function as a disinfectant. The two shades are workable, but this has limited appeal.

☹ **Tea Tree Face Mask** *($15 for 3.85 ounces)* has a tiny bit of tea tree oil, so the name isn't nonsense, but is otherwise a standard clay mask that's a good option for normal to oily skin. Some of the thickening agents in this mask may be problematic for use on blemished skin. Of greater concern is the inclusion of Calophyllum inophyllum seed oil, which is derived from a species of evergreen tree. Research has shown this ingredient is cytotoxic (kills cells) and although it may have antibacterial properties for acne, there are better ingredients to use for this purpose (Sources: *Journal of Photochemistry and Photobiology*, September 2009, pages 216-222; and *Phytochemistry*, October 2004, pages 2,789-2,795).

THE BODY SHOP VITAMIN C PRODUCTS

☺ **Vitamin C Energizing Face Spritz** *($18 for 3.3 ounces)* omits the grapefruit oil but leaves the fragrant orange oil, and its vitamin C content is paltry. This average toner is more akin to spraying perfume on the face than anything really helpful.

☹ **Vitamin C Re-Texturizing Peel** *($24 for 1.7 ounces)* lists alcohol and polyvinyl alcohol as main ingredients, making this peel-off peel too drying and irritating for all skin types. This also contains several citrus oils that only add to the irritation from the alcohol.

☹ **Vitamin C Cleansing Face Polish** *($16 for 3.3 ounces)* contains grapefruit and orange oils, making this substandard scrub too irritating for all skin types.

☹ **Vitamin C Micro Refiner** *($25 for 2.5 ounces)* contains grapefruit and orange oils, making this substandard scrub too irritating for all skin types.

☺ **Vitamin C Eye Reviver** *($22 for 0.5 ounce)* isn't much for vitamin C but is still a decent water- and silicone-based moisturizer for slightly dry skin anywhere on the face. The orange flower water just provides fragrance and can be a problem for use around the eyes, though there's only a tiny amount present.

☺ **Vitamin C Intensive Night Treatment** *($24 for 1 ounce)* contains a significant amount of vitamin C (ascorbic acid) in a nonaqueous base with a silky finish. Vitamin E is on hand as well, and the only detriment is the inclusion of orange oil. A more robust ingredient listing would have made the name "intensive" really mean something.

☹ **Vitamin C Moisturizer SPF 15** *($20 for 1.7 ounces)* has the right stuff when it comes to broad-spectrum sun protection, but also contains grapefruit oil. The chemical constituents of grapefruit oil are known to cause contact dermatitis and phototoxic reactions when skin is exposed to sun. Although this product provides sun protection, why risk a reaction when so many effective sunscreens are available without problematic extras?

☺ **Vitamin C Plus Time Release Capsules** *($28 for 28 capsules)* isn't pure vitamin C as claimed because there are several ingredients in these silicone-filled capsules, including fragrant orange oil and fragrance components, that aren't the best for skin. This is an intriguing way to supply skin with stable doses of vitamin C (ascorbic acid) but overall it's not as elegant as Elizabeth Arden's Ceramide Time Complex Capsules, which, while without vitamin C, supply skin with a greater array of beneficial ingredients than this product, and without adding potential irritants.

☹ **Vitamin C Skin Boost** *($26 for 1 ounce)* contains grapefruit and orange oils, neither of which provides a positive boost for skin. This serum is not recommended.

☹ **Vitamin C Lip Care SPF 15** *($8 for 0.15 ounce)* lacks the UVA-protecting ingredients of titanium dioxide, zinc oxide, avobenzone, Tinosorb, or Mexoryl SX, and is not recommended.

THE BODY SHOP VITAMIN E PRODUCTS

☺ **Vitamin E Cream Cleanser** *($14 for 6.7 ounces)* is a very standard, cold cream-style cleanser that can work well for someone with normal to dry skin. It does contain fragrance and fragrance components that are potentially irritating, though less so in a rinse-off product like this. The amount of vitamin E is insignificant.

☹ **Vitamin E Gentle Cleansing Wipes** *($14 for 25 wipes)* are water- and castor oil-based cleansing wipes that, while effective for removing makeup, contain fragrant irritants of linalool, eugenol, and limonene, among others. With the abundance of cleansing wipes available, most for less money, there is no reason to use these and subject skin to irritation.

☹ **Vitamin E Soap** *($8 for 4.5 ounce bar)* is standard bar soap, and no amount of vitamin E will make it less drying for any skin type.

☺ **Vitamin E Face Mist** *($16 for 3.2 ounces)* is a very basic toner with a minor amount of vitamin E, almost to the point of making the name embarrassing. It's an OK option for normal to dry skin, and contains fragrance in the form of rose water.

☺ **Vitamin E Cream Exfoliator** *($20 for 2.5 ounces)* contains some problematic fragrant components (eugenol among them) that downgrade an otherwise excellent topical scrub for dry to very dry skin. This is still worth considering since it is rinsed from skin so quickly.

☺ **Vitamin E Eye Cream** *($17 for 0.5 ounce)* is a basic but decent moisturizer for slightly dry skin around the eyes or elsewhere on the face. Vitamin E makes more than a cameo appearance in this product, and in this amount is much more likely to be effective as an antioxidant. This eye cream is fragrance-free.

☺ **Vitamin E Facial Day Lotion SPF 15** *($14.50 for 2.5 ounces)* has an in-part titanium dioxide sunscreen in a rather boring base formula that's mostly aloe and thickeners. The vitamin E content is minuscule and no other antioxidants are included.

☹ **Vitamin E Facial Oil** *($22 for 0.5 ounce)* could've been a superb option for very dry skin if only several fragrant oils hadn't been included. The *Bosweliia carterii* (olibanum), *Pelargonium Graveolens* (rose geranium), vetiver, and lavender oils are a distinct problem for all skin types, as are fragrance chemicals of linolool, limonene, and citronellol. You'd be better off skipping this fragrant problem and treating very dry skin to pure olive or evening primrose oils instead.

☺ **Vitamin E Illuminating Moisture Cream** *($18.50 for 1.7 ounces)* is an average moisturizer for normal to dry skin that's mostly water, thickener, water-binding agent, shea butter, pH adjuster, and wax. The jar packaging won't help keep the meager amount of vitamin E stable.

☺ **Vitamin E Moisture Cream** *($16 for 1.8 ounces)* is nearly identical to the Vitamin E Illuminating Moisture Cream, and the same review applies. The fact that this product is a Body Shop best-seller means a lot of people aren't giving their skin everything it needs to look and feel its healthy best.

☺ **Vitamin E Moisture Serum** *($20 for 1 ounce)* shortchanges skin on vitamin E and other antioxidants, and ends up being a basic, lightweight, water- and silicone-based serum that's an acceptable, though hardly exciting, option for normal to dry skin. There is nothing about this serum that is not easily replaced by myriad alternatives.

☺ **Vitamin E Nourishing Night Cream** *($18 for 1.7 ounces)* covers some of the basics in terms of what makes a great moisturizer, but some isn't enough, and the jar packaging won't keep the tiny amount of vitamin E in here stable once the product is opened.

☺ **Vitamin E Sink-In Moisture Mask** *($18.50 for 3.38 ounces)* is worth considering by those with dry to very dry skin due to its effective blend of glycerin, silicone, plant oils, and skin-identical ingredients. It's a shame the jar packaging doesn't help keep the vitamin E stable, but without question this will make dry skin look and feel better, and it does not need to be rinsed from skin.

☹ **Vitamin E Lip Care Stick SPF 15** *($8 for 0.15 ounce)* does not contain the UVA-protecting ingredients of titanium dioxide, zinc oxide, avobenzone, Tinosorb, or Mexoryl SX, and is not recommended.

THE BODY SHOP WISE WOMAN PRODUCTS

☺ **Wise Woman Luxury Cleanser** *($17.50 for 6.75 ounces)* is primarily a blend of water with several nonvolatile plant oils. The detergent cleansing agents are present in minor amounts, though the oils certainly work to remove makeup. This is a good option for dry to very dry skin not prone to blemishes; you may need a washcloth for complete removal.

☹ **Wise Woman Softening Toner** *($17.50 for 5.4 ounces)* has some fancy-sounding ingredients and some of them are beneficial for dry skin, but not in the tiny amounts used in this overall boring toner. It contains mostly water, slip agents, witch hazel, castor oil, and preservative.

☹ $$$ **Wise Woman Eye Cream** *($24 for 0.5 ounce)* is an aloe-based moisturizer that contains more witch hazel than beneficial ingredients, though not enough to be irritating. This is an OK, slightly emollient formula whose most intriguing ingredients are listed after the preservative, so they don't count for much.

☹ $$$ **Wise Woman Regenerating Day Cream** *($32 for 1.7 ounces)* isn't suitable for daytime because it does not carry an SPF rating (though sunscreen agents are the second- and fifth-listed ingredients). Why The Body Shop included broad-spectrum protection without going through the testing necessary to establish an SPF rating is a mystery, and leaves this as an unwise choice for any woman. Moisturizer-wise, it doesn't break any new ground and is best suited for normal to dry skin. The antioxidants are sullied by jar packaging.

☹ **Wise Woman Regenerating Night Cream** *($36 for 1.7 ounces)* would have been a slam-dunk for dry to very dry skin were it not for jar packaging that hinders the effectiveness of the antioxidant-rich plant oils and the inclusion of irritating lavender oil.

☹ $$$ **Wise Woman Vitality Serum** *($36 for 1.7 ounces)* is built around the ingredient lactobacillus clover flower extract. Lactobacillus is a type of aerobic bacteria that produces large amounts of lactic acid as it ferments with carbohydrate sources. There is some research indicating that taking supplements of lactobacillus (it is also considered a probiotic) may help reduce skin allergies and forms of dermatitis. However, substantiated research on topical application of lactobacillus is nonexistent, though it likely functions as a water-binding agent. Clover flower has no research proving its mettle for aging skin, though it may be sensitizing. There is little reason to consider this serum compared to superior options from Olay, Neutrogena, Clinique, and Paula's Choice.

☺ **Wise Woman Intensive Firming Mask** *($20.50 for 3.4 ounces)* is a very good moisturizing mask for normal to dry skin. It is not ultra-creamy or lush, so it will leave those with very dry skin wanting more. The film-forming agent in this mask can make skin look firmer temporarily, but this is a minor cosmetic improvement; no one will think you've had anything lifted. Still, in terms of moisturizing ability and some elegant ingredients, this is worth considering.

OTHER BODY SHOP SKIN CARE PRODUCTS

☺ **Camomile Gentle Eye Make-Up Remover** *($14.50 for 8.4 ounces)* is a simple formula that removes makeup with gentle detergent cleansing agents. The amount of chamomile is likely too small to have a soothing effect, but it's a plus that this makeup remover is fragrance-free. Still, this becomes a superfluous product when you realize that it's basically a watered down cleanser. Their previous formula, which contained silicone, was better.

✓ ☺ **Camomile Waterproof Eye Make-Up Remover** *($14.50 for 3.3 ounces)* doesn't contain much chamomile, but is in fact an excellent lotion-type eye-makeup remover. It works swiftly to remove even stubborn waterproof mascara, and is fragrance-free. This is best applied before washing with a water-soluble cleanser.

☹ **Skin Focus Re-Texturizing Peel** *($20 for 1.67 ounces)* has a low enough pH to allow the salicylic acid to exfoliate (peel) skin, but the amount in this product is 0.5% or less, meaning the results are limited. More of an issue is that alcohol is the second ingredient—and there's enough bergamot oil on hand to cause irritation without any benefit for skin.

☺ **Honey & Oat 3-In-1 Scrub Mask** *($16.50 for 3.6 ounces)* uses natural ingredients such as oat bran for its scrub action, kaolin (clay) for its absorbency when used as a mask and honey for its moisture-binding ability (though this will be minimal due to the inclusion of clay), which is a big part of this scrub mask's appeal. It's a novel option for those with normal to dry skin looking for a close-to-natural scrub. Used as a mask, it may end up confusing skin because it is overall too emollient for oily skin and too absorbent for dry skin. It's not a "triple action" time-saving product, but when used gently is a serviceable scrub.

☹ **Camomile Moisturising Eye Supplement** *($17.50 for 0.5 ounce)* doesn't contain enough of chamomile in this water- and silicone-based serum to even make a bland cup of tea, never mind that chamomile isn't an ingredient for reducing puffy eyes. The witch hazel water has constricting effects, and stands a better chance of slightly reducing puffy eyes, but that's at the expense of irritating already-inflamed skin. This product will have no effect on puffiness related to aging (when the fat pads beneath the eye begin slipping from their support system). Considering the price and questionable benefit, this product is not recommended.

☹ **Blue Corn 3 in 1 Deep Cleansing Scrub Mask, for Normal/Oily Skin** *($16.50 for 4.2 ounces)* has been around for years and, although it has some positives (the convenience of an absorbent mask that has a slightly abrasive quality so you can exfoliate as you rinse), it's more harmful than helpful for skin because of the volatile fragrant oils it contains.

☹ **Lavender Chamomile Facial Blotting Tissues** *($10 for 65 sheets)* are blotting tissues steeped in plant oils, which is odd because who needs oil on oil blotting papers? Odd becomes irksome when you see that one of the oils is lavender, and that's a problem for skin.

☺ **Natural Powder Facial Blotting Tissues** *($10 for 65 sheets)* work to mattify skin by depositing a sheer layer of talc, clay, and absorbent minerals each time you blot. The finish may need some slight blending to avoid a too-powdered look, but these certainly work to tame shine.

☺ **Powder-Free Facial Blotting Tissues** *($10 for 65 sheets)* are standard, powder-free blotting papers that are a quick, convenient way to absorb excess oil before touching up your makeup.

☺ **$$$ Seaweed Ionic Clay Mask** *($22 for 4.2 ounces)* does indeed contain several types of seaweed, but seaweed cannot detoxify skin. The ionic properties attributed to the clay content are bizarre because clay is merely an absorbent, whether ions are involved or not. This mask is an OK yet needlessly pricey option to use on oily skin or oily areas. The amount of alcohol (it's the fifth ingredient) is not likely to be problematic, but along with the fragrance and artificial coloring agents this formula is just disappointing.

☹ **Warming Mineral Face Mask** *($16.50 for 5.1 ounces)* contains a mineral that warms when it is mixed with water, but that has no special benefit for skin beyond feeling pleasant. That's fine, but what's not is the inclusion of irritating ginger oil and cinnamon bark oils, joined by several fragrance components, including problematic eugenol.

☺ **Born Lippy Balms** *($8 for 0.3 ounce)* are standard castor oil- and lanolin-based lip balms that are available in a variety of fruit flavors. Never mind the fact that fruit-flavored balms encourage lip-licking and create the need to reapply the product frequently, more important is that not all of the flavors are recommended. The ones to avoid due to irritating fragrance components are Mango Peach and Strawberry. Exotic Passionfruit, Raspberry, and Watermelon do not contain these problematic ingredients and are recommended.

✓☺ **Cocoa Butter Lip Care Stick** *($8 for 0.15 ounce)* is an excellent lip balm that contains a thoughtful blend of nut oils, wax, olive oil, and, as the name states, cocoa butter. An added bonus is several anti-irritants, which makes this lip balm a step above most others.

✓☺ **Hemp Lip Protector** *($8 for 0.15 ounce)* has a different assortment of beneficial ingredient for dry lips than the Cocoa Butter Lip Care Stick, but is just as effective and equally recommended.

☹ **Lip Butter** *($8 for 0.3 ounce)* has a buttery-smooth texture and can ably take care of dry, chapped lips. However, it is available in several flavors and all but one of them contain irritating fragrance components. The flavor to consider is Coconut. None of the others are recommended.

☹ **Lip Scuff** *($12 for 0.14 ounce)* has been reformulated again and although the abrasive particles are gentler on lips, this oil-based, lipstick-style exfoliant contains spearmint and peppermint oils along with the irritating menthol derivative menthyl lactate. What a shame; this could have been one of the best lip exfoliants available. As is, chapping will be diminished but lips will be irritated, which, surprise, leads to more chapping.

☹ **Stop Violence in the Home Lip Care Stick** *($8 for 0.15 ounce)* should be renamed "Stop the Irritation," because that's what your lips are subjected to once this peppermint oil-infused stick balm is applied. The proceeds from this product support a good cause, but there are ways to be charitable without irritating your lips.

THE BODY SHOP MAKEUP

FOUNDATION: ✓☺ **All in One Face Base** *($20)* has been reformulated and is better than ever! This talc-based, pressed-powder foundation has an amazingly silky application that provides a natural matte finish and light coverage. Few powders look this natural on skin, and it does a great job of minimizing pores and controlling excess oil. The one caution is that the third ingredient is cornstarch, which can contribute to breakouts by "feeding" the bacteria that trigger them. However, your skin may not react in that manner, so don't let that stop you from trying this. The six shades are best for fair to medium skin tones and all of them are soft and neutral. All in One Face Base is best for normal to slightly dry or slightly oily skin.

✓☺ **Flawless Skin Protecting Foundation SPF 25** *($25)* is a cream-to-powder foundation that has a more powdery finish than other foundation options in this category. Those with normal to oily skin will find this foundation's formula works quite well, providing medium coverage and a natural-looking matte finish. Add to that the sun protection provided by the in-part titanium dioxide sunscreen and this foundation is a home run. The shade range favors those with light to medium-dark skin tones, but all of the options are good.

☺ **$$$ Nature's Minerals Foundation SPF 25** *($25)* boasts formidable broad spectrum sunscreen protection from titanium dioxide, which makes this loose powder a very good option amid the crowded selection of mineral makeup. The drawback is that the coverage is quite sheer with a hint of shimmer (thanks to the mica), and doesn't build to anything more than that without becoming cakey and dry. As such, this product would work best as added SPF protection over foundation with sunscreen, or even dusted atop a good, SPF-rated tinted moisturizer. The six shade options are hit-and-miss, and though the nearly-translucent Shade 1 produces nothing more than a veil-like glow to skin, Shades 2-4 prove to be workable hues for medium skin tones. Avoid the ashy Shade 5, and light-to-medium skin tones could consider super-warm Shade 6 as a bronzing option with the added bonus of an SPF! Thanks to the inclusion of kaolin, this powder foundation will work well for normal to oily skin. It is not recommended for dry skin due to the absorbent nature of the ingredients.

☺ **$$$ Moisture Foundation SPF 15** *($23)* certainly delivers on its promise of moisture and, therefore, is definitely too emollient for skin that's even slightly oily. The silky consistency is that of any good rich moisturizer and it won't run or dribble out of its airtight pump. Once applied, that emollience produces a lovely dewy finish, but then, unfortunately, it turns greasy and settles into lines within minutes. As if that weren't issue enough, the limited shade range provides suitable options only for lighter skin tones, because Shade 5 goes on too peach and Shade 6 wears too orange (incidentally, the darker Shades 7 and 8 aren't even available in most stores, but can be found online). There's no question that this foundation will deliver moisture and UVA protection in the form of zinc oxide, but with such light coverage and that unpleasantly greasy finish, it's doubtful this will do more to flatter and even your complexion than any good tinted moisturizer with an SPF 15+ would.

☺ **Oil-Free Foundation SPF 15** *($23)* gets its sunscreen partly from titanium dioxide. Although that's great news for this matte finish foundation, the high amount (and likely the grade) of titanium dioxide used lends a slightly chalky finish that is difficult to soften. If you want an oil-free, medium to full coverage foundation and are amenable to this one's finish (the chalkiness is coupled with a soft shimmer) it may be worth a look. The predominantly yellow-based shades are quite good and include options for fair to dark skin tones. Shades 05 and 06 may be too gold for medium skin tones but are still worth testing.

☺ **Ultra Smooth Foundation** *($18.50)* is aptly named because this is indeed one smooth foundation! The initially thick texture blends well, leaving a powdery matte finish. Unfortunately, the finish, while feeling matte, remains slick on the skin. That means someone with oily skin or oily areas will find this foundation easily slips, fades, and may make large pores more apparent. What a shame, because the shade selection has some very good choices for those with fair and dark skin. This is a potential option for someone with normal to dry skin, but those skin types may not like the matte feel.

CONCEALER: ☹ **Concealer Pencil** *($11)* is a thick, creamy concealer packaged as a thick pencil that needs regular sharpening. This covers well and blends better than expected, but the greasepaint-like texture creases easily and the shades aren't anything to get excited about. Considering the number of amazing concealers available in all price ranges, this isn't worth an audition.

☹ **Flawless Skin Protecting Concealer** *($16.50)* is a creamy stick concealer that provides sheer coverage, which limits its appeal, as does the fact that the formula is prone to creasing into lines. Anyone who wants to cover dark circles or red spots or who has wrinkling around the eyes will find this concealer a huge disappointment. It sets into wrinkles immediately and accentuates them rather than camouflaging them. The inclusion of African baobab oil is marketing hype and provides no benefit. When I came across the testers at the store this concealer was listed on the display as having an SPF of 25; however, neither the labeling nor the Web site listed sunscreen actives, and The Body Shop's customer service personnel could not give me a list of sunscreen actives, adamantly stating that it did not contain any sunscreen. Therefore, this product cannot be counted on to provide any sun protection.

☺ **Ultra Smooth Liquid Concealer** *($12)* has an accurate name because this silicone-enhanced liquid concealer dispensed from a tube is very smooth. Its ultralight texture blends to a silky finish that, unfortunately, never sets completely. That leads to slippage into lines under the eyes and less than ideal coverage that fades before it should. It comes in three excellent neutral shades, but this is only one to consider if you need minor coverage and are willing to tolerate some creasing.

POWDER: ✓ ☺ **Pressed Face Powder** *($18.50)* has an admirably silky, talc-based texture that is minimally dry. In fact, the oils in this pressed powder and the smooth, non-powdery finish it provides make it a good choice for those with normal to dry skin. The four shades are remarkably neutral and meant for light to medium skin tones only.

☺ **Loose Face Powder** *($16)* has a silky, airy, talc-based texture and a drier-than-usual finish that is ideal for normal to very oily skin. Shades 01, 02, and 03 are neutral flesh tones perfect for fair to medium skin, while shade 05 is a sheer bronze color with gold shimmer, which tends to flake. Apparently The Body Shop hasn't had a loose powder for years, and customer demand made them reconsider—and what they produced is well worth an audition!

BLUSH AND BRONZER: ☺ **Bronzing Powder** *($18.50)* possesses a wonderfully smooth texture that applies evenly—a critical point for bronzing powder. Even better, both of the shades allow you to create a convincing tan effect. The 01 shade is matte and best for fair to light skin, while shade 02 is for light to medium skin and has a subtle amount of shine.

☺ **Cheek Blush** *($14.50)* is an odd product. It begins slick and so is tricky to blend, and then stays that way, so it always has some movement. Here's the odd part: The sheer, shimmer-laced colors have a stain effect on skin, so the color itself stays where you blend it. This product is best for normal to dry skin types that don't mind shimmering cheeks.

☺ **Pearly Lip & Cheek Stain** *($14)* is a dual-purpose product that produces lovely, natural color beneath a slightly moist, pearly finish that can be applied to either lips or cheeks and is available in only one shade: a gold-flecked pink. As a lip color, it's nothing extraordinary (in fact, even the salesperson couldn't distinguish it from a similarly colored Liquid Lip Color product), but it's workable as a cheek stain. Surprisingly, the sole color option proves flattering on most skin tones and sets nicely without any greasiness beyond its intended "pearl" luminescence.

☺ **Sheer Sun Gel** *($14.50)* is a very standard but good bronzing gel that feels light and dries fast, so blending must be quick. The translucent color is convincing and relatively long-lasting. It is best for medium skin tones looking for a touch of sun without the damage actual tanning causes.

☺ **Cheek Color** ($15.50) is a large-size traditional powder blush, reminiscent of the size and packaging of M.A.C.'s powder blushes. This has a soft texture and a dry but smooth application that imparts very sheer, see-through color. All of the shades shine, but Golden Pink and Hazelnut are ultra-shiny and are not recommended for daytime. The shine among the remaining understated shades is, well, understated!

☺ **$$$ Nature's Minerals Bronzing Powder** *($21)* comes packaged in a plastic screw-top container like many mineral powder products, only this one includes a fine mesh screen to help sift and contain the loose powder to avoid waste not to mention mess. This packaging strategy is smart, but it backfires when chunks of powder accumulate and become trapped above the screen—so either way, there's wasted product and mess! And that's a shame, because the powder itself has a smooth texture that applies easily to create an even bronze effect. The minerals at work here are illite and mica, and like nearly all products involving mica, there's a good amount of sparkle to contend with, especially in Warm Sandstone, the lighter of the two shades.

EYESHADOW: ☺ **Cream Eye Color** *($12)* is a find if you want a sheer, shimmer-infused eyeshadow that has a soft, lightweight, cream-to-powder texture and a silky, creaseless finish that stays put (so does the shine). The shade selection favors warm nudes and steely silver-to-blue cool tones, but if you find an appealing hue and want to experiment beyond powder eyeshadows, why not?

☺ **Eye Colors** *($12)*. The collection of over 20 Eye Colors feels silky and blends beautifully, but here's the frustration: All of the shades, even the dark ones, go on extremely sheer. Talk about subtle color! And these do not build that well, so you're pretty much stuck with no intensity and a light wash of color that stands a good chance of fading even before you leave your house. If you're looking for very soft color, these are worth a peek, but watch out for the glittery shades because they do not apply as smoothly and the glitter tends to flake. The non-glittery but still shiny shades don't have this trait. If you're shopping for matte options, you'll need to look elsewhere.

☺ **Eye Shimmer** *($12)* doesn't apply as smoothly as the Eye Colors, but it's not worth downgrading to an unhappy face rating. The small selection of shades is all about shine, and they serve their purpose with minimal flaking despite slightly uneven application.

☹ **Eye Lustre Pearls** *($16.50)* are small pots filled with two shades of shimmery powder beads. Meant to be applied separately or blended together (the little jars have no divider), these beads provide lots of shimmer, but very little pigment. The color flakes very easily and ends up all around (and in) the eye, which only accentuates any wrinkles in that area. Add to those drawbacks the fact that each of the three color options is either too blue, green, or pink to look good on almost anyone and you have a truly "why bother?" or "what were they thinking?" product.

EYE AND BROW SHAPER: ✓ ☺ **Liquid Eyeliner** *($13.50)* has an excellent soft, but firm, brush that is adept at drawing a thin, continuous line and a fast-drying formula that minimizes the risk of smearing, plus its wearability has improved since it was last reviewed, making it deserving of a Paula's Pick rating.

☺ **$$$ Brow & Liner Kit** *($18)* combines a brow powder and powder eyeshadow to use as liner in one petite compact. The circular component houses a cleverly designed dual-sided brush, but regrettably the brow brush is too stiff (and deposits too much product if your brows are thin) and the eyeliner brush is too floppy for precise control. Still, both powders go on smoothly and are pigment-rich. Each also has a touch of shine, but it's barely noticeable on skin. The three duos include options for all brow colors except shades of red or auburn.

☺ **Brow & Lash Gel** *($14)* is a standard clear gel that works to groom brows and barely enhance lashes. It will feel sticky unless applied lightly, but it doesn't take much to achieve a groomed look.

☺ **Eye Definer** *($11)* is a routine pencil in terms of the inevitable sharpening, but it does glide on and is minimally creamy, which means there's a low risk of smudging or fading. Avoid shade 07, which is blue.

☹ **Brow Definer** *($10)* has a smooth, not-too-stiff texture but applies unevenly, depositing even color followed by dots and specks of color, plus the tip breaks off quickly. Under the assumption that I was experimenting with old testers, I used this pencil at other Body Shop stores, all with the same result. That's reason enough to avoid it.

LIPSTICK, LIP GLOSS AND LIPLINER: ✓ ☺ **Lip Line Fixer** *($11)* marks the return of a former Body Shop favorite, though the name has been changed. Lip Line Fixer was No Wander in its first incarnation, and this remains a very good automatic, retractable lip pencil whose colorless formula puts an invisible border around the mouth that stops lipstick from feathering into lines. It worked brilliantly as No Wander, and works just as well today. Keep in mind that as effective as this pencil is, it won't completely stop greasy, overly slick lipsticks or lip glosses from traveling into lines around the mouth.

☺ **Colourglide Lip Color** *($12.50)* is an emollient, creamy lipstick whose colors have a good stain but you really need to layer them to get much impact. They're best for someone who wants light to moderate coverage and a slightly glossy finish. The oil-based formula will quickly move into lines around the mouth so if that describes your predicament move on to other lipsticks. Otherwise, the shade range is extensive with a pleasing array of cream and shimmer finishes.

☺ **Hi-Shine Lip Treatment** *($13)* is billed as a treatment because it contains marula oil, but this plant oil isn't a special or essential ingredient for lip care, it's just another emollient plant oil. This is otherwise a standard viscous gloss and offers a wet-looking, high-shine finish with a slightly sticky feel. All of the colors are very sheer.

☺ **Lip Color** *($14)* feels smooth, goes on light, and is truly a very nice opaque, mildly creamy lipstick. There are some striking nude and attractive bright colors available, although the overall shade selection isn't huge.

☺ **Liquid Lip Color** *($14)* feels smooth yet slippery and offers a glossy, minimally sticky finish. The shades go on softly but builds well if more intensity is desired; think of it as a lip gloss with a bit more pigment than the norm.

☺ **Sheer Lip Shine** *($14.50)* is moderately sheer, imparting less color than traditional lipstick but more than many lip glosses (and similarly-textured sheer lipsticks). It offers an emollient feel and glossy finish without excess slickness, and the shades are mostly inviting.

☺ **Shimmer Hi-Shine Lip Treatment** *($13)* is identical in every respect to the original version, except that a couple of shades have a shimmer finish that may be more to your liking.

☹ **Lip Care** *($14)*. Lip Care is a very ordinary, but nevertheless emollient, lipstick-type lip balm that has a particularly glossy finish. It will soothe dry skin quite nicely.

☹ **Lip Gloss Dots** *($10)* has a strange name for what amounts to a standard, thick lip gloss packaged in a pot. The color intensity is deceptively sheer, even for the deepest shades, and it is sticky enough to be bothersome (assuming sticky lip gloss bothers you).

☹ **Lip Liner** *($10)* is a standard, but quite workable, lip pencil that features some versatile colors. If this did not need to be sharpened it would earn my Paula's Pick rating for its texture and application, but convenience is important too when it comes to makeup application.

☹ **Lip & Cheek Stain** *($14)* is an exceptionally sheer, gel-based stain that comes in one pink-berry color. This stays sticky on the skin, and is not preferred to similar versions from Origins or Benefit.

☹ **Stay On Lip Color** *($14.50)* doesn't measure up to the estimable Max Factor Lipfinity or M.A.C.'s Pro Longwear Lipcolour. The dual-sided packaging includes a lip color applied with the wand applicator and a clear gloss at the other end to add shine (and comfort). The shades have been whittled down to two, and each goes on opaque and takes too long to dry. Once the lip color has set, you will immediately feel your lips become dry and tight, which is where the clear top coat comes in. It provides the requisite glossy finish, but it can't overcome the dry, slightly grainy feel of the lip color underneath. After a short time (less than an hour in my case, but your experience may vary) the glossy effect and the smooth feel were gone, and the lip color began to flake and peel off—and I hadn't even tried to eat with this on yet! I rarely refer to a makeup product as "abysmal," but the word is applicable here.

MASCARA: ☺ **Super Volume Mascara** *($14)* is a reworking of The Body Shop's former Volumizing Mascara, and although it is a distinct improvement this mascara's performance doesn't fall into the "super" category. It builds average length and thickness in equal measures, and has a slightly uneven application that requires a bit more patience—but the results may be worth it if you want a reliable mascara that doesn't take lashes too far.

☺ **Waterproof Mascara** *($14)* was redone as well, and it lengthens lashes and provides a hint of thickness without clumps, leaving lashes with a soft curl. It is waterproof.

☺ **Define and Lengthen Mascara** *($14)* is the same as it was when I last reviewed it: a boring mascara that builds minimal length and definition even after considerable effort. It's OK for a natural look, but that's about it.

☺ **Double Intensity Mascara** *($18)* is The Body Shop's contribution to the double-ended primer and mascara category. The promise of these products is that by first applying a primer you will be rewarded with lashes that are thicker and fuller than you would get by applying mascara alone. In this case, you'll get some length, but not much volume and no discernible thickness. The primer applies smoothly with minimal clumping, as does the mascara. The product wears well with no flaking or smudging, but the effect is ho-hum, so why bother with two steps? For volume and drama, you're better off opting for a more impressive mascara (there are many to be found at the drugstore and cosmetic counters) and applying enough coats to build the beautiful lashes you desire.

FACE AND BODY ILLUMINATING/SHIMMER PRODUCTS: ☺ **Glow Enhancer** *($14)* is a liquid shimmer that casts an ethereal pink glow that is apparent but still understated. It is easy to apply and control, and dries to a matte (in feel) finish.

☺ **Shimmer Sun Gel** *($14.50)* has a different formula than the Sheer Sun Gel. It has more slip so blending doesn't have to be as quick, and instead of getting a bronze color you get a sheer medium gold that leaves a very shiny finish. The best news is the shine lasts, though it can rub off a bit on clothing.

☺ **Shimmer Waves** *($22)* presents "waves" of shiny pressed powder colors in one compact. Although the powder has a dry, grainy feel, it goes on smoothly and clings better than expected. The finish is best described as moderate shimmer, and is an option for evening glamour.

☺ **Tinted Glow Enhancer** *($14)* has the same basic characteristics as the Glow Enhancer, but comes in four sheer, flesh-toned tints. Each imparts a very soft glow to skin that would actually be acceptable even in daylight. However, this works best applied over or mixed with a foundation to delicately highlight skin.

☺ **$$$ Brilliance Powder** *($22)* packages loose shimmer powder in a cylindrical component with an attached brush. A push button shoots powder onto the brush, ready for application. Although the powder adds lots of shine to skin and clings well, the brush is somewhat stiff and uncomfortable to use.

☺ **$$$ Brush-On Beads** *($21)* has been part of The Body Shop makeup line for years, but I don't understand why these shiny powder beads have maintained such an indispensable status in this line. In any event, this is still the same as it ever was, and it works well for a sparkling peachy brown effect, or use Brush-on Buff as a soft highlighting powder. The beads allow for very sheer color application, but if they break you're left with an uneven application with chunks of powder.

☺ **Lightening Touch** *($14)* has been around for years and is available in two sheer shades. It's an OK highlighting option with a soft shimmer finish, but doesn't illuminate the skin in the same beguiling way as superior options from Giorgio Armani and Lorac.

☹ **$$$ Matte & Shimmer Cheek Color** *($17.50)*. Here's a riddle: What do you get when you combine matte powder with shimmery powder? Give up? The answer is… Slightly less shimmery powder! Why someone thought this was a good idea is a mystery because the single palette of two shades in one compact has two sides that are shiny and two that are matte, but there is no brush that would enable you to choose one over the other, so both get swirled on together. The two color options are Pink & Gold (which appears quite orange) and Bronze & Gold (which, ironically, is more pink than golden bronze). Both have a grainy texture that immediately settles into lines and flakes easily. If you're dead-set on a shimmer powder, L'Oreal offers a suitable shimmer bronzing powder that's worth checking out instead of this one.

☹ **Radiant Highlighter** *($14)* should be named "Sparkling Highlighter" because its glimmering finish isn't subtle nor is this a great way to highlight skin. If you're looking to add an ethereal, whitish sparkling shine to skin this is a product to consider; however, it doesn't make wrinkles less apparent as claimed. Radiant Highlighter is fragrance-free.

☹ **Body & Leg Shine** *($18.50)* is a problematic addition to The Body Shop's ever-expanding bronzing line. The deodorant-like stick meant to glide easily over skin, and it does indeed glide, but the result looks more like greasy glitter than true bronzer, causing the skin to appear almost dirty rather than tanned (and given the product's inherent stickiness, dirt and lint will no doubt stick to you in no time). Both shades have this problem, appearing dingy once applied, and the lighter tone deposits far more coppery glitter than actual tint. The deeper shade, though less glittery, had the added issue of the grease-like waxy product grabbing to even the fine hairs on the upper arm, so it also makes body hair appear cakey and dark. No thanks!

☹ **Shimmer Cubes** *($22)* are described as "four cute blocks of earthy, shimmery color" but end up being anything but cute. The blocks are not fastened to the main component, which is a poor choice given how easily these could break if dropped. In addition, each shade is grainy and the shine tends to flake.

☹ **Shimmer Cubes Sparkle** *($22)* is nearly identical to the Shimmer Cubes except the shine comes from multicolored, prismatic pigment. Otherwise, the same negatives apply.

BRUSHES: ☺ **The Body Shop Brushes** *($10.50-$26)* are each composed of synthetic hair and most of them are supremely soft and beautifully shaped. The best of the bunch (notable for their ability to hold and accurately deposit color) include: **Eyeliner Brush** *($10.50)*, **Face & Body Brush** *($26)*, **Foundation Brush** *($23)*, **Slanted Brush** *($18)*, **Retractable Blusher Brush** *($22)*, and **Blusher Brush** *($24)*. The less appealing or unnecessary brushes include the rubber-tipped **Line Softener** *($10.50)*, **Brow & Lash Comb** *($10.50)*, **Lipstick/Concealer Brush** *($14.50)*, and **Eyeshadow Blender Brush** *($18)*, which is nicely shaped but doesn't have enough give to apply color evenly. The **Mini Brush Kit** *($18.50)* is a small, portable brush set that includes a built-in mirror and a brush to apply powder, blush, eyeshadow, and lipstick.

It's not the best to tote for applying a full makeup, but is ideal to keep in your purse or office for quick touch-ups. ☺ **Brush Roll** *($17)*. This is a nylon brush satchel that will hold 10-12 standard-size makeup brushes. The Velcro® closure and thin nylon material don't lend much weight to this product, nor do they give the impression of being long-lasting, nor is the material easy to clean. Also of note, the inside lining is marked repeatedly in neon green with the phrase "made with passion." Whether true or not, some are likely to find it distracting every time they open the roll to access the brushes.

SPECIALTY PRODUCTS: ☺ **Skin Primer Matte It** *($14)* is a fragrance-free, silicone-based primer with a slightly viscous texture that melts into skin, leaving a silky, imperceptible soft matte finish. It is an option for normal to oily skin and aids with foundation application. Despite my enthusiasm, there are lightweight moisturizers and serums whose ingredient roster bests this and supplies skin with a wide range of ingredients it needs to look its best. Those with sensitive, oily skin may want to check this out, though.

☺ **Nature's Minerals Blotting Tissues** *($10 for 65 sheets)* use a blend of titanium dioxide and clay to absorb excess oil and leave a slight powder finish. Beyond the titanium dioxide, a token amount of minerals are included but they offer no special benefit to skin. It's curious that mica is included in these tissues, because this mineral pigment is typically used to add shine— just the opposite of what you want oil-blotting papers to do!

☺ **Matte It Face & Lips** *($14)* is a basic silicone serum that contains a tiny amount of aloe and chamomile to reinforce The Body Shop's natural persona. This has a silky finish and will allow for smooth application of foundation, but the type of silicone used is too slick to provide significant shine control.

☺ **Skin Primer Moisturize It** *($14)* is sold as a primer able to provide a moisturizing base prior to applying foundation, but it doesn't deliver. Someone with dry skin will find this is not the least bit moisturizing, though it does leave a very smooth finish. This has a very thin texture that's easy to apply, and it sets quickly to a subtle glow finish. Given the lack of intriguing ingredients in the formula, this isn't worth strong consideration over several other primers or, better yet, a serum loaded with beneficial ingredients.

BOOTS

BOOTS AT-A-GLANCE

Strengths: Inexpensive; some great cleansers, including a few without fragrance; all sunscreens provide sufficient UVA protection; a couple of good scrubs; well-formulated self-tanning lotions; a smoothing, soothing lip balm; the only mass-market makeup line with testers for almost every product; great return policy on makeup at Target, if you save your receipt; mostly impressive foundation shades; very good powders; powder blush; great sheer lipstick; the Botanics Gloss; a handful of good mascaras.

Weaknesses: Abundance of ordinary formulas; Botanics line products contain few botanical ingredients; Time Dimensions line lacks sunscreen and provides more shine than proven antiaging formulas for skin; repetitive formulas and a penchant for including the good stuff in amounts too small to be all that helpful; majority of products are surprisingly average; no AHA or BHA products; no products to help battle blemishes or lighten skin discolorations; jar packaging; foundations are more expensive than the competition, but do not best them;

No7 and Botanics makeup products have several similarities, except the Botanics include plant extracts that have no impact on performance; mostly disappointing eyeshadows; average to poor eye, brow, and lip pencils; inferior makeup brushes; superfluous or just plain unattractive specialty products.

For more information about Boots, call (866) 752-6687 or visit www.boots.com or www. Beautypedia.com.

BOOTS SKIN CARE

BOOTS BOTANICS PRODUCTS

☺ **Botanics Complexion Refining Deep Clean Mousse** *($8.99 for 5 ounces)* is a basic but good water-soluble cleanser for all skin types except very oily. The liquid-to-foam action may be your preference, but it has no advantage over non-foaming cleansers.

☺ **Botanics Moisturising Deep Clean Foam** *($6.99 for 5 ounces)* is similar to the Botanics Complexion Refining Deep Clean Mousse, but the higher concentration of glycerin makes it more moisturizing and best for normal to dry skin. The tiny amount of sodium lauryl sulfate in both of these cleansers is not cause for concern.

☹ **Botanics Quick Fix Cleansing Wipes** *($6.99 for 30 wipes)* work very well to remove makeup and leave skin refreshed, but they're not the best for on-the-go cleansing without water because one of the preservatives can be irritating if left on skin. The same goes for the fragrance components linalool and benzyl salicylate. These are recommended only if you rinse your skin after using them.

☹ **Botanics Skin Brightening Cleanser** *($6.99 for 8.4 ounces)* won't brighten skin, but it can be a good cleansing lotion for normal to very dry skin. The mineral oil doesn't rinse easily without the aid of a washcloth.

☺ **Botanics Skin Brightening Deep Clean Gel** *($6.99 for 5 ounces)* is a very good water-soluble cleanser for normal to oily skin. It removes makeup and won't leave skin feeling stripped.

☹ **Botanics Soothing Eye Make-Up Remover** *($5.99 for 5 ounces)* is a silicone-in-water dual-phase makeup remover that works well to take off all types of makeup. This is labeled as suitable for even the most sensitive skin, but the preservative 2-bromo-2-nitropropane-1,3-diol can be problematic (Source: *Handbook of Cosmetic and Personal Care Additives*, 2nd Edition, volume 1, Synapse Information Resources, 2002). Almay and Neutrogena sell the same type of makeup remover with more gentle preservatives.

☹ **Botanics Complexion Refining Toner** *($7.99 for 5 ounces)* is a water-based toner that contains two kinds of clay, which allows it to have a matte finish. Including castor oil is inappropriate, but the amount is small, making this an OK option for normal to oily skin.

☹ **Botanics Organic Face Rosewater Toner** *($7.99 for 5 ounces)*. This is little more than eau de cologne disguised as skin care. Water, alcohol, and rose oil do not add up to good skin care any more than a martini flavored with a liqueur adds up to a balanced diet or is healthy for your brain. Ironic that alcohol can pass as good for skin under the heading "organic", when the only thing that alcohol does is cause irritation, dryness, and free-radical damage!

☹ **Botanics Skin Brightening Toner** *($6.99 for 8.4 ounces)* contains enough alcohol to be irritating, and the sole plant extract, horsetail, has constricting properties that are not helpful for skin. The amount of AHAs is too low for exfoliation to occur.

☺ **Botanics In Shower Facial Polish** *($7.99 for 3.3 ounces)* is an OK scrub with cleansing ability for normal to oily skin. It loses points for the amount of ginger root it contains, along with several potentially irritating fragrance components.

☹ **Botanics Organic Face Smoothing Face Polish** *($8.99 for 3.3 ounces)*. This water- and oil-based scrub has a deceptively thick texture that thins out considerably and doesn't feel very oily on skin. Ground cranberry seeds are the abrasive agent, and their uneven size and shape means you stand a good chance of doing more harm than good to your skin because they can damage the skin barrier, which reduces the skin's ability to keep moisture in and protect from the environment. Despite the natural ingredients, this isn't preferred for those with dry skin; it'd be better to use a washcloth or scrub with synthetic polyethylene beads or just a washcloth and your daily cleanser.

☺ **Botanics Purifying Face Scrub** *($7.99 for 2.5 ounces)* is a greasy scrub that contains apricot seeds and walnut shells as the abrasive agent. These are not preferred to polyethylene beads, but the mineral oil helps protect skin from their rough edges.

☺ **Botanics Day Moisture Cream SPF 12** *($8.99 for 1.69 ounces)* improves slightly on the Botanics Complexion Refining Day Moisturising Lotion SPF 12 reviewed below, but the similarities still keep it from earning a happy face rating.

☺ **Botanics Day Moisture Lotion** *($8.99 for 2.5 ounces)* is similar to the Botanics Complexion Refining Light Night Cream below, but this version comes in better packaging. That's a plus, but still doesn't elevate this above average status.

☹ **Botanics Eye and Lip Correction Serum** *($14.99 for 0.5 ounce)* claims to make dark circles and puffiness around the eyes "a thing of the past in just 4 weeks," but you're in for a disappointing experience if you believe it. This is a simple blend of mostly water, glycerin, mineral oil, slip agent, emollient, silicones, film-forming agent, and preservative. These ingredients cannot fade dark circles or reduce puffiness any more than an accountant can perform laser eye surgery.

☺ **Botanics Complexion Refining Light Night Cream** *($13.99 for 1.69 ounces)* is an unremarkable lightweight moisturizer for normal to dry skin. The jar packaging won't keep the two antioxidants in it stable during use.

☺ **Botanics Complexion Refining Day Moisturising Lotion SPF 12** *($12.99 for 2.5 ounces)* has merit due to its in-part avobenzone sunscreen, but the SPF rating is below the benchmark set by most major medical organizations, and the base formula for normal to dry skin is, well, really basic. This does contain potentially irritating fragrance components.

☺ **Botanics Face Lift Firming Cream SPF 10** *($13.99 for 1.69 ounces)* has a better base formula than any of the Boots Botanics sunscreens; what a shame the SPF 10 with avobenzone is too low for daytime use. This is an option if you have normal to dry skin and are willing to pair this with a foundation rated SPF 15 or greater.

☺ **Botanics Face Renewal Cream SPF 15** *($13.99 for 1.69 ounces)* is nearly identical to the Botanics Face Lift Firming Cream SPF 10, except that this one has a better SPF rating and a change in antioxidants. Unfortunately, jar packaging won't keep them stable during use, though this is an option for normal to dry skin.

☺ **Botanics Intensive Nourishing Serum** *($14.99 for 1 ounce)*. Labeling this a serum is not accurate because texture- and formula-wise it is best described as a traditional moisturizer for normal to dry skin not prone to breakouts. Skin will get some antioxidant benefit from the olive oil it contains, but the amount of vitamin C is unimpressive and not enough to be part of the company's so called "brightening complex" that this is supposed to contain. This isn't a bad moisturizer for the money, but it doesn't live up to the claims on the label and is outpaced by many other well-formulated products for about the same cost.

☺ **Botanics Moisturising Eye Cream** *($13.99 for 0.84 ounce)* is a very basic moisturizer for normal to dry skin anywhere on the face. The amount of mica leaves a noticeable shine on skin. Grape seed oil is a great antioxidant, but the jar packaging won't let it maintain its potency during use.

☺ **Botanics Night Moisture Cream** *($13.99 for 1.69 ounces)* is an OK lightweight moisturizer for normal to slightly dry skin. The amount of grape seed oil is impressive, but the jar packaging won't keep its antioxidant elements stable during use.

☹ **Botanics Organic Face Hydrating Day Cream** *($12.99 for 3.3 ounces)*. This very fragrant moisturizer contains several plant oils that are excellent for dry skin. Unfortunately, the jar packaging won't keep the antioxidants stable after opening and the fragrant oils and fragrance chemicals will only irritate skin. I have no doubt that the ingredients in this product are mostly organic, but not every organic ingredient is worthwhile for your skin. Given the formula, you would be better off using a tiny bit of pure olive oil on your dry skin; after all, it's the second ingredient in this emollient cream.

☺ **Botanics Organic Face Super Balm** *($8.99 for 3.2 ounces)*. This simply formulated, emollient, and all-natural moisturizer is a good choice for treating very dry skin anywhere on the body, but it is best for stubborn dry areas like heels, cuticles, and elbows. Simple isn't bad for skin, but the jar packaging won't keep the air-sensitive oils in this product stable.

☺ **Botanics Radiance Beauty Balm** *($14.99 for 1.3 ounces)* provides a visual pick-me-up because the mica leaves a shiny finish. That can help make dull, dry skin look livelier, but the main ingredients in this balm are standard, and what's lacking makes this nothing more than an average option.

☺ **Botanics Radiance Renewal Night Serum** *($15.99 for 1 ounce)* is a very good, ultralight moisturizer for normal to oily skin. It contains bilberry extract as the main antioxidant, and it does have anti-inflammatory benefits. The citrus extracts and sugarcane do not function as AHAs, but do contribute to this serum's water-binding properties. However, the citrus is potentially irritating, and that keeps this serum from earning a Paula's Pick rating.

☺ **Botanics Responsive Moisture Lotion** *($9.99 for 2.5 ounces)* claims to be responsive in the sense that it moisturizes where needed, but also helps minimize excess oil to keep skin shine-free. Don't bet on it; moisturizing and absorbent ingredients don't separate on skin, each going to where they're needed most (how would they know where to go?). The amount of zinc oxide this contains does lend a soft matte finish, but that also keeps the emollients from being as moisturizing as they could be. One of the antioxidants has a positive effect on skin while the other has a negative effect (not every plant with antioxidant ability is great for skin), so they cancel each other out. That leaves you with an unimpressive moisturizer for normal to slightly dry or slightly oily skin not prone to blemishes.

☺ **Botanics Smoothing Facial Serum** *($11.99 for 1 ounce)* contains one "botanic," which in this case is a tiny amount of horse chestnut extract. I can think of several other botanical ingredients that would have made this silicone-based serum for all skin types more intriguing, but it does contain a dusting of antioxidant vitamins. Nothing in this serum can purify skin or make it feel clearer. Skin can look clearer, but how can it feel clearer?

☺ **Botanics Soothing & Calming Eye Base** *($8.99 for 0.27 ounce)* contains a tiny amount of soothing licorice extract, but is otherwise a bland blend of thickeners, mineral oil, aluminum starch, and several waxes. The iron oxide pigments provide a bit of sheer color and coverage, but I wouldn't choose this over a great liquid or cream concealer.

☺ **Botanics Ultimate Lift Eye Gel** *($13.99 for 0.5 ounce)* is so basic and boring that the name is embarrassing. This won't lift skin in the least; it's just water, slip agents, plant extract, film-forming agent, and preservatives. It's not even exciting that this is one of the only Boots products that is fragrance-free.

☺ **Botanics Conditioning Clay Mask** *($8.99 for 4.2 ounces)* is a very standard but good clay mask that is an option for oily to very oily skin. It is fragrance-free and the sole plant extract, burdock root, has soothing properties.

☹ **Botanics Complexion Refining Clay Mask** *($8.99 for 1.69 ounces)* is a below-standard clay mask due to the amount of irritating isopropyl alcohol. It cannot draw out "even the most deep-rooted impurities"—you won't see a marvelously clear complexion after use, and your skin may feel uncomfortably dry.

☺ **Botanics Vitamin Recovery Mask** *($6.99 for 1.69 ounces)* contains an inconsequential amount of vitamin E, and lacks significant amounts of ingredients that allow dry skin to recover (that is, restore a healthy barrier function so skin can repair itself). This is barely passable as a decent mask for normal to slightly dry skin.

✓ ☺ **Botanics Organic Face Lip Balm** *($6.99 for 0.33 ounce)* is a very good emollient (and notably greasy) lip balm that is 100% natural and includes lanolin. It is fragrance- and colorant-free, and doesn't contain any irritants, which is great. The greasy nature of this balm makes it best for use at night because it makes a mess, whether paired with lipstick or by itself, something you wouldn't want during the day.

BOOTS EXPERT PRODUCTS

✓ ☺ **Expert Anti-Blemish Cleansing Foam** *($5.29 for 5 ounces)* is a basic, but very good, water-soluble cleanser for all skin types. It is fragrance-free and works well to remove excess oil and makeup. There isn't anything about this cleanser that makes it preferred for blemish-prone skin, but it's not a cleanser those dealing with blemishes shouldn't consider, either.

✓ ☺ **Expert Sensitive Cleansing & Toning Wipes** *($4.49 for 30 wipes)* are steeped in a mild cleansing solution that's fragrance-free and ideal for those with dry, sensitive skin—including those dealing with rosacea (though the rubbing of facial cloths on skin can exacerbate rosacea symptoms, so use caution). These cloths remove most types of makeup (eye makeup is trickier, especially waterproof formulas) and are a great on-the-go solution for using while traveling or to remove makeup before exercising.

✓ ☺ **Expert Sensitive Gentle Cleansing Lotion** *($4.49 for 6.7 ounces)* is a very standard but exceptionally gentle detergent-free cleansing lotion for dry, sensitive skin. Most users will find a washcloth is necessary for complete removal. This works beautifully to take off makeup, including waterproof formulas, without drying or stripping skin. Although the formula is essentially a liquid cold cream, this deserves a Paula's Pick rating due to its value for sensitive, easily irritated skin. The price is great, too!

✓ ☺ **Expert Sensitive Gentle Cleansing Wash** *($4.49)*. This cleanser is a gentle, very basic formula that is a good option for sensitive skin whether it's oily or dry. The formula is so mild that it isn't much for makeup removal, but is fine for those who wear minimal makeup or for use as your morning cleanser. It is fragrance- and colorant-free.

☺ **Expert Sensitive Gentle Eye Makeup Removal Lotion** *($5.49 for 6.7 ounces)* is a basic, oil-based eye makeup remover anyone can use. The formula is quite greasy and requires a separate cleanser to avoid a residue, but it works fine to remove all types of eye makeup. It is fragrance-free.

☹ **Expert Sensitive Gentle Eye Makeup Removal Pads** *($5.49 for 60 pads)* are soaked in an oily base that works to remove makeup (including waterproof formulas) but not without leaving a greasy film that must be washed off. The simple formula is fragrance- and preservative-free (the lack of water means preservatives aren't essential). This is similar to using plain mineral oil on a cotton pad, except it costs a lot more.

☺ **Expert Sensitive Gentle Refreshing Toner** *($3.99 for 6.7 ounces)* is an exceptionally basic, gentle toner whose fragrance-free formula is suitable for all skin types, including sensitive skin. It would be rated higher if it contained a selection of skin-identical ingredients and at least one antioxidant of note.

☹ **Expert Anti-Blemish Toner** *($4.29 for 6.7 ounces)* isn't expert at anything except perhaps causing needless irritation and excess free-radical damage due to the amount of alcohol it contains.

✓☺ **Expert Sensitive Gentle Smoothing Scrub** *($5.49 for 3.3 ounces)* is a simply formulated but very gentle fragrance-free scrub. It is suitable for all skin types, including sensitive (assuming your sensitive skin can tolerate a gentle scrub). The sheer, gel-like formula rinses cleanly and doesn't contain extraneous ingredients skin doesn't need. Well done!

☹ **Expert Anti-Blemish Night Moisturizer** *($4.99 for 1.69 ounces)* lists alcohol as the second ingredient. That's not a helpful or "expert" ingredient for any skin type, blemishes or not. Alcohol can trigger oil production in the pore lining, too. Definitely a product to leave on the shelf!

☺ **Expert Sensitive Anti-Blemish Serum** *($7.99 for 1 ounce)*. This water-based serum contains mostly water, glycerin, the plant extract willow bark, and preservative. Willow bark is not considered an effective anti-acne ingredient, though it has anti-inflammatory properties. There is no research proving willow bark is helpful for those with oily skin either. Consider this a very basic serum whose few interesting ingredients are present in amounts too small to matter.

☺ **Expert Anti-Redness Serum** *($7.99 for 0.84 ounce)*. There are some great ingredients in this serum that all skin types can benefit from, including ceramides and anti-irritants. Unfortunately, most of them are present in paltry amounts your skin won't notice. That leaves us with moisturizer (it's definitely more of a moisturizer formula than a serum) that's an OK emollient option for normal to dry skin not prone to blemishes. It is fragrance-free.

☺ **Expert Anti-Blemish 2-in-1 Scrub and Mask** *($5.79 for 3.3 ounces)* is an OK scrub option for normal to dry skin. Polyethylene is the scrub agent, and it's buffered by the oil so there's less chance of overdoing it. The oil makes this scrub more difficult to rinse than most others. It is a poor choice for blemish-prone skin for two reasons: willow bark has minimal blemish-busting activity (and even less in a product that's rinsed from skin) and acne cannot be scrubbed away. In fact, scrubbing active acne lesions can cause further redness and risk spreading acne-causing bacteria to areas of the face that may not have breakouts.

☺ **Expert Scar Care Serum** *($7.99 for 1.6 ounces)*. This silicone-based serum doesn't contain any ingredients capable of eliminating scars. However, massaging this over scars or skin anywhere on the body will result in a silky softness that can improve skin's appearance. Any scar reduction seen from the use of this product (such as color or length of scar) is purely coincidental. In many cases, skin continues to remodel and heal after a scar forms. That means the scar will continue to improve with time, regardless of what you use. Keeping scars protected from sunlight and treating skin with a well-formulated serum or moisturizer (this Boots product doesn't quite meet that standard) will go a long way toward encouraging the most productive healing and best-looking outcome.

☺ **Expert Sensitive Hydrating Eye Cream** *($6.99 for 0.67 ounce)* is a very basic emollient eye cream for dry skin. It can be used anywhere on the face, though its fragrance-free, gentle formula is a plus for use near the sensitive eye area. Expect this to moisturize skin, but that's all. The formula doesn't contain a single state-of-the-art ingredient.

✓ ☺ **Expert Sensitive Hydrating Moisturizer** *($4.99 for 1.6 ounces)* is a gentle, fragrance-free formula that's suitable for sensitive or rosacea-affected skin (that is why it earned a Paula's Pick rating) but doesn't offer skin any beneficial extras such as antioxidants or cell-communicating ingredients. This is only recommended if you have dry, sensitive skin that does better with less. The choice of jar packaging is not a concern for this moisturizer.

✓ ☺ **Expert Sensitive Hydrating Serum** *($7.49 for 1.6 ounces)*. Although labeled a serum, this product's formula is much closer to a moisturizer. It contains some good, though standard, slip agents and emollients and is also fragrance-free. That's the best I can state, though this is an unquestionably safe option for those with dry, sensitive skin and/or rosacea (which is why it's rated a Paula's Pick). It works quite well under makeup, but be sure your foundation includes an SPF rating of 15 or greater.

✓ ☺ **Expert Sensitive Light Moisturizing Lotion** *($5.99 for 6.7 ounces)*. You can completely ignore the oily skin claims for this moisturizer. This isn't a product anyone with oily skin should be using because the oil and triglyceride it contains will contribute to making skin even oilier. This is a basic, bare-bones moisturizer for normal to dry skin that's sensitive or affected by rosacea. Its merit for sensitive skin is why it is rated a Paula's Pick. All other skin types should be using something else because this formula completely lacks beneficial extras.

✓ ☺ **Expert Sensitive Restoring Night Treatment** *($6.99 for 1.69 ounces)* is a bland, very basic fragrance-free moisturizer that is only recommended if you have dry skin that's prone to sensitivity or you're struggling with rosacea and need a basic moisturizer to help keep skin smooth. This moisturizer's value for sensitive skin is why it's rated a Paula's Pick. If sensitive skin isn't your concern, this isn't your moisturizer.

☺ **Expert Sensitive Soothing Eye Gel** *($5.49 for 0.5 ounce)*. This fragrance-free gel moisturizer is suitable for slightly dry skin anywhere on the face, but it couldn't be more basic and ho-hum. There's no reason to consider this over using plain glycerin or aloe vera gel as a moisturizer.

☹ **Expert Shine Control Instant Matte** *($5.99 for 0.5 ounce)*. This water-based mattifying fluid lists alcohol as the second ingredient. It is not recommended due to the dryness and irritation this much alcohol causes. Alcohol can degrease the skin, but it also triggers oil production in the pore lining, so the oil will be back in no time and likely worse than before.

☺ **Expert Shine Control Lotion** *($5.99 for 3.38 ounces)*. This lightweight moisturizer's oil-control claims are a joke. The second ingredient is a thickening agent that is incapable of keeping skin matte for eight minutes, let alone eight hours as claimed! At best, this is an OK fragrance-free moisturizer for slightly dry skin. The amount of alcohol is potentially cause for concern.

☺ **Expert Shine Control Papers** *($4.49 for 50 sheets)* are imbued with chalk (calcium carbonate), which has absorbent properties and will leave a fresh matte finish. You may find you don't need to follow up with powder after using these blotting papers.

BOOTS NO7 PRODUCTS

✓ ☺ **No7 Beautifully Balanced Purifying Cleanser, for Oily/Combination Skin** *($7.99 for 6.6 ounces)* is a slightly fluid, fragrance-free, water-soluble cleanser that is suitable for its intended skin type. The smaller amount of detergent cleansing agent doesn't allow for complete removal of makeup, but this is an option as a morning cleanser or for those who wear minimal makeup.

✓ ☺ **No7 Soft & Soothed Gentle Cleanser, for Normal/Dry Skin** *($7.99 for 6.6 ounces)* is a good detergent-free cleansing lotion for its intended skin types. The fragrance-free formula is very gentle, yet removes makeup easily (though you may need a washcloth to avoid leaving a residue of mineral oil).

☺ **No7 Gentle Foaming Facial Wash, for All Skin Types** *($8.99 for 5 ounces)* is similar to the Boots Botanics Moisturising Deep Clean Foam, but with fewer bells and whistles (which just end up being rinsed down the drain anyway). Otherwise, the same review applies.

☹ **No7 Quick Thinking 4 in 1 Wipes** *($6.99 for 30 wipes)* are nearly identical to the Boots Botanics Quick Fix Cleansing Wipes, and the same review applies. The tiny amount of witch hazel included is not cause for concern.

☹ **No7 Cleanse & Care Eye Make-Up Remover** *($7.99 for 3.3 ounces)* is nearly identical to the Boots Botanics Soothing Eye Make-up Remover, save for a smaller size and the addition of some plant extracts, none of which help remove makeup. Otherwise, the same review (and concern) applies.

☹ **No7 Beautifully Balanced Purifying Toner, for Oily/Combination Skin** *($7.99 for 6.6 ounces)* lists alcohol as the second ingredient, which makes this toner too drying and irritating for all skin types; plus alcohol can cause free-radical damage.

☹ **No7 Soft & Soothed Gentle Toner, for Normal/Dry Skin** *($7.99 for 6.6 ounces)* provides skin with a tiny amount of soothing agents, but is otherwise a lackluster fragrance-free formula that merely helps remove the last traces of makeup and leaves normal to dry skin soft.

☺ **No7 Radiance Revealed Exfoliator, for All Skin Types** *($9.99 for 2.5 ounces)* is a good fragrance-free scrub for dry to very dry skin. The water- and mineral oil–based formula contains a small amount of polyethylene beads for a gentle polishing, but this doesn't rinse as well as water-soluble scrubs.

☺ **No7 Total Renewal Micro-Dermabrasion Exfoliator** *($14.99 for 2.5 ounces)* has a similar base and is recommended for the same skin types as the No7 Radiance Revealed Exfoliator, for All Skin Types. However, the abrasive agent is alumina, and as such this scrub can be grittier and potentially too abrasive unless used with great care. This does rinse better than the aforementioned scrub.

☹ **No7 Advanced Hydration Day Cream SPF 12** *($14.99 for 1.69 ounces)* provides sufficient UVA protection via its in-part avobenzone sunscreen, but the SPF rating is disappointing because you cannot use this as your only source of daily sun protection. Another letdown is that this day cream for normal to dry skin contains just a dusting of several state-of-the-art ingredients, including ceramides and phytosphingosine.

☹ **No7 Advanced Hydration Day Fluid** *($14.99 for 1 ounce)* is an OK moisturizing lotion for normal to slightly dry or slightly oily skin. It lacks antioxidants, and the amounts of skin-identical ingredients found in healthy skin are in very short supply.

☹ **No7 Advanced Hydration Night Cream** *($15.99 for 1.69 ounces)* is a standard lightweight moisturizer for normal to slightly dry skin. Jar packaging is irrelevant because this does not contain any air- or light-sensitive ingredients. The truly elegant ingredients round out the ingredient list, but that's not where you want to see them, especially in a moisturizer labeled "advanced."

☺ **No7 Calm Skin Redness-Relief Gel** *($19.99 for 1 ounce)*. This is better described as a moisturizer than as a gel because the thickeners and emollients it contains don't combine to create a gel texture or finish. It's a fairly average product that achieves some silkiness from the silicones. Regrettably the anti-irritants it contains, which could help squelch redness, are present in such negligible amounts they are pretty much useless; ditto for the range of skin-identical ingredients. It's good that this product is fragrance-free, but it is not a good choice if your goal is combating persistent redness.

☺ **No7 Intensive Line Filler** *($17.99 for 0.67 ounce)* is very similar to the No7 Refine & Rewind Intense Perfecting Serum reviewed below, except here you get less product and it is packaged in a tube instead of a bottle with built-in pump applicator. This formula differs because it has a slightly thicker texture and it includes mineral pigments (what the company refers to as "light-diffusing particles"), but otherwise the same comments apply. I can think of many other products whose state-of-the-art formulas are a better way to treat aging skin.

☺ **No7 Lifting & Firming Day Cream SPF 8** *($19.99 for 1.69 ounces)* tries to seem more state-of-the-art than it is, but doesn't get off to a grand start because of its low SPF rating (though avobenzone is included for UVA protection). Boots claims this will firm skin in just two weeks, but this product doesn't contain ingredients that will restore youth, and the low amount of peptides and antioxidants is a letdown, as is the choice of jar packaging. And this is supposed to be their most advanced formula?!

☺ **No7 Lifting & Firming Eye Cream** *($19.99 for 0.5 ounce)* provides moisture to slightly dry skin and has a silky texture, but that's the extent of this eye cream's abilities. Once again, the amount of intriguing ingredients is depressingly small.

☺ **No7 Lifting & Firming Night Cream** *($19.99 for 1.69 ounces)* is nearly identical to the No7 Lifting & Firming Eye Cream, except this is more emollient for dry skin. Otherwise, the same review applies.

☺ **No7 Moisture Quench Day Cream, For Normal/Dry Skin** *($12.99 for 1.69 ounces)* fails to impress because the majority of its formula is ho-hum, and the good stuff that shows up at the end of the ingredient list is too little, too late. Consider this a decent choice for dry skin, but realize that there are several superior formulas available elsewhere.

☺ **No7 Moisture Quench Day Fluid, For Normal/Dry Skin** *($12.99 for 3.3 ounces)* is the lotion version of the No7 Moisture Quench Day Cream, for Normal/Dry Skin, and other than being better suited for normal to dry skin and not using jar packaging, the same review applies.

☺ **No7 Moisture Quench Night Cream, for Normal/Dry Skin** *($12.99 for 1.69 ounces)* is a standard emollient moisturizer for dry to very dry skin. Someone with normal skin will likely find this too rich. And someone shopping for a brilliantly formulated moisturizer not packaged in a jar will be disappointed.

☺ **No7 Protect & Perfect Beauty Serum** *($21.99 for 1 ounce)*. This serum reigns above every other Boots product in terms of reader curiosity. It seems there is intense interest in whether or not the claims made for this product and the media attention paid to it are true. Why the hullabaloo? A television documentary that aired in the United Kingdom in March 2007 featured the results of a blind test that compared the efficacy of this serum to tretinoin, the active ingredient in Retin-A and Renova. The research was carried out by scientists at the

University of Manchester, with the conclusion that this Boots serum was just as effective at stimulating collagen production as tretinoin, yet costs considerably less. That sounds great until you learn that Boots paid for the research, which means they had a vested interest in making sure the study made their product look great. Also, because the study was done "blind" instead of double-blind, the researchers knew who was getting which treatment. This type of study isn't as reliable as double-blind studies because, especially when money is at stake, there is a natural bias toward making sure the product in question comes out in the best possible light. "Our studies show" is a major attention-getting technique used in cosmetic advertising and press releases. Studies are great and vital to understanding how skin works and what helps skin work better, but not all studies are created equal and one study is not definitive of anything. Further, a study paid for by the company selling the product is ALWAYS circumspect. It's not that the study may not be valid, but the bias is present from the beginning and that must always be taken into consideration. More to the point, any legitimate research would include the negative studies as well or compare other products from other lines (not just the one from the company paying for the study). No one has even seen a cosmetics company tell you about the studies they did where the product tested didn't work or where products from other companies worked as well. From my perspective that would be even more fascinating information but it will be a cold day in hell before that kind of data is ever offered up by a cosmetics company.

One more point: comparing a product to tretinoin in a short period of time is just absurd. Tretinoin works over time (there's abundant research about that); it initially makes the skin worse due to the irritation it can cause, such that over time there is no way to know what the results would have been. This is a great example of how media hype can generate tremendous interest in (and resulting sales of) a product. It reminds me of the frenzy after ads for StriVectin-SD appeared in *Parade* magazine with the tag line "Better than Botox!" Beauty chat rooms were quick to crown this serum as an antiaging powerhouse, simply on the basis of media attention alone. It's not that this serum isn't worth purchasing, but I wouldn't recommend anyone consider it over tretinoin or several other serums whose formulas outpace this one. Protect & Perfect Beauty Serum is silicone-based and contains a small amount of vitamin C as sodium ascorbyl phosphate (which research has shown is not as effective as ascorbic acid, though it is more stable). A nearly insignificant amount of vitamin A (as retinyl palmitate, not retinol as claimed) and other antioxidants hardly makes this an antiaging product worth any amount of frenzy. Its vitamin C content and other attributes are not even worth mild enthusiasm when you consider that several companies offer serums that are infinitely more state-of-the-art. Examples include serums from Estee Lauder Perfectionist, Clinique Repairwear, Olay Regenerist, MD Skincare by Dr. Dennis Gross, Dr. Denese's Hydroshield products, and various options from Skinceuticals. And if you're looking for peptides (or hope that the ones used in this Boots serum will spell certain doom for your wrinkles), this isn't the product that will flood your skin with them. In fact, there are more preservatives than peptides in this fragrance-free serum.

Despite my dispelling the hype this product generated (and remember, it all began with funding from Boots, and no one else has reproduced the results from their "study"), it can be a good serum-type moisturizer for all skin types, and the silicones make skin feel wonderfully silky. This product comes in translucent glass packaging that will compromise the stability of the vitamin C and vitamin A unless this is constantly kept away from light. By the way, there is plenty of substantiated, published research indicating that topically applied vitamin C can stimulate collagen production, but so can a lot of other ingredients (for example, any sunscreen comes to mind), but you would need more vitamin C than what is in this Boots serum. (Sources: *Journal of Cosmetic Dermatology*, June 2006, pages 150-156; *Pharmaceutical Development and Technology*, November 2006, pages 255-261; *Dermatologic Surgery*, July 2005, pages 814-817; and *Experimental Dermatology*, June 2003, pages 237-244). Keep in mind that one skin care ingredient is never enough for skin, just like one type of food (like broccoli) doesn't make for a healthy diet. It is the combination of healthy substances that is truly the best for skin; there isn't one miracle ingredient to be found anywhere. And by the way, even Boots doesn't believe their own claims or they wouldn't be selling a dozen+ products making the same promises about getting rid of wrinkles. If the one they launched works, what are all the others for?

☺ **No7 Protect & Perfect Day Cream SPF 15** *($19.99 for 1.7 ounces)* doesn't list active ingredients and, therefore, it cannot be relied on for adequate sun protection. This contains several sunscreen ingredients, but a product sold in the United States must follow FDA regulations for over-the-counter drug products, and Boots isn't doing that. However, even if they modify the labeling so that it follows regulations, this jar-packaged moisturizer will be a resounding disappointment for anyone hoping there is truth behind its claims of being a fantastic moisturizer for younger-looking skin. Any of the daytime moisturizers with sunscreen from Olay are preferred to this.

☺ **No7 Protect & Perfect Eye Cream** *($19.99 for 0.5 ounce)*. This lightweight, silky eye cream doesn't contain exceptional levels of any state-of-the-art ingredients and it does not have any ability to chase dark circles and puffiness away. Puffy eyes and dark circles do not have a cosmetic solution, unless they are the result of using particularly badly formulated products around your eyes that actually are causing the puffiness and darkness, in which case you could stop using them. This cream contains a smattering of peptides and some antioxidants, but even combined, the amount is likely too small to make much difference for eye-area skin, plus none of them have any research showing they can improve problems around the eyes.

☺ **Protect & Perfect Intense Beauty Serum** *($22.99 for 1 ounce)*. Boots lauded this product based on the results of a 12-month study they performed. The results were that 70% of the "volunteers" using this product showed a "marked improvement" in the appearance of their sun-damaged skin. That's hardly surprising, given that this serum contains some ingredients that can help sun-damaged skin look better, just like countless other serums and moisturizers. Regardless, the study claim is bogus because this so-called study wasn't published or peer-reviewed. We don't know if it was done double-blind, if the effect of the Boots serum was compared with the effect of other products, or even if the participants were using other products at the same time. For example, if they were using sunscreen during the test period, that would have had far more impact than this serum as far as the results go. As is, this "study" is meaningless and poses more questions than answers, but it does make for great marketing headlines that I'm sure the media splashed all over the place.

In short, there is no real evidence that this is *the* serum everyone with sun-damaged skin needs. Based on the ingredient list, this isn't anything special for anyone's skin. It's remarkably similar to Boots No7 Protect & Perfect Beauty Serum—the very same one that caused a frenzy a few years back because it was said to work as well as tretinoin without the irritation. If that serum (which the company still sells) is so remarkable, why do they need another version with a nearly identical formula? The logical answer is that they want to continue the marketing hype of its progenitor and sell more product using this thinly veiled pseudoscience. Don't fall for it; this serum pales in comparison to many others, including several from Olay and Neutrogena.

The only intense thing about it is the name, not what it does for aging skin. Note that this serum is sold in Canada as No7 Refine & Rewind Beauty Serum.

☺ **No7 Protect & Perfect Night Cream** *($19.99 for 1.7 ounces)*. How important does Boots consider the Protect & Perfect complex in this moisturizer? Not very, or even slightly. If they did, the key antiaging ingredients would amount to more than a mere dusting. As is, your skin is getting more fragrance and preservative than antioxidant vitamins and peptides. Moreover, those ingredients won't remain potent for long due to the jar packaging. This ends up being an average moisturizer for normal to dry skin.

☺ **No7 Radiant Glow Beauty Lotion** *($15.99 for 1 ounce)* is a respectable lightweight moisturizer with shine for normal to slightly dry skin. It is fragrance-free and works well under makeup, but comparably speaking, doesn't best several moisturizers from Olay or Dove.

☹ **No7 Rebalancing Day Gel, for Oily/Combination Skin** *($12.99 for 1.69 ounces)* will not revitalize skin with green tea and seaweed because those ingredients are barely present. This is merely a boring gel moisturizer that's suitable for its intended skin types. It's nice that fragrance was omitted, but why aren't more beneficial ingredients added?

☹ **No7 Rebalancing Night Fluid, for Oily/Combination Skin** *($12.99 for 3.3 ounces)* is a skin-confusing mix of slip agent, silicone, zinc oxide, emollients, clay, talc, and wax. It's too light and absorbent for dry skin, yet too potentially troublesome for oily skin or oily areas. I suppose it's OK for normal skin, but overall it's an unimpressive formula.

☹ **No7 Refine & Rewind Intense Perfecting Serum** *($21.99 for 1 ounce)* is said to work little miracles on your skin day by day, but the only miracle is how amazingly silky the silicones in here can make your skin feel. Silicones are hardly unique to this serum, and while it should be loaded with antioxidants, skin-identical substances, and cell-communicating ingredients, it either comes up short or contains such a tiny amount that your skin (and wrinkles) won't notice. The form of vitamin C is sodium ascorbyl phosphate. Although it has antioxidant ability like other forms of vitamin C, research has shown that it is not as effective as ascorbic acid (pure vitamin C) despite being more stable (Sources: *Skin Pharmacology and Physiology*, July-August 2004, pages 200-206; and *International Journal of Pharmaceutics*, April 2003, pages 65-73). That's not to say it does not have benefit for skin; it most certainly does. It's just that this doesn't appear to be the ideal form of vitamin C to include in a serum with claims like those Boots is making. By the way, the pro-retinol referred to on the label is not retinol, but rather retinyl palmitate, which is not the same thing.

☹ **No7 Reviving Eye Gel** *($11.99 for 0.5 ounce)* is nearly identical to the Boots Botanics Ultimate Lift Eye Gel, except this version adds a couple of silicones for a silky texture. It remains an unexciting product that is minimally helpful for slightly dry skin. The amounts of witch hazel and horse chestnut are too small for skin to notice, for better or worse.

☹ **No7 Time Resisting Day Cream SPF 12** *($19.99 for 1.69 ounces)* deserves credit for its in-part avobenzone sunscreen, but the base formula for normal to slightly dry skin offers little of substance for skin. The mica provides a soft shine finish and, while Boots talks up this sunscreen's antioxidant complex, the amount of antioxidants is likely too small for skin to gain any benefit.

☹ **No7 Time Resisting Night Cream** *($19.99 for 1.69 ounces)* does not contain retinol as claimed (retinyl palmitate is not the same thing), and ends up being another plain emollient moisturizer for normal to dry skin. It is far less elegant than the moisturizer options from many other drugstore lines, including Olay, Dove, Pond's, and Neutrogena.

☺ **No7 Intensive Moisture Face Mask** *($19.99 for 3.3 ounces)* is an exceptionally standard moisturizing mask for dry to very dry skin. What you get for your money isn't worth the cost, but this will cover the basics in terms of making dry skin feel smoother and comfortable.

☹ **No7 Pamper & Peel Radiance Mask** *($19.99 for 1.69 ounces)* is a traditional peel-off mask that contains polyvinyl alcohol, which means it is too irritating for all skin types.

☺ **No7 Deeply Moisturising Lipcare** *($6.99 for 0.33 ounce)* is a somewhat sticky but emollient lip balm that is an option if you need such a product and prefer a glossy finish. Including several ceramides was a good idea, but the amounts in this product—well, they don't amount to much.

☺ **No7 Protect & Perfect Lip Care** *($7.99 for 0.33 ounce)* is mostly style with little substance. The core ingredients will help moisturize lips and make them feel silky, but the complex referred to in this product's claims won't do anything to repair signs of aging around the mouth. This is a decent, waxy, lanolin- and Vaseline-based, lightweight lip moisturizer, but that's about it.

☺ **No7 Sunless Tanning Quick Dry Tinted Lotion, for Face and Body** *($14.99 for 6.6 ounces)* is available in two formulas. The Light/Medium version is a water-based lotion with a tiny amount of emollients, while the Medium/Dark formula is silicone-based and omits the emollient. The latter is best for normal to oily skin, while the former is preferred for normal to dry skin. Both self-tanners turn skin color via dihydroxyacetone and the slower-acting erythrulose, and are tinted so you can see where they've been applied. Each also contains soothing chamomile oil, though in an amount that's likely too small to have much, if any, effect on skin. Still, these are good, inexpensive self-tanning lotions.

BOOTS TIME DIMENSIONS PRODUCTS

✓☺ **Time Dimensions Conditioning Cleansing Cream** *($8.99 for 6.7 ounces).* is nearly identical to the No7 Soft & Soothed Gentle Cleanser, for Normal/Dry Skin, and the same review applies.

☺ **Time Dimensions Deep Cleansing Wipes** *($6.99 for 30 wipes)* work well to cleanse normal to very dry skin, and are fairly adept at removing makeup (waterproof formulas will withstand these wipes). The amount of plant extracts is very small, and they won't reduce the visible signs of aging any more than a steady diet of cheesecake will encourage weight loss.

☺ **Time Dimensions Clarifying Facial Exfoliator** *($9.99 for 5 ounces)* is very similar to the No7 Radiance Revealed Exfoliator, for All Skin Types, except this version has greater cleansing ability because it contains sodium laureth sulfate. Otherwise, the same review applies. This version ends up being a better value than the No7 scrub.

☺ **Time Dimensions Brightening Facial Balm** *($16.99 for 1 ounce)* is a fluid moisturizer whose silicone content will make all skin types feel silky while the mica imparts a noticeable shine. The amount of antioxidants and peptides is disappointing, and certainly doesn't make this a top choice for improving skin of any age.

☺ **Time Dimensions Instant Eye Reviver** *($14.99 for 0.33 ounce)* is similar to but with more ingredients than the Boots Botanics Moisturising Eye Cream, and the same basic comments apply. The addition of petrolatum makes this product more moisturizing than the Botanics version, but the amounts of the extra ingredients are mere dustings, so cannot be counted on for a healthy skin boost.

☺ **Time Dimensions Intensive Restoring Treatment** *($18.99 for 1 ounce)* is neither intensive nor restorative. This is a simple, light-textured lotion with a lot of mica for a shiny finish.

Vitamin A and peptides are supposed to be major players here, but their presence amounts to a non-speaking, walk-on part in a movie, not the "top billing" your skin needs to look and feel its best.

☺ **Time Dimensions Nourishing Eye Cream** *($18.99 for 0.5 ounce)* is a below-standard lightweight moisturizer for slightly dry skin anywhere on the face. The mica leaves a soft shine finish, but this has nothing to do with boosting collagen or elastin, or reducing fine lines or puffiness in the eye area.

☺ **Time Dimensions Rejuvenating Day Moisturiser** *($16.99 for 1.69 ounces)* is a thicker version of the Time Dimensions Nourishing Eye Cream, except this version doesn't contain mica. Otherwise, the same basic comments apply.

☺ **Time Dimensions Restoring Night Moisturiser** *($17.99 for 1.69 ounces)* contains a teeny-tiny amount of antioxidants and peptides, features jar packaging, and is otherwise very similar to the Time Dimensions Rejuvenating Day Moisturiser.

☺ **Time Dimensions Softening Line Smoother** *($17.99 for 0.5 ounce)* is merely a blend of silicones and slip agents whose texture is meant to serve as a sort of spackle for superficial lines and wrinkles. It works marginally well, but how long the effect lasts depends on how much you move your face. At least this is an option for those who want to try such a product but don't want a shiny or sparkling finish.

☹ **Time Dimensions Instant Lip Plumper** *($9.99 for 0.27 ounce)* is perhaps the most irritating lip plumper being sold today. Most such products contain one or two irritants that cause lips to swell slightly by virtue of irritation. Boots uses menthol (a lot of it), spearmint oil, eugenol, clove oil, pepper extract, methyl eugenol, and cinnamon. All I can say, besides "buyer beware," is "Ouch!" And Boots calls this product a "special treat"!?

BOOTS MAKEUP

FOUNDATION: ✓ ☺ **No7 Intelligent Balance Mousse Foundation** *($13.99)* is an outstanding, feather-light mousse foundation for normal to very oily skin. The sponge-like texture blends seamlessly over skin, leaving a smooth matte finish without a hint of flatness. The powdery silicones (which comprise the bulk of this nonaqueous formula) do a good job of keeping excess shine in check, although this foundation's finish can magnify dry areas, so be sure to prep your skin beforehand. You'll enjoy sheer to light coverage that holds up surprisingly well throughout the day, except for very oily areas, which will require some blotting and perhaps a powder touch-up or two. The only drawback (well, aside from there being no shades for dark skin tones) is the jar packaging, which isn't the most sanitary way to use makeup. However, because this is a nonaqueous product (note that any water in a product increases the risk of bacterial growth), problems will be minimal. One other comment about the jar packaging: once you're about halfway through this foundation, the relatively narrow opening makes it more difficult to get product out. All of the shades are very good, and finish lighter than they appear, but Target offers testers for the Boots No7 line, so seeing if one of the shades will work for you is convenient.

✓ ☺ **No7 Soft & Sheer Tinted Moisturiser SPF 15** *($11.99)* is a great find for those with normal to dry skin! Titanium dioxide is partially responsible for UVA protection, while the creamy-smooth texture applies and blends beautifully, providing sheer coverage and a fresh, moist finish. All three shades are recommended.

✓ ☺ **No7 Stay Perfect Foundation SPF 15** *($13.99)* makes reference to the skin-strength-ening ceramides it contains, but the amount of them in this silky liquid foundation is barely a dusting. Although this isn't skin care disguised as makeup, it contains an in-part titanium dioxide sunscreen, feels nearly weightless, and sets to a smooth matte finish. Sheer to light coverage is obtainable and the overall formula is best for normal to very oily skin. Among the eight mostly great, neutral shades, the only one to avoid (due to its orange tone) is Truffle.

☺ **No7 Intelligent Balance Foundation SPF 12** *($13.99)* contains octinoxate and tita-nium dioxide for broad-spectrum sun protection, and is one of those foundations that claim to know where skin is oily and where it is dry, releasing the appropriate moisturizing or absorbent ingredients where needed most. The claim is bogus, but the fluid texture has a smoothness that makes blending a pleasure, though you don't have much time before this sets to a true matte finish. Best for normal to oily skin, this provides light to medium coverage without looking artificial, and among the six shades, only Walnut is suspect for being slightly peach (but it's still worth a try). This would be rated a Paula's Pick if the SPF rating were 15 or greater.

☺ **Botanics Fresh Face Tinted Moisturiser** *($8.99)* is a fragrant tinted moisturizer whose omission of sunscreen is odd, given that its competitors typically include this for the 3-in-1 benefit many women love. Still, it has a great lightweight but creamy texture, very sheer cover-age, and a natural finish from either of its two shades.

☺ **No7 Lifting and Firming Foundation SPF 15** *($14.99)* gets its sun protection partly from titanium dioxide, though it would be better if a higher percentage were included (1.6% is low). This is otherwise a very silky liquid foundation for those with normal to oily skin seeking medium coverage and a non-powdery matte finish. Seven of the eight shades are recommended; Truffle is too peach for its intended range of skin tones. Do I need to state that this won't lift or firm skin in the least?

☺ **No7 Radiant Glow Foundation SPF 15** *($10.49)* is remarkably similar to the No7 Lifting and Firming Foundation SPF 15, right down to the number of shades and advice to avoid Truffle. This version doesn't contain as much mica, which is strange because that pigment provides a "glow," but the Lifting and Firming Foundation isn't shiny.

☺ **No7 Stay Perfect Foundation Compact SPF 15** *($15.99)* is a traditional cream-to-powder makeup with an in-part titanium dioxide sunscreen. The creamy texture sets quickly to a powder finish, owing to the fact that aluminum starch is the second ingredient. This is best for normal to slightly oily skin not prone to blemishes, and provides light to medium cover-age. Each of the six shades is soft and neutral, though options for fair and dark skin tones are lacking. The crescent-shaped sponge accompanying this foundation is almost useless; a full-size circular sponge works much better.

☺ **No7 True Identity Foundation** *($12.49)* is a foundation no superhero should be without, lest their true identity be revealed! OK, not really, but the attempt at humor was a lead-in to what is an amazing foundation—if you need barely any coverage. The silicone- and talc-based formula feels silky, provides a real-skin finish, and has a hint of color. It is best for normal to oily skin, and all four shades are great (but again, this is not one to pick if you need coverage beyond what strategically placed concealer provides).

☺ **Botanics Complexion Refining Foundation** *($12.99)* begins slightly creamy, but sets to a nearly weightless matte finish suitable for normal to oily skin. Coverage goes from sheer to light, and each of the eight shades is a winner (there are options for someone with fair skin, too). The only drawback is the inclusion of volatile fragrance components, which can cause irritation.

The Reviews B

☺ **No7 Mineral Perfection Foundation** *($13.99).* Boots' contribution to the glut of mineral makeup doesn't bring anything new to the table, unless you happen to believe that ruby, amethyst, and sapphire powders are great for skin (they're not); even if they were, the trace amounts in this product translate into a nothing for skin. Aside from the gimmick, this loose-powder foundation has a silky texture that's nearly weightless. It provides sheer to almost medium coverage and leaves a sparkling shine finish. Boots includes a brush with a stubby handle but full-size head, and it's much better than the applicators that accompany several other mineral makeups on the market. The one drawback to this otherwise very good powder is the colors, each of which goes on darker than it looks and errs on the peach side rather than being neutral. There are no shades suitable for fair to light skin tones. Avoid Buff and note that all shades of this foundation can easily appear streaky if it isn't carefully blended.

☹ **No7 Colour Calming Makeup Base** *($9.99)* has a strong green tint that doesn't correct a reddened complexion; it just substitutes one problem for another, and the light lotion texture, while easy to apply, doesn't do a thing to make the green color less apparent.

CONCEALER: ☺ **Botanics Complexion Refining Concealer Stick** *($9.99)* is a find for those who prefer lipstick-style concealers and are not using them to cover blemishes (because the ingredients that keep this in lipstick form can contribute to clogged pores). It blends very well, leaves a satin-smooth finish, and poses just a slight risk of creasing into lines around the eye. Only two shades are available, one of which (Sweet Ginger) will be too peach for some, so this is recommended only if you have light skin.

☺ **Botanics Totally Concealed** *($7.99)* is a good liquid concealer available in three workable shades. It has enough slip for targeted blending, and sets to a matte finish that remains slightly tacky and only minimally creases into lines. This does not provide total coverage as the name implies, but offers enough camouflage for minor imperfections.

☺ **No7 Radiant Glow Concealer** *($12.99)* functions best as a highlighter because it brightens shadowed areas, but provides minimal coverage. The finish feels matte but has a slight shine to it, which works to a subtle extent to reflect light away from dark areas. You push a button at the bottom of the pen-style component, and the product is fed onto a built-in synthetic brush. There are better versions of this product from Estee Lauder (Ideal Light) and Yves Saint Laurent (Touche Eclat Radiant Touch), but both cost twice as much.

☹ **Expert Anti-Blemish Concealer Duo** *($5.99).* This dual product features an anti-acne fluid on one end and a concealer on the other. The Blemish Lotion is loaded with alcohol and will be of precious little help against acne; the Concealer has a thick, occlusive texture that is no match for today's best concealers. I guarantee your acne will not improve or be convincingly hidden if you choose to try this product.

☺ **No7 Quick Cover Blemish Stick** *($9.99)* lists its first ingredient as chalk and, as expected, looks chalky on skin. This lipstick-style concealer contains wax-like ingredients that are not recommended for use on blemishes, though it does provide sufficient coverage. Still, each of the four shades tends toward pink and peach tones, and overall this has more strikes than positives.

POWDER: ✓☺ **No7 Perfect Light Loose Powder** *($11.99)* has a feather-light texture and seamless, dry finish. The aluminum starch- and talc-based formula is excellent for normal to oily skin because it absorbs well without looking chalky or thick. Although Boots advertises four shades on their Web site, the Target stores I visited consistently sold only two, both of which are sheer and recommended. Bonus points are deserved because the packaging for this loose powder works great to minimize mess.

✓ ☺ **No7 Perfect Light Portable Loose Powder** *($12.99)* has the same formula and review as the No7 Perfect Light Loose Powder, except this comes in a portable container that includes a built-in brush. Powder is dispensed onto the brush for quick touch-ups on-the-go, and the brush itself is quite nice; not incredibly dense, but soft and shaped well for its intended purpose.

☹ **No7 Perfect Light Pressed Powder** *($11.99)* has a texture that feels waxy and dry at the same time. That not only makes application with a brush difficult (the powder doesn't pick up easily) but also creates a heavy appearance on skin. The finish is made even more obvious because each of the shades has a slight pink or peach tone.

☹ **Botanics Lighter Than Air Loose Powder** *($12.99)* has an accurate name, but although the feel is weightless, the finish is unnaturally dry and lends a flat, overly powdered appearance to skin, even when applied sheer. Moreover, this powder has a strong scent and contains volatile fragrance components. Why consider this when there are so many great powders without this one's drawbacks?

BLUSH AND BRONZER: ☺ **No7 Natural Blush Cheek Colour** *($8.99)*. No7 Natural Blush Cheek Colour isn't the silkiest powder blush around, but is a definite option for those who prefer soft colors that apply sheer, build well (if more color is desired), and come in a selection of very good matte shades.

☺ **Botanics Cheek Colour** *($8.99)* is very similar to the No7 Natural Blush Cheek Colour, except each shade has a soft shine and the formula includes walnut shell powder and apple extract. Neither additive makes a big difference in performance, so the same review applies.

☺ **No7 Blush Tint Cream Blush** *($9.99)* presents cream blush in stick form, and you get a surprisingly small amount of product. Still, this goes on easily, blends well, and provides a sheer wash of translucent color with a slightly moist finish. It is best for normal to dry skin not prone to blemishes.

☺ **No7 Sun Kissed Bronze Shimmer Powder Compact** *($11.99)* is a dual-sided powder bronzer that features light and medium colors, both with a soft shine. This has a good, smooth texture but works best as blush because neither shade has enough depth to register as a bronze-y color on skin.

☺ **No7 Mineral Perfection Blush** *($9.99)*. This loose-powder blush is mica-based, and because mica is a mineral, the name fits. Mica shows up in most powder blushes, so having it headline here doesn't make this a unique product in any way. Boots includes a minibrush, but it's too scratchy for comfortable use. Applied with a better brush, this goes on evenly and imparts a soft wash of color. The two shades are best for fair to light skin tones, and each has enough shine to make them too much for daytime wear, but they're fine for evening glamour. Keep in mind that this can be a messy way to apply blush.

☹ **Instant Sunshine Smooth-On Bronzer** *($11.99)*. This spray-on bronzer has the advantage (some would say disadvantage) of drying quickly, but that trait comes from skin-damaging alcohol. The amount of alcohol makes this bronzer a problem for all skin types, and it is not recommended.

EYESHADOW: ☺ **Botanics Eye Colour** *($3.99)* has a much smoother, silkier texture and application than either of the No7 eyeshadow products. The shade selection includes some almost matte nude and brown tones alongside shiny blues and greens that are best left alone. The Botanics Personal Eyes Magnetic Compact is sold separately and can house three eyeshadows. Colors can be rotated as needed because they are held in place by a magnet.

☹ **No7 Stay Perfect Eye Mousse** *($7.99)* has a light-as-mousse texture but so much slip that controlled blending becomes an issue. Once set, this tends to last with minimal creasing, though because the shine is intense it's not for the wrinkled set. Only a tiny dab is needed, and again, blending must be done carefully or this will slide all over the eye area.

☺ **No7 Stay Perfect Eye Shadow Single** *($5.99)* has a smooth but dry texture that applies better than expected but can be tricky to blend with other colors (it doesn't have much movement after the initial application). The range of colors allows for some good pairings, but every color has strong shine, so these aren't for women with wrinkles or a sagging eye area.

☹ **No7 Mineral Perfection Eye Shadow Palette** *($8.99)*. These eyeshadow trios are mica-based, and because mica is a mineral, the name is apropos, yet the formula is nothing unique or different when compared with hundreds of other eyeshadows. Although the powder eyeshadows in these sets have a smooth texture, their waxy nature disrupts color pickup on the brush, so application doesn't go past sheer; even the darker colors barely register on skin. Still, these can work for a soft eyeshadow design and the Rose and Topaz trios are decent. Avoid the too colorful Breeze and Heather trios unless you're looking for a blatant and very noticeable effect that's far from eye design.

☹ **No7 Stay Perfect Eye Shadow Palette** *($7.99)* products have a different formula that's inferior to that of the No7 Stay Perfect Eye Shadow Single. It is unusually dry, flakes all over the place, and tends to sit on top of skin rather than mesh with it (owing to its lack of smoothness). Further, most of the color combinations either lack depth, are too pastel, or are contrasting.

☹ **No7 Stay Perfect Smoothing & Brightening Eye Base** *($6.99)* is a pink-tinted cream meant to function as an anchor so eyeshadow lasts longer. The thick, creamy formula does just the opposite—your eyeshadows won't make it to lunch without fading, creasing, or smearing, and the pink color is obvious enough to interfere with any eyeshadow color used over it. Stay away from this product if you want your eye makeup to stay perfect!

EYE AND BROW SHAPER: ☺ **No7 Liquid Eye Liner** *($8.99)* comes in inkwell packaging and features a thin, flexible brush that works well; if only the color deposit weren't so sheer. That means successive layers are needed to build color, which increases the chance of smearing. This dries quickly, but will fade before long, so overall it doesn't compare favorably with liquid liners from L'Oreal and Almay, to name just two.

☺ **Botanics Eye Definer** *($5.99)* is a very standard eye pencil that needs routine sharpening and is available in classic colors. This applies easily and feels almost powdery but is still slightly prone to smudging.

☺ **No7 Amazing Eyes Pencil** *($6.99)* needs sharpening but other than that this is quite good, and preferred to the Botanics Eye Definer. It glides on swiftly, deposits strong color (which is what you want for eye lining) that can be softened with the built-in sponge tip, and stays in place. The only issue is minor fading, which will be a deal-breaker only for those with oily eyelids.

☹ **No7 Beautiful Brows Pencil** *($6.99)* won't create beautiful brows unless your definition of that includes flaking color and matted brow hairs from this substandard pencil's waxy texture and finish. This is one of the worst brow pencils I've ever come across. Great colors, though.

LIPSTICK, LIP GLOSS, AND LIPLINER: ✓ ☺ **Botanics Lip Gloss** *($7.99)* earns its rating because it has a superior smooth texture, moisturizes lips without feeling goopy, isn't sticky, and provides a beautiful selection of sheer to moderate colors, each with a sexy gloss finish and subtle shimmer.

✓ ☺ **No7 Sheer Temptation Lipstick** *($9.99)* feels rich and emollient, and while the colors look quite bold in the tube, each goes on sheer, as the name states. This has a glossy finish yet isn't too slippery, and the colors are great. If you want sheer lip color, what more could you ask for?

☺ **No7 High Shine Lip Gloss** *($7.99)* is a traditional sheer lip gloss applied with a sponge tip attached to a wand. It feels smooth and is non-sticky and has a less extreme gloss finish than the No7 Lip Glace.

☺ **No7 Lip Glace** *($9.99)* comes in a tube and is a standard, thick lip gloss with a slightly sticky finish and wet, glossy shine. Some of the colors go on sheer, while others go on more intense and imbue lips with sparkles. That's why it's good that the Boots display includes testers.

☺ **No7 Mineral Perfection Lipstick** *($9.99)*. Minerals play a minor role in this lipstick, other than the mica that gives almost every shade in this small collection a slight shimmer. This is otherwise a very standard, lightweight cream lipstick with a smooth, slick finish. It will travel into lines around the mouth, but if that's not an issue for you, this is a viable lipstick. The color payoff is moderate.

☺ **No7 Stay Perfect Lip Lacquer** *($9.99)* is Boots' version of the long-wearing lip paint first made famous by Max Factor. Just like that company's Lipfinity, this two-part product includes a lip paint and a clear top coat to ensure a glossy finish and comfortable wear (the lip paint used by itself makes lips feel dry). Although this version doesn't have the same impressive longevity as Max Factor's (or Cover Girl's, or those from Estee Lauder and M.A.C.), I was pleasantly surprised that not once in several hours of wear did I feel compelled to apply more top coat. Perhaps I should have, as this might have "protected" the color from fading so much; but at least when that occurred it did so evenly rather than peeling or flaking off. All in all, this is worth a look despite the fact that it does not keep color looking perfect for eight hours as claimed.

☺ **No7 Stay Perfect Lipstick** *($9.99)* feels much better and more modern than the Botanics Lipstick. It has a lightweight texture and smooth, creamy finish that remains a bit slick, so this will migrate into lines around the mouth. If that is not a concern, this is definitely worth auditioning.

☺ **No7 Moisture Drench Lipstick** *($9.99)* is a standard, but good, cream lipstick. Each of the attractive colors provides moderate coverage and a soft, moisturizing finish. Several shades provide a dimensional shimmer, which can create the illusion of fuller lips.

☺ **Botanics Lip Liner** *($6.99)* applies easily but has an emollience that makes it prone to smearing and traveling into lines around the mouth. This needs-sharpening pencil works best when applied all over lips and blended with a gloss for a soft, stained effect.

☹ **Botanics Lipstick** *($7.99)* has an unappealingly thick, waxy texture that's a far cry from the elegantly smooth creaminess of countless other lipsticks. This isn't much for color either, requiring several coats to register beyond sheer, but that only makes this lipstick feel worse.

☹ **No7 Line & Define Lip Pencil** *($6.99)* is a decent automatic, retractable lip pencil available in a small assortment of mostly versatile shades. Although this applies easily, the finish feels (and stays) tacky, and the colors, while initially rich, fade too quickly.

MASCARA: ☺ **Botanics Volumising Mascara** *($6.99)* ranks as the best non-waterproof mascara from Boots. You'll enjoy equal parts length and thickness without clumps or smearing, resulting in moderately dramatic, beautifully separated lashes.

☺ **No7 Lash & Brow Perfector** *($7.99)* is a clear mascara that works best as a lightweight brow gel. Although application is wetter than most, this does not feel sticky or stiff once it dries, yet it holds brows neatly in place. Used as mascara, you'll get a smidgen of emphasis, but that's it.

☺ **No7 Maximum Volume Waterproof Mascara** *($7.99)* is much better than its non-waterproof partner, but its one drawback is that it is minimally waterproof (your eyes getting misty won't cause this to budge, but don't go into the pool with the expectation this will stay put). It is otherwise a very good lengthening and thickening mascara that builds well without getting too dramatic, and it doesn't clump. Removing this takes just a water-soluble cleanser.

☺ **No7 Lash 360°** *($7.99)* is an entry whose odd brush is the only point of difference. Unfortunately, the variable bristles, which are thicker and shorter in the center of the brush and longer on the ends, don't translate into unique lash effect. You'll find this allows for ample length and slight thickness without clumps, along with great lash separation, just like many other recommended mascaras. It leaves lashes soft and is easy to remove with a water-soluble cleanser. That's all good news, but again, this wasn't a necessary addition to Boots' already-crowded lineup of mascaras.

☺ **No7 Super Sensitive Mascara** *($7.99)* has fewer ingredients than most mascaras, although that's not a guarantee that someone with sensitive eyes won't have a problem (and the bulk of this formula consists of ingredients found in most mascaras). Still, this has a very clean application that lets you build impressive length and some thickness with zero clumps. As a bonus, it leaves lashes very soft and doesn't flake.

☺ **Botanics Lash Defining Mascara** *($6.99)* winds up being merely average and is an option only if you want to barely enhance your lashes because you're already satisfied with they way they look minus mascara.

☺ **No7 Longer Lashes Mascara** *($7.99)* is a decent lengthening mascara that doesn't do a thing to build even a hint of thickness. It wears well and removes easily, but this is an option only if slightly longer lashes are your sole requirement.

☺ **No7 Maximum Volume Mascara** *($8.99)* is below average if you were banking on the name translating into copiously thick lashes. This does little to enhance lashes in any respect, but is OK if you want a minimalist look.

☺ **No7 Ultimate Curl Mascara** *($7.99)* has a great name but the performance of this boring mascara is far from "ultimate." You'll get negligible length, no thickness whatsoever, and minimal curl.

☹ **Botanics Waterproof Mascara** *($6.99)* is not recommended at any price unless you want minimal length, sparse definition, and no thickness regardless of how many coats you apply. It is waterproof and comes off with a water-soluble cleanser, but so what?

BRUSHES: ☺ **No7 Brushes** *($5.99-$8.99)*. No7 Powder Brush is an OK powder brush that isn't as soft as most others, but isn't terrible either. Its floppiness doesn't make for controlled application, but it works in a pinch. No7 Blusher Brush should be softer, but it is the appropriate shape and, for the money, works well. Spending a bit more for Sonia Kashuk's brushes (also sold at Target) will get you better performance and higher quality. The No7 Eye Brush is also inferior to those from Kashuk's line, but is still functional and preferred to the sponge-tip applicators that accompany most powder eyeshadows.

☹ **No 7 Retractable Lip Brush** *($6.99)*. No 7 Retractable Lip Brush has the retractable benefit, but so do many other lip brushes whose brush heads aren't so ridiculously small. It would take way too long for someone to apply lip color with this, even if they have thin lips.

FACE AND BODY ILLUMINATING/SHIMMER PRODUCTS: ☺ **No7 Sun Kissed Bronze Shimmer Pearls** *($11.99)* are multicolored powder beads packaged in a jar. You swirl a brush over the beads and apply a sheer layer of powder, which creates a peachy tan color and provides a radiant finish. Although gimmicky, this is a good way to perk up a sallow complexion and add a soft, non-sparkling shine.

☺ **Botanics Shimmer Pearls** *($12.99)* are identical to the No7 Sun Kissed Bronze Shimmer Pearls, except there are more pink and peach beads, so the result is a soft blush color that applies sheer and leaves a subtle shine.

☺ **No7 High Lights Illuminating Lotion** *($12.99 for 1 ounce)* is a standard lightweight shimmer lotion that applies easily and sets to a matte (in feel) finish that stays put. The shine is moderate and not sparkling or glittery, making it a good choice for evening makeup. The pale, opalescent pink color works best on fair to light skin tones.

☺ **Instant Sunshine Shimmer Gel** *($11.99).* Based on the name and appearance of this product, you'd think it was a bronzing gel, but it isn't. Instead, this lightweight, silky gel imparts incredibly sheer tan color and a lot of sparkling shine. This is shine that gleams and won't be anyone's definition of subtle (OK, maybe a Vegas showgirl would find this a tad soft). This shine has merely average ability to cling, so expect flaking and a gradual diminishing of the shine impact. Shimmer Gel is fragrance-free.

SPECIALTY PRODUCTS: ☺ **No7 Mattifying Makeup Base** *($9.99 for 1.3 ounces)* creates a solid, long-lasting matte finish with silicones, clay, and a tiny amount of alcohol (likely too low to cause irritation). This is a very good (colorless) option to use prior to foundation if you have oily to very oily skin. It is not rated a Paula's Pick because other companies (including mine) sell better versions of this product; better because they mattify skin and control excess shine while supplying oily skin with beneficial ingredients it needs.

BORGHESE (SKIN CARE ONLY)

BORGHESE AT-A-GLANCE

Strengths: Good cleansers; a handful of impressive moisturizers (with and without sunscreen), including eye creams (though you don't need a separate eye cream; a well-formulated face moisturizer will do); and some well-formulated serums.

Weaknesses: Expensive; some of the SPF-rated products do not provide sufficient UVA protection; jar packaging is common; toners with irritating ingredients; the Fango mud products aren't even remotely the miracle they're made out to be; no effective AHA or BHA products; no products to address skin discolorations or acne; several products contain more fragrance than skin-beneficial ingredients.

For more information about Borghese, call (866) 267-4437 or visit www.borghese.com or www.Beautypedia.com.

BORGHESE CREMA STRAORDINARIA PRODUCTS

☹ **$$$ Crema Straordinaria Sapone Creme Extraordinaire Foaming Cleanser** *($35.50 for 6.7 ounces)* is little more than liquid soap. The third ingredient is potassium hydroxide and that is about as drying and irritating as it gets for a cleanser.

☺ **$$$ Crema Straordinaria Tonico Creme Extraordinaire Balancing Softening Toner** *($35.50 for 8.4 ounces).* Despite a fantastic-sounding name and the claims of ultimate clarity and extraordinary balancing properties, this is just a simplistic, fairly ordinary toner. It contains a few bells and whistles and isn't overly fragrant, but it's hardly anything to rave about.

✓ ☺ **$$$ Crema Straordinaria Da Giornio SPF 25** *($66 for 1.7 ounces).* Supposedly this daytime moisturizer with an in-part avobenzone sunscreen is worth the cost because it contains Borghese's Stratopeptide Energizing Complex. Aside from the clever marketing name (there is no such complex except in the mind of Borghese's marketing staff), what this contains is a tiny amount of palmitoyl tetrapeptide 7, a type of peptide, the same peptide found in many other products. There's no proof that any peptide has any ability to affect wrinkles. Peptides are fragile ingredients, hard to keep stable, and easily break down as they are absorbed into the skin. Particularly bothersome are the dual claims that this product provides oxygen to skin, while also offering antioxidant protection. That's contradictory, because oxygen encourages free-radical damage. However, not to worry: this product doesn't provide extra oxygen to skin. The good news is that this daytime moisturizer for normal to dry skin contains a bevy of potent antioxidants and some good cell-communicating ingredients. I'm concerned, however, that users will be less likely to apply this liberally due to the cost, but the formula deserves a top rating.

☺ **$$$ Crema Straordinaria Essenza Revitalizing Serum** *($96 for 1.4 ounces)* is mostly slip agents and smoothing film-forming agents similar to what you find in many hairsprays. They make skin feel temporarily tighter, but it's strictly a cosmetic effect. The amount of alcohol is cause for concern (alcohol causes free-radical damage, dryness, and irritation), as is the number of fragrant plants and fragrance chemicals. When you consider that the most beneficial ingredients are barely present, this isn't a product for anyone.

☺ **$$$ Crema Straordinaria Eye Treatment** *($61 for 0.5 ounce)* is an ordinary though emollient eye cream that can make dry skin anywhere on the face look and feel better. However, it cannot tighten, lift, and lighten skin as claimed. Since when do fatty acids, plant oils, and wax have those abilities? They don't, and there isn't any research indicating otherwise. This contains fragrant hibiscus extract and a smattering of antioxidants that won't remain potent for long due to the jar packaging, which makes this an expensive way to get average results.

☺ **$$$ Crema Straordinaria Night Treatment** *($76 for 1.7 ounces)* is a curious formula, and not just because of its too-good-to-be-true claims. It's meant to be applied at night, but it contains a sunscreen ingredient (octinoxate) that skin doesn't need in the evening, especially considering that it's a synthetic sunscreen ingredient that has the potential for causing irritation. It also contains some elegant, state-of-the-art ingredients, but many of them are light- and air-sensitive and so will degrade after opening due to the jar packaging. This could have been an interesting moisturizer for dry skin, but if you're after peptides, you can get a very good peptide-enriched moisturizer from Olay for a lot less money, and in better packaging.

BORGHESE KIRKLAND SIGNATURE PRODUCTS

☺ **$$$ Pure Moisturizing Cleanser** *($16.99 for 7 ounces).* This cleanser, exclusive to Costco stores, is a gentle, water-soluble lotion suitable for normal to dry skin. It removes makeup easily but you may need to use a washcloth to eliminate a residue. This absolutely doesn't qualify as an "herbal infused" formula; that's just marketing copy so consumers think it is more natural than it really is—this formula is about as natural as polyester. The package also includes an additional 3-ounce travel-size cleanser.

☺ **Advanced Age-Defying Wrinkle Defense Serum** *($26.99 for 1.7 ounces).* For a serum that touts its peptide as being able to repair damaged skin, Borghese certainly didn't include much of it in this product. This silicone-enriched serum has the requisite silky texture along with Vaseline and several nonfragrant plant oils for moisture. It would be rated a Paula's Pick and highly recommended for dry skin if it did not contain potentially troublesome horsetail (*Equisetum arvense*) and buckbean (*Menyanthes trifoliata*) extracts. This fragranced serum is exclusive to Costco stores.

☺ **Age-Defying Protective Eye Cream & Restorative Night Cream** *($26.99 for 2.2 ounces)*. Sold exclusively at Costco stores, this is a "package deal" for those seeking an eye cream and a nighttime moisturizer (which you shouldn't be looking for because there is no reason to use an eye cream; there is no research showing that the eye area needs something different from what the face needs). The Age-Defying Protective Eye Cream is a good moisturizer for dry skin anywhere on the face. Two things keep it from earning a happy face rating. First, it's packaged in a jar, so the antioxidants it contains won't remain effective. Second, it contains the plant extract *Menyanthes trifoliata*. Also known as buckbean, this plant contains bitter chemicals that may cause skin irritation. It has no known benefit for skin, but oral consumption can lead to digestive tract irritation and vomiting (Source: www.naturaldatabase.com). The Restorative Night Cream is packaged in a jar, so the effectiveness of its antioxidants will be compromised after opening. It also contains several plants that are known irritants, though these are joined by beneficial plant ingredients, so they likely cancel each other out, but that isn't helpful for skin. Why have anything in a product that irritates skin when research tells us that irritation causes collagen to break down and hurts the skin's protective outer barrier? With some minor formula adjustments and airtight packaging, this duo could have been a value-priced option for managing dry facial skin.

☺ **Age-Defying Protective Moisture Lotion SPF 15** *($21.99 for 3.4 ounces)*. Forget the helpful ingredients in this daytime moisturizer for normal to oily skin; the active ingredients cannot protect skin from the entire UVA range of sunlight because the actives don't include the UVA-protecting ingredients of titanium dioxide, zinc oxide, avobenzone (also called butyl methoxydibenzylmethane), Tinosorb, or Mexoryl SX; as such, this is not recommended.

BORGHESE FANGO PRODUCTS

☺ **$$$ Fango Active Mud for Face and Body** *($61 for 17.6 ounces)* is an extremely standard, inactive clay mask that contains bentonite, slip agent, and plant oils as the primary ingredients. The mix of absorbent clay (bentonite) and oils will leave skin more confused than nourished, and this formula is absolutely not capable of unclogging pores. By the way, whether sourced from Tuscany or Topeka, minerals in clay are not a cure-all or even all that helpful for your skin. Clay serves only to temporarily absorb oil from skin and provide some exfoliation, but there are other ways to achieve that without layering on a mask and sitting around waiting for it to dry. Plus, it's what you do every day for skin care that truly makes a difference for skin, just like eating healthy only once a week or exercising only once a week isn't going to make much of a difference for your health.

☺ **$$$ Fango Brillante Brightening Mud Mask for Face and Body** *($61 for 17.6 ounces)*. This is a very expensive clay mask masquerading as a specialty spa treatment. You're getting far more fragrance than beneficial ingredients and the plant oils it contains will hinder the absorbent nature of the clays and likely confuse your skin. Strangely, this contains several sunscreen ingredients, perhaps to enhance the appearance of this over-glorified, clear jar-packaged mask. By the way, whether sourced from Tuscany or Topeka, minerals in clay are not a cure-all or even all that helpful for your skin. Clay serves only to temporarily absorb oil from skin and provide some exfoliation, but there are other ways to achieve that without layering on a mask and sitting around waiting for it to dry. Plus, it's what you do every day for skin care that truly makes a difference for skin, just like eating healthy only once a week or only exercising once a week isn't going to make much of a difference for your health.

☹ **Fango Delicato Active Mud for Delicate Dry Skin** *($61 for 17.6 ounces)*. This mask is completely wrong for anyone dealing with dry, sensitive skin. The amount of clay is not what dry skin needs. (Talk about making dry skin worse—let's suck out any remaining moisture that's there!) This also contains a veritable who's who of irritating fragrant oils, including peppermint, grapefruit, and bergamot. Avoid this overpriced, underwhelming mud mask at all costs!

OTHER BORGHESE SKIN-CARE PRODUCTS

☺ **$$$ Crema Saponetta Cleansing Creme** *($32.50 for 6.7 ounces)* is an extremely drying water-soluble foaming cleanser that lists potassium hydroxide way too high up on the ingredient list to be considered a healthy option for skin. The ingredients that create all the foam are also too drying for most skin types. Collagen and hyaluronic acid are included, but those ingredients won't fuse with your skin and make it look younger, plus in a cleanser they are just rinsed down the drain or wiped off. It almost goes without saying that there are less expensive, less irritating cleansers for oily skin at the drugstore.

☺ **$$$ Effetto Immediato Spa-Comforting Cleanser** *($30.50 for 6.7 ounces)* is a good water-soluble cleansing lotion for normal to dry skin. It removes makeup well but may require a washcloth to ensure a makeup-free result. Nothing about this formula makes it more spa-worthy than any other cleansing lotion or worth the money. This is about as standard a cleansing formula as you can get. The few bells and whistles added (e.g., collagen and hyaluronic acid) are nice in a moisturizer, but in a cleanser they are just rinsed down the drain.

☹ **Gel Delicato Gentle Makeup Remover** *($30.50 for 8.4 ounces)*. Although this product is reasonably effective at removing most types of makeup, it isn't a gentle option in the least. That's because it contains fragrant plants that can cause irritation and salts that ideally shouldn't be used in a product that gets so close to the eyes. Add to this the cost and there's no reason to choose Gel Delicato over makeup removers from Almay, L'Oreal, Paula's Choice, or Neutrogena.

☹ **$$$ Effeto Immediato Spa Soothing Tonic for Sensitive Skin** *($29 for 8.4 ounces)* is a mixed bag. It includes some beneficial plant extracts and helpful skin-identical ingredients on the one hand, and irritating plants and fragrance on the other. Knowing this, and considering the steep price, it's easy to relegate this to the "why bother?" list. In addition, several of the ingredients in this toner are inappropriate for sensitive skin.

☹ **Tonico Minerale Stimulating Tonic** *($29 for 8.4 ounces)* does stimulate skin, but only by irritating it with alcohol and witch hazel distillate, which is the most concentrated form of extract from this plant. Alcohol serves only to stimulate free-radical damage, redness, and dry skin's surface as it increases oil production in the pore. Want more trouble? This product also causes further irritation and cell death because of the lavender and peppermint oils it contains.

☹ **Esfoliante Delicato Gentle Cleanser and Exfoliant** *($26 for 3.5 ounces)* is loaded with irritating, drying ingredients, including problematic detergent cleansing agents, and with numerous fragrant plant oils, including peppermint. It is absolutely not recommended. The few beneficial ingredients included are just rinsed down the drain. Labeling this "great for all skin types" is like suggesting cigarettes are great for all lungs!

☺ **$$$ Pelle Rinnovo Skin Renewal Polish** *($48.50 for 1.9 ounces)* is a standard, over-priced scrub that includes alumina as the abrasive agent, similar to what's used in professional microdermabrasion treatments. The alumina is buffered by olive oil and corn oil, which makes it somewhat less abrasive and suitable for normal to dry skin not prone to breakouts. Although this does manually exfoliate skin and can leave it feeling smooth and soft, it also can be difficult to rinse without the aid of a washcloth. Knowing this, you're better off exfoliating skin with your regular cleanser and a washcloth. Better still would be to apply a well-formulated AHA or BHA product on a regular basis because the research on the benefits of those two topical, leave-on exfoliants is extensive.

☺ **Intensivo Tonico Age Defying Facial Pads** *($51 for 30 pads)* are soaked in a toner-like solution said to offer antiaging benefits. The formula contains the AHA alternative gluconolactone, which can be helpful. However, it also contains the irritating menthol derivative menthyl lactate along with eucalyptus, which completely negates Borghese's claim that these pads are non-irritating. Those ingredients are exceptionally irritating, and irritation causes collagen to break down and hurts the skin's protective outer barrier. There are many effective AHA products to consider over this poor entry, such as those from Alpha Hydrox to NeoStrata and Paula's Choice.

☺ **Botanico Eye Compresses** *($51 for 60 compresses).* This rather ordinary, poorly formulated product is a toner-like solution steeped onto pads you're directed to place over your eyes to smooth, cool, and refresh this area. The second ingredient is witch hazel, a plant whose tannin content has a constricting effect on skin and whose alcohol content can cause irritation and free-radical damage. In other words, this isn't a pick-me-up for eyes or a way to reduce wrinkles. The pads contain some helpful plant extracts and skin-identical ingredients, but they are only an afterthought in comparison to the amount of witch hazel, and that combination isn't good for skin.

☺ **$$$ Complesso Intensivo Intensive Age Defying Complex** *($71.50 for 1.7 ounces)* is very similar to Borghese's Advanced Age-Defying Wrinkle Defense Serum, which is part of the company's line sold at Costco stores under the Kirkland Signature brand. The Costco version costs one-third the price of Borghese's main line serum, so there's no question which one you should buy, but there isn't much reason to buy either. This isn't the most sophisticated serum around because it contains only a few helpful ingredients, though it does include an impressive amount of vitamin C (ascorbic acid)—but skin needs more than a one-note product. It also contains two potentially problematic plant extracts: horsetail leaf and *Menyanthes trifoliata*. Neither is present in an amount that is cause for concern, but the formula would be better without them.

☺ **$$$ Crema Intensiva Intensive Firming Creme** *($76.50 for 1 ounce)* is a very standard emollient moisturizer for dry skin. It isn't any more intensive than lots of standard moisturizers at the drugstore because the good ingredients that are present won't remain stable due to the jar packaging. The "cellular complex" Borghese refers to is incapable of reversing skin laxity (sagging skin) and there's no proof to the contrary.

☺ **$$$ Crema Occhi Intensiva Intensive Eye Creme** *($66.50 for 0.5 ounce).* In some respects, this is a more elegant formula than Borghese's Crema Intensiva Intensive Firming Creme. However, it's not without its problems. Foremost is the jar packaging, which means the numerous antioxidants won't remain active once this product is open and in use. The formula also contains a few potentially irritating plant extracts as well, though they are less of a concern than the shortcoming of the jar packaging. What a shame; this product could do a lot for dry skin if the packaging were better.

☹ **Cura Di Vita Protettivo Protective Moisture SPF 15** *($44 for 1.7 ounces)* lacks the UVA-protecting ingredients of titanium dioxide, zinc oxide, avobenzone (also known as butyl methoxydibenzoylmethane), Tinosorb, or Mexoryl SX and is not recommended. It also contains far more fragrance than it does antiaging ingredients, which is a further disappointment.

☺ **$$$ Cura-C Anhydrous Vitamin C Face Treatment** *($67.50 for 1.7 ounces)*. We know that vitamin C, especially in the form of ascorbic acid, is a light- and air-sensitive ingredient (Source: *Critical Reviews in Food Science and Nutrition*, April 2009, pages 361-368). Why Borghese doesn't know this is a good question because the vitamin C present in this serum will become useless shortly after opening because of the jar packaging. It's also not good news that this serum-like moisturizer contains several fragrance chemicals known to cause irritation. Skinceuticals and MD Skincare by Dr. Dennis Gross offer much better and stably packaged products with vitamin C if that's the ingredient you're after.

☺ **$$$ Cura-C Vitamin C Eye Treatment** *($45 for 0.5 ounce)*. In contrast to Borghese's Cura-C Anhydrous Vitamin C Face Treatment, this nonaqueous product comes in opaque tube packaging and omits the fragrance chemicals that can cause irritation (a nice change of pace for Borghese). The silicone-based formula is wonderfully silky and contains stabilized vitamin C along with a beneficial plant oil. It also is fragrance-free, which all adds up to a good formula, but it is still a one-note product. Skin is a complex organ and requires far more than just vitamin C. Think about it like your diet; if you ate only oranges or took vitamin C supplements you wouldn't last very long.

☺ **$$$ CuraForte Moisture Intensifier** *($66.50 for 1.7 ounces)*. For the money, this moisturizer aimed at those with dry skin is a big letdown. It contains mostly water, silicone, slip agents, mineral oil, olive oil, and fragrance. That's hardly exciting and will leave your skin wanting more. The most exciting ingredients are listed after the fragrance, which is never a good sign. As for the claims—any moisturizer, even those that cost a fraction of the price, can increase skin's capacity to hold moisture by 200% as Borghese asserts. I would argue, however, that increasing skin's capacity to hold moisture by 200% would be a bad thing because healthy skin has only 30% water and adding more would cause skin cells to break down.

☹ **Dolce Notte Re-Energizing Night Creme** *($53.50 for 1.8 ounces)* is supposed to encourage cell turnover (i.e., to prompt exfoliation) while you sleep, but it doesn't contain a single ingredient capable of doing that. Instead, nestled in an exceptionally ordinary emollient base are several fragrant plant oils that cause irritation, which is not related to healthy, normal exfoliation. This pricey moisturizer is not recommended.

☺ **$$$ Energia Firming Wrinkle Cream** *($51.50 for 1.7 ounces)*. Once again, a very good moisturizer from Borghese is compromised due to the unfortunate choice of jar packaging. That means that for your money you're getting little more than standard emollients to help ease dry skin. It's depressing that such an antioxidant-rich formula won't remain potent for long. In better packaging, this moisturizer would be a slam dunk for those not put off by its price. As is, you should consider any of the well-packaged moisturizers from Estee Lauder, Clinique, Paula's Choice, or Cosmedicine before this.

☹ **Equilibrio Equalizing Restorative** *($44 for 1.7 ounces)* is not equalizing and the oil-free claim is misleading. It does contain some absorbent ingredients that have the ability to help control surface shine, but the effect is countered by the emollient thickeners that also are present, and which only make your skin feel more oily. The biggest offenders are the fragrant plant oils, which make Equilibrio Equalizing Restorative too irritating for all skin types (irritation stimulates the oil gland to make more oil).

✓ ☺ **$$$ Fluido Protettivo Advanced Spa Lift for Eyes** *($46.50 for 1 ounce)*. If this product is such an advanced way to lift aging skin around the eyes, why does Borghese sell so many other products making the same claims? Which one is the real deal? As it turns out, none of them are authentic choices if you're hoping wrinkles and sagging skin will become distant memories. But don't let that get you down—this is still a moisturizer worth considering. The fragrance-free formula is excellent for treating normal to dry skin to a host of intriguing ingredients, including several antioxidants, skin-identical substances, and cell-communicating ingredients. It is one of Borghese's best moisturizer formulas, and although it's marketed as an eye cream, you can use it anywhere on your face. This comes in a frosted glass bottle with a pump dispenser. Keep the bottle away from light sources to protect the integrity of the antioxidants.

☺ **$$$ Insta-Firm Advanced Wrinkle Relaxer** *($51 for 1 ounce)* is about as boring and ordinary as it gets. Almost any moisturizer at the drugstore in the $5 range would outdo this one. The big-deal ingredient in this lightweight, water-based serum is acetyl hexapeptide-3. Claims for this peptide are that it works like Botox, and it shows up in dozens of products claiming to relax expression lines; however, it doesn't work like that. Think of it this way: not even Botox works like Botox if it's rubbed on skin instead of injected into the muscles responsible for expression lines. Moreover, if this peptide really did reduce muscle contractions, it would do so regardless of where you applied it. For example, if you apply it with your fingers, it eventually would reduce muscle contractions in your fingers, too, which means you wouldn't be able to grip items or do everyday tasks such as typing or cooking. Luckily, that's not the case, but the implications are frightening!

☹ **Siero Intensivo Intensive Firming Serum** *($86.50 for 1.5 ounces)* contains some intriguing ingredients and has a moist, silky texture, but in many respects it's a real burn for both your skin and your pocketbook. A major ingredient in this formula is benzyl alcohol, a drying alcohol typically used in small amounts as part of a product's preservative system. In tiny amounts, it doesn't pose a problem for skin, but larger amounts, as is the case here, it can cause dryness, irritation, and free-radical damage (Sources: *Cutis*, July 2008, pages 75-77; and *Journal of Pharmaceutical Sciences*, October 2003, pages 2128-2139). The risk of irritation isn't worth it and there are plenty of other serums to consider that are beautifully formulated and free of needless irritants.

☹ **Splendide Mani Smoothing Hand Creme SPF 8** *($30.50 for 7 ounces)*. The SPF rating on this hand cream is embarrassingly low because your hands are constantly exposed to sun and need as much or more sun protection than any other part of the body. Even worse is that the active ingredient doesn't provide sufficient UVA protection. This also contains fragrant oils that will irritate skin—not what I'd consider a "splendide" choice!

BURT'S BEES

BURT'S BEES AT-A-GLANCE

Strengths: One good, non-irritating lip balm; budget-priced (it's always a letdown when you pay too much for lackluster and ineffective products); good lip gloss; complete ingredient lists for every product are available on the company's Web site.

Weaknesses: Pervasive use of irritating ingredients, all of which have documentation proving their problematic nature for skin (and lips); average to poor sunscreens; no effective antiblemish products; poor selection of cleansers; antioxidants sullied by reliance on jar packaging.

For more information about Burt's Bees, call (866) 422-8787 or visit www.burtsbees.com or www.Beautypedia.com.

BURT'S BEES NATURAL ACNE SOLUTIONS PRODUCTS

☺ **Natural Acne Solutions Purifying Gel Cleanser** *($10 for 5 ounces)* is a very good water-soluble cleanser for all skin types. The detergent cleansing agents are quite gentle and so are not especially adept at removing makeup, but those who wear minimal to no makeup won't find this to be an issue. The active ingredient is 1% salicylic acid, but its blemish-busting effect is limited when it's in a product that's quickly rinsed from skin. The salicylic acid isn't derived from willow bark as claimed, so this product shouldn't be construed as a natural alternative to other anti-acne cleansers. Willow bark contains salicin, a chemical that can be converted via enzymes into salicylic acid when ingested, but not when applied topically (Source: www.naturaldatabase.com). Including salicylic acid and willow bark in this product is a way to make a claim about natural effectiveness while including a synthetic ingredient that has all the research showing it has benefit for skin.

☹ **Natural Acne Solutions Pore Refining Scrub** *($10 for 4 ounces)*. This topical scrub is a mess on several counts. The main issue is that it contains several plant oils that are inappropriate for anyone struggling with blemishes. Secondary issues include the thick, creamy texture and the fact that it doesn't rinse without leaving a waxy film on skin (it really feels awful over oily areas). The active ingredient is salicylic acid, but it has minimal chance of being helpful due to this scrub's brief contact with skin (not to mention it has all those oils to work through before it can touch your skin). From any direction, this is a serious problem for blemish-prone skin, wrapped in the hope that going "natural" will take better care of you.

☹ **Natural Acne Solutions Daily Moisturizing Lotion** *($10 for 2 ounces)*. This lightweight lotion has an odor reminiscent of chlorine and citronella, so we're not off to a good start if your olfactory sense is especially acute. It's also a letdown that the main ingredient is sunflower oil, which someone with blemish-prone skin does not need—yet the company claims this product controls oil! How? By adding more? That's like telling an obese person they'll slim down by consuming more calories and not exercising! The theory that oily skin is producing too much oil because it needs more has no basis in fact. Skin makes oil because of androgens (male hormones).

Adding to the misinformation is the fact that this contains 1% salicylic acid as its active ingredient, a decidedly unnatural ingredient (so much for a natural solution for acne), but the pH of 5 prevents it from exfoliating skin or from affecting the bacteria that cause acne. Last, this has an unappealing waxy, tacky finish on skin that is far from representative of how today's best moisturizers (those with and without salicylic acid) feel.

☹ **Natural Acne Solutions Targeted Spot Treatment** *($10 for 0.26 ounce)*. This may contain several natural ingredients, but many of them are nothing more than an assault on skin that's already reddened and inflamed from acne. The main ingredient is alcohol, which not only is irritating but also stimulates oil production in the pore lining. (How ironic that it is indeed natural, but once again, natural as a skin-care category doesn't tell you anything about whether or not a product has benefit for your skin.) If that weren't bad enough, you're also getting a potent dose of lemon peel oil and lesser, but still problematic, amounts of other irritating plants, including eucalyptus. The only thing targeted about this product is the potential problems it will generate on your skin.

BURT'S BEES NATURALLY AGELESS PRODUCTS

☺ **Naturally Ageless Intensive Repairing Serum** *($25 for 0.5 ounce)* consists of a blend of oils, most of which are helpful for dry to very dry skin, but dry skin and wrinkles are not associated so the "ageless" claim is unwarranted. It is also mislabeled as a serum; it is really more an oil mix and the oils in this product are easily replaced by those available in any health food store, and then you won't have to risk irritation from the bitter-orange and rose oils this product contains.

☺ **Naturally Ageless Line Diminishing Day Lotion** *($25 for 2 ounces)* is an unsuitable choice for daytime unless your foundation contains a sunscreen rated SPF 15 or higher and you apply it evenly to your face. This moisturizer is an average option for normal to dry skin. The amount of antioxidant-rich pomegranate (supposedly "packed" into this formula) is less than the amount of denatured alcohol, which causes free-radical damage, dryness, and irritation.

☺ **Naturally Ageless Line Smoothing Eye Creme** *($25 for 0.5 ounce)* is an emollient moisturizer for dry skin, but one that's not advised for use around the eyes because the amount of alcohol it contains can be potentially irritating and drying. The formula overall is boring, lacking state-of-the-art ingredients, and the jar packaging won't keep the minimal amount of antioxidants in this product stable.

☺ **Naturally Ageless Skin Firming Night Creme** *($25 for 2 ounces)* wastes its few antioxidants because of the poor choice of jar packaging, which won't keep them stable. Otherwise, it's a basic, emollient moisturizer for normal to dry skin not prone to blemishes. The fact that it includes more denatured alcohol than it does state-of-the-art ingredients is disappointing at any price, and nothing about this moisturizer is skin-firming. This does contain fragrance.

OTHER BURT'S BEES SKIN-CARE PRODUCTS

☹ **All-In-One Wash** *($5 for 4 ounces)* is sold as a gentle formula suitable for cleansing face, hair, and body—yet this is as gentle for skin as exfoliating with sandpaper thanks to the inclusion of irritating fragrant oils including lime, peppermint, and spearmint.

☹ **Baby Bee Buttermilk Soap** *($5 for 3.5-ounce bar)* has some gentle ingredients, including oatmeal flour, but this is still standard-issue bar soap and is not recommended over cleansing baby's skin with a water-soluble, fragrance-free body wash.

☹ **Garden Carrot Complexion Soap** *($8 for 4-ounce bar)* is standard-issue bar soap that also contains irritating cinnamon powder, and is not recommended for any skin type.

☹ **Garden Tomato Complexion Soap** *($8 for 4-ounce bar)* has tomato powder but that's of little consequence in a drying bar soap, and lycopene (the red pigment in tomatoes) has no ability to balance skin's pH as claimed.

☹ **Lemon Poppy Seed Facial Cleanser** *($8 for 4 ounces)*. Lemons and poppy seeds make for good muffins, but adding lemon oil to a cleanser is only asking for trouble, and there's a significant amount of it in here, too.

☹ **Orange Essence Facial Cleanser** *($8 for 4.34 ounces)* has more than orange essence; it irritates skin with orange and rosemary oils and is not recommended. It isn't even a very good cleanser, making it a waste of time and money.

☹ **Poison Ivy Soap** *($8 for 2-ounce bar)* is standard, drying bar soap that adds irritation to its drying base thanks to pine tar and balsam leaf. Both will lessen the itch of poison ivy, but they do so as counter-irritants (meaning their stimulus is more irritating than the poison ivy itself).

⊗ **Soap Bark & Chamomile Deep Cleansing Cream** *($8 for 6 ounces)* contains several problematic ingredients for skin, especially for use around the eyes, and is not recommended.

⊗ **Garden Tomato Toner** *($12 for 8 ounces)* lists alcohol as the second ingredient, which makes this toner too drying and irritating for all skin types. The alcohol in this toner also serves to stimulate oil production in the pore.

⊗ **Rosewater & Glycerin Toner** *($12 for 8 ounces)* lists alcohol as the second ingredient, which makes this toner too drying and irritating for all skin types. The alcohol in this toner also serves to stimulate oil production in the pore.

⊗ **Citrus Facial Scrub** *($8 for 2 ounces)* is an inelegant scrub whose abrasive agents are composed of nutshells whose uneven shape can cause tiny tears in the skin during use (in contrast, perfectly rounded polyethylene beads polish skin without this effect). Although the nutshells aren't the best, they don't make this product a poor contender. What makes it a bad formula are the nutmeg and clove powders, which only serve to provide fragrance and irritate skin.

⊗ **Peach & Willowbark Deep Pore Scrub** *($8 for 4 ounces)* contains an appreciable amount of sodium borate. Also known as borax, this ingredient has a drying effect on skin due to its alkaline pH. It is fine in small amounts, but that's not the case here, making this a scrub to avoid.

☺ **Baby Bee Skin Creme** *($10 for 2 ounces)* is a basic, oil-based moisturizer for dry skin of any age, though its jar packaging compromises the stability of the antioxidant vitamin E.

☺ **Beeswax & Royal Jelly Eye Creme** *($15 for 0.25 ounce)* contains a tiny amount of royal bee jelly (in powder form), but this ingredient, despite tempting folklore, has no established benefit for skin. It can cause contact dermatitis, though the amount of it in this product likely negates that possibility (Source: www.naturaldatabase.com). This is otherwise a boring moisturizer consisting mostly of plant oil, glycerin, and beeswax. It's an OK option for dry skin anywhere on the face.

☺ **Beeswax Moisturizing Creme** *($15 for 2 ounces)* is described as a lightweight formula but it contains too much oil to make that claim a reality. This is a good, basic moisturizer for dry skin but definitely lacks state-of-the-art ingredients.

☺ **Beeswax Moisturizing Night Creme** *($15 for 1 ounce)* is primarily plant oil, water, wax, and aloe. It serves its purpose for dry skin, but also leaves skin wanting more.

⊗ **Carrot Nutritive Day Creme** *($15 for 2 ounces)* doesn't make sense for daytime because it lacks sun protection; it also contains enough balsam peru to cause irritation and has the potential to cause a phototoxic reaction due to its volatile components (Source: www.naturaldatabase.com).

☺ **Carrot Nutritive Night Creme** *($15 for 1 ounce)* contains a much smaller amount of balsam than the Carrot Nutritive Day Creme, but its jar packaging compromises the effectiveness of the antioxidant plant oils that compose the bulk of this moisturizer.

⊗ **Chemical-Free Sunscreen SPF 15** *($15 for 3.46 ounces)* leaves out synthetic sunscreen actives (though there's nothing wrong with those ingredients) and relies on titanium dioxide for sun protection. That's great, but the many fragrant volatile oils in this product are a considerable problem. Of particular concern is the balsam oil, which can cause a phototoxic reaction (Source: *The British Journal of Dermatology*, September 2002, pages 493-497).

☺ **Chemical-Free Sunscreen SPF 30** *($15 for 3.5 ounces).* The name of this product infuriates me because, technically, everything is a chemical. Every object, substance, and, yes, even natural ingredients, are composed of various chemicals. That's scientific fact, but I digress: labeling a skin-care product "chemical-free" is a strong hook for many consumers, and the word "chemical" sounds frightening to most. This sunscreen contains only titanium dioxide as the active ingredient, and comes in an emollient, oil-rich formula suitable for dry to very dry skin. The amount of fragrance is surprisingly high, and makes this mineral sunscreen a poor choice for sensitive skin. Without so much fragrance and minus the comfrey extract, this would earn a better rating.

☹ **Evening Primrose Overnight Creme** *($18 for 1 ounce)* has more problematic than beneficial oils for skin, including lavender, rose, and ylang-ylang. Otherwise it differs little from the Carrot Nutritive Night Creme above.

☹ **Marshmallow Vanishing Creme** *($18 for 1.5 ounces)* contains too many emollients to vanish immediately into skin as claimed. Although this has ingredients that are great for very dry skin, the rosemary oil makes it too irritating to consider over better formulations.

☹ **Radiance Day Creme** *($18 for 2 ounces)* contains several irritating or problematic ingredients, including comfrey, spearmint, and lemon oil. It is not recommended.

☺ **Radiance Day Lotion SPF 15** *($18 for 2 ounces).* This mineral sunscreen contains an effective blend of titanium dioxide and zinc oxide for broad-spectrum sun protection. The creamy, borderline greasy base formula is recommended only for dry skin not prone to blemishes. Royal jelly doesn't have miraculous benefits for skin, so just ignore the claims for this ingredient. It would be better for you if Burt's Bees had included some potent antioxidants, but this is really just an average moisturizer with sunscreen. By the way, this isn't an all-natural product, although it's fairly close if you want to stretch your definition of what constitutes natural.

☹ **Radiance Eye Creme** *($18 for 0.5 ounce)* contains the same offending ingredients as the Radiance Day Creme and is also not recommended. Using lemon oil around the eyes is never a good idea.

☹ **Radiance Night Creme** *($18 for 2 ounces)* contains the same offending ingredients as the Radiance Day Creme and is also not recommended.

☹ **Repair Serum** *($18 for 1 ounce)* won't repair skin but will damage skin cells due to its high content of lavender oil. Components in lavender oil have been shown to cause skin-cell death when applied topically (Source: *Cell Proliferation*, June 2004, pages 221-229).

☺ **Royal Jelly Eye Creme** *($18 for 0.5 ounce)* shares the same basic formula as most of the Burt's Bees moisturizers that combine a non-volatile plant oil with glycerin and beeswax to benefit dry skin. The amount of royal jelly is minuscule, but that's fine because it isn't a must-have ingredient for skin.

☹ **Pore-Refining Mask** *($8 for 1 ounce)* is just clay with fragrance and fragrant plant extracts, including peppermint. It has absorbent properties, but is too potentially irritating to make it worth considering over numerous other clay masks.

☹ **Doctor Burt's Herbal Blemish Stick** *($8.50 for 0.3 ounce)* proves without a doubt that Burt should stick to beekeeping instead of doctoring. With alcohol as the main ingredient and irritating fragrant oils of juniper, lemon, and eucalyptus, this only serves to make blemished skin look worse and to impede skin's healing process.

☺ **Doctor Burt's Res-Q Ointment** *($5.99 for 0.6 ounce)* is a rich, oil-based balm that contains some restorative ingredients for dry to very dry skin. The tiny amounts of fragrant plant extracts don't add to the benefit, but they're on target with the natural image this company espouses. The jar packaging hinders the antioxidant properties of the olive oil and vitamin E.

☹ **Aloe & Linden Flower After Sun Soother** *($10 for 6 ounces)* has more irritating than soothing properties for skin thanks to the comfrey extract and citrus oils it contains. Pure aloe vera gel would be a much better option.

☹ **Beeswax Lip Balm Tin** *($3 for 0.3 ounce)* is the company's most popular product, but it isn't one I'd recommend because it contains irritating peppermint oil.

☹ **Beeswax Lip Balm Tube** *($3 for 0.15 ounce)* is a waxy version of the Beeswax Lip Balm Tin, and also contains peppermint oil.

☺ **Honey Lip Balm** *($3 for 0.15 ounce)* is a shea butter–based lip balm that contains a nice array of ingredients to make dry, chapped lips look and feel better. The comfrey root is a minor cause for concern, so this is overall a very good lip moisturizer.

☹ **Lifeguard's Choice Weatherproofing Lip Balm** *($3 for 0.15 ounce)* contains peppermint oil, and the lifeguard who chooses this is in for lip irritation along with sun damage since this balm lacks active ingredients (the titanium dioxide is not listed as such).

☺ **Replenishing Lip Balm With Pomegranate Oil** *($3 for 0.15 ounce)* has pomegranate oil, which is great, and it has been reformulated to eliminate the plant irritants that kept it from earning a happy face rating. The reformulation is a good lip balm capable of taking care of chapped lips. Note: the ingredient list for this product matches what is on Burt's Bees current packaging for this lip balm. You may find different ingredient statements on the company's Web site. The company confirmed that the ingredient list on their site is inaccurate and will be updated.

BURT'S BEES MAKEUP

☹ **Lip Shimmers** *($5)* are sheer, glossy lipsticks that apply well but irritate lips with a potent mix of peppermint and rosemary oils.

☹ **Radiance Lip Shimmer** *($5)* is identical to Burt's Bees regular Lip Shimmer, except the Radiance versoin has a stronger shimmer. Neither product is recommended because they contain irritating peppermint and rosemary oils. Those ingredients are natural, but also proof that just because an ingredient is natural doesn't make it better for skin (or, in this case, lips).

✓ ☺ **Super Shiny Lip Gloss** *($7)*. This lip gloss in a tube has a simple, irritant-free formula that glides over lips, producing a soft gloss finish with subtle shimmer. Completely non-sticky, this is Burt's best gloss by far, and one of the better lip gloss options at the drugstore. The small shade range is sheer to translucent, so these work well alone for a hint of color or can be applied over just about any shade of lipstick.

CARGO (MAKEUP ONLY)

CARGO AT-A-GLANCE

Strengths: Some good foundations; excellent lip glosses; several bronzing options; great eyeshadow sets (though not every color combination is recommended); some high-performance mascaras; the liquid eyeliner; a handful of innovative products that nicely distinguish Cargo from other makeup lines.

Weaknesses: A few otherwise good products are marred by an abundance of fragrance; no foundations with sunscreen; limited selection of brushes; the Blu-Ray concealer isn't worth the money; standard to below-standard pencils and lipstick; several items are overpriced for what you get.

For more information about Cargo, call (416) 847-0700 or visit www.cargocosmetics.com or www.Beautypedia.com.

CARGO BLU-RAY PRODUCTS

☹ **Blu-Ray Concealer** *($28)*. You may be intrigued by this product because it promises to be a concealer and wrinkle eliminator in one package. (Doesn't that sound enticing?) Well, it certainly doesn't eliminate wrinkles, and you can test that for yourself by dabbing and blending this over any wrinkle on your face; the reality is it will look more pronounced with this concealer than without—makeup always has that effect, despite the industry's claims to the contrary. As a concealer, this is a subpar option that isn't worth the price, even if it were only $1. The thick-textured liquid is dispensed from a pen-style applicator onto an angled sponge tip. It provides moderate coverage, but also tends to look too obvious, plus it creases into lines and magnifies large pores. This isn't "high definition makeup" in the least! If anything, using this concealer instead of countless others is akin to tossing out your flat screen TV in favor of a black-and-white analogue set with a rabbit-ear antenna!

☺ **$$$ Blu-Ray Pressed Powder** *($30)*. The ingredients in this talc-based pressed powder differ little from those of most other pressed powders, so it is merely marketing finesse that this is called "high definition makeup." However, today's best powders in all price ranges offer the same benefits as this one—it will make your skin look polished and refined, even up close. The company offers only one shade, which they maintain works for all skin tones, but the depth of color and yellow tone work best for light to barely medium skin tones. Darker skin tones will not be happy with this, not in the least, because it can look off, particularly on fair and tan or deep complexions. This powder has a smooth, dry texture and sheer matte finish that melds well with skin, making it look dimensional rather than flat and powdered. That's great news, but there are many other powders that have risen to the top but that also offer more than one shade, and with a better price tag.

✓☺ **$$$ Blu-Ray Blush/Highlighter** *($24)*. Available in a single warm pink shade, this is a pressed-powder blush/highlighter. The solo shade is certainly limiting, but it's versatile enough to work for fair to medium skin tones. More blush than highlighter, the pink hue enlivens skin and has a gorgeous smooth finish that looks completely natural. The shine comes in the form of tiny gold particles, and they cling quite well to skin. This product's shine is understated enough that it is suitable for daytime wear.

☺ **$$$ Blu-Ray Bronzer** *($30)* has a superfine texture and silky application that lends itself to a natural-looking matte finish. The problem is that the single shade veers toward slightly orange (which is most apparent on lighter skin tones) and doesn't quite replicate a sun-kissed look. As for this being a high-definition product, it isn't at all distinctive from many other talc-based pressed bronzing powders I've reviewed favorably, but it certainly doesn't look too powdery or flat on skin.

☺ **$$$ Blu-Ray High Definition Lip Gloss** *($24)*. You're said to get "picture-perfect results" using this plumping lip gloss. A peptide is included, in the tiniest amount imaginable, for the plumping part, so those hoping for larger lips will be disappointed. But then, peptides in any amount have no effect on plumping lips, so it wouldn't happen even if a large amount were included. What can happen with this product is that your lips may swell slightly from the mint flavoring because mint can cause temporary irritation, which results in minor swelling. But, as is true with any lip gloss, lips look larger due to the light-reflective quality that glosses impart. You can test this yourself: examine your lips without gloss and then apply some—and you'll see they have a dimensional quality that makes them appear a bit larger. Getting past the high-definition marketing reveals this to be a thin-textured, slick lip gloss that has a non-sticky, wet-look shine. The shades are attractive—too bad the price isn't as enticing.

☺ $$$ **Blu-Ray Mascara** *($20)*. "Wow" is an apt word to describe the swift results this outstanding mascara provides. You apply it with a serrated comb rather than with a traditional nylon-bristle brush, and it quickly extends lashes to nearly ridiculous lengths. It is also easy to reach the base of the lashes for extra emphasis and depth, and clumps aren't an issue. You can build thickness with successive coats, but this mascara's primary strength is length, length, and more lash-fluttering length. In addition, it's easy to remove. With all this praise, you ask, why isn't this rated a Paula's Pick? In a word: fragrance. For inexplicable reasons, this mascara is strongly scented, and it is certainly not one to consider if you have sensitive, watery eyes. Most mascaras omit fragrance, or at least keep it subtle. I have no idea why Cargo added this much fragrance; it isn't even typical in French-formulated mascaras, and French companies use fragrance like water!

☺ $$$ **Blu-Ray High Definition Mattifier** *($24)* is a very good silicone-based cream that feels feather-light and sets to a silky matte finish that leaves a slight sheen. It isn't as absorbent as the mattifiers from Clinique or Smashbox, so someone with very oily skin will want to try those before Cargo's option. Despite the Blu-Ray name, this mattifier doesn't make skin more highly defined—pores and other minor flaws are still plainly visible. However, it works to keep mild to moderately oily skin in check and has a bit of benefit from a small amount of antioxidants. This product works well under foundation, too.

☺ $$$ **Blu-Ray Polishing Cloths** *($15 for 20 cloths)* are meant to be used with your facial cleanser (or alone) to exfoliate skin. They're sort of like a high-tech washcloth—each small, reusable cloth is composed of tiny microfibers that lightly abrade skin. In fact, these cloths are much gentler than most scrubs, but you can still overdo it if you're not careful. They work quite well to remove dead skin cells and traces of built-up makeup, leaving your skin smooth and polished. Consider this a clever alternative to scrubs and washcloths, but ignore the claim that using these "prevents blackheads and acne" because that won't happen; you can't scrub away blemishes or blackheads. In fact, trying to scrub away acne will only make matters worse.

CARGO PLANTLOVE PRODUCTS

☺ $$$ **PlantLove Loose Mineral Foundation** *($30)*. This mica- and cornstarch-based loose powder (cornstarch isn't a mineral, it's a food product) feels silky and slightly creamy. It applies smoothly and finishes matte with a hint of shine. You'll get sheer coverage and the range of shades is beautifully neutral for those with light to medium skin. This certainly is the least tidy method of applying foundation, and the packaging doesn't help control the potential mess. In terms of it being a natural origin product, the majority of the formula meets that claim. Some of the ingredients begin as natural sources, but are converted via chemical processes to become cosmetic ingredients (you wouldn't want to use them in their natural, raw state), but that's why Cargo uses the term "plant origin" instead of the term "all natural." This mineral powder foundation is best for normal to oily skin not prone to blemishes because the cornstarch and rice powder can feed the bacteria that trigger acne.

☺ $$$ **PlantLove Pressed Powder** *($30)* is a mica- and oil-based pressed powder with a slightly thick texture and an application that's heavier than that of most pressed powders. Best for normal to dry skin not prone to blemishes, it leaves a satin finish and comes in a small but workable range of shades. The formula is about as close as you can get to a pressed powder that remains easy to work with and is aesthetically pleasing.

☺ $$$ **PlantLove Blush** *($28)* is a standard pressed-powder blush with a smooth yet dry texture and soft application. The core ingredients show up in almost every powder blush being sold. Cargo added a selection of plant oils to make this sound as if it's a cut above the rest in the natural category, but it isn't. However, the oil content makes this blush ill-suited for those with oily, breakout-prone skin. The pastel and rose tones are enticing, and all shades except Rose have varying degrees of shine.

☺ $$$ **PlantLove Baked Bronzer** *($28)* has a texture that's drier than usual, which hinders getting the stuff on evenly. This is full of natural ingredients, but the core ingredients are commonly found in pressed powders throughout the cosmetics industry. Cargo just added some plant ingredients to go along with the theme for this sub-brand. One more thing: the sole shade isn't bronze or capable of mimicking a tan; it's a rosy tan shade that most women will prefer as blush.

☺ $$$ **PlantLove Eye Shadow** *($20)* is marketed as being inspired by nature for its formula as well as its, um, colorful colors. If you can look past the blues, purples, and green shades, you'll find some attractive brown tones as well as soft mauves, golds, and peach tones. These powder eyeshadows have a dry, powdery texture that is the result of being pressed so softly, but they blend well if applied in sheer layers. The core ingredients are the same ones that show up in most powder eyeshadows. Cargo added some plant ingredients to go along with this sub-brand's theme, but there is nothing more plant-like about these eyeshadows than there is about any other cosmetic brand's eyeshadows.

☹ $$$ **PlantLove 100% Natural Origin Eye Pencil** *($16)*. This slightly creamy eye pencil is easy to apply and sets quickly to a long-wearing finish that resists smearing or fading. If it did not require routine sharpening, it would've earned a happy face rating. Avoid the Khaki shade; it's too green.

☹ $$$ **PlantLove Botanical Lipstick** *($20)*. Get this: the outer paper carton of this lipstick is made of flowers that have been pressed into paper and embedded with seeds. Instead of discarding the packaging, you can plant it and, with standard care, flowers will grow. Now that's environmentally friendly! Cargo claims the lipstick itself is made entirely of corn, but a quick glance at the ingredient list disproves that claim; corn can do many things, but you can't turn corn into sunflower, apricot, or jojoba oils. This lipstick is composed almost entirely of plant oils and natural waxes, so it ought to appeal to anyone seeking to avoid synthetic ingredients. Unfortunately, this happens to be one of the greasiest lipsticks around. It practically slides right off your lips and onto your face. The shimmer-infused colors are mostly pretty pastels and vivid brights, but this lipstick travels into lines around the mouth immediately and wears away almost as fast. The plants are plentiful and the packaging concept admirable, but you're buying lipstick for its overall performance on your lips, right?

☹ **PlantLove Lip Gloss** *($20)* is a castor oil-based gloss that comes in a tube with a wand applicator. Most glosses don't contain castor oil as a main ingredient (it's more common with lipsticks), but I suspect that's what gives this such a rancid odor. Every tester I tried at our local Sephora store had the same "off" smell, and the testers were fresh; the PlantLove line had been on display for only about a week. This gloss contains fragrance, too, so the rancid odor was even strong enough to get past the added perfume.

☺ **$$$ PlantLove Lip Liner** *($16)* is a very standard creamy lip pencil that demands routine sharpening to keep its point. The oil-based formula doesn't stay in place as well as silicone- or wax-based lipliners, so expect fading and, potentially, smearing, especially if you combine this with a greasy lipstick or slick lip gloss.

☹ **PlantLove Lip Balm** *($20)*. This emollient, waxy lip balm has what it takes to protect lips from dryness and chapping. The majority of the formula is natural, too, so Cargo isn't far from the truth with its claims. Of concern is the inclusion of bergamot oil, a citrus plant oil that contains a constituent known as bergapten, which can cause a phototoxic reaction when lips are exposed to sunlight. Considering you can get this lip balm's best qualities from many other products that omit bergamot oil, this one isn't worth the risk.

☹ **PlantLove Baked Illuminator** *($28)*. This marbleized pressed powder with shimmer is a mess. It's a mess to apply, the swirled colors tend to look splotchy on skin, and the finish is somehow dull rather than illuminating. Sephora (where Cargo is primarily sold) sells lots of pressed shimmer powders that handily outperform this one. By the way, the only thing that makes this product plant-like is the addition of some plant oils, none of which are exclusive to this product.

OTHER CARGO MAKEUP PRODUCTS

FOUNDATION: ✓ ☺ **One Base Concealer + Foundation in One** *($24)* comes packaged in a tube with an angled sponge-tip applicator wand affixed. It feels light and silky and is easy to blend over a small area. It sets to a satin matte finish that looks believably natural and stays in place well. Coverage is light to medium, so it's not quite up to the level of the camouflage you'd get from a typical concealer. However, if you don't need significant coverage and are simply try-ing to mask minor flaws or redness, this works really well. One Base works as either foundation or concealer, but ideally you'd want to use a foundation that matches your skin exactly and a concealer that's a shade or two lighter. The available shades are quite good; only 03 should be considered carefully due to its slight peach cast.

☺ **$$$ Wet/Dry Foundation** *($32)*. This pressed-powder foundation has the requisite smooth texture and an even, sheer application to provide a soft matte finish. The emollient ingredients make it best for normal to dry skin; those with oily areas will find it doesn't control shine all that well. Almost all of the shades are exemplary, particularly for those with fair to medium skin tones. Shade 70 will be too gold for many medium skin tones, but is still worth considering. Avoid the darkest shades (80 and 90) because both are slightly ash, despite an impressive depth of pigment.

☹ **$$$ Foundation, Oil-Free** *($32)*. The packaging for this creamy liquid foundation leaves much to be desired; instead of packaging it in a standard squeeze tube or plastic bottle, Cargo opted to put it in a soft plastic bag, sort of like a medical IV drip bag, but prettier. Because the bag is soft, it's very easy to dispense much more foundation than you need, and there's no put-ting it back. What were the marketing people thinking? Packaging aside, this foundation has a couple of other significant drawbacks: it can look a bit too noticeable on skin (keep in mind that I'm comparing its appearance with today's best foundations—and at this price you should expect no less) and it is intensely fragranced. In fact, this contains several fragrance chemicals that can cause irritation, which is a serious ding when you consider that most foundations omit such ingredients. If you decide to try this anyway, the formula and matte finish are best for normal to oily skin. Foundation, Oil-Free provides medium coverage and is relatively easy to blend. Among the shades, consider F30 carefully and avoid F60 and F80—whose skin is this peach? Shades F90 and F100 are beautiful for deeper African-American skin.

POWDER: ☹ **$$$ Liquid Powder** *($22)* claims to provide the effect of loose powder with the convenience of a tube. Liquid Powder shouldn't replace anyone's traditional loose or pressed powder, and those with oily skin will note that the sparkles make their oily areas look greasier. This is an OK option if you want a sheer shine product that has a matte (in feel) finish. Otherwise, don't bother.

BLUSH AND BRONZER: ✓ ☺ **$$$ Multi-Mix Bronzer** *($28)*. I was instantly impressed with this lightweight, fragrance-free bronzing gel. The water-based formula is easy to apply and you have enough time to blend it accurately before it sets. Color-wise, you get a sheer, golden tan with a faint hint of shine. It is one of the best bronzing gels around, and suitable for all skin types. Special note: this formula doesn't make large pores look dotted with color, though generally speaking anyone with large pores and oily skin should stick with bronzing powders.

☺ **$$$ BeachBlush** *($26)* presents four stripes of colors that produce one uniform shade when blended together. It has a beautifully smooth texture and even application, but the amount of shine makes it a tricky choice for daytime wear (and a must-avoid if you have oily skin and don't want it to look oilier). The range of shades includes options for fair to medium skin tones.

☺ **$$$ Blush** *($24)*. Blush is one of the key items Cargo is known for, and it's not hard to see why. Their powder blushes have an enviably smooth, almost creamy texture that's easy to apply and meshes well with skin. The only drawback is shine, which most of the shades have in spades. The shiny shades are too distracting for daytime wear, but are a workable option for evening makeup. The best daytime shades are Catalina, Prague, and Tonga. Of course, you know that Rimmel, Sonia Kashuk, Almay, and everyone in between at the drugstore have gorgeous options for one-quarter the price.

☺ **$$$ Bronzer** *($25)* is an incredibly smooth, almost creamy-feeling pressed bronzing powder that is a breeze to apply. The colors resemble various degrees of tan skin, but almost all of them are waylaid by an abundance of shimmer. The amount of shimmer limits their use, at least in terms of day-to-day professional makeup, but this bronzer is fine for evening or special-occasion makeup when all systems are "go" for maximum shimmer. Those looking for a bronzed finish with minimal shine should consider Medium Matte.

☺ **$$$ SuedeBlush** *($24)*. This talc-based pressed-powder blush has an even smoother, lighter texture than Cargo's regular Blush and BeachBlush, but the marbleized colors really up the ante in terms of shine. You actually get more shine than color from this blush, and the strong, almost metallic-looking shimmer is overpowering for daytime makeup (or natural lighting). As with most of the shiny blushes that apply and wear as well as this one, it's best reserved for evening wear and best avoided altogether if you have oily skin.

☺ **$$$ The Big Bronzer** *($32)* is Cargo's answer to the question of how to improve on their original pressed powder bronzer. Making it bigger was as creative as they got, along with a really sleek, snazzy compact with a mirror. The golden tan color of this suede-smooth bronzing powder is beautiful. However, the strong shimmer finish it has won't make anyone think you've gotten your tan from the sun. Application is flawless and it layers expertly for more color (and shine), but the effect this bronzing powder has is best reserved for evening or special-occasion makeup. It works well to highlight the décolleté, but keep in mind that this powder will come off on clothing. Note that the formula for The Big Bronzer is slightly different from that of Cargo's original Bronzer.

☺ **$$$ Matte BeachBlush** *($26)* is a powder blush that's available in one color, and it's a collection of four stripes (deep peach, apricot, bronze, and golden tan) in one tin. Sweeping a blush brush over these stripes results in one uniform color on skin, a soft, fleshy peach. It is matte as claimed, but the result isn't as blush-like as it should be. In fact, the color won't show up well on medium to dark skin tones and can make some lighter skin tones look drab.

EYESHADOW: ✓☺ **$$$ Essential Eyeshadow Palette** *($32)*. Now this is how to assemble an eyeshadow collection! Arranged in a large compact are four complementary shades of ultra-smooth powder eyeshadow. Each shade is cleverly marked to indicate where it should be placed (e.g., brow bone, lid) and although you don't have to follow those guidelines, novices will appreciate the help. Each shade is a pleasure to blend and applies softly, yet is buildable for those who desire more intensity. There are no 100% matte shades; instead, you'll find each has some amount of shine, with the majority defaulting to low-glow shimmer. All of the sets are highly recommended; the darkest shade in each works great used with a damp eyeliner brush.

☺ **$$$ EyeBase** *($20)* is meant as a primer for eyeshadow. The pen-style component is outfitted with a synthetic brush applicator that dispenses a lightweight concealer. It provides sheer to light coverage and sets to a tenacious matte finish. You will find that eyeshadows apply easily and last longer using this product, but the same statement is true if you prep your eyelids with a good matte-finish concealer. EyeBase works well, but most will find it superfluous. The single shade is a soft peach that looks best on light to medium skin tones.

☹ **$$$ EyeBronzer** *($22)*. Housed in an inkwell-style package, you apply this loose-powder eyeshadow with a pointed sponge tip that picks up more color every time you plunge it into the base to recap. The mica-based powder is very shiny and has a texture that glides over skin with minimal flaking. The color is golden peach, not bronze, and as such its appeal is limited.

☺ **$$$ EyeLighter** *($17)* is a dual-sided pencil-like product that houses a shimmery powder eyeshadow in both ends. Both ends are equipped with a sponge-tip applicator to apply powder to the inner and outer corners of the eye. The goal is to widen and brighten the eyes with strategic placement of shimmer, a makeup trick you see on countless magazine covers. Cargo states that one of the two powders is matte, but both are shiny. One is shinier than the other, but the less shiny shade doesn't pass for matte by any standard—well, except for Cargo's. The sponge tips make it easy to apply powder to the corners of the eye, and the effect, while not subtle, definitely adds sparkle to the eyes. All three shades (white, gold, and pink) are workable, with gold being the most flattering.

☹ **$$$ Color Eyeshadow Palette** *($28)*. Color is definitely the name of the game for these pressed-powder eyeshadow palettes! From the colorful packaging to the mostly odd mix of shades inside these quad sets, you're given few choices to successfully shape and shade the eye. The eyeshadows themselves have a fairly smooth, dry texture and unusually sheer application/color deposit. They blend well and the shine in each shade clings well enough. But among the many quads, the only workable ones are Baja, Bermuda, and Shanghai; the others are too colorful or contrasting to make the purchase a safe bet.

EYE AND BROW SHAPER: ✓☺ **$$$ Liquid Liner** *($22)* happens to be one of the best, easiest-to-use liquid liners you're likely to find. Packaged like a felt-tip pen, the applicator has a narrow point so you can get an ultra-thin line. Alternatively, you can use the side of the brush for a thicker line. In either case, application is even and pigment-rich, the formula dries quickly, and it stays in place exceptionally well. Only one shade is available, but unless you have very pale skin, you can't go wrong with classic black!

☺ **$$$ SmokyEye Eyeliner Duo** *($28)*. Looking to create a sultry, smoky eye but don't know where to start? This kit may be your solution. It includes tone-on-tone shades of a cream-to-powder and powder eyeshadow, both of which have shine, although the shine is not over the top. Smoky eyes demand precise, controlled application to the lid and just above the eye's crease. Each product in this kit has minimal slip but is still blendable. You apply the cream-to-powder shadow first, and then top with the powder shadow for added intensity and long-lasting results. The best duos are Budapest, Katmandu, and Brazil. Skye and Barcelona are not recommended unless you want an unnaturally colorful interpretation of a smoky eye design.

☹ **$$$ High Pigment Eye Pencil** *($16)*. These standard pencils are standard only because they require routine sharpening and because the pigment they deposit isn't much greater than what's typical. Where these excel is in their ultra-smooth application and soft powder finish, which remains smudge- and smear-proof unless you have oily eyelids, in which case you're better off using silicone-enhanced gel eyeliners. If you're OK with routine sharpening, these are recommended. But you should know there are automatic pencils at the drugstore that cost less and perform just as well, such as Cover Girl Outlast. Note: the Brown shade is laced with shine.

☹ **$$$ Wet/Dry Eyelining Palette** *($32)*. Assembled in a sleek compact no bigger than a credit card are eight shades of powder eyeshadow meant for eyelining. Two of the eight shades are bold blue hues, while another is bright purple; none of these three is recommended as an eyeliner. The remaining shades are variations on brown and black, and work great as eyeliner. The powders have a dry texture that isn't as easy to work with as it should be, although they're still workable. Dry application is sheer and somewhat muddy looking; wet application looks better and is preferred.

LIPSTICK, LIP GLOSS, AND LIPLINER: ✓ ☺ **$$$ Classic Lip Gloss** *($22)* has a luxuriously smooth texture and a moist finish that takes excellent care of your lips while imparting sheer, glossy color. The colors look imposing when viewed in their clear packaging (equipped with an applicator wand), but they apply nearly translucent and lack even a hint of stickiness. Another well-executed lip gloss from Cargo!

✓ ☺ **$$$ High Intensity Gloss** *($22)* is an excellent brush-on lip gloss whose colors have more intensity than standard glosses but not as much intensity as a regular lipstick. Overall results are still on the sheer side, so this is fine for the color-shy. The smooth texture moisturizes without feeling too slippery, while the glossy finish doesn't leave a trace of stickiness.

✓ ☺ **Lip Gloss Duo** *($14)* has a liquid-cream, minimally sticky texture that feels great on the lips. Each generous tin features two shades and the duos are mostly beautiful. You're definitely getting your money's worth with generously sized portions of two complementary shades!

✓ ☺ **$$$ Lip Gloss Quad** *($16.80)*. If you love Cargo's classic tin-packaged Lip Gloss Duo, you'll also appreciate having four shades in one tin. Each sheer color is separated by a divider, and they have the same liquid-cream texture and super-smooth, non-sticky finish. The color combinations are great; all have a glossy finish and some shades add shimmer to the mix for a heightened effect.

☺ **Daily Gloss** *($12)*. If you find the concept of jar-packaged lip gloss unhygienic, then you can consider DailyGloss, where you get 30 individually wrapped applications of gloss (packaged like pills in a foil blister pack) along with a disposable lip brush. Each set of gloss offers three shades so you can change things up each day. The concept is gimmicky and more inconvenient than useful, but the gloss inside is great due to its ultra-smooth texture and non-sticky finish.

The Reviews C

☺ **Lip Pencil** *($14)*. Available in only two shades, this needs-sharpening lip pencil is neither too dry nor too creamy. It applies well and then blends well if you desire to soften the line. For the money, this isn't worth considering over less expensive pencils at the drugstore that don't require routine sharpening.

☺ **Reverse Lipliner** *($14)*. Cargo makes much ado about this needs-sharpening pencil, but the fuss is all posturing; this is truly a lackluster product to say the least. It's claimed to add definition and fullness to the lip line while also being perfectly suited to pair with any lip gloss. It is supposed to lock gloss color in place and prevent feathering, but this palm oil–based pencil does neither. Two flesh-toned shades are available. You're supposed to apply this outside your natural lip line to create an "invisible" border around the mouth, but unless your skin matches one of the pencils, the line won't be invisible. Lip glosses will slip right past this pencil, making things only slightly better than if you didn't use a liner at all. Still, there are better pencils to consider if you're prone to lipstick feathering into lines around the mouth.

MASCARA: ☺ **$$$ SupersEyes Mascara** *($18)*. The name of this mascara conjures up images of large, fluttering lashes that are beautifully thickened and ready to be noticed. The results don't quite measure up to the expectations, but it's still a good mascara. The dual-sided brush allows for even, clump-free application that produces good length and a modest amount of thickness, primarily at the roots of the lashes. This wears well and removes easily, but its performance doesn't propel it to Paula's Pick status.

☺ **$$$ TexasLash Mascara** *($20)*. The name for this large-brushed mascara is enticing, but the results aren't going to be as vast and expansive as the state of Texas. If anything, the large brush is tricky to work with, especially for the small lashes at the eye's inner corner. With patience you'll get good length and moderate thickness, but nothing that makes this a must-have. It wears well without flaking and is easy to remove, yet the price and less-than-outstanding results won't make you want to do the Texas Two-Step!

☺ **$$$ Better Than Waterproof Mascara** *($20)*. The name for this mascara is tied to Cargo's claims that it technically isn't waterproof mascara, but wears like one so you don't have to worry about lashes getting wet or moisture causing the formula to smear. If you find that confusing, don't worry, it is confusing and just false. It isn't better than waterproof, it just isn't waterproof, it's water soluble. The claim is just silly. This easily comes off with plain water and gentle pressure. As a regular mascara (which is all it is) the application is initially too heavy but it can be thinned out easily enough, resulting in modestly long lashes with a hint of thickness. The formula is heavy on film-forming agents, so lashes tend to get stuck together more than they do with a wax-based mascara formula. The film-formers also make lashes feel dry and slightly stiff.

BRUSHES: ☺ **Eyelining Brush** *($18)*. This long-handled brush has an angled head composed of natural hair. It works for eyelining if you don't want a thin line, but its density makes it best suited for filling in and shaping eyebrows. This is a good choice if you're in need of a high-performance, reasonably priced eyebrow brush.

☺ **$$$ SmokyEye Brush** *($32)*. This firm-yet-flexible natural-hair eyeshadow brush is designed to make it easy to create the classic smoky eye. It works well, but depending on your preference and technique, lots of eyeshadow brushes can be used for this purpose. The unique handle of this brush makes it easy to hold, but its chunky, weighted design means it won't fit into most brush rolls. The tip of SmokyEye Brush works well to apply a wider swatch of powder eyeshadow along the lash line.

☺ **Covered Lip Brush** *($17)* comes equipped with a cap, a feature many lip brushes lack. The bristles are synthetic and are great for applying lipstick or gloss. The problem is that the brush has a squared tip cut straight across, so it doesn't hug the contours of the lips (or the mouth's corners) as well as a rounded or pointed lip brush. Most will find this brush too difficult to work with.

☹ $$$ **Essential Brush Kit** *($32)* is deceptively named because it omits many truly essential brushes. All you get are two dual-sided eyeshadow brushes tucked in a small clutch bag. The brushes are functional and, for the most part, shaped well, and the price isn't bad either. But this is worth considering only if you need a travel set of small eyeshadow brushes and are willing to pack your other brushes (e.g., powder, blush, lipstick, concealer) separately.

SPECIALTY PRODUCTS: ☹ **Lash Activator** *($35)* is supposed to promote "lash vitality," whatever that's supposed to mean. It is said to contain special ingredients that result in better-looking lashes. The thing is, because this product is essentially a thinly disguised mascara, that claim is true. Applying this does result in lashes that look better. But you can get even better results for a lot less money from countless other mascaras. There is nothing in Lash Activator that gives it an edge over standard mascaras. The so-called special ingredients are barely present. At best, this is just an average mascara. It can be applied over other mascaras without much trouble, but really, why bother?

CAUDALIE PARIS (SKIN CARE ONLY)

CAUDALIE PARIS AT-A-GLANCE

Strengths: Good cleansers; an excellent scrub for dry skin; airtight packaging; a good lip balm and moisturizing mask; one truly state-of-the-art moisturizer for dry skin (one is better than none).

Weaknesses: Expensive; mundane to irritating serums, moisturizers, and eye creams; limited sun protection options; no AHA or BHA products; no products to lighten skin discolorations; several products contain irritating plant extracts.

For more information about Caudalie Paris, call (866) 826-1615 or visit www.caudalie.com or www.Beautypedia.com.

CAUDALIE PARIS PULPE VITAMINEE PRODUCTS

☺ $$$ **Pulpe Vitaminee Energizing Cream, for Normal to Dry Skin** *($55 for 1.3 ounces)* is more impressive than most of Caudalie's moisturizers, and is a good option for normal to slightly dry skin not prone to blemishes. Skin is treated to lightweight emollients, plant oils, and a decent blend of antioxidant plant extracts. This contains a small amount of fragrance components that may prove irritating.

☺ $$$ **Pulpe Vitaminee Energizing Fluid, for Normal to Combination Skin** *($55 for 1.3 ounces)* is a lighter, thinner-textured version of Caudalie's Pulpe Vitaminee Energizing Cream, for Normal to Dry Skin. This version is indeed preferred for normal to combination skin that's slightly oily. Contrary to claim, however, this is not "remarkably effective" at reducing sagging skin; in fact, it cannot affect sagging in the least. Skin-care products cannot affect the physiological reasons behind sagging skin, plus this contains no sun protection.

CAUDALIE PARIS VINEXPERT PRODUCTS

☺ **$$$ Vinexpert Anti-Ageing Serum Eyes and Lips, For Skin Lacking Vitality** *($70 for 0.5 ounce)* is terribly overpriced and is actually a nearly do-nothing water-based serum for normal to slightly oily skin. The amount of witch hazel is potentially irritating, and all of the intriguing ingredients are listed after the preservative. Nothing in this serum can diminish puffiness or dark circles, either.

☺ **$$$ Vinexpert Firming Serum, For Skin Lacking Vitality** *($79 for 1 ounce)* has a barely discernible tightening effect on skin; however, the effect is only temporary, and strictly cosmetic. This is otherwise an embarrassingly overpriced water-based serum whose bitter-orange and rose flower water can cause irritation. Very few ingredients beneficial for skin are included (though I have no clue what ingredients skin needs for vitality; what does "Skin Lacking Vitality" mean anyway?), but this serum is not a total waste of money.

☺ **$$$ Vinexpert Night Infusion Cream, for Skin Lacking Vitality** *($68 for 1 ounce)* is a lightweight cream moisturizer for normal to dry skin, but its regenerating action is limited unless you believe that grape seed oil is the only antioxidant to seek. It's a worthwhile ingredient for skin, but its effect in this product is likely offset by the amount of fragrance and the potentially irritating fragrance components it contains. I can think of much better products for skin, including several products from Olay, Clinique, and Estee Lauder.

☹ **Vinexpert Radiance Day Fluid SPF 8, For Skin Lacking Vitality** *($68 for 1 ounce)* is described as a sunscreen, but for this amount of money, and given the low SPF number (SPF 15 is the minimum recommended by the American Academy of Dermatology and the Skin Cancer Foundation) and the lack of active ingredients listed, you have to wonder whether the executives spent too much time swigging wine and not enough time researching what sunscreen needs to do. Hint: The purpose of sunscreen is not to make your skin smell like a floral vineyard!

CAUDALIE PARIS VINOPERFECT PRODUCTS

☺ **$$$ Vinoperfect Day Perfecting Cream SPF 15, For All Skin Types** *($68 for 1 ounce)* provides UVA protection with an in-part avobenzone sunscreen, and is formulated in a lightweight cream base ideal for normal to dry skin. (Someone with oily skin will find this too heavy, so the "all skin types" designation should be ignored.) This contains a smattering of antioxidants and interesting water-binding agents, but is not rated a Paula's Pick because most of the really intriguing ingredients are listed after the fragrance.

☺ **$$$ Vinoperfect Night Correcting Cream, for All Skin Types** *($68 for 1 ounce)* claims to work overnight at diminishing dark spots and tightening pores, yet the ingredients in this cream show up in almost all of Caudalie's other moisturizers, which seems to mean that they do all those other things, too, right? Wrong! This standard, overpriced moisturizer for normal to dry skin contains nothing that can fade the faintest freckle, nor can it tighten pores (triglycerides and shea butter are not what pores need if they are clogged or engorged with too much oil). The tartaric and malic acids are present in amounts too low for them to function as AHAs, and the pH of 4.4 wouldn't permit exfoliation anyway.

☺ **$$$ Vinoperfect Radiance Serum, for Skin Lacking Vitality** *($79 for 1 ounce)* has such an average formulation that the price just seems to be in bad taste. This contains mostly water, slip agents, emollient, thickener, vitamin E, plant extracts, fragrance, and film-forming agent. The small amount of grape extract means that this product likely has minimal antioxidant ability—and what about skin-identical substances, cell-communicating ingredients, or an anti-irritant or two? All of those are hallmarks of state-of-the-art serums, which this product certainly is not.

✓ ☺ $$$ **Vinoperfect Radiance Revealing Mask** *($42 for 1.3 ounces)*. Although overpriced, this is a very good moisturizing mask for dry to very dry skin. It contains an impressive amount of antioxidant-rich grape seed oil, and should ideally be left on skin overnight rather than rinsed off after 10 minutes. The applicator brush helps exfoliate skin as you apply the mask. There are some AHA ingredients in this mask, but none of them are present in the amounts needed to ensure exfoliation.

CAUDALIE PARIS VINOPURE PRODUCTS

☺ $$$ **Vinopure Matte Finish Fluid, For Combination Skin** *($49 for 1.3 ounces)* contains a frustrating combination of beneficial and irritating ingredients for its intended skin type. The sage leaf water doesn't get this off to a great start because sage can be a skin irritant. This is an OK moisturizing fluid with some good antioxidants, but it absolutely cannot regulate oil production. Its texture and finish are soft matte, and it works well under makeup; however, the matte feel doesn't have any effect on what's happening in your skin's oil glands.

☹ **Vinopure Purifying Concentrate, For Combination Skin** *($39 for 0.5 ounce)* irritates skin with lemon, balm mint, and eucalyptus oils—none of which can work "deep down to balance combination skin," though it can hurt your skin's healing process and work against collagen production. Avoid this product unless your goal is to create skin problems rather than find solutions.

☹ **Vinopure Purifying Mask, for Combination Skin** *($40 for 1.6 ounces)* is a standard clay mask wrapped up in one of the longest ingredient lists you're likely to see. The odd mix of absorbents and emollient, oily, or wax-based thickeners is bound to be confusing for your skin. Contrary to the claim, this mask cannot regulate oil production, something that is controlled by hormones and not affected by products like this. Moreover, the bergamot, lavender, clary, and sandalwood oils are all irritating for any skin type.

CAUDALIE PARIS VINOSOURCE PRODUCTS

☺ $$$ **Vinosource Anti-Wrinkle Nourishing Cream** *($49 for 1.3 ounces)* impresses with its lightweight yet creamy texture and antioxidant-rich formula, which is also imbued with other helpful ingredients for dry skin, including borage oil, olive esters, and glycerin. Although not quite on par with today's best moisturizers, it is one of the better formulas from Caudalie and, like all of their moisturizers, the opaque tube packaging will help keep the antioxidants stable during use.

☹ **Vinosource Moisturizing Concentrate, For Dry Skin** *($39 for 0.5 ounce)* contains rosewood and palmarosa oils along with other fragrant irritants such as eugenol, limonene, and citral. None of these are suitable for dry skin; you'd be better off applying pure grape seed oil or jojoba oil instead to treat dry skin, instead of wasting your money on this product.

✓ ☺ $$$ **Vinosource Riche Anti-Wrinkle Ultra Nourishing Cream** *($50 for 1.3 ounces)* is an even better formula than Caudalie's impressive Vinosource Anti-Wrinkle Nourishing Cream above. This version ups the ante with more emollients and a greater amount of antioxidants, plus some cell-communicating ingredients. It is an excellent, albeit pricey, moisturizer for dry to very dry skin. Although this contains fragrance, it does not contain the potentially sensitizing fragrance components that are present in many other Caudalie moisturizers.

☺ **$$$ Vinosource Moisturizing Cream-Mask Face and Eyes, for Dry Skin** *($40 for 1.6 ounces)* is a glycerin-rich mask for dry skin, and supplies an impressive amount of antioxidant grape seed oil, which makes this a decent option for skin.

OTHER CAUDALIE SKIN-CARE PRODUCTS

☺ **$$$ Cleansing Water Face and Eyes, For All Skin Types** *($12 for 3.4 ounces)* is a very standard liquid makeup remover that contains a tiny amount of oil and a soothing agent. It works as well as any, but isn't as adept at removing waterproof formulas as are makeup removers that contain silicone or more oil than this one. Their claim about "micelle" water being able to capture dirt like tiny magnets is true, but that is true of any detergent-based makeup remover. Micelle technology is simply one way of explaining how a detergent cleansing agent combines with water and interacts with oils to clean any surface, including skin. That technology is not by any means unique to this product.

☺ **$$$ Gentle Cleanser Face and Eyes, For Normal To Dry Skin** *($26 for 6.7 ounces)* would be better classified as "gentle" if it didn't contain fragrance, but it is still an effective, detergent-free cleansing lotion for normal to dry skin not prone to blemishes. It will remove makeup and rinses fairly well, though you may find you need a washcloth for complete removal. This cleanser does not protect your skin from free radicals—that is impossible. Even to come close to achieving that, you'd have to be in an environment without oxygen, which would mean you couldn't breathe, and that wouldn't be good! There isn't any product anywhere that can stop free-radical damage; at best we can only reduce the impact. Further, in a cleanser, any ingredient that is going to provide any protection from free radicals is just rinsed down the drain.

☺ **$$$ Instant Foaming Cleanser** *($26 for 5 ounces)* is a standard water-soluble cleansing gel suitable for its intended skin type. The price is out of line for what you get, but it works well and won't leave your skin feeling tight or dry. This does contain fragrance.

☹ **$$$ Grape Water, for All Skin Types** *($8 for 1.6 ounces)* is an incredibly simple toner that contains only grape water. You might as well mist your skin with pure grape juice, because at least that isn't diluted, and it certainly costs less than this. Either way, it takes more than grapes to give your skin what it needs to look its best.

☺ **$$$ Gentle Buffing Cream, for Sensitive Skin** *($35 for 1.6 ounces)* is an excellent scrub for normal to very dry skin not prone to blemishes. It would be gentler (and better for sensitive skin) without the fragrance, but in terms of abrasiveness and ingredients that cushion skin as you scrub, this is quite mild.

☹ **$$$ 1st Wrinkle Serum** *($59 for 1 ounce)*. This water-based serum is supposed to reverse the first signs of aging. If it could do that, Caudalie wouldn't need to sell so many other antiwrinkle/firming products making the exact same claim, but of course they do. This serum contains some intriguing ingredients for skin, but none of them are capable of reversing aging. What's most disappointing is that most of the intriguing ingredients are listed after the preservatives, so they don't count for much. This is an average, overpriced serum for normal to dry skin.

☹ **Beauty Elixir, for All Skin Types** *($15 for 1 ounce)* lists alcohol as the second ingredient, making it too drying and irritating for all skin types; plus alcohol causes free-radical damage and cell death. Even if this were alcohol-free, it contains several irritating plant oils that will leave your skin less than beautiful. This would be a terrible aftershave for men, so ignore that selling point, too.

☺ **$$$ Contour Cream Eyes and Lips, For Sensitive Skin** *($53 for 0.5 ounce)* is an OK fragrance-free moisturizer for normal to dry skin. This has a slightly matte finish, which can work well under the eyes if you need to use a lighter moisturizer in that area but don't want to encourage concealer slipping into lines around the eye. Overall this just doesn't contain enough state-of-the-art ingredients to warrant spending this kind of money. It doesn't even contain much grape extract for that matter.

☹ **Energizing Concentrate, For Sensitive Skin** *($39 for 0.5 ounce)* makes about as much sense for sensitive skin as making sure someone who's trying to lose weight has a second helping of dessert! Although the triglyceride and nut oil base are decent basics (albeit ordinary) for very dry skin, the inclusion of several fragrant plant oils makes this too irritating and completely incapable of providing "antiaging protection."

☺ **$$$ Fresh Complexion Tinted Moisturizer** *($39 for 1 ounce)* is a lightweight, fluid tinted moisturizer suitable for normal to slightly dry skin. Both of the shades are too peachy pink and each imparts shine from mica (which is why it is not recommended for oily areas, unless you want to look extra shiny). The formula will leave your skin wanting more; it really is boring, and highly fragranced as well (smelling more like eau de cologne than skin care), which makes this less desirable when compared with far better tinted moisturizers from Aveda, Bobbi Brown, and Neutrogena (and their options include the added benefit of a broad-spectrum sunscreen).

☺ **$$$ Premieres Vendanges Moisturizing Cream** *($40 for 1.3 ounces)* is a basic moisturizer for normal to dry skin, but it's inappropriate for sensitive skin due to the amount of fragrance and the potentially sensitizing fragrance components it contains. Antioxidant-wise, you're limited to grapes and a tiny amount of vitamin E.

☺ **$$$ Teint Divin Self Tanner Face** *($39 for 1 ounce)* is a very good self-tanner for dry to very dry skin, but the price is just silly. It contains dihydroxyacetone to turn skin tan, the same ingredient that's present in almost every self-tanner sold today, from L'Oreal to Neutrogena and Coppertone, and for a fraction of the price—just take a look at how tiny this container is! This is a good self-tanner, but absolutely not worth wasting money on. It does contain fragrance.

☺ **$$$ Lip Conditioner** *($12 for 0.14 ounce)* is a standard, mineral oil– and wax-based lip balm that contains a nice array of emollients that can help lips feel smooth, soft, and comfortable, but labeling this "antioxidant-rich" is definitely an exaggeration.

☹ **Contouring Concentrate** *($35 for 2.5 ounces).* You may be enticed by this product's claim of being the only 100% natural anti-cellulite treatment, but here's what you need to know: while this product is indeed 100% natural, it is no more a treatment for cellulite than a concealer is a treatment that will change skin discolorations. None, and I mean none, of the ingredients in this oil-based "concentrate" are capable of changing one dimple of cellulite on your thighs. Whether the ingredients are synthetic or natural, there is nothing you can rub on your legs to change or improve cellulite. With this product, what you will be giving to your skin is irritation caused by several potent fragrant oils, which cause collagen to break down, and that doesn't improve the appearance of skin. Perhaps the resulting inflammation may make cellulite appear less obvious, temporarily (maybe minutes), but the damage being done to your skin will gradually weaken its support structure.

☹ **Firming Concentrate** *($35 for 2.5 ounces).* This body product is supposed to be a firming and toning treatment for skin on the neck, chest, arms, and stomach. A "significant tightening effect" is promised, but absolutely cannot be delivered. Instead, this emollient lotion subjects skin to a host of potent irritants, including spearmint, balsam resin, and peppermint oil. None of these ingredients can firm skin or make it tighter in any way, shape, or form, unless irritating skin is someone's definition of tighter skin. If anything, continually massaging such irritants on your skin will lead to collagen breakdown and loss of firmness.

CETAPHIL (SKIN CARE ONLY)

CETAPHIL AT-A-GLANCE

Strengths: Inexpensive; their original, often-recommended Gentle Skin Cleanser; mostly fragrance-free products; affordable and widely available; offers complete ingredient lists on its Web site.

Weaknesses: No anti-acne products; no state-of-the-art moisturizers; limited sunscreen options (and a line with a focus on gentle should offer at least one mineral sunscreen for sensitive skin).

For more information about Cetaphil, call (817) 961-5000 or visit www.cetaphil.com or www.Beautypedia.com.

☹ **Antibacterial Gentle Cleansing Bar** *($4.49 for 4.5 ounces)* is a standard bar cleanser with the antibacterial active ingredient triclosan. This bar cleanser contains ingredients that impede rinsing and that won't make breakouts any better. It is not preferred to Cetaphil's water-soluble cleansers.

☺ **Daily Facial Cleanser for Normal to Oily Skin** *($7.99 for 8 ounces)* is a standard, detergent-based cleanser that can work for most skin types except dry to very dry skin. It removes makeup nicely, far better than the original Cetaphil Gentle Skin Cleanser, and doesn't irritate the eyes or dry out the skin. It does contain fragrance, which seems a misguided idea for this company.

☺ **Gentle Cleansing Bar** *($4.49 for 4.5 ounces)* is similar to Dove's original Beauty Bar and is a soap-free bar cleanser. It's an OK option for use from the neck down, but the sodium tallowate and sodium palm kernelate may clog pores and exacerbate breakouts.

✓ ☺ **Gentle Skin Cleanser** *($7.99 for 8 ounces)* is a dermatologist favorite that has remained the same for years, and that's a good thing! This fragrance-free, ultra-gentle cleanser is very good for normal to dry skin that is sensitive or prone to skin conditions such as eczema or psoriasis. The non-lathering, lotion formula rinses well without the aid of a washcloth, and the tiny amount (less than 1%) of sodium lauryl sulfate does not cause dryness or irritation (a question I'm often asked). The only significant drawback of this cleanser is it does not remove makeup very well. However, it has its place as a morning cleanser or for those who use minimal makeup.

☺ **Daily Advance Ultra Hydrating Lotion, for Dry, Sensitive Skin** *($10.79 for 8 ounces)* isn't all that advanced, but it is a good option for dry to very dry skin types needing a bland yet effective moisturizer to ease and prevent dryness. The sole antioxidant is vitamin E (not too inventive and rather lonely), but the amount is more reasonable than what's seen in many expensive moisturizers that brag about their vitamin E content (Lancome, I'm looking at you). This claims to be fragrance-free, but contains fragrance in the form of farnesol, an alcohol whose floral odor contributes to the smell of many essential oils, including citronella. Farnesol in this small amount isn't likely to cause problems, but its presence makes the company's fragrance-free claim inaccurate. Compared to Cetaphil's longstanding Moisturizing Cream, Daily Advance Ultra Hydrating Lotion has a creamier texture and slightly greasy feel on skin.

☺ **Daily Facial Moisturizer SPF 15 with Parsol 1789** *($11.50 for 4 ounces)* is a good, avobenzone-based sunscreen in a standard moisturizing base that is OK for someone with normal to dry skin. The product is fragrance-free; adding antioxidants and a broader array of ingredients that mimic the structure and function of healthy skin would make this good daytime moisturizer superior.

☺ **UVA/UVB Defense SPF 50 Facial Moisturizer for All Skin Types** *($13.99 for 1.7 ounces)* is a fluid moisturizer that contains an in-part titanium dioxide sunscreen for reliable UVA protection. I take issue with their claim that the UV filters chosen are an "optimum blend" because that isn't the case. The blend is fine, but the combination of actives isn't unique to this product, nor is it the only one to provide such a high level of sun protection. Another questionable claim is that this is non-irritating. If titanium dioxide were the only active, I would agree with the claim, but that's not the case. It's disingenuous to state that your sunscreen is non-irritating when it contains sunscreen actives that people can (and sometimes do) react to. That's the reality, though it doesn't mean such sunscreens should be avoided (many people can tolerate any sunscreen active); just be aware there is the potential for a skin reaction. A couple more observations: Although this is recommended for those with normal to dry skin, it absolutely isn't nongreasy as claimed. Also, the amount of titanium dioxide lends a slight white cast that cannot be blended away (though it's much less noticeable than that of many other mineral sunscreens). Considering that this is a new product for Cetaphil, it's disappointing that they neglected antioxidants. A token amount of vitamin E is all that's included, which won't help this product compete with others at the drugstore that offer a range of potent antioxidants. Still, this deserves a happy face rating for its sun protection ability, for its acceptable aesthetics, and because it is fragrance-free.

☺ **Moisturizing Cream** *($12.99 for 16 ounces)* is a thicker version of the Moisturizing Lotion, although this product really is fragrance-free; it's an excellent choice for dry to very dry skin that is sensitive. The tiny amount of vitamin E is likely inconsequential for skin, and this moisturizer would be rated higher if it contained more antioxidants and a cell-communicating ingredient such as lecithin.

☺ **Moisturizing Lotion** *($11.99 for 16 ounces)* claims to be fragrance-free but it contains farnesol, an ingredient whose chief function is adding fragrance to a product (Source: *International Cosmetic Ingredient Dictionary and Handbook*, 11th edition, 2006, page 864). This is a good, basic moisturizer for normal to dry skin anywhere on the body. It contains mostly water, glycerin, thickeners, nut oil, silicone, vitamin E, preservatives, fragrance, and film-forming agent.

☺ **Therapeutic Hand Cream** *($7.99 for 3 ounces).* Cetaphil is known for crafting basic, gentle moisturizers, but basic is not enough, especially when you consider that companies like Olay, Aveeno (a select few products), and CeraVe all have launched reasonably priced, state-of-the-art body products containing skin-identical ingredients and antioxidants. Cetaphil's beyond-ordinary formula leaves much to be desired. It isn't bad, just bland, sort of like a chocolate cake without the sugar and icing.

The Reviews C

CHANEL

CHANEL AT-A-GLANCE

Strengths: Hmmm ... sleek and occasionally elegant packaging; almost all of the sunscreens contain avobenzone for UVA protection; one very good Age Delay serum; a handful of good cleansers and topical scrubs; two fantastic foundations with sunscreen; some very good concealers; several good mascaras; a sheer lipstick with sunscreen that includes avobenzone; all of the powder eyeshadows have superb textures; some elegant shimmer.

Weaknesses: Expensive, with an emphasis on style over substance; overreliance on jar packaging; antioxidants in most products amount to a mere dusting; terrible anti-acne and oily skin products; almost all of the Micro-Solutions products are hardly what the doctor ordered, yet priced to be in line with professionally administered cosmetic corrective treatments; no products to address sun- or hormone-induced skin discolorations; mediocre to poor eye pencils and brow-enhancing options; extremely limited options for eyeshadows if you want a matte finish.

For more information about Chanel, call (800) 550-0005 or visit www.chanel.com or www.Beautypedia.com.

CHANEL SKIN CARE

CHANEL BEAUTE INITIALE PRODUCTS

☹ **Beaute Initiale Serum Energizing Multi-Protection Concentrate** *($85 for 1 ounce)* promises to be "a true concentrate of energy for skin," but the only concentrated result you can count on from this hapless serum is irritation. Alcohol is the second ingredient, and what follows is about as intriguing for skin as learning that cars can go forward and backward. If you're in the market for a state-of-the-art serum in this price range, every option from MD Skincare by Dr. Dennis Gross or Dr. Denese is preferred to this one.

☺ **$$$ Beaute Initiale Energizing Multi-Protection Eye Cream SPF 15** *($70 for 0.5 ounce)* includes avobenzone for sufficient UVA protection, yet this sunscreen active and the other (octinoxate) are not the best for use around the sensitive eye area. Although this deserves credit for providing broad-spectrum sun protection, the base formula for normal to dry skin is seriously lagging behind even the typically average eye cream options from Lancome.

☹ **Beaute Initiale Energizing Multi-Protection Cream SPF 15** *($75 for 1.7 ounces)* includes avobenzone for sufficient UVA protection, but the second ingredient in this needlessly expensive sunscreen is alcohol. As such, it is too drying and irritating for all skin types. Even without the alcohol, the overall formula is very disappointing and a terrible way for women just beginning to assemble a skin-care routine to give their skin a boost of anything helpful. Well, there is the sun protection—but lots of products provide that without alcohol, and for a lot less money.

☹ **Beaute Initiale Energizing Multi-Protection Fluid Healthy Glow SPF 15** *($75 for 1.7 ounces)* doesn't contain alcohol like the other Beaute Initiale moisturizers, but it does contain the menthol derivative menthyl lactate, which doesn't make it a better product. Any glow you experience from this daytime moisturizer for normal to dry skin is from irritation. There are plenty of in-part avobenzone sunscreens to consider before this one, including those from Olay Regenerist and Estee Lauder DayWear.

☹ **Beaute Initiale Energizing Multi-Protection Fluid SPF 15** *($75 for 1.7 ounces)* is similar to the Beaute Initiale Energizing Multi-Protection Cream SPF 15, except this has a fluid texture and includes more silicone than alcohol. That makes it slightly less irritating and drying, but, once again, you're getting a disappointingly mundane formula for the money.

CHANEL HYDRAMAX + ACTIVE PRODUCTS

☺ **$$$ Hydramax + Active Serum Active Moisture Boost** *($80 for 1 ounce)* features (according to Chanel) a "powerful formula" that "performs at the source of dehydration," but somehow the ad copy didn't mention that this product contains a high amount of alcohol (it's the third ingredient). When alcohol is listed before such skin-identical ingredients as glycerin and sodium PCA, it means your dry skin won't get the moisture boost it deserves. This product does contain a strong, lingering fragrance.

☺ **$$$ Hydramax + Active Creme, Active Moisture Cream** *($65 for 1.7 ounces)* continues Chanel's tradition of offering beautifully packaged moisturizers that are long on claims that the formulas cannot live up to. This is a decent moisturizer for normal to dry skin, but vitamin E is the only significant antioxidant and elegant skin-identical ingredients are absent, so you're not getting your money's worth. The few intriguing ingredients are listed well after the preservatives and fragrance, making them inconsequential.

☹ **Hydramax + Active Active Moisture Gel Cream** *($70 for 1.7 ounces)*. Chanel markets this moisturizer exclusively for those with normal skin. Regardless of skin type, this product is not recommended due to the amount of skin-damaging alcohol. Alcohol causes free-radical damage, irritation, and dryness, and can stimulate oil production in the pore lining, none of which are good for skin. Estee Lauder and Clinique offer much better lightweight moisturizers.

☹ **Hydramax + Active Serum Active Moisture Tinted Lotion SPF 15** *($55)*. Sigh. For the price Chanel is charging, this should be an amazing tinted moisturizer in every respect. As is, the sunscreen leaves skin vulnerable to UVA damage because it does not contain the active ingredients of titanium dioxide, zinc oxide, avobenzone, Mexoryl SX (ecamsule), or Tinosorb. Adding to that serious problem is the base formula, which is as basic as it gets and is overly fragranced to boot. The texture is creamy and the finish soft and radiant from each of the three very sheer shades, but come on! Stila, Bobbi Brown, Estee Lauder, Shiseido, and many other brands offer far better tinted moisturizers that don't leave your skin vulnerable to UVA damage (and treat it to at least a smattering of state-of-the-art ingredients).

CHANEL MICRO SOLUTIONS PRODUCTS

☺ **$$$ Micro Solutions Refining Peel Program** *($250 for 0.63 ounce)* is shocking, and not in a good way, at least not if you're at all concerned about spending way more than you need to for an effective skin-care product. In what essentially amounts to a hamburger with Kobe beef pricing, Chanel has produced an 8% glycolic acid serum, packaged in three stacked plastic trays, each containing seven single-use mini-tubes of product. The product's pH of 3.8 does ensure exfoliation, and the water and silicone base feels exceptionally light and silky, but the price is outrageous! Chanel positions this system as equivalent to a professional AHA peel, "without the drawbacks," but the amount of glycolic acid doesn't even come close to what is used in a professional setting, where AHA concentrations range from 20% to 40% and up. For what Chanel is charging, you could get a professional AHA peel and purchase one of the effective 8% AHA products from Alpha Hydrox, Neutrogena, or Paula's Choice, and end up with better results. Micro Solutions Refining Peel Program deserves a happy face rating because it is an effective exfoliant, but it is absolutely not worth even a fraction of its price. In fact, it's almost insulting that Chanel didn't include other state-of-the-art ingredients in this formula, especially anti-irritants. By the way, Chanel's labeling of this product as "ultra-gentle" isn't accurate for many reasons, primarily due to the effective AHA component, which can be irritating for lots of women, and also because of the unnecessary amount of fragrance.

☺ $$$ **Micro Solutions Refining Peel Program Advanced** *($275 for 0.63 ounce)* is nearly identical to the Micro Solutions Refining Peel Program, except this slightly more expensive version contains 10% glycolic acid. That will theoretically produce better results, but the trade-off is increased risk of irritation. This kit will not approximate the results obtainable from a series of doctor-performed AHA peels, but it is a good, albeit exceedingly pricey, AHA product.

☹ **Micro Solutions Wrinkle Neutralizing Treatment** *($185 for 0.05 ounce)* is a kit that comes with a wrinkle massaging tool and a gel-texture serum that's applied afterward, left on overnight, and rinsed in the morning. I don't quite know how to describe the absurdity of this "treatment," but I'll do my best. Chanel's "tool" (a plastic device with a rubber massaging piece that resembles an inverted "C" similar to Chanel's logo) is supposed to relax expression lines and lift wrinkles before you apply the gel. The kit comes with instructions on how to carefully massage your wrinkles, depending on whether or not they are vertical or horizontal lines, or crow's feet around the eyes. These instructions are meaningless, because nothing about this tool (or massaging wrinkles in any possible way) will relax or change expression lines or prep wrinkles for treatment with the gel. If anything, manipulating or pulling the skin too much will eventually lead to sagging, and that certainly won't make a wrinkle less apparent! You may be wondering, forgetting the inane massage tool for a moment, if there is something special about this gel. There isn't. It's a water- and alcohol-based liquid that also includes film-forming agents (like those found in hairstyling products), meager amounts of plant extracts, and a tiny amount of two forms of vitamin C. There is enough alcohol that it has a constricting effect on skin, not to mention its irritation potential. This and the tightening effect of the film-forming agents may make wrinkles look less obvious, but the effect is at best fleeting and in the long run problematic to the health of your skin. Chanel labels this kit a "dermatologist-based procedure," but no self-respecting dermatologist would offer patients such a baseless, useless treatment under the guise of reducing the appearance of wrinkles.

CHANEL PRECISION PRODUCTS

☺ $$$ **Gel Purete Rinse-Off Foaming Gel Cleanser** *($45 for 5 ounces)*. The good news: this is an efficient water-soluble cleanser for normal to oily skin. The bad news: the price is positively ridiculous. Paying this much for something you can get at the drugstore for less than ten dollars (and the same size container) is ludicrous, and advised only if you steadfastly refuse to cleanse your face with anything but a Chanel product. By the way, the plant extracts in this cleanser offer no special benefit to combination skin, nor are they any more adept at removing pollutants from skin than any other cleanser.

☺ $$$ **Lait Confort Creamy Cleansing Milk** *($45 for 5 ounces)* is a standard, insanely overpriced, detergent-free cleansing lotion suitable for dry to very dry skin that's not prone to breakouts. It removes makeup easily and feels silky, but likely will require a washcloth to ensure you're not leaving residue behind. Tulip extract isn't capable of removing pollutants from skin, and lily extract isn't hydrating. Even if those plants had such properties, the amount of them in this product is minuscule. (I have to say: I hate giving happy face ratings to absurdly expensive products like this one.)

☺ **$$$ Mousse Confort Rinse-Off Foaming Cleanser** *($45 for 4.2 ounces)* is a standard, exceptionally overpriced cleanser that can be too drying for most skin types. The potassium-based cleansing agents aren't as prevalent as they are in some other foaming cleansers, which makes this a slightly gentler option, but it would be important to keep this away from the eye area. It does remove makeup and rinses cleanly, but that is hardly unique or worth this amount of money.

☺ **$$$ Mousse Douceur Rinse-Off Foaming Mousse Cleanser** *($45 for 5 ounces)* produces copious, mousse-like foam, but the potassium-based ingredients responsible for creating all the foam can be needlessly drying for skin. This removes makeup easily and rinses cleanly, but there are gentler foaming cleansers for normal to oily skin to consider, from Neutrogena, Dove, and L'Oreal, none of which have this Chanel cleanser's price tag.

☺ **$$$ Lotion Confort Silky Soothing Toner** *($45 for 6.8 ounces)*. The core ingredients in this toner for normal to dry skin lend a silky texture and smooth finish on skin. However, the formula doesn't make it worth the inflated price. Several of the intriguing ingredients are listed after the preservative, and there's no proof anywhere that tulip extract combats pollutants or that lily extract hydrates skin as Chanel claims. Furthermore, what pollutants are they referring to that require a special ingredient anyway, especially tulips?

☹ **Lotion Douceur Gentle Hydrating Toner** *($45 for 6.8 ounces)*. "Gentle" and "hydrating" are not the words I'd choose to describe this alcohol-laden toner. It is a problem for all skin types because alcohol causes dryness, irritation, and free-radical damage, everything that a smart skin-care routine is designed to avoid.

☹ **Lotion Purete Fresh Mattifying Toner** *($45 for 6.8 ounces)* contains some intriguing ingredients for skin, including unique water-binding agents. However, the beneficial ingredients are trumped by the amount of skin-damaging alcohol Chanel included. Alcohol can degrease the skin and leave it temporarily matte, but the resulting irritation stimulates skin's oil glands to produce more oil, so in almost no time oily skin is back and worse than before.

☺ **$$$ Gommage Microperle Eclat Extra Radiance Exfoliating Gel** *($45 for 2.5 ounces)* is a minimally abrasive, fairly gentle topical scrub whose oil content makes it preferred for dry to very dry skin. The exfoliating agent is pearl powder, but that in and of itself has no special benefit for skin compared with other scrub ingredients. What a shame to grind up pearls for this effect when a washcloth would have the same benefit.

☺ **$$$ Gommage Microperle Hydration Gentle Polishing Gel** *($45 for 2.5 ounces)* is similar to the Gommage Microperle Eclat Extra Radiance Exfoliating Gel above, minus the prevalence of oil and some thickeners. It is preferred for normal to oily skin but still contains enough plant oil to be potentially problematic for blemish-prone skin.

☺ **$$$ Gommage Microperle Purete Deep Purifying Exfoliating Mousse** *($45 for 2.5 ounces)* contains polyethylene beads as the abrasive agent, making it a more traditional exfoliating gel than the other Chanel Precision scrubs. The oil content makes this best for normal to dry skin, and helps keep the witch hazel from causing irritation.

☹ **Purete Ideale Serum Intense Refining Skin Complex** *($75 for 1 ounce)* gets its matte finish from silicone and alcohol, but the amount of alcohol here, along with witch hazel, makes this water-based serum too drying and irritating for all skin types. Alcohol won't balance oil production because oil production is controlled by hormones, and topically applied products like these have no effect on what's happening hormonally. However, applying alcohol-based products to skin can stimulate oil production in the pore lining.

☺ **$$$ UV Essentiel Protective UV Care SPF 30** *($48 for 1 ounce)* contains an in-part zinc oxide sunscreen, but that's where the good news stops because you don't get anything else for what amounts to little more than a mundane overpriced sunscreen. The denatured alcohol that's included is an exceedingly irritating and skin-damaging ingredient, and it's especially a concern because it's listed before any of the intriguing ingredients. This daytime moisturizer has a light, fluid texture and soft matte finish those with normal to oily skin will appreciate, but other than the sun protection it offers there is nothing of significance to extol.

☹ **Purete Ideale Serum T-Mat Shine Control** *($40 for 1 ounce)* lists alcohol as the second ingredient, followed by witch hazel. It is too drying and irritating for all skin types and not recommended over superior products such as Clinique Pore Minimizer Instant Perfector. This much alcohol causes excess oil production in the pore lining, too.

☹ **Purete Ideale Blemish Control** *($38 for 0.5 ounce)* has enough beeswax and other thickeners to make blemishes worse; the salicylic acid is not present in an amount that's effective, and even if it were, the pH of this lotion puts it out of its efficacious range.

☹ **Masque Destressant Eclat Anti-Fatigue Gel Mask** *($50 for 1.7 ounces)* lists alcohol as the second ingredient, which isn't exactly a "luxurious time-out for tired, lackluster skin." If anything, this gel mask will cause dryness and irritation while providing minimal benefit.

☺ **$$$ Masque Destressant Hydratation Nourishing Cream-Gel Mask** *($50 for 1.7 ounces)* is said to imbue skin with a sense of serenity, but serenity is a state of mind, not something skin can experience, so the claim is silly. There are some great-for-dry-skin ingredients in this mask, but many of them are listed after the alcohol (and at least the amount of alcohol is not cause for concern). It's an OK mask but vastly overpriced for what you get.

☺ **$$$ Masque Destressant Purete Purifying Cream Mask** *($50 for 2.5 ounces)* is a basic clay mask for normal to oily skin (those with very oily skin would want something more absorbent). The thickening agents (including beeswax) may be problematic for blemish-prone skin, but this does the job in terms of absorbing surface oils without overdrying the skin.

CHANEL RECTIFIANCE INTENSE PRODUCTS

☺ **$$$ Rectifiance Intense Eye Retexturizing Line Correcting Eye Cream** *($72 for 0.5 ounce)* is not capable of taking care of eye-area woes. The really interesting ingredients (including those that serve as a protein source for skin) are listed well after the preservatives, meaning they're barely present. All in all, this is just another average option for normal to dry skin for an above-average amount of money.

☺ **$$$ Rectifiance Intense Nuit Retexturizing Line Correcting Night Cream** *($92 for 1.7 ounces)* works beautifully to keep dry to very dry skin moisturized and smooth. The jar packaging is inconsequential given the paltry amount of antioxidants in this product, but its blend of silicone, thickeners, nut oil, and proven emollients makes it worth considering if your budget allows (though to be clear, better moisturizers are available that cost much less). This does contain fragrance.

☺ **$$$ Rectifiance Intense Retexturizing Line Correcting Cream SPF 15** *($86 for 1.7 ounces)* makes claims identical to those of the Rectifiance Intense Retexturizing Line Correcting Fluid SPF 15 below, and contains the same in-part avobenzone sunscreen. It comes in a standard, but effective, moisturizing base suitable for normal to dry skin, but if you were hoping your $86 would buy you an appreciable amount of state-of-the-art ingredients, you would be mistaken. A relatively small number of antioxidants and skin-identical ingredients are here, but in amounts too tiny to matter for skin.

☹ **Rectifiance Intense Retexturizing Line Correcting Fluid SPF 15** *($86 for 1.7 ounces)* is supposed to contain "a micro-protein complex [that] slows down the deterioration of the Extra-Cellular Matrix, the supporting cushion essential for skin firmness and elasticity." That's a fancy, scientific-sounding way to say that this product prevents the breakdown of collagen and other elements of skin's support structure, such as elastin and fibronectin; however, the minuscule amounts of amino acids, plant extracts, and protein in this fluid aren't up to that task. What is suspect about this product is the third ingredient, alcohol, which is problematic because it can break down skin, not reinforce it. Chanel should have bragged that it is the in-part avobenzone sunscreen in this product that can benefit the underlying portion of your skin by preventing it from assault by ultraviolet rays from the sun—but it is the rare cosmetics company that brags about their sunscreens. An effective sunscreen with UVA-protecting ingredients can prevent the breakdown of collagen and other elements present in the extracellular matrix. The base formula is primarily water, silicones, and alcohol. All of the intriguing, state-of-the-art ingredients are listed after the preservative, so they are a mere dusting, which won't do your skin much good. Considering the formulary issues and the price, there's no logical reason to select this sunscreen over dozens of better-formulated, less expensive alternatives.

☺ $$$ **Rectifiance Intense Serum Retexturizing Line Corrector** *($105 for 1 ounce)* contains Chanel's typical token amount of intriguing ingredients, and basically relies on fanciful claims to convince women they can "outsmart time" with this silicone-laden serum. Water and several forms of silicone comprise the bulk of the formula, followed by some slip agent and preservative. Silicone isn't a bad ingredient for skin, but it's not an antiaging miracle and there is no reason to spend this much for it when Olay, Neutrogena, Clinique, Estee Lauder, and Aveeno offer similar but better serums for much less money.

CHANEL SUBLIMAGE PRODUCTS

☺ $$$ **Sublimage Essential Regenerating Cream "Texture Supreme"** *($375 for 1.7 ounces).* Chanel wants you to know that although they sell numerous antiwrinkle, skin-firming products, this one is the real deal. It's the ultimate, according to their marketing copy, which of course explains why the price is so completely out of synch with reality, even though the formula is far from state-of-the-art. Just as with their other Sublimage products, you're supposed to believe that vanilla fruit oil and Chanel's special fractionation process are the key to vanquishing everything that keeps skin from looking youthful. (Fractionation is strictly a chemical process, not a miracle of any kind, and certainly not unique to Chanel.) Admittedly, this emollient moisturizer for dry skin has a rich, elegant texture that feels great, but almost all of the ingredients creating that texture are as standard as it gets. Perhaps most frustrating is that the effectiveness of the few antioxidants and plant extracts that are included will be compromised due to the jar packaging, which won't keep them stable for very long. For what Chanel is charging, you should expect the most airtight packaging available (along with an attractive pair of gold earrings). Enough said, other than that there are no words fit for print to describe what a tremendous waste of money this moisturizer is.

☺ $$$ **Sublimage Essential Regenerating Cream (Texture Universelle)** *($375 for 1.7 ounces)* is one of those products that cause me to throw up my hands and say "I give up!" We are asked to believe that the vanilla plant in Madagascar (where most of the world's vanilla comes from), coupled with Chanel's exclusive "polyfractioning" technique (polyfractioning isn't a word found in any dictionary—rather it is a term coined by Chanel), is the key to restoring firm, radiant, youthful skin. According to Chanel, polyfractioning is a new process that isolates the active ingredients from a plant, paring down millions of molecules to just a handful. Even if that were true, the concept of obtaining the active component from a plant is hardly new, and it's definitely not unique to Chanel. Considering its price, this product contains a minuscule amount of vanilla oil (there's more fragrance and preservative in it than there is of the supposedly wrinkle-fighting ingredient). All in all, this ends up being just a very emollient moisturizer for dry to very dry skin. It contains several ingredients that make dry skin feel smoother and softer, but so do hundreds of other moisturizers that wouldn't dare charge this much. The air-sensitive ingredients in this product (antioxidants and the vanilla) will become almost instantly useless once you open it, thanks to the unwise choice of jar packaging. Putting your faith and dollars in this product won't bring you any closer to a wrinkle-free face—and personally I'd rather devote these funds to new shoes or a night at the theater or an investment toward my face-lift.

☹ **$$$ Sublimage Eye Essential Regenerating Eye Cream** *($175 for 0.5 ounce)* doesn't carry the same sticker shock as the Sublimage Essential Regenerating Creams, but is still outrageously priced for what amounts to a standard emollient moisturizer for dry skin anywhere on the face. It contains mostly water, glycerin, emollient thickening agents, canola oil, film-forming agent, wax, more film-forming agent, a cell-communicating ingredient, silicone, preservatives, and a tiny amount of vanilla oil and antioxidants (which are rendered ineffective due to jar packaging). You don't have to spend even one-third this much to get a good moisturizer, and in this case, unless you believe the claims, why would you?

☹ **$$$ Sublimage Serum Essential Regenerating Concentrate** *($400 for 1 ounce)*. As if the prices and claims for Chanel's range of Sublimage moisturizers weren't high enough, we now have this overly expensive, but underwhelming, truly ordinary serum. I can't imagine how anyone at Chanel could be so crass. This is merely a blend of standard ingredients, beginning with water (you'd think for $400 they would eliminate the least expensive ingredient in any cosmetic product) and including what Chanel deems the star attraction, vanilla. $400 for a tiny amount of vanilla! Unbelievable! Apparently, this serum gets immediate must-have status because of the precious vanilla water and vanilla oil it contains. It should be noted, however, that the vanilla oil is listed after the preservative, while the vanilla water (vanilla tea) is more prominent—again, for the money, Chanel shouldn't be diluting the alleged good stuff. Is there any reason to believe vanilla in any form can regenerate skin and provide "unprecedented results" for wrinkles? Not according to any published research. In fact, some forms of vanilla can cause contact dermatitis and skin sensitivity, and as you might expect, that would become only more likely in a product that contains concentrated amounts of it, as this serum claims. The lack of supporting evidence for vanilla makes this serum a ludicrous investment—nothing else it contains is unique and you're getting no special benefit for the money. But, without question, some people will buy this on the basis of its price and name brand status but it just ends up being a complete waste of money. If you really want Chanel, look to their makeup and fragrances rather than their antiwrinkle skin care.

CHANEL ULTRA CORRECTION PRODUCTS

☺ **$$$ Ultra Correction Creme Restructuring Anti-Wrinkle Firming Cream SPF 10** *($105 for 1.7 ounces)* has an SPF rating that falls short of the minimum recommended by the National Cancer Institute and the American Academy of Dermatology, although it does include an in-part avobenzone sunscreen. The base formula falls short, too, offering skin little more than a bland mixture of water, glycerin, plant extract, slip agents, canola oil, and silicone. It is an OK option for normal to slightly dry skin if you're willing to pair it with another sunscreen or foundation with sunscreen rated SPF 15 or greater.

☺ **$$$ Ultra Correction Eye Restructuring Anti-Wrinkle Firming Eye Cream** *($85 for 0.5 ounce)* is just an emollient, creamy moisturizer that can moisturize dry skin anywhere on the face. An ingredient referred to as Adhesioderm (I am not making this up) is the alleged wrinkle reducer, but it's not listed as one of the ingredients, and there is no other information beyond what Chanel wants you to believe about it. I won't even get into the second part of this product, referred to as the Life Cycle Regenerator! Anyone who knows how to interpret an ingredient list would likely find these "pay no attention to the man behind the curtain" claims far-fetched, but there is no question that consumers are taken in by this, as are Chanel salespeople, who speak of this product so highly you would swear it was a packaged fountain of youth (Ponce de Leon should be pulling up to a counter any minute). This is not a bad product, and it will soften, smooth, and hydrate the skin. But anything beyond that is not within the realm of possibility, despite claims to the contrary. Chanel left the fragrance out of this product, but did add mica, which will add a subtle shimmer to the skin.

☺ **$$$ Ultra Correction Nuit Restructuring Anti-Wrinkle Firming Night Cream** *($115 for 1.7 ounces)* encourages you to be firm, look young, and, while you're at it, go ahead and use this product to "correct every sign of age." You're to believe this standard emollient moisturizer has the ability to resculpt and firm skin as you sleep while Chanel's exclusive "Life Cycle Regenerator" attacks wrinkles and restores "the look of youth." It's all fiction (someone on Chanel's marketing team must be a great storyteller), because all this product will do is restore a soft, smooth feel and appearance on normal to dry skin. The amount of vitamin E is next to nothing, so the jar packaging, which is attractive, doesn't really make a difference in this case (form over function is rarely a good idea, especially in skin care).

☺ **$$$ Ultra Correction Restructuring Anti-Wrinkle Firming Lotion SPF 10** *($105 for 1.7 ounces)* contains an in-part avobenzone sunscreen, but providing the optimum SPF is as crucial for the skin as the UVA-protecting active ingredient, and SPF 10 just doesn't cut it. Apart from the low SPF, this product claims to have ingredients that firm and resculpt the skin "as if surface skin is bonded to its support system." Here's a news flash: Surface skin already is bonded to its support system—the dermis and subcutaneous layer of fat. It is the lower layers of skin (including facial ligaments, muscles, bone, fat, and collagen) that deteriorate with age and years of unprotected sun exposure, and none of those can be affected in any way by this product. Along with the enticing claims comes Chanel's "unique resculpting massage," which supposedly relaxes facial muscles "contracted by aging." Yet facial muscles do not contract with age, they simply diminish in mass and lose their tension. It is this process, coupled with the fact that the skin continues to grow as the muscles and bone break down and the fat pads break through the lax muscles, that eventually leads to sagging. That can be corrected with plastic surgery, but not by massage of any kind. (If massage could build muscles, then bodybuilders could forgo lifting all those heavy weights and just get massages all day long.) The aluminum starch in this product will leave a slight matte finish, and makes this best for normal to slightly dry skin.

☹ **Ultra Correction Serum Restructuring Lift Complex** *($180 for 1.7 ounces)* lists alcohol as the second ingredient. That's not only irritating to skin, but, given the price of this product, insulting to consumers. It does not contain a single ingredient capable of firming skin—and definitely not in the paltry amounts Chanel used (as usual, there's more fragrance than anything genuinely intriguing).

☹ **$$$ Ultra Correction Total Eye Revitalizer** *($125)* comprises a roll-on serum and an eye patch, both designed to lift and firm eye-area skin. The serum is mostly water, glycerin, film-forming agents, and starch; the patches are basically a lightweight, water-based solution with ultra-small amounts of truly state-of-the-art ingredients. Used alone or as a pair, this gimmicky duo won't lift or firm in the least, though the amount of film-forming agent can have a temporary tightening effect. It's up to you to decide if that's worth more than $100, but don't say I didn't warn you.

☹ **$$$ Ultra Correction Lip Restructuring Anti-Wrinkle Lip Contour** *($65 for 0.5 ounce)* is said to contain, like the Firming Eye Cream, the Adhesioderm complex, but Chanel doesn't explain what it is or what it does. Perhaps a surgical-sounding name is necessary when your antiaging product contains nothing of significance to restore firmness or rejuvenate the lips. This is merely water, plasticizing thickener, talc, wax, silicone, and several thickeners, along with a tiny amount of vitamin E and lesser amounts of soothing plant extracts and antioxidants. At best, this is an overpriced lip balm, but the talc keeps it from being all that moisturizing.

CHANEL ULTRA CORRECTION LIFT PRODUCTS

☹ **$$$ Ultra Correction Lift Lifting Firming Day Cream SPF 15** *($150 for 1.7 ounces)*. This daytime moisturizer with an in-part avobenzone sunscreen follows the same pattern as many other Chanel products: Showcase a star ingredient, in this case something called elemi PFA; attach an antiaging claim to it; then include just a dusting of it in the formula and don't bother to mention that there's no research anywhere proving it lifts skin. But wait, there's less: They not only include a mere dusting of their allegedly superior ingredient (elemi PFA), but also package the product in a jar so that if it did have any potency it will be diminished once the product is opened. Add a lot of fragrance to those disappointments and this doesn't shape up to be a brilliant choice for anyone's skin, regardless of age or amount of sagging. For more information about elemi PFA, please see the review for Chanel's Ultra Correction Lift Sculpting Firming Concentrate.

☹ **$$$ Ultra Correction Lift Lifting Firming Day Fluid SPF 15** *($150 for 1.7 ounces)* is the lotion version of Chanel's Ultra Correction Lift Lifting Firming Day Creme SPF 15, and overall the same review applies. This daytime moisturizer with an in-part avobenzone sunscreen follows the same pattern as many other Chanel products: Mention a star ingredient, in this case elemi PFA; attach an antiaging claim to it; then include just a dusting of it in the formula and don't bother to mention that there's no research anywhere proving it lifts skin. The exception for this version is that this isn't packaged in a jar, but that doesn't change the paltry amount of exciting ingredients. This is about as ordinary and dated a moisturizing product as you will find. Given the wafting amount of fragrance, this doesn't shape up to be a brilliant choice for anyone's skin. For more information about elemi PFA, please see the review for Chanel's Ultra Correction Lift Sculpting Firming Concentrate.

☺ **$$$ Ultra Correction Lift Lifting Firming Night Cream** *($165 for 1.7 ounces)*. This moisturizer has an emollient texture that will feel great on dry skin. However, the price is absurd for what amounts to a completely ordinary, ho-hum formulation. Aside from a pathetic amount of state-of-the-art ingredients, the little it does contain won't remain stable due to the jar packaging. There are hundreds of moisturizers whose textures are as nice as this one, but whose formulas provide a well-rounded assortment of ingredients that dry skin needs to look and feel its best. Chanel includes more fragrance than intriguing plants and peptides, and for what they're charging those ingredients should be up front and center. None of the ingredients in this moisturizer can stimulate building blocks in skin so it becomes lifted and firmer. Besides, Chanel sells over a dozen other products claiming the same thing; if those really worked to lift skin, then why create the Ultra Correction line?

As is true for all of the Ultra Correction products Chanel is selling, this one contains elemi PFA as the showcased miracle ingredient. It isn't. For more information about this substance, see the review for Chanel's Ultra Correction Lift Sculpting Firming Concentrate.

☹ **Ultra Correction Lift Sculpting Firming Concentrate** *($165 for 1 ounce)*. Unbelievable! Products like this make me want to scream, not only because of their exorbitant cost, but also because the formulas are so undeserving of your dollars and attention. This product wouldn't be worth it even if it were free!

This water-based serum lists alcohol as the second ingredient, which means it will cause dryness, irritation, and free-radical damage. Of course, it cannot lift or sculpt an aging face in any way, shape, or form—unless you count the tightening effect from the film-forming agents (think hairspray for your face) as a remarkable benefit—it isn't, and the effect is strictly cosmetic. Even fragrance is listed before anything of real benefit for skin.

Of course, Chanel's claims are tied to yet another "star" ingredient they've unearthed (of course, it has to be a plant), something called elemi PFA, an extract from the Manila elemi plant (*Canarium luzonicum* gum). It's supposed to restore tensin, a protein substance that regulates other substances to help keep skin structure intact (Source: *The International Journal of Biochemistry & Cell Biology*, January 2004, pages 31-34). Whether or not elemi PFA can effect tensin or any other part of the skin is something you have to take Chanel's word for because there is no research showing that to be true. Even if it happened to be true, however, there are lots of substances that can help keep skin intact; Chanel doesn't have the miracle, magic bullet that your skin must have to do this, not any more than any other cosmetic does. Overall, this is a poorly formulated product you should just ignore.

OTHER CHANEL SKIN-CARE PRODUCTS

☺ **$$$ Demaquillant Yeux Intense Gentle Biphase Eye Makeup Remover** *($32 for 3.4 ounces)* is a standard, but good, water- and silicone-based makeup remover. It makes short work of long-wearing makeup, including waterproof mascara, but so do similar removers from Neutrogena, Almay, Maybelline New York, and Paula's Choice.

☹ **Eclat Originel, Maximum Radiance Cream** *($55 for 1.7 ounces)* lists alcohol as the second ingredient, and at that level it is one of the last things you want to apply to skin if your goal is to boost radiance. Looking past the water-and-alcohol base reveals a lightweight moisturizer that contains several worthy ingredients for skin, including silicones, shea butter, glycerin, and good skin-identical ingredients. However, they won't be as effective in a product that lists alcohol before them, and as such this moisturizer is not recommended.

☺ **$$$ Creme N⁰ 1, Skin Recovery Cream** *($210 for 1.7 ounces)* is merely a standard moisturizer for normal to slightly dry skin, and its meager antioxidant content is diminished by jar packaging. The name is misleading, because in terms of what it takes to create a state-of-the-art moisturizer, this formula wouldn't even crack the top 50.

CHANEL MAKEUP

FOUNDATION: ✓ ☺ **Mat Lumiere Long Lasting Soft Matte Makeup SPF 15** *($54)* presents a new breed of matte-finish makeup; the only cons are how fleeting the matte-finish can be over oily areas. Otherwise, this fluid, ultra-smooth foundation is a pleasure to blend. It provides medium to almost full coverage and leaves skin looking what is best described as luminous matte. That means this isn't as reflective or moist-feeling as foundations with a satin finish, but it also isn't powdery matte like most traditional oil-free liquid foundations. Mat Lumiere is definitely a consideration for those with normal to slightly oily or slightly dry skin, and its sunscreen is pure titanium dioxide, which is excellent. Among the range of 11 shades are several beautiful options. Porcelaine 0.5 is great for fair skin, while Chestnut 8.0 is a very good dark shade. The shades to avoid due to overtones of orange or peach include Natural 4.0, Cedar 6.0, and Walnut 7.0. Ginger 3.0 and Soft Honey 5.0 are slightly peach, but may work for some medium to tan skin tones.

☺ **$$$ Lift Lumiere Firming and Smoothing Fluid Makeup SPF 15** *($65)*. Described as being more than a foundation, Chanel wants you to know they have created "the consummate skin-caring makeup." That sounds great, but the ingredient list doesn't support the boast. In terms of texture, this has a beautifully silky feel and includes a broad-spectrum sunscreen with an in-part titanium dioxide base, but that's only a start when it comes to ultimate skin-caring makeup. Where are the antioxidants and cell-communicating ingredients? How about some anti-irritants or skin-identical ingredients like ceramides or hyaluronic acid? They're not here, save for a teeny-tiny amount of plant oil and plant extracts with antioxidant ability. That doesn't add up to being worth $65. Even though this is a long way off from being skin-caring makeup, you can count on reliable sun protection, supremely smooth application, and an attractive satin matte finish suitable for normal to slightly dry or slightly oily skin. Coverage begins at medium and can be built to nearly full camouflage, although doing so produces a heavier look that is not easily softened. The majority of shades are neutral and ideal for fair to medium skin tones. Avoid the following shades because they are too pink, orange, or rose to look convincing: Natural Beige, Naturel, and Tawny Beige. One more point: it goes without saying that this foundation won't firm skin in any noticeable way, though it definitely creates the illusion of smooth, even-toned skin.

☹ **$$$ Pro Lumiere Professional Finish Makeup SPF 15** *($54)* falls short due to its lack of sufficient UVA protection. It does have a smooth, fluid texture that applies creamy and sets to a soft satin finish providing medium to full coverage. Blending isn't difficult but, because this foundation doesn't set that quickly, it is more time-consuming than some others. Best for normal to dry skin, Pro Lumiere Professional Finish Makeup SPF 15 comes in 11 shades, with no options for dark skin tones. Most of the shades are quite good, but avoid Cool Beige and Natural Beige (both are too pink) and be wary of Caramel, which has a tendency to turn peach.

☹ **$$$ Teint Innocence Naturally Luminous Fluid Makeup SPF 12** *($47)* has an SPF rating that's below the benchmark for daytime protection, and lacks the UVA-protecting ingredients of titanium dioxide, zinc oxide, avobenzone, Tinosorb, or Mexoryl SX. That's a letdown, because this foundation has a beautiful silky texture that blends flawlessly to a soft matte finish suitable for normal to oily skin. It provides light to almost medium coverage, and layering doesn't net significantly more camouflage. The 13 shades present better options for fair to light skin tones than for dark skin tones, though the darkest shades are recommended. The following shades are slightly pink or peach and should be considered carefully: Naturel 4.5, Soft Bisque 2.5, and Soft Honey 7.0. Avoid Natural Beige 3.5; it is noticeably pink.

☺ $$$ **Teint Innocence Compact Naturally Luminous Compact Makeup SPF 10** *($56)* disappoints because it does not contain the UVA-protecting ingredients of titanium dioxide, zinc oxide, avobenzone (also known as butyl methoxydibenzoylmethane), Tinosorb, or Mexoryl SX. Of course, the SPF rating is too low for sufficient daytime protection so opting to use this requires another product rated SPF 15 or greater. What's sad about the sunscreen deficiency is that this is otherwise a top-notch cream-to-powder foundation. It blends over skin impeccably and provides medium coverage that perfects without looking artificial. The moist, slightly thick finish is best for normal to dry skin not prone to blemishes. Almost all of the shades are neutral, with the best ones being those designed for fair to medium skin tones. Wheat is slightly peach but may work for some skin tones while Walnut is noticeably orange and should be avoided. This would have earned a happy face rating if it had the right UVA-protecting ingredients and was rated SPF 15 or greater.

☺ $$$ **Vitalumiere Satin Satin Smoothing Fluid Makeup SPF 15** *($54)* had almost everything going for it, but Chanel inexplicably didn't include UVA-protecting ingredients. The liquid texture is irresistibly smooth, and blends with ease to a light-to-medium coverage satin finish. But using words like "vibrant" and "young" to describe this is disingenuous considering the incomplete sunscreen (and Chanel knows better because many of their sunscreens do include UVA-protecting ingredients). Still, for those with normal to dry skin willing to pair this with a good sunscreen, the 11 colors present some impressive options. The only shades to avoid due to rose or peach tones are Soft Bisque, Cool Bisque, Natural Beige, and Tawny Beige.

☺ $$$ **Double Perfection Compact Matte Reflecting Powder Makeup SPF 10** *($50)* has merit as a silky-feeling, easy-to-blend, talc-based pressed-powder foundation. Its sunscreen is pure titanium dioxide, but why Chanel stopped at SPF 10 is a frustrating mystery. The ultralight, non-powdery finish puts skin in its most polished light, but be aware that any dry spots will be magnified with this type of makeup. Ideal for normal to very oily skin, it comes in 14 superb shades for fair to dark (but not very dark) skin. If you opt to use this product as an adjunct to a foundation with sunscreen or regular sunscreen rated SPF 15 or higher, it earns a happy face rating.

CONCEALER: ✓ ☺ $$$ **Correcteur Perfection Long Lasting Concealer** *($40)* is an updated version of Chanel's longstanding Quick Cover concealer. I am pleased to report that the update is an across-the-board improvement. This concealer has a gorgeously smooth, lightweight texture that blends easily and doesn't crease into lines or magnify their appearance. It has a soft, satin matte finish that lasts and won't make the under-eye area look dry or cakey. Among the mostly excellent neutral shades, be careful with Beige Petale; it is too peach for some medium skin tones. One more note: this concealer contains fragrance; that's not a deal-breaker, but the formula would be better without it.

✓ ☺ $$$ **Eclat Lumiere Highlighter Face Pen** *($40)*. Housed in a click-pen component with a built-in synthetic brush applicator, this is a beautiful highlighter. Whether you choose the golden or beige rose shade (which isn't rose at all), you'll get a soft, slightly creamy texture that's a pleasure to blend and sets to a soft matte finish complete with a subtle glow. The finish is ideal for highlighting around the eyes, down the bridge of the nose, or the top of the cheekbones. This is thicker and easier to control than Yves Saint Laurent's popular Radiant Touch product.

☺ $$$ **Pro Lumiere Correcteur Professional Finish Concealer** *($40)* has a texture that Chanel refers to as "velvety-smooth," and that's correct. This liquid concealer is housed in a pen-style container with a built-in synthetic brush applicator. It blends very well, with just enough slip, and sets to a satin matte finish that provides moderate but natural-looking coverage. The finish presents a small risk of creasing into lines around the eyes, but this is much less apparent if you set it with a loose or pressed powder. All five shades are recommended, and best for fair to tan skin tones. Overall, this is a good compromise if you think true matte-finish concealers are too dry and creamy concealers are too emollient.

☺ $$$ **Vitalumiere Satin Satin Smoothing Creme Concealer** *($40)* has a lush, creamy texture and is presented in packaging that looks elegant on your vanity. A true cream concealer, it has sufficient slip and is easy to blend, while also providing substantial coverage that builds well without caking. The moist finish lends itself to creasing unless blended very well and set with powder, which is this concealer's only drawback (well, that and the steep price). All three shades are beautiful, though they only cover fair to barely medium skin tones.

☹ $$$ **Lift Lumiere Concealer Smoothing and Rejuvenating Eye Contour Concealer** *($45)*. I had to wonder what Chanel was thinking when they created this well-intentioned but poorly conceived concealer. First, a concealer is intended, as the name implies, to provide appreciable coverage—this one doesn't. Second, a concealer should be easy to blend (which this is) and stay in place once it has set—this one doesn't. Chanel's new concealer, which doesn't lift anything, begins creamy and stays that way, so it begins creasing into lines and fading in short order and that continues throughout the day. You can set the concealer with pressed powder, but that doesn't help because the powder tends to stick to this emollient concealer, leading to skin that looks matte on top but "crinkled" underneath. Another sour note is the packaging. Although generously sized, the pump bottle dispenses way too much product even when you're being extra careful, so a lot gets wasted (and at this price, wasting even a drop of concealer isn't the goal). This concealer actually works best as a sheer- to light-coverage foundation for those with dry skin or dry patches. It conceals minor flaws reasonably well, but there are dozens of other concealers that outperform this and its three mediocre shades.

☹ **Estompe de Chanel Corrective Concealer** *($34)* is a creamy, lipstick-style concealer with light coverage and poor colors that can easily crease into lines around the eye. Trying to achieve additional coverage creates a heavy, caked appearance and you have to wonder, after all these years, who is still buying such an inferior concealer?

POWDER: ✓ ☺ $$$ **Poudre Universelle Libre Natural Finish Loose Powder** *($52)* has an extremely fine, sifted texture and a soft matte finish that looks beautiful on skin. It is talc-based and comes in three very good, sheer colors. Do you need to spend this much money for a superior loose powder? No, but if you're swayed by Chanel, this won't disappoint.

☺ $$$ **Poudre Universelle Compact Natural Finish Pressed Powder** *($44)* has a finely milled texture and a sheer, dry finish. This talc-based powder comes in only two shades, suitable for fair to light skin, but they're both good.

☺ $$$ **Poudre Cristalline Ultra-Fine Translucent Powder with Deluxe Puff** *($60)* is a finely milled, very sheer white loose powder meant to set makeup and create a "weightless veil effect." It is barely perceptible on skin, yet makes it look polished, and it tempers shine (though it also adds a soft shine due to the subtle sparkles it contains). The Chanel makeup artist indicated this was a limited edition product, but also said it may become part of Chanel's line after the spring season. Either way, it's an indulgence and not necessarily worth purchasing over many other weightless loose powders that cost significantly less. As for the puff, I wouldn't call it "deluxe"—it's just big and fluffy and hard to control (watch out for your eyes and hair). Loose powder almost always looks best when applied with a brush.

☺ **$$$ Poudre Douce Soft Pressed Powder** *($50)* is a silky, slightly dry-textured, talc-based powder that imparts sheer color and a soft shine finish. Only two shades are available, but the color deposit is so minimal that it makes them versatile for fair to medium skin tones, assuming you don't enjoy the shiny finish. The included compact-sized brush is better than most, but that doesn't completely justify the price of this powder.

BLUSH AND BRONZER: ☺ **$$$ Joues Contraste Powder Blush** *($42)*. This is Chanel's pressed-powder blush, and unless you are shopping for a matte-powder blush, it's a winner. The texture and application are suede-smooth, with plenty of pigmentation, so a little goes a long way. Every shade has at least a soft shine, and the following shades have a sparkling shine that's a bit too much for daytime wear: Mocha, Orchid Rose, and Tempting Beige. The brush provided is terribly small and the wrong shape for applying a soft wash of color to cheeks.

☺ **$$$ Soleil Tan de Chanel Bronzing Makeup Base** *($48)* is best used as a sheer bronzing cream for cheeks and other key areas of the face, such as temples or the eye contour. I wouldn't take Chanel's advice and apply this balm-like bronzing base all over your face because the color change is noticeable enough that you'd need to apply it to your neck and hands, too, and that's never a good idea for day-to-day makeup. The soft golden tan color works best for light to medium skin tones, and it has a satin powder finish that looks great.

☺ **$$$ Soleil Tan de Chanel Moisturizing Bronzing Powder** *($50)*. Labeling this a moisturizing blush must have been a mistake (either that or Chanel's marketing department never saw or tried the product) because it is not moisturizing in the least. This is a dry powder blush that is almost a bit too powdery for seamless application. Each shade has enough pigment so that it's best to start with a sheer application, and you can layer from there. Among the shades, the most attractive and versatile are Desert Bronze and Terre Ambre, each of which has a subtle sparkling shine. It nearly goes without saying that there are equally good and better bronzing powders at the drugstore.

☺ **$$$ Les Tissages de Chanel Blush Duo Tweed Effect** *($45)*. No one wants a tweed pattern on their cheeks, so it's a good thing the name for this powder blush has to do with the tweed appearance of the blush itself. Unfortunately, that's its most intriguing element; otherwise, this is a very standard blush with shine that's not worth the expense, and isn't in the same league as Chanel's other powder blush.

EYESHADOW: ☺ **$$$ Irreelle Duo Silky Eyeshadow Duo** *($40)* has a beautifully smooth application with slightly softer colors than what you'll find in Chanel's quad and single eyeshadows. Shine is a fact of life with Chanel shadows, but at least they paired some good colors, including Brun-Express and Desert Rose.

☺ **$$$ Les 4 Ombres de Chanel Quadra Eyeshadow** *($56)* has been the backbone of Chanel's eyeshadow collection for years, and they have maintained its enviably silky, utterly blendable texture and wonderfully even application. It is a pleasure to work with these shadows, but working with the colors is another story! In most of these quads, three of the four shades are intensely shiny. Either that, or the selected shades are too contrasting to create an attractive, enhancing eye design. The Spices quad has stronger but workable colors. Without such intense shine, these would easily merit a Paula's Pick rating. For an equally impressive texture and application with less obvious shine, consider Dior's 5-Colour Eyeshadow.

☺ **$$$ Lumieres Facettes Iridescent Effects for Eyes** *($56)* is a quad eyeshadow set that provides copper, peach, and bronze shades, each with a smooth texture and iridescent finish. You should apply it sheer and build from there because these shadows tend to grab if overdone. In addition, it's not a look those with wrinkles around the eye can pull off well. Given the price, be sure you love and will use every shade in the set.

☺ **$$$ Ombre Essentielle Soft Touch Eyeshadow** *($28.50)* consists of single eyeshadows packaged lavishly in the typical Chanel style, complete with their logo embossed on the powder shadow. The formula is accurately described as a creamy-feeling powder, and it applies beautifully—though this is best applied in sheer layers to avoid flaking. You'll find these are pigment-rich, blend smoothly, and their intensity lasts through the day. The matte shades are few and far between, but if shiny eyeshadows are what you want and the price doesn't faze you, this is highly recommended based on its application and longevity. Avoid the green-tinged Bambou, unless you're wearing eyeshadow for shock value.

☹ **$$$ Ombre d' Eau Fluid Iridescent Eyeshadow** *($32)* really is a fluid eyeshadow that comes in a small glass bottle. The biphase formula must be shaken before use (the pigments settle to the bottom of the bottle), but it applies surprisingly easily and evenly. You have only a few seconds to blend this shadow correctly because the formula dries fast and, once dry, stays put—no smudging, flaking, or smearing. It really is an innovative formula and a fun new way to experiment with eyeshadow, but the colors! Only Sand and Source resemble shades that you could use to shape and shadow the eye. The other colors are so bright or pastel they would look out of place as part of a sophisticated eye design. Every shade is intensely shiny, so use these sparingly for evening makeup and avoid them altogether if you have any amount of wrinkling or crepey skin in the eye area.

☹ **$$$ Base Ombre A Paupieres Professional Eye Shadow Base** *($32)* is essentially a cream-to-powder concealer for the eyelids, sold with the claim that it prolongs eyeshadow wear while also brightening eyes. Eye Shadow Base is packaged in a click pen with a brush applicator, and comes in two shades, a fleshy peach tone and the shiny Lumiere Bright. This product does blend well and sets to a matte (in feel) finish, but so do many other concealers, most of which cost less than this.

EYE AND BROW SHAPER: ☺ **$$$ Stylo Yeux Waterproof Long-Lasting Eyeliner Waterproof** *($28)* is indeed waterproof. In fact, this automatic, retractable pencil puts on eyeliner that is nearly budge-proof; it takes considerable effort to remove. However, it applies easily and it lasts, its creamy texture and finish belie its longevity, and it is best for creating a moderately thick rather than thin line. Avoid the various green, blue, and purple shades unless you're going for shock value.

☺ **$$$ Ecriture de Chanel Automatic Liquid Eyeliner** *($34)* is packaged in a click-pen applicator and has a decent, flexible brush. Problems arise when too much liquid liner is dispensed (which happens fairly often), so you wind up wasting a lot of product. It applies a bit too wet, so don't blink or it will smear, though dry time remains fast. Once set, this wears well but you have to be OK with the fact that each shade has a shiny finish. Given the price and the difficult-to-avoid dispensing of excess product, this is one to consider with caution.

☺ **$$$ La Ligne de Chanel Professional Eyeliner Duo** *($45)*. Unless you're a fan of cake eyeliner and want two variations on black (with shine) in one compact, there's little reason to get enthusiastic about this duo, especially given the price. Tools are provided so you can achieve a liquid liner or smoky eye effect, but full-size brushes are preferred to the tiny ones that accompany this product. I can't imagine why someone would choose this over the selection of excellent, easy-to-use gel eyeliners available, many of which also have shine.

☺ **$$$ Le Crayon Khol Intense Eye Pencil** *($27)* is a standard pencil that's about as intense as reading the funny pages on Sunday morning. The pencil's creamy texture has a soft powder finish and the colors are quite soft, meaning you need several applications before you get what most consider an intense line.

☺ **$$$ Le Crayon Yeux Precision Eye Definer** *($28)* is a very expensive, utterly standard pencil that has a soft texture, a slightly dry finish, and an angled sponge tip for blending. Nothing is extraordinary here except the price, and it isn't justified by the performance.

☺ **$$$ Le Crayon Sourcils Precision Brow Definer** *($28)* is a needs-sharpening pencil that has a texture and application a step above most brow pencils, and it includes a brush to comb through brows. This goes on softly, has a dry, smooth finish, and would have been rated a Paula's Pick if sharpening weren't required. If you decide to try this, the Taupe shade is great for blondes (but not platinum or very light blonde brows).

☺ **$$$ Le Sourcil de Chanel Perfect Brows** *($65)* is a set of three powdered brow colors (taupe, medium brown, and brownish black), minitweezers, and a grooming brush in one sleek compact. The intent is for women to mix and match the three shades to achieve their "Perfect Brow," but this ends up being useless for anyone with light hair (which means all blondes), who could maybe use the lightest color; and what are brunettes supposed to do with two dark colors, one of which will undoubtedly make the brows look severe? I could go on, but you get the idea. I admit that the concept has merit, because no one's brows are all one color, but there are dozens upon dozens of suitable brow powders and eyeshadows that perform beautifully and aren't so insultingly expensive.

☹ **Aqua Crayon Eye Colour Stick** *($23.50)* is Chanel's only automatic eye pencil, but since it isn't retractable, winding up more than you need becomes an issue. The tip remains dull and rounded, making it impossible to draw a thin line. Yet it's the creamy, fleeting texture that is the main reason to skip this pencil altogether.

☹ **Forme Sourcils Brow Shaper** *($32)* is only available in clear. There are no shades for brunettes, light blondes, or redheads, and even though it does keep brows in place, it also tends to glob onto the hairs and flake once it's dried. Origins' Just Browsing is a far superior option.

LIPSTICK, LIP GLOSS, AND LIPLINER: ✓ ☺ **$$$ Aqualumiere Sheer Colour Lipshine SPF 15** *($28.50)* is one of a handful of lipsticks whose sunscreen offers adequate UVA protection. This features an in-part avobenzone sunscreen in a silky, weightless, but still creamy-feeling lipstick. All of the colors are gorgeous, though none are all that sheer. For a medium-coverage lipstick with an effective sunscreen, this wins high marks. If only the price weren't so "Chanel." Watch out for the shades with large glitter particles, as these tend to feel grainy as the lipstick wears off. However, to maintain sun protection, you should be reapplying it often anyway, especially if you are spending more than a couple of hours outdoors.

✓ ☺ **$$$ Aqualumiere Gloss High-Shine Sheer Concentrate** *($27)*. If you're going to splurge on lip gloss, it should be on one like this ultra-smooth entry. Easily Chanel's best lip gloss, this applies like liquid silk and enlivens lips with sheer yet exciting color that has more staying power than standard lip gloss (though it still doesn't last nearly as long as lipstick). The high gloss finish is completely non-sticky, while the shade selection is gorgeous and not at all overwhelming.

☺ **$$$ Creme Gloss Lumiere Brush-On Creme Lip Colour** *($32)* is a lipstick/lip gloss hybrid that's housed in a sleek click-pen applicator with a built-in synthetic brush. The thick, viscous texture applies smoothly and imparts a color intensity that's in between a standard lipstick and a sheer gloss. All told, this stays in place quite well, but at the cost of slight stickiness.

☺ **$$$ Rouge Allure Luminous Satin Lip Color** *($30)* promises alluring color and sensational comfort, and it does deliver—but so do many other creamy lipsticks that cost much less than this one. The semi-opaque, shimmer-infused shades slip over lips and feel comfortably light, but the slight amount of stain doesn't promote longevity, so frequent touch-ups are necessary. As usual, Chanel's shade range is an enticing blend of traditional and fashion-forward hues, so you won't be disappointed there. However, I'd think twice about spending this much on lipstick. Chanel made a considerable price leap here for no reason other than status.

☺ **$$$ Rouge Hydrabase Creme Lipstick** *($28.50)* has an excellent creamy, slightly greasy texture and a splendid variety of opaque colors. This traditional cream lipstick is not worth the price when compared with less expensive options. But do women buy Chanel for performance or for the image it evokes?

☺ **$$$ Rouge Double Intensite Ultra Wear Lip Colour** *($34)* is poised as Chanel's answer to the question some women must be asking: "Max Factor's Lipfinity and Cover Girl's Outlast work really well, but isn't there a similar product that costs a lot more?" Mirroring the same concept introduced by the aforementioned products (i.e., a lip color that dries to a matte, unmovable finish, accompanied by a clear gloss that doesn't disturb the color to create a comfortable finish), Rouge Double Intensite Ultra Wear Lip Colour is a formidable option for those looking for long-wearing lip color. The shade selection is smaller than those of competing brands, but each shade is quite attractive, with colors that are complimentary to light and dark skin tones (the dark shades are very dark, so test them before purchasing). It does wear well throughout the day (and night), but as with similar products, it requires regular reapplication of the glossy top coat to keep lips from feeling dry and chapped.

☺ **$$$ Aqua Crayon Lip Colour Stick** *($25)* is an automatic, nonretractable lip pencil that applies well and has good pigmentation to ensure long wear. It's not as creamy as it used to be, and so is a better (though needlessly pricey) option than it once was.

☹ **$$$ Glossimer** *($27)* has a sumptuous name and a bevy of sparkling colors, but that does little to make this very standard, thick, and sticky gloss a top contender. Glossimer just isn't as nice as many newer glosses in all price ranges.

☹ **$$$ Le Crayon Gloss Sheer Lip Colouring Pencil** *($25)*. The price for this belowstandard, needs-sharpening pencil is ludicrous for what you get. The "luminous transparency" Chanel mentions is just another way to state that this is a sheer lip pencil. It has a very greasy consistency that glides on easily, but the effect is, as you can imagine, short-lived. You'll be left wondering why you bothered with this instead of just slicking on some lip gloss.

☹ **$$$ Le Crayon Levres Precision Lip Definer** *($28)* needs sharpening, and despite some versatile colors that are sure to please, this doesn't distinguish itself from many other pencils that cost less. The built-in brush is a nice touch, but not enough to justify the expense.

MASCARA: ✓ ☺ **$$$ Inimitable Waterproof Mascara** *($30)* impresses in every respect, which it should at this price! The rubber-bristled, spiky-looking brush quickly thickens and

lengthens lashes for outstanding definition without clumps. It wears without flaking or smearing, and is very waterproof (you will need an oil- or silicone-based remover when it's time to
take this off).

✓ ☺ **$$$ Exceptionnel De Chanel Intense Volume and Curl Mascara** *($30)*. With
promises of intense volume and sensational curl, does this mascara deliver? Yes and no. Those
hoping for intense curl will be disappointed (though you can always curl lashes beforehand),
but if you let go of that expectation this ends up being an exceptional mascara if you crave
thick, dense lashes. The wetter-than-usual application needs some smoothing with a separate
lash brush for best results, but the payoff is worth it. True to claim, this wears without smudg-
ing or flaking, and removes with a water-soluble cleanser. It is worth mentioning that you don't
need to spend this much money for a fantastic mascara, but if you choose to do so and want
dramatic lashes, you will be pleased.

☺ **$$$ Inimitable Mascara Multi-Dimensionnel** *($30)* is an impressive mascara, but not
superior to many others. You'll achieve length and thickness in nearly equal measures, but nei-
ther is extraordinary and there are some clumps along the way (which can be brushed through
without incident). This wears all day without a flake or smear, and keeps lashes remarkably soft
and with a slight curl. Note: Based on the brush style and rubber bristles, you should know that
similar results are obtainable from Cover Girl's Lash Exact Mascara.

☺ **$$$ Mascara Base Lash Enhancing Base** *($24)* is one of the few pre-mascara lash prim-
ers that make a noticeable difference. The formula differs from most mascaras, and it applies
smoothly without making lashes look too coated. Applying mascara afterward allows for slightly
enhanced definition and more length. I'd argue that you can get even better results by using a
superior mascara, but for those who like the idea of primers, this is a good one to consider.

☹ **$$$ Extracils Super Curl Lengthening Mascara** *($30)*. They have to be joking with
the "super" part of the name, but it isn't too funny considering the price of this below-average
mascara. You will achieve some length and lashes will be cleanly separated, but curl is practically nonexistent, as is thickness. Chanel (and many other lines) have done better with their
other mascaras.

BRUSHES: ✓ ☺ **$$$ Eyeshadow Brushes** *($27-$30)*. Chanel offers several eyeshadow
brushes, and all of them are worth considering if you don't mind the expense. The **#3 Eyeshadow
Crease Brush** is particularly good, as is the **#12 Contour Shadow Brush**. The **#11 Quick
Shadow Brush** is flat, wide, and well-shaped to apply a powder eyeshadow to the entire eyelid
area with ease. Less impressive but still worth considering for those with money to burn are the
#5 Precise Liner Brush and the **#2 Eye Shadow Brush**. Avoid the ☹ **#4 Shadow/Liner Brush**
($27), which is not only overpriced, but also poorly shaped for its intended purposes.

✓ ☺ **$$$ Face/Cheek Brushes** *($34-$52)*. Chanel's powder and blush brushes comprise
their category of face brushes, and they're not quite as elegant as I was hoping. The **#6 Powder
Brush**, which costs over $50, isn't worth it though there's no denying it's soft and works well to
deposit powder. The **#7 Blush Brush** is merely average and also not worth its price. The **#10
Contour Brush** is worth considering, as is the excellent, sumptuously soft **#8 Touch-Up Brush**.
If you're keen on trying a synthetic brush to paint on your foundation and can somehow master
the technique, Chanel's **#16 Foundation Brush** is an excellent option. It's soft, well-shaped,
and has enough give to fit the contours of the face.

☺ **$$$ Brow/Eyeliner Brushes** *($26-$28)*. Chanel's long-handled brow and eyeliner brushes are
a mostly impressive lot, though none of them are worth the price. Still, if designer brushes are what

you're after, you can check out their "push liner" brush, which is synthetic, and their **#9 Eyelash/ Brow Definer**, a dual-sided brush that features a lash comb with metal teeth (so use caution).

FACE AND BODY ILLUMINATING/SHIMMER PRODUCTS: ✓ ☺ $$$ **Brilliance Pur Sheer Brilliance** *($45)* is a generous (for Chanel) sized bottle of liquid shimmer that can be used anywhere, though it's recommended for the face, with or without foundation. It imparts a subtle shine that makes skin look luminous rather than laced with sparkles, and remains one of the top liquid shimmer products around.

☺ $$$ **Base Lumiere Illuminating Makeup Base** *($42)* works to promote smooth skin and leaves a silky feel that isn't the least bit heavy. Sold as a foundation primer, it does facilitate application of makeup, but so do many other lightweight, silicone-based gels and serums. So, while the effect is nice, you don't necessarily need another step in your routine to achieve results.

☺ $$$ **Soleil Lame Tinted Bronzing Gel** *($40)* turns out not to have the texture of a gel. Rather, it's an opaque lotion that feels very light and imparts sheer, peachy bronze color with a soft shimmer finish. The formula blends very well and leaves a bit of a glow that's perfectly suitable for daytime. The sole shade is best for fair to almost medium skin tones.

SPECIALTY PRODUCTS: ☹ $$$ **Le Blanc de Chanel Sheer Illuminating Base** *($45)*. This lightweight foundation primer-type product is basically talc suspended in a moisturizing base. It adds a whitish glow to skin (mica adds some shine), but this is an awfully expensive way to net this ordinary cosmetic effect! This doesn't compete well with other primers or even with the many illuminating products sold from several makeup artist brands. It's needlessly expensive and extraneous. Your payout is far more than the payoff you'll get.

CLARINS

CLARINS AT-A-GLANCE

Strengths: Wide selection of effective, broad-spectrum sunscreens; excellent range of self-tanning products; some good cleansers and gentle topical scrubs; superb foundations and powders; very good powder blush; an ideal brow pencil; wonderfully creamy lipsticks; great lipliner and mascaras.

Weaknesses: Overpriced; pervasive reliance on jar packaging; most products have more fragrance than beneficial plant extracts; poor toners; an overabundance of average moisturizers; no effective products for lightening discolorations or treating acne; no AHA or BHA products; disappointing eye pencils; average eyeshadows and makeup brushes.

For more information about Clarins, call (866) 252-7467 www.clarins.com or www. Beautypedia.com.

CLARINS SKIN CARE

CLARINS ADVANCED EXTRA-FIRMING PRODUCTS

☺ $$$ **Advanced Extra-Firming Day Lotion SPF 15, for All Skin Types** *($78 for 1.7 ounces)* doesn't disappoint with its in-part avobenzone sunscreen and silky, lightweight lotion base. However, for the money, this supplies skin with almost no extras beyond basic sun protection, and any firming benefit would have to be accidental, because none of the ingredients in this daytime moisturizer have that effect. It is best for normal to slightly oily or slightly dry skin.

☺ **$$$ Advanced Extra-Firming Eye Contour Cream** *($58 for 0.7 ounce)* is an extension of Clarins' previously released "extra firming" products, but this version is an "advanced" formula accompanied by a higher price tag, most likely due to the claim that it is specially designed for the eye area. If this is Clarins' idea of an advanced formula, then I assume their chemists are still using textbooks dating back at least a decade or two. Far from being a "revolutionary night-time treatment," this water-based moisturizer has a temporary tightening effect on skin, thanks to the amount of absorbent rice starch it contains and a significant amount of film-forming agent. (Neither of these ingredients is beneficial or helpful for dry skin.) The truly beneficial ingredients are few and far between, including tiny amounts of the plant extracts Clarins always boasts about, but that isn't unique to this product. For an absurd amount of money, you're getting mostly water, thickener, glycerin, rice starch, slip agent, film-forming agent, preservatives, and vitamin E. Not very exciting, and in no way should this be considered a state-of-the-art antiaging moisturizer for the eyes or elsewhere.

☹ **$$$ Advanced Extra-Firming Eye Contour Serum** *($58 for 0.7 ounce)* makes the same claims and has the same non-advanced formulary issues as the Advanced Extra-Firming Eye Contour Cream, except this has a serum texture and omits the rice starch. It still has enough film-forming agent to produce a temporary tightening effect on skin, and the silica lends a drier finish, but this type of effect can eventually make the eye area look dry and more wrinkled. This product does not contain anything that can lift or regenerate skin.

☹ **$$$ Advanced Extra-Firming Neck Cream** *($80 for 1.7 ounces)* claims to be the ultimate firming neck treatment, but that's about as true as saying Ivory soap is the ultimate cleanser. This product contains mostly water, silicone, thickeners, slip agent, preservative, and fragrance. None of it is firming, but it will make dry skin look and feel smoother. That's probably not what you were expecting for $80, but it's the truth.

CLARINS BRIGHT PLUS PRODUCTS

☺ **$$$ Bright Plus Brightening Cleansing Mousse** *($32 for 5.1 ounces)* cannot reduce the appearance of dark spots any more than drinking coffee will make teeth whiter. This is an overpriced but effective water-soluble cleanser that contains mostly water, several detergent cleansing agents, and lather agent. It is best for normal to oily skin.

☺ **$$$ Bright Plus Gentle Brightening Exfoliator** *($34 for 1.7 ounces)* has the properties of a cleanser, topical scrub, and clay mask all in one product, with the clay and its absorbency being the dominant quality. This is an interesting option for someone with normal to oily skin, but is best used in the morning because this much clay isn't going to help remove makeup. Nothing in this product will reduce the appearance or occurrence of dark spots.

☹ **Bright Plus HP Brightening Peel** *($44 for 4.2 ounces)* lists alcohol as the second ingredient, so it is too drying and irritating for all skin types. The amount of AHAs (glycolic and tartaric acids) is far too low for them to function as exfoliants, and that also goes for the BHA (salicylic acid). In addition to the alcohol, this contains several fragrance chemicals that also irritate skin. The fact that this product is positioned as being suitable for "fragile skin" is further testament to how much Clarins doesn't know about good skin care.

☺ **$$$ Bright Plus HP Firming Brightening Serum** *($68 for 1.06 ounces)* is a lighter, less emollient version of the Bright Plus HP Repairing Brightening Night Cream reviewed below, and although it cannot fade a freckle or reduce the appearance of discolorations, it is an OK, ordinary moisturizer for normal to slightly dry or slightly oily skin.

☹ **Bright Plus HP Protective Brightening Day Lotion SPF 20** *($59 for 1.7 ounces)* promises radiant, matte skin all day long, but the amount of alcohol in this daytime moisturizer with an in-part avobenzone sunscreen is irritating. Further, the amount of soothing plant extracts is minimal while fragrance wafts, and none of this is helpful for skin or worth the expense.

☺ $$$ **Bright Plus HP Repairing Brightening Night Cream** *($65 for 1.7 ounces)* is a good moisturizer for normal to dry skin but does not contain a single ingredient that will work to fade sun-induced skin discolorations. This mundane, pricey formulation is a dim light for day or night, though the vitamin C will be preserved thanks to airless jar packaging.

☺ $$$ **Bright Plus HP Intensive Brightening Mask** *($32 for 2.24 ounces)*. In the case of this mask, the packaging is supposed to make you think you're getting potent, individually packaged "doses" of a special treatment, but you're not. The brightening effect comes from titanium dioxide, while the rice starch and clay promote a matte finish (an odd trait for a moisturizing mask, and one that likely will confuse dry or oily skin). The tiny amounts of plants (a common characteristic of Clarins products) have minimal impact on skin. This mask contains a lot of fragrance and also includes several fragrance chemicals that are potential irritants. In the end, this product's brightening effect is simply cosmetic; there is nothing intensive about it. Consider it a superfluous option for normal to slightly dry or slightly oily skin.

☹ **Bright Plus HP On-The-Spot Brightening Corrector** *($35 for 0.34 ounce)* lists alcohol as the second ingredient and that makes this product too irritating and drying for all skin types. In addition, none of the ingredients can fade sun or age spots, and the pH of the product is too high for the tiny amount of salicylic acid it contains to function as an exfoliant.

☹ **Bright Plus HP Intensive Brightening Botanical System with Snow Lotus** *($155 for 1.2 ounces)*. The goal of this two-step system is to "brighten tired-looking skin" and restore "a luminous and healthy-looking glow in just 3 weeks." How is this supposed to be accomplished? Step 1 involves applying **Age Control Concentrate**. A cursory look at the ingredient list reveals what a joke the name of this product is. It's mostly water and alcohol, the latter of which is age-promoting, not reversing. Other than tiny amounts of vitamins C and E, there is nothing positive about this product. It contains a large amount of fragrance and is laced with fragrance chemicals known to cause irritation. What a slap in the face to women looking to take the absolute best care of their skin, regardless of cost! Step 2 is the **Brightening Concentrate**, a bland yet silky moisturizer that contains a tiny amount of vitamin C, most certainly not enough to affect skin discolorations. Again, the amount of fragrance is cause for concern, as is the inclusion of several fragrance chemicals known to be irritating. Used separately or alone, there is no reason to believe either of these products will do much more than make skin feel smoother while inciting inflammation and irritation: two things that lead to increased signs of aging. And who wants to pay good money for that?

CLARINS EXTRA-FIRMING PRODUCTS

☺ $$$ **Extra-Firming Age Control Lip & Contour Care** *($36 for 0.7 ounce)* is a lightweight lotion that contains mostly water, film-forming agent, silicone, glycerin, emollient, and more silicones. The peptide and plant extracts are barely present, and although this can provide moisture and a temporary smooth appearance to lips and the surrounding area, it won't firm them.

☺ $$$ **Extra-Firming Day Cream, for All Skin Types** *($78 for 1.7 ounces)* is a very boring, exceedingly overpriced concoction of water, emollients, glycerin, slip agents, aluminum starch, preservative, and fragrance. The amount of plant extracts (none of which have a firming effect) and peptide is so small as to be nearly inconsequential for skin. This is too emollient for all skin types; it is best for normal to dry skin not prone to breakouts.

☺ **$$$ Extra-Firming Day Cream, Special for Dry Skin** *($78 for 1.7 ounces)* is a more emollient version of the Extra-Firming Day Cream, for All Skin Types above, and as such is preferred for dry to very dry skin. That preference doesn't change the fact that this is an overall mundane formula with an undeserved price.

☺ **$$$ Extra-Firming Day Lotion SPF 15** *($78 for 1.7 ounces)* ends up being one of the better daytime moisturizers from Clarins thanks to its in-part titanium dioxide sunscreen and more interesting mix of lightweight emollients, silicones, and soothing plant extracts. This won't firm skin in any noticeable way, but is a good option for those with normal to slightly oily skin.

☺ **$$$ Extra-Firming Eye Contour Cream** *($58 for 0.7 ounce)* has more of a lotion than cream texture, but it contains some intriguing skin-identical ingredients, antioxidant soy, and emollient peanut oil. Antioxidants are present but in very limited supply, making this a not-quite state-of-the-art option for slightly dry skin anywhere on the face. The product contains fragrance in the form of orange fruit extract.

☺ **$$$ Extra-Firming Eye Contour Serum** *($52.50 for 0.7 ounce)* is a lighter, serum version of the Extra-Firming Eye Contour Cream above, but the amount of fragrant *Rosa gallica* flower extract and pineapple can be a problem for use around the eyes.

☹ **$$$ Extra-Firming Night Cream, for All Skin Types** *($86 for 1.7 ounces)* is the help Clarins maintains skin over age 40 needs (if you're 38 or 39 you'll have to stay away), and purports to lift, firm, and tighten skin each night. The formula is similar to, but more boring than, that of the Extra-Firming Day Cream, for All Skin Types, and absolutely not worth the price. Any facial moisturizer from Eucerin is better than this, and Eucerin isn't all that great! This product is heavily fragranced.

☹ **$$$ Extra-Firming Night Cream, Special for Dry Skin** *($84 for 1.7 ounces)* contains a smattering of plants, but is primarily a water- and mineral oil–based moisturizer joined by several thickeners, glycerin, shea butter, and peanut oil. It will take good care of dry to very dry skin, but it won't make it firmer. It's interesting that although some Clarins products contain mineral oil, I have dealt with several salespeople from this line who love to speak of the alleged evils of this ingredient, ignoring (or oblivious to) the fact that Clarins uses it. Just to be clear, mineral oil is not harmful or suffocating to skin in the least and it doesn't deserve its reputation as a problematic ingredient.

☹ **Extra-Firming Tightening Lift Botanical Serum** *($78 for 1 ounce).* The firming and tightening sensation you get from this water-based serum comes from tapioca starch, an ingredient you can buy at the grocery store for pennies per use. The rest of this product is mostly slip agents, anti-irritant, gel-based thickener, pH adjuster, and fragrance. The amount of peptide is so small it's a joke, and that minuscule amount pales in comparison to the amount in other products with peptides (if that's what you're after), including Olay Regenerist and Olay Definity. Moreover, Clarins included pepper extract (listed as *Capsicum annuum* fruit), a needless irritant that interferes with the soothing action of the oat kernel extract, essentially canceling it out. If you want to spend this much money on an antiaging serum, your skin will be much better served with options from Estee Lauder, Laura Mercier, or MD Skincare by Dr. Dennis Gross. Even the overly fragrant serums from Dior and Chanel best this embarrassing formula.

☺ **$$$ Extra-Firming Facial Mask** *($47 for 2.7 ounces)* is sold to reinforce the benefits of the other Extra-Firming products, but is similar enough that using it will only do what the others products accomplish, which is the basic task of making skin softer and smoother. This is an OK mask for dry to very dry skin not prone to breakouts; it would be rated higher if it contained less fragrance and added some soothing ingredients.

☺ **$$$ Extra-Firming Lip & Contour Balm** *($37 for 0.45 ounce)*. I don't know how the folks at Clarins can sleep at night knowing they've blended mineral oil with waxes, made ridiculous firming claims, and then charged way too much money for a product whose contents comprise some of the least expensive cosmetic ingredients available. Yes, this lip balm will reduce chapping and dryness, but it cannot make lips appear any fuller or younger looking than any other lip balm or Vaseline for that matter. The simple act of moisturizing lips with any helpful ingredient will make them look younger and fuller (moist lips look fuller than dry, cracked lips). This contains cosmetic pigments to reflect light away from lips, which can (cosmetically) make them appear fuller. However, any shimmering lip gloss has the same effect. In short, I can't discredit this product for being ineffective on dry lips, but I encourage you to ignore the antiaging claims and realize you don't have to spend anywhere near this amount of money to have smooth, soft lips. As an example, Neutrogena Lip Nutrition Lip Balm, Vanilla Replenish works beautifully and is far better formulated!

☺ **$$$ Extra-Firming Lip & Contour Gentle Exfoliator** *($23 for 0.6 ounce)* blends mineral oil (a non-plant ingredient Clarins uses way more often than they like to admit, and their counter personnel continually admonish it as a terrible ingredient) and sugar, which does indeed work as a gentle exfoliant. Of course, part of the gentleness depends on the user not applying too much pressure, but if you take care, the result is flake-free, smoothed lips. Clarins also included some fragrance chemicals (and fragrance itself), which aren't the best for lips. More important, you can create this product at home by blending any nonfragrant oil with a small amount of sugar. Mix until a paste is formed, and gently massage this over your lips, then rinse with warm water. You can also use a soft baby's toothbrush to gently exfoliate dry, flaky skin from lips. By the way, regardless of the method, exfoliating lips isn't going to make them firmer, "extra plump" or otherwise.

CLARINS HYDRAQUENCH PRODUCTS

☹ **HydraQuench Cooling Cream-Gel, for Normal to Combination Skin or Hot Climates** *($48 for 1.7 ounces)* lists alcohol as the second ingredient. That certainly explains the cooling effect of this "anti-heatwave" gel (clearly this line is aimed at menopausal women or women afraid global warming is hurting their skin), but it also makes this too drying and irritating for all skin types, regardless of the climate (and alcohol triggers more oil production in the pore lining). Plus the effect is transient at best, lasting only a few seconds, and then it's long gone. There is no reason to subject your skin to this misguided, overly fragranced product.

☺ **$$$ HydraQuench Cream, for Normal to Dry Skin** *($48 for 1.7 ounces)* claims to satisfy the needs of everyone who has normal to dry skin, regardless of temperature variations or climate. Yet this boring moisturizer definitely leaves your skin wanting more beneficial ingredients. It certainly isn't a barometer for skin exposed to varying temperatures or climate shifts; if that were true, the same could be said for countless other moisturizers because the ingredients Clarins used to create this product are at best described as commonplace. In addition, the jar packaging won't keep the smattering of antioxidants stable during use, and you have to tolerate a lot of fragrance, a trait seen throughout the Clarins line. Regarding the claim that this moisturizer is able to address all the needs of normal to dry skin: No way! What about the need for sunscreen, stable packaging, and state-of-the-art ingredients that help create and maintain healthier skin? All of that is missing here; it's only the claims and sales pitch that could make you think you're getting more—more than you really are.

☹ $$$ **HydraQuench Intensive Serum Bi-Phase, for Dehydrated Skin** *($58 for 1 ounce)* is a water-based serum that contains some good emollients and water-binding agents, along with a type of Peruvian nut oil whose fatty acid content is helpful for normal to dry skin. I wouldn't consider this a slam-dunk solution for dehydrated skin in unforgiving climates, but it's a decent, albeit ordinary, serum-type moisturizer for normal to slightly dry skin (assuming you pair it with a sunscreen or foundation with sunscreen for daytime use).

☹ $$$ **HydraQuench Lotion SPF 15, for Normal to Combination Skin or Hot Climates** *($48 for 1.7 ounces)* contains avobenzone to provide sufficient UVA protection, and comes in a lightweight base with an odd mix of absorbents (aluminum starch) and emollients (shea butter). It is likely to leave those who have normal to dry skin wanting more moisture and those with normal to oily or combination skin feeling it is too heavy. Although this contains some helpful ingredients to reinforce healthy skin, it isn't nearly as advanced as the best daytime moisturizers from the Lauder companies, Neutrogena, or Olay.

☹ $$$ **HydraQuench Rich Cream, for Very Dry Skin or Cold Climates** *($48 for 1.7 ounces)* is simply a more emollient version of Clarins' HydraQuench Cream, for Normal to Dry Skin. Adding mineral oil and shea butter does make this better for dry to very dry skin, and the emollients can indeed help protect your skin when subjected to cold weather. However, that benefit isn't by any means unique to this product, which is actually a pretty ordinary moisturizer even with their list of plant extracts (with unproven benefits), which cannot help skin defend itself from climate changes. The claim is based on the fact that the plants can survive dramatic climatic extremes, and Clarins wants you to believe that extracts from these plants can transfer that benefit to your skin. Just because a plant can survive under extreme climatic conditions in its native environment doesn't mean the mechanisms that allow it to do so are transferable to your skin, especially when you consider that the plants are harvested and processed and then teeny amounts of them are added to a cosmetic product.

CLARINS LINE PREVENTION MULTI-ACTIVE PRODUCTS

☹ $$$ **Line Prevention Multi-Active Day Cream, for All Skin Types** *($64 for 1.7 ounces)* is supposed to "regulate daily stresses responsible for premature aging," but without sunscreen, that claim is as reliable as a June snowstorm in Miami! This is yet another mundane moisturizer from Clarins whose formula follows their pattern of standard thickeners and emollients followed by fragrance and tiny amounts of several plant extracts (some beneficial, some problematic, and some with unknown or unproven properties). The helpful plant ingredients (antioxidants) are compromised by jar packaging, making this a lesser consideration and assuredly not one to choose if your concern is forestalling wrinkles.

☹ $$$ **Line Prevention Multi-Active Day Cream, for Dry Skin** *($64 for 1.7 ounces)* is an inappropriate choice for daytime unless you're willing to pair this standard moisturizer with an effective sunscreen. Calling this daytime product "Line Prevention" and not including a sunscreen is sort of like calling chocolate cake a diet food. This is a moisturizer you can easily pass up in favor of products with better formulations, though it has some benefit for normal to dry skin.

☹ $$$ **Line Prevention Multi-Active Day Cream-Gel, for All Skin Types** *($64 for 1.7 ounces)* is also an inappropriate option for daytime use unless you pair it with an effective sunscreen. This is a light-textured moisturizer that is an OK option for normal to slightly dry skin. Most of the plant extracts that Clarins plays up are listed after the preservatives, so they don't count for much. One of the main plant extracts (*Pinus lambertiana*) may have skin-sensitizing properties (Source: Botanical Dermatology Database, http://bodd.cf.ac.uk/index.html).

☺ **$$$ Line Prevention Multi-Active Day Lotion SPF 15** (*$64 for 1.7 ounces*) has a price that is insulting when you consider that the only significant thing this moisturizer has going for it is an in-part avobenzone sunscreen. If no one else was using this UVA sunscreen in their products, Clarins would have a unique product on their hands—but that's not the case. If anything, Line Prevention Multi-Active Day Lotion SPF 15 is mundane and ordinary. And because this is Clarins, there are lots of plant extracts thrown in for show that are not very effective for skin care. What seems to be a priority is the fragrance. Aside from that, there are plenty of sunscreens available at the drugstore with far more in the way of state-of-the-art ingredients, and that cost much less, too.

☺ **$$$ Line Prevention Multi-Active Night Cream** (*$72 for 1.7 ounces*) is a better formulation than the Line Prevention Multi-Active Night Lotion below, and the fragrance is less prominent on the ingredient list. This is an OK moisturizer for normal to dry skin, but lacks any state-of-the-art ingredients that would help justify the price. It almost goes without saying that this product is not able to forestall the appearance of first lines, nor can it offer protection against free-radical damage, since it lacks significant antioxidants.

☺ **$$$ Line Prevention Multi-Active Night Lotion** (*$72 for 1.7 ounces*). Clarins claims that using this will help avoid the appearance of first lines, but without a sunscreen that's a dubious claim. This lackluster formula consists primarily of water, film-forming agent, silicones, and fragrance. This has considerably more fragrance than most of the other ingredients, but no effective skin-identical ingredients or antioxidants. There is no reason to consider this moisturizer over the far more elegant options available from Estee Lauder, Clinique, or Chanel, to name just a few.

☹ **Line Prevention Multi-Active Serum** (*$69 for 1 ounce*) lists drying, irritating alcohol as the second ingredient, while claiming to keep skin looking younger longer. How insulting, and to top that off there isn't a significant amount of a single interesting ingredient in this serum. Any of the serum options from Olay, Neutrogena, or Aveeno beat this one hands down.

CLARINS SUPER RESTORATIVE PRODUCTS

☺ **$$$ Super Restorative Day Cream** (*$110 for 1.7 ounces*) is another fairly standard moisturizer from Clarins with the usual assortment of wow-factor claims, including smoothing wrinkles, helping skin feel "lifted," and restoring a youthful appearance. If you have dry, dehydrated skin, any moisturizer can make skin look younger and feel smoother, so where are the state-of-the-art ingredients to justify the hefty expense? There are barely enough to mention. To make matters worse, Super Restorative Day Cream isn't the best choice for daytime because it lacks a sunscreen, and there is no recommendation on the label to make sure you use sunscreen in addition to this product.

☺ **$$$ Super Restorative Decollete and Neck Concentrate** (*$100 for 1.7 ounces*) purports to reduce visible signs of aging on the neck and chest because of the "high-performing plant extracts" it contains. The plant extracts must be able to exert stellar performance at minuscule concentrations, however, because that's all you're getting in this wolf-in-sheep's-clothing moisturizer disguised as a specialty treatment. Plenty of emollients and skin-silkening agents are on hand to make normal to dry skin look and feel better, but none of the plants can affect pigmentation (age spots from sun damage) or restore the elegant, feminine qualities to an aged-looking décolletage. If anything, the volatile fragrance components in here can cause irritation, and possibly make the chest and neck look blotchy and red. What would have made this product truly super is a blend of potent antioxidants, an AHA for exfoliation, and broad-spectrum sunscreen to protect these oft-exposed areas and prevent further damage.

☹ **$$$ Super Restorative Day Cream SPF 20** *($102 for 1.7 ounces)* has an in-part titanium dioxide sunscreen, but that's the only positive element of this vastly overpriced, overhyped moisturizer. Nothing about it is a restorative treatment for aging skin, and some of the fragrance components can be a problem on skin that's exposed to sunlight.

☹ **$$$ Super Restorative Night Wear** *($118 for 1.7 ounces)* is nearly identical in emollient feel and performance to the Super Restorative Day Cream above, and the same basic comments apply. There is no logical reason to charge more for this product than for the Day Cream, but this would still be illogically priced even if it cost only $20. The various types (and tiny amounts) of algae it contains cannot promote a brighter, more even-toned complexion. Actually, all of the played-up plant extracts—and a few antioxidants too—are listed after the fragrance, so they don't add up to much of anything, and the jar packaging will reduce what little potency may be present.

☹ **$$$ Super Restorative Serum** *($130 for 1 ounce)* is one of Clarins' most expensive skin-care products, but this is also a classic case of a product's name, price, and marketing agenda not adding up to what's inside the bottle, which, for all intents and purposes, is just another moisturizer. The Clarins sales staff would no doubt blanch at that statement, as most of the counter personnel I spoke to treated this product as if it were the fountain of youth, yet they clearly must be entranced by their company's assertions, because nothing in this product can firm, lift, restore, or tone the skin. This product contains mostly water, slip agents, thickeners, emollient, silicone, film-forming agent, water-binding agent, fragrance (lots of fragrance), several plant extracts (all present in minute amounts), caffeine, preservatives, and coloring agents. Clarins tends to favor exotic-sounding plants over state-of-the-art skin-care ingredients such as antioxidants or anti-irritants. Obviously, although that is undeniably enticing to some consumers, it doesn't help skin and it often causes undue irritation. There is no reason to consider this product an antiaging treatment option. If you're shopping for moisturizers at the department store and want a selection of modern, elegant formulas, your skin and pocketbook would be better off exploring the options from Estee Lauder, Chanel, or Clinique before just about anything Clarins offers.

☹ **$$$ Super Restorative Total Eye Concentrate** *($78 for 0.53 ounce)* promises to banish all manner of under-eye skin complaints, from puffiness to crow's feet. Yet all it can do is moisturize the skin, and at most temporarily reduce the appearance of wrinkles. Although this isn't what I would consider a cutting-edge formula, it will make skin look smoother and feel softer. It contains mostly water, silicone, glycerin, thickeners, emollient, preservative, plant extracts, and the tiniest amount of peptides you're likely to find in a skin-care product. Nothing in this eye cream will protect skin from pollution, a claim Clarins is fond of making for many of their moisturizers and specialty items.

OTHER CLARINS PRODUCTS

☹ **Cleansing Milk with Alpine Herbs, for Dry or Normal Skin** *($29.50 for 7 ounces)* is a basic cleansing lotion that rinses decently but contains some problematic plant extracts, including arnica, St. John's wort, and *Melissa* (balm mint), along with fragrance components that are irritating for skin, including eugenol and linalool. This is not recommended for any skin type.

☹ **Cleansing Milk with Gentian, for Combination/Oily Skin** *($29.50 for 7 ounces)* contains a lot of sage extract, way too much fragrance, and lesser but still potentially problematic amounts of fragrance components, including eugenol. This is not recommended because even without the irritants it is way too emollient for its intended skin type.

☺ **$$$ Extra-Comfort Cleansing Cream, for Dry or Sensitized Skin** *($42 for 7 ounces)* is a rich, cold cream–style cleanser for dry to very dry skin. It is not recommended for sensitized skin due to its fragrance and the presence of fragrance components. This requires use of a washcloth for complete removal.

☹ **Gentle Foaming Cleanser for Normal or Combination Skin** *($29 for 4.4 ounces)*. The amount of potassium hydroxide in this cleanser is cause for concern and disqualifies this from being a gentle formula. The potassium hydroxide, combined with some of the other main ingredients, makes this closer to a drying soap than to a gentle water-soluble cleanser. In addition, all of the intriguing plant extracts are wasted in a cleanser because they are just rinsed down the drain, and the fragrance is so potent this product ends up being far more problematic than dozens of other cleansers with fragrance. All told, this is a terrible cleanser and the tight dry feeling it leaves on skin is not good skin care for anyone.

☹ **Gentle Foaming Cleanser for Combination or Oily Skin** *($29 for 4.4 ounces)*. The backbone of this foaming cleanser is nearly identical to the Clarins Gentle Foaming Cleanser for Normal or Combination Skin above. As such, the same review applies.

☺ **$$$ Gentle Foaming Cleanser for Dry or Sensitive Skin** *($29 for 4.4 ounces)* replaced Clarins' former Gentle Foaming Cleanser, but it isn't an improvement in any way, shape, or form. By no means is this a bad cleanser, but the fragrance and preservatives it contains shouldn't be in a product meant for sensitive skin. Best for normal to dry skin, this water-soluble foaming cleanser has a lotion-like texture that removes makeup well, if you can stand the amount of fragrance (which sensitive skin definitely should not risk). Another issue is the price, which is significantly higher than that of any cleanser I recommend from the drugstore. You're not getting extra benefits with this Clarins cleanser, other than the prestige and French flair the brand espouses.

☹ **One-Step Facial Cleanser** *($32 for 6.8 ounces)* lacks cleansing agents and is sort of a modified silicone-based makeup remover. The amount of orange-fruit water makes this ill-advised for use around the eyes, and several of the fragrance components will prove irritating because this product is not intended to be rinsed from skin.

☺ **$$$ One-Step Gentle Exfoliating Cleanser** *($35 for 4.4 ounces)* is a standard, but good, water-soluble cleanser that contains gentle detergent cleansing agents. Plant cellulose provides a mild exfoliating effect, and is fine for occasional use by all skin types—just use caution and avoid massaging this over blemishes. Clarins claims this cleanser purifies and smooths the skin with natural botanicals, but their presence is sparse and mainly provides an orange-tinged fragrance. Actually, the ratio of synthetic to natural ingredients in this product is 5:1, which pretty much nullifies any credibility for the botanical claim.

☹ **Pure Melt Cleansing Gel, for All Skin Types** (*$32 for 3.9 ounces*) is supposed to veil skin in gentleness, but if that's the case, why did Clarins choose the preservatives methylchloroisothiazolinone and methylisothiazolinone (Kathon CG) for this residue-leaving, emollient, oily cleanser? Both preservatives are known for their sensitizing potential, and are not the best choice for a cleanser whose oil and emollient ingredients remain on your skin even after rinsing. This will remove any kind of makeup easily, but the ingredients Clarins used to do that are incredibly commonplace.

☺ **$$$ Water Comfort One-Step Cleanser, for Normal to Dry Skin** (*$30 for 6.8 ounces*) is a water- and solvent-based cleanser that contains gentle cleansing agents and, aside from fragrance, no problematic ingredients. That's a positive step since this product is meant to be a convenient cleanser that does not require rinsing. It is an option for normal to slightly dry skin, but is not adept at removing long-wearing or waterproof makeup.

☹ **Water Purify One-Step Cleanser, for Combination or Oily Skin** (*$30 for 6.8 ounces*) is a cleanser that doesn't require rinsing, but contains peppermint extract, which may feel refreshing but winds up irritating skin unless you rinse thoroughly, which isn't the point of this otherwise gentle cleanser.

☺ **$$$ Gentle Eye Make-Up Remover Lotion** (*$26 for 4.32 ounces*) is an exceptionally standard water-based makeup remover that contains a lot of fragrant rose water along with soothing cornflower water. The rose water isn't the best for use around the eyes, making this not preferred to less costly options that omit fragrant additives.

☺ **$$$ Instant Eye Make-up Remover** (*$26 for 4.32 ounce*) is a standard, silicone-in-water, dual-phase fluid that works very well to remove stubborn makeup and waterproof mascara. The rose flower water is primarily fragrance, and doesn't make this preferred to less expensive silicone-based removers from Almay or Neutrogena, among others.

☹ **Expertise 3P** (*$42 for 3.5 ounces*) contains mostly water, rosemary water, slip agent, salt, water-binding agent from bacteria, detergent cleansing agent, plant extracts, gum-based thickener, pH-adjusting agent, preservative, and more slip agents. Can any of these ingredients protect skin from the "accelerated aging effects of all indoor and outdoor pollution," especially electromagnetic waves? Not in the least. Such logic is on par with thinking that a steady diet of cheese pizza will fulfill all of your nutritional needs. Clarins heralds this product as a worldwide first, and it is—though that doesn't mean it's an innovative, must-have product whose time has come. Rather, it just has an eccentric, something-else-to-be-afraid-of marketing angle. Electromagnetic radiation (low- or high-frequency electrical currents, also called electromagnetic fields [EMF]) has been around since the birth of the universe; light is its most familiar form. Electromagnetic radiation includes radiation from magnets, the sun, cell phones, X-rays, radios, televisions, heat lamps, and on and on. Tiny electrical currents are even present in the human body due to the chemical reactions that occur as part of normal bodily functions, even in the absence of external electric fields. For example, nerves relay signals by transmitting electrical impulses. Most biochemical reactions, from digestion to brain activity, are associated with the rearrangement of charged (electric) particles. Even the heart is electrically active—an activity a doctor can trace with the help of an electrocardiogram. You have to wonder what would happen if Expertise 3P could protect us from all that! There is concern about EMFs, though it's not so much from computer monitors, which are truly a minor source. However, the World Health Organization, after reviewing more than 25,000 research papers on the topic, concluded that there is no negative biological consequence associated with low-level electrical currents. Therefore, there is no need to "protect" skin with a "snake-oil" product like this one. The unhappy face rating has little to do with the product's formula, which ends up being that of a very ordinary toner. Rather, it pertains to the false claims that may stir a sense of unease in women who sit down in front of their computers every day.

☺ **$$$ Extra-Comfort Toning Lotion, for Dry or Sensitized Skin** *($30 for 6.8 ounces)* is a fairly basic toner but it does contain some decent ingredients for dry skin. The problem is that the really beneficial ingredients are listed after the preservative and the fragrant ingredients, so there's little chance this will be what sensitized skin needs.

☹ **Toning Lotion with Iris, for Combination or Oily Skin** *($26.50 for 7 ounces)* lists witch hazel as the second ingredient and contains a lesser but still worrisome amount of iris root extract.

☺ **$$$ Toning Lotion, for Dry or Normal Skin** *($26.50 for 7 ounces)* is an OK toner for normal to dry skin, but does not distinguish itself from several less expensive options. It contains some good skin-identical ingredients, but leaving the fragrance components on the skin after daily use isn't the best idea.

☺ **$$$ Gentle Exfoliating Refiner** *($28.50 for 1.7 ounces)* is a good, basic creamy scrub that contains cellulose as the abrasive agent. That is indeed gentle and makes this a good, though pricey, scrub for normal to dry skin.

☺ **$$$ Gentle Facial Peeling** *($30 for 1.4 ounces)* uses paraffin (a wax) to gently exfoliate skin. You apply this cream-textured product to skin, and as you massage it in the paraffin balls up, taking dead skin cells with it for a smooth result. Clarins maintains that regular use of this product helps skin "breathe better," but the wax can leave a film that clogs pores, so that claim is nonsense. A product like this is best for exfoliating dry trouble spots such as elbows, knees, and heels. A water-soluble topical scrub is better for the face.

☺ **$$$ Beauty Flash Balm** *($45 for 1.7 ounces)* is an extremely average moisturizer that contains absorbent rice starch, which can be problematic for dry skin. It temporarily makes skin feel tighter, but that's about all the flash you'll get.

☹ **Contouring Facial Lift** *($67 for 1.7 ounces)* lists alcohol as the second ingredient, and that makes this serum too irritating for all skin types. Nothing in this product will minimize signs of slackened skin.

☺ **$$$ Double Serum Generation 6** *($94 for 1.06 ounces)* is a dual-phase product that Clarins sells as "the complete answer to age-control." It certainly isn't complete—what about sunscreen, something that's key to antiaging and not present in this serum? And what about the dozens of other products Clarins sells, all claiming a subtle variation on that theme? Reading the ingredient list for both the Hydro Serum and Lipo Serum, neither one has any wow-factor ingredients. In fact, both contain mostly common ingredients that show up in hundreds of other moisturizers (and some serums), including other options from Clarins. The Hydro (referring to water) Serum is mostly water, glycerin, starch, slip agents, preservative, and film-forming agent. Plant extracts and a peptide are barely present, certainly not in an amount your skin will derive great benefit from. The Lipo (lipid, as in fat) portion adds dry-finish solvents, oils, vitamin-based antioxidants, and emollients to the mix, along with a lot of fragrance, making it the more interesting of the two, but still not enough to warrant the investment. Of course, they're dispensed as one and applied to skin, so you're getting a mix of beneficial, questionable, and very fragrant ingredients. How this is the answer to age control is anyone's guess, but it's an OK moisturizing serum for dry skin—just keep it away from the eye area due to the potent fragrance.

☺ **$$$ Energizing Morning Cream** *($59 for 1.7 ounces)* has a very long ingredient list, parts of which read like a trip through your grocer's produce department. Tiny amounts of pineapple, kiwi, and orange won't energize skin, and this remains another ho-hum, jar-packaged moisturizer that's a poor choice for daytime unless you're willing to pair it with a sunscreen or a foundation with sunscreen. The formula is suitable for normal to dry skin.

☹ **$$$ Eye Contour Balm, for All Skin Types** *($48 for 0.7 ounce)* is an exceedingly ordinary moisturizer that would be OK for dry skin. However, it lacks any state-of-the-art ingredients for skin, and a couple of the fragrance components can be irritating for use around the eyes.

☹ **$$$ Eye Contour Balm, Special for Dry Skin** *($48 for 0.7 ounce)* contains mostly water, mineral oil, thickeners, water-binding agent, silicone, plant oils, antioxidants, mica (adds shine), and preservatives. This is a good moisturizer for dry skin but it isn't special, although it is preferred to the All Skin Types version.

☹ **$$$ Eye Contour Gel** *($48 for 0.7 ounce)* is primarily water, slip agent, and the pH-adjusting and emulsifying ingredient triethanolamine. It is fragrance-free, but other than feeling refreshing due to its gel texture it has minimal benefit for skin around the eyes.

☹ **$$$ Eye Revive Beauty Flash** *($46 for 0.7 ounce)* is supposed to be an emergency treatment to relieve dark circles, puffiness, and fine lines around the eyes. It's a basic moisturizer with a standard combination of mostly water, thickener, slip agents, glycerin, antioxidant olive leaf, emollient, film-forming agent, and preservative. It will take care of dry skin around the eyes, but calling this a "one-of-a-kind treatment" is akin to thinking tap water is a rare beverage.

☹ **Face Treatment Oil, Blue Orchid, for Dehydrated Skin** *($48 for 1.4 ounces)* contains a lot of irritating patchouli oil as well as irritating rosewood oil and several volatile fragrance components, making this about as good for dehydrated skin as massaging it with sandpaper!

☹ **Face Treatment Oil, Lotus, for Combination Skin** *($48 for 1.4 ounces)* contains rosemary, geranium, and clary oils, all of which are irritating to skin and do not provide a soothing or rebalancing benefit for combination skin. This oil-based product cannot tighten pores; if anything, this much oil can lead to clogged pores, which will enlarge their appearance.

☹ **Face Treatment Oil, Santal, for Dry or Extra Dry Skin** *($48 for 1.4 ounces)* contains a lot of sandalwood and lavender oils, along with more fragrance and problematic fragrance components. This is akin to applying perfume to your face and is not recommended.

☺ **$$$ Gentle Day Cream, for Sensitive Skin** *($59 for 1.7 ounces)* isn't more gentle than most Clarins moisturizers and the fact that it contains fragrance shows they're not taking the needs of truly sensitive skin seriously. Still, this can be a good moisturizer for normal to dry skin not prone to blemishes, and most of the plant extracts are soothing and anti-inflammatory, which is a nice change of pace.

☺ **$$$ Gentle Night Cream, for Sensitive Skin** *($69 for 1.7 ounces)* is nearly identical to the Gentle Day Cream, for Sensitive Skin, and its higher price isn't justified. Either option is best for normal to dry skin not prone to blemishes.

☹ **$$$ Hydra-Matte Lotion, for Combination Skin** *($39.50 for 1.7 ounces)*. This glycerin-enriched fluid does not contain skin-repairing ingredients, at least not any that can't be found in hundreds of other moisturizers. Fragrance and preservatives are listed before all of the plant extracts (some of which are soothing) and antioxidants, so the latter don't count for much.

☹ **Pore Minimizing Serum** *($47 for 1 ounce)* leaves skin with a soft matte finish, but the amount of alcohol here means this isn't the best for any skin type. None of the plant extracts in this serum have any effect on pores. Even if they did, the amount of each is minuscule when compared with the amount of fragrance. Clinique's Pore Minimizer products are much better than this.

☺ **$$$ Renew-Plus Night Lotion** *($65 for 1.7 ounces)* is said to contain a retinol precursor activated by plant extracts, but retinyl palmitate is not the precursor to retinol, nor can it be activated by plants to become retinol; even if it could, they'd be moving in the wrong direction, since retinol and retinyl palmitate require special enzymes in skin to convert them to all-trans retinoic acid. Even if this was a slam-dunk process, there's barely any vitamin A in this moisturizer. It is a decent formulation for normal to dry skin and contains some helpful plant oils and a couple of good antioxidants.

☹ **Skin Beauty Repair Concentrate for Sensitive Skin** *($59 for 0.5 ounce)* is an emollient fluid that contains irritating lavender and marjoram oils. Talk about adding fuel to the fire! Topically applied lavender oil can cause skin cell death (Source: *Cell Proliferation*, June 2004, pages 221-229).

☹ **Ultra-Matte Rebalancing Lotion, for Oily Skin** *($39.50 for 1.7 ounces)* lists alcohol as the second ingredient, which means this won't rebalance anything. The alcohol will irritate skin and generate more oil production in the pore lining, which is exactly what those struggling with oily skin don't need. This product also contains a significant amount of fragrance; the most helpful ingredient, green tea, is listed last.

☺ **$$$ Younger Longer Balm** *($99 for 1.7 ounces).* What a great, succinct name. No question as to what this product is supposed to do! Clarins goes off the deep end with claims for this product, especially with their statement that it "maintains proper functioning of skin nerve endings." What we apply to our skin can indeed affect nerves in our skin—just touching your skin affects the nerve endings, but "proper functioning"? My question is: How do your nerve endings behave improperly? By reacting? If anything, the nerve endings in skin may be adversely affected by the amount of fragrance in this moisturizer for normal to dry skin. For the money, you're not getting anything special; all of the intriguing ingredients are listed after the fragrance, as is typical of Clarins. Moreover, without a sunscreen, this doesn't hold much promise of keeping your skin looking younger for even one second longer. All in all, this product is really disappointing, at least if you're expecting protection from free radicals and a reduction in broken capillaries. For less money, you'd be wise to consider any of the non-jar–packaged moisturizers from Clinique or Estee Lauder.

☺ **$$$ Skin-Smoothing Eye Mask** *($46 for 1.05 ounces)* does not contain ingredients unique to the eye area, and the amount of rice starch may prove too drying. Nothing in this product will minimize dark circles or puffiness either. This has moisturizing qualities, but is not preferred to several other masks and moisturizers.

☺ **$$$ Pure and Radiant Mask** *($28.50 for 1.7 ounces)* contains more moisturizing ingredients than absorbents, which may leave combination to oily skin confused rather than purified. This mask is best for normal to slightly dry skin, but for the money it's a rather superfluous product. Contrary to claim, the thickening agents this mask contains can clog pores.

☹ **Blemish Control** *($22.50 for 0.34 ounce)* has a roll-on applicator that may seem convenient, but this product contains too much alcohol and too little of anything even remotely capable of minimizing blemishes. Wintergreen and volatile fragrance components make this even more troublesome for inflamed, reddened skin.

☺ **$$$ Moisture Replenishing Lip Balm** *($24 for 0.46 ounce)* is a mineral oil–based lip balm that contains an effective blend of emollient thickeners and helpful plant extracts. It's a pricey way to care for dry, chapped lips, but will do the job if you decide to splurge. The amount of peptide is so small as to be inconsequential.

☹ **Stretch Mark Control** *($49 for 6.8 ounces)* purports to prevent stretch marks from forming and to reduce the appearance of stretch marks that are less than two years old. How it goes about doing this isn't explained, and rightly so, because it isn't possible. Stretch marks are broken elastin fibers in the subcutaneous (lower) layers of skin, coupled with collagen bundles trying to correct the damage. The problem happens because not all of the pieces of the "building materials" are there, resulting in the familiar white lines that, in most people, are slightly raised, though they may also be indented. Aside from topical application of prescription tretinoin, no other topical product is backed by any evidence it can prevent stretch marks or measurably reduce their appearance. And even tretinoin's results aren't that impressive, unless you consider a 20% length reduction wow-inducing (Source: *Advances in Therapy*, July/August 2001, pages 81-86). This product is principally body lotion with a selection of plant extracts, none of which have a shred of research proving their mettle against stretch marks. Clarins' use of *Empetrum nigrum* fruit juice is actually a problem for skin. This plant, also known as crowberry or poke-weed, has components (especially the root) that are toxic to skin cells. In fact, ingesting only ten crowberries can be fatal to an otherwise healthy adult (Source: www.naturaldatabase.com). This product will have zero effect on stretch marks, but may cause skin problems.

☹ **Body Shaping Supplement** *($77 for 1.68 ounces)*. Sigh. Here we have another product aiming to diminish fat deposits and cellulite (how many of these can the cosmetics industry launch before women learn that none of these ever change a dimple anywhere on the body? This time it's sold as an additive you can mix with your regular body moisturizer, sort of like adding liquid vitamins to your food—except this isn't the least bit nutritious (read: beneficial) for skin. Clarins makes drug-like claims by stating that applying this product blocks the formation of new adipocytes (fat cells), which it absolutely cannot do. It also cannot reduce unwanted curves by stimulating fat removal. Besides, cellulite is unrelated to fat content, over 85% of all women have cellulite and a good percentage of those are normal weight. The major ingredients in this product are water, alcohol, slip agents, and caffeine. None of these can affect the formation or size of new fat cells, nor can they dissolve existing pockets of fat. If such simple ingredients could do this, then who would be fat? Think about it: A few too many pints of ice cream late at night and all we have to do to fix the damage is massage our skin with alcohol and caffeine? It's not possible, and Clarins should be ashamed of itself for proffering such a product without a modicum of proof concerning its effectiveness.

☹ **High Definition Body Lift** *($65 for 6.9 ounces)*. What is in this "high definition" product? Mostly water, alcohol, slip agents, caffeine, fragrance, and irritating menthol. The only ingredient of note that's related to cellulite reduction is caffeine, which is popular in cellulite-related products because caffeine contains theophylline (Source: *Progress in Neurobiology*, December 2002, pages 377-392), which is a modified form of aminophylline, a pharmaceutical that once was thought to reduce cellulite (Source: *Yale New Haven Health Library, Alternative/Complementary Medicine,* www.yalenewhavenhealth.org). However, there is no substantiated research proving theophylline can affect cellulite, and researchers have disproved aminophylline's claimed impact on cellulite. The second reason caffeine may show up in cellulite products stems from research showing it to have benefit for weight loss, but that's only when you drink it, not when you rub it on your thighs. Regardless, if you want to believe caffeine is the answer, make a toner of your own with leftover coffee or consider products (equally silly, but cheaper) by RoC and Aveeno.

High Definition Body Lift won't get your thighs ready for close-up photos, although you may notice a temporary tightening sensation from the alcohol. Unfortunately, all the alcohol is doing is irritating your skin and causing free-radical damage. The menthol is just there so your skin will tingle and you'll think the product is working. Clarins has reformulated and re-launched their Body Lift product numerous times, and none of them have worked even remotely like the claims suggest. If any of them did, you'd have to ask yourself why Clarins never keeps one of them around for long. One more technical point: Research has shown that when caffeine and its derivatives are formulated in a gel vehicle (such as this product) the caffeine was not effective in reducing the size of fat cells in vitro (meaning not on people, but in a petri dish). Also, when sodium benzoate was added to the formula, the caffeine was rendered ineffective (Source: *Journal of Cosmetic Dermatology*, March 2008, pages 23-29). Guess what? High Definition Body Lift contains sodium benzoate. That means even if caffeine could work, it wouldn't in this product formulated by Clarins.

CLARINS SELF-TANNING PRODUCTS

☺ **After Sun Moisturizer with Self Tanning Action** *($30 for 5.3 ounces)* is sold to prolong and enrich a natural tan, a choice that is infuriating from a company with so many products that claim to forestall aging and wrinkles, because getting a tan from the sun is what causes the wrinkles in the first place. (Well, perhaps that's job security for Clarins?) Despite the lack of ethics involved in encouraging tanning, this is a good self-tanning lotion that contains dihydroxyacetone (DHA) and a small amount of erythrulose, an ingredient similar to DHA that develops color at a slower rate.

☹ **$$$ Delicious Self Tanning Cream** *($42 for 3.9 ounces)* could not be a more basic self-tanning lotion if it tried, and labeling this as having "skin-nourishing benefits" is like labeling M&Ms as health food. Like most self-tanners, this turns skin color with dihydroxyacetone. A secondary self-tanning agent (erythrulose) is in here as well, so your color will continue to develop after the initial tan appears within hours. That's nice, but many other self-tanners offer this perk, and few dare to charge as much as Clarins. If you want a Clarins self-tanner, they offer several options more elegant than this.

☺ **Intense Bronze Self Tanning Tint, for Face and Decollete** *($32 for 4.2 ounces)* is a tinted self-tanner so you'll get instant sheer bronze color and a longer-lasting "tan" once the dihydroxyacetone has time to work its magic on skin. Alcohol is the third ingredient listed, but it's unlikely to cause irritation because of the small amount relative to the ingredients that precede it. This product's cotton-pad applicator is a nifty inclusion, but for best results you'll still want to blend it into your skin with your fingers.

☺ **Liquid Bronze Self Tanning, for Face and Decollete** *($32 for 4.2 ounces)* is a very silky self-tanning lotion that can be used anywhere on the body. It turns skin tan with dihydroxyacetone and a lesser amount of the self-tanning ingredient erythrulose.

☺ **Radiance-Plus Self Tanning Body Lotion** *($42 for 5.3 ounces)* has a color result similar to that of the Radiance-Plus Self Tanning Cream-Gel reviewed below, but in a more emollient lotion base. This version may be used on the face if desired, and is best for normal to dry skin.

☺ **$$$ Radiance-Plus Self Tanning Cream-Gel** *($52 for 1.7 ounces)* is a lightweight, silicone-enhanced moisturizer with a lesser amount of the self-tanning ingredient DHA. That means less color, so this can be a good option for fair skin tones or times when you want a hint of sunless tan rather than that "day at the beach" look.

☺ **Self Tanning Instant Gel** *($32 for 4.4 ounces)* contains dihydroxyacetone to turn skin tan, along with a tiny amount of erythrulose, all in a silky lotion base that doesn't feel thick or greasy. Clarins states there's no need to wait before dressing once this is applied, but I'd play it safe and wait at least 30 minutes to avoid streaks and stained clothing.

☺ **Self Tanning Milk SPF 6** *($32 for 4.4 ounces)* has an in-part avobenzone sunscreen, but the SPF rating makes it too low for daytime protection. Given that most people don't apply self-tanner daily, formulating one with a sunscreen is an odd choice. This product is recommended as a standard, creamy self-tanner, though its active ingredient, dihydroxyacetone, is found in many self-tanning products that cost less than this.

CLARINS SUN PRODUCTS

☺ **$$$ Sun Care Spray Radiant Oil Low Protection SPF 6, for Body and Hair** *($30 for 5 ounces)* is an emollient, spray-on sunscreen that contains avobenzone (3%) for sufficient UVA protection. The SPF rating on the label is too low for it to provide sufficient protection, and as a result this sunscreen for dry skin is difficult to recommend. It can be an option for hair that's dry or exposed to the elements, but keep in mind we have no reliable information or standards to determine how much sun protection you're getting when sunscreen is applied to hair. But, if the FDA gets a peek at the SPF claim and the label that says it works on hair, they won't be happy, because hair-care products worldwide are not allowed to carry an SPF rating.

☹ **Sunscreen Cooling Gel Rapid Tanning SPF 8** *($34 for 6.8 ounces)* achieves sufficient UVA protection from its in-part avobenzone sunscreen, but the SPF rating, according to the American Academy of Dermatology and the Skin Cancer Foundation, is too low for daytime protection, and the base formula is primarily alcohol, which makes this drying and irritating.

☺ **$$$ Sun Control Stick Ultra Protection SPF 30, for Sun-Sensitive Areas** *($26 for 0.17 ounce)* is an emollient, oil-based sunscreen stick that includes titanium dioxide for UVA protection. It's a good choice for use over dry to very dry areas of skin, or areas such as the scalp or top of the ears, assuming you feel the need to overspend on sun protection.

☺ **$$$ Sunscreen Cream High Protection SPF 30, 100% Mineral Filters, for Children** *($30 for 4.32 ounces)* is indeed a good option for kids because it provides gentle, broad-spectrum protection with titanium dioxide and zinc oxide. The creamy lotion formula is fine for adults too, particularly those with normal to dry skin. This would be a slam dunk for sensitive skin if it did not contain fragrance, and would be even better for all skin types if it contained some established antioxidants. However, it is still worth considering.

☺ **$$$ Sunscreen Cream High Protection SPF 30, for Sun-Sensitive Skin** *($30 for 4.32 ounces)* has too many synthetic active ingredients and too much fragrance to make it a safe bet for sensitive skin, but it does include titanium dioxide for sufficient UVA protection. This water-resistant sunscreen has a silky-smooth finish that doesn't feel too thick, and is best for normal to slightly dry or slightly oily skin.

☹ **Sunscreen Smoothing Cream-Gel Rapid Tanning SPF 10** *($37 for 6.8 ounces)* has a name that should not be taken seriously, because the sunscreen agents in this product, which include avobenzone, are not designed to allow skin to tan rapidly, nor do you want your skin to tan (well, at least not if you want to keep it healthy and youthful). Regardless of the ethical issue of a company selling dozens of antiwrinkle products alongside items like this that encourage tanning, the amount of alcohol in this sunscreen makes it a poor choice for skin of any color.

☺ **Sunscreen Soothing Cream Progressive Tanning SPF 20** *($37 for 6.8 ounces)* is said to ensure an even, long-lasting tan, which is an unethical claim for any cosmetics company to make, especially one with as many antiaging products as Clarins. Still, this in-part titanium dioxide sunscreen is a great option for normal to slightly dry or slightly oily skin. It is very similar to the Sunscreen Cream High Protection SPF 30, for Sun-Sensitive Skin.

☺ **Sunscreen Spray Gentle Milk-Lotion Progressive Tanning SPF 20** *($29 for 5.2 ounces)* leaves skin wanting more in terms of antioxidants (fragrance got higher priority in this sunscreen), but it's an easy-to-apply, alcohol-free sunscreen spray that includes 3% avobenzone for UVA protection. The water-resistant formula is best for oily to very oily or breakout-prone skin. It may be applied to face or body (but don't spray it directly on your face).

☹ **Sunscreen Spray Oil-Free Lotion Progressive Tanning SPF 15, for Outdoor Sports** *($30 for 5.2 ounces)*. Clarins should be ashamed of selling so many products that encourage tanning from the sun. Ignoring this issue (which I can't; I just want to scream!), this in-part avobenzone sunscreen suffers from an alcohol base that makes it too drying and irritating for all skin types.

☺ **$$$ Sunscreen Spray Radiant Oil Intensive Tanning SPF 4, for Body and Hair** *($28 for 5.1 ounces)* includes avobenzone for UVA protection, but SPF 4 is a pathetic rating unless your time outdoors is very brief. Ignoring the "intensive tanning" part of this product's name, it's a nonaqueous, triglyceride- and silicone-based spray that can make hair look greasy, and it's not recommended for skin unless you're willing to pair it with a sunscreen that meets trustworthy dermatology guidelines for daytime protection.

☹ **Sun Tinted Gel SPF 10** *($27.50)*. This merely OK bronze-tinted gel is not recommended because its SPF rating is too low (most medical associations recommend a minimum of SPF 15) and it does not contain the UVA-protecting ingredients of titanium dioxide, zinc oxide, avobenzone, Tinosorb, or Mexoryl SX.

☺ **$$$ Sun Wrinkle Control Cream Ultra Protection SPF 30, for Sun-Sensitive Skin** *($29.50 for 2.7 ounces)* is a good, though ordinary, in-part titanium dioxide sunscreen in a moisturizing cream base suitable for dry to very dry skin. It is oil-free as claimed, but the thickening agents are a poor fit for oily or blemish-prone skin. And by the way, all skin types and all skin colors are sun-sensitive!

☺ **$$$ Sun Wrinkle Control Cream Very High Protection SPF 15, for Face** *($29.50 for 2.6 ounces)* has a misleading name because no one familiar with sunscreen chemistry would consider SPF 15 to be "very high protection." This in-part titanium dioxide sunscreen has a smooth lotion base that lacks any bells or whistles (the antioxidants are window dressing only), but it is suitable for normal to dry skin.

☺ **$$$ Sun Wrinkle Control Eye Contour Care Ultra Protection SPF 30** *($28 for 0.7 ounce)* contains only titanium dioxide as the active ingredient, making this a gentle, nonstinging option to use around the eyes. The base formula isn't exciting, but it is fragrance-free—a rarity for Clarins!

☹ **After Sun Gel Ultra Soothing** *($30 for 5.3 ounces)* lists alcohol as the second ingredient, which isn't the least bit soothing, especially if you're dealing with sunburn.

☹ **After Sun Moisturizer Ultra Hydrating** *($32 for 7 ounces)* doesn't improve Clarins' track record of producing average moisturizers. This is an OK option for dry skin, sun-exposed or not, but doesn't best what's available at the drugstore from Curel, Olay, or even Lubriderm.

☹ **$$$ After Sun Replenishing Moisture Care for Face** *($36 for 1.7 ounces)* should be loaded with antioxidants and ingredients that mimic the structure and function of healthy skin—but it's not, which makes this a poor choice for after-sun care. This is a lot of money, too, for what amounts to water, thickeners, silicone, and talc.

CLARINS MAKEUP

FOUNDATION: ✓☺ **$$$ Extra Firming Foundation** *($42)* doesn't contain a single ingredient capable of firming skin, extra or otherwise (tiny amounts of mushroom and algae extracts do not firm skin). That doesn't stop this foundation from being a top choice for someone with normal to dry skin. Its texture and application are creamy smooth, setting to a soft matte finish that remains slightly moist to the touch, which provides a healthy glow. You can attain medium to full coverage, but it looks best when blended on lightly (over a sunscreen if you're using it during daylight hours). The range of shades has some impressively neutral options for fair to medium skin, as well as Clarins' only selection of truly dark foundation shades (Mahogany, Camel, and Chestnut).

✓☺ **$$$ Truly Matte Foundation SPF 15** *($37.50)* has an utterly accurate name! This fluid is a beautiful, silky liquid foundation that provides sun protection solely from titanium dioxide, which helps contribute to its powdery, long-wearing matte finish. Even better, this provides light to medium coverage while looking surprisingly skinlike. Someone with very oily skin will be pleased with the application and finish, not to mention the sun protection, because that means you wouldn't have to layer products. Drawbacks include a strong scent and the fact that the darkest shades tend to look a bit dull due to the amount of titanium dioxide and the dry finish of the silicones. Among the 15 shades (Clarins' largest selection) are options for fair to dark (but not very dark) skin tones. Most of the shades are very good; the ones to avoid are the slightly peach Ginger, Real Honey, and Hazelnut, the slightly pink Sunlit Beige, and the orange-tinged Nutmeg.

✓☺ **$$$ Express Compact Foundation Wet/Dry** *($37)* has a supremely silky, talc-based texture and blends seamlessly to a natural matte finish that makes skin look dimensional, not dry and powdery. The eight outstanding shades provide sheer to light coverage, but there are no options for dark skin tones. It can be used wet for more coverage, but apply it carefully or you'll risk streaking.

☺ **$$$ Super Restorative Tinted Moisturizer SPF 20** *($77)*. This creamy tinted moisturizer with a pure titanium dioxide sunscreen has a beautiful smooth texture that feels luxurious and enlivens dull skin with sheer, luminescent color. Each of the four shades has a peach to orange cast, but the sheerness makes it a non-issue except for the darkest shade (05 Tea). The formula sets to a satin matte finish that remains slightly moist to the touch. As for the claims, all I can say is they are as inflated as Goldie Hawn's lips in *The First Wives Club* (remember that scene? It's one of my favorites)! In order to justify the expense of what amounts to a good tinted moisturizer with sunscreen, Clarins claims this replenishes and lifts the complexion. The only skin-lifting you'll see is if you do a handstand while applying this (thus causing sagging facial skin to go in the opposite direction) and its replenishment ability is not reflected in a state-of-the-art formula. All of the intriguing ingredients are present in the tiniest amounts, so calling this super restorative is not accurate. For less money and a better formula, check out the tinted moisturizers from Bobbi Brown, Neutrogena, or even from Perricone M.D. Cosmeceuticals before this option.

☺ **$$$ True Radiance Foundation** *($37.50)* supposedly distinguishes itself from other foundations with its gold pigments, which Clarins describes as "enhancing luminosity while maximizing the power of surrounding light." The only luminosity you will see is from the glittery gold particles in the foundation. You have to look closely to see them, but catch your skin in the right light, and there they are. That doesn't make this modestly creamy foundation a poor choice, but you should know you're getting shine, not maximizing the power of light. Beginning moist and blending impeccably, this sets to a satin matte finish and provides light to medium coverage. It does an excellent job of enhancing skin tone rather than concealing it. Because of this feature, you shouldn't use True Radiance Foundation if you have many flaws to hide. But those with minor flaws (including redness) who also have normal to slightly dry or slightly oily skin should take a closer look. Ten shades are available for light to dark (but not very dark) skin, with only a few to avoid. Praline 06 and Tender Gold 10 are slightly peach, so consider them carefully. Sunlit Beige 08 can turn pink, but is still an option for light skin tones, while Tender Ivory 07 and Soft Ivory 03 are wonderful neutral shades. Clarins typically has take-home samples of this foundation, which gives you an excellent opportunity to audition it all day and in natural (not department-store) lighting.

☺ **$$$ Super Restorative Foundation SPF 15** *($56)*. Taken on its own merits as a foundation with an in-part titanium dioxide sunscreen, this is a beautifully done option for normal to dry skin. The initially creamy texture becomes lighter (in feel) as you blend, and it sets to a gorgeous satin matte finish that enlivens skin rather than making it look like a layer of makeup intended to mask it. You'll get medium coverage that's ideal for evening out your skin tone and reducing minor flaws. All in all, this is excellent—and there isn't a bad shade in the bunch. Now, to the over-the-top claims that are likely the reason some women may be willing to spend this much money on a foundation even when there are perfectly beautiful foundations available for less than half the price: Clarins wants you to believe you can fight aging and wrinkling with this foundation, but the only antiaging element in this foundation is its sunscreen, which is the same for any well-formulated foundation with sunscreen. This makeup isn't restorative on any level other than sunscreen, and it doesn't contain any ingredients capable of lifting skin. It also is not a specialized formula for those over the age of 50. Such a ridiculous notion won't go away, but please don't shop for skin-care or makeup products based on the number of candles on your birthday cake—age is not a skin type. Such claims rarely lead you to the products you really need, especially if you're in your 50s and still struggling with breakouts, oily skin, rosacea, blackheads, whiteheads, or overly sensitive skin. The ingredient list for this foundation is similar to that of many others I've reviewed favorably (and for less money, but I already mentioned that). Clarins included a lot of fragrance, which keeps this from earning a Paula's Pick rating, and the allegedly "super-restorative" plant extracts are but a dusting, so you're left with the unsung heroes of today's best foundations: silicones and silicone polymers. These are what create the silky, unbelievably smooth textures and finishes that, when combined with modern pigment technology, result in foundations that look more skin-like than ever.

☺ **$$$ Instant Smooth Foundation** *($37)*. This soft-textured whipped mousse foundation goes on creamy and transforms almost instantly to a silky, weightless matte finish that gives skin an attractive dimensional quality. Coverage is sheer to modestly medium, meaning this isn't for anyone with a noticeably uneven skin tone or dark discolorations. The silicone-heavy formula is best for normal to slightly dry or slightly oily skin. Those with oily skin will see shine in short order (the formula contains vegetable oil), while those with dry skin won't really get the moisture Clarins promises; but this does go on smooth. Almost all of the shades are worth considering by those with fair to slightly tan skin tones. Avoid 05, which is too peach. Shades 0 and 1.5 are remarkably neutral. Note: As with many Clarins products, this has a strong fragrance. Those looking for a similar foundation for a lot less money should consider Maybelline New York's Dream Matte Mousse Foundation or Cover Girl's TruBlend Whipped Foundation. A mid-priced option available at Target is the Boots No7 Intelligent Balance Mousse Foundation.

☺ $$$ **Hydra-Care Tinted Moisturizer SPF 6** *($42)* has an embarrassingly low SPF. This is a sheer, silicone-based moisturizer that would be fine for normal to dry skin. Of the four shades, the best are Bisque and Gold. Amber is too peach and Copper is too orange, but they may work for darker skin tones. This is absolutely not recommended as your sole source of daytime sun protection.

☺ $$$ **True Comfort Foundation SPF 15** *($37.50)* would have been a great foundation in almost every respect except for sun protection—an omission that prevents it from earning a better rating. Without titanium dioxide, zinc oxide, avobenzone, Tinosorb, or Mexoryl SX listed as an active ingredient, you need to pair this makeup with another sunscreen that contains UVA-protecting ingredients. If you have normal to dry skin and don't mind the aforementioned pairing, you will be pleased with this foundation's lightweight yet creamy texture, its superb blendability, and its satin finish, which lends a radiant glow to skin. Coverage goes from light to medium and nine of the ten shades are remarkably neutral, although there are no options for darker skin. Only Tender Gold and Chestnut stand out as being a bit too peach, though they may be options for medium and tan skin tones.

CONCEALER: ☺ $$$ **Instant Light Perfecting Touch** *($30)* is an agreeably smooth concealer that nicely diffuses dark circles and minor flaws. It is easy to blend, doesn't have too much slip, and sets to a soft matte finish (with sparkles) that poses only a minimal risk of creasing into lines around the eye. There are three shades (best for fair to light-medium skin), and although each starts out a bit pink they soften once the product dries. Use caution with the click-pen and brush applicator, because it is easy to dial up more concealer than you need, and there's no way to put it back.

☺ $$$ **Instant Light Eye Perfecting Base** *($24.50)* comes packaged in a click-pen applicator with a built-in synthetic brush tip. Housed inside is a smooth liquid concealer that blends well, evening out the appearance of skin on the eyelid or under-eye area. This has a crease-free matte finish that adds a touch of shine to skin, though not distractingly so. Both shades are good, but they are best for fair to light skin tones. Although this is an impressive product, it is superfluous if you're already using an excellent concealer in the eye area.

POWDER: ✓ ☺ $$$ **Loose Powder** *($35)* comes in a generous container and has a silky, feather-light texture and a sheer, dry application that looks beautiful and feels weightless on the skin. The two sheer shades are good, each with a satin finish—meaning this is best for those with normal to dry skin who want to avoid a true matte finish.

☺ $$$ **Powder Compact** *($30)* has a very silky, ultra-fine texture and a dry, non-powdery finish. The talc-based formula comes in three sheer shades appropriate for fair to light skin.

☺ $$$ **Shine Stopper Powder Compact** *($30)* comes in only one shade, but this talc-based pressed powder applies nearly translucently, so it can work for a range of skin tones. It is adept at tempering shine without looking thick or powdery, and offers a sheer, dry finish. The only caution is the amount of rice starch it includes. Although not irritating, this food-based ingredient can feed the bacteria that cause blemishes. The salicylic acid in this powder cannot exfoliate skin (even if it could, the amount Clarins includes is nearly insignificant).

BLUSH AND BRONZER: ✓ ☺ **$$$ Powder Blush Compact** *($29.50)* impresses with its finely milled silky texture and smooth application. The selection of sheer, warm-toned shades are quite flattering and matte, but it struck me as odd that some classic pink and rose colors are absent.

✓ ☺ **$$$ Multi-Blush** *($28.50)* is an excellent option for cream-to-powder blush. The formula is very easy to blend, and all but one of the colors are beautiful. Avoid Tender Raspberry because it's intensely fuchsia and not easy to soften to a more flattering tone.

☺ **$$$ Bronzing Duo Compact** *($35)*. Housed in an attractive gold compact are two complementary shades of pressed powder bronzer. Each has a soft, smooth texture that applies sheer and even, imparting subtle color and shine. The duo has a minor intensity that works best on fair to light skin tones. Financially, the pressed-powder bronzer from Wet 'n' Wild is even better and costs less than five dollars.

☺ **$$$ Bronzing Powder Compact** *($36)* is a standard, really overpriced, pressed bronzing powder with the requisite smooth yet dry texture and shiny (not overly so) finish. All of the shades apply sheer and can be difficult to build should you want more color. Morning Sun is OK for fair skin, but applies as a peachy blush rather than a true bronze or tan color.

EYESHADOW: ✓ ☺ **$$$ Single Eye Colour** *($20)*. I wish this eyeshadow were available in a wider range of workable shades, because its very smooth texture applies beautifully without flaking. Color saturation is on the sheer side, with the exception of the dark brown and black shades, both of which are suitable for eyelining. Most of the colors are shiny, and there are some purples and greens to avoid. The almost-matte, easy-to-blend options include Vanilla Beige, Mocha Mousse, and Totally Black. Overall, this is a great eyeshadow to check out if your budget permits, although you don't need to spend this much for a quality powder eyeshadow.

☹ **$$$ Colour Quartet for Eyes** *($40)*. The compact for these eyeshadow quads is gorgeous; too bad the color combinations (most of which are pastel-oriented) aren't. Each powder eyeshadow in the sets has a smooth, dry texture that deposits color somewhat unevenly and with some minor flaking. Every shade is also shiny, so we're talking maximum spotlight on less-than-taut or wrinkled eye-area skin. If you're angling for Clarins eyeshadows, the colors they sell singly are much better.

☹ **$$$ Soft Cream Eye Colour** *($20)* comes in aluminum tubes, each containing a concentrated amount of very shiny cream-to-powder eyeshadow. A little of this product goes a long way, and each shade blends out sheer, leaving a hint of color (and lots of shine) behind. Because this product remains somewhat slick, applying it evenly takes practice, and it does have a tendency to settle into creases. If this concept appeals to you, consider M.A.C.'s Paint or Paint Pot first—you'll get a broader selection of shades and budge-proof, crease-resistant wear.

EYE AND BROW SHAPER: ☺ **$$$ Liquid Eye Liner** *($26)* has a long, thin brush. That makes it harder to control, but once you get the hang of it the formula lays down color well (if a bit wet), and it dries quickly. Wear time is more than respectable, but the more-trouble-than-it-needs-to-be brush keeps this from earning a Paula's Pick rating.

☹ **$$$ Eyeliner Pencil with Sharpener** *($23)* is a black, standard, slightly creamy eye pencil that comes with its own sharpener. It's functional and has only a slight tendency to smear, but the price is prohibitive considering the equally good eye pencils available at the drugstore.

☹ **$$$ Waterproof Eyeliner Pencil** *($23)* has a tenacity that can survive swimming and tears, so it is waterproof—but you have to tolerate sharpening it, and a finish that remains tacky to the touch. It's an OK occasional-use option, but there are smoother, silicone-based eye pencils that are also waterproof, even though they may not advertise that fact.

☹ **Eye Liner Pencil** *($23)* is a standard pencil with substandard attributes. This soft-textured pencil glides on but is too creamy for it not to smudge and smear, though the built-in sponge-tip applicator facilitates smudging and smearing if you use it

☹ **Eye Shimmer Pencil** *($21)* is nearly identical to the Eye Liner Pencil, except that the few available shades have a strong shimmer finish that detracts from rather than enhances the eyes.

LIPSTICK, LIP GLOSS, AND LIPLINER: ✓ ☺ **$$$ Joli Rouge** *($23.50)*. "Joli" is a French word that means attractive, and this luscious cream lipstick certainly has its attractive qualities. Exceptionally moisturizing, smooth, and pigment-rich, the colors glide on easily and leave a beautiful cream finish that doesn't veer toward being too glossy or slick. Be careful because this is creamy enough to bleed into lines around the mouth, but if that (and this lipstick's price tag) isn't an issue for you, it is one of the best cream lipstick options at the department store.

✓ ☺ **$$$ Colour Quench Lip Balm** *($20)* shows Clarins has its act together for lip gloss, too. This tube-packaged gloss feels wonderfully emollient and keeps lips smooth while leaving a non-sticky, wet-look finish. The juicy colors offer varying degrees of intensity, so those looking for sheer and more intense shades are well served. If you're going to splurge on lip gloss, this option is money well spent!

✓ ☺ **$$$ Retractable Lip Definer** *($22.50)* will make those prone to lipstick feathering into lines around the mouth happy because this automatic, retractable lipliner applies smoothly without smearing, setting up a solid boundary to keep traveling lipstick from crossing the border. As a bonus, it is minimally prone to fading. The only disappointment here is the small selection of shades, of which three are dark brown tones that won't work with softer lipstick colors.

☺ **Joli Rouge Brilliant** *($23.50)* is similar to Clarins' Joli Rouge Perfect Shine Sheer Lipstick reviewed below, minus the glitter (which is a plus) and with a slightly greater color payoff. As a result, this lipstick feels smoother, lasts a bit longer, and feels great from first application to the inevitable touch-up. The colors are beautiful worn alone or applied over an opaque lipstick when you want a glossy finish.

☺ **$$$ Gloss Appeal** *($21)* is a lip gloss whose deep, bold colors may look imposing at first glance, but that actually go on watercolor sheer. The slightly thick texture feels balm-like but isn't sticky, and leaves an attractive gloss finish with a blend of gold and silver shimmer.

☺ **$$$ Instant Light Lip Perfector** *($20)* is simply a shimmering lip gloss available in two sheer shades (pastel pink and peach). It has a smooth, non-sticky texture and a sheer, glossy finish. Clarins suggests using this under lipstick, but that only leads to a messy application that takes more time to neaten than just applying gloss after lipstick.

☺ **$$$ Lip Colour Tint** *($20)* works beautifully to impart soft color to lips along with a smooth texture that's creamy without being overly slick. The shade range is enticing, and many of the shades have a flattering soft shimmer finish to highlight lips. This is worth a look if you prefer shopping for lipsticks at the department store!

☺ **$$$ Joli Rouge Perfect Shine Sheer Lipstick** *($23.50)*. This very sheer, glossy lipstick has the distinction of maintaining a glossy look without being too slick or slippery. Instead, you get an emollient texture that offers a soft wash of translucent color. The color fades within an hour, but that's the nature of most sheer, glossy lipsticks. The main drawback is that each shade is imbued with glitter particles that, while not garish, feel grainy as this lipstick's finish wears off. You can get better results with the sheer, glittery lipsticks from Wet 'n' Wild for less than $4.

☺ **$$$ Lip Liner Pencil** *($23)* is a standard pencil that has an easy-to-apply texture, but it needs sharpening and doesn't hold a candle to many other automatic lip pencils.

MASCARA: ✓ ☺ **$$$ Pure Curl Mascara** *($24)* is a superior lengthening mascara, but no more so than any other good mascara. Where this mascara sets itself apart is in how well it lifts and curls lashes. You'll get even better results using it with an eyelash curler (though that's only needed if your lashes grow straight or slant down), but even on its own you will be impressed.

✓ ☺ **$$$ Wonder Waterproof Mascara** *($23.50)*. The "wonder" of this mascara is how well it lengthens and separates lashes without clumping or smearing, yet remains waterproof while keeping lashes soft. This is a top department store mascara for those who need a long-wearing formula that isn't nearly as harsh on lashes as many waterproof formulas. Taking this off requires an oil- or silicone-based makeup remover.

☺ **$$$ Wonder Volume Mascara** *($23.50)* provides substantial lash enhancement without being too dramatic, and the formula wears well without making lashes feel brittle. It is similar to Clarins Pure Volume Mascara, except it doesn't have the same curling effect and it goes on a bit heavier (but without clumps or smearing).

☺ **$$$ Wonder Length Mascara** *($23.50)* works well to make lashes longer, though not without a slightly uneven application and not with the same extensive elongation as several superior drugstore mascaras. The real wonder is how Clarins gets women to spend this much on an average mascara! Those who prefer the style of brush offered by Clarins should consider Maybelline New York Lash Discovery Mascara instead.

☺ **$$$ Double Fix Mascara Waterproofing Seal** *($21)* is sold as a waterproofing top coat for use with non-waterproof mascaras. It works, but applying this over mascara isn't always flattering because—depending on which mascara you're wearing—it either clumps lashes together, makes them look spiky, or creates a wet look that may not be to your liking. Why bother with this (and the extra expense) when there are dozens of excellent waterproof mascaras available?

BRUSHES: ☺ **$$$ Clarins Brushes** *($20-$38)*. The majority of Clarins Brushes are decent, but they pale in comparison to what most makeup artistry lines sell for the same amount of money. The hair quality isn't up to par, nor are the brush shapes as elegantly functional as they could be, all of which makes this small brush collection one to consider carefully, if at all.

SPECIALTY PRODUCTS: ✓ ☺ **$$$ Instant Light Complexion Perfector** *($32)* is a unique primer that feels weightless and leaves skin silky-smooth. The uniqueness comes from the subtle opalescent shine of this fluid product. You'll get a low-glow shine that enhances the complexion by making it look luminous without obvious sparkles. The matte (in feel) finish provides an excellent base to apply foundation over, and this works well to optically minimize darkness in shadowed areas (although a good concealer or other highlighters can do so, too).

☺ **$$$ Instant Smooth Perfecting Touch** *($30 for 0.5 ounce)* calls itself "the modern, magic makeup base" and has "innovative line-filling technology" that claims to do all sorts of astounding things for skin. Reading the description, you might be curious how you ever got away with wearing makeup before this jar of wonder arrived. As it turns out, this is nothing more than a multiple silicone primer whose spackle-like texture and silky finish do work (temporarily) to fill in superficial wrinkles and large pores. How long the effect lasts depends on your skin type and, in the case of wrinkles, how expressive you are. The pale pink color adds a subtle luminous quality to skin, but that's camouflaged if you follow it with foundation. It's an option for a silky-feeling pre-makeup moisturizer, but not as impressive as silicone-based serums loaded with antioxidants and other skin-beneficial ingredients (and Clarins did not include any).

CLE DE PEAU BEAUTE

CLE DE PEAU BEAUTE AT-A-GLANCE

Strengths: None of note among skin-care items; even the best products are not worth the money when compared with superior versions from other lines that cost slightly to considerably less; foundations that provide excellent coverage without looking heavy; a magnificent concealer; good highlighting powder and eyeshadows; one good mascara.

Weaknesses: Too many to list, but major ones include: average to ineffective moisturizer and serum formulas; no sunscreens; no products to address acne; several products sold as nourishing or antiaging that douse skin with alcohol or other irritants; makeup products rated as average that are definitely not worth the investment.

For more information about Shiseido-owned Cle de Peau, visit www.cledepeaubeaute.com or www.Beautypedia.com.

CLE DE PEAU BEAUTE SKIN CARE

☺ **$$$ Cleansing Cream (Creme Demaquillante)** *($70 for 4.2 ounces)* has a lot going for it in terms of being a cushiony-rich cleansing cream for dry to very dry skin. It removes makeup easily and rinses decently (a washcloth is needed for complete removal), but then look at the price! There's no reason to spend this much money on such a small amount of cleanser, but if you do this shouldn't disappoint.

☹ **Cleansing Lotion (Lotion Demaquillante)** *($70 for 6.7 ounces)* lists alcohol as the second ingredient, and that makes this shockingly basic cleanser a no-go for all skin types.

☹ **$$$ Deep Cleansing Oil (Huile Demaquillante)** *($60 for 1.3 ounces)* is a mineral oil–based cleanser that also contains silicones and a tiny amount of alcohol and vitamin E. I am almost speechless that a company is charging $60 for just over 1 ounce of mineral oil. This will remove makeup quickly, but regardless of your budget, so will plain Johnson's Baby Oil ($4.99 for 20 ounces). One more thing: Cle de Peau's claim that this oil diminishes the appearance of coarse or darkened pores is a falsehood.

☺ **$$$ Gentle Cleansing Foam (Mousse Nettoyante Tendre)** *($60 for 3.3 ounces)* is a basic foaming cleanser that is water-soluble and an option for normal to oily skin. Its name would make more sense without the fragrance.

☺ **$$$ Refreshing Cleansing Foam (Mousse Nettoyante Fraiche)** *($60 for 3.3 ounces)* is nearly identical to the Gentle Cleansing Foam above, and the same review applies. The fragrance might seem refreshing, but it won't do your skin any favors.

☺ **$$$ Absolute Eye Makeup Remover (Demaquillant Pour Les Yeux Absol)** *($38 for 2.5 ounces)* is a silicone-in-water makeup remover that is very similar to considerably less expensive options from Almay, Neutrogena, and Clinique. It works quickly and efficiently, but so do the others.

☹ **$$$ Gentle Balancing Lotion (Lotion Tendre)** *($95 for 5 ounces)* contains enough alcohol to be potentially irritating, and makes the price insulting. The sugar-based skin-identical ingredients are a nice addition, but the plant-based antioxidants are scant when they should be front and center.

☹ **Refreshing Balancing Lotion (Lotion Fraiche)** *($95 for 5 ounces)* lists alcohol as the second ingredient and otherwise takes a "too little" approach to adding truly beneficial ingredients for skin.

The Reviews C

☹ **Intensive Treatment (Soin Intensif)** *($135)* is sold as a weekly treatment to exfoliate and nourish skin instead of just using your usual nighttime skin-care lineup. The **Lotion Intensive** is an alcohol-laden toner with barely a dusting of intriguing ingredients for skin; the **Essence Intensive** is a slightly creamy moisturizer similar to most of those in the Cle de Peau line. It contains some antioxidants and cell-communicating ingredients, but not in amounts that are likely to benefit skin, making them relatively useless. Last is the **Intensive Mask**, which is mostly slip agent and film-forming agents with a small amount of absorbents and alcohol. Nothing in these products exfoliates skin, nor are any of them "intensive." It's just another gimmicky, superfluous kit that is dressed up as a specialized solution for aging skin.

☹ **Micro-Refining Treatment (Soin Micro-Lissant)** *($200)* begins the first of many examples of Cle de Peau's ludicrous pricing of mediocre to downright poor formulations. This two-step system includes Exfoliator and Mask. The **Exfoliator** uses silica beads and cellulose to function as a topical scrub, and contains enough alcohol to be problematic. The **Mask** (the kit includes six two-piece masks) is mostly water, glycerin, thickener, and alcohol. The tiny amount of plant extracts and silk powder have no research proving their benefit for skin, and that's the least you should expect at this price.

☹ **Anti-Age Spot Serum (Serum Anti-Taches Brunes)** *($145 for 1.3 ounces)* lists alcohol as the second ingredient, which is a real burn for skin and the pocketbook. All of the exotic-sounding plant extracts and the form of vitamin C included don't have an established track record of lightening skin discolorations. Cle de Peau wants you to think their cellular ion-channel technology can inhibit the formation of melanin (skin pigment), but there is no research showing that to be the case. And what about the inflammation and free-radical damage the alcohol causes?

☹ $$$ **Clarifying Emulsion (Emulsion Eclat)** *($110 for 1.7 ounces)* is supposed to be an exfoliating moisturizer but does not contain ingredients that are capable of removing or dissolving dead skin cells. It barely passes as a moisturizer due to its lackluster formula, which is primarily water, slip agent, silicone, thickener, alcohol, and the water-binding agent xylitol. Antioxidants are present, but not in an amount your skin will notice.

☹ **Clarifying Serum (Serum Eclat)** *($110 for 2.5 ounces)* could not be a more mundane serum, which makes the price outrageous. It contains mostly water, glycerin, alcohol, slip agents, and preservative, and is not recommended unless you enjoy wasting money.

☹ $$$ **Energizing Essence (Essence Energisante)** *($130 for 2.5 ounces)* is a water- and silicone-based serum whose truly interesting ingredients are barely present, so they don't count for much. Any serum from Olay, Clinique, Neutrogena, or Estee Lauder easily bests this formula.

☺ $$$ **Eye Contour Balm Anti-Wrinkle (Baume Contour Des Yeux Anti-Rides)** *($130 for 0.5 ounce)* is a very good emollient moisturizer that's suited for dry skin around the eyes or elsewhere. It contains more antioxidants, the cell-communicating ingredient retinol, and skin-identical ingredients than the other Cle de Peau Beaute products, although the price is absurd given that better formulations are available from other companies for a lot less.

☺ $$$ **Eye Contour Essence Anti-Dark Circles (Essence Contour Des Yeux Anti-Cernes)** *($115 for 0.5 ounce)* does not contain any ingredients that improve the appearance of dark circles unless they are accompanied by dry skin. In that case, they'll look better—because the same benefit can be had by applying any emollient ingredient to dry skin around the eyes. It's a decent moisturizer for slightly dry skin, but once again the really intriguing ingredients are in very short supply.

☹ **$$$ Energizing Cream (Creme Energisante)** *($145 for 3.3 ounces)* is an OK moisturizer for normal to dry skin, but the energizing element will only occur if you happen to get hyped from spending this amount of money on a single skin-care item (and an unexciting one at that).

☹ **$$$ Enriched Nourishing Cream (Creme Soyeuse)** *($130 for 1 ounce)* claims to improve the appearance of lines overnight, but does that no better than any other ordinary moisturizer, because that is what this product is—an extremely ordinary, standard moisturizer. The ingredients responsible for the "enriched" name are present in such tiny amounts that your skin has every right to feel shortchanged, and what little potency they had will quickly deteriorate in the jar packaging.

☺ **$$$ Enriched Protective Cream (Creme Protectrice Soyeuse)** *($110 for 1 ounce)* contains appreciable amounts of sunscreen ingredients, but does not sport an SPF rating. You'd think Cle de Peau could bankroll the required SPF testing given what a skin-care routine from them costs the consumer, but that's not the case. This is otherwise another ho-hum, severely overpriced moisturizer that's an OK option for normal to slightly oily skin.

☺ **$$$ Enriched Protective Emulsion (Emulsion Protectrice Soyeuse)** *($120 for 1.7 ounces)* is similar to the Enriched Protective Cream, but with a thicker texture better suited for normal to slightly dry skin. Otherwise the same comments apply.

☺ **$$$ Gentle Nourishing Emulsion (Emulsion Tendre)** *($130 for 2.5 ounces)* has a price that should reward the consumer with a moisturizer that goes above and beyond state-of-the-art, but ends up barely meeting minimum requirements. This isn't a problematic moisturizer, just unbelievably boring for the money. It's an OK option for normal to dry skin, but nothing I'd encourage you to choose over countless other options.

☺ **$$$ Gentle Protective Emulsion (Emulsion Protectrice Tendre)** *($110 for 1.7 ounces)* contains mostly water, slip agent, sunscreen, glycerin, skin-identical ingredients, avobenzone, and Vaseline. This lightweight lotion is not SPF-rated and so it cannot be relied on for daily sun protection. It is another lackluster moisturizer for normal to slightly oily skin (though the sunscreen agents don't coincide with the "gentle" portion of the name).

☹ **Intensive Wrinkle Correcting Cream (Creme Intensive Correctrice Rides)** *($167 for 1 ounce)* contains an insignificant amount of retinol, although the packaging will keep it stable. Even so, the alcohol and peppermint content of this no-action product are cause for concern. Oddly, a few of the plant extracts in this moisturizer are used medicinally to treat urinary tract infections and female reproductive organ anomalies. What that has to do with wrinkles is anyone's guess!

☺ **$$$ Massage Cream (Creme de Massage)** *($118 for 3.4 ounces)* promises a delightful sensation and magnificent result, both adjectives that don't accurately describe this substandard yet very emollient moisturizer for dry to very dry skin. The chief ingredients (squalane, water, and Vaseline) are found in dozens of moisturizers costing significantly less than this product.

☹ **Oil Balancing Essence (Essence Equilibrante)** *($58 for 2.5 ounces)* contains too much alcohol to balance oil, but it will help degrease oily skin (at the expense of causing irritation which, ironically, triggers more oil production so oily skin will quickly worsen). The amount of astringent zinc phenosulfate is also cause for concern, as is the presence of sage oil.

☹ **Oil Balancing Gel (Gel Equilibrant)** *($58 for 1 ounce)* lists alcohol as the second ingredient, along with menthol and camphor. Oddly enough, this product does contain the anti-irritant dipotassium glycyrrhizate (from licorice), but that doesn't have a chance against the potent skin sensitizers included in this formulation. The alcohol in this product will trigger more oil production in the pore lining, making oily skin worse.

☹ **Refreshing Nourishing Emulsion (Emulsion Fraiche)** *($130 for 2.5 ounces)* contains enough alcohol to be anything but nourishing for skin (when was the last time someone called a martini nourishment?). This is a poorly formulated moisturizer that provides minimal benefit at an insulting price.

☹ **Refreshing Protective Emulsion (Emulsion Protectrice Fraiche)** *($110 for 1.7 ounces)* is similar to the Refreshing Nourishing Emulsion above, except this adds some sunscreen ingredients to the mix, although it carries no SPF rating. Otherwise, the same review applies.

☺ **$$$ Revitalizing Emulsion (Emulsion Revivifiante)** *($145 for 1.3 ounces)* claims to protect the skin from signs of sagging, but it cannot do that. This water- and silicone-based moisturizer will feel silky and leave a lightweight smooth finish, but when it comes to beneficial skin-care ingredients, it didn't just miss the boat—it missed the dock, too.

☺ **$$$ Smoothing Base for Lines SPF 26** *($72)*. This moisturizer with an in-part titanium dioxide sunscreen is sold as a pre-makeup cream meant to enhance foundation. If you're using a well-formulated daytime moisturizer with sunscreen (or you have oily skin and your foundation is rated SPF 15 or greater), then you don't need to add a product like this. Used under foundation, it feels creamy without being slick and it leaves a silky finish that illuminates skin, but also leaves a faint white cast; some may interpret the white cast as a brightening effect, but it is really more mask-like in appearance. This is an intriguing product for those with normal to dry skin not prone to blemishes, but, like every Cle de Peau product, the price is out of line for what you get.

☺ **$$$ Smoothing Base for Pores SPF 24** *($72)*. Just like any moisturizer with a soft matte finish and soft spackle-like texture, this helps temporarily minimize the appearance of pores, but once the oil gets going it can slip and pool in the pores unless you touch up during the day. It adds the benefit of an in-part titanium dioxide sunscreen, so you could use this with a matte-finish foundation that doesn't contain sunscreen; however, if you have oily skin you won't appreciate the extra layer on your face. (Cle de Peau wants you to use this as a foundation and a moisturizer!) Application is smooth, but that doesn't help this foundation go on any better than other silky moisturizers. Smoothing Base for Pores does differentiate itself slightly because it does a relatively good job of absorbing excess oil, but that effect doesn't last the day. This is not the answer for someone struggling with oily skin.

☹ **Soothing Essence (Essence Apaisante)** *($88 for 5 ounces)* lists alcohol as the second ingredient and also contains menthol and its derivative menthyl lactate. And this is supposed to be soothing?!

☹ **The Cream (La Creme)** *($500 for 1 ounce)* is one of many so-called "prestige" moisturizers with stratospheric prices. Before I get into the details of this product, suffice it to say that this product is poorly formulated and absolutely not worth even a fraction of the price. The former version of this product contained the skin-lightening agent arbutin, making it effective for those seeking an ultra-pricey product to handle discolorations. This version is arbutin-free and, considering the cost, free of anything else that justifies the price. The bulk of the formula is water, glycerin, slip agent, Vaseline, emollient thickeners, and jojoba oil. Does any of that sound like it can deliver "unparalleled age-defying benefits" to your skin? Hardly, and this is a poor choice for daytime because it doesn't provide sun protection. Further, the choice of jar packaging means the antioxidants (including a decent amount of vitamin C) will become ineffective shortly after the product is opened. This cream has an elegant texture, but its sensation on skin doesn't translate into a sensational formula that's worth parting with hundreds of dollars.

☺ **$$$ Facial Contour Treatment (Traitement Visage Remodelant)** *($135)* is a two-step kit designed to treat puffiness by "encouraging the skin's healthy fluid exchange balance," which in turn will make skin more resistant to becoming puffy. The **Anti-Puffiness Massage Gel** contains a blend of water, the emollient squalane, slip agents, thickeners, and vitamin E, along with meager amounts of plant extracts, none capable of reducing puffy skin. The second portion is the **Cooling Mask**, which doesn't cool skin with menthol but does contain alcohol and a hairspray-like film-forming agent that can temporarily smooth skin and make it feel tighter. None of the ingredients in either product can control skin's fluid balance, although the alcohol in the Cooling Mask may cause some superficial dehydration. Although this duo won't work as claimed, I suppose it can be a somewhat soothing experience for those with money to burn.

☹ **Translucency Mask (Masque Transparence)** *($118 for 3.4 ounces)* is a standard peel-off facial mask that lists polyvinyl alcohol (a hairspray fixative) as the second ingredient, followed by utterly ordinary ingredients that don't come close to offering anything to rationalize the product's price. This is an unsatisfactory choice for any skin type.

☹ **Lip Contour Treatment (Soin Levres)** *($48 for 0.14 ounce)* reigns as one of the most expensive lip balms in existence, it not ever. Although this emollient stick will moisturize and help keep dry, chapped lips protected, it will not prevent and correct signs of aging because it contains no sunscreen. Further, the orange and peppermint oils promote irritation, which promotes chapped lips, making this an expensive mistake.

CLE DE PEAU BEAUTE MAKEUP

FOUNDATION: ✓ ☺ **$$$ Refining Fluid Foundation SPF 24** *($118)* was Cle de Peau's first foundation with sunscreen, and I am pleased to report that it includes titanium dioxide for sufficient UVA protection. In addition to the sunscreen, this has a wonderfully smooth, fluid texture that blends well (though it takes more time than many liquid foundations) and sets to a satin-matte finish with a hint of luminescence. Calling this a "treatment foundation" is stretching the truth because it does not contain any ingredients that aren't also found in similar water- and silicone-based foundations. Tiny amounts of vitamin E and green tea do not add up to an antiaging bonanza for skin, nor do they justify this foundation's hefty price. Still, for those with normal to slightly dry or slightly oily skin inclined to overspend on makeup, this medium to almost full coverage option may prove appealing. Among the eight shades, P10 is too pink and B10 is too peach. Shade B20 is slightly peach, but workable, while the rest of the shades are well-suited for light to medium skin tones.

☺ **$$$ Color Control Foundation** *($90)* includes white and bronze shades that Cle de Peau recommends using to deepen or lighten any of the foundation colors, or for contouring and highlighting the face. These two extras are an option (and much better than standard color correctors), but before you drop almost $200 for two bottles of foundation, please remember that the existing foundation colors should work just fine on their own and that any special shading or highlighting can be achieved with considerably less expensive products. This formula is good for normal to oily skin. Using it over dry skin can be tricky because it tends to accentuate the dryness; however, an emollient sunscreen underneath can help it go on more easily.

☺ **$$$ Cream Foundation SPF 18** *($118)*. I won't even try to explain why the price tag for this foundation is so ridiculous. Other than claims and marketing exaggeration, no matter how you look at it, this is just a good foundation; ironically, it isn't even a great foundation.

This cream foundation is packaged in a cylindrical component that resembles a tube of deodorant. When you remove the cap you press down on the sides to dispense a small amount of foundation. It's a cute dispensing system, but it offers no advantage or preferred control for application.

Despite the "cream" in the name, this has a lightweight, silky texture. It blends readily yet sets to a soft matte finish that can look heavy if you aren't careful. If you want medium to full coverage this is an option. It also contains a high amount of titanium dioxide (it's the sole active ingredient for the SPF) that contributes to the overall opacity and thickness you'll experience. Most of the shades are exemplary and include options for fair to light skin tones. Watch out for slightly pink B20 and slightly peach B30. There are no shades for tan to dark skin tones. By the way, Cle de Peau advisors will tell you this foundation has significant skin-care benefits. It doesn't, at least not if you compare its ingredients with those of several other less expensive foundations, most of which are sold without fanfare for skin-care benefits. But, at this price, Cle de Peau had to come up with some claim why there is an advantage to spending over $100 (or even $20 for that matter) on a foundation.

☺ $$$ **Creamy Powder Foundation** *($77.50)* is an incredibly standard but undeniably smooth, talc-based powder foundation. It applies easily and quite sheer, with a satin finish. The ten shades are very good, but B10, B20, B30, and B40 can turn peach if used on oily skin. For the money, this is not as impressive as the powder foundation options from Lancome, L'Oreal, Chanel, Estee Lauder, Clinique, and Laura Mercier.

☺ $$$ **Silky Cream Foundation** *($118)* was designed to be a lighter alternative to the Teint Naturel Cream Foundation reviewed below. It has a similar consistency and comes in the same type of jar packaging, but provides less intense coverage for a more natural finish. "Natural" is a relative term here, because although this foundation feels exceptionally light and silky on skin, it still has enough pigment and opacity to provide medium coverage, and its somewhat powdery finish isn't the best if you have any dry areas—though its mica content does provide a soft glow. The water- and silicone-based formula contains enough absorbents (including talc) to keep oily areas matte for longer than usual. Eight shades are offered, with no options for tan to dark skin. The only colors to skip are P10, which is too pink, and the too-peach B10.

☺ $$$ **Teint Naturel Cream Foundation** *($110)* has its strong points but there is no doubt the price is out of line, and nothing in this foundation makes it exceptional or even remotely worth the money. (You'd think that for over $100 they would have included a sunscreen or some state-of-the-art ingredients.) It is just a very good silicone- and talc-based makeup that goes on very smoothly and dries to a silky matte finish. What is unique about the formulation is that it's densely pigmented. That can be good in the sense that a little goes a long way, but it can also be problematic if you want sheer or light coverage. This foundation can be mixed with a moisturizer to thin out the coverage if desired, and that may be a good idea, since using it at full strength results in such intense camouflage that it isn't what anyone would call "natural." The formula is best for normal to oily skin, and comes in ten shades, of which the following are slightly pink or peach, but not worth dismissing altogether: B10, B20, and B30.

CONCEALER: ✓ ☺ $$$ **Concealer** *($70)* is exceptional. This twist-up stick concealer has a light, smooth texture that glides over the skin and offers substantial but (almost) imperceptible coverage in three excellent shades, best for fair to light skin. The soft matte finish poses little risk of creasing, and the only thing that's disconcerting about this is the prohibitive price. As a suggestion, Maybelline's Instant Age Rewind Double Face Perfector works brilliantly for a fraction of the cost.

☺ **$$$ Brilliant Enhancer** *($62)* is a very good fluid highlighter that you dispense from a pen-style component and apply with a built-in synthetic brush. The texture is smooth and sets to a nearly weightless, sheer finish that leaves a soft, sparkling shine. Despite these pleasant attributes and an even application, there is no need to spend this much money to add shine to skin. For half the price and equally good results, try Lorac Luminizer shade Pearl L1. For less than ten dollars, try Maybelline's Instant Age Rewind Double Face Perfector.

☹ **$$$ Refining Corrector for Lines** *($50)* is sold as "a translucent, hydrating concealer," which is sort of like wearing sunglasses that are minimally tinted. In other words, what's the point? This isn't a concealer at all; it's an eye cream that has an emollient feel and noticeably dewy finish. Applying makeup over this can cause it to slip into wrinkles around the eye, not to mention shorten its wear time. If you're looking for an eye cream, consider the non-jar-packaged options from Estee Lauder before this moisturizing but lackluster formula.

POWDER: ✓ ☺ **$$$ Luminizing Relief Powder** *($45)* is meant to "create great sculptural effects," but that's just a fancy way of saying these pressed powders can be used for contouring (shade 32) or highlighting (shade 31). Both have shine but also an enviably silky texture, and they apply flawlessly, with minimal flaking (of the shine, not the color itself—that goes on evenly). Although pricey, both shades work well for their intended purpose if you have fair to medium skin. The included brush is compact, but the hair is sable, so it's not your standard throwaway applicator.

☹ **$$$ Contour Defining Powder** *($75)* provides your choice from one of four sets of two powders (Are you confused yet?) that are snapped into an elegant compact that also holds two brushes. The texture of these pressed powders is super fine, so it looks incredibly natural on skin, although color deposit is minimal, which is not what you want from a product meant to contour. Only one true tan tone is offered, and it barely registers even on porcelain skin tones. The other shades (peach, yellow, pink, white) have nothing to do with contouring and are actually better for highlighting. This confounding product has tactile benefits, but fails to impress if you're looking to shape and shade your face.

☹ **$$$ Perfect Enhancing Powder** *($55)* is a product that has some versatility, but it shouldn't be used as an allover finishing powder because the four colors aren't true skin tones. The pale pink and pale yellow pressed powders are workable for highlighting or using as eyeshadow base, while the pale gold and bronze tones can work as a blush combination or for eyeshadows. All have a silky texture, but aren't as smooth as the Luminizing Relief Powder, and are not worth the money unless you can honestly see yourself using one of the shades over a standard blush or eyeshadow.

☹ **$$$ Translucent Pressed Powder** *($80)* is talc-based, has a superfine texture, and comes in a single shade that is supposedly translucent but can look pink on light skin and ashen on dark skin. The powder has a refined finish with a noticeably drier feel. For a comparable texture and more than one shade, consider the powders from Sonia Kashuk, L'Oreal, or Laura Mercier.

☹ **$$$ Translucent Loose Powder** *($100)* is talc-based, has a superfine texture, and comes in a single shade that is supposedly translucent but can look pink on light skin and ashen on dark skin. This slightly shiny powder has a refined finish. For a comparable texture and more than one shade, consider the powders from Sonia Kashuk, L'Oreal, or Laura Mercier.

BLUSH: ☹ **$$$ Cheek Color Duo** *($45)* includes a regular powder blush and a sheer highlighting shade. Application is sheer, the colors are pastel-ish, and the finish is soft matte with a hint of shine. There isn't really much to write about these ordinary blushes. If you are a Cle de Peau Beaute fan maybe you have a reason to waste your money, but if not, move on, these blushes are absolutely not worth the price.

EYESHADOW: ☺ **$$$ Eye Color Quad** *($75)* has a beautifully soft texture reminiscent of powdered sugar. The colors aren't tightly pressed, so pickup with a brush is easy, though you've got to pay attention to not go overboard during application. The eyeshadows blend easily and color deposit is moderate. The formula contains enough oil to make slight creasing and fading an issue. With so many good qualities, why the neutral face rating? Because every quad has at least one shade whose glittery shine flakes all over the place. There are some enticing color combinations, but at this price, an eyeshadow should be 110% perfect.

EYE AND BROW SHAPER: ☺ **$$$ Eye Liner Pencil** *($30)*. This automatic, retractable pencil's best part is its luxurious, weighty component. The pencil itself is as standard as it gets, with a soft but firm texture and even application. It has a soft powder finish that doesn't smudge, but the color payoff is soft, so you must layer it to build intensity. Although this pencil performs well and deserves a happy face rating, you absolutely do not need to spend anywhere near this much for a great eye pencil. The drugstore has so many options, it makes this one silly by comparison.

☺ **$$$ Eyebrow & Eyeliner Compact** *($70)*. Do not mistake the happy face rating as somehow justifying the price tag. The price tag is an insult and only those who like throwing money down the toilet should take notice. There is nothing exceptional about this product, which contains a powder brow color and powder eyeliner along with an ivory shade of powder eyeshadow to highlight the brow bone. The brow and eyeliner powders have a smooth, non-powdery texture that allows for even application. Because the colors go on softly, the eyeliner powder is best used wet. Every product in this compact casts a subtle shine on skin. Only light brown and dark brown color combinations are offered, but all told you can use considerably less expensive products to get the same results that this one provides.

☹ **Intensifying Cream Eyeliner** *($60)* is a very expensive way to apply cream eyeliner that never sets to a long-wearing finish. Instead, it remains creamy and tends to smudge and fade within hours. The colors are mostly odd because each has a metallic sheen and is laced with sparkles. Even the Cle de Peau makeup artist freely admitted that he dislikes the colors and steers his clients interested in this type of eyeliner to the superior options from M.A.C. or Bobbi Brown. I suggest the same thing!

LIPSTICK, LIP GLOSS, AND LIPLINER: ☺ **$$$ Lip Gloss** *($47)* doesn't have any issues other than its price, which becomes ridiculous when you consider the number of equally good non-sticky glosses that impart sheer color without feeling thick. This lip gloss includes a brush applicator.

☺ **$$$ Lip Liner Pencil** *($25)* is an automatic, retractable lip pencil that has a creamy, just-right texture, although precise application is hindered by the wider-than-usual pencil tip. The pencil case includes a very good lip brush; the only oddity is the small selection of shades, most of which don't easily complement Cle de Peau's lipsticks.

☺ **$$$ Extra Silky Lipstick** *($50)* is housed in a click pen-style component, but there's actually a lipstick inside instead of color being dispensed onto a built-in brush applicator. Beyond the packaging novelty, this is a great lipstick, but the price tag is nothing more than a marketing ploy. Yes, the colors are attractively sheer and you get a finish so glossy your lips look positively drenched in shine, but it doesn't last and quickly travels into lines around the mouth. It is an understatement to say that there are plenty of very good glossy lipsticks for a fraction of this price from lots of other brands.

☺ **$$$ Lipstick** *($55)* is available in Cream or Sheer formulas, which are slick, greasy-feeling lipsticks that are less than desirable by comparison to today's top cream and sheer lipsticks. Either formula, but especially the glossy Sheer, will make a beeline into lines around the mouth. A review of the ingredients shows that your money isn't buying anything not found in hundreds of other lipsticks.

MASCARA: ☺ **$$$ Volume Mascara** *($45)* ably builds noticeable length and some thickness without clumping or smearing. You absolutely do not have to spend this much money for a good mascara, but if you're set on Cle de Peau, this is the one to purchase. One last point: With either mascara, avoid the blue and violet shades, which are none too subtle.

☹ **$$$ Lengthening Mascara** *($45)*. Talk about underwhelming! For $45, a mascara should not only make your lashes look their absolute best, it should cook dinner, too! This overpriced mascara has a thin application that does little to enhance lashes, although it does apply neatly without a clump or flake in sight. This does not come off with a water-soluble cleanser, but removes well with a silicone-based makeup remover.

BRUSHES: ☺ **$$$ Brush Set** *($300)* is one of the most expensive brush sets I know of, yet it's incomplete and the brushes aren't nearly as luxurious and foolproof as you'd expect given the price. Included are a Powder, Concealer, Blush, and Highlighter brush. Nothing for brows, eyelining, or eyeshadow—brushes that any makeup artist considers essential. The leather case is great, but the brushes themselves are what matter most. This set's shortcomings don't add up to a wise investment, and at this price tag it is nothing less than a waste of money.

CLEAN & CLEAR (SKIN CARE ONLY)

CLEAN & CLEAR AT-A-GLANCE

Strengths: Inexpensive; an excellent 10% benzoyl peroxide product; some very good cleansers.

Weaknesses: The majority of products contain irritating fragrant extracts, alcohol, menthol, menthyl lactate, or other problematic ingredients; no broad-spectrum sunscreens; below-average moisturizers; one of the worst lines for assembling an effective anti-acne routine.

For more information about Clean & Clear, call (877) 754-6411 or visit www.cleanandclear.com or www.Beautypedia.com.

CLEAN & CLEAR ADVANTAGE PRODUCTS

☹ **Advantage Acne Cleanser** *($6.99 for 5 ounces)* contains 2% salicylic acid in a base with a pH of 4, but because this cleanser is quickly rinsed away, the BHA will have little or no impact on the skin. In addition, this cleanser contains sodium C14-16 olefin sulfonate as its main cleansing agent, which makes it too drying for all skin types, plus the cinnamon and cedar extracts are irritating. For an "advanced formula," this is quite a letdown.

☹ **Advantage Acne Clearing Astringent** *($4.49 for 8 ounces)* lists alcohol as the main ingredient, and also contains irritating cinnamon and cedar bark extracts. None of this is helpful for acne-prone skin, or for any skin for that matter. The alcohol will trigger oil production in the pore lining, making oily skin worse.

☺ **Advantage Oil-Free Acne Moisturizer** *($7.49 for 4 ounces)* is an OK lightweight moisturizer for normal to oily skin. The 0.5% concentration of salicylic acid isn't that helpful for blemishes, and it's not effective in this product given that its pH is above 4. The cinnamon and cedar bark extracts pose a risk of irritation.

☹ **Advantage Acne Control Kit** *($20.19)* is supposed to make fighting acne as easy as 1-2-3, but each of the products in this misguided kit has its share of problems. The **Advantage Acne Control Cleanser** contains 10% benzoyl peroxide, a concentration that can be quite drying, although it won't have time to work because it is rinsed quickly from your skin. A larger problem is the drying detergent cleansing agent sodium C14-16 olefin sulfonate along with menthol, neither of which helps combat blemishes, and which just add irritation and inflammation to skin. Step 2 is the **Advantage Acne Control Moisturizer**, which is nearly identical to the Advantage Oil-Free Acne Moisturizer reviewed above. Last is the **Advantage Fast Clearing Spot Treatment**, which contains 2% salicylic acid, but also enough alcohol to cause irritation and prompt more oil production, and the irritation is not reduced by the inclusion of cinnamon and cedar bark extracts. In short, there is little reason to expect relief from acne with this kit, and every reason to expect irritated, reddened skin.

☹ **Advantage Acne Spot Treatment** *($6.99 for 0.75 ounce)* is a 2% salicylic acid gel with a pH of 3.2, so it can exfoliate the skin's surface and inside the pore lining. That's great, but the alcohol base is problematic, especially when combined with the cinnamon and cedar bark extracts here. You would fare better with Neutrogena's BHA products.

☹ **Advantage Invisible Acne Patch** *($10.99 for 0.07 ounce)* seems a convenient way to zero in on blemishes and zap them overnight with 2% salicylic acid. However, the BHA is suspended in a solution of alcohol along with irritating cedar and cinnamon bark extracts, making it a problem product for all skin types.

CLEAN & CLEAR DEEP ACTION AND DEEP CLEANING PRODUCTS

☹ **Deep Action Cream Cleanser, Oil-Free** *($5.99 for 6.5 ounces)* contains menthol and is not recommended for any skin type.

☹ **Deep Action Cream Cleanser, Sensitive Skin** *($5.99 for 6.5 ounces)* contains menthol and is not recommended for any skin type. Without it, this would be an appropriate cleanser for sensitive skin.

☹ **Deep Action Refreshing Gel Cleanser, Oil-Free** *($4.99 for 8 ounces)* is just another poorly formulated water-soluble cleanser that assaults your skin on two fronts: the drying detergent cleansing agent sodium C14-16 olefin sulfonate and the inclusion of menthol plus menthyl lactate, a derivative of menthol. The minty sensation is not akin to your skin being cleansed deeply, it simply means your skin is being irritated.

☹ **Deep Cleaning Astringent** *($4.99 for 8 ounces)* contains 2% salicylic acid but the pH is too high for it to function as an exfoliant. Even with its pH in the correct range, the amount of alcohol in this anti-acne toner makes it a problem for all skin types.

☹ **Deep Cleaning Astringent, Sensitive Skin** *($5.19 for 8 ounces)* has been reformulated so it is less irritating than before, but that's not good enough for your skin, especially if it is sensitive. The amount of alcohol remains problematic while the amount of salicylic acid (plus this toner's pH) isn't going to be helpful for those struggling with breakouts. Even though the amount of alcohol was reduced, it can still trigger more oil production in the pore lining, and that's not what oily skin needs.

☹ **Deep Action Exfoliating Scrub** *($4.99 for 5 ounces)*. Because this cleanser-scrub hybrid contains the irritating ingredient menthol, it is not recommended. Without it, Clean & Clear would have had a very good scrub for normal to oily skin.

CLEAN & CLEAR MORNING BURST PRODUCTS

⊗ **Morning Burst Detoxifying Facial Cleanser** *($5.99 for 8 ounces)*. The claims for this cleanser are contradictory: on the one hand, it's supposed to oxygenate skin to remove impurities, but on the other hand it contains antioxidant-filled beads that burst as you cleanse (antioxidants work against oxygen to prevent it from damaging cells; clearly Clean & Clear assumes their consumers wouldn't notice this incongruity). As it turns out, this isn't an oxygenating experience for skin, and that's a good thing. The bad part of this very basic cleanser is the inclusion of irritating menthyl lactate (a form of menthol). Clean & Clear, as well as Neutrogena and Aveeno (all owned by Johnson & Johnson), all have better cleansers to consider.

⊗ **Morning Burst Facial Cleanser** *($6.49 for 8 ounces)* is a below-standard water-soluble cleanser that "wakes you up" with an irritating dose of menthol and the menthol derivative menthyl lactate, which leaves your face tingling after rinsing. Without those troublemakers and an assortment of irritating plants, this would've been a great cleanser for oily skin.

⊗ **Morning Burst Shine Control Facial Cleanser** *($6.49 for 8 ounces)* wants you to wake up radiant, but after washing with this problematic cleanser you'll only be waking up irritated. It contains menthol and menthyl lactate along with irritating citrus extracts, and is not recommended.

⊗ **Morning Burst Detoxifying Facial Scrub** *($5.99 for 5 ounces)*. This standard cleansing scrub cannot oxygenate skin (which is good, because adding oxygen to skin causes free-radical damage), but it will irritate it thanks to the inclusion of the menthol derivative menthyl lactate. This is not a wise way to get your morning skin-care routine off to a good start.

⊗ **Morning Burst Facial Scrub** *($6.49 for 5 ounces)* is a standard scrub that contains polyethylene (plastic) beads as the scrubbing agent. It also contains menthyl lactate, a form of menthol that instantly makes this scrub too irritating for all skin types.

⊗ **Morning Burst Shine Control Facial Scrub** *($6.99 for 5 ounces)* has the same problem as the Morning Burst Facial Scrub above, and the same review applies.

⊗ **Morning Glow Moisturizer SPF 15, Oil-Free** *($6.49 for 4 ounces)* contains a form of menthol that can cause skin to tingle (not glow) with irritation, and that is unquestionably a problem. Without it, this in-part avobenzone sunscreen would have been highly recommended as a basic, lightweight, affordable sunscreen for normal to slightly oily skin.

☺ **Morning Burst Oil Absorbing Sheets** *($5.49 for 50 sheets)* are thin plastic polypropylene sheets. They work decently to absorb excess oil and perspiration, but the mineral-oil additive won't keep skin as shine-free as other options. These are fragranced, too.

CLEAN & CLEAR SOFT PRODUCTS

☺ **Soft Purifying Cleanser** *($6.99 for 5 ounces)* is a combination cleanser/scrub product suitable for normal to oily or slightly dry skin. Clean & Clear is marketing this product to teens, but adults can benefit from it as well. The amount of salicylic acid is too low for it to exfoliate, while the fruit and sugarcane extracts don't function like AHAs; not to mention that all of these ingredients will be rinsed from your skin before they have a chance to work.

⊗ **Soft In-Shower Facial** *($6.99 for 5 ounces)* is a slightly creamy scrub that contains polyethylene (plastic beads) as the abrasive agent. This product attempts to go beyond a mere scrub by promising to provide a one-minute facial for skin. Coupled with the steam from your shower, it is supposed to deep clean pores while fruit acids exfoliate skin. The fruit certainly doesn't exfoliate, but the glycolic acid in this product could have if the pH were lower and if

The Reviews C

you left it on your skin for more than a minute. However, doing so would only cause further irritation from the menthol in this well-intentioned but poorly formulated product.

☺ **Soft Oil-Free Day Moisturizer SPF 15** *($8.49 for 4 ounces)* is recommended as a good daytime moisturizer for normal to oily skin. UVA protection is assured thanks to an in-part avobenzone sunscreen, and this product has a light texture that doesn't leave your skin looking greasy. It contains a few notable antioxidants, though their concentration in this product is a mystery because Clean & Clear listed the inactive ingredients alphabetically rather than in descending order of amount. Listing them like that is permissible for over-the-counter drugs, which is how sunscreens are classified, but it doesn't help consumers know the relative amounts of what they are really putting on their faces.

☺ **Soft Oil-Free Night Moisturizer** *($8.49 for 4 ounces)* doesn't contain oil, but the main thickening agent (cetearyl alcohol) isn't necessarily a get-out-of-jail-free card for those trying to avoid blemishes. Still, this product has a lightweight, silky texture and contains approximately 3% glycolic acid at a pH that permits exfoliation to occur. There are better moisturizers with AHA to consider if exfoliation is your goal, but this fits the bill as a basic moisturizer for normal to slightly oily skin.

OTHER CLEAN & CLEAR PRODUCTS

☹ **Continuous Control Acne Cleanser** *($6.49 for 5 ounces)* contains 10% benzoyl peroxide, but this topical disinfectant is of little use to skin because it is quickly rinsed off. The menthol in this unusually creamy cleanser makes it too irritating for all skin types.

☺ **Continuous Control Acne Wash, Oil-Free** *($6.99 for 6 ounces)* lists 2% salicylic acid as its active ingredient, but any benefit it might have is rinsed down the drain, making this ineffective against acne. It is recommended as a standard water-soluble cleanser for oily to very oily skin.

✓ ☺ **Daily Pore Cleanser, Oil-Free** *($5.49 for 5.5 ounces)* is a very good water-soluble cleanser/scrub hybrid for oily to very oily skin. It removes makeup easily and rinses cleanly. This is definitely one of Clean & Clear's better cleansers!

☺ **Foaming Facial Cleanser, Oil Free** *($5.49 for 8 ounces)* is recommended if you prefer a water-soluble cleanser with copious foaming action. The foam has no cleansing ability, but the impression it gives is one some consumers prefer, and in the case of this product is not irritating or drying. The antibacterial agent triclosan is listed as an active ingredient, but its effect in cleansing products that are quickly rinsed from skin is negligible.

✓ ☺ **Foaming Facial Cleanser, Sensitive Skin** *($5.49 for 8 ounces)* is not only Clean & Clear's best cleanser, thanks to its gentle yet very effective water-soluble formula, but is also one of the best beauty buys at the drugstore. It would be even better without fragrance, but that's a minor concern. This cleanser removes makeup easily and is suitable for all skin types except very dry.

☺ **Makeup Dissolving Facial Cleansing Wipes, Oil-Free** *($5.99 for 25 wipes)*. These soft-textured cleansing wipes are a great way to remove makeup and refresh skin. They're particularly useful for travel because they almost always make it through airport security in your carry-on luggage. They are capable of removing long-wearing or waterproof formulas, though wipes aren't the best method for gently removing mascara. A liquid makeup remover applied with a cotton pad or swab gives you greater control and less pulling.

☹ **Makeup Dissolving Foaming Cleanser, Oil-Free** *($5.99 for 6 ounces)* definitely has a strong foaming action, but its main detergent cleansing agent (sodium C14-16 olefin sulfonate) makes it too drying and irritating for all skin types. Clean & Clear offers gentler yet still effective cleansers, as do its sister companies Neutrogena and Aveeno (all owned by Johnson & Johnson).

☺ **Soothing Eye Makeup Remover, Oil-Free** *($5.99)* is a simply formulated but very good fragrance-free eye-makeup remover. The dual-phase formula contains silicones to dislodge makeup and it works beautifully, even on waterproof formulas. The only reason this is not rated a Paula's Pick is due to my concern that the amount of benzyl alcohol may be problematic. This ingredient is used in many makeup removers, but typically in much lower amounts, where its irritation potential is not an issue.

☹ **Cooling Daily Pore Toner** *($4.69 for 8 ounces)* lists alcohol as the second ingredient, so it will make oily skin worse by triggering more oil production to flood the pore lining. This also contains a form of menthol for a cooling (and irritating) effect on skin. The glycolic and salicylic acids won't exfoliate skin due to the too-high pH of this toner.

☹ **Dual Action Moisturizer, Oil-Free** *($6.49 for 4 ounces)* has a pH that allows its 0.5% salicylic acid to exfoliate skin, but half a percent won't be effective and the menthyl lactate in this moisturizer causes undue irritation.

☺ **Shine Control Moisturizer, Oil-Free** *($6.49 for 4 ounces)*. Shine Control Moisturizer, Oil-Free is an exceptionally basic moisturizer that leaves a slight matte finish, but lacks ingredients capable of absorbing oil. Actually, it also lacks any ingredients necessary to create a state-of-the-art moisturizer!

✓☺ **Persa-Gel 10, Maximum Strength** *($5.89 for 1 ounce)* remains a very potent, fragrance-free topical disinfectant for blemishes. It contains 10% benzoyl peroxide, the maximum amount approved for over-the-counter sales. Although this amount can be drying and potentially irritating, this is an option for stubborn cases of acne.

☺ **Oil-Absorbing Sheets** *($5.29 for 50 ounces)* are an interesting twist on the standard oil-absorbing papers. These are more like soft plastic sheets with a slight rubbery feel. They work well enough, but it takes several of them to make a difference, just as it does with any of the more standard oil-absorbing papers.

☹ **Blackhead Eraser** *($19.99)*. This aptly named product is a small, battery-powered device meant to erase blackheads. Supposedly, it does this thanks to the device's vibrating motion coupled with pads steeped in a solution that features 1% salicylic acid as the active ingredient. First, you insert the included battery into the bottom of the device, affix the base, and attach one of the included cleansing pads. Wet the pad, then turn the device on; with the device vibrating, you move it around your face in a circular motion. It's nice to think you can just scrub blackheads away, but that just isn't possible. And if you have raised acne lesions along with blackheads, this device can be too aggressive, causing the pimples to rupture and become more inflamed, and potentially causing scarring. Scrubbing your skin with this device or even with a plain washcloth may remove the top layer of the blackhead, but the root of it is still deep in the pore lining well beyond the reach of any scrub or abrasive action, which means the original problem will surface again before long. What about the 1% salicylic acid solution? When properly formulated, salicylic acid can penetrate into the pore lining and help eliminate the oil, whose buildup is what causes blackheads. The downside of this product is that the pH is greater than 5, which means the salicylic acid won't function as an exfoliant. Completely separate from the pH issue is that this cleansing solution also contains menthol, an ingredient that is always a problem for skin, and even more so when it's part of a system that involves manipulating the skin under the pretense of scrubbing blackheads away.

CLEARASIL

CLEARASIL AT-A-GLANCE

Strengths: Inexpensive; effective topical disinfectants with 10% benzoyl peroxide; a good BHA option for those who prefer pads; a decent selection of water-soluble cleansers and scrubs.

Weaknesses: As is true for most anti-acne lines, irritating ingredients with no benefit for skin take precedence; no sunscreens (just because you have acne doesn't mean sun protection falls by the wayside); no lower-strength benzoyl peroxide products (10% has a higher chance of causing irritation than 2.5% and 5% versions).

For more information about Clearasil, call (866) 252-5327 or visit www.clearasil.com or www.Beautypedia.com.

CLEARASIL STAYCLEAR PRODUCTS

☺ **StayClear Acne Fighting Cleansing Wipes** *($5.19 for 32 ounces)* cleanse skin and remove makeup while depositing 2% salicylic acid. The pH of 2.9 permits exfoliation, making these wipes a worthwhile option for those battling blemishes. The only caution is to avoid using them around the eye area.

☺ **StayClear Daily Face Wash** *($5.29 for 6.5 ounces)* is a somewhat harsh, water-soluble foaming cleanser because of the inclusion of alkaline potassium stearate and other cleansing agents that aren't the best for skin unless it is very oily.

☺ **StayClear Daily Face Wash, Sensitive Skin** *($5.29 for 6.5 ounces)* is nearly identical to the Daily Face Wash above, minus a couple of nonessential ingredients, but the same basic comments apply. It is too drying for someone with sensitive skin, though it is fragrance-free.

☺ **StayClear Oil-Free Gel Wash** *($5.29 for 6.78 ounces)* is a good water-soluble cleanser for normal to oily skin, whether blemishes are a concern or not. The active ingredient of 2% salicylic acid won't be active on skin because it is rinsed off before it has a chance to work, so don't count on it for exfoliation. Salicylic acid shouldn't be used to cleanse around the eyes.

☺ **StayClear Skin Perfecting Wash** *($5.29 for 6.78 ounces)*. This cleanser-scrub hybrid contains 2% salicylic acid as the active ingredient. However, unless you're willing to leave this on your skin for several minutes (which is not recommended) the exfoliating benefit of the salicylic acid will be rinsed down the drain. The amount of the synthetic scrub ingredient polyethylene is low, so this functions best as a cleanser with a mild scrub effect. Note that you should not use this over acne lesions; you can't scrub acne away and using topical scrubs can irritate the lesions and prolong healing time. In the long run, there are far better products for acne-prone skin than this one.

☹ **StayClear Daily Pore Cleansing Pads** *($4.99 for 90 pads)* contain skin-irritating alcohol and menthol, making these 2% salicylic acid pads too irritating and drying for all skin types—plus the pH is too high for the BHA to function as an exfoliant.

☹ **StayClear Acne Control Deep Cleansing Scrub** *($4.79 for 5 ounces)* is a topical scrub that's medicated with 2% salicylic acid, but its brief contact with skin and the product's pH keep it from working to fight blemishes. The menthol in this scrub does not make it preferred over other options, and the amount of sodium lauryl sulfate is potentially drying.

☺ **StayClear Daily Facial Scrub** *($5.29 for 5 ounces)* contains salicylic acid as the active ingredient. However, unless you're willing to leave this on your skin for several minutes (which is absolutely not recommended), the exfoliating benefit of the salicylic acid will be rinsed down the drain. The synthetic scrub ingredient polyethylene allows for manual exfoliation, which is OK, but be careful using this over acne lesions because acne cannot be scrubbed away and its presence has nothing to do with skin being too dirty.

☺ **StayClear Adult Care Acne Treatment Cream** *($5.99 for 1 ounce)* contains 2% resorcinol along with 8% sulfur, both topical disinfectants that can be effective against acne-causing bacteria. The trade-offs are that resorcinol can be exceedingly irritating and drying to skin (Source: *Contact Dermatitis*, April 2007, pages 196-200), and sulfur, while less irritating, can cause superficial dryness. Still, this may be a worthwhile option for someone with acne whose blemishes have not responded to benzoyl peroxide, salicylic acid, or prescription options.

✓ ☺ **StayClear Tinted Acne Treatment Cream** *($6.29 for 1 ounce)* provides 10% benzoyl peroxide in an absorbent base with a sheer peach tint and matte finish. This provides minor camouflage, but the peach tinge can draw more attention to the blemish than you want. Still, this is a potent disinfectant that puts the kibosh on acne-causing bacteria.

✓ ☺ **StayClear Vanishing Acne Treatment Cream** *($6.29 for 1 ounce)* is identical to the Tinted Acne Treatment Cream, minus the tint. That makes this option more versatile for daytime use with makeup, though this much benzoyl peroxide is best reserved for blemishes that have been unresponsive to lower strengths.

CLEARASIL ULTRA PRODUCTS

☺ **Ultra Daily Face Wash** *($8.99 for 6.78 ounces)*. Labeling this a "next generation face wash" is a bit like labeling Frank Sinatra a contemporary pop star. This is really an antiquated formula that brings nothing new to those with acne. The 2% salicylic acid is the active ingredient, but it's of little use in a cleanser because of its brief contact with skin before being rinsed down the drain. This is otherwise a very standard water-soluble foaming cleanser suitable for normal to oily skin. It is fine for those struggling with acne; it just doesn't offer any special benefit.

☹ **Ultra Gel Wash** *($5.29 for 6.78 ounces)* could have been a great option for normal to oily skin, but it contains menthol. Menthol is never appropriate in any skin-care product because it causes irritation, which in turn inhibits skin's ability to heal and can stimulate oil production in the pore.

☹ **Ultra Deep Pore Cleansing Pads** *($8.99 for 90 pads)* contain 2% salicylic acid as the active ingredient, but the pH of the solution they are soaked in is too high for exfoliation to occur. Even within the right pH range, these pads wouldn't be recommended because of their alcohol and hydrogen peroxide content. Both of those ingredients cause free-radical damage, which impedes skin's ability to heal, plus they cause irritation, which stimulates oil production in the pore. Talk about a double whammy of problems for anyone's skin.

☺ **Ultra Acne Clearing Scrub** *($8.79 for 5 ounces)* contains 2% salicylic acid (BHA), but the real exfoliating benefit comes from the polyethylene beads because this scrub, just like any other scrub, won't be left on the skin long enough for the BHA to have an effect, even though its pH of 3.6 is low enough for exfoliation to occur. It's a decent scrub option, but the sodium lauryl sulfate makes it less enticing than similar options from Neutrogena or Olay. Leaving it on the skin is an option, but not one I would encourage, given that there are better ways to get the benefits of BHA.

☹ **Ultra Acne Solution System** *($24.99)* comprises four items in a kit designed to address the causes of and help combat facial acne. The **StayClear Daily Face Wash** is a medicated cleanser with 2% salicylic acid, but this anti-acne wonder works best when left on the skin. It is otherwise an average cleanser/scrub hybrid that contains the irritant menthol, so we're not off to a good start. Step 2 involves the **StayClear Daily Toner**, but with alcohol as the second ingredient it's also a problem for all skin types, but especially oily skin because alcohol triggers excess oil production in the pore lining. Things begin looking up with the **StayClear Daily Lotion**, a 0.5% BHA lotion with a pH of 2.3. The pH allows the salicylic acid to exfoliate skin, but is considerably more irritating than a pH of 3 or 4, which is a safe pH range for skin and salicylic acid. The only product that deserves consideration is the **Quick Start Treatment Cream**. This is a simply formulated 10% benzoyl peroxide lotion that has a slightly absorbent matte finish. Ten percent benzoyl peroxide is a potent disinfectant for blemishes, and in general it is best to start with lower strengths to see if those work for you without pronounced side effects such as dryness or flaking. All told, with three out of four products in this system faltering, the only conclusion is to ignore this kit and keep in mind that separate benzoyl peroxide products are available from Clearasil, Neutrogena, and other drugstore lines.

☺ **Ultra Rapid Action Treatment Cream** *($9.99 for 1 ounce)* is a very good topical disinfectant for those struggling with stubborn acne. It is available in colorless ("Invisible") and tinted versions, and both have the same formula, including 10% benzoyl peroxide as the active ingredient. The amount of benzoyl peroxide is potent, and you should consider it only if your acne hasn't responded to lower concentrations of this over-the-counter drug. Benzoyl peroxide is the gold standard as a starting point in treating acne. This product also contains gluconolactone, an AHA-type exfoliant. That is helpful for skin, but salicylic acid is a far better exfoliant for oily or acne-prone skin because it also has antibacterial and anti-inflammatory properties.

☹ **Ultra Tinted Acne Treatment Cream** *($9.99 for 1 ounce)* is nearly identical to the Ultra Vanishing Acne Treatment Cream below, except this version has a sheer peach tint. It's too peach to use on its own during the day, but can look convincing if a neutral foundation is applied afterward.

☹ **Ultra Vanishing Acne Treatment Cream** *($9.99 for 1 ounce)* combines 10% benzoyl peroxide with enough glycolic acid to exfoliate skin, which this product's pH of 3.6 allows. However, according to a cosmetics chemist I interviewed, benzoyl peroxide's stability can be negatively affected at this pH level, causing it to break down into benzoic acid (which has no effect on acne). This product's combination of actives sounds intriguing, but their effectiveness may be inhibited by the unknowns about what happens when they are combined. Further, glycolic acid isn't preferred to salicylic acid for acne.

☹ **Ultra PImple Blocker Pen** *($10.47 for 0.06 ounce)*. The pen concept of this product is clever because lots of consumers with acne want to zero in on their blemishes and zap them away. Treating acne in this manner can be effective, but treating the entire face is better than spot treating because then you are working on preventing blemishes from occurring in the first place, plus the same ingredients that zap zits help reduce them as well. What is pathetic about this terribly formulated product is that the second ingredient is alcohol. And it also contains menthol. Alcohol causes free-radical damage and irritation, and menthol adds to the irritation. Those two ingredients not only hurt the skin's ability to heal but also stimulate oil production in the pore. This product is an ultra problem for anyone's skin.

CLINIQUE

CLINIQUE AT-A-GLANCE

Strengths: One of the best selections of state-of-the-art moisturizers and serums loaded with ingredients that research has shown are of great benefit to skin; excellent sunscreens; good selection of self-tanning products; some very good cleansers and eye makeup removers; some unique mattifying products; a large but wholly impressive selection of foundations, many with reliable sun protection (and shades for darker skin tones); good concealers; some remarkable mascaras; much-improved eyeshadows; loose powder; all of the blush products; some brilliant lipsticks, lip gloss, and the Quickliner for lips; gel eyeliner; priced lower than most competing department-store lines.

Weaknesses: The three-step skin-care routine, because of the bar soaps and irritant-laden clarifying lotions; jar packaging downgrades several otherwise top-notch moisturizers; incomplete routines for those prone to acne; skin-lightening products with either unproven or insufficient levels of lightening agents; the pressed-powder bronzer, liquid eyeliner, and brow pencil disappoint; lip plumper; one truly awful mascara; Clinique Medical's doctor-oriented, professional product positioning is just bizarre.

For more information about Clinique, owned by Estee Lauder, call (800) 419-4041 or visit www.clinique.com or www.Beautypedia.com.

CLINIQUE SKIN CARE

CLINIQUE ACNE SOLUTIONS PRODUCTS

☹ **Acne Solutions Cleansing Bar for Face and Body** *($12.50 for 5.2 ounces)* contains 2% salicylic acid, which is good for acne but useless in a rinse-off product. Beyond that, this bar soap is a poor choice for all skin types, blemishes or not, as it may be irritating and drying to skin.

☹ **Acne Solutions Cleansing Foam** *($17.50 for 4.2 ounces)* would have been an excellent liquid-to-foam cleanser for normal to oily skin, but the peppermint is a problem and salicylic acid's benefit in a cleanser is minimal at best because it is rinsed from skin before it can penetrate into the pore lining. This cleanser does contain some very good (and some unique) water-binding agents, but again, their impact on skin won't be great and the peppermint remains a problem.

☹ **Acne Solutions Clarifying Lotion** *($13.50 for 6.7 ounces)* doesn't improve on Clinique's long-standing Clarifying Lotions. This version still contains a lot of alcohol and a lesser but still potentially problematic amount of witch hazel. Without those, it would be an excellent toner for all skin types, though the 1.5% salicylic acid cannot exfoliate due to the pH of this toner.

☺ **Acne Solutions Post-Blemish Formula** *($13.50 for 0.07 ounce)* claims to gently fade the appearance of post-inflammatory hyperpigmentation—those pesky red or brown marks left over for a period of time after a blemish has healed. However, other than the smattering of anti-irritants, nothing in this lightweight lotion (dispensed through a click-pen precision applicator) will hasten the fading of these unsightly marks. That's because the main "ingredient" necessary to fade post-blemish marks is time. The typically red or pink pigmentation you're seeing is a remnant of your skin's healthy immune response to the blemish, and for most skin types and skin colors it tends to linger long after the blemish is gone. The marks will fade, but it can often take 12 months or longer. If you don't have that kind of patience (and who does?), a better option for speeding up the fading of this type of discoloration is to use a topical exfoliant (a pH-effective AHA or BHA product works well) or a tretinoin product (available by prescription). It is also critical that you wear sunscreen daily to prevent more damage that will impede the skin's healing process. Finally, when new blemishes appear, take steps to treat skin gently while using effective blemish-battling products, and, whatever happens, do not pick at them and make scabs—that is a surefire way to damage skin further, resulting in darker and longer-lasting post-inflammatory hyperpigmentation. Bottom line: This Clinique product won't make matters worse, but it won't help things either, and as such is relegated to "why bother?" status.

☺ **Acne Solutions Clearing Moisturizer, Oil-Free** *($16 for 1.7 ounces)* is one of the most state-of-the-art benzoyl peroxide lotions available today. It contains 2.5% of this topical disinfectant, an excellent amount to apply all over acne-prone skin. The lightweight lotion base feels silky and contains oodles of good-for-skin ingredients, including green tea, acetyl glucosamine, and many soothing plant extracts. The only misstep (one that prevents this product from earning a Paula's Pick rating) is the addition of peppermint extract. The amount is so small as to very likely be a non-issue for skin, but why include it at all when it has no benefit for acne-prone skin?

✓ ☺ **Acne Solutions Emergency Gel Lotion** *($13.50 for 0.5 ounce)* remains an outstanding topical disinfectant for blemish-prone skin with 5% benzoyl peroxide and a good group of anti-inflammatory agents.

☹ **Acne Solutions Body Treatment Spray** *($19.50 for 3.4 ounces)* is a spray-on BHA product that lists 2% salicylic acid as the active ingredient. The pH of this spray won't permit exfoliation to occur, while the amount of alcohol can cause dryness and irritation.

☹ **Acne Solutions Spot Healing Gel** *($13.50 for 0.5 ounce)* lists alcohol as the main ingredient, and in this amount it can cause severe irritation and trigger oil production in the pore lining. Although Spot Healing Gel also contains 1% salicylic acid, the pH is too high for it to function as an exfoliant, leaving your skin irritated and still blemished.

CLINIQUE MEDICAL PRODUCTS

Clinique partnered with the health care company Allergan (of Botox fame) to formulate skin-care products sold exclusively through a physician's office (the line is not available on Clinique's Web site or at Clinique counters at this time, which contributes to the exclusivity angle both companies are hoping to translate into patient sales). There are no ingredients in this or any of the other Clinique Medical products that are not found in products sold outside your physician's office, though it is gratifying to know that Clinique has stepped up its game in the BHA category.

☺ **$$$ Probiotic Cleanser** *($27.50 for 5 ounces)*. In an attempt to have this product be viewed as a new type of cleanser separate from other Clinique cleansers, Clinique added the probiotic lactobacillus ferment to this very standard detergent-free cleansing lotion. According to Clinique, this strain of "friendly" bacteria (also known as acidophilus) can restore the skin's bacterial balance. If that's the case, however, there is no published research to support it or prove that this bacterium is an advantageous ingredient in a cleanser. Moreover, skin doesn't need any strain of bacteria, friendly or not, to naturally restore its bacterial balance; it is capable of doing that on its own. That fact is in contrast to certain medical conditions where oral consumption of lactobacillus may prove helpful to recolonize bacterial strains that serve to enhance health. Besides, even if lactobacillus were a helpful topical ingredient, in a cleanser it is just rinsed from the skin before it has a chance to work. What does make this cleanser different is that it lacks detergent cleansing agents and is fragrance-free, which makes it good for dry to very dry skin that is also sensitive; on the other hand, the lack of detergent cleansing agents also reduces its makeup-removing potential. One more comment: Despite the positives for this cleanser, there isn't anything remotely medical about it, not any more than Dr. Weil adding mushroom extracts to a few Origins products (another Lauder corporation, like Clinique) makes them medical—that's just marketing hype to ignore.

✓ ☺ $$$ **Skin Conditioning Treatment** *($65 for 1 ounce)* ranks as one of the most expensive BHA products I have ever recommended for normal to slightly dry or oily skin, but if you're willing to spend more than you need to for results, you'll find it effective, though definitely not a must-have. The silky, cream-gel texture makes skin look very smooth and it provides light hydration. The formula contains approximately 1% salicylic acid (Clinique would not confirm the amount, and for this price they should) and with a pH of 3.6 you will definitely benefit from exfoliation. Clinique positions this as a medically enhanced product (whatever that means, because the formula is not medical in any way, shape, or form) capable of balancing skin's bacteria, yet it doesn't contain anything that can do that; perhaps they're basing their assertion on salicylic acid's antibacterial properties. But salicylic acid isn't about balancing bacteria—what it can do is kill the bacteria that can cause blemishes. As for the medical positioning, chalk it up to marketing rather than to any special benefit that warrants the cost.

☺ **Daily SPF 38** *($38 for 1.7 ounces)* is no more potent than any other product with a similar or higher SPF rating, nor does it hold special promise for anyone considering a cosmetic corrective procedure. It's just a good daily moisturizer with sunscreen and UVA protection provided by avobenzone. Those with normal to slightly dry or slightly oily skin will fare best with this product. Anyone with sensitive skin (whether the sensitivity is ongoing or the temporary result of a cosmetic corrective procedure) should know that the synthetic active ingredients are not preferred over the gentler mineral-based sunscreens (titanium dioxide and zinc oxide).

☺ $$$ **Optimizing Treatment Cream** *($85 for 1.7 ounces)* is positioned as elite because of the Clinique Medical brand name (which is ironic considering that Clinique started out and continues to market itself as a dermatologist-tested line of products) yet it doesn't raise the bar for moisturizer formulas from Clinique or anyone else. This is just a good but needlessly expensive emollient moisturizer for normal to dry skin. Like most Clinique moisturizers, this contains several antioxidants; however, their presence isn't as impressive as the amount/blend of antioxidants in Clinique's Super Rescue moisturizers, all of which sell for half the price of the Optimizing Treatment Cream. There is nothing medically oriented about this moisturizer (or any other of the Clinique Medical products) beyond the brand name on the box. As for the patent-pending probiotic technology said to balance skin's bacteria, don't count on it or any potential results adding up to a superior skin-care product because there is no research supporting the claim. The whole probiotic concept for Clinique Medical works best as a marketing differentiator rather than as meeting a bona fide skin need that no other line can match. (Lest we forget, Clinique's sister company Estee Lauder also includes forms of probiotics in their Advanced Night Repair products.)

✓ ☺ $$$ **Recovery Week Complex** *($65 for 1 ounce)* is a very thick but silky moisturizer intended to protect dry skin while improving barrier function. Of course, it is also positioned as being the ideal product to use after laser, AHA peel, or microdermabrasion treatment to help the compromised skin heal faster. Whether you have an in-office procedure or not, this moisturizer delivers the goods to improve the appearance and feel of uncomfortably dry skin. The formula isn't terribly exciting for the money, but it contains greater amounts of antioxidants and skin-identical ingredients than any of the other Clinique Medical products. This formula also contains several cell-communicating ingredients, and the plant ingredients are known to reduce inflammation, which should help ease redness. Price notwithstanding, this is recommended for those with sensitive, dry, or rosacea-affected skin; it's certainly more elegant than several other sensitive skin-geared moisturizers.

CLINIQUE CX PRODUCTS

Please note: Clinique CX products can only be found exclusively at Neiman Marcus, Saks Fifth Avenue and Bergdorf Goodman.

☺ **$$$ CX Soothing Cleanser** *($5 for 4.2 ounces)* doesn't provide much cleanser for the money, but it is indeed gentle and does contain soothing ingredients. Completely without detergent cleansing agents, it instead uses a blend of emollients, plant oils, and silicones to dissolve makeup. It does not contain any irritants (not even fragrant plant extracts), so it should be fine for dry to very dry skin that is also sensitive, easily irritated, or dealing with rosacea. The oils do not make this easy to rinse completely, so you may need a washcloth. A lighter, but still gentle, and considerably less expensive alternative to this cleanser is Clinique's Comforting Cream Cleanser.

✓ ☺ **$$$ CX Antioxidant Rescue Serum** *($135 for 1 ounce)* is a water- and aloe-based lightweight serum that contains some formidable antioxidants, cell-communicating ingredients, skin-identical substances, and soothing agents. It is ideal for all skin types and can definitely minimize visible signs of irritation and help skin repair a compromised barrier. Despite this praise, you should know that the Lauder companies have several other serums with similar formulas and benefits, none of which cost this much money. In fact, Clinique's own Repairwear Deep Wrinkle Concentrate for Face and Eyes is just as good in terms of state-of-the-art ingredients, yet costs half as much.

☺ **$$$ CX Protect Base SPF 40** *($55 for 1.69 ounces)* claims to be exceptionally gentle, but two of the four active sunscreen ingredients don 't fit that description. Not that they're a problem, it's just that a sunscreen designed for sensitive skin should only contain the mineral sunscreens titanium dioxide and/or zinc oxide. This product contains those actives too, in a moisturizing base suitable for normal to dry skin. It contains some very good soothing agents, but fewer antioxidants than many other Clinique moisturizers. Two types of lecithin are on hand for their cell-communicating abilities, with the iron oxide and mica mineral pigments bringing a radiant glow to skin.

☺ **$$$ CX 24-Hour Eye System** *($115 for 1 ounce)*. This eye duo is said to provide relief from almost every major eye-area concern. Where have we heard this before? Yes, from practically every other eye cream, gel, or serum sold today. Phase 1 of this duo is the **Day & Night Eye De-Ager**. It's a brilliantly formulated emollient eye cream that contains the key ingredients skin needs to look and feel its best (but that doesn't mean they'll chase away wrinkles). The problem is that Clinique packaged this in a jar, so the effectiveness of several light- and air-sensitive ingredients will be diminished. This eye cream contains titanium dioxide and mica to brighten and add soft shine to the eye area; maybe that's what Clinique means by their "evens skin tone" claim, but a concealer does a much better job if discoloration is a concern.

Phase 2 is the **CX Daily Eye Protector SPF 15**. With titanium dioxide as the sole active, this is a wonderful sunscreen to use around the sensitive eye area. The base formula is enhanced with silicones, and has a texture that works to temporarily fill in superficial lines (not the wrinkles you can still see when your face is expressionless). A small amount of antioxidants and a skin-identical ingredient are also included, along with mineral pigments to visually brighten and add soft shine to the eye area. Once again, jar packaging will render the antioxidants less and less effective with repeated use.

For the money, this fragrance-free system squanders several important ingredients thanks to the jar packaging, and, despite some outstanding attributes, isn't worth the investment.

☺ **$$$ CX Soothing Moisturizer** *($65 for 1.7 ounces).* Unfortunately this very nicely formulated moisturizer comes packaged in a jar, which means that the really helpful antioxidant ingredients won't last very long once you open and start using it. The other ingredients make it a decent choice for dry to very dry skin that needs a rich, protective moisturizer, and it is completely fragrance-free. Were it not for the non-airtight packaging that compromises the effectiveness of the antioxidants, this product would have merited a Paula's Pick rating.

CLINIQUE PORE MINIMIZER PRODUCTS

☺ **$$$ Pore Minimizer Thermal-Active Skin Refiner** *($28.50 for 2.5 ounces)* is Clinique's version of their parent company Estee Lauder's Idealist Micro-D Deep Thermal Refinisher. The two products are remarkably similar and both claim to open pores to free clogging debris; however, pores cannot be opened or closed like window blinds. Lauder's product has more of a microdermabrasion-at-home marketing slant, whereas the Clinique version positions itself as a "mini-spa for pores." Both products contain the scrub ingredient polyethylene (ground-up plastic) as the exfoliating agent, along with the inorganic salt calcium chloride, which is where the "thermal" part comes in. When calcium chloride is mixed with water (Clinique's directions state that you should use this product on damp skin) it causes an exothermic reaction. Simply put, that's a chemical reaction—in this case, between water and calcium chloride—that generates heat. This is merely a nifty science project, however, and has no benefit for skin. Heat of any kind does not help minimize pores. In reality, the warm sensation is there just to give the impression that the product is doing something. It is actually the action of massaging scrub particles over the skin that loosens debris (dead skin cells and oil) from the surface of your pores, allowing it to be rinsed away. That will make skin feel smoother and look more even-toned, and can temporarily make pores smaller—but only because the buildup of dead skin cells and oil has been reduced. Almost any topical scrub or even just a washcloth does this; I no longer recommend baking soda as a scrub. In contrast, chemical exfoliants such as glycolic and salicylic acids surpass topical scrubs because they exfoliate more evenly and thoroughly and with no abrasion. Nevertheless, Pore Minimizer Thermal-Active Skin Refiner will produce smoother, more even-toned skin with consistent use. You don't need to spend this much money to get such results, but there is nothing in this product that is harmful to skin. The pH of 5 prevents the salicylic acid in this product from functioning as an exfoliant.

✓ ☺ **Pore Minimizer Instant Perfector** *($17.50 for 0.5 ounce)* comes in two shades, but the color itself barely registers on the skin. Rather, this product is designed to mattify the skin and create a silky-smooth surface by filling in large pores and absorbing excess oil. This irritant-free formula does just that, and beautifully, too. No, it does not have a long-lasting effect on reducing pore size or holding back every drop of excess oil, but it is a smart product to add to your routine if oil control is an issue. When paired with an ultra-matte foundation (preferably one that has a built-in SPF 15), this can be a formidable option for keeping skin matte most of the day. This can also be applied (carefully) over makeup to absorb oil rather than dusting on more powder.

☺ **Pore Minimizer Refining Lotion** *($19.50 for 1.4 ounces)* is a water- and silicone-based fluid lotion that also contains a good deal of film-forming agent (which can temporarily make pores look smaller) along with alcohol and the absorbents silica and talc. Clinique claims that, with ongoing use, this product makes the pore walls stronger, but nothing in this formula supports that claim. If anything, daily exposure to the high amount of film-forming agent and alcohol can cause chronic irritation and stimulate oil production, and that won't strengthen pores in the least.

☹ **Pore Minimizer T-Zone Shine Control** *($14.50 for 0.5 ounce)* contains several dry-finish ingredients (such as silicones) that can indeed leave a lasting matte finish on the skin. Unfortunately, they are joined by irritants such as denatured alcohol, witch hazel, and clove extract, and that means this product is not recommended for any skin type. The alcohol content can trigger more oil production in the pore lining.

☺ **Pore Minimizer Oil-Blotting Sheets, for Combination Oily to Oily Skin** *($14.50 for 50 sheets)* are standard powder-free blotting papers that work as well as most to soak up excess oil and perspiration. Reducing surface oil will make pores appear smaller, but that benefit isn't unique to this product.

CLINIQUE REDNESS SOLUTIONS PRODUCTS

✓☺ **$$$ Redness Solutions Soothing Cleanser** *($20.50 for 5 ounces)* is an emollient cleansing lotion that is a fantastic option for those with dry, sensitive skin because it lacks detergent cleansing agents. The emollients and silicone are what remove makeup, though they can impede rinsing and might make it necessary to use a washcloth. This cleanser contains several anti-irritants that are beneficial for all skin types, and because the formula doesn't rinse easily, some of the soothing agents will be left on skin, which is good. The claim that this can make skin smoother with mild exfoliation is inaccurate; there are no exfoliating ingredients in this fragrance-free cleanser. Overall, this should prove a helpful option for those with rosacea and/or dry skin.

✓☺ **Redness Solutions Daily Protective Base SPF 15** *($17.50 for 1.35 ounces)* gets the gentle sunscreen right with its pure titanium dioxide and zinc oxide blend. The base formula is similar to that of Clinique's City Block Sheer Oil-Free Daily Face Protector SPF 25, which is also suitable for someone with sensitive, reddened skin (and that's why this earns a Paula's Pick rating). Both products contain some very good water-binding agents, skin-identical substances, and antioxidants. However, it is worth noting that the aforementioned Clinique City Block Sheer offers skin a greater complement of bells and whistles. The only advantage of the Redness Solutions is its sheer green tint (if you consider that a plus). When applied to skin, the green tint becomes a pale flesh tone that provides a bit of coverage. If you have superficial, minor redness, you'll notice it is less apparent, but that would be true for any tinted moisturizer, too. Anyone with lingering or persistent redness (such as occurs with rosacea) will want to pair this with a foundation that supplies at least medium coverage. One more thing: The finish of this product is matte, but also somewhat chalky. It can lend a flat appearance to skin that someone who is not bothered with oiliness may not like.

☺ **$$$ Redness Solutions Daily Relief Cream** *($39.50 for 1.7 ounces)* is nearly identical to Clinique's former, very expensive CX Redness Relief Cream. The Redness Solutions version is an equally impressive soothing moisturizer for dry, reddened skin—but the jar packaging remains. That means the plethora of antioxidants (Clinique is rarely stingy with such ingredients) is not going to be of much ongoing benefit once the product is opened. What a shame! This is an overall brilliant moisturizer formula, but any major benefits are lost due to the poor packaging decision.

✓ ☺ **Redness Solutions Urgent Relief Cream** *($30 for 1 ounce)* is a throwback to Clinique's former Exceptionally Soothing Cream for Upset Skin. That was also a well-formulated moisturizer whose active ingredient was 0.5% hydrocortisone. Cortisones are definitely capable of reducing inflammation, itching, and signs of redness. However, ongoing, long-term use isn't wise because of the eventual effect of hydrocortisone, which is collagen destruction. For occasional use to calm reddened, itchy skin this cream is a very good option, though not any better than some of the far less expensive products available at the drugstore (and some of those have double the concentration of hydrocortisone that this product does). While the drugstore versions are not as elegantly formulated or loaded with anti-irritants and skin-identical substances as Clinique's version, such substances are extraneous and need not be a consideration for an effective hydrocortisone product. Outside of the added expense, occasional use of this product comes down to whether or not you want a hydrocortisone cream with an elegant, silky texture or you want something more basic. From my perspective, there is no reason to use a more expensive hydrocortisone product because you would only be using it intermittently and over spot areas. For regular allover use, you should use products that have more state-of-the-art ingredients.

CLINIQUE REPAIRWEAR PRODUCTS

☹ $$$ **Repairwear Day SPF 15 Intensive Cream** *($48.50 for 1.7 ounces)* is an excellent, in-part zinc oxide sunscreen in a moisturizing base that's characteristic of the best moisturizers from Clinique, but it also has jar packaging. That means the many light- and air-sensitive ingredients in this product will be compromised once you begin using it. Some of the plant extracts can be problematic, but they are present in small amounts and the beneficial plant extracts and cell-communicating ingredients have them outnumbered. Clinique maintains that Repairwear "helps block and mend the look of lines and wrinkles," though that's true only to the extent that an effective sunscreen, which this product contains, can prevent further skin damage. As well-formulated as this product is, please don't be fooled into thinking it can repair your skin and eliminate wrinkles, or you're bound to be disappointed. The fact that this is described as an intensive cream may make you think it is for very dry skin, but it's actually best for normal to dry skin.

☹ $$$ **Repairwear Day SPF 15 Intensive Cream Very Dry Skin Formula** *($48.50 for 1.7 ounces)* is a more emollient, dry-to-very-dry-skin-appropriate version of the Repairwear Day SPF 15 Intensive Cream above, and the same basic comments apply, including those about the poor choice of jar packaging.

✓ ☺ $$$ **Repairwear Deep Wrinkle Concentrate for Face and Eyes** *($55 for 1 ounce)* lists 72 ingredients, so it's reasonable to suppose that at least a few of them might be helpful for your skin—yet how much of any one ingredient is actually in here in a level that is beneficial for skin is questionable. After all, the contents can only add up to 100%. Claiming to deal with "wrinkles at their base" and to "jump-start natural collagen production," this antiaging product is one many baby-boomer consumers will take seriously. Despite the somewhat misleading claims (shared by dozens of other products), this product is as state-of-the-art as it gets. What a remarkably elegant formula! Just as advanced as most of Clinique's Repairwear products that aren't packaged in jars, its formula includes effective and abundant antioxidants, skin-identical ingredients, cell-communicating ingredients, potent anti-irritants, fatty acids, plant oil, and smoothing film-forming agents. It really is a brilliant formula that has the potential to significantly improve the health and appearance of skin. Will it vanquish wrinkles? No, at least not those related to years of unprotected sun exposure. But it will help skin help itself to an improved, smoothed appearance, thus making earlier damage less apparent. That is reason enough to highly recommend this fragrance-free product. One more comment: The serum texture makes this a suitable product for oily skin looking to benefit from topical antioxidants without making skin feel slick or too moist.

☺ $$$ **Repairwear Intensive Eye Cream** *($38.50 for 0.5 ounce)* has a lot going for it in terms of its plentiful antioxidant content—that's why the choice of jar packaging was a bad one, because these ingredients won't remain potent once the product is opened and used repeatedly. It's a good emollient eye cream for dry skin, but opaque tube packaging would have made it a slam dunk.

☹ $$$ **Repairwear Intensive Night Cream** *($48.50 for 1.7 ounces)* is an elegant formulation that covers all the bases when it comes to a modern combination of emollients, skin-identical ingredients, antioxidants, and cell-communicating ingredients—yet the effectiveness of several of those ingredients is compromised due to the jar packaging. This does contain a jasmine oil–derived fragrance in the form of methyldihydrojasmonate, which refutes Clinique's 100% fragrance-free assertion.

☹ $$$ **Repairwear Intensive Night Cream Very Dry Skin Formula** *($48.50 for 1.7 ounces)* is a richer, creamier version of the Repairwear Intensive Night Cream above, and the same basic comments apply. This product's jar packaging won't allow "24-hour antioxidant protection" as claimed. And besides, I wonder how they determined that, given that we don't know with certainty how long topically applied antioxidants can protect skin.

☹ $$$ **Zero Gravity Repairwear Lift Firming Cream, for Combination Oily to Oily Skin** *($52.50 for 1.7 ounces)* promises an instant firming sensation, but a sensation isn't the same as an actual result, and about all this moisturizer will do instantly is make skin feel smoother and softer. That won't help skin stand up to gravity's downward assault, but then again, no skin-care product can do that. As is true for most Clinique moisturizers, this is loaded with antioxidants, cell-communicating ingredients (including retinol), and ingredients that mimic the structure and function of healthy skin. The problem with this product is twofold: jar packaging won't keep the buzz-worthy ingredient stable during use and the inclusion of alcohol (it's the sixth ingredient) prior to any antioxidant is a letdown because alcohol causes free-radical damage. Considering the price and aforementioned detriments, this moisturizer is a tough sell. The mineral pigments in this product lend a soft glow to skin.

☹ $$$ **Zero Gravity Repairwear Lift Firming Cream, for Dry Combination Skin** *($52.50 for 1.7 ounces)* makes the same claims as the Zero Gravity Repairwear Lift Firming Cream, for Combination Oily to Oily Skin, but omits the alcohol and contains several thickeners to create a creamier texture suitable for normal to dry skin (not combination skin, assuming part of this combination includes oily areas). It's still unfortunate that so many light- and air-sensitive ingredients are prone to breaking down quickly once this jar-packaged moisturizer is opened.

☹ $$$ **Zero Gravity Repairwear Lift Firming Cream, for Very Dry to Dry Skin** *($52.50 for 1.7 ounces)* has a surprisingly lighter texture than the Zero Gravity Repairwear Lift Firming

Cream, for Dry Combination Skin above, despite being labeled for very dry skin. The glycerin, plant oil, and emollient thickeners are certainly capable of making any degree of dry skin look and feel better, but the state-of-the-art efficacious ingredients (numerous antioxidants and several cell-communicating ingredients, including retinol) won't last for long once this jar-packaged moisturizer is opened. It is doubtful their presence in this product will stimulate collagen production even a little; in stable packaging, that would be another story.

☺ $$$ **Repairwear Intensive Lip Treatment** *($25 for 0.14 ounce)* functions as a soft spackle for lines on and around the lips. The very thick, lipstick-style balm has several emollients to condition lips, and also contains film-forming agents and waxes that temporarily fill in lines. The addition of peppermint may make you think the product is doing something special, but it's just especially irritating, which isn't great for routine use. Smaller amounts of antioxidants and cell-communicating ingredients are included, but not enough to justify the cost or make this a revolutionary treatment for lip lines.

CLINIQUE SUPERDEFENSE PRODUCTS

☹ $$$ **Superdefense SPF 25 Age Defense Moisturizer, for Combination Oily to Oily Skin** *($42.50 for 1.7 ounces)* was a replacement for Clinique's former Superdefense SPF 25 for Combination to Oily Skin. The sunscreen is still in-part avobenzone, so the UVA portion is covered (and the avobenzone is stabilized by octocrylene, another active sunscreen ingredient). Also like the previous formula, the product is loaded with antioxidants, water-binding agents, and cell-communicating ingredients. The silky-textured formula is ideal for its intended skin types because it supplies light hydration and skin-beneficial ingredients without potentially problematic thickening agents. The problem? Once again, Clinique relies on jar packaging, which compromises the effectiveness and stability of all the ingredients you're paying extra for. Antioxidants can help "insulate skin from visible signs of aging," but they need to be protected from light and air if you're going to get any benefit from applying them to skin. The choice of jar packaging takes this daytime moisturizer from "super" to "average," and that's not a great way to face each day.

☹ $$$ **Superdefense SPF 25 Age Defense Moisturizer, for Dry Combination Skin** *($42.50 for 1.7 ounces)* is similar to but slightly more emollient than the Superdefense SPF 25 Age Defense Moisturizer, for Combination Oily to Oily Skin above, and the same comments apply.

☹ $$$ **Superdefense SPF 25 Age Defense Moisturizer, for Very Dry to Dry Skin** *($42.50 for 1.7 ounces)*. The same packaging-related inadequacy that sullies Clinique's other Superdefense daytime moisturizers is present here, too. Between that and the core formula (including the in-part avobenzone sunscreen) the same comments apply. The difference is that this cream-textured substantive product is well-suited for its intended skin types.

CLINIQUE SUPER RESCUE PRODUCTS

Note: All of Clinique's Super Rescue Antioxidant Night Moisturizers are fragrance-free and suitable for sensitive skin.

✓☺ $$$ **Super Rescue Antioxidant Night Moisturizer, for Combination Oily to Oily Skin** *($42.50 for 1.7 ounces)* is a slightly reformulated version of Clinique's former Continuous Rescue Antioxidant Moisturizer for Combination Oily to Oily Skin, and the claims are the same: using this will protect your skin from free-radical damage and help make it stronger. It's true that antioxidants applied topically (and consumed as part of a healthy diet) do much to diffuse and reduce free-radical damage, but it isn't physically possible to stop free-radical damage in its entirety. Antioxidants have their place in skin-care products, but they are not an all-out rescue from or an impervious shield against free-radical damage. Super Rescue is suitable for normal to combination skin, but is probably too heavy for oily skin or really oily areas. It contains some great emollients, silicone, slip agents, several antioxidants, Vaseline, cell-communicating ingredients, and soothing plant extracts. The only frustrating element is that half of the really intriguing ingredients are listed after one of the preservatives, which means that they're basically window dressing. However, even without considering the mere dustings of those ingredients, this fragrance-free moisturizer is still antioxidant-packed, and it is recommended for normal to slightly dry or slightly oily skin. What's more, Clinique kept the opaque tube packaging that debuted with the Continuous Rescue Antioxidant Moisturizer, which means the many light- and air-sensitive ingredients will remain stable during use.

✓☺ $$$ **Super Rescue Antioxidant Night Moisturizer, for Dry Combination Skin** (*$42.50 for 1.7 ounces*) is an outstanding blend of water, silicone, thickeners, shea butter, fatty acids, glycerin, antioxidants, cell-communicating ingredients, and skin-identical ingredients. In short, this fragrance-free moisturizer takes advantage of what solid research has shown is necessary to create a truly state-of-the-art moisturizer. What's more, Clinique kept the opaque tube packaging that debuted with the Continuous Rescue Antioxidant Moisturizer (off which this product is based), which means the many light- and air-sensitive ingredients will remain stable during use. This moisturizer is suitable for normal to dry skin; it is too emollient for use over oily areas.

✓☺ $$$ **Super Rescue Antioxidant Night Moisturizer, for Very Dry to Dry Skin** (*$42.50 for 1.7 ounces*) is the richest of Clinique's three Super Rescue Antioxidant Night Moisturizers, and is appropriate for dry to very dry skin. Interestingly, this version contains greater amounts of antioxidants known for their potent anti-inflammatory effect. That attention to detail can help dry skin repair itself because the less inflammation skin endures, the better it is able to strengthen itself and repair damage. Some of the intriguing ingredients aren't present in amounts large enough to provide much benefit to your skin, but there are enough bells and whistles in this moisturizer to compensate for that. It is great news that Clinique kept the opaque tube packaging that debuted with the Continuous Rescue Antioxidant Moisturizer (off which this product is based), which means the many light- and air-sensitive ingredients will remain stable during use.

CLINIQUE TURNAROUND PRODUCTS

☺ $$$ **Turnaround Instant Facial** (*$36.50 for 2.5 ounces*) is a water- and silicone-based scrub that contains diatomaceous earth (ground-up porous rock composed of the skeletons of sea creatures) to manually scrub skin. The formula also features salicylic acid, but the pH is too high for it to function as an exfoliant. Even if it worked in this manner, you're not going to gain much benefit from the 5 minutes this product is supposed to be left on skin before rinsing. Not to mention that scrubbing the skin for 5 minutes is just plain excessive, and potentially damaging to the skin. Consider this an expensive face scrub that can be difficult to rinse because of the silicones (though ironically the silicones help buffer skin from the abrasiveness of the diatomaceous earth). The bells and whistles Clinique added look good on the label, but antioxidants, anti-irritants, and cell-communicating ingredients are most effective in leave-on products; rinsing them down the drain doesn't help your skin. Turnaround Instant Facial is best for normal to dry or slightly oily skin. As you may have guessed by now, 5 minutes with this scrub isn't the equivalent of a facial, though used too aggressively this may cause instant irritation!

✓ ☺ **$$$ Turnaround Concentrate Visible Skin Renewer** *($37.50 for 1 ounce)* contains what Clinique refers to as "an advanced cocktail of exfoliants," but the only ingredient that has substantiated research behind it to support that claim is salicylic acid. Although salicylic acid is present in this silky-smooth lotion at approximately 1%, the pH of 5 limits its ability to exfoliate. Clinique has taken a cue from parent company Estee Lauder and included acetyl glucosamine, which they believe is an effective non-acid exfoliating agent, although there is still no substantiated research proving this ingredient's effectiveness as an alternative to AHA or BHA exfoliants. It does have excellent water-binding properties for skin, and complements the other skin-beneficial ingredients in this product quite well. Although this product won't "renew" skin, it is an outstanding, well-packaged, lightweight moisturizer that contains several antioxidants, vitamins, cell-communicating ingredients, and anti-irritants. It is fragrance-free and best suited for those with normal to oily skin. Fans of Estee Lauder's Idealist take note: Turnaround Concentrate Visible Skin Renewer is incredibly similar, right down to its light texture and silky finish.

☹ **$$$ Total Turnaround Visible Skin Renewer** *($36 for 1.7 ounces)* cannot exfoliate skin because the amount of salicylic acid is too low and the pH of the product is too high. It's an option for someone with normal to slightly oily skin looking for a silky, lightweight moisturizer. The antioxidants will be diminished by jar packaging, but the cell-communicating ingredients will fare better. The mica and titanium dioxide lend a radiant finish to this moisturizer; but be sure you like this before applying it over shine-prone areas.

☹ **$$$ Turnaround Radiance Peel Once-a-Week System** *($55)*. This weekly two-part system is a great example of an extraneous product. Phase 1 is the **Radiance Peel**, which is packaged in eight vials, each intended for a single use (so the set offers eight treatments). The liquidy Radiance Peel is mostly alcohol and its salicylic acid is wasted because the product's pH is too high for it to work as an exfoliant. If you're using the Clinique Clarifying Lotions 1-4, adding the Radiance Peel essentially gives your already-damaged skin a double dose of alcohol-fueled irritation, free-radical damage, and excess oil production. After inflaming your skin with Phase 1, you're invited to rinse the Peel and apply Phase 2, the **Calming Cream**. This is a well-formulated moisturizer that's packaged to keep the antioxidants it contains stable during use. It is fragrance-free and contains anti-irritants that really do have a calming effect on skin—and your skin will need to be calmed after applying the Radiance Peel! Because one part of this system is terrible for skin and one part is great for dry to very dry and sensitive skin, I assigned it a neutral face rating. The Radiance Peel is absolutely not recommended, while the Calming Cream would earn a very good rating if it were available separately.

☺ **$$$ Turnaround Body Smoothing Cream** *($28.50 for 5 ounces)* contains urea as the main moisturizing agent. In addition to urea's moisturizing properties, it is also a keratolytic (exfoliating) agent when its concentration exceeds 40%. That's likely not the case with this product, though, as I said, the urea still has value for its moisturizing abilities (Source: *Dry Skin and Moisturizers Chemistry and Function*, CRC Press, Loden and Maibach, 2000, pages 243-247). You may be wondering if the salicylic acid in this product makes it an effective option for a BHA body lotion. Regrettably, it doesn't, because this product's pH is well above the range that will allow exfoliation to occur. Still, this is an effective moisturizer with a silky texture that can benefit dry skin. It contains some good antioxidants, though not the same impressive range that you see in many of Clinique's other facial moisturizers. If you're looking to spend less for an outstanding body lotion, consider the Paula's Pick-rated options from Olay's Quench line (reviewed on www.Beautypedia.com) or, for very dry skin, CeraVe Moisturizing Lotion.

CLINIQUE YOUTH SURGE PRODUCTS

☺ **$$$ Youth Surge SPF 15 Age Decelerating Moisturizer, Combination Oily to Oily** (*$48.50 for 1.7 ounces)* is said to leverage sirtuin technology to tackle lines and wrinkles. Before I discuss sirtuins and skin, it is worth asking what the company means by "leverage." By stating in their ads that their product is "Leveraging sirtuin technology," they could mean gaining advantage from this technology, paying to use this technology, or, really, whatever they want it to mean. It doesn't say the technology is making a difference and changing the structure of your skin. Look closely at the claims for the Youth Surge products and you'll see that every statement they make is a purely cosmetic claim. "Visible effects" could mean anything—visible effects of what? "Seem to evaporate" doesn't mean that lines and wrinkles will really go away, it could mean that water evaporates, and the word "seems" doesn't mean it is actually happening. "Skin gains strength" is a strange claim that might lead you to believe it will build collagen or appear more taut, but it could really mean just about anything you want it to mean. That's the art of cosmetics ad copy.

Now, back to sirtuins. Sirtuins are proteins that are involved in regulating biological processes by controlling the chain of events that cause these processes to occur, which is why they're often referred to as information regulators. The antiaging connection has to do with their potential to regulate cellular processes responsible for aging. It is believed that if certain sirtuins can be modified to work against the mechanisms of aging, the results might be visible on skin: think fewer wrinkles, less sagging, and greater resiliency. Although sirtuin manipulation has no research showing it can affect wrinkles, that certainly didn't stop Clinique from jumping on the youthful skin connection and parlaying the research about sirtuins and degenerative diseases into skincare products. And what about all of Clinique's other "de-agers" that don't contain sirtuins? Are they of lesser value for skin because they're behind the times? Should Clinique stop selling those? What seems promising is that topical application of specific sirtuins derived from yeast (in this case *Saccharomyces lysate*) and the antioxidant resveratrol (in this case from the root of the plant *Polygonum cuspidatum*) seems to have a protective effect on skin in the presence of oxidative and ultraviolet light stress. However, more research is needed before I'd suggest anyone run out and look for products that increase sirtuin activity in their skin. Plus, we don't know the risk associated with manipulating sirtuins, whether they might have negative side effects. The problem is twofold. First, there is limited research showing how much and what type of sirtuin is needed topically to cause desirable cellular changes leading to younger-looking skin. Plus, the bioavailability of a topically applied source of sirtuins is questionable given that we don't know how efficiently they penetrate intact skin. (Testing skin cells in a lab setting with concentrated doses of ingredients that stimulate sirtuins is an entirely different story from actual use.) Second, and an even bigger concern, is that whenever normal cellular processes are manipulated, you run the risk of causing a potential overproliferation of cells, which is the blueprint for cancer. In other words, how would the sirtuin-influenced cells know when too much of a good thing becomes a health-threatening problem? How long is too long to keep skin cells active? How much manipulation of biological processes starts a cascading negative chain of events (Sources:

Current Medicinal Chemistry, 2008, pages 1887-1899; *Journal of Drugs in Dermatology*, June 2007, pages 14-19; *Nature Reviews: Drug Discovery*, June 2006, pages 493-506)? As has become standard for Clinique, this daytime moisturizer with sunscreen includes reliable UVA protection (from titanium dioxide, though a higher percentage would be preferred) and is loaded with antioxidants, cell-communicating ingredients, and, to a lesser degree, skin-identical substances. Unfortunately, jar packaging won't keep the majority of these state-of-the-art ingredients stable during use. Youth Surge's sunscreen is the only "age decelerating" effect you can rely on, but I'd advise you to look for equally impressive formulas in better packaging. If you decide to try this anyway, it's best for normal to dry skin; those with oily skin will find it way too creamy.

☺ **$$$ Youth Surge SPF 15 Age Decelerating Moisturizer, Dry Combination** *($48.50 for 1.7 ounces)* is very similar to the Youth Surge SPF 15 Age Decelerating Moisturizer, Combination Oily to Oily, and the same basic comments apply. Those with combination skin (meaning oily and dry areas) will find this to be too emollient for their oily areas—and sunscreen needs to be applied all over.

☺ **$$$ Youth Surge SPF 15 Age Decelerating Moisturizer, Very Dry to Dry** *($48.50 for 1.7 ounces)*. This daytime moisturizer with sunscreen includes reliable UVA protection (from avobenzone) and is loaded with antioxidants, cell-communicating ingredients, and, to a lesser degree, skin-identical substances. Unfortunately, jar packaging won't keep the majority of these state-of-the-art ingredients stable during use. Youth Surge's sunscreen is the only "age decelerating" effect you can rely on, but I'd advise you to look for equally impressive formulas in better packaging. If you decide to try this anyway, it is best for normal to dry skin. Those with very dry skin will likely prefer the Youth Surge formula for Dry Combination skin. For details on the claims behind this product, refer to the review above for Youth Surge SPF 15 Age Decelerating Moisturizer, Combination Oily to Oily.

OTHER CLINIQUE SKIN-CARE PRODUCTS

✓☺ **$$$ Comforting Cream Cleanser** *($18.50 for 5 ounces)* is an excellent lotion-type cleanser for normal to dry skin that is close to being water-soluble, but still requires the use of a washcloth for complete removal. This would be an option for normal to dry or sensitive skin, and it is truly fragrance- and irritant-free. Clinique claims you can tissue this off, but is anyone still using tissues to remove their cleanser? If they are, they should stop!

☺ **Extremely Gentle Cleansing Cream** *($26 for 10 ounces)* is standard-issue cold cream and is recommended only for very dry skin not prone to breakouts. It removes makeup easily but also leaves skin feeling greasy and coated.

☹ **Facial Soap Extra Mild** *($11 for 5.2-ounce bar)* may be mild, but it's still standard bar soap and as such can be needlessly drying and irritating to skin. If you prefer bar cleansers, Dove's original Beauty Bar is actually a better formulation.

☹ **Facial Soap Mild** *($11 for 5.2-ounce bar)* is a less emollient version of the Facial Soap Extra Mild, and the same review applies.

☹ **Facial Soap Oily** *($11 for 5.2-ounce bar)* contains a high amount of menthol and sodium borate, both of which are irritating to skin.

☹ **Foaming Mousse Cleanser** *($20 for 4.2 ounces)* is a liquid-to-foam cleanser containing potassium-based cleansing agents that give this seemingly benign cleanser a pH of 9, which is way too alkaline for any skin type because it can cause unnecessary dryness and a tight feeling, similar to what you get from bar soap.

✓☺ **Liquid Facial Soap Extra Mild** *($15 for 6.7 ounces)* is not necessarily water-soluble due to its oil content, but it is an excellent option for someone with dry to very dry skin. A true lotion cleanser, it does not contain any detergent cleansing agents, and so is actually a smart choice for someone with sensitive or easily irritated skin (and infinitely better for skin than any of Clinique's bar soaps). The oil content helps dissolve makeup, including mascara, but you'll need a washcloth for complete removal. One nice touch is the anti-irritants, although they are not as beneficial here as they are in leave-on products.

✓☺ **Liquid Facial Soap Mild Formula** *($15 for 6.7 ounces)* is a standard, but good, water-soluble cleanser for normal to slightly dry or slightly oily skin. Despite its name, it is completely soap-free, and contains gentle but effective detergent cleansing agents and skin-smoothing skin-identical ingredients to prevent skin from feeling dry or tight. It is also completely fragrance-free and does a good job of removing makeup.

☹ **Liquid Facial Soap Oily Skin Formula** *($15 for 6.7 ounces)* is similar to the Liquid Facial Soap Mild Formula, but loses points for the senseless inclusion of menthol. This irritant has no benefit for skin, oily or not. What a shame, because without the menthol this would have been a slam-dunk recommendation for normal to oily skin.

☹ **Rinse-Off Foaming Cleanser** *($18.50 for 5 ounces)* produces copious, creamy foam, but the potassium-based cleansing agents can be drying for most skin types, and the inclusion of eucalyptus, pine, lemon, and lavender makes this too irritating for everyone and unsuitable for use around the eyes.

✓☺ **$$$ Take The Day Off Cleansing Balm** *($27 for 3.8 ounces)* is a modern-day version of a classic cleansing cream. It contains emollients and plant oil to dissolve makeup, and is capable of removing stubborn or waterproof formulas. This is best for dry to very dry skin or sensitive skin not prone to breakouts.

✓☺ **$$$ Take The Day Off Cleansing Milk** *($25 for 6.7 ounces)* is a silky, lightweight cleansing lotion whose solvent does dissolve makeup quickly and easily. This doesn't rinse completely without the aid of a washcloth, but is nevertheless a very gentle option for those with normal to dry, sensitive skin. It is truly fragrance-free. This would also be a prime choice for someone with dry skin and rosacea.

☹ **Wash-Away Gel Cleanser** *($18.50 for 5 ounces)* would be recommended as a very good water-soluble cleanser if it didn't contain eucalyptus, lavender, lemon, and pine—none of which have a single benefit for skin, but all of which can cause irritation.

☺ **$$$ Naturally Gentle Eye Makeup Remover** *($16.50 for 2.5 ounces)* is indeed gentle, but also oily enough to make it difficult to rinse from the eye area or eyelashes. It is an option, but Clinique's Take the Day Off Makeup Remover for Lids, Lashes & Lips below is less messy, easier to rinse, and effectively removes all types of eye makeup. An interesting side note on this product is that it contains sialyllactose, a complex carbohydrate that is derived from human milk and urine. It's not formally listed as a cosmetic ingredient, but is a sugar-based emulsifier that is a component of human tears. The idea was to add ingredients to this eye makeup remover that mimic human tears. Ironically, the sesame oil in the formula, while gentle, is assuredly not a component of natural human tears, and like any oil it can cause temporary blurred vision if it gets into the eye.

☺ **Rinse-Off Eye Makeup Solvent** *($16.50 for 4.2 ounces)* is a basic, no-frills eye-makeup remover that contains mild detergent cleansing agents to dissolve makeup. It does not contain extraneous ingredients that may irritate the eye.

✓ ☺ **$$$ Take The Day Off Makeup Remover for Lids, Lashes & Lips** *($17.50 for 4.2 ounces)* is a very good silicone-in-water, dual-phase remover that makes quick work of even the most stubborn foundations, lipsticks, and waterproof mascaras. It is Clinique's most efficient makeup remover and may be used before or after cleansing.

☹ **Clarifying Lotion 1** *($11.50 for 6.7 ounces)* lists alcohol as the second ingredient, and that makes this toner too irritating for all skin types. The alcohol this contains will trigger oil production in the pore lining.

☹ **Clarifying Lotion 2** *($11.50 for 6.7 ounces)* is an alcohol-based toner that also contains witch hazel and menthol. The Clinique salespeople may claim that the alcohol is "cosmetics-grade," which sounds nice but doesn't make this product any less irritating. The alcohol this contains will trigger oil production in the pore lining.

☹ **Clarifying Lotion 3** *($11.50 for 6.7 ounces)* is similar to Clarifying Lotion 2, but with less alcohol and no menthol. It's still way too irritating and drying, even for oily skin. The alcohol this contains will trigger oil production in the pore lining.

☹ **Clarifying Lotion 4** *($11.50 for 6.7 ounces)* is nearly identical to Clarifying Lotion 3, and the same review applies.

☺ **Mild Clarifying Lotion** *($11.50 for 6.7 ounces)* puts all of Clinique's other Clarifying Lotions to shame with its alcohol-free formula that contains 0.5% salicylic acid at an effective pH of 2.9. Although a higher concentration of salicylic acid would be more effective for someone battling blemishes and blackheads, this is a step in the right direction and contains some very good skin-identical ingredients.

☺ **$$$ Moisture Surge Face Spray Thirsty Skin Relief** *($20 for 4.2 ounces)* is a very good spray-on, alcohol-free toner. This is a good choice for all skin types, including oily or blemish-prone skin that has minor dry patches.

☺ **$$$ 7 Day Scrub Cream Rinse-Off Formula** *($17.50 for 3.4 ounces)* rinses decently, but may still require use of a washcloth for complete removal. It also contains polyethylene as the scrub agent, and is an option for normal to slightly dry skin not prone to blemishes.

☹ **Exfoliating Scrub** *($17.50 for 3.4 ounces)* is Clinique's most abrasive topical scrub and also its most irritating, thanks to menthol.

☺ **$$$ Advanced Stop Signs Eye Preventive Cream SPF 15** *($33.50 for 0.5 ounce)* is a creamy, initially greasy-feeling moisturizer that contains zinc oxide as its primary sunscreen agent, a gentle choice for use around the sensitive eye area. There is a synthetic sunscreen agent also, but the small amount should not be a problem for use near the eyes. While the zinc oxide leaves a slight whitish cast on the skin, this can be considered a benefit because it creates a brightening effect under the eye that can soften the appearance of dark circles. Beyond the sunscreen, the moisturizing base for this elegant formula contains several emollients and skin-identical ingredients. There's also a range of antioxidants (in greater amounts than in the original version of this eye cream), but the jar packaging won't keep them stable once the product is opened. This is still a good option for those with normal to dry skin, or someone with oily skin experiencing dryness around the eyes. Although it is not necessary to purchase a separate sunscreen for the eye area, if your favorite sunscreen tends to cause stinging or burning when applied near the eye area, a product like this one may be the solution. Despite the claims made for this product, Advanced Stop Signs Eye Preventive Cream SPF 15 won't make an existing wrinkle revert back to smooth, unlined skin, but it absolutely can reduce the risk of future wrinkles (to some extent) and shield skin from further environmental damage.

☹ **$$$ All About Eyes** *($28.50 for 0.5 ounce)* remains one of Clinique's most popular items, and its silicone-based formula leaves skin very smooth and silky. It contains some outstanding ingredients to fortify skin and allow it to repair itself, but many of these are compromised by packaging that exposes them to light and air. Clever cosmetic pigment technology changes the way light is reflected off shadowed areas, temporarily improving the appearance of dark circles (sort of like a concealer but without coverage).

☹ **$$$ All About Eyes Rich** *($28.50 for 0.5 ounce)* is an emollient version of the original All About Eyes above, but unlike that product, whose silkiness is largely due to its silicone base, All About Eyes Rich contains several emollients, chiefly shea butter. It is indeed a moisture-rich product and is preferred for dry to very dry skin around the eyes or elsewhere on the face. It cannot diminish dark circles or puffy eyes as claimed. The usual roster of antioxidants, anti-irritants, and ingredients that mimic the structure and function of healthy skin are present, but the antioxidants won't remain potent for long given the jar packaging. The packaging keeps it from earning a higher rating, but this is still an unquestionably emollient moisturizer, even though its base formula doesn't contain anything that's exclusively "all about eyes."

☹ **$$$ Anti-Gravity Firming Eye Lift Cream** *($33.50 for 0.5 ounce)* is a good emollient moisturizer for dry skin anywhere on the face, but its formula isn't as elegant as that of All About Eyes Rich. Jar packaging brings this product's score down considerably, and to boot the overall formula has fewer antioxidants than many Clinique moisturizers.

✓ ☺ **City Block Sheer Oil-Free Daily Face Protector SPF 25** *($17.50 for 1.4 ounces)* protects skin from sun damage with its actives of titanium dioxide and zinc oxide. The lightweight but still moisturizing base is best for those with normal to dry or sensitive skin, including those dealing with rosacea. Clinique has included a very good blend of antioxidants and cell-communicating ingredients. As such, this is highly recommended for those seeking a gentle sunscreen. It is slightly tinted to offset the whitening effect from the amount of mineral sunscreens it contains.

☹ **$$$ Comfort On Call Allergy Tested Relief Cream** *($39.50 for 1.7 ounces)* is not as impressive as Clinique's Super Rescue or Repairwear moisturizers. The active ingredient is 1% dimethicone (a silicone), an amount found in hundreds of other moisturizers (particularly those at the drugstore, and for far less money) and in hundreds of other serums that don't opt to position this silicone as an active ingredient. It is classified as a skin protectant, just as are zinc oxide or petrolatum when labeled as active ingredients. This contains a smattering of anti-irritants, but because all of them are plant-based and Clinique opted for jar packaging (again), their potency and that of the few antioxidants will be quickly compromised. Sensitive skin deserves better than this, and Clinique knows it. Any Clinique moisturizer rated Paula's Pick would be preferred to Comfort On Call. Despite the marketing claims, this is not first aid for skin living "in a world of irritants."

☺ **Dramatically Different Moisturizing Gel in Tube** *($12.50 for 1.7 ounces)* is more a lotion than a gel, but does feel quite light and silky on the skin. It does not contain any oils or heavy thickening agents, and this fragrance-free moisturizer is appropriate for normal to slightly dry or slightly oily skin. The only issue I have with the product is its meager antioxidant content (though it has some great anti-irritants). Most of Clinique's moisturizers are brimming with state-of-the-art ingredients, but this one, though certainly effective for its intended skin types, is plain by comparison—yet dramatically better than their original and still incredibly popular lotion.

☺ **Dramatically Different Moisturizing Lotion** (*$22.50 for 4.2 ounces*) is the same as it always was: a basic, mundane, out-of-date, yellow-colored moisturizer built around mineral and sesame oils. It's an option for dry skin and is fragrance-free, but, other than its reasonable price tag, there is nothing else attractive or beneficial about this product.

☺ **$$$ Even Better Skin Tone Corrector** (*$39.50 for 1 ounce*) is a product many will be tempted to try, and why wouldn't they be—this product claims to erase discolorations from sun damage and acne in four to six weeks. Supposedly, Clinique's multi-level approach targets pigment problems (including redness from acne) and exfoliates those unsightly marks away. In terms of exfoliation, this contains less than 0.5% salicylic acid (confirmed by Clinique via email; that's why it's not listed as an active ingredient), which is a meager amount at best. However, no matter the amount, the pH of 4.4 prevents it from functioning as an exfoliant. The tiny amount of acetyl glucosamine doesn't exfoliate either (and there's no substantiated research proving otherwise), but it likely has merit as a water-binding agent. I don't know how Clinique can position this serum as a skin-lightening product because the only ingredients it contains that have that potential aren't present in impressive amounts, and research into these ingredients (mulberry root and ascorbyl glucoside) is not conclusive, nor have concentration protocols been established for skin-care products. What you may notice from using this silky-textured serum is an improvement in your skin's appearance because of its moisturizing benefits, and that's about it. Although the plant extracts it contains don't have a solid history of efficacy for eliminating hyperpigmentation from sun damage and acne, they do have antioxidant potential. Couple that with the soothing agents and skin-identical substances Clinique included and you have yourself a very good serum for normal to very oily skin, and the price isn't terribly high either. This isn't quite as impressive as Clinique's Repairwear serum or Lauder's Perfectionist [CP+] Wrinkle Lifting Serum, but both of those cost considerably more. As long as you don't expect this serum to banish discolorations, you likely won't be disappointed with its performance. In fact, the acne-prone may find that using a product like this to keep skin in a healthier state may result in faster fading of red marks (post-inflammatory hyperpigmentation) from blemishes. Even Better Skin Tone Corrector is fragrance-free but does contain artificial coloring agents.

☹ **$$$ Moisture On-Line** (*$38 for 1.7 ounces*) is an OK option for normal to dry skin, but some of its ingredients will degrade due to jar packaging. By the way, this product's claim to trigger skin's ability to build and hold moisture can be attributed to any well-formulated moisturizer.

☹ **$$$ Moisture Surge Extended Thirst Relief** (*$34 for 1.7 ounces*). Jar packaging will ensure that the antioxidants this contains won't remain potent after the product is opened, and the amount of peptide is rather small, which isn't what most people would consider impressive. Promising to never let skin go thirsty again (which is odd because it takes much more than water to replenish dry skin), this silicone-enhanced moisturizer ends up being an OK option for normal to slightly dry or slightly oily skin, but Clinique definitely sells better moisturizers.

☺ **Super City Block Oil-Free Daily Face Protector SPF 40** (*$17.50 for 1.4 ounces*) contains titanium dioxide and zinc oxide for UVA protection, along with a couple of synthetic sunscreen actives. The potential for angelica extract to cause a phototoxic reaction is inhibited both by the amount of it in this product and the sunscreen actives. Most of the really interesting ingredients are present in minor amounts, making this less impressive than Clinique's City Block Sheer Oil-Free Daily Face Protector SPF 25.

The Reviews C

☹ **Deep Cleansing Emergency Mask** *($19.50 for 3.4 ounces)* is a standard clay mask that also contains absorbent cornstarch and an ineffective amount of salicylic acid. The menthol doesn't help and makes this not worth considering over several other clay masks.

☺ **$$$ All About Lips** *($20 for 0.41 ounce)* theoretically smooths and fills in superficial lip lines and lines around the mouth with silicones and film-former, but I would test this out before spending the money. Even if it does have an impact, which is merely temporary and quickly undone if you follow with lipstick or gloss (the product's performance largely depends on leaving it undisturbed), it will be convincing only for the most superficial of lines. This also contains salicylic acid, but not in an amount that will exfoliate skin around the mouth—and it is too drying for use on lips, but that won't be a problem if you follow with lipstick or gloss.

☹ **Superbalm Lip Treatment** *($11.50 for 0.25 ounce)* has a lot going for it if you're looking for an emollient lip balm that provides a glossy finish with minimal stickiness. Several ingredients in this balm are aces for keeping lips smooth and soft. However, this is not recommended over similar lip balms (or even plain Vaseline, which is the main ingredient in Superbalm Lip Treatment) because Clinique added spearmint, grapefruit, and other problematic plants.

CLINIQUE SELF-TANNERS

☺ **$$$ Self Sun Body Airbrush Spray** *($20 for 4.2 ounces)* is a good aerosol, spray-on self-tanner that, true to claim, produces a fine mist from any angle. It's a convenient option for covering hard-to-reach areas, but you still need to blend it over your skin to avoid streaks and blotches. Just like almost all self-tanners, this contains the ingredient dihydroxyacetone (DHA) to turn skin tan. It also contains erythrulose, another self-tanning ingredient that works slower than DHA. The combination can be longer lasting and if you have used a self-tanner with these two ingredients it's worth a test run. The small amount of alcohol in this product is unlikely to cause irritation or dryness, though it does help this self-tanner set quickly. Self Sun Body Airbrush Spray is fragrance-free.

✓☺ **$$$ Self Sun Body Daily Moisturizer, Light-Medium** *($20 for 5 ounces)*. It's true that this self-tanning lotion for normal to dry skin contains dihydroxyacetone (DHA), the same ingredient that shows up in almost every self-tanner being sold because DHA is what turns skin a golden tan color. What propels this product to my highest rating is the fact that it has an elegant texture laced with beneficial extras that your skin needs. It's also fragrance-free, which makes it a better option for those with sensitive skin. My only issue is with Clinique's claim that this product won't cause acne. There are no standards for that claim and it can be attached to any product, so it's meaningless. (Heck, Crisco vegetable shortening could claim to be "non-acnegenic" in terms of cosmetic regulation requirements.) In theory, the triglycerides that comprise the bulk of this formula are capable of clogging pores. That doesn't mean they will, but as with all such ingredients, the potential is there for those prone to acne.

✓☺ **$$$ Self Sun Body Daily Moisturizer, Medium-Deep** *($20 for 5 ounces)*. Except for a higher amount of the self-tanning ingredient dihydroxyacetone, this product is nearly identical to Clinique's Self Sun Body Daily Moisturizer, Light-Medium above. As such, the same review applies.

☺ **$$$ Self Sun Body Tinted Lotion, Light-Medium** *($20 for 4.2 ounces)* is a very good lightweight self-tanning lotion suitable for all skin types. The Light-Medium designation means there is less of the self-tanning ingredient dihydroxyacetone (DHA) in this product, and less DHA means it will turn your skin a deep shade of tan only after a few applications. This particular product is tinted with caramel so you get instant color along with the lasting color that develops after a few hours. Although Clinique's non-acnegenic claim is meaningless (it has no legal definition or requirement), the texture of this product does make it a safer bet for those prone to blemishes. It is fragrance-free, too. The mica this contains adds a slight shimmer to skin.

☺ $$$ **Self Sun Body Tinted Lotion, Medium-Deep** *($20 for 4.2 ounces)* is a very good lightweight self-tanning lotion suitable for all skin types. The Medium-Deep designation means there is more rather than less of the dihydroxyacetone (DHA) self-tanning ingredient in this product; more DHA means your skin will turn a deeper shade of tan faster. This particular product is tinted with caramel so you get instant color along with the lasting color that develops after a few hours.

☺ $$$ **Self Sun Face Tinted Lotion** *($18.50 for 1.7 ounces)*. Although there is nothing about this formula that makes it better for the face than the body, it is still a great, silky-textured option for all skin types. You get instant sheer color from the tint this has, and your self-tan color develops within hours thanks to dihydroxyacetone, the same ingredient that shows up in most self-tanning products. This deserves consideration also because it is fragrance-free. The mica this contains adds a slight shimmer to skin.

CLINIQUE SUN PRODUCTS

All of Clinique's new sunscreens (in their sun-care line, not in their "regular" facial-care line) claim to use what the company refers to as SolarSmart technology. This technology is supposed to trigger a repair mechanism in skin to help prevent signs of aging. What they're really referring to are the antioxidants in this sunscreen; the claim is basically just a new way of stating what we've known for some time—antioxidants added to sunscreens help boost the efficacy of the active ingredients while also helping skin defend itself against sun damage (Sources: *Clinics in Dermatology*, November-December 2008, pages 614-626; and *Photochemistry and Photobiology*, July-August 2006, pages 1016-1023). That doesn't mean that Clinique's latest sun-care products are superior to others that also contain antioxidants, although that could certainly be inferred from the claims they're making.

✓☺ **Sun SPF 30 Face Cream** *($17.50 for 1.7 ounces)* is an outstanding sunscreen formula for normal to dry skin. It contains a wide range of antioxidants and cell-communicating ingredients as well as stabilized avobenzone for UVA protection. I disagree with Clinique that this sunscreen is gentle enough for sensitive skin. Without question, the active ingredients it contains can absolutely be sensitizing for all skin types, although that doesn't mean they shouldn't be considered or that they don't have value when it comes to protecting skin from sun damage. Anyone with sensitive, reactive skin should stick with sunscreens whose only active ingredients are titanium dioxide and/or zinc oxide. This sunscreen is fragrance-free and contains mica, a mineral pigment that leaves a slight shimmer on skin. Its formula is a bit tricky to use with makeup, but it works well if you prefer pressed-powder foundations over creams or liquids.

✓☺ **Sun SPF 50 Face Cream** *($17.50 for 1.7 ounces)* is similar to the Sun SPF 30 Face Cream reviewed above, and the same basic comments apply. Keep in mind that SPF 50 is probably too much (there aren't that many hours of daylight in most parts of the world) but if you tend to be someone who doesn't apply sunscreen liberally, this will help assure that you get enough sunscreen ingredients on your skin in any case to at least equal an SPF 20 or so, depending on how much you apply. This sunscreen is fragrance-free.

The Reviews C

☺ **$$$ Sun Advanced Protection SPF 45 Stick** *($17.50 for 0.21 ounce).* This emollient, nonaqueous sunscreen stick provides UVA protection with avobenzone. Although it doesn't contain oils, the wax and emollients that keep this in stick form can certainly contribute to clogged pores. Although the active ingredients in this sun stick are great, I don't advise using it in the eye area unless you know you're not sensitive to the sunscreen agents. Most people should tolerate this well using it on lips, the bridge of the nose, tops of the ears, and other vulnerable areas prone to sun damage due to neglectful application.

✓☺ **Sun SPF 30 Body Cream** *($20 for 5 ounces)* is identical to Clinique's Sun SPF 30 Face Cream, only you get more for your money with the body version. You can use either one on facial skin, too, and the same comments made for the Face version also apply here.

✓☺ **Sun SPF 50 Body Cream** *($20 for 5 ounces)* is identical to Clinique's Sun SPF 50 Face Cream, only you get more for your money with the body version. You can use either one on facial skin, too, and the same comments made for the Face version also apply here.

✓☺ **Sun SPF 15 Face/Body Cream** *($20 for 5 ounces)* is an outstanding sunscreen formula for normal to oily skin. It contains a wide range of antioxidants and cell-communicating ingredients as well as stabilized avobenzone for UVA protection. I disagree with Clinique that this sunscreen is gentle enough for sensitive skin. Without question, the active ingredients it contains can absolutely be sensitizing for all skin types, although that doesn't mean they shouldn't be considered or that they don't have value when it comes to protecting skin from sun damage. Anyone with sensitive, reactive skin should stick with sunscreens whose only active ingredients are titanium dioxide and/or zinc oxide. This sunscreen is fragrance-free and contains mica, a mineral pigment that leaves a slight shimmer on skin.

☹ **Sun SPF 25 Body Spray** *($20 for 5 ounces).* Although this spray-on sunscreen contains avobenzone for sufficient UVA protection, its base formula is mostly alcohol, which makes it too drying and irritating for skin. Alcohol also causes free-radical damage, and for some reason this Clinique sunscreen is woefully short on antioxidants to help offset that damage. This product is not recommended. Those looking for spray-on sunscreens should consider the better options from Coppertone and Paula's Choice.

CLINIQUE MAKEUP

FOUNDATION: ✓☺ **Superbalanced Compact Makeup SPF 20** *($28)* is a beautiful cream-to-powder foundation with a brilliant in-part zinc oxide sunscreen. As with all cream-to-powders, this is best for someone with normal to slightly oily skin. The matte, slightly powdery finish of Superbalanced Compact Makeup SPF 20 will magnify any dry areas, so if that's an issue be sure to moisturize before application. This foundation blends easily and builds from sheer to medium coverage that does not appear heavy. Its soft, creamy texture sets quickly and feels very light on skin. There are 11 mostly stellar shades, including options for fair and dark (but not very dark) skin. The only shades to use caution with are Warm Buff (slightly peach) and Cream Chamois (slightly peach). Although it cannot make good on its claim to control oil and hydrate dry areas, this is still an exceptional choice if you prefer cream-to-powder makeup with sunscreen.

✓☺ **$$$ Dewy Smooth Anti-Aging Makeup SPF 15** *($22.50)* is definitely smooth, with a silky, silicone-based texture that feels amazing and blends without a hitch. Titanium dioxide is not only the sunscreen agent, but also lends an opacity that allows this makeup to provide medium to almost full coverage with a satin matte finish that feels slightly moist. This does not make skin look dewy or drenched in moisture, but it is still a great option for normal to dry skin. Beyond the sunscreen, there is nothing antiaging about the formula. Ignore the marketing hype and you'll be left with a superior foundation that comes in mostly gorgeous colors for very light to dark skin. Use caution with Beige Petal, which is slightly peach. By the way, although Repairwear Anti-Aging Makeup SPF 15 has more bells and whistles, Dewy Smooth is much easier to blend and doesn't look as heavy, which makes it a better option.

✓☺ **Perfectly Real Makeup** *($22.50)* is a near-perfect choice for those who want a smooth, lightweight foundation that fulfills its promise of looking as natural as possible. This foundation has a slightly creamy texture that quickly morphs into a soft matte finish once it's blended. Clinique states that Perfectly Real Makeup "feels like nothing at all." It isn't quite that light—you will notice it's there—but your skin will look improved without appearing made-up. It provides sheer to light coverage, so you still need a concealer for red spots or dark circles. The matte finish makes this product preferable for normal to oily skin. It can definitely exaggerate any dry spots, so it's important for your skin to be completely smooth before application. Almost all of the shades are gorgeous, neutral options with no strong overtones of peach, pink, ash, or rose. The only shades to consider avoiding are 28, 34, and 36, each of which can be too peach for its intended skin tones. There are options for very light skin, as well as some beautiful darker shades, but watch out for shade 46, which has a slight tendency to turn ashy on the skin.

✓☺ **$$$ Perfectly Real Compact Makeup** *($22.50)* is a talc-based pressed-powder foundation with wow-factor silkiness. It glides over skin and doesn't look the least bit heavy, even when applied with the included sponge. Those with normal to slightly dry or oily skin will enjoy the smooth matte finish and light, buildable coverage. Much like the Perfectly Real Makeup, the range of 20 shades is brilliant. Those with fair to medium skin will find neutral option after neutral option. The only potential problem shades are 116 (too yellow), 120 (slightly peach), and the darkest shade, 148, which looks slightly ash for the depth of its intended skin tone. Your skin won't look "believably perfect," but will look even and polished. A caveat: those with melasma or rosacea will likely want more coverage than this foundation provides, but its texture is so light that it could be brushed over a medium- to full-coverage liquid foundation without detriment.

✓☺ **Repairwear Anti-Aging Makeup SPF 15** *($28.50)* continues Clinique's Repairwear lineup as the company's first makeup to feature their so-called line-blocking, line-mending technology. Lines (wrinkles) will indeed be forestalled thanks to this foundation's titanium dioxide sunscreen, but the "mending" part is open to interpretation. This makeup does contain many of the same antioxidants and skin-beneficial ingredients as Clinique's Repairwear skin-care products, but just how much such ingredients will improve wrinkles is not established. As for the makeup itself, it is incorrectly described as "luxuriously moisturizing." It has an initially creamy texture that smooths over skin, blending to a satin matte finish, but it won't thrill those with extremely dry skin, and ends up being far better for normal to moderately dry skin. Coverage is substantial, but with this level of camouflage the trade-off is a makeup that looks (but doesn't feel) heavier on skin. It would be an excellent choice for those battling redness from rosacea. Not only are such mineral-based sunscreens extra gentle, but also the amount of coverage they offer (when combined with pigments) will tone down excess redness—assuming you choose your shades carefully.

Clinique hit a stumbling block in regard to shades, however. Although there are some great choices among the 11 options, Porcelain Beige, Sand, and Nutty are too pink, rose, peach, or yellow to recommend, so choose carefully. This foundation does not include shades for dark skin, although Alabaster is an option for fair skin.

✓ ☺ $$$ **Superfit Makeup Oil-Free Long Wear** *($20.50)* has long been a favorite of mine to recommend for those with oily skin. It's been in Clinique's foundation lineup for several years and was re-launched in 2008 after some minor formulary tweaks. The ingredient list changed very little from that of the original formula; mostly they added a polymer complex and removed parabens, which is something the Lauder companies are doing across the board. Although minimal, the changes are good news because they mean this is still a formidable foundation for normal to very oily skin. It does an impressive job of keeping excess shine in check without breaking down and making skin look spotty. Superfit has a beautifully fluid, silky texture that blends easily and sets to a soft matte finish. It's a great medium-coverage foundation for those who don't want to "feel" their makeup, which is basically everyone, but especially those with oily skin! There are 15 shades available, and in some respects the shade selection has improved a bit from the original lineup. Champagne is too pink, Shell is slightly peach, and Toffee Bronze is a tricky color for dark skin tones with oily skin due to its tendency to turn slightly orange. Spicy will be too copper for some, but is still worth considering, and Petal leaves a slight peach cast that limits its versatility for light skin tones.

✓ ☺ **City Stick SPF 15** *($22)* is a very good stick foundation to consider and the SPF is excellent, with pure titanium dioxide as the only active ingredient. The coverage is sheer to medium, with a definite silky powder finish. As is true for any cream-to-powder foundation, the powder element can be drying for someone with dry skin, and the cream part can be greasy for someone with combination to oily skin, so that makes this one best for those with normal to slightly dry or slightly oily skin. Of the five shades, the only one to watch out for is Beige Twist, which can be too peach for most skin tones.

✓ ☺ **Almost Powder Makeup SPF 15** *($22.50)* has a buttery smooth texture that slips on like a second skin and blends to a seamless satin-matte finish with a hint of sparkling shine. This feels incredibly light for a pressed-powder foundation capable of sheer to medium coverage, and you get brilliant sun protection from 13% titanium dioxide (in addition, there's a synthetic sunscreen active, something you don't typically see in a product being sold as mineral makeup). Almost all eight shades are soft and neutral; Deep Honey may be too orange for some skin tones, while Deep is slightly ash, probably due to the amount of titanium dioxide. Deep Golden is best for tan skin tones, which is about as dark as the shade range goes. Whether applied with a sponge for medium coverage or a brush for a sheer look, this is an outstanding powder foundation with sunscreen.

✓ ☺ **Almost Makeup SPF 15** *($20.50)* is a very sheer foundation with a broad-spectrum titanium dioxide sunscreen, making it ideal for sensitive skin. It is definitely not akin to traditional foundation, and is available in several great shades, although it lacks a color for dark skin. The product's moist finish is best for normal to dry skin.

☺ $$$ **City Base Compact Foundation SPF 15** *($22.50)* isn't as elegant as Clinique's Superbalanced Compact Makeup SPF 20 reviewed above, but is a consideration for those with normal to slightly dry skin. It's a classic cream-to-powder makeup with an initially creamy application and soft powder finish that doesn't hold up well over oily areas. Except for Porcelain Beige and Almond Beige, the shades are excellent and would work for a wide range of skin tones, from light to dark, but not for someone with very light or very dark skin. The SPF 15 sunscreen contains titanium dioxide as the only active ingredient.

☺ **Moisture Sheer Tint SPF 15** *($27)* has a satin-smooth texture and slightly creamy application that sets to a minimally moist finish. This product is aptly named, as it provides sheer, almost nonexistent coverage. Its sunscreen is in-part titanium dioxide, but it's at a level of only 1%, which may be too low to provide sufficient UVA protection for long days outdoors. Three shades are available, and the best among them are Fair and Neutral. Beige is good but may be too yellow for medium skin tones. All told, Moisture Sheer Tint is a good option for someone with normal to slightly dry skin seeking sheer coverage.

☺ **$$$ Superbalanced Powder Makeup SPF 15** *($34.50)*. Surprise, Clinique is in the mineral makeup game too. Given that other Lauder-owned brands also offer various forms of mineral makeup, it was a foregone conclusion that Clinique would join the fray. So how does their contribution stack up? Overall, reasonably well. It's great that the sunscreen is pure titanium dioxide, and the base formula does indeed contain minerals (including talc, which many mineral makeup brands routinely yet unjustly eschew and berate). Clinique opted to package this mineral makeup in a jar that includes a sifter which shaves off powder as you rotate the sifter. The powder is actually in solid form but dispenses loose as you turn the sifter. Although this seems clever and allows the user to control how much powder is dispensed, it does little to minimize the mess inherent to loose powders. Application-wise, this powder's slightly creamy texture goes on smoothly and provides sheer to medium coverage with a soft matte finish. It is best for normal to slightly dry or slightly oily skin; those with pronounced oily areas will find this isn't absorbent enough, while noticeably dry areas will be magnified. You may be tempted to try this foundation because it claims to help absorb oil while maintaining skin's moisture balance, but it absolutely cannot do that. The main ingredients are absorbent by nature and even though Clinique includes some emollient ingredients, they cannot overcome the absorbency of the titanium dioxide, talc, and mica—though they do keep this powder from being as absorbent as it could be, which is why those with oily skin won't be pleased. As for the shades, almost all of them are excellent but the medium to dark shades (there are no options for very dark skin tones) tend to look slightly chalky unless applied sheer. Natural 6 and Natural 7 suffer a bit from being slightly peach, but are still worth considering.

☺ **Supermoisture Makeup** *($22.50)*. The claims for this foundation are truly clever—extolling that it's a makeup that thinks it's a moisturizer. It supposedly contains a special time-release technology that places powerful moisturizing agents where and when skin needs them most. I wouldn't count on that, since a makeup doesn't have a radar-like ability to detect dry spots and respond accordingly, while holding back over the oily areas. Still, this creamy liquid foundation is definitely worth considering by those with dry to very dry skin. It has a soft, slightly whipped texture that glides over skin, provides light to medium coverage, and leaves skin visibly hydrated with a soft shimmer glow (the Clinique consultant insisted there wasn't any shimmer, but it's there). Those with very dry skin who want to apply more than the standard amount of foundation will notice increased coverage. The collection of 17 shades is mostly impressive, offering good colors for fair to dark skin tones. Bisque, Warm Caramel, and Golden suffer from being slightly peach; Honeycomb is too orange; and Amber veers a bit too copper, but may be workable for some darker skin tones.

☺ **Clarifying Powder Makeup** *($22.50)* is a wonderfully smooth-textured, talc-based powder foundation, especially if you have normal to oily skin. This applies impeccably and leaves a natural matte finish that looks smooth and even, rather than dry or powdery. The four shades are soft and neutral, but best for fair to medium skin only.

☺ **Soft Finish Makeup** *($20.50)*. Soft Finish Makeup is quite similar to Clinique's Balanced Makeup Base (reviewed below) in terms of consistency and coverage, but this one has a silicone-enhanced slip and is slightly sheerer than the Balanced. It's a good foundation for normal to very dry skin but does not have a special ability to make lines and wrinkles less obvious. Of the seven shades, most are beautifully neutral. Soft Bisque is slightly peach, while Soft Porcelain is too pink, and Soft Honey should be considered with care.

☺ **Stay-True Makeup Oil-Free Formula** *($20.50)*. Stay-True Makeup Oil-Free Formula now ranks as one of Clinique's oldest foundations, and remains a satisfactory option for those with normal to very oily skin who want an oil-absorbing matte finish. It has a slightly thick texture that blends well despite its lack of slip and it provides medium coverage. Definitely a traditional but worthwhile matte makeup. Among the available shades, avoid Stay Neutral, Stay Porcelain, and Stay Golden due to their overtones of pink or peach.

☹ **$$$ Superbalanced Makeup** *($20.50)*. Superbalanced Makeup is Clinique's top-selling foundation worldwide (Source: www.elcompanies.com), in no small part because it claims to provide moisture and absorb oil when and where needed—a skin-care dream many women share. However, this ends up doing neither job very well. There is no way a product can differentiate between the oily parts of your face and the dry parts. The absorbent ingredients in it will soak up any oil they come in contact with (including the moisturizing ingredients in this product or in the one you applied to your skin) and the moisturizing ingredients will get deposited over areas you don't want to be moisturized. With Superbalanced Makeup, you get a silicone-in-water liquid that provides light to medium coverage with a smooth, matte-finish foundation that is best for someone with normal to slightly dry or slightly oily skin. Someone with any amount of excess oil would not be happy with the finish or with how it wears during the day. The shades have been refined a bit since this foundation was last reviewed, and a few of the poor colors are gone. Still, compared to several other Clinique foundations, the palette isn't as neutral. The following colors are best avoided by most skin tones: Light, Cream Chamois, Ivory, Linen, Neutral, Vanilla, Porcelain Beige, Sunny, and Honeyed Beige. Alabaster and Breeze are the best neutral shades if you have fair skin, while Amber and Clove are attractive dark shades.

☺ **Balanced Makeup Base** *($20.50)* is Clinique's oldest foundation, and the three shades that remain are likely there to placate the consumers who just aren't ready to give this up. It is best for those with dry to very dry skin. The mineral oil-based consistency is emollient and creamy, and it applies well, leaving a natural finish. The coverage is light to medium, but I encourage you to explore Clinique's other liquid foundation options before this.

☺ **Work-Out Makeup All Day Wear** *($20.50)* is a creamy, water-resistant foundation that provides medium coverage and a rather heavy application, though it does hold up well. The problem is that three of the four shades are too pink or rose to look natural. Cloud is the sole recommended shade, but this is not one of Clinique's better foundations.

☹ **Clarifying Makeup Clear Skin Formula** *($20.50)* has too many drawbacks to make it a workable foundation for those with blemished, oily skin. Alcohol is the third ingredient, followed closely by witch hazel and, further down the list, clove extract. None of these ingredients is helpful for skin, and when you consider that the formula tends to separate as well as ball up on skin that has any sort of lightweight moisturizer or serum applied, it's a no-brainer to avoid.

CONCEALER: ✓ ☺ **$$$ All About Eyes Concealer** *($15.50)* is a state-of-the-art concealer formula thanks to the inclusion of pentapeptides, antioxidants, and elegant skin-identical ingredients. It has a smooth, creamy texture and concentrated pigmentation. A little goes a long way and provides good coverage with minimal slip. The seven shades present mostly true skin-color options, though Light Neutral (the palest shade) is too yellow for most fair skin and Medium Beige is too bright yellow. The others are superb and include options for darker skin. Clinique claims this is recommended for disguising dark circles, and it does indeed work very well for that purpose, without looking thick or cakey.

☺ **$$$ Instant Light Eye Perfecting Base** *($24.50)* comes packaged in a click-pen applicator with a built-in synthetic brush tip. Housed inside is a smooth liquid concealer that blends well, evening out the appearance of skin on the eyelid or under-eye area. This has a crease-free matte finish that adds a touch of shine to skin, though not distractingly so. Both shades are good, but they are best for fair to light skin tones. Although this is an impressive product, it is superfluous if you're already using an excellent concealer in the eye area.

☺ **Advanced Concealer** *($14)* comes in a squeeze tube and goes on like a thick cream, but quickly dries to a powder. Coverage is very good without looking heavy. This comes in two excellent shades, Matte Light and Matte Medium. The fine print: This concealer works only if the skin under your eyes is smooth; any dry or rough skin will look worse because of this product's powdery finish.

☺ **Line Smoothing Concealer** *($14)* promises an instantly firmer look and is said to contain ingredients to "bridge" wrinkles, making them less apparent. Neither claim becomes reality, but this is still a very good liquid concealer with a smooth, even application, the right amount of coverage for most flaws, and a semi-matte finish that leaves a bit of a glow. I suppose it's that glow that helps reflect light away from wrinkles, but the visual trickery is minor, at least if you have the kind of lines that don't disappear when your face is motionless. Of the mostly neutral shades, only Medium Honey (which is bright peach) and Deep Honey (an unattractive ochre hue) should be avoided.

☺ **$$$ Airbrush Concealer** *($19.50)* is housed in a pen-style applicator; you rotate the base to feed concealer onto the built-in brush tip. It offers a smooth (though too sheer to provide any amount of concealing) application that has an airy, silky texture and sets to a natural matte finish. Two of the three shades are the main issue here, because Fair is too pink and Medium is undeniably peach. Neutral Fair is great. Despite the shade issues, this concealer is so sheer that the misguided colors get toned down. By the way, the finished effect on the skin is not akin to airbrushing a photo, where flaws are eliminated. If anything, even minor flaws will still be visible with this concealer, but, to Clinique's credit, they do describe this as being sheer, so it still deserves a happy face rating for those looking more for a highlighter/enhancer than for significant coverage.

☹ **Quick Corrector** *($14)* comes in a tube with a wand applicator and has a fluid, slightly moist application. It smooths on easily and covers well, though the unstable, minimally matte finish can translate into creasing around the eyes. Avoid Medium, which is too pink.

☹ **City Cover Compact Concealer SPF 15** *($14)* is one of the few concealers that have a reliable SPF 15 with UVA protection. The two colors are quite workable for fair to light skin and capable of almost full coverage. The problem is that this has a creamy consistency that will crease before you're out the door. If the sun protection appeals to you, make sure you try this at the counter first and see how it wears over time.

POWDER: ✓ ☺ **$$$ Blended Face Powder & Brush** *($19)* is one of the best talc-based loose powders available, and is available in an attractive array of colors. This has a light, supple finish that clings well without caking and doesn't look dry or dull skin's natural glow. Of the eight shades, use caution with Transparency 2 (pale pink but goes on sheer) and Transparency Bronze (nice color, but too shiny, though it's an option for evening sparkle). The finish this powder leaves is best for normal to dry skin. The Invisible Blend shade goes on translucent but not too white, so it is indeed suitable for most skin tones looking for a powder that tempers shine without adding color. One more point: toss the brush; it doesn't apply powder well, feels scratchy, and sheds too much.

☺ **$$$ Soft Finish Pressed Powder** *($19)* is intended by Clinique to be used for drier skin, and that makes sense, as this talc-based formula has a creamier, silky feel and smooth, even coverage. The light-diffusing claims are bogus, and this is down to two shades, so your choices are limited.

☺ **$$$ Stay Matte Sheer Pressed Powder Oil-Free** *($19)* ranks as Clinique's top-selling powder. It's a good, talc-based powder with a slightly dry, powdery, sheer finish. The absorbency of this powder is ideal for oilier skin types, but it isn't as refined as the pressed powders from Bobbi Brown, M.A.C., Stila, or even Clinique's own Clarifying Powder Makeup. The shades are beautiful and there are some good options for light and dark skin tones.

☺ **$$$ Superpowder Double Face Powder** *($19)* is a standard, talc-based pressed powder with a smooth, soft texture. It can be used alone or as a regular finishing powder. There are eight very sheer shades, all terrific. Interestingly, Clinique is now advising against using this product wet—a wise direction!

☹ **$$$ Gentle Light Powder and Brush** *($22.50)* is a talc-based loose powder that is exceptionally light and soft, yet infused with enough shine to make a chorus of Las Vegas showgirls sparkle with envy. The four shades are beautiful, but this shiny powder clings poorly to skin.

☹ **$$$ Redness Solutions Instant Relief Mineral Powder** *($32.50)* purports to "measurably reduce redness on contact," and this claim is somewhat true. The minerals present in this loose powder (mica, bismuth oxychloride) don't make it anything special (nor do they have redness-reducing properties), but this powder's soft yellow color does help reduce the appearance or redness on the face. Nothing in this formulation will actually reduce the redness caused by rosacea; it will simply help to conceal the appearance of redness. If anything, I am concerned that the amount of potentially irritating grapefruit peel extract may make redness worse. Despite that ingredient misstep, this is a good loose powder for use to help even out skin tone and set makeup. Clinique is dancing on a fine line with its claims for this product, but as long as you have reasonable expectations, you'll find this a fine option for a loose powder. Toss the small antibacterial brush that's included with this powder. It's too rough to be used on anyone's skin, much less those who are already suffering from sensitivity issues.

BLUSH AND BRONZER: ✓ ☺ **$$$ Blushwear Cream Stick** *($18.50)* is a twist-up, sleekly packaged blush. Basically a cream-to-powder blush in stick form, it is easy to blend over moist skin and provides a soft wash of color that looks quite natural. Each of the pastel shades has a touch of shine, but the effect is a subtle glow rather than obvious sparkles. Blushwear Cream Stick is an excellent option for those with normal to dry skin who don't wish to use powder blush.

☺ **$$$ Blushing Blush Powder Blusher** *($18.50)* has the smoothest texture and best color deposit of all of Clinique's powder blushes, but each shade is laden with shine (on most shades, the shine is metallic-looking rather than a soft shimmer). This powder blush is otherwise very workable and easy to blend, but this much shine is best reserved for nighttime glamour.

☺ **$$$ Almost Bronzer SPF 15** *($28.50)*. This pressed bronzing powder contains titanium dioxide as the active ingredient, so it is capable of providing sufficient broad-spectrum protection. The talc-based formula has a smooth, dry texture that applies sheer and leaves a soft shine finish. I wish the colors were better; they appear tan, but they apply peachy, which almost makes this better as blush. The sunscreen element serves as a helpful adjunct to your foundation or moisturizer with sunscreen, but if you use it alone you'll have to apply way too much over your entire face to get the SPF protection of 15. A brush is included, and although it's not preferred to a full-size powder or blush brush, it's usable.

☺ **$$$ Quick Blush** *($21.50)* is sold as a powder blush and brush in one, and it is. A tiny disc of pressed-powder blush is housed in the base of the product's cap. You twist the opposite end before opening, which deposits a small amount of color onto the built-in (and surprisingly good) blush brush. The concept is practical and great for on-the-go use, but all of the shades go on so sheer you need several applications to get noticeable color. This ends up being an OK option for a very subtle blush effect, but only if you have fair to light skin.

☺ **$$$ Soft Pressed Powder Blusher** *($18.50)* is decently silky but almost too sheer. Color deposit is minimal and requires successive layers to register on most skin tones (and forget about it showing up at all on dark skin). All of the shades are shiny and the shine tends to flake, making this less enticing than the powder blushes from M.A.C., Stila, or Clarins.

☹ **True Bronze Pressed Powder Bronzer** *($23.50)* has a dry, grainy texture and somewhat spotty, sheer application with shine. It isn't nearly as impressive as it should be, and is not worth considering even though the tan shades are a balanced mix without too much red or copper.

EYESHADOW: ✓☺ **Colour Surge Eye Shadow Duo** *($17.50)* has an ultra-smooth texture and application that is Clinique's best ever. Several sets contain two shiny colors, albeit in mostly workable combinations. The deeper shades apply smoothly and are an option for creating a shiny, smoky, evening eye makeup. There are some blue-toned duos to watch out for, but the odd pairing of purple with pale gold (in the Beach Plum duo) is actually quite attractive. Matte duos were launched for spring 2008, and all of them are worthwhile with an enviably silky texture and matte finish.

✓☺ **$$$ Colour Surge Eye Shadow Quad** *($25)* has the same velvety texture and swift-blending application as Clinique's single and duo Colour Surge Eye Shadows, which is good news! Quads make sense if the shades are well-coordinated, and that is indeed the case with three of the six sets available. Teddy Bear is a beautiful group of nude and earth tones, Spicy combines bronzes, gold, and taupe-rose shimmer for those who can pull off shiny eyeshadow (though the effect is more shimmery than glittery), and Choco-Latte is beautiful. The other quads are more difficult to work with because they're slightly mismatched, not to mention that the blue tones won't serve to shape and shade the eye, which is the purpose of eyeshadow. Ignore the applicators that come with this set and stick with full-sized professional eyeshadow brushes for best results.

✓☺ **Colour Surge Eye Shadow Stay Matte** *($14)*. Despite the "matte" in the name of this powder eyeshadow, each shade leaves a hint of shine. The shine is little enough to almost be a non-issue, but those shopping for a completely matte option should know that this isn't it. The smooth texture and strong pigmentation (strong for Clinique, as many of their eyeshadows are quite sheer) make for lasting impact. Application is smooth with no flaking, and several of the shades work well for creating the classic smoky eye. Martini is a medium olive-green tone that's muted enough to not be distracting and that works quite well with warm brown or caramel tones.

✓ ☺ **Colour Surge Eye Shadow Soft Shimmer** *($14)* offers a splendid texture and sublimely silky colors that blend beautifully, and although the shine (shimmer) isn't what I consider "soft," the finish is appropriate for daytime makeup if you have unwrinkled eyelids and a smooth under-brow area. The small shade selection is impressive, with only a few pastel tones that you should consider carefully.

☺ **Colour Surge Eye Shadow Super Shimmer** *($14)* is nearly identical to the Colour Surge Eye Shadow Soft Shimmer, except this version has more shine. As such, it's best reserved for evening or special occasion makeup. The shine in these shadows has a greater tendency to flake, which is why this is not rated as a Paula's Pick. However, the flakiness is minimal compared to that of most other eyeshadows with this much shine.

☺ **$$$ Colour Surge Eye Shadow Trio** *($21.50)* has a very soft, silky texture and an even, although sheer, application that builds well for a greater "surge" of color. Depending on the trio, the finishes vary from satin matte to soft shine. Totally Neutral and Come Heather are great sets; Ebb and Flow has a greenish shade that's tricky to use, although the color isn't unattractive. The color payoff isn't as noticeable as Clinique's other Colour Surge eyeshadows; perhaps they scaled back for the trios.

☺ **Quick Eyes Cream Shadow** *($15)* is sold for women in a hurry, but the reality is that a liquid eyeshadow simply takes longer to apply than a powder shadow. So, you'll need more time, but if you're looking for an alternative to powder eyeshadow, this semi-liquid cream shadow is a very good option. It offers enough initial slip to make precise blending easy, and sets to a budge-proof and crease-proof finish replete with lots of shine. The shade selection favors light to medium brown and bronze tones, which is ideal for most women. It is best to dab this on with the sponge-tip applicator, then use a brush to blend.

☺ **Touch Base for Eyes** *($14)* is one of the better cream-to-powder eyeshadows. This comes in a compact that must be kept closed tightly or the product will dry out and be useless. However, it might dry out even if you follow that guideline, so recommending this is risky. Test this at the counter, but be forewarned that every shade (even the flesh-toned Canvas and Canvas Light) is shiny. This no longer fills the bill for a truly matte eyeshadow base.

☹ **$$$ Pair of Shades Eyeshadow Duo** *($17.50)* represents Clinique's older eyeshadow formula, with a slightly powdery application and sheer colors that aren't for anyone who wants to use eyeshadow to shape and shade the eye. Of the duos that remain, all but one (No-Show Taupes) have glaring shine. They remain an OK option for sheer eyeshadow if you have fair to light skin.

EYE AND BROW SHAPER: ✓ ☺ **Brush-On Cream Liner** *($14.50)* is a densely pigmented cream-gel eyeliner packaged in a glass jar. The formula applies easily (similar to liquid eyeliner) and sets to a long-wearing finish that won't smear, smudge, or flake even if oily eyelids are a problem. It may seem like a bonus that Clinique included a brush, but unless you want a thick line, you'll want to experiment with fine-tipped options. Among the four shades, Black Honey is shiny and the remainders are classic black, brown, and gray. As with all products of this nature, it must be recapped tightly after each use to prevent the product from drying out.

☺ **Superfine Liner for Brows** *($13)* is an automatic, nonretractable, very thin brow pencil that works well to softly accent and fill in brows for those who prefer pencils to powder. It applies without dragging or feeling thick, and has a slightly tacky powder finish that lasts with minimal fading and no smearing. The five shades are excellent, and include options for blondes and redheads.

☺ **Brow Shaper** *($15)* is a powder brow color that comes in four excellent shades, though now each of them has shine, which is a bit over the top. The texture is slightly heavy, but these blend onto the brow quite well, even though the brush that comes packaged with them is too stiff and scratchy. For the money, a matte, brow-toned eyeshadow would work just as well and could also double as an eyeshadow; Brow Shaper is too heavy for eyeshadow.

☺ **$$$ Cream Shaper for Eyes** *($14.50)* is a very soft-textured eye pencil. The saleswomen who demonstrated this for me commented that caution is warranted because the tip breaks so easily. The good news is that you need only minimal pressure to get a smooth line of color, though it may take some practice before you get the hang of it. This needs-sharpening pencil goes on creamy and stays creamy, yet (this is the best part) barely smudges. Each shade is infused with shimmer, which should raise a red flag if your eyelids are wrinkled. Otherwise, the glow these pencils provide can be subtly effective. It is best for defining eyes and then smudging the effect for a smoky look, and is not recommended as a lower-lid liner if you have allergies or watery eyes, both of which promote smearing with a creamy pencil like this.

☺ **$$$ Kohl Shaper for Eyes** *($15.50)* is a standard pencil that needs sharpening (though a cleverly concealed built-in sharpener is included), but has a great smooth application that doesn't skip, so drawing one continuous line is a breeze. Once it sets, the creaminess is gone, and it barely moves or smudges. As usual, a classic black shade is available, but all of the other shades have a black base, which makes the blue-toned options acceptable because they come across as deep navy, appearing almost black.

☺ **Quickliner for Eyes** *($14.50)* is a standard automatic pencil that provides a smooth, no-tugging application and is very easy to smudge before it sets. Because this stays creamy, its wear time is compromised and every shade goes on too soft for quick definition.

☹ **Brow Keeper** *($15)* is a substandard brow pencil that comes in only two colors. It has a slick texture and slightly creamy, sticky finish that prompts smudging and fading.

☹ **Eye Defining Liquid Liner** *($14.50)* has an uneven application, takes too long to dry (which encourages smearing), and its brush isn't the best for precise application.

LIPSTICK, LIP GLOSS, AND LIPLINER: ✓☺ **High Impact Lipstick SPF 15** *($14)*. This cream lipstick comes with the selling point of having it all, and Clinique is almost right. I am thrilled that the sunscreen is in-part zinc oxide, so broad-spectrum protection is assured (If only Clinique would follow suit with their other lipsticks and glosses with sunscreen!). This also has a beautifully creamy texture that feels neither greasy nor thick. It sets to a soft cream finish and provides medium coverage. Where they went slightly astray, at least in terms of the "have it all" claim, is that the colors aren't full coverage, which compromises their longevity. Most of them have a good stain, but this will wear off the same as most cream lipsticks—it won't maintain a just-applied look for eight hours, even if you avoid lipstick-wrecking activities such as eating and drinking. However, taken as a creamy lipstick with effective sunscreen, there is no question this wins high marks, and the shade range is wonderful. Those who love cool-toned red shades should check out Red-y to Wear!

✓☺ **Long Last Soft Shine Lipstick** *($14)* has a luscious feel and smooth, even application with opaque coverage. It is nicely creamy without being greasy or too glossy. The color selection is extensive, with equally impressive pale and deep shades.

✓ ☺ **Long Last Soft Matte Lipstick** *($14)* has a very small shade selection but all are beautiful. This smooth-textured lipstick feels great, provides opaque coverage, and has a satin matte finish that holds true to the "long last" part of this lipstick's name.

✓ ☺ **Superbalm Moisturizing Gloss** *($13.50)* comes in a squeeze tube and is an emollient, balm-like lip gloss that moisturizes while imparting sheer, juicy color and a minimally sticky feel. It's a good way to condition lips while adding a hint of color, and some of the shades have a slight shimmer for a glistening effect.

✓ ☺ **Quickliner for Lips** *($14)* is an automatic, nonretractable pencil that must have been improved (the Clinique salespeople weren't sure) because it now has a super-smooth, just-right creamy application that doesn't feel thick or waxy but does a great job of keeping lipstick from feathering into lines around the mouth. The shade range is gorgeous and easy to coordinate with just about any Clinique lipstick. Just keep in mind that their greasier and glossy formulas aren't for those prone to lipstick feathering.

✓ ☺ **$$$ Vitamin C Smoothie Antioxidant Lip Colour** *($17.50)* is an antioxidant-rich lip color that comes housed in a click-style pen with a splay-proof brush applicator. That's great news not only because it produces superior results, but because it also keeps the antioxidants stable. At the counter this was described to me as a lipstick-lipgloss hybrid, and I'd tend to agree with that description because the product imparts creamy, sheer-to-medium color that doesn't feel heavy or sticky in the least, but does leave a healthy shine with the kind of staying power you may not expect from something with a glossy finish. The eight versatile colors are lovely, and the formula impressive. All told, it's another winner from Clinique!

☺ **Colour Surge Butter Shine Lipstick** *($14)* goes on quite thick and feels considerably more greasy than creamy. It has a glossy finish and comes in an attractive selection of shades seemingly based on best-sellers from Clinique's vast lipstick library—but this will bleed into lines around the mouth almost as soon as you apply it, and its longevity is cut short by the extra-emollient formula. It isn't a bad lipstick by any means, just one to approach with caution if you're prone to lipstick feathering and/or want long-lasting color. Those without this problem but with chapped lips should stop by the Clinique counter to explore this lipstick!

☺ **Different Lipstick** *($14)* is one of Clinique's older lipstick formulas and has long since stopped being "different." It comes in a classic range of colors with some pretty neutrals and pastel brights. This is not as long-lasting as any of Clinique's lipsticks rated as Paula's Picks.

☺ **Almost Lipstick** *($14)*. This Clinique classic has been whittled down to one shade, the company's best-selling Black Honey. True to claim, it is a flattering color for most skin tones (although it looks imposingly dark in the tube). This remains a smooth, sheer lipstick that provides a soft gloss finish.

☹ **Long Last Glosswear SPF 15** *($14)*. It's hard to make an unappealing lip gloss, but Clinique has managed to create one of the most undesirable glosses in recent memory. Not only does the sunscreen leave lips vulnerable to UVA damage, but the texture is inordinately thick and uncomfortably sticky. This comes close to feeling like you've painted a mix of maple syrup and glue on your lips, and then allowed it to dry. Each sparkle-infused shade (all go on much softer than they look in the tube) provides a vinyl-like shine, but other glosses do that also, and without the unpleasant aesthetics of this. For better results, check out glosses from Dior, M.A.C., or others from Clinique.

☹ **Full Potential Lips Plump and Shine** *($17.50)* is said to have a triple-plumping action and promises to keep the plumpness going for hours. The trio of plumping agents are all of the irritating kind, and include peppermint, capsicum (pepper), and ginger root oils. None of them are good news for lips, especially if this is a product you intend to use routinely. It's otherwise a standard, slightly thick lip gloss with a sticky finish and an attractive selection of sparkle-infused colors. This lip-plumping product ends up being more irritating than similar options.

MASCARA: ✓☺ **High Impact Mascara** *($14)* is simply fantastic and is on my short list of favorite mascaras. If you're looking for mascara that quickly builds substantial length and substantial thickness while defining lashes without clumping, this is a must-try. It wears well throughout the day and is easily removed with a water-soluble cleanser, qualities that make it even more ideal.

✓☺ **Lash Doubling Mascara** *($14)* does a very good job of living up to its name, as this quickly builds lots of length and a fair amount of thickness with ease. The formula sweeps on with no clumps or smearing—each lash is well defined—so unless you're looking for all-out drama, this is an outstanding choice.

☺ **Lash Power Mascara Long Wearing Formula** *($14)* is a great waterproof mascara that stays on through any precipitation or amount of eye tearing, and is surprisingly easy to remove (it comes off with very warm water, followed by your regular cleanser). Application-wise, the small, pointed brush allows you to reach and elongate every lash, providing clean definition. Thickness and volume are harder to come by because it's a gel-based formula. Those looking for lash separation with length and worry-free long wear are this mascara's target audience.

☺ **Long Pretty Lashes Mascara** *($14)* has an accurate name, as this mascara produces lots of length and does so without clumping, smearing, or flaking. The clean, quick application does not produce any thickness, so it's not as all-out impressive as High Impact Mascara. Still, if length is what you're after, this is well worth trying!

☺ **Gentle Waterproof Mascara** *($14)* is a bit of a misnomer, as waterproof mascara in general is hard on lashes for both wear and removal. It is best for creating moderately long, well-defined lashes; thickness is slow going and peters out before reaching anything too dramatic.

☹ **High Impact Curling Mascara** *($14)* is misnamed; it should be called No Impact, No Curl Mascara. This mascara goes on wet and smears easily if you're not careful. It will separate and lengthen lashes, but it doesn't provide much thickness and it has zero curling effect. If you want curled lashes that last, you will need to use a lash curler. The curved brush also makes application to the lower lashes needlessly difficult. While this mascara doesn't flake, it does begin to smudge underneath the eyes after a few hours of wear, leaving you with dark under-eye circles. Clinique's original High Impact Mascara is highly preferred over this.

☹ **Naturally Glossy Mascara** *($14)* is a basic mascara that builds some length and minimal thickness, though it leaves lashes feeling dry and stiff due to the film-forming agents and the amount of PVP (an ingredient used in many hairstyling gels) it contains.

☹ **Lash Building Primer** *($13)* is nothing to get excited about. This will only impress you if it is used with a mediocre to poor mascara. In that case, you could expect to see increased length and thickness that would not be possible using the inferior mascara alone. However, when paired with a superior mascara, such as any rated a Paula's Pick, you won't notice much, if any, difference between using the primer and mascara together or simply applying two coats of the mascara.

☹ **High Definition Lashes Brush Then Comb Mascara** *($14)* is really bad, and that's not something I see too often with new mascaras. The dual-sided brush features comb-like teeth on one side and standard mascara bristles on the other. You're directed to use the bristled portion first to build thickness, then comb through lashes for length and added drama. Neither side works well, though at least the brush side doesn't leave lashes clumped together and spiky-looking. This is one of the few mascaras that require more effort to apply and neaten than the results merit.

BRUSHES: ☺ **The Brush Collection** *($13.50-$32.50).* Most of these brushes are full, well-shaped, and functional for their intended purpose. The prices are similar to most other brushes at the department store. All feature elegant handles that are neither too long nor too short, though no brush cases are currently available. The best options from the main collection are the Blush Brush, Concealer Brush, Eye Shadow Brush, Eye Contour Brush, and Eye Definer Brush, which is preferred for defining brows rather than eyelining. Adding a unique marketing element to their new brushes is Clinique's assertion that the brush hairs are treated with a long-lasting antibacterial agent to keep them hygienic. That could very well be possible, but it seems Clinique doesn't quite believe it either because they still advise you to clean your brush monthly for hygienic purposes, and the makeup artists at the counter clean the brushes with alcohol after each use. It's also important to keep in mind that the kind of bacteria that grow on brushes aren't the kind associated with breakouts, so the antibacterial claim won't help that aspect of your skin's appearance.

☺ **Powder Foundation Brush** *($32.50)* is designed to apply Clinique's powder foundations or it may also be used to apply loose powder. The density of brush hair (from goat) and the cut of the brush allow the user to apply more powder than usual, which will enhance coverage. Some experimentation is needed, as it can be easy to overdo and end up looking too powdered.

☹ **Bronzer/Blender Brush** *($32.50)* is incredibly full and a bit unwieldy, but is an option for applying powder to large areas of skin.

☹ **Eye Shader Brush** *($20)* is very soft and full, making it too large for most eyes, and is best for applying a wash of color to the entire eye area.

☹ **Powder Brush** *($30)* is quite soft and full, but a bit more density would make it easier to control.

FACE AND BODY ILLUMINATING/SHIMMER PRODUCTS: ✓ ☺ $$$ **Fresh Bloom Allover Colour** *($29.50)* started as a limited edition seasonal product but ended up becoming a permanent part of Clinique's makeup line, and for good reason! This pressed shimmer powder is outstanding. It has a buttery smooth texture and nearly foolproof application that adds soft, sheer colors and a radiant finish that enlivens skin without overdoing the sparkles. It is excellent used over blush, on its own as a cheek color/highlighter, or dusted over other smaller areas. All of the colors are beautiful.

☺ $$$ **Up-Lighting Liquid Illuminator** *($22.50)* may seem like the latest and greatest when it comes to shimmer, but the four sheer shades in this lightweight lotion don't break any new ground for radiant shine. Each applies smoothly and imparts a hint of color and shine that can be layered for more intensity. Flesh and bronze tones are sold alongside a peach and rosy pink shade, the latter two best used as blush rather than applied all over. The good news is that the shine clings well and the color lasts—though keep in mind the effect of both is subtle. This isn't the best if you want something more noticeable, say, for special occasion evening glamour.

SPECIALTY PRODUCTS: ☹ **Makeup Brush Cleanser** *($12.50 for 8 ounces)* will remove excess oil and pigment, but washing your brushes with a standard shampoo would work better than using this formulation. Makeup Brush Cleaner is primarily water, alcohol, and detergent cleansing agent, designed to be misted on and tissued off. There is no question this fast-drying formula works in between routine brush cleansing (especially if you need to use the same brushes on multiple people or you want to use one brush to apply two contrasting colors), but most women will find it an unnecessary addition to their makeup accessories. Also, the alcohol can be drying and can degrade the brush hair over time.

COPPERTONE

COPPERTONE AT-A-GLANCE

Strengths: A few effective basic sunscreens with various but typically lightweight textures (especially the Ultra Sheer); all recommended sunscreens are also water-resistant; inexpensive, which should encourage liberal application and reapplication; reliable self-tanners tailored to various skin tones.

Weaknesses: The majority of their sunscreens lack sufficient UVA-protecting ingredients, even though Coppertone clearly knows about this and routinely reformulates.

For more information about Coppertone, call (866)-288-3330 or visit www.coppertone. com or www.Beautypedia.com.

COPPERTONE KIDS PRODUCTS

☹ **Kids Continuous Spray SPF 50** *($10.49 for 6 ounces).* Although this provides plenty of avobenzone for sufficient UVA protection, the amount of alcohol is incredibly irritating and drying to skin of any age. There are plenty of spray-on sunscreens that do not contain alcohol—and this is far from a hypoallergenic formula that would be ideal for kids!

☹ **Kids Continuous Spray SPF 70+** *($10.99 for 8 ounces).* Parents may think the continuous spray action of this in-part avobenzone sunscreen is a quick and convenient way to protect their kids from sun exposure. However, the fine mist, which sprays from any angle, propels a hefty amount of skin-damaging alcohol onto your kid's skin, and that's not the way to set them up for a lifetime of healthy skin-care habits. Given the number of broad-spectrum sunscreens that don't have this drawback, Kids Continuous Spray SPF 70+ is not recommended. Also worth mentioning is that the SPF 70 is overkill. There isn't enough daylight for this SPF rating to make sense, and the amount of sunscreen ingredients needed to obtain this level of protection (based on time, not quality) can cause skin irritation.

☹ **Kids Sunblock Stick SPF 30** *($5.99 for 0.6 ounce)* lacks the UVA-protecting ingredients of titanium dioxide, zinc oxide, avobenzone, Tinosorb, or Mexoryl SX, and is not recommended.

☺ **Kids Sunscreen Lotion SPF 50** *($9.99 for 8 ounces)* has an in-part avobenzone sunscreen to ensure sufficient UVA protection and comes in a smooth, water-resistant lotion base suitable for normal to slightly oily skin. The tiny amount of vitamin E is likely ineffective at providing much, if any, antioxidant protection.

☺ **Kids Sunscreen Lotion SPF 70+** *($10.99 for 8 ounces)* is an in-part avobenzone sunscreen that comes in a lightweight base suitable for all skin types, and it contains a handful of notable antioxidants. If you're on a budget you should definitely consider this water-resistant sunscreen. It is fragrance-free. Also worth mentioning is that the SPF 70 is overkill. There isn't enough daylight for this SPF rating to make sense, and the amount of sunscreen ingredients needed to obtain this level of protection (based on time, not quality) may cause skin irritation.

COPPERTONE NUTRASHIELD PRODUCTS

☺ **NutraShield Faces SPF 70+ with Dual Defense** *($10.99 for 3 ounces).* The goal of this Coppertone sunscreen is to provide broad-spectrum sun protection enriched with antioxidants to further help skin. For the most part, they achieve that goal. I wish they'd included greater amounts of antioxidants, but some are better than none when it comes to giving skin a boost before it will be exposed to sunlight. As far as sun exposure goes, this in-part avobenzone sunscreen for normal to slightly dry or slightly oily skin has you well protected, though the SPF rating is needlessly high. Consider that SPF 70 means you can stay in the sun for 1,400 minutes without turning pink. (The formula is: 20 minutes [before you would normally turn pink in the sun without sunscreen] x 70 = 1,400 minutes.) There are only 1,440 minutes in a day, so that works out to be almost 24 hours of protection, which is way more time than the average person's skin sees the sun anywhere in the world. That doesn't mean this isn't a sunscreen to consider, just that its SPF rating is a bit much. On the other hand, given the fact that most people tend to under-apply sunscreen, it can be construed as a positive because at least you will be getting a lot more sunscreen ingredients on your skin even if you don't apply it liberally.

☺ **NutraShield SPF 30 with Dual Defense** *($10.99 for 6 ounces)* is worth a try if you have normal to oily or blemish-prone skin and are looking for a water-resistant sunscreen with a lightweight finish. Stabilized avobenzone is on hand for sufficient UVA protection and the fragrance isn't intrusive. Aside from vitamin E, the antioxidant content of this sunscreen is minuscule; a greater amount would've earned this product a Paula's Pick rating.

☺ **NutraShield SPF 70+ with Dual Defense** *($10.99 for 6 ounces)* is identical to Coppertone's NutraShield Faces SPF 70+ with Dual Defense, except you get twice as much product for the same price, and the same review applies.

COPPERTONE OIL FREE PRODUCTS

☺ **Oil Free Faces Lotion SPF 30** *($9.99 for 3 ounces)* is oil-free but its absorbent base isn't hydrating. This is a great choice for oily to very oily skin. Avobenzone provides UVA protection, and the fragrance-free, water-resistant lotion feels light and applies easily. It would be rated a Paula's Pick if the antioxidants weren't such an afterthought.

☺ **Oil Free Lotion SPF 30** *($11.19 for 8 ounces).* Although this includes not a single bell or whistle for extra skin-care benefits (the tiny amount of vitamin E doesn't count), it is a good, basic sunscreen that's water-resistant, and it includes avobenzone for UVA protection. This is best for normal to oily skin, and can be applied to the face.

☹ **Oil Free Lotion SPF 15** *($11.19 for 8 ounces)* is yet another Coppertone sunscreen that lacks the UVA-protecting ingredients of titanium dioxide, zinc oxide, avobenzone, Tinosorb, or Mexoryl SX, and is not recommended.

COPPERTONE SPORT PRODUCTS

☹ **Sport Continuous Spray SPF 15** *($9.99 for 6 ounces)* may spray continuously, but lacks the UVA-protecting ingredients of titanium dioxide, zinc oxide, avobenzone, Tinosorb, or Mexoryl SX and also contains 80% alcohol. This sunscreen is not recommended.

☹ **Sport Continuous Spray SPF 30** *($9.99 for 6 ounces)* has the same drawbacks as Coppertone's Sport Continuous Spray SPF 15 above, and is not recommended.

☹ **Sport Continuous Spray SPF 50** *($10.99 for 6 ounces).* It is gratifying that this spray-on sunscreen contains avobenzone for sufficient UVA protection, but terrible that the base formula is primarily alcohol. The spray-on sunscreens from Paula's Choice or Kinesys are preferred to this.

☹ **Sport Continuous Spray SPF 70+** *($10.99 for 6 ounces)*. Other than featuring a higher concentration of active ingredients to achieve its greater SPF rating, this spray-on sunscreen is nearly identical to Coppertone's Sport Continuous Spray SPF 50 above.

☺ **Sport Faces SPF 50** *($6.99 for 4 ounces)* is a good but very basic sunscreen that includes avobenzone for reliable UVA protection. It is water-resistant (not waterproof as claimed because that implies you don't need to reapply this after water activity). As for the hypoallergenic claim, there is no way that a sunscreen with this many active ingredients could ever make good on that claim. A percentage of people will always be allergic or sensitive to high percentages of sunscreen actives, no two ways about it. This formula is best for normal to oily skin.

☹ **Sport Lotion SPF 30** *($9.99 for 8 ounces)* lacks the UVA-protecting ingredients of titanium dioxide, zinc oxide, avobenzone, Tinosorb, or Mexoryl SX and is not recommended. Not very sporty, is it?

☹ **Sport Lotion SPF 50** *($9.99 for 8 ounces)* lacks the UVA-protecting ingredients of titanium dioxide, zinc oxide, avobenzone, Tinosorb, or Mexoryl SX and is not recommended.

☺ **Sport Quick Cover Lotion Spray SPF 30** *($9.99 for 6 ounces)* includes avobenzone for reliable UVA protection, and is nearly identical to many of the other in-part avobenzone sunscreen sprays from Coppertone. Skin-beneficial extras are in very short supply, but this has what it takes to provide broad-spectrum, water-resistant (not waterproof, as claimed; you'll still need to reapply this after swimming or perspiring heavily) coverage.

☹ **Sport Spray SPF 30** *($9.99 for 7 ounces)*. A lack of sufficient UVA protection coupled with an enormous amount of drying, irritating alcohol makes this spray-on sunscreen a must to avoid, at least if you care about the health of your skin.

☹ **Sport Stick SPF 30** *($5.49 for 0.6 ounce)* is identical to the company's Kids Sunblock Stick SPF 30 reviewed above. As such, it is not recommended.

☺ **Sport Sunscreen Lotion SPF 70+** *($10.99 for 6 ounces)* is identical to Coppertone's Kids Sunscreen Lotion SPF 70+ reviewed above. As such, the same review applies.

☹ **Sport Lotion SPF 15** *($9.99 for 8 ounces)* lacks the UVA-protecting ingredients of titanium dioxide, zinc oxide, avobenzone, Tinosorb, or Mexoryl SX and is not recommended.

COPPERTONE SUNLESS PRODUCTS

☺ **Gradual Tan Continuous Spray** *($9.69 for 6 ounces)* is a very basic but good spray-on self-tanner that turns skin color slowly with the ingredient erythrulose and a tiny amount of faster-acting dihydroxyacetone. It is suitable for all skin types except sensitive (because it contains fragrance).

☺ **Gradual Tan Moisturizing Lotion** *($10.29 for 9 ounces)*. This lightweight self-tanning lotion turns skin a subtle tan color thanks to the low amount of the self-tanning agent dihydroxyacetone it contains. It is fine for normal to dry skin and a good choice for those who've never tried a self-tanner or want just a hint of color.

COPPERTONE TANNING PRODUCTS

☹ **Dry Oil Continuous Spray SPF 10** *($9.99 for 6 ounces)*. Not only does this unethical product encourage tanning, it leaves skin vulnerable to UVA damage and contains so much alcohol skin that can't help but be dry and irritated.

☹ **Dry Oil Continuous Spray SPF 4** *($9.69 for 6 ounces)* is very similar to the Dry Oil Continuous Spray SPF 10 above, and the same review applies.

☹ **Lotion SPF 4** *($8.99 for 8 ounces).* The SPF rating is embarrassingly low, the formula lacks sufficient UVA-protecting ingredients, and it encourages tanning. I'm surprised it doesn't come with a pack of cigarettes, too.

☹ **Lotion SPF 8** *($10.49 for 8 ounces)* shares the same concerns and missteps as the Lotion SPF 4 above, and the same review applies.

COPPERTONE ULTRAGUARD PRODUCTS

☹ **Ultraguard Continuous Spray SPF 30** *($9.99 for 6 ounces)* is very similar to the other poorly-formulated spray-on versions from Coppertone. The right UVA-protecting ingredients are absent, and the amount of alcohol is exceedingly drying and irritating to skin. It is not recommended.

☹ **Ultraguard Continuous Spray SPF 50** *($9.99 for 6 ounces).* It is consistently maddening that Coppertone's sunscreens go back and forth between offering skin sufficient UVA protection or leaving skin vulnerable to UVA damage. Thankfully this product gets it right with its in-part avobenzone sunscreen—but that's the only good news. The amount of alcohol in this sunscreen is too irritating and drying for all skin types.

☹ **Ultraguard Continuous Spray SPF 70+** *($10.99 for 6 ounces).* Save for slightly less alcohol and an additional active ingredient to ensure a higher SPF rating, this drying, irritating sunscreen is nearly identical to Coppertone's Ultraguard Continuous Spray SPF 50. It is not recommended.

☺ **Ultraguard Lotion SPF 30** *($9.49 for 8 ounces)* is a basic, but good, broad-spectrum sunscreen for normal to slightly dry skin. UVA protection is assured with avobenzone, which is great because several Coppertone sunscreens completely ignore this issue. The tiny amount of vitamin E is not going to impact skin for the better.

☺ **Ultraguard Lotion SPF 50** *($10.99 for 8 ounces)* is nearly identical to Coppertone's Kids Sunscreen Lotion SPF 50, reviewed above, and the same review applies.

☺ **Ultraguard Lotion SPF 70+** *($10.99 for 8 ounces)* is identical to Coppertone's Kids Sunscreen Lotion SPF 70+ reviewed above, and the same review applies.

☺ **Ultraguard Quickcover Lotion Spray SPF 30** *($9.99 for 6 ounces)* is a good spray-on sunscreen lotion for normal to oily skin. It includes avobenzone for sufficient UVA protection, but is not waterproof as claimed. The accurate description is water-resistant, because this will need to be reapplied after prolonged immersion in water or perspiring.

☺ **Ultraguard Quickcover Lotion Spray SPF 50** *($10.99 for 6 ounces)* is a good, spray-on sunscreen lotion for normal to oily skin. It includes avobenzone for sufficient UVA protection, but is not waterproof as claimed. The accurate description is water-resistant, because this will need to be reapplied after prolonged immersion in water or perspiring.

☹ **Ultraguard Continuous Spray SPF 15** *($9.99 for 6 ounces)* is very similar to the other poorly-formulated spray-on versions form Coppertone. The right UVA-protecting ingredients are absent, and the amount of alcohol is exceedingly drying and irritating to skin. It is not recommended.

☹ **Ultraguard Lotion SPF 15** *($9.99 for 8 ounces)* lacks the UVA-protecting ingredients of titanium dioxide, zinc oxide, avobenzone, Tinosorb, or Mexoryl SX and is not recommended.

COPPERTONE WATER BABIES PRODUCTS

☺ **Water Babies Lotion SPF 50** *($10.99 for 8 ounces)* is nearly identical to Coppertone's Kids Sunscreen Lotion SPF 50 above, and the same review applies.

☺ **Water Babies Lotion SPF 70+** *($10.99 for 8 ounces)* is not for babies, but it is a great sunscreen. This fragrance-free sunscreen is identical to Coppertone's Kids Sunscreen Lotion SPF 70+ reviewed above. As such, the same review applies.

☺ **Water Babies Lotion Spray SPF 50** *($10.99 for 8 ounces)*. Coppertone uses the same sunscreen formulas repeatedly, and this is no exception. Except for the name, this is identical to the company's Kids Quick Cover Lotion Spray SPF 50. As such, the same review applies.

☺ **Water Babies Pure & Simple Lotion SPF 50** *($10.99 for 8 ounces)* contains zinc oxide and is fragrance-free, which gets things off to the right start. However, zinc oxide is joined by other active ingredients that aren't the best for a baby's skin. This sunscreen is fine for kids past their toddler years or for adults, but it isn't quite as impressive as several others from Coppertone.

☺ **Water Babies Quick Cover Lotion Spray SPF 50** *($10.99 for 6 ounces)* is nearly identical to Coppertone's Kids Quick Cover Lotion Spray SPF 50 reviewed above, and the same review applies. This is absolutely not a mild, non-irritating formula as claimed!

☹ **Water Babies Stick SPF 30** *($4.99 for 0.6 ounce)*. This wax-based sunscreen stick feels thick and occlusive, but more important, it doesn't provide sufficient UVA protection and can be quite sensitizing on an infant's skin. It is not recommended.

COVER FX

COVER FX AT-A-GLANCE

Strengths: Broad range of foundation shades for those seeking moderate to full coverage; good primer; most of the products are fragrance-free; very good brushes at an attractive price.

Weaknesses: Expensive overall; some of the foundations with sunscreen leave skin vulnerable to UVA damage; average mineral makeup (loose powder form); lip balm/lipstick contains irritants; mixed bag of good and bad products; really exaggerated claims.

For more information about Cover FX, call (866) 424-3332 or visit www.coverfx.com or www.Beautypedia.com.

COVER FX MAKEUP

MAKEUP REMOVER: ☺ $$$ **Clean FX Make Up Cleansing Solution** *($28 for 3.34 ounces)* is a standard gentle makeup remover whose efficacy is enhanced by silicone and a mild detergent cleansing agent. It works to remove all types of makeup, including waterproof mascara. The fragrance-free remover is suitable for all skin types; however, you don't have to spend this much to get an effective product. For example, Neutrogena and Almay offer equally effective, equally gentle options for a lot less money.

FOUNDATION: ✓ ☺ $$$ **Powder FX Mineral Powder Foundation** *($32)* is the pressed-powder (and preferred) version of Cover FX's Mineral FX Pure Mineral Foundation SPF 15 reviewed below. The differences are that this has a much smoother, talc-based texture, no sunscreen, and a sheer matte finish that has a subtle shine. Also worth mentioning is how well this pressed-powder foundation blends—it has a natural affinity for skin and leaves it looking smoothed and refined. The shade range is good, and includes options for very fair to tan skin.

The Reviews C

The darkest B shades, such as Warm Walnut, Burnished Mahogany, and Warm Espresso, should be tested carefully to make sure they don't turn ash on your skin (otherwise, they're attractive shades); E40 Peach Taupe is slightly peach and should also be considered carefully, while M80 Deep Mocha is ash and best avoided. This foundation is recommended for normal to oily skin (assuming you don't mind a slight shine).

☺ **$$$ Skin Tint FX Moisturizing Treatment & Tint SPF 30** *($42)*. In a line whose foundations are built largely around providing significant coverage, this sheer tint is a welcome change of pace. The sunscreen includes titanium dioxide and zinc oxide among other active ingredients (though for sensitive skin the synthetic ingredients should have been left out; you can easily achieve great SPF protection with only zinc oxide and titanium dioxide, which present no risk of irritation), and the formula contains some state-of-the-art ingredients. The very light, fluid texture can be tricky to dispense from the pump (it tends to squirt out forcefully) and it has lots of slip during blending. You must shake the bottle well before each use to keep the ingredients blended and to provide the intended soft powder finish, which is ideal for normal to slightly oily skin. True to its tint name, this provides sheer coverage. Among the small selection of shades are some good neutral tones for fair to slightly tan skin tones. M Light is slightly peach but still worth considering, while C Deep is noticeably peach and best avoided. Overall this could have been better; there are less expensive options from Neutrogena and Olay that are better formulated and blend easier, but this still deserves consideration.

☺ **$$$ Natural FX Water Based Liquid Foundation SPF 15** *($40)* is designed to be a more wearable, lighter version of Cover FX's Total Coverage Cream Foundation SPF 30, reviewed below. It certainly is easier to work with and has some great attributes. Unfortunately, one of those attributes is not reliable sun protection from UVA rays because it lacks active ingredients that cover the entire UV spectrum, which is disappointing. This water- and silicone-based foundation has a fluid texture that requires shaking before each use because it separates when it sits in the container. In fact, several of the testers I used at the counter had separated, even though they were new (in some cases they were brand new, and I had to peel the safety seal away to dispense the product). Once shaken well, however, this has a beautiful silky texture that slips over skin easily and sets to a lightweight satin finish that provides light to medium buildable coverage. Unlike many foundations, this is pigment-rich, so a little goes a long way. However, if you don't apply this liberally, it will compromise the amount of sun protection you get (although you'll still need to pair this with an effective sunscreen rated SPF 15 or greater that contains UVA-protecting ingredients because, applied liberally or not, this foundation won't cut it for sufficient UVA protection). The formula is best for normal to slightly dry or slightly oily skin. There are 20+ shades, many of which are quite good and well-suited to a wide range of skin tones. The colors to avoid due to overtones of peach, orange, or rose include C30 Rose Bisque (may be OK for some), C40 Rose Wheat, C60 Pink Almond, C80 Rosewood, E30 Peach Beige, and E40 Peach Taupe. Consider M40 Honey carefully, and realize that M90 Deep Mocha isn't as dark as the name suggests.

☺ **$$$ Mineral FX Pure Mineral Foundation SPF 15** *($37)*. I always find it odd when companies advertise and promote one of their powder foundations because it is talc-free, and then turn around and also advertise their products that contain talc. If you're going to denigrate an ingredient, then be consistent—don't contradict your stance by also formulating products that contain it. (In the case of talc, it is a brilliant and desirable cosmetic ingredient). This loose-powder "mineral" makeup contains 20% zinc oxide and 20% titanium dioxide, so broad-spectrum sun protection is assured, and that's great. Of course, that level of mineral pigments, along with the absorbent powders in this makeup, results in a dry texture that can also make your skin appear dry. Perhaps that's why the company added a shimmer finish to this silky-textured powder? The packaging makes it relatively easy to dispense powder onto the built-in sponge and then buff it over your skin. Coverage is in the medium range and it can be layered for more camouflage, but doing so increases the odds that this will look too opaque and chalky. All told, this isn't the best loose-powder mineral makeup around, though the sun protection element and most of the 20+ shades are commendable. If you opt to try this, avoid the following shades: C60 Pink Almond (slightly pink, may be OK for some light skin tones); E40 Peach Taupe (slightly peach but may work for some medium skin tones); E60 Desert Peach; and the ashen M80 Deep Mocha. E60 Porcelain is excellent for very fair skin.

☺ $$$ **Total Coverage Cream Foundation SPF 30** *($42)* is the Cover FX foundation that put this company on the map, so to speak—but is it worth your attention? Definitely not if you want sun protection from your foundation because this does not contain sufficient UVA-protecting ingredients. This is also a bad choice if you have blemish-prone skin; the waxes and emollients it contains can contribute to clogged pores (labeling this foundation noncomedogenic is an extreme example of how misused this term has become). More akin to greasepaint than traditional foundation, this thick cream compact foundation drags if you apply it over bare skin. Application improves when you moisturize your skin beforehand, and this has a moist finish that absolutely must be set with powder (which adds to its already thick appearance). The only reason to consider this heavy-duty foundation is if you need major coverage, such as for birthmarks, melasma, persistent redness, or flat facial scars. Although it looks more natural on skin than some other full-coverage foundations (such as original Dermablend), it still is not natural by anyone's definition—you will absolutely look like you're wearing foundation. Part of what keeps this foundation from looking better on skin is the shocking number of poor shades. There are more than 40 shades available, which is certainly a lot of options, but the number of workable shades is considerably less. The following shades are not recommended because they are overly peach, orange, copper, pink, or rose: B15 Honey Ginger, B25 Warm Walnut, B45 Burnished Mahogany (may be OK for some Native American or Polynesian skin tones), C20 Pink Cream, C40 Rose Wheat, C50 Rose Sand, C60 Pink Almond, C80 Rosewood, E50 Warm Taupe, E60 Desert Peach, E80 Rich Tan, and M80 Deep Mocha. There are some excellent shades for very fair skin, including E0 Porcelain and M10 Bone, and some impressive colors for dark to very dark skin, including B65 Warm Espresso and M70 Mocha. The E and M ranges of shades tend to be the safest bets in terms of neutral to warm beige tones. When all is said and done, although this is a tenacious makeup in terms of wear (and washing this off requires an oil, cold cream, or silicone-based makeup remover) and provides ample coverage, it isn't the best look for full-face makeup unless you have something glaring or significant to hide. Otherwise, consider this best as a cream concealer that requires careful blending and, again, it must be set with powder to avoid creasing and to prolong wear.

POWDER: ☺ $$$ **Setting FX Loose Setting Powder** *($32)* is a feather-light, mica- and silica-based dry-finish loose powder designed to set any Cover FX cream or liquid foundation. One "colorless" shade is available, and it goes on translucent enough to work for most fair to medium skin tones. On darker skin tones, it will slightly change the way the foundation shade "reads" on skin, so a different skin tone–matching powder is advised. Otherwise, this is a good, sheer loose powder that is best for normal to oily skin.

The Reviews C

☺ **$$$ Matte FX Oil Absorbing Pressed Powder** *($22)*. Best described as a blotting powder for oily skin, this talc- and cornstarch-based powder has a smooth, dry texture and sheer matte finish that effectively absorbs excess shine. In a counterintuitive move, this pressed powder deposits a small amount of sparkling shine on skin, a point to be aware of if your goal is to temper shine, which is how most people use pressed powder. Three shades are available: Light is best for fair skin; Medium is slightly peach and should be considered carefully; Dark is slightly rose and won't work for most dark skin tones.

BLUSH AND BRONZER: ☺ **$$$ Bronzed FX Bronzing Powder** *($28)*. You'd expect this to be capable of providing a tanned appearance to skin, but only two of the five shades come close to meeting that goal, and even those do it only marginally well. This is best as a shiny blush, and the shine has modest cling. The texture and application are very smooth and even, while the colors have a sheer vibrancy that enlivens cheeks. Pink Topaz and Golden Peach are best for fair to medium skin tones, while Garnet is suitable for tan to dark skin tones, assuming you want shiny cheeks.

BRUSHES: ☺ **Brushes** *($14–$36)*. The Brushes from Cover FX don't present many options, but those available are mostly excellent. The **#110 Concealing Brush** ($14) is synthetic and workable, but many will find it too small for ease of use in covering dark circles. The **#120 Layering Brush** ($20) is a synthetic brush that works best to apply and blend eyeshadow; the **#130 Foundation Brush** ($32) costs less than many others, and is excellent for its intended purpose (this brush is also synthetic); also worth considering is the natural-hair **Cream Foundation Brush** ($36), though this is best for applying powder to the T-zone or applying contour rather than using it with cream-based products. For detail work with foundation, the pointed, dense, synthetic-hair **Precision Foundation Brush** ($32) is definitely worth auditioning.

FACE AND BODY ILLUMINATING/SHIMMER PRODUCTS: ☺ **$$$ Radiant FX Luminescent Powder** *($32)*. Shiny loose powders aren't hard to come by, so when you're charging this much you'd better have an exemplary option. Despite a weightless sheer texture, that's not the case here. The two shades are workable, but the shine has minimal cling and the packaging wasn't well thought out—powder gets everywhere once the seal is removed, and the cap is difficult to secure, which increases the risk of spillage in your makeup bag. This has too many strikes against it to warrant much consideration, especially if you want the luminous effect to last instead of ending up on your clothes.

SPECIALTY PRODUCTS: ☺ **$$$ Clearprep FX Matte Foundation Primer and Anti-Shine Treatment** *($39)* has a nearly weightless matte finish that's made more intriguing for blemish-prone skin because it contains 1% salicylic acid. The pH of 4 is borderline for exfoliation to occur, but some people will benefit from this product. The ingredient mix is mostly winning for those with oily, blemish-prone skin, but there are some setbacks. The inclusion of citrus extracts and a small amount of fragrant neroli oil aren't good news for any skin type, but at least there's a potentially effective amount of the anti-irritant willow bark to counter these unnecessary additions. The texture and finish of this primer facilitate makeup application, and it's good that Cover FX added some beneficial extras for skin. This would be rated a Paula's Pick if it did not contain the aforementioned fragrant plant ingredients.

☺ **$$$ Skinprep FX Treatment and Priming Serum** *($45 for 1 ounce)*. This silicone-based primer contains some intriguing ingredients, including emollient squalane, vitamin-based antioxidants, and a couple of cell-communicating ingredients. Just like all silicone-laden primers or serums, it makes skin feel very silky, it isn't heavy, and it facilitates a smooth makeup application.

The company's claim that this serum is fragrance-free is inaccurate because it contains fragrant neroli oil. As such, it is not recommended for sensitive skin. In addition, neroli oil can cause photosensitivity in those with fair skin (Source: www.naturaldatabase.com). Beyond the faulty fragrance-free claim, this is a good, though pricey, serum for normal to dry skin.

☺ **$$$ Brush Cleanser** *($13 for 7.9 ounces)* is simply a water- and alcohol-based solution that works to remove makeup, facial oil, and perspiration from brushes. It is essentially a watered-down shampoo, and for the long-term softness and durability of your makeup brushes, occasional cleansing with a shampoo instead of a potentially drying product like this is preferred.

☹ **FX Lip Treatment & Tinted Lustre SPF 15** *($24)*. This dual-sided lip balm and lipstick not only leaves lips vulnerable to UVA damage because it does not contain active ingredients that cover the entire UV spectrum, but also causes irritation due to the peppermint oil that was included. The claim that the "blend of peptides" is supposed to restore youthful density and volume to lips is a joke, and it's not because the formula contains only one peptide (What blend were they referring to?). Rather, there is no research anywhere showing that peptides can restore aging lips to their once-plump state.

COVER GIRL (MAKEUP ONLY)

COVER GIRL AT-A-GLANCE

Strengths: Inexpensive and widely available; a hugely improved selection of foundations, several with reliable sunscreen; good concealers; enviable pressed powders; some fantastic mascaras; mostly great eyelining options; a vast selection of lip color options, from the long-wearing Outlast to sheer lip glosses.

Weaknesses: The older foundations are seriously lacking; the newer Advanced Radiance foundation has great texture but disappointing SPF rating; Professional Loose Powder; powder blush and eyeshadows; terrible makeup brushes; all of the "Clean" products contain irritating ingredients.

For more information about Cover Girl, owned by Procter & Gamble, call (800) 426-8374 or visit www.covergirl.com or www.Beautypedia.com.

COVER GIRL CG SMOOTHERS PRODUCTS

FOUNDATION: ✓☺ **CG Smoothers AquaSmooth Makeup SPF 15** *($9.99)* is an ultralight, silicone-to-powder compact makeup that smooths easily onto the skin and dries to a soft, powdery matte finish. As with similar foundations, quick, deft blending is key: these formulas dry fast, and are not easy to move once they do. The sunscreen is all titanium dioxide, so even sensitive skin should be able to wear this, though the formula and finish are best for normal to slightly oily skin: dry skin will only look more noticeable with this type of foundation. Although the formula contains waxes, the amount is small enough that it's unlikely to be a problem for blemish-prone skin. The 15 shades offer light to medium coverage. The ones to avoid due to overtones of pink or peach are Natural Ivory, Medium Light, Warm Beige, Natural Beige, Creamy Beige, and Toasted Almond. The remaining shades feature some excellent options for light and dark skin tones.

☺ **CG Smoothers All Day Hydrating Makeup** *($7.77)* isn't all that hydrating. In fact, the talc content (it's the fourth ingredient) gives this sheer-to-medium-coverage foundation a soft matte, slightly powdery finish suitable for someone with normal to oily or combination skin. The range of 15 shades is impressive, and the packaging now permits you to see the color, although it's still best to test it on your skin. The following colors are too pink, rose, or peach for most skin tones: Natural Ivory (just slightly pink), Natural Beige, Medium Light, Warm Beige, Creamy Beige, and Toasted Almond. Soft Sable is a beautiful color for dark skin tones. This is fragrance-free.

☺ **CG Smoothers SPF 15 Tinted Moisture** *($7.59)* is an exceptionally sheer moisturizer that imparts the smallest amount of color to the skin. The four shades are all worth considering, but keep in mind these are very sheer, so dark circles or red discolorations will require a concealer. This is fragrance-free, with a lightweight lotion texture and minimally moist finish. The sunscreen is in-part zinc oxide, making this product appropriate for normal to slightly dry or slightly oily skin. The formula could certainly be more state-of-the-art, especially for older women, but it's recommended as a reliable tinted moisturizer with broad-spectrum sunscreen.

CONCEALER: ☹ **CG Smoothers Concealer** *($6.25)* is a standard, lipstick-style concealer that doesn't go on as greasy as it appears and provides good coverage with minimal creasing. However, four of the six shades are on the peach side, and the coverage is opaque enough for that to be a problem for some skin tones. Neutralizer is OK, but Illuminator is too whitish pink for even very light skin. This concealer is not recommended for use over blemishes or blemish-prone areas.

POWDER: ☺ **CG Smoothers Pressed Powder** *($6.25)* comes in six suitably neutral colors that leave a subtle, shiny finish on skin. The talc- and mineral oil-based formula is best for normal to dry skin. It leaves a satin finish yet isn't quite as silky as Cover Girl's TruBlend Pressed Powder and Advanced Radiance Age-Defying Pressed Powder.

COVER GIRL CLEAN PRODUCTS

EYE-MAKEUP REMOVER: ☹ **Clean Makeup Remover for Eyes and Lips** *($4.53 for 2 ounces)* is mineral oil–based and yet this fluid, greasy lotion doesn't remove long-wearing makeup nearly as well as a silicone-based remover. It's an OK option for standard lipsticks that may leave a stain, but is far too greasy to use around the eyes or to remove mascara.

FOUNDATION: ☹ **Clean Makeup Fragrance Free** *($5.99)* mercifully omits the sickly sweet scent that is present in the original Clean Makeup formula, as well as the irritating extracts. Unfortunately, most of the 15 shades are just too strongly peach, pink, or rose for most skin tones. The only four shades worth considering are Ivory, Classic Ivory, Soft Honey, and Classic Tan.

☺ **Clean Makeup Oil Control** *($5.93)* is an oil- and fragrance-free liquid foundation that I suppose was Cover Girl's attempt to modernize their original Clean Makeup. It's nice that the irritants and overpowering fragrance were omitted, but the shades still suffer from a preponderance of rose, pink, peach, and orange tones. The foundation itself isn't as silky-smooth as it could have been, and its matte, slightly powdery finish tends to look a bit chalky in the lighter shades. It's an OK light-coverage option for normal to oily skin, but the only worthwhile shades are Ivory, Classic Ivory, Buff Beige, and Creamy Natural.

☹ **Clean Makeup** *($5.99)* is the original Cover Girl foundation (launched in 1961) that hasn't yet been discontinued despite the fact that it has a dated, basic formula that contains clove, menthol, camphor, and eucalyptus, which are extremely irritating for skin, comes in colors that are largely unusable for any skin tone, and has fragrance that is intrusive. This must be selling well, however, or why would they keep it for so many years? Yet all that means is that there are thousands of women wearing an irritating foundation whose colors haven't kept pace with the vast majority of foundations available, including those from Cover Girl.

POWDER: ☺ **Clean Pressed Powder Fragrance-Free** *($5.99)* isn't "cleaner" than any of the other pressed powders in the Cover Girl line. It's a standard talc-based powder with a smooth application and soft, slightly dry finish suitable for normal to oily skin. The 15 shades fare much better than those for the Clean Makeup, with the only missteps being Classic Beige, Warm Beige, Creamy Beige, and the borderline-peach Soft Honey.

☹ **Clean Pressed Powder for Normal Skin** *($5.99)* is almost identical to its fragrance-free counterpart, but this one includes eucalyptus oil and camphor, both of which are very irritating even in small amounts. It also has a medicinal-sweet fragrance that will enter a room before you do.

COVER GIRL EXACT PRODUCTS

EYESHADOW: ☹ **Exact Eyelights Eye Brightening Eyeshadow** *($7.49)* is a collection of four different powder eyeshadow palettes that are designed to "enhance and brighten" your natural eye color, be it blue, brown, green, or hazel. An interesting concept, but not even one of the four palettes offers workable options that could reasonably complement its corresponding eye color. Instead, Cover Girl included shades that match these eye colors outright (and it's never a good idea to match your eyeshadow to your eye color). Of the four color options, only the palette for brown eyes contains workable shades for any eye color. Consider that moot, however, because the eyeshadow formula is Cover Girl's oldest, and as such has an unpleasantly dry texture, imparting extremely sheer color that flakes away almost as fast as it's applied.

EYE AND BROW PRODUCTS: ☺ **Exact Eyelights Eye Brightening Liner** *($6.99)* intends on enhancing eye color with colors that just don't make any sense. Radiant Sapphire for blue eyes? The best strategy for playing up eye color is to do so with contrasting color, not an exact match. But if you just ignore Cover Girl's recommended pairings, you'll be rewarded with an automatic, retractable eyeliner available in interesting shade options that goes on smoothly and has incredible staying power—though for a pencil liner, it does set fast and isn't forgiving if you want to blend it. Of the four options, the ones with the most baffling names are best: Vibrant Pearl is a smoky black and Vivid Ruby, a deep brown.

☺ **Line Exact Liquid Liner Pen** *($6.79)* offers precision application from a felt-tip-style pen that is easier to work with than liquid liners that apply with a long, thin brush. The formula dries quickly, so smearing and smudging are not an issue. So why the neutral face? Primarily because this tends to wear unevenly and is prone to fading—so the intense line you begin the day with looks like a shadow of its former self by lunchtime.

MASCARA: ☺ **Lash Exact Mascara** *($8.05)* has a unique brush that appears spiky, almost resembling cactus bristles, yet it turns out that the brush does an amazing job of making lashes thick with minimal effort. It's not much for creating length, but if thickness without clumps is what you're after, this is highly recommended and a welcome addition to Cover Girl's gradually-getting-better mascara lineup.

☺ **Lash Exact Waterproof Mascara** *($7.99)* has the same rubber-bristled brush as the original (non-waterproof) Lash Exact Mascara. Cover Girl claims that this special brush has the advantage of allowing you to easily reach every lash, but lots of mascara brushes have that capability. It's more about the size of the brush than what the bristles are made of. In any event, this is an admirable waterproof mascara that builds long lashes quickly along with moderate thickness. You'll notice some minor clumping, especially with lashes at corners of the eye, but that's easily remedied with the brush. This wears all day without a flake or smear, and must be taken off with a silicone- or oil-based remover.

☺ **Volume Exact Mascara** *($7.99)* is riding the success of Cover Girl's popular Lash Exact Mascara, and compared to the progenitor, this formula (also with a rubber-bristle brush) thickens lashes even more and keeps them well-defined with only minor clumping. Successive coats smooth things out, but, oddly, don't make lashes much longer. Some length is attainable, but this is really best as a thickening mascara, and it wears beautifully.

☺ **Volume Exact Waterproof Mascara** *($8.05)* isn't as impressive as the non-waterproof version of Volume Exact, but it works if what you're after is a clean application, soft definition, and a trusty waterproof formula. Lashes never look too coated or too heavy, regardless of how many coats you apply. The downside is that lashes never get beyond moderately long, and thickness is on the mild side. Depending on what you want out of a mascara, those can be good or bad traits.

☹ **Exact Eyelights Eye Brightening Waterproof Mascara** *($7.99)*. The concept behind this mascara is that you get waterproof protection while adding a brightening shimmer to your lashes (as if any other part of the face needed more shimmer products). The brightening effect is really subtle, and ends up being a bit annoying because the sparkle particles tend to flake throughout the day. This mascara has a thin, uneven application that takes patience to get what never amounts to more than modest length and no thickness. It's waterproof as stated, but so what? There are lots of waterproof mascaras that handily outperform this, and you can get the brightening effect from eyeliner or eyeshadow instead.

☹ **Exact Eyelights Mascara** *($7.49)*. Ads featuring pop singer Rihanna tout this mascara's chief selling point, which is that it makes eyes appear to glisten, and that's because it contains shimmer pigments. Your eyes won't glisten or sparkle with this mascara, but they may become slightly irritated because the shiny particles flake slightly. The other novel feature of this mascara is that its shades are made to correspond with various eye colors. If you notice any difference it will be subtle; for the most part, these are all soft black mascara lightly tinted with either blue, olive green, copper, or aubergine for a really, really slight effect. As for length and thickness, both are respectable, without a single clump or smear, though not to the same impressive extent as Cover Girl's formidable Lash Blast Mascara. This is worth a trial run if you don't want the dramatic lashes Lash Blast provides and are curious to see if the slight color and sparkle effect will enliven your eyes a bit (or make them red and irritated due to the flaking).

COVER GIRL LASH BLAST PRODUCTS

✓☺ **Lash Blast Mascara** *($8.69)* ranks as Cover Girl's most expensive mascara to date, but the performance won't disappoint and it still costs much less than the best department-store mascaras. The oversized, rubber-bristled brush seems imposing at first, but allows you to be surprisingly nimble when defining, lengthening, and slightly thickening your lashes. You're left with a full, dramatic, clump-free sweep of softly fringed lashes that look gorgeous and last all day. Fans of Lash Exact and Volume Exact Mascara should give this strong consideration; it gives a greater payoff in less time, and combines the best attributes of its predecessors into one superior mascara.

☺ **Lash Blast Luxe** *($7.99)* comes with a giant rubber-bristle brush, just the original Lash Blast Mascara—a brush that some will love and others will instantly dislike. The differences between Lash Blast Luxe and the original Lash Blast are that the new version is infused with shimmer and it does not enhance thickness the way the original did. The shiny lash effect is very subtle, so aside from the reduced thickness (and remember, thickness is what catapulted the original Lash Blast to a Paula's Pick) this mascara is quite similar. The large plastic brush makes it difficult to get an even application on smaller lashes, but once on, Lash Blast Luxe lengthens and separates lashes well with minimal clumping. It doesn't do much for thickness, but it will wear well for hours with no flaking. Removal is easy with a cleanser or an eye-makeup remover.

☺ **Lash Blast Waterproof Volume Mascara** *($8.39)* proves that it really is the marriage of a brush and mascara formula that creates a perfect union of beautiful lashes (a problem often discussed among cosmetics chemists who formulate makeup). Cover Girl's original (non-waterproof) version of Lash Blast Mascara is arguably their best mascara (at least if you want gorgeously thick, elongated lashes without a clump in sight). Although the waterproof version has the same spiky, rubber-bristle brush, the results aren't as impressive due to the differences in the formulas. Yes, this is waterproof (and requires an oil- or silicone-based remover when you're ready for it to come off), but it requires a lot more work to get close to "lush, volumized lashes." It outperforms many lackluster waterproof mascaras, but doesn't jump to the head of the class. Despite its shortcomings, Lash Blast Waterproof Volume Mascara still deserves consideration for the times when you need waterproof mascara that provides equal parts length and thickness.

COVER GIRL OUTLAST PRODUCTS

EYE AND BROW PRODUCTS: ✓☺ **Outlast Smoothwear All-Day Eyeliner** *($6.99)* is an automatic, silicone-based retractable pencil that features a built-in sharpener, a nice option when you need to sharpen the point to allow you to draw on a thinner line. I was very impressed with how well this pencil goes on and how, once set, it wears fairly well without a trace of smudging or smearing. Some fading does occur, especially by the end of the day, but for the most part this is a slam-dunk recommendation as one of the best eye pencils available at the drugstore. One caution: removing this requires more than a water-soluble cleanser. OK, two cautions: avoid Sage, because this shade of green eyeliner isn't pretty on anyone, especially if you want to be taken seriously.

LIPSTICK, LIP GLOSS, AND LIPLINER: ✓☺ **Outlast All-Day Lipcolor** *($9.99)* is identical in every respect to Max Factor's Lipfinity. Both products feature a liquid color you apply to lips (make sure they're clean, dry, and free of any flakes), let set for a moment or two, then apply a glossy top coat for comfortable wear and shine. Outlast wears about the same as Lipfinity, which is to say extraordinarily well. As long as you can commit to regularly applying the moisturizing top coat, you'll be rewarded with feel-good color that lasts through most meals (oily salad dressings or fried foods are this lip color's undoing), and it doesn't come off on cups or people (so go ahead and freely kiss the ones you love). The only minor areas where Cover Girl's Outlast bests Max Factor's Lipfinity are price (Outlast typically costs $1-$2 less) and shade selection.

✓☺ **Outlast Smoothwear All-Day Lipcolor** *($10.30)* is similar to Cover Girl's regular Outlast All-Day Lipcolor, but with less pigment and the trade-off of a shorter wear time, although Cover Girl claims both products last ten hours. This has the same formula and technology as original Outlast—the only difference is the level of pigment in each color. If you thought the first round of Outlast colors was too bold or intense, consider this sheer option so you can experience one of the best long-wearing lipsticks available. Yes, you need to reapply the Conditioning

Moisturecoat at regular intervals to avoid lips that feel desert dry, but the color itself really does stay put, and that is what makes this type of long-wearing lip color so unique.

☺ **Outlast Double LipShine** *($10.30)* is a sheerer, glossier version of Cover Girl's Outlast Smoothwear All-Day Lipcolor. The same application steps are called for, meaning you apply a coat of color, wait for it to set, then brush on the glossy top coat for shine and comfortable wear. The big claim here is that this product lasts longer than the leading lip gloss (whatever product that is, it wasn't identified), with up to ten hours of wear. Although the color does last for hours (with regular touch-ups to the top coat to keep lips from feeling parched), it doesn't last evenly for more than a couple of hours. You'll likely notice some fading, especially toward the inner portion of the lips, while the border retains stronger color, sort of like when your lipstick wears off before the lipliner. It's not a deal-breaker, and there's no question this product wears longer than a regular lip gloss, but it isn't fail-safe and does require maintenance to keep up appearances.

☺ **Outlast Lipstain** *($7.49)* has packaging that resembles a felt-tip marker. The pointed-tip applicator makes precise application easy, but as with most lip stains the watery color distributes unevenly and will need to be blended with a fingertip or lip brush. Also, the sheer colors apply brighter than they appear on the packaging, so choose carefully. Once this stain sets, it wears well on its own and provides a matte base for gloss. If you've been using BeneTint as your lip stain, give Outlast Lipstain a try—you won't be disappointed. Neither will your wallet!

☺ **Outlast Smoothwear All-Day Lipliner** *($6.90)* is a very good automatic, retractable lip pencil. It glides on with a creaminess that is smooth but easy to control, and does its job of staying put, defining the lip line without migrating into creases or fading before your lipstick does. The shade selection isn't as extensive as it is for Cover Girl's Outlast Lipcolor, but most of the colors are versatile.

COVER GIRL QUEEN COLLECTION PRODUCTS

FOUNDATION: ☺ **Natural Hue Liquid Makeup** *($6.99)* is a standard, but good, lightweight oil-free foundation for normal to oily skin. As part of Cover Girl's Queen (Latifah) Collection, the shade range is designed for women with dark skin tones. For the most part, the colors are spot-on (though it's a shame there are no testers). Be careful with the orange-tinged Golden Honey and Amber Glow; Rich Mink and True Ebony are gorgeous for very dark skin tones. Regardless of shade, you get sheer to light coverage and a soft matte finish. This must be blended carefully to avoid an uneven appearance.

☹ **Natural Hue Compact Foundation** *($8.69)* is a classic cream-to-powder foundation, but in this case, classic isn't a positive thing. Lots of brands offer better cream-to-powder formulas, including Clarins and M.A.C., both lines that offer shades for women of color. Cover Girl's contribution has a waxy yet smooth texture that has OK initial slip but sets almost too quickly to a powdery finish that can appear greasy. What's worse, most of the colors are terrible. They're either too orange, too copper, or too red. The few worthwhile shades include Rich Mink and Warm Caramel. If you opt to try this, it's best for normal to slightly dry skin that's not prone to blemishes.

POWDER: ☹ **Natural Hue Minerals Pressed Powder** *($8.19)* contains mica, a mineral that, along with the talc base, gives credibility to this product's name. It has an unusual texture that's smooth yet waxy, and the result is minimal powder deposit and poor shine control. You'll get a sheer satin finish that doesn't look overly powdered, but doesn't do much to enhance skin tone or downplay large pores, either. Oddly, the shade selection doesn't go as dark as the foundations that are part of Cover Girl's Queen Collection. Every color goes on lighter and softer than it appears in the compact, and all except Light Bronze 1 are recommended.

BRONZER: ☺ **Natural Hue Bronzer** *($8.19)* is described as a mineral-enriched formula, and it is. The minerals are talc and mica, and they show up in the majority of bronzing powders sold today. This is a standard pressed bronzing powder that has a smooth, dry texture and soft application (too soft, in fact, for the darker skin tones it's intended for). The shades aren't that impressive; only Ebony Bronze is recommended, though this won't register on most dark skin tones.

EYESHADOW: ☺ **1-Kit Eye Shadow** *($2.99)* is a collection of eyeshadow singles designed to complement dark skin tones, and most of the shades have enough impact to do just that. The texture is smooth yet slightly dry, with an even application that resists streaking or flaking and is quite blendable. All of the shades have shine that's best described as slightly metallic. Avoid the very green Emerald and blue After Midnight. Black Tie works great as a powder eyeliner for most skin tones.

☹ **Eyeshadow Quads** *($4.99)* comes in two quad sets of color combinations that are difficult to work with, and one (Blue Notes) isn't flattering on any skin tone. You never see Queen Latifah (the celebrity spokesperson and namesake of Cover Girl's Queen Collection) sporting such colors in ads or on magazine covers, and you shouldn't, either.

EYE AND BROW PRODUCTS: ☺ **Eye Liner** *($4.59)* doesn't require sharpening, but it isn't retractable, so be careful with how much of the tip you expose at once. It has a smooth, creamy application that deposits color evenly, though I expected these to be more pigmented given that this pencil is designed for dark skin tones. Once set, the formula stays put and is minimally prone to fading. Avoid the ashen Grey Khaki; the navy Midnight Blue is OK if because it's more of a bluish-black.

LIPSTICK AND LIPLINER: ✓ ☺ **Lip Gloss** *($5.49)* is a superior lip gloss that is outfitted with a sponge-tip applicator. It applies smoothly, imparts sheer, shimmering color, and hasn't a trace of stickiness. The shade range is well-suited to those with darker skin tones, though each color goes on softer than it appears in the package. Consider this a best beauty buy!

✓ ☺ **Vibrant Hue Color** *($6.29)* is described as a rich, creamy lipstick and it is. One swipe and you'll appreciate how indulgent this feels, yet it isn't greasy or too slick. It's a very good, classic cream lipstick whose riveting colors have enough pigmentation to last beyond that first cup of coffee. Women of all skin tones can enjoy these bolder colors, none of which goes on as opaque as it appears.

☺ **Lasting Lip Pencil** *($6.29)* is an automatic, retractable lipliner that is identical to Cover Girl's Outlast Smoothwear Lip Liner above, and the same review applies: it glides on with a creaminess that is smooth but controllable and does its job of staying put. This pigmented pencil won't fade before your lipstick does, and comes in a workable range of shades to pair with bold lipstick hues.

☺ **Vibrant Hue Shine** *($6.29)* is a good, standard sheer lipstick that provides a high-gloss shimmer finish. The brown-toned range of colors was designed for African-American skin tones, but is versatile enough for all skin tones, assuming you don't mind brown-toned shades (plum and mauve tones are available too).

MASCARA: ☺ **Volume Mascara** *($6.39)* doesn't do anything exceptionally well, but it doesn't falter enough to warrant an average rating. It deserves a happy face rating for its ability to lengthen, separate, and moderately thicken lashes without clumps, smears, or flakes. Wearability is great, and this removes easily with a water-soluble cleanser.

The Reviews C

COVER GIRL TRU AND TRUBLEND PRODUCTS

FOUNDATION: ✓ ☺ **TruBlend Liquid Makeup** *($9.39)* is a reformulated version of Cover Girl's original TruBlend Foundation, and the biggest differences are the thinner texture and reduced coverage. The original formula dispensed somewhat thick and then softened eventually, feeling quite light upon application and providing even coverage. This reformulation remains a formidable makeup that exemplifies just how natural a foundation can look on skin. Procter & Gamble's pigment technology allows this makeup to cover minor flaws and even your skin tone without looking obvious (though just to be clear, no one will think you've gone barefaced). This is indicative of what today's best foundations can accomplish, and although this is a very good foundation, Cover Girl's version isn't the only choice. The tricky aspect of this particular makeup is choosing a shade. That's true for any foundation, but Cover Girl tends to have more unnatural colors than its competitors, especially L'Oreal. Some of the lightest TruBlend shades go on an unattractive grayish pink, while others in the medium skin-tone range are blatantly pink to rose. None of the following shades is recommended: Natural Ivory 415 (Cover Girl maintains this is the shade that actress Drew Barrymore wears in their ads, but there is no way this would match her skin tone), Classic Beige 430, Medium Light 435, Natural Beige 440, Creamy Beige 450, and Toasted Almond 470. The other nine shades are worth considering, and include options for fair and dark skin tones. Cover Girl's numbering system of 1 through 6 is designed to make it easier for you to pair the products in the "Tru" line of products with each other. However, if you don't want to remain exclusive to this range of products (which is probably wise), it becomes a superfluous rating system.

✓ ☺ **TruBlend Whipped Foundation** *($9.60)* has a delicately whipped, slightly creamy texture that floats onto skin and feels gossamer light. Blending progresses very well and it sets to a natural matte finish with a hint of luminosity (not the sparkling or shiny kind). As with Cover Girl's original TruBlend Foundation, most of this version's shades are versatile, meaning you will likely find that, because of the pigment technology they use, you can wear two or three shades without looking unnatural. Among the 15 colors are excellent options for fair to dark skin tones. The only shades to avoid due to overtones of pink, peach, or copper are Natural Ivory, Creamy Beige, Toasted Almond, and Natural Beige (after all, whose skin resembles these shades?). This silicone-in-water foundation is best for normal to slightly dry or slightly oily skin. It's workable for those with dry skin provided you apply a moisturizing sunscreen first.

✓ ☺ **TruBlend Minerals Pressed Mineral Foundation** *($9.39)* isn't a traditional "mineral" foundation because it does not contain the types of minerals (such as bismuth oxychloride or zinc oxide) that show up in the niche, overly hyped mineral makeup lines. It is predominantly mica and talc, which are, in fact, minerals, so the name isn't misleading. In contrast to standard mineral makeup, this pressed-powder foundation has a buttery smooth texture that blends seamlessly with skin, producing a non-sparkling natural matte finish. Layering it for more coverage results in a drier-looking finish, but this doesn't feel as thick as many other mineral makeups. It is a very good option for normal to oily skin prone to blemishes. There are six shades available, most of which resemble real skin tones. Be careful with Natural Beige—unless blended on sheer, it is simply too pink. One more thing: The brush that comes packaged with this powder is too small for practical use, and doesn't feel great on skin either.

☺ **TruBlend Microminerals Foundation** *($11.99)* is packaged with a powder brush on the top and a mineral powder foundation on the bottom. The included brush is cheap, feels rough, and is not recommended for applying powder. It also splays when you try to replace it into its storage cap, thus damaging the bristles. This mineral powder, which Cover Girl advertises as being "5 times finer than other leading mineral foundations," is nothing more than a standard blend of talc and mica, something found in countless other powders. It goes on sheer and dry and provides minimal coverage. The powder packaging is messy because the narrow opening of the sifter/dispenser makes it nearly impossible to get powder out without also getting it all over your vanity. That's a lot of hassle for a below-average mineral foundation. If you're still dying to try this foundation, be aware that every shade except 405 Ivory tends toward orange. Really, if you want "mineral" in the name of your product, consider Neutrogena's Mineral Sheer with SPF 20; it has every benefit this one doesn't.

CONCEALER: ☺ **TruConceal Concealer** *($7.49)* is identical in every respect except in name to Cover Girl's longstanding Invisible Concealer. That means the formula still lags behind what most other mainstream makeup companies are doing with their concealers, and the shades still aren't impressive. Among the six choices, the only good ones are TruConceal 5 and 6. Shade number 1 may work for some fair skin tones, but will be too pink for others. Invisible Concealer is still in stores and is still being showcased on Cover Girl's Web site next to this new option, but I suspect this will soon change.

POWDER: ✓ ☺ **TruBlend Pressed Powder** *($7.99)* continues the remarkable pigment technology introduced with Cover Girl's TruBlend Foundation. This talc-based powder has a silky-smooth, slightly thick texture that meshes so well with skin you won't know you're wearing powder. Instead, the skin looks refined and finished rather than pasty or dry, an effect that is flattering on all skin types. Six very good shades are available, and they're versatile enough to work for many skin tones within their respective range. Somehow, the pigments in this powder simply enhance skin without changing its natural color. This is good news, because it means you're not likely to make a mistake choosing a shade—just pick something that looks close to your skin tone and you should be all set (unless skin is very fair or dark, in which case you should turn to the pressed-powder options from L'Oreal or Revlon before Cover Girl TruBlend).

☺ **TruBlend Naturally Luminous Loose Powder** *($7.99)* gets its luminosity from the finely milled sparkles it contains, though they don't cling well to skin so the luminous finish is short-lived. This is otherwise an airy, dry-textured, talc-based loose powder that imparts very sheer color from its four shades (most of which look brazenly peach to orange in the container but not on skin). Its soft finish looks fairly natural on skin, too, and it's a good option if you need a sheer loose powder but don't require lots of oil absorption.

☺ **TruBlend Microminerals Finishing Veil** *($10.99)* is supposed to provide an air-brushed finish when used over Cover Girl's TruBlend Microminerals Foundation. The formulas of these two loose powders are nearly identical; the Finishing Veil is practically colorless and provides a sheer satin finish. Although it does enliven the complexion (especially if your powder foundation is too matte), most will find it superfluous. The included brush is scratchy and tends to splay when you recap the product, which isn't helpful; you can easily discard the brush without missing it. In terms of "minerals," this talc-based powder is no more mineral laden than anyone else's.

BLUSH AND BRONZER: ☺ **TruBlend Naturally Luminous Blush** *($8.09)* has the exact same formula as the TruBlend Naturally Luminous Loose Powder, except this version comes in two sheer blush shades, neither of which does much to impart noticeable cheek color. This is best used as a highlighting powder paired with a standard powder blush, though the two shades are limited to those with fair to light skin.

☺ **TruBlend Naturally Luminous Bronzer** *($7.99)* has the exact same formula as the Tru-Blend Naturally Luminous Loose Powder, except this version comes in two sheer, bronze-toned shades, both suitable for fair to medium skin tones. The shine is more apparent with this powder when compared with the other two TruBlend powders, and it has the same problem of not clinging well. However, the sheer hint of tan can be attractive and the shine isn't so distracting as to make this an evening-only product.

☺ **TruBlend Microminerals Bronzer** *($10.99)* has a nearly identical formula to that of Cover Girl's other TruBlend Microminerals products. It is talc-based and applied with a built-in brush that most of you will find too scratchy (plus the brush splays whenever you replace the cap that it's attached to). The powder itself provides more shine than bronze color, and the shine tends to cling poorly. At best, this is a messy way to use an average bronzing powder. In terms of "minerals," this powder is no more mineral laden than anyone else's.

☹ **TruBlend Microminerals Blush** *($11.49)* comes in the same terrible packaging as the other TruBlend Mineral products. It includes the same shoddy brush, which is too scratchy to use on the face and splays when you try to put it back in the lid; plus the messy sifter bottom with a small opening that makes getting to the blush without making a mess on your bathroom counter an unnecessary challenge. If all this doesn't deter you, the dry, powdery texture of this shimmery blush will. The minerals in this product are primarily mica and talc, which you can find in dozens of other, far better powder blushes. Pass on this dud from Cover Girl and select any number of better options available from L'Oreal Paris, Jane, or Rimmel.

☹ **TruCheeks Blush** *($7.49)* shares the same formula as Cover Girl's longstanding Instant Cheekbones. That means you get a somewhat dry, flaky texture that applies very sheer (you really need to layer this to get a color payoff) and includes colors for blushing and highlighting the cheek area. What's most unsettling and almost noxious is the Noxzema-like smell from the ingredients camphor, clove oil, menthol, and eucalyptus, all of which are skin irritants; I know of no other blush outside the Cover Girl line that uses them—which makes everyone else's powder blushes automatically preferred to this one.

LIPSTICK: ☺ **TruShine Lipcolor** *($6.99)* is a moderate-coverage, smooth cream lipstick with a soft gloss finish. The selling point is Cover Girl's claim that the shade range matches 97% of skin tones. That's not surprising, nor is it a marvel of chemistry, because the selection of warm and cool tones coordinates well with a multitude of skin tones and colors. Basically, the shade range is a can't-go-wrong mix of classic neutrals, reds, pinks, plums, and coral hues, most offset by a slight shimmer finish. The deeper shades have more staying power thanks to their pigmentation, while the pastel shades tend to fade quickly. The slippery finish of this lipstick ensures movement into lines around the mouth, but if that's not an issue for you, this is yet another cream lipstick to consider.

OTHER COVER GIRL PRODUCTS

FOUNDATION: ☺ **Fresh Complexion Pocket Powder** *($7.77)* maintains that it will provide "fresh coverage that lasts," but they should have inserted the adjective "sheer" because this talc-based, pressed-powder foundation barely registers on the skin in terms of coverage. It does have a velvety texture that never looks dry or powdery, but the finish almost leaves a glow on the skin: not something those with oily skin have on their makeup checklist. It's best for normal to dry skin that doesn't need to hide anything, but you won't net any lasting shine control with this product. The 15 shades present some visibly pink and peach colors, but the sheerness makes the color almost irrelevant. The ones to use with caution are Buff Beige, Natural Beige, Medium Light, and Classic Beige. Fair to light skin tones have the best chance of finding a perfect shade, while dark skin tones should look elsewhere.

☺ **Advanced Radiance Age-Defying Liquid Makeup SPF 10** *($11.99)* gets its sunscreen rating partially from titanium dioxide, so it's sad that the SPF number is too low to rely on for daytime protection. Even more disturbing is Cover Girl's "restores youthful appearance" claims, which would have resonated better with an SPF 15 sunscreen. There is no question you'll be impressed with the airy-yet-creamy texture of this smooth-blending foundation. It blends on easily, providing sheer to light coverage and a radiant finish that enlivens the skin's appearance. Despite the creamy feel, this isn't the best formula for someone with dry skin because the base of silicone and glycerin combined with talc won't be enough to make dryness look or feel better. However, this is an option if you pair it with a moisturizing sunscreen rated SPF 15 or higher. Cover Girl's selection of 14 shades is mostly impressive and includes choices for fair to dark (but not very dark) skin tones. The following shades are best avoided due to overtones of peach, pink, and red: Natural Ivory (which has enough pink to qualify as a blush), Classic Beige, Natural Beige, Creamy Beige, and Toasted Almond. This foundation does contain the Olay ingredients (remember, Cover Girl and Olay are owned by Procter & Gamble) niacinamide and palmitoyl pentapeptide-3, which is a nice touch, but what a shame the SPF rating falls short of the desired SPF 15.

☺ **Ultimate Finish Liquid Powder Makeup** *($7.77)* is a below-standard, very dated cream-to-powder foundation. It smooths on OK but the high amount of aluminum starch octenylsuccinate causes it to dry almost instantly, and it can feel uncomfortably matte. Ultimately, this is workable only for those with oily skin not prone to blemishes, because the waxlike thickeners in this product certainly won't promote clear skin. The 15 shades are packaged so you can see the color, but remain a mixed bag; eight of them are too glaringly peach, pink, or rose for most skin tones, so you should avoid Natural Ivory, Creamy Natural, Classic Beige, Medium Light, Warm Beige, Creamy Beige, Natural Beige, and Toasted Almond. Soft Sable and Tawny are worthwhile shades for darker skin tones, but Cover Girl's AquaSmooth Makeup SPF 15 or their Advanced Radiance Age-Defying Compact Foundation are assuredly preferred to this.

☹ **Cover Girl & Olay Simply Ageless Foundation SPF 22** *($14.99)*. Just when I thought I'd seen everything, Olay and Cover Girl (both owned by Procter & Gamble) have launched a foundation with both companies' names on the label. Wow! I wonder if Olay is positioning itself to combine the two lines under one name, sort of like the name change Olay did several years back when it went from Oil of Olay to just Olay. Other than that I have no idea what this marketing maneuver is about. But marketing is not the reason to buy a product. This new foundation is supposed to combine the benefits of Olay Regenerist Serum in a foundation with sunscreen. The claim is that it can stay suspended above wrinkles, covering them evenly without seeping into lines and not clogging pores. Well, don't count on it. The only two redeeming qualities of this foundation are (1) the spokesperson is Ellen DeGeneres (though clearly she's being paid a lot of money for this endorsement, and I doubt that she could possibly believe this product has any merit), and (2) the sponge that's included in the packaging is good for blending. Seriously, that's it; it's all downhill from there. This cream foundation blended with Olay Regenerist serum is all gimmick and hype. The creamy texture is difficult to blend, even with the included sponge, feels greasy on the skin, and sets easily into lines and wrinkles, leaving your face with a heavy and cakey made-up look. If this doesn't clog pores, I don't know what will. Cover Girl & Olay Simply Ageless Foundation SPF 22 isn't recommended for any skin type.

☹ **Simply Powder Foundation** *($7.77)* claims it "covers like a liquid," and it may seem convenient to get that benefit from a powder. Don't bother. This talc-based pressed-powder foundation goes on unevenly, looks chalky, and isn't nearly as silky as Cover Girl's superior TruBlend Pressed Powder. The shades are also mostly problematic, because with the texture and finish this has, even the neutral options just don't look convincing on skin.

CONCEALER: ☺ **Fresh Complexion Concealer** *($5.50)* is the only Cover Girl concealer to seriously consider. It has a wonderful, lightly creamy texture and a soft application that provides almost too much slip. Although blending this concealer takes a bit more time, the natural matte finish and smooth coverage are worth it. This wouldn't be my top choice if your main concern is great coverage, but those with minor imperfections should check it out. Of the four colors, only Natural Beige is too pink to purchase, but be careful with the slightly pink Creamy Beige, too.

☺ **Invisible Concealer** *($4.53)* has a formula and mostly poor colors that have caused it to fall out of favor as a recommended concealer. It provides adequate coverage but has a somewhat tacky finish that isn't as elegant as today's best liquid, wand-applicator concealers. Among the five shades, only the darker ones (Honey and Tawny) are workable.

POWDER: ✓ ☺ **Advanced Radiance Age-Defying Pressed Powder** *($8.05)* has a formula, texture, and finish that are identical to those of the TruBlend Pressed Powder, so the same basic comments apply. Six shades are available, and there's not a bad one in the bunch. Both this and the TruBlend Pressed Powder are wonderful for all but very oily skin—because that will need more shine control than these powders are capable of providing.

☺ **Fresh Look Pressed Powder** *($5.99)* deserves a compliment for its smooth texture and lightweight matte finish, but tends to look dry on skin, creating a flatness that doesn't translate to a fresh complexion. It's best dusted on sheer, and is a reasonably good option for those with oily skin, plus all six colors are soft and neutral.

☹ **Professional Loose Powder** *($5.50)* comes in six mostly well-conceived shades and has a fine texture, but that is canceled out by the pointless inclusion of eucalyptus, camphor, clove oil, and menthol—four potent irritants—and the sickly sweet fragrance.

BLUSH AND BRONZER: ☺ **Cover Girl & Olay Simply Ageless Sculpting Blush** *($10.99)* continues the marriage of Olay and Cover Girl in one product, which in this instance paid off. Olay's contribution of niacinamide and acetyl glucosamine certainly goes well beyond what a standard cream-to-powder blush can offer, and in this case these ingredients (neither of which are air/light-sensitive) will indeed give skin an extra boost. Better still, the product works quite nicely as a blush, coming in four versatile shades that are best suited for light to medium skin tones. Housed in a flat, jar-like package, the product applies a bit greasy, but this allows adequate time for blending (the product's claim of "sculpting" seems a stretch, especially considering the tones all hover around pink and peach). Once it sets to a soft powder finish, the results are natural and lasting—though not "ageless," of course!

☺ **Cheekers Bronzer** *(4.29)* This pressed bronzing powder comes in one shade: Golden Tan, which is too gold to look convincing as bronzer. The slightly waxy texture isn't the greatest, but it applies OK and leaves a shiny finish.

☺ **Tanfastic Bronzer** *($6.53)* is a pressed, talc-based bronzing powder that comes in two sheer tan shades best for fair to light skin. The dry texture isn't as elegant as many others, likely due to the calcium silicate (the second ingredient) that compromises chances for attaining a silkier feel. It's an OK option, but the bronzing powders from Wet 'n' Wild are nicer and cost less (though Cover Girl's price is nothing to scoff at).

☹ **Cheekers** *($4)* are finally updated in a palette of contemporary shades, but have a terribly dry, flaky texture that sweeps on unevenly, creating a blotchy look.

☹ **Classic Color Blush** *($5.69)* is a powder blush that comes in four shades that, although vivid, blend on sheer. These are fairly powdery, and the color intensity is too soft for darker skin tones.

☹ **Instant Cheekbones** *($5.50)* has three colors in one compact—a blush tone, a contour color, and a shiny highlighter. The colors for these and for the single blush version, Cheekers, finally are an updated palette of contemporary shades, but have a terribly dry, flaky texture that sweeps on unevenly, creating a blotchy look.

EYESHADOW: ☹ **Eye Enhancers 1-Kit Shadows** *($3.49)* have a nonsense name because one color (or one of anything) does not make a kit. Each shade has a smooth, unusually dry texture that imparts sheer color, but not without some flaking and skipping during application. Again, these apply very sheer—even the black shade goes on almost translucent. Compared to powder eyeshadows from L'Oreal, Sonia Kashuk, and Jane, these really aren't worth considering.

☹ **Eye Enhancers 3-Kit Shadows** *($5.49)* have some potentially workable color combinations (and some real duds), but also have the same formula and application issues as the Eye Enhancers 1-Kit Shadows.

☹ **Eye Enhancers 4-Kit Shadows** *($5.49)* have some potentially workable color combinations (and some real duds), but also have the same formula and application issues as the Eye Enhancers 1-Kit Shadows.

EYE AND BROW PRODUCTS: ☺ **CG Eyeslicks Gel Eyecolor** *($5.49)* consists of chubby pencils that go on somewhat wet, which means they glide on easily, and then the color dries to a matte (in feel) finish that doesn't budge or smear all day. Because of the wider pencil head, you can't draw a thin line. In addition, all of the shades are shiny, so these are best used on smooth, taut eyelids for a shadowy effect or on the under-brow area to highlight. Oddly, despite budge-proof wear, this comes off immediately with just water, so don't get caught in the rain!

☺ **Perfect Point Plus** *($4.99)* is an automatic eye pencil that glides on easily without being greasy, and it maintains a consistent, sharp point. Chestnut is a great shade as an auburn eyeliner, but Midnight Blue is best avoided. Avoid using the smudge tip—it's not well made and can change your eye makeup look from smoky to messy.

☹ **Brow and Eye Makers** *($2.99)* feature two short pencils that are the same color. You're supposed to use one for eyes and one for brows, but the dry, waxy texture makes both of them more appropriate for use as a brow pencil, albeit not a very good one. That's because application can be painful and the finish is tacky enough to be bothersome.

☺ **Perfect Blend Eye Pencil** *($4.53)* hasn't changed since it was last reviewed. It remains a standard but good pencil that goes on slightly drier than most others and has decent staying power. There are six shades, and all come with a sponge tip to ease blending. Avoid Cobalt Blue.

LIPSTICK AND LIPLINER: ☺ **Continuous Color Lipstick** *($5.70)* is available in a Creme or Shimmer finish, with the Creme version being preferred for its smoother texture and the fact that the shimmer in the Shimmer version tends to feel grainy as the lipstick's creaminess wears off. Both formulas feel emollient and last decently without feathering into lines around the mouth.

☺ **IncrediFULL Lip Color** *($6.99)* follows a trend in the cosmetics industry in which makeup products are positioned as going beyond what is typically expected for their category. This lipstick is a great example. Rather than just positioning it as a creamy, "all-day moisturizing" lipstick with rich color, Cover Girl's angle is to address the needs of women concerned with lips that become thinner with age. IncrediFULL is said to plump lips and add volume, and they even go so far as to proclaim it enhances the natural lip line! The ingredients allegedly responsible for such effects are vitamin E and various B vitamins, including niacinamide. This lipstick also contains an appreciable amount of glycerin, which helps attract moisture to the lips and keep it there, temporarily making them appear fuller. The amount of vitamins in this lipstick is negligible relative to the other standard ingredients, and vitamins won't add volume to lips, at least not in any way close to what collagen or hyaluronic acid dermal injections can accomplish. But that doesn't mean this isn't a worthwhile lipstick. It has a wonderfully creamy feel and imparts opaque color that doesn't feel thick or greasy, although the formula is slick enough to feather into lines around the mouth. The shade selection favors pinks and reds, so unless you're looking for soft, sheer colors, most of the options are attractive.

☺ **LipSlicks Lipgloss** *($3.99)* is a basic, emollient, castor oil–based sheer lipstick with some very shiny shades, all in packaging that makes getting it on the lips very tricky for anyone with thin lips.

☺ **Wetslicks Fruit Spritzers** *($5.93)* smell and taste like fruit, and all of the sheer, shimmer-infused shades coat lips with a juicy shine and non-sticky, thick-but-smooth texture. This tube lip gloss is an option if you're looking for soft, sparkling colors; however, the flavor may make you lick your lips more often, which means more frequent touch-ups (not to mention that ingesting extra lip gloss isn't necessarily the best idea).

☺ **Wetslicks Lip Gloss** *($5.93)* is a gloss to consider if you're a fan of sparkly lip gloss and prefer a smooth, non-goopy texture that doesn't make lips feel like they're coated in caramel.

☹ **Wetslicks AmazeMint** *($6.25)* comes in some enticing, shimmer-infused sheer colors, but the advertisement about it containing Crest peppermint oil is not to be taken lightly! This irritating gloss tingles immediately and keeps on tingling, a sure sign that your lips are being irritated. The mint aroma is also unmistakable, and may entice you to continually lick your lips—not a good idea. By the way, Crest is another of the many brands (including Cover Girl) that are owned by Procter & Gamble.

MASCARA: ☺ **Fantastic Lash Mascara, Curved Brush** *($6.99)* marks one of the few times where I noticed the curved brush makes a difference for the better. With some effort, you can build long, reasonably thick lashes with minor, easily fixed clumping. It also leaves lashes softly curled, and wears well, making it Cover Girl's overall best mascara.

☺ **Professional Mascara Classic Look Curved Brush** *($4.99)* makes lashes longer but not the least bit thick. It separates and defines without clumping, though it takes a bit of practice with the curved brush to get an even application.

☺ **Professional Remarkable Washable Waterproof Mascara** *($4.99)* applies evenly and builds good length with minimal thickness. It isn't as waterproof as others, withstanding only a little water (such as a light rain) and breaking down underwater—so swimmers and criers will have to look elsewhere. True to its name, it does wash off easily—but that's the trade-off for a formula that isn't as waterproof as most others.

☺ **Professional Super Thick Lash Mascara** *($5.29)* does well as a lengthening mascara, easily elongating lashes without clumps. Despite the name, it builds modest thickness, but is best as a lengthening mascara that leaves lashes softly fringed.

☺ **Professional Waterproof Mascara** *($4.99)* has a formula that applies easily and with some effort builds noticeable length and minimal thickness. Best of all, it really does hold up when wet yet is easy to remove, coming off almost completely with just a water-soluble cleanser.

☺ **Fantastic Lash Mascara** *($6.90)* claims to provide five times the volume of ordinary lashes, which would really be fantastic, but it doesn't deliver. Instead, it excels at creating long (but not impressively long), separated lashes. If you want truly fantastic mascara, you'll have to look to L'Oreal or Maybelline, because Cover Girl's options fall short of fantastic.

☺ **Marathon Waterproof Mascara** *($5.49)* is Cover Girl's most impressive waterproof mascara in terms of how tenaciously waterproof it is, but the lengthened, wet look it creates isn't for everyone, and there's some clumping along the way. This is extremely difficult to remove, even with an oil- or silicone-based remover. It definitely turns your nightly cleansing routine into a marathon of its own.

☺ **Professional Mascara Classic Look Straight Brush** *($4.99)* has an easier-to-wield wand than the curved version (though I suspect some women like curved brushes, whereas I find them awkward), but this version builds lengthy lashes unevenly and needs more fine-tuning than it should.

☺ **Professional Natural Lash Mascara** *($5.33)* is just a clear, boring mascara that does incredibly little to enhance lashes, and is best used as a soft-finish brow gel. Cover Girl claims this mascara is smudgeproof, but this claim is meaningless—the product is clear, so what difference does it make if some smudging occurs?

☹ **Fantastic Lash Waterproof Mascara** *($6.99)* is fantastically mediocre for length and thickness, although it is waterproof. Still, there are plenty of waterproof mascaras (including others from Cover Girl) that do not flake and smear the way this one does, making Fantastic Lash Waterproof Mascara one to ignore.

BRUSHES: ☺ **Eyeshadow Brush** *($4.53)* isn't the most versatile due to its thickness, and if you're only going to offer one eyeshadow brush, it should be flatter and a bit more pointed for better control and blending. This remains an OK option for applying allover or soft crease color.

☹ **Large Blush Brush** *($4.99)* is a poorly constructed brush that is not recommended because the bristles are too soft and too sparse, making color placement and control an issue.

☹ **Powder Brush** *($5.69)* is cut straight across rather than domed or tapered, a shape that tends to work against the natural contours of the face and makes it easy to overpowder.

DARPHIN PARIS (SKIN CARE ONLY)

DARPHIN PARIS AT-A-GLANCE

Strengths: Lauder's influence on this line has resulted in only a few improved products; there are some good cleansers; some worthwhile serums and moisturizers.

Weaknesses: Very expensive; no products to address acne or pigmentation issues; only one sunscreen and it has problems; jar packaging for products that contain air- and light-sensitive ingredients.

For more information about Darphin Paris, owned by Estee Lauder, call (866) 880-4559 or visit www.darphin.com or www.Beautypedia.com.

DARPHIN PARIS AROVITA PRODUCTS

☺ **$$$ Arovita C Energic Firming Cream** *($110 for 1.7 ounces)* is an emollient moisturizer for dry skin that contains some very good skin-identical ingredients, but the vitamin C and other antioxidants won't last long after this jar-packaged product is opened. As expected, this will not firm skin. One of the main plant extracts is morinda (listed as *Morinda citrifolia*). You may be more familiar with this plant's common name of noni (it is sold as a juice and in supplement form with dozens of unsubstantiated health-related claims). There is no research proving morinda can help aging skin in any way, but it doesn't appear to be a cause for concern either, at least when it comes to topical application.

☺ **$$$ Arovita C Line Response Cream** *($110 for 1.7 ounces)* is actually a much more exciting formula than the Arovita C Energic Firming Cream, so it's that much more disappointing that jar packaging limits the effectiveness of the light- and air-sensitive powerhouse ingredients that are in here. Given the poor packaging choice, this ends up being a needlessly pricey moisturizer for normal to dry skin.

☺ **$$$ Arovita C Line Response Firming Serum** *($125 for 1 ounce)* is a serum version of the Arovita C Line Response Cream. It contains some noteworthy antioxidants, skin-identical ingredients, and cell-communicating ingredients, but its translucent glass bottle packaging means the vitamin C and other antioxidants are subject to deterioration unless this is kept stored in a dark place and away from sources of natural light. It is suitable for normal to slightly dry skin that is not prone to breakouts.

☺ **$$$ Arovita C Line Response Fluid** *($110 for 1.7 ounces)* is very similar to the Arovita C Line Response Firming Serum above, and the same review applies.

☹ **Arovita Eye and Lip Contour Gel** *($85 for 1 ounce)* contains several fragrance components that can be irritating to skin, but especially so when used around the eyes. This water- and jojoba oil–based gel is not recommended.

DARPHIN PARIS CLEAR WHITE PRODUCTS

☺ **$$$ Clear White Brightening and Hydrating Cream** *($120 for 1.7 ounces)* costs a lot of money for a product that contains only a small amount of ingredients capable of lightening sun-induced skin discolorations. Even more troubling is the jar packaging, because routine exposure to light and air won't keep the many plant extracts and vitamin C derivative this contains stable during use. This is merely an overpriced moisturizer for normal to dry skin; any whitening you get is accidental. If you're serious about lightening skin discolorations, you should consider over-the-counter or prescription products that contain hydroquinone or arbutin (in stable packaging, of course).

☺ **$$$ Clear White Brightening and Soothing Serum** *($140 for 1 ounce)* definitely shows Lauder's influence on Darphin since they acquired the company. Many of the ingredients Lauder includes in their other products (which cost less than those from Darphin) also are included in this serum—but can any of them lighten skin discolorations? Although this silicone-enhanced serum comes in stable, opaque packaging, the plant extracts and vitamin C ingredient (ascorbyl glucoside) have limited research pertaining to their effectiveness on hyperpigmentation. The amount of ascorbyl glucoside in this serum may be effective, but for the money, I'd remain skeptical of the results and would rather invest in a prescription for Tri-Luma (which costs less than this and has a good deal of published research showing it works). At least with Tri-Luma you're getting a reliable skin-lightening agent coupled with a retinoid that not only helps the skin-lightening agent work better, but also stimulates collagen production for younger-looking skin. This serum does contain fragrance that may cause irritation.

DARPHIN FIBROGENE PRODUCTS

☺ **$$$ Fibrogene Line Response Nourishing Balm** *($150 for 1.7 ounces)* has an astronomical price for what amounts to an overly fragranced, very emollient, basic moisturizer for dry to very dry skin. Ingredients such as shea butter, glycerin, and vegetable oil are worthwhile for making dry skin a thing of the past, but they cannot deter signs of premature aging as claimed and they are standard in dozens of less expensive options. The only product that can legitimately make the claim of deterring premature "aging" is sunscreen (because the sun is the only thing that causes premature aging), and sunscreen is something this product lacks. Beyond the faulty antiaging claims, it deserves mention that the many fragrant components in this product can be irritating, and that's not what dry skin (or any skin for that matter) needs to look and feel better. And again, the price is way (way) out of line for what you get. If shea butter is your thing, consider the many less expensive shea-butter-loaded products from L'Occitane. Those looking to spend a lot less for a good moisturizer for very dry skin should consider CeraVe Moisturizer at the drugstore.

☹ **Fibrogene Line Response Nourishing Cream** *($150 for 1.7 ounces).* Without even saying a word about the price or formula, a major offense of this dry-skin moisturizer is the jar packaging. For $150, you should expect and get a product packaged to keep its light- and air-sensitive ingredients stable. Packaging aside (though it can never be disregarded when it comes to making a decision about great skin care), this moisturizer has a richly emollient texture and contains a roster of beneficial ingredients, but there are troubling ingredients as well. The problematic ingredients include several fragrance chemicals known to cause irritation and an assuredly irritating amount of fragrant coriander oil. Coriander can cause a phototoxic reaction in the presence of sunlight and is also known to cause contact dermatitis (Source: www. naturaldatabase.com). Coriander may contribute a pleasant fragrance to this moisturizer, but it's not going to help your skin.

☹ **Fibrogene Line Response Nourishing Serum** *($165 for 1 ounce)* is a product with a texture much closer to a moisturizer than a serum, and contains several beneficial ingredients that show Lauder's influence on Darphin's formulas (Estee Lauder Corporation acquired the brand a few years ago). Unlike many Lauder moisturizers this contains several volatile fragrance chemicals known to cause irritation. It also contains an assuredly irritating amount of fragrant coriander oil. Coriander can cause a phototoxic reaction in the presence of sunlight and is also known to cause contact dermatitis (Source: www.naturaldatabase.com). How important is an "exquisitely scented" product if the fragrance isn't doing your skin any favors? From a marketing point of view I suspect Lauder's execs figured scent was more important than the quality of the product.

DARPHIN PARIS HYDRASKIN PRODUCTS

☺ **$$$ Hydraskin Intensive Moisturizing Serum** *($90 for 1 ounce)* contains mostly water, slip agents, plant oil, glycerin, gemstone extract, antioxidants, water-binding agents, preservative, vitamin E, film-forming agents, fragrance, and potentially irritating fragrance components. It's an OK lightweight moisturizer for normal to oily skin, but for the money not nearly as elegant as the serum-type moisturizers from Estee Lauder or Clinique.

☺ **$$$ Hydraskin Light** *($85 for 1.7 ounces)* is a good lightweight, silicone-enhanced moisturizer for normal to slightly oily skin, but the jar packaging won't keep the plant-based antioxidants stable once the product is opened. This does contain potentially irritating fragrance components.

The Reviews D

☹ **Hydraskin Night** *($90 for 1.7 ounces)* contains irritating horsetail extract (listed by its Latin name of *Equisetum arvense*) as well as irritating fragrance components of eugenol, isoeugenol, linalool, and geraniol, among others.

☺ **$$$ Hydraskin Rich** *($85 for 1.7 ounces)* works well for dry to very dry skin, but so do many other moisturizers that not only cost less but use packaging that will keep the antioxidants stable while excluding potentially irritating fragrance components.

DARPHIN PARIS INTRAL PRODUCTS

☺ **$$$ Intral Cleansing Milk** *($50 for 6.7 ounces)* is a lighter version of Darphin's Cleansing Aromatic Emulsion, and is better suited for those with normal to slightly dry skin not prone to breakouts. This still ends up being a lot of money for a standard detergent-free cleansing lotion.

☺ **$$$ Intral Toner** *($50 for 6.7 ounces)* is a basic, alcohol- and fragrance-free toner that contains some good water-binding and soothing agents. It is recommended for normal to dry skin, but so is Neutrogena Alcohol-Free Toner.

☺ **$$$ Intral Redness Relief Recovery Cream** *($90 for 1.7 ounces)* is a well-intentioned moisturizer, but it isn't the boon for sensitive, reddened skin it's made out to be. Darphin's Intral Mask is a much better choice because it omits fragrance and contains a far better mix of ingredients, or you can look to several fragrance-free products from drugstore lines like CeraVe or Eucerin. This moisturizer is nothing more than an ordinary option for normal to dry skin, but relief is not what it provides, and the price is out of line for what you're (not) getting. Talk about not getting relief!

☺ **$$$ Intral Redness Relief Soothing Serum** *($110 for 1 ounce)*. The selection of plant extracts in this water-based serum is mostly helpful for sensitive skin. Peony root extract is slightly suspect due to its potential to cause contact dermatitis, but the root contains a chemical (paeoniflorin) that has anti-inflammatory activity, including promoting collagen, although this effect has not been tied to topical application (Source: www.naturaldatabase.com). Darphin includes some good skin-identical ingredients and antioxidants, but a serum designed for sensitive skin shouldn't contain fragrance or coloring agents as this one does. The formula isn't impressive enough to warrant its price tag or a Paula's Pick rating. It can be used by all skin types except sensitive.

☺ **$$$ Intral Soothing Creme** *($90 for 1.7 ounces)* is designed for sensitive skin, but isn't as "exceptionally gentle" and "non-irritating" as it could've been. It contains fragrant plants and a fragrance chemical (citronellol) that has the potential to cause irritation. Another questionable, but likely innocuous, ingredient is peony root. The root contains a chemical (paeoniflorin) that has anti-inflammatory activity, including promoting collagen production, although this effect has not been tied to topical application (Source: www.naturaldatabase.com). This moisturizer is good for dry skin but there are better, less expensive moisturizers to consider from various department store and spa lines.

☺ **$$$ Intral Mask** *($65 for 1.7 ounces)* is a good, albeit pricey, moisturizing mask for dry to very dry skin. It is loaded with helpful emollients, soothing plants, and water-binding agents. It is also fragrance-free, which is highly unusual for a Darphin product. To get your money's worth, it's best to leave this mask on your skin as long as possible (overnight is fine) rather than remove it after several minutes, because in essence this is just a good moisturizer.

DARPHIN PARIS PREDERMINE PRODUCTS

☹ **Predermine Cream** *($185 for 1.7 ounces)* has the most rudimentary base formula that ends up being an overpriced showcase for tiny amounts of skin-identical ingredients and some problematic plant extracts, along with 14 volatile fragrance component ingredients that add up to trouble for most skin types.

☹ **Predermine Serum** *($325 for 1 ounce)* doesn't contain a single ingredient that even remotely justifies its price, nor can anything in this product boost natural collagen production better than other products. It's an average water-based serum that contains problematic horsetail, jasmine, and iris extracts along with over a dozen fragrance components, most of which are considered skin sensitizers. I don't know whom to recommend this to except those who like spending a lot for a potentially troublesome return on their investment.

☺ **$$$ Predermine Wrinkle Corrective Serum** *($205 for 1 ounce)* is one of the best formulations in Darphin's lineup, with ingredients that mimic the structure and function of healthy skin. Although this product deserves its rating because of the plethora of state-of-the-art ingredients it contains, you should know that nearly identical products are available from Clinique's Repairwear line and from Estee Lauder's Perfectionist line. Along with Darphin, these are all Lauder-owned lines. Whichever product you purchase will produce good results, but won't eliminate wrinkles. If anything, Darphin's option ends up being less impressive because of the volatile fragrance components it contains (a factor that also keeps it from earning a Paula's Pick rating).

☹ **Predermine Mask** *($85 for 1.7 ounces)* is a below-standard, ridiculously expensive clay mask that irritates skin by including iris and horsetail extracts.

DARPHIN PARIS STIMULSKIN PRODUCTS

☺ **$$$ Stimulskin Plus Eye Contour Cream** *($135 for 0.5 ounce)* has some wonderful ingredients for dry to very dry skin around the eyes or elsewhere on the face, but the antioxidants are compromised by jar packaging. Similarly rich moisturizers are widely available for much less money.

☺ **$$$ Stimulskin Plus Firming Smoothing Cream** *($240 for 1.7 ounces)* is similar to, but with fewer bells and whistles than, the Stimulskin Plus Firming Smoothing Cream, for Dry Skin below, and the same basic comments apply. For over $200, the least you should expect is packaging that will keep the retinol stable.

☺ **$$$ Stimulskin Plus Firming Smoothing Cream, for Dry Skin** *($240 for 1.7 ounces)* is loaded with state-of-the-art skin-care ingredients, but the potency of most of them (including retinol) is significantly diminished because of the jar packaging. Even if the packaging were better, however, the fragrant oils are potentially irritating, making this a less desirable option at any price.

☺ **$$$ Stimulskin Plus Intensive Face Lifting Complex** *($370 for 1 ounce)* may sound like a face-lift in a bottle, but doesn't come even a little bit close. This serum contains mostly water, slip agents, castor oil, silicone thickener, skin-identical ingredients, fragrant plant extracts (none capable of lifting or firming skin), antioxidants, alcohol, preservatives, and fragrance. Several of the fragrance components are potentially irritating to skin, and keep this product from earning a better rating. Even without them, this serum pales in comparison to any offered by other Lauder-owned companies.

The Reviews D

☺ **$$$ Stimulskin Plus Rejuvenating Lifting Serum** *($310 for 1 ounce)* is very similar to the Stimulskin Plus Intensive Face Lifting Complex, except with a lower price and more skin-identical ingredients. Otherwise, the same review applies.

OTHER DARPHIN PARIS PRODUCTS

☹ **Azahar Cleansing Micellar Water, All-In-One French Cleanser** *($50 for 6.7 ounces)* has minimal cleansing ability and offers a hefty dose of irritation to your skin (and eyes, if this cleanser gets too close to them) from the bitter-orange oil it contains. The French angle is nothing more than marketing; the French don't know any more about cleansing than any other nationality. And the price! What a joke! There is nothing in this cleanser that makes it worth even $10, let alone $50.

☺ **$$$ Cleansing Aromatic Emulsion** *($50 for 4.2 ounces)* contains tiny amounts of plant extracts, but is overall a very standard water- and mineral oil–based cleanser for normal to dry skin. The aromatic element of this cleanser is what you're paying for, but that's not what's removing makeup or cleansing the skin. This rinses without the need for a washcloth.

☺ **$$$ Purifying Foam Gel, for Combination Oily Skin** *($50 for 4.2 ounces)* contains tiny amounts of plant extracts, none of them problematic. Nothing about this standard water-soluble cleanser is more purifying than most others; it's just an effective, albeit overpriced, option for normal to oily skin.

☺ **$$$ Refreshing Cleansing Milk** *($50 for 6.7 ounces)* is nearly identical to the Intral Cleansing Milk, save for a change in plant extracts, which have no bearing on skin but add fragrance to this cleansing lotion. Otherwise, the same review applies.

☺ **$$$ Rich Cleansing Milk** *($50 for 6.7 ounces)* is actually lighter than the other Darphin Cleansing Milks, although its oil content makes it unsuitable for breakout-prone skin. There are some intriguing antioxidants in this cleanser, but their benefit is quickly rinsed down the drain. It's an otherwise standard cleansing lotion that requires the use of a washcloth for complete removal and is best for normal to slightly dry skin. And the rich price tag? Sheer nonsense!

☹ **Gentle Eye Make-Up Remover** *($45 for 5.1 ounces)* contains fragrant plant extracts with no established benefit for skin and fragrance components, including eugenol and geraniol, neither of which is gentle or suitable for use in the eye area.

☺ **$$$ Exfoliating Foam Gel** *($50 for 4.2 ounces)* is a very standard cleanser/scrub hybrid that contains polyethylene (plastic) beads as the abrasive agent. Although this is workable for normal to oily skin, there is no reason to choose this over topical scrubs from the drugstore unless you steadfastly believe Darphin has all the answers.

☹ **Mild Aroma Peeling** *($55 for 1.7 ounces)* is a paraffin-based mechanical scrub that is a poor option for all skin types because it contains irritating sandalwood oil.

☹ **Purifying Toner** *($50 for 6.7 ounces)* lists alcohol as the second ingredient, which is a shame because this is otherwise a well-formulated toner for all skin types.

☹ **Refreshing Toner** *($50 for 6.7 ounces)* contains a high concentration of fig fruit extract, which is known to cause contact dermatitis due to its psoralen content. Psoralens may also cause reactions when skin is exposed to sunlight.

☺ **$$$ Rich Toner** *($50 for 6.7 ounces)* contains a hefty amount of antioxidant black tea ferment, but the translucent packaging won't keep it potent unless it is kept away from light sources. That's the most exciting aspect of this standard but good (and overpriced) toner for normal to dry skin.

☹ **8 Flower Nectar** *($150 for 0.5 ounce)* is an oil-based product whose main ingredients are indeed helpful for restoring smoothness and lubrication to dry or very dry skin. However, due to the many fragrant oils and fragrant components in this "rare aromatic composition," your skin would be better served with just plain jojoba or sunflower oil (not to mention the money you'll save!). In the long run, this product is more eau de cologne than it is a skin-care product.

☹ **Aromatic Purifying Balm** *($80 for 0.5 ounce)* is a rich blend of hazel seed and vegetable oil along with beeswax and several irritating fragrant oils, including sage, thyme, and lavender. It smells divine, but the fragrant oils are very irritating to skin and won't reduce the appearance of skin imperfections as claimed. If anything, they can make matters worse.

☹ **Aromatic Renewing Balm** *($80 for 0.5 ounce)* is an oil- and wax-based balm that would be much better for any degree of dry skin if the fragrant citrus oils were left out. They certainly make this an aromatic experience, but applying this much fragrance to skin is irritating, not renewing. If this were a cologne it would get high ratings, but fragrance does not make for good skin care.

☹ **Chamomile Aromatic Care** *($80 for 0.5 ounce)* contains several irritating fragrant oils and fragrance components (such as eugenol) that make this a poor choice for all skin types, especially the product's targeted audience of consumers with blotchy, irritated skin.

☺ **$$$ Dark Circles Relief and De-Puffing Eye Serum** *($75 for 0.5 ounce)* would be a good way to see if a product with peptides will work for you, although there is no research proving peptides' mettle for vanquishing dark circles or puffy eyes. The prominence of passion-flower extract in this water-based serum looks impressive—if only it had documented benefit for skin. Research surrounding passionflower's potential benefit for skin did not involve the type Darphin uses, nor did that research have to do with eye-area cosmetic woes. The volatile fragrance components in this gel keep it from earning a higher rating, and may be a problem when this is applied near the eyes.

☹ **Jasmine Aromatic Care** *($105 for 0.5 ounce)* contains several irritating ingredients for any skin type, including limonene, orange oil, and rosewood oil. Rather than risk irritation, why not just treat your dry skin to pure sweet almond oil, which is the main ingredient in this fragrant moisturizer?

☺ **$$$ Lifting and Firming Eye Serum** *($80 for 0.5 ounce)* is an interesting blend of water, slip agents, tree pulp extract (likely functioning as a thickener because there is nothing but anecdotal evidence to support its usefulness for skin care), and some very good skin-identical ingredients and antioxidants. Darphin even left out fragrance components, which is a breath of fresh air given that almost every other product in the line literally stinks with fragrance. This is a worthwhile product for all skin types looking for a lightweight serum. It is not recommended for dry skin around the eyes (you'll want something emollient).

☹ **Myrrh Aromatic Care** *($80 for 0.5 ounce)* follows the same path as most of Darphin's Aromatic Care products and assaults the skin with several irritating volatile oils, including lavender, myrrh, and balsam. This sunflower oil–based moisturizer is not recommended.

☹ **Niaouli Aromatic Care** *($80 for 0.5 ounce)* has the same base as the Myrrh Aromatic Care above, but irritates skin with a potent blend of rosemary, bitter-orange, and lavender oil, among other problematic ingredients. Plain sunflower seed oil is distinctly preferred to this product.

☹ **Rose Aromatic Care** *($80 for 0.5 ounce)* contains irritating volatile fragrant oils, including bay, as well as fragrance components that are not helpful for skin. Using plain sunflower or almond oil to moisturize very dry skin is preferred.

The Reviews D

☺ **$$$ Skin Mat Balancing Serum** *($85 for 1 ounce)* is a water-based serum that contains about 1% salicylic acid, but the pH of 4.7 prevents it from working optimally as an exfoliant, and at this price that's the least you should expect. Although there are some good anti-irritants in this product, it lacks ingredients capable of making good on its claim of absorbing excess oil. The plant extracts it contains do nothing to reduce the appearance of pores, making this lightly moisturizing serum an expensive letdown.

☺ **$$$ Skin Mat Matifying Fluid** *($85 for 1.7 ounces)* is a fairly standard, lightweight moisturizer that helps create a matte finish due to the silicone it contains. The slip agents and thickeners won't keep skin matte for long, but will hydrate slightly dry skin. Although there are some good skin-identical ingredients in this product, it's an overall unimpressive formula for the money and absolutely will not reduce excess oil.

☺ **$$$ Soothing Eye Contour Mask** *($75 for 1 ounce)* would warrant a Paula's Pick rating if it did not contain potentially problematic fragrance components. It's a lightweight gel mask that contains some helpful and truly soothing ingredients as well as antioxidants, plus the cell-communicating ingredient niacinamide. It's an option for all skin types needing mild hydration around the eyes or elsewhere on the face.

☹ **Tangerine Aromatic Care** *($80 for 0.5 ounce)* contains a trio of irritating plant oils, including orange, orange peel, and grapefruit peel. Skip the irritation and the potential for phototoxic reactions and use plain sunflower or jojoba oil if your skin is very dry.

☺ **$$$ Vitabalm** *($25 for 0.12 ounce)* ends up being one of the most expensive castor oil–based, lipstick-style lip balms around—but it certainly takes good care of dry, chapped lips. Vitabalm does contain fragrance.

☺ **$$$ Vital Protection Age Defying Protective Lotion SPF 15** *($120 for 1.7 ounces).* The SPF rating on this product cannot be relied on because no active ingredients are indicated, a truly strange misstep for a major cosmetics company such as Darphin. The formula contains titanium dioxide, but unless it is listed as active, you can't bank on it for reliable sun protection. By the way, titanium dioxide isn't a "100% natural" filter. The process used to create the titanium dioxide that is included as a sunscreen and the manner in which it's coated to be aesthetically pleasing are not all-natural processes. The formula contains other synthetic sunscreen ingredients also, but again, they're not listed as active. I am also concerned about the number of fragrance chemicals in this moisturizer, all of which are known to be irritating.

☺ **$$$ Vital Protection Age Defying Soothing Lotion** *($120 for 1.7 ounces)* is a moisturizer designed as an after-sun solution to help repair damaged skin. This lofty claim is something any well-formulated "moisturizer" can do; the question is how much repair, which no one can answer. The emollients and fatty acids in this lotion can help restore a damaged or compromised skin barrier. It also contains several plant-based antioxidants and other antioxidants and some cell-communicating ingredients. The problem is how unsoothing this moisturizer becomes when you realize the number of fragrance chemicals it contains. None of them are abundantly present individually, but even small amounts of them are not what irritated, sun-damaged skin needs to repair itself, and combined they account for a larger percentage. For the money and a good, but not outstanding, formula, this doesn't deserve better than a neutral face rating.

☹ **Skin Bronze Self-Tanning Face & Body Tinted Cream** *($50 for 4.2 ounces)* contains the volatile fragrance components eugenol, linalool, and others. The potential for irritation makes this otherwise standard self-tanning lotion not worth considering over hundreds of others, most selling for under $20.

☹ **Skin Bronze Self-Tanning Face Tinted Gel** *($50 for 1.7 ounces)* has the same problems as the Skin Bronze Self-Tanning Face Tinted Gel above, and the same review applies.

☹ **Soleil Plaisir, Protective Face Cream SPF 30** *($50 for 2.6 ounces)* provides broad-spectrum sun protection and includes avobenzone for UVA protection, but the formula lacks ingredients of interest to justify the price, although it does have a silky-smooth texture. A larger problem is the inclusion of many potent fragrance components, including eugenol. Plenty of sunscreens avoid these irritants, leaving this one not worth considering.

☺ **$$$ Hydrating Kiwi Mask** *($60 for 1.7 ounces)* is a very good, though needlessly expensive, moisturizing mask for normal to dry skin. The packaging will help keep the plant-based antioxidants stable, but it would be better if this product did not contain so many volatile fragrance components.

☺ **$$$ Instantly Radiant** *($65 for 0.05 ounce)* costs an off-putting amount of money for what amounts to primarily water, silicone, thickeners, and talc. The talc, titanium dioxide, and zinc oxide combine to cosmetically brighten the eye area, but this effect is attainable from careful use of any good concealer.

☹ **Overnight Refining Lotion** *($50 for 0.5 ounce)* is a problematic anti-acne lotion that contains a host of irritating ingredients, including alcohol, witch hazel, and the fragrant oils of lemon, sage, thyme, and lavender. In addition, none of the ingredients in this product can reduce blackheads or pore size; in fact, because irritation can trigger increased oil production, this kind of formula actually will make matters worse, including causing dry skin and free-radical damage.

☹ **Purifying Aromatic Clay Mask** *($55 for 1.7 ounces)* has far too many irritating fragrant oils to make it an option for any skin type. Bergamot, lavender, lemon, orange, and cypress present far more problems than benefits for skin.

☹ **Purifying Targeted Gel** *($50 for 0.5 ounce)* is supposed to be Darphin's "luxurious answer to an un-glamorous skincare problem," that being acne. Before you get carried away by the luxury aspect (which is only tied to this brand's faux prestige, not its skin-care expertise), you need to know that using this product is guaranteed to harm your skin. It contains an irritating amount of alcohol along with too many fragrant plant oils to name. None of them can do anything for skin other than cause more problems, such as irritation and redness. Plus, irritation can trigger increased oil production and the alcohol causes free-radical damage.

DDF
DOCTOR'S DERMATOLOGIC FORMULA
(SKIN CARE ONLY)

DDF AT-A-GLANCE

Strengths: Several good water-soluble cleansers; every sunscreen includes sufficient UVA-protecting ingredients; some truly state-of-the-art moisturizers and serums; a few good AHA and skin-lightening options; a good benzoyl peroxide topical disinfectant.

Weaknesses: Expensive; products designed for sensitive skin tend to contain one or more known problematic ingredients; several irritating products based on alcohol, menthol, or problematic plant extracts; more than a handful of average moisturizers, many in jar packaging.

The Reviews D

For more information about DDF, call 1-800-818-9770 or visit www.ddfskin.com or www. Beautypedia.com.

DDF DOCTOR'S DERMATOLOGIC FORMULA ADVANCED PRODUCTS

☺ **$$$ Advanced Micro-Exfoliation Cleanser** (*$46 for 6 ounces*). There really isn't anything advanced about this overpriced cleanser. Calling this an advanced cleanser is like calling a typewriter an advanced word processing system. This is mostly a mixture of water, wax, Vaseline, glycerin, and mineral oil, so it is little more than an old-fashioned cold cream base. A basic emollient cleanser that is recommended only for dry to very dry skin, this has a mild scrub action from the rice bran wax it contains, but the emollient base makes it difficult to rinse completely. DDF added some potent antioxidants and cell-communicating ingredients to this product, and because some of it remains on the skin due to the poor rinsability, you may in fact get some benefit from them, but that's a stretch. There are far better ways to get beneficial ingredients to the skin.

☹ **Advanced Eye Firming Concentrate** (*$88 for 0.5 ounce*). I would love to give this product a better rating. It is beautifully formulated, though the caffeine has no special benefit for the eye area, despite the association with waking someone up. However, the jar packaging wastes all the air-sensitive ingredients, including vitamin A and the peptides. It is also important to point out that the eye-area claim and the idea it requires a higher price tag is just silly; it doesn't contain any special ingredients exclusively for skin around the eyes. I am a bit concerned that the preservative dmdm hydantoin (a formaldehyde-releasing ingredient) may be a problem, but the small amount used is likely not troublesome. This contains titanium dioxide and mica for a cosmetic brightening effect, but firming is just a joke, and again, the jar packaging renders it unacceptable.

☺ **$$$ Advanced Firming Cream** (*$130 for 1.7 ounces*). I'm not going to dispute that this is, in fact, an advanced formula for dry skin. What's not advanced is the jar packaging, which will lead to the light- and air-sensitive ingredients deteriorating shortly after you begin using this moisturizer. The claims are mostly nonsense; for example, simply hydrating skin isn't going to improve its firmness and the turmeric plant cannot completely protect skin from free-radical damage. It's a good antioxidant, but not the one we should all be using to the exclusion of others. The claim of neutralizing 82% of free radicals is an in vitro claim, not an ongoing effect given skin's continual exposure to the environment. Aside from the claims, this would have gotten a great recommendation if the packaging would help you get the good stuff delivered to your skin.

☺ **$$$ Advanced Moisture Defense** (*$105 for 1.7 ounces*). What a shame jar packaging keeps this daytime moisturizer with sunscreen from earning a high rating because it is a very well-formulated moisturizer. It contains avobenzone for sufficient UVA protection and has a silky base that's loaded with the cell-communicating ingredient niacinamide. The formula also contains several impressive antioxidants, and that's where the jar packaging starts to rain on the parade because all of these state-of-the-art ingredients deteriorate in the presence of air when the package is opened. A great formula is meaningless if it's not in packaging that keeps the most delicate yet effective ingredients stable during use.

OTHER DDF DOCTOR'S DERMALOGIC FORMULA PRODUCTS

☺ **$$$ Blemish Foaming Cleanser** (*$32 for 6.6 ounces*) is a standard liquid-to-foam cleanser that contains mostly water, detergent cleansing agents, lather agent, and pH-adjusting agents. Salicylic acid is listed as an active, but its contact with skin is too brief for it to affect blemishes.

The token amount of azelaic acid won't impact blemishes even a little. The same can be said for the plant extracts, some soothing and some irritating—but none present in an amount great enough to be a problem or to exert a benefit. This is a good, though pricey, option for normal to oily skin.

☺ $$$ **Brightening Cleanser** *($35 for 8.5 ounces)* is similar to DDF's Blemish Foaming Cleanser, except the azelaic acid is replaced by glycolic acid and the plant extracts are those known (at least in vitro) to have a skin-lightening effect. However, none of these ingredients will be helpful in a cleanser because it's rinsed from the skin before the ingredients can affect pigmentation. This won't lighten, brighten, or exfoliate skin, but it's a good water-soluble cleanser for normal to oily skin.

☺ $$$ **Cellular Cleansing Complex** *($46 for 6 ounces)* is a very expensive version of the original Cetaphil Gentle Skin Cleanser. The big-deal claim is that this is formulated with enzymatic exfoliators. Although enzymes are present (listed as papain), they are unstable ingredients that don't exfoliate skin as efficiently as an AHA or BHA product does. Even if they were equal, the exfoliating benefit wouldn't occur unless you left this cleanser on skin for several minutes or longer, and that's not how most people wash their faces. This is a good lotion-style cleanser for normal to dry skin, but assuredly not worth the extra money compared to Cetaphil.

☹ **Glycolic 5% Exfoliating Wash** *($35 for 8.5 ounces)* is a detergent-based water-soluble cleanser that contains 5% glycolic acid and is formulated in the correct pH for it to exfoliate, but its contact with skin is too brief for it to provide much benefit because cleansers are rinsed off the skin. Add to that the inclusion of spearmint oil (which does nothing but irritate skin) and this expensive cleanser is one to leave on the shelf; it's better to use your money for a far better-formulated product.

☺ $$$ **Non-Drying Gentle Cleanser** *($32 for 8.5 ounces)* is billed as ultra-mild, and for the most part, it is. The detergent cleansing agent is one typically seen in "no more tears" baby shampoos and it is fragrance-free. This is a semi-water-soluble cleanser most suitable for normal to slightly dry skin.

☹ $$$ **Salicylic Wash** *($35 for 8.5 ounces)* omits the peppermint oil present in DDF's Glycolic 5% Exfoliating Wash, and contains 2% salicylic acid instead of an AHA. However, both its brief contact with skin and the pH of the base still prevent exfoliation. This is otherwise a very standard, water-soluble cleanser for normal to oily skin. It should be kept away from the eye area.

☹ $$$ **Sensitive Skin Cleansing Gel** *($32 for 8.5 ounces)* is a standard detergent-based water-soluble cleanser for normal to oily skin. It is not a slam dunk for sensitive skin (including rosacea) because of the potentially irritating plant extracts and preservatives it contains.

☺ $$$ **Wash Off Cleanser** *($30 for 8.5 ounces)* contains a tiny amount of coltsfoot extract, which can be problematic in leave-on products due to its alkaloid content. Because this is a rinse-off, water-soluble cleanser it shouldn't be a problem for most skin types.

☹ **Aloe Toning Complex** *($32 for 8.5 ounces)* contains an amount of comfrey extract that makes it potentially problematic for all skin types. Please refer to the *Cosmetic Ingredient Dictionary* on www.Beautypedia.com for detailed information on why comfrey is a problem for skin.

☺ $$$ **Glycolic 10% Exfoliating Moisturizer** *($50 for 1.7 ounces)* contains 10% glycolic acid at a pH of 3.6, making it an effective exfoliant. The lightweight, silicone-enhanced lotion base is suitable for normal to slightly dry skin. Although it contains some great antioxidants and the packaging will keep them stable, the amount of each is so small as to be almost nonexistent.

☹ **$$$ Glycolic 10% Exfoliating Oil Control Gel** *($48 for 1.7 ounces)* has a pH of 4.1, which limits the effectiveness of the 2% salicylic acid and 10% glycolic acid it contains. There isn't any other reason to consider this gel, and for the money it doesn't best options from Neutrogena, Alpha Hydrox, or Paula's Choice.

☹ **Glycolic 10% Toning Complex** *($35 for 8.5 ounces)* contains alcohol and menthol, and is not recommended for any skin type. What a shame, because this is otherwise a well-formulated 10% glycolic acid toner.

☹ **Glycolic 5% Daily Cleansing Pads** *($35 for 56 pads)* lists alcohol as the second ingredient followed soon after by menthol and witch hazel, all of which make these pads too irritating for all skin types.

☹ **$$$ Ultra-Lite Peel, with Elm Extract** *($42 for 1 ounce)* is designed as a leave-on peel product for sensitive skin, and the chief exfoliant is arginine. Arginine is an amino acid that functions as an antioxidant and may have wound-healing properties, but there is no research showing it to be an exfoliant (Sources: *Journal of Surgical Research*, June 2002, pages 35-42; *Nitric Oxide*, May 2002, pages 313-318; *European Surgical Research*, January-April 2002, pages 53-60; and www.naturaldatabase.com). The exfoliant in this product is approximately 1% salicylic acid, and the pH is low enough for it to function in that manner. However, alcohol precedes it on the list and makes this a less appealing BHA option due to the kickback from irritation. Elm extract has no research establishing its benefit for skin when applied topically.

☹ **$$$ Acne Scrub** *($35 for 8.5 ounces)* is a polyethylene-based (plastic bead) scrub. Benzoyl peroxide is listed as an active ingredient, but its effect will be limited because this product is rinsed from skin shortly after being applied. This cleansing scrub is best for oily to very oily skin.

☹ **$$$ Clarifying Enzyme Complex** *($32 for 2 ounces)* is a thick, water- and wax-based facial scrub with polyethylene beads that act as the abrasive agent. The tiny amount of papain (enzyme) won't exfoliate skin, but the mechanical process of massaging the polyethylene beads over skin will. There is only one study demonstrating papain as an effective exfoliant, but it used only a pure concentration (Source: *Archives of Dermatological Research*, November 2001, pages 500-507). This formula is only for dry to very dry skin and is not the easiest to rinse.

☹ **$$$ Bio-Molecular Firming Eye Serum** *($88 for 0.5 ounce)* is a lightweight, water-based serum that contains several antioxidants (most in tiny amounts) whose effectiveness is compromised by clear packaging. The peptides and other cell-communicating ingredients have merit and somewhat justify this product's price, but they're not enough to make this worth the investment unless you don't mind overspending for an eye-area product that's best for slightly dry skin.

✓ ☺ **$$$ C3 Plus Serum** *($68 for 0.5 ounce)* is an excellent product if you're looking for a fragrance-free serum that combines the antioxidant benefits of vitamin C with the skin-enhancing benefits of peptides. Packaged in an airtight opaque bottle to keep the antioxidants stable, C3 Plus Serum also contains a nice complement of skin-identical ingredients, making it worthwhile for someone with oily or blemish-prone skin who wants an antioxidant-rich product. Traditionally, ascorbic acid (the form of vitamin C in this product) has been considered difficult to stabilize. However, new placebo-controlled research shows that a 3% concentration of ascorbic acid (which this product contains) in an emulsion can produce positive results in skin within a short period of time. This means that although the ascorbic acid will break down faster than more stable forms of vitamin C, some immediate efficacy is obtained when the formulation is correct (Source: *Skin Pharmacology and Physiology*, July-August 2004, pages

200-206). Assuming that your skin-care routine includes an effective sunscreen—and without it all the antioxidants in the world will have minimal positive impact on your skin—this is a good product to consider, especially if you'd like to see what the vitamin C and peptides combination can do for your skin.

☹ **$$$ Cellular Revitalization Age Renewal** *($130 for 1.7 ounces)* makes all manner of cellular repair claims tied to the company's proprietary complex of proteins and peptides. However, there isn't much of those high-tech ingredients in this emollient moisturizer for dry to very dry skin, and several of the beneficial ingredients will be compromised by jar packaging. The phytoestrogen ingredients in this product cannot control skin symptoms associated with menopause. If you were intending to explore the potential antiwrinkle benefits of copper, this product contains barely a dusting of it.

✓ ☺ **$$$ Daily Protective Moisturizer SPF 15** *($40 for 1.7 ounces)* has a larger concentration of antioxidants and is a superior option, when compared to other DDF sunscreens. The base formula is best for normal to slightly dry skin. This sunscreen is fragrance-free.

☹ **$$$ Dramatic Radiance TRF Cream** *($100 for 1.7 ounces)* is a fairly standard moisturizer whose formula is quite mundane for the price. It contains mostly water, glycerin, emollients, slip agents, silicones, shea butter, film-forming agent, several more thickeners, antioxidants, plant oil, and preservatives. It purports to change the way skin utilizes oxygen in an effort to restore "youthful suppleness and elasticity," but does not accomplish that goal. How can a product change the way skin handles oxygen? And does that increase free-radical damage? The claims are the only mildly interesting part of this product, and the only dramatic element of this moisturizer for normal to dry skin is the price.

☹ **$$$ Erase Eye Gel** *($48 for 0.5 ounce)* is a decent serum whose film-forming agent will make skin appear temporarily smoother. There is nothing in this formulation that will minimize dark circles or puffiness.

☹ **$$$ Mattifying Oil Control UV Moisturizer SPF 15** *($42 for 1.7 ounces)*. I'm glad this daytime moisturizer with sunscreen claims to control "exterior" (meaning surface) oil because that's plausible, although that's true for any product that contains oil-absorbing ingredients. No skin-care product can control oil production beneath the skin's surface because that process is almost exclusively governed by hormones. That said, this product isn't as matte as the name states, though it does provide UVA protection courtesy of avobenzone and it also contains some good antioxidants. I'm concerned, however, that there might be enough of the pH-adjusting ingredient triethanolamine to present the potential for irritation; plus, this also contains some fragrant irritants (e.g., ginger) that have no benefit for skin. The amount of witch hazel also isn't good news. All told, this is a tough one to balance out with a rating. It doesn't provide a lasting matte finish and it doesn't contain an impressive complement of beneficial ingredients. It's a questionable product for normal to oily skin, and with so many great products out there, this one can stay on the shelf.

✓ ☺ **$$$ Mesojection Healthy Cell Serum** *($84 for 1 ounce)* is sold as a topical substitute for a procedure known as mesotherapy. This treatment, which according to research is not medically sound, is most commonly used to dissolve fat and improve the appearance of cellulite via injections that contain either homeopathic or pharmaceutical substances. Strangely, there isn't necessarily any consistency in the range of mesotherapy procedures, and the cocktail of ingredients varies from practitioner to practitioner, which makes this treatment very hard to evaluate. The most commonly used substance is phosphatidylcholine, but it also is frequently combined with deoxycholate. A handful of studies have shown that this can successfully reduce fat when injected into the skin, with one study demonstrating this effect for the under-eye area. Theoretically, the reduction of subcutaneous fat may be caused by inflammatory-mediated cell death and resorption. What does any of this have to do with skin? DDF is hoping that the effects associated with the injection of potentially helpful substances will correlate with the effects of topical application of this water-based serum. They state that this product's technology allows for 85% more potent antioxidant activity to be delivered to the deepest layers of the skin's surface (that's really not so deep, since it's still the surface of skin, but it sounds impressive, doesn't it?). But there is no published research to confirm that this antioxidant has any "mesojection" (who came up with that deceptive term?) impact or any benefit whatsoever. Other than this overblown marketing angle, the good news is that it does contain impressive amounts of several antioxidants, in a base that is suitable for normal to dry skin. The amount of salicylic acid is too low for it to be efficacious, although this serum has a pH that would allow it to exfoliate if more were included.

✓☺ **$$$ Nourishing Eye Cream** *($48 for 0.5 ounce)* is an outstanding fragrance-free moisturizer for slightly dry skin around the eyes or anywhere on the face. It contains a thoughtful blend of emollients, skin-identical ingredients, silicone, antioxidants, and plant oil.

☺ **$$$ Nutrient K Plus** *($58 for 1 ounce)* is supposed to be the answer for those dealing with broken capillaries because it contains vitamin K (phytonadione). There is lots of research pertaining to vitamin K's circulation-enhancing benefit when it's consumed orally, but this has not been demonstrated for topical application (Source: www.naturaldatabase.com). There is no reason to believe this lackluster moisturizer will have a visible effect on broken capillaries.

✓☺ **$$$ Retinol Energizing Moisturizer** *($88 for 1.7 ounces)* presents retinol along with several antioxidants in a slightly emollient lotion base suitable for normal to dry skin. This well-packaged product contains some beneficial fatty acids and nonvolatile plant oils that go beyond merely moisturizing skin. If you're going to splurge on a moisturizer, this product won't prove to be a letdown (provided you keep your expectations in check about it making you look years younger).

✓☺ **$$$ Protect and Correct UV Moisturizer SPF 15** *($60 for 1.7 ounces)* is an in-part avobenzone sunscreen that makes claims similar to those of Olay's Definity brand, and the formulation isn't that much different either. That's not surprising given that Olay owner Procter & Gamble is now at the helm of DDF, too. Of course, because DDF is a "dermatologist-developed" line sold in upscale stores, the price point is much higher than that of Olay. But the good news is you're getting a well-formulated daytime moisturizer that is suitable for normal to dry skin. The amount of niacinamide will likely have a positive impact on skin discolorations, and the formula does include several antioxidants (though only a couple are present in meaningful amounts). The amount of mica in this moisturizer with sunscreen leaves a soft shimmer on skin that, to some extent, can indeed make it look "translucent," but you can get that result from any cosmetic that contains soft-shine ingredients. The Olay equivalent of this product is Definity Correcting Protective Lotion with SPF 15, though it should be stated that DDF's version has a few more bells and whistles.

☺ **$$$ Protective Eye Cream SPF 15 Plus** *($50 for 0.5 ounce)* has a great SPF number although the creamy base formula is lackluster and unimpressive. This product includes some intriguing ingredients, but they are present in such minute amounts as to be almost inconsequential for skin. There are less expensive, more impressive sunscreens available from Neutrogena,

Clinique, and Olay, to name a few. By the way, there is nothing about this product that makes it better for the eye area.

☹ **Redness Relief** *($52 for 1 ounce)* positions itself as a botanically based treatment to soothe reddened or hypersensitive skin. I'm always suspicious of such claims because so many botanical ingredients tend to be problematic for skin, and that turns out to be the case here, too. Although DDF included some very good anti-irritants (all plant-based), they also added *Ranunculus ficaria* extract. This weed may have antibacterial and antifungal properties, but applied topically it can cause irritation and possibly photodermatitis (Source: www.naturaldatabase.com).

unrated **RMX Essential** *($200 for 3.75 ounces)* caused quite a stir when it launched in Sephora stores in 2006, mostly because of its regimented usage instructions and lofty price. The original RMX lineup included the Essential version as well as RMX Intense ($550) and RMX Maximum ($1,000). The latter two were discontinued because, according to a Sephora insider, they were "ahead of their time." That's funny, because most cosmetics companies are trying to outdo the competition with ahead-of-time products. I'm fairly certain the real reason the Intense and Maximum versions disappeared is because, quite simply, consumers weren't buying into the absurd price and accompanying inane claims. So that leaves RMX Essential at a comparatively cheap $200. After delving into this product's formulation, it leaves far more questions than answers, which is why it didn't get a rating. Do not make the mistake of thinking this is medicine or the high cost is equal to proof or evidence that it is the best formulation out there—it isn't. There is no published research to prove that this product will change your skin so it will never be the same again, but who really knows? You have to take Dr. Sobel's word for it because, other than that, there are no studies to rely on. From an ingredient standpoint, there's a little bit of everything in RMX Essential. It contains several popular peptides (cell-communicating ingredients), ingredients that mimic the structure of skin, and antioxidants. Lots of these ingredients are clearly intriguing, but they are by no means unique to this formula. If the amount of these substances is meant to be the strong suit, there's no indication of how much of any ingredient you are actually putting on your skin; you just have to take the company's word for it that these ingredients are "concentrated."

As far as cell-communicating ingredients, this product contains basically palmitoyl oligo-peptide, acetyl hexapeptide, and palmitoyl pentapeptide-3, all described in my online *Cosmetic Ingredient Dictionary*. Most of the research that cosmetics companies rely on for their "belief" in the value of peptides is performed by the manufacturers of the ingredients. Independent research about how peptides affect wrinkles when applied topically is practically nonexistent (Source: *International Journal of Cosmetic Science*, June 2005, page 155). Whether peptides ever get to the skin cell and have an impact there is just not known. Many researchers feel that they don't (peptides are notoriously unstable and easily broken down by enzymes in the skin), but obviously there are those researchers who do. One thing that is known, at least, is that they are beneficial as skin-identical ingredients. All in all, $200 for two months' worth of RMX Essential packets is a lot of money for guessing.

The second ingredient in RMX Essential is colostrum, which is the thick yellowish fluid secreted by the mammary glands during the last weeks of pregnancy and the first days after a baby is born, before actual milk is produced by the breast. (The source of colostrum used in supplements and skin-care products is primarily bovine.) Colostrum is a highly nutritious substance, loaded with proteins, immunity-building substances, and growth factors. Primarily, colostrum is about antibodies and growth factors to help the infant fight viruses and bacteria and to jump-start the growth of muscle, bone, and tissue. A small amount of research shows that colostrum can have benefit when applied topically for wound healing, but there is also research that shows it is not helpful. Either way, wrinkles and aging skin are not wounds (getting cut by a knife isn't related in any way to the slow process of how skin comes to be wrinkled and look older), so the little research that has been done does not relate to anything claimed on the label of this product (Sources: *Indian Journal of Pediatrics*, July 2005, pages 579-581; *Cells Tissues Organs*, January 2000, pages 92-100; *Australasian Biotechnology*, July-August 1997, pages 223-228; and *Journal of Dermatologic Surgery Oncology*, June 1985, pages 617-622). Further, if you're supposed to believe that colostrum's growth hormone content can impact your skin, then you would also have to believe that other constituents of colostrum would also have an effect. A major component of colostrum is a laxative to help newborns, whose digestive tracts are not fully formed. Anyone for a laxative while they fight wrinkles?

Farther down on the ingredient list is something called glycoproteins-Y28. It is nowhere to be found, whether in a search of medical journals, in the International Nomenclature of Cosmetic Ingredients (INCI, a compendium of cosmetic ingredients), or in an Internet search. Glycoproteins are fairly well understood, but exactly what the Y28 designation stands for is unknown. Most likely it's a specific receptor site on the cell that this ingredient is destined for, but that's just a guess because there is no way to know (Source: *Archives of Biochemistry and Biophysics*, June 1998, pages 232-238). In general, glycoproteins are cell-to-cell communicating ingredients created when a protein links with a carbohydrate. In the body, glycoproteins play a critical role in the way various systems recover from internal and external stresses; they also are fundamentally involved in cellular repair, among other functions. Beyond that, studies on whether they can affect skin as a cell-communicating ingredient when applied topically just aren't anywhere to be found in science (Sources: www.glycoscience.com; www.anatomyatlases.org; and *Journal of Immunology*, November 1, 2000, pages 5295-5303, and September 1991, pages 1614-1620). What we do know is that glycoproteins function very well as ingredients that mimic the structure of skin. When combined with saccharides, glycoproteins form polysaccharides and glycosaminoglycans (hyaluronic acid) that help keep skin cells and the skin's framework intact. As high-tech as this RMX formula is, it contains retinyl palmitate instead of retinol or retinaldehyde. Here, the research is fairly clear: in the skin retinyl palmitate does not convert to retinoic acid—the active, beneficial form of vitamin A—as readily as retinol or retinaldehyde. That's important, because retinoic acid is the substance that can communicate with a skin cell to tell it to function normally (Sources: *Skin Pharmacology and Physiology*, May-June 2004, pages 124-128; *European Journal of Pharmaceutics and Biopharmaceutics*, May 2000, pages 211-218; and *Journal of Investigative Dermatology*, September 1997, pages 301-305).

One more ingredient that stands out is prasterone (dehydroepiandrosterone, DHEA), a naturally occurring prohormone that in the body is converted primarily to androgens (male steroids) and, to a lesser degree, estrogens. As an oral supplement, DHEA is controversial because long-term use has been associated with women developing secondary masculine traits, liver damage, disrupted menstrual cycles, and defects in fetuses, and, for men, with decreased sperm count. More superficial risks include hair loss, acne, and weight gain. When applied topically, it is possible that DHEA can increase collagen production and prevent collagen destruction by decreasing matrix metalloproteinases (MMP), but the research about this is extremely limited and the studies that do exist were done on only a handful of people (Sources: *Drug Delivery*, September-October 2005, pages 275-280; *Journal of Endocrinology*, November 2005, pages

169-196; *Journal of Investigative Dermatology*, November 2005, pages 1053-1062, and February 2004, pages 315-323; *Gynecological Endocrinology*, December 2002, pages 431-441; www.fda.gov; and www.mayoclinic.com/health/dhea/NS_patient-dhea).By now you probably see what I mean about this being a hard product to review. For example, I still can't decide with any certainty whether it is worth any amount of money. And I can't give you an answer because there is simply no way to know. The ingredients appear to be helpful for skin, but how much more helpful than other combinations, or in exactly what capacity, remains a mystery. As skin-care formulations get more technical, it would be nice if they came with more than just the formulator's word on their reliability. Without research to point the way (and in the cosmetics industry, products launch well before research has proven their effectiveness, as was the case with this one), it is all speculation and conjecture. Still, this product does have some state-of-the-art ingredients and may be worth a try by those with unlimited skin-care budgets.

☺ **$$$ Silky C** *($78 for 1 ounce)* is a very good nonaqueous serum that silkens skin with silicones while treating it to stabilized vitamins C and E. The antioxidant content of this serum isn't quite as prodigious as DDF's C3 Plus Serum.

☹ **$$$ Wrinkle Relax** *($88 for 0.5 ounce)*. Is there any mistaking what this product is supposed to do? DDF touts its combination of two "non-toxic antiaging peptides" as being able to prevent lines formed from facial expressions. One of the peptides is palmitoyl tetrapeptide-7, which has no research proving it works in any capacity similar to Botox (it's a good ingredient, just incapable of relaxing expression lines). The same is true of the main peptide, acetyl hexapeptide-8. In the end, this serum's peptides have water-binding properties and can function as cell-communicating ingredients (assuming enzymes in the skin don't break them down before they reach their target), but this product is overpriced for what you get—and not even Botox works like Botox when applied topically, rather than being injected into the skin.

✓ ☺ **$$$ Wrinkle Resist Plus Pore Minimizer Moisturizing Serum** *($85 for 1.7 ounces)*. You may recall that Procter & Gamble, the giant consumer goods company that owns the Olay brand, now also owns DDF. As I expected, DDF's newest products are straight out of P&G's Olay brand, and DDF is now offering a version of Olay's Regenerist serums. The difference? You guessed it: Price! Whether you pay $80 for DDF's serum or $20 for one from Olay, you'll be getting a very good serum that treats skin to smoothing silicone, glycerin, cell-communicating ingredients (niacinamide and peptides), plus notable antioxidants. This version from DDF has pigments for a slight shimmery finish, but in my estimation that doesn't make it worth considering over the considerably less expensive version from Olay (and Olay offers a fragrance-free version). Still, if you're loyal to DDF, I can't dispute that this is an impressive formula for normal to slightly dry or slightly oily skin, but then again, so is Olay's.

☺ **Ultra-Lite Oil-Free Moisturizing Dew SPF 15** *($40 for 1.7 ounces)* is a daytime moisturizer for normal to dry skin, and the best thing about it is its in-part avobenzone sunscreen. Considering the main thickening agent is polyethylene, labeling this "ultra-lite" is misleading. Moreover, the amount of antioxidants and other specialty ingredients is paltry, especially for the money.

☺ **$$$ Ultra-Lite Oil-Free Moisturizing Dew** *($38 for 1.7 ounces)* contains some ingredients that support the name, but the amount of wax and thickeners doesn't make this a slam-dunk solution for those battling blemishes. This is one of the less impressive DDF moisturizers, whose antioxidant content is almost too minor to matter. It's an OK option for normal to slightly oily skin.

☺ **$$$ Benzoyl Peroxide Gel 5%, with Tea Tree Oil** *($28 for 2 ounces)* is a simply formulated but effective topical disinfectant for blemish-prone skin. The amount of tea tree oil is

The Reviews D

not enough to function as a disinfectant (it just adds fragrance), but the benzoyl peroxide takes care of that on its own.

☺ $$$ **Discoloration Reversal-Pod** *($72 for 0.45 ounce).* Discoloration Reversal-Pod shows DDF owner Procter & Gamble is sharing its packaging and formulary information with one of their latest acquisitions. That's hardly surprising (most companies do this after acquiring a new company), but as consumers you should realize that this product is remarkably similar to P&G brand Olay's Regenerist Eye Derma-Pod. Please refer to that product's review for a description of the unique packaging and method of application (keeping in mind that DDF's version is meant for use on the entire face, but Olay's can be used that way, too). The main difference between the two is that DDF included significantly more antioxidants and the potential skin-lightening ingredient undecylenoyl phenylalanine. This ingredient was researched by P&G and, according to a report on www.pgbeautyscience.com, it works "as an MSH (melanin-stimulating hormone) antagonist, preventing the melanin synthesis from starting. In vitro testing shows that the combination of undecylenoyl phenylalanine, N-acetyl glucosamine, and niacinamide show an additive effect in reducing melanin production without damaging skin cultures." That sounds great, but what about how it performs on intact human skin? And how much of it is needed to work for discolorations? We don't know, and there isn't a shred of other research proving undecylenoyl phenylalanine is as effective as P&G claims. For now, the consumer is the guinea pig on this one, and so I wouldn't bank on superb results or give up skin-lightening agents with a long history of efficacy, such as hydroquinone. Still, if you don't mind the pod-style packaging and application method (it is at best awkward and the applicator is not the most sanitary), the solution dispensed onto the pads is loaded with good-for-skin ingredients, including glycerin, vitamin E, and niacinamide. You may want to try Olay's version first, given that the skin-lightening agent in DDF's option has almost no research proving its worth (and again, who knows if DDF includes enough for it to be effective, assuming it really is). As long as you don't expect this product to make good on its name, it is an option as a serum for all skin types.

☺ $$$ **Daily Matte SPF 15** *($40 for 1.7 ounces)* is a good, fragrance-free, basic, matte-finish sunscreen for normal to oily skin. It includes an in-part titanium dioxide sunscreen and leaves a silky finish. Several antioxidants are part of the formula, but in amounts so small it's unlikely they'll have much impact on skin.

✓ ☺ $$$ **Daily Organic SPF 15** *($36 for 1.7 ounces)* claims the antioxidants it contains provide complete protection from free radicals, but that's impossible because there is no way any amount of antioxidants can shield skin from all sources of oxidative damage. (For example, how do you block oxygen without dying? And there is no sunscreen ingredient that can block every ray of the sun.) This is an excellent, fragrance-free "mineral" sunscreen whose actives are titanium dioxide and zinc oxide. It is recommended for sensitive skin that is normal to dry or struggling with rosacea.

☺ **Enhancing Sun Protection SPF 30** *($32 for 4 ounces)* provides broad-spectrum sun protection with its titanium dioxide and zinc oxide sunscreen ingredients, and comes in a tinted moisturizing base for normal to dry skin. Although this is a very good sunscreen, it's disappointing that the antioxidants are barely present and that the formula isn't too exciting when compared to options from Clinique or Estee Lauder. This product is fragrance-free.

✓ ☺ **Matte Finish Photo-Age Protection SPF 30** *($32 for 4 ounces)* is a good, in-part titanium dioxide sunscreen for normal to slightly oily skin, though the main thickening agent keeps it from being matte for long. More important than the short-lived matte finish is the fact that this sunscreen has a nice array of antioxidants and a soothing agent. This is a good example of a sunscreen that goes beyond the basics.

✓☺ **Moisturizing Photo-Age Protection SPF 30** *($32 for 4 ounces)* is preferred for normal to slightly dry skin and contains an impressive blend of antioxidants, though half of those are listed after the preservatives. The lightweight moisturizing base, with its in-part titanium dioxide sunscreen, will work well under makeup. This product is fragrance-free.

☺ **Organic Sun Protection SPF 30** *($32 for 4 ounces)* is an antioxidant letdown compared to the other DDF sunscreens, though this titanium dioxide and zinc oxide sunscreen has merit for normal to dry skin. It's not the best for sensitive or rosacea-affected skin because it is fragranced, and it's a shame that the many antioxidants are present in such minuscule amounts.

☺ **$$$ Fade Cream 15** *($40 for 1.7 ounces)* is an effective skin-lightening product that contains 2% hydroquinone. However, you should ignore the claim that it "protects as if you were wearing an SPF 15 because it contains a sunscreen." There are sunscreen ingredients in this product, but they're not listed as actives, and these ingredients won't keep skin shielded from the full spectrum of UVA rays. In particular, the product does not have an SPF rating, and you have to wonder if the FDA knows about this—because making this claim about sun protection without an SPF rating would not make any regulatory board in the world very happy. There isn't anything else to extol beyond the hydroquinone, which makes this a pricier option while offering no incentives to justify the cost.

☹ **Fade Gel 4** *($56 for 0.5 ounce)* contains alcohol, lemon oil, and lime oil, all of which are very irritating to skin, especially when combined with active ingredients (hydroquinone in this case) that may make skin more sensitive.

☹ **Glossy Lip Treatment SPF 15** *($19 for 0.25 ounce)* contains peppermint oil, which makes it too irritating for routine use.

☺ **$$$ Intensive Holistic Lightener** *($52 for 0.5 ounce)* is an effective AHA product with dubious skin-lightening ability. The sensible packaging and pH-correct formula permit the glycolic acid to function as an exfoliant. The inclusion of salicylic acid and azelaic acid (other agents that can help pigmented areas look better) will also impart some benefit.

☺ **$$$ Intensive Hydration Mask** *($32 for 2 ounces)* is a wonderfully rich mask for dry to very dry skin and it's fragrance-free, but you can get a similar benefit from applying plain safflower oil or sesame oil (the main ingredients after water in this mask) to dry skin and then washing it off after several minutes.

☹ **Sulfur Therapeutic Mask** *($38 for 4 ounces)* is a standard clay mask that also contains 10% sulfur. Sulfur is a topical disinfectant that is very irritating and highly alkaline, and can cause problems for skin.

DECLEOR (SKIN CARE ONLY)

DECLEOR AT-A-GLANCE

Strengths: None of note.

Weaknesses: Expensive; pervasive use of volatile essential oils that have limited to no benefit for skin and are known irritants; almost all the sunscreens lack the right UVA-protecting ingredients; no product to address acne or skin discolorations; inappropriate jar packaging.

For more information about Decleor, call (888) 414-4471 or visit www.decleor.com or www.Beautypedia.com

DECLEOR AROMA PURETE PRODUCTS

☹ **Aroma Purete Matt Finish Skin Fluid** *($43 for 1.69 ounces)* is a silicone-enriched moisturizer that has mattifying properties, but irritates skin with *Cananga odorata* flower oil. Also known as ylang-ylang, this oil has research demonstrating its relaxing quality when inhaled, but that's how most essential oils are best enjoyed (Source: *Phytotherapy Research*, September 2006, pages 758-763).

☹ **Aroma Purete Instant Purifying Mask** *($43 for 1.69 ounces)* contains a high amount of ylang-ylang oil, which can be irritating to skin (Source: www.naturaldatabase.com). This is otherwise a very standard clay mask that is easily replaced by many others that not only omit problematic ingredients but also cost much less.

☹ **Aroma Purete Matifying Powdered Blotting Papers** *($25 for 48 sheets)* are talc-imbued papers that also contain cornstarch, pigment, and lots of fragrance, including ylang-ylang oil. Considering the potential for irritation and the exorbitant price, these are not recommended.

DECLEOR AROMA WHITE PRODUCTS

☺ **$$$ Aroma White Brightening Treatment Lotion** *($38 for 8.4 ounces)* is a fairly basic gel-textured toner that contains more fragrant orange and kiwi water than mulberry extract. The latter is the only ingredient in this product that can have an effect on melanin production, but there isn't enough of it here to bring a benefit for hyperpigmented skin.

☺ **$$$ Aroma White Brightening C+ Essence** *($78 for 0.99 ounce)* only contains vitamin C in the sense that some of the plant extracts in this serum are a natural source of it. However, it's doubtful the vitamin C content is still viable once the extract has been processed; pure, stabilized forms of vitamin C are preferred. There's no compelling reason to consider this treatment kit, particularly since the antioxidants are compromised by non-opaque bottles, making it more a waste of money than anything else.

☹ **Aroma White Brightening Matifying Fluid SPF 15** *($55 for 1.69 ounces)* lacks the UVA-protecting ingredients of titanium dioxide, zinc oxide, avobenzone, Tinosorb, or Mexoryl SX and is not recommended.

☺ **$$$ Aroma White Brightening Make Off Cream, Face and Eyes** *($36 for 5 ounces)* won't help unevenly pigmented skin in terms of lightening discolorations, but this is a good, irritant-free cleansing cream for dry to very dry skin. It requires a washcloth for complete removal, but does remove makeup well.

☺ **$$$ Aroma White Brightening Night Cream** *($67 for 1.69 ounces)* is a good emollient moisturizer for dry to very dry skin, though its jar packaging compromises the stability of the few antioxidants present. The tiny amount of mulberry extract won't lighten skin one iota, so this is not the moisturizer to choose if you're looking to fade sun- or hormone-induced discolorations.

☺ **$$$ Aroma White Brightening Purifying Mask** *($48 for 1.69 ounces)* is a standard clay mask dressed up with claims of preventing dark spots and featuring a list of plant oil and extracts that are no match for an over-the-counter skin-lightening product that contains hydroquinone. Not only that, but a mask is designed for occasional use and is rinsed off, and not even proven skin-lightening agents would work if you were following that routine.

☺ **$$$ Aroma White Brightening Spot Corrector** *($35 for 0.5 ounce)* lists active ingredients that aren't regulated as such, including roman chamomile. There is no evidence that any of Decleor's self-proclaimed "actives" will correct dark spots and pigment imperfections, or help prevent new spots from forming. This is basically clay, thickeners, and cornstarch along with a form of vitamin C not known to be effective on discolorations, and the plant extracts this product contains aren't helpful for that either.

DECLEOR AROMESSENCE PRODUCTS

☹ **Aromessence Angelique Night Balm** *($69 for 1 ounce)* has an oil-based, emollient texture that those with very dry skin will love, but your skin won't appreciate the irritation from the rosemary, geranium, and angelica oils (the latter is phototoxic, so it's good this is recommended for nighttime use).

☹ **Aromessence Angelique Nourishing Concentrate** *($68 for 0.5 ounce)* is mostly hazel seed, wheat germ, and avocado oils, all of which are available separately at health food stores and are a far better choice than this overpriced "concentrate" and its irritating fragrant oils of rosemary, geranium, and angelica.

☹ **Aromessence Essential Balm** *($69 for 1 ounce)* contains irritating basil, bitter-orange, and neroli oils and is not recommended. This very fragranced balm would make a much better candle than skin-care product! Basil oil has mutagenic properties and its active constituents (concentrated in the oil) are bad news for skin (Source: *Natural Medicines Comprehensive Database*, 2006).

☹ **Aromessence Iris Night Balm** *($76 for 1 ounce)* contains fragrant geranium oil as well as lavender oil, and the latter is capable of causing skin-cell death when applied topically (Source: *Cell Proliferation*, June 2004, pages 221-229).

☹ **Aromessence Iris TimeCare Concentrate** *($84 for 0.5 ounce)* claims to redefine features, but you can take that to mean causing visible irritation and possibly contact dermatitis from the litany of problematic fragrant volatile oils it contains.

☹ **Aromessence Neroli Comforting Concentrate** *($68 for 0.5 ounce)* is similar to the Aromessence Iris TimeCare Concentrate above, only with a different blend of problematic oils.

☹ **Aromessence Rose D'Orient Night Balm** *($69 for 1 ounce)* absolutely won't reduce signs of irritation given the number of volatile plant oils it contains. Routine use of this product is likely to cause irritation and inflammation.

☹ **Aromessence Rose D'Orient Soothing Concentrate** *($68 for 0.5 ounce)* is similar to the Aromessence Iris TimeCare Concentrate above, only with a different blend of problematic oils.

☹ **Aromessence Ylang-Ylang Night Balm** *($69 for 1 ounce)* is not recommended because it contains irritating ylang-ylang and basil oils.

☹ **Aromessence Ylang-Ylang Purifying Concentrate** *($68 for 0.5 ounce)* smells divine, but the blend of ylang-ylang, geranium, rosemary, and bay oils won't do your skin one bit of good, and none of these oils can control sebaceous (oil) gland secretions.

☹ **Aromessence Repairing After-Sun Balm, for Face** *($38 for 0.5 ounce)* is a rich balm that contains several beneficial plant oils. That's the good news. The bad news is this also contains a litany of irritating fragrant plant oils, all of which are not helpful for skin, whether it has been exposed to sunlight or not. If anything, the texture of this balm is not what you should be putting on skin if it has been reddened or otherwise inflamed by the sun. A sheer, water-based gel is preferred because thick products like this can trap heat and push a sunburn's damaging effects deeper into skin.

☹ **Aromessence Solaire Protection Booster, for Face** *($63 for 0.5 ounce)* contains what Decleor refers to as a "cocktail of essential oils that work in synergy to increase cells' natural defenses against sun damage," but that's completely false. Sunflower, rice bran, and wheat germ oil will keep skin from drying out in the sun, but won't prevent sun damage. Further, the volatile components geranium oil and rose oil are irritating to skin.

☹ **Aromessence Lip Balm** (*$26 for 0.33 ounce*) won't nourish lips as claimed because the nourishing ingredients are impeded by the irritants lemon, orange, and cinnamon oils.

☹ **Aromessence White Brightening Concentrate** (*$81 for 0.5 ounce*) contains fragrant rose and orange oils along with lemon peel, all of which are irritating to skin and all of which have no positive effect on pigmentation.

DECLEOR EXPERIENCE DE L'AGE PRODUCTS

☺ $$$ **Experience De L'Age Triple Action Eye And Lip Cream** (*$64 for 0.5 ounce*) contains problematic iris extract and herbs such as *Bupleurum falcatum* root, which do not have established safety records for topical application (Source: www.naturaldatabase.com). This creamy moisturizer has some beneficial ingredients for dry skin, but it's not an antiwrinkle product with "corrective action" and is very overpriced for what you get. The fragrance components it contains are best kept away from the eyes and mouth.

☺ $$$ **Experience De L'Age Triple Action Light Cream** (*$100 for 1.69 ounces*) has a lighter texture than the Experience De L'Age Triple Action Eye and Lip Cream, but makes similar claims and contains the same problematic and questionable plant extracts. The base formula is an OK moisturizer for normal to slightly dry or slightly oily skin.

☺ $$$ **Experience De L'Age Triple Action Rich Cream** (*$100 for 1.69 ounces*) is a more emollient (but not "rich") version of the Experience De L'Age Triple Action Light Cream, but makes the same claims and has the same problematic plant extracts. It's an option for normal to dry skin, but the jar packaging won't keep the antioxidants stable.

☹ **Experience De L'Age Triple Action Gel Cream Mask** (*$46 for 1.69 ounces*) is a silky-textured mask that would be better without the problematic iris extract and irritating menthol derivative.

DECLEOR EXPRESSION DE L'AGE PRODUCTS

☹ **Expression De L'Age Radiance Smoothing Cream** (*$80 for 1.69 ounces*) has an elegantly smooth texture and treats normal to dry skin to several helpful ingredients, among them shea butter and retinol (in stable, airless packaging). Some of the plant extracts can be irritating, while the bitter-orange and neroli oils are definitely cause for concern. Given the drawbacks, this isn't a top moisturizer with retinol to consider, especially when Alpha Hydrox, DDF, Estee Lauder, and Neutrogena offer less expensive versions that do not contain extraneous irritants.

☹ **Expression De L'Age Relaxing Eye Cream** (*$56 for 0.5 ounce*) has the same pros and cons as Decleor's Expression De L'Age Radiance Smoothing Cream (above), and is not recommended. This contains a tiny amount of retinol and other antioxidants in stable, airless packaging, but the amount of fragrant plant oils is cause for concern, especially in a product meant to be applied near the eyes. By the way, the floral waters and sweet clover cannot reduce dark circles, puffiness, or sagging skin around the eyes. If that's all it took to ameliorate these problems, you could whip up your own blend of these fragrant ingredients without having to tolerate this product's unjustified price.

DECLEOR HARMONIE PRODUCTS

☺ **$$$ Harmonie Soothing Eye Contour Gel** *($38 for 0.5 ounce)* has a lotion texture and is actually an impressive formula for normal to dry skin. It contains rose oil and a couple of problematic plant extracts, but in amounts unlikely to cause problems. You should still keep this away from the eye area.

☹ **Harmonie Delicate Soothing Emulsion** *($67 for 1.69 ounces)* begins as one of Decleor's more intriguing moisturizer formulas, but quickly heads in the wrong direction due to the inclusion of irritating (not calming, as claimed) lavender, thyme, bitter-orange, rose, and marjoram oils. This is one to steer clear of if you have sensitized, reddened skin—unless you want to make matters worse.

☹ **Harmonie Essentielle Ultra Soothing Cream** *($68 for 1.69 ounces)* contains the same potent cocktail of irritating essential oils as the Harmonie Delicate Soothing Emulsion, and the same review applies.

☹ **Harmonie Gentle Soothing Cream** *($70 for 1.69 ounces)* contains the same potent cocktail of irritating essential oils as the Harmonie Delicate Soothing Emulsion, and the same review applies.

☹ **Harmonie Gentle Soothing Mask** *($45 for 1.69 ounces)* contains the same group of irritating essential oils as the Harmonie Delicate Soothing Emulsion, and is equally problematic for all skin types, particularly "reactive skin," for which Decleor specifically designed this product.

DECLEOR HYDRA FLORAL PRODUCTS

☹ **Hydra Floral Deeply Hydrating Eye Contour Gel-Cream** *($43 for 0.5 ounce)* has a delicate, gel-cream texture, but its main ingredients are orange fruit and peppermint leaf water, which, though diluted, are still far too irritating to use around the eyes. (Decleor claims these plant ingredients make up 10% of the product, which is really depressing news if true.) Farther down the list are fragrant neroli oil and other fragrant components, such as amyl cinnamal, linalool, and limonene—all problematic ingredients for skin, and incapable of diminishing dark circles and puffiness. If anything, the irritating ingredients in this moisturizer will create, not ease, puffy eyes.

☹ **Hydra Floral "Flower Nectar" Moisturising Cream** *($58 for 1.69 ounces)* lists orange fruit and peppermint leaf water as the main ingredients, as well as neroli oil and several fragrance chemicals. This product is absolutely not recommended for any skin type.

☹ **Hydra Floral "Fresh Flower" Moisturising Emulsion** *($57 for 1.69 ounces)* contains the same irritating ingredients mentioned for Decleor's other Hydra Floral products, and is not recommended. Even without the irritants and the many fragrant components, this is an incredibly boring moisturizer formula for the money.

☹ **Hydra Floral "Flower Petals" Eye and Lip Moisturising Mask** *($42 for 1 ounce)* completes the progression of irritation that will result from combined or continued use of this line of products. Putting this much peppermint, orange, and neroli on your lips is almost as bad as using it near your eyes, and none of these ingredients (or any other ingredient in the product) can alleviate dark circles or puffiness—if anything, irritating ingredients make matters worse.

☹ **Hydra Floral "Flower Essence" Moisturising Mask** *($42 for 1.69 ounces)* doesn't improve in any way on the other Hydra Floral products reviewed because it contains the same group of irritating ingredients, albeit in a more emollient base. How any of these products is supposed to protect skin from pollution is beyond me, so don't count on that or any other significant benefit.

DECLEOR NUTRI-DELICE PRODUCTS

☹ **Nutri-Delice Delicious Ultra-Nourishing Cream** *($58 for 1.69 ounces)* is a very emollient, water- and oil-based moisturizer that would be much better for dry skin if the ceramide content were increased and the irritating angelica oil eliminated. This oil contains chemical constituents that can be phototoxic, including bergapten, imperatorin, and xanthotoxin. Although some of the components of angelica oil have antioxidant ability, it is a risky ingredient to use on skin if you are going to expose your skin to sunlight (Sources: www.naturaldatabase. com; and *Journal of Agricultural and Food Chemistry*, March 2007, pages 1737-1742). That news is neither nourishing nor delicious.

☹ **Nutri-Delice Delightful Extreme Protection Cream** *($65 for 1.69 ounces)* is similar to the Nutri-Delice Delicious Ultra-Nourishing Cream above, and the same review applies.

☹ **Nutri-Delice Meltingly Soft Nourishing Cream** *($56 for 1.69 ounces)* is similar to the Nutri-Delice Delicious Ultra-Nourishing Cream above, and the same review applies.

☺ **$$$ Nutri-Delice Nourishing Cereal Mask** *($42 for 1.69 ounces)* includes cereal grains such as oatmeal and wheat germ in a water-and-oil base suitable for dry to very dry skin. The tiny amount of angelica oil is unlikely to be a problem, provided you rinse this mask from your skin and don't wear it in the presence of sunlight. This is a decent mask but it's more a do-nothing than anything resembling nourishment for skin.

OTHER DECLEOR PRODUCTS

☹ **Cleansing Cream** *($36 for 8.4 ounces)* is a cold cream–style cleanser that contains irritating angelica and geranium oils. That's not as much of an issue in a rinse-off product, but given the number of cleansers for normal to dry skin that don't contain potentially problematic ingredients, why choose this one?

☹ **Cleansing Gel** *($36 for 8.4 ounces)* contains peppermint leaf water as a main ingredient as well as irritating (but delicious-smelling) ylang-ylang oil, making it a poor choice for all skin types.

☹ **Cleansing Milk** *($36 for 8.4 ounces)* contains lavender and bitter-orange oils, both of which are irritating and only serve to add fragrance.

☹ **Cleansing Water** *($36 for 8.4 ounces)* contains several irritating fragrant oils and has a formula that ranks below average for overall cleansing ability.

☹ **Foaming Cleanser** *($36 for 6.7 ounces)* has merit as a water-soluble cleanser, but the irritating lavender and bitter-orange oils serve only to damage the skin's hydrolipidic film, which this cleanser is supposed to protect.

☺ **$$$ Eye Makeup Remover Gel** *($28 for 5 ounces)* is an OK option to remove eye makeup if you prefer water-based gels and aren't trying to take off waterproof formulas. (It takes more effort than it's worth to remove such makeup with this type of product; silicone- or oil-based removers work much faster.) The minor red flags for this product include fragrant orange flower water and a couple of fragrance ingredients that aren't the best for applying to eye-area skin.

☹ **Fresh Hydrating Mist** *($23 for 5.07 ounces)* irritates skin with lavender and bitter-orange oils and is otherwise a very boring, overpriced spray-on toner.

☹ **Matifying Lotion** *($36 for 8.4 ounces)* lists peppermint leaf water as the second ingredient and also contains fragrant ylang-ylang oil and extracts of cinnamon and ginger. This is a recipe for potpourri, not a skin-care product to tackle oiliness.

☹ **Tonifying Lotion** *($36 for 8.4 ounces)* won't rebalance skin, but it will irritate it thanks to the amount of lavender and bitter-orange oil.

☹ **Phytopeel Natural Exfoliating Cream** *($43 for 1.69 ounces)* contains lemon peel, lavender, thyme, and marjoram oils, all of which would serve much better in a salad dressing than as something to apply to skin.

☹ **Purete Exfoliante Natural Micro-Smoothing Cream** *($40 for 1.69 ounces)* contains black pepper oil and menthol, which makes no sense from any skin-care point of view and is just really bizarre. It also uses coconut shell powder as the abrasive agent, which, while natural, has uneven surfaces that can cause micro-tears in skin.

☹ **Alpha Morning Alpha Hydrating Cream SPF 12** *($57 for 1.69 ounces)* does not contain the UVA-protecting ingredients of titanium dioxide, zinc oxide, avobenzone, Tinosorb, or Mexoryl SX, and is not recommended. That's a shame, because the pH of 4 allows the glycolic and lactic acids to function as exfoliants—yet you definitely do not want to wear this during daylight hours.

☹ **Aroma Sun Protective Anti-Wrinkle Cream SPF 15, for Face** *($36 for 1.69 ounces)* lacks the UVA-protecting ingredients of titanium dioxide, zinc oxide, avobenzone, Tinosorb, or Mexoryl SX, and is not recommended.

☹ **Aroma Sun Protective Anti-Wrinkle Cream SPF 30, for Face** *($36 for 1.69 ounces)* lacks the UVA-protecting ingredients of titanium dioxide, zinc oxide, avobenzone, Tinosorb, or Mexoryl SX, and is not recommended. Not to mention that the antiwrinkle claim is bogus.

☹ **Baume Excellence Regenerating Night Balm** *($89 for 1 ounce)* is indeed 100% natural; though this greasy balm is also proof that natural isn't automatically what's best for your skin. None of the natural ingredients in this balm are specific to the needs of mature skin because mature skin (a nice way to say old skin, but it is always left as some undefined age group—does it start at 48, 49, 50, 55?) can have needs that run the gamut, from oily to dry or blemish-prone. Mature skin doesn't equal dry skin, but dry skin is what this balm is designed to combat. However, along with the soothing oils, it also contains several irritating fragrant oils as well as waxes that can cause clogged pores and lead to a complexion that looks dull. If you need extra oil for your dry skin, a little plant oil, like olive or evening primrose, would work great and cost a fraction of this product's price tag.

☺ **$$$ Excellence De L'Age Sublime Regenerating Cream** *($110 for 1.69 ounces)*. There are lots of intriguing, skin-beneficial ingredients in this product, although they should be present in more generous amounts considering the price. There are numerous plant extracts and some of them have documented benefit for skin, but many have unknown or questionable benefit. There are also some, such as iris root extract and *Boswellia carterii* (frankincense), that are irritating; that's not great, but not terrible either. What this absolutely won't do is live up to the claims on the label. This won't regenerate skin or improve skin density (whatever that means). It also doesn't contain ingredients that will lighten discolorations. It's a very good moisturizer for dry skin, but it isn't cutting-edge or worth the price tag. If anything, a moisturizer at this price should be redefining, not approaching state-of-the-art.

☺ **$$$ Excellence De L'Age Regenerating Eye and Lip Cream** *($74 for 0.5 ounce)* is said to be specially formulated for the eye and lip area, but the ingredients don't support that. For example, why did they include problematic iris extract and herbs such as *Bupleurum falcatum* root, which do not have established safety records for topical application (Source: www.natu-raldatabase.com). This creamy moisturizer has some beneficial ingredients for dry skin, but it's not an antiwrinkle product with "lipofilling technology" and is quite overpriced for what you get. The fragrance components it contains are best kept away from the eyes and mouth.

☺ $$$ **Hydrotenseur Eye Contour Firming Serum** *($52 for 0.5 ounce)*. Other than some standard skin-identical ingredients, there isn't much to write about this water-based serum. It's OK for a quick fix, but shortchanges the eye area by omitting antioxidants.

☹ **Prolagene Energising Gel** *($53 for 5.07 ounces)* claims to be a complete skin-care treatment, working to smooth imperfections that are both natural and accidental. It cannot do that, and is a very basic, watery gel formula that contains irritating osmanthus oil.

☹ **Soin Du Soir Night Repair Cream** *($52 for 1.69 ounces)* is a below-standard emollient moisturizer because it contains irritating bitter-orange oil and bitter-orange wax. Nothing in this moisturizer is capable of repairing skin, day or night.

☹ **Source D'Eclat 10-Day Radiance Powder Cure** *($37 for 0.33 ounce)* is a two-part product where you mix a vitamin C powder (pure ascorbic acid) with a glycol-based serum, apply it, and then your complexion becomes radiant. Vitamin C is mentioned as a skin stimulator, but the real stimulation (and irritation) comes from the citrus oils in the serum, and volatile fragrance components such as eugenol and limonene don't make matters any better.

☹ **Source D'Eclat Instant Radiance Moisturiser** *($56 for 1.69 ounces)* contains several problematic ingredients for skin, including citrus oils, oak root, and volatile fragrance components. The radiance comes from the mineral pigments mica and titanium dioxide, but you can get that effect from many other products that don't subject skin to irritation.

☹ **Vitaroma Wrinkle Prevention and Radiance Face Emulsion** *($68 for 1.69 ounces)* continues Decleor's pattern of emollient moisturizers infused with irritating essential oils. This product's offending ingredients include citronella and rose moschata oils.

☹ **Vitaroma Wrinkle Prevention Eye Contour Cream** *($45 for 0.5 ounce)* lists several of its most intriguing ingredients (vitamin E, retinol, lecithin) well after problematic ones such as geranium and citronella oils, neither of which is appropriate for skin around the eyes (or anywhere else on the face).

☹ **Clay and Herbal Cleansing Mask** *($42 for 1.69 ounces)* doesn't break any new ground in terms of clay masks, but will irritate skin with arnica and horsetail extracts.

☹ **Nourishing Lip Treatment** *($23 for 0.14 ounce)* contains cinnamon oil as well as problematic fragrance components, including eugenol and linalool. Plain Vaseline would be a much better, and much less expensive, lip moisturizer.

☹ **Source D'Eclat Radiance Revealing Peel-Off Mask** *($42 for 1.69 ounces)* contains two types of drying alcohol as the main ingredients, along with irritating citrus oils and other problematic plant extracts.

DECLEOR AROMA SUN PRODUCTS

☹ **Aroma Sun SPF 8 Hydrating Self-Tanning Milk, for Face & Body** *($36 for 4.2 ounces)* is one of two Decleor sunscreens that get the issue of UVA protection right, thanks to its in-part avobenzone sunscreen. Unfortunately, this self-tanner's sunscreen rating is too low and you're not likely to apply such a product daily or liberally. Plus the fragrant oils can cause irritation.

☹ **Aroma Sun SPF 10 Hydrating Tinted Self-Tanning Gel-Cream, for Face** *($36 for 1.69 ounces)* contains avobenzone like the Aroma Sun SPF 8 Hydrating Self-Tanning Milk, for

Face & Body above, but it also contains volatile fragrant oils to irritate skin and a pepper resin that makes matter worse, especially if applied around the eyes.

☹ **Aroma Sun Anti-Sunburn Refreshing Gel-Cream, for Face & Body** *($36 for 4.2 ounces)* should not be applied to skin anywhere on the body because of the number of irritating volatile oils it contains. This is far from a refreshing experience for your skin, but your nose will be pleased with the scent.

☹ **Aroma Sun Express Hydrating Self-Tan Spray, for Body** *($36 for 5 ounces)* is a spray-on self-tanner that lists alcohol as the second ingredient and also contains a significant amount of irritating volatile plant oils.

☹ **Aroma Sun High Protection Sun Stick SPF 25, for Lips & Sensitive Areas** *($21 for 0.26 ounce)* lacks the UVA-protecting ingredients of titanium dioxide, zinc oxide, avobenzone, Tinosorb, or Mexoryl SX, and is not recommended. Even if it had sufficient UVA sunscreen ingredients, this contains problematic fragrant oils that would make it hard to recommend.

☺ **$$$ Aroma Sun Protective Beautifying Mist SPF 8, for Face & Body** *($36 for 5 ounces)* lacks the UVA-protecting ingredients of titanium dioxide, zinc oxide, avobenzone, Tinosorb, or Mexoryl SX, and is not recommended. Moreover, the SPF rating is too low for daytime protection.

☹ **Aroma Sun Protective Hydrating Spray SPF 20, for Face & Body** *($36 for 5 ounces)* lacks the UVA-protecting ingredients of titanium dioxide, zinc oxide, avobenzone, Tinosorb, or Mexoryl SX, and is not recommended.

☹ **Aroma Sun Protective Hydrating Spray SPF 30, for Face & Body** *($36 for 5 ounces)* lacks the UVA-protecting ingredients of titanium dioxide, zinc oxide, avobenzone, Tinosorb, or Mexoryl SX, and is not recommended.

☹ **Aroma Sun Protective Hydrating Sun Milk SPF 15, for Face & Body** *($36 for 4.2 ounces)* lacks the UVA-protecting ingredients of titanium dioxide, zinc oxide, avobenzone, Tinosorb, or Mexoryl SX, and is not recommended.

DERMALOGICA (SKIN CARE ONLY)

DERMALOGICA AT-A-GLANCE

Strengths: Good eye-makeup remover; a combination AHA/BHA product; a couple of commendable moisturizers.

Weaknesses: Expensive; almost every category has one or more products that contain irritating ingredients with no established benefit for skin; poor sunscreens.

For more information about Dermalogica, call (800) 831-5150 or visit www.dermalogica.com or www.Beautypedia.com

DERMALOGICA AGE SMART PRODUCTS

☹ **AGE Smart Skin Resurfacing Cleanser** *($37 for 5.1 ounces)* is an acidic water-soluble cleanser whose lactic acid content has the ability to exfoliate skin; that is, if you leave it on your skin for at least several minutes. Doing that, however, would only increase the irritation potential of this cleanser, a result of the many fragrant oils, other fragrant components, and the detergent cleansing agents it contains. And getting this cleanser anywhere near your eyes would be a problematic experience!

⊗ **AGE Smart Antioxidant Hydramist** *($37 for 5.1 ounces)* winds up being a very disappointing, poorly formulated toner! The amount of peptides, vitamin C, green tea, and water-binding agents is impressive and somewhat justifies the product's price, but the addition of rosewood, clove, and lemon peel oils is a mistake. These ingredients make this toner too irritating for all skin types, and negate any soothing effects the beneficial ingredients might have. By the way, there is no research anywhere showing that the peptides Dermalogica includes in this toner can prevent signs of aging associated with the creation of advanced glycation end-products (AGE). Advanced glycation end-products are abnormal, cross-linked, and oxidized proteins that might play a role in the aging process. That oxidation process also involves sugars, particularly in the form of glucose, which are one of the primary ways the body gets its fuel for producing energy and "get-up-and-go" power. But glucose also can, through an enzymatic trigger, attach itself to proteins anywhere in the body, forming "glycated" substances that damage tissue by making it stiff and inflexible. AGEs directly affect the surface layers of skin as well as structures beneath the surface, such as collagen and elastin. What is still unknown, despite ongoing research, is whether topical application of ingredients can disrupt the internal creation of AGEs. For now, that claim is still wishful thinking.

⊗ **AGE Smart Multivitamin Thermafoliant** *($48 for 2.5 ounces)*. Dermalogica has taken an everything-but-the-kitchen-sink approach to exfoliation, and as usual with their products, the results backfire as they make several formulary mistakes. Let's begin by discussing the thermal reaction alluded to in the product's name, which is nothing more than a high school student's science class project. When two of the ingredients in this product, polyethylene glycol and baking soda, are mixed with water, heat is released (you start the reaction when you splash your face with water). The fleeting heating sensation may psychologically feel good, but it isn't doing anything to help your skin (if anything, making your skin too warm can lead to problems). The real exfoliating component of this product consists of abrasive magnesium oxide crystals, which provide manual exfoliation as you massage them over your skin (just like any scrub). This also includes an AHA (lactic acid) and BHA (salicylic acid). Although the latter ingredients are present in a potentially functional amount, the alkaline pH of this product keeps them from exfoliating, not to mention that they are rinsed down the drain before they can have any effect on your skin. Dermalogica included some emollient plant oils to protect your skin during the scrubbing process, but they also added several fragrant oils and fragrance chemicals that do nothing but irritate skin. Rosewood, lemon peel, and clove oils are not what you want to expose your skin to, especially when it is about to be scrubbed. One more point: There is a lot of retinol in this product, but this antiwrinkle ingredient is wasted in a product that you rinse from your skin.

☺ **$$$ AGE Smart Dynamic Skin Recovery SPF 30** *($61 for 1.7 ounces)* deserves credit for combining an in-part avobenzone sunscreen with several state-of-the-art ingredients known to help skin look and function better. This would have rated a Paula's Pick if it did not contain problematic feverfew extract along with several irritating fragrant oils. The oils are present in meager amounts, but why include them at all?

✓ ☺ **$$$ AGE Smart Map-15 Regenerator** *($85 for 0.3 ounce)* ranks as one of the few Dermalogica products that does not assault skin with irritating fragrant oils. That's a plus, and there is every reason (other than the price, that is) to consider this an excellent way to treat your skin to the benefits of stabilized vitamin C. The "Map" in this product's name stands for magnesium ascorbyl phosphate, a form of vitamin C that research has shown to be beneficial for skin (Sources: *Photochemistry and Photobiology*, June 1998, pages 669-675; and *Journal* *of Pharmaceutical and Biomedical Analysis*, March 1997, pages 795-801). Dermalogica purports to use 15% of this ingredient, which means it can also have skin-lightening ability. The silicone-enhanced powder-to-lotion texture is unique, and skin is also treated to some good water-binding agents and additional antioxidants, all without a hint of fragrance. This does not contain hyaluronic acid as claimed; rather, it contains the salt form (sodium hyaluronate) of this ingredient. That's fine, but the company shouldn't call out an ingredient that isn't really in the product. Map-15 Regenerator is suitable for all skin types, but those with rosacea may not be able to tolerate the amount of vitamin C it contains.

☺ **$$$ AGE Smart Multivitamin Power Firm** *($48 for 0.5 ounce)* contains mostly silicones, thickeners, vitamin E, vitamin A, antioxidants, anti-irritant, plant oils, plant extracts, and vitamin C. It's a good antioxidant serum for all skin types, but has no special benefit (and is not emollient enough) for the lips. Although this is a very good formulary, it's not as impressive as the top serum options from Lauder-owned lines.

☺ **$$$ AGE Smart Super Rich Repair** *($75 for 1.7 ounces)* is sold as the company's "most intense, super-concentrated cream." Super Rich Repair is indeed an emollient, oil-rich moisturizer, even if it is packaged so that the effective ingredients won't stay stable. Plus the antioxidants in here are present only in very small amounts. (In fact, there's more preservative than state-of-the-art ingredients, a ratio that isn't good news, considering the premium price of this moisturizer.) So much for being super. Another issue is the inclusion of several essential oils, including sandalwood, eucalyptus, cedarwood, and geranium, which all work in opposition to the anti-irritants, and that means the two types of ingredients cancel each other out. All in all, this moisturizer will certainly make dry to very dry skin feel better, but for the money and because of the needless inclusion of fragrant irritants, you'd be better off considering state-of-the-art (and non-jar–packaged) formulas from Clinique, SkinCeuticals, or Paula's Choice.

☺ **$$$ AGE Smart Renewal Lip Complex** *($25 for 0.06 ounce)* is a somewhat unconventional lip balm because it has a lighter texture than standard wax- or oil-based balms. Both of those substances (wax and oil) show up in Renewal Lip Complex (which is good because they help keep lips moist and have tenacity) along with vitamin E, emollients, plant oil, and some peptides. It is the peptides that Dermalogica claims are responsible for preventing signs of aging caused by AGEs, but there is no proof they can do this. We do not know yet whether applying small amounts of ingredients that inhibit AGEs in a petri dish or on cultured cells can do the same thing in a cosmetic product. Realistically, this balm will keep lips smooth and help prevent chapping, but that's all you can legitimately rely on.

DERMALOGICA CHROMAWHITE TRX PRODUCTS

☺ **$$$ ChromaWhite TRx Tri-Active Cleanse** *($38 for 5.1 ounces)* is a creamy standard detergent-based, foaming cleanser that has lots of potential for those with dry to very dry skin. However, it isn't any more adept at lifting dulling skin cells than any other cleanser; if anything, the emollients in this product impede rinsing, which means more dead skin cells remain than are washed away. The whitening name and brightening claims are meaningless, too, and it's worth noting that this product does not contain enzymes or peptides as claimed. It does contain fragrant ylang-ylang oil, listed by its Latin name *Cananga odorata*. Including ylang-ylang is not great news because fragrant extracts are not good skin care, but the amount is likely too low to be problematic. Consider this a worthwhile cleanser for dry skin, but not a specialized brightening product.

☹ **ChromaWhite TRx Powerfoliant2** *($65 for 0.6 ounce)* is an ultra-expensive product that is nothing more than a gimmicky cleanser that adds AHAs and enzymes to the mix. You combine a small amount of cleansing powder with a liquid mixture that contains lactic acid and you then wash your face with it. Exfoliation will occur, too, but only if you leave it on your skin for several minutes, and that is not a good idea. There are many reasons not to leave this on your skin, including the fact that the product contains irritating grapefruit peel oil and detergent cleansing agents, which you should never leave on your skin because doing so is just too irritating and compromising to the skin's barrier. Using a separate cleanser and a well-formulated, leave-on AHA product is not only less expensive, but also much better for your skin.

☺ **$$$ ChromaWhite TRx C-12 Concentrate** *($90 for 1 ounce)*. This water- and silicone-based serum's only unique ingredient is oligopeptide-34, an ingredient that allegedly is responsible for improving skin clarity and treating discolorations. It comes from raw material supplier Caragen, and the only information pertaining to its efficacy also comes from Caragen, which makes it not much to go on. You can consider the claim unsubstantiated and completely biased. All in all, this is just an ordinary (and I mean really ordinary) serum for normal to dry skin, with nothing to offer for skin discolorations or any other skin concern. For the health and appearance of your skin you should opt for a product whose lightening ingredients have a better track record than those that Dermalogica chose. For the same amount of money you can get a prescription for Tri-Luma, a hydroquinone/tretinoin product with copious research proving its efficacy for treating skin discolorations, including melasma. Or, in the cosmetic realm, for this kind of money, selecting a product loaded with antioxidants (especially vitamin C given its role in mitigating sun-induced skin discolorations), cell-communicating ingredients, and skin-identical ingredients, which this one sorely lacks, would be far better!

☺ **$$$ ChromaWhite TRx Pure Light SPF 30** *($60 for 1.7 ounces)*. It's wonderful that this daytime moisturizer with sunscreen contains titanium dioxide and zinc oxide in a silky, lightweight base formula with some very good antioxidants and a cell-communicating ingredient. What rains a bit on this parade is (1) the lack of substantiated research about the peptide that Dermalogica claims will treat discoloration and (2) the inclusion of fragrant, but irritating, ylang-ylang oil (listed by its Latin name *Cananga odorata*). There isn't much of this fragrant oil present, but its inclusion means that what would've been a brilliant sunscreen is instead just a very good sunscreen for sensitive skin. Those with sensitive skin that reacts to this product should likely blame it on the ylang-ylang oil.

☺ **$$$ ChromaWhite TRx Pure Night** *($75 for 1.7 ounces)*. Although there is a lack of serious research that the peptide in this product will lighten skin discolorations, this is, for the most part, an outstanding moisturizer for dry to very dry skin. It contains a copious amount of antioxidants (including some that rarely show up in other products), cell-communicating niacinamide, and skin-conditioning emollients. The only drawback (and the reason this is not rated a Paula's Pick) is the inclusion of ylang-ylang oil, listed by its Latin name *Cananga odorata*. Although the small amount present is not likely to cause irritation, it serves no purpose for skin and contains potentially irritating fragrance chemicals.

✓ ☺ **$$$ ChromaWhite TRx Extreme C** *($85 for 0.3 ounce)* would be an interesting way to experiment with stabilized vitamin C, given its liquid powder form. The form of vitamin C is magnesium ascorbyl phosphate. Based on its concentration, there is reason to believe you will see some improvement in skin discolorations, although the research is clear that the results will not be as impressive as what you'd get from a hydroquinone-based product. It's good that there are other antioxidants, a cell-communicating ingredient, and some skin-identical ingredients included, too, because without them this would have been a one-note product not worth its price. Although this is still on the extremely pricey side (you're only getting 0.3 ounce, making this about $250 per ounce), it's a good formula in stable packaging. This product is suitable for all skin types.

DERMALOGICA CLEAN START PRODUCTS

☹ **Clean Start Wash Off** *($20 for 6 ounces)* makes impossible claims; no skin-care product can regulate oil production because oil production is primarily a function of androgens, male hormones that everybody has. Any aesthetician who believes the claim needs to go back to Skin Physiology 101. In addition, the main cleansing agent is sodium lauryl sulfate, which poses a high risk of skin irritation. That, plus the inclusion of lavender and orange oils, makes this cleanser too drying and irritating for all skin types.

☹ **Clean Start All Over Clear** *($18 for 4 ounces)*. The claim that this product controls oil production is completely bogus, although it does briefly eliminate it from the surface of the skin, something that most cleansers or toners do. This spray-on toner contains the most potent (and irritating) form of witch hazel (the distillate, which is mostly alcohol) as well as fragrant oils that cause irritation. Alcohol also causes free-radical damage, but the irritation stimulates oil production in the pore, which is hardly a control mechanism. Some of the ingredients in this toner are helpful for skin, but not nearly as much as they could be given that they are commingled with irritants.

☹ **Clean Start Ready, Set, Scrub** *($21 for 2.5 ounces)*. Skin will be off to an irritating start if you opt to use this scrub/clay mask hybrid product. It contains fragrant plant oils with known cell-damaging properties and irritation potential as well as several forms of menthol, which adds to the irritation. Numerous scrubs outperform this one without needlessly irritating skin in the process.

☹ **Clean Start Brighten Up SPF 15** *($24 for 2 ounces)* lacks the UVA-protecting ingredients of titanium dioxide, zinc oxide, avobenzone (also known as butyl methoxydibenzoylmethane), Tinosorb, or Mexoryl SX and is not recommended. Also, nothing in this formula is capable of refining or purifying pores. If anything, the triglyceride base can contribute to clogged pores.

☹ **Clean Start Welcome Matte SPF 15** *($24 for 2 ounces)* lacks the UVA-protecting ingredients of titanium dioxide, zinc oxide, avobenzone (also known as butyl methoxydibenzoylmethane), Tinosorb, or Mexoryl SX and is not recommended. Using this product instead of a sunscreen that provides sufficient UVA protection will get your skin off to an unhealthy start. Even if this did contain reliable UVA-protecting ingredients, it also has several irritating plant oils, and irritation increases oil production in the pore. This product is 100% incapable of banishing breakouts and cleaning pores. The small amount of salicylic acid and the pH won't allow any exfoliation to occur; the other aspects of the formula make it somewhat matte, but that doesn't hold up as the day goes by.

☹ **Clean Start Bedtime for Breakouts** *($22 for 2 ounces)* is supposed to be your bedtime answer for preventing breakouts before they surface and lead to a series of bad skin days. It contains 2% salicylic acid as the active ingredient, but the pH of this product is too high for exfoliation to occur. Even if the pH was within range, the base formula contains camphor, which is exceedingly irritating and will increase oil production in the pore. Some of the plant extracts have antibacterial action, but, with the exception of tea tree oil, none of them have convincing research proving their effectiveness against acne-causing bacteria (Sources: *Phytomedicine*, August

2007, pages 508-516; *Pharmazie*, March 2005, pages 208-211; and *African Journal of Medicine and Medical Sciences*, September 1995, pages 269-273). As for the tea tree oil being useful, the amount this product contains is too low for it to have a positive impact on breakouts.

☺ $$$ **Clean Start Hit the Spot** *($22 for 0.3 ounce)* is similar to Dermalogica's Clean Start Bedtime for Breakouts, but it bests that product because it omits irritating camphor and includes a much greater amount of anti-irritants. That's helpful for inflamed skin, but this still isn't much of a spot treatment for breakouts because it doesn't contain the ingredients necessary to kill acne-causing bacteria or to exfoliate dead skin cells. Oleanolic acid, a component of plants, is present and has a mild antibacterial potential, but the ingredients it was compared with (none are in this product) did much better (Source: *Phytomedicine*, August 2007, pages 508-516). I certainly wouldn't choose this gel-based product over a well-formulated product with benzoyl peroxide.

☺ $$$ **Clean Start Smart Mouth Lip Shine** *($16 for 0.3 ounce)*. Other than the fact that it contains a small amount of fragrance chemicals, this is a well-formulated lip moisturizer. Its smooth texture is lighter than traditional oil-based balms, though it still works to prevent chapping and keep lips soft. Kudos to Dermalogica for not adding the irritants such as mint or menthol that they add to their other Clean Start products!

DERMALOGICA MEDIBAC CLEARING PRODUCTS

☹ **MediBac Clearing Skin Purifying Wipes** *($16 for 20 wipes)* contain balm mint (*Melissa*), witch hazel, and camphor, all of which are irritating to skin. The amount of salicylic acid isn't sufficient for exfoliation, and the pH wouldn't allow that to happen even if it contained a decent amount.

☹ **MediBac Clearing Skin Wash** *($32 for 8.4 ounces)* contains a small amount of salicylic acid, which is rinsed from skin before it can affect blemishes, and the main detergent cleansing agent is drying, irritating sodium C14-16 olefin sulfonate. This also lists several irritating plant extracts rather high up on the ingredient list, making it an all-around bad choice.

☹ **MediBac Clearing Concealing Spot Treatment** *($31 for 0.5 ounce)* contains 5% sulfur, a potent disinfectant that can be unusually drying and irritating for skin. This also contains a large amount of witch hazel and other irritants, including camphor and cinnamon bark.

☹ **MediBac Clearing Overnight Clearing Gel** *($42 for 1.7 ounces)* has a pH of 4, which is borderline for allowing its 2% salicylic acid to exfoliate skin. While some exfoliation will occur, which is good, this product contains several irritating plant extracts and oils, including sage, rosemary, and citronella. Camphor is also in the mix. That's really disappointing, because without the copious amounts of irritants this would have been an above-average BHA option for all skin types.

☹ **MediBac Clearing Clearing Mattifier** *($40 for 1.3 ounces)* contains 2% salicylic acid, yet the pH of 4.7 doesn't allow it to function as an exfoliant. The silicones in this product leave a soft matte finish, but the amount of cinnamon bark extract is cause for concern, making this unhelpful BHA product a poor option—not to mention an expensive one, considering that several products can provide a matte finish just like this one does.

☹ **MediBac Clearing Oil Control Lotion** *($35 for 2 ounces)* contains 1% salicylic acid at an effective pH of 3.6, but this is not recommended because it also contains irritating balm mint, camphor, and menthol. What a shame! And none of the plant extracts in this lotion can have any effect on skin's oil production.

☹ **MediBac Clearing Sebum Clearing Masque** (*$40 for 2.5 ounces*) is a clay mask that contains several menthol derivatives as well as menthol itself, which makes it too irritating for all skin types. Menthol has no effect on oil production or absorption, and the pH of 4.5 prevents the salicylic acid from clearing "congested follicles." As for follicle cleaning, that is classic "spa talk," and has nothing at all to do with clogged pores or any other pore problem.

OTHER DERMALOGICA PRODUCTS

☹ **Dermal Clay Cleanser** (*$31 for 8.4 ounces*) is an odd mixture of plant oil, clay, detergent cleansing agents, thickeners, and several irritating plant extracts. This concoction won't help oily or "congested" skin, but could very well make matters worse, mostly because it doesn't rinse well.

☺ **$$$ Essential Cleansing Solution** (*$31 for 8.4 ounces*) is a cold cream–style cleanser that is an option for dry to very dry skin, but it's not so enticing owing to the inclusion of a few potentially irritating plant extracts.

☹ **Precleanse** (*$33 for 5.1 ounces*) is marketed as "the professional's deep cleansing weapon," but is nothing more than a mix of trigylceride with several nonvolatile plant oils. Also included are two forms of lavender and forms of citrus that serve to fragrance the product and irritate skin. For the money, irritant-free jojoba or olive oil is preferred.

☹ **Special Cleansing Gel** (*$31 for 8.4 ounces*) contains irritating essential oils of lavender and balm mint (*Melissa*) and is neither recommended nor the least bit special.

☹ **Ultracalming Cleanser, for Face and Eyes** (*$31 for 8.4 ounces*) contains lavender as a chief ingredient, which prevents this otherwise well-formulated cleansing lotion from being ultra-calming or recommended.

☺ **$$$ Soothing Eye Makeup Remover** (*$22 for 4 ounces*) is a standard, but good, detergent-based eye-makeup remover that is free of fragrance and the irritating plant extracts Dermalogica puts in their facial cleansers.

☹ **Multi-Active Toner** (*$28.50 for 8.4 ounces*) is multi-irritating because it contains lavender, balm mint, pellitory, arnica, and ivy. None of these ingredients are humectants (as Dermalogica asserts) and they certainly are not "skin-repairing."

☹ **Soothing Protection Spray** (*$31 for 8.4 ounces*) is supposed to protect skin from reactive ozone, which is impossible. Perhaps they made that claim to skirt the fact that this toner irritates, not soothes, skin with lavender oil and the menthol derivative menthoxypropanediol.

☹ **Daily Resurfacer** (*$65 for 0.51 ounce*) is an extremely expensive, somewhat gimmicky way to exfoliate skin, and its exfoliating benefit is dubious. Enclosed in a jar are almost three dozen packets of a liquid solution and a presoaked sponge designed to fit on your index finger. You're directed to massage this in circular motions over skin, with no need to rinse. The solution has in its base a bitter-orange extract, which is a fragrant extract and a skin irritant, so things aren't off to a good start. Salicylic acid (BHA) is included, at about a 1% concentration, but the AHAs touted on the label are sugarcane and apple extracts, neither of which are true AHAs that can exfoliate skin, or at least not with any supporting research. Either way, the pH of this solution is too high for exfoliation to occur, so you're left hoping the sponge applicator will be abrasive enough to do the job. (It isn't, but that's a good thing.) Making matters worse, especially because the product remains on the skin, is grapefruit peel oil. This citrus oil can cause contact dermatitis and phototoxic reactions due to its volatile chemical constituents (Source: www.naturaldatabase.com).

The Reviews D

☹ **Gentle Cream Exfoliant** *($34.50 for 2.5 ounces)* ends up being Dermalogica's idea of gentle, but that includes irritants such as sulfur and lavender oil. Who's formulating these products and marketing them so disingenuously?

☺ **$$$ Skin Renewal Booster** *($45 for 1 ounce)* is a 10% AHA and 0.5% BHA product whose pH of 3.6 is great for exfoliation. The aloe base is excellent for all skin types, though this does contain some thickeners that may be a problem for blemish-prone skin. Skin Renewal Booster contains a few fragrant plant extracts, but in amounts unlikely to cause a problem. Finally, the packaging of this product will help keep the retinol stable.

☹ **$$$ Daily Microfoliant** *($49 for 2.5 ounces)* costs a lot for what amounts to cellulose, talc (the exfoliants in this cleansing scrub), detergent cleansing agents, plant extracts, and irritating essential oil of grapefruit peel. There is no reason to choose this over a standard topical scrub, or just using a washcloth with your water-soluble cleanser.

☹ **$$$ Skin Prep Scrub** *($29 for 2.5 ounces)* is a detergent-based, water-soluble cleanser that contains cornmeal as the scrub agent. It would probably be better to just use cornmeal from the grocery store if you want a cornmeal scrub, because then at least you wouldn't be applying some of the irritating plant extracts that are present in this product, including arnica and ivy. Although these ingredients are probably present in such small amounts that they don't have much effect on skin, why are they in here at all?

☹ **Active Moist** *($36 for 1.7 ounces)* contains lavender and arnica, both problematic ingredients for skin. This is otherwise a very bland, lightweight moisturizer lacking any state-of-the-art ingredients to justify its price.

☹ **$$$ Barrier Repair** *($36 for 1 ounce)* is a silicone-based moisturizer that also contains some vitamin E, plant oils, vitamin C, and anti-irritants. The silicone feels silky on skin and this would be an option for someone with normal to dry skin. It is not rated higher because the antioxidants are in such short supply.

☹ **Climate Control** *($30 for 0.75 ounce)* cannot shield skin from environmental pollutants or protect it from reactive ozone (ozone is bad to breathe, too, so how does this moisturizer protect us from that?). It's an oil- and wax-based formula that would have been recommended for dry to very dry skin if it did not contain geranium oil and lavender.

☹ **Extra Firming Booster** *($45 for 1 ounce)* has an irritating bitter-orange flower base and only makes skin feel firmer because of the PVP (a hairstyling film-forming agent) it contains. The ylang-ylang oil can cause contact dermatitis and itchy skin, which isn't what you want from any product.

☹ **Extra Rich Faceblock SPF 30** *($48 for 1.7 ounces)* would have been an excellent, in-part zinc oxide moisturizing sunscreen for normal to dry skin, but it contains irritating essential oils of sandalwood, eucalyptus, and geranium. Without these troublesome ingredients, this would be highly recommended due to its antioxidant and cell-communicating ingredient content.

☹ **Gentle Soothing Booster** *($45 for 1 ounce)* could have earned highly recommended status due to its roster of genuinely soothing plant extracts. However, the St. John's wort (*Hypericum*) extract can cause severe phototoxic reactions on sun-exposed skin, and that's hardly gentle (Source: www.naturaldatabase.com).

☹ **$$$ Intensive Eye Repair** *($45 for 0.5 ounce)* should not be used around the eyes because the first ingredient is fragrant rose extract. It is an OK moisturizer for normal to dry skin elsewhere on the face, though the arnica extract is present in an amount that may prove irritating to sensitive or reactive skin.

☺ **$$$ Intensive Moisture Balance** *($38 for 1.7 ounces)* lists rose extract as the first ingredient, which makes this a very fragranced moisturizer whose blend of thickeners, silicone, aloe, and antioxidants is fairly good. Without the rose extract this would have rated a Paula's Pick; it includes the cell-communicating ingredient lecithin and does not contain any irritating plant extracts or oils. Those with normal to dry skin may want to consider it.

☹ **Multivitamin Power Concentrate** *($52 for 45 capsules)* has antioxidant finesse and a nonaqueous formula, but it's sabotaged by irritating citrus oils of lime, orange, and grapefruit. This is a dangerous product to apply to skin if it will be exposed to sunlight.

☹ **Oil-Free Matte Block SPF 20** *($45 for 1.7 ounces)* includes titanium dioxide for UVA protection and comes in a lotion base that contains some good antioxidants. Unfortunately, it also contains enough grapefruit peel oil to be irritating and possibly cause a sensitizing reaction on sun-exposed skin.

☹ **Power Rich** *($175 for 1.5 ounces)* promises a pharmaceutical-strength formula that will show a difference after just one week. This rose flower– and silicone-based serum isn't powerful or rich, and it doesn't contain ingredients that have a pharmaceutical quality. It does irritate skin with essential oils of jasmine, ginger, and grapefruit.

☹ **Sheer Moisture SPF 15** *($39 for 1.5 ounces)* includes zinc oxide for UVA protection, but has a lavender base and contains lavender oil. This sunscreen also contains English walnut oil (listed as *Juglans regia*), which, when applied topically, can cause yellow to brown skin discolorations and contact dermatitis (Source: www.naturaldatabase.com).

☹ **Sheer Tint Redness Relief SPF 15** *($39 for 1.3 ounces)* does not provide skin with sufficient UVA protection, and in addition it's a problem that a sheer, moisturizing tint designed to reduce redness contains sensitizing lavender oil as well as the fragrance components limonene and linalool.

☹ **Skin Hydrating Booster** *($53 for 1 ounce)* lists balm mint (*Melissa*) as the main ingredient and also contains lavender oil, making this far too irritating for all skin types.

☹ **Skin Smoothing Cream** *($37 for 1.7 ounces)* contains a potentially irritating amount of arnica as well as sensitizing ylang-ylang oil. Even if you wanted to tolerate these ingredients, the moisturizer is an overall boring formula with a paltry amount of antioxidants.

☺ **$$$ Total Eye Care SPF 15** *($39 for 0.5 ounce)* lists only titanium dioxide as the active ingredient, making this a gentle sunscreen to use around the eyes. Iron oxides, talc, and mica provide a brightening effect to shadowed areas, while lightweight emollients moisturize. The formula lacks significant amounts of antioxidants and interesting skin-identical ingredients, but is an option for normal to dry skin.

☺ **$$$ Intensive Moisture Masque** *($38 for 2.5 ounces)* has some good ingredients for dry to very dry skin, and includes antioxidant vitamins. However, the antioxidants are best left on skin and the titanium dioxide (the second ingredient) creates a strong whitening effect that isn't what you'd want to wear all day. Not to mention that the orange oil can cause irritation.

☹ **Multivitamin Power Recovery Masque** *($40 for 2.5 ounces)* includes some very good plant oils and antioxidants, but those are countered by irritating plant extracts as well as the potent menthol derivative menthoxypropanediol, making this impossible to recommend for any skin type.

☹ **Skin Hydrating Masque** *($35 for 2.5 ounces)* is based around irritating bitter-orange flower extract and also contains irritating ivy, pellitory, and arnica extract, all of which cancel out the effect of the anti-irritant plant extracts in this well-intentioned but problematic mask.

The Reviews D

☹ **Skin Refining Masque** *($34 for 2.5 ounces)* contains the same irritating plant extracts as the Skin Hydrating Masque, but makes matters worse by adding menthol and sage to the mix. There are many clay masks that absorb oil and refine skin's texture without causing undue irritation.

☹ **Special Clearing Booster** *($41 for 1 ounce)* is a needlessly expensive topical disinfectant with 5% benzoyl peroxide as the active ingredient. This water-based solution is not recommended because it contains St. John's wort, sage, lemon, and ivy.

☹ **Sheer Tint Moisture SPF 15** *($40 for 1.3 ounces)*. Although this tinted moisturizer includes an in-part zinc oxide sunscreen and comes in three sheer colors, the base formula contains pure lavender oil. Although it may smell soothing, lavender oil can be a skin irritant and a photosensitizer (Sources: *Contact Dermatitis*, August 1999, page 111; and *Family Practice Notebook*, www.fpnotebook.com/DER188.htm). Research also indicates that components of lavender, specifically linalool, can be cytotoxic, meaning that topical application causes skin-cell death (Source: *Cell Proliferation*, June 2004, pages 221-229). In addition, the fragrance constituents in lavender oil oxidize when exposed to air; this not only makes lavender oil a pro-oxidant, but also increases its irritancy on skin (Source: *Contact Dermatitis*, September 2008, pages 143-150). Lavender oil is a must to avoid if you care about the health of your skin.

☺ **$$$ Treatment Foundation** *($35)*. Dermalogica describes this as skin care disguised as makeup, but there's not much to extol about this formula in terms of genuine skin-care benefits. The ingredients it contains aren't a treat for skin; the minuscule amount of vitamins doesn't count. The foundation itself dispenses thick but blends smoothly and feels lighter than you might think. It provides medium coverage and a smooth matte finish suitable for normal to slightly oily skin. The shades aren't the best because most of them leave an odd grayish cast on skin. Shades 1G, 2G, and 3G aren't as affected by this oddity and those are the recommended colors should you decide to try this foundation.

DERMALOGICA SUN PRODUCTS

☹ **After Sun Repair** *($31 for 3.4 ounces)* contains far too many irritating plant extracts and essential oils to be even slightly capable of repairing sun-exposed skin. If anything, the irritant potential of the essential oils will further damage skin and negatively affect the healing process.

☹ **Multivitamin Bodyblock SPF 20** *($35 for 4.2 ounces)* contains avobenzone for sufficient UVA protection, but also has lavender oil, which can irritate skin and cause skin-cell death (Source: *Cell Proliferation*, June 2004, pages 221-229).

☹ **Solar Defense Booster SPF 30** *($43 for 1 ounce)* contains avobenzone, so this one has good UVA protection! However, it also contains balm mint and lemon extracts plus lavender oil, all skin irritants.

☹ **Solar Defense Wipes SPF 15** *($22 for 15 wipes)* not only lack the correct UVA-protecting ingredients, but also contain balm mint and several irritating essential oils, including spearmint.

☹ **Solar Shield SPF 15** *($12 for 0.28 ounce)* is an emollient sunscreen in stick form that lacks the UVA-protecting ingredients of titanium dioxide, zinc oxide, avobenzone, Tinosorb, or Mexoryl SX. Making matters even worse is the inclusion of menthol and grapefruit oil.

☹ **Super Sensitive Faceblock SPF 30** *($45 for 1.7 ounces)* contains lavender oil, which is completely unsuitable for "super sensitive" skin. It's good that the active ingredients are only titanium dioxide and zinc oxide, and the formula has some well-researched antioxidants and soothing agents, but the lavender oil trumps them all.

☹ **Ultra Sensitive Faceblock SPF 25** *($30 for 1.7 ounces)* lists balm mint as the first ingredient, which may make skin ultra-sensitive and irritated. This completely titanium dioxide sunscreen also assaults skin with several ouch-inducing essential oils, including thyme, rosewood, and orange.

☹ **Waterblock Solar Spray SPF 30** *($38 for 4.2 ounces)* leaves skin vulnerable to UVA damage because it lacks titanium dioxide, zinc oxide, avobenzone, Tinosorb, or Mexoryl SX. It also contains irritating balm mint extract and grapefruit peel oil.

DHC

DHC AT-A-GLANCE

Strengths: Several inexpensive products; many fragrance-free products; complete product ingredient lists on their Web site; several worthwhile cleansers and makeup removers; an effective AHA product; every sunscreen provides UVA protection; antioxidant olive oil and olive leaf extract are present in many products.

Weaknesses: Mostly unexciting toners; an effective BHA product that regrettably contains an irritant; no skin-lightening options with a roster of proven ingredients; huge assortment of products, many with repetitive or gimmicky formulas; products with nanoparticles of silver (completely useless for skin), which can cause permanent skin discoloration (who wants to absorb silver into their skin given that it can be toxic when consumed?).

For more information about DHC, call (800) 342-2273 or visit www.dhccare.com or www. Beautypedia.com.

DHC SKIN CARE

☺ **Cleansing Foam** *($9 for 2.1 ounces)* is a standard, foaming water-soluble cleanser that is a good option for normal to oily skin, as the amount of potassium hydroxide makes it potentially drying for those with normal to dry skin. I disagree with their claim that this formula is "gentle enough for multiple daily cleansings," because it isn't, not to mention that washing your face more than twice daily is not only unrealistic for most people, but also incredibly drying and stripping for skin. Frequent cleansing doesn't improve skin, and with these ingredients, it can disrupt the skin's protective barrier.

✓ ☺ **Cleansing Milk** *($24 for 6.7 ounces)* is an excellent, detergent-free cleansing lotion for dry to very dry or sensitive/rosacea-prone skin. It removes makeup easily, but you'll have to use a washcloth to avoid leaving a film on your skin.

☺ $$$ **Deep Cleansing Oil** *($25 for 6.7 ounces)* is said to be the company's most popular product the world over, but the formula doesn't support the claim. The olive oil–based formula is blended with a surfactant/emulsifying agent (sorbeth-30 tetraoleate) that provides greater cleansing ability than oils alone (which aren't really that cleansing, but can remove makeup) and also helps make this oil easier to rinse than you might expect, though it can still leave a film. The rosemary oil is a potential irritant, especially when used around the eyes, but this is still a workable option.

☺ $$$ **Face Wash** *($28.50 for 6.7 ounces)* would earn a Paula's Pick rating if it did not contain fragrant rosemary oil (which isn't "rejuvenating" as claimed). The amount is small enough that it isn't likely cause for concern, but you should be extra careful using this water-soluble

The Reviews D

cleanser around the eyes. The detergent-based formula removes makeup easily and is best for normal to oily skin.

✓☺ **Make Off Sheets** *($7.50 for 50 sheets)* are cotton wipes soaked in a lightweight water-soluble cleanser. These are fragrance-free, and are an option for all skin types. The only issue is that these tend to be ineffective for removing long-wearing or waterproof makeup.

☹ **Mild Soap** *($15.50 for 3.1 ounces)* is mild in name only. This is a very standard bar soap formula that can be too drying for all skin types, not to mention that it leaves a residue on skin that can build up and make for a dull-looking complexion.

☺ **$$$ Olive Soap** *($22 for 3.1 ounces)* is a soap-free bar cleanser that contains detergent cleansing agents buffered by olive oil and glycerin. Although this is better than traditional soap, it can be drying for dry or sensitive skin, and isn't preferred to a good water-soluble cleanser.

☺ **Pure Soap** *($10.50 for 2.8 ounces)* is very similar to DHC's Olive Soap, except this version has less olive oil and a lighter texture, making it suitable for oily skin. It is fragrance-free, but still not preferred to an effective and gentle water-soluble cleanser.

☹ **Q10 Facial Film** *($11 for 40 sheets)* consists of dry sheets steeped in a dehydrated cleansing solution that is activated by mixing with water. They can be too drying and irritating for all skin types because the main ingredient is sodium lauryl sulfate (which is listed on the label as sodium laurate, another name for sodium lauryl sulfate, something that perhaps the company was trying to hide).

☺ **Salicylic Acne Wash** *($14.50 for 4 ounces)* cannot banish acne blemishes because its active ingredient (2% salicylic acid) is rinsed down the drain along with the rest of it before it has a chance to work. This is otherwise a very ordinary cleanser/scrub hybrid for normal to oily skin. Keep in mind that acne cannot be scrubbed away, nor can blackheads. In fact, using a scrub over acne lesions can worsen the inflammation and slow the healing process.

✓☺ **Soft Touch Cleansing Oil** *($14 for 5 ounces)* is a light cleansing oil that removes makeup with oil-like ingredients and emollients and a relatively small amount of actual oil (olive). It is fragrance-free and is a gentle, reliable option for normal to dry skin not prone to blemishes.

☺ **Washing Powder** *($10 for 1.7 ounces)* is a detergent-based powder that forms a water-soluble, foaming cleanser when mixed with water. The amount of papain is much too small to provide enzymatic exfoliation, not to mention that papain is an unreliable ingredient for exfoliating skin because it has stability issues. If the novelty of this is appealing, it's a good fragrance-free option for normal to oily skin.

✓☺ **Eye Make-Up Remover** *($11 for 3.7 ounces)* is a very standard, fragrance-free, detergent-based makeup remover that works as well as any, but is notably gentle.

☹ **$$$ Acerola 100** *($22.50 for 1 ounce)* does contain a minute amount of acerola, which is a source of vitamin C; however, acerola included in a cosmetic is unlikely to be a good source of vitamin C because much of the vitamin is destroyed during the drying and processing (Source: www.naturaldatabase.com). Plus, for the money, there is not enough of the showcased ingredient present to maintain healthy skin; the skin is more complicated than that, just like vitamin C isn't the only vitamin you need in your diet. This is just a bare-bones fragrance-free toner for normal to dry skin.

☺ **Acerola Lotion** *($17 for 3.3 ounces)* is similar to DHC's Acerola 100, except this version offers skin some good water-binding agents and a tiny amount of placental protein, an animal-derived ingredient that some of you may wish to avoid. Acerola is a poor source of vitamin C because of how it is processed (which likely destroys the vitamin C content that it had when in pure form), but this is still a decent toner for normal to dry skin. It contains fragrance in the form of peony extract.

☺ **$$$ Alpha-Arbutin White Lotion** *($42 for 3.3 ounces)* contains mostly water, slip agents, water-binding agent, plant extract, alpha-arbutin, more water-binding agents, pH adjusters, and fragrant flower extracts. Alpha-arbutin has some research showing it can lighten skin discolorations, but the research was on a 5% concentration, while this product has less than a 2% concentration. Hydroquinone is still the ingredient with the most research showing efficacy for skin-lightening, but as an alternative, a 5% alpha-arbutin product is an option. It's just that this product isn't it.

☺ **Balancing Lotion** *($22 for 6 ounces)* contains less than 1% glycolic acid, which is a shame, because this toner's pH of 3.9 would have allowed exfoliation to occur if the AHA were present at a higher concentration. As is, this toner underwhelms, and also contains two problematic plant extracts (horsetail and lemon), making it a "Why bother?" for any skin type.

☺ **$$$ Ceramide Quick** *($28 for 4 ounces)* doesn't actually contain any ceramides. It's just a simple, fragrance-free "toner" that contains mostly water, slip agent, glycerin, soybean seed extract, placental protein, and preservative. It's OK, but there is little about this product that can restore ceramide levels to your skin, at least not any more than any other simple moisturizer can.

☺ **$$$ Mild Lotion** *($34 for 6 ounces)* is merely water, glycerin, slip agent, cucumber juice, placental protein (an ingredient many cosmetics companies no longer use due to pressure from animal rights advocates), and preservatives. The price is insulting for what is nothing more than an exceedingly ordinary toner.

☺ **$$$ Olive Leaf Lotion** *($38 for 4 ounces)* is a boring, overpriced toner for all skin types. While it's good that they omitted fragrance, there isn't much to extol here, unless you believe olive leaf extract is the best antioxidant around (which, of course, it isn't).

☺ **$$$ Q10 Lotion** *($36 for 5 ounces)* is a water-based toner that contains some good anti-irritants and water-binding agents along with a tiny amount of antioxidants, including ubiquinone (coenzyme Q10). Much is known about the antioxidant activity of Q10 when ingested, but there is only a small amount of in vitro research demonstrating its effect on skin cells. From what's known, it appears that ubiquinone not only has antioxidant activity that allows it to protect skin from sun damage, but also can inhibit MMP-1, a matrix metalloproteinase that causes collagen breakdown (Sources: *Journal of Cosmetic Dermatology*, March 2006, pages 30-38; *Biofactors*, 2005, pages 179-185, and 1999, pages 371-378). Note that the Biofactors studies were conducted by researchers working for Beiersdorf, and one of their brands (Nivea) sells products that contain ubiquinone. More important, the concentration of ubiquinone used in the studies was likely much greater than the tiny amount present in skin-care products, including this one. As long as you don't expect this toner to keep your skin looking wrinkle-free, it's a suitable option for normal to dry skin.

☺ **$$$ Q10 Water Mist** *($29 for 5 ounces)* is an unimpressive, overpriced toning mist that contains mostly water, slip agent, anti-irritant, and preservative. The amount of ubiquinone (coenzyme Q10) is too insignificant for your skin to notice (see the review of the Q10 Lotion above for a brief description of the research on this ingredient). It is fragrance-free.

☹ **Rose Toner** *($21 for 3.3 ounces)* is more eau de cologne than toner, and with alcohol as the second ingredient, it is too drying and irritating for all skin types. Nothing in this toner is helpful for skin "plagued by blemishes."

The Reviews D

☹ **Rose Water** *($22 for 5 ounces)* is a nearly do-nothing-but-smell-floral concoction of water, rose water, slip agents, and preservatives. Wearing perfume is one thing, but it certainly is not skin care.

☹ **Salicylic Acne Toner** *($14.50 for 5.4 ounces)* contains 2% salicylic acid as an active ingredient, but the pH is above 4, so it will not function very well, if at all, as an exfoliant. This is otherwise a below-average toner whose rosemary oil content can irritate skin.

☹ **Skin Softener** *($32 for 3.3 ounces)* contains a high amount of coltsfoot extract, a plant whose chemical constituents are considered carcinogenic and toxic when administered orally, and it has no documented benefit for skin (Source: www.naturaldatabase.com).

☹ **Soothing Lotion, For Drier Skin** *($19 for 6 ounces)* contains alcloxa, an ingredient that has constricting properties, which is certainly not helpful for dry skin, and it can be irritating. The glycolic acid is present at too low a concentration to exfoliate skin, but the pH of 4.4 would inhibit that from occurring anyway. DHC makes other toners that actually are deserving of being labeled "soothing," but this one isn't.

☺ **$$$ White Lotion** *($29 for 3.3 ounces)* is an OK toner for normal to dry skin, assuming that you believe cucumber juice is a helpful skin-care ingredient. The amount of botanical ingredients in this product that can potentially "brighten" skin is teeny, so this would not be the toner to use if skin discolorations or dullness are concerns.

☺ **Renewing AHA Cream** *($39 for 1.5 ounces)* contains a blend of 10% AHAs (mostly lactic acid) and the pH of 3.8 allows exfoliation! The lightweight lotion base is great for normal to dry skin, and this contains antioxidant olive oil along with a couple of impressive water-binding agents.

☺ **Salicylic Face Milk** *($19 for 2 ounces)* contains 2% salicylic acid and has a pH of 3.8, so exfoliation will occur. Although this is an effective BHA product for blemishes and blackheads, it also contains a couple of troublesome ingredients (rosemary oil and perilla extract). Neither is present in significant amounts, however, so this is still worth considering as a BHA product for normal to slightly dry or slightly oily skin.

☺ **$$$ Facial Scrub** *($16.50 for 3.5 ounces)* is a substandard scrub for normal to dry skin because the abrasive agent is apricot seed powder. This is not preferred to polyethylene or jojoba beads, which are spherical, because the apricot seed powder particles may have sharp edges that leave your skin with microscopic, skin-damaging scratches. The potassium-based ingredients add unnecessary dryness, making this less preferred to most other facial scrubs.

☺ **Acerola Cream** *($23 for 1.4 ounces)*. DHC boasts about the antioxidant content of this moisturizer for normal to dry skin, but then neglect to use air-tight packaging to keep them stable. The jar packaging allows the antioxidants to deteriorate after opening, but that isn't a big issue because there aren't many antioxidants in this product anyway. This is an OK moisturizer, but forget about any benefits from the acerola (a type of cherry that's rich in vitamin C), which could have been helpful if a larger amount were included and if it were in better packaging.

☺ **Acerola Gel** *($17 for 1.4 ounces)* contains a bit of acerola and little else. This is a mediocre gel moisturizer for normal skin. Acerola is not a wonder ingredient for skin; plus, the manner in which it is processed and packaged depletes any potential efficacy.

☹ **Alpha-Arbutin White Cream** *($45 for 1.2 ounces)* claims to be a one-of-a-kind skin-lightening product because it contains alpha-arbutin. However, this potential skin-lightening agent isn't unique to this product or to DHC. Alpha-arbutin can block the pathways involved in causing melanin to form, but this product doesn't contain the 5% concentration that has been shown in some research to be effective. Plus, the jar packaging DHC uses will not keep this ingredient stable! Although this has much going for it as a moisturizer for dry to very dry skin, it is not recommended because it contains silver, which can cause a permanent bluish discoloration to skin (Source: www.naturaldatabase.com).

☹ **Alpha-Arbutin White Milk** *($42 for 2.7 ounces)* contains more mulberry root than alpha-arbutin, but both have in vitro research demonstrating their potential effectiveness for lightening skin discolorations. Although this product comes in stable packaging (unlike DHC's Alpha-Arbutin White Cream), it is still a risky choice for skin because of its silver content (and I'd be suspicious of the placental protein in here, too, particularly if it is from a bovine source).

☺ **Antiox C** *($34.50 for 1.4 ounces)* is worth considering if you have normal to dry skin and are looking for a stably packaged moisturizer with stabilized vitamin C. The vitamin C and the olive oil are the only antioxidants of note in this moisturizer. The inclusion of anti-irritant licorice is thoughtful, and the formula is fragrance-free.

☺ **Ceramide Cream** *($33 for 1.4 ounces)* doesn't contain any ceramides; if it did they would have to be listed because ceramides are individual ingredients, not delivery systems like liposomes. Unfortunately, this moisturizer for normal to dry skin will see its antioxidants break down shortly after the jar is opened, and that's not good news.

☺ **Ceramide Milk** *($29 for 2.7 ounces)* is a standard lightweight yet emollient moisturizer for normal to dry skin. The formula does not list any ceramides, which makes the name misleading. Although this contains antioxidants (mostly from olive oil), the translucent bottle packaging demands careful storage to keep it protected from exposure to light. Ceramide Milk is fragrance-free.

☺ **Concentrated Eye Cream** *($31.50 for 0.7 ounce)* is a basic, lightweight eye cream whose rosemary leaf extract content (while a good source of antioxidants) may be too irritating for use near the eyes. None of the plants in this cream can diminish drooping skin or lighten dark circles. In fact, the antioxidant potency of these plants is lessened due to jar packaging, making this a merely average option for normal to slightly dry skin.

☺ **Dual Defense SPF 25** *($27 for 3.5 ounces)* is a good, fragrance-free daytime moisturizer for normal to slightly dry or slightly oily skin. The active ingredients include titanium dioxide for UVA protection, while the base formula works well under makeup. The only antioxidant of note is olive oil, yet it is present in an efficacious amount, and DHC left the fragrance out.

☺ **$$$ EGF Cream** *($89 for 1.2 ounces)* claims to combat signs of aging with a peptide linked to epidermal growth factors. I think it's a good thing the peptide in question is barely present. Why? Because the research examining the topical effects of epidermal growth factors has been short term and concerned primarily with their effect on wound healing. Wrinkles and discolorations (common signs of aging) are not wounds, and although the claim that you can "heal" a wrinkle like a wound by treating it with growth factors is good theory, the research hasn't been done to prove such efficacy. In theory, epidermal growth factors (hormones that induce skin-cell production), when applied topically, may trigger repair mechanisms in skin that have become faulty due to age and sun damage (DNA damage caused by sun exposure). However, theory isn't fact. The problem is, we don't know for sure which growth factors work best, how much is needed, and whether or not long-term use is safe (Sources: *Skin Research and Technology*, August 2008, pages 370-375; and *The Surgeon*, June 2008, pages 172-177). In addition, it's well known that epidermal growth factors administered orally as an adjunct or alternative to chemotherapy cause a variety of skin problems, from rashes to acne (Source: *Clinical Journal of*

Oncology Nursing, April 2008, pages 283-290). In short, until more is known about formulary protocols for epidermal growth factors in skin-care products, I don't advise using them as part of your antiaging skin-care routine, no matter how small an amount is in the product. Although the small amount means that it is probably not going to have any effect at all, pro or con, why take the risk? As mentioned, this DHC moisturizer claims to contain a peptide classified as an epidermal growth factor, but that designation isn't clear in any research; rather, it appears to be strictly a marketing claim. That leaves you with an emollient moisturizer whose plant oil and antioxidant efficacy will suffer due to the jar packaging (after all those claims, using jar packaging is just plain stupid). This ends up being a grandiose-sounding product that's essentially just a basic moisturizer that doesn't outpace many lesser priced options.

☹ **Emollient Balm** *($33 for 3.3 ounces)* is a basic emollient moisturizer for normal to dry skin not prone to breakouts. It contains some good, if gimmicky, water-binding agents and the primary antioxidant is olive oil. The translucent glass bottle means this should be stored away from light to keep the antioxidants stable during use. The amount of retinol is too small to matter, while the addition of coltsfoot extract is potentially problematic.

☹ **$$$ Extra Concentrate** *($40 for 1 ounce)* plays on the popular myth that topically applied collagen can add to the collagen content of wrinkled, sun-damaged skin. It doesn't work that way, but most of the ingredients in this "concentrate" have hydrating ability. The plant extracts include a mix of anti-irritants and irritants, so in effect they cancel each other out.

☹ **Extra Nighttime Moisture, For Everyone's Skin** *($32.50 for 1.5 ounces)* is not for everyone—those with acne-prone skin will not appreciate the oil content of this moisturizer. It is otherwise a basic, minimal frills moisturizer for normal to slightly dry skin. The jar packaging will compromise the antioxidant potential of the olive oil; the other antioxidants are present in amounts too small for skin to benefit.

☹ **Eye Bright** *($21.50 for 0.52 ounce)* is mostly water and cucumber juice with slip agents and the plant *Isodonis japonicus*, whose terpene content can be irritating to skin, especially around the eyes. You'd be better off using plain, fresh cucumber slices to soothe the eye area, though that home remedy isn't all it's cracked up to be either!

☹ **Eye Off-Shade** *($19 for 0.21 ounce)* tries to convince you it is the solution for dark, puffy eyes, but it contains not a single ingredient that can alleviate either condition. The plant extracts referred to as brightening agents are present in the tiniest amounts imaginable, while the crux of the formula relies on placental protein. Growth factors from animal and human placentas appear to play a role in wound healing, but that is completely unrelated to the cause of dark circles or puffy eyes.

☹ **$$$ Eye Treatment Essence Peptides** *($39.50 for 1 ounce)* wants you to believe the tiny amount of peptides it contains will stimulate collagen production to rejuvenate skin's support structure. There is no proof peptides can do this, though they appear to have worth as cell-communicating ingredients, assuming that enzymes in the skin don't destroy them before they reach their target cells. Even so, the peptide content of this product is really disappointing, and it is otherwise a do-nothing gel for normal to oily skin.

☺ **$$$ Eye Wrinkle Stick** *($36 for 0.07 ounce)* is a very good, fragrance-free, balm moisturizer for dry to very dry skin. It contains some very effective emollients and a couple of antioxidant plant oils (though the amount of vitamin-based antioxidants is likely too small for skin to notice). This stick will soften the appearance of wrinkles, especially lines resulting from dry, irritated skin, but how it goes about making eyes look more awake (as claimed) is a mystery, unless by that DHC means the satin finish this leaves reflects light from skin better than when it is dry.

☹ **Fermented Soy Milk Essence** *($31 for 1 ounce)* contains fermented soybean extract as one of the main ingredients, but there is zero research qualifying this ingredient as an "age-defying wonder." Besides, if it's that amazing, how come DHC doesn't include it in their numerous other moisturizers and serums? The research done on fermented soy does show that the ingredients used in the fermentation process cause volatile compounds to form (sesquiterpenes and ethanol, among them). That means this is not an ingredient you'd want to use on your skin, especially given its unproven efficacy (Source: *International Journal of Food Microbiology*, January 2007, pages 133-141).

☹ **Matte Cream** *($28 for 1.4 ounces)* is supposed to mattify skin to reduce "beauty meltdowns" from excess oil production. The stearic acid won't make your skin feel matte at all, while the amount of absorbent kaolin is too small to keep excess shine at bay for more than an hour. Lastly, the garlic bulb extract in this can cause serious skin irritation, and has no benefit for oily skin, and the silver can cause discoloration. Who was in charge of creating this product?!

☹ **Neck Treatment Essence Peptides** *($39.50 for 1 ounce)* is a ridiculously ineffective product to consider if you're concerned about slackening skin on the neck. First, there is no research proving any peptide can shore up and tighten loose skin (and the amount of peptides in this product is embarrassingly low); second, there is far more preservative than interesting ingredients in this product; and third, nothing in this formula can improve the appearance of sun-damaged skin on the neck or décolleté. All this adds up to is a waste of time and money.

☹ **Olive Leaf Cream** *($38 for 1.4 ounces)* is an emollient moisturizer that indeed does contain olive oil, which can be a beneficial, nonirritating plant oil for dry skin. However, the moisturizing goes astray because of the pointless inclusion of menthol, which is irritating, and jar packaging, which won't keep the olive-based antioxidants stable during use.

☺ **$$$ Olive Leaf Extract** *($45 for 1 ounce)* is simply olive leaf extract with slip agents and a preservative. The olive leaf is a source of antioxidants, but I could find no independent substantiation that olive leaf supplies coenzyme Q10 to skin as DHC claims, and this coenzyme (also known as ubiquinone) is not listed on the ingredient statement. This is an awfully pricey way for anyone with any type of skin to see how olive leaf works for them. I'd rather see you using a product that has a cocktail of antioxidants rather than a one-note product like this.

☺ **Olive Leaf Milk** *($38 for 2.7 ounces)* claims to be the daytime moisturizer for environmentally damaged (including sun-damaged) skin. What a joke! This contains nothing that's not also in most of DHC's other moisturizers, and without a sunscreen it is an impractical choice for daytime use (unless your foundation is SPF 15 or greater and you apply it evenly and liberally). This is a good moisturizer for normal to dry skin that relies on olive oil and extract as its main antioxidants. It does contain a tiny amount of the cell-communicating ingredient lecithin. Olive Leaf Milk contains fragrance in the form of floral extracts.

☺ **Olive Virgin Oil** *($39 for 1 ounce)*. At first I thought this was a joke, but it isn't. This is pure virgin olive oil. Even if virgin olive oil were a great skin-care ingredient (and it does have benefits for dry skin), why would you bother buying this from a cosmetics company for such an absurd amount of money, as opposed to buying the exact same thing from a grocery store for a fraction of the price? Olive oil is a good antioxidant moisturizing oil for dry skin, but that's about it. DHC does their best to convince consumers that this offering is somehow special and superior to the olive oil you'd use for cooking, but it absolutely is not.

☹ **Platinum Nanocolloid Lotion** *($27 for 4 ounces).* With a name like this product has, you'll either wonder what in the world it's supposed to do or assume that the mystery behind the name must mean an antiwrinkle miracle is in store. "Nanocolloid," what does that mean? Regrettably, the answer is depressing rather than enlightening. This toner-like product contains mostly water, slip agent, and alcohol. Alcohol causes free-radical damage, irritation, and dryness. This also contains a small amount of other problematic ingredients, including the plants angelica and arnica, both irritants, and pure silver, which can cause a permanent bluish discoloration on skin (Source: www.naturaldatabase.com).

☹ **Platinum Silver Nanocolloid Cream** *($25 for 1.5 ounces)* makes claims that have no substantiated research behind them, and also contains several plant ingredients that are a distinct problem for skin, including angelica, arnica, and perilla. In addition, it contains silver, which can cause bluish skin discolorations, and platinum powder, which has no benefit for healthy, intact skin. The silver is even more of a problem if DHC is serious about it being nano-sized, as this will enhance its penetration into the skin, which is not a good thing.

☹ **Platinum Silver Nanocolloid Milky Essence** *($25 for 2.7 ounces)* contains several plant ingredients that are a distinct problem for skin, including angelica, arnica, and perilla. This also contains silver (supposedly nano-sized), which can cause bluish skin discolorations, and platinum powder, which has no benefit for healthy, intact skin.

☺ **$$$ Protein Gel** *($38 for 1 ounce)* cannot protect moisture levels in the dermis, because no moisturizer can reach this deeper layer of skin. This is a simple mix of water, slip agent, water-binding agent, antioxidants, and preservative. It's about as exciting as Monday morning after a fun weekend, but it is a passable gel for oily skin if you're not expecting much beyond lightweight moisture.

☺ **$$$ Q10 Cream** *($45 for 1 ounce)* contains more antioxidants than what DHC typically puts in their moisturizers, which makes it all the more shameful that jar packaging was chosen. You're paying a hefty price for this moisturizer for normal to dry skin, but most of what you're paying for will be wasted as the antioxidants degrade in the jar packaging. I also am concerned that the silver in this product may be a problem for skin, though only a small amount is present.

☺ **Q10 Eye Cream** *($24 for 0.88 ounce)* has a texture similar to DHC's Q10 Cream, but has a more well-rounded formula and packaging that will keep the many antioxidants it contains stable. The drawback is that most of the antioxidants (and the alpha-arbutin, which doesn't lighten dark circles) are present in meager amounts, unlike in the aforementioned Q10 Cream. That's disappointing, but this is still a good fragrance-free moisturizer for dry skin anywhere on the face.

☺ **Q10 Milk** *($36 for 3.3 ounces)* would be rated a Paula's Pick if the majority of the antioxidants weren't listed after the preservative. As is, Q10 Milk is a good-but-should've-been-better moisturizer for normal to oily skin, including sensitive or blemished skin. It is fragrance-free.

☺ **Q10 Neck Cream** *($24 for 0.88 ounce)* contains the same ingredients as the DHC Q10 Eye Cream, and holds no special benefit for skin on the neck. How odd that nearly identical formulas are positioned for two different areas, but undoubtedly there are some women who will buy into that foolishness. The best neck cream a person can use is a well-formulated sunscreen that provides sufficient UVA protection. No neck-area products I've ever seen can forestall aging, slackening skin if sun protection isn't used daily.

☺ **$$$ Retino A Essence** *($36 for 0.51 ounce)* contains a very small amount of vitamin A as retinyl palmitate. It is otherwise a lightweight, silky moisturizer for normal to slightly dry skin not prone to blemishes. If you're looking for a vitamin A product, there are better options from Neutrogena, among other brands.

☺ **Rich Moisture, For Normal to Drier Skin** *($29.50 for 3.3 ounces)* is a good emollient moisturizer for dry skin, but one that must be stored away from light to protect the antioxidant action of the olive oil. There's a minuscule amount of royal jelly, which sounds good and can be an emollient, but it serves no great purpose for skin care.

☹ **Rose Treatment Oil** *($25 for 1.6 ounces)* is an olive oil–based moisturizer that contains some good emollients, vitamin E, plant extracts, and rose hip extract. It's an option for dry to very dry skin, but does not list the fragrant (and potentially irritating) rose otto oil referred to in the claims. Given this product's fragrance and the fact that the fragrance isn't listed on the ingredient statement, this product isn't too appealing.

☹ **$$$ Royal Jelly Extract** *($39.50 for 1 ounce)* is merely water with slip agents, royal jelly protein, and preservatives. If you believe all the claims attributed to royal jelly, there's nothing I can say to deter you from purchasing this product. According to the compiled research, how-ever, there is little evidence of this ingredient's benefit, whether applied topically or consumed in supplement form.

☹ **Suncut Q10 30+** *($16.50 for 1 ounce)* contains several active ingredients, including 20% zinc oxide and almost 6% titanium dioxide. UVA protection is assured, but the amount of aforementioned mineral sunscreens will leave your skin with an unmistakable bluish-white cast. Moreover, the amount of alcohol in this silky lotion is cause for concern, especially given its prevalence over any of the antioxidants in this sunscreen.

☹ **Suncut Q10 30+ Light Lamé** *($17 for 1 ounce)* contains several active ingredients, including 20% zinc oxide and almost 6% titanium dioxide. UVA protection is assured, but the amount of these mineral sunscreens will leave an unmistakable bluish-white cast on your skin. The amount of alcohol in this sunscreen is very disappointing, and makes it not worth considering (and why they added a lamé-like shimmer is just plain weird).

☺ **Tocophero E Cream** *($29 for 1.2 ounces)* contains an impressive amount of vitamin E along with some other known antioxidants. However, jar packaging won't keep them stable during use, relegating this to ho-hum status as a moisturizer for normal to dry skin not prone to blemishes.

☺ **Velvet Skin Coat** *($21)* is said to be a DHC customer favorite, and it's not hard to see why: its silky, silicone-based formula leaves all skin types feeling incredibly soft and smooth. It can minimally fill in pores and superficial lines and help facilitate makeup application. The problem is in how basic the formula is—the blend of silicones and a tiny amount of olive oil isn't nearly as impressive as similar primer/line filler–type products from lines such as Good Skin, Estee Lauder, Smashbox, and even the Regenerist serums from Olay. All of these can make your skin feel equally silky, yet they offer several more beneficial ingredients. This DHC product is an option if you need a lightweight moisturizer or want to try a basic foundation primer; it's just not as noteworthy as competing products. It is worth mentioning that, with the exception of Olay, DHC's Velvet Skin Coat is among the least expensive options in this category.

☺ **$$$ Vitamin C Essence** *($38 for 0.84 ounce)* is a very good lightweight, fragrance-free serum with stabilized vitamin C (magnesium ascorbyl phosphate) as the second ingredient. Al-though really a one-note product for all skin types, it is a formidable option for those interested in seeing what a vitamin C-exclusive product can do for their skin.

☺ **Water Base Moisture** *($16.50 for 2 ounces)* is a simple, ultralight moisturizer for normal to oily skin. It supplies some skin-identical substances and other water-binding agents such as placental protein and serine, along with tiny amounts of anti-irritants. Although inexpensive, your skin deserves more than this can provide.

☹ **White Cream** *($34 for 1.4 ounces)* doesn't stand a chance of whitening your skin because the vitamin C and plant extracts in here that have that capability (though the efficacy of the plants is questionable, especially given the mere dusting of them in this product) will quickly deteriorate once this jar-packaged moisturizer for normal to dry skin is opened. How sad, because in an opaque, airless package this would have been a fantastic option.

☺ **White Sunscreen SPF 25** *($23.50 for 1 ounce)* has more pros than cons. The pros include titanium dioxide and zinc oxide as active ingredients, making this a potential option for sensitive skin. It also has a lightweight, silky texture and absorbent matte finish suitable for oily skin, and it works well under makeup. The cons include a slight white cast from the amount of mineral sunscreen ingredients and the inclusion of silver, which has potentially unpleasant, permanent side effects for skin. The amount of silver is barely worth mentioning, but it really should not be included in skin-care products.

☹ **$$$ Wrinkle Essence** *($43 for 0.67 ounce)* is no more the "essence of youthful skin" than cosmetic surgery is the best solution for personal relationship issues. This blend of water with slip agents and water-binding agents is about as unexciting as it gets. Almost all of the ingredients appear in myriad DHC products, making this an expensive extra that can be ignored, mostly because it doesn't work as claimed.

✓ ☺ **Wrinkle Filler** *($27 for 0.52 ounce)* doesn't fill wrinkles in the same way some silicone-based primers can, and would be better described as an oil-based moisturizer for dry to very dry skin that is also sensitive. Antioxidant benefit is provided from the olive and rice oils along with vitamin E. This also contains an impressive amount of a licorice-based soothing agent, and is fragrance-free.

☹ **Acne Spot Therapy** *($12.50 for 0.52 ounce)* contains 3% sulfur as the active ingredient, which makes this too drying and irritating for all skin types. A couple of the plant extracts are also irritating and lack efficacy for acne-prone skin, but sulfur is the main concern.

☺ **Alpha-Arbutin White Mask** *($12 for 5 sheets)* is a gimmicky sheet-style mask you place over your face and remove after several minutes. The amount of alpha-arbutin is inconsequential for lightening skin discolorations, not to mention that this ingredient is best left on skin to work, which makes it silly to include it in a short-term application product meant for occasional use.

☺ **$$$ Alpha-Arbutin White Powder** *($20.50 for 0.17 ounce)* is meant as a spot treatment for small areas of discoloration. The amount of alpha-arbutin is potentially effective, but there isn't a lot of research proving this is the best skin-lightening agent to choose. Still, if you're curious and will diligently wear a sunscreen as well, this is an option for all skin types and may be used with any other skin-care product.

☺ **Eyelash Tonic** *($13 for 0.21 ounce)* does not contain a single ingredient that can discourage lash breakage or create a "more robust lash line." Instead, this contains problematic plant extracts, including comfrey and watercress. Interestingly, the main plant ingredient, *Swertia japonica*, is one of several herbs listed as plant sources for a substance that helps inhibit the conversion of testosterone to its more potent form, dihydrotestosterone, which causes men to lose their hair. That fact is unrelated to keeping eyelashes from falling out (men who go bald typically don't lose their eyelashes along with scalp hair), and the fact remains that there is no proof this plant extract has any effect, pro or con, on eyelashes.

☺ **Lip Cream** *($7.50 for 0.05 ounce)* is an emollient, lanolin-based lip balm packaged in a lipstick-style container, making for a portable, convenient way to keep dry, chapped lips to a minimum. This is fragrance-free, and contains antioxidant olive oil, too, putting it above many other balms.

☹ **Q10 Mask** *($14 for 4 sheets)* is a gimmicky sheet meant to work as a mask; you place it over your face and then remove it after several minutes. The water-based formula is OK for normal to oily skin, but if you were hoping to get a megadose of coenzyme Q10 (ubiquinone), keep shopping—it is barely present in this formula, and is of little use to skin when used short-term. Plus, it is not the only ingredient skin needs (any more than it is the only vitamin needed in your diet).

☹ **Revitalizing Moisture Strips: Eyes** *($8 for 6 strips)* consist of crescent-shaped paper strips that you moisten and affix to the under-eye area, hoping they'll impart "brightness and vibrancy to weary-looking eyes." About the only thing these strips impart is irritation, which results from a high amount of salt-based film-forming agents and starch. And while the irritation is occurring, your skin is also being constricted by alcloxa; there is very little going on that is actually helpful, let alone revitalizing. This is one to ignore!

☹ **Revitalizing Moisture Strips: Mouth** *($9.50 for 6 strips)* share the same application method and formulary inadequacies as DHC's Revitalizing Moisture Strips: Eyes. That means little benefit to skin around the mouth, but lots of irritation from the salt-based film-forming agent and the constricting alcloxa.

☹ **Revitalizing Moisture Strips: Neck** *($11 for 6 strips)* share the same application method and formulary inadequacies as DHC's Revitalizing Moisture Strips: Eyes. That means little benefit to skin on the neck, but lots of irritation from the salt-based film-forming agent and constricting alcloxa. The tartaric acid can also be irritating.

☺ **$$$ Mineral Mask** *($35 for 3.5 ounces)* is a standard clay mask containing enough water-binding agents to help offset the clay content that can make skin feel too dry or tight. It is a good option for normal to oily skin.

☺ **Tourmaline Pack** *($35 for 3.5 ounces)* is a standard clay mask that contains a lot of tourmaline, which DHS maintains energizes skin and delves deep into pores to rid them of embedded impurities. It sounds like a marvelous mask, which makes you wonder why DHC needs so many other masks, none of which contain tourmaline. The truth is the whole notion is bogus, and the only revving-up your skin will see is from the irritation possible due to the inclusion of capsicum (pepper) extract.

☺ **Vitamin C White Stick** *($22 for 0.05 ounce)* is a lip balm for aging lips; its main ingredient is ascorbyl tetraisopalmitate, a form of vitamin C with limited research pertaining to its antioxidant ability (Sources: *International Journal of Pharmaceutics*, October 2007, pages 181-189; and *Photochemistry and Photobiology*, May-June 2006, pages 683-688). Because this is not an acidic form of vitamin C, it shouldn't cause irritation. However, it isn't the all-in-one antiaging savior DHC makes it out to be; it's just a potentially effective antioxidant for skin. This is otherwise a standard wax-infused lip balm that puts a slight white cast on lips due to the zinc oxide it contains.

DHC MAKEUP

FOUNDATION: ☺ **Q10 Liquid Foundation SPF 15** *($17.50)*. The name of this foundation is intended to highlight the presence of the antioxidant coenzyme Q10. Technically known and listed on the packaging as ubiquinone, the amount of it in this foundation is insignificant (it's listed well after the preservative). Although the Q10 isn't going to "fight fine lines," this thin-textured, fluid foundation with titanium dioxide for sun protection is worth auditioning if you have normal to oily skin and want a satin matte finish with sheer to light coverage. There are 14 shades available, and the mostly good selection includes options for fair to dark skin tones. Pink Ocher 01 and Pink Ocher 02 are slightly pink, but may work for some fair skin tones (they're not nearly as strongly pink as the same-named shades in DHC's Q10 Cream Foundation). The Natural Ocher range is most impressive, with the exception of Natural Ocher 05, which is too orange. Other problem shades are Pink Ocher 03 and Pink Ocher 04. Note: this foundation is so thin that you need to take care when dispensing it to ensure you don't overdo it.

☺ **Q10 Cream Foundation SPF 18** *($17.50)*. Obviously, the name of this foundation is designed to highlight the presence of the antioxidant coenzyme Q10. Technically known and listed on the packaging as ubiquinone, the amount present in this foundation is insignificant (it's listed well after the preservative). Although the Q10 isn't going to "fight fine lines," this creamy foundation with titanium dioxide and zinc oxide for sun protection has merit. It slips over skin and blends quite well, but blending must be thorough to prevent it from looking too heavy or chalky (the chalkiness results from the titanium dioxide and zinc oxide, which are great sun protection but don't have the most natural-looking finish). It sets to a satin matte finish capable of providing light to moderate coverage, not quite the full coverage DHC touts. The formula is best for normal to dry or sensitive skin not prone to blemishes. Among the 14 shades, there are some very good options for fair to dark skin tones. The shades to avoid due to overtones of pink, peach, or copper include Pink Ocher 01, Pink Ocher 02, Pink Ocher 03, Pink Ocher 04 (are you sensing a pattern here?), and Natural Ocher 06 (may be OK for some dark skin tones). The Natural Ocher range is great for most light to barely medium skin tones, while the Yellow Ocher range is best for medium skin tones (though some of the shades will be too yellow unless your skin tone is olive or you're of Asian descent).

☹ **Q10 Moist Color Base SPF 30+** *($17)*. The sun-protecting ingredients of this tinted moisturizer are the best part: a blend of titanium dioxide and zinc oxide totaling over 33% of the formula. That amount of those two actives ensures great broad-spectrum protection! As you may already know, there is a downside to such formulations: that amount of titanium dioxide and zinc oxide lends a heavy, chalky look to the product. Although it has an impressive silicone-based texture that blends easily and sets to a moist finish suitable for normal to dry skin, getting it to look sheer and natural isn't easy. An additional problem, which makes matters worse, is the fact that four of the five shades are "color-correcting." Pink, Apricot, and Green are out because they cannot correct skin color. Yellow is an option for select medium skin tones, but Beige is the only real skin shade (and is excellent). Although the sun protection is stellar and the overall formula is good, the appearance of this product on skin keeps it from earning a happy face rating.

POWDER: ✓ ☺ **Q10 Face Powder** *($17)* is a talc-based powder with a beautifully airy texture that gives skin a polished look without being the least bit dry or powdery. Recommended for all but very oily skin, this powder's four shades are nearly interchangeable. All go on translucent, including the Yellow and Pink options, both of which have a barely discernible shimmer that the Transparent shades lack. Despite the name, the amount of coenzyme Q10 (listed by its technical name, ubiquinone) is too small to be of any benefit for your skin.

BLUSH: ✓☺ **Face Color Perfect Pro Cheek** *($9)* is a surprisingly impressive powder blush for normal to dry skin! It has a very smooth, non-powdery texture that supplies concentrated color (begin with a sheer application) and leaves a satin-smooth, non-flat finish to enliven cheeks. The shade range is small but has some attractive options for fair to medium skin tones. Each shade is infused with shimmer that translates to a soft, minimally sparkling glow on skin. Note that the price of this product is only for the powder; for an additional price, you can purchase DHC's Face Color Perfect Pro Case, which holds an additional blush that also must be purchased separately.

EYESHADOW: ✓☺ **Eye Shadow Moon** *($6)* is DHC's single eyeshadow option, and is every bit as worthwhile as the eyeshadow formula of the company's Eye Shadow Perfect Pro (though the formulas are slightly different). This eyeshadow applies smoothly and covers well, with noticeable color impact from one stroke of the brush. Every shade has some amount of shine, and for most the shine is quite pronounced, so this isn't recommended for a less-than-taut eye area because shiny eyeshadows enhance the appearance of wrinkles. The Misty Khaki shade looks greener than it applies, which is a good thing (no one should wear vivid green eyeshadow unless they're the Wicked Witch of the West). Avoid the Misty Navy and tricky-to-work-with Misty Bordeaux.

✓☺ **Eye Shadow Perfect Pro** *($21)*. This eyeshadow set features three shades for shaping and shading the eyes, along with a thin strip of powder eyeliner. Shine is the name of the game here, but for those who prefer shiny eyeshadows these have a sumptuous, almost creamy texture that is a pleasure to apply and blend. Color payoff (including for the dark eyelining shade) is sheer, but the formula builds well and the shine tends to stay in place. Each of the sets is well coordinated, though what's available is limited, to say the least.

☺ **Eyeliner Perfect Pro Powder** *($7)* must be used with DHC's Eyeliner Perfect Pro Holder, available for purchase separately. It would have been far better and more logical if DHC just provided a product you could use without assembling anything. What you end up with is an inadequate pointed sponge-tip applicator, and it's a poor way to apply powder eyeshadow. A regular eyeshadow and eyeliner brush is distinctly preferred, but this setup is passable for a soft, diffused effect.

EYE AND BROW PRODUCTS: ✓☺ **Eyeliner Perfect Pro Pencil** *($7)*. Before I comment on the pencil itself, please note that the price for the pencil does not include an attachment to hold the pencil—it is just for the pencil head. I know that sounds strange, but that's the way it's sold, and you definitely need the attachment piece for the pencil to work. Why DHC doesn't offer this as an assembled pencil is odd, but you can purchase their Eyeliner Perfect Pro Holder for an additional price, so the cost is basically equivalent to that of other eyeliner pencils sold at the drugstore. If you don't mind the contrivance, you'll find this a superior automatic eye pencil for drawing thin, precise lines that last.

☺ **Eyeliner Pencil** *($6)*. If it weren't for the fact that this pencil needs routine sharpening, it would be rated a Paula's Pick. Application is smooth and even, and the slightly creamy texture sets to a long-wearing powder finish that beautifully resists smudging and smearing. If you don't mind sharpening and prefer basic brown and black for eyeliner, this is a pencil to purchase!

☺ **Eyebrow Perfect Pro Pencil** *($5.50)* is an automatic, retractable eyebrow pencil that requires you to purchase DHC's Eyebrow Perfect Pro Holder + Brush for an additional price (the brush is nothing more than a small mascara head) if you want to use this as an intact, complete pencil. The combined price isn't bad, and although this pencil has a powder finish that stays in place, it's tough to apply and tends to hurt because you must use so much pressure to define your brows. Far better powder brow pencils are available from the drugstore at this price, or for less.

☺ **Eyebrow Perfect Pro Powder** *($7.50)* is applied with a pointed sponge-tip applicator that touches a reservoir of powder every time you take it out of its case. You can use this alone or elongate it to normal pencil size by purchasing DHC's Eyebrow Perfect Pro Holder. This is an OK way to softly define brows with powder, but a pencil with a powder finish is more versatile, especially if you need to better define your brows without adding much thickness or color.

LIPSTICK & LIPLINER: ✓ ☺ $$$ **Lip Color Perfect Pro Creme** *($20)* is sold by itself in a lipstick tube or you can purchase a sleek refillable case at an additional cost. True to its name, this is a creamy lipstick. It feels lush and moisturizing on lips while imparting full color and a soft sheen finish. It isn't nearly as slick as DHC's Lip Color Perfect Pro Long Last, and as a result it lasts longer! One drawback: DHC offers only three shades, which is definitely limiting.

☺ $$$ **Lip Color Perfect Pro Long Last** *($21)* is sold by itself in a lipstick tube or you can purchase a sleek refillable case at an additional cost. The slick, creamy formula feels lighter than traditional cream lipsticks, and imparts rich color with a satin finish. The slickness doesn't dissipate, and as a result this won't be anyone's go-to cosmetic when you want a long-lasting lipstick. This is recommended if you don't mind routine touch-ups and you find one of the few shades DHC offers appealing.

☺ **Moisture Care Lip Gloss** *($9)* is a very standard tube lip gloss that imparts sheer, juicy-looking color with the requisite glossy finish. It is minimally sticky and, despite some strange-looking shades, goes on nearly translucent. (There's a colorless version, too, just in case you're concerned about the orange and yellow shades offered.)

☺ **Moisture Care Lip Gloss Shimmer** *($9)* is identical to DHC's Moisture Care Lip Gloss, except that these shades include a soft shimmer and each imparts a bit more color. Those differences may be your cup of tea, but neither gloss is exceptional enough to warrant purchasing via mail order instead of gloss-shopping at your local drugstore.

☺ $$$ **Lip Color Perfect Pro Shimmer** *($20)* is sold by itself in a lipstick tube or you can purchase a sleek refillable case for an additional cost. It has a smooth, lightweight cream texture and, true to its name, a shimmer finish. Actually, the finish is more glittery than shimmery and that's this lipstick's weak point: the emollient feel wears off and the shiny particles tend to feel grainy. So many cosmetics lines offer smoother shimmer finishes, there's no reason to settle for a grainy feel.

MASCARA: ✓ ☺ $$$ **Mascara Perfect Pro Double Protection** *($17.50)*. There isn't anything about this mascara that makes it more "pro" than any other great mascara, but wow, does it produce copious length and thickness without clumps! The polymer-based formula forms tiny tubes around each lash. Initial application is wet, but if you're careful this won't smear as it sets and then it's locked in place until you use water and gentle pressure to loosen the tubes (no cleanser needed). It's quite impressive that this stays on when you splash your face, but then comes off with plain water and slight agitation. One more comment: this dries quickly, so if any comb-through is needed, be swift.

FACE AND BODY ILLUMINATING SHIMMER PRODUCTS: ✓ ☺ **Face Color Perfect Pro Highlighter** *($9)* comes in three workable shades, each with a sheer, buttery smooth texture that leaves a soft glow on skin. All work quite well as pressed highlighting powders, but the shade intensity makes it best for fair to light skin tones. Note that the price of this product is only for the powder, not for the case; for an additional price, you can purchase DHC's Face Color Perfect Pro Case, which also holds an additional blush or Pro Highlighter that you also must purchase separately. All told, this is shine done right!

DIOR

DIOR AT-A-GLANCE

Strengths: Every sunscreen offers sufficient UVA protection; a handful of outstanding cleansers and makeup removers; some extraordinary foundations, some of which include sunscreen; the liquid concealer; very good loose powder, powder blush, and powder eyeshadows; some great mascaras; brow gel; elegant creamy lipsticks and several good lip glosses.

Weaknesses: Expensive; lackluster moisturizers and serums that contain more fragrance and preservatives than elegant ingredients; irritating toners and self-tanners; ordinary masks; lack of products to address the needs of those with blemishes or skin discolorations; some foundations with SPF ratings that are too low; mostly average makeup brushes.

For more information about Dior, call (212) 931-2200 or visit www.dior.com or visit www. Beautypedia.com.

DIOR SKIN CARE

DIOR CAPTURE PRODUCTS

☹ **Capture Totale Rituel Nuit, Multi-Perfection Nighttime Soft Peel** *($80 for 3.4 ounces)* lists alcohol as the second ingredient, which makes this product too irritating for all skin types. The amount of salicylic acid is way too small and the pH is way too high for it to be effective as an exfoliant, making this a complete waste of time and money.

☹ **$$$ Capture R60/80 Filler Intense Deep Wrinkle Filler** *($69 for 0.67 ounce)*. So what do the numbers R60/80 mean? According to Dior's Web site, the R60 stands for 60% reduction in wrinkles after just one hour following application and 80 represents the claim that "After 1 month: 80% of women surveyed noticed a visibly younger-looking appearance." In addition, all of Dior's Capture R60/80 products contain their patented C.U.R.E. complex; the letters stand for Cutaneous Ultra-Revitalizing Extract. Dior does not reveal what specific ingredients make up this complex, but the ones on the label are not exactly earthshaking or even vaguely as unique as the name attributed to them. Further, in every Capture R60/80 product, the beneficial ingredients are listed well after the fragrance and preservatives, meaning that the amounts present are most likely not enough to deliver much, or at least no more than any other supposed antiwrinkle product. This water- and silicone-based serum makes skin feel silky and contains film-forming agents to smooth superficial wrinkles, but that's about it.

☹ **$$$ Capture R60/80 First Wrinkles Smoothing Eye Creme** *($52 for 0.5 ounce)* contains an amount of film-forming agent that may prove irritating for use around the eyes, plus it's a really boring formula.

☹ **$$$ Capture R60/80 Nuit Enriched Wrinkle Night Creme** *($86 for 1.7 ounces)* is a standard, jar-packaged emollient moisturizer for dry skin. Its creamy texture shortchanges skin of many essential ingredients it needs, and it contains more fragrance and preservatives than antioxidants or skin-identical substances.

☺ **$$$ Capture R60/80 XP Ultimate Wrinkle Restoring Creme** *($100 for 1.7 ounces)*. Is it just me or does the name for this moisturizer state that your wrinkles will be restored in an ultimate way? That's how I interpreted it, but I'm sure that's not what Dior meant (maybe it's a translation problem from French to English). This product is part of what Dior refers to as "21st century anti-wrinkle skincare" that was inspired by "revolutionary research." (They have to say it's "revolutionary" because just showing us the research, which they don't do, wouldn't sound nearly as exciting.) Maybe they didn't want to show us the actual research because their formula for this very standard moisturizer is about as far from revolutionary as it gets. This breaks no new ground for skin care; instead, it's the type of below-standard, mundane moisturizer I've come to expect from Dior, regardless of how they carry on about their alleged breakthroughs. It's mostly water, glycerin, thickeners, emollients, silicone, and preservatives; the smattering of plant extracts and antioxidants are clearly an afterthought and are barely present. Even if more of the "21st century" ingredients were in here, the jar packaging won't help keep them stable once you begin using this moisturizer. The only ingredient worth further comment is phosphatidyl-choline. It is the active ingredient in lecithin, and it does have benefit for skin as a water-binding agent and helping other ingredients penetrate skin better. In the case of this product, however, enhancing the penetration isn't necessarily a good thing, because Dior included several sensitizing fragrance chemicals that are best left out of any skin-care products, especially one claiming to be "revolutionary." The only effect this product will have on your wrinkles is to temporarily plump them, just like any moisturizer can do for less than $10 in a very big container at the drugstore. Knowing that, the price Dior is asking becomes utterly obnoxious.

☹ **Capture R60/80 XP Ultimate Wrinkle Restoring Serum** *($120 for 1.7 ounces)*. Unbelievable, but true, this absurdly priced serum consists primarily of water, slip agents, and preservative. Dior actually has the gall to refer to this as "21st century skin care." The lack of any state-of-the-art ingredients for the price is insulting. If they really believe a fraction of what they claim, then no one at Dior has even read a fashion magazine, much less any medical or science journal, in the past 30 years. Even fashion magazines offer information Dior knows nothing about. Calling this product the reinvention of wrinkle care is akin to replacing your Toyota hybrid with a Model-T Ford or Edsel! I won't comment further other than to say that this serum is a terrible waste of time and money. OK, one more comment, because I never thought I'd say this: you'd be better off buying a serum from Chanel than this one from Dior (though serums from many other lines best what both of those companies have produced recently).

☺ **$$$ Capture R60/80 Yeux Wrinkle Eye Crème** *($54 for 0.51 ounce)* is basically a hybrid of the other two Dior Ultimate Wrinkle Crèmes, with a silky texture that's in between a cream and a lotion. Although this feels quite nice, the formulation lacks worthwhile amounts of antioxidants, skin-identical ingredients, and anti-irritants, and there is little reason to consider this a special formulation for the eye area. It contains mostly water, film-forming agent, emollient, slip agent, a long list of thickeners, preservatives, fragrance, plant extracts, and the tiniest amount of vitamin C and glycosaminoglycans (water-binding agent) imaginable.

☺ **$$$ Capture R60/80 XP Yeux Wrinkle Restoring Eye Crème** *($80 for 0.5 ounce)* is part of what Dior refers to as "21st century anti-wrinkle skincare" that was inspired by "revolutionary research." (They've got to say it's "revolutionary" because just showing us the research, which they don't do, wouldn't sound nearly as exciting.) Maybe they didn't want to show us the actual research because their formula for this very standard moisturizer is about as far from revolutionary as it gets. This breaks no new ground for skin care; instead, it's the type of below-standard, mundane moisturizer I've come to expect from Dior, regardless of how they carry on about their alleged breakthroughs. It's mostly water, glycerin, thickeners, emollients, silicone, and preservatives; the smattering of plant extracts and antioxidants are clearly an afterthought and are barely present. The amount of film-forming agent in this eye cream can have a temporary tightening and smoothing effect on skin, but the benefit is more tactile than antiwrinkle. Beyond the film-former, which some may find irritating when used around the eyes, this contains mostly thickeners and preservative with nary an interesting ingredient to be found. The amount of fragrance chemicals in this eye cream is troubling because their presence increases the risk of irritation for any part of the face but especially the eye area. Considering that fact and the ridiculous cost, this isn't an eye cream you should even wink at. There are so many superior moisturizers to consider that you can use anywhere on your face and that really do have antiaging properties, rather than this poorly conceived, antiquated formulary.

☹ $$$ **Capture Totale Haute Nutrition Rich Crème** *($125 for 1.7 ounces)* has a silky texture and contains some beneficial emollients for dry skin, but it's way overpriced for what you get. The plant oils and tiny amounts of antioxidants won't remain potent for long due to the jar packaging, which is disappointing at any price point. The youth-promoting plants Dior boasts about that are in this product have no research proving they can make skin look younger, by one day or even by one minute. Besides, they're present in token amounts in this moisturizer, which is typical for Dior's skin-care products. This contains several fragrance chemicals known to cause irritation.

☹ $$$ **Capture Totale Multi-Perfection Concentrated Serum** *($135 for 1 ounce)* is an average water- and silicone-based serum that contains enough film-forming agent to make skin look smoother temporarily. For the money, it is not preferred to the truly state-of-the-art serums from Olay, Paula's Choice, Estee Lauder, or Neutrogena.

☹ $$$ **Capture Totale Multi-Perfection Crème** *($120 for 1.7 ounces)* is supposed to correct all the visible signs of aging, but since there's no sunscreen here you can forget about making your wrinkles or dark spots look any better. It's a standard, emollient moisturizer for normal to dry skin that contains far more fragrance than legitimate bells and whistles (and the jar packaging won't help keep the tiny amount of antioxidants stable once this is opened).

☹ $$$ **Capture Totale Multi-Perfection Eye Treatment** *($80 for 0.5 ounce)* attributes its Multi-Perfection name to its alleged ability to correct wrinkles, discolorations, and dark under-eye circles. Considering the price, it would be rewarding if this product really were a "totale" treatment for eyes, but it's not. As with most Dior moisturizers, including those meant for the eye area, it is inadequately formulated—all of the interesting ingredients are listed well after the preservative and fragrance, which means they are barely present. Interesting or not, none of the ingredients in this product will prolong skin's youthful appearance, nor is it soothing as claimed. It's just a lightweight, water- and silicone-based moisturizer with enough film-forming agent to make the eye area look temporarily smoother.

☹ $$$ **Capture Totale Rituel Nuit, Multi-Perfection Intensive Night Restorative** *($130 for 1.8 ounces)* takes a cue from competitor Chanel's ultra-pricey Sublimage Essential Regenerating Cream, claiming that its rare, revitalizing plant, longoza, is "grown only in Madagascar" and, therefore, must have phenomenal benefits for aging skin. Why is it that such ingredients never seem to show up in Peoria or Houston? Why only in exotic locales? Are exotic plants automatically better for skin? The mystique makes it sound like you're buying something unique or special. The marketing myths about plants or rare species of seaweed, from remote countries or islands where they're gathered by tribal harvesting practices, and on and on, seem never-ending. Speaking of marketing nonsense, Longoza is actually a city in Madagascar, and the plant of that name appears to be a form of wild ginger. Yet it's not present anywhere in this product. That's OK, though, because there's no evidence that any species of ginger can "turn back the clock" for your skin. This ends up being a silky-textured but basic moisturizer that contains mostly water, glycerin, silicone, slip agent, film-forming agent, emollients, alcohol, more film-forming agent, salt, preservative, and fragrance. It's a mediocre option for normal to slightly dry skin.

☹ $$$ **Capture Totale UV Protect SPF 35** *($52 for 1 ounce)* is a daytime moisturizer with an in-part avobenzone sunscreen and has a silky, lightweight texture and smooth finish that those with normal to slightly dry or slightly oily skin will appreciate. This is an expensive way to get sun protection, and because you have to apply all sunscreens liberally to get the SPF benefit on the label, you have to ask yourself how liberally you'll apply this, knowing that if you apply it correctly you'll be replacing it fairly often, and that could add up to spending more than $600 per year on a facial sunscreen. I wish I could tell you that the price is justified because this product is brimming with state-of-the-art ingredients, but it isn't. The mica adds a subtle glow to skin, but that's a cosmetic effect, and all of the antioxidants are listed after the preservative and fragrance, making them merely a dusting.

DIOR DIORSNOW PRODUCTS

☹ **DiorSnow Sublissime Whitening Radiance Foaming Cleanser** *($31 for 3.6 ounces)* won't whiten skin one iota, and ends up being a foaming cleanser that's potentially drying due to the amount of alkaline potassium hydroxide it contains. It also contains the irritating menthol derivative menthoxypropanediol, and is not recommended.

☹ $$$ **DiorSnow Sublissime Whitening Lotion Moisture** *($48 for 6.8 ounces)* is a water-based toner for normal to dry skin that contains the vitamin C ingredient ascorbyl glucoside. Various forms of vitamin C have been shown to lighten sun-induced skin discolorations, but there is little research demonstrating ascorbyl glucoside has that ability (Sources: *Skin Research and Technology*, May 2006, pages 105-113; and *Dermatologic Surgery*, July 2005, pages 814-817). Removing the vitamin C from this toner's formula would result in a very basic, overpriced option. For the money, you're better off investing in a vitamin C serum or in a skin-lightening product with hydroquinone than this toner. It isn't a bad product, just overpriced for what you get.

☹ $$$ **DiorSnow Pure Whitening Moisturizing Creme** *($65 for 1 ounce)* pales in comparison to the best moisturizers from Estee Lauder, Clinique, and Olay. The amount of vitamin C is encouraging, but the jar packaging won't keep it or the couple of other antioxidants in the product stable. Once again, nothing in this moisturizer will impact skin discolorations.

☺ $$$ **DiorSnow Sublissime UV Ultra-Protective Whitening UV Base SPF 50 PA +++** *($45 for 1 ounce)* is an in-part titanium dioxide sunscreen with a fluid texture and soft matte finish suitable for normal to oily skin. The additional titanium dioxide and mineral pigments mica and iron oxides create a subtle whitening and brightening effect. This product contains no ingredients capable of lightening skin discolorations other than the protection the sunscreen offers them, which is true for any well-formulated sunscreen that is used religiously.

☹ **$$$ DiorSnow White Reveal Essence** *($110 for 1.7 ounces)* is a water-based serum with a beguiling description, but you're not getting a well-proven ingredient for your money. Dior includes ascorbyl glucoside as the key whitening agent in this product. Various forms of vitamin C have been shown to lighten sun-induced skin discolorations, but there is little research demonstrating that ascorbyl glucoside has that ability (Sources: *Skin Research and Technology*, May 2006, pages 105-113; and *Dermatologic Surgery*, July 2005, pages 814-817). If you removed the vitamin C from this formula, the result would be a very basic, overpriced option. For the money, you're better off investing in a vitamin C serum with proven forms of this vitamin or skin-lightening product with hydroquinone.

☺ **$$$ DiorSnow Pure UV Ultra-Whitening Spot Corrector SPF 50 PA+++** *($42 for 0.63 ounce)* contains almost 20% titanium dioxide, along with other sunscreen actives, which assures you of significant broad-spectrum sun protection. Sold as a spot treatment, this whitens skin cosmetically (the titanium dioxide and iron oxides provide concealer-like coverage) and is best paired with a skin tone-correct foundation. This is an OK, though very expensive, option for normal to oily skin not prone to blemishes. With its fragrance components, this product should be kept away from the eye area.

☹ **DiorSnow Pure Whitening Skin Repairing Essence** *($85 for 1.7 ounces)* lists alcohol as the second ingredient, which makes it too irritating for all skin types. Immediately after the alcohol is the stable vitamin C derivative magnesium ascorbyl phosphate. Research into magnesium ascorbyl phosphate's ability to lighten skin via inhibition of melanin is scientifically promising (Sources: *Phytotherapy Research*, November 2006, pages 921-934; *Skin Research and Technology*, May 2002, page 73; and *Journal of the American Academy of Dermatology*, January 1996, pages 29-33). These studies used 3% and 10% concentrations, respectively—and although this Dior product may meet that criterion, the alcohol makes this potentially effective skin-lightening product an irritating proposition.

DIOR HYDRACTION PRODUCTS

☹ **HydrAction Deep Hydration Radical Serum** *($69 for 1.7 ounces)* contains too much alcohol to be hydrating or capable of giving skin an "extra moisture boost." It also contains fragrance components that can irritate skin, and that won't help it look radiant or healthy.

☹ **$$$ HydrAction Deep Hydration Rich Crème** *($53 for 1.7 ounces)* is an acceptable moisturizer for normal to dry skin, but is easily replaced by less expensive and better formulated products.

☺ **$$$ HydrAction Deep Hydration Skin Tint SPF 20** *($38 for 1.7 ounces)* wins points for its in-part titanium dioxide sunscreen, but the application leaves something to be desired. The creamy, slippery texture takes its time to set, and it remains moist to the touch. That means this tinted moisturizer is best for normal to dry skin, and is a decent option if you're seeking sheer to light coverage plus built-in sunscreen. Among the four shades, three are good and suitable for fair to medium skin tones. Shade #4 is very peach, and the sheerness doesn't dissipate this unnatural overtone.

☹ **$$$ HydrAction Deep Hydration Sorbet Crème** *($35 for 1 ounce)* is a lightweight, refreshing, cream-gel moisturizer that's an OK option for normal to oily skin. It contains a dusting of antioxidants, but the jar packaging won't keep them stable.

☹ **HydraAction Hydra-Protective UV Milk SPF 20** *($54 for 1.7 ounces)* is a daytime moisturizer with an in-part zinc oxide sunscreen that cannot quench dryness because it lacks emollient ingredients and because of the amount of alcohol, which causes free-radical damage and irritation and that is not good for skin. Between the formulary deficiencies and the paltry amount of truly helpful ingredients (independent of the sunscreen actives), this is an expensive mistake for all skin types.

☹ **$$$ HydrAction Visible Defense Hydra Protective Eye Crème SPF 20** *($47 for 0.5 ounce)* is a "highly protective" moisturizer only because of the sunscreen and only as long as you apply it liberally, but there is little else to say about this overpriced product. Dior calls this product "legendary," but the only conceivable way HydrAction has the status of being legendary is that the company believes their own exaggerations and hype, because there's nothing about the formula that is uniquely beneficial for skin. This can be an OK moisturizer for slightly dry skin, but it is not recommended for use in the eye area because it contains a synthetic sunscreen active that can be sensitizing for eye-area skin, and this potential is increased because of the numerous fragrance chemicals also present. Plus, the jar packaging won't keep the dusting of antioxidants stable once you open and begin using this eye cream (which you really shouldn't do given the number of superlative products for the face or the eye that you can use instead).

☹ **$$$ HydraAction Visible Defense Hydra-Protective Light Crème SPF 20** *($54 for 1.8 ounces)*. The good news is that this daytime moisturizer for normal to slightly dry skin contains an in-part titanium dioxide sunscreen. The bad news is the boring base formula, which contains more fragrance than intriguing ingredients. Plus, what small amounts of exciting ingredients this does contain will be wasted due to the jar packaging.

☹ **$$$ HydrAction Deep Hydration Intensive Mask** *($34 for 2.5 ounces)* is a standard moisturizing mask for normal to dry skin. Almost any moisturizer at the drugstore can take this product's place, as it pretty much covers the basics (though it does so with lots of fragrance).

☹ **$$$ HydrAction Deep Hydration Pore Reducing Treatment** *($35 for 0.67 ounce)* smooths skin's texture with its mixture of glycerin and silicones. However, since alcohol is the second ingredient, this will also irritate, and the fragrance components compound this side effect.

DIOR L'OR DE VIE PRODUCTS

☹ **$$$ L'Or de Vie La Crème** *($350 for 1.7 ounces)*. Let me say from the start that reviewing any product with this price tag just makes me hate the cosmetics industry. It is such a blatant joke I can't imagine how the marketing people and chemists involved in this product sleep at night. OK, having had my little tirade, the claim that this moisturizer combines the best antiaging ingredients with the powers of L'Or de Vie is true only in the mind of Dior; there is no research proving any of that claim is true. And, for this amount of money there should be some proof somewhere because prescription medications that cost far less require piles of documentation. L'Or de Vie is supposedly a unique French vine that is harvested at its peak and goes through a multi-step purification process to extract every bit of this vine's regenerative essence. The vine doesn't have regenerative properties for skin, but if you're going to charge such an outlandish amount of money for what amounts to a basic moisturizer, then you need this kind of story for support. As usual for Dior products, the intriguing ingredients comprise very little of the formula. There are some good ingredients in this moisturizer, but none of the proven ones are unique to Dior, nor are they present in amounts that come close to justifying the price. Bottom line: this falls far short of offering a selection of "the best" antiaging ingredients. It's little more than a vastly overpriced moisturizer for dry skin. Even more pathetic, the jar packaging will render the few antioxidants this does contain ineffective shortly after the product is opened.

☹ **$$$ L'Or de Vie La Crème Yeux Eye Cream** *($195 for 0.5 ounce)*. With a claim of providing "unprecedented antioxidant protection," you'd expect this eye cream to be brimming with a who's who of today's most well-researched, proven antioxidants. Well, it isn't; not even close. It contains nothing to eliminate dark circles or signs of fatigue or stress. Eye creams from Olay or Clinique run circles around this formula. In addition, this moisturizer cannot protect "against the forces of age and time" any more than a tent will protect you from a hurricane. For your money (whether you have a lot of it or are on a budget), all you get is an elegant texture and breathtakingly beautiful packaging, but neither of those things offer special benefits or help your skin function like younger skin. What your skin really needs to look and feel its best comes up short in this product. There are some interesting antioxidants and several peptides in the formula, but the jar packaging isn't going to keep them stable during use. This cream contains mica and iron oxide to cast a reflective glow on skin, but that is strictly a cosmetic effect, which you can get from far less pricey products. One more point: there is absolutely nothing in this product special for the eye area, and there is also no published research in the world indicating that eye-area skin needs anything different from skin elsewhere on your face. If it's good for your face, it's good for the eye area; if it's bad for the eye area, it's bad for your face. This one is just boring and overpriced for both areas.

☺ **$$$ L'Or de Vie L'Extrait** *($370 for 0.5 ounce)*. What could possibly be in this product that prices out to $740 per ounce? Absolutely nothing! This lavishly packaged serum claims to be "the most powerful antioxidant treatment available without a prescription." Never mind that the comparison is nonsense because there are no prescription antioxidant products; so, in essence, that would make any product containing antioxidants more powerful than a prescription product that doesn't exist. Even if the marketing claim weren't so completely inane this formula is nearly void of antioxidants. How ironic is that? This is as mundane a moisturizing formula as any you can buy at the drugstore for a fraction of this insulting price. The minute amount of antioxidants Dior chose for this "L'Extrait" couldn't be more common: vitamin E and grape extract. They're as basic to moisturizing formulas as you can get; this product is no more exotic than Corn Flakes. The only really impressive part of the product is the packaging, and no matter how much disposable income you have, you shouldn't be spending it on such chicanery. The formula also contains several fragrance chemicals known to cause irritation and it contains alcohol. As you may have guessed, these irritants undermine what little effectiveness the antioxidants in this serum have.

OTHER DIOR PRODUCTS

☺ **$$$ Cleansing Gelee, for Face, Lips and Eyes** *($32 for 6.7 ounces)* is a fluid cleanser that contains cleansing agents typically found in eye-makeup removers. This product removes makeup quite well, but the fragrance components can be problematic for use around the eyes, which limits its appeal.

☺ **$$$ Cleansing Milk, for Face and Eyes** *($29 for 6.7 ounces)* shouldn't be used around the eyes because of the volatile fragrance components it contains, but is otherwise an innocuous lotion cleanser for normal to dry skin. You'll need a washcloth for complete makeup removal.

☺ **$$$ Cleansing Water, for Face and Eyes** *($29 for 6.7 ounces)* is a standard but effective water-based makeup remover. It is not adept at removing long-wearing or waterproof makeup, but is a fine water-soluble option for removing other types of makeup.

The Reviews D

☺ **$$$ Rinse-Off Cleansing Foam** *($29 for 5.3 ounces)* has merit if you prefer foaming cleansers, but the amount of potassium hydroxide is potentially drying and makes this Foam best for oily skin. Needless to say, Neutrogena and L'Oreal sell similar cleansers for considerably less money.

✓ ☺ **$$$ Self-Foaming Cleanser** *($29 for 5 ounces)* is a very good all-around cleanser for all skin types. Gentle but effective cleansing agents combine with skin-softening ingredients to remove makeup and leave skin satin-smooth. If you're going to splurge on a Dior cleanser, make it this one.

✓ ☺ **$$$ Duo-Phase Eye Make-Up Remover** *($26 for 4.2 ounces)* is an excellent, fragrance-free, silicone-enhanced makeup remover that may be used around the eyes or anywhere on the face. The price should give you pause (Almay and Neutrogena sell similar products for under $10), but this is still recommended.

☹ **Energizing Toner** *($29 for 6.7 ounces)* lists alcohol as the second ingredient and contains insignificant amounts of helpful ingredients for any skin type.

☹ **Matifying Toner** *($29 for 6.7 ounces)* contains too much alcohol and also irritates skin with camphor and menthol. The inclusion of castor oil is odd for a toner that claims to mattify skin and minimize pores.

☺ **$$$ Soothing Toner, Alcohol-Free** *($29 for 6.7 ounces)* contains a tiny amount of soothing ingredients and ends up being a truly ho-hum, overpriced toner for normal to dry skin.

DIOR BRONZE PRODUCTS

☹ **Dior Bronze Self-Tanner Natural Glow, Body** *($31 for 4.4 ounces)* lists alcohol as the second ingredient, and contains the same ingredient (dihydroxyacetone) found in most self-tanning products. Knowing this, why subject your skin to irritation from this much alcohol?

☹ **Dior Bronze Self-Tanner Natural Glow, Face** *($29 for 1.8 ounces)* contains far too many potentially irritating fragrance components to make it worth choosing over countless other self-tanning products, not to mention the needlessly high price for a very basic formula.

☹ **Dior Bronze Self-Tanner Shimmering Glow, Body** *($31 for 4.5 ounces)* is similar to the Dior Bronze Self-Tanner Natural Glow, Face above, and the same review applies.

☺ **$$$ Dior Bronze Sun Powder Spray** *($60)*. The price makes this an indulgent product to consider, but wow, is it ever a cool way to get an instant, natural-looking spray-on tan. Not a self-tanner, this is akin to body makeup that sets quickly and resists rubbing off. (Well, you can rub it off if you rub hard, but that's easily avoided.) The fine mist is surprisingly easy to control and provides even coverage with a soft matte (in feel) finish plus a hint of shine. Both shades are excellent, but Light Tan is preferred for, surprise, lighter skin tones. The formula is suitable for all skin types except sensitive (due to the fragrance).

DIOR MAKEUP

FOUNDATION: ✓ ☺ **$$$ DiorSkin Forever Compact Flawless & Moist Extreme Wear Makeup SPF 25** *($42)* is a terrific, mica-based pressed-powder foundation with an in-part titanium dioxide sunscreen. This applies easily, feels wonderfully silky, and leaves a sheer matte finish that can provide sheer to light coverage. That means you can add this to the very short list of pressed powders with sunscreen that not only blend like a second skin, but also come in a gorgeous range of neutral shades, though there are no options for dark skin. Note: Each shade applies lighter than it appears in the compact, and Dark Beige 050 may be too peach for some tan skin tones. All skin types can use this foundation with success.

☺ **$$$ DiorSkin AirFlash Mist Makeup** *($60)* is an aerosol foundation that can be tricky to use, but with a little patience the results are rewarding. The coverage you get depends on your application. Spraying it in your hand at close range and then applying to the face will net medium to full coverage that looks surprisingly natural, and is far less messy than holding it 12 inches or more from your face (as the Dior makeup artist I spoke to recommended). Either way it provides a sheer veil of color and coverage. Once sprayed on, AirFlash dries, well, in a flash—so blending must be quick. Luckily, this blends evenly and sets to a long-wearing, silky matte finish that will require more than a water-soluble cleanser to remove. Only four shades are available, with options for fair to medium skin, but each one is excellent. Although this is pricey, it is a unique twist on liquid foundations (even those that are silicone-based) and does indeed feel weightless, which is ideal for oily to very oily skin. By the way, since this foundation can get on your clothing or hairline as you spray it (especially given that you should keep your eyes closed when doing so), it is best applied before dressing, with your hairline protected by a towel or headband, because if you aren't careful it can get all over. The mist this produces is ultra-fine, but some spotting can occur when spraying from the distance that Dior recommends, and do make sure the opening doesn't clog or a mess will ensue.

☺ **$$$ Capture Totale Foundation SPF 15** *($75)*. If you're wondering why this foundation is so expensive, let me make it absolutely clear that it has nothing to do with the formula and everything to do with marketing. You're being sold an image, not a better product. This foundation is part of Dior's Capture Totale brand, whose items are even more overpriced than other brands in the Dior collection. What is totally disappointing is that the Capture Totale products in their entirety have much better packaging than they do formulas. Despite the formulary shortcomings, Dior claims that this foundation contains the Capture Totale's antiaging ingredients, giving you more of what Dior thinks is best for aging skin, which realistically isn't good thinking for your skin. Although this foundation has many positive tactile traits, those hoping it will combine antiaging ingredients with their daily makeup will be disappointed. The water- and silicone-based formula contains more talc, salt (sodium chloride), fragrance, and preservatives than anything approaching an antiaging ingredient. Besides, the plant extracts Dior includes in their Capture Totale products haven't a shred of research proving their efficacy in the tiny (really, really tiny) amounts Dior uses. The good news is that this foundation for normal to dry skin has an in-part titanium dioxide sunscreen, a creamy texture that blends easily, and a mostly attractive range of shades. Among the mostly neutral colors, Peach 023 is aptly named and best avoided, and Honey Beige 040 is also too peach to recommend. The silky, moist finish conceals flaws and enhances skin tone, which is what you want a liquid foundation to do—you just don't need to spend this much for these results. Foundations with sunscreen from L'Oreal, Estee Lauder, and Clinique are preferred, unless you enjoy spending too much money on your makeup.

☺ **$$$ DiorSkin Eclat Satin** *($42)* is Dior's foundation for those with dry skin, and it delivers—with a creamy, moisturizer-like texture that has a natural affinity for skin. It provides medium to almost full coverage, yet does so without looking thick or cakey and leaves an attractive dewy finish. Six shades are available, but watch out for the slightly peach #400 and avoid #402, which is glaringly rose. The fact that this foundation is highly fragranced keeps it from earning a Paula's Pick rating.

The Reviews D

☺ **$$$ DiorSkin Forever Extreme Wear Flawless Makeup SPF 25** *($42)* is a very silky, fluid foundation that comes with some strong pros and cons. The pros include that it is suitable for oily to very oily skin due to its texture and smooth, long-wearing matte finish. It also provides medium to almost full coverage without looking artificial, and the sunscreen includes titanium dioxide for UVA protection. The major cons include the fact that alcohol is the third ingredient and that six of the 10 shades are noticeably peach, rose, or orange. Dior, what happened? All of your other newer foundations present a palette that's mostly neutral and beautiful! If you're willing to risk the irritation and free-radical damage the alcohol may cause, the best shades to consider are Ivory 010, Linen 021, Peach 023 (which isn't peachy), and Sand 031.

☹ **$$$ DiorSkin Nude Natural Glow Hydrating Makeup SPF 10** *($45)*. It's unfortunate that this otherwise impressive foundation has an SPF rating that's below the standard recommended by all major health organizations. SPF 10 isn't terrible, but SPF 15 or greater is preferred and for the money why not? Even more to the point, why doesn't Dior know that? The fluid texture of this foundation has an elegant slip that makes blending a breeze, and the satin matte finish looks incredibly skin-like. It provides sheer to light coverage, but layers well for trouble spots, although you'll still need a concealer to mask red spots or dark circles. Dior's shade range has improved over the years, but despite their efforts, some duds remain. The following shades are blatantly rose, orange, or peach and are not recommended: Rosy Beige, Dark Beige, Medium Beige, and Honey Beige. The Dark Brown shade is slightly copper, but may work for some skin tones. Ivory is slightly pink, but again, may be workable for some fair skin tones. This foundation is best for normal to slightly oily skin. This would have rated a happy face if its SPF rating was 15 or greater.

☹ **$$$ DiorSkin Sculpt Line-Smoothing Lifting Makeup SPF 20** *($53)* contains nothing that will make lines look smoother, at least not any more so than any other foundation, but that cosmetic effect is a poor substitute for wrinkle prevention, which is where an effective sunscreen comes in. Unfortunately, this antiaging makeup misses the mark by not including the UVA-protecting ingredients of titanium dioxide, zinc oxide, avobenzone, Tinosorb, or Mexoryl SX. That's truly a shame, because it has a creamy-smooth texture and a beautiful application perfect for those with normal to dry skin who prefer a slightly moist finish and medium to full coverage. Six of the nine shades are excellent, with Ivory 010 being a prime choice for very fair skin. Rosy Beige 032 is too peach, Honey Beige 040 is slightly rose, and Dark Beige 050 is noticeably rose. In terms of sculpting or lifting, don't count on such benefits, especially with insufficient sun protection. This does contain a tiny amount of peptides, but they're listed after the preservative, meaning their benefit to skin will be minimal at best. There are enough positives to make this worth considering, but not over similar foundations that get the critical issue of sun protection right.

☹ **DiorSkin Nude Natural Glow Fresh Powder Makeup SPF 10** *($45)* is a loose-powder foundation with a gossamer-light texture and silky, sheer application. Things go awry with the finish, however, which casts an ethereal, whitish glow. This is apparent with all of the shades, despite their perceptible depth of color when viewed in the package. If that isn't odd enough, for some reason Dior chose to add the potent menthol derivative menthoxypropanediol to the formula. Between that, the strange way each shade "reads" on skin, and the low SPF rating, this isn't recommended.

CONCEALER: ✓☺ **$$$ DiorSkin Sculpt Lifting Smoothing Concealer** *($30)* has a price that should give you pause, but there's no denying that this is a formidable concealer that is worthy of your attention. The silky, silicone-enhanced formula begins slightly thick, but blends very well. It has minimal slip, so it does a great job of staying precisely where you place it, drying to a satin matte finish that provides significant coverage. Dark circles and redness are easily erased, but this concealer never looks too thick and it creases only minimally. It comes in three superb shades, though only for fair to medium skin tones. Forget about the sculpting and lifting claims because they are mere fantasy, but the rest is as real as it gets.

POWDER: ☺ **$$$ DiorSkin Pressed Powder** *($35)* is also talc-based and has an expectedly heavier (but still natural-looking) application when compared with its loose counterpart. It isn't the most absorbent powder, so those with very oily skin will not be satisfied, but for all other skin types this is recommended, and all three shades are very good.

☺ **$$$ DiorSkin Loose Powder** *($42.50)* is a talc-based powder with a silky, finely milled texture and satin matte finish suitable for normal to dry skin. All three shades go on almost translucent, so there's no need to worry about getting the color exactly right. This does come with a worthwhile brush instead of the more typical powder puff.

BLUSH AND BRONZER: ✓☺ **$$$ DiorBlush** *($38)* will not disappoint, given its sublime texture and application. In a word, DiorBlush is superlative, and most of the available colors are excellent, with several soft choices that apply evenly. Each shade is infused with shine, but it's not too intrusive. This blush has that extra something that pushes it above and beyond the best, and, comparing French lines, Dior's powder blush puts Lancôme's to shame.

✓☺ **$$$ Dior Bronze Matte Sunshine SPF 20** *($40)* is, admittedly, an expensive talc-based pressed bronzing powder. However, if the price doesn't deter you, it performs quite well. The sunscreen is in-part titanium dioxide, so this can serve as a helpful adjunct to an SPF-rated product applied to your entire face, something you wouldn't want to do with a bronzing powder. But remember, you must apply it liberally to achieve the SPF rating on the label. This has a sublimely silky texture that goes on beautifully smooth, leaving a dimensional matte (yes, this is a matte bronzing powder) finish. Dior has created a top-notch bronzing powder with sunscreen whose only drawback, as mentioned, is the price. The best shades are Amber Matte and Honey Matte.

✓☺ **$$$ Pro Cheeks Ultra-Radiant Blush** *($30)* has a spongy texture that turns into an airy cream-to-powder blush that's a cinch to apply and blend. In fact, if you're new to this type of blush this is almost foolproof, and the translucent colors look remarkably natural. (It's still blush, though, so "natural" is a relative term.) Among the four shades, the only non-blush tone is Limelight, which is opalescent, very pale pink, and best for highlighting, if you use it at all.

✓☺ **$$$ Bronze Harmonie de Blush** *($42)* is an attractive pressed bronzing powder featuring multiple colors in one compact. The idea is to swirl the brush over the entire cake, which transfers an even application of sheer bronze tones to your skin. The texture is wonderfully smooth and the sheer colors leave a soft shine finish. This is worth exploring if you normally combine powder blush and bronzer.

☺ **$$$ Dior Essential Bronzing Powder** *($40)* is a monumental improvement over Dior's former pressed bronzing powder. Not only have the texture and application been improved, but also the range of four colors now resembles golden, tan, and bronze tones rather than the former version's peachy orange hues. The only drawback is the shine. Each shade is imbued with large sparkling particles that tend to flake off. It's not a huge drawback, but a bronzing powder at this price should be as close to perfect as possible.

☺ **$$$ Sunshine Tones** *($42)* is a pressed-powder blush/bronzer that includes four shades (two for blush, one bronze tone, and one highlighter) in a compact. Dior has offered this type of product for years, and some women will indeed find it convenient. You have the option of using each color individually (a tricky feat given there are no dividers between the stripes of color) or sweeping a brush over the whole powder cake for one uniform color. Either way you'll get decent pigmentation and noticeable shine, which makes this best for evening wear.

EYESHADOW: ✓ ☺ **$$$ 1-Colour Eyeshadow** *($24.50)* has a formula different from that of the 5-Colour Eyeshadow Compact reviewed below, but it's still enviably silky, almost creamy. The application is excellent, as is the color saturation, making these single shadows a pleasure to work with. The drawback for those with wrinkles is the amount of shine. If wrinkles aren't a concern and you want shine, there are some attractive brown, gray, and off-white shades to consider (and the requisite blue and green shades to ignore).

✓ ☺ **$$$ 2-Colour Eyeshadow** *($35)* carries on the tradition Dior established long ago of offering powder eyeshadows with an ultra-fine, supremely silky texture that feels almost creamy and blends superbly. The vast majority of Dior's eyeshadows are replete with shine, and that carries on here, too. Each duo features a light and dark complementary or tone-on-tone blend, so as long as you avoid the blue, bright pink, and lime green duos the combinations are all pretty much can't-go-wrong. However, unless your eye area is perfectly smooth and unwrinkled, these are too shiny for daytime wear. Younger women who are not yet dealing with visible signs of aging on their eyelids (such as the models Dior tends to use in their eye-makeup ads) can use these shadows with abandon. The best pairings are Diorchic, Diorgraphic, and Diorwild. The talc-free formula can be used wet or dry, with wet application intensifying the color (often to a flattering effect).

✓ ☺ **$$$ 5-Colour Eyeshadow Compact** *($54)* represents Dior's classic eyeshadow offering and has been around almost from this line's inception. The texture of these is like powdered sugar and although the formula puts emollience before absorbent ingredients like talc, it doesn't crease. Each shade applies very smoothly, doesn't flake, and provides more coverage (and definitely has a stronger color payoff) than most powder eyeshadows. The ongoing problem is Dior's often contrasting or overly trendy color combinations. Sadly, these tend to outnumber the workable sets, though the following are worth considering: Beige Massai, Incognito, Night Dust, Sweet Illusion, and Tender Chic. All of these are predominantly shiny, but if that's your thing the shine goes on softer than in the past and clings beautifully. It's still too shiny for wrinkled or drooping eyelids, but younger women with the means to afford these eyeshadow sets will be impressed.

☺ **$$$ DiorShow Eyecolor** *($30)* is packaged in a click pen with a built-in synthetic brush applicator. The formula is creamy-slick, but blends to a finish that feels matte and looks shiny. In fact, shine is the name of the game here because you'll see more of that than color. Use caution when dispensing, as this tends to get slightly chunky if you don't clean the brush between uses. Overall this is more novelty than practical, and doesn't surpass Dior's shiny powder eyeshadows.

☺ **$$$ Eye Show** *($30)* has the same formula and texture characteristics as Dior's Pro Cheeks Ultra-Radiant Blush, but it doesn't translate as well to eyeshadow. The trend-driven colors are difficult to work with and all are infused with chunky shine that looks more flashy than classy. Used as directed, these tend to crease quickly and, unlike the blush, the colors fade easily, leaving behind bits of sparkles. This is minimally waterproof.

EYE AND BROW PRODUCTS: ✓ ☺ **$$$ DiorShow Brow Fixing Gel** *($17)* is a standard, lightweight brow fixative. The brush is excellent, with both long and very short bristles, so every hair will be tamed, and this has a minimally sticky finish that's a step above similar brow-taming products.

☺ **$$$ DiorLiner Precision Eyeliner** *($30)* is a long-lasting liquid liner that comes with a good brush that makes even application easy. The bottom of the pen houses the liquid and you have to click the base to feed the brush. If Dior sold refills, this would be an option; since they don't, this is absurdly overpriced for what you get, though still deserving of a happy face rating.

☺ **$$$ Sourcils Poudre Powder Eyebrow Pencil** *($25)* remains one of the better standard brow pencils, even though an automatic, twist-up brow pencil or a powder eyeshadow with a thin brush is easier to use to create realistic eyebrow definition. This product has a soft powder texture that fills in and defines brows without looking heavy (no Joan Crawford arches here!) and comes in three beautiful shades suitable for blonde to medium brown brows. The mascara brush at the opposite end of the pencil is a nice touch for softening the result.

☺ **$$$ Style Liner** *($30)* is an inkwell-style liquid eyeliner that applies better and dries faster than Dior's Liquid Eyeliner. The thin, flexible brush is the perfect length for controlled application, and you'll find this doesn't chip or smear once dry. If only the colors were better! Still, a classic black option is available and is the only shade I recommend unless you want a space-age iridescent finish.

☹ **$$$ Crayon Eyeliner** *($25)* is a standard though quite creamy pencil that makes smearing almost a certainty. Perhaps that's why a smudge tip was included, as this only works for smoky eyes, preferably when set with a coordinating powder eyeshadow.

☹ **$$$ Crayon Eyeliner Waterproof** *($25)* needs routine sharpening, but does have a soft, creamy application. The finish, though waterproof, feels tacky, so consider this a special occasion pencil and know that it's not recommended over automatic pencils that stay put, such as Cover Girl's Outlast version.

☹ **$$$ DiorShow Brow** *($17)* puts the spotlight on your brows thanks to its glitter-infused tinted-gel formula. The dual-sided brush is great at allowing you to create a softer or more defined effect, and the shine tends to cling to brow hairs rather than flake onto the eyelid. Although this is worth considering if you want glossy-looking, glitter-infused brows, the finish feels somewhat dry and stiff, though it does keep unruly hairs in place. The two shades include sheer blonde and brunette.

LIPSTICK AND LIPLINER: ✓ ☺ **$$$ Crème de Gloss** *($25.50)* has a smooth, non-sticky application that looks beautiful on the lips. Before you get too excited, though, know that this creamy gloss/lipstick hybrid wears more like a gloss than a lipstick and it will bleed into lines around the mouth if you have any. Using a lipliner will help with this problem as well as extend the wear time between applications. All of the colors have subtle shimmer and they are all beautiful; I can't imagine most women not finding a shade to covet. For the money, the wear time should be longer, but if you're a Dior lip gloss fan, you will be very happy with Crème de Gloss.

✓ ☺ **$$$ RougeLiner Automatic Lip Liner** *($25)* is obviously expensive for a lip pencil. However, it never needs sharpening, is retractable, and has a beautifully smooth application. Another strong point is how long-lasting the color is: some of the shades have such a strong stain they take considerable effort to remove! It is definitely an excellent lip pencil to consider if you feel the need to spend in this range. If not, Almay, Clinique, and Origins have equally good options for less money.

☺ **$$$ Dior Addict Lipstick** *($24.50)* has a soft, creamy texture and a slightly greasy-feeling finish. That may feel great, but it doesn't help in the longevity department. The majority of the colors are fine, with most having an iridescent or soft shimmer finish.

☺ **$$$ Dior Addict Ultra-Gloss** *($24.50)* has an emollient, lanolin-based formula that is great for dry lips and provides a smooth, glossy finish that isn't sticky. The sheer- to light-coverage colors are a tantalizing mix, with options for the color-shy and for those with a flair for the dramatic. It's not the ultimate gloss, but at least those prone to overspending won't be disappointed!

☺ **$$$ Rouge Dior Replenishing Lipcolor** *($27)* makes all sorts of claims in terms of long wear and amplified color technology, but for all the hype this is nothing more than a standard, but good, creamy lipstick. It offers enticing shades with medium opacity and a soft glossy finish. The pigments in this lipstick are more concentrated than usual, which means the colors last longer. However, you'll likely be ready for a touch-up before then because the glossy finish is short-lived.

☹ **$$$ Dior Addict High Shine** *($24.50)* is a standard, slightly greasy sheer lipstick with a sparkling, glossy finish that feels slippery. The shade range offers choices from the softest nude to bright, vibrant pinks and corals. However, this lipstick is more style than substance (the attractive holographic packaging alone costs vastly more than the lipstick), and it doesn't really offer anything special or unique for your lips. As with all sheer lipsticks, these won't last long before you need a touch-up. Note also that the glitter particles tend to stick around long after the color has faded, so it would be best to cover the entire lip area with a lipliner beforehand.

☹ **$$$ Dior Contour Lipliner Pencil** *($25)* is a standard, creamy-finish lipliner that comes in a dwindling array of colors (almost all of which are brown-based) and has a lipstick brush at one end. It's exceptionally overpriced for what you get, but it does the job.

☹ **DiorKiss Luscious Lip-Plumping Gloss** *($19.50)*, regrettably, isn't recommended due to the irritants it contains. In addition to lemon peel oil (which can cause a phototoxic reaction when lips are exposed to sunlight), a major ingredient in this smooth-textured non-sticky lip gloss is methyl hydrogenated rosinate. This ingredient has many functions, including as a thickening and flavoring agent (all of these glosses are flavored after coffee beverages or cocktails) and as a fragrance. Its inclusion, combined with the lemon peel oil, only increases the risk of irritation. There are many outstanding lip glosses that work just as well as this one but without the problem ingredients.

MASCARA: ✓ ☺ **$$$ DiorShow Iconic Mascara** *($27)*. Fashion trends, fashion designers, and red-carpet celebrities play a big role in selling this mascara (as they do for many cosmetics and other objects of desire). That's where the Iconic name comes from, along with this mascara's backstage legacy of creating outrageously long, curved lashes. The unique rubber-bristled brush does a fantastic job of extending and curling every last lash, all without clumps. This doesn't build the wow-factor thickness of the original DiorShow Mascara, but has a cleaner, more precise application that refuses to falter (and gets incrementally better) with successive coats. Those looking for just as much length and curl but with lots of thickness should check out Cover Girl's hard-to-beat Lash Blast Mascara or L'Oreal's Lash Architect Mascara, both of which cost one-fourth what Dior is charging for Iconic Mascara.

✓ ☺ **$$$ DiorShow Waterproof Mascara** *($24)* is Dior's best waterproof mascara to date. Although the brush is enormous and can be difficult to work with, you will find it produces copious length and respectable thickness without clumps or smears. The formula is tenaciously waterproof, but easier than most to remove, making this highly recommended if your mascara budget extends to Dior's price point.

☺ **$$$ DiorShow Black Out Spectacular Volume Intense Black-Kohl Mascara** *($24)* has a large brush that is similar to but more spiral-shaped than the original DiorShow Mascara. It can be difficult to control and apply evenly, but with patience this builds dramatically thick, full lashes. This is also one of the blackest mascaras I've tried; the color really makes an impact. You'll appreciate how soft this keeps lashes, plus it wears beautifully yet removes easily with a water-soluble cleanser. A less cumbersome brush would have earned this a higher rating.

☺ **$$$ DiorShow Mascara** *($24)* has one of the largest brushes I've ever seen on a mascara wand, which makes it a bit tricky to work with, and nearly impossible to reach the small lashes near the eye's inner and outer corners, but with patience and practice every lash can be covered. The payoff is extraordinarily long, thick lashes with minimal to no clumping, and beautiful separation. Beyond the cumbersome brush, the only caveat with this mascara is its potent fragrance. There is no reason for mascara to contain fragrance, but then again, this is Dior.

☹ **DiorShow Iconic Extreme Waterproof Mascara** *($27)*. This mascara produces prodigious length quickly and cleanly, of that there's no denying. Thickness is minimal, but it builds decently if you have the patience to apply several coats. Lashes are left with a soft curl that lasts. Despite these impressive traits and the fact that this won't flake, it isn't waterproof. Simply splashing your eyes with a bit of water causes the formula to break down and run. Didn't anyone at Dior test this product before they decided to label it waterproof?

☺ **$$$ DiorShow Unlimited Ultra-Lengthening Curving Mascara** *($24)* actually thickens better than it lengthens, and nothing about its performance deserves "ultra" status. Application tends to be a bit uneven and slightly wet, so you'll get some smearing unless you're meticulous (or wipe down the wand beforehand). It wears well and does leave lashes softly curled, but all in all, if Dior mascaras are your thing, consider their superior DiorShow Iconic before this.

FACE AND BODY ILLUMINATING/SHIMMER PRODUCTS: ✓ ☺ **$$$ DiorSkin Shimmer Star** *($43)* is an ideal find for those who want a soft, glowing sheen rather than "look at me!" sparkles. The super-smooth texture makes it a joy to apply, and it blends evenly to a finish that's tailor-made for highlighting skin. The multiple tones in this pressed shimmer powder are best swirled together with your brush so they come off as one uniform shade on skin. Amber Diamond is preferred for light to medium skin tones, while all skin tones can use Rose Diamond for strategic highlighting.

☺ **$$$ Skinflash Radiance Booster Pen** *($33)* promises "professional lightworks in a flash." What this really ends up being is merely a click-pen applicator set up so that you need to twist the base of the component to feed product onto the attached synthetic brush. This produces a flesh-toned liquid that at first appears to be a concealer. Yet once it's applied to skin it practically vanishes into it, providing minimal coverage as it sets to a natural matte (in feel) finish. Basically, this is a sheer highlighter with a touch of shimmer to help light reflect more evenly off skin. To some extent, this can soften minor flaws and subtle discolorations. It is best for creating soft highlights under the eye, on the brow bone, and down the bridge of the nose, and the fact that this blends so well into skin makes it a pleasure to work with, especially if you're attempting a complex highlighting/contouring makeup application. Three shades are available, and though each is initially pink or peach, they "neutralize" once blended. The effect this product provides can be created with less expensive concealers (just make sure the color you select is at least one shade lighter than your skin tone or the highlighting effect won't work).

☹ **Diorskin Radiant Base SPF 20** *($40)* is a flesh-toned liquid highlighter that contains an in-part titanium dioxide sunscreen. It has a sheer, fluid texture that feels weightless on skin and imparts a subtle glow while helping to slightly (and I mean slightly) blur minor imperfections. The problem is the amount of alcohol—it's a main ingredient and you'll smell it as soon as you blend Radiant Base on skin. Given the number of highlighting liquids without problematic ingredients, there's no reason to choose this.

BRUSHES: ☺ **$$$ Dior Brushes** *($25-$52)*. The small collection of Brushes is respectable but by no means perfect or worthy of must-have status. Given Dior's vast selection of makeup, it's surprising their brush choices (especially for eye makeup) are so limited. The brushes to consider include the **DiorShow Blush Brush** ($35), which is better than the flimsy **DiorShow Powder Brush** ($52). Also good are the **DiorShow Eyeshadow Brush** ($25), and the synthetic-hair **DiorShow Foundation Brush** ($32), which is not as large as many others, making it easier to reach tight spaces.

DOVE (SKIN CARE ONLY)

DOVE AT-A-GLANCE

Strengths: Inexpensive; some state-of-the-art water-soluble cleansers and moisturizers; available in every major drugstore and mass-market store.

Weaknesses: A few products with low SPF ratings; problematic ingredients in some products designed for sensitive skin; many bar cleansers; the Pro-Age line is overall disappointing; their best products tend to be discontinued while the average to poor ones remain.

For more information about Dove, call (800) 761-3683 or visit www.dove.com or visit www.Beautypedia.com.

DOVE COOL MOISTURE PRODUCTS

☹ **Cool Moisture Beauty Bar** *($3.99 for 2 bars)* is a standard bar cleanser that contains a combination of detergent cleansing agents and ingredients found in traditional soap. This makes for a drying experience that doesn't rinse well, and it is not recommended.

✓☺ **Cool Moisture Facial Cleansing Cloths** *($6.49 for 30 cloths)* are a convenient way to cleanse skin, especially when you're on the go. The sturdy cloths are steeped in a gentle water-soluble cleansing solution that's suitable for all but very oily skin. The amount of cucumber and green tea isn't significant, and what counts most is how well these work to refresh skin and remove makeup.

✓☺ **Cool Moisture Foaming Facial Cleanser** *($6.49 for 6.76 ounces)* is an excellent water-soluble cleanser for all skin types except very dry. It produces a soft lather, removes makeup well, and rinses easily.

DOVE PRO-AGE PRODUCTS

☹ **Pro-Age Beauty Bar** *($3.99 for 2 bars)* is a standard bar cleanser that is soap-free, but the ingredients necessary to keep it in bar form can still clog pores and impede rinsing. The "fine exfoliants" in this beauty bar are no match for the superior combination of a water-soluble body wash and washcloth, or a standard body scrub.

☺ **Pro-Age Foaming Facial Cleanser** *($5.99 for 5 ounces)* is a very good, water-soluble cleanser for normal to dry skin, but nothing in it is capable of "optimizing surface cell turn-over," a process that slows down as skin ages. This product will leave skin feeling clean, soft, and smooth, but supplying moisture via a cleanser is not a tremendous antiaging benefit or something that's unique to this product.

☺ **Pro-Age Day Moisturizer SPF 15** *($11.99 for 1.7 ounces).* Pro-Age Day Moisturizer SPF 15 is actually a disappointing product from Dove, although it does not leave your skin vulnerable to UVA damage. An in-part zinc oxide sunscreen is included, and the base formula has a lightweight texture and silky finish. The letdown is that Dove's other facial moisturizers are full of ingredients that mimic the structure and function of healthy skin as well as several antioxidants. Those ingredients are in short supply here, and that's not a plus for aging skin. This is a worthwhile daytime moisturizer for normal to slightly dry skin, provided you don't mind a soft shimmer finish, but its positioning for skin of "advancing age" isn't reflected in the formulation here.

☺ **Pro-Age Eye Treatment SPF 8** *($11.99 for 0.5 ounce)* includes an in-part zinc oxide sun-screen, but the SPF rating is woefully low. In addition, the only antioxidant is a tiny amount of olive oil, making this inappropriate for anyone concerned with forestalling the signs of aging.

☺ **Pro-Age Rich Night Cream** *($11.99 for 1.69 ounces)* doesn't contain significantly rich ingredients, but instead has a lightweight cream texture built around silicones and glycerin. The amount of olive oil is decent but its effectiveness is compromised by jar packaging. The inclusion of the cell-communicating ingredient linolenic acid is a nice touch, but once again this formula should have had more stacked in its favor to address the needs of aging skin.

DOVE SENSITIVE SKIN PRODUCTS

☹ **Sensitive Skin Beauty Bar** *($3.99 for 2 bars)* is similar to Dove's other Beauty Bars and is not recommended. This option is particularly troublesome for anyone with sensitive skin because it contains fragrant rosewood, cedarwood, and rose oils.

☺ **Sensitive Skin Facial Cleansing Cloths** *($6.49 for 30 cloths)* must be water-activated before use. Once wet, they allow you to swiftly cleanse skin with a gentle combination of glyc-erin and water-soluble cleansing agents. Ideally, you'll want to splash your face with water to complete the process because you don't want to leave cleansing ingredient residue on your skin. These fragrance-free cloths are a safe bet for sensitive skin, unless you know you're sensitive to one or more of the preservatives; Dove could've used a gentler blend in that regard.

☺ **Sensitive Skin Facial Lotion** *($7.49 for 4.05 ounces)* has some terrific ingredients to create and maintain healthy skin, including ceramides, anti-irritants, antioxidants, and linolenic acid. However, it is not suitable for sensitive skin because it contains fragrant coriander oil. This oil's linalool content can cause contact dermatitis (Source: www.naturaldatabase.com), and although there's not much of it in this product it's enough to keep it from earning a higher rating.

OTHER DOVE PRODUCTS

☹ **Beauty Bar, Pink** *($3.99 for 2 bars)* is standard-issue, no-frills bar soap. Yes, it does contain a detergent cleansing agent and moisturizing stearic acid, but the overall effect on skin is still drying, and it doesn't rinse easily.

☹ **Beauty Bar, White** *($3.99 for 2 bars)* is a standard-issue bar cleanser that contains elements of traditional soap with detergent cleansing agents. Despite some moisturizing ingredients, the overall effect on skin is drying and the soap leaves a residue that is difficult to rinse, so expect it to impede the performance of other, leave-on skin-care products.

☺ **Energy Glow Skin Vitalizer Facial Cleansing Pillows** *($4.79 for 14 pillows)* are dual-sided "pillows" infused with a cleansing solution that is activated by water. Sweeping either side over your skin prompts a scrub-like effect that renders skin soft and smooth. The formula is suitable for all skin types except oily or sensitive. Be sure to rinse any remaining cleanser with water because you don't want to leave it on your skin.

☹ **Nutrium Cream Oil Beauty Bar** *($3.99 for 2 bars)* is similar to the almost all of the other Beauty Bars from Dove. That means its combination of traditional soap and detergent cleansing agents is too drying for all skin types, plus it doesn't rinse well and the residue impedes the performance of leave-on skin-care products.

☹ **Gentle Exfoliating Beauty Bar** *($3.99 for 2 bars)* is a standard bar cleanser that does not contain any exfoliant ingredients (the former version did). It is very similar to Dove's other Beauty Bars, and as such is not recommended.

☺ **Gentle Exfoliating Daily Facial Cleansing Pillows** *($4.99 for 14 pillows)* are nearly identical to the Energy Glow Skin Vitalizer Facial Cleansing Pillows above, and the same review applies.

☺ **Gentle Exfoliating Foaming Facial Cleanser** *($5.99 for 6.76 ounces)* is a creamy-textured product that's recommended for those with normal to dry skin looking for a water-soluble cleanser/scrub hybrid.

☺ **Deep Moisture Facial Lotion SPF 15** *($7.49 for 4.05 ounces)* is a good lightweight day-time moisturizer with an in-part avobenzone sunscreen. The lack of antioxidants is disappointing but this contains some great skin-identical ingredients. It is best for normal to oily skin.

☺ **Skin Vitalizer Facial Cleansing Massager** *($12.49)* is a battery-operated, hand-held cleansing tool designed for use with Dove's Cleansing Pillows. It provides a "powered" cleansing and exfoliation that I suppose goes beyond what manual cleansing can do, but all in all this isn't a must-have if you're using another exfoliating product (such as a topical scrub, a washcloth, or, better yet, a well-formulated AHA or BHA product, something Dove doesn't offer).

DR. BRANDT (SKIN CARE ONLY)

DR. BRANDT AT-A-GLANCE

Strengths: Provides complete ingredient lists on the company Web site; some novel products in the Laser Lightning Line; a good sunscreen.

Weaknesses: Expensive; overwhelming number of products that contain irritating ingredients with no established benefit for skin; no products to comprehensively address acne or oily skin; nearly every Pores No More product is a disappointment; jar packaging.

For more information about Dr. Brandt's products, call (800) 234-1066 or visit www.drbrandtskincare.com or www.Beautypedia.com.

DR. BRANDT ANTI-IRRITANT PRODUCTS

☺ **$$$ Anti-Irritant Comforting Cleanser** *($40 for 4 ounces)* is an overall well-formulated, albeit needlessly pricey, cleanser for dry to very dry skin. It is capable of removing makeup, but is not recommended for use around the eyes (or for skin experiencing signs of irritation) because it contains fragrant ylang-ylang oil (listed by its Latin name *Cananga odorata*). Brandt should know perfectly well that fragrance is a problem for sensitive skin, but he includes it anyway. Knowing that, you have to ask yourself how seriously does he take any skin care need you might have? All told, despite its aforementioned effectiveness, this doesn't compete favorably with classic Cetaphil Gentle Skin Cleanser or other options such as Neutrogena Extra Gentle Cleanser or CeraVe Hydrating Cleanser. $40 for 4 ounces? How can there be women fooled by this hype and insanity? This formula isn't worth $10.

☹ **$$$ Anti-Irritant Laser Relief** *($85 for 1.7 ounces)*. The notion that skin-care products can mimic the effects of laser treatments on skin is nothing less than ridiculous, but when such products are created and endorsed by a dermatologist it becomes downright ludicrous. Dr. Brandt has had success with other products he sells that claim to work like microdermabrasion and Botox injections, so why not add another one that misleads consumers on faux-laser treatments too? The big to-do about Anti-Irritant Laser Relief is that it reduces redness and soothes irritated skin. What's so disappointing is that, for the money, you're not getting much in the way of anti-irritants. The amount of green tea extract is impressive, and without question this antioxidant also has anti-irritant properties. But unlike the previous version of this product, additional anti-irritants aren't included, at least not in amounts that reddened skin is likely to notice. The inclusion of fragrant ylang-ylang oil (listed by its Latin name of *Cananga odorata*) is not good news for sensitive skin. There isn't much of it in this product, but Brand should know better than to add any amount of fragrance to a product designed for skin already dealing with redness and irritation.

☹ **$$$ Anti-Irritant Soothing Moisturizer** *($65 for 1.7 ounces)* is an ultra-soothing moisturizer for sensitive skin. It has been formulated with pumpkin seed extract to promote relief to sensitive skin, shea butter to replenish moisture, and glistin, a bipeptide, to repair and protect skin cells from damage.

DR. BRANDT BLEMISHES NO MORE PRODUCTS

☹ **Blemishes No More Intensolution** *($35 for 3.7 ounces)*. The only thing this anti-acne product does intensely is irritate skin. It contains a hefty amount of alcohol along with menthyl lactate, and, in a lesser amount, pure menthol. Irritation not only damages skin but also stimulates an increase in oil production in the pore. Salicylic acid is present, but not in an amount those with acne will find helpful. It's incredibly frustrating that such a poorly formulated product comes from a dermatologist who should have done some research before putting his name on a product.

☹ **Blemishes No More Oil-Free Hydrator** *($35 for 1.7 ounces)* would've been an acceptable lightweight option for oily, acne-prone skin experiencing minor dryness if it did not contain witch hazel and various forms of menthol. Those ingredients only irritate skin, which is damaging and increases oil production in the pore. Another disappointment is that the low amount of salicylic acid won't have any effect on blemishes. The claims for this product are as overblown and contrived as it gets in the world of cosmetics. Brandt's "Active Impurity Shield" is likely just a blend of silicone-enhanced film-forming agents. So what? They cannot protect skin from acne-causing bacteria that are naturally present in skin, and none of the ingredients in this product have significant antibacterial action.

☺ **$$$ Blemishes No More Redness Relief** *($35 for 1 ounce)*. I haven't a clue why Dr. Brandt formulated a moisturizer for acne-prone skin with this much plant oil, but he did. Unlike mineral oil, whose molecular structure is too large to penetrate the pore lining, many plant oils have a smaller molecular size that allows such penetration. When a person is already dealing with excess oil and a faulty pore lining that isn't shedding debris as it should, you don't want more oil gumming up the process. The main anti-irritant in this moisturizer is green tea. Others are included, but likely not in amounts large enough to help relieve red skin. Although this isn't a safe bet for blemish-prone skin, it's an OK option for normal to dry skin, although it's really just a waste of money. This contains fragrance in the form of *Cananga odorata* (ylang-ylang) oil.

☹ **Blemishes No More Cleansing Pads** *($25 for 60 pads)* are an expensive way to effectively irritate skin while doing very little to reduce blemishes. As a dermatologist who no doubt has seen his share of patients struggling with acne, Brandt should know better. Then again, this is the same doctor who believes skin-care products can perform like lasers and Botox, but all the while his practice thrives on performing those same cosmetic corrective procedures. The various parts of the witch hazel plant and the amount of alcohol spell irritation and dryness for skin, while the menthol adds to those side effects. Irritation damages skin and increases oil production. This is a really insulting product for blemish-prone skin, to say the least!

☹ **Blemishes No More Spot Blotter & Concealer** *($25 for 0.35 ounce)* is a thick-textured concealer stick with a dry matte finish that claims to do everything possible to control acne, from inhibiting bacterial growth to controlling oil production. None of that is evident from the formulation, however. The amount of titanium dioxide in this formula can contribute to clogged pores, while the clay tends to exacerbate even minor dry spots. Brandt's Active Impurity Shield is certainly no superhero ready to vanquish blemish-causing foes. It appears to be a blend of silicone with film-forming agents, but none of them have documented evidence that they can keep acne-causing bacteria from affecting skin. Any lightweight liquid concealer with a soft matte finish will do a much better job of camouflaging breakouts and redness than this product.

DR. BRANDT FLAWS NO MORE PRODUCTS

☺ **$$$ Flaws No More r3p Cream, for Normal to Dry Skin** *($125 for 1.7 ounces)* makes me sigh heavily, but not because it's a bad product. Rather, the price is astonishing for what amounts to a relatively standard but effective moisturizer for normal to slightly dry skin. It cannot make good on its claims for exfoliation because it contains no ingredients that would make that happen. Coming from a dermatologist, this is a moisturizer you should expect to be brimming with state-of-the-art ingredients such as antioxidants and those that mimic the skin's intercellular matrix; alas, that isn't the case. These ingredients are present in this product, but barely, serving as little more than window dressing. This cream does contain acetyl hexapeptide-3, an ingredient that is present in many products claiming to topically reduce muscle contractions, and that use phrases like "similar to Botox." Such claims are not made here, but you should be aware that this ingredient is incapable of exerting any muscle-relaxing effect on skin, nor is it exclusive to high-end doctors' lines. The other two peptides serve as skin-identical ingredients, but they are present in amounts so small that any benefit to skin is likely negligible. This product contains fragrance in the form of lavender oil, but contains less of it than other Brandt products.

☹ **Flaws No More r3p Eye, for All Skin Types** *($80 for 0.5 ounce)* has a lush, emollient texture and contains several ingredients that are brilliant for dry to very dry skin. The antioxidants won't last for long once this jar-packaged eye cream is opened, while the lavender oil is toxic to skin cells and definitely not an ingredient that should be applied near the eye.

DR. BRANDT HOUSE CALLS PRODUCTS

☹ **Microdermabrasion for Face** *($75 for 1.7 ounces)* doesn't deserve consideration over the multitude of other topical scrubs claiming to mimic the effects of microdermabrasion because they use the same crystals. Brandt's version is quite abrasive, and even without this issue, Neutrogena's version is very effective and one-third the price.

☹ **Contour Effect** *($185 for 1.7 ounces)* not only has a ridiculous price tag, but also shortchanges skin by including only meager amounts of exciting ingredients and then further reducing their efficacy with jar packaging. Contour Effect is supposed to restore volume and plumpness to aging skin while boosting cells' energy (which declines with age and years of sun exposure). Although this moisturizer has an elegant, silky texture based largely on silicone technology, its unique ingredient, *Bacopa monniera* (also known as brahmi), has zero research pertaining to its benefit for skin. There's quite a bit of research examining oral consumption of this herb, but even that doesn't have anything to do with its ability to restore the diminishing substances (such as fat pads and collagen) whose loss causes skin to slacken and droop. Further, the inclusion of lavender oil causes skin-cell death; how is that supposed to rev up cellular energy? Your money is much better spent on dermal fillers that really do restore volume and plumpness to aging skin (an alternative Brandt would likely not admit, even though he offers such procedures in his practice).

☹ **Crease Release, with GABA** *($150 for 1 ounce)* is a basic emollient moisturizer that claims to rapidly reduce wrinkles with gamma amino butyric acid (GABA). Please refer to the *Cosmetic Ingredient Dictionary* on www.Beautypedia.com for detailed information on this ingredient. GABA cannot and does not work as Dr. Brandt claims, and this moisturizer irritates skin because it contains the allergenic fragrance component eugenol. Eugenol is a standard substance used to test for skin allergies, and has a deleterious effect on skin's immune cells (Sources: *Molecular Immunology*, March 2007, ePublication; and *Biological Chemistry*, September 2006, pages 1201-1207).

DR. BRANDT LASER LIGHTNING PRODUCTS

☺ **$$$ Laser Lightning Foaming Cleanser, for All Skin Types** *($45 for 8 ounces)* is a good though very expensive cleanser for normal to dry skin. Slightly lathering but not completely water-soluble because of the amount of castor oil, this will cushion dry skin and remove makeup easily. The tiny amount of mandarin orange peel oil is not likely to cause problems. By the way, nothing in this cleanser will help fade freckles or dark spots, nor does it have anything to do with lasers.

☺ **$$$ Laser Lightning Toner, for All Skin Types** *($45 for 8 ounces)* has a fairly standard backbone for a toner for normal to dry skin. Things get more interesting with the inclusion of ingredients such as the plastic polymer polypropylene tetraphthalate and the alanine amino acid component aminoethylphosphinic acid; the trouble is that these ingredients have no effect on lightening skin discolorations, whether they're laser-precise or not (and there is absolutely nothing laser-like about this product). Brandt also includes fullerenes in this product and this is where this toner gets its potential for lightening skin discolorations. A fullerene is a cage-like, hollow molecule composed of hexagonal and pentagonal groups of carbon atoms which can have other elements attached to them. That means there can be various forms and adaptations of a fullerene, though "fullerenes" is the term defined in the latest *International Cosmetic Ingredient*

Dictionary and Handbook. There is one study that compared the effects of a fullerene deriva-tive (C60-fullerene) with the effects of arbutin and vitamin C (L-ascorbic acid). It revealed that C60-fullerene has an inhibitory effect on melanin production in the presence of UVA radiation. The study also demonstrated that this fullerene derivative was better at inhibiting melanin formation than arbutin or L-ascorbic acid, although the publication did not reveal the concentrations that were used in the study. (Source: *Archives of Dermatological Research*, August 2007, pages 245-257). Whether or not Brandt used this specific fullerene derivative (C60) is not known, and one study isn't much to go on (not when the tried-and-true skin-lightening agent hydroquinone has volumes of research attesting to its efficacy). All in all, this product is at best a leap of faith and definitely not better then staying out of the sun and being diligent about using a mineral-based sunscreen. Still, if your budget allows, this is a novel way to approach skin lightening and it may have benefit. The inclusion of a tiny amount of orange peel oil isn't great, but such a small amount is unlikely to be much of a problem for skin.

    unrated **Laser Lightning Day Lotion, For All Skin Types** *($90 for 1.7 ounces)* is positioned as an alternative skin-lightening product that eschews the gold standard hydroquinone in favor of ingredients known as fullerenes. Please refer to the review of Dr. Brandt's Laser Lightning Serum (below) for an in-depth discussion of fullerenes. The bottom line is that fullerenes are potentially effective, but risky, to use and Brandt doesn't reveal what type his products contain. This product contains some helpful antioxidants and skin-identical substances, but until more is known about how fullerenes function on skin, you don't need to be Brandt's guinea pig for this product. This also contains the ingredient diacetyl boldine for its potential ability to suppress excess melanin (skin pigment) production. However, there is no independent, peer-reviewed research supporting this ingredient's use for lightening skin discolorations.

    unrated **Laser Lightning Night Cream, For All Skin Types** *($110 for 1.7 ounces)* is a slightly emollient, silky-textured moisturizer that would be an option for normal to dry skin if not for the potential unknowns and the risk associated with fullerenes. The only positive research that exists for a specific fullerene (C60) mentioned its antioxidant capability and that it seems to interrupt the expression of tyrosinase, an oxidizing enzyme in skin that triggers melanin production—but this was only when cultured human cells were exposed to UVA light. We don't know if fullerenes work against discoloration if, say, skin is protected by a sunscreen. Would blocking UVA rays from damaging skin render the fullerene incapable of stopping excess melanin production? Or can fullerene absorb into skin (versus being added to a petri dish) and have a similar effect? Moreover, the manner in which fullerenes work to block melanin production in the presence of UVA radiation is not fully understood, not to mention that the sole study was performed using a pure concentration of the fullerene, not the tiny amount used in this product meant for application to intact skin. Another concern: research has shown that when applied to epidermal skin cells, fullerenes "decrease cell viability and initiate a pro-inflammatory response." (Sources: *Aesthetic Plastic Surgery*, November-December 2007, pages 711-718, and *Toxicology In Vitro*, December 2006, pages 1313-1320). Considering the cost, the unknowns, and the use of jar packaging, I wouldn't hang my skin-lightening hopes on this product—and it has nothing to do with the way lasers work to fade discolorations from sun damage (Source: *Archives of Dermatological Research*, August 2007, pages 245-257).

    unrated **Laser Lightning Serum, for All Skin Types** *($110 for 1 ounce)* has a water-based serum texture and bases its lightening ability around the ingredient fullerene. A fullerene is defined as a cagelike, hollow molecule composed of hexagonal and pentagonal groups of atoms. Their major element is carbon, and fullerenes constitute the third form of carbon after diamond and graphite. Various fullerene molecules exist. There is one study that compared a fullerene derivative (C60-fullerene) to arbutin and vitamin C (L-ascorbic acid). It revealed that C60-fullerene has an inhibitory effect on melanin in the presence of UVA radiation. Therefore, over time and with diligent use of sunscreen, its ongoing use should fade sun-induced skin discolorations and prevent new discolorations from appearing. The study also demonstrated that this fullerene derivative was better at inhibiting melanin formation than arbutin or L-ascorbic acid, though the concentrations used in the study were not revealed (Source: *Archives of Dermatological Research*, February 28, 2007, ePublication). Whether or not Brandt used this fullerene derivative is not known, and one study isn't much to go on (especially when the tried-and-true skin-lightening agent hydroquinone has volumes of research attesting to its efficacy). It is also important to point out that there is research showing fullerenes to be extremely risky (Source: *Environmental Health Perspectives*, July 2004, pages 1058-1062). With so many questions about this ingredient left unanswered, this serum is best left on the shelf. You need not be a guinea pig for anyone.

DR. BRANDT LINELESS PRODUCTS

☹ **Lineless Foaming Cleanser, for All Skin Types** *($40 for 3.5 ounces)*. The air-activated foaming qualities of this fairly average cleanser may intrigue you, but they have no bearing on how clean your skin will be after using this or on how well it can remove makeup. This ends up being an incredibly expensive way to cleanse and also to irritate your skin, thanks to the hefty amount of tangerine oil. None of the citrus oils are good for skin, and they're especially problematic if they come into contact with the eyes.

☹ **Lineless Tone, for Normal to Dry Skin** *($40 for 8 ounces)* lists witch hazel as the second ingredient, which negates the effect of the anti-irritants that follow, as does the inclusion of lavender oil.

☹ **Lineless Anti-Glycation Serum** *($90 for 1.5 ounces)* claims to address the effects of glycation on skin cells. Advanced glycation end-products (AGEs) are abnormal, cross-linked, and oxidized proteins that might play a role in the aging process. That oxidation process also involves sugars, particularly in the form of glucose, which is one of the primary ways the body gets its fuel for producing energy and "get up and go" power. This is because glucose can also, through an enzymatic trigger, attach itself to proteins anywhere in the body and form "glycated" substances that damage tissue by making it stiff and inflexible. AGEs directly affect the surface layers of skin as well as structures beneath the surface, such as collagen and elastin. What is still unknown, despite ongoing research, is whether topical application of ingredients known to disrupt the internal process AGEs go through to damage normal proteins (including collagen) can have any effect on skin. Brandt's serum is claiming to prevent the effects of glycation while strengthening the collagen and elastin fibers, but for now, that claim is still wishful thinking. A couple of ingredients do stand out for their potential role in mitigating the effects of AGEs: carnosine and prolinamidoethyl imidazole. Both of these ingredients have demonstrated potent antioxidant ability, but there is no conclusive research pertaining to their use in cosmetic formulations meant to combat AGEs, so whether or not they'll really work for that purpose is a leap of faith (Sources: *Life Sciences*, April 2006, pages 2343-2357; and *Pathologie-biologie*, September 2006, pages 396-404).Even if this serum could put a stop to AGEs and therefore slow the skin's aging process, this product contains lavender oil, which has been proven to cause skin-cell death (Source: *Cell Proliferation*, June 2004, pages 221-229). That error alone makes this pricey serum not worth considering, as any potential AGE-mitigating benefit from the aforementioned ingredients isn't worth the irritation the lavender oil can cause.

☹ **Lineless Cream, Age-Inhibitor Complex, for All Skin Types** *($100 for 1.7 ounces)* contains irritating lavender oil (which doesn't inhibit one second of aging), and lists most of its antioxidants well after the preservatives, meaning they're barely present. Even if there were greater amounts, Brandt's choice of jar packaging will quickly render them ineffective.

☺ **$$$ Lineless Eye Cream, for All Skin Types** *($60 for 0.5 ounce)* is a very good moisturizer for dry skin around the eyes, or anywhere on the face. It contains mostly water, emollients, plant oil, green tea, silicones, anti-irritant plant extracts, aloe, more plant oil, skin-identical ingredients, and preservatives. The inclusion of geranium oil isn't ideal, but the amount is unlikely to be a problem.

☹ **Lineless Gel** *($100 for 1.7 ounces)* is a water-based gel that, according to the company, is supposed to contain concentrated levels of the antioxidants green tea and grape seed. If that's true, then the amount of alcohol in this gel is even more concentrated because it's listed before them, and it poses a significant problem for all skin types. Alcohol damages skin and the irritation it causes promotes increased oil production in the pore. Between the alcohol, the fragrant geranium oil, and the obnoxious price for what amounts to a skin-damaging product, this is not recommended.

☹ **Lineless Infinite Moisture, for All Skin Types** *($65 for 1.7 ounces)* is a mixed bag of what to include and what not to include when formulating a skin-beneficial moisturizer. This product begins well, with an emollient and several good skin-identical ingredients, but begins to unravel with the addition of guarana and kola nut extracts, each in higher-than-usual amounts. Guarana is an herb that contains two-and-a-half times more caffeine than coffee, has constricting properties on skin, and is a skin irritant. Kola nut has plenty of caffeine as well, but of greater concern is its amine content, which can form nitrosamines—potential carcinogens that are not something you want to routinely (if ever) apply to your skin (Source: *Food and Chemical Toxicology*, August 1995, pages 625-630). This product also contains irritating geranium and ylang-ylang oils, which have no place in a moisturizer except to add fragrance. What a shame, because this is otherwise an excellent, well-packaged moisturizer for normal to slightly dry skin.

☺ **$$$ Lineless Lines No More** *($55 for 0.35 ounce)*. You'd think that if any of Dr. Brandt's Lineless products worked even a little, his Botox and dermal filler appointment book would dwindle with each passing week. That's not the case, the guy's still in business and statistically, the number of Botox and dermal filler injections is increasing exponentially around the world year after year. None of the evidence, especially not the research showing these products don't stop lines in any fashion, doesn't stop Brandt from launching more products promising to do what only cosmetic corrective procedures can. This wrinkle filler-type product has a lotion texture that does little to fill in lines, unless they're the superficial kind caused by dryness (which can be remedied by almost any moisturizer). Nothing in this product can add volume to skin—to do that, you absolutely need dermal fillers. Other than the skin-identical ingredient lecithin, there is nothing special about this formula, at all and the showcased peptide in this formula palmitoyl tripeptide-3, has limited research proving it can boost collagen production (Source: *International Journal of Cosmetic Science*, June 2005, pages 155-160). Besides, there are lots of ingredients that can boost collagen production; it doesn't take this one to do it even if there were more research. This does contain a potentially irritating amount of ylang-ylang oil (listed by its Latin name *Cananga odorata*). This specialty skin-care product is really Useless, not Lineless for all skin types.

☺ **$$$ Lineless Liquid Synergy, for All Skin Types** *($70 for 1.7 ounces)* is sold as a premoisturizer to be applied before your regular night cream. What always strikes me as odd about these prep kind of products is why the company can't figure out how to make the cream good enough to not need a second step. On the positive side, this product is well designed and the claims reflect exactly what a well-formulated moisturizer should do. That is, it contains ingredients that mimic the structure of skin to help it behave in as healthy a manner as possible by supplying key ingredients to improve barrier function. With a blend of silicones the application has a silky-smooth finish, but that's about all there is to this pricey product; not bad, but not great, and not worth the price. Even the preservative phenoxyethanol is listed before some of the intriguing water-binding agents and helpful ceramides, which means that those bells and whistles barely make a sound. In the long run, this doesn't lend any improvement to a well-formulated moisturizer that should contain the ingredients in this product plus much, much more.

☹ **Lineless Vitamin C Serum** *($75 for 1 ounce)* is a silky, silicone-based serum that contains an impressive amount of antioxidant grape seed oil. That's great but considering this serum's price, you should expect (and get) a lot more. And without a doubt, this contains ingredients no one's skin needs, including cell-damaging lavender oil and grapefruit peel oil, a citrus oil that can make skin more sun-sensitive while causing irritation.

DR. BRANDT PORES NO MORE PRODUCTS

☹ **Pores No More Cleanser** *($35 for 8 ounces)* contains irritating sodium lauryl sulfate along with lavender and rosemary oils, making this cleanser a problem for any skin type.

☹ **Pores No More Moisture** *($42 for 3.5 ounces)* contains lavender and rosemary oils, both volatile substances with more detriments than benefits for skin.

☹ **Pores No More Pore Effect** *($55 for 1.7 ounces)* is said to stimulate cellular turnover, but it doesn't contain ingredients capable of doing that. It will, however, irritate skin because it contains lavender and rosemary oils.

☹ **Pores No More Poreless Gel** *($55 for 1.7 ounces)* lists witch hazel as the second ingredient, and also contains potentially irritating levels of film-forming agents as well as the menthol derivative menthyl lactate. The fact that such a poor concoction is from a dermatologist is just embarrassing.

☹ **Pores No More Pore Refiner** *($45 for 1 ounce)* blends multiple silicones (possibly more than I've ever seen in a single product) and has a spackle-like texture that works to a minor extent to fill in large pores and help keep skin matte (matte skin automatically makes pores look smaller). It would be wholeheartedly recommended if Brandt hadn't included skin cell-damaging lavender oil. Mattifying products from Smashbox and Clinique are preferred to this one, and they cost much less, too.

☺ **$$$ Pores No More Vacuum Cleaner** *($45 for 1 ounce)* has a name that makes it sound like you can suck pores right off your face, but that's impossible. It's really a blend of the good, bad, and ugly when it comes to skin care. The absorbent base can keep surface oils at bay, which makes pores appear smaller temporarily. However, the amount of alcohol means that there is the potential for free-radical damage and irritation, which increases oil production in the pore. This also contains skin cell–damaging lavender oil. Glycolic and salicylic acids are present, but they cannot function as exfoliants because the pH of the product is too high. This is an expensive way to keep skin matte; a pressed powder would work just as well and also would even your skin tone.

DR. BRANDT TIME ARREST PRODUCTS

⊗ **Time Arrest Creme** *($100 for 1 ounce)*. Dr. Brandt claims that his Time Arrest products contain age-reversing technology in the form of platinum, which is the angle he uses to try to justify the ridiculous price tags for these products. My question is: What about the other anti-aging products Brandt sells, such as Lineless and those claiming to work like Botox, lasers, and face-lifts? If those worked as claimed, why is the Time Arrest line needed? And why does Brandt himself keep busy performing countless cosmetic corrective procedures if all it takes to reverse aging are his skin-care products? I could go on, but suffice it to say this Creme isn't anyone's age-reversing answer. It has a lush, silky texture and contains some impressive water-binding agents, but nothing that warrants the cost or that justifies the outlandish claims. Platinum, whether attached to a peptide chain or not, cannot prevent skin from sagging or restore a "sculpted look" to the face. These kinds of claims from a physician are just embarrassing. What really hurts this product is the inclusion of skin cell–damaging lavender oil (Sources: *Contact Dermatitis*, September 2008, pages 143-150; and *Cell Proliferation*, June 2004, pages 221-229). For that reason, plus the completely fabricated claims that lack a shred of substantiation, this moisturizer is not recommended. By the way, what limited research there is on topical use of platinum has shown that it causes skin-cell death, which isn't what you want if your goal is to look younger (Source: *Skin Pharmacology*, volume 4, 1991, pages 169-174).

⊗ **Time Arrest Eye Serum** *($85 for 0.5 ounce)* fails to impress beyond mild applause and deserves a round of boos because it contains skin cell-damaging lavender oil along with platinum. Platinum has no benefit for aging skin, although there is limited research showing that it, like lavender oil, has cytotoxic properties (Sources: *Contact Dermatitis*, September 2008, pages 143-150; *Cell Proliferation*, June 2004, pages 221-229; and *Skin Pharmacology*, volume 4, 1991, pages 169-174).

⊗ **Time Arrest Face Fluid** *($90 for 1 ounce)* is an overpriced, water-based serum that fails to impress on almost any criterion of good skin care because it contains skin cell–damaging lavender oil along with platinum, which has no benefit for aging skin. Platinum, however, does have limited research showing that it, like lavender oil, is cytotoxic (Sources: *Contact Dermatitis*, September 2008, pages 143-150; *Cell Proliferation*, June 2004, pages 221-229; and *Skin Pharmacology*, volume 4, 1991, pages 169-174). The amount of film-forming agent (hairspray-type ingredient) in this serum can have a temporary tightening effect on skin, but that won't reverse time, provide lift, or enhance facial volume and it is a standard effect you can get from lots of products containing acrylates. All of those claims are beyond silly, especially for a physician.

⊗ **Time Arrest Laser Tight** *($85 for 1.3 ounces)*. I imagine lots of people who want to avoid cosmetic corrective procedures will be tempted by this product's claims of firming and tightening skin while adding fullness and preventing sagging. Lots of women will think that if a physician promises results that are similar to the results of expensive medical treatments, then he must be telling the truth. That faith will prove at best disappointing. No skin-care product can address age- and sun damage-related changes such as sagging skin or loss of facial volume. Those physiological changes, which everyone will experience to some extent, can be remedied only with cosmetic corrective procedures. Time Arrest Laser Tight has nothing to do with lasers; the best it will do is make skin smoother and softer while supplying some antioxidants and skin-identical ingredients. That's noteworthy, but like so many of Brandt's formulas, one or more irritants get in the way of the benefits. In this case, he added the menthol derivative menthone glycerin acetal as well as lavender oil, which increases free-radical damage and causes cell death when applied topically (Sources: *Contact Dermatitis*, September 2008, pages 143-150; and *Cell Proliferation*, June 2004, pages 221-229). The resulting irritation leads to collagen breakdown and inflammation, which is not the way to look younger or take great care of your skin, at any age.

☹ **$$$ Time Arrest V-Zone Neck Cream** *($60 for 1.7 ounces)* offers no special benefit for the thin skin on the neck. It is merely an emollient moisturizer for dry skin anywhere on the body. The jar packaging won't keep the plant-based antioxidants stable during use, and this contains fragrant geranium oil, which isn't a helpful addition. As for the platinum, there is no research proving it has a positive effect on aging skin, whether on the face, around the eyes, or on the neck.

DR. BRANDT SUN PRODUCTS

☺ **$$$ UV SPF 30** *($32 for 4.2 ounces)* is a good in-part avobenzone sunscreen in a lightweight yet moisturizing base suitable for normal to dry skin. Extras include the cell-communicating ingredient lecithin along with small amounts of antioxidants, but you should expect more in a product at this price point. It contains fragrance in the form of orange peel oil, though the amount is likely too small to cause problems for skin. One thing to be very aware of is that you must apply sunscreen liberally to achieve the SPF rating on the label, and 4.2 ounces isn't going to last very long. There are more impressive formulations you can consider for a lot less money!

DR. DENESE NEW YORK

DR. DENESE NEW YORK AT-A-GLANCE

Strengths: Several well-formulated serums and moisturizers that are reasonably priced; a very good matte-finish, tinted sunscreen with zinc oxide; uses well-researched, proven ingredients that truly benefit skin, and uses them in higher concentrations than most skin-care lines.

Weaknesses: Some problem cleansers and toners; inclusion of unnecessary irritants such as lavender oil and menthol; limited options for sun protection; a few gimmicky, multistep kits that are easily replaced by other products in her line.

For more information about Dr. Denese New York, call QVC at (800) 345-1515 or visit www.drdenese.com or www.Beautypedia.com.

DR. DENESE NEW YORK SKIN CARE

☹ **DermaClean Gentle BHA Cleanser** *($19 for 8 ounces)* does contain BHA (salicylic acid), but the amount is not specified, although the pH of 3.2 will permit exfoliation. The inherent problem with including BHA in a cleanser is that it is not left on the skin long enough to have an optimal effect because it is quickly rinsed off your skin and down the drain. The main problem with this otherwise well-formulated cleanser is the high amount of lavender oil, which is irritating to skin and should not get anywhere near the eyes or mucous membranes (Source: *Cell Proliferation*, June 2004, page 221). Contrary to claim, the vitamins in this cleanser do not exfoliate.

☺ **$$$ Hydrating Cleanser** *($22 for 6 ounces)* is a simply formulated, detergent-based cleanser that contains borage oil to soften skin and facilitate makeup removal. The big-deal ingredients that supposedly justify the price are coenzyme Q10 (CoQ10), vitamin A, and vitamin E. The vitamins are barely present in this cleanser and the CoQ10 is completely absent, which is strange. However, even if they were present, neither the CoQ10 nor the other vitamins can have a positive effect on the skin because, when they are included in a cleanser they are rinsed off before they have a chance to have any impact. So, paying extra for such bells and whistles isn't necessary. Regardless, this is still a good cleanser for normal to slightly dry skin.

☹ **Pore Refining Toner** *($19 for 8 ounces)* is a water- and aloe-based toner that would have been much better for skin if it didn't include irritating witch hazel, lavender oil, and several citrus extracts. This toner does contain AHAs, but the pH of 6 prevents them from functioning as exfoliants. This product is not recommended.

☺ **$$$ Microdermabrasion Cream** *($35 for 4 ounces)*. Unlike most microdermabrasion scrubs, which contain aluminum oxide crystals, Dr. Denese opted to use pumice, one of the more abrasive scrub agents available. The base formula has sufficient oil and emollients to prevent the pumice from being too rough on skin, but between this and the various AHA peels in this line, we're talking potential exfoliation overload. This product also contains small amounts of several irritating plant extracts. If you're looking for a topical scrub, the microdermabrasion-in-a-jar versions from Neutrogena, Susan Lucci's Youthful Essence, Clinique, and Olay Regenerist are better and less expensive. But remember, simply using a washcloth with your cleanser can easily net the same results.

☹ **Advanced Firming Facial Pads** *($35 for 60 pads)* contain 10% glycolic acid and have a pH of 3.8 to ensure efficacy (this was confirmed by the company and our own testing). Interestingly, although menthol is no longer listed on the ingredient statement, these pads have a noticeable mint smell and definitely cause your skin to tingle while providing an intense cooling sensation. The tingle can occur with use of an effective AHA product (which this qualifies as), but the cooling effect is not indicative of how AHAs should feel. My research assistant called the company to ask about this discrepancy, and was told that the pads do, in fact, still contain menthol. Therefore, they are still not recommended. The addition of a couple of peptides doesn't change the fact that these pads add extra irritation to the skin and still have poor aesthetics.

☺ **$$$ Damage Reversal Pads** *($45 for 60 pads)* contain a solution of 2% hydroquinone in a water base with an effective amount of glycolic acid. However, because these pads are packaged in a jar, the hydroquinone will quickly become inactive, as will the arbutin and antioxidants; what a shame. At best, this is a pricey way to exfoliate skin with AHA.

☺ **Baggage Lost Puff Reducing Eye Gel** *($25 for 1 ounce)* is a lightweight moisturizer that doesn't contain anything that can noticeably reduce puffiness or dark circles under the eye. Classic "deflating" ingredients such as cucumber show up, but no topical ingredient or blend can address the cause of age-related puffy eyes. The second ingredient, sweet almond seed extract, has soothing properties—nice but not a cure-all for under-eye woes.

☹ **Cellular Firming Serum** *($64 for 1 ounce)* has a formula that is nothing if not intriguing, because it contains a blend of AHAs and BHA as well as the skin-lightening ingredients arbutin and kojic acid. It also contains hydroquinone PCA, although that isn't the same as hydroquinone because it does not have the ability to lighten skin. Dr. Denese claims this product tingles when applied to skin, and attributes this tingling to the alpha lipoic (thioctic) acid. However, it's more likely that the combination of alcohol with glycolic and lactic acids is what causes the sensation, and that isn't great for skin. It is true that at the appropriate pH, AHA or BHA products may cause slight tingling or stinging due to the manner in which they work on skin. But you want to avoid the additives, such as alcohol, that add to this irritation. This serum has a lot going for it, but it fails to successfully combine the benefits of exfoliation and skin lightening without causing excess irritation.

☹ **Contouring Serum with Stem Bio-Technology** *($64.32 for 1 ounce).* You can ignore the claims about this serum being able to lift key parts of the face based on its "plant stem cell technology." If this were the answer for skin, then Dr. Denese should at least be telling you that all of her other products don't work as well and you shouldn't buy them.

Here is what you're supposed to absorb. The showcased ingredient, Domestica Fruit Cell Culture, is touted by the manufacturer, and by the cosmetics companies that have thrown it into their formulas, as being able to restore skin. The Domestica Fruit Cell Culture is claimed to be from a rare Swiss apple tree (of course it has to be rare; the marketing story wouldn't be nearly as interesting if the apple tree were in Seattle or Chicago) and is based on plant callus cells. Plant callus cells are formed when a plant is wounded. The cells surrounding the wound turn back into stem cells, meaning they change and become cells that can produce wound-healing plant tissue. After the wound has healed, these callus cells remain stem cells (they are totipotent) and can continue to make whatever cells the plant needs. The Swiss apple tree in question also has substances that give the tree longevity. That's really good news for the plant, but whether or not it is good news for your skin is simply a guessing game, supported only by the in vitro research performed by the ingredient manufacturer, who claims that it shows some protective benefit. Even if this ingredient has some protective potential for skin cells, then the same would be true of hundreds of ingredients, from sunscreens to antioxidants and cell-communicating ingredients such as retinol or niacinamide. This is not a miracle or the new must-have ingredient for skin. There simply isn't any published research showing benefit or even demonstrating that there are no risks. There are several helpful ingredients for skin in this serum, but none of them will contour the face or result in a tighter, lifted appearance, at least not any more than other well-formulated "moisturizers." Despite the helpful ingredients, this isn't recommended because it contains the sensitizing preservative methylisothiazolinone. Another caution is the amount of antioxidant alpha lipoic acid. Although this can be a good ingredient for skin, topical application of high concentrations can cause burning, stinging sensations or produce a rash (Source: *British Journal of Dermatology,* October 2003, pages 841-849).

☺ **Doctor's Night Recovery Cream** *($39.50 for 2 ounces)* is an excellent formula for those with dry to very dry skin. It includes fatty acids, ingredients that mimic the structure and function of healthy skin, plant oils, anti-irritants, many antioxidants, and cell-communicating ingredients, including retinol. Unfortunately, the jar packaging means that many of these ingredients (especially the retinol) won't remain stable once the container is open and exposed to air. With improved packaging, this would be one of the best moisturizer formulas money can buy.

☺ **$$$ Firming Facial Age Corrector Cream** *($43.50 for 1.7 ounces)* is a lushly textured moisturizer for normal to dry skin that contains several beneficial ingredients for skin. Unfortunately, those ingredients (which include retinol) won't remain potent for long due to the jar packaging. I was hoping Denese would update her packaging to reflect this need, but she's seemingly ignored the issue or even worse, doesn't care or doesn't know about it. That means the good stuff you're paying for isn't going to be around for long once you open this product, exposing it to air, and introduce bacteria into the container that deteriorate the good ingredi-

The Reviews D

ents. All you're left with is an overpriced moisturizer. Also, the amount of glycolic acid in this product is too low for it to exfoliate skin, plus the product's pH isn't within the correct range for that to occur.

☺ **$$$ Firming Facial Age Corrector Eye Cream** *($36.82 for 0.5 ounce)* makes claims of being able to exfoliate skin, but none of its ingredients can do that. This product is mostly water, gel-based thickener, some peptides, and what Denese describes as botanical stem cell extract from apple. I couldn't find a shred of research about botanical stem cells from apples, but apple extract certainly has antioxidant ability, just like all fruits (and Dr. Denese's customer service and public relations people couldn't provide any either). Absurdly, we're meant to believe a plant stem cell can stimulate our stem cells. (That would make research into stem cells far less political if it involved plants instead of human sources of stem cells from fetuses. Now why didn't politicians and scientists all over the world think of that? All they had to do was call Dr. Denese or watch her home shopping appearances.) None of the peptides in this product have independent, peer-reviewed research proving their antiwrinkle, elasticity-boosting prowess, so you're left to take Dr. Denese's word for it (or the doctor's marketing department; you pick who you think is pulling the wool over your eyes). This can be a good lightweight gel moisturizer for slightly dry skin, but the inclusion of fragrant lavender extract means it's best to avoid using it in the eye area. One thing to keep in mind: using this product isn't going to correct anyone's age—the concept is silly because it implies that women get to an age where their age is "wrong" or incorrect and needs to be fixed.

☺ **$$$ Hyaluronic Wrinkle Filler Serum and Cream** *($59)* is a two-part system—but for the life of me I can't figure out why these products needed to be separated. The decision seems to be more marketing caprice than necessity. Step 1 is a serum, which consists solely of water, vitamin B5, slip agent, preservative, skin-identical ingredients, and more preservatives. Step 2 is a silicone-based cream that contains some skin-identical ingredients and a small amount of antioxidants. The products are said to work in tandem to reduce creases, but since the ingredients in the serum could have easily been added to the cream, why bother splitting them up? The system does constitute an effective moisturizer for normal to slightly dry or slightly oily skin, but compared to other Denese products it's disappointingly short on antioxidants. The skin-identical ingredients can temporarily plump skin, reducing the appearance of creases, but neither these ingredients nor the effect are unique to this product.

☹ **$$$ HydroShield Eye Fix Duo** *($30 for 2 0.5-ounce jars; 1 ounce total)*. The Denese line sells several products for the eye area, but if any of them worked as claimed, you'd only need one, right? This unnecessary option includes two products: one for the upper eye area and one for the skin beneath the eye. **Upper Eye Lid Care** is a creamy moisturizer that contains some very good antioxidants and cell-communicating ingredients, but the jar packaging will reduce their potency after opening. The **Under Eye Care** is a silicone-based serum that has a mild, spackle-like effect on superficial lines. It contains some good antioxidants and mineral pigments that provide a cosmetic brightening effect. Unfortunately, this product is also packaged in a jar, so the antioxidants won't do much for your skin. This isn't a great solution or fast fix for "the total eye area," or any area of the face for that matter.

✓☺ **$$$ HydroShield Eye Serum** *($44 for 0.5 ounce)* contains silicone, antioxidants, ceramides, retinol, several fatty acids, and preservatives. This fragrance-free serum is an outstanding formulation that is recommended for all skin types. It may be used around the eyes or anywhere on the face. Its lightweight texture and matte finish make it well-suited for those with oily skin looking for the benefits of antioxidants and retinol without heaviness. This is a product any dermatologist would be proud of!

☺ **$$$ HydroShield Hydrating Dream Cream** *($40 for 1.7 ounces)* may seem like a dream cream because of the silky-smooth texture that makes skin feel amazing, but it's a crying shame that most of the state-of-the-art ingredients in this moisturizer for dry skin will see their efficacy suffer due to the jar packaging. Dr. Denese supposedly is a research-oriented physician and it's her research that led to the creation of these products. That doesn't explain why she routinely overlooks the importance of packaging as it relates to formulas containing light- and air-sensitive ingredients (exposure to air deteriorates all plant extracts, vitamins, antioxidants, peptides, and on and on). It's also disappointing that this product contains fragrance and coloring agents, because a physician should know both are common sources of skin allergies (with fragrance being the bigger offender) and have no value as skin-care ingredients.

✓☺ **$$$ HydroShield Neck Serum** *($44.50 for 1 ounce)* is yet another well-formulated silicone-based serum with retinol from Dr. Denese. It holds no special benefit for skin on the neck, so you certainly can use it on the face and/or around the eyes, and anywhere else on the body for that matter. It contains an exciting blend of silkening silicones with retinol, skin-identical ingredients, cell-communicating ingredients, and antioxidants. It also is fragrance-free, though the retinol content (and retinol in general) makes it iffy for someone with sensitive skin. Otherwise, this is suitable for all skin types except very oily. The tiny amount of clover flower extract is not likely to be a problem for skin.

☺ **$$$ HydroShield Ultra Moisturizing Face Serum** *($69 for 1 ounce)* contains a brilliant assortment of ingredients, including skin-silkening silicone, ceramides, cell-communicating ingredients, and vitamins, and all without added fragrance or irritants. What a shame the latest frosted-glass packaging will compromise the stability of the retinol and also hinder the effectiveness of the antioxidants. This is only recommended if you're willing to store it in a cool, dark place to minimize retinol-degrading light exposure.

✓☺ **$$$ Neck Saver Serum** *($34 for 1 ounce)* is a brilliantly formulated serum that can be used on the face or from the neck down. It contains a blend of silicones, antioxidants, retinol, ceramides, several cell-communicating ingredients, plant extracts (a couple with undetermined benefit for skin), and preservatives. The clover extract in this serum adds fragrance.

☺ **$$$ RestorEyes Eye Cream** *($45 for 0.5 ounce)* is an even better formulation than the HydroShield Eye Serum, so why the neutral rating? Jar packaging. Thanks to that poor choice, the many antioxidants in this product (plus its retinol) will be useless shortly after the product is opened. This is still a good option for a silky-textured, normal-to-dry-skin moisturizer anywhere on the face.

✓☺ **$$$ SPF 30 Defense Day Cream** *($34 for 1.5 ounces)* features an in-part zinc oxide sunscreen and is slightly tinted to offset the white cast this ingredient can leave on skin. The product is described as being able to "intensely hydrate" the skin, but the inactive ingredients don't support this claim because they are primarily dry-finish silicones, aloe, and talc. The jar packaging won't keep the antioxidants in the formula stable during use, so avoid that option (available in a 2-ounce size). Instead, go for the larger, 4-ounce size packaged in an opaque tube or, if your budget is limited, they also offer a 1.5-ounce tube for $32.50. This fragrance-free sunscreen is best for normal to slightly oily skin not prone to blemishes. It feels wonderful and is tenacious, so be sure you remove it with a washcloth and/or silicone-based makeup remover.

✓ ☺ **SPF 30 Neck Defense Day Cream UVA/UVB** *($32.25 for 2 ounces)* is an excellent daytime moisturizer with sunscreen for normal to dry skin, whether it's used on the neck or face. UVA protection is provided by avobenzone, and the formula contains retinol along with antioxidants and cell-communicating ingredients. The jasmine extract is a fragrant additive that should've been left out, but the amount is so small that it's unlikely to be cause for concern (plus the extract isn't as problematic for skin as the pure oil would be).

☺ **$$$ Triple Strength Eye Wrinkle Smoother** *($49.50 for 0.5 ounce)* is similar to but more emollient and less exciting than the Triple Strength Wrinkle Smoother below. Peptides are present in lesser quantities than its partner product, and the group of ingredients said to reduce dark circles (including hesperidin methyl chalcone and vitamin K) don't have substantiated research proving they work for this purpose. This is still a worthwhile product for use around the eyes or elsewhere on the face, and is best for normal to dry skin.

☹ **Triple Strength Neck Wrinkle Smoother** *($36.50 for 2 ounces)* isn't specific to the neck, and contains mostly water, chelating agent, glycerin, plant oils, and emollients suitable for dry to very dry skin. The jar packaging means that the many antioxidants and retinol won't remain stable during use, though most of them are present only in meager amounts anyway.

✓ ☺ **$$$ Triple Strength Wrinkle Smoother** *($54 for 2 ounces)* won't help reduce lines resulting from facial expressions, but it is an elegant moisturizer for normal to dry skin. It contains mostly water, film-forming "opacifying" agent, thickener, several peptides, shea butter, skin-identical ingredients, retinol, anti-irritant, antioxidants, preservatives, and fragrance. The opaque tube packaging helps keep the light- and air-sensitive ingredients stable. The level of acrylate film-forming agent in this moisturizer does lend a slight tightening and "firming" effect to skin, but this tactile benefit is temporary and incapable of keeping expression lines at bay. Dr. Denese states in her book that this product has "three times the Oligopeptide of the industry standard." That sounds impressive, but is less so when you consider that there is no industry standard for this ingredient, nor any independent research showing it has antiwrinkle efficacy on skin. Nevertheless, this moisturizer does have a higher amount of peptides than many competing products and they can, in theory, function as cell-communicating ingredients.

☹ **$$$ Vitamin C Line Filling Radiance Cream** *($38 for 1 ounce)*. Curse the jar packaging that is this product's downfall! In better packaging (such as an airless jar or an opaque tube with a pump dispenser) this would be an affordable way to treat normal to dry skin to an antioxidant-rich moisturizer with a beautifully silky texture. The silkiness doesn't depend on the packaging, so you'll still get a beautifully smooth texture and finish, but nearly all of the beneficial ingredients in this product (including retinol) will deteriorate with the repeated exposure to light and air. By the way, vitamin C plays only a minor role in this formula; Vitamin E is present in a much greater amount, so the name isn't logical.

☺ **$$$ Wrinkle Rest Expression Line Peptide Concentrate** *($100 for 1.7 ounces)* is a silicone- and glycerin-based serum that primarily claims to moisturize skin by infusing the top layers with lipids (fats). However, it doesn't contain any lipids, and the peptides aren't as concentrated as they are in other Denese products. This contains an ingredient listed as pinacolyl-trans retinoate, which the company making it says is a retinol derivative. The only information about this ingredient (trade name RETexture Granactive RD-101) comes from the manufacturer, which is about as reliable as McDonald's saying hamburgers are nutritional powerhouses. It likely has antioxidant ability similar to other forms of vitamin A, but there's no proof it is as efficacious as tretinoin (Retin-A) without the irritation. This serum won't put wrinkles to rest, but is a good option for normal to slightly dry skin.

☺ **$$$ Wrinkle Rx Extreme Pro-Peptide Gel** *($64.50 for 1.7 ounces)* Denese's company is very excited about this gel-textured serum, claiming it is "the one" for tackling expression lines, be they around the eyes, between the brows, or on the forehead. The expression lines are supposedly eliminated thanks to the peptides and vitamin C this serum contains, but this isn't Botox in a bottle. There is no substantiated research proving that any of the peptides in this product can relax expression lines, and the same goes for the apple stem cell technology Denese brags about (but that's a good thing, because if this stem cell worked as claimed it could cause more problems than benefits). Despite the claims being more fantasy than reality, this is actually an exceedingly well-formulated serum that can, to some extent, help mitigate signs of aging and stimulate collagen production. The amount of vitamin C is impressive, as is the retinol. The serum is loaded with peptides, which have theoretical cell-communicating ability, and antioxidants are plentiful. Its only drawback (and what keeps it from earning a Paula's Pick rating) is the inclusion of bitter-orange oil. There isn't much of it in the product, but its presence is still discouraging. Still, this is recommended if you have normal to oily skin and aren't expecting deep wrinkles to vanish. It will likely prove to be too active for those with sensitive skin.

✓ ☺ **$$$ 15 Day SkinScience Booster Program** *($74.76 for 15 0.07-ounce tubes; 1.05 ounces total).* This kit sells itself as a concentrated program to boost your skin-care routine, but analyzing the ingredient lists for both steps in this duo doesn't reveal anything that you can't find in many other products, from this brand as well as from other lines. However, that fact doesn't change the efficacy of these formulations.

Step 1 is a great blend of silicones with antioxidants, retinol, and lecithin. Denese makes a big deal about the retinol being encapsulated, but lots of companies use retinol in this form because it reduces the risk of irritation and allows the retinol to work better. And what about her other products with retinol, where she doesn't make claims about the encapsulation? Are those no good despite claims to the contrary?

Step 2 is a moisturizer that supposedly contains "advanced peptides" to improve deep expression lines, but peptides of any kind have no legitimate research showing they are effective for skin over and above other ingredients. It's also supposed to firm skin with a "never-before-seen rate of effectiveness." However, "never-before-seen rate of effectiveness" is a meaningless claim. Who hasn't seen this rate of effectiveness? The Denese team? What research and what effectiveness are they talking about? Admittedly, this is a very good moisturizer for normal to very dry skin, but that's about it. It contains several key ingredients that skin needs to look and feel great, but the peptides and ceramides have no research proving their unprecedented firming action or any effect on tightening and defining skin, and those ingredients are not unique to this product anyway.

Both steps are packaged in single-use plastic vials designed to be used over a 15-day course of treatment. This seems very structured and medicinal, but the formulas, while impressive in their own right, tell another story. This "program" is deserving of a Paula's Pick rating for its formulary attributes and packaging, but it isn't an essential kit if your regular skin-care routine is supplying the same types of ingredients seen in these products.

☹ **$$$ Lash Faker Eyelash & Brow Enhancer** *($38.75 for 0.2 ounce).* Is this reasonably priced lash enhancer the way to obtain hydrated, fuller-looking lashes and eyebrows? No, absolutely not. This is merely a cosmetic without any capacity to change one hair on your face. The ingredients in this product will moisturize and condition eyelashes and brow hair, but that's about all you can expect and that won't change how they look in the least. Do not confuse this product with those that contain prostaglandin analogues, the class of ingredients included in some lash-enhancing products that actually do have an effect on lash growth and their resulting length and color. This ordinary formula isn't unique to Dr. Denese, either; you can find the exact same product in the Model Co. line's Lash + Brow on Sephora's Web site. If your expectation is simply to apply a blend of conditioning agents to make lashes and brows softer, this will work. If you want longer, thicker lashes without using mascara then you'll need to use one of the lash-enhancing products that contain drug ingredients whose side effects include lash growth and darkening. An example of such a product is Peter Thomas Roth's Lashes to Die For, reviewed on this site.

✓ ☺ $$$ **Glow Younger Clear Self-Tanner for Face and Body** *($32 for 6 ounces)*. This fragrance-free self tanner is a wonderful option for all skin types. It feels light and silky, absorbs quickly, and supplies skin with small amounts of several cell-communicating ingredients, which is more than what most self-tanners provide. Ignore the wrinkle-reducing claims, but consider this an above-average self-tanner.

☹ **SPF 25 Hand Defense Cream UVA/UVB** *($11 for 1 ounce)* has an in-part avobenzone sunscreen and retinol, with only one drawback: the inclusion of chaulmoogra oil, a plant oil that can cause skin irritation (Source: *PDR for Herbal Medicines*, 1st Edition, Medical Economics Company, Inc., 1998). Otherwise, it would have been an intriguing option for dry hands, and including sunscreen in a hand cream is a very good idea. Unfortunately, the aforementioned oil doesn't make this a hand cream with sunscreen worth considering, especially knowing that some people are sensitive to the synthetic sunscreen actives chosen as well as to the retinol.

DR. DENESE NEW YORK MAKEUP

FOUNDATION: ☺ $$$ **Age Corrector Firming & Retexturizing Foundation** *($31.50)*. If the name isn't a giveaway, this liquid foundation is designed with antiaging in mind. It is said to instantly firm skin while giving skin instant perfection. Admittedly, the formula is laced with several ingredients that typically show up in antiwrinkle products, but none of them have a miracle firming or tightening effect on skin. This foundation also contains stem cells from apples, but there is no proof that apple stem cells are the answer for wrinkles. The real reason to consider this foundation is for its silky texture and air-brushed matte finish. You'll get sheer to light coverage and a formula that does a good job of not slipping into lines, although it can crease a bit under the eyes if not blended well. Only three shades are available, and they're not the most neutral. Medium has a peach cast that's hard to soften, but it may work for some skin tones. Light is too dark for fair skin but OK for light skin. If one of the shades works for you, this foundation is best for normal to slightly dry or slightly oily skin.

☺ $$$ **Foundation Faker** *($28)* is a one-shade-fits-all solution to "improve skin's overall appearance." It's a good thing the single shade goes on sheer, because it has a peachy tone that looks 100% obvious on fair to light skin tones and does nothing on darker skin tones. The cream-to-powder texture feels light and blends easily, setting to a satin matte finish. This is best for medium skin tones dealing with normal to slightly dry skin that's not prone to breakouts. All told, most people will have better results using a foundation that offers more than one color.

CONCEALER: ☺ **Body Perfect Concealer** *($28.50)* is a generously sized concealer (it comes in a 2-ounce tube) with a nonaqueous, silicone-based formula that has a silky texture and smooth, even application. It's meant to conceal spider veins and discolorations on legs, hands, and chest, but you can apply it to the face as well. Overall, it's better at covering smaller discolorations than applying over a roadmap of spider veins. It doesn't conceal purplish vari-cose veins at all. This blends readily and provides very good coverage, but it isn't opaque like Dermablend, and it lasts. The silicone base provides a relatively budge-proof and water-resistant finish. I wish more than two shades were offered because what's available will work only for those with light to medium skin tones.

☺ $$$ **Damage Reversal Treatment Stick** *($28 for 0.16 ounce)* is the only concealer I know of that contains hydroquinone as an active ingredient. Denese opted for a 1.5% concentration, which won't be as effective as traditional 2% versions, but is still worth considering as a skin lightening and concealing product in one. The dual-sided component includes two shades of lipstick-style cream concealer. Both shades are neutral and work well on light skin tones used separately or blended together. The texture is thick and this doesn't have much slip, but it covers well and stays in place. It is fragrance-free.

☹ $$$ **Smart Concealer Duo Compact for Eyes & Face** *($24)* is also known as Smart Concealer Duo Compact for Face and Eyes. Housed in a sleek compact are two creamy conceal-ers, each with its own formula. The Eye Concealer has a smoother texture and applies easier, though is slightly prone to creasing into lines under the eye; the Face Concealer has a thicker, drier texture that can feel heavy and doesn't provide what most would consider natural-looking coverage. The full-size brush that's included is useful, though synthetic bristles would've made it even better. Unfortunately, the shades for each of the three sets aren't the easiest to work with. Light and Medium are slightly peach while Tan is slightly rose-toned.

POWDER: ☹ $$$ **HydroShield Hydrating Treatment Powder** *($23)* isn't hydrating in the least! Talc is the first ingredient, but the second is an acrylic, the third is boron nitride, and then there are other absorbing ingredients. Calling this hydrating is akin to calling a tricycle a car. You'll find this has a smooth, dry texture that provides a sheer matte finish, although the finish doesn't feel hydrating at all. The colors veer toward being too warm, so each has an overtone of peachy gold that's tricky to soften. If you decide to try this, it's best for normal to oily skin. There is a tiny amount of cell-communicating ingredients and an antioxidant, but the container won't keep them stable. It also contains polytetrafluoroethylene (PTFE), also known as Teflon.

BRONZER: ☺ $$$ **SunShield Anti-Aging Bronzer** *($25)* isn't adept at giving skin a sun-kissed glow. Instead, it's best as a pressed-powder blush with shine. The medium peach color has a soft gold shimmer finish that, applied sparingly, casts an attractive glow on cheeks. The name for this product is misleading because it doesn't provide any sun protection. Still, this is worth considering if you want a peachy blush with shine, although there are lots of less expensive options and better color options available for less than half this price at the drugstore.

EYE AND BROW PRODUCTS: ☹ $$$ **Triple Strength Eye Brightener** *($30)* a pale, peachy pink color (almost all of Denese's makeup products have a peach tinge) that works to highlight (OK, "brighten") skin under the eyes or on the eyelid. The liquid highlighter product is dispensed from a pen onto a synthetic brush, though getting the product to brush on evenly is a challenge because of the haphazard way it is dispensed. The Triple Strength part of the name refers to the company's wrinkle-smoothing peptide technology. However, the formula is short on antiaging ingredients. In fact, the finish of this highlighter will magnify wrinkles unless applied sheer. This product doesn't hold a candle to the much less expensive Maybelline New York's Instant Age Rewind Double Face Perfector.

LIPSTICK, LIP GLOSS AND LIPLINER: ☹ **Lip Firm Gloss SPF 15** *($11)* lacks the UVA-protecting ingredients of titanium dioxide, zinc oxide, avobenzone, Tinosorb, or Mexoryl SX, and is not recommended.

MASCARA: ☺ **Lash Faker Mascara** *($12)* quickly lengthens lashes while providing appreciable thickness, all without clumping or flaking. Lashes are left soft and slightly curled, and this mascara doesn't smear during wear. The price isn't terrible, either!

FACE AND BODY ILLUMINATING/SHIMMER PRODUCTS: ☺ **Sheer Glow Face Brightener with Pro-Peptide Factor** *($24.50)* produces a glow that isn't what most people would consider sheer. This lightweight lotion provides a moderate amount of peachy gold shimmer anywhere it's applied. It looks best when mixed with a moisturizer or liquid foundation because then the shine is downplayed and you get what the product name states, a sheer glow. For some reason, the sunscreen ingredient ethylhexyl methoxycinnamate is a major ingredient in this product. Although that's not a bad thing, you should use caution if applying this near your eyes, and certainly do not apply it to your eyelid area due to the risk of irritation if the sunscreen ingredient gets into your eyes.

E.L.F. (EYES LIPS FACE)

E.L.F. AT-A-GLANCE

Strengths: Inexpensive; lip gloss with broad-spectrum sunscreen; praiseworthy powder blush and eyeshadows; brow gel/clear mascara; oil-blotting papers are a steal; great brushes in the Studio line; complete ingredient lists are provided on the company's Web site.

Weaknesses: Mostly average formulas in smaller packaging than what's typical; terrible concealer; limited options for foundation; average to not-worth-it-at-any-price brushes (in E.L.F.'s main line).

For more information about E.L.F., call (800) 231-4732 or www.eyeslipsface.com or www.Beautypedia.com.

E.L.F. MINERAL MAKEUP

FOUNDATION: ☺ **Mineral Foundation SPF 15** *($5)* is one of the least expensive loose powder mineral foundation's available, and it's mostly impressive for the money. In the plus column are its titanium dioxide and zinc oxide active ingredients. The formula is also fragrance-free so it's great for sensitive or rosacea-affected skin. It also feels and looks lighter than many competing mineral makeups yet provides medium coverage. In the minus column are its shiny finish imbued with sparkles, its component (because it plays up the messy element of loose-powder foundation), and the fact that three of the five shades (Warm, Dark, and Deep) are terrible. The Fair shade is slightly pink but workable, while the Light shade fares best. This mineral makeup has its strong points, but its drawbacks significantly limit its appeal.

CONCEALER: ☺ **Mineral Concealer SPF 15** *($5)* has a formula that's identical to E.L.F.'s Mineral Foundation SPF 15. Its loose-powder texture is messy to apply as concealer (dusting it all over as a powder foundation is easier) and it suffers from almost the same shade issues as the Foundation: the Fair, Dark, and Deep shades don't resemble real skin tones and look either too peach, ghostly, or ashen. Warm and Light fare best, but that certainly limits this product's appeal. If you decide to try this, it has a smooth, soft texture that provides moderate coverage and leaves a shiny finish. This is dry enough to emphasize lines around the eyes. The average rating is due to this product's difficulty of use and overall performance as a concealer. The Mineral Foundation functions better for its intended purpose.

POWDER: ☺ **Mineral Booster** *($5)*. This cornstarch-based loose powder is designed to be worn alone or over one of E.L.F.'s Mineral Foundations. Results are supposed to be a "photo finishing touch," but let's get real here: this is just a sheer, translucent loose powder! It doesn't have any magic soft focus qualities that make it a must-have for picture-perfect skin. Besides, if mineral makeup is so great, why does it need a "booster" product like this? At best, this matte finish powder is best for oily skin because it is so absorbent. It is not recommended for use on breakout-prone skin because cornstarch can feed the bacteria that causes blemishes.

BLUSH: ☺ **Mineral Blush** *($5)*. If you can tolerate the messiness inherent with loose powder blush packaged in a standard jar with a non-closable sifter, this is a very good option to consider. The colors are soft and beautiful, and include muted and bright shades, each with a soft glow finish. Application is smooth and even, while the overall texture is dry due to the minerals it contains.

EYESHADOW: ☺ **Mineral Eyeshadow** *($3)* is a mica-based loose-powder eyeshadow that has a markedly dry texture that applies surprisingly smooth. The shade range is extensive and presents some beautiful options whether you want to go with soft or bold colors. All of them have shine, and many have shiny particles that tend to flake. Others omit the shiny particles and leave a metallic sheen instead. The company claims this formula is hydrating, but it absolutely isn't. No powder can be hydrating because the ingredients composing a powder are absorbent by nature. This eyeshadow also will not "minimize the appearance of fine lines." Just the opposite is true: the shiny finish these have will emphasize lines. However, those without lines in the eyes and who have a preference for loose-powder eyeshadow may want to give this affordable option a go.

☺ **100% Pure Mineral Eyeshadow Set** *($12)* includes three Mineral Eyeshadows, two brushes, an eye pencil, and pencil sharpener. Sets are available for various eye designs, including one built around classic brown tones and one for doing smoky eyes. Each boxed kit comes with instructions for how to do the eye design it's supposed to allow the user to accomplish. The eyeshadow has a soft, smooth texture that feels dry but blends surprisingly well. Each shade has a modest to strong degree of shine, ranging from sparkling to metallic, so none of these sets are for wrinkled eyes. The eyeshadow brushes are quite good and are well-shaped for their intended purpose. As for the eye pencil, it has a stiff texture that hurts to apply and, even worse, it needs almost constant sharpening (perhaps that's why they included a sharpener; it's built into the pencil's cap). Overall, if you're a fan of loose-powder eyeshadow and shine, this set is a worthwhile investment.

☹ **Mineral Eyeshadow Primer** *($3)* is a liquid eyeshadow primer that goes on slick and takes way too long to set. The result is sheer coverage and a translucent peach cast that feels tacky to the touch once it finally dries. The finish isn't the easiest to apply shadows over, and this isn't preferred to a good matte finish liquid concealer.

EYE AND BROW SHAPER: ☹ **Mineral Eye Liner** *($3)*. This automatic, retractable eye pencil has a trace amount of minerals, but minerals are absolutely not key to an eyeliner's performance. This pencil has an oily-based formula that's noticeably greasy. It glides on, but tends to smear and fade quickly.

LIPSTICK, LIP GLOSS, AND LIPLINER: ✓☺ **Mineral Lip Gloss** *($3)* is a standard lip gloss that has a thin but moisturizing texture, smooth application, and soft gloss finish that doesn't feel the least bit sticky. The mineral oil–based formula includes a well-edited selection of versatile shades, including a colorless option (Crystal Clear). It is also fragrance- and flavor-free. Well done and wonderfully affordable!

✓ ☺ **Mineral Lipstick** *($5)*. This creamy lipstick is composed of natural oils and waxes, most of which show up in other lipsticks, though this one does have an edge if you're looking for a formula that's all natural and doesn't contain fragrance. It has a smooth, slightly stiff texture that feels creamy and not the least bit slippery, so it tends to wear well and fade evenly. Color payoff is great and the shade range presents several enticing options.

☺ **Mineral Lip Liner** *($3)* is an oil-based, automatic, retractable pencil that applies smoothly but is too creamy to last. It does an OK job of defining lips but cannot stop lipstick or gloss from bleeding into lines around the mouth. The price is great, but performance is what counts most, and that's where this pencil becomes a letdown.

BRUSHES: ☺ **Kabuki Brushes** *($5-$8)*. Whether you choose the Kabuki Face Brush or Kabuki Body Brush, you'll get a reasonably soft option for applying mineral powder or any other loose powder in your makeup wardrobe. The lack of a handle can make either brush tricky to use, but with practice, it isn't so bad. For the money, although these are a bit floppy, they're workable for applying powder to large areas.

☺ **Brush Kit** *($10)* includes the Total Face Brush, Bronzing Brush, Defining Eye Brush, Brow Comb & Brush, Lip Defining Brush, and a synthetic fabric carrying case. With the exception of the Defining Lip Brush, all of them are too stiff, scratchy, or simply not dense enough for a beautiful makeup application. The lip brush does not come with a cap, but may be worth it given the low cost of this kit.

FACE AND BODY SHIMMER/ILLUMINATING PRODUCTS: ✓ ☺ **Mineral Glow** *($8)*. This illuminating loose mineral powder is excellent. It has a soft, smooth texture that applies and adheres well without flaking. Like all loose powders, this can come off on clothing, so use caution if you're applying this from the neck down. Both shades are attractive and cast a subtle glow wherever they're applied. The shades work best for fair to light skin tones.

☺ **Mineral Glow Kit** *($15)* contains one shade of E.L.F.'s Mineral Glow along with a Kabuki Body Brush and synthetic fabric carrying case. The Mineral Glow powder has a beautifully soft, silky texture and even application. Whether you choose the pale, fleshy glow of Shimmer or the soft peachy tan of Bronzed, the results are attractive and case a soft glow on skin. Either powder is a great way to wear subtle shine day or night, and flaking isn't a problem. As for the Kabuki Body Brush that's included, it's OK but many will find it not soft enough or be annoyed at how easily the hairs shed. If you don't want the brush or the case, Mineral Glow is sold separately. This kit earns a happy face rating, but the Mineral Glow powder deserves a Paula's Pick rating.

SPECIALTY PRODUCTS: ☺ **Starter Kit** *($20)* contains the company's **Mineral Foundation SPF 15**, **Mineral Concealer SPF 15**, a **Mineral Blush**, two makeup brushes, and a carrying case composed of durable synthetic fabric. The mineral foundation and concealer both have the same formulas. Each provides sun protection via titanium dioxide and zinc oxide. Both have a silky, sheer texture and lightweight finish that doesn't look as heavy or opaque as many other mineral makeups. Unfortunately, the foundation and concealer contain a lot of shine, so you get a finish that feels matte but looks shimmery with colorless sparkles. Someone with oily skin won't be happy with the finish either product provides. Another issue with the foundation and concealer is that the concealer tends to be a darker shade than the foundation, or it is tonally off. In essence, the pairings aren't that workable but either product can be brushed on as a loose-powder foundation and you can use a liquid or cream concealer where needed. The blush is similar to the foundation and concealer, except it doesn't contain titanium dioxide or zinc oxide. That allows it to go on softer and more sheer, but it still leaves cheeks quite shiny. As for the brushes, forget about them. Both are poor examples of quality makeup brushes and don't do a great job of applying these loose powders neatly. There are five Starter Kits available, from Fair to Deep. The foundation and concealer in the Dark and Deep sets have a slight ashen cast, while the blush isn't dark enough to show up well.

E.L.F. STUDIO MAKEUP

MAKEUP REMOVER: ☺ **Makeup Remover Cleansing Cloths** *($3)* contain a silicone and emollient blend that works quite well to remove makeup, including waterproof formulas. The fragrance-free formula is a nice change of pace, too, not to mention the price! These cloths would earn a Paula's Pick rating if they didn't contain the Kathon CG blend of preservatives. Because these preservatives are irritating if left on skin, you'll need to rinse after using these cloths.

CONCEALER: ☹ **Corrective Concealer** *($3)* isn't a product any professional makeup artist would have in his or her kit. You get two shades of peach concealer, one pastel pink color, and a mint green shade. Although these have a light cream texture, coverage is sparse and they remain creamy enough to crease and fade in short order. Don't bother!

☹ **Under Eye Concealer & Highlighter** *($3)* is a dual-sided liquid concealer with a matte finish and a complementary liquid highlighter that has a fluid texture and a bit too much slip. Although the color pairings are workable and the concealer provides OK coverage, both formulas contain sensitizing preservatives not recommended for use in leave-on products. They definitely pose a risk of irritating delicate skin around the eyes.

☹ **Concealer Pencil & Brush** *($3)* is a dual-sided pencil with one end being a cream concealer and the other being a firm brush for blending. The pencil is medicated with 2% salicylic acid but the nonaqueous formula prevents a pH from being established, so this has no effect on acne. Even if it did, the waxes and oils in this formula are absolutely not what anyone struggling with acne should be applying to their breakouts. Not only does the concealer end look too thick and heavy on skin, but all of the colors veer toward peach.

POWDER: ☺ **Translucent Matifying Powder** *($3)* is a talc-based pressed powder that's available in only one shade. It is supposed to go on translucent, but instead leaves a soft pink cast that works best on fair to light skin tones. The powder has a silky texture and fine, natural-looking finish on skin. It isn't the best for keeping skin matte, but is suitable for all skin types, provided you have a light skin tone, too.

BLUSH AND BRONZER: ☺ **Contouring Blush & Bronzing Powder** *($3)*. Housed in one compact is a pressed-powder blush and pressed bronzing powder. Both products leave a shiny finish and share the same talc-based formula. The colors look best when blended together using the golden brown bronzer first and the peachy-pink blush next. The bronzing powder is suitable for contouring light to medium skin tones, but generally speaking, it isn't a great idea to contour with a shiny powder (you want contour to be subtle). The shiny finish affords a shimmer that lasts and sparkling particles that have a slight tendency to flake.

☺ **Bronzer** *($3)* is a mica- and talc-based pressed bronzing powder that includes four squares of color (without dividers) in one compact. Swirled together with a brush, the colors come off as one uniform bronze shade. All three of the Bronzers are recommended, though this isn't rated a Paula's Pick due to its drier-than-usual texture. It finishes matte, which is unusual for bronzing powders.

EYESHADOW: ☺ **Shimmering Palette (aka Shimmer Palette)** *($3)* includes four shades of pastel cream-to-powder eyeshadows in one compact. These have a unique texture that begins creamy and slick but sets to a noticeably dry powder finish replete with shine. The pastel tones go on so softly you're left with a lot of shine, though the finish does keep it on skin quite well; if only the highlighting effect wasn't so obvious.

☹ **Eye Transformer** *($3)* is nothing more than a quad set of pastel-tinged shiny eyeshadows. Each has a dry texture that flakes during application and none of the shades are that attractive whether worn alone, mixed together, or applied to "transform" other shades of eyeshadow. No matter how you slice it, this isn't a transformation for the better!

☹ **Eye Primer & Liner Sealer** *($3)* includes an oil-based eye primer on one end and a water-based liquid on the other. The flesh-toned eye primer winds up like a lipstick and has a thick, creamy texture that covers poorly. Its oil base doesn't improve eyeshadow application or wearability, and it looks obvious on skin. The Liner Sealer takes too long to dry and ends up removing a portion of whatever you've used to line your eyes … and this is supposed to be helpful?

EYE AND BROW SHAPER: ☺ **Eyebrow Treat & Tame** *($3)* is a dual-sided product that offers a tinted brow gel (labeled as "Tame") on one end and a clear, brush-on, "regrowth treatment" on the other. The sheer brow gel works great and comes in three very good colors for dark blonde to medium brown brows. The brush-on clear gel doesn't contain anything capable of stimulating hair growth, so ignore that claim. It functions best as a brush-on setting gel for unruly brows, and it has a non-sticky finish. Definitely one of the better products from E.L.F. Studio.

☺ **Eyebrow Kit** *($3)* features a pressed brow powder and creamy brow tint in one compact. The brow powder is silky and works well to fill in and define brows with soft color. The creamy brow tint, which is incorrectly labeled as a gel, is oil-based and imparts soft color that goes on sheer. The sheerness is good because the brow tint's hue is considerably darker than the brow powder. Used together, this is a smart way to enhance brows and help keep stray hairs in place. The limited shades are best for light to medium brown eyebrows.

☺ **Eyeliner & Shadow Stick** *($3)* is a dual-sided automatic pencil that provides a twist-up cream shadow stick on one end and an eyeliner pencil on the other. Both sides are retractable and both formulas are wax-based, so they don't have the greatest textures around, but what are you expecting for a few dollars? As it turns out, the ultra-shiny, sparkling Shadow Stick isn't easy to blend and imparts way too much shine for daytime wear. The Eyeliner has a nice glide to it but it is also shiny, this time leaving a metallic finish that works against the sparkling finish of the Shadow Stick. This is merely an OK product for those looking to try a cream shadow with a decent pencil liner.

☹ **Eyebrow Lifter & Filler** *($3)* is a dual-sided, slightly chunky pencil that includes a brow pencil on one end and a creamy highlighter on the other. The pinky peach color and thick texture of the highlighter are wholly unattractive and the product tends to sit on top of skin, looking very artificial. The brow pencil isn't terrible, but it has a soft, creamy texture that isn't preferred to brow pencils that have a smooth, dry texture and powder finish.

LIPSTICK, LIP GLOSS, AND LIPLINER: ☺ **Lip Liner & Blending Brush** *($3)* includes just what the name states, housed in a dual-ended pencil cartridge. The Lip Liner is a wind-up, retractable pencil with a creamy texture and easy application. The Blending Brush is flexible, nicely tapered, and works well should you wish to soften the result from the Lip Liner. Only one shade is offered, but it's one many women will find quite wearable.

☺ **Lip Definer & Shaper** *($3)* is a dual-sided pencil with one end being a lipliner and the other being a pale peach highlighter to emphasize the cupid's bow of the lips. The lipliner is very creamy and tends to bleed outside the lip line and fade quickly. Also, the color is a drab mauve-brown that gives lips a deadened look. The highlighter is quite shiny but has a much better texture and finish than the liner. Still, only half of this duo is good and both ends need routine sharpening.

MASCARA: ☺ **Lengthening & Volumizing Mascara** *($3)*. Fuller, thicker lashes are something this mascara is incapable of providing. It goes on evenly but very thin, so at best you'll get modest length without clumps or smearing. It wears well and is easy to remove, but contains two preservatives (methylisothiazolinone and methylchloroisothiazolinone), which are not recommended for use in leave-on products due to their irritation potential.

☺ **Waterproof Lengthening & Volumizing Mascara** *($3)* builds modest length and hints at some thickness, but never progresses beyond average regardless of how many coats are applied. The formula is waterproof and removes easily with a water-soluble cleanser. It also wears well without flaking, and is an OK option if you're not one for much lash impact.

BRUSHES: ✓☺ **11 Piece Studio Brush Collection** *($30)* includes every brush E.L.F. Studio offers. All of the brushes in this set are also sold separately for $3 each, so with the kit's 11 brushes you're essentially getting the carrying case plus one brush for free. The zippered case is made of a soft synthetic fabric that has room for every brush in the set. As for the brushes themselves, they are each made of synthetic Taklon hair and are surprisingly good considering their low cost. Each one is exquisitely soft and well made, with sleek handles that feel great. It's really hard to believe such quality brushes are so darn cheap! The best brushes in the set (and again, all of the brushes are sold individually) are the Complexion Brush, Small Smudge Brush, Concealer Brush (though I prefer one with a more pointed tip), Small Precision Brush (great for lining the eyes when a smoky eye design is being done), and the Small Angled Brush (which works great for brows or eyelining). Fans of applying foundation with a brush should check out the Angled Foundation Brush. The Contour Brush isn't the best and the Powder Brush is cut straight across, which isn't the easiest way to dust on loose or pressed powder (this type of cut makes it easy to over-powder).

☺ **Blush Brush** *($3)*. For the money, this synthetic hair blush brush is more than respectable. It has a good shape and is extremely soft plus it picks up and holds color well. Ideally, it should be denser and the hairs should be a bit longer to cover the full cheek area (someone with large cheeks or a full face will find this brush way too small). However, if the size and cut works for you, the price cannot be beat.

☺ **Eyelash Curler** *($3)*. Whether you need a mini eyelash curler to handle the corner lashes or a regular sized one to take on a full row of eyelashes, these metal curlers with a rubber strip work as well as any to make lashes look uplifted and fringed. These curlers aren't of the same craftsmanship as those from, say, Shu Uemura, but they cost a lot less.

☺ **Kabuki Brushes** *($5-$8)*. E.L.F. Studio offers a Face Kabuki Brush and a Body Kabuki Brush. Both are composed of synthetic Taklon fiber and feel wonderfully soft. They're not as dense as many other Kabuki brushes I've seen, but they're shaped well and do a good job of applying loose or pressed powder in even, sheer layers. I don't buy the antibacterial claims made for these brushes, so these should be washed every few months or so depending on frequency of use. At the very least, you need to remove the facial oils that can build up on brushes over time.

☺ **Makeup Artist Brush Belt** *($15)* is a brush carrying case composed of a soft synthetic leather that's flexible enough to wrap around your waist. That's exactly how it's meant to be used, and it comes equipped with adjustable straps so you can secure this to your waist area while doing your own or someone else's makeup. It can hold over a dozen brushes of various sizes, and is a great buy for those who have need for this type of product.

FACE AND BODY SHIMMER/ILLUMINATING PRODUCTS: ☺ **Complexion Perfection** *($3)* is a mica-based shiny pressed powder that includes four sheer, pastel shades in one compact. The shine is moderate but this has a dry texture and, as such, the results don't last long, not to mention the pastel finish is trickier to work with.

SPECIALTY PRODUCTS: ☺ **Mini Makeup Collection** *($15)*. If you love E.L.F.'s Studio makeup, this kit is right up your alley. You get nine shades of eyeshadow, one cream eyeshadow, blush, bronzer, brow powder, mini eye pencil, mini applicators, and lots of lip gloss in one small, square plastic box. The cream eyeshadow is mostly useless because it deposits almost no color, but the powder eyeshadows, each quite shiny, are smooth with the medium to dark shades having a good color deposit. There are two green shades that are best avoided. The eye pencil and mini applicators are a joke, but the brow powder, powder blush, and bronzing powder are fine (though the blush and bronzer are shiny). Not everything in this kit is brilliant, but it remains a good value overall, assuming you have full-sized brushes already!

☹ **Lip Primer & Plumper** *($3)*. Half of this dual-sided product is an oil-based cream concealer for lips and the other half is a clear lip balm. The concealer portion (labeled "primer") is supposed to function as a lip base for your lipstick to keep color from smudging. It doesn't do that. Instead, it places a thick, opaque layer over lips that interferes with lipstick application and doesn't keep it in place. The lip balm doesn't list any plumping ingredients, but smells strongly of cinnamon, which will plump lips via strong irritation. This is one to leave on the shelf!

E.L.F. SUGAR KISS MAKEUP

EYESHADOW: ☹ **Sparkle Eye Duo** *($2)*. This powder eyeshadow duo is clearly designed for kids or pre-teens who find the cutesy packaging and bright colors appealing. It isn't a great introduction to makeup because the creamy-feeling powder tends to fade quickly and it creases a bit, and did I mention the colors?

LIPSTICK, LIP GLOSS, AND LIPLINER: ☺ **Heart Lip Tint** *($1)* is housed in a compact and must be applied with a fingertip (not the most sanitary option) or a lip brush. It feels moist yet light and offers a soft cream finish. The Light Purple shade actually goes on fuchsia. This offers light coverage and isn't nearly as slick as many lip glosses.

☺ **Perfect Glossy Gift** *($4)* contains four tubes of lip gloss for a value price. The gloss has a rich, creamy texture that feels smooth and slick. It imparts sheer color and a shimmer or sparkling finish depending on the shade. The only drawback is that the tubes do not have any sort of applicator, so you have to squeeze the gloss out and then dab on lips with your finger or a brush. That makes these glosses an inconvenient option for on-the-go use.

☺ **Super Glossy Lip Shiner** *($2)* is packaged in a squeeze tube and you get two shades in each package, so that works out to be one dollar per tube of gloss. Is this a true beauty bargain? Yes, provided you want sheer colors infused with lots of sparkles that cling to lips long after the glossy feel and finish have worn away. You also have to accept a sweet, candy-like fragrance, but if these issues are non-issues for you, go for it!

☺ **Glitter Lip Glaze** *($2)* is a very standard, smooth lip gloss whose candy-scented shades impart almost no color but leave behind a glossy, glittery sheen. Kids and pre-teens will love it; adults will wonder why they bothered.

☺ **Hyper Shiny Lip Gloss** *($1)*. Almost all of the glosses from E.L.F.'s Sugar Kiss line are nearly identical, and this one is no exception. It's a sheer, candy-scented gloss that imparts minimal color but lots of glittery shine. It isn't sticky, but the glittery begins to feel grainy shortly after application. I suppose it's handy that this is packaged in a click-pen applicator with a built-in brush, but so are many other glosses that best this, though they do cost more.

☺ **Lip Color Trio** *($2)*. Housed in one compact with a brush that sheds immediately are three sheer, greasy lip glosses. They smell artificially fruity and impart a glossy finish that's not sticky, but that's about it. Adults will likely find the scent and packaging too cloying for their taste.

☺ **Lip Gloss Tin** *($1)* is a sheer red gloss that's flavored like cherry candy, which will only encourage youngsters who try this to lick their lips, ingesting the gloss in the process. You also have to apply this stuff with your fingers, unless you're willing to carry a lip brush with you.

☺ **Lip Liner Pencils** *($1)*. This set of lip pencils is the cheapest option around for lining your lips! You get two pencils that require routine sharpening, but who cares at this price (and E.L.F. includes a sharpener)? The pencils apply easily but are too creamy to keep lipstick from bleeding into lines around the mouth. If that's not an issue for you and you're not expecting hours of worry-free wear, check this out.

MASCARA: ☺ **Daring Mascara Duo** *($2)* gets you two mascaras (it's a dual-sided product) for an insanely low price. I wish this was the value mascara champ of all time, but its performance is no better than average and it can make lashes feel stiff, sort of like what styling gel does on your hair. It doesn't thicken lashes at all and is best for natural definition.

BRUSHES: ☺ **Eye Shadow Brush Set** *($2)*. One of the three brushes in this inexpensive (OK, it's downright cheap) brush set is great, while the other two are unnecessary. The superfluous brushes include a pointed smudger and a standard sponge-tip applicator, which doesn't apply powder shadow nearly as well as a brush. The smudger tool has its uses, but in this case, the rubber tip tends to drag over skin.

E.L.F. MAKEUP

MAKEUP REMOVER: ☺ **Eye Makeup Remover Pads** *($1)* offer a very gentle, fragrance-free formula infused onto small round pads. They produce a slight lather and should be rinsed from the skin (or used before cleansing), but they work well to remove non-waterproof makeup.

FOUNDATION: ☺ **Shielding Hydrotint SPF 15** *($1)* does not list active sunscreen ingredients on the carton or product itself, so this cannot be relied on for sun protection. It has a strong fragrance and a sheer texture that gives minimal coverage, providing a satin matte finish that is best for those with normal to dry skin. Among the four shades, only Tone 3 should be avoided. However, this product is not recommended for its sunscreen.

CONCEALER: ☹ **All Over Cover Stick** *($1)* is a very tiny stick foundation with an unattractively thick, greasy texture that blends decently but still looks heavy on skin (sort of like theatrical greasepaint). The waxlike thickening agents put acne-prone skin on the fast track for more blemishes, and two of the three shades are very peach. It does not contain a single "active natural" ingredient, and is in no way preferred to any other stick foundation.

☹ **Tone Correcting Concealer** *($1)* has a silky, moist texture that never sets, so this liquid concealer is prone to fading and creasing. That's not good news, especially when combined with its spotty coverage and three fairly peach colors.

POWDER: ☺ **Clarifying Pressed Powder** *($1)* claims to help treat and prevent breakouts, but it contains absolutely nothing that is capable of doing that. This is a very good, talc-based pressed powder with enough mineral oil and petrolatum to create a satin-smooth texture that's best for normal to dry skin. It applies sheer, all four colors are great, and it leaves a satin matte finish that doesn't look the least bit powdery. The Tone 3 and Tone 4 shades function as bronzing powders for light to medium skin tones.

BLUSH AND BRONZER: ☺ **Custom Face** *($1)* is a group of smooth-textured powder colors meant for use anywhere on the face. However, the small shade range makes it ideally suited for use as a blush. Dusting pink, peach, or rose tones all over your face would look odd, and only one of these shades (Bronzed) is appropriate as eyeshadow. All of them have some amount of shine, with Coy being almost matte. The color saturation is stronger than that of the Custom Eyes or Custom Lips products, but it can be applied sheer.

☺ **Natural Radiance Blusher** *($1)* is a pressed-powder blush with a smooth, slightly thick texture that applies evenly and imparts sheer color with a soft glow for a soft shine finish. The pigmentation of the shades is best for fair to medium skin tones; layering produces a slightly greater color payoff.

☺ **All Over Color Stick** *($1)* is a tiny, twist-up color stick meant for use anywhere on the face. The sheer, shimmer-infused colors are best for highlighting features, such as the brow bone or top of the cheekbone, and the fragrance-free formula is best for normal to dry skin. This product is not emollient enough to use on your lips (nor are the colors well-suited for lips) and applying it to your eyelid or crease area guarantees creasing due to the moist finish.

☺ **Healthy Glow Bronzing Powder** *($1)* is a talc-based pressed bronzing powder with an initially smooth texture that can apply unevenly because it tends to grab onto your skin. Its dry finish (enhanced by clay) also makes it difficult to blend. The Sunkissed shade is a rosy bronze tone with shimmer that can work for light to medium skin tones, while Warm Tan is more versatile. The Luminance shade isn't bronze-toned at all, and is best for highlighting with a shimmer finish, assuming you have the patience to deal with this product's application and blending issues.

EYESHADOW: ☺ **Brightening Eye Color** *($1)* presents a selection of eyeshadow quads packaged with sponge-tip applicators, which should be tossed out. These quads are an amazing value for the money, especially if you prefer sheer colors and don't mind shine (every quad has some amount of shine, but none are outright glittery). They have a reasonably smooth texture and apply evenly, and every set has at least one shade that can serve as powder eyeliner. The best sets include Matte Mauve (it's almost matte), Butternut, Drama, and Nouveau (the olive-green shade in this one goes on khaki and blends well with the other colors). You can find eyeshadows that last longer and have a texture that's more elegant, but you'll pay a lot more for the privilege.

☺ **Custom Eyes** *($1)* are powder eyeshadows sold singly so that you can customize a quad set of your own. The compact holds four colors, and it can also hold the Custom Lips and Custom Face shades. These eyeshadows have a different formula than the Brightening Eye Color. They're powder-free and based on oil and waxes, which result in a smooth, creamy-feeling texture that applies like a powder, but unfortunately are also prone to creasing and fading, especially if your eyelids are oily. These are still worth testing because they blend well and go on sheer. The best shades (all with some amount of shine) are Pink Ice, Wisteria, Mocha, Ivory, Dusk, and Moondust.

EYE AND BROW SHAPER: ☺ **Brightening Eye Liner** *($1)* is a basic, creamy eye pencil that needs routine sharpening. It applies smoothly and remains creamy enough to smudge slightly, so it's best for smoky eye designs where you intend to soften the line rather than keep it solid. Classic shades are available; the Gilded shade has a metallic shine.

☺ **Eye Widener** *($1)* is a creamy, standard pencil with a sharpener built into the cap. You're instructed to stroke the pencil along the upper lash line and on the inside rim of the lower lash line to create the illusion of larger eyes. This is a theatrical makeup technique that tends to look obvious in person (and in daylight), not to mention the risk of putting a cosmetic product so close to the eye itself. This is an OK option as a soft white shimmer pencil for the upper lash line.

LIPSTICK, LIP GLOSS, AND LIPLINER: ✓☺ **Super Glossy Lip Shine SPF 15** *($1)* wins as the best product from E.L.F. because nowhere else will you find a supremely smooth, non-sticky lip gloss with gorgeous sheer colors and excellent sun protection courtesy of its in-part titanium dioxide sunscreen. Pink Kiss, Candlelight, Goddess, and Mauve Luxe have a soft metallic finish, while Angel is a colorless shade with flecks of glitter (definitely not a sophisticated look). The remaining colors have a soft shimmer and all of them have a fruity scent and taste. At this price, why not buy all the shades?

☺ **Custom Lips** *($1)* are pans of lip color that you add to a compact. You can add up to four shades, or you can mix and match with E.L.F.'s Custom Eyes and Custom Face shades. These have a thick texture with a slight slip and minimally emollient finish. Every color, even the deep reds and plums, applies very sheer. The only issue with this product is that it requires finger application, unless you're willing to tote a lip brush.

☺ **Hypershine Lip Gloss** *($1)* has a combination of thickness and slickness that's unusual, but it applies smoothly and leaves a non-sticky, moderately (not hyper) glossy finish. The click pen with brush applicator works well and, though this gloss offers only a small selection of shades, they go on nearly transparent, making these a safe bet to apply over any color of lipstick.

☺ **Hypershine Mini Cell Phone Lip Gloss Charms** *($5)* are sold as mini versions of the Hypershine Lip Gloss. They have a different formula that's more emollient but not glossier. The set presents eight glosses with an overcap that can be attached to any shade, so it can be worn as a charm (or added to a key ring). This is primarily a teen-appeal product, but is an option for adults who want a tiny gloss to tuck into an evening bag.

☺ **Luscious Liquid Lipstick** *($1)* is a standard, slightly thick lip gloss housed in a click-pen applicator that includes a built-in synthetic brush. The mineral oil–based formula feels smooth and has a strong vanilla/mint fragrance though it doesn't make lips tingle, which is good. The mostly sheer colors are fine.

☺ **Therapeutic Conditioning Lip Balm** *($1)* is an emollient, oil-based stick lip balm that comes in assorted fruit flavors. It's very basic and doesn't impart much gloss, and the fruity element of each shade can be cloying.

☺ **Feather Proof Moisturizing Lip Liner** *($1)* has a formula that's way too greasy to prevent feathering, and it needs routine sharpening. This is an OK lip pencil that comes in a mostly pink-tinged range of shades, but spending a bit more at the drugstore will open the door to several superior lip pencils.

☹ **Plumping Lip Glaze** *($1)* is a waxy-feeling, dual-sided lip gloss that contains a lot of menthol, which plumps lips by virtue of irritation but ends up being too irritating for frequent use (and touch-ups with this very sheer gloss would definitely be frequent).

MASCARA: ✓ ☺ **Wet Gloss Lash & Brow Clear Mascara** *($1)* houses the same clear gel formula in a dual-sided, dual-brush component. One end is for eyebrows (and the brush is suitable for brow application) and the other for lashes (with an equally suitable brush). The gel applies smoothly, is non-sticky, and does a great job of grooming brows or providing slight lash enhancement while leaving a subtle glossy finish. All this for $1? Sold!

☺ **Earth & Water Mascara Duo** *($1)* has a New Age-y name that doesn't really explain the fact that this is a dual-sided mascara. One side is regular mascara, the other is waterproof. The regular mascara is surpassingly good, allowing quick and dramatic lengthening of lashes with minimal clumps and delivering a long-lasting finish. In contrast, the waterproof version (which has the same brush as the regular mascara) goes on thin, doesn't build much length, doesn't thicken, and is only mildly waterproof. Although not equally impressive, for the price, even half of this mascara is a beauty steal.

BRUSHES: ☺ **E.L.F. Brushes** *($1)*. All of E.L.F.'s brushes are sold individually. As you may have expected, the quality isn't top of the line. What's missing from many of them is soft, dense hair that allows precision application of color and expert blending. Still, some of these are surprisingly good for the money (they beat any pre-assembled brush set from major drugstore lines). The ones to consider are the Eyelash and Brow Wand, Brow Comb and Brush, Defining Eye Brush (best for shadow, not for applying powder eyeliner), and the synthetic Eyeliner Brush.

☺ **Mechanical Eyelash Curler** *($1)* is so named because the handle is spring-loaded and must be kept together with the included plastic clasp. This is a standard, workable eyelash curler and is worth a try, but only if your lashes don't curl well on their own from use of an outstanding mascara. Still, this costs next to nothing and can be nice to have around if you ever decide to try a lash curler.

☹ **Professional 5-Piece Brush Collection** *($10)* includes basic brushes for powder, blush, and eyeshadow, but none of them are good enough to make this your primary brush set, even though the price is right.

☺ **Professional 9-Piece Master Set** *($15)* includes the Total Face Brush, Blushing/Bronzing/Blending Brush, Foundation Brush, Defining Eye Brush, Blending Eye Brush, Smudge Eye Sponge, Eyelash/Brow Wand, Brow Comb/Brush, and Lip Defining Brush, all packaged in a deluxe roll-up case. A couple of the tools are great, but the rest are average to poor, making this a sketchy set to consider.

☺ **Professional Complete Set** *($9)* includes nine brushes that cover all the basics from powder to lashes and eyelining options, all packaged in a tri-fold case. Most of the brushes are below average and no match for pricier options, but this can work if you need a second set for casual makeup.

FACE AND BODY SHIMMER/ILLUMINATING PRODUCTS: ☺ **Shimmering Facial Whip** *($1)* comes in a tiny tube and dispenses as a lotion that tends to drag a bit during application. It sets to a slightly moist finish that imparts gleaming shimmer that's too strong for daytime unless blended very well. Most of the sheer shades are best for the cheeks or for highlighting lips; Toasted and Citrus are good options for eyeshadow, but be sure to set this with a powder eyeshadow to avoid creasing.

SPECIALTY PRODUCTS: ✓ ☺ **Shine Eraser** *($1)* is the best value around for oil-blotting papers. These powder-free sheets work quickly to mop up excess shine before touching up with powder. They are supposedly infused with green tea extract, which the company says will retexture skin to mask facial imperfections, but, of course, this does no such thing.

☺ **Natural Lash Kit/Dramatic Lash Kit** *($1)* is a good, inexpensive way to experiment with false eyelashes. Both kits present a full set and include a tiny tube of adhesive, which is convenient. The kits are aptly named based on the results they provide, although getting false eyelashes to look natural isn't an easy feat.

ELIZABETH ARDEN

ELIZABETH ARDEN AT-A-GLANCE

Strengths: Moderately priced; some excellent serums (including the ceramide capsules) and moisturizers; good cleansers for normal to dry skin; good makeup remover; good concealer, pressed powder, eyeshadow, and lipsticks.

Weaknesses: No products for those battling blemishes; no skin-lightening products; no AHA or BHA products or topical scrubs; several products whose sunscreen lacks sufficient UVA protection; none of the foundations with sunscreen provide sufficient UVA protection; lackluster eye and brow pencils; some problematic lip color products; mediocre brushes; jar packaging.

For more information about Elizabeth Arden, call (800) 326-7337 or visit www.elizabetharden.com or www.Beautypedia.com.

ELIZABETH ARDEN SKIN CARE

ELIZABETH ARDEN CERAMIDE PRODUCTS

☹ **$$$ Ceramide Purifying Cream Cleanser** *($27 for 4.2 ounces)* is a basic, water- and mineral oil–based cleansing lotion that contains barely any ceramides. The tiny amount of sandalwood oil isn't great for skin or for use in the eye area, but is not likely a cause for concern. This will require a washcloth for complete removal and is suitable for normal to dry skin.

☹ **Ceramide Purifying Toner** *($27 for 6.7 ounces)* lists alcohol as the second ingredient and also contains some potentially irritating plant extracts, all of which undermine the effectiveness of the ceramides and other skin-identical ingredients in this misguided toner.

✓ ☺ **$$$ Ceramide Advanced Time Complex Capsules Intensive Treatment for Face and Throat** *($65 for 60 capsules)* have been a hallmark of Arden's Ceramide line for years, and they remain a good choice if you're looking for a silky, silicone-based serum that contains some beneficial ingredients for normal to dry skin types not prone to breakouts. The silicone is joined by emollients, lipids, ceramides, plant oil, and antioxidant vitamins, all packaged to ensure potency before use. The drawback to these capsules is that you must use all the contents each time, because leaving them open is not only potentially messy, but also will allow these antioxidants to quickly degrade.

☹ **Ceramide EyeWish Eye Cream SPF 10** *($45 for 0.5 ounce)* not only has an SPF rating that's too low for daytime protection, but also leaves skin vulnerable to UVA damage. UVA rays cause wrinkles, so this product's shortage of protection in that regard isn't what's needed to keep eye-area wrinkles at bay.

☺ **$$$ Ceramide Gold Ultra Lift and Strengthening Eye Capsules** *($52 for 60 capsules)* is a silicone-based serum packaged in capsules that are housed in a jar container (the jar packaging is irrelevant here). The capsules contain many impressive ingredients, including ceramides, several antioxidants, and cell-communicating ingredients. All of these can help improve skin cell production, but none are capable of lifting skin that has begun to sag. One problem in an otherwise exemplary formula is the amount of witch hazel extract. This is not a great ingredient for skin, especially around the eyes, and unfortunately, there is more of it in these capsules than there is of the aforementioned beneficial ingredients. Still, the extract form of witch hazel isn't as bad as the distillate or pure form—but it's enough to keep this product from earning a Paula's Pick rating.

✓ ☺ **$$$ Ceramide Gold Ultra Restorative Capsules** *($68 for 0.95 ounce)* are an interesting way to provide normal to very dry skin with a short but very effective roster of ingredients that can restore a healthy skin-barrier function, all while supplying elements that skin needs to look and feel its best. Cell-communicating ingredients and skin-restoring ceramides join two forms of antioxidant vitamin A as well as some vitamin E. As claimed, these capsules are fragrance- and preservative-free. They are definitely a consideration for those dealing with eczema or rosacea (assuming your rosacea-prone skin is not also oily).

☹ **$$$ Ceramide Moisture Network Night Cream** *($59 for 1.7 ounces)* takes the "everything but the kitchen sink" concept, and, well, includes the sink! With over 90 ingredients, this moisturizer doesn't leave any stone unturned when it comes to providing dry skin with emollients, oils, skin-identical ingredients, antioxidants, ceramides, plant extracts, and even a few anti-irritants. But is that better for skin? It definitely isn't from the standpoint of allergic reactions, because it stands to reason that the more ingredients a product contains, the greater the likelihood that your skin will react to one or more of them. The other downside to packing so many ingredients into a moisturizer is that, aside from the ingredients that create the product's texture and finish, you're only getting tiny amounts of them (the ingredients can only add up to a 100% total content). It is unknown whether tiny amounts of several ingredients (such as antioxidants or anti-irritants) are better for skin than larger amounts of just a few. And even the antioxidants in this moisturizer are subject to quick deterioration due to jar packaging. This Arden product isn't without its flaws because it does contain balm mint extract and some fragrant components (linalool, hexyl cinnamal), which can spell trouble for skin, but the amounts used are likely too small to be cause for concern.

☹ **Ceramide Plump Perfect Eye Moisture Cream SPF 15** *($48 for 0.5 ounce)* lacks the UVA-protecting ingredients of avobenzone, titanium dioxide, zinc oxide, Tinosorb, or Mexoryl SX, and is not recommended. None of the ingredients in this eye cream can combat puffiness. If anything, applying the synthetic sunscreen agents in this product too close to the eyes can cause puffiness (and irritation).

☹ **$$$ Ceramide Plump Perfect Moisture Cream SPF 30** *($65 for 1.7 ounces)* doesn't disappoint with its in-part avobenzone sunscreen and SPF rating, but for the money the base formulation is disappointing. It contains mostly water, slip agent, emollient, silicones, glycerin, and preservative—not a bad ordinary roster for taking care of normal to dry skin and offering great sun protection. But considering the price tag, the exciting state-of-the-art ingredients (ceramides, antioxidants, anti-irritant plant extracts, and skin-identical ingredients) should be present in more than just a dusting. This is still a good option for a daytime moisturizer for normal to dry skin, but it's not as enticing as other options with stable packaging and a larger amount of skin-beneficial substances.

☺ **$$$ Ceramide Plump Perfect Targeted Line Concentrate** *($65 for 0.5 ounce)* has a lot of wonderful things going for it, including a supremely silky texture and nearly weightless finish suitable for all skin types. The pump-dispensed serum is packed with antioxidants and ingredients that mimic the structure and function of healthy skin, as well as lesser amounts of a couple of cell-communicating ingredients. The only drawback keeping it from earning a Paula's Pick is the volatile fragrance components, which can be irritating. Their presence is minimal, but they ding this product relative to similarly well-formulated serums from Estee Lauder, Olay, and Clinique.

☹ **$$$ Ceramide Time Complex Moisture Cream** *($52 for 1.7 ounces)* should have better packaging to keep its antioxidants stable. There are several state-of-the-art ingredients in this product, but with sodium chloride (salt) as the fourth ingredient, they won't impact skin in the manner they should.

☹ **Ceramide Time Complex Moisture Cream SPF 15** *($52 for 1.7 ounces)* lacks the UVA-protecting ingredients of titanium dioxide, zinc oxide, avobenzone, Tinosorb, or Mexoryl SX, and is not recommended.

☺ **$$$ Ceramide Plump Perfect Firming Facial Mask** *($58 for 4 masks)* consists of cloth masks steeped in a moisturizing solution that includes lightweight hydrating agents, several ceramides, a peptide, cell-communicating ingredients, stabilizers, and preservatives. Although this fragrance-free product has some impressive attributes, you're not getting much for your money considering that only four single-use masks are included.

☹ **Ceramide Plump Perfect Lip Moisture Cream SPF 30** *($27.50 for 0.5 ounce)* has a lot going for it, starting with an effective, in-part avobenzone sunscreen in an emollient base that includes ceramides and shea butter, and packaging that keeps light- and air-sensitive ingredients stable. In order to plump up your lips, though, peppermint, balm mint, and menthol were added, even though they merely cause irritation and do not make lips perfect, just chapped, dry, and inflamed. What a shame, because this is otherwise a great sunscreen option for lips.

☹ **$$$ Ceramide Plump Perfect Firming Body Souffle** *($49.50 for 6.8 ounces)*. There is nothing in here that can firm skin. Claims aside, Arden has quite an intriguing body moisturizer on its hands, with too many problems for skin, which is so frustrating given how promising a product this could have been. The crux of the formula is the glycerin and shea butter, but it's odd to see cornstarch so high on the ingredient list. (Likely it's used as a thickening agent, but its absorbent nature negates some of the moisture you'd get from the ingredients listed before it.) It is also enriched with several skin-identical ingredients (chiefly ceramides) and many antioxidants, which is wonderful. Where this derails is with jar packaging and the inclusion of several fragrance chemicals known to cause irritation. For the money, you should expect airtight, or at least opaque, packaging and the absence of ingredients that put skin at risk of irritation without imparting a benefit (pleasing your nose with scent or aroma is rarely good for your skin). Regrettably, the beneficial ingredients are wasted due to the jar packaging.

ELIZABETH ARDEN INTERVENE PRODUCTS

☺ **INTERVENE 3-in-1 Daily Cleanser Exfoliator Primer** *($21.50 for 5 ounces)*. This copiously foaming cleanser does a much better job of cleansing skin than exfoliating it. The scrub particles are polyethylene beads, but their presence in this product isn't as prominent as in many other (less expensive) cleanser/scrub options available at the drugstore. Consider this a good cleanser for normal to oily skin. It's capable of removing makeup, but the scrub particles aren't for use over the eye area.

☺ **$$$ INTERVENE Eye Pause & Effect Moisture Eye Cream** *($42 for 0.5 ounce)* has an unbelievably silky texture that's laced with several beneficial antioxidant ingredients for skin around the eyes or elsewhere. That's why it's so disappointing that jar packaging was chosen; it won't help keep these ingredients stable during use, and that makes this just another moisturizer for normal to slightly dry skin whose best attributes are compromised. Arden's claim that this eye cream will delay future signs of aging (with continued use, of course) is inaccurate. The only product that can legitimately make that boast is a sunscreen, which this cream lacks.

☺ **$$$ INTERVENE Pause & Effect Moisture Cream SPF 15** *($55 for 1.7 ounces)* deserves credit only for its innovative name and its in-part avobenzone sunscreen. The Intervene portion of the name is meant to describe how it can interrupt the aging process and the wrinkles associated with that process. Arden goes beyond basic antiaging claims and states that this product also "helps minimize imbalances in the look of skin caused by fluctuating hormonal and protein levels." Arden doesn't explain what these imbalances are or how this product corrects these problems, so it may be as simple as addressing the dryness that can accompany postmenopausal skin, benefits that aren't specific to this product but rather are common to all moisturizers. Although this is an effective sunscreen in a lightweight moisturizing cream base, it contains a fair amount of narcissus bulb, which may cause contact dermatitis, while having no established benefit for skin. Red clover is present to minimize skin symptoms of menopause, but its benefit when applied topically has not been proven (Sources: www.naturaldatabase.com; and *Contact Dermatitis*, August 1997, pages 70-77). Although some worthwhile ingredients appear farther down on the ingredient list, many of them will be compromised by this product's jar packaging. In the end, this is a costly sunscreen, not a wrinkle intervention.

☺ **$$$ INTERVENE Pause & Effect Moisture Lotion SPF 15** *($55 for 1.7 ounces)* is similar to the Intervene Pause & Effect Moisture Cream SPF 15, and also includes an in-part avobenzone sunscreen. The primary differences are in texture (with this one being a thin but substantial lotion) and packaging (with this product featuring an opaque bottle that will keep its antioxidants stable). Although the latter feature is positive, the presence of problematic narcissus bulb is too great to ignore, and makes this an iffy proposition for skin, even though the sunscreen portion is right-on.

☺ **$$$ INTERVENE Stress Recovery Night Cream** *($49.50 for 1.7 ounces)*. Lots of products are sold with the promise of revitalizing skin while you sleep, and here's one more to add to this overcrowded category. For the most part, this is a relatively unimpressive moisturizer. It has the requisite silky texture and some mica that adds a soft shine to your skin, but it's disappointing that several state-of-the-art ingredients will have their potency muted due to jar packaging. An intriguing ingredient in this product is Teprenone, which is described as an active ingredient whose multiple functions include limiting skin-cell senescence (cell death). As it turns out, this ingredient is a drug that Arden appears to be using off-label (meaning it is really a pharmaceutical), which my research indicates is against FDA regulations. Teprenone is the brand name for a drug known as geranylgeranylacetone, which is used to treat gastric ulcers and is being researched as an option for slowing age-related hearing loss (Sources: *Brain Research*, May 2008, pages 9-17; and *Digestion*, October 2007, pages 215-224). What do hearing loss and ulcers have to do with aging skin? One of the key ways geranylgeranylacetone works is by influencing heat shock proteins. These proteins help other proteins interact as they should at the cellular level, which affects many systems in the body. Heat shock proteins are most active during times of stress, such as exposure to cigarette smoke and exposure to sunlight. When heat shock proteins are reduced (which is ultimately what you want because that means reducing inflammation), cells appear to live longer. I suppose Arden theorized that geranylgeranylacetone (as Teprenone) may also have a helpful effect when applied topically. After all, the skin is a source of heat shock proteins, and it is certainly exposed to enough stressful situations that an ingredient to help these proteins function more efficiently would be a benefit. However, there's no research proving that topically applied geranylgeranylacetone has any effect on heat shock proteins within skin. Moreover, as previously mentioned, Arden is using a drug ingredient in a cosmetic product, which means the consumer is the guinea pig. For that reason, Intervene Stress Recovery Night Cream is not a product I can recommend, though the formula doesn't deserve an unhappy face rating.

☺ **$$$ INTERVENE Timefighting Radiance Serum** *($49.50 for 1 ounce)*. With only a few missteps, this water-based serum is a very good option for normal to slightly dry skin. It's no more concentrated than several other well-formulated serums, so ignore that attempt to make Intervene seem as though it's the only answer for your aging skin. However, it's a worthwhile serum that can help smooth the appearance of lines and encourage a healthy barrier function, although reversing the hands of time is not in its bag of tricks. The downsides to this serum are a couple of potentially irritating plant extracts (clover and narcissus) along with some fragrance chemicals that can be troublesome for all skin types, especially sensitive skin or skin affected by rosacea. Their inclusion isn't a deal-breaker for this serum, but they do keep it from earning a Paula's Pick rating.

ELIZABETH ARDEN MILLENIUM PRODUCTS

☹ **Millenium Revitalizing Tonic** *($28 for 5 ounces)* is an antiquated toner formula, and is nothing short of an assault on skin thanks to the amount of alcohol it contains. Menthol is on hand to promote further irritation, and truly beneficial ingredients are barely present. This is not recommended.

☺ **$$$ Millenium Day Renewal Emulsion** *($62.50 for 2.5 ounces)* is neither essential nor any sort of "treatment" for dry skin. The lack of sunscreen makes it inappropriate for daytime use unless your foundation is rated SPF 15 or greater. Otherwise, this is an average emollient moisturizer with zero frills. Jar packaging isn't an issue because this product doesn't contain light- or air-sensitive ingredients.

☺ **$$$ Millenium Eye Renewal Crème** *($45 for 0.5 ounce)* is described as a "lavish concentration of emollient ingredients," which is going too far, but without question this is an emollient, almost greasy eye cream. Unfortunately, it's also a dated formula that fails to take advantage of what we've learned skin needs and can benefit from. Dry skin needs more than just oil and wax-like thickeners to look and feel its best, so this eye cream comes up short.

☺ **$$$ Millenium Night Renewal Cream** *($88.50 for 1.7 ounces)* is a very boring emollient moisturizer that barely covers the basics of making dry skin look and feel better. The price is insulting for what you get, and the formula is completely lacking any state-of-the-art ingredients. It's no better than an average option for dry skin.

ELIZABETH ARDEN PREVAGE PRODUCTS

☺ **$$$ Prevage Anti-Aging Night Cream** *($125 for 1.7 ounces)* attempts to carry on the theme that idebenone is the best antioxidant to exert an antiaging, reparative effect on skin. The research hasn't shown that to be the case, at least not in comparison to a wide range of antioxidants. A study funded by Allergan (the company that owns Prevage and has a licensing deal with Elizabeth Arden to retail certain products bearing the Prevage name) demonstrated that idebenone exerted greater antioxidant activity than several commonly used antioxidants, including vitamin C and green tea. But the comparison was relatively small, and I stated that although the results put idebenone on top, it was premature (and shortsighted) to instantly deem it the "best" antioxidant available. Indeed, a recent study comparing idebenone and L-ergothioneine showed that the latter outperformed idebenone in free radical-scavenging ability and protecting cultured skin cells from UVA damage (Source: *Journal of Cosmetic Dermatology*, September 2007, pages 183-188). I suspect if other comparison studies were conducted, similar results would be found. None of this means idebenone is not worth considering or that it's ineffective. Rather, it isn't the only game in town when it comes to selecting a skin-care product with antioxidants. Don't dismiss this product's antioxidant stability because it is packaged in a jar. As it turns out, the packaging is innovative due to the fact that it uses an airless jar with one-touch dispensing. This moisturizer has many state-of-the-art traits but a more balanced approach to antioxidants would have been better, not to mention a more consumer-friendly price.

☺ **$$$ Prevage Anti-Aging Treatment** *($155 for 1.7 ounces)* continues the carefully orchestrated launch of Prevage, which was first marketed to physicians and is now available in what is termed an "over-the-counter" version, marketed under the Elizabeth Arden name. Arden partnered with Allergan, the company that makes Prevage, to create a product that contains the "powerful" antioxidant idebenone (listed on the ingredient list as hydroxydecyl ubiquinone). What is the difference, you ask, between the dermatologic version and the one sold at the Arden counter? The original Prevage formula is billed as "physician-strength" and contains 1% idebenone, while Arden's cosmetics-counter version contains 0.5% idebenone. The physician-strength angle is bogus because idebenone is not a drug of any kind, nor is it regulated or akin to any type of prescription treatment. There is no reason it can't be sold in any retail channel. Such positioning and exclusivity is clever marketing on Allergan's part (the company also distributes Botox and markets the M.D. Forte skin-care line). The intense curiosity about this product has been nothing short of amazing, with most women asking me if idebenone really is the best antioxidant available. The study that showed idebenone has the antioxidant muscle to surpass others involved only 30 subjects, and compared idebenone to vitamins C and E, alpha lipoic acid, coenzyme Q10, and kinetin. The study did not, however, compare the effects of idebenone to many of the hundreds of other potent antioxidants that commonly appear in other skin-care products, nor did it compare the effects of idebenone with the effects of a combination of antioxidants. Perhaps a cocktail of antioxidants would far surpass idebenone—we don't know. Interestingly, a study comparing the protective effect of idebenone on sun-exposed skin found it ineffective compared to topical application of vitamins C and E with ferulic acid, but this study was conducted in part by Dr. Sheldon Pinnell, whose SkinCeuticals line sells an antioxidant serum with those very ingredients (Source: *The Journal of Investigative Dermatology*, May 2006, pages 1185-1187). The world of antioxidants is far more complex than the mere handful that Allergan compared to idebenone. To date, there are still no published, peer-reviewed studies that support idebenone's alleged superiority. This does not mean idebenone is not a valid antioxidant for skin. Given what we know about how ubiquinone performs in the body, it is definitely not a throwaway ingredient. What is fairly certain, however, is that it is neither the best nor most potent antioxidant around. Comparing Allergan's original Prevage formula to Arden's is like comparing night and day. Arden's water-in-silicone version is silky-smooth, and with a formula that's nearly identical to that of Allergan's "medically positioned" (however inaccurate that is) Prevage MD. Both Prevage products are water-in-silicone serums that contain several skin-friendly ingredients, including glycerin, phospholipids, green tea, sodium hyaluronate, and algae. Which Prevage product to choose isn't a tough decision, given that efficacy levels for idebenone have not been established. The fact that Arden's product contains 50% less than the original Prevage is inconsequential, and there is no research proving that 1% idebenone is preferred to Arden's 0.5%. Is Arden's readily available version worth the money? Despite its elegant formula, the answer is "no." Considering that idebenone is not the definitive antioxidant and that many companies are producing antioxidant serums and lotions that contain a cocktail of antioxidants, Arden's price point is undeservedly high. The product is a worthwhile option, and the formula is suitable for all skin types—unless you're sensitive to fragrance. But money-wise, lots of companies have antioxidant-loaded products that cost less (in some cases, much less) and, due to their blend of antioxidants, potentially offer skin a greater complement of benefits. One last note: The mica in both Prevage products lends a slight shimmer to skin, which the companies describe as enhancing skin's radiance; it's just a glitter-effect, nothing more.

✓ ☺ **$$$ Prevage Eye Anti-Aging Moisturizing Treatment** ($98 for 0.5 ounce) provides less product than the original Prevage, yet the price ends up being much higher on an ounce-per-ounce comparison basis. Good thing it is a more impressive formula! Claiming to be "anti-everything" that you don't like about the skin around your eyes, it is mostly a blend of silicones with sea water and algae. Lesser amounts of several antioxidants (including idebenone, listed as hydroxydecyl ubiquinone) and cell-communicating ingredients are included, but the good news is that the small amount of each adds up to a significantly beneficial product for slightly dry skin anywhere on the face. Don't count on this serum-type product to banish dark circles or deflate puffiness, but do count on it to provide skin with an array of excellent ingredients to help it look its best. The mica and titanium dioxide pigments add a soft shine to skin, but the effect on dark circles pales in comparison to the camouflage a good concealer can provide.

☺ **$$$ Prevage White Concentrated Brightening Serum** ($125 for 1 ounce). The combination of soy, stabilized vitamin C, and one other infrequently used potential skin-lightening agent (explained below) in this serum may indeed produce a satisfactory level of lightening with diligent use (and religious daily use of a sunscreen). This water-based serum has an elegant texture and its packaging is airtight, which is exactly what you want to see because it will keep the light- and air-sensitive ingredients stable during use. A small part of this formula is devoted to the potential skin-lightening ingredient octadecenedioic acid. This ingredient has some research indicating it has a secondary effect in interrupting melanin (skin pigment) transfer, and it also is an anti-inflammatory. The research is limited, appears to have been done by companies with a vested interest in the ingredient, and no concentration protocols were established (Sources: *International Journal of Cosmetic Science*, August 2006, pages 263-267, and April 2005, pages 123-132). However, paired with the soy and vitamin C, both of which have more convincing research than octadecenedioic acid, the combination is likely to produce more promising results. However, it is not necessary to spend this much money for an effective skin-lightening product. If anything, those considering a lightening product in this price range should also speak to their dermatologist about a prescription for Tri-Luma, especially if you have stubborn discolorations that haven't responded well to over-the-counter lighteners. Alternatively, you could buy an over-the-counter hydroquinone-based product because hydroquinone has a huge amount of research showing it to be effective in improving skin discolorations.

☺ **$$$ Prevage Body Total Transforming Anti-Aging Moisturizer** *($135 for 6.8 ounces).* Prevage continues to plod along, still maintaining that its star antioxidant (idebenone) is the most powerful one under the sun and, therefore, the only one you need, and, of course, that it's worth the extreme price tag. This body moisturizer, with its eyebrow-raising price, makes all manner of claims to try to make you believe it isn't just another moisturizer for your body from the neck down. No, sir! Making claims that should be preceded by a "step right up folks" invite, Prevage's body lotion is said to remedy scars, reduce discolorations, tackle cellulite, and, in short, "totally transform" your skin in just six weeks. Regrettably, there is nothing in this moisturizer that can perform any of those feats over and above what many other body moisturizers offer. You will not see one change in cellulite or skin discolorations, and scars may improve as they would with any moisturizer, but not in six weeks as claimed, or even in six years, even if you took a nightly bath in this stuff. What you get is a lightweight formula effective for most cases of dry skin, though someone with eczema or very dry, itchy skin will likely find this not moisturizing enough. It does contain some intriguing antioxidants, including idebenone (listed as hydroxydecyl ubiquinone, a synthetic form of coenzyme Q10), but the superiority studies Prevage and parent company Elizabeth Arden refer to compared idebenone to only five other antioxidants. Given the vast number of antioxidants in use (plus those yet to be discovered), how can a cosmetics company conclude that they're using the best? In addition, their studies didn't look at improvements related to scarring, cellulite, or skin discolorations. Interestingly, idebenone has taken a backseat to the red grape antioxidant compound resveratrol. A comparison study measuring idebenone and resveratrol's antioxidant ability showed the latter to be 17 times stronger (Source: *Journal of Cosmetic Dermatology*, March 2008, pages 2-7). Despite its incorrect labeling as the "best" antioxidant, there is not and likely never will be a "best" in this category. In terms of skin lightening, the only skin-lightening ingredient of note in this formula is octadecenedioic acid, which has some research indicating a secondary effect in interrupting melanin (skin pigment) transfer. The questionable part is that the research is limited, appears to have been done by companies with a vested interest in the ingredient, and there were no concentration protocols established (Sources: *International Journal of Cosmetic Science*, August 2006, pages 263-267, and April 2005, pages 123-132). All in all, this body moisturizer is a very expensive way to obtain smoother, softer skin with a slight shimmer (from mica). That shimmer is the only real lightening effect you'll see, but that's a cosmetic effect, not skin care, and you'll still need a sunscreen if your legs see daylight. In the long run and in the short run, any of the body lotions from Olay Quench best this formula and have a comparable texture. The overall formula for Prevage Body deserves a happy face, but that doesn't change the fact that I find the claims misleading and inaccurate, and there are far better options to consider.

OTHER ELIZABETH ARDEN PRODUCTS

☺ **$$$ 3-in-1 Daily Cleanser Exfoliator Primer** *($21.50 for 5 ounces)* is a copiously foaming cleanser that does a much better job of cleansing skin than exfoliating it. The scrub particles are polyethylene beads, but their presence in this product isn't as prominent as in many other (less expensive) cleanser/scrub options available at the drugstore. Consider this a good cleanser for normal to oily skin. It's capable of removing makeup, but the scrub particles aren't for use over the eye area.

☺ **$$$ Hydra-Gentle Cream Cleanser, for Dry/Sensitive Skin** *($19.50 for 5 ounces)* would be better for its targeted sensitive-skin customer if it did not contain fragrance; however, this is a very good, silky cleansing lotion that removes makeup and does not contain detergent cleansing agents.

✓ ☺ $$$ **All Gone Eye and Lip Makeup Remover** *($16 for 3.4 ounces)* is an impressive, fast-acting, water- and silicone-based makeup remover. The lack of fragrance and the inclusion of an anti-irritant make this a cut above many others.

☺ $$$ **Hydra-Splash Alcohol-Free Toner, for All Skin Types** *($19.50 for 6.8 ounces)* contains mostly water, slip agent, algae, soothing agent, witch hazel, skin-identical ingredients, plant oil, and emollients. It's a good option for normal to dry skin and would rate a Paula's Pick without the witch hazel.

☹ **Peel & Reveal Revitalizing Treatment** *($32 for 1.7 ounces)* contains two forms of drying, irritating alcohol as the main ingredients and the jar packaging will make the many antioxidants unstable shortly after the product is opened. Finally, several of the plant extracts (horsetail, orange, and lemon among them) are irritating to skin.

☹ **Bye Lines Anti-Wrinkle Serum** *($45 for 1 ounce)* contains a significant amount of coriander oil, so it's not so much "bye lines" as "hello irritation." The main fragrance component of this oil is linalool, which can cause allergic reactions and make skin more sensitive to sunlight (Source: *Herbal Drugs and Pharmaceuticals*, Medpharm GmbH Scientific Publishers, 1994).

☹ **Daily Moisture Lotion SPF 15** *($39 for 1.7 ounces)* lacks the UVA-protecting ingredients of titanium dioxide, zinc oxide, avobenzone, Tinosorb, or Mexoryl SX, and is not recommended.

☹ **Eight Hour Cream Intensive Daily Moisturizer for Face SPF 15** *($35 for 1.7 ounces)*. Arden's original Eight Hour Cream has been around for decades, though it's little more than glorified, overhyped Vaseline. I imagine Arden is hoping that revitalizing this product's image will spike interest in other Arden products. Whether or not their marketing idea proves worthwhile, it doesn't change the fact that this daytime moisturizer with sunscreen is better left on the shelf. It doesn't provide sufficient UVA protection because its only active ingredient is oxybenzone. As an approved active ingredient, oxybenzone protects against a partial range of UVA light, but it doesn't offer as much protection as avobenzone, titanium dioxide, zinc oxide, Mexoryl, or Tinosorb. Several other active ingredients (including avobenzone, listed by its chemical name of butyl methoxydibenzoylmethane) are listed as "other" ingredients, which mean you cannot count on them for protection. With some minor formulary changes, this could've been a very good option for those with normal to dry skin. As is, it's not recommended.

☺ **Eight Hour Cream Skin Protectant** *($17 for 1.7 ounces)* lands on many fashion magazines' "best of beauty" lists for its long-standing history and versatility. However, it's just a blend of emollients with fragrance, salicylic acid (incapable of exfoliating in this product), plant oil, vitamin E, and preservatives. (So much for the validity of the "best" lists in fashion magazines!) Plain Vaseline, which makes up the bulk of this formula, would work just as well.

☺ **Eight Hour Cream Sun Defense for Face SPF 50** *($30 for 1.7 ounces)*. Here's an oddity: Arden's Eight Hour Cream Intensive Daily Moisturizer for Face SPF 15 lacks great UVA protection, but contains several antioxidants and skin-identical ingredients that are great for skin. For some unknown reason this product provides great UVA protection, but lacks antioxidants and other essential extras for the face. The SPF 50 deserves praise for providing ample sun protection, but at this price, antioxidants, skin-identical ingredients, and cell-communicating ingredients should be standard.

✓ ☺ $$$ **Extreme Conditioning Cream SPF 15** *($38.50 for 1.7 ounces)* provides UVA protection with its in-part avobenzone sunscreen and comes in an emollient, silky, antioxidant-

The Reviews E

enriched base. The opaque pump bottle will keep the light- and air-sensitive ingredients stable, so this is an all-around exceptional daytime moisturizer for normal to dry skin.

☹ **First Defense Advanced Anti-Oxidant Cream SPF 15** *($39 for 1.7 ounces)* is a more emollient version of the First Defense Advanced Anti-Oxidant Lotion SPF 15, and also includes an in-part avobenzone sunscreen. The same formulary issues (that is, the intriguing ingredients are listed after the preservative) apply here, too, though this formula adds irritating grapefruit juice, which serves no purpose in a sunscreen other than to cause irritation and possibly a photosensitizing reaction.

☺ **$$$ First Defense Advanced Anti-Oxidant Lotion SPF 15** *($39 for 1.7 ounces)* is a good, though standard, sunscreen lotion that contains avobenzone for UVA protection. The water- and silicone-based lotion leaves skin feeling silky and moist, but all of the interesting skin-identical ingredients and, most important, the antioxidants are minimally present. Actually, the more than 40 ingredients show up in short supply here, which means that you essentially get a whole lot of nothing. Arden claims that the carnosine and wolfberry plant extract are proven to outperform vitamins A, C, and E at neutralizing skin-damaging free radicals. Yet if that's true, there is no substantiated research to support it. Carnosine has a good amount of promising research concerning its antioxidant benefit when taken orally, but compared to the piles of research on topical use of the three aforementioned vitamins, information on topical use of carnosine is scarce. As for the wolfberry, there isn't much of it in here to extol, and there is insufficient reliable information about its effectiveness whether it's used topically or consumed (Source: www.naturaldatabase.com).

☺ **$$$ Good Night's Sleep Restoring Cream** *($38 for 1.7 ounces)* is designed to be used at night, yet contains three sunscreen ingredients, which is unnecessary and can cause irritation. This rich-textured cream contains a frustrating blend of problematic and helpful plant extracts. The helpful plants have antioxidant properties, but won't remain stable once this jar-packaged product is opened. The amount of lavender extract is unlikely to cause problems, but if you're interested in this plant's sleep-inducing effect, a far better method would be to inhale lavender essential oil or potpourri before bedtime.

☺ **$$$ Good Morning Skin Serum** *($34 for 0.5 ounce)* is a silicone-based serum that contains several plant extracts, some of which can have antioxidant properties for skin and some that can be skin irritants. The teeny amount of mulberry is not enough to inhibit melanin production. What this product lacks is a significant quantity of skin-identical ingredients, which would have made this a far better way to say good morning for skin.

☹ **Matte Moisture Lotion, Oil Free** *($34 for 1.7 ounces)* has a matte finish thanks to the amount of alcohol and talc it contains. There are less irritating ways to keep skin shine-free than with an alcohol-laden moisturizer, and this also contains some potentially irritating plant extracts. Ironically, the alcohol will stimulate oil production in the pore!

☺ **$$$ Moisture Shield Lotion SPF 15** *($62 for 1.7 ounces)* is a good, though needlessly expensive, daytime moisturizer with sunscreen for normal to dry skin. Sufficient UVA protection is provided by avobenzone and the base formula feels silky and hydrates well. It contains good emollients and a nice selection of antioxidants and skin-identical ingredients.

☺ **$$$ Overnight Success Cellular Renewal Serum** *($49 for 1 ounce)* promises to resurface and regenerate skin's appearance, giving your skin enhanced clarity and a less blotchy appearance. Yet the best thing this serum has going for it is that its silicone base will leave skin feeling exceptionally silky. In terms of enhanced clarity, there is nothing in the product that can make skin clearer. However, because silicone can even out your skin's texture, you may perceive more clarity. This is because of how silicone functions on skin: smooth-textured skin is better able to reflect light, which does improve its appearance, but that's a cosmetic effect, not an antiaging breakthrough. Arden wisely filled this serum with several very good skin-identical ingredients and antioxidants, ingredients you should expect to see in any serum (or moisturizer), especially in this price range. Even better, packaging for this product will ensure that the antioxidants remain stable during use. The inclusion of the Australian flower extract *Centipedia cunninghamii* (also known by its less appealing garden name, old man weed) is curious, because it is commonly used as a medicinal remedy for colds and chest pain (Source: www.naturaldatabase.com). Reliable, substantiated information about this extract's effect on skin doesn't seem to exist. The extract does not appear to be harmful or irritating, but there are no proven studies pertaining to its usefulness as an antiwrinkle ingredient. My one complaint about this product is its intense fragrance. I don't often comment on a specific skin-care product's scent, but this serum's perfumey scent lingers on the skin long after it has been absorbed. Both Clinique and my line have similar products that are fragrance-free and less expensive, but this product is definitely an option for all but sensitive skin types seeking either a lightweight moisturizer or antioxidant product.

☺ **$$$ Perpetual Moisture 24 Cream** *($42 for 1.7 ounces)* is another moisturizer in which the effectiveness of the many antioxidants is compromised by jar packaging. However, a larger offense is Arden's decision to include balm mint extract, which poses a risk of irritation for skin. The amount is likely too small to be a problem, but this otherwise nicely done moisturizer for normal to dry skin would be better without it.

☺ **$$$ Perpetual Moisture 24 Lotion** *($42 for 1.7 ounces)* is a lighter-weight version of the Perpetual Moisture 24 Cream, and is packaged in an opaque pump bottle, which better preserves the effectiveness of its antioxidants. This is a mostly outstanding moisturizer for normal to slightly dry or slightly oily skin. It would earn a Paula's Pick rating if not for the balm mint extract. Regarding Arden's claims that this product "preempts moisture loss at its source," that is merely a standard for any well-formulated moisturizer. It should indeed contain ingredients that keep moisture in skin (preventing moisture loss) and draw moisture to the skin's surface. This Arden product contains essential ingredients that do just that.

☺ **Velva Moisture Film** *($43 for 6.7 ounces)* is a very dated moisturizer recommended for combination or oily skin. The thickeners and lanolin make it inappropriate for these skin types, particularly if breakouts are a concern. Actually, this formula makes Clinique's boring Dramatically Different Moisturizing Lotion look like a state-of-the-art product, which isn't saying much.

☺ **$$$ Visible Difference Refining Moisture Cream Complex** *($52 for 2.5 ounces)* has been in the Arden line for years, which means customers are still buying it. It's a jar-packaged, very standard moisturizer for normal to dry skin that contains a tiny amount of antioxidants and doesn't compete favorably with today's state-of-the-art moisturizers.

☹ **Eight Hour Cream Lip Protectant Stick SPF 15** *($17 for 0.13 ounce)* won't protect lips from the sun's UVA rays because it lacks any of the UVA-protecting ingredients of titanium dioxide, zinc oxide, avobenzone, Tinosorb, or Mexoryl SX. In addition, the sheer colors can't provide the physical-type block that opaque lipsticks offer, so this product is not recommended.

ELIZABETH ARDEN MAKEUP

FOUNDATION: ☺ **$$$ Pure Finish Mineral Powder Foundation SPF 20** *($37.50).* Arden's edge with their mineral makeup lies in their packaging. Rather than putting a loose

The Reviews E

powder in a standard jar with a sifter, the powder is in semi-solid form. You rotate the outside of the sifter to "shave" off (and push up) the desired amount of loose powder. From there, you simply swirl your brush in the powder, tap off the excess, and blend on skin. The mica-based powder has a silky, dry texture that adheres well, but it tends to grab on any excess moisture. If you opt to try this, it's best applied over bare skin or a matte-finish serum or moisturizer. This foundation is best for those with normal to slightly oily skin. Once applied, it sets to a powdery satin matte finish with a bit of shine. Sun protection is from pure titanium dioxide, but unless you apply this liberally (which results in a very powdered look), you likely won't get the SPF rating on the label. When brushed on, this provides light to barely medium coverage; it isn't as opaque as many other mineral makeups. Most of the colors are great, but consider shades 7 and 8 carefully; both are slightly ash on dark skin tones.

☺ **$$$ Ceramide Plump Perfect Makeup SPF 15** *($39.50)* has many positive attributes, but for a foundation purporting to reduce the appearance of wrinkles, its cardinal error was not including a sunscreen that offers UVA-protecting ingredients. This is otherwise a modern formula that does include ceramides, though it takes more than that to create radiant, healthy-looking skin. The silky texture blends easily, providing medium coverage and leaving a soft matte finish. Ten shades are available, with some enticing options for light to medium skin tones. Avoid Honey, Cameo, Mocha II, and Bisque, and avoid this foundation altogether if you're looking for reliable sunscreen protection.

☺ **$$$ Flawless Finish Bare Perfection Makeup SPF 8** *($32)* is actually an impressive foundation suitable for normal to dry skin, other than its shortcoming of having a way too low SPF without adequate UVA protection. With a smooth, moist texture and satin finish capable of delivering sheer to light coverage, it's worth a look, but it's not recommended over foundations that go the distance to protect skin with SPF 15. There are 15 shades to consider, including a couple of good options for darker skin tones. The shades that should be avoided due to overtones of peach, orange, or pink are Bisque, Cameo, Honey, Mocha II, and Fawn. Buff is slightly peach but may work for some light skin tones.

☺ **$$$ Flawless Finish Dual Perfection Makeup SPF 8** *($32)* is a talc-based pressed-powder foundation with a silky feel and a very smooth finish. The SPF rating is embarrassingly low—by itself this is a no-no for daytime—but it is part titanium dioxide, so if you pair it with an effective SPF 15 sunscreen it would add some extra protection. The formula works best for someone with normal to slightly dry or slightly oily skin, and most of the 12 colors are excellent. The only ones that should be avoided due to their peach casts are Buff and Cameo.

☺ **$$$ Flawless Finish Mousse Makeup** *($32)* is the original mousse foundation. It's packaged in a metal can that uses a propellant to distribute an airy, bubbly, flesh-toned foam, which blends on better than you might expect, though you might end up wasting some product until you get used to the dispensing method. Coverage is sheer, and the texture has enough slip to allow for adequate blending. This dries to a soft matte finish and is an option for normal to slightly oily or dry skin. If you're prone to breakouts, you will appreciate the absence of potentially pore-clogging thickening agents in this formula. Thirteen shades are on hand, including some great colors for fair skin tones, but avoid Melba, Bisque, and Natural. Champagne and Ginger are slightly pink, and should be considered carefully.

☺ **$$$ Flawless Finish Radiant Moisture Makeup SPF 8** *($29)* is an elegant, moisturizing foundation for those with normal to very dry skin. What a shame the sunscreen lacks adequate UVA-protecting ingredients and that the SPF rating is pitifully low. This somewhat thick, creamy makeup provides medium coverage and a moist finish that can look thick if not blended carefully. The 11 shades include some notable neutral options; the ones to avoid due to peach or pink tones are Bisque, Cameo, Honey, Mocha II, and Fawn.

☺ $$$ **Flawless Finish Sponge-On Cream Makeup** *($32)* has been part of Arden's makeup lineup for years, but that's not necessarily a good thing. This fairly thick and somewhat greasy petrolatum- and mineral oil–based compact makeup is only for someone with dry skin. It starts out very thick and moist, providing medium to full coverage with a creamy, opaque finish. It blends well enough, but most women don't need this much coverage, and the fragrance is quite strong. Those who are loyal to this makeup may want to reconsider what they want from a foundation. Of the 11 shades, the following are too pink, orange, or peach: Vanilla, Softly Beige, Porcelain Beige, Toasty Beige, Gentle Beige, and Toasty Rose.

☺ $$$ **INTERVENE Makeup SPF 15** *($36)* is another look-younger-now foundation whose antiaging claims are immediately discredited because the sunscreen does not provide sufficient UVA protection, one of the most significant aspects of keeping skin young. Arden, come on! Everything else about this foundation (well, almost everything—some of the shades are duds) is outstanding, from its silky-smooth texture that provides light moisture to its satin finish suitable for normal to dry skin. Coverage goes from light to medium, and this offers plenty of time to blend before it sets. If you decide to try this (and doing so requires you to pair it with a broad-spectrum sunscreen rated SPF 15 or greater), the shades to avoid include Soft Sand and Soft Cognac. Soft Shell and Soft Cameo are borderline pink and should be considered carefully.

☹ $$$ **Sheer Lights Illuminating Tinted Moisturizer SPF 15** *($28)* leaves your skin vulnerable to UVA damage because it does not contain the UVA-protecting ingredients of titanium dioxide, zinc oxide, avobenzone, Tinosorb, or Mexoryl SX. That's a shame, too, because this sheer, tinted moisturizer with soft shimmer comes in stable packaging and has an antioxidant-rich formula that's ideal for normal to dry skin. Each of the four shades veers toward being too pink or peach, but the sheerness negates this fact.

CONCEALER: ✓ ☺ **Flawless Finish Concealer** *($16)* remains an excellent wand-applicator type concealer with a lightweight, smooth texture and an opaque, soft matte finish that poses almost no risk of creasing. The three colors are superbly neutral, and best for fair to medium skin. Surveying Arden's entire makeup collection, this is one of a handful of items that is really worth your attention (and money).

POWDER: ☺ $$$ **Ceramide Skin Smoothing Loose Powder** *($30)*. This talc-based loose powder contains several ceramides, but in a powder I'm skeptical that the benefits of those ingredients are helpful given that the packaging isn't airtight. For aesthetics, it has an obviously shiny finish. The Arden makeup artist commented on how much she loves the sparkles in this powder. I mentioned that her skin wasn't sparkling and asked her if she was wearing this powder. She said, no, because she prefers a matte finish. Interesting! I suspect this woman, who had some amount of wrinkling, knows that shine makes wrinkles more noticeable. Hopefully, she shares that information with other women who have wrinkles. If you're OK with or want a very shiny loose powder, this does have a gossamer texture, weightless finish, and comes in four workable shades that go on translucent.

☺ $$$ **Flawless Finish Pressed Powder** *($24.50)* appears to have been improved, because it now competes nicely with other talc-based pressed powders that leave a silky, sheer, real-skin finish rather than looking dry or chalky. It comes in five shades, though each is so sheer the

The Reviews E

color is almost a non-issue. One more thing: this deposits so minimally on skin that someone with very oily areas will be disappointed and need to find a more absorbent powder.

BLUSH AND BRONZER: ☺ **$$$ Color Intrigue Cheekcolor** *($22)* is a collection of pressed-powder blushes, each with a slightly dry, grainy texture and sheer, blendable application. Every shade has some amount of shine, but the truly underwhelming texture doesn't make this worth considering over blushes rated with a happy face or greater.

☹ **Color Intrigue Bronzing Powder Duo** *($32)* is a talc-based, pressed-powder bronzer that features two shiny colors in one compact. Each shade has a dry, slightly grainy texture but sheer application. The overall performance doesn't come close to matching the price, and this makes it not worth considering over countless other bronzing powders.

EYESHADOW: ✓☺ **Color Intrigue Eyeshadow** *($15)* is ideal. Each shade has a wonderful, satin matte, non-powdery finish and a texture that blends and layers beautifully. Every shade has at least a touch of shine, but the good news is the shiniest shades leave more of a sheen than glitter or sparkles, and these shadows don't flake. The almost-matte options include Teak, Urban, Vanilla, and Wheat.

✓☺ **$$$ Color Intrigue Eyeshadow Duo** *($24.50)*. This powder eyeshadow has a very smooth texture and beautifully even application that blends well and provides ample color saturation. Each duo has shine, but in most cases it's more of a soft sheen than all-out sparkles. Regrettably, most of the color pairs aren't the easiest to work with. The best duos are Pink Clover and Autumn Leaves.

☺ **Color Intrigue Palette Eyeshadow Quad** *($30)* shares the same formulary and application traits as the single Color Intrigue Eyeshadow, but here you get four shades in one compact. I wish the color combinations were more thoughtful; the quads I saw weren't the easiest shades to work with, and every one was very shiny. The shades tend to change seasonally, so keep your eyes open for an attractive grouping where you can realistically use more than two colors!

☹ **Eye-Fix Primer** *($21.50)* is supposed to be a sheer cream for the eyelid to prevent makeup creasing; it's basically water, silicone, talc, and wax. Forget this boring, superfluous product and just use the Flawless Finish Concealer, which would work as well, if not better, than this product.

EYE AND BROW SHAPER: ☺ **$$$ Color Intrigue Gel Eyeliner with Brush** *($22.50)*. Arden is finally in the gel eyeliner game, but how does their contribution (which is pricier than most) compare? In most respects, quite well. The silicone-based formula glides on just as well as other gel eyeliners, and sets to a smooth, long-wearing finish. Arden's brush works beautifully to apply a thin or thick line though some will wish the handle was longer (it's not a throwaway brush and helps explain the higher cost compared to similar gel eyeliners where you'd have to purchase the brush separately). If you opt to try this, the best shades are black and brown. The pearl finish shades can be fun for evening glamour, but the shine particles tend to flake off during wear.

☹ **Color Intrigue Eyeliner** *($16)* wins points for being an automatic, retractable pencil with an easy-glide application, but because it stays creamy you'll find that it fades and smears easily. All of the shades have a slight to strong metallic finish, which can be a fun departure, though perhaps too distracting for day-to-day wear. If you decide to try this, it works best to create a smoky eye, rather than a long-lasting line.

☺ **Smoky Eyes Powder Pencil** *($16)* is definitely powdery, and best used to draw a thick line that you then smudge for a smoky appearance; otherwise this will smudge on its own. It needs routine sharpening but applies without pulling or tugging—always a plus.

☹ **Dual Perfection Brow Shaper and Eyeliner** *($18)* has a dry, grainy texture and is meant to be used wet, yet once dry the powder tends to flake. There are much easier, longer-lasting ways to shape and define the eyebrow and line the eye.

LIPSTICK, LIP GLOSS, AND LIPLINER: ✓ ☺ $$$ **Ceramide Plump Perfect Lipstick** *($21.50)* contains a tiny amount of palmitoyl pentapeptide, not enough to plump lips (though even a large amount of this peptide lacks reliable research confirming its plumping prowess). Despite that letdown, there's no denying that this is a remarkable cream lipstick. The colors are riveting, the texture sublime, and the non-greasy, non-slippery finish lasts longer than many other creamy lipsticks. As an added bonus, the formula is rich in ceramides and antioxidants—a rarity in lipstick formulas at any price.

✓ ☺ $$$ **Color Intrigue Lipstick** *($19.50)* comes in almost two dozen shades, each with beguiling names such as Seduction, Entrapment, and Drama. The color selection favors bolder, shimmer-infused colors, and includes some decadent reds and rich browns. As for the lipstick itself, it is creamy-smooth without feeling a bit slick or greasy. This is one of the few creamier lipsticks that won't immediately creep into lines around the mouth, and it sets to a semi-matte finish that allows for reasonably long wear (it helps that these lipsticks have lots of pigment, too!).

☺ $$$ **Exceptional Lipstick** *($19.50)* is a great name for what is a standard, but good, creamy lipstick. These all tend to have a slight to strong glossy finish and enough stain to allow for longer wear. The color range is smaller than ever due to the newer (and better) Color Intrigue Lipstick.

☺ **High Shine Lip Gloss** *($15)* doesn't distinguish itself as a "must-have" lip gloss, but it's a workable option with a medium-thick texture and slightly sticky finish. The sheer shades are infused with sparkles, and luckily they don't make lips feel grainy as the moisturizing effect wears off.

☺ **Lip Definer** *($16)* is an automatic, nonretractable pencil that goes on smoothly and sets to a semi-matte finish that does a reasonable job of keeping lipstick from feathering into lines around the mouth.

☹ **Smooth Line Lip Pencil** *($16)* is a standard, needs-sharpening pencil that slides over lips without tugging or skipping. It is more creamy than greasy, and would have been rated higher if routine sharpening weren't required. Arden included a lip brush on the opposite end of the pencil, and it's surprisingly good.

☹ **Crystal Clear Lip Gloss** *($14)* is a very thick, sticky gloss that is flavored with spearmint, which tastes nice but can be irritating for the lips.

MASCARA: ✓ ☺ $$$ **Ceramide Lash Extending Treatment Mascara** *($20)*. Arden is playing up this mascara by mentioning their ceramide complex, which is said to lengthen, define, and revitalize lashes. Although the formula contains some ingredients not seen in many other mascaras, the ceramides compose only a small part of the total package. They likely have some conditioning benefit for lashes, but this isn't lash revitalization in a tube and ceramides can't grow or change lashes in any way. The ingredients that lengthen and define lashes are standard and, of course, the brush plays an even more important role in how mascara applies than almost any other part of the product. In this case, claims notwithstanding, you will be impressed with the clean, swift application that lengthens and separates lashes evenly. Unless you were trying for mondo thickness, I can't imagine someone being disappointed with this mascara's performance, and it leaves lashes feeling soft. It is definitely one of Arden's best mascaras in a long time!

The Reviews E

☺ **$$$ Double Density Maximum Volume Mascara** *($19)* is a mascara whose name conflicts with the actual results you'll notice. This isn't a poor mascara—far from it. But if your definition of "dramatically" thickened lashes is textbook, you'll see that this mascara is primarily about clump-free lengthening. You will get some thickness, with effort, but not an effect most people would call dramatic. This mascara is worth trying if your expectations are not as lofty as Arden's claims.

☹ **Lash Optimizer Primer with Conditioners** *($15)* contains hydrated silica as a main ingredient. That's not a bad thing, but since this is absorbent by nature, it negates any conditioning benefit stated in the product name. This ends up being another superfluous lash primer; it makes very little difference if you are already using an outstanding mascara (and if you aren't, why not?), and a slightly discernible difference with average mascaras. The concept of lash primers (or anything primer-related) appeals to many women; if a lash primer is what you want, consider Smashbox's Layer Lash Primer, which produces good results and really is conditioning.

BRUSHES: ✓☺ **Face Powder Brush** *($28)* is an exceptionally soft and dense synthetic hair brush, designed to be used with Arden's Pure Finish Mineral Powder Foundation. It's ideal for applying all types of loose powder, mineral or not. The slightly angled cut allows the brush to easily fit the contours of the face. As a bonus, Arden includes a tiny version of this brush that's meant to be stashed in the component for their Pure Finish Mineral Foundation. It's so small as to be impractical, but I suppose it's OK in a pinch.

☺ **Multipurpose Brush #3** *($20)*. Professional application tools aren't this line's strong point, which may explain why their brushes are neither displayed nor advertised. The Multipurpose Brush #3 is a decent option, but not worth considering over the impressive (if for nothing more than the number of choices) from M.A.C.

SPECIALTY PRODUCTS: ☹ **$$$ Lip-Fix Cream** *($20)* is supposed to prevent lipstick from feathering. Packaged in a tube, it goes on like a moisturizer and must dry before you put on your lipstick, which is not convenient for touch-ups during the day. Anti-feathering products that come in lipstick or lipliner forms mean there's no waiting between applications, and you don't need to remove what you have on to reapply more, and those options make Arden's version less enticing.

ESTEE LAUDER

ESTEE LAUDER AT-A-GLANCE

Strengths: Some of the most state-of-the-art moisturizers and serums around; excellent sunscreens and self-tanning products; some good cleansers, toners, and makeup removers; excellent retinol product; several categories of makeup excel, including some extraordinary foundations (that include beautiful shades for darker skin tones), concealers, powders, blush, and eyeshadows; a mostly good selection of eye, brow, and lip pencils; their long-wearing lip color and some of the lipsticks are supremely good.

Weaknesses: Several items are highly fragranced; incomplete and/or problematic products for anyone battling blemishes; no effective AHA or BHA products; many of the Re-Nutriv products are priced too high given similar, less expensive options from Lauder; some of the sunscreens and foundations with sunscreen lack sufficient UVA protection; the mascaras; the brushes aren't on par with those from other Lauder-owned lines, such as Bobbi Brown or M.A.C.; some superfluous specialty products and problem pencils; jar packaging.

For more information about Estee Lauder, call (877) 311-3883 or visit www.esteelauder. com or www.Beautypedia.com.

ESTEE LAUDER SKIN CARE

ESTEE LAUDER ADVANCED NIGHT REPAIR PRODUCTS

✓ ☺ **$$$ Advanced Night Repair Concentrate Recovery Boosting Treatment** *($85 for 1 ounce)* serves as a partner product to Lauder's enduring Advanced Night Repair serum and their Advanced Night Repair Synchronized Recovery Complex. This concentrated version (supposedly with five times the amount of patented recovery complex than the original Advanced Night Repair) is meant to be used for three weeks, after which you revert to your usual routine of applying original Advanced Night Repair. Considering that the price for the Concentrate is double that of the original Advanced Night Repair, you may wonder if this allegedly more potent version is worth the upgrade. It turns out that the formulas are similar in some ways, but the differences are notable enough to definitely make Advanced Night Repair Concentrate the superior product, and not only for three weeks. Its silicone content gives the Concentrate a silkier texture than the original, but the big difference is in the larger amount of antioxidants Lauder packed into the Concentrate version. This is enough of a difference to consider the original antiquated. Whether or not the extras are worth the money is up to you. Clinique's Repairwear Deep Wrinkle Concentrate for Face and Eye is just as well-formulated, as is Estee Lauder's Perfectionist [CP+] Wrinkle Lifting Serum. A major ingredient in the Advanced Night Repair Concentrate and in the original Advanced Night Repair is bifida ferment lysate. The bifida portion refers to bifidobacteria, a strain of bacteria found in the human body and believed to provide immune protection and prevent gastrointestinal problems (in other words, it's a friendly strain of bacteria). How does it relate to skin care? Claims made for this ingredient are that it can do for the face what it does for the body, enhance the immune system and decrease bad bacteria. There is no published information establishing that to be true. Oral consumption of this bacteria (it is often present in yogurt and can be purchased in supplement form) has a couple of studies that show it can be of benefit in helping with infant eczema, but that's about it when it comes to skin (Source: www.naturaldatabase.com).

☺ **$$$ Advanced Night Repair Eye Recovery Complex** *($48.50 for 0.5 ounce)*. The kicker with this moisturizer is that it claims to address pretty much every eye-area skin-care woe you can think of, from puffiness to dark circles, wrinkles, and environmental damage. It sounds like the ultimate choice for eyes, but we've all heard this song before with countless other Lauder eye products that have come and gone, from Uncircle to Unline to Eyezone, along with a vast selection from the ten other lines under Lauder's ownership. Still, skin-repairing claims aside, this is indeed a very good, silicone-based moisturizer that would take good care of dry skin anywhere on the face. It contains mostly water, silicones, emollients, thickeners, anti-irritants, antioxidants, skin-identical ingredients, vitamins, film former, and preservatives. Unfortunately, the antioxidants lose potency once this jar-packaged product is opened.

☺ **$$$ Advanced Night Repair Protective Recovery Complex** *($46.50 for 1 ounce)* is the original Night Repair product, and although this water-based serum has some very good ingredients for all skin types, it just isn't as exciting as Lauder's superior Advanced Night Repair Concentrate Recovery Boosting Treatment or their Perfectionist [CP+] Wrinkle Lifting Serum. Lauder recommends it as an essential for all skin types, but it isn't—at least not anymore.

☺ **$$$ Advanced Night Repair Synchronized Recovery Complex** *($74.50 for 1.7 ounces).* Lauder's longstanding Advanced Night Repair product has finally been updated, and the company is sparing no expense to advertise the update. With its new name, it's natural to think that this updated version goes beyond its predecessor. The original version had definitely become a dated formula; several other serums from Estee Lauder and other Lauder-owned brands handily surpass it in terms of giving skin a wide breadth of beneficial ingredients. The Synchronized Recovery Complex bears striking formulary similarities to the original Advanced Night Repair product. Both have the same base formula consisting of water, a type of friendly bacteria (bifida ferment lysate), slip agents, and thickener. The Synchronized Recovery Complex adds three new ingredients, which are discussed below. Needless to say, this serum isn't a must-have for anyone's skin and certainly doesn't break new ground for state-of-the-art products or for Lauder, either. I suspect Lauder simply realized (though what took them so long is anyone's guess) that their original Night Repair product was getting long in the tooth, especially when compared with their other offerings, and needed an update. One of the new ingredients is *Arabidopsis thaliana*, a small flowering plant that has in-vitro research showing its protein fragments may enhance the skin's ability to protect itself from UVB damage. Preliminary research also suggests it may function as a cell-communicating ingredient; however, research on intact human skin is lacking and this plant is far from the only ingredient to offer these potential benefits (Sources: *Biochemistry*, April 2008, pages 4583-4596; and *FEBS Letters*, July 2007, pages 3356-3362). Tripeptide-32 is another new ingredient in this serum, and it also has research showing it, like many other peptides, has theoretical cell-communicating ability. It's theoretical because getting a peptide to reach its target site within the skin is difficult due to the presence of enzymes in skin that work to break down the peptide before it has a chance to work as claimed. However, tripeptide-32 appears to have a protective effect against proteins that damage cells, though there is no research proving it works when applied in small amounts to intact human skin (Sources: *Neuroscience Letters*, Volume 419, 2007, pages 247-252; and *Folia Pharmacologica Japonica*, Volume 129, 2007, page 18P). Still, it's a step in the right direction and clearly shows Lauder put some thought into this redo. The last new ingredient of note is lactobacillus ferment, another strain of friendly bacteria. Although this ingredient has multiple health benefits when consumed orally, there is no research proving its merit for topical application on skin (Source: www.naturaldatabase.com). All told, although this serum is an improvement over Lauder's original Advanced Night Repair product (and deserving of a happy face rating), it doesn't join the ranks of today's best serums and doesn't have what it takes to make good on its dramatic, reparative claims. This fragrance-free serum is suitable for all skin types, and leaves a slightly tacky finish on skin.

ESTEE LAUDER DAYWEAR PRODUCTS

☺ **$$$ DayWear Plus Multi Protection Anti-Oxidant Crème SPF 15, for Dry Skin** *($38.50 for 1.7 ounces)* has an in-part avobenzone sunscreen that would be an excellent choice as a daytime moisturizer for dry skin were it not for jar packaging that limits the long-term effectiveness of the antioxidants. It does contain some good skin-identical ingredients and the familiar DayWear cucumber fragrance, but what a shame the antioxidants won't last long.

☺ **$$$ DayWear Plus Multi Protection Anti-Oxidant Crème SPF 15, for Normal/Combination Skin** *($38.50 for 1.7 ounces)* leaves out the petrolatum found in the DayWear Plus for Dry Skin and instead uses silicones for a lighter-feeling, creamy emulsion. This formula is indeed suitable for normal to combination skin, and contains an in-part avobenzone sunscreen. Unfortunately, it is packaged in a clear jar, which will quickly negate the benefits of including such an inspired variety of antioxidants. This does contain fragrance.

☺ **$$$ DayWear Plus Multi-Protection Anti-Oxidant Lotion SPF 30, for Normal/ Combination Skin** *($38.50 for 1.7 ounces)* is another well-formulated, well-packaged sunscreen from Estee Lauder. The active ingredients include titanium dioxide and zinc oxide for UVA protection, and the lightweight lotion texture slips on without a trace of the white cast typical of mineral sunscreens (the formula includes synthetic sunscreens, too). This product is loaded with antioxidants, cell-communicating ingredients, and ingredients that mimic the structure and function of healthy skin. The only drawback is the fragrance, which is stronger than it needs to be. For a daytime moisturizer available at the department store, this runs circles around what Lancome, Clarins, and Chanel have to offer in the way of sunscreens, and Lauder's price point offers better protection for your budget as well. Another job well done, and it is indeed appropriate for normal to combination skin types.

✓ ☺ **$$$ DayWear Plus Multi Protection Anti-Oxidant Lotion SPF 15, for Oily Skin** *($38.50 for 1.7 ounces)* has a fluid, non-greasy texture and a lightweight feel on the skin. This is not a matte-finish sunscreen, and there's no way to guarantee it won't cause breakouts (this is true of all sunscreens), but it is worth auditioning if you have oily skin and have not been able to find a daytime moisturizer with sunscreen that works for you. The packaging will definitely keep the many antioxidants stable much longer than the jar-packaged DayWear Crèmes, and this also contains some intriguing cell-communicating ingredients.

✓ ☺ **$$$ DayWear Plus Multi Protection Anti-Oxidant Moisturizer Sheer Tint Release Formula SPF 15, for All Skin Types** *($38.50 for 1.7 ounces)* has an in-part avobenzone sunscreen, which makes for great UVA protection from this lightly emollient lotion. The soft tan tint looks great over a variety of skin tones, and is a believable color for those with fair skin if they want to pull off a slightly tan look. Coverage is sparse, and, like the other DayWear Plus products, this includes a nice array of antioxidants and some cell-communicating ingredients. Lauder's opaque tube packaging for this product ensures that the antioxidants remain stable. Although the sunscreen is the same, the base formulation is different from those of the other DayWear Plus products, and is best for normal to slightly dry or slightly oily skin.

✓ ☺ **$$$ DayWear Plus Multi Protection Tinted Moisturizer SPF 15** *($35 for 1.7 ounces)* combines an in-part avobenzone sunscreen with an antioxidant-rich lotion that's beautifully suited for normal to dry skin. Coverage is sheer, just as it is for most tinted moisturizers, while the finish is satinlike. What makes this Lauder moisturizer different is the very good assortment of skin-friendly ingredients that take it above and beyond what some other tinted moisturizers with sunscreen provide. Among the four neutral-to-yellow shades, the only tricky one is Medium, and even that is still worth trying to see if it works for you.

ESTEE LAUDER HYDRA BRIGHT PRODUCTS

☺ **$$$ Hydra Bright Skin-Tone Perfecting Lotion, for Normal/Combination Skin** *($40 for 1.7 ounces)* beckons you with promises of seeing glowing skin and a flawless radiance, along with a dramatic reduction in discolorations (though Lauder uses the word "appear," which is a clever way of stating that the product doesn't necessarily eliminate discolorations, it just makes them less apparent—that isn't a change in skin, just a temporary camouflage). Will you be "guaranteed to glow" with this product? I don't see how that's possible, since the formula doesn't include any glow-enhancing pigments such as mica. The formula itself isn't as impressive as other Lauder moisturizers and serums (but that's saying a lot, because Lauder offers some of the best formulas around). It has a silky, lightweight lotion texture suitable for normal to oily skin, but the usual roster of skin-identical and cell-communicating ingredients are present in only meager amounts. Several antioxidants are included at levels amounting to more than a dusting, which keeps this moisturizer from earning a neutral face rating. None of these antioxidants have documented evidence of their skin-lightening ability. The only ingredient that has any research pertaining to that is mulberry, but the amount Lauder uses in this product isn't likely to lighten even a faint freckle. However, there are enough positive attributes about the formula itself to make it worthwhile as a moisturizer. If skin discolorations are a concern, you will need another product that contains ingredients that are proven to fade them because this one falls way short.

☺ $$$ **Hydra Bright Skin-Tone Perfecting Moisturizer Crème SPF 15, for Normal/Combination Skin** *($40 for 1.7 ounces)* provides UVA protection with avobenzone and would have been an outstanding daytime moisturizer for normal to slightly dry or slightly oily skin if jar packaging not been used. Among the Lauder Hydra Bright products, this version contains the best blend of state-of-the-art ingredients skin needs to look and feel healthy—but most of what you're paying for won't last long once this product is opened and in use. Come on Lauder! Enough with the jars! You're not doing your customers any favors; you're only shorting the benefits of your typically excellent moisturizer formulas!

☹ $$$ **Hydra Bright Skin-Tone Perfecting Moisturizer Crème, for Normal/Combination Skin** *($40 for 1.7 ounces)* contains more mulberry root extract than any of the other Hydra Bright Skin-Tone Perfecting products Lauder offers, which means that, at least based on limited in vitro research, it stands a remote chance of having a positive effect on skin discolorations. At least it would stand a chance if Lauder had chosen better packaging. As is, once you open this jar the potency of the plant extracts and antioxidants begins to deteriorate. There are enough antioxidants in this product to want to salvage them with better packaging, while the amount of cell-communicating and skin-identical ingredients is, by comparison, nearly insignificant. This silicone-enhanced moisturizer isn't the best for combination skin, especially if it is prone to breakouts. It is preferred for normal to dry skin, but the choice of packaging really should be a deal-breaker.

☹ $$$ **Hydra Bright Skin-Tone Perfecting Moisturizer Crème, for Dry Skin** *($40 for 1.7 ounces)* is the cream version of Lauder's Hydra Bright Skin-Tone Perfecting Lotion, for Normal/Combination Skin. It makes the same radiance-boosting, skin discoloration–banishing claims, but cannot deliver on the latter. Although this contains a heftier amount of antioxidants and cell-communicating ingredients, the jar packaging won't keep them potent once you begin using the product. That's a shame, because in many ways (although not for skin discolorations), this is a state-of-the-art moisturizer for its intended skin type.

ESTEE LAUDER IDEALIST PRODUCTS

☹ $$$ **Idealist Dual-Action Refinishing Treatment** *($49.50 for 2.5 ounces)* purports to combine the benefits of microdermabrasion with a 30% glycolic acid (AHA) peel, but it is really just a scrub with a fancy name. Interestingly, the formula doesn't contain any AHAs; instead, it contains acetyl glucosamine and salicylic acid, which is beta hydroxy acid (BHA). Acetyl glucosamine doesn't have convincing research proving its exfoliating ability (only the Lauder companies seem to think it works in this manner), and the salicylic acid cannot exfoliate because the product pH is well above 4. The pH is above 4 because the main ingredient is magnesium sulfate, which when mixed with water forms a solution with a pH of approximately 6 (Source: www.drugs.com). The warming sensation on your skin is the result of a chemical reaction that occurs when magnesium sulfate is mixed with water. The warmth may feel nice and may make you think it's doing something for your skin, but it doesn't do a thing; it's just a high school chemistry class demonstration. Lauder claims this product opens pores, but pores cannot be opened and closed like window blinds, although this myth perpetuates like so many others. If anything, the heat this product generates can cause capillaries to surface and that can be a problem. In no way is this product similar to any 30% AHA peel; in fact, it isn't even close to being a good scrub. The silicone in this product makes it difficult to rinse, but it does leave a smooth finish.

☺ $$$ **Idealist Pore Minimizing Skin Refinisher** (*$46.50 for 1 ounce*) is Lauder's all-in-one solution to problems such as large pores, flaky skin, redness, and, of course, fine lines. It launched in Summer 2007 as a replacement for the company's original (and very popular) Idealist Skin Refinisher. What's the difference? Well, Lauder is now claiming that this product makes pores appear one-third smaller, instantly, and that this version contains three times more acetyl glucosamine than the original formula. It does indeed contain more acetyl glucosamine, but is that an advantage? Derived from sugar, acetyl glucosamine doesn't have known exfoliating properties (Lauder claims it helps unglue the bonds that hold dead skin cells to the surface, something a well-formulated AHA or BHA product accomplishes). Acetyl glucosamine's primary constituents are mucopolysaccharides and hyaluronic acid. Found in all parts of the skin, it has value as a water-binding agent and is effective (in high concentrations) for wound healing. There is also research (*Cellular-Molecular-Life-Science*, 53(2), February 1997, pages 131-140) showing that chitins (also known as chitosan, which is composed of acetyl glucosamine) can help in the complex process of wound healing. However, that is a few generations removed from acetyl glucosamine being included in a skin-care product. Procter & Gamble has published research on the skin-lightening effect of acetyl glucosamine when used at concentrations of 2% or more in combination with niacinamide (such as in their Olay Definity moisturizers), but although Lauder is likely using that amount, they left out niacinamide (Source: *Journal of Cosmetic Dermatology*, March 2007, pages 20-26). There are some notable ingredients in Idealist Pore Minimizing Skin Refinisher, but in terms of making skin look better and pores appear smaller, it does so mostly by cosmetic trickery. For example, the strong silicone base instantly makes skin look smoother, so it reflects light better, and it can temporarily fill in large pores and superficial lines. Cosmetic pigments (iron oxides, mica, and titanium dioxide) provide a brightening effect, imparting a "glow" to your skin. Beyond the light show, plant-based anti-inflammatory ingredients help minimize minor redness and antioxidants such as green tea help keep skin protected from free-radical damage. What's not good news is the inclusion of lavender and orange along with the fragrance components limonene and linalool. They're present in a greater amount than in the original Idealist, and may be potentially irritating, which keeps this product from earning a Paula's Pick. If you decide to give this a go, it is best for normal to oily skin.

✓☺ $$$ **Idealist Refinishing Eye Serum** (*$48 for 0.5 ounce*) is similar to the original Idealist product above, but the formula is updated to capitalize on the latest skin-care ingredients. Included in this water- and silicone-based gel-cream are long-proven emollients (petrolatum), several antioxidants (the packaging will keep them stable), state-of-the-art skin-identical ingredients, and anti-irritants. It won't minimize puffiness or significantly brighten the eye area, but it will protect skin and help it function more normally. This would be even better without the fragrance, but that's a minor complaint for such a thoughtfully formulated product. By the way, this can be used anywhere on the face—there is nothing in this product that makes it unique for the eye area.

ESTEE LAUDER NUTRITIOUS PRODUCTS

☹ **$$$ Nutritious Purifying 2-in-1 Foam Cleanser** *($18 for 4.2 ounces)* contains some plant oil and extracts that are nutritious when consumed as part of a healthy diet, but have no effect when massaged over skin and quickly rinsed off. Some of the potassium-based cleansing agents in this product are constituents of soap and as such they can be drying unless your skin is oily to very oily. This cleanser is an effective makeup remover.

☹ **$$$ Nutritious Vita-Mineral Infusing Eye Gel** *($32 for 0.5 ounce)*. Lauder's Nutritious sub-brand is their attempt to offer customers products that contain more natural ingredients than what they typically include in their other brands. Like many cosmetics companies, Lauder routinely includes natural ingredients in their products, many of which are helpful for skin. In the case of this lightweight gel moisturizer, almost all of the plants fall into that helpful category. The concern is that a couple of the plants (such as rosemary and tangerine) pose a risk of irritation for skin, and this risk increases when they're in a product meant for use in the eye area. Ironically, even though this eye gel has "mineral" in its name, the only mineral in the formula is manganese, and it's barely present. Manganese isn't a must for skin, but if you're going to position this product as containing minerals, they deserve more prominence. There are several antioxidants in this formula, including from plant sources. However, the jar packaging Lauder chose won't keep them stable during use, which is disappointing. This is otherwise a fairly standard gel moisturizer that isn't worth considering over Philosophy Eye Believe Deep Wrinkle Peptide Gel.

✓ ☺ **$$$ Nutritious Vita-Mineral Radiance Serum** *($40 for 1 ounce)* is very similar to other water-based serums from Lauder-owned brands. The mix of bells and whistles differs between the serums, with Lauder's Nutritious containing more food-based ingredients such as soy, pomegranate, and corn. However, both serums are shining example of how to formulate a state-of-the-art product that treats all skin types to many of the ingredients they need to maintain and ensure healthy functioning. Antioxidants and cell-communicating ingredients are present in appreciable amounts, which is what you want to see in a serum at any price point. This serum cannot increase natural cell turnover, so don't mistake it for an exfoliant.

☺ **Nutritious Vita-Mineral Moisture Gel Crème** *($36 for 1.7 ounces)* is a silky-textured, water-based moisturizer suitable for normal to slightly dry or slightly oily skin housed in a jar package. The packaging ends up negating the potency of the pomegranate and other antioxidants that make more than a cameo appearance in this product. In better packaging, this moisturizer would be highly recommended.

✓ ☺ **Nutritious Vita-Mineral Moisture Lotion** *($36 for 1.7 ounces)* isn't any more "nutritious" for your skin than any other well-formulated moisturizer, but it contains the usual Lauder assortment of beneficial ingredients. Skin is treated to a lightweight, slightly creamy texture that is best for those whose complexion is normal to dry (this is too emollient for oily areas). Several antioxidants are included, plus cell-communicating ingredients and some intriguing water-binding agents. The minerals in this product are scant and do not offer protection against irritants (my goodness, what claim isn't attached to minerals these days?), but the combination of ingredients in this moisturizer will strengthen skin's barrier and help it to become healthier.

✓ ☺ **$$$ Nutritious Vita-Mineral Lip Treatment** *($22 for 0.5 ounce)*. Think of this as a super-charged lip gloss that goes above and beyond other lip glosses; that is, it adds shine while preventing moisture loss. Although pricey, this balm-like gloss contains an impressive amount of vitamin E along with other antioxidants and some cell-communicating ingredients. The minerals are present, too, but there's no evidence they have any special revitalizing effect on lips or on skin anywhere else on the body. Nutritious Vita-Mineral Lip Treatment is fragrance-free, which makes it even more appealing, at least from the standpoint of not applying ingredients that may irritate lips.

ESTEE LAUDER PERFECTIONIST PRODUCTS

✓ ☺ **$$$ Perfectionist [CP+] Wrinkle Lifting Serum** *($80 for 1.7 ounces)* is a formidable option for all skin types. Interestingly, Lauder dropped the emphasis on works-like-Botox-without-painful-injections claims they made for the previous version of Perfectionist. Now, they're asking you to believe that this is their most effective wrinkle-fighting formula ever (if that's the case, why are they also selling numerous other ultra-pricey antiwrinkle products in their Re-Nutriv line or La Mer line?), because it begins stimulating collagen production in just two hours. There's no proof of that (Lauder never makes their research available for public scrutiny), but we do know that when skin is protected from sun damage and treated to the ingredients it needs to restore and defend itself, it will make plenty of healthy collagen on its own (skin loves making collagen and would do so in a controlled manner if we would just stop preventing that from taking place). It's not as though you can begin using this serum and within weeks your skin will have generated so much collagen that even the deeper, etched wrinkles will be a thing of the past. Besides, if this serum were as adept at generating collagen as claimed that would eventually be to your skin's detriment; too much collagen can result in bumpy skin that doesn't move naturally. Don't forget, excess collagen production is the basis of many scars, including surgical incision scars and deep wounds. Lauder still plays on the topical Botox claim, but in a far more subtle way. They've toned down the rhetoric about those awful "needles" and "injections." Instead, this version of Perfectionist is supposed to visibly immobilize lines with its "flexible elastomer," which is a fancy way of saying this silicone-based serum contains a polymer that works to temporarily fill in superficial lines by forming a flexible, invisible mesh (sort of like a girdle) on your skin's surface. Such technology and ingredients aren't unique to Lauder; you'll find it in similar serums that make firming or lifting claims; however, the effect is always temporary and how long it lasts depends on how expressive you are. Despite some antiaging claims that still qualify as over-the-top, there's no question that this is a sophisticated formula that does an excellent job of combining and supplying skin with a wide complement of beneficial ingredients. Some of those ingredients can notably improve your skin's appearance, and, yes, reduce the signs of aging, including, to some extent, wrinkles. If you're looking for peptides, this serum contains them, but they're certainly not front and center. Perhaps this is Lauder's way of acknowledging that peptides aren't the antiwrinkle wonder many companies make them out to be. They do have theoretical cell-communicating ability, but whether or not they can last in skin long enough to penetrate to where they could do the most good is unlikely. This serum does contain mineral pigments that cast a subtle glow, but that is a cosmetic effect not a skin-care benefit.

☺ **$$$ Perfectionist Correcting Concentrate for Deeper Facial Lines/Wrinkles** *($42 for 0.11 ounce)* is packaged in a pen-style applicator with an angled tip that supposedly allows you to zero in on your most troublesome expression lines and wrinkles. You're likely wondering if what gets dispensed can really relax lines and reduce the look of wrinkles. Forget about the relaxing part, because nothing in this product is capable of that feat. Lauder uses acetyl hexapeptide-3, also known as argireline, for this alleged effect, but it has never been proven to work as claimed. Even Botox doesn't relax wrinkles when applied topically, as opposed to being injected. This water- and silicone-based formula will help temporarily to smooth and fill in lines and wrinkles, making them look less apparent. It's a cosmetic effect, similar to what you get with lots of moisturizers. What's most exciting about this product is that it is jam-packed with ingredients that are beneficial to skin, including several antioxidants, cell-communicating ingredients, anti-irritants, and a plethora of ingredients that mimic the structure and function of healthy skin. So how come this Perfectionist product was not rated a Paula's Pick? In a word, alcohol. Although not present in an amount significant enough to cause irritation, it's listed before the many state-of-the-art ingredients, an unwelcome blemish on an otherwise spotless formulation. Perfectionist Correcting Concentrate is best for normal to dry skin, and is fragrance-free.

☺ **$$$ Perfectionist Correcting Concentrate for Lip Lines** *($35 for 0.08 ounce)* is meant to be the product to correct any flaws around your lips. The claims are literally mouth-watering: "In as fast as 1 week, the fine lip lines around your mouth look remarkably reduced as our exclusive BioSync Complex quickly strengthens skin's suspension and amplifies natural collagen levels. By Month 1 and beyond, deep vertical lip lines look lifted away, helping redefine the contours around your lips so they appear fuller, softer, more sensual." A great story, but it's just mumbo jumbo—it never says anything substantive. Lauder is careful never to state that the vertical lines around the lips will be eliminated, removed, gone forever, or done away with. Rather, they will only look lifted away, an optical illusion at best and one that doesn't have to be structural. What does "amplifies natural collagen levels" mean anyway? Any moisturizer can help skin build collagen, so that isn't unique to this concoction. Like any moisturizer, the effect is hardly unique and is bound to be short-lived unless you make a concerted effort to keep your mouth perfectly still all day long, which isn't realistic. The happy face rating pertains to this product's overall formulation as an aid to making skin around the lips look better, not to Lauder's claims.

☺ **$$$ Perfectionist Power Correcting Patch for Deeper Eye Lines/Wrinkles** *($100 for 8 pairs)*. I remember a few years ago when a cosmetic chemist I know first showed me this kind of patch. He said, "These are going to be the next big thing" and then he laughed, adding "and these are the biggest do-nothing products since astringents with alcohol." He was right. The claims for Lauder's eye-area patches are much longer than the ingredient list, which is little more than water, film-forming agents (think hairspray), slip agent, thickener, a peptide, more slip agent, and preservative. The claims of reducing wrinkles via "micro-current" energy sound intriguing, but are completely bogus. There are no micro-currents being generated by these ordinary ingredients. What you might experience is your skin feeling smoother after the patch dries and you peel it off; sort of like peeling glue off the back of your hand when you were in grade school. The effect is temporary at best, and not helpful in the least. Looking at the price, you're spending $12.50 per pair to put hairspray around your eyes. Lauder offers far better products than this. Think twice, and then once more, before you invest in these gimmicky patches.

ESTEE LAUDER RE-NUTRIV PRODUCTS

☺ $$$ **Re-Nutriv Intensive Hydrating Crème Cleanser** *($39 for 4.2 ounces)* is an emollient, creamy cleanser for dry to very dry skin. It's pricey for what you get, but will hydrate and remove makeup efficiently (though not without the aid of a washcloth).

☹ $$$ **Re-Nutriv Crème** *($85 for 1.7 ounces)* is a very emollient, mineral oil–based moisturizer for dry skin. It does contain some good skin-identical ingredients and antioxidants, but jar packaging won't keep the antioxidants stable.

☹ $$$ **Re-Nutriv Intensive Lifting Crème** *($160 for 1.7 ounces)* is a good moisturizer with lots of good skin-identical ingredients, antioxidants, and anti-irritants, but there is nothing in it that will lift skin anywhere, and the price is nothing less than obscene given the ingredient list and jar packaging. Estee Lauder charges a lot less for other moisturizers that have a similar ingredient list and are appropriately packaged to keep the light- and air-sensitive ingredients stable during use.

☹ $$$ **Re-Nutriv Intensive Lifting Eye Crème** *($85 for 0.5 ounce)* is a very emollient eye cream for dry to very dry skin, but it won't lift skin or reduce dark circles. It comes up comparably short in antioxidants, but even if they were there in abundance, jar packaging wouldn't keep them stable once the product is opened.

☹ $$$ **Re-Nutriv Intensive Lifting Crème for Throat and Décolletage** *($100 for 1.7 ounces)* is a good emollient moisturizer for dry skin that contains a good mix of plant oils, skin-identical ingredients, and a small amount of antioxidants. There is nothing in this formulation that makes it better for the throat and chest area than for the face, and the jar packaging is disappointing.

✓ ☺ $$$ **Re-Nutriv Intensive Lifting Serum** *($180 for 1 ounce)* boasts it is Lauder's "ultimate" antiaging/repair formula, which you'd think would leave the hundred-plus other antiaging/repair products the Lauder company sells unnecessary and superfluous. But aside from that realization, does this live up to that lofty assertion? It isn't all that ultimate in the least. Without question, there are some extraordinary ingredients in this product that can make a difference in the health, resilience, and appearance of skin. The packaging is such that the many antioxidants and the cell-communicating ingredient retinol will remain stable during use, but you don't need to spend this much to get the advantageous ingredients that make this product a winner. Lauder's Perfectionist [CP+] Wrinkle Lifting Serum and their Advanced Night Repair Concentrate Recovery Boosting Treatment offer similar benefits (albeit with different textures), and Clinique has equally impressive options in their Repairwear line. The base formula of this Re-Nutriv serum is preferred for normal to dry skin.

✓ ☺ $$$ **Re-Nutriv Intensive Softening Lotion** *($40 for 8.4 ounces)* is an incredibly well-formulated toner that's chock-full of helpful ingredients for all skin types, including antioxidants and cell-communicating ingredients. If you're going to spend a lot of money on a toner, this option has visible rewards! One caution: Lauder included gold in this product, likely to reinforce their marketing of Re-Nutriv as luxury skin care. If you have metal allergies (such as to nickel), this may be a problem; research has shown those with nickel allergies often have a similar though less-intense response to skin contact with other metals, including gold (Source: *Clinical and Experimental Immunology*, December 2006, pages 417-426).

☺ $$$ **Re-Nutriv Re-Creation Day Crème SPF 15 and Re-Creation Night Crème** *($900 for 3.4 ounces)* tries to justify its astonishingly high price by not only being a two-piece set, but also by showcasing the fact that these products are "endowed with tomorrow's science, including eight U.S. and international patents pending." Lauder's idea of tomorrow's science includes using "a wealth of rare plants and minerals known to create life, respond to natural stresses, and promote longevity." That point deserves additional explanation, because it sounds amazingly helpful. It is true that countless plants have internal support systems that allow them to survive and in many cases thrive, despite constant exposure to the elements and sunlight, but that doesn't translate to humans. The natural systems that a growing plant uses to sustain itself are built around antioxidants and other cellular ingredients responsible for defending a plant from environmental aggressors. Yet that process in a living plant doesn't explain what happens when a portion of it is uprooted, extracted, and chemically treated to be mixed into a cosmetic product. The plant extracts used in the products below have antioxidant capability, but they cannot transfer their own life-sustaining benefits to your skin, so please don't think that this Re-Nutriv duo is the antiwrinkle answer we've all been waiting for. Further, patents have nothing to do with proof of efficacy. Patent law is about establishing a unique ingredient or group of ingredients that can't be used by anyone else. That doesn't mean the ingredients work or have any purpose whatsoever; in a cosmetic, it is all marketing hype and legalese that has nothing to do with the well-being of your skin. Turning to the products, **Re-Nutriv Re-Creation Day Crème SPF 15** includes avobenzone for UVA protection and has a silky, lightweight cream texture suitable for normal to slightly dry skin. However, jar packaging spells an unstable future for the many antioxidants in this product (one more example of how antioxidants from plants are subject to deterioration when removed from their living source), which is a major misstep from a product costing $450. All you'll be getting is an elegantly textured daytime moisturizer with sunscreen—and how liberally are you going to apply this product knowing its cost is equivalent to a monthly automobile payment? **Re-Creation Night Crème** is not only disappointing due to jar packaging, but also, for the money, it lacks many of the state-of-the-art ingredients found in dozens of other Lauder moisturizers. Talk about insulting a consumer's intelligence! Yes, there are some unusual species of seaweed in this moisturizer, but the other antioxidants and cell-communicating ingredients are also found in other products that wouldn't dare charge this much (and seaweed is not a cure-all for aging skin, nor is it an expensive ingredient to include in a product). In summation, this duo is more dour than dynamic, and won't give skin of any age a new lease on life.

☺ **$$$ Re-Nutriv Lightweight Crème** (*$85 for 1.7 ounces*) is an emollient but overall lackluster formula compared to most other Lauder moisturizers, including those selling for half this price. The "Lightweight" portion of the name is misleading due to this moisturizer's oil content.

☹ **$$$ Re-Nutriv Revitalizing Comfort Crème** (*$120 for 1.7 ounces*) is another Lauder moisturizer for dry skin that contains dozens of light- and air-sensitive ingredients subject to deterioration once this jar-packaged product is opened. This has merit, but why would you want to spend so much for ingredients that won't remain stable?

☺ **$$$ Re-Nutriv Revitalizing Comfort Eye Crème** (*$65 for 0.5 ounce*) is similar to the Re-Nutriv Intensive Lifting Eye Crème below, and the same review applies. This is a very emollient eye cream for dry to very dry skin, but it won't lift skin or reduce dark circles. It comes up comparably short in antioxidants, but even if they were there in abundance, jar packaging wouldn't keep them stable once the product is opened. In some respects, this is a better formula, but it doesn't deserve more than a neutral face rating because of jar packaging.

☺ **$$$ Re-Nutriv Ultimate Lifting Eye Crème** (*$100 for 0.5 ounce*) promises to be "the most extravagant eye care you've ever experienced." Well, along with ignoring that, you can also ignore this product's claims of reducing the appearance of dark circles and puffiness—even today's best skin-care formulations cannot effectively remedy these common complaints. This product is remarkably similar to Lauder's Re-Nutriv Intensive Lifting Eye Crème, and once again jar packaging makes this a less desirable option. The texture feels extravagant, but it won't perform as claimed. This product is fragrance-free.

✓ ☺ $$$ **Re-Nutriv Ultimate Lifting Serum** *($200 for 1 ounce)* claims to be the ultimate repair product, which is odd because so do several other Lauder products. You have to wonder, if they are all advertised as ultimate, how do you know which one really is the best? It's not this option, but only because of its prohibitive price. There is much to applaud about this formula, whose chief antioxidant is pomegranate. Another major ingredient is a species of mushroom known as *Inonotus obliquus*, which has no research pertaining to its benefit for skin. However, one study demonstrated its anti-tumor capability when one if its triterpenoid extracts was applied to mouse skin (Source: *Bioorganic and Medicinal Chemistry*, January 2007, pages 257-264). Other antioxidants and cell-communicating ingredients are present, along with some plant extracts that have no established benefit for skin, but nevertheless provide the "everything-but-the-kitchen-sink" image to make you think it is jam-packed with good-for-skin ingredients. Although this is an impressive product, it isn't worth considering over Lauder's Advanced Night Repair Concentrate, Perfectionist [CP+] Wrinkle Lifting Serum, or Lauder-owned Clinique's Repairwear Deep Wrinkle Concentrate for Face and Eyes. If you choose to splurge on this option, at least you can do so knowing you're getting a well-formulated product.

☹ $$$ **Re-Nutriv Ultimate Youth Eye Crème** *($100 for 0.5 ounce).* First things first: For $100, you shouldn't have to deal with an eye cream packaged in a jar. Not only does hygiene become an issue, but in addition almost all of the state-of-the-art ingredients Lauder included will lose their efficacy because of consistent exposure to light and air, which causes the air-sensitive ingredients (think plants, vitamins, antioxidants, and the like) to deteriorate after opening. It may seem impressive and cost-worthy that this eye cream contains pearl powder, gold, and a "Youth Molecule" (that's how Lauder describes the form of the antioxidant resveratrol included in this product), but it's meaningless on two fronts: pearl powder and gold have no special benefit for skin and although resveratrol is a potent antioxidant, it is neither a youth-restoring miracle nor the best antioxidant available. But, all of that is moot because of the aforementioned jar packaging, which means the potency of the resveratrol and the many other antioxidants in this eye cream will rapidly degrade after opening.

☹ $$$ **Re-Nutriv Ultimate Lifting Crème** *($250 for 1.7 ounces)* wants to endow your skin with amazing powers, but this isn't a Superhero secret—it's just another well-formulated moisturizer for normal to dry skin that includes many antioxidants (though not as many as some less expensive Lauder moisturizers), which won't last long once this jar-packaged product is opened. The radiance and "next generation optical effects" come from the pearl powder, mica, and titanium dioxide in the formula. This isn't futuristic, it's a commonplace way to manipulate the way light reflects off skin and is found in many other products, including Lauder's antioxidant-rich, well-packaged Spotlight Skin Tone Perfector. What would really make this the ultimate moisturizer is opaque, pump-bottle packaging and even greater amounts of antioxidants.

☹ $$$ **Re-Nutriv Ultimate Youth Crème** *($175 for 1 ounce)* carries a price tag that by itself should give you pause, but likely won't because statistically, consumers are spending more money on luxury skin-care products like this than ever before, even at the expense of other necessities. Of course, Lauder has a story and claims to support this product's price tag, and it begins with what they refer to as a "Youth Molecule" and "the prestige of 23 patents pending worldwide," all to help your skin look younger now and "far into the future." We've heard this song before, just the lyrics are slightly different this time. Patent-pending may sound impressive (and 23 of them? My goodness!), but that has nothing at all to do with whether or not the formula works as claimed (patents have nothing to do with efficacy, just use). What is worth some explanation is their Youth Molecule, which Lauder refers to as Resveratrate. The company maintains it "is a more potent, stable and time released form of Resveratrol, and was shown by in vitro testing to provide 6 times more protection from environmental damage, more than doubling the survival rate of skin cells." Resveratrol, derived from red grapes, is indeed a potent antioxidant (Sources: *Journal of Cosmetic Dermatology*, March 2008, pages 2-7; *Photochemistry and Photobiology*, January 23, 2008, Epublication; and *Experimental Dermatology*, September 2006, pages 678-684). How does resveratrol compare to Lauder's Resveratrate? According to the scientists who discovered this molecule, "while resveratrol is effective, it has limited solubility and instability in high concentrations. Resveratrate, however, is said to allow the molecule to penetrate deeply into the skin creating a reservoir for the skin to draw upon." That sounds promising, but it doesn't explain why Lauder ignored the need to keep this ingredient and the many other antioxidants in Re-Nutriv Ultimate Youth Crème protected from light and air exposure. A moisturizer this loaded with antioxidants demands opaque, non-jar packaging, but Lauder didn't go that route. That means you're essentially paying top dollar for what amounts to a silky, emollient moisturizer for dry to very dry skin. Lauder goes on to claim their Resveratrate molecule interacts with a protein in our skin (SIRT1, one of seven identified sirtuins in mammals that seem to have some amount of genetic control over how we age) and this interaction prolongs the life span of epidermal cells. But if you think about it, prolonging the life span of our skin cells doesn't net younger-looking skin. All that really means (assuming the technology works, which is doubtful in the case of this product) is that anyone using this cream (and it is marketed to women over age 40) will see the skin cells they have now last longer. Is that healthy? Not if the person's epidermal cells are sun-damaged or dry or irritated, and none of this addresses the numerous other factors of aging that are seen in skin. And of course, prolonging the life of any cell may lead to problems as we interfere with the body's pre-programmed system of replacing old cells with new ones. The bottom line is that the antiaging technology supposedly built into this product has limited research proving its worth, and if it is effective, the choice of jar packaging negates any benefit your skin cells may have received.

☺ **$$$ Re-Nutriv Intensive Lifting Mask** *($70 for 1.7 ounces)* is a very good moisturizing mask for normal to dry skin, but for the money, the formula cannot compete with Lauder's superior, less expensive Resilience Lift Extreme Ultra Firming Mask.

☺ **$$$ Re-Nutriv Intensive Soothing Hand Creme** *($45 for 3.4 ounces)* has a beautifully smooth, emollient texture that works great to make dry, rough hands feel and look immensely better. Most of the plant extracts it contains are helpful for skin, but some (e.g., *Coleus forskohlii*) are potentially problematic. Lauder also included gold in this hand cream, but it and other precious metals are known to cause contact dermatitis, and gold doesn't convey any benefit to skin. On balance, this hand cream contains many more beneficial ingredients than troublesome ones, and deserves consideration if you don't mind spending more than necessary to treat dryness. Some of the plant ingredients have the potential to lighten skin discolorations, but only if you pair this hand cream with a sunscreen rated SPF 15 or greater that contains the right UVA-protecting ingredients.

ESTEE LAUDER RESILIENCE LIFT PRODUCTS

☺ **$$$ Resilience Lift Extreme Overnight Ultra Firming Crème** *($75 for 1.7 ounces)* is supposed to use exclusive nighttime technology to lift and firm skin by "taking advantage of skin's own restorative rhythms," but if that's true, then the same claim can be applied to most of Lauder's moisturizers. This formula doesn't distinguish itself from the pack, and includes a similar complement of antioxidants, cell-communicating ingredients, emollients, and ingredients that mimic the structure and function of healthy skin. It's a shame an otherwise superior moisturizer for normal to dry skin has jar packaging to hinder the effectiveness of its antioxidants.

☹ **Resilience Lift Extreme Ultra Firming Crème SPF 15, for Dry Skin** *($70 for 1.7 ounces)* lacks the UVA-protecting ingredients of titanium dioxide, zinc oxide, avobenzone, Tinosorb, or Mexoryl SX, and is not recommended.

☺ **$$$ Resilience Lift Extreme Ultra Firming Crème SPF 15, for Very Dry Skin** *($70 for 1.7 ounces)* provides the UVA protection missing in the Resilience Lift Extreme Ultra Firming Crème SPF 15, for Dry Skin, but the amount of titanium dioxide (0.9%) may still leave skin vulnerable to UVA damage. This is otherwise an exceptionally emollient formula whose many antioxidants are at risk for quick deterioration due to jar packaging.

☺ **$$$ Resilience Lift Extreme Ultra Firming Eye Crème** *($50 for 0.5 ounce)* is similar to, but has a lighter texture and fewer bells and whistles than, the Re-Nutriv Intensive Lifting Eye Crème above, and the same basic comments (including jar packaging) apply. The "luminizing optics" are just cosmetic pigments that reflect light from skin, cosmetically minimizing shadowed areas around the eye.

✓☺ **$$$ Resilience Lift Extreme Ultra Firming Lotion SPF 15, for Normal/Combination Skin** *($70 for 1.7 ounces)* bests the other Resilience Lift Extreme moisturizers with sunscreen, not only because it contains more titanium dioxide for UVA protection, but also because it has much better packaging. As a result, this is a winning option for normal to dry skin (it's not the best for use over oily areas, so isn't appealing for combination skin) provided you aren't hooked by the lifting and firming claims, which won't materialize. What this does do is provide reliable sun protection in an elegant moisturizing base that contains a state-of-the-art mix of antioxidants and cell-communicating ingredients. Liberal application is necessary to ensure protection, so you have to be OK with replacing this fairly often to avoid putting your skin at risk for sun damage, but other than that caveat, go for it.

✓☺ **$$$ Resilience Lift Extreme Ultra Firming Mask** *($40 for 2.5 ounces)* takes an everything-but-the-kitchen-sink approach to skin care, and includes almost every major emollient, antioxidant, water-binding agent, skin-identical substance, and cell-communicating ingredient I've ever heard of. It's certainly a powerhouse formula for dry to very dry skin and is best left on as a moisturizer rather than used occasionally as a mask to be rinsed off. This mask is supposed to revitalize skin with advanced lifting and firming technology, but it can't do that. It doesn't even contain ingredients that create a temporary tightening effect and that are often used in products to convince you that your skin really is being firmed and lifted. However, as long as you're not banking on this product being a face-lift in a tube, it is without question a formidable moisturizer that treats dry skin to a bevy of ingredients that will improve its feel and appearance.

ESTEE LAUDER TIME ZONE PRODUCTS

☺ **$$$ Time Zone Anti-Line/Wrinkle Eye Creme** *($43.50 for 0.5 ounce)* is the eye-area counterpart to Lauder's overhyped Time Zone moisturizers. Other than being more emollient, there is nothing about it that makes it specially formulated for the eye area. The claims mention that this eye cream is "so powerful" that every woman showed a reduction in the look of lines and wrinkles. This sounds mighty impressive until you realize that simply improving the look of lines and wrinkles, which any moisturizer will do, is a cosmetic effect. Not to mention how many times we've heard this before about countless other products the Lauder corporation sells. What Lauder and most other cosmetics companies know, women never tire of being hit with the same claims over and over and over again. As usual for most Lauder moisturizers, this is loaded with beneficial ingredients, including many antioxidants and cell-communicating ingredients. Unfortunately, it shares the all-too-common trait of jar packaging, which means those exciting, air-sensitive ingredients won't remain potent for long after opening. In this case, that can be construed as a good thing. Why? Because Lauder included a potentially irritating amount of rosemary and tangerine extracts, and irritation isn't what you want for skin anywhere, especially on the face.

☹ **$$$ Time Zone Line & Wrinkle Reducing Moisturizer SPF 15 Dry Crème** *($58 for 1.7 ounces)*. Every time Lauder launches a new line of antiwrinkle moisturizers, the questions come pouring in. Women don't seem to make the connection that just a couple months before, Lauder was lauding (pun intended) another group of antiwrinkle products with astonishing claims. Now that those products have had their day in the fashion magazines and their marketing impact has waned, it's time to promote another group, even though the claims differ little between them. I suppose the curiosity about the Time Zone products comes from the attention-getting claim that they take 10 years off the look of your skin in 4 weeks. That would certainly grab my attention, but if you stop and think, it really isn't a claim we haven't heard before, from Lauder and numerous other lines. If skin is rough and dry and you put a moisturizer on you're going to look younger, but you don't need this product to achieve that. Examining the ingredient list for this product reveals that it truly isn't different from most other daytime moisturizers with sunscreen, sold by Lauder and other companies. So do all of those take 10 years off, too? It was an interesting experience at the Estee Lauder counter asking several sales representatives what made the Time Zone products different or more special when compared to Lauder's DayWear, Re-Nutriv, and Resilience Lift brands. They stumbled about and really couldn't come up with a good answer, finally just saying that it was a good product. My advice? Ignore the decade-erasing claim because it won't show up in the mirror no matter how long you use this product. It provides sufficient sun protection (which is the only legitimate wrinkle-reducing claim that can be made for this product) and it has a creamy texture suitable for normal to dry skin. However, and this is the key reason why you shouldn't spend money on this product, the jar packaging undermines the effectiveness of the numerous antioxidants Lauder included. Just like many of their moisturizers, the overall formula is incredibly sophisticated and chock-full of potentially beneficial ingredients—if only they were packaged to retain their potency once you opened this product and started using it!

☹ **$$$ Time Zone Line & Wrinkle Reducing Moisturizer SPF 15 Normal/Combination Crème** *($58 for 1.7 ounces)* is a daytime moisturizer with an in-part avobenzone sunscreen, and is similar to but slightly less emollient than Estee Lauder's Time Zone Line & Wrinkle Reducing Moisturizer SPF 15 Dry Crème above. As such, the same review and comments apply.

By the way, this is only suitable for combination skin if you do not apply it to oily areas (yet not doing so leaves those areas vulnerable to sun damage, so you'd be better off using a lighter weight moisturizer).

✓ ☺ **$$$ Time Zone Line & Wrinkle Reducing Moisturizer SPF 15 Normal/Combination Lotion** ($58 for 1.7 ounces). It was an interesting experience at the Estee Lauder counter to ask several sales representatives what made the Time Zone products different or more special when compared to Lauder's DayWear, Re-Nutriv, and Resilience Lift brands. They stumbled about and really couldn't come up with an answer, finally just saying that it was a good product. My advice? Ignore the decade-erasing claim because it won't show up in the mirror no matter how long you use this product. It provides sufficient sun protection (which is the only legitimate wrinkle-reducing claim that can be made for this product) and it has a creamy texture suitable for normal to dry skin. However, unlike Lauder's other Time Zone moisturizers, which are packaged in jars, this is packaged in an opaque pump bottle. That means that in addition to an in-part avobenzone sunscreen, you're getting lots of antioxidants, cell-communicating ingredients, and some decent water-binding agents and they will remain stable once you start using it. The base formula isn't as light as many with combination skin would prefer, but it's acceptable and certainly worth a trial run. Despite my enthusiasm for the formula and the packaging, as I mentioned, there isn't much difference between the Time Zone daytime moisturizers and those with sunscreen from Lauder's other sub-brands. If you're using DayWear or Resilience Lift with good results, there's no need to try Time Zone—it isn't the one group of Lauder products finally telling you the truth about youth in a bottle. And keep in mind that any well-formulated daytime moisturizer with sunscreen can do what this product claims to do (and I don't mean subtracting 10 or more years from your face): it can protect your skin from sun damage while allowing it to repair past damage (to an extent) and can encourage a healthy barrier function so your skin is better able to defend itself against future signs of aging. Now that's the kind of time zone I'd prefer to live in, and Lauder doesn't have a corner on this arena!

ESTEE LAUDER VERITE PRODUCTS

✓ ☺ **$$$ Verite LightLotion Cleanser** ($23.50 for 6.7 ounces) is an emollient, cold cream-style cleanser that is an option for someone with dry, sensitive, or reddened skin not prone to breakouts. Its merit for sensitive skin earns it a Paula's Pick rating.

☺ **$$$ Verite Calming Fluid** ($60 for 1.7 ounces) is a fragrance-free, lightweight moisturizing lotion that's sort of a stripped-down version of other Lauder moisturizers. It contains significantly fewer antioxidants, and the soothing agents should have been more prominent. Still, it's an option for normal to slightly oily skin and leaves a silky finish.

☺ **$$$ Verite Moisture Relief Crème** ($50 for 1.7 ounces) is a standard, slightly emollient moisturizer for normal to slightly dry skin. The jar packaging won't keep the minor amount of antioxidants stable once opened, but it is fragrance-free.

✓ ☺ **$$$ Verite Special EyeCare** ($37.50 for 0.5 ounce) is a very emollient, water-based moisturizer that contains a good mix of skin-identical ingredients, antioxidants, and cell-communicating ingredients. Like all Verite products, this is fragrance-free.

OTHER ESTEE LAUDER PRODUCTS

☺ **$$$ Perfectly Clean Light Lotion Cleanser** ($23 for 6.7 ounces) is a water-based emollient cleansing lotion that does not contain detergent cleansing agents, so it is a good option for dry to very dry skin. This product can do a reasonably good job of removing makeup, but you may need to pair it with a washcloth or wipe it off altogether to ensure complete removal.

☺ $$$ **Perfectly Clean Splash Away Foaming Cleanser** *($19 for 4.2 ounces)* lists alkaline and drying potassium myristate as the main cleansing agents, so this will be a problem cleanser for all skin types except very oily. It does remove makeup completely, but is nearly akin to washing with standard bar soap.

☺ $$$ **Soft Clean Moisture Rich Foaming Cleanser** *($19 for 4.2 ounces)* is a creamy, cushiony cleanser whose potassium-derived cleansing base can produce a copious foam, although that has little to do with a product's cleansing abilities. This can be a good, water-soluble cleanser for normal to slightly dry or slightly oily skin. It contains more fragrance than Lauder's other cleansers.

☺ $$$ **Soft Clean Tender Crème Cleanser** *($19 for 4.2 ounces)* is a standard cleansing cream for normal to dry skin. It does not contain detergent cleansing agents, but it can remove most types of makeup without the aid of a washcloth. Used around the eyes (to remove eye makeup or mascara), it can leave a greasy film that is not preferred, especially when compared with a silicone-based makeup remover or water-soluble cleanser. For the money, you may want to try Dove Pro-Age Foaming Facial Cleanser over this pricier option.

☹ **Sparkling Clean Oil-Control Foaming Gel Cleanser** *($23 for 6.7 ounces)* is a somewhat drying water-soluble cleanser that would have been an option for oily skin, but the inclusion of irritating menthyl lactate makes it a less than sparkling option.

☹ **Sparkling Clean Purifying Mud Foam Cleanser** *($19 for 4.2 ounces)* is a water-soluble foaming cleanser that contains soap-based potassium myristate as its main cleansing agent. It can be drying for all but very oily skin, especially with the "mud" (clay) thrown in. The deal-breaker is the addition of irritating menthyl lactate, which won't purify skin in the least.

☺ $$$ **Gentle Eye Makeup Remover** *($15.50 for 3.4 ounces)* is a very standard, but effective, fragrance-free, detergent-based eye-makeup remover. Several less expensive versions at the drugstore easily replace this, but it's an option if you want to spend more.

☺ $$$ **Take It Away LongWear Makeup Remover Towelettes** *($17.50 for 45 towelettes)* feature a formula that is remarkably similar to that of the Gentle Eye Makeup Remover, only steeped into disposable towelettes. This product is not adept at removing long-wearing or waterproof makeup and ideally should be rinsed from skin because, left on, the detergent cleansing agent can be drying.

☺ **Take It Away Total Makeup Remover** *($22 for 6.7 ounces)* is a water-and-wax concoction with a lotion texture that does an efficient job of removing most makeup without irritating skin.

☹ $$$ **Perfectly Clean Fresh Balancing Lotion** *($19.50 for 6.7 ounces)* is a very standard toner that lists alcohol as the second ingredient, and that makes this too drying and irritating for all skin types, not to mention the alcohol will stimulate oil production in the pore lining. It cannot "balance" skin, and the exotic plant extracts are a mix of irritants and anti-irritants, which means that basically they cancel each other out.

☺ $$$ **Soft Clean Silky Hydrating Lotion** *($19.50 for 6.7 ounces)* is one of the most original and skin-beneficial toners in the Estee Lauder line, and would be a great option for normal to dry skin. It is alcohol-free and contains mostly water, silicone, thickener, slip agent, plant extracts (including fragrant floral extracts), skin-identical ingredients, an emollient, an anti-irritant, Vaseline, film-forming agent, fragrance, and preservatives. The tiny amount of caffeine is unlikely to be a problem, but this toner is a bit too fragrant for someone with very sensitive skin.

☹ **Sparkling Clean Mattifying Oil-Control Lotion** *($19.50 for 6.7 ounces)* lists alcohol as the second ingredient, which is drying and irritating for skin, plus it stimulates oil production in the pore lining. This also contains the alkaline ingredient barium sulfate, which is a potential skin irritant. Keep in mind that you can't "dry up" oil because it isn't wet. Drying ingredients also negatively affect skin cells, and that doesn't help skin in the least. Many better mattifying options are available, with one of the more interesting versions being Smashbox's Anti-Shine.

✓ ☺ **$$$ Fruition Extra Multi-Action Complex** *($73 for 1.7 ounces)* contains a blend of synthetic hydroxy acids along with salicylic acid (BHA), but the total amount is very likely less than 1%, and the pH of 4.1 is just above the acceptable range for exfoliation to occur. So why the excellent rating? Although this won't exfoliate skin to the same degree that a well-formulated AHA or BHA product will, the silky lotion formula has a potent amount of antioxidant green tea and contains several other well-researched antioxidants as well as soothing agents, plus a cell-communicating ingredient. It is an excellent moisturizer for slightly oily to oily skin (I know, I know, Lauder positions this as a treatment product, but at its heart it is just a well-formulated moisturizer).

☺ **$$$ So Polished Exfoliating Scrub** *($22 for 3.4 ounces)* could also be named "So Expensive Exfoliating Scrub" because, although it's an effective topical scrub option for normal to oily skin, it differs little from those available in the drugstore for one-third the price.

☹ **$$$ Age-Controlling Crème** *($63.50 for 1.7 ounces)* has jar packaging and is one of Lauder's oldest moisturizers. Antioxidants are in short supply, but my goodness is this emollient! It would be very effective for someone with painfully dry skin.

☹ **Clear Difference Advanced Oil-Control Hydrator** *($32.50 for 1.7 ounces)* lists alcohol as the second ingredient, and that makes this otherwise fine moisturizer a problem for all skin types. This product does not contain ingredients that can keep skin "hydrated inside, perfectly matte outside." Rather, the predominance of alcohol keeps the moisturizing ingredients from doing their job and stimulates oil production in the pore lining. How unfortunate, because the price is downright affordable (for a Lauder moisturizer, anyway) and this contains some excellent skin-identical ingredients (though few antioxidants).

☺ **$$$ Estoderme Emulsion** *($30 for 4 ounces)* is an emollient moisturizer for dry skin that contains some good skin-identical ingredients and antioxidants, though not to the extent of several other options from Lauder.

☹ **Eyzone Repair Gel** *($38.50 for 0.5 ounce)* contains the preservatives methylisothiazolinone and methylchloroisothiazolinone (Kathon CG), which are contraindicated for use in leave-on products due to their sensitizing potential (Sources: *Contact Dermatitis*, November 2001, pages 257-264; and *European Journal of Dermatology*, March 1999, pages 144-160).

☹ **$$$ Hydra Complete Multi-Level Moisture Eye Gel Crème** *($38.50 for 0.5 ounce)*. Just like most of Lauder's moisturizers, whether they're sold for use in the eye area or not, this one has a beautifully silky texture and contains an impressive amount of antioxidants along with some notable skin-identical and cell-communicating ingredients. Unfortunately, those ingredients (which skin needs) won't remain potent once this product is in use because of the jar packaging. You're left with a moisturizer for slightly dry skin anywhere on the face, but that's it. The algae extract in this eye cream won't reduce puffiness over time. If it could, why not just use the pure substance on skin instead of the tiny amount in this product?

☹ **$$$ Skin Perfecting Crème Firming Nourisher** *($38 for 1.7 ounces)* is an OK moisturizing cream for normal to slightly dry skin. There is no reason to consider this one over hundreds of other more modern formulas (with better packaging).

☺ **$$$ Spotlight Skin Tone Perfector** *($32 for 1.7 ounces)* provides a soft, radiant glow thanks to the cosmetic pigments it contains. They won't make skin look perfect in every light, but can enliven dull, sallow skin, and the silicone-enriched moisturizing base contains some reliable antioxidants and soothing agents.

☹ **Swiss Performing Extract** *($42 for 3.4 ounces)* is another long-time moisturizer from Lauder, and although it is based around emollient, antioxidant grape seed oil and comes in stable packaging, the fragrance components (including eugenol), which are not present in many other moisturizers in this line, are irritating.

☹ **Body Performance Anti-Cellulite/Anti-Fluid Advanced Visible Contouring Serum** *($52.50 for 6.7 ounces)* is another anticellulite gel that lists alcohol as the second ingredient, so expect dryness, irritation, and free-radical damage, because that's what you get from alcohol. This also contains two types of menthol and several plant extracts that have the potential to cause irritation. These assaults may make dimpled skin look temporarily better due to the swelling action they cause, but with daily use, these ingredients break down skin's support structures; so, eventually your cellulite will be even more apparent.

☺ **$$$ Body Performance Firming Body Creme** *($37.50 for 6.7 ounces)* is a surprisingly simple (for Lauder) yet elegant body moisturizer formula. It contains some good emollients, a form of silicone, several antioxidants, and a cell-communicating ingredient. Unfortunately, the jar packaging inhibits the long-term effectiveness of the ingredients you're paying extra for because they all are air sensitive and won't stay stable once you've taken the lid off. As for the consumer testing results, is it really that impressive to find out that 98% of women said their skin felt moisturized after using this product? The same seemingly enthusiastic statistic could be attributed to lots of moisturizers, or even to plain Vaseline.

✓ ☺ **$$$ Body Performance Naturally Radiant Moisturizer** *($35 for 6.7 ounces)* is an emollient self-tanning lotion for the body that browns skin with dihydroxyacetone, as with most self-tanning products. The difference? This option includes several skin-beneficial ingredients that are missing from most self-tanners, and that elevates its status.

☺ **Bronze Goddess Sun Indulgence Lotion for Face SPF 30** *($22 for 1.7 ounces)* is a tinted sunscreen with shimmer that contains avobenzone for sufficient UVA protection. Because the Bronze Goddess products are all about the seduction of tropical, exotic scents, this product is highly fragranced. It contains the usual assortment of beneficial ingredients we've come to expect from Lauder, but their effect on skin will be limited because the skin has to defend itself from the irritation caused by the amount of fragrance and the many fragrant plants in this product. This isn't one of Lauder's better sunscreens, but it's an acceptable option for normal to slightly dry skin.

☹ **Lip Conditioner SPF 15** *($16.50)* is basically a lipstick without pigment, but the fact that it does not contain the UVA-protecting ingredients of titanium dioxide, zinc oxide, avobenzone, Tinosorb, or Mexoryl SX makes it not worth considering.

ESTEE LAUDER MAKEUP

FOUNDATION: ✓ ☺ **$$$ Nutritious Vita-Mineral Loose Powder Makeup SPF 15** *($33.50)*. Minerals abound in this loose-powder foundation with a pure titanium dioxide sunscreen, but guess what—the main mineral is talc, a mineral that is present in almost any loose or pressed powder you'll come across. Clearly, Lauder doesn't want to denigrate talc the way many other mineral makeup lines choose to do, and that's great. In fact, the talc in this formula has a superfine texture that, combined with the silicone-based binding agents, creates this powder makeup's gossamer application and seamless finish. This is an outstanding "mineral makeup" that's more sheer than all the others I've reviewed to date. It glides over skin, blurring slight imperfections and leaving a faint shiny finish (the predominant finish is matte, making this best for normal to oily skin). Because this powder is used as an adjunct to your moisturizer or liquid foundation with sunscreen, you will get great added protection. On its own, however, you'd really have to pile it on to get the stated level of protection, and doing that would lend a slightly ashen look to every shade of this powder foundation. So, if you consider this a great finishing powder with sunscreen you're apt to love it. Avoid the Intensity 8.0 shade because it's too ash to look natural One more comment: the "nutritious" ingredients in this loose-powder foundation include antioxidant vitamins and plant extracts. They're an intriguing addition, but the packaging for this product won't keep them stable during use.

✓ ☺ **$$$ Resilience Lift Extreme Ultra Firming Crème Compact Makeup SPF 15** *($34.50)* deserves every bit of praise I am going to heap on it. Simply put, this is one of the best, if not the best, cream foundation I've seen in years. Lauder has crafted a compact foundation with an in-part titanium dioxide sunscreen that has an extraordinarily smooth texture. As such, it is a dream to blend, and sets to a natural matte yet slightly moist finish capable of providing medium to nearly full coverage without looking waxy or mask-like. The formula is best for normal to dry skin not prone to blemishes, and comes in 16 shades, almost all of which are recommended. Consider Outdoor Beige and Cognac carefully, and avoid the too peach Shell Beige. Cashew is a great neutral for medium skin tones, while Teak and Walnut are superb dark shades. Bravo!

☺ **$$$ Re-Nutriv Intensive Lifting Makeup SPF 15** *($65)* is elegantly packaged in a frosted-glass jar complete with golden cap and trim, and includes a titanium dioxide sunscreen. In contrast to the pricier Re-Nutriv Intensive Lifting Crème Makeup SPF 15, this has a silkier, silicone-based formula that blends down to a satin matte finish that is not at all emollient—nor something those with dry skin would enjoy. It's best for those with normal to slightly dry or slightly oily skin seeking medium coverage and a whatever-it-may-cost makeup. The ten shades are impressively neutral, with the exceptions being Outdoor Beige and Auburn, both of which are too rose to look convincing. This foundation is not capable of lifting the skin, but it will lift lots of money from your bank account.

☺ **$$$ Re-Nutriv Ultimate Lifting Crème Makeup SPF 15** *($80)* is Lauder's most expensive foundation, and your first question may be, "Is it worth the money?" Although this creamy foundation has a lot going for it, the answer is "no." It has a titanium dioxide–based sunscreen, which is great for protecting skin, but so do countless other foundations that cost significantly less. Lauder goes on and on about the skin-care technology behind this foundation, but it won't lift skin in the least. The base formula isn't nearly as exciting as many of their well-formulated moisturizers, plus the jar packaging won't keep the antioxidants in here stable. Texture-wise, this is extra rich, almost to the point of being greasy. It slides over skin and is easy to blend, but doesn't ever set, so you're left with a creamy finish that must be set with powder. You'll get medium coverage without much effort, and it's hard to get less than that, even if you apply a sheer layer (but don't do that because you'll cheat your skin of the sun protection it needs). Ten shades are available, and most of them are very good. Avoid the too-rose Outdoor Beige and Auburn. Based on the emollience of this foundation, I recommend it only for someone with dry to very dry skin, assuming you're willing to pay the exorbitant price.

☺ **$$$ Re-Nutriv Ultimate Radiance Makeup SPF 15** *($80)* is one of the most expensive foundations sold in department stores, and the extra expense gets you a lavish silver box (which you'll recycle or discard) and a pretty, though standard, frosted-glass bottle that complements other makeup products in the Re-Nutriv line. But, given that none of that paraphernalia goes on your face, it is a waste and not what you should pay attention to. The foundation itself includes an in-part titanium dioxide sunscreen, just like lots of other foundations. That's the only antiaging element you can count on, but it doesn't have to cost this much. Ultimate Radiance Makeup has a slightly creamy texture reminiscent of a lightweight moisturizer. It blends easily and sets to a radiant finish suitable for normal to dry skin. Lauder salespeople like to point out that this foundation is different because it contains precious gemstones, but adding ruby, gold, or sapphire powder to makeup doesn't bestow a special benefit on skin of any age, not to mention that the amount is so trivial as to be nothing more than a dusting. If you want gem stones to be your best friend, save your money and buy the real deal in the form of a piece of jewelry, which you can afford if you don't buy this foundation. The small range of shades is mostly neutral, though a few have a slightly pink cast. Fresco is too peach for most medium skin tones. Although this foundation deserves a happy face rating, I must say that Lauder sells other foundations that are just as good (or better) for almost one-third the price.

☺ **$$$ Double Wear Light Stay-in-Place Makeup SPF 10** *($33.50)* misses being assigned a happy face rating because its SPF rating is below the benchmark for daytime protection. The sole active sunscreen ingredient is titanium dioxide, which is present in an amount that suggests a higher SPF rating was attainable—so why Lauder assigned a paltry SPF 10 is odd. This fluid foundation isn't as sheer as the description states. Yes, it feels much lighter than Lauder's original Double Wear foundation, but it loses none of its predecessor's formidable staying power. Application is smooth, but blending must be swift because it sets quickly to a long-wearing matte finish (applying it to small areas at a time works best). This really does stay on like few other foundations do, whether you're perspiring or simply have oily skin. Coverage is light to medium—trying to apply this sheer still nets noticeable coverage, so don't mistake this for a tinted moisturizer, because it isn't. There are only six shades, but all of them are very good. Regrettably, the lightest shade, Intensity 1.0, will be too dark for most fair skin tones (a fact the Lauder salesperson bemoaned—she was disappointed they didn't create a shade for her light skin). I suspect if this becomes a hot seller Lauder will expand the range of shades (and perhaps increase the SPF rating? Please?). For daytime wear, this is best for those with normal to very oily skin who want a budge-proof foundation but are willing to apply a sunscreen rated SPF 15 or greater first. One more comment: the strong matte finish of this foundation tends to magnify large pores. I compared this in a split-face test with Lauder's Equalizer Makeup, and the difference was obvious (but Equalizer isn't the best for very oily skin and doesn't have Double Wear's longevity).

☺ **$$$ Double Wear Stay-in-Place Makeup SPF 10** *($33.50)* is great—at least when it comes to a terrific matte finish that doesn't move. If you have normal to oily skin, you'll be impressed with the application and the way it holds up over a long day, and the texture isn't as thick and hard to move as it once was. The SPF is too low for it to be your sole source of daytime protection, but it is pure titanium dioxide. If you have oily skin and want to give this a try, pair it with one of Neutrogena's matte-finish sunscreens with UVA protection. There are several shades offered. Shell and Ecru are excellent for fair skin, and darker skin tones are well-served, too. The shades to steer clear of due to pink, orange, or peach tones are Suede, Rich Cocoa, and Rich Ginger (though this may be a workable option for dark skin tones).

☹ **$$$ Equalizer Smart Makeup for Combination Skin SPF 10** *($33.50)* is similar in concept to Lauder-owned Origins' Stay Tuned Balancing Face Makeup and Clinique's Super-balanced Makeup. All of these foundations make the same improbable claim of being able to moisturize dry areas while absorbing oil from oily areas. How a product could hold back its moisturizing ingredient from one area while absorbing oil or moisture from another is a mystery, and in fact it doesn't work—which you will be able to tell immediately after your first application. All claims aside, Equalizer leapfrogs over Stay Tuned and Superbalanced by adding an all titanium dioxide–based sunscreen. The SPF 10 is a shame because it's not enough for daytime protection, and brings this foundation's rating down compared to similar versions. Equalizer has a very silky, light texture, offering sheer to medium coverage with a soft, slightly powdery finish that is best for those with normal to slightly oily skin. The powder finish will exaggerate any dry spots, so address those before application. The majority of shades are wonderful. Pearl is a gorgeous shade for very fair skin, while Nutmeg, Truffle, and Mocha are beautiful, non-ashy dark shades. Avoid the Vanilla, Rich Fawn, and Copper due to overtones of peach or rose.

☺ **$$$ Fresh Air Makeup Base** *($24.50)* is an old-fashioned liquid foundation exclusively for oily skin. It blends on lighter than you might expect and sets quickly to a strong, clay-based matte finish, similar to Clinique's Stay True Makeup Oil-Free Formula, which is actually the better foundation, especially considering Fresh Air's uninspired shades.

☺ **$$$ Futurist Age-Resisting Makeup SPF 15** *($34.50)* leaves out the most important antiaging weapon anyone can have: sunscreen with sufficient UVA-protecting ingredients! How disappointing that a foundation with such a superlative texture and luminous finish has this as its major flaw. Almost as upsetting is that the base formula was modified to include several state-of-the-art ingredients (if ever there was a foundation that functions like skin care, this is it), yet Lauder didn't improve the deficient sunscreen element. Sigh! If you have normal to dry skin and are prepared to wear a sunscreen underneath, you will get a great medium-coverage foundation. Unusual for Lauder is that half of the 16 available shades are too rose, orange, or copper for most skin tones: Fawn, Pale Almond (slightly pink), Tender Cream, Cool Sand, Golden Petal, Cameo, Sunlit Topaz, and Bare Beige are best avoided, or at the very least auditioned carefully.

☺ **$$$ Maximum Cover Camouflage Makeup for Face & Body SPF 15** *($29.50)* has a more fluid texture, with enough slip to make controlling the application tricky. It doesn't provide as much coverage as the name indicates (this isn't Dermablend), but it does cover well, provides a titanium dioxide sunscreen, and blends to a solid matte finish. The range of four shades is limited but commendable, with only Creamy Tan being a bit too peach. A Green Corrector shade is also offered, but it's intensely green and will make it extremely obvious that you are wearing an odd shade of makeup, even when mixed with a flesh-toned shade.

☺ **$$$ Nutritious Vita-Mineral Makeup SPF 10** *($33.50)*. Estee Lauder, why only an SPF 10 in this otherwise great foundation? Nutritious Vita-Mineral Makeup SPF 10 is a sheer liquid foundation that blends beautifully into the skin. The satin finish and sheer coverage of this makeup make it a great option for a more natural look, and fans of tinted moisturizer will love the ease with which this foundation applies and wears. But alas, for complete daytime wear, you will need to apply a moisturizer or primer with an SPF 15 or higher beforehand. If you're willing to take the extra step, this foundation is recommended for those with normal to slightly dry or slightly oily skin. There are currently only six shades available, but the range is good enough to offer options for light to dark skin tones. By the way, despite the mineral name, minerals make up only a small amount of this foundation. This would earn a happy face rating if the SPF were 15 or greater.

☺ **$$$ Resilience Lift Extreme Ultra-Firming Makeup SPF 15** *($34.50)* doesn't provide an ultra- or even a mildly firming benefit. If anything, the lack of sufficient UVA-protecting ingredients leaves skin vulnerable to sun damage, which encourages loss of firmness. As with most new foundations, this has a lush, silky texture that slips on like a second skin and blends very well. Its radiant satin finish makes normal to dry skin look much better, which makes the lack of UVA protection even more disappointing. If you are willing to wear an effective sunscreen underneath this foundation, there are some excellent options among the 15 shades, including colors for dark (but not very dark) and fair skin. The following colors are too pink, peach, or copper for most skin tones: Outdoor Beige, Pale Almond, and Rich Cocoa. Ivory Beige is slightly pink but may work for some fair skin tones; ditto for Shell Beige, although it has a slightly peach cast.

☹ **Country Mist Liquid Makeup** *($24.50)* is a holdover from several years ago. It is a standard, no-frills, emollient foundation for normal to dry skin that comes in disappointing colors and is not worth considering. Even the Lauder salespeople I spoke with were embarrassed this foundation was still around, and were reluctant to even show it to me.

☹ **Double Matte Oil Control Makeup SPF 15** *($33.50)* does not offer the UVA-protecting ingredients of titanium dioxide, zinc oxide, avobenzone, Tinosorb, or Mexoryl SX, and also has other undesirable traits (including the irritant balm mint and a preponderance of peachy shades), which make it a poor choice for all skin types. Revlon's ColorStay foundations are much better for someone with oily skin that needs a long-wearing matte finish and excellent sun protection.

☹ **Lucidity Light-Diffusing Makeup SPF 8** *($33.50)* does not include the UVA-protecting ingredients of titanium dioxide, zinc oxide, avobenzone, Tinosorb, or Mexoryl SX and its SPF is much too low for adequate daytime protection. In addition, this has become a dated liquid foundation with few redeeming qualities. It was once recommended, but given its shortcomings, it doesn't deserve serious consideration over many other foundations with better textures that get the sunscreen issue right.

CONCEALER: ☺ **$$$ Resilience Lift Extreme Ultra-Firming Concealer SPF 15** *($20)* protects skin from sun damage with an all-titanium dioxide sunscreen, which also makes this a gentle choice to use around the eyes (it also lacks fragrance, another plus). The sun protection is commendable, but this creamy, supremely smooth stick concealer has two strikes against it: coverage is barely passable and it creases almost immediately. The creasing can be minimized by setting the concealer with powder, but that step often makes wrinkles stand out more. This is a workable option if you don't need much coverage but want moisture and sun protection around your eyes. Each of the four shades is recommended, though options for dark skin tones are absent. As for the ultra-firming and lifting claims, they're not to be had from using this product. Blending this on your skin won't result in less sagging, no matter how much you apply.

☺ **$$$ Smoothing Crème Concealer** *($20)* comes in a squeeze tube, so be cautious of dispensing too much. It has a soft, creamy texture and a natural finish that allows for medium coverage with minimal chance of creasing. This can easily look too thick and heavy if not blended well; with practice, you'll find it a workable option. Among the six shades, Smooth Ivory is only for very fair skin, and Smooth Medium may be too peach for some skin tones. The remaining shades are great, including Smooth Extra Deep for dark skin tones.

☺ **$$$ Double Wear Stay-in-Place Concealer SPF 10** *($20)* is a liquidy, ultra-matte concealer that provides nearly opaque coverage and includes a titanium dioxide sunscreen. I am a bit surprised the SPF stopped at 10 (which is why this did not earn a happy face rating) because the active ingredient list has titanium dioxide at 17%. That should be equal to more than an SPF 15, but perhaps Lauder thought a higher SPF would be off-putting for use around the eyes. That's not the case from my perspective, though—I'd welcome it. This formula has minimal slip and dries quickly to a matte finish that won't budge, so blending must be precise.

☹ **Re-Nutriv Intensive Concealing Duo** *($38)* They have to be kidding about this being "the ultimate" concealer! This is one of the thickest, greasiest concealers around, and although it provides sufficient coverage, it looks heavy and creases endlessly. You get two colors in one very elegant-looking mirrored compact, the idea being to use the lighter shade to disguise dark circles and the darker shade to conceal other flaws. Mixing the shades is an option, and one that works best given the peachy pink tone present in two of the three available duos. The Light/Medium Duo has the best shades, but this is not a creamy concealer I'd encourage you to try.

POWDER: ✓ ☺ **$$$ AeroMatte Ultralucent Pressed Powder** *($26)* directs you to "finish flawlessly" because "AeroMatte is so soft and air-light sheer, all you see is skin." And that's really true with this amazing, talc-based powder. AeroMatte has a supremely silky, cashmere-like texture that is a pleasure to work with because it never leaves skin looking too powdered or dry. It is available in eight neutral-toned shades, including options for darker skin (these options also work well as bronzing powder on light to medium skin tones). Lauder recommends this powder for all skin types, a point with which I almost concur. Someone with very oily skin will want a powder more absorbent than this, and the cornstarch in this formula may present a problem for those battling blemishes. Otherwise, it is highly recommended, although it's a good idea to apply it with a powder brush rather than the included applicator.

☺ **$$$ Lucidity Translucent Loose Powder** *($30)* is now talc-free and has an intriguing texture that's difficult to describe because Lauder opted not to use talc alternatives such as mica and cornstarch. The texture is very light and feels weightless and smooth on skin. It leaves a soft, radiant shine, which is supposed to downplay wrinkles but doesn't really have that effect. Still, this is recommended for normal to dry skin and it comes in six beautiful shades, including options for dark (but not very dark) skin.

☺ **$$$ Re-Nutriv Intensive Comfort Pressed Powder** *($50)* is also talc-based and shares the same level of silkiness as the Re-Nutriv Intensive Smoothing Powder reviewed below. Because this version is pressed, it offers more coverage and a longer-lasting matte (in feel) finish. The shine is toned down compared to the loose version, but still visible. All told, this is a very good, though pricey, powder for normal to very dry skin. It doesn't look the least bit powdery, and comes in four excellent shades.

☺ **$$$ Re-Nutriv Intensive Smoothing Powder** *($50)* has a supremely silky, almost creamy-feeling, talc-based texture. It meshes perfectly with skin and leaves a polished finish complete with a noticeable amount of shine. I suppose that part is what Lauder hopes will distract you from noticing that your wrinkles aren't really smoothed, but at least it's not blatant sparkles. If you're going to spend too much money on a loose powder, this is definitely one of the better ones to consider. All four shades are soft and neutral, imparting just a hint of color.

☺ **$$$ Double Matte Oil-Control Pressed Powder** *($26)* has a talc- and silica-based formula. The texture is similar to that of the Lucidity Translucent Pressed Powder reviewed below, but with an even drier, slightly chalky finish. Although that can be a problem for some skin tones, a powder this dry is a boon for those with very oily skin. All of the shades are good, and include options for dark (but not very dark) skin.

☺ **$$$ Lucidity Translucent Pressed Powder** *($26)* has a talc-based formula that goes on smoothly but quite dry. It leaves skin looking powdered and doesn't do a thing to soften the appearance of lines, but that's not a realistic quality to look for in powder anyway. The six sheer shades tend to be a bit peach or pink, but that's not really noticeable on skin. I wouldn't choose this over the superior AeroMatte Ultralucent Pressed Powder.

BLUSH AND BRONZER: ✓ ☺ **$$$ Signature Satin Crème Blush** *($26)*. Lauder has a history of producing enviable cream-to-powder blushes, and this option continues that tradition. The exquisite texture applies smoothly, setting to a silky-soft powder finish that feels slightly moist. Ideal for normal to dry skin, the colors go on translucent and build well if you want more intensity. The only drawback is the limited range of shades, but hopefully they will remedy that. By the way, what's available now contains only traces of shine, so this is suitable for daytime makeup.

☺ **$$$ Bronze Goddess Soft Matte Bronzer** *($30)* may not make you feel worthy of goddess status, but if it will keep you from tanning, it's worth the investment! This pressed-powder bronzer doesn't have the smoothest texture around, but it's still worthwhile and does apply evenly, leaving a soft shine. The single shade is a realistic tan color that's neither too red nor too orange, but it's best for light to medium skin only.

☺ **$$$ Signature Silky Powder Blush** *($26)* replaced Lauder's Tender Blush, and I'm disappointed to report it's a step backward. Whereas Tender Blush was incredibly silky and a breeze to apply, Signature Silky Powder Blush is smooth but noticeably drier, though it does have an even application. Between this and Tender Blush, the latter had a better color payoff—you'll need to experiment with Signature Silky Powder Blush because its pigmentation can be tricky when more color is desired (all of a sudden it can look like you went overboard with the blush brush). For the money, this isn't worth strong consideration over the best powder blushes at the drugstore from Jane, Rimmel, L'Oreal, or Cover Girl (their TruBlend blush).

EYESHADOW: ✓ ☺ **Pure Color EyeShadow** *($17.50)* is remarkable. It has an enviable silkiness and ultra-smooth texture that meshes with skin rather than looking like powder sitting on top of it. Each shade is packaged in a flat compact that includes a built-in mirror and throwaway sponge-tip applicator. None of the shades sold singly are truly matte, but the almost-matte options (which have a slight reflective quality suitable for daytime wear) include Sand Box, Chocolate, Mink, Ivory Box, Plum Pop, and Slate.

☺ **$$$ Double Wear Stay-in-Place ShadowCreme** *($17.50)* is a very good cream-to-powder eyeshadow that's housed in a cumbersome glass pot. Application is impressive: it has just the right amount of slip to allow for smooth, controlled blending. Its crease-free finish is matte in feel, but appearance-wise it's shiny as all get-out. Those with wrinkles around the eye won't appreciate how this cream shadow magnifies them, but if that doesn't apply to you (or you only blend this on the brow bone), then this is recommended.

☺ **$$$ Double Wear Stay-in-Place Shadowstick** *($17.50)* is a twist-up, retractable cream-to-powder eyeshadow in stick form. Because the texture of this sets quickly to a powder finish replete with shine, it is best used to shadow or highlight small areas (depending on the shade chosen). The colors are mostly in the pale pastel to neutral range, and are suitable for most skin tones. They will fade slightly, but are fairly resistant to creasing, making them a viable alternative to powder eyeshadows.

☺ **Double Wear Stay in Place Eyeshadow Base** *($15)* looks like a pale peach cream concealer in its glass pot, but applies silky-smooth and almost colorless. The powdery solvents and clay that comprise the bulk of this formula lend a matte base to eyelids, and this works well to enhance eyeshadow application and longevity. Although this works as claimed (it even kept a cream eyeshadow crease-free all day), you can get the same results by applying a matte-finish concealer (such as Lauder's Double Wear Stay-in-Place Concealer SPF 10) before brushing on your eyeshadow. If you don't like the look of concealer on your eyelid area (though I can't imagine why you wouldn't), this Eyeshadow Base may be worth auditioning.

☹ **$$$ Signature Silky Eyeshadow Duo** *($25)*. These shadows apply super sheer and silky-smooth. The color wears for hours without creasing, but the application is so sheer that it's nearly impossible to get any color payoff without a great deal of layering and effort. Also, each of the duos has varying shades of shimmer, and many of them have only one natural-looking shade, making the combination relatively unsuitable for a daytime look. Overall, the texture and wear-time is commendable, but these shadows don't have anything else going for them. Lauder offers better powder eyeshadows than this.

☹ **$$$ Signature Eyeshadow Quad** *($35)*. All the same pros and cons of the Estee Lauder Signature Silky Eyeshadow Duo reviewed above apply here, with the exception of less shimmer, so you can use some of the quads reliably for daytime makeup. However, you will still need to layer heavily due to the super-sheer application of these shadows. For the money, you'd do better at the drugstore. If you really must try these, avoid Arctic Night altogether; the purple shades can create an overdone makeup look.

EYE AND BROW SHAPER: ✓ ☺ **$$$ Double Wear Zero-Smudge Liquid Eyeliner** *($19.50)* is an excellent liquid liner with a precision felt tip that applies color evenly and easily. This takes several seconds to set, but once it does, it won't move until you're ready to take it off. An interesting twist to this liner is that all of the shades have a slight glossy finish. Most of the shades are classics, but they do have a touch of sparkle that's not distracting. I still prefer the application and ultra-long wear of the gel eyeliners (interestingly, Lauder doesn't offer such a product yet, though most of its other brands do), but this is indeed a top choice for fans of liquid eyeliner.

☺ **$$$ Automatic Brow Pencil Duo** *($23.50)* comes in the same elegant, refillable packaging as the Automatic Eye Pencil Duo, but instead of the sponge tip you get an angled brow brush. The pencil has a dry but smooth texture that applies evenly without being too thick or greasy, nor does it deposit too much color at once. The shade selection includes options for blondes and redheads, but the brow brush is too stiff and scratchy for consistent, comfortable use.

☺ **$$$ Automatic Eye Pencil Duo** *($23.50)* is a standard, twist-up, retractable pencil in an elegant container that features a pointed sponge tip for softening and blending. Although pricey, the refills are a bargain and then you have the sexy container. The formula sports a drier finish than in the past, making these less prone to smearing or fading. The Plumwood shade is an attractive alternative to traditional black or brown liner.

☺ **$$$ Brow Setting Gel** *($16)* comes in a sheer brown or colorless shade and does a good job of taming brows without looking or feeling heavy or making brow hairs stiff. A slight residual stickiness is apparent, but that's from the film-forming agent that works to keep stray hairs in place. The Brunette shade is so sheer that almost anyone can use it; only those with very light blonde brows would find it unappealing.

☺ **$$$ Artist's Eye Pencil** *($19)* is a standard pencil with a smooth, slightly creamy application that sets to a relatively solid finish that goes the distance. The pencil includes a sponge tip

The Reviews E

for softening the line, and the "artist" portion comes into play with the movable rubber gripper. This accessory is designed to provide more control during application, but isn't really needed and it can be a problem if it slides as you're drawing a line. Several shades are available.

☺ $$$ **Brow Perfecting Duo** *($26)*. Housed in a sleek compact are a pressed brow powder, clear brow wax (the company describes it as a gel, but it is more akin to a lightweight wax), and a mini dual-ended applicator that includes an angled brow brush and spoolie wand to groom brows. The powder portion is sheer and matte, so you get minor definition and soft fill-in of sparse areas. Those looking for greater definition or emphasis will prefer a more pigmented powder or brow pencil. The brow wax goes on smoothly and doesn't make brow hairs feel thick or gummy, but it's not adept at controlling unruly brow hairs unless you apply a lot, which isn't the best look (think 1940s and 1950s a la Joan Crawford or Elizabeth Taylor). The tools, while small, are better than average and functional (though not preferred to full-size applicators). Only two shades are available, and they're best for dark blonde to light brown brows. Considering Lauder's global reach, this shortcoming is strange. For about half as much money, Clinique's Brow Shaper is a better option unless you want sheer color. Looking to spend even less? Consider using a matte powder eyeshadow for brow filling, such as those from Jane, Physicians Formula, or L'Oreal.

☺ $$$ **Double Wear Stay-in-Place Eye Pencil** *($19)*. Longevity is this pencil's strongest trait, but to enjoy that you'll have to be OK with the fact that this needs routine sharpening and that the formula will dry out unless you tightly recap the pencil after each use. Application is slightly creamy and sets quickly to a smudge-proof finish. There are some purple, green, and blue shades to avoid due to their brightness and intensity. This would earn a happy face rating if not for the routine sharpening issue.

LIPSTICK, LIP GLOSS AND LIPLINER: ✓ ☺ $$$ **Double Wear Stay-in-Place Lip Duo** *($24)* has a formula, application process, and performance identical to that of (Lauder-owned) M.A.C.'s Pro Longwear Lipcolour. As such, this and M.A.C.'s version take first place as the best long-wearing lip colors on the market although, for this category of lip products, the term "best" is relative. We've tested every major contender in this group, from the original Max Factor Lipfinity to copycat versions from Cover Girl, L'Oreal, Lancome, Maybelline New York, Revlon, and Smashbox. Most of them have similar positive attributes and all of them wear longer than traditional lipsticks (even those with a matte finish). Lauder and M.A.C.'s versions excel because they have the smoothest textures and the most even wear. When the color starts to fade (and exactly when that occurs depends greatly on the type of food you eat), it does so without chipping or flaking. In addition, the glossy top coat feels light and is completely non-sticky, while others run the gamut from thick and syrupy to super-slick. There are drawbacks to be sure, such as needing to routinely reapply the top coat to ensure comfortable wear, but that's a much simpler task than touching up lipstick, where in most cases you need a mirror (especially if you wear reds or other strong colors). Speaking of color, Lauder's shade selection is smaller than M.A.C.'s, but there's not a bad one in the bunch!

✓ ☺ $$$ **Double Wear Stay-in-Place Lipstick** *($22)*. Wow, this is a truly matte lipstick! It goes on surprisingly creamy and then dries down to a long-wearing, non-slip finish. No worry about slippage into lines around the mouth, that's for sure. For those who are used to creamy or glossy lipsticks, you will not be happy with this one, but if you would like to stop using lipsticks that quickly run into lines, then this should be high on your list. Because this has a dry finish, you may be tempted to apply a gloss over it, but that negates the benefit of a matte lipstick and the same potential problems will ensue. Lauder's shade range is beautiful and every color provides full coverage.

✓ ☺ **$$$ Signature Hydra Lustre Lipstick** *($19.50)* is a very good cream lipstick that doesn't feel too slick or slippery and as a result has reasonably good staying power. This remains comfortably creamy with a moist finish that's not noticeably glossy. The shade range is enticing, and offers your choice of cream, shimmer, or very sparkly finishes. Yes, this is pricey; but if you're going to spend this much for lipstick, you should be buying those that go the distance, and this one fills the bill!

☺ **$$$ High Gloss** *($16)* is "all you really need to shine," at least if you only want shiny lips. This tube lip gloss has a smooth, slightly thick feel with a minor amount of stickiness. High Gloss is exactly the finish you'll get from each of the sheer shades, including a colorless option and several with shimmer. The only caveat is the strong fragrance; make sure you're OK with that before you purchase!

☺ **$$$ Pure Color Gloss** *($18)* carries over the opulent packaging of its lipstick predecessor, but the formula itself, while good, is nothing spectacular. It feels relatively light and applies smoothly with its sponge tip, leaving a moist, glossy finish. The only significant point of difference is that the colors have more intensity than your average lip gloss.

☺ **$$$ Pure Color Long Lasting Lipstick** *($22)* is too creamy to make good on its long-lasting claim, but the colors are richly luxurious and this has a beautifully smooth application that feels creamy without being greasy. It isn't too slick either, which means there's much less chance of it feathering into lines around the mouth, although that will occur if paired with lip gloss. The shade selection is enticing and the component opulent—you'll want to touch up in public with this one!

☹ **$$$ All-Day Lipstick** *($17.50)* is extremely creamy, bordering on greasy, with medium coverage and no stain to speak of. It does not hold a candle to any of the other Lauder lipsticks reviewed, and absolutely does not last all day (actually, it barely makes it through coffee breaks).

☹ **Tender Lip Balm SPF 15** *($14)* has a lot going for it, including a beautifully smooth texture that moisturizes and provides a soft gloss finish without being thick, sticky, or gloppy. The selection of sheer colors, while small, is still bound to please. Unfortunately, the sunscreen leaves lips vulnerable to UVA damage because it doesn't contain any of the five ingredients that protect the entire UVA spectrum (avobenzone, zinc oxide, titanium dioxide, Tinosorb, or Mexoryl SX), so it isn't a good choice for daytime wear (assuming you're purchasing this for all of its selling points, including sun protection).

☹ **$$$ Artist's Lip Pencil** *($18.50)* has a much better texture and longer-lasting finish than the Automatic Lip Pencil Duo, but the fact that it needs sharpening and has an inferior built-in lip brush keeps it from earning a better rating. If you're intrigued, the shade range is expansive. Like the Artist's Eye Pencil, it comes with a movable rubber gripper; I don't think it's too useful, but your experience may differ.

☹ **$$$ Automatic Lip Pencil Duo** *($23.50)* is a standard, twist-up, retractable lipliner, but the tip of the pencil comes out of a wider-than-normal opening, which makes it too thick to be capable of drawing a thin outline around the mouth. That's not a deal-breaker, but what you may not like is that this pencil stays creamy, diminishing its longevity. The built-in lip brush is a nice touch, but not enough to warrant a happy face rating.

MASCARA: ✓ ☺ **$$$ Double Wear Zero-Smudge Lengthening Mascara** *($19.50)* is Lauder's version of sister company Clinique's Lash Power Mascara. Both have similar formulas and claims about long, smudge-proof wear regardless of heat, humidity, or level of activity. Although I liked Clinique's contribution, Lauder's is even better. Their version has a different, larger brush whose shape and bristle layout allows for equal measures of length and thickness (Clinique's Lash Power isn't much for building thicker lashes). This is easily one of Lauder's most impressive mascaras, and it wears tenaciously. The bonus, at least compared to other long-wearing/waterproof mascaras, is how easy this is to remove. Warm water and agitation alone will do it, but for best results you should follow with your regular cleanser or makeup remover. Great job, Lauder!

✓ ☺ $$$ **Sumptuous Bold Volume Lifting Mascara** *($19.50)*. Initially unimpressive due to its uneven application, which tends to deposit too much mascara to the outer lashes, this gives way to smooth results and supremely long lashes that are assuredly defined and flutter-ready. Want more? Successive coats not only smooth through minor clumps, but also build appreciable thickness. The formula wears without smearing and flaking, and removes easily with a water-soluble cleanser. Lauder has officially upped its game with this mascara!

☺ $$$ **Projectionist High Definition Volume Mascara** *($19.50)* has a great unconventional name, and it also comes with the benefit of producing pronounced lashes. Although results with this mascara are good overall, getting there can be a messy proposition. Length outshines thickness here, but with successive coats it builds reasonably dramatic, defined lashes. Expect minor clumping and a slightly uneven deposit of mascara that requires careful comb-through and you won't be disappointed.

☺ $$$ **TurboLash All Effects Motion Mascara** *($32)*. Lauder's priciest mascara gets its turbo-charge association from the battery-powered brush. The idea is that the small wristwatch-style battery (which you insert into the cap and plug in prior to first use) powers the bristles so they vibrate during application. This is said to enhance the application process by not only depositing more mascara in a calibrated manner, but also quickly smoothing out clumps for foolproof results. The problem is getting the unit to work properly! I went through two of them and couldn't get either unit to work despite following the battery insertion instructions exactly. Nothing happened: no whirring bristles, no motorized sound, nothing to make me feel like the price was justified. Not wanting to deal with the malfunction any more than I already had, I decided to try the mascara without the "turbo" boost. As is turned out, this is an excellent lengthening and curling mascara that works quickly to produce dramatic results. There was some minor clumping, but otherwise lash separation was excellent, and the formula doesn't flake. You don't have to spend this much money (or even spend close to it) for similar results, but, inoperability aside, this is an option and further evidence that Lauder's mascaras are improving.

☺ $$$ **Lash XL Maximum Length Mascara** *($21)* won't become any mascara-lover's new favorite for all-out length, but it does do a respectable job of defining and moderately dramatizing lashes without clumping or flaking. Its lengthening abilities don't qualify as maximum, but this does make lashes perceptibly longer with just a few strokes, and builds some thickness, too.

☺ $$$ **MagnaScopic Maximum Volume Mascara** *($21)* supposedly makes lashes 300% thicker. Lauder even refers to it as "the fast track to thick lashes." If that's the case, then it must be a poorly traveled track, because thickness was hard to come by even after successive applications—and there were clumps along the way. Where MagnaScopic really excels (beyond its clever name) is for lengthening and long wear. If you're willing to put up with a slightly uneven application and have the patience it takes to separate clumped lashes, this is a good (but not great) option. If thickness and truly maximum volume are your mascara mantra, consider Clinique's High Impact Mascara or L'Oreal's Lash Architect Mascara.

☺ **$$$ More Than Mascara** *($21)* is less than adequate, at least if you're expecting a payoff of substantial length with some thickness, because this mascara provides neither. In terms of this being a "moisture-binding" formula, it doesn't contain much that makes it different from countless other mascara formulas, though it does leave lashes feeling soft.

☺ **$$$ Lash Primer Plus** *($18.50)* is sold as a pre-mascara conditioning base for lashes, but that is an unwarranted step given the industry-wide availability of superlative one-step mascaras. The formula closely matches that of most mascaras, save for the addition of a tiny amount of nut oils.

FACE ILLUMINATING PRODUCTS: ☺ **$$$ Ideal Light Brush-On Illuminator** *($24.50)* is sold as a concealer and radiance-reviving product in one. The click-pen applicator feeds product onto a synthetic brush tip. This makes spot application easy, but it is possible to dispense too much product, and there's no way to put it back. This concealer works better as a highlighter due to its sheer texture. Coverage is not sufficient enough to hide darkness under the eyes, camouflage redness, or blur sun-induced discolorations. It layers well for areas that do need more coverage, but why bother when a standard concealer does that with considerably less product? As a highlighter, this product adds a soft-focus effect to skin, sets to a satin matte finish, and actually works better when paired with a regular concealer (applied afterward). You can dab it on to highlight under the eyes, the brow bone, or bridge of the nose. Seven shades are offered, and the only one to be careful with is Medium Deep, which is slightly peach. Soft Pink has a name that may raise concerns, but although it is pink-based, it applies so sheer that it's not a bad choice for fair skin.

BRUSHES: ☺ **$$$ Estee Lauder's Brushes** *($20-$42)* were updated in fall 2009 and although they're better than the last collection in terms of shape, density, and softness, they're still not as elegant, functional, or attractive as those from Lauder-owned M.A.C., Bobbi Brown, or Aveda. At Lauder's price points, I expected but didn't observe higher quality. Still, they have improved and if you're keen on exploring brushes with the Lauder logo, the best ones to consider are the **Foundation Brush 1** *($32)*, **Powder Foundation Brush 3** *($42)*, **Powder Brush 10** *($42)*, **Blending Shadow Brush 25** *($27)*, and **Concealer Brush 5** *($23)* which is preferred for powder or liquid eyeshadow application.

☺ **$$$ Makeup Brush Cleanser** *($15 for 7.9 ounces)* is a basic, water- and alcohol-based cleanser that does remove makeup and oil buildup from brushes, but it's best for someone who needs to clean their brushes quickly because they are using them on multiple people. For your personal brush collection, occasional washing with a gentle shampoo is all you need to keep them in good shape—it does not require a specialized product.

EUCERIN (SKIN CARE ONLY)

EUCERIN AT-A-GLANCE

Strengths: Inexpensive and widely distributed; gentle, fragrance-free cleansers.

Weaknesses: Anti-redness products that added questionable ingredients instead of increasing the anti-inflammatory agents; nothing for acne-prone skin; jar packaging.

For more information about Eucerin, call (800) 227-4703 or visit www.eucerin.com or www.Beautypedia.com.

EUCERIN AQUAPHOR PRODUCTS

✓ ☺ **Aquaphor Gentle Wash for Baby** *($5.99 for 8 ounces)*. The main detergent cleansing agent in this fragrance-free body wash isn't the gentlest around for a baby's skin, but it's a fine option for adults. Fragrance-free body washes are rare, so this one definitely deserves consideration by those with sensitive skin. It makes a suitable shampoo for babies and kids.

✓ ☺ **Aquaphor Healing Ointment** *($5.99 for 1.75 ounces)*. There isn't much to this classic ointment, but without question it's a gentle formula that does a formidable job of protecting skin that is dry, cracked, or irritated. Aquaphor Healing Ointment may be used anywhere on the face, including the lips. It is excellent for severely dry hands and feet. The price and size mentioned in this review refers to the tube. Aquaphor also comes in a larger jar, but this tends to be messier. This deserves a Paula's Pick rating due to its value for compromised skin and as an aid for sensitive skin.

☺ **Aquaphor Baby Healing Ointment** *($6.99 for 3 ounces)*. This ointment is nearly identical to the original Aquaphor Healing Ointment, and it's just as basic and effective at protecting very dry skin from moisture loss and reducing dryness. However, the dated formula of Vaseline, mineral oil, and wax lack the state-of-the-art ingredients that can repair the skin's barrier so it can function more like normal skin. The formula is exceptionally gentle and doesn't contain fragrance or coloring agents. A larger size is available in a jar, and is also recommended, although the tube packaging is easier to use and more sanitary.

☺ **Aquaphor Original Ointment** *($17.99 for 14 ounces)*. This version of the popular Aquaphor range isn't as well-formulated as the Aquaphor Baby Healing Ointment, but that isn't saying much. This one lacks the beneficial extras like panthenol, glycerin, and the anti-irritant bisabolol. Still, the greasy emollients of Vaseline and mineral oil, along with wax to keep it holding tight to your skin, do a good job of protecting skin from moisture loss and easing dryness. There's just no compelling reason to consider this over the Healing Ointment.

EUCERIN REDNESS RELIEF PRODUCTS

✓ ☺ **Redness Relief Soothing Cleanser** *($8.99 for 6.8 ounces)* is a gentle, fragrance-free, water-soluble cleansing gel whose simple formula is ideal for those with sensitive, easily irritated skin. It contains licorice root extract, a good anti-irritant, but considering the amount of it here and the limited time it's in contact with your skin, it will not lead to "immediate redness relief." The good news is that this cleanser isn't apt to make persistent facial redness worse. It is best for normal to slightly dry or slightly oily skin.

☺ **Redness Relief Daily Perfecting Lotion SPF 15** *($14.99 for 1.7 ounces)* deserves praise for including titanium dioxide for sufficient UVA protection, but there are problems with this formula, especially for those with reddened, easily irritated skin. The active ingredients are two synthetic sunscreens, which, while generally well tolerated, are not the best for someone with sensitive skin. Eucerin would have been wise to use just titanium dioxide and/or zinc oxide as the active(s). Another issue is the inclusion of denatured alcohol. There's not a lot of it in the product, but for someone with red, sensitive skin, it's cause for concern. The alcohol is more prevalent than the played-up licorice extract, which is present in such a small amount its soothing benefit to skin is negligible. Finally, this lotion is tinted mint green in an effort to cancel facial redness. Such color-correction rarely looks convincing, but in this case it's so sheer as to be barely noticeable on skin, so it doesn't matter one way or the other. This moisturizing sunscreen is an OK option for normal to dry skin that is not affected by redness or sensitivity, but it's certainly not what current research indicates is a state-of-the-art formula.

☺ **Redness Relief Soothing Moisture Lotion SPF 15** *($14.99 for 1.7 ounces)* is very similar to the Redness Relief Daily Perfecting Lotion SPF 15 above, except this option is not tinted. Otherwise, the same review applies, including the comment about the amount of alcohol.

☺ **Redness Relief Soothing Night Creme** *($14.99 for 1.7 ounces)* doesn't have much to it, though it is fragrance-free, which is great for sensitive skin. Given what we know about what skin needs to look and feel healthy, whether it is sensitive or not, this jar-packaged moisturizer lacks interest. Consisting primarily of water, glycerin, panthenol, and triglycerides, it's an extremely simple, slightly emollient formula for normal to slightly dry skin. What's missing are antioxidants, cell-communicating ingredients, and a more sophisticated mix of ingredients that mimic the structure and function of healthy skin. It does contain licorice extract for its anti-irritant properties, but given the small amount, I am skeptical that someone with persistent redness or rosacea will notice their symptoms abating. Still, if you're curious, this bland formula shouldn't make reddened, sensitive skin worse.

OTHER EUCERIN PRODUCTS

✓☺ **Gentle Hydrating Cleanser** *($6.99 for 8 ounces)* contains the essential ingredients necessary to create a detergent-based, water-soluble cleanser that is suitable for all skin types, except very dry. The fragrance-free formula is truly gentle, removes makeup well, and doesn't leave a residue on skin. What more could you ask for?

☺ **Calming Creme Daily Moisturizer** *($8.49 for 8 ounces)* is a very basic body moisturizer for normal to dry skin. It contains skin-soothing oatmeal, but lacks antioxidants or any other interesting ingredient for skin. It's cheap, but that's not enough for skin. Plus the dmdm hydantoin preservative isn't the best for sensitive or eczema (atopic dermatitis)–prone skin.

☺ **Everyday Protection Face Lotion SPF 30** *($9.99 for 4 ounces)*. The two things this daytime moisturizer for normal to dry skin has going for it are its in-part mineral sunscreen (titanium dioxide and zinc oxide with other actives) and a fragrance-free formula. The synthetic sunscreen actives, while important, don't qualify this product as non-irritating, so this isn't a surefire bet for those with sensitive skin or rosacea. It is also disappointing that antioxidants are completely absent. Still, this provides reliable broad-spectrum sun protection in a creamy base and ends up being an affordable, though unexciting, option.

☺ **Extra Protective Moisture Lotion SPF 30** *($9.99 for 4 ounces)* is a good, basic, fragrance-free daytime moisturizer for normal to dry skin not prone to blemishes. The in-part titanium dioxide and zinc oxide sunscreens keep skin well shielded from the sun, while the silicone-enhanced formula doesn't feel too heavy or tacky. What's missing are antioxidants to help boost skin's natural defenses, and that's what keeps this from earning a higher rating.

☹ **Q10 Anti-Wrinkle Sensitive Skin Lotion SPF 15** *($10.99 for 4 ounces)* does not contain the UVA-protecting ingredients of titanium dioxide, zinc oxide, avobenzone, Tinosorb, or Mexoryl SX, and is not recommended. No antioxidant around can make up for an omission like this, at least if your goal is to keep skin from wrinkling and sagging.

☺ **Q10 Anti-Wrinkle Sensitive Skin Creme** *($11.42 for 1.7 ounces)* contains some well-documented antioxidants in a light yet creamy base formula. Unfortunately, jar packaging won't keep the antioxidants stable, leaving you with an average choice for normal to dry skin.

☺ **Everyday Protection Body Lotion SPF 15** *($10.29 for 13.5 ounces)* is a lighter-weight, but still moisturizing version of Eucerin's Everyday Protection Face Lotion SPF 30 above. In this case, the SPF rating is lower, but it still provides UVA protection via its in-part titanium dioxide sunscreen. Cost-wise, it's quite a value as an allover sunscreen. Those with normal to

The Reviews E

dry skin will find this works well as a facial moisturizer, too, though it is short on the bells and whistles that many other facial moisturizers with sunscreen do provide. Unlike the facial version of this product, Eucerin included an antioxidant (vitamin E) in this version.

☹ **Calming Itch-Relief Treatment** *($8.49 for 6.8 ounces).* The active ingredient in this "treatment" is menthol. It serves as a counter-irritant, which means the irritation the menthol produces is stronger than the irritation (such as itching) that you're trying to remedy. The base formula is a standard, fragrance-free lotion, but using menthol on itchy, dry skin on a regular basis isn't the answer if your goal is to heal the skin's barrier and prevent further damage.

FLIRT (MAKEUP ONLY)

FLIRT AT-A-GLANCE

Strengths: Inexpensive; excellent concealer; good options for powder and powder blush; mascaras; the lip color product selection is plentiful without being overwhelming.

Weaknesses: Foundation and lip tint with sunscreen lack sufficient UVA protection; most categories have at least two mediocre products; the brushes are unremarkable.

For more information about Flirt, owned by Estee Lauder and sold exclusively at Kohl's, call (866) 343-5478 or visit www.flirtcosmetics.com or www.Beautypedia.com.

MAKEUP REMOVER: ☺ **See-Ya Makeup Remover** *($10 for 4.2 ounces)* is a very standard, but effective, detergent-based makeup remover. Flirt claims this removes waterproof mascara, too, but it doesn't do as good a job as the dual-phase makeup removers with silicone. This is fragrance-free.

FOUNDATION: ☹ **Act Natural Light & Sheer Foundation SPF 15** *($12)* would be a great option for a basic foundation that imparts light coverage with a silky-smooth, somewhat matte finish. However, this SPF 15 product lacks the UVA-protecting ingredients of titanium dioxide, zinc oxide, avobenzone, Tinosorb, or Mexoryl SX, and is not recommended, despite its impressive color selection.

CONCEALER: ✓☺ **Pretty Easy Quick Cover** *($10)* is suitably named, as this foundation/concealer is a pretty easy, quick way to apply foundation with almost no chance of making a mistake. I am generally very skeptical of cream-to-powder foundations. Often, they either go on and feel too dry and look flaky, go on too creamy and look greasy, or just appear thick on the skin if not blended with diligence. That isn't true for this twist-up cover stick with skin-accurate shades. It goes on effortlessly, with a silky smoothness that immediately dries to an exceptionally soft powder finish, providing light to medium coverage. Now if only they gave you more product! The 0.17 ounce is stingy at best, but that also means it won't take up much room in your makeup bag. The colors are great and the tester units will help you choose the best one to match your skin tone.

☹ **Glamouflage Healer/Concealer Anti-Acne Formula with Salicylic Acid** *($10)* is meant to double as a concealer, while also providing the exfoliating and anti-irritant benefit of salicylic acid. The pH of this product, however, is too high for it to be effective as an exfoliant. Plus, you don't want to put salicylic acid around your eye area—as an active ingredient it is not good for the thinner skin there anyway—so you would have to use another concealer for the eye area. Instead of this concealer, consider a well-formulated gel, lotion, or toner that contains salicylic acid—that's a far better way to treat acne.

POWDER: ☺ **Love & Matteness Oil-Free Pressed Powder** *($12)* comes in several attractive shades that go on fairly sheer and smooth. For a pressed-powder option, you may just love it.

BLUSH AND BRONZER: ☺ **Big Deal Lip & Cheek Tint** *($10)* isn't a big deal for the cheeks or lips. It is merely a twist-up, creamy stick blush that you can use on your lips, though the size of the applicator means it will be far handier for the cheeks. It works, but cream blushes aren't for everyone and there are lots of superior options around for your lips.

☺ **Bring on the Bronze Bronzing Powder** *($12)* is more impressive and less expensive than the similar bronzer from Flirt's sister brand, American Beauty. The smooth texture of this talc-based pressed powder applies evenly and clings well, yet imparts minimal color. If you want a noticeably bronze look, you'll need to apply a lot of this. Still, those seeking a softer, translucent look will be pleased, and both shades are good. Foxy Bronze has obvious shine, while Golden Minx has a subtle sheen that's suitable for daytime wear.

☺ **Peek-A-Blush Sheer Powder Cheek Color** *($12)* is a standard powder blush that has an attractive, smooth application. The 20 colors are a mix of shiny and matte, and they all go on evenly when used with a good blush brush.

☺ **I'm Whipped Cheek Mousse** *($12)* is a sheer, mousse-textured, slightly creamy blush. Each shiny shade glides over skin and blends well, but can be a bit tricky to control. The soft wash of color and strong shine make this best for younger skin looking for more cheek gleam than color.

EYESHADOW: ☺ **Dreamy Eyes Eyeshadow** *($10)* has a soft, even application that can be a bit powdery—but not enough to detract from the wide array of color choices with a selection of matte and shiny shades. One word of warning: this eyeshadow compact is one of the trickiest to open I've ever encountered. Even after I figured it out, sliding one compartment out, it still wasn't easy to figure out how to open the lid. Give me good old reliable M.A.C. packaging any day!

☺ **I'm Whipped Eyeshadow Mousse** *($12)* has a soft, mousse-like texture that's a bit too creamy for its own good. The creaminess of the silicone-based formula leads to creasing and fading, making each sparkle-infused color short-lived, although they are easy to apply.

EYE AND BROW SHAPER: ☺ **Opening Line Liquid Eyeliner** *($11)* is an easy-to-apply eyeliner that goes on in a solid line of obvious color that dries quickly and leaves dramatic definition around the eyes, without flaking or smudging during the day. You can't really soften the line once it's on, so what you draw is what you get.

☺ **Look of Love Eye Pencil** *($10)* is a standard eye pencil that is creamy enough to make it easy to apply. It glides right on, and can be smudged to soften the line. The color range of over a dozen shades has a little bit of everything, from exotic to standard. As far as the brows go, there are colors that would work, but the texture is a bit too creamy for a realistic appearance. This does need sharpening, which isn't convenient, and with all the twist-up eye pencils available that don't need sharpening, there is no reason to bother with one that makes you do all the work.

LIPSTICK, LIP GLOSS AND LIPLINER: ☺ **Candy Stripes Glossy Lip Palette** *($14)* This compact-sized palette offers five thin strips of lip gloss. Each has a wonderfully smooth and non-sticky texture, and leaves a rich, glossy finish without a high-mirror shine. The shades range from creamy pink to glittery champagne and are not separated within the palette, which allows for creative mixing of colors. The only drawback is that the size and design of the palette definitely necessitates a lip brush (which isn't included) in order to avoid messy and unsanitary fingertip application.

☺ **Chickstick Smooth & Shiny Lipcolor** *($10)* can only be described as a traditional creamy lipstick. The best thing is the name—too bad the name alone doesn't make for a great lipstick. It's worth checking, but it doesn't warrant accolades.

☺ **Flirt-Tinis Swirled Lipshine** *($12)* is a very emollient, sheer lip gloss applied with a built-in brush applicator that leaves lips with the requisite glossy finish. Stickiness isn't an issue and the colors are soft enough to work over almost any lipstick. What's odd is that there are only two shades—although both are enticing with their swirl patterns (which come off as one color on lips).

☺ **Glamourazzi Extreme Lip Lacquer** *($12)* definitely leaves lips looking lacquered, although you have to tolerate a sticky finish from this pen-style lip gloss with a built-in synthetic brush. Tenacity is this product's strong suit, but it also compromises how comfortable a gloss-like product can feel. The trade-off is apparent, but if you want longer wear than standard lip gloss and like bolder, shimmer-infused colors that still apply translucent, give this a try.

☺ **Plushious Liquid Velvet Lipcolor** *($10)* is just a traditional gloss, and not all that different from Squeeze Me Super Shiny Lipgloss below. The assortment of 24 colors is attractive, but all in all this is just gloss with a very plushy name.

☺ **Squeeze Me Super Shiny Lipgloss** *($10)* is a tube lip gloss with a soft plastic applicator that smooths effortlessly over the skin, leaving vivid iridescence and an emollient, moist, non-sticky feel when applied. It is more a traditional gloss than anything else, and gives only a hint of color on the lips. For a minimalist color look with lots of shine and lots of colors to choose from, this will do nicely.

☻ **Draw Attention Lip Pencil** *($10)* isn't a unique lip pencil by any means, despite a good basic selection of eight workable lip shades that glide on beautifully. It also needs sharpening, which makes it less desirable than the numerous other options that don't need to be sharpened.

☻ **High Wattage Intense & Creamy Lipcolor** *($10)* offers an odd variety of features. It can be intense and creamy, but also sheer and glossy, or matte and soft, or glittery and uneven, depending on the color! Unless you try this on before buying, you will have no idea what you are going to find once you get it home and apply it.

☹ **Tint-A-Licious Lip Color Lipsheer SPF 15** *($10)* is a disappointment in that it lacks the UVA-protecting ingredients of titanium dioxide, zinc oxide, avobenzone, Tinosorb, or Mexoryl SX. Other than that, this is just a standard, glossy, lip color that is not delicious in the least.

MASCARA: ☺ **Big Flirt Thickening Mascara** *($10)* is not a mascara you can count on for much thickening, although it scores well in the lengthening department. It takes a bit of work to build the look you want, but it doesn't clump in the least and won't flake all day long, no matter how often you flutter your lashes. Easily washed off, this is a mascara to consider.

☺ **Clear Deal 3-in-1 Lash/Glosser/Primer/Brow Groomer** *($9)* is a mascara wand in a hard, tubelike container holding a clear gel that feels more like a styling product than a mascara (and the ingredients read more like that, too). It does work well to shape brows and keep them in place without adding any color or thickness. As a mascara primer, this extra step would seem necessary only if you are using a poorly performing mascara. If you have a great mascara, why use two steps when you only need one? But for a truly natural look to your lashes, with just a teeny bit of accent, this would do the trick.

☺ **Far Out Lengthening Mascara** *($11.50)* replaces the usual brush with a slightly C-shaped comb that has short, serrated "teeth." Although it looks odd, you can create really long, dramatic lashes with this mascara. Trying to build thickness can get messy (a lot of mascara gets deposited at lash roots), but with agile comb-through, lashes end up long, defined, and softly curled.

☺ **$$$ Lash-A-Delic Fast Defining Mascara** *($14)* is a supremely good mascara to help you achieve lots of length without a clump in sight. A few coats take lashes from blah to wow, and you'll get some thickness, too. After all that praise, there is a fly in the ointment: It tends to flake during wear.

BRUSHES: ☺ **Flirt Everywhere Brush Kit** *($12)* has a great price tag, but the brushes are mediocre. You get two eyeshadow brushes (which are really too small for easy application), a standard brow/eyelash comb, and brushes for blush and powder that have an average texture and density. In comparison to other brushes, these fall short.

☺ **Total Flirt Eye Brush Kit** *($8.50)* comes with two eyeshadow brushes, an eyeliner brush, and a standard brow/eyelash comb. The brushes are workable and have a lovely soft feel, but they are too soft and floppy for controlled application.

FRESH

FRESH AT-A-GLANCE

Strengths: fresh provides complete product ingredient lists on their Web site; some good facial cleansers; the sunscreens provide sufficient UVA protection and contain antioxidants; excellent bronzing powders; one good mascara.

Weaknesses: Very expensive; very fragrant; several products contain potent plant irritants; limited sunscreens; boring below-standard toners and masks; no viable exfoliant options (at least if you're aiming to avoid extraneous irritation); no products to manage acne or reliably lighten skin discolorations; the lip balm with sunscreen does not provide sufficient UVA protection; overpriced beyond reason; no matte eyeshadow options.

For more information about fresh, call (800) 373-7420 or visit www.fresh.com or www. Beautypedia.com.

FRESH SKIN CARE

☹ **Cleansing Balm with Lemon Oil** *($38 for 4 ounces)*. Lots of cleansers contain soothing or helpful plant extracts, but not this one. Instead, your skin is exposed to peppermint, citrus, and fragrant oils that cannot control combination or oily skin in any way, shape, or form. This overpriced cleanser is not recommended.

☺ **$$$ Cucumber Cleansing Foam** *($48 for 4.1 ounces)*. Although ridiculously overpriced, this is still a very good water-soluble cleanser for normal to dry skin. It foams slightly and works well to remove makeup without stripping skin. It does not contain fragrance, but it does contain fragrant plant extracts.

☺ **$$$ Soy Face Cleanser** *($38 for 5.2 ounces)* is based around rose water, which is little more than eau de cologne and potentially irritating, though the risk isn't too great in a rinse-off product like this one is. This is otherwise a fairly gentle water-soluble cleanser for normal to dry skin, though it's very fragrant. The small amount of soy makes it hardly worth including it as part of the name, but it's of little consequence anyway in this product because the soy is just rinsed down the drain before it can have any benefit. And the price? Get real! There is absolutely nothing in this product that isn't easily replaced (and improved upon) by far less expensive cleansers available at the drugstore, from CeraVe, Olay, or Neutrogena.

☹ **Umbrian Clay Treatment Bar** *($38 for 7.8 ounces)* is just fuller's earth, which is mainly alumina, silica, iron oxides, lime, magnesia, and water, and it is not unique in the least. Fuller's earth is used as an absorbent and thickening agent in many cosmetics, and all claims pertaining to it being an important aid for skin conditions like eczema and acne are folklore, not backed up by any research. If anything, the ingredients in this cleanser will make matters worse for sensitive or dry skin. fresh maintains that this soap can reduce oiliness (which it temporarily will do because of its drying nature, and almost any cleanser removes oil from the surface of skin after rinsing), shrinks pores (wishful thinking), and reduces breakouts (which is way beyond the capabilities of this brick of clay).

☺ **$$$ Rose Marigold Floral Water** *($35 for 8.6 ounces)* is essentially eau de cologne for your face and offers next to no benefit beyond the pleasing scent of roses. If that were enough to make for good skin care, then we would be back in the days of rose water for about $2 at the drugstore. That wasn't good skin care years ago and it still isn't today.

☹ **Appleseed Brightening Exfoliant** *($60 for 3.4 ounces)* is an excessively priced scrub (how anyone could be convinced that this is worth even a fourth the price is beyond me) that contains pomegranate seed powder as the abrasive agent. Although this is a natural ingredient, seeds are not the preferred method for gently scrubbing skin because they have an uneven shape that can cause microscopic tears in the skin. The amount of coconut alcohol and the unusually high amount of fragrance make this more irritating than brightening, and at this price you should expect the absolute best scrub ever. As is usually the case, a washcloth used with your cleanser does a better, and more gentle, job.

☹ **Appleseed Resurfacing Kit** *($145)* is designed to prepare skin for exfoliation and provide soothing protection afterward, but this trio of products is far from the perfect solution for achieving smooth, exfoliated skin. The **Appleseed Activator** *(1.7 ounces)* is simply a water-soluble cleanser that contains glycolic acid. The pH of the cleanser is too high for exfoliation to occur, and even if it were within range for efficacy, the glycolic acid isn't in contact with skin long enough to have much benefit because it is just rinsed down the drain (and leaving a cleanser on your skin longer to get some benefit would leave detergent cleansing agents on the skin way too long). This product doesn't prep skin for exfoliation any better than any other standard water-soluble cleanser (which is all this is). Next is the **Appleseed Peel** *(1.7 ounces)*, a water-based liquid that contains approximately 3% glycolic acid, yet, as with the Activator, the pH is too high to permit exfoliation. The Peel contains several potentially irritating citrus ingredients along with a lot of fragrance. In order to convince you the product is working, this peel also contains the menthol derivative ethyl menthane carboxamide (which is interesting, because it is a synthetic ingredient, while fresh touts their use of natural ingredients). All this Peel will really do is irritate your skin and provide negligible benefit. The final step after rinsing the Peel is to apply the **Appleseed Soother**, which is nothing more than a moisturizer for normal to dry skin. It is far from an impressive formula, containing mostly water, emollients, and a heaping amount of fragrance. The iris and rosemary, and the presence of several fragrance chemicals, make this potentially irritating, degrading the effectiveness of the antioxidants in this moisturizer. In summation, this exfoliation kit pales in comparison to simply adding a well-formulated AHA or BHA product to your existing routine. Those who insist on spending this much money for smoother skin should seriously consider a professional AHA or BHA peel instead of products like these.

☺ **$$$ Sugar Face Polish** *($55 for 4.2 ounces)* has a main ingredient of sugar (in this case sucrose), and despite being coupled with some emollient ingredients, this facial scrub remains too abrasive for use on the face. It's better to use sugar scrubs like this one from the neck down, where the skin is a bit more resilient to manual abrasion. The fact that this scrub contains strawberry fruit may increase its "natural" appeal, but it doesn't do your skin any favors. Whether used as a mask or scrub, this is an average, yet very costly, way to exfoliate normal to dry skin.

☹ **Anise Day Serum** *($85 for 1 ounce)* contains anise, a helpful ingredient for skin because of its antioxidant properties, but its fragrant components can cause irritation, which doesn't make it the most desirable choice to build a serum around (Source: www.naturaldatabase. com), especially considering the number of antioxidant options that are available that do not have the potential for irritation. This product is better described as a lightweight moisturizer rather than a serum, and although it contains several impressive ingredients for dry skin, it also contains potentially irritating plant extracts, including iris, myrrh, and several fragrance chemicals. If you're looking to spend in this price range for an outstanding serum, consider those from Estee Lauder, Clinique, or MD Skincare by Dr. Dennis Gross before this far-from-advanced concoction.

☺ $$$ **Appleseed Brightening Essence** *($95 for 1 ounce)*. Mulberry root and vitamin C are what fresh says will lighten and brighten areas of skin discoloration, but I suspect that the amount of these ingredients isn't enough for them to have a significant lightening effect. It's likely that the amount of mulberry extract is too low for it to be useful, and the form of vitamin C included (ascorbyl glucoside) has limited research demonstrating its effectiveness at inhibiting melanin production. Other forms of vitamin C are preferred, such as ascorbic acid or magnesium ascorbyl phosphate (Sources: *Phytotherapy Research*, November 2006, pages 921-934; *International Journal of Dermatology*, August 2004, pages 604-607; and *Journal of the American Academy of Dermatology*, January 1996, pages 29-33). Ascorbyl phosphate is present in this serum, but again, the amount is likely too low for it to have any visible benefit. This is otherwise an OK yet not-worth-the-expense serum-type moisturizer for normal to dry skin.

☺ $$$ **Black Tea Age-Delay Cream** *($125 for 1 ounce)* contains a wide complement of beneficial plant extracts and antioxidants, more so than many other fresh products. The problem is the jar packaging, which rapidly reduces the potency of all of the ingredients for which you're paying a premium; at this price, an antioxidant-rich moisturizer packaged in a jar is just insulting. As for the name and the claims, black tea ferment cannot firm skin or reduce wrinkles to a significant degree. Moreover, there is no evidence that the Chinese lychee that's present can boost collagen production. Research shows that not only is lychee highly oxidative (which means its protective components break down quickly when the cut plant is exposed to air), but also it is a tannin-rich fruit, and tannins are irritating due to their constrictive action on skin (Source: *Journal of Agricultural and Food Chemistry*, December 2000, pages 5995-6002).

☹ **Creme Ancienne** *($250 for 3.5 ounces)*. I had to step away from my computer for a moment before writing about this offensively priced, badly formulated product. Composed primarily of meadowfoam seed oil, this is no more the ultimate moisturizer for face and body than a unicycle is the ultimate mode of transportation! On the ingredient list, fragrant ingredients follow the meadowfoam seed oil, along with wax (Yes, wax, for $250!) and irritating fragrant oils. The vitamin E and chamomile are helpful, but again, for the money, and by any professional standards, these are not the ultimate ingredients for aging skin; at best they are meager options for beneficial skin care. Meadowfoam seed oil is a good, nonfragrant moisturizing oil for dry skin, but it shows up in many less expensive moisturizers, including several from Aveda. Even if this product were well-formulated, the jar packaging makes it even more pathetic (as if that were possible). What were these people thinking?

☺ **$$$ Elixir Ancien** *($250 for 1.7 ounces)* is less problematic for skin than fresh's Creme Ancienne, although it still carries an absurd price for what you get—basically an emollient serum for dry to very dry skin not prone to blemishes. Aside from a tiny amount of myrrh and rosemary extracts, there are no irritating ingredients in this product. Although it is helpful for dry skin, you can get the same benefit for a lot less money by applying plain jojoba, olive, or wheat germ oils to your skin. Knowing that, does it really matter that this Elixir is hand-blended in a Czechoslovakian monastery. I mean really, ask yourself: Does that make any difference to you? I didn't think so!

☹ **Lotus Eye Gel** *($48 for 0.5 ounce)* has a lightweight lotion texture suitable for slightly dry skin anywhere on the face, although the inclusion of irritating lemon peel oil is a big problem, especially if you intend to use this in the eye area. This product is not recommended.

☺ **$$$ Mamaku Night Serum** *($85 for 1 ounce).* I don't know where the mistaken notion that skin-cell division occurs more at night came from, because skin cannot tell time and new skin cells are constantly being formed and shed. But as you might expect, that doesn't stop many a cosmetics company from attaching the "cell division occurs at night" claim to their products. Mamaku Night Serum is no exception. This water-based serum contains mostly slip agent, emollient, and film-forming agent. The mix of plant extracts it contains has both beneficial and irritating properties, so they're essentially at odds with each other and end up not doing much for skin. None of this is worth the money, and there is nothing in this serum that can enhance skin's regenerative ability, assuming that your skin is already doing fine on its own. At best, this is an average option for normal to slightly dry skin, but its price is unjustified.

☺ **$$$ Repair and Restore Face Balm, Extra Rich for Dry Skin** *($95 for 1 ounce)* is a very good moisturizer for dry skin anywhere on the face, aside from the inclusion of a few problematic plant extracts. The potentially irritating plant extracts aren't the reason for the neutral face rating; rather, the jar packaging is. Considering the amount of antioxidants (including an impressive amount of green tea oil) in this moisturizer, jar packaging is a real letdown. Couple that with an above-average price and the letdown becomes a major disappointment. This also contains several fragrance chemicals that can be irritating, though without question there are several helpful ingredients in this poorly packaged moisturizer.

☹ **Repair and Restore Face Balm, Normal to Combination Skin** *($95 for 1 ounce).* Jar packaging, several plant irritants (including lemon peel oil), and irritating fragrance chemicals make this a terrible choice for any skin type. Those with combination skin where oily skin is a concern should be aware that the thickeners and plant oil in this moisturizer aren't going to make your oily skin happy.

☺ **$$$ Soy Face Cream** *($42 for 1 ounce)* contains a core ingredient that will do a good job helping dry skin look and feel better, which is great. What's not so great is the amount of fragrance, which is much more prominent than the soy and several other truly beneficial ingredients; that's not a smart formula decision (fragrance is not skin care). Considering the cost and a formula that's closer to perfume than to really outstanding skin care, this doesn't deserve better than a neutral face rating. Note: This product is available exclusively at Sephora.

☺ **$$$ Top Protection Layer SPF 20** *($48 for 1 ounce).* The fact that this facial moisturizer with sunscreen contains avobenzone for UVA protection is good; but the lavender water base (eau de cologne is not good skin care) and the oxygenating claims are not. Thankfully, lavender water is not as troublesome for skin as lavender oil (it mostly adds fragrance) and fresh did not include any oxidizing ingredients in this product. Instead, they include several antioxidants, which are great for skin that's exposed to sunlight. This is a good, though needlessly pricey, option for normal to dry skin not prone to breakouts. Unless your skin is very dry, you shouldn't need to pair this with another moisturizer (definitely not if you're using a moisturizing foundation).

☺ **$$$ Umbrian Clay Face Lotion, Oil-Free** *($65 for 1.7 ounces)*. Those with combination to oily skin will likely find their skin doesn't respond well to this confusing blend of emollients and absorbent. The fuller's earth has absorbent properties, but those properties are compromised, and in all likelihood negated, by the emollient, oil-like ingredients listed before it. The plant extracts are the typical fresh mix of beneficial and problematic, which will only confuse skin further. This is best for normal to dry skin; but for the money, countless other formulas "best" this one.

☺ **$$$ Anise Wrinkle Eraser** *($55 for 0.5 ounce)*. Even a line like fresh that celebrates the "traditions of beauty" feels the need for a works-like-dermal-fillers product (definitely not traditional). However, this Wrinkle Eraser doesn't cut it compared with most others, including those that sell for $20 to $30 less. Yes, fresh has formed a silky blend of silicones that help this product serve as a soft spackle for minor wrinkles, but unlike similar products, fresh's contains a potentially irritating amount of myrrh and anise, two plants that skin does better without. Due to those ingredients and the higher price, this Wrinkle Eraser (which doesn't really erase lines, but will temporarily reduce their appearance) isn't the one to choose. The amount of the ingredients that may have "long term wrinkle-reducing benefits" is meager, and if you don't use sunscreen daily then you can forget about any amount of wrinkle reduction!

☹ **Black Tea Instant Perfecting Mask** *($85 for 3.4 ounces)*. Instant perfection from any skin-care product is a tempting promise and an all-too-frequent claim, but it's also one that is always too good to be true. Even the best skin-care routine isn't going to get your skin to a "perfect" state, not ever, though if you stick with it, over time you will see steady improvements and healthier skin. Can you expect the same from weekly use of this mask? No such luck. Beyond the fact that what you do daily for your skin counts much more than what you do occasionally, this mask contains several problematic ingredients. From rose flower oil to the potent menthol derivative menthoxypropanediol, this product is a problem for all skin types and is not recommended. The exorbitant price doesn't even deserve comment, especially because my jaw is still on the floor in shock.

☺ **$$$ Rose Face Mask** *($55 for 3.5 ounces)* is an utterly boring formula. The main ingredient is rose flower water, which is mostly alcohol and fragrance, and that is just plain bad for skin. The skin-beneficial ingredients are listed after the preservative, which means you're getting a scant amount of them, at best. At this price, the showcased ingredients should play a much larger role. However, even if those ingredients were plentiful, the jar packaging won't keep them stable once this product is opened.

☹ **Umbrian Clay Face Treatment** *($48 for 3.4 ounces)* is designed to be used as a cleanser, mask, or spot treatment for blemishes. No matter which way you use it, the effect is supposed to be detoxifying and neutralizing—in fact, it is neither. First, skin doesn't need to be detoxified; there is no research proving otherwise, and no one in the cosmetics industry has ever identified what toxins they claim to be removing from skin or how much is being removed with a product like this. What utter nonsense! Second, this is mostly absorbent fuller's earth and lavender water, which makes the price insulting. Fuller's earth is used as an absorbent and thickening agent in lots of cosmetics; all claims pertaining to it being an important aid for skin conditions like eczema and acne are folklore, and are not based on any research anywhere. When it comes to improving matters for those prone to blemishes and blackheads, fuller's earth is certainly no match for benzoyl peroxide, salicylic acid, and a good clay mask without fragrant irritants and film formers.

☹ **Sugar Lip Treatment SPF 15** *($22.50 for 0.15 ounce)* is an over-fragranced lip balm with sunscreen that lacks the UVA-protecting ingredients of titanium dioxide, zinc oxide, avobenzone (also known as butyl methoxydibenzoylmethane), Tinosorb, or Mexoryl SX and is not recommended.

✓ ☺ **$$$ Sunshield Face and Body SPF 30** *($48 for 5.1 ounces)*. For a company that focuses its marketing on natural contents, it's surprising to note that their sunscreens contain synthetic (though very effective) active ingredients. Given their positioning and fresh's claims, it seems logical to me that they would include titanium dioxide and zinc oxide for their "natural" qualities, but then again, the cosmetics industry is not known for its logic. This ends up being a very good antioxidant-rich sunscreen for normal to dry skin. UVA protection is ensured thanks to avobenzone and the company couples this with other actives known to enhance avobenzone's stability, which is great. Although it doesn't make water-resistant claims, this product does contain ingredients that help the actives adhere to skin when immersed in water (as with any sunscreen, be sure to reapply this after swimming or toweling off). However, I am slightly concerned that the price of this sunscreen may discourage liberal application (which is essential for getting the amount of protection stated on the label); this product is actually inexpensive when compared with all of the fresh facial moisturizers that do not contain sunscreen. Perhaps the best part of this well-formulated sunscreen is that it does not contain a single irritating plant extract. Too bad more fresh products don't follow this one's lead; if they did, there would be a lot more products to recommend.

FRESH MAKEUP

FOUNDATION: ☹ **$$$ Umbrian Clay Freshface Foundation SPF 20** *($42)* disappoints from the get-go because it does not contain active ingredients that provide sufficient UVA protection, plus the amount of actives listed on the active ingredient list doesn't add up to the SPF on the label. The lightweight base formula is a strange mix of dry-finish silicone, plant oil, and wax along with sea water, which has no superior benefit for skin. Blending this on is tricky, and it never seems to mesh with skin, so the result is you look like you're wearing foundation instead of looking like you have even, natural skin tone. The shade range is quite neutral and offers options for fair skin tones, but this really has too many drawbacks to make it worth choosing over dozens of other foundations. By the way, whether "clay" comes from Umbria, Italy, or Detroit, Michigan, clay is clay. The location doesn't change how this makeup ingredient impacts the skin.

CONCEALER: ☹ **$$$ Umbrian Clay Absolute Concealer** *($22)*. Umbrian clay has nothing to do with creating better makeup, as this creamy concealer quickly proves. Clay is clay, no matter where it comes from. In this case, regardless of how long you struggle to blend it into place, this concealer won't set. It remains moist and prone to creasing, not to mention fading, as the day goes by (actually within the first hour of wearing it). The colors are mostly impressive, but aren't enough to make this a concealer to choose over lots of others, including the better ones from inexpensive lines like L'Oreal and Avon.

POWDER: ☺ **$$$ Face Luster** *($45)*. According to fresh, you can use Face Luster pressed powder either as a sheer coverage foundation when applied with the included sponge or as a finishing powder to set makeup when applied with a powder brush. While the first two listed ingredients in this powder (talc and mica) are minerals, the very sheerness of this pressed powder makes it best for use as a finishing product to set makeup, not as a foundation. When applied with a sponge as a mineral foundation, the powdery, dry finish will only draw attention to fine lines and wrinkles, and eventually will look thick or pool in oily areas of the skin. However, when applied with a brush over foundation and concealer, its sheer coverage sets makeup nicely without cakiness. The shade selection is small, but the colors and finish are so sheer that most skin tones will likely be able to make use of more than one shade.

BLUSH AND BRONZER: ✓ ☺ **$$$ Here Comes the Sun Face Palette** *($45)* comes in a plastic case with a mirror and three somewhat shallow pans that hold two face lusters and one peachy pink blush. The colors are sheer but buildable, and the effect is natural and glowy without being too obvious or shiny. It's absurdly pricey and the colors are unoriginal, but the portability and convenience make it worth considering, that is, if you don't mind being embarrassed about spending this much money on such a standard product.

✓ ☺ **$$$ Marbella Gold and Tunisian Bronze Face Lusters** *($45)*. Each of these pressed bronzing powders is sheer and beautiful. Both shades have some shimmer and apply sheer enough to be used by those with light to medium skin tones. There is no reason to spend this much for what amounts to nothing more than an ordinary bronzer (Wet 'n' Wild makes a great one for a fraction of the price, as do other lines), but if you're a Fresh devotee and want a bronzer with shimmer, these powders won't disappoint. Basic products priced like this make me wish I had a different rating system that included a category for great products that are insultingly overpriced!

☺ **$$$ Blush Cream** *($28)* is an overpriced, relatively standard cream blush that applies and blends easily. The color goes onto the skin more sheer than it appears in the compact, but a little still goes a long way. Apply sparingly and you'll be rewarded with beautiful color and all-day wear. This blush is best suited for those with normal to dry skin not prone to blemishes.

☺ **$$$ Blush Powder** *($28)*. There is absolutely no reason to spend this much for any blush. All you get with this option from Fresh is a standard powder blush. It is the best option from Fresh for those with normal to oily skin not prone to blemishes. Like its Blush Cream counterpart, these powder shades apply more sheer than they appear in the compact. The two available colors will work for those with fair to medium skin tones looking for a natural blush that wears well throughout the day.

EYESHADOW: ☹ **$$$ Eye Shadow Trios** *($32)*. Each of the colors in these eyeshadow trios has shimmer. The shadows apply much more sheer than they appear in the palette and thus the shimmer may not be an issue for some (this isn't glittery, just shiny), but there are no matte options available for those who don't want to have a glowing eye design. The sheerness of the application and the inclusion of shimmer also make these trios a poor choice for use as eyeliner when applied wet with a brush. Oh, and the price, it's just silly for what you get, because the product doesn't begin to compare with products from myriad lines such as M.A.C., Jane, Rimmel, Sonia Kashuk, and on and on!

EYELINER: ☺ **$$$ Satin Liner Palette** *($45)*. Fresh Makeup has a penchant for gauging what's in their customers' checkbooks. There is no reason, from any perspective (except for Fresh, which is laughing at women who buy into their marketing hype), to pay this much for eyeliner. Aside from the ridiculous price, the three metallic cream shadows in the Satin Liner Palette are acceptable only for those who want a dramatic look. Each of the shiny and shimmery shades (Sienna, Olive, and Coal) applies smoothly and once dry, they stay put. The included brush works OK, but application is easier and more precise with a better eyelining brush. It's a shame Fresh doesn't offer this product in other colors for those who want something other than a metallic liner. However, there are plenty of excellent, non-metallic liquid liners available at the drugstore, and some very good cream eyeshadows, too, such as those from Revlon and L'Oreal HIP.

LIPSTICK, LIP GLOSS AND LIPLINER: ☺ **$$$ Fresh Lipstick** *($22)* comes in a range of beautiful sheer shades. Those prone to lip color bleeding into lines will need to use a liner with this lipstick due to its moisturizing formula, which causes the lipstick to travel into lines around the mouth and to fade easily. Even if lip lines are not a problem for you, it's recommended that you use a lipliner to give this lipstick more staying power.

☺ **$$$ Lip Shine** *($20)* is a $20 lip gloss that should cost half the price. The formula is slick and non-sticky with a color range that is shimmery and sheer. There is nothing wrong with this gloss (hence the happy face rating), but there's nothing special about it either.

☺ **$$$ Sugar Lip Gloss** *($18)* is a non-sticky gloss that comes in a range of beautiful shimmery colors. But once again with Fresh, there is no reason to pay this much for what amounts to a standard, shiny, sheer gloss that you will need to reapply often throughout the day.

☺ **$$$ Gloss Absolute** *($24)* would have been rated higher but for the fact that you must either carry a lip brush with you or use your finger for application. Neither option is as convenient or sanitary as using the built-in applicator that comes with myriad glosses. Other than that inconvenience, these shiny glosses are more accurately described as tinted balms. Each shade applies much more sheer than it appears in the compact and each has some shimmer. Nothing in this formulation will plump the lips, and that's a good thing, because plumping lips almost always involves exposing them to irritants.

☹ **Lip Pencil Duo** *($22).* These dual-ended lipliners are standard pencils that need sharpening. The need for sharpening and the hardness of these pencils, which makes application difficult, mean this is a lipliner you can easily pass up.

MASCARA: ☺ **$$$ Supernova Mascara** *($25)* lengthens beautifully and doesn't clump or flake. The jet black color is very glossy, leaving you with dark, full, soft lashes. The formulation applies a bit wet, so you do need to let it dry for a moment, otherwise it can smudge. Once dry, Supernova Mascara wears well throughout the day. For the money and performance, consider Maybelline's The Colossal mascara, an extraordinary mascara for only 1/3 the price of this version from fresh.

☺ **$$$ Firebird Mascara** *($26)* is a truly overpriced option for those who want natural-looking lashes and aren't hoping for much added length, volume, or curl, as if those were the reasons anyone would buy mascara! The large brush makes it tricky to reach the smaller lashes, but application is otherwise easy, with very little clumping and no smudging. This mascara wears well and removes easily with any makeup remover, but it's really so average you're well advised to save your money and buy any of the better options available at the drugstore.

FACE AND BODY ILLUMINATING PRODUCTS: ☺ **$$$ Satin Luster Face Palette** *($45)* is a mirrored three-pan palette that contains three Satin Lusters for highlighting the face. Each of the three shades (China Pearl, Peach Butterfly, and Winter Rose) is a shimmery, sheer illuminating cream that can be used anywhere on the face. They blend easily, giving the skin a flattering glow. A little goes a long way, so while the palette is overpriced, it will last you a long time.

☺ **$$$ Twilight Freshface Glow** *($36)* is a lightweight illuminating lotion that works well either as a primer or as a facial highlighter. From the tube, it dispenses a pearlescent white, but when applied it gives a very pretty and subtle luminescence that's slightly pinkish and that will flatter most skin tones. The slight bit of shimmer this product has gives the skin a healthy glow. A little goes a long way, so while the cost is high, the 1-ounce tube will last you for quite a while. It's worth noting that Sephora's "Tricks of the Trade" Perfection Primer is nearly identical to this and only half the price.

☹ **$$$ High Noon Freshface Glow** *($36)*. Describing High Noon Freshface Glow as a sheer liquid bronzer is inaccurate. This pale orange-tinted lotion is best described as a facial illuminator. The sheer shimmer it provides means that it will work only for the fairest of skin tones, assuming you have a preference for apricot-hued makeup. High Noon can be used to highlight the face, and it blends easily, but it will not plump up the skin as promised by Fresh. There are some antioxidants included in the formula, but at $36 for 1 ounce, you should be getting more, a lot more.

SPECIALTY PRODUCTS: ☹ **$$$ Imperial Bedroom Face Palette** *($55)* is a mirrored five-pan palette that consists of eye, cheek, and lip colors meant to "capture the behind-the-curtain, forbidden sensuality of imperial aristocracy." Wow! Now that kind of spin outdoes any snake oil sales pitch I've ever heard. In actuality, this color array has both shimmery and sheer shades, which are pretty enough, but not awe-inspiring or aristocratic in the least. In fact, they're pretty ordinary. The five products in the palette include two very sheer, shimmery eyeshadows that you must apply sparingly to avoid shimmer overload; one cream liner that applies easily and wears well, but also has shimmer; a face highlighter with shimmer (not a surprise), which is easy to blend; and for the lips a single gloss that looks dark in the pan but applies sheer and wears away too quickly. If you're not a fan of shimmer, don't waste your money on this overpriced grouping. Even if you do like shimmer, use the shades sparingly. Wearing all the colors at once will leave your face looking way too shiny, almost to the point of looking greasy.

☹ **$$$ Island Reverie Face Palette** *($55)* is a mirrored five-pan palette that consists of three small powder eyeshadows, a bronzer, and a blush. All of the powder products in this palette are very sheer, so if you want any amount of color, you're not going to get it without a lot of layering, which will end up making your face look over-powdered. The shadows are shimmery and the blush and bronzer are unattractive shades of pink and orange, although their sheerness can be forgiven when you consider the not-so-good colors. In general, this palette has more negatives than positives and you would be better served buying Fresh's Here Comes the Sun Face Palette because it has better colors and costs less. However, there's no reason at all to spend your money on any of the overpriced products in the Fresh makeup line.

☺ **$$$ Rose FreshFace Primer** *($36)* is a creamy white primer with a consistency that closely resembles that of a lightweight lotion. It's a good option for those with normal to dry skin who don't like, or cannot use, silicone-based primers. It blends well on skin without leaving any residual stickiness, though it isn't nearly as silky as most primers. Those with drier skin may need to use an additional moisturizer before applying the primer. One possible drawback of this formulation is the rose smell, the result of rose water, which is eau de cologne, not a skin-care ingredient. The fragrance is not overwhelming, but its presence is unmistakable. For the money, this doesn't begin to compare to well-formulated serums or lightweight moisturizers, which also function as "primers."

GARNIER NUTRITIONISTE (SKIN CARE ONLY)

GARNIER NUTRITIONISTE AT-A-GLANCE

Strengths: Well-formulated moisturizers with and without sunscreen (well, those in non-jar packaging); an intriguing serum.

Weaknesses: Lack of sufficient UVA protection from the sunscreens; mostly irritating cleansers; no products for blemish-prone skin; no products to address uneven skin tone or skin discolorations; ineffective BHA products; jar packaging.

For more information about Garnier Nutritioniste, call (800) 370-1925 or visit www. garniernutritioniste.com or www.Beautypedia.com.

GARNIER NUTRITIONISTE NUTRI-PURE PRODUCTS

☺ **Nutri-Pure Detoxifying Cream Cleanser, Oil-Free** *($5.99 for 6.7 ounces)* is a water-soluble cleanser with a slightly creamy texture. Adding nutrients (antioxidants) to a cleanser is somewhat of a waste because they are rinsed from skin before they can exert a benefit. In this case, there's more fragrance than nutrients. Although this won't detoxify skin (nor does skin need to be detoxified), it is an effective option for normal to slightly dry or slightly oily skin. The tiny amount of peppermint extract is unlikely to cause irritation.

☹ **Nutri-Pure Detoxifying Gel Cleanser** *($5.99 for 6.7 ounces)* is a very fragrant water-soluble cleanser that contains enough peppermint extract to cause irritation. This is paired with the potent menthol derivative menthoxypropandediol, which only compounds the irritation and is problematic for use around the eyes. The dermatologists behind this line should have known better, but perhaps the cooling effect was created so consumers think the product is working to detoxify their skin, but that's not what's happening.

☹ **Nutri-Pure Detoxifying Wet Cleansing Towelettes, Oil-Free** *($6.49 for 25 towelettes)* have minimal cleansing ability (they don't remove mascara, as claimed) and end up being irritating to skin thanks to the amount of peppermint steeped in each cloth. If you're a fan of cleansing cloths or wipes, Olay, Dove, and Pond's have much better options for around the same price.

☹ **Nutri-Pure Daily Exfoliating Gel Cleanser** *($6.49 for 5 ounces)*. Although this cleanser/scrub hybrid has its strong points, they're weakened by the inclusion of several problematic ingredients, including the drying cleansing agent TEA-lauryl sulfate and an irritating amount of peppermint, not to mention the menthol, which cannot deep clean or refine pores as claimed.

☺ **Nutri-Pure Microbead Cream Scrub, Oil-Free** *($6.49 for 5 ounces)* is a creamy facial scrub that contains polyethylene as the abrasive agent. The exfoliating granules are larger and, as such, can be a bit rough on skin even in the creamy base of this scrub. The amount of peppermint isn't terrible, but the tingling sensation it causes is concerning, and doesn't make this scrub preferred to most others.

GARNIER NUTRITIONISTE SKIN RENEW PRODUCTS

☺ **Skin Renew Anti-Puff Eye Roller** *($13.49 for 0.5 ounce)*. The best part of this product is the metal roller-ball applicator, which glides along the curvature of the under-eye area with ease, depositing a thin layer of water-based liquid. The two ingredients associated with reducing puffiness and dark circles are escin (a component of horse chestnut), due to its circulation-stimulating abilities, and caffeine, due to its constricting abilities. Regrettably, neither ingredient's association with reducing puffy eyes has any solid research to support the claim, although both are notable antioxidants (Source: www.naturaldatabase.com). This does have a temporary smoothing and tightening effect on skin, but not to the extent that puffy eyes will be visibly deflated. The mica casts a slight shimmer on skin, which reflects light away from dark circles, but a concealer would work much better. At best, this is a novel way to apply a light film of moisture-binding agents and antioxidants to skin. The fragrance-free formula is suitable for all skin types.

☺ **Skin Renew Anti-Sun Damage Daily Eye Cream SPF 15** *($12.99 for 0.5 ounce)*. The fact that this eye cream provides broad-spectrum sun protection is all that's needed to support the anti-sun damage claim, but that doesn't mean this is a product to slather around your eyes. Many people find the active ingredients in this product sensitizing when applied close to the eyes, so in that sense, mineral sunscreens (titanium dioxide and/or zinc oxide) would be preferred. So, if you can tolerate the active ingredients just fine, would this be recommended? Yes, but only for its sun-protecting ability; when it comes to your face, your skin really needs more. I would encourage you to seek out another SPF-rated product for daytime whose base formula provides far more for preventing wrinkles and environmental damage than this one does, such as antioxidants, cell-communicating ingredients, and skin-identical ingredients. This eye cream also loses points because it contains a potentially irritating amount of alcohol and offers precious little in the way of proven anti-sun damage ingredients (sunscreen actives excluded). This contains cosmetic pigments that leave a shiny finish on skin, but those mineral pigments aren't reversing sun damage; they're just minimally camouflaging it. By the way, the commercials for this product are maddeningly misleading and hyperbolic!

☺ **Skin Renew Anti-Sun Damage Daily Moisture Lotion SPF 28** *($13.49 for 2.5 ounces)* provides avobenzone for sufficient UVA protection, which is great. This lotion-textured, soft matte-finish daytime moisturizer is a good choice for those with normal to oily skin prone to breakouts. Garnier even included a noteworthy blend of antioxidants in packaging that keeps them stable. This would be rated a Paula's Pick if it didn't contain a small amount of irritating fragrance components (linalool, limonene, geraniol, and citral). The salicylic acid does not function as an exfoliant, so any fading of sun spots or discolorations will result from the simple act of keeping your skin protected from sun damage every day, possible with any well-formulated sunscreen.

☺ **Skin Renew Awakening Face Massager** *($12.99 for 1.7 ounces)*. This product is a water-based serum housed in a component with a roller-ball applicator. The idea is to massage the ball over facial skin, releasing the serum and encouraging a healthy glow by stimulating skin's circulation. The roller ball (or any other form of skin manipulation) will stimulate circulation, but that's not necessarily a good thing. Overstimulating skin's circulation can lead to broken capillaries and redness. Indeed, those with rosacea don't need a stitch of stimulation unless they want to exacerbate rosacea's most telling symptom—redness. What about the serum itself? It contains too much alcohol to be helpful for any skin type (alcohol causes free-radical damage and cell death), and that's disappointing given the handful of helpful ingredients that follow it. If your skin is looking dull and tired, a well-formulated exfoliant and exercise program will net improvements that this product cannot begin to approach.

☺ **Skin Renew Daily Anti-Fatigue Eye Cream** *($13.49 for 0.5 ounce)* claims to boost surface cell regeneration to diminish dark circles and puffiness. This lightweight moisturizer not contain ingredients capable of doing that, and even if it did boost skin-cell turnover (regeneration), that isn't going to help dark circles or puffiness in any way. The amount of salicylic acid in this product isn't enough to exfoliate skin. It's a good option for slightly dry skin anywhere on the face and includes more than token amounts of antioxidants. Used around the eyes, the mica and titanium dioxide will cosmetically blur the appearance of dark circles by reflecting light from shadowed areas.

☺ **Skin Renew Daily Regenerating Moisture Cream** *($13.99 for 1.7 ounces)* has a formula that bests most of those from Lancome's moisturizer collection (remember, L'Oreal owns Lancome and Garnier), which makes the choice of jar packaging unfortunate because it won't keep the vitamins and antioxidants stable after the product is open. As is, it's an OK option for normal to slightly dry skin. The salicylic acid is not present in an amount great enough to exfoliate, and the fragrance components at the end of the ingredient list pose a slight risk of irritation.

☺ **Skin Renew Daily Regenerating Moisture Lotion** *($13.99 for 2.5 ounces)* is similar to, but has a thinner texture than, the Skin Renew Daily Regenerating Moisture Cream, and also has packaging to keep its antioxidants stable during use. The glycerin- and silicone-enriched formula is ideal for normal to slightly oily skin and leaves a soft matte finish. This would rate a Paula's Pick were it not for tiny amounts of the fragrant additives linalool, limonene, and geraniol. One more thing: the pH of this moisturizer is too high for the salicylic acid to function as an exfoliant.

☹ **Skin Renew Daily Regenerating Moisture Lotion, SPF 15 Sunscreen** *($13.99 for 2.5 ounces)* lacks the UVA-protecting ingredients of titanium dioxide, zinc oxide, avobenzone, Tinosorb, or Mexoryl SX, and is not recommended. Even with sufficient UVA protection, the base formula is a step down from the Skin Renew Daily Regenerating Moisture Lotion.

☺ **Skin Renew Daily Regenerating Serum** *($13.99 for 1.7 ounces)* makes skin feel very silky thanks to the amount of silicone it contains. Also on hand are appreciable levels of antioxidants and some interesting skin-identical ingredients. This serum's main drawback is its potentially irritating fragrance components (linalool, limonene), and for that and some minor formulary reasons, it is not preferred to serums from Olay Regenerist or Neutrogena Healthy Skin. Once again, the amount of salicylic acid and the pH of this product won't permit exfoliation to occur.

☺ **Skin Renew Overnight Regenerating Cream, Night** *($13.49 for 1.7 ounces)* doesn't contain ingredients that can renew skin in terms of exfoliation, but the isohexedecane and silicones will make your skin feel very smooth. This not-quite-state-of-the-art moisturizer is an option for normal to oily skin, but not a very impressive one. It contains a smattering of antioxidants but that's about it. This does include a tiny amount of fragrance components.

GARNIER NUTRITIONISTE ULTRA-LIFT PRODUCTS

☺ **Ultra-Lift Anti-Wrinkle Firming Eye Cream** *($14.99 for 0.5 ounce)* doesn't (surprise!) contain any ingredients capable of lifting or noticeably firming skin, but it's an elegant formula with a silky cream texture and a good amount of antioxidant vitamin A (as retinyl palmitate). The other intriguing ingredients are present in lesser amounts, but include some effective skin-identical ingredients and passion fruit oil, which supplies skin with several essential fatty acids and adds a soft fragrance to this moisturizer that's best for normal to dry skin anywhere on the face.

☺ **Ultra-Lift Anti-Wrinkle Firming Moisture Cream** *($15.89 for 1.6 ounces)* is similar to the Ultra-Lift Anti-Wrinkle Firming Eye Cream above, except this version has a thicker texture and less silky finish. It is minimally fragranced and overall a worthwhile moisturizer for normal to dry skin. Its fortifying action on surface skin cells will not result in a deep-lifting action, as claimed. Such lifting and tightening of slackened skin is the essence of an artful, medically precise, surgeon-performed face-lift—nothing a moisturizer can match.

☹ **Ultra-Lift Anti-Wrinkle Firming Moisture Cream, SPF 15** *($15.89 for 1.6 ounces)* continues L'Oreal's (parent company of Garnier) frustrating predilection for selling sunscreens that lack sufficient UVA-protecting ingredients. They know better, and have for years, so products like this are in no way deserving of a purchase or even a second glance.

☺ **Ultra-Lift Anti-Wrinkle Firming Night Cream** *($15.89 for 1.7 ounces)* contains several ingredients that are necessary to make dry to very dry skin look and feel better, including glycerin and shea butter. Although those and the thickening agents in this moisturizer serve dry skin well, the product's jar packaging compromises the effectiveness of the antioxidants, and that's ultra-disappointing.

☹ **Ultra-Lift Anti-Wrinkle Firming Serum** *($14.99 for 1.7 ounces)* lists alcohol as the third ingredient, which is detrimental for skin and cancels out any beneficial effect the antioxidants in this serum may have had. If you want a serum from Garnier, their Skin Renew Daily Regenerating Serum is the one to choose.

☺ **Ultra-Lift Daily Targeted Deep Wrinkle Treatment** *($14.99 for 1 ounce)* is said to target deep wrinkles at their source, but that's not possible because deep wrinkles (the kind you see after years of sun damage and facial expressions) have their source in the dermis, beyond where moisturizers can really have an impact. This is simply a good moisturizer, although the formula is relatively impressive coming from a L'Oreal company, but that's not saying much. It's best for normal to dry skin. Although this won't lift skin or secure its support structure (that requires a surgical procedure), it supplies emollients, antioxidants, and mineral pigments to optically brighten skin and add a soft shine. That adds up to a product that creates some glow (shiny ingredients will do that) and, of course, it will make skin softer—but this truth is radically different from what the claims say it will do!

☹ **Ultra-Lift Glow Anti-Wrinkle Firming Moisture Cream SPF 15** *($14.99 for 1.6 ounces)* lacks the UVA-protecting ingredients of titanium dioxide, zinc oxide, avobenzone, Tinosorb, or Mexoryl SX, and is not recommended. This inconsistency about sunscreen that even some of the major brands keep demonstrating is nothing short of maddening (especially from a L'Oreal corporation that has a patent on a popular UVA-protecting ingredient, which they brag about in other products they sell)!

☹ **Ultra-Lift Pro Deep Wrinkle Cream SPF 20** *($17.99 for 1.6 ounces)* is supposed to be a daily treatment targeting deep wrinkles and loss of firmness, but with only one exception, it's another resounding disappointment for L'Oreal-owned Garnier. The sole bright spot is this daytime moisturizer's in-part avobenzone sunscreen. The sun protection it provides will prevent further damage to skin, but the rest of the product is a joke when it comes to improving the appearance of aging skin. Yes, it feels silky, but the amount of alcohol it contains is likely to cause irritation and free-radical damage, while the amount of state-of-the-art ingredients pales in comparison to the amount of fragrance. This contains shimmery pigments to give skin a glow, but please don't mistake that cosmetic effect for any sort of skin treatment, because it absolutely isn't a treat.

☹ **Ultra-Lift Pro Deep Wrinkle Dual Eye** *($17.99 for 0.5 ounce).* Most cosmetic companies sell several types of eye-area moisturizers, often with the claims that they'll banish dark circles, deflate puffiness, and, of course, reduce wrinkles. Garnier decided that women need two eye-area moisturizers: one for the eyelid area and one for the under-eye area. I wonder how they explain the preponderance of the other eye creams they sell, each with claims similar to this one, but for some unexplained reason to be used all around the eye. It's all utter nonsense. A well-formulated moisturizer, no matter how it is labeled, can be used all around the eye area. This waste-of-money product is packaged in a single jar with a divider between the two products. The Eye Gel is meant to be used in the under-eye area, and is said to reduce puffiness. Let me tell you, it could not be a more basic, useless formula even if it wanted to be, because it already has hit bottom. All you'd be getting is little more than water, slip agents, gel-based thickener, and coloring agent. The tiny amount of escin (a component of the horse chestnut plant) is not going to be enough to reduce inflammation that leads to puffy eyes, and it has zero effect on age-related puffiness that results from the fat pads beneath the eye shifting. It does have antioxidant potential, but not in the jar packaging used here because it won't keep the air out. The Eye Cream feels silky because of its silicone content, and although glycerin is a great moisturizing ingredient, the amount of alcohol in this moisturizer negates some of its benefit. Although the eye cream contains a few good moisturizing ingredients, none of them are capable of lifting droopy skin around the eyes, nor are they the least bit firming. It's nice that this product isn't expensive, but it is so ordinary and there are so many better options to consider.

☺ **Ultra- Lift Pro Deep Wrinkle Roller** *($17.99 for 1.7 ounces)* is a lightweight fluid housed in a roller-ball applicator that claims to firm and lift skin for increased definition. It would be great if the roller ball allowed you to massage sagging skin back into place, because it's certain that the formula won't be of any help. This product contains mostly water, slip agents, silicone, wax, plant oil, and fragrance (linalool). Almost all of the intriguing ingredients are barely present, which makes this more of a gimmick than an intelligent way to improve the appearance of aging skin. It would be great if we could just roll our winkles away and cancel that appointment with the cosmetic surgeon, but it's not possible.

GIORGIO ARMANI

GIORGIO ARMANI AT-A-GLANCE

Strengths: For skin-care products there are none; the makeup is a very different story: outstanding foundations, superb powder textures, a brilliant shimmer fluid, great primers; perfect bronzers; a neutral palette make this line a must-see.

Weaknesses: Expensive; lack of options to address most consumers' skin-care needs; foundations with sunscreen that do not provide sufficient UVA protection; mascaras that aren't as impressive as they should be.

For more information about Giorgio Armani, owned by L'Oreal, call (877) ARMANI-3 or visit www.giorgioarmanicosmetics.com or www.Beautypedia.com.

GIORGIO ARMANI SKIN CARE

☺ **$$$ Mineral Cleansing Balm** *($65 for 5 ounces)* is an emollient cleanser that begins as a balm but transforms to a slick, oily feel once massaged onto your skin. It removes all kinds of makeup easily, but the price is outrageous for what amounts to thickener, water, glycerin, alcohol, and some minerals (very common ones—you'd think that for this much money they could find at least one exotic mineral). This does not rinse well without the aid of a washcloth, and is recommended only for those with normal to dry skin not prone to breakouts, and who also have money to burn and desire everything Armani. Mineral Cleansing Balm does contain fragrance.

☺ **$$$ Mineral Cleansing Foam** *($65 for 5 ounces)* is an exceptionally standard water-soluble foaming cleanser for normal to oily skin. This is no more a mineral bath for your face than just soaking it in salt water would be (salt, aka sodium chloride, is the fifth ingredient in this cleanser), and I wouldn't recommend that as a way to "maintain the moisture balance of the skin." Almost any water-soluble cleanser at the drugstore is preferred to this overpriced option.

☹ **$$$ Mineral Cleansing Milk** *($65 for 5 ounces)* ranks as one of the most expensive bottles of water and mineral oil you're likely to find (of course most consumers wouldn't notice). The mineral oil is the only "mineral" aspect of this pricey, detergent-free cleansing milk for normal to dry skin. This is fragrance-free and removes makeup easily, but that isn't worth the investment when there are similar cleansers available at the drugstore that perform just as well. A bottle of mineral oil from the drugstore for $4 would do the exact same thing.

☹ **$$$ Mineral Soothing Lotion** *($80 for 5 ounces)* almost leaves me speechless. Eighty dollars for an embarrassingly paltry formula of mostly water, slip agents, gel-based thickener, and preservatives. The tiny amount of water-binding agents and antioxidants is little consolation for an utterly ordinary toner that barely makes it to mediocre status. Clearly, the folks behind Armani know a lot more about creating makeup than they do about skin care!

☹ **$$$ Crema Nera** *($275 for 1.7 ounces).* In an attempt to justify the outrageous price for this product, Armani's marketing team has concocted a story of heroic proportions. This "cell regenerating cream" was supposedly inspired by Giorgio Armani's trips to Pantellaria, an Italian island between Sicily and Tunisia. Somehow Armani discovered that the petrified lava from this island's volcanoes contains everything needed to "nearly perfectly recapture the earth's rejuvenating secrets." (Ah, so the fountain of youth is really in Italy.) So basically what they're asking you to swallow is that fossilized lava can somehow generate new skin cells and restore radiance to aging skin. According to an article in the August 2007 issue of fashion magazine *W*, L'Oreal (Armani's owner) researchers studied obsidian (volcanic rock) on this island and worked with experts on volcanoes at Naples' Vesuvian Observatory. The minerals sodium, potassium, silica, and iron are claimed to be collectively responsible for oxygenating skin (which by the way generates free-radicals) and helping skin to absorb water (something the top dead layers do exceptionally well all on their own if there is enough moisture in the environment). In short, those minerals or any lava are useless topically on skin and absorbing water is only a small part of what makes skin healthy. This water- and silicone-based moisturizer does contain all of those minerals, but none of them are capable of achieving skin-perfecting results, including regenerating cells. There is a tiny amount of salicylic acid, but certainly not enough to prompt exfoliation (now that would have been really helpful for skin). Beyond all of the nonsense claims and useless input from volcanic experts, this is a shockingly boring formula whose only redeeming value is a silky, elegant texture. The fifth ingredient is paraffin, as in paraffin wax, and the other thickening agents that make up the bulk of this product are as inexpensive as it gets. There are a few token antioxidants in here, but whatever slight benefit they may have provided is lost because of jar packaging. Armani stated that his goal was "to have one cream for a lifetime …. I want one product that does everything." Lots of women feel that way, too, but there is no product that can fill that bill (who knows what new discoveries lay around the corner?) and this product doesn't even come close to making a valid attempt. Crema Nera falls drastically short of being an all-encompassing product for anyone's skin: it does not contain sunscreen, is inappropriate for blemish-prone skin, won't be emollient enough for very dry skin, and lacks ingredients that reinforce skin's structural components. On top of all that, the fragrance and fragrance components can be problematic for sensitive skin. When all is said and done, Crema Nera is the skin-care version of a red carpet fashion faux pas.

☹ **$$$ Crema Nera Obsidian Mineral Restoring Serum** *($250 for 2.5 ounces)*. The nicest thing I can say about this serum is that if you believe the claims about the effects of the obsidian minerals it contains, then I have a bridge in New York I'd like to sell you. The main ingredients in this uber-expensive product include water (which is about as cheap as it gets as far as cosmetic ingredients go), slip agents, nonfragrant plant oil, alcohol, thickeners, silicone, and Vaseline. This is a formula that is more nonsense and problems than anything else. None of the volcanic minerals in this serum live up to the assertions on the label. This serum supposedly is "designed to effectively combat deep wrinkles," but it's completely incapable of doing that. Choosing this serum over several better formulas that cost drastically less isn't something I recommend, even if you love wasting money.

GIORGIO ARMANI MAKEUP

FOUNDATION: ✓ ☺ **$$$ Designer Shaping Cream Foundation SPF 20** *($65)* earns a place on the ever-growing list of uber-pricey foundations, but at least there is a lot to love about this particular option. Its higher-than-usual sunscreen is in-part titanium dioxide, and this is one of the creamiest yet lightweight foundations for dry to very dry skin you're likely to find. Its emollient texture feels decadently silky and blends very well, though it takes time to set to a soft satin finish. Dry skin is left with a radiant glow, while coverage stays in the medium range. The range of 12 shades is, by and large, quite neutral. The only shades to be careful with are the slightly peach #6 and slightly orange #9.5. Shade #2 is gorgeous for fair skin, and those with light to just-medium skin have several excellent choices. The silk fibers and oil in this foundation do not contour skin, so don't mistake this for a face-lift in a jar (though that's likely how the lofty price was determined). It is a rich yet not heavy-feeling cream foundation with a superb blend of ingredients to replenish dry skin while leaving a soft glow.

✓ ☺ **$$$ Luminous Silk Foundation** *($58)* is the foundation every Armani makeup artist I spoke to raves about. It's not hard to see why, because this liquid foundation has a fluid, ultra-smooth texture that floats over the skin and dries to a natural, slightly matte finish with a faint hint of shine. For light coverage and an unbelievably skin-like result that comes in 15 mostly gorgeous colors for fair to dark skin, this foundation is tough to beat. The only misstep is shade 0, which is pure white and tends to look ashen. Luminous Silk Foundation is best for normal to slightly dry or slightly oily skin.

☹ **$$$ Designer Compact Foundation SPF 22** *($65)* has several strengths that could have come together to create one of the best cream-to-powder foundations I've ever seen, hands down. So what's the kryptonite that weakens this otherwise super foundation? A sunscreen whose actives do not provide sufficient UVA protection. Considering the cost of this foundation, that's almost unforgivable. If you can look past the sunscreen mistake, you'll find this silicone-based makeup (in cumbersome, heavy packaging. Who said designer chic has to be weighty?) has one of the smoothest textures around, and a finish that's so skin-like it has to be seen to be believed. Armani includes a flat, fan-like synthetic brush to apply it, but a regular sponge works better; the brush tends to apply the product in streaks, forcing you to smooth those out with your fingers. The formula provides light to barely medium coverage and has a soft powder finish best for normal to slightly oily skin. Despite how natural this looks while concealing minor imperfections and improving skin tone, it can exaggerate dry areas just like most cream-to-powder makeups. Among the six mostly neutral shades Armani offers, only number 7 suffers from being slightly ash. Finally, I disagree with the company's claim that this provides 12 hours of moisture comfort. The only legitimately moisturizing ingredient is jojoba oil, and there isn't enough of it in this foundation to please someone with dry skin. This would have earned a Paula's Pick rating if not for the sunscreen deficiency.

☺ **$$$ Face Fabric Second Skin Nude Makeup SPF 12** *($45)*. While this foundation does have an innovative texture, it has an antiquated sun protection factor of 12 (it should be a minimum of SPF 15 by the standards of medical associations around the world), and it does not contain the right UVA-protecting ingredients. Armani doesn't have a good track record for foundations with sunscreen, and this continues their disappointing trend. If sunscreen is not an issue for you (because your daytime moisturizer is rated SPF 15 or greater and contains the right UVA-protecting ingredients), then this foundation is best described as a primer with color. Most foundation primers are silicone-based (as this Armani foundation is) and leave a weightless, silky matte finish that slightly fills in large pores and superficial lines. That's exactly how this foundation functions, except that it also contains pigments that provide sheer to light coverage and contribute to its very skin-like natural appearance. This foundation is best for normal to oily skin because the powdery silicones it contains will magnify even the smallest amount of dry skin—one of the reasons the Armani makeup artist I spoke with commented that people either love or hate this foundation. It simply isn't forgiving of even the tiniest speck of dry skin. There are nine shades available, two of which have shimmer and are best used as a highlighter (shade 8) or shiny peach-tinged bronzer (shade 9). Shades 1-7 are flesh-toned without shimmer, and all but one are recommended; avoid shade 5, which is noticeably peach. With a higher SPF rating and the right UVA-protecting ingredients, this foundation really would be something to consider, because on the right skin types it really can look like a second skin.

☺ **$$$ Hydra Glow Foundation SPF 15** *($57)* continues Armani's trend of creating foundations with exceptional textures and a shade range that almost perfectly defines neutral. The bad news is that the sunscreen does not contain the UVA-protecting ingredients of titanium dioxide, zinc oxide, avobenzone, Tinosorb, or Mexoryl SX. Considering the high price, that oversight is particularly egregious, because protecting your skin from the detrimental effects of UVA radiation is just too important to ignore. If you have normal to dry skin and are willing to pair this foundation with an effective sunscreen, it has a fluid, slightly creamy application that provides medium coverage and a slightly moist finish, which lends a subtle, non-sparkling glow to skin. The amount of coverage it provides isn't what I would call natural, so you can ignore Armani's claims that this foundation looks like "a second skin." Hydra Glow Foundation SPF 15 is available in ten shades and, with one exception (shade 6.5 is a yellow tone that can turn a bit too olive), they are beautifully neutral.

☹ **Lasting Silk UV Foundation SPF 20** *($58)*. Every time Armani launches a new foundation I get lots of requests to review it. That's to be expected, because many of their foundations have exquisite textures and an exemplary range of shades. Coupled with modern pigment technology, Armani's foundations are among the best. Sadly, the trend doesn't continue with their Lasting Silk formula. Although UVA protection is assured thanks to the in-part titanium dioxide sunscreen, alcohol is the third ingredient. Sometimes, depending on the formula, that isn't an issue, but in this case, you can smell the alcohol and feel its tingle on your skin—and that's never a good sign because alcohol causes free-radical damage, triggers oil production in the pore lining, and irritates skin, which is not silky, but rather rough and unpleasant on skin.

The Reviews G

This liquid foundation has a sheer, fluid texture that blends well and sets to a satin matte finish, but so do many other foundations that don't cause the problems this one does. For significantly less money and no irritation, consider L'Oreal True Match Super Blendable Makeup SPF 17 (L'Oreal owns Giorgio Armani).

CONCEALER: ☺ **$$$ High Precision Retouch** *($35)* is a liquid concealer applied with the type of long, thin brush usually reserved for liquid eyeliners. You can indeed be precise with the brush, but it's not the best for covering large areas, such as darkness under the eye. Its fluid texture provides medium coverage and blends decently, but because it never really sets, it won't last long before fading and creasing. The four shades are mostly very good, though 4.5 is slightly bright for medium skin tones.

☺ **$$$ Master Corrector** *($35)* is a series of color-correcting liquids packaged in slim, shapely components and outfitted with a precision brush applicator. The thin, light texture is easy to blend, but the four colors are too obvious on skin, so you end up substituting one color "flaw" for another. The Green shade is less green than most, but doesn't look convincing unless you blend it with another color. The Yellow option is so yellow that it's almost jaundiced. Pink and Orange are workable but only if carefully applied and deftly blended. I suspect most women won't want to bother with this product. I know I wouldn't.

POWDER: ✓ ☺ **$$$ Luminous Silk Powder** *($44)* is an outstanding talc-based pressed powder whose pigments and talc are finely milled so you get a silky, sheer application that meshes with skin and provides a matte finish that's not powdery or dry. Note that this powder is laced with a tiny amount of sparkles, but their subtlety makes this suitable even for daytime wear. Each of the eight shades is recommended, and there are options for fair to dark (but not very dark) skin. If you're going to spend top dollar on a pressed powder, you should be looking at products like this (but you also should be aware that L'Oreal and Maybelline offer competitive pressed powders at the drugstore for one-fourth the price). And if you want to shop at the department store, know that Lancome's Color Ideal Precise Match Skin-Perfecting Pressed Powder has a formula that's nearly identical to this Luminous Silk Powder (L'Oreal owns both Lancome and Giorgio Armani).

✓ ☺ **$$$ Micro-fil Loose Powder** *($48)* has an airy, ultra-fine texture and a seamless finish that is incapable of looking too dry or powdery on skin. The three colors are excellent, though each one leaves a very soft sparkle—something those with oily skin will not be thrilled with, but that those with dry skin will find attractive.

BLUSH AND BRONZER: ✓ ☺ **$$$ Bronze Mania Skin Tint** *($55)*. The Armani makeup line does several things well, and making good bronzing products is definitely one of them! This liquid bronzer is exceptional, especially its range of four convincing colors suitable for a range of skin tones. Dispense it carefully, though, because it's very fluid and a little goes a long way. Blending is best done by dabbing it on your face in dots of color, then blending together using small circular motions. The sheer tint sets to a translucent matte finish and layers well if additional color is needed. Admittedly, you don't need to spend this much for a good liquid bronzer (Benefit has a good option that costs half as much, or Maybelline has a bronzing mousse that produces beautiful results for less than $10), but those who decide to splurge will be rewarded with one of the best bronzing products at the department store.

✓ ☺ **$$$ Bronze Mania Summer Foundation** *($55)*. This sheer, ultra-silky foundation is a remarkable way to add soft golden bronze color to skin. Both shades are excellent and utterly believable, and each has a soft matte finish. Summer Foundation is sheer enough to be applied all over, but you will want to blend downward onto the neck. The good news is that this makeup doesn't transfer to clothing easily. Despite that plus, most will find this works best in place of bronzing gel or powder. It applies beautifully over bare skin or foundation.

✓ ☺ **$$$ Body Tints Bronzer** ($75). Armani knows how to do beautiful bronzing products, and this fluid gel exemplifies their expertise. Blending must be quick and purposeful because this sets quickly, but the result is a gorgeous natural tan finish that works for most skin tones, including fair skin. This feels nearly weightless and stays in place well, although you may notice some color transfer to clothing or furniture, so keep that in mind when applying. An indulgent product to be sure, but one that does produce a convincing tan without exposing skin to sunlight. Note that the "tan" you get from this product doesn't supply sun protection, so you'll still need to apply a product rated SPF 15 or greater.

☺ **$$$ Blending Blush Duo** ($60). This is a cream-to-powder blush and highlighter in one compact. Both formulas are supposed to morph into a fluid when they come in contact with your skin, but that doesn't happen. The blush and highlighter blend easily and supply soft color with a delicate powder finish. You'll notice subtle sparkles, so keep that in mind if you don't want shiny cheeks. Shade 3 is an attractive peach/bronze duo for summer.

☺ **$$$ Sheer Bronzer** ($48) is a collection of three bronzing powders, each with a silky but dry texture that is tightly pressed, so the application is sheer. These brush on evenly and leave a soft, shimmering finish. It's not as natural as a true tan (which doesn't glisten), but the believable colors compensate for that. Shade #1 is tricky because it tends to look a bit too brown, but it works as a soft contour color.

☺ **$$$ Sheer Blush** ($42) is a good powder blush with a silky, dry texture and smooth application that imparts minimal color. For this amount of money, you should expect (and get) a bigger color payoff. As is, the palette of nude and soft pastel tones provides a bit too much shine for daytime wear.

EYESHADOW: ✓ ☺ **$$$ Maestro Eye Shadow Quads** ($58). Armani's eye for smart color coordination is apparent in this excellent collection of powder eyeshadow quads. The texture is very smooth and it blends on slightly creamy, leaving a soft satin finish. Each shade goes on softer than it looks in the compact, but they layer well for enhanced shading. Every quad is recommended except number 1, which is mostly obvious blue tones that are not for everyday use, that's for sure. One more note: the colors have dividers between them and the strips are wide enough to accommodate regular-size eyeshadow brushes, which is a nice touch.

☺ **$$$ Eye Shadow** ($28) features an impressively smooth texture that is a pleasure to work with. The shades apply sheer and don't allow you to build much color intensity, though they cling well to skin. All of the shades have some amount of shine (typically a soft shimmer), with the following being almost matte: 6, 7, 12, 21, and 39. Numbers 1, 15, and 27 are too blue, green, or lilac to recommend.

☺ **$$$ Maestro Eye Shadow** ($28) is said to be an irresistible invitation to play with color, but I think many women would find the price of these single pressed-powder eyeshadows easy to resist! Still, these do have an extremely silky texture that blends beautifully. The collection of shades tends to emphasize sparkling shine, despite claims that there are matte and satin shades (the only matte shades I saw were numbers 9, 11, and 16). Oddly, almost all of them apply more sheer than they look, including the darker browns and grays. Also, the tester unit is not labeled in a way that makes it easy to tell which finish you're viewing. In contrast, lines such as Laura Mercier, Chanel, and NARS have much more user-friendly eyeshadow tester units.

EYE AND BROW SHAPER: ☺ **$$$ Maestro Liquid Eye Liner** *($30)* is packaged like a fountain pen, and its brush allows for a precise, controlled application. The dry time is average; ideally, liquid eyeliner should dry faster than this to reduce the chance of smearing. However, once set, this has a matte finish and stays in place really well. You don't need to spend this much for a great liquid eyeliner, but those so inclined most likely won't be disappointed.

☺ **$$$ Eye Brow Defining Pencil** *($26)* needs sharpening, but for those who don't mind the inconvenience, this has a smooth, dry application and soft powder finish that really stays in place. The three shades present no options for dark brown or red/auburn brows, a strange oversight from a line of this nature.

☺ **$$$ Smooth Silk Eye Pencil** *($26)* is a standard pencil (in that it needs regular sharpening), but otherwise it has a wonderfully silky application that sets to a reasonably solid finish. For the money, this is above average, though it's not preferred to automatic pencils. Unless you're interested in using an eye pencil for shock value, avoid numbers 3 and 6.

LIPSTICK, LIP GLOSS AND LIPLINER: ✓ ☺ **$$$ Armanisilk Lipstick** *($25)* is a very good cream lipstick that, true to its name, has a silky texture. It manages to be creamy without feeling overly slick or greasy, and has a soft cream finish (some shades are imbued with shimmer). It is one of the better lipsticks at the department store, though you can find equally silky lipsticks from Max Factor and L'Oreal (Armani's owner) at the drugstore.

✓ ☺ **$$$ Lip Shimmer** *($26)* is a splurge, but one you may not mind making if a fantastic lip gloss tops your list of makeup must-haves. This elegant, lightweight, and completely non-sticky lip gloss is applied with a brush and comes in a beautiful selection of colors, each with varying degrees of shimmer.

✓ ☺ **$$$ Midnight Lip Shimmer** *($26)* is similar to Armani's Lip Shimmer, but is applied with a sponge-tip applicator instead of a brush and the colors are bolder with a strong iridescent finish. Otherwise, the same texture comments apply.

☺ **$$$ Lip Wax** *($26)* is essentially a thick, waxy lipstick melted into a pot, described as a modern version of lip color. Applied with a brush (which must be purchased separately) or a clean fingertip, this has a balm-like texture and leaves lips with a soft wash of color. Depending on how much you apply, the finish varies from soft matte to low-glow sheen. As for how modern this is, I suspect many women will find it a step backward because it isn't as convenient as popping open a lipstick and slicking it on lips.

☺ **$$$ Shine Lipstick** *($25)* is suitably creamy and offers an attractive glossy finish that's a step above Armani's Sheer Lipstick. The color range is remarkably well-edited and includes some stunning reds. The stain these shades leave give this lipstick a longevity boost that is most welcome.

☹ **$$$ Sheer Lipstick** *($25)* has a moisturizing but greasy feel, although it isn't so slick it slides right off your lips. As the name states, the colors are sheer. They provide no stain, so you're paying top dollar for a lipstick that likely won't make it past the morning commute.

☺ **$$$ Smooth Silk Lip Pencil** *($25)*. This needs-sharpening lip pencil feels creamy without being slick and applies smoothly. Pigmentation is stronger than usual, so each of the attractive shades has a good stain and impressive staying powder. This would earn a happy face rating if it didn't require routine sharpening. It goes without saying that there are hundreds of lip pencils for less than half the price that perform as well, if not better, than this one.

MASCARA: ✓ ☺ **$$$ Soft Lash Mascara** *($26)* is an admirable lengthening mascara that does not clump or flake and allows you to define lashes quickly, plus it layers effortlessly. It isn't much for thickness, but remains a superior lengthening mascara.

☺ **$$$ Eyes to Kill Mascara** *($28)*. This mascara promises weightless volume, but once you brush on several coats, lashes take on a distinctly heavy feel that differs from the feel you get with most mascaras. Interestingly, this mascara's component and cap are surprisingly heavy, too. If these trade-offs don't bother you, Eyes to Kill Mascara produces strikingly dramatic results. With just a few strokes, lashes are amazingly long, thick, and slightly curled. Even if you're careful during application, some clumping is inevitable; however, it is easy to smooth through and this mascara wears well throughout the day. Results are comparable to wearing false eyelashes, but this is easy to remove with a water-soluble cleanser.

☺ **$$$ Sparkling Mascara Top Coat** *($26)*. I have to admit that at first glance I thought this product was silly. I mean, come on—it's a glittery top coat for mascara. I pictured it being a mess to apply and envisioned the glitter flaking all night. Imagine my surprise when none of that happened. Instead, this sheer top coat applies smoothly over mascara (no dragging whatsoever) and leaves a sparkling finish that, applied softly, adds that special touch to evening or glamour makeup. Armani routinely offers this in translucent black with silvery glitter, and rotates other shades seasonally.

☹ **$$$ Maestro Instant Volume Mascara** *($26)* is another comb mascara. Although it does create instant volume, the best-looking result required more work than a mascara should. The variegated mini-combs deposit a lot of mascara on lashes, but their layout doesn't allow for even application. Therefore, brushing through lashes with a clean mascara wand is necessary to make things look clean yet full. If you're curious to try this type of mascara, L'Oreal's Volume Shocking Mascara is half the price and has a much better application.

☹ **$$$ Soft Lash Primer** *($25)* is essentially a mascara without color, and it builds a waxy base coat on which to apply a regular mascara. A product like this is superfluous if you are already using an excellent mascara, and there are plenty of those to be found for significantly less money than this primer.

FACE AND BODY ILLUMINATING/SHIMMER PRODUCTS: ✓☺ **$$$ Fluid Sheer** *($58)* is similar in texture and application to Armani's Luminous Silk Foundation, but is meant to "sculpt" and "illuminate" the complexion. For a touch of radiant shine or to softly highlight or shadow your features in the evening, these are fine and they blend well with foundation or moisturizer. The shade range presents potential options for blush, contour, or bronzing—and, of course, highlighting. Best of all, the shine effect doesn't flake and stays in place on all but the oiliest skin.

✓☺ **$$$ Light Master Primer** *($55)* is a thin-textured fluid that imparts skin with a subtle lit-from-within glow. Its texture is light and silky, and it leaves a minimally moist finish. Applied under foundation, it helps enliven the complexion and adds heightened dimension to skin. It may also be used over foundation to highlight key areas. The light-show claims that Armani makes for this primer are over-the-top, but if you're shopping Armani for primers and don't mind the expense for a cosmetic facial pick-me-up, this is worth a trial run.

BRUSHES: ☺ **$$$ Giorgio Armani Brushes** *($24-$55)* offer a functional, well-assembled brush collection without any glaring omissions, though the price point doesn't make them preferred to less expensive brushes. **The Face Brush** *($55)* and **Blush Brush** *($43)* are full, soft, and luxurious (which they should be at this price), while the **Large Eye Contour Brush** *($40)* and **Blender Brush** *($47)*, which Armani recommends for applying foundation, are also standouts for their versatility. ☹ **$$$ Lip Brush** *($24)* is too standard for the money, and because it's a nonretractable brush and without a cap, portability is a problem.

SPECIALTY PRODUCTS: ☺ **$$$ Fluid Master Primer** *($55)* spreads easily over skin and leaves a beautifully silky finish. You're not getting anything extra for your money, other than the Armani name. This clear, silicone-based primer doesn't "hold" makeup better than most others, and its formula is comparable to silicone-based primers from many other brands, from Lancome to Smashbox.

GLOMINERALS (MAKEUP ONLY)

GLOMINERALS AT-A-GLANCE

Strengths: Very good loose- and pressed-powder mineral foundations; gentle makeup remover; great bronzing gel, blush, and eyeshadow options; the brow powder; fantastic cream lipstick; Liquid Lips; mostly good makeup brushes.

Weaknesses: Not distributed well and salons that stock this line rarely have all of the products; none of the foundations offer sun protection, which is uncommon for a mineral makeup line; the liquid foundations look too heavy and opaque on skin; average loose and pressed powders; specialty makeup products that are below standard and not worth the cost.

For more information about gloMinerals, call (800) 496-8007 or visit www.glominerals.com or www.beautypedia.com.

MAKEUP REMOVER: ✓ ☺ **gloEye Make Up Remover** *($14 for 4 ounces)* is a standard detergent-based eye makeup remover that's suitable for all skin types. It is fragrance-free, does not contain needless irritants, and removes all but the most stubborn waterproof makeup.

FOUNDATION: ☺ **$$$ gloPressed Base Powder Foundation** *($39)* is the pressed (and less messy) version of gloMinerals' gloLoose Base Powder Foundation. Like the Loose version, this has a mica base and an application that feels silky and slightly creamy, but sets to a dry matte finish. It feels remarkably smooth and offers a soft, non-sparkling glow to skin. If you have lines or wrinkles, be sure to check the application in daylight because any amount of shine can make wrinkles more obvious. Overall, this is one of the better pressed-powder mineral foundations due to its superior texture, application, and blendability, but regrettably it doesn't contain sunscreen. It also manages to not look flat or dull on skin, although overdoing this definitely results in a powdery appearance that accentuates lines. This is still highly recommended for fans of mineral makeup who have normal to slightly dry or oily skin. The shade selection is excellent. Most of the colors are neutral to slightly warm (yellow/gold) and are suitable for most fair to dark skin tones. The darkest shades (those in the Cocoa range) are worth a look because this mineral foundation doesn't look ashen.

☺ **$$$ gloLoose Base Powder Foundation** *($37)* is a mica-based mineral foundation that promises a dewy finish, but doesn't provide it. It cannot make good on the dewy finish claim because most of the ingredients are extremely absorbent and not moisturizing in the least. However, the mica base does lend a shiny finish some may misconstrue as dewy. Be cautious if you have wrinkles because any amount of shine can make wrinkles more obvious, so be sure to check this in the daylight. Texture-wise, this feels quite silky and it blends on with a slight creaminess that quickly changes to a dry matte finish (matte in feel, the sparkling shine remains evident). This provides light to medium coverage when brushed on, and approaches full coverage if buffed on with a sponge. Sponge application results in a heavier look and feel, but that's the trade-off for extra coverage with most mineral-based foundations, and this one is no exception. The shade selection is extensive and mostly neutral and there are options for light to tan skin tones. There are no shades you need to avoid, which is reassuring. As for the claims about this being special due to the antioxidants it contains—they won't provide any benefit, for the following two reasons: one, the product comes in clear jar packaging, which means these air-sensitive ingredients won't remain stable, and two, there is only a tiny amount of antioxidants in the formula. This is best for normal to oily skin, provided you don't mind the shiny finish.

☹ **$$$ gloProtective Liquid Foundation Matte II** *($30.50)* is a liquid foundation the company claims to have created for oily skin. It is available only in four shades, but all of them are neutral and will work for most medium skin tones. The problem is this foundation's heavy appearance on the skin. It has an opacity that provides considerable coverage, but the trade-off is a finish that doesn't look as natural as that of today's top foundations, and the matte finish, while nice, doesn't last very long.

☹ **$$$ gloProtective Liquid Foundation Satin II** *($36.50)*. This silky liquid foundation comes in a tube. Even using only a small amount will provide considerable coverage. gloMinerals describes the coverage range as sheer to full, but this foundation cannot be blended out sheer—there's too much pigment and opacity from the titanium dioxide, so it stays noticeable and has a rather thick appearance on the skin. The thick appearance is this foundation's main downfall. It feels uncomfortably dry on skin and the matte finish looks flat and artificial, at least compared with today's best liquid foundations. If you decide to try this anyway (as mentioned, it is useful if you need significant, heavy coverage), you'll want to avoid the slightly pink Beige Light and the slightly peach Natural. The dark shades in the Cocoa range look too ashen and are not recommended.

☺ **$$$ gloSheer Tint Base** *($32)* is a standard, lightweight tinted moisturizer that's suitable for normal to slightly dry skin. It blends well without much slip and sets to a satin matte finish while providing sheer coverage. Note that this product's matte finish feels progressively drier the longer it's on, so this supplies zilch moisture and will absorb whatever moisture is already present. In the long run, it will only make the dry areas of your face drier. This contains a couple of sunscreen ingredients, but because they're not listed as active, you cannot rely on this moisturizer for sun protection. The shade range includes options for light to tan skin tones and all of them are workable.

CONCEALER: ☺ **$$$ gloCamouflage** *($22)* is a standard creamy concealer with a smooth, emollient texture. The triglyceride base allows for smooth blending, while the waxes contribute to this concealer's thickness and opacity. It provides excellent coverage, but poses a risk of creasing into lines around the eyes unless set with powder. This is too emollient for use over breakouts, but works great to conceal pronounced redness, brown discolorations, and dark circles. All of the shades are very good.

☺ **$$$ gloBrightener Highlight Concealer** *($16)* is a good liquid concealer whose texture is thin and whose coverage is on the sheer side. Its sole light neutral shade is best used to highlight or to cover areas that require only minor camouflage. This blends easily and has a satin-smooth finish that you should set with powder to avoid creasing into lines.

☹ **$$$ gloBlemish Stick** *($18)* is a twist-up, retractable stick concealer whose sole bright spot is excellent coverage. The trade-off for this much coverage is a heavy appearance on skin, seeping into lines, and a thick, greasy texture that shouldn't be used over blemishes. There are two shades: Light is acceptable, while Medium is slightly peach.

☹ **$$$ gloConcealer Under Eye** *($30)* is a dual-sided cream concealer that offers two shades in one component. It blends on smoothly and has a slightly slick yet creamy texture. Once set, this has a soft powder finish that's short-lived, so expect this to crease into lines and slip into large pores. The shades are a mixed bag; most are too pink, peach, or orange to look convincing under the eyes. The only workable duo is Golden.

POWDER: ☺ **$$$ gloMatte Finishing Powder** *($33.50)*. This mica-based pressed powder comes in one shade, a soft, pale fleshy peach. It has a dry, dusty texture that goes on sheer and provides a dry matte finish without looking cakey. The shade limits its appeal to those with light or dark skin tones; actually, even someone with a neutral skin tone should test this before purchasing because it can have a strange color effect.

☺ **$$$ gloPerfecting Powder** *($33.50)* is similar to the gloMatte Finishing Powder above, except that this one comes in a more neutral shade that enhances its versatility. The texture is still dry, but not as dusty and flyaway as that of the gloMatte Finishing Powder. It provides a strong matte finish and is best applied sheer to avoid a chalky appearance.

BLUSH AND BRONZER: ✓ ☺ **$$$ gloSheer Tint Base Bronzing Gel** *($30)* is an excellent bronzing gel. It not only produces a believable tan color for light to medium skin tones, but also has a silky, lotion-like texture that blends beautifully and sets to a soft, slightly moist finish. You get a translucent bronze color with a subtle glow that isn't the least bit sparkly, all from a formula that's suitable for all skin types.

☺ **$$$ gloBlush** *($25)* is a standard pressed-powder blush. It has a smooth although noticeably dry texture, but it applies evenly and deposits a soft color. The shade range is impressive for a line of this size, although each shade has some amount of shine. The obviously shiny shades are best for evening glamour rather than daytime makeup.

☺ **$$$ gloBlush Duo** *($27)* is similar to the regular gloBlush reviewed above, except here you get a powder blush and complementary tone of highlighting powder in one compact. The blush has modest shine; the highlighter has strong shimmer. The pairs are fine, but this much shine is best for evening makeup.

☺ **$$$ gloGolden Bronzing Stick** *($22)* provides a soft wash of golden tan color with a hint of copper shimmer. It looks quite nice, but the oil- and wax-based formula is only for those with dry to very dry skin that's not prone to blemishes. The finish feels thick and slightly moist and leaves skin with a subtle glistening appearance.

☺ **$$$ gloCream Blush** *($25)* begins creamy thanks to the formula's emollient main ingredient, but it sets to a soft matte finish due to the amount of clay and titanium dioxide. Although this is not a true cream blush (someone with dry skin won't be happy with the finish), it allows controlled blending and produces long-lasting color that has more pigmentation than a standard powder blush. gloCream Blush is best for normal to slightly dry skin that's not prone to blemishes.

☹ **$$$ gloBronze** *($38.50)*. This sheer, mica-based pressed bronzing powder comes in an attractive soft tan color, but its unusually dry texture gets in the way of smooth application and makes blending difficult. It leaves a soft shine, which helps offset the dry finish, but still, for the money, there are lots of bronzing powders that outperform this.

☹ **$$$ gloTint for Cheeks & Lips** *($14)* is a sheer, water-based gel blush that sets quickly, so blending must be lightning fast. The rosy color has a soft fuchsia undertone that works best as a lip stain. Used on cheeks, it's too easy to make a mistake that leads to a blotchy, streaky result. Note: If you use this as a lip tint, you should follow it with a lip balm or gloss to leave lips comfortable.

EYESHADOW: ☺ **$$$ gloEye Shadow** *($18)* is a pressed eyeshadow that comes in a large range of shades, most with some degree of shine. The texture is smooth yet dry, but not too dry, so this applies fairly well and provides more coverage than eyeshadows typically do. The best shades among the fairly extensive selection include Bamboo, Blackberry, Diamond, Eggplant, Fawn, Harvest, Haze, Honey, Kona, Mink, Orchid, Twig, Sand Pebble, and Sea Shell.

☺ **$$$ gloEye Shadow Trio** *($29.50)* has a formula that is slightly different from that of the gloMinerals gloEye Shadow above. The formula difference translates into a smoother application that blends better and feels a bit silkier. Most of the trios are workable color combinations, but all of them have a moderate to strong degree of shine. It's good news that the shine doesn't flake, but bad news if you have wrinkles or sagging in the eye area, because this much shine will call attention to such signs of aging.

☺ **$$$ gloReflection Cream Eye Shadow** *($20)* is not a cream eyeshadow, so the name is either a mistake or just strange. It is more accurately described as a liquid eyeshadow that doesn't feel the least bit creamy, during blending or after it sets. Despite the misleading name, this is a very good way to apply shiny eyeshadow that lasts. There's enough slip to make controlled blending easy, and the shine remains virtually flake-free for hours. Gilded Bronze and Golden Pearl are the most versatile shades.

☺ **$$$ gloSmoky Eye Kit** *($36)* is a set of four powder eyeshadows that range from light to dark. The idea is to follow the step-by-step instructions to create the perfect smoky eye. The eyeshadow formula differs slightly from that of other gloMineral powder shadows, and the result is a smooth, dry texture that applies evenly and sheer enough so that you can gradually build color. Best of all is how well the shadows in this kit blend, although it's a shame each shade is shiny, because all-out shine isn't required for the perfect smoky eye.

☺ **$$$ gloLid Primer** *($24)* is a cream concealer meant for use on the eyelids. The thick texture softens on skin so blending isn't difficult, and this doesn't get slick so you can control placement easily. The single shade is best for fair to medium skin tones, and it not only provides coverage but also lightens and brightens the eye area prior to eyeshadow application. This tends to crease if you have oily eyelids, but if that is not an issue, this is worth trying if you're not pleased with how your foundation or concealer works to prime the eyelid and under-brow area.

☹ **gloLoose Eye Shadow** *($15).* This loose-powder eyeshadow is quite messy to use, even though the company packaged it to minimize the mess. I ordered this directly from gloMinerals, and it arrived with shiny powder all over the outside of the container and inside the outer carton. After cleaning the mess up, I used it, making a mess of things once more. If you can tolerate the mess, this mica-based powder has a soft, silky texture and slightly dry finish. Pigmentation is strong, as is the shiny finish. Unless applied very sheer, this amount of shine is best for evening makeup only.

EYE AND BROW SHAPER: ☺ **$$$ gloBrow Powder Duos** *($24).* This matte-finish brow powder is one of gloMineral's sleeper products. In one compact you get two shades separated by a divider. You can mix to create a custom shade or use whichever one matches your brow hair best. These apply smoothly, don't flake, and impart rich color, but a little goes a long way.

☺ **$$$ gloPrecision Eye Pencil** *($16)* is a standard slightly creamy, needs-sharpening eye pencil. Application is smooth and it sets to a soft powder finish that doesn't smudge, although it is slightly prone to fading. Some of the shades have a shimmer or metallic finish, so choose carefully. The Peach and Silver Lilac shades are poor choices for defining the eyes.

☹ **$$$ Metallic gloEye Pencil** *($16)* is a very standard, creamy eye pencil whose shades offer a metallic finish. The look isn't for everyone, and it is distracting for professional daytime makeup. This pencil needs routine sharpening.

☺ **$$$ gloBrow Gel** *($17)* is an average, utterly ordinary option to tame unruly brow hairs. It's available in Clear or sheer shades for brown or dark blonde brows. The main drawback is that it takes too long to set and can gum up brows if not applied precisely.

☺ **$$$ gloPrecision Brow Pencil** *($16)* is easy to apply and has a smooth, powder-like texture that allows you to "feather in" color between the brows for natural-looking results. The colors are great, too. This would be rated a Paula's Pick if not for the sharpening requirement; there are just too many good screw-up pencils to bother with the extra effort of sharpening.

☺ **$$$ gloCream EyeLiner** *($19)* is a standard cream eyeliner that applies easily and imparts deep, defining color but isn't reliable when it comes to long wear. The finish remains slightly creamy, while the emollients in the formula make this cream eyeliner prone to fading and smudging. It is not recommended over the long-wearing gel-cream eyeliners available from brands such as Bobbi Brown, M.A.C, or Paula's Choice.

☺ **$$$ gloLiquid Eye Liner** *($16)* has a good brush, but the color deposit is uneven and a bit too sheer, which makes layering mandatory. Dry time is slow, which increases the chance that this will smear before it sets. As for wearability, this doesn't flake, but the colors will fade before you're ready to remove it.

LIPSTICK, LIP GLOSS, AND LIPLINER: ✓ ☺ **gloLiquid Lips** *($14.75)*. Think of this tube lip gloss as a product that combines the smooth texture and shiny finish of a gloss with the color intensity of traditional lipstick. The color saturation is rich and the glossy, wet finish is attractive without feeling sticky or syrupy. This is an excellent product, but one to avoid if you're prone to lip color bleeding into lines around the mouth.

✓ ☺ **$$$ gloLip Stick** *($16.50)*. What a surprise that a cosmetics line known for their mineral makeup offers such an outstanding cream lipstick! This has a beautifully smooth application that feels lush and creamy without being slippery. You get full color, a soft cream finish, and impressive wear from any of the enticing shades. gloMinerals also offers a colorless version of this product, labeled **Lip Treatment**. Whichever shade you choose, this is a remarkable lipstick that deserves strong consideration.

☺ **$$$ gloSheer Lip Stick** *($17)* is a standard, but good, sheer cream lipstick. You get soft color and an even application that does not feel too slippery and does not provide a strong glossy finish. The range of shades is limited, but all go on brighter than they appear.

☺ **gloGloss** *($15.50)* is a standard, but good, lip gloss with a wand applicator. It feels moderately smooth and emollient without a trace of stickiness. The shade range is superb, with sheer and light coverage options and varying degrees of shimmer.

☺ **$$$ gloGlaze Lip Polish** *($22)* is a rather unexciting dual-sided lip gloss. You get two colors in one component, and both are quite sheer. The texture is closer to that of a thin lip balm than a lip gloss, and the finish is shiny but not glaringly so. Not bad, but not exceptional either, and the fragrance is unusually potent.

☺ **$$$ gloPrecision Lip Pencil** *($17)* has a smooth application that, once set, tends to stay in place quite well, so there's no need to worry about smudging. The pencil requires routine sharpening and the finish feels a bit tacky, which is a definite drawback. The shade range favors darker berry and brown tones, but it coordinates well with the gloMinerals lipstick palette. The brush on the other end of this pencil is good, but once this pencil sets, it cannot be blended.

☹ **gloRoyal Lip Crayon** *($16)* needs routine sharpening (the company sells a special sharpener separately), but in addition the pencil tip is soft and tends to squish, both during use and while sharpening. Add to that the greasy texture and glitter-infused finish that feels grainy on lips within an hour. This is a lip crayon to leave in the box!

☹ **Mint Balm SPF 15** *($12)*. Not only is this lip balm awkward to use because of the large size of the component, but also the sunscreen does not provide sufficient UVA protection, despite the SPF 15 claim. Moreover, the formula contains peppermint oil, which gets your lips tingling from irritation on contact and will make chapped lips worse.

☹ **gloLip Plumper** *($16)*. Put this slightly thick but smooth lip gloss on and within moments you'll feel the burn from the pepper extract. The offending ingredient (listed by its Latin name *Capsicum frutescens*) plumps lips by virtue of irritation, and it leaves a lingering burning sensation that intensifies the longer you keep this on your lips. The plumping is minimal, and I doubt most women will find the burning sensation tolerable, especially considering the merely OK and very temporary results. In addition, the irritation will make chapped lips worse.

MASCARA: ☺ **$$$ gloVolumizing Mascara** *($19)* is a very good thickening mascara. It goes on slightly heavy, but isn't messy, and within a few strokes you have thick, separated lashes. Successive coats build a bit more length, but the real reason to go for this one is the lush, dramatic lashes it creates. This removes easily with a water-soluble cleanser.

☺ **$$$ gloLash Lengthening Mascara** *($16)* isn't a very impressive mascara. It makes lashes moderately long and keeps them soft, but application tends to be a bit uneven and the formula smears readily. Even when I was being extra careful during application, it was impossible to not get some mascara on my eyelid and in the under-brow area. That's disappointing and necessitates lots of clean-up before this looks presentable.

☺ **$$$ gloLash Thickener & Conditioner** *($16)* is a standard colorless lash primer that adds bulk to lashes prior to applying mascara. This primer makes a noticeable difference if paired with an average mascara, but the real question is why would anyone settle for an average mascara when there are so many outstanding options? Paired with a great mascara, this primer makes little difference when compared with simply applying another coat or two of mascara.

BRUSHES: The ☺ **Brushes** *($8.50-$37)* from gloMinerals don't distinguish themselves in any significant way, but almost all of the brush options match the status quo and work just fine for their intended purpose. The **Cream Blush** *($28)* brush doesn't work as well as dabbing and blending cream blush with your fingers, while the **Fan Brush** *($16)* is not an essential brush for anyone. The various brushes for applying eyeshadow and eyeliner are worth a look, and the price range of these brushes makes them somewhat of a value compared with brushes from several department store makeup lines.

☺ **$$$ Mini Travel Brush Kit** *($60)* includes six of gloMineral's makeup brushes, most of which are workable and well shaped. A powder brush is included, but there's not one to apply blush and/or bronzer, a strange omission. The kit is nice, but I suspect most consumers will do better assembling their own kit from this line's extensive collection of brushes.

☺ **Brush Cleaner** *($12)* is just isopropyl alcohol with several fragrant plant extracts. The alcohol will remove excess oil and cosmetic pigments from your brushes, but repetitive use will make the brush hairs dry and brittle. This isn't preferred to washing your brushes with a gentle shampoo; however, it is a quick way to clean and sterilize brushes between uses on multiple people.

FACE AND BODY ILLUMINATING/SHIMMER PRODUCTS: ☺ **$$$ gloDust 24K** *($36.50)* is a loose powder that's loaded with shine. You get a moderate shimmer from the base pigment (either bronze, gold, or silver) in each shade plus a crystalline sparkling finish that makes skin look glistening and slightly wet. This powder's blend of shine doesn't last long, but it's an OK option to dust on for evening makeup. It isn't as flyaway as several other shiny loose powders, but it still sheds.

☺ **$$$ gloHighlighter** *($16)*. Rather than being subtle, this sheer liquid highlighter produces an obviously shiny finish even when blended on sheer. Available in one pale pink shade, the shiny finish gives skin an icy, ethereal crystalline glow that looks more alien than fresh-faced and radiant. This contains a tiny amount of antioxidants (not enough for skin to notice) and comfrey extract, a plant that can cause problems for skin (though likely not in this small amount).

☺ **$$$ gloShimmer Brick** *($31.50)*. Housed in one compact are four individual pans of pressed shimmer powder. They feel creamy at first, but set to a dry matte finish that's loaded with shine. The shiny particles don't cling well, and the powder overall has a dry feel, which means it doesn't mesh well with skin. In this price range, you can find better shimmer products form Bobbi Brown or Laura Mercier.

SPECIALTY PRODUCTS: ☺ **gloExfoliating Lip Wand** *($15)* isn't a lip scrub as described in the gloMinerals catalog. Rather, it's a pale peach-tinted (and peach scented) lip balm in stick form. It is supposed to contain wax microcrystals that exfoliate lips on application, but this goes on smoothly and doesn't feel the least bit grainy, which is not what you'd expect from a product claiming to exfoliate lips. The good news: this is an emollient lip balm with a soft gloss finish.

☺ **$$$ gloFace Primer** *($23)* is a very standard silicone-based primer in terms of its silky texture and slight ability to fill in superficial lines and large pores. It contains some good antioxidants, but the clear glass bottle packaging doesn't shield them from light, so they will degrade. This would be rated higher if it came in opaque packaging and omitted the fragrant sandalwood extract, which isn't going to do your skin any favors. For slightly more money, consider the primer from Giorgio Armani or go for an antioxidant-packed serum such as those from Dr. Denese New York.

☹ **gloMoist Hydration Mist** *($17.50 for 2 ounces)* is a waste of time and money because the formula is chiefly water and preservatives, and a formaldehyde-releasing preservative at that. It contains a tiny amount of anti-irritants and water-binding agents and is fragranced with irritating geranium oil. Don't bother with this—it is a mistake for any skin type.

☹ **gloEye Revitalize** *($22)*. This sheer, pale pink fluid is designed to be dabbed on the under-eye area (along the orbital bone) for an instant pick-me-up. Its invigorating action comes from the inclusion of several irritating plants, including oils of eucalyptus and peppermint. These ingredients aren't good for skin anywhere on the body, but around the eyes? No way!

GOOD SKIN

GOOD SKIN AT-A-GLANCE

Strengths: Reasonable prices; several state-of-the-art moisturizers and serums; superb cleansers; some well-rounded sunscreens that go beyond just protecting skin from sunlight; hand cream with sunscreen; one awesome foundation; powder blush; loose powder; loose shimmer powder.

Weaknesses: A few sunscreens with paltry amounts of UVA-protecting ingredients; some problematic anti-acne products and a lack of topical disinfectant for blemishes; the makeup items with sunscreen lack sufficient UVA-protecting ingredients; the anti-acne foundation and concealer; the mascara; jar packaging.

For more information about Good Skin, owned by Estee Lauder and sold exclusively at Kohl's, call (866) 352-8338 or visit www.goodskindermcare.com or www.Beautypedia.com.

GOOD SKIN SKIN CARE

GOOD SKIN ALL BRIGHT PRODUCTS

✓ ☺ **All Bright Moisture Cream** *($24.50 for 1.7 ounces)* has a compelling assortment of state-of-the-art ingredients covering every category that could make your skin happy, along with a wonderful silky texture. There's only one misstep, but it's barely worth mentioning. In essence, this is a very good moisturizer for normal to dry skin—just don't count on it to improve skin discolorations. Mulberry extract and glycyrrhetinic acid (a derivative of licorice) have only a small amount of research showing them to have benefit in this regard, and this research included only a handful of participants who applied those ingredients at high concentrations (Sources: *International Journal of Dermatology*, April 2000, pages 299-301; and *Skin Lightening and Depigmenting Agents*, www.emedicine.com/derm/topic528.htm).

✓ ☺ **All Bright Moisturizing Sunscreen SPF 30** *($12 for 1.7 ounces)* can be relied on for sufficient UVA protection. It also has an array of beneficial ingredients for skin, and that all adds up to a decent daily sunscreen. It isn't the best formula for sensitive skin, but a well-formulated sunscreen of any kind is the first line of defense to improve the appearance of skin discolorations—and prevent them in the first place. Yeast is a good water-binding agent, but has zero effect on discolorations.

☺ **All Bright Spot Treatment** *($16 for 0.5 ounce)* is supposed to dramatically dissolve dark spots and discolorations because of the yeast ferment and fruit extracts it contains. The amount of fruit extracts is barely worth mentioning, and although there's a considerable amount of yeast extract, there is no research aligning it with any measure of skin-lightening ability. In the end, this is a lightweight, serum-like moisturizer for normal to slightly dry skin.

GOOD SKIN ALL CALM PRODUCTS

✓ ☺ **All Calm Creamy Cleanser** *($15 for 6.7 ounces)* is indeed creamy and fairly emollient, so you need a washcloth to be sure you remove all of it and get all your makeup off as well. A blend of thickeners, plant oils, and silicones makes this extremely helpful for someone with dry skin, regardless of whether your skin is sensitive or not.

☹ **All Calm Soothing Toner** *($15 for 6.7 ounces)* is a simple blend of water, slip agents, glycerin, skin-identical ingredients, anti-irritants, and an antioxidant. It isn't a particularly exciting formulation, but it has potential for normal to dry skin. The lavender extract keeps it from earning a higher rating.

✓ ☺ **All Calm Gentle Sunscreen SPF 25** *($12 for 1.7 ounces)* is aptly formulated for someone with sensitive skin. The sunscreen base is purely titanium dioxide and zinc oxide, which means you get excellent sun protection with almost no risk of irritation. It also has a wonderful silky feel with a nice array of impressive, state-of-the-art ingredients. While it does contain coloring agents to lessen the white appearance of the sunscreen ingredients on skin, it is fragrance-free. This one is a winner!

☹ **$$$ All Calm Moisture Cream** *($24.50 for 1.7 ounces)* contains some good soothing agents and antioxidants, but since these ingredients are light- and air-sensitive, their potency is compromised by the jar packaging. This ends up being a decent option for normal to dry skin, but better packaging would have made it so much better!

✓ ☺ **All Calm Moisture Lotion** *($24.50 for 1.7 ounces)* is a silky, lotion-textured moisturizer with a smattering of skin-identical ingredients, anti-irritants, and antioxidants. It's definitely a great moisturizer for someone with sensitive skin, which is why it's rated a Paula's Pick. Those with normal to dry skin that's not overtly sensitive will likely want to find better options for a moisturizer.

GOOD SKIN ALL FIRM PRODUCTS

☹ **All Firm Moisture Cream SPF 15** *($24.50 for 1.7 ounces)* does contain the UVA-protecting ingredient titanium dioxide, but in a concentration of less than 1%, which is not enough to make it reliable for protecting skin from the full spectrum of the sun's damaging rays. It does have an impressive array of ingredients that would make it noteworthy for skin, but putting these unstable ingredients in jar packaging means that any benefit from them is time-limited due to the way they decompose on contact with air. That, together with the less-than-exciting sunscreen ingredients, means this is a product that can stay on the shelf.

✓ ☺ **All Firm Rebuilding Serum** *($26 for 1 ounce)* is a good, lightweight moisturizer with a very good mix of interesting state-of-the-art ingredients. This is definitely helpful for skin, and the weightless texture works for many skin types. Just don't expect to see firmer skin anytime soon.

GOOD SKIN ALL RIGHT PRODUCTS

☹ **All Right Medicated Cleanser** *($12 for 4.2 ounces)* contains 1% salicylic acid, but it's in a cleanser, so the exfoliating acid is rinsed down the drain before it has an opportunity to benefit the skin. The inclusion of peppermint wrecks an otherwise good, water-soluble cleanser for normal to oily skin.

☹ **All Right Purifying Toner** *($12 for 6.7 ounces)* has alcohol and witch hazel headlining the ingredient list, so the only thing "all right" about this product is the name. The 1.5% salicylic acid it contains is a good exfoliant, but the risk of irritation, redness, and dryness posed by the other ingredients means it isn't worth the price of admission. The alcohol will trigger oil production in the pore lining, which is anything but purifying!

☺ **All Right Portable Anti-Acne Swabs** *($6.50 for 12 swabs)* are intended to provide a way to precisely apply salicylic acid (BHA) directly to a blemish without getting it on the surrounding skin. The stem of the cotton swab contains a liquid solution of 2% salicylic acid, and when you break the tip the fluid flows into it, ready to apply to the blemish-prone area. The pH of 3.6 ensures the salicylic acid will work as intended. Although BHA can help disinfect and reduce inflammation (salicylic acid is both an antibacterial agent and an anti-irritant, since it is closely related to aspirin), it can also work preventively to keep breakouts from happening in the first place. With this product, however, you don't get enough to apply all over, you barely get enough for even a couple of blemishes. This ends up being a fairly pricey way to treat acne, unless you happen to be the lucky person who gets only one or two pimples a month.

☹ **All Right Spot Treatment** *($8.50 for 0.5 ounce)* is a 1% salicylic acid topical exfoliant that would be a slam-dunk recommendation if it didn't contain menthol, which only serves to irritate skin.

☹ **All Right Mattifying Gel** *($12 for 0.5 ounce)* could have been a contender for helping someone with a minor blemish problem, thanks to its 0.5% salicylic acid content, but the alcohol listed prominently in second place on the ingredient list makes the potential for irritation, dryness, and excess oil production more likely, and that doesn't help any skin type.

☺ **All Right Oil-Free Lotion** *($17.50 for 1.7 ounces)* is a 0.5% salicylic acid lotion with a pH of 3.8, so it will provide minor exfoliation (1% salicylic acid is preferred). The small amounts of antioxidants and anti-irritants are a thoughtful touch, and this does have a smooth texture with a decent matte finish for someone with normal to oily skin.

OTHER GOOD SKIN PRODUCTS

☺ **Clean Skin Foaming Cleanser** *($12.50 for 6.7 ounces)* is a standard but good detergent-based, water-soluble cleanser for normal to oily skin. It leaves skin feeling clean but not too dry; this would be rated higher if not for the amount of grapefruit extract it contains.

✓☺ **Perfect Balance Gel Cleanser** *($12.50 for 6.7 ounces)* does have a very good balance going for it, just as the name says. The effective assortment of gentle detergent cleansing agents makes it a very good water-soluble cleanser for someone with normal to oily or combination skin.

✓☺ **Soft Skin Creamy Cleanser** *($12.50 for 6.7 ounces)* is a very good emollient cleanser for dry skin that contains a nice blend of emollients, plant oils, and silicone. You may need to use a washcloth to be sure it is all rinsed off, but all in all this is an excellent product.

☹ **$$$ Citra-Peel, High Intensity Resurfacing Peel** *($32)* is an odd, and rather disappointing, two-step system. Step 1 is **Resurface**, which comes in a jar of 30 pads soaked in water, citric acid, slip agents, lime extract, and preservatives. Citric acid can exfoliate, but it isn't the best way to go about it; far more preferred are glycolic, lactic, or salicylic acid. This would be an option, however, if it weren't for the lime extract, which doesn't do much but add a risk of irritation. Step 2 is **Restore,** another jar package with 30 pads that are basically soaked in water and sodium bicarbonate (baking soda) plus some anti-irritants. That's OK, but there really isn't any reason to raise the pH of the skin that high, when all you really need to do is rinse your face with water after waiting a period of time to remove Step 1. Water does the job far better than the baking soda. But still, when it comes to exfoliation, a leave-on product is easier to use and less complicated than this one. This isn't a terrible product, just not the best way to exfoliate skin.

☺ **$$$ Lumecin Overnight Brightening Gluco-Protein Treatment** *($44.50 for 1.3 ounces).* I wouldn't describe this product as "revolutionary" as Good Skin claims it is, but in the world of cosmetics, such a word does attract attention. Without mincing words, what you will find is an intriguing product to consider if you're looking for an exfoliant that combines approximately 0.5% salicylic acid with the polyhydroxy acid gluconolactone (used to a greater extent in NeoStrata products). The pH of 4 ensures some exfoliation will take place, but not to the extent you'd get with a higher concentration of salicylic (or glycolic) acid at a slightly lower pH. This contains some plant extracts that have limited research about their ability to lighten skin discolorations, but the small amounts present in this product probably won't give you the results you'd like to see in the mirror. Of more interest is the ingredient acetyl glucoasamine because there is some in vitro research showing this to be an effective inhibitor of melanin synthesis. Interrupting this process (or pathway) before discoloration surfaces is how acetyl glucosamine is believed to function. The rub is that this research has been carried out only by Procter & Gamble, the company that owns Olay, and their Definity line contains acetyl glucosamine. That means it isn't much to go on, as P&G stands to gain from their own studies, not to mention that how an ingredient behaves on skin cultures in a Petri dish can be quite different from how it works on intact skin. Still, taken as a lightweight, mild BHA product, this is an option for normal to slightly dry or slightly oily skin. The texture is fluid and it sets to a soft matte finish; plus, your skin is treated to some beneficial extras, including antioxidants and soothing agents.

☺ **$$$ Microcrystal Skin Refinisher** *($25 for 1.7 ounces)* is a lotion-style scrub that contains alumina as the abrasive agent. Alumina has a texture akin to salt, which makes this fairly gritty and scratchy, so be extra careful if you decide to give it a try. A handful of antioxidants and anti-irritants are included, but will be rinsed off before they can have any effect. For manual exfoliation, this is a pricey and perhaps overly rough scrub; gentler options are definitely available.

✓ ☺ **Polished Skin Gentle Exfoliator** *($14 for 3.4 ounces)* comes in a gel formulation that is, indeed, quite gentle, and for exfoliation it works well. Because the base doesn't have other cleansing agents, you wouldn't want to rely on this alone for cleansing; you'd need to use it after using a water-soluble cleanser.

☹ **All Hydrated Moisture Cream** *($24.50 for 1.7 ounces)* has many formulary positives, but the overriding negative is that jar packaging will render several of the most helpful ingredients ineffective shortly after you begin using this. The fragrance-free, silky-finish formula is suitable for normal to dry skin not prone to blemishes.

✓ ☺ **Clean Skin Oil-Free Lotion SPF 15** *($16 for 1.7 ounces)* is a very good moisturizer for someone with normal to oily skin who needs a reliable sunscreen with UVA-protecting ingredients. With an impressive 3% avobenzone, this one fills the bill for the kind of sun protection skin needs. It is appropriately lightweight, with a slight matte finish (though it won't hold up all day). It has a decent amount of ingredients that mimic skin structure, a cell-communicating ingredient, antioxidants, and anti-irritants. It is also fragrance-free and coloring agent-free. Now that's what I'm talking about!

☺ **$$$ Eyliplex-2, Eye Lift + Circle Reducer** *($39.50 for 0.68 ounce)* is a two-part product that is all about making eyes tighter, brighter, less wrinkled, and—what a shock—younger-looking. Why the need for two different products for what amounts to one concept for making the under-eye area look better, you ask? It's marketing shenanigans, and has nothing to do with good skin care. The **Fast Acting Day Gel** is supposed to lift and tighten and the **Long Lasting Night Balm** is supposed to reduce dark circles and make skin firmer. Aside from the fact that these two products are in jar packaging, which won't keep the interesting ingredients stable, the two-part product doesn't add any special benefit, and the claims are just exaggerated to the max. If the day version had sunscreen, this would be a different discussion, but that isn't the case, and is a huge misstep. If you're going to ask women to use two different products, then you should at least give them a reason why they should do that. The Fast-Acting Day Gel is nicely formulated, with an impressive array of skin-identical ingredients, cell-communicating ingredients, and antioxidants. It even has a lightweight application that is fine if the eye area isn't dry. Regrettably, the packaging sets this formula back in the Dark Ages. The Long-Lasting Night Balm has many of the strengths of the gel, only in a far more emollient base. But from a formulary perspective, there is no reason to use this at night rather than during the day. Actually, if you have dry skin around your eyes, this would work far better than the Gel version anyway. Ultimately, this entire discussion is for naught because the packaging is such an utter disappointment.

☺ **$$$ Instant Lightening Eye Cream** *($21 for 0.5 ounce)* has a fairly matte finish and isn't the best if you have dry skin around your eyes. The "instant lightening" claim relates to the inclusion of mica, which adds a small amount of shine, and titanium dioxide, which adds a teeny amount of whiteness, but that won't fool anyone. None of the other ingredients can instantly or even slowly lighten the eye area. Other than that, this does contain a decent group of state-of-the-art ingredients, but they would have worked so much better for lots of women if the base had a nicer texture.

☺ **$$$ Perfect Balance Moisture Lotion SPF 15** (*$16 for 1.7 ounces*) contains 1.2% titanium dioxide for UVA protection, which is going in the right direction, but it's still not a big enough improvement to warrant an all-star rating. All the best state-of-the-art ingredients are present in this product, and it does have a light silky feel that makes it a wonderful option for someone with normal to dry or combination skin.

☺ **$$$ Sculptinex Instant ReSculpting Face Treatment** (*$44.50 for 1.4 ounces*). Here's another product essentially claiming to be a face-lift in a tube. The promise of "instant sculpting" is one that many women who are dealing with a less-than-taut visage will find appealing. But, applying a skin-care product cannot undo what time, genetics, sun damage, hormonal changes, bone loss, muscle movement, and gravity have caused. The backbone of this dubious treatment is a film-forming agent that forms a flexible, mesh-like "net" over the skin. As it sets on your skin, you may feel a slight tightening sensation. But if you look closely, sagging skin won't be lifted in the least; it's just a tactile sensation meant to convince you the product is working. The statistics from clinical studies for this product seem enticing, but good luck seeing them (the company would not release them, which is typical), so this ends up being marketing artifice rather than a real study. You're left to take Good Skin's word for it that your skin will be 51% firmer after two months of use. Beyond the talk of firming and sculpting, is there any reason to consider this serum? It contains several intriguing ingredients that have value for skin, but for a Lauder-owned line, the Sculptinex isn't quite as impressive as similar products from other Lauder-owned lines, such as Clinique Repairwear or Lauder's own Perfectionist brand. Many of the state-of-the-art extras in this product are listed after the preservative, and as such don't have much impact on skin. Still, this is a good formula overall, and it has a cosmetic tightening and smoothing effect some may enjoy. (Just keep in mind that your skin isn't really being sculpted or lifted back into place.) By the way, this doesn't contain the antioxidant resveratrol, as claimed, at least not according to the ingredient list.

☺ **Smooth-365 Intensive Clarity + Smoothing Peptide Serum** (*$42.50 for 1.7 ounces*) ranks as the most expensive Good Skin product, but is it worth the investment? Said to perfect "the overall quality of our skin's appearance right now and into the future" gets things off to a questionable start. That's because without a sunscreen, this cannot prevent sun exposure from making your appearance imperfect. This silicone-based serum will make all skin types feel wonderfully silky, and it contains some good antioxidants and mulberry root extract, which can have a positive impact on skin discolorations (though likely not in the amount used in this product). There is only one peptide in this product, and the amount used is rather small. Although this is an option, it is not as well-rounded or state-of-the-art as Good Skin's Tri-Aktiline Instant Deep Wrinkle Filler.

✓☺ **$$$ Tri-Aktiline Instant Deep Wrinkle Filler** (*$39.50 for 1 ounce*) is supposed to help eliminate wrinkles, frown lines, brow lines, and lines around the eye, leaving you flawless, lineless, and, presumably, expressionless. Not to worry. This water- and silicone-based serum doesn't come close to achieving its goals (and, of course, Good Skin's "stringent tests" establishing efficacy were neither available for review nor published). Although it won't send wrinkles and expression lines packing, it does provide a dose of antioxidants, sophisticated skin-identical ingredients, and cell-communicating ingredients, and it comes in packaging that will keep them stable. It has what it takes to promote and maintain healthier skin, and does so without adding fragrance, always a plus. You'll only be disappointed if you believe the wrinkle-eliminating claims. Those with realistic expectations should definitely consider this product, though its texture is best for normal to slightly dry or slightly oily skin.

☺ **$$$ Smoothing Lifting Eye Cream** *($21 for 0.5 ounce)* is far more emollient than the Instant Lightening Eye Cream, and would be preferred by those who tend to have drier skin in the under-eye area. It also has an impressive range of antioxidants, ingredients that mimic skin structure, cell-communicating ingredients, and anti-irritants, which made this a strong contender as a Paula's Pick. But why, oh, why, did they have to package it in a jar? These smart-to-include ingredients are all air-sensitive, and the jar packaging will render them ineffective in a short time. Sigh! Very disappointing! By the way, the Good Skin Web site poses the following question: "Do I really need to use a separate eye cream, or will my everyday moisturizer do?" The answer they provide is: "The skin around the eyes is more fragile than that of the face, and therefore requires more delicate formulas specifically targeted for the area." My response is: while the skin around the eye does have some differences from the skin on the rest of the face—in thickness and in the number of oil glands present—I've yet to see an eye cream, including this one, that is formulated in any way that makes it "unique" for the eye area only. In reality, skin anywhere on the body requires the same, skin-friendly ingredients to improve cell production, generate healthy collagen, and make skin feel silky-smooth.

☺ **Soft Skin Moisture Cream SPF 15** *($16 for 1.7 ounces)* does contain titanium dioxide for UVA sun protection, but not very much. A 1% concentration is disappointing, but not terrible. A higher concentration would have provided far better UVA protection. All in all, this is a reliable, emollient moisturizer for normal to dry skin. The assortment of antioxidants, ingredients that mimic skin structure, and cell-communicating ingredients is impressive, but several of these ingredients will be compromised once this jar-packaged product is opened.

☺ **$$$ Megabalm Ultra Soothing Lip Treatment** *($9.50 for 0.24 ounce)* is a standard, Vaseline-based lip balm that will take good care of dry, chapped lips. The tiny amount of sage leaf is unlikely to be irritating. This does contain coloring agent.

GOOD SKIN MAKEUP

FOUNDATION: ✓☺ **All Firm Makeup** *($16)* is the best foundation in Good Skin's makeup collection. The fluid texture blends very well, feels silky, and leaves a gorgeous, natural-looking smooth matte finish. This is meant to soften the appearance of lines and wrinkles, but it cannot do that. It will provide light to medium coverage without looking or feeling heavy, and the formula does contain some intriguing extras such as peptides and several cell-communicating ingredients. There are 12 shades, most of which are suitably neutral and appropriate for fair to dark (but not very dark) skin tones. Consider Level 4 Warm and Level 5 Cool carefully because of their peachy-pink tones, and avoid the obviously pink Level 4 Cool and rosy-copper Level 6 Cool. All Firm Makeup is best for normal to slightly dry or slightly oily skin.

☹ **All Right Makeup** *($15)* doesn't deserve its name because the alcohol-laden formula is far from all right. Other irritants added to this foundation for acne-prone skin include eucalyptus and clove, neither of which are the least bit helpful. The 0.5% amount of salicylic acid is hardly enough to provide exfoliating benefits; there are better BHA products available. This foundation also has an unpleasant texture, separates easily, and has an uncomfortably dry finish.

CONCEALER: ☹ **Two Perfect Eye Concealer Duo** *($15)* is a dual-sided product in which one end is a liquid concealer and the other is a pale yellow "corrector" for dark circles. Both formulas have enough slip to make blending easy and they provide moderate coverage with a matte finish. The concealer portion doesn't look as flawless as it should; even a slight over-application can create a too-opaque finish that calls attention to itself. Furthermore, half of the six shades are too orange or peach to consider, those being Level 3, Level 4, and Level 5. Level 6 is slightly copper but may work for some dark skin tones, while the yellow "corrector" shade is the same regardless of its partner color (which won't look good on medium to dark skin tones).

☹ **All Calm Redness Tamer** *($15)* is merely an emollient, green-tinted concealer that doesn't contain anything that can calm down what might be causing your skin to be red. Besides, green doesn't cover red, and you end up with a noticeably green cast to the area you are trying to cover.

☹ **All Right Anti-Acne Concealer** *($12)* lists 0.5% salicylic acid as an active ingredient, which is an amount most won't find effective enough (and it's ineffective in this concealer because of its pH above 4). This tube concealer has a very dry, difficult-to-blend texture and finish that causes the lighter shades to appear chalky, while the darker shades are too peach or orange to consider. The final strike is the inclusion of drying, irritating sulfur.

POWDER: ✓ ☺ **Totally Natural Loose Powder** *($16)* has an absolutely beautiful, smooth texture that sets makeup and makes skin look refined rather than dry and powdered. The finish is so skin-like, it's difficult to believe this is a talc-based powder. It is best for normal to dry skin (someone with oily skin won't appreciate the finish), and all four shades are sheer and highly recommended. This powder, like all Good Skin makeup, is fragrance-free.

☺ **Sheer Color Finishing Powder** *($15)* is a very standard talc-free pressed powder. Kaolin (clay) is used instead of talc or mica, and although this results in a drier finish, application remains smooth and even. Best for normal to very oily skin, this powder's six shades are mostly great; only Level 4 suffers from being a bit pink, but is still worth considering.

BLUSH: ✓ ☺ **Naturally Cheeky Powder Blush** *($15)* rates as another winner from Good Skin. This pressed-powder blush has an exceptionally smooth texture, applies beautifully, and allows you to build intensity without looking oversaturated. Although the palette of shades is great, each has some amount of shine. The almost-matte options include Pink Lotus, Spring Rose, Tuscan Sun, Golden Ginger, and Plum Crush.

EYESHADOW: ☺ **Smooth Color Eyeshadow Duos** *($14.50)* are powder eyeshadows whose texture and application is disappointing compared to the eyeshadow options from Estee Lauder and Clinique (Lauder owns Good Skin). Most of the duos have pairings that are closer to tone-on-tone than complementary colors with one shade being suitable for crease color, which creates shadow and depth. The only pairs worth considering (if you're OK with a less-than-smooth texture) are Nutmeg Spice and Natural Stone.

LIPSTICK AND LIP GLOSS: ☺ **Megabalm Tinted Lip Gloss** *($9.50)* is a sheer lip balm in a tube. It has a smooth, emollient feel and provides a wet-looking gloss finish that's only slightly sticky. The shade range is small but good, and each looks darker in the tube than it does when applied to lips.

☹ **Creamcolor Lipstick SPF 15** *($12.50)* has an unusually greasy texture and its sunscreen leaves lips vulnerable to UVA damage because it does not contain titanium dioxide, zinc oxide, avobenzone, Tinosorb, or Mexoryl SX.

MASCARA: ☺ **Lash Lengthening Mascara & Conditioner** *($12.50)* is a dual-sided mascara, with one end being traditional mascara and the other a lash conditioner. The latter is a joke because the amount of alcohol in this clear "primer" will only leave lashes feeling dry. Applying it before the mascara doesn't enhance its results. The mascara itself does a decent job of making lashes longer and defined, but doesn't hold a candle to superior, less expensive mascaras at the drugstore.

ISOMERS (SKIN CARE ONLY)

ISOMERS AT-A-GLANCE

Strengths: Complete ingredient lists are available on the company's Web site and on shopnbc.com; many fragrance-free products; several products are reasonably priced (but many are overpriced and the price isn't related to the formula, so be careful); a good AHA product; some good moisturizers and serums; a good self-tanner; very good hydroquinone-free skin-lightening product; most products come in packaging that helps keep the light- and air-sensitive ingredients stable.

Weaknesses: An overabundance of antiwrinkle serums, when only one well-formulated product is ever needed; only one sunscreen (that's ridiculous given the number of "antiwrinkle" products they sell); some products contain controversial ingredients, such as the drug teprenone or ingredients said to stimulate human stem cells; the lip-plumping and lash-enhancing products; greasy eye makeup remover; incomplete options for managing acne.

For more information about Isomers, call (416) 787-2465 or visit www.isomers.ca or www. Beautypedia.com.

ISOMERS ABSOLUTES PRODUCTS

☺ **$$$ Absolutes Co-Complex 3-Spray** *($50 for 4.06 ounces)* is a very good, though overpriced spray-on toner for those with sensitive skin. It contains a good amount of the anti-irritant madecassoside (gotu kola nut extract) along with a small amount of skin-identical ingredients. I would be tempted to give this a bigger happy face if the price weren't so out of line with the formula. It isn't the most state-of-the-art toner around, but it is fragrance-free and that's a nice change of pace. By the way, don't spray this at your face because you don't want the preservatives in this product to get in your eyes or mouth.

✓ ☺ **Absolutes Anti Redness Serum** *($29.99 for 1 ounce)* is, in many ways, a much better formulation than Isomers' expensive Advanced Fortifying Serum with Essenskin below, which for some unknown reason costs a lot more. This formulation is rich in skin-identical ingredients, has antioxidants, and helps restore and maintain a healthy skin barrier. The result is skin that's more resistant to irritation, which reduces signs of sensitivity (assuming you're not using other irritating skin-care products), and builds collagen—all the good stuff skin needs. This fragrance-free serum is excellent for normal to dry skin and, as mentioned, great for sensitive skin, including those with rosacea.

☺ **Absolutes Chito-Firm Skin Lifting Serum** *($34.75 for 2.03 ounces)* is a vial of serum that is supposed to "hold skin firm" when it has become inelastic. It can't. Having said that, however, I realize that it will take a lot of willpower to resist, especially for those who are susceptible to this kind of advertising ruse, which makes this product sound like a girdle for your face. The second ingredient in this serum is dipalmitoyl hydroxyproline, a good skin-identical ingredient (i.e., water-binding agent), but it can't firm skin. The only information about its skin-firming ability comes from companies selling products that contain this ingredient. There is no reliable, published research documenting this ingredient as being capable of lifting sagging skin and keeping it in place. At best, this is an interesting serum that treats skin to some good water-binding and skin-identical ingredients, but that's it. One more point: it does contain a tiny amount of glycolic acid, but it's too small an amount for exfoliation. All skin types can use this, and it is fragrance-free.

☺ **$$$ Absolutes Co-Complex 3 Cream an Ally for the Skin** *($75 for 1 ounce)* is a basic emollient moisturizer whose price is absurd for what you get. Isomers included a good anti-irritant, some plant-based water-binding agents, and a cell-communicating peptide, but those ingredients show up in dozens and dozens of products that not only cost much less but also have more complex and enhanced formulas. This fragrance-free product is suitable for dry, sensitive skin, but don't settle for less when your skin can have so much more (and for less money, which is the only "less" you should tolerate).

☺ **Absolutes Eye Serum Intensive Treatment** *($30 for 1 ounce)* is merely a lightweight gel moisturizer suitable for slightly dry skin anywhere on the face. It doesn't contain any ingredients capable of firming skin around the eyes, though the carrageenan extract forms a slight film on skin that may give users the perception of firmness, but that's about a gum resin, not a skin-care benefit. Other than that, it contains a small amount of skin-identical ingredients and a peptide, but not enough to get excited about.

☺ **Absolutes Wrinkle Defense Cream with Matrixyl and Green Tea** *($40 for 3.04 ounces)* is a standard, slightly emollient moisturizer that contains the Matrixyl peptide complex, something many other cosmetics companies use as well. There is no substantiated proof that Matrixyl has antiwrinkle benefit, but, like all peptides, it has theoretical cell-communicating ability and helps skin hold moisture. The antioxidants in this cream are a nice addition, but they won't remain effective long due to the jar packaging.

☺ **$$$ Absolutes Wrinkle Viper Cream** *($35 for 0.51 ounce)*. Those not keen on the serum texture of Isomers' Absolutes Wrinkle Viper Skin Smoothing Serum below can try their antiwrinkle luck with the cream version of the product. This is yet another works-like-Botox product from Isomers. They sell so many of these, but if any of them worked, only one would be necessary. As is, none of them work as claimed because the peptides they contain do not mimic the effects of Botox. There's no reason to spend money on this moisturizer unless you want to ignore facts and go for the fantasy that using this may actually reduce expression lines caused by repeated muscle contractions. In the long run, what you are actually putting on your face is mostly water and a hair spray-type acrylate, which isn't the best for anything except your hair.

☺ **$$$ Absolutes Wrinkle Viper Skin Smoothing Serum** *($49.99 for 1 ounce)*. "Wrinkle Viper"? Does that mean this serum is poised to attack wrinkles with snake-like precision? Is it youthful venom in a bottle? Nope. This is just another works-like-Botox serum from Isomers. This product doesn't work as claimed because the peptides it contains do not mimic the effects of Botox. For further comment on this issue, see the Absolutes Wrinkle Viper Cream above.

ISOMERS AUSTRALIAN HARVEST PRODUCTS

☺ **Australian Harvest Daily Control Cream with Tea Tree Extract** *($29 for 4.06 ounces)* contains approximately 3% glycolic acid at a pH of 3.8, so some exfoliation will occur. Those struggling with breakouts would do better with a higher concentration of glycolic acid or, better yet, salicylic acid (BHA), which has properties that make it better for fighting blemishes. The amount of tea tree oil in this AHA moisturizer for normal to dry skin isn't high enough for it to function as a topical disinfectant against acne-causing bacteria. Research indicates that 5% tea tree oil is necessary for that, and this product contains barely 1%. The tea tree oil does lend a medicinal smell to this product, but smelling like medicine doesn't make it medicine.

☺ **Australian Harvest Daily Control Serum with Tea Tree Extract** *($12.50 for 0.5 ounce)* is an interesting serum with potential benefit for blemish-prone skin. The amount of tea tree oil is likely enough to allow it to function as a topical disinfectant, but the amount of salicylic acid is likely less than 0.5%. That means that despite this serum's pH of 3.7, it is an option only for those with mild acne. This is worth considering as an alternative to benzoyl peroxide, but you would absolutely want to start with a benzoyl peroxide product, because benzoyl peroxide is the gold standard, anti-acne active ingredient and there is a ton of research proving its efficacy.

☹ **$$$ Australian Harvest Daily Cleanser with Tea Tree Extract** *($35 for 16.32 ounces)* is a cleanser with glycolic acid, a teeny amount of salicylic acid, and tea tree oil that is supposed to keep blemishes away and prevent acne. It cannot do that, and is actually fairly ineffective at cleansing because they chose thickening agents over cleansing agents, which is not the best for oily or blemish-prone skin. The glycolic and salicylic acids are of little use in a cleanser because their benefit is rinsed down the drain before they have a chance to exfoliate or, in the case of salicylic acid, to provide benefit by virtue of its antibacterial properties. The same goes for the tea tree leaf oil; it does lend a medicinal smell to this cleanser, but smelling medicinal doesn't mean it's medicine. This harvest will reap your skin no rewards.

ISOMERS INTELLISOME PRODUCTS

☺ **Intellisome Sebu-Monitor** *($35 for 1.86 ounces)* is a water-based, fragrance-free moisturizer that is supposed to monitor sebum (oil) levels in the dermis, but how it's to do that is a mystery. In fact, a skin-care product can't do that. Beyond the suspect claim, this product is incapable of keeping skin matte because it doesn't contain absorbent ingredients. The zinc gluconate, given the tiny amount offered here, can't have an impact on acne, and there is little research showing that it could have an effect even if there were more of it. The tropolone included is potentially risky because tropolone is a growth hormone, and you don't want to use a cosmetic product that contains an ingredient without published research and that might negatively affect your skin.

☺ **$$$ Intellisome Skin Stacker** *($85 for 1 ounce)* is all about triggering collagen production, and Isomers claims this water- and silicone-based serum can do that because of the peptides it contains. This has a very silky texture and is suitable for all skin types, but research related to the collagen-stimulating claims for the peptides simply isn't there, at least not in substantiated form. Lipotec, the company that sells this peptide to cosmetics companies, published the results of its study on in vitro collagen stimulation using tripeptide-10. That's fine, but given that no one has duplicated or expanded on Lipotec's single study, you're left to take their word for it (Source: *International Journal of Cosmetic Science*, April 2008, pages 97-104). It's possible that certain peptides, if bioengineered correctly so they don't break down before reaching their target, can play a significant role in antiaging products. For now, however, what we know for certain is that they function as water-binding agents and, theoretically, could have cell-communicating ability. If you're curious to see how peptides will work for you, there are plenty of less expensive products to consider (I'd start with Olay Regenerist).

☹ **$$$ Intellisome Synchronizer Cell Renewing Complex** *($75 for 1.86 ounces)* makes claims that sound like an all-in-one miracle worker for aging skin, but aside from one ingredient (hexanoyl dipeptide-3 norleucine acetate), the fragrance-free formula is commonplace. The unique ingredient, hexanoyl dipeptide-3 norleucine acetate, supposedly is what provides all of the look-younger action this serum promises. Not surprisingly, the only research about this peptide comes from the company that sells it to cosmetics manufacturers. That isn't good news, because, of course, they're going to present their ingredient blends in the best light. Where's the independent research to verify that this peptide does everything Isomers says it can? Given that you cannot rely on this serum to work as claimed and that there are plenty of serums that make skin feel silky, this isn't a product I'd encourage anyone to purchase.

ISOMERS ONE AND ONE 3000 PRODUCTS

☺ **$$$ One 3000 Cream with Liquid Crystal Technology** *($80 for 1.86 ounces).* If this is the "one" cream to address multiple skin needs, then why does Isomers sell so many other moisturizers, all with similar claims? This option combines ingredients of several other Isomers moisturizers, including various peptides, mineral ferments, and emollients. It's a decent moisturizer for normal to dry skin, but it comes up short for the money. Where are the antioxidants and skin-identical ingredients? Including them would have made this a well-rounded formula that would get you more for your money. The claims may seem fascinating ("liquid crystals able to target multiple skin-care needs"), but the reality is that this is just another moisturizer with peptides, and there are hundreds of such products on the market.

☺ **$$$ One 3000 for Eyes** *($59.99 for 1 ounce)* is an eye-area moisturizer meant to address every concern you may have with the skin around your eyes. Puffiness, dark circles, wrinkles, even hooded brow: it seems there's nothing this cream cannot undo. Although this "one" product cannot alleviate all of the eye-area woes it claims to, it does contain some impressive water-binding agents and cell-communicating ingredients. There is every reason to believe this fragrance-free eye-area moisturizer will improve dry skin around the eyes, soften the appearance of wrinkles, and perhaps even stimulate collagen production. It's not going to eliminate all signs of aging, but it is an overall well-formulated product.

☺ **$$$ One 3000 for Face** *($99.99 for 1.86 ounces)* is a blend of water-binding agents and peptides that has a lightweight texture and the ability to plump skin, which reduces the appearance of wrinkles. Of course, lots of moisturizers and serums have this ability, so there's no reason to overspend on this fragrance-free serum. They claim that this peptide, acetyl hexapeptide-8, will work like Botox by relaxing the muscles responsible for expression lines; however, it doesn't work like that, and that's a good thing, because how would it know which muscles to relax? If it worked as claimed, applying this all over your face would likely result in drooping skin because all of your facial muscles would be relaxed. Although I don't recommend investing in this product, it is suitable for all skin types.

☺ **$$$ One for Eyes** *($49.99 for 1 ounce)* is nearly identical to Isomers' One 3000 for Eyes above. As such, the same review applies.

☹ **$$$ One Freeze for Expression Lines** *($69.99 for 1 ounce)* is another works-like-Botox product from Isomers. I guess the others don't work as well as claimed; otherwise, why would they need this version, too? The silicone-enriched formula makes skin feel wonderfully smooth, but the peptides it contains are not capable of targeting "facial skin contractions" to "prevent the formation of horizontal and vertical frown lines," as well as other expression lines. Cosmetic surgeons aren't going out of business or seeing their Botox or dermal-filler clientele diminish, and that's because products like this don't work. The texture of this product has a slight (really slight) "filling" effect on expression lines, but it doesn't freeze muscles to prevent those lines from being etched deeper into skin. Remember, not even Botox works like that if you rub it on your skin rather than have it injected into key muscles. This serum doesn't deserve better than a neutral face rating because, for the money, it doesn't contain much of what skin needs to look and feel its best (think antioxidants and skin-identical ingredients).

☺ **$$$ One Intellisome Complex** *($99.90 for 1.86 ounces)* is very similar to Isomers' Intellisome Skin Stacker above, except it contains an additional peptide that has no substantiated research proving that it works as claimed. This serum doesn't qualify as "an intensive workhorse blend" unless you want to overlook the fact that the efficacy of the bells and whistles is not confirmed by any independent research. And this is a very expensive bet to place, especially when you consider that skin needs much more than this product provides.

ISOMERS R SERIES PRODUCTS

☹ **$$$ R Series B5 Skin Hydration Serum** *($69 for 1 ounce)* contains such a scant amount of vitamin B5 (panthenol) that this water-based serum isn't worthy of its name. It's a simple blend of water, skin-identical ingredients, fatty acid, and preservatives. The price is out of line for what you get, but it's a decent serum for normal to dry skin.

☹ **$$$ R Series Gemmotherapy Cream** *($60 for 1.86 ounces)* isn't an intensive cream as described. This moisturizer for normal to dry skin contains a standard roster of thickening agents and plants, including aloe, soy, and wild yam. It's fragrance-free, but the ingredients offer no special benefit for "changing" (read: menopausal) skin. Wild yam doesn't work the same way topically that it does when consumed orally in terms of providing skin with hormonal benefit (Source: www.naturaldatabase.com).

☺ **$$$ R Series Intensive Serum with Soy DNA** *($69 for 1 ounce)*. Whether this product contains soy DNA or not (it doesn't appear to), you don't want plant DNA interacting or interfering with your skin's DNA. Doing so could lead to a host of problems, including DNA mutation that might result in cancer. This is merely another water-based serum from Isomers, a line overloaded with serums, all proclaiming to have the antiwrinkle answers. Soy and wild yam do not have the same benefit for menopausal skin when they are applied topically rather than consumed orally. The soy has some antioxidant benefit, but there are a few other intriguing ingredients in this fragrance-free serum that elevate it above average, so that's the most you can expect.

☹ **$$$ R Series Pur Face High Potency Soy DNA** *($160 for 1.86 ounces)* is supposed to be for women over the age of 40 who are experiencing skin changes from menopause. This overpriced serum contains various forms of soy and wild yam, ingredients that show up in many skin-care products marketed to menopausal women. Although there is research pertaining to oral consumption of soy and wild yam helping to balance estrogen levels, the same effect hasn't been demonstrated for these ingredients when applied topically (Sources: *International Journal of Toxicology*, volume 23, 2004, pages 23-47; and *Climacteric*, June 2001, pages 144-150). Soy has antioxidant and anti-inflammatory benefit when applied to skin and also (to a limited extent) can help skin recover from sun damage. However, lots of products contain soy and aren't sold at such an off-putting price (think Aveeno at the drugstore). This serum has benefit for all skin types, but it's certainly not all-encompassing. Soy isn't the only gainful ingredient available, and no single ingredient (or multiple forms of it) is capable of providing everything aging skin needs, whether menopause is an issue or not.

OTHER ISOMERS PRODUCTS

☺ **$$$ Double Duty Cleanser** *($20 for 4.06 ounces)* is a fairly gentle cleansing lotion that does a good job removing most types of makeup. It is preferred for normal to dry skin because of the fatty acids that are up front on the ingredient list. The tiny amounts of lactic and salicylic acids don't function as exfoliants. Even if they could, that benefit would be gone before it could happen because this product is rinsed off. This contains fragrance in the form of lavender extract.

✓☺ **\$\$\$ Foaming Facial Cleanser** *($20 for 4.06 ounces)* is a very good fragrance-free water-soluble cleanser for all skin types. It is somewhat similar to but stronger than the basic formula of many baby shampoos. Foaming Facial Cleanser rinses easily and doesn't leave skin feeling stripped or dry. If only the price weren't so high. Note that Isomers does occasionally offer larger sizes for a value price, so if you're tempted, check to make sure you are getting the most bang for your buck!

☹ **\$\$\$ Makeup Remover** *($10 for 2.03 ounces)* is merely emollient thickeners with preservatives. It has a fluid texture, but is very greasy. The ingredients definitely break down makeup, including waterproof mascara, but you can get the same effect for a lot less money using plain mineral oil or, better yet, a water-based makeup remover that won't leave a greasy residue on your skin. This should not be used by someone with oily, combination, or blemish-prone skin.

☹ **\$\$\$ Moisture Mist with Minerals** *($22 for 4.06 ounces)* is a very basic spray-on toner suitable for all skin types. It isn't as impressive as Isomers' Absolutes Co-Complex 3 Spray, but it also costs significantly less. There is also nothing in this product associated with earth minerals, unless you consider the salt component of sodium lactate and sodium hyaluronate to be a mineral. Isomers' attempt to cash in on the craze for all things mineral is good marketing, but it's not helpful for your skin. By the way, sodium lactate is the salt form of lactic acid, but in that form it has almost no ability to exfoliate skin.

☺ **\$\$\$ Daily Exfoliating Serum** *($30 for 2.03 ounces)* contains an effective concentration of glycolic acid. Most likely it's 8-10%, although the company wouldn't divulge the exact percentage; I'm not sure why it needs to be a secret, because there is nothing secretive about glycolic acid. Nonetheless, this lightweight fluid will exfoliate because the pH is within the range of effectiveness. Salicylic acid is present, too, though most likely at 0.5%, not the best for effective exfoliation. Consider this an effective, fragrance-free AHA product for all skin types.

☹ **\$\$\$ Duo Derm Exfoliation Set** *($25)* includes an AHA serum and a separate topical scrub in this two-product kit. The pairing is strange because one form of exfoliation is enough for anyone's skin. Moreover, there's no question that using a well-formulated AHA or BHA product offers skin greater benefit than using a scrub. In this set, the **Alpha Renewing Serum** with glycolic acid has a pH that's well above 4, so forget about any exfoliation benefit. That leaves you relying on the **Microderm Polish Cream**, which is a standard, slightly creamy scrub that polishes skin with synthetic polyethylene beads (which isn't what's used during microdermabrasion treatments, but even so, the particles used in microdermabrasion have nothing to do with how a scrub exfoliates skin). The Polish Cream is a good scrub and is formulated without fragrance, but it's the only reason to consider this set. Ultimately, you can find similar scrubs, plus a really effective AHA product, at the drugstore for less money.

☹ **Perfecting Lotion** *($29.99 for 4 ounces)* contains lactic acid (AHA) and salicylic acid (BHA) in a combined amount that would allow some exfoliation to occur—if only the pH were within the correct range. Because it isn't, this is nothing more than an average moisturizer for dry skin. It isn't even close to being the perfect solution it's made out to be.

☺ **Manual Microderm Cleanser** *($10 for 4 ounces)* is positioned as a cleanser with exfoliating benefits, but it's really a scrub masquerading as a cleanser. It doesn't contain ingredients capable of cleansing skin, but it does contain polyethylene beads for gentle exfoliation. The plant oil and shea butter keep this from rinsing as easily as many other scrubs, but it is an option for those with dry to very dry skin. One other thing: this has no relation to a microdermabrasion treatment, any more than a tricycle is related to a car.

☺ **$$$ Accelerated Recovery Serum** *($130 for 0.91 ounce)*. For a ridiculous amount of money, you're getting a water-based serum that's mostly glycerin, algae (*Entermorpha compressa* is a type of algae), and a plant resin with one study showing that it protected mouse skin from tumor formation in the presence of UVB radiation (Source: *Nutrition and Cancer*, 2000, pages 73-77). Vitamin C is included, too, but not in an amount that makes this serum worth the cost or that delivers concentrated "age-defying" benefits. This serum contains some good water-binding agents and peptides, but again, nothing that justifies the cost or choosing it over several other well-formulated serums. If you decide to go for this, it can be used by all skin types.

☹ **$$$ Acetyl Hexapeptide-8 15% Solution** *($39.50 for 0.5 ounce)* contains a water-based extract of linseed along with the touted acetyl hexapeptide-8 and preservatives. The peptide is supposed to target deep lines formed by repetitive facial expressions, but there is no substantiated research to support those claims. This isn't a "works-like-Botox" product, and if it were, it would be cause for concern. Why? Because if acetyl hexapeptide-8 could affect muscles that control facial expression, what would happen if you applied too much of it? Would your face droop or become expressionless? And what about losing muscle control in your fingers, with which you'd apply this serum? Remember, not even Botox works like Botox when it is applied topically rather than injected, and that's a good thing. This is a one-note serum with nothing to offer skin but a lot of hype and marketing nonsense.

☹ **$$$ Advanced Fortifying Serum with Essenskin** *($65 for 1 ounce)* is a serum Isomers supposedly developed to target thin, fragile skin that's "mature." Apparently, the company believes that skin reaches this state due to nutrient deficiencies, which doesn't explain why someone in their 20s or 30s who has a poor diet doesn't have thin, sagging skin, too. Not to mention there is no research showing "mature" skin needs anything different from "immature" skin. In fact, there is nothing in this product of particular interest for anyone at any age. Nothing in this serum can add density to skin or help keep it from sagging. Skin becomes thinner and sags due to a combination of sun damage, fat loss, collagen depletion, bone loss, and age. No skin-care product, especially not one as mundane as this, is capable of replenishing your skin to combat all those factors that contribute to what we call "aged" or "mature" skin. At best, this is an average serum for dry skin.

☺ **$$$ Carnosine + Antioxidant Complex** *($39.99 for 1 ounce)* is a good emollient moisturizer for dry skin. It contains carnosine, an amino acid that has antioxidant and anti-inflammatory properties as well as the potential to inhibit advanced glycation end-products (AGE), which are believed to play a role in how skin "ages." Other antioxidants are included, too, and the formula is fragrance-free. By the way, there isn't any substantiated research proving carnosine is 250 times more powerful than the antioxidant idebenone, as claimed in the marketing material for this product.

☹ **$$$ Copper-P Concentrate Serum** *($49.95 for 1 ounce)* is one of Isomers' less impressive serums, but Isomers has so many serums with various antiwrinkle claims, I have no idea how their customers decide which one to use. The only interesting aspects of the formula are that it contains palmitoyl oligopeptide (an ingredient that shows up in several less expensive products, including many from Olay) and some yeast ferments. Although interesting, this peptide isn't, and yeast ferments aren't the antiwrinkle miracles they're made out to be—not even close. The mineral ferments in this serum have no research proving they enhance skin's firmness.

☹ **$$$ Desert Youth 4X with Ectoin** (*$59.99 for 1 ounce*). Here's a serum that's said to protect skin from the harmful environment and harsh chemicals. It doesn't contain sun protection ingredients, however, so forget about the most important means of protecting your skin from the environment, and what harsh chemicals are they referring to? If your skin is in contact with harsh chemicals, you need to call 911, not use this product. Overall this product is a one-note song and your skin truly needs a symphony. There is nothing about this product that warrants the claim about it being a "revolution in skin care." The only unique aspect of this product is a single ingredient called ectoin, which has some research indicating that it helps protect skin from DNA damage caused by sun exposure (Sources: *Journal of Photochemistry and Photobiology*, April 2008, pages 24-34; and *Skin Pharmacology and Physiology*, September-October 2004, pages 232-237), but that's true of many antioxidants and skin-identical ingredients. A single ingredient is never the answer for skin; skin is complex and needs a sophisticated blend of antioxidants, skin-identical ingredients, and cell-communicating ingredients. There isn't much else to say about this product other than it is fragrance-free and suitable for all skin types.

☺ **Fast Lift Eye Serum** (*$29.99 for 1 ounce*) is very similar to Isomers' Absolutes Eye Serum Intensive Treatment above. As such, the same review applies: this is merely a lightweight gel moisturizer suitable for slightly dry skin anywhere on the face. It doesn't contain any ingredients capable of firming skin around the eyes, though the carrageenan extract forms a slight film on skin, but that isn't a skin-care benefit. This can quickly make the skin around your eyes feel firmer, but your skin isn't actually being firmed. It contains a small amount of skin-identical ingredients and a peptide, but overall nothing to get excited about.

☺ **Hydrafirm Plus** (*$29.99 for 4.06 ounces*) is a basic, exceedingly mundane moisturizer that comes with claims that apply to almost any moisturizer. Basically, all that's being said is that skin will be smoother and wrinkles will be less apparent. That's good, but it isn't good news that this contains arnica extract, a potential skin irritant, although the small amount is unlikely to be problematic. Still, there's no compelling reason to consider this moisturizer over many at the drugstore.

☺ **$$$ Matrixyl 3000 Rejuvenation Serum** (*$49 for 1 ounce*). This water-based serum makes skin feel smoother and temporarily firmer due to a film-forming agent. Your skin isn't actually being firmed, and the peptides in this product don't have reliable research pertaining to their antiwrinkle benefit. The peptides theoretically could have cell-communicating ability and they do work as water-binding agents, but that's not enough if your skin needs rejuvenation after years of sun damage and neglect.

☺ **$$$ Matrixyl Wrinkle Defense Serum** (*$39 for 1 ounce*) should only be considered if you're interested in seeing if the claims attached to the Matrixyl peptide blend are true. Several Olay Regenerist products that contain this peptide (and others) are available for less money, but I wouldn't label this product as being too expensive, plus it's fragrance-free. However, skin needs more than peptides, so this serum is a one-note option that isn't as exciting as they make it sound.

☺ **$$$ Moisture Rich Antarcticine Cream** (*$50 for 1.86 ounces*) has one ingredient that differentiates it from the others Isomers sells. They want you to believe that the bacteria *Psuedoaltermonas* ferment can help your skin tolerate extreme cold. The story goes that this strain of bacteria was discovered in mud by explorers on an expedition to Antarctica (because, as we all know, mud from the New Jersey shore couldn't possibly be beneficial for skin). Testing revealed that the bacteria contain a glycoprotein that helps it retain water. So now, making a big leap, the cosmetic ingredient manufacturer Lipotec is touting it as a miraculous ingredient. First, there are lots of plant extracts that contain glycoproteins. Second, and more important, there is absolutely no evidence anywhere that this bacteria can help skin. It can't defend against cold anymore than it can preserve collagen and elastin in skin. It's all nonsense.

☺ **Neck and Chin Firming with Essenskin and Ovaliss** *($49.99 for 4.06 ounces)* is a basic emollient moisturizer for normal to dry skin. It doesn't contain a single ingredient capable of firming the neck or chin. (Are they really saying now that the chin needs its own moisturizer?!) This contains a small amount of intriguing ingredients, but not enough to warrant a purchase or to believe even a fraction of the claims for this product.

☺ **$$$ NRG Serum with Adenosine Triphosphate** *($34.99 for 2 ounces)* is a good, lightweight serum that treats all skin types to an intriguing skin-identical ingredient (glycosaminoglycans) and cell-communicating ingredient (adenosine triphosphate). The problem is, like many Isomers products, the whole isn't worth the sum of its parts. Skin needs more from a serum than what this provides, although they are on the right track and it isn't a waste of money. It's just not as stellar as the marketing language would lead you to believe. NRG Serum is fragrance-free.

☹ **$$$ R Pur Eyes** *($35 for 0.34 ounce)* was formulated with ingredients meant to address the aging effects seen when the lower eyelid area becomes puffy as a result of the fat pads beneath the skin shifting. Don't believe it for a second. No skin-care product can remedy this common eye-area concern. Once the fat pad has shifted and the skin has slackened, the only way to fix it is cosmetic surgery, and in most cases, surgically correcting this eye-area issue nets astonishing results. None of the plants in this product are capable of addressing what happens when fat pads beneath the skin shift. The various forms of soy have antioxidant benefit, but none of the other plants have any established benefit for skin. Oddly, two of the main plant extracts in this product are used in products sold to increase sexual motivation. What that has to do with aging skin around the eyes is anyone's guess! All told, this isn't nearly as elegant or state-of-the-art as eye creams from the Estee Lauder-owned lines.

☹ **$$$ Renovage Youth Precursor Complex** *($60 for 1 ounce)* is primarily a standard moisturizer for normal to dry skin. I say "primarily" because it contains one ingredient in an amount that deserves explanation: Teprenone. It's described as an active ingredient whose multiple functions include limiting skin-cell senescence (cell death). As it turns out, this ingredient is a drug that Isomers appears to be using off-label (meaning it is really a pharmaceutical), which my research indicates is against FDA regulations. Teprenone is the brand name for a drug known as geranylgeranylacetone, which is used to treat gastric ulcers and is being researched as an option for slowing age-related hearing loss (Sources: *Brain Research*, May 2008, pages 9-17; and *Digestion*, October 2007, pages 215-224). What do hearing loss and ulcers have to do with aging skin? One of the key ways geranylgeranylacetone works is by influencing heat-shock proteins, which helps other proteins interact as they should at the cellular level, which in turn affects many systems in the body. Heat-shock proteins are most active during times of stress, such as exposure to cigarette smoke and exposure to sunlight. When heat-shock proteins are reduced (which is ultimately what you want because that means reducing inflammation), cells appear to live longer. I suppose the folks behind Isomers theorized that geranylgeranylacetone (as Teprenone) may also have a helpful effect when applied topically. After all, the skin is a source of heat-shock proteins, and it certainly is exposed to enough stressful situations that an ingredient that could help these proteins function more efficiently would be a benefit. However, there's no research proving that topically applied geranylgeranylacetone has any effect on heat-shock proteins in skin. Moreover, as previously mentioned, Isomers is using a drug ingredient in a cosmetic product, which means the consumer is the guinea pig. For that reason, this isn't a moisturizer I can recommend, though it doesn't deserve an unhappy face rating.

☺ **Shine Less Oil Control Blotting Cream** *($19.99 for 1.86 ounces)* contains a tiny amount of silica, an absorbent ingredient that, if present in the right formula, has a dry, powder-like finish on skin. Isomers uses standard thickening agents to create this product's lotion texture, and the result isn't what anyone with oily skin would find mattifying. Shine control is minimal and short-lived; those with oily skin should check out the absorbent products form Smashbox (Anti-Shine is marvelous) or Clinique's Pore Minimizer line.

☺ **$$$ Sirtuin Telomore Supporting Concentrate** *($199.99 for 1 ounce)* is Isomers' most expensive product, and of course it comes with scientific claims tied to supporting the activity and repair of genes in our skin. The interesting thing is this serum doesn't contain a single ingredient not seen in other products from Isomers, or in products from numerous other cosmetics lines. At the very least, Isomers, when pushed, would have to admit (but they won't) that this product is a waste of money when so many of their other less expensive serums contain roughly the same assortment of ingredients. The ingredient Teprenone deserves further explanation and is described above in the review for Renovage Youth Precursor Complex.

☺ **$$$ Stem Genesis** *($75 for 1 ounce)* is supposed to make skin look younger because it contains stem cells from a species of Swiss apple. The entire issue of stem cells as they relate to skin care is in its infancy, and suffice it to say there is no substantiated proof anywhere that stem cells from fruit (whether an apple or pomegranate or grape) can somehow prompt stem cells in human skin to act younger. The miracle ingredient in this case is *Malus domestica* fruit cell culture (Isomers has so many of these "miracle" ingredients; they just keep putting them in different products instead of all together in one product). There is no substantiated, published research proving this has any effect on stem cells in our skin. Instead, the bulk of the information comes from Mibelle Biochemistry, the company that developed and is selling it. (What a shock!) According to information from the company, in vitro and in vivo tests performed by Mibelle have suggested that the ingredient, PhytoCellTec (*Malus domestica*) boosts the production of human stem cells, protects human stem cells from stress, and decreases wrinkles. In vitro, when the extract was applied to human stem cells from umbilical cord, it was found to increase the number of the stem cells in culture. Furthermore, the addition of the ingredient to umbilical cord stem cells appeared to protect the cells from environmental stress such as UV light. Mibelle got these results in a laboratory setting under controlled conditions, so what the results would be on intact, healthy human skin is difficult to predict. Not to mention that umbilical cords love to make stem cells all on their own. Further, the big unknown when using ingredients to signal stem cells in skin is how to control the proliferation of unwanted cell growth. Assuming that stem cells in skin could be stimulated by topical application of skin-care products, how would the cells know when to stop producing? Uncontrolled, overproduction of cells is the blueprint for cancer, a fact that seems to be ignored in the literature that promotes stimulation of stem cells with cosmetics products. As for real-world applications, Mibelle did conduct an experiment that involved 20 participants applying a cream with 2% of this rarified apple extract to wrinkles around their eyes. After four weeks of twice daily application, wrinkle depth was reduced by 15%. That's not much when you consider that 85% of the wrinkle was still there, and still apparent. Plus, the study was neither comparative nor double-blind. Who knows if a cream with 2% vitamin E or green tea might have performed even better? Because all of the research on this ingredient comes from the company promoting it, you have to look at it with a great deal of skepticism—or at least acknowledge that its efficacy is a stretch and the potential unknowns are scary. Other than the rare apple extract, there isn't much in this serum that doesn't show up in most of Isomers' other serums. If this is the ultimate product to promote a youthful appearance, why is the company still selling so many other products making the same claims? Although there are some efficacious ingredients in this serum, the unknowns surrounding topical application of ingredients that may trigger stem cells in skin makes it impossible to recommend, and there's just too much of this stem cell culture here to make it risk-free. You don't need to be any cosmetics company's guinea pig.

☺ **$$$ Sunshine Serum** *($39.99 for 1 ounce)* is designed to supply vitamin D to skin so you don't have to expose your skin to sunlight, which is one way the body can obtain adequate levels of this critical vitamin. Isomers used two forms of this fat-soluble vitamin, but there's no evidence that they can penetrate skin and enter the bloodstream, which is what you want to happen. Nor do they explain why taking vitamin D supplements or consuming vitamin D–rich foods is or is not preferred. Although this serum isn't a replacement for maintaining adequate vitamin D levels via supplements or foods, it contains several helpful ingredients for skin, including ceramides and essential fatty acids. Antioxidants are included, too, which is not common for serums from Isomers. The plant *Boerhavoa diffusa* has no research pertaining to its benefit for skin, but it may have anti-inflammatory properties.

☺ **$$$ Time Freeze** *($49 for 1 ounce)* is similar to, but less expensive than, their One Freeze for Expression Lines above. They make the same claims about a reduction in expression lines here, too. Therefore, the same review applies. The silicone-enriched formula makes skin feel wonderfully smooth, but the peptides it contains are not capable of targeting expression lines. Cosmetic surgeons aren't going out of business or seeing their Botox or dermal filler clientele decrease because of products like this. The texture of this product has a slight (really slight) "filling" effect on expression lines, but it doesn't freeze muscles to prevent those lines from being etched deeper into skin. Remember, not even Botox works like that if you rub it on the skin rather than have it injected into key muscles. This serum doesn't deserve better than a neutral face rating because, for the money, it doesn't contain much of what skin needs to look and feel its best.

☹ **$$$ Uncircle Neck Firming Treatment** *($40 for 4.06 ounces)* is very similar to Isomer's Neck and Chin Firming with Essenskin and Ovaliss product above and the same review applies. I mean, really, two neck products from the same line making the same claims; how does the company explain this? The amount of arnica extract isn't cause for concern, though the product would be better without it.

☹ **$$$ Under Eye Gelee for Puffiness** *($34.99 for 1 ounce)* has a gel texture that certainly won't make under-eye puffiness any worse, but it doesn't contain ingredients that can alleviate puffy eyes either. The peptides are an interesting addition, but at best they'll help hydrate skin and, theoretically, they could have cell-communicating ability. However, they can't tell your cells to stop being puffy; that's about fat deposits and edema. In the long run, all you're really getting is water, glyceryl, and a hair spray–type ingredient, which is not the best as a base formula for the eye area.

☺ **$$$ Vitamin C Serum Map + E High Potency Blend** *($39.99 for 1 ounce)* is a good plant-based serum that contains stabilized vitamin C along with vitamin E. (I suspect the plant is an aqueous solution because water is not on the ingredient list.) These two antioxidants work well together, though I must say that this could have been a multifaceted product had the formula been expanded to include other ingredients that skin needs. Those looking for an affordable vitamin C serum should check this out.

☺ **$$$ Vitamin K Serum with MDI Complex** *($34.99 for 2 ounces)* is a good-but-could-have-been-so-much-better plant-based serum that contains a skin-identical ingredient along with a cell-communicating ingredient. (I suspect the plant is an aqueous solution because water is not part of the ingredient list.) Vitamin K (phytonadione) has never been proven to reduce under-eye circles or circulation when applied topically. If it really worked as well as some cosmetics companies claim, no one would have dark circles and everyone's veins would be perfect. The titanium dioxide and mica in this serum cast a shiny whitish glow on skin, which can make dark circles less apparent. However, that effect is strictly cosmetic and can be bested by skillful application of any good concealer.

☺ **Tan Trick Self Tanner** *($14.50 for 4.06 ounces).* What a great name for a very standard self-tanning lotion. Just like almost every self-tanner sold today, it turns skin brown with the ingredient dihydroxyacetone. This deserves credit for being fragrance-free. It is suitable for normal to dry skin.

☺ **TanGlo** *($14.50 for 5 ounces)* is a body moisturizer with a tiny amount of the self-tanning ingredient dihydroxyacetone. Using this daily allows you to develop a subtle "tan," but because the amount of the tanning ingredient is so low, the effect is softer than the effect of a regular self-tanner. The formula contains no bells or whistles to speak of, but it's fine for normal to dry skin. You can find less expensive versions of this type of product from Olay, Dove, and Jergens.

☺ **Sunscreen with UV Pearls SPF 20** *($14.50 for 4.06 ounces)* is the only sunscreen in the Isomers line. They sell more antiwrinkle serums and moisturizers than just about any other cosmetic line I can think of, but sun protection, which is the real key to maintaining youthful skin, is relegated to one product. Unbelievable! At least the company's sole sunscreen is a good one. It includes an in-part zinc oxide sunscreen in a moisturizing base suitable for normal to dry skin. Regrettably, antioxidants are in short supply, but at least they included some. On the upside, the price is reasonable and the formula is fragrance-free. Isomers maintains that the active ingredients are encapsulated so they don't penetrate skin. Whether or not this is true doesn't guarantee that someone with sensitive skin won't have a reaction to this product.

☺ **$$$ Clay Mask Deep Action Toning & Purifying** *($25 for 3.04 ounces)* is a very standard clay mask that is a good, though pricey, option for oily skin. The ingredient hexyl nicotinate is a vasodilator that has been shown to increase circulation at concentrations as low as 0.1%, which is likely the amount this mask contains. Increasing circulation to the skin's surface isn't necessarily a benefit, however, and this product has no effect on purifying skin or absorbing excess oil. Still, it's likely not a problem in an occasional-use product like this.

☹ **$$$ Enzyme Peel Serum Acid Free Exfoliation** *($43.50 for 1.86 ounces).* How this serum is supposed to peel or deep clean skin is a mystery. It doesn't contain any ingredients capable of doing that, though it is gentle. The main benefit you'll get is smoother, softer skin, something that any moisturizer and most toners can provide, which means you should consider this a superfluous product.

☺ **Eyelash Protein Conditioning Treatment** *($18)* is a brush-on lash product that is just a blend of conditioning agents along with a thickener, a slip agent, preservatives, and silicone. It will make lashes softer and, if they're dry, will improve their appearance. Most women will do just fine without a product like this, but there's nothing to be concerned about if you're curious to try it.

☺ $$$ **Lip Firming Serum** *($20 for 0.51 ounce)*. Isomers believes lips need a serum, too, so they've created this water- and aloe-based product. Although this conveys no special benefit to lips, its ingredients supply antioxidants and also have a lightweight moisturizing ability. (This isn't close to a lip balm or gloss.) Despite claims of containing micro-collagen, no form of collagen is on the ingredient list. This fragrance-free serum isn't a must-have, but it can be used for slightly dry skin anywhere on the face, including the lips.

☹ $$$ **Mini Lift** *($19 for 0.27 ounce)*. I'm glad Isomers describes this product as providing "cosmetic" skin tightening, because that's all it does. No lifting whatsoever is taking place. Believing this product is similar to a face-lift is like saying building an airplane is the same as being a passenger on one. This product contains a starch-based ingredient and a film-forming agent that, together, temporarily make skin feel tighter. However, no one will think you've had work done or that you look the least bit younger, so buyer beware.

☺ **Moisture Mask** *($12 for 1.86 ounces)* is a good, inexpensive, lightweight gel mask that is suitable for all skin types experiencing minor dryness. The fragrance-free formula is gentle and rinses well, but there's no reason you can't leave this on your skin overnight.

☺ $$$ **Skin Brightening Complex II** *($40 for 1 ounce)*. The good news is that this fragrance-free skin-brightening complex contains an impressive amount of niacinamide, a B vitamin known to interrupt the pathway of melanin production. Daily use of this skin-lightening product coupled with an effective sunscreen rated SPF 15 or greater should result in a reduction in sun-induced discolorations. Niacinamide also has other benefits for skin, such as increasing its production of ceramides. The other ingredient of note that research has shown to be a potentially effective option for fighting discolorations is licorice root extract. However, it's the niacinamide that stands the greatest chance of making the product effective. This product is best for normal to dry skin not prone to blemishes.

☹ $$$ **Stem Genesis Extreme Eyelash Enhancer** *($35.75 for 0.27 ounce)* is a specialty product that is supposed to enhance eyelashes so they appear thicker and longer. The short story is that it doesn't contain ingredients that are capable of making lashes longer, thicker, or darker. This doesn't begin to compare to products that contain prostaglandin analogues, a class of ingredients known to promote eyelash growth and color. You're better off asking your doctor about a prescription for Latisse, because that's a lash-enhancing product you can count on to work as claimed. By the way, this product contains a fruit cell culture from a species of apples that Isomers believes stimulates stem cells in our skin. There are too many unknowns surrounding this concept to make it something consumers should experiment with, and there's no evidence that stimulating stem cells results in better eyelashes anyway.

☹ $$$ **Trace Elements Wrinkle Release Complex for Expression Lines** *($25 for 0.51 ounce)* is another product from Isomers claiming to be a treatment for expression lines—it isn't. The peptide it contains absolutely does not have a Botox-like effect on the muscle contractions that form expression lines and, therefore, wrinkles. The ingredient, which has a very long name—polydodecanamideaminium triazadiphenylethenesulfonate—is a synthetic polymer the manufacturer says diffuses light. It may do that, but not to an extent that your expression lines will seem soft-focused.

☹ **Lip Balm** *($12 for 0.51 ounce)* is a very good lip balm but is packaged in a jar, which will not keep the antioxidants stable during use. It's also not good that this contains lavender extract, an ingredient that imparts fragrance but has no benefit for lips. If you don't mind a lavender scent and the jar packaging, this will keep dry lips soft, smooth, and protected from moisture loss.

✓☺ **Lip Exfoliating Balm** *($8 for 0.17 ounce)* is a very good, emollient scrub for lips. It contains polyethylene as the abrasive agent and, coupled with the moisturizing ingredients, is a gentle way to remove dry, dead skin from lips. Bonus: it's fragrance-free, too.

☺ **$$$ Maxi-Lip II** *($20 for 0.27 ounce)* is a lip serum that is really more of a lip moisturizer and, although it contains several ingredient that keep dry lips at bay, it also contains the irritant methyl nicotinate. This increases circulation to the lips by virtue of irritation; that is why your lips feel warm and tingly when you apply it. Maxi-Lip II is an OK product for occasional use (it slightly plumps lips, though the effect is temporary), but it is too irritating to use daily.

JAN MARINI SKIN RESEARCH, INC.

JAN MARINI SKIN RESEARCH, INC. AT-A-GLANCE

Strengths: Most of the products are fragrance- and colorant-free; excellent AHA and retinol options, including an AHA combined with sunscreen; the water-soluble cleansers.

Weaknesses: Expensive; some categories contain ingredients (growth factors, hormones, and interferon) with unreliable track records or whose long-term risks, if any, remain unknown; sunscreens that lack sufficient UVA-protecting ingredients; jar packaging; Marini Lash isn't as exciting as Marini's former lash-enhancing products.

For more information about Jan Marini Skin Research, Inc., call (800) 347-2223 or visit www.janmarini.com or www.Beautypedia.com.

JAN MARINI SKIN RESEARCH, INC. SKIN CARE

JAN MARINI AGE INTERVENTION PRODUCTS

☺ **$$$ Age Intervention Transitions Face Lotion** *($89 for 1 ounce)* is made to sound like a specialized, targeted treatment product for older women struggling with acne, but ends up being a mixed bag of effective, questionable, and irritating ingredients. The effective portion is the 1% salicylic acid and the pH of 4, which allows this lightweight lotion to exfoliate and help dislodge blackheads. The questionable ingredient is something Marini refers to as Spirolac. This is followed by a long chemical name, and there isn't a shred of information available about this ingredient. The Spirolac name is similar to the name of the prescription drug spironolactone (Aldactone), which is an orally administered anti-hypertension medication sometimes prescribed to women with stubborn or cystic acne because it regulates androgens (male hormones), which have a causative role in acne. Although the similarity of the names may make you think that Marini included a drug in this cosmetic product—which is not permissible—in actuality the chemical name for Spirolac doesn't match the chemical name of the drug spironolactone. So it's just a way to make you associate this product with a prescription drug. And even if it did contain the drug, there is no research showing topical application of spironolactone helps with acne. In contrast, oral doses have benefit (and some risks) due to the balancing effect on hormones (Sources: *Journal of the American Academy of Dermatology*, January 2008, pages 60-62; *Advances in Dermatology*, 2007, pages 155-163; and *Journal of Cutaneous Medicine and Surgery, Supplement,*

2004, pages 11-15). The lack of research on Spirolac (including its safety) is reason enough to view this product with suspicion. In addition, this product contains a form of resorcinol, which can be irritating and drying to skin, as well as a tiny amount of arnica and Spanish pellitory (*Anacylus pyrethrum*), which also can cause irritation. There are some intriguing, skin-beneficial ingredients in this BHA lotion, but the amounts are likely inconsequential for skin, while the unknowns about Spirolac (and the product's price) make it an uneasy recommendation, in spite of it being an effective BHA product.

☺ **$$$ Age Intervention Eye Cream** *($64 for 0.5 ounce)* is a very emollient eye cream that contains some excellent nonvolatile plant oils and very good water-binding agents. Lots of antioxidants are included, but they won't remain stable for long once this jar-packaged product is opened. This is an option for dry to very dry skin, but the unknowns surrounding long-term use of products with hormones and interferon are a cause for concern.

☹ **$$$ Age Intervention Face Cream** *($77 for 1 ounce)* is very similar to the Age Intervention Eye Cream, except this has a few more bells and whistles. Otherwise, the same comments apply.

☹ **$$$ Age Intervention Face Serum** *($77 for 1 ounce)* is a water- and oil-based serum that contains some great water-binding agents and lesser amounts of antioxidants. Although it is an option for normal to slightly dry skin, the concerns about long-term application of interferon and hormones remain.

☺ **$$$ Age Intervention Peptide Extreme Facial Serum** *($89 for 1 ounce)*. With each new product launch, Jan Marini's claims get more and more over the top; they've begun to propel into outer space and are setting ever higher the standard for cosmetic hype and absurdity. For this product, Marini repeatedly uses words such as "concentrated," "proprietary," and "extraordinary," well aware that consumers will very likely think it is the answer to aging skin they've been seeking. Of course, in the field of cosmetics, many products are exalted as miracles, and this one is no exception. Is there anything behind the astounding claims for this serum? Well, Marini included a good nonfragrant plant oil, several peptides, some skin-identical ingredients, and a smattering of antioxidants. However, none of the ingredients are unique to her line; you'll find similar and, in some cases, even better serums from competing lines. Moreover, none of these ingredients are going to bring about a dramatic change in your skin "on every [or any] measurable level." And, of course, there are no published studies showcasing these measurable results. For a product that boasts of superior status, it's disappointing to see that several of the key antiaging ingredients are listed after the preservatives, meaning they don't count for much. As for the peptides in this serum, all of them have theoretical cell-communicating ability, assuming they remain intact on their journey into the skin. Remember, naturally occurring enzymes in skin tend to break down peptides before they reach their target, although even when that happens they can still have a moisturizing benefit for skin. Keep in mind that all of the peptides in this serum are found in other products, too. That doesn't make this Marini product bad, but it certainly doesn't make it unique or worth the exalted descriptions, either. The peptide blend Marini chose for this serum doesn't have any substantiated research indicating it rejuvenates skin in the manner the company claims; the only information about these peptides comes from the company that sells them. There is every reason to consider this serum if you have normal to dry skin and want a lightweight product to smooth and hydrate while supplying some potentially state-of-the-art ingredients. Although this isn't the best serum around and the fantasyland claims are unproven, Marini deserves credit for combining peptides with other beneficial ingredients and packaging them in an airtight container to ensure stability during use.

☺ **$$$ Age Intervention Enlighten Facial Lotion** (*$89 for 1 ounce*) contains the emollient kojic dipalmitate as the main lightening agent in this "composition." This ingredient is not the same as pure kojic acid, a skin-lightening agent that Marini and other companies use as a substitute for hydroquinone in their products. Although kojic acid isn't the most reliable skin-lightening agent, it does work. However, it has some negative research associated with it in terms of causing problems for skin. Hydroquinone has some negative research as well, but considerably more positive research (including safety and toxicity studies) to support its efficacy and ongoing use. In contrast, kojic dipalmitate has only one published study, and that merely examined how to detect the ingredient in cosmetic products, not whether or not it actually worked to lighten skin discolorations (Sources: *Talanta*, April 2008, pages 407-411; *Analytical Biochemistry*, June 2002, pages 260-268; and *American Journal of Clinical Dermatology*, September-October 2000, pages 261-268). Still, because kojic dipalmitate is related to kojic acid, it may have some lightening effect, but it's not a sure thing, and for the price Marini is charging, you should expect a product that lightens. The other skin-lightening agent used here is hexylresorcinol. This ingredient is considered an antimicrobial agent, and the only research pertaining to its effect on melanin (skin pigment) has to do with treating fresh shrimp during processing to prevent black spots (melanosis) that would undoubtedly decrease their visual appeal at the local seafood counter (Sources: *Journal of Food Science*, April 2008, pages S124-S133; and *Journal of Food Protection*, January 2005, pages 98-104). This is definitely a novel blend of skin-lightening agents, but it is a stretch that either one will be the answer to your skin discoloration issues, as human skin cells and the skin of dead shrimp are not exactly related. I certainly wouldn't choose this option over products with tried-and-true skin-lightening ingredients, even those derived from plant extracts such as arbutin or bearberry. There isn't a wealth of research on those ingredients either, but at least there is some. Marini also references the retinol in this product as being capable of suppressing excess melanin production, but that ability isn't reflected in the body of research for this vitamin A ingredient, at least not when used by itself and not when compared to tretinoin (the active ingredient in Renova and Tri-Luma). Instead, retinol's role in skin lightening tends to be more as a co-factor when paired with skin-lightening agents such as hydroquinone, vitamin C, or glycolic acid (Sources: *Cutis*, December 2007, pages 497-502; and *Cosmetic Dermatology*, January 2005, *Supplement: "Revisiting Retinol"*). In the end, this skin-lightening product isn't all that enlightening.

unrated Age Intervention Regeneration Booster (*$225 for 1.5 ounces*) is said to be an "extraordinary new skin care compound [that] captures the emerging science of topical telomerase enzyme as a realistic science-based option for dramatically younger looking skin." Telomerase is an enzyme that appears to be responsible for creating what are called immortal cells, and immortality sounds like a good thing. The dark side is that telomerase appears to be responsible for the unchecked growth of cells seen in human cancers. Telomerase levels appear to be carefully maintained in normal body tissues, but the enzyme is reactivated in cancer, where immortal cells are likely required to maintain tumor growth (Source: *Science*, 1994, volume 266, pages 2011-2015). Further, the authors of an article published in *Nature* (June 15, 2000) have this to add: "scientists report that using telomerase to extend the life-span of human tissue culture cells ... may present some level of cancer risk...." Additionally, other research has revealed that telomerase is capable of maintaining itself if its environment is correct. If that's not the case, however, differentiation can occur and that may negatively affect other cells, such as fibroblasts.

Telomerase may also play a causative role in the formation and development of melanoma, the deadliest form of skin cancer (Sources: *Ontogenez*, March-April 2007, pages 105-119; and *Collegium Antropologicum*, January 2007, pages 17-22). That's not good news for skin, something that Marini conveniently leaves out of her company's information.

The bottom line is that the telomerase enzyme is not the antiwrinkle answer. There is only one potentially convincing piece of research on the role of telomerase in preventing skin from further aging, and it's not a slam-dunk or without cause for concern. The study examined using telomerase to extend the life span of fibroblasts (cells that contribute to the building of connective fibers, including collagen). The problem is that the study was done in vitro, and involved adding telomerase to dermal fibroblast cells and then monitoring these cells for behavioral changes. The results showed that telomerase kept fibroblast cells alive, and as such may reverse the manner in which cell reproduction slows down as we age. How this applies to stimulating telomerase activity on intact, healthy skin is an unknown, and assuming it will work just as this study showed is a leap of faith (Source: *Experimental Cell Research*, August 2000, pages 270-278). Moreover, keep in mind that doing or using something that causes telomerase activity to increase in the body (which normally regulates telomerase on its own) may lead to the unchecked growth of cells that won't die—the basis for most types of cancer. Because these vials contain telomerase enzyme and we don't know how this actually works on skin (for better or potentially worse), it is left unrated. The water- and oil-based fluid is loaded with peptides, ceramides, plant oil, silicones, and emollients that help restore a healthy barrier to dry skin. The peptides have theoretical cell-communicating ability, while other cell-communicating ingredients and antioxidants play supporting roles (though antioxidants aren't present in amounts that justify this product's price). Despite these positives, the inclusion of telomerase and several growth factors make this Age Intervention product too potentially risky to consider—and you don't want to be any skin-care company's guinea pig. For more information on the various growth factors, please refer to the Cosmetic Ingredient Dictionary at www.Beautypedia.com.

☺ **$$$ Age Intervention Regeneration Facial Mask** (*$90 for 1 ounce*). Marini has created a clay mask that goes above and beyond a standard clay mask but, as you'll see, is not without its peccadilloes. It not only absorbs excess oil, but also provides slight exfoliation thanks to its glycolic acid content and the borderline pH of 4.1 that enables it to be effective. The mask is also loaded with helpful ingredients, including potent antioxidants and cell-communicating ingredients. Ideally, you want those ingredients in leave-on products rather than in masks, which you rinse off. However, every little bit helps so long as your skin-care routine includes the aforementioned ingredients in products meant to stay on skin. This mask is an acceptable addition, assuming the price doesn't make you gasp! This product would be rated better if it did not contain arnica and pellitory extracts, neither of which is helpful for skin, and if it weren't packaged in a jar, which won't keep the antioxidants stable during use. But really, I ask you, $90 for a mask—in any economy, that is just foolish!

JAN MARINI ANTIOXIDANT PRODUCTS

☺ **$$$ Antioxidant Daily Face Protectant, SPF 30, Waterproof** (*$48 for 2 ounces*) includes avobenzone for UVA protection. The amount of avobenzone (1%) is disappointing for a sunscreen rated SPF 30, but at least this is an improvement over the previous version, which left skin vulnerable to UVA damage. In terms of antioxidants, this product still comes up short; however, it contains some excellent water-binding agents and is an option for normal to slightly dry skin.

☺ **$$$ Antioxidant Daily Face Protectant Tinted, SPF 30, Waterproof** *($51 for 2 ounces)* is a good, slightly moisturizing, water-resistant sunscreen that contains avobenzone for sufficient UVA protection. Despite the name, the only antioxidant is yeast extract (incorrectly listed by its trade name Nayad S). This has a sheer tint and soft shimmer that would work for light to medium skin tones.

☺ **$$$ Recover-E** *($44.50 for 1 ounce)* contains vitamin E and a few other antioxidants, but they won't remain stable once this jar-packaged, otherwise bland moisturizer, is opened.

☺ **$$$ Skin Silk Protecting Hydrator** *($44.50 for 1 ounce)* is a standard, slightly emollient moisturizer for normal to dry skin that's not prone to blemishes. The antioxidant plant oils won't retain potency once this jar-packaged product is opened.

☹ **Body Block SPF 30, Waterproof** *($28 for 4 ounces)* lacks the UVA-protecting ingredients of titanium dioxide, zinc oxide, avobenzone, Tinosorb, and Mexoryl SX, and is not recommended. This also does not contain a single notable antioxidant.

JAN MARINI BENZOYL PEROXIDE PRODUCTS

☺ **$$$ Benzoyl Peroxide 2.5% Wash** *($30 for 8 ounces)* is a cleanser and, because a cleanser is washed away, the benzoyl peroxide (the effective ingredient), which should stay on the skin to work, will be rinsed down the drain. This is otherwise a standard, but good, water-soluble cleanser for all but very dry skin.

☹ **Benzoyl Peroxide 5%** *($30 for 4 ounces)* is a topical disinfectant listing 5% benzoyl peroxide as the active ingredient. That's great, but the amount of sodium lauryl sulfate makes an already potentially drying product far more likely to cause problems. This does not compare favorably with leave-on benzoyl peroxide products from the drugstore.

☹ **Benzoyl Peroxide 10%** *($30 for 4 ounces)* is nearly identical to the Benzoyl Peroxide 5%, except this contains a 10% concentration. The same concerns apply: the amount of sodium lauryl sulfate makes an already potentially drying product far more likely to cause problems. This does not compare favorably with leave-on benzoyl peroxide products from the drugstore.

JAN MARINI BIOGLYCOLIC PRODUCTS

✓ ☺ **$$$ Bioglycolic Bioclean Cleanser** *($29 for 8 ounces)* is a good option for a water-soluble cleanser for all skin types. It removes makeup easily, is fragrance-free, and doesn't contain a single potentially problematic ingredient, making it a top choice. This cleanser does not contain any AHAs, and that's just fine because their benefit would be wasted in such a product.

☺ **$$$ Bioglycolic Facial Cleanser** *($29 for 8 ounces)* differs from the Bioglycolic Bioclean Cleanser because it contains glycolic acid and has a minimalist cleansing base. Unless you're willing to leave this on skin, it's not the best idea if you want to get the benefits of glycolic acid. It is an OK cleanser for normal to slightly dry or slightly oily skin, but should not be used around the eyes or to remove eye makeup.

☺ **$$$ Bioglycolic Oily Skin Cleansing Gel** *($29 for 8 ounces)* is similar to the Bioglycolic Facial Cleanser, but with a higher amount of detergent cleansing agent and a lesser amount of glycolic acid. Otherwise, the same basic comments apply.

☺ **$$$ Bioglycolic Cream** *($67 for 2 ounces)* is a pricey but effective option for normal to dry skin that needs an AHA product. Glycolic acid is the second ingredient listed, and the pH of 3.2 allows it to exfoliate. This would be rated higher if it did not contain comfrey extract, which can be problematic for skin once it is absorbed.

☺ **$$$ Bioglycolic Eye Cream** *($41 for 0.5 ounce)* goes beyond just being an eye cream with AHA (it contains glycolic acid at about 10% with a pH of 3) by claiming to have an effect on the fat pockets of the lower eyelids. Supposedly, this cream contains ingredients that can induce lipolysis (a process that allows fat cells to be released from areas resistant to fat metabolism), so it also minimizes under-eye bags to "re-contour" the eye area. One of the ingredients in this eye cream, methylsilanol theophyllinacetate alginate (trade name: Theophyllisilane C) shows up in a few anti-cellulite products. However, there is no research anywhere proving it can affect fat cells in skin when applied topically. Consider this an AHA moisturizer and disregard all the other claims.

☹ **Bioglycolic Facial Lotion** *($51 for 2 ounces)* has a pH of 3 so the sufficient amount of glycolic acid will exfoliate skin. This product doesn't offer much else, and the inclusion of a significant amount of comfrey makes it a problem for all skin, and definitely not preferred to the AHA products from Alpha Hydrox, Pond's, or Neutrogena.

✓ ☺ **$$$ Bioglycolic Facial Lotion SPF 15** *($52 for 2 ounces)* omits the comfrey found in the Bioglycolic Facial Lotion and protects skin from sun with a pure titanium dioxide sunscreen. The combination of sun protection and an effective amount of glycolic acid at a pH of 3.2 makes this a winning, triple-duty product for normal to dry skin.

☹ **Bioglycolic Sunless Self-Tanner** *($28 for 4 ounces)* contains approximately 2% glycolic acid, which is too small an amount to exfoliate. The pH of this self-tanner (it contains dihydroxyacetone to darken skin, just like hundreds of other self-tanning products) is 2.6, making it too irritating for all skin types.

☺ **Bioglycolic Lightening Gel** *($41 for 2 ounces)* contains a potentially effective amount of AHAs at a pH of 3.2 to permit exfoliation. The skin-lightening agent is kojic acid, but it is not preferred to other options, such as hydroquinone or stabilized vitamin C. If anything, kojic acid has research pointing to stability issues in skin-care products (Sources: *Bioorganic and Medicinal Chemistry Letters*, June 2004, pages 2843-2846; and Journal of Cosmetic Science, March-April 2004, pages 139-148). This is still an option as an AHA product for normal to oily skin.

☺ **$$$ Bioglycolic Bioclear Cream** *($58 for 1 ounce)* contains about 8% to 10% AHA and about 1% BHA in a fairly basic, lightweight moisturizing formula. It would work well for exfoliation for someone with normal to dry skin. BHA can exfoliate both in the pore and on the surface of skin, while AHA concentrates on the surface. In some ways it is redundant to have both, but some people find that better for their skin type. This also contains azelaic acid (a component of grains such as wheat, rye, and barley), which has been shown to be effective for a number of skin conditions when applied topically in a cream formulation at a 20% concentration (Source: *International Journal of Dermatology*, December 1991, pages 893-895). However, other research suggests that azelaic acid is more irritating than hydroquinone when mixed with glycolic acid or kojic acid (Source: *eMedicine Journal*, www.emedicine.com, November 5, 2001, volume 2, number 11). Regardless, this product contains far less than 20% azelaic acid, so it is hard to say what, if any, effect it would have on skin. The group of potentially irritating plant extracts in this product makes it less desirable.

☺ **$$$ Bioglycolic Bioclear Lotion** *($58 for 1 ounce)* is a stripped-down version of the Bioglycolic Bioclear Cream, and ends up being a better choice because it eliminates the problematic plant extracts and simply exfoliates skin with a pH-correct combination of 2% salicylic acid and 8% to 10% glycolic acid, all in a fragrance-free gel base.

☺ **Bioglycolic Acne Gel I** *($41 for 2 ounces)* contains alcohol and lavender oil, which make it too irritating for all skin types. The alcohol will stimulate oil production in the pore lining, which only makes skin oilier.

☺ **Bioglycolic Acne Gel II** *($41 for 2 ounces)* has the same problems as the Bioglycolic Acne Gel I above, and the same review applies.

JAN MARINI C-ESTA PRODUCTS

☺ **$$$ C-ESTA Cleansing Gel** *($29 for 6 ounces)* is a basic, but good, water-soluble cleanser for all skin types. It does contain fragrance.

☹ **$$$ C-ESTA Cream** *($79 for 1 ounce)* contains a good amount of vitamin C in the form of ascorbyl palmitate, but the jar packaging won't keep this light- and air-sensitive ingredient stable during use, and there isn't much else to extol about this product.

☹ **$$$ C-ESTA Eye Contour Cream** *($45 for 0.5 ounce)* does not contain a single ingredient backed by any evidence to show that it can diminish dark circles via vasodilation. And actually, you don't want to encourage vasodilation, because dilating veins encourages more blood to flow to an area, and it is this expansion of blood vessels and pooling of blood beneath thin under-eye skin that has a darkening effect, resulting in dark circles. So, if anything, you'd want to reduce the blood flow to the area. However, in this case it's moot, because this product doesn't contain ingredients that can cause vasodilation. In fact, there are no topical ingredients that can accomplish that without being problematic for skin. This jar-packaged moisturizer has a lot of vitamin C, but it won't remain stable once the product is opened.

☺ **$$$ C-ESTA Eye Repair Concentrate** *($59 for 0.5 ounce)* contains a good amount of vitamin C in a serum texture and in packaging that will keep the vitamin C stable. Other than that, there's one significant water-binding agent in this product, and the other goodies appear after the preservatives. It is an option for normal to slightly dry skin.

☺ **$$$ C-ESTA Serum** *($79 for 1 ounce)* combines effective water-binding agents with vitamin C and silicone plus a tiny amount of vitamin E. This is a well-designed, well-packaged product if you're curious to try a vitamin C serum.

☺ **$$$ C-ESTA Serum, Oil Control** *($79 for 1 ounce)* lacks any absorbent ingredients needed to control excess surface oil. It also can't regulate oil production, something that is not possible with a topical product, but this is a good lightweight moisturizer with vitamin C and green tea for normal to oily skin.

☺ **$$$ C-ESTA Facial Mask** *($57 for 2 ounces)* promises face-contouring results, but just delivers light moisture, soothing agents, and the antioxidant capability of vitamin C. This is a good mask for normal to dry skin, but to obtain the most benefit, leave it on overnight.

☺ **$$$ C-ESTA Lips** *($45 for 0.5 ounce)* assumes that none of the other C-ESTA products can be used around the mouth, so now you have one just for the lips and skin in that immediate area. This isn't necessary. There are no ingredients in here that are unique or special for the lip area. The formula is almost identical to the other C-ESTA products for skin, and the same comments apply.

JAN MARINI ENZYME PRODUCTS

☹ **$$$ Clean Zyme** *($28 for 4 ounces)*. Despite all the fancy words about how papaya (source of the enzyme papain) works on skin, there is no research showing it to have exfoliating properties on skin, and definitely none showing it to be preferred over AHAs or BHA. The Web site www.naturaldatabase.com states that there is insufficient reliable information to support the effectiveness of papaya (also known as green papaya, which is how Marini lists it). Note: Persons allergic to latex, kiwi, or figs are very likely to have a negative reaction to papain, the enzyme component of papaya (Source: *Clinical and Experimental Allergy: Journal of the British Society for Allergy and Clinical Immunology*, August 2004, pages 1251-1258).

☺ $$$ **Skin Zyme** *($44 for 2 ounces)* lists green papaya concentrate as the main ingredient, followed by plant oil, thickeners, slip agent, preservative, honey, vitamin E, and fragrance. The enzyme component of papaya is not a reliable way to exfoliate skin, though some people may notice a slight benefit, and the other ingredients in this product will make skin feel smooth.

☺ $$$ **Day Zyme** *($45 for 1 ounce)* is similar to the Skin Zyme, only without the plant oil and in a base that's better for those with oily skin. It contains a citrus fragrance.

☺ $$$ **Night Zyme** *($44.50 for 1 ounce)* is very similar to the Skin Zyme, only with added ginger, which can be a skin irritant when applied topically, though the amount in this product is unlikely to have that effect.

JAN MARINI FACTOR-A AND FACTOR-A PLUS PRODUCTS

☺ $$$ **Factor-A Cream** *($51 for 1 ounce)* is an emollient moisturizer for dry to very dry skin. It contains some very effective water-binding agents, but, if you're to believe the ingredient list, no retinol (or any other form of vitamin A). The jar packaging won't keep the antioxidants stable once opened, and some of the plant extracts can be irritating (though there's not much of them in here).

✓ ☺ $$$ **Factor-A Eyes for Dark Circles** *($78 for 60 capsules)* are single-use capsules and a great way to get the benefits of retinol, as it can remain very stable in this kind of packaging. The silicone base lends a pleasant application and silky finish, while the antioxidants green tea and vitamin C lend support. Marini claims the vitamin K in this serum addresses the cause of dark circles, but there is no published research to support topical application of vitamin K for that purpose. This is still an excellent retinol/antioxidant product for all skin types.

☺ $$$ **Factor-A Lotion** *($48 for 1 ounce)* is a relatively standard but worthwhile moisturizer for normal to dry skin that contains more retinyl palmitate than retinol, but at least the packaging will keep the retinol stable. It also contains vitamins C and E and a tiny amount of niacinamide.

☹ **Factor-A Plus Cream** *($51 for 1 ounce)* features what the company calls Factor A Plus Complex, which should be listed as retinol—and whatever else is in this complex. (One consistent pattern in Marini's line is failing to meet FDA regulatory ingredient labeling guidelines.) The complex may also contain glycolic acid. Marini claims it does contain glycolic acid, but it is not listed separately, and it should be. The product has a pH of 3, but without knowing if glycolic acid is really in the product, I wouldn't bank on this for exfoliation. Further, the retinol will deteriorate because of the jar packaging. Adding a selection of irritating plant extracts doesn't make for delicious icing on this already flavorless cake.

☹ **Factor-A Plus Lotion** *($48 for 1 ounce)* lists alcohol as the second ingredient, making this too irritating for all skin types. The AHAs in this product are not as helpful for acne-prone skin as BHA (salicylic acid) would be.

✓ ☺ $$$ **Factor-A Plus Mask** *($81 for 2 ounces)* is an intriguing, well-formulated mask for normal to oily skin. The 2% salicylic acid will exfoliate skin thanks to the pH of 3.2, while antioxidants, soothing agents, and cell-communicating ingredients provide benefit. Given the number of bells and whistles in this product, it would be a waste to rinse it after only a few minutes; there is nothing in this fragrance-free product that cannot be left on skin overnight, and that's what you should do to get the most benefit.

JAN MARINI TRANSFORMATION PRODUCTS

☹ **$$$ Transformation Face Cream** *($78 for 1 ounce)*. The big-deal ingredient in this product is transforming growth factor (TGF beta-1). The claims for the actions of this ingredient are at best exaggerated, and its effectiveness is not established in skin-care products. This also contains some good water-binding agents and a small amount of antioxidants, but jar packaging won't keep them stable. It does contain fragrance and, despite the claims, there are no peptides listed.

☹ **$$$ Transformation Eye Cream** *($58 for 0.5 ounce)*, like Marini's Transformation Face Cream above, contains TGF beta-1, and the same comments apply. This one also contains sugarcane extract, but that is not an AHA and, even if it were, the pH is not appropriate for exfoliation. This version does contain a more impressive mix of water-binding agents and antioxidants, but the choice of jar packaging means the ingredients won't stay stable after it's opened.

☹ **Transformation Serum** *($78 for 1 ounce)* contains a high amount of transforming growth factor, but there are so many unknowns about this ingredient that applying so much of it is a potential risk for skin. The effective water-binding agents won't have much benefit on skin due to the presence of several irritating plant extracts, including comfrey, arnica, ivy, and pellitory.

JAN MARINI MAKEUP

MASCARA: ☹ **Marini Mascara Performance Mascara** *($80)*. Normally I'd rate a mascara that performs as this one does just average, but not this time. That's because who in their right mind would pay $80 for mascara that's at best average to below average? You can get astonishingly great mascaras at the drugstore for less than $8, so why the big step-up in price here? It's because, according to Jan Marini, this mascara contains a proprietary peptide blend (the same one included in the company's Marini Lash product) that "gives you the darkest, lushest looking, thickest and densely defined lashes ever." Of course, all of those boasts can be attributed to the cosmetic effect that any good mascara would have, but this one doesn't qualify as a good mascara. Application is uneven, it does a poor job of adding thickness, and it takes far too long to attain what is best described as modest length. In addition, the formula tends to make lashes feel brittle and dry at the end of the day. What about the proprietary peptides meant to make your lashes grow? There is no substantiated research proving they have even a small impact on lash growth, thickness, or color. If anything, this product and Marini Lash are supposed to replace the lash-enhancing products they used to sell that contained a prescription drug ingredient that really worked, but that ended up being confiscated by the FDA. Believing any of the claims about this product merely means you would be taking Marini's word for it because there is no research showing peptides have any benefit for growing lashes—and after the former lash growth problems she went through (which was a terrible financial fiasco) and the fact that she deceived consumers about what was really in her products until the FDA stepped in, she's not one I'd consider a good source of information (if nothing else, she's certainly biased).

SPECIALTY PRODUCTS: ☹ **$$$ Marini Lash** *($160 for 0.23 ounce)*. I have to admit, Jan Marini has nerve! After the well-publicized news reports of the issues surrounding her two previous eyelash-growth products (Age Intervention Eyelash and Age Intervention Eyelash

Conditioner, of which $2 million in inventory was confiscated by the FDA, and the latter she renamed to coincide with the toned-down cosmetic claims), she rebounded with what she claims is another pace-setting lash product, but this one should keep her out of the FDA's sights and prevent another smackdown. Of course, Marini Lash is being advertised as not containing prostaglandins, the active ingredient in her other versions that got her into hot water with the FDA and saw her company facing a potential lawsuit from Allergan (who developed their own eyelash growth product [Latisse] but went about it the right way in terms of seeking FDA approval). While Marini was selling the earlier versions of eyelash products, the company never admitted that they contained drug ingredients being used off-label, and now they're advertising the lack of prostaglandins! See what I mean about nerve? As I previously reported, these drugs (such as latanoprost, bimatoprost, and travoprost) are used to treat eye health problems such as glaucoma or ocular hypertension. One of the common side effects of using eye drops containing prostaglandin analogues is eyelash growth and darkening (Sources: *Clinical and Experimental Ophthalmology*, November 2006, pages 755-764; www.nlm.nih.gov/medlineplus/druginfo/medmaster/a602027.html; http://dermatology.cdlib.org/93/commentary/alopecia/wolf.html; www.medscape.com/viewarticle/443657; and *Drugs of Today*, January 2003, pages 61-74). It wasn't much of a stretch to assume that topical application of a very low dose of these drugs might have a similar effect, and I can attest to the fact that Marini's previous Age Intervention Eyelash products definitely worked; my lashes have never been so long and thick—I'm routinely asked if I am wearing false eyelashes! So how does Marini Lash stack up? Well, unless Marini simply didn't list the eyelash growth ingredient this time around, the latest version is a poor substitute for its predecessor. The "proprietary peptides" and "other essential factors" (talk about a phrase that says everything and nothing; I mean, if they are essential, then tell us what they are!) have no research proving they can stimulate lash growth or density. I'm sure Marini will insist otherwise, but until information on these peptides is peer-reviewed and published, given the company's track record of being dishonest about what they used in previous versions, can you really trust them to be forthcoming? I wouldn't bank on Marini Lash being able to provide "the eyelashes of your dreams." At best, the water-binding and conditioning agents in this brush-on product will help make lashes softer, but that's about it. The ending to what became an undoubtedly stressful time for Marini and Company isn't a happy one (their former Age Intervention Eyelash products accounted for over 30% of the line's revenue), at least not for consumers expecting Marini Lash to perform as well (or better) than either of the preceding Age Intervention Eyelash products. Interestingly, there are other eyelash growth products still being sold that contain prostaglandin analogues. Although I have not personally tried these (with the exception of mascaras, I rarely review products from the perspective of personal experience—all that would tell you is how I liked the product, and preferences vary widely, as does personal experience—I almost exclusively prefer facts and research). You may want to consider Revitalash, Peter Thomas Roth Lashes to Die For, MD Lash Factor, and Lilash. Of course, you can also talk to your doctor about a prescription for Latisse. All of these are pricier options, but they should work as claimed due to the prostaglandin analogues they contain.

By the way, you may have heard or read that prostaglandin analogues can cause eye darkening or reduced vision. These warnings apply to prostaglandin analogues used in eye drop form, not for topical application to the lash line. It's certainly plausible that some of the ingredient will get in your eye as a matter of course, but the risk of suffering from the aforementioned side effects is slim (Sources: www.nlm.nih.gov/medlineplus/druginfo/medmaster/a602030. html; www.rxlist.com/cgi/generic/bimatoprost_ad.htm; and www.medicinenet.com/travoprost-ophthalmic_solution/article.htm).

JANE IREDALE

JANE IREDALE AT-A-GLANCE

Strengths: Pom Mist toner; lip balm with SPF 15; the makeup is mostly excellent, particularly the powder-based products, which include Iredale's contribution to mineral makeup; several impressive makeup brushes.

Weaknesses: Two problematic toners; many of the claims made for these products are not supported by solid research; the Circle/Delete and Zap/Hide concealers, poor eye pencils; Lip-Colours SPF 18 contain irritating peppermint; some superfluous specialty products.

For more information about Jane Iredale, call (800) 762-1132 or visit the Web site at www.janeiredale.com or www.Beautypedia.com.

JANE IREDALE SKIN CARE

☹ **Balance Antioxidant Hydration Spray** *($17.50 for 2 ounces)* was formulated "specifically to help balance the skin's oil production and pH," but nothing in this toner can have that effect, plus the skin handles it's own pH fairly well via sweat and oil production. (After all, oil production is regulated internally by hormones, so external factors have only a negligible influence.) Further, this toner contains irritating tangerine extract as a major ingredient, as well as myrrh. Tangerine can be a skin irritant (though the extract is not as potent as the oil), and myrrh can cause contact dermatitis due to its volatile components, though it does have anti-inflammatory benefits (Source: www.naturaldatabase.com). However, myrrh is not worth seeking out over several other plants whose soothing benefits are not offset by the potential for sensitization.

☹ **Dot the i** *($22 for 50 swabs)* is a set of cotton swabs with hollow tubes filled with a pre-measured amount of makeup remover. A clever concept, but for some inexplicable reason, Iredale added ingredients like lavender water and radish root, which are irritating and extremely problematic for skin, around the eyes or elsewhere. If the packaging concept of this product appeals to you, consider the options from Swabplus, available for a lot less money and with a better ingredient list, found at beauty supply stores.

☹ **D2O Hydration Spritz** *($17.50 for 2 ounces)* lists *Cananga odorata* extract (ylang-ylang) water as the main ingredient, which isn't hydrating at all; it's fragrant and irritating. The myrrh extract is also a problem, which is a shame because this toner has some very good water-binding agents. The heavy water has no established benefit for skin.

✓ ☺ **$$$ Pom Mist** *($17.50 for 2 ounces)* is an antioxidant-laden toner that also contains some good water-binding agents and the cell-communicating ingredient lecithin. It is highly recommended for all skin types and is fragrance-free.

☺ **$$$ Facial Blotting Papers** *($11 for 100 sheets)* are average blotting papers because they simply don't absorb oil as well as several other options. Perhaps this is because the papers are made from flax seeds, which are themselves somewhat oily, but whatever the reason, standard tissue paper works better, as do the blotting papers composed of polypropylene (a plastic-like substance).

✓ ☺ **Lip Drink SPF 15** *($11.60)* contains a pure zinc oxide sunscreen and has a plant oil–based formula that is wonderfully conditioning for lips. I disagree with Iredale's claim (and there is no research to prove it) that petrolatum-based lip balms put users on a "continual drying cycle," but that doesn't change the fact that this is a very well-formulated lip balm. The only potential caution is the lemon peel oil, but there's only a tiny amount of it in here and it's unlikely to be a problem.

☺ **$$$ More Lip Lip Plumper** *($18 for 0.25 ounce)* is made for those who have some trepidation about collagen or hyaluronic acid lip injections, and promises to give you "the same full pout without the pain." All this emollient lip balm does is swell lips temporarily with ginger root oil. Ginger root oil can be irritating, so proceed with caution; products like this should be used only occasionally—and the results are not comparable to what's possible with cosmetic lip injections.

☺ **$$$ Sugar & Butter Lip Exfoliator/Plumper** *($24)* is a dual-sided product that features an oil-based stick with brown sugar crystals to exfoliate lips and a sheer pink shimmer lipstick designed to plump them. The scrub portion definitely takes care of dry, flaky skin on the lips yet can feel too abrasive unless used very gently. Iredale encourages users to eat the sugar crystals rather than rinsing them (nothing in this portion of the product is harmful to ingest), but that encourages lip-licking, which begins the dryness/chapping cycle anew. This is further aggravated when you apply the Lip Plumper, because it contains mint and ginger (listed on the box as "flavor") that cause a cooling, tingling sensation; lips become inflamed from the irritation. This type of product isn't the best for routine use due to the irritation it causes. And the amount of product you get is really tiny, which doesn't justify the price.

JANE IREDALE MAKEUP

JANE IREDALE MINERAL MAKEUP

FOUNDATION: ✓ ☺ **$$$ Amazing Base Loose Minerals SPF 20** *($42)* contains titanium dioxide and zinc oxide as the active sunscreen ingredients and these definitely contribute to the powder's opacity, cling, dry finish, and long-wearing capabilities. This loose-powder foundation is talc-free and has a very smooth texture that tends to get drier in feel and appearance the longer it's worn. You can use it dry or can mix it with a moisturizer to approximate a liquid foundation or to allow for easier application over drier skin. (Keep in mind, however, that mixing it will diminish the powder's sunscreen properties.) Either method can be messy, which is true for any loose-powder application, and that's a definite drawback. Amazing Base provides medium to full coverage. The smooth, dry texture and comparatively lighter finish (though it still looks like powder makeup) with a faint bit of shine is preferable to many other mineral makeups. It is much less shiny than the bareMinerals foundation from bare escentuals. Most of Iredale's 15 shades are superbly neutral, but some go on a bit lighter or darker than they appear, so testing them on your skin is imperative. The only shade to be careful of, due to its slight peach-rose tone, is Honey Bronze. This version lacks any colors for darker skin tones. Despite some minor drawbacks discussed above, this is still worthy of a Paula's Pick rating because it is great for sensitive or rosacea-affected skin.

✓ ☺ **$$$ PurePressed Pressed Minerals SPF 20** *($48)* is a pressed-powder version of the Amazing Base, except this one is more matte and not as thick, so oilier skin will be less likely to experience a heavy, caked look once the skin's oil and the powders mix. The sunscreen is pure titanium dioxide and zinc oxide. The same basic comments made for Amazing Base apply here as well; however, this offers a considerably more tidy application and a broader range of shades, including some exemplary options for darker skin tones. These are richly pigmented and, as a result, do not look as ash or gray on deeper skin tones like many other powders can. Of the 24 shades, the only ones to consider avoiding are Honey Bronze, Butternut, and Teakwood. The vast majority of skin-true shades here are gorgeous, just as they are for the Amazing Base.

☺ **$$$ Liquid Minerals** *($46 for 1.01 ounces)* combines "light-diffusing, soft focus" minerals with "ingredients that replenish the cellular layers of the epidermis." That sounds tempting until you realize that lots of ingredients in liquid foundations (such as glycerin and cholesterol) offer this benefit. This non-powder entry from Iredale is a bit tricky to dispense from its pump applicator, but does have a silky, water-light texture and does provide a smooth, sheer-coverage matte finish. The minerals (pigment) are encapsulated and dispense somewhat chunky, which makes blending a bit more difficult. However, once you get the hang of it, this foundation applies well with a sponge or synthetic brush. Among the 18 shades, a few (Golden Glow, Autumn, and Honey Bronze) are a bit too peach for some medium skin tones, but are still worth considering. Warm Sienna is slightly gold, while the rest of the shades are beautifully neutral and appropriate for fair to dark skin. This is a much lighter alternative to either of the powder-based mineral foundations and, although it contains some great water-binding agents, the matte finish makes it best for normal to slightly oily or oily skin.

POWDER: ✓ ☺ **$$$ Amazing Matte Loose Powder** *($31)* comes in one shade, and although it's translucent it still looks best on fair to light skin. This talc-free, mica- and rice starch–based powder looks beautiful on the skin and provides a dry, matte finish that does a good job of keeping excess shine (oil) in check. The mica lends a subtle glow to skin without being at all sparkly, making the strong matte finish look more natural. This is an impressive product for oily to very oily skin; the only caution has to do with using rice starch (a food-based ingredient) over blemishes.

☺ **$$$ Brush-Me Matte** *($46)* involves a loose powder housed in a component that's affixed with a powder brush for convenient, on-the-go application. The brush is quite good, and the closure mechanism keeps the bristles from splaying and the mess to a minimum. The powder has a fine, dry texture that mattifies skin while imparting subtle sparkle (not exactly what oily skin needs). It goes on translucent, and as such is suitable for all skin colors. Note that the second listed ingredient in this powder is rice starch, a food ingredient that can feed the bacteria that contributes to acne.

☹ **$$$ PureMatte Finish Powder** *($36)* feels matte and has a light, dry texture oily skin will love, but it contains more shine than both of Iredale's foundation powders. There is one shade, and it's suitably neutral, although limited to light skin. Rice starch is not an ideal ingredient to use over blemishes.

BLUSH AND BRONZER: ✓ ☺ **$$$ PurePressed Blush** *($26)* has a silky texture that goes on exceedingly smooth. The color range is impressive, offering equally good options for light and dark skin tones, but note that each shade has a touch of shine.

☹ **$$$ Sunbeam Bronzer** *($46)* is a very expensive pressed bronzing powder that features four segments of color: pale pink, rose, bronze, and copper. The result when all are swirled together with a brush is a soft rosy bronze tone that looks best on light to medium skin tones. The powder has a smooth, dry texture and is best brushed on sheer, because more than a sheer application results in the powder grabbing and looking uneven on skin.

EYESHADOW: ✓ ☺ $$$ **PurePressed Eye Shadows** *($17.50)* are sold as singles and have a formula and application identical to the PurePressed Blush, which is great. Each shade applies evenly without flaking or skipping, and tends to go on color-true. Note: The eyeshadow shades that still list bismuth oxychloride as the first ingredient feel drier and don't apply as smoothly. Look for the shades that list titanium dioxide and dimethicone as the main ingredients. Each shade has at least a slight amount of shine, but it is downplayed to a soft glow in many of the shades. The shiniest shades tend to deposit the least amount of color, and are best for highlighting the brow bone.

OTHER JANE IREDALE MAKEUP

FOUNDATION: ☺ **Dream Tint Moisture Tint SPF 15** *($36)* is a gentle, fragrance-free formula with sun protection that comes solely from titanium dioxide; it contains a couple of antioxidants, too. But I wouldn't consider this a dream tinted moisturizer unless almost no coverage is on your checklist. However, if very sheer coverage is what you're looking for, this is worth checking out. This dispenses like a fluffy cream, and quickly liquefies as you blend, setting to a finish that looks matte but feels slightly moist. It is best for normal to slightly dry or slightly oily skin. There are several shades available, most of which are very good, and even the not-so-good shades are acceptable because this product goes on so sheer that no one, including you, will notice. The Peach Brightener and Lilac Brightener are tricky to work with because both place an unnatural hue on skin. Although they're sheer enough to be a minor issue, these shades should be sampled first. Dream Moisture Tint SPF 15 would be suitable for sensitive skin.

☹ $$$ **Absence Oil Control Primer SPF 15** *($35.50)* seems to be, according to the claims, the product those with overactive oily skin have been searching for—yet the formula doesn't give much credibility to the oil-control and regulating claims. Although it's nice that the sunscreen is pure titanium dioxide and zinc oxide, some of the major ingredients (including candelilla wax and fatty acids from macadamia nut oil) in this cream-to-powder primer won't help oily skin. The colorless base of the original Absence slips over skin and sets to a matte finish, but those with truly oily skin will find it doesn't last as long as they'd like. The Absence 2 shade has a sheer peach tint (not tan, as described) that is borderline problematic for medium skin tones. Both versions are an OK option if your foundation doesn't contain sunscreen and you want to prep your skin with a matte-finish product; just don't expect it to regulate your skin's oil production.

CONCEALER: ☺ $$$ **Disappear** *($24)* is positioned as "the ultimate in camouflage creams" and is designed to conceal tattoos. It doesn't provide that much coverage, but does a great job concealing minor redness and other bothersome discolorations. The semi-liquid consistency has just enough slip to blend well, and once dry, its matte finish stays put. The formula contains several antioxidants, but the "blemish control botanicals" are a far cry from tried-and-true anti-blemish actives such as benzoyl peroxide or salicylic acid. Iredale maintains that the green tea extract in this concealer combats acne, but research does not support this assertion when green tea extract is applied topically instead of consumed in the diet. All four shades are outstanding and best for fair to medium/tan skin.

☺ $$$ **Active Light Under-Eye Concealer** *($25)* is a thick liquid concealer dispensed from a click-pen applicator and applied with a built-in synthetic brush. The smooth texture blends readily and provides nearly full coverage with a slightly flat, opaque finish. Creasing is minimal and the formula contains several skin-friendly ingredients—though it includes too many waxes for use over breakouts. The major problem is with the colors, half of which look nothing like skin and, when used over dark circles, essentially trade one discoloration problem for another. Avoid shades 4, 5, and 6, all of which are too pink or peach. Shades 1, 2, and 3 are yellow-toned options, but only for very fair to light skin to tones. This is not preferred to Estee Lauder's Ideal Light Brush-On Illuminator.

☹ **Circle/Delete** *($29)* comes in a pot with two colors; one is a lighter tone, the other a medium tone. The texture is quite thick and creamy, and you will get opaque coverage. This will definitely crease, and applying one of the mineral powders over it tends to look heavy and obvious. All of the colors are a far cry from real skin tones, and blending them is tricky.

☹ **Enlighten Concealer** *($28)* is a creamy concealer available in a single shade that is blatantly orange. Supposedly, this color is the key to erasing the look of dark circles, bruising, and hyperpigmentation (brown spots). The opacity of this concealer will provide coverage of those skin issues, but the resulting color is awful. The tiny amount of arbutin in this product is likely insufficient to lighten discolorations, plus the packaging chosen won't keep it stable during use.

☹ **Zap&Hide Blemish Concealer** *($25)*. I admire the concept behind this dual-sided product packaged to resemble a smaller-than-usual lipstick. The **Zap** portion is a colorless balm designed to disinfect the cause of a blemish, while the **Hide** portion is a cream concealer meant to camouflage unsightly redness from the blemish. Things begin to unravel from there. The Zap portion is based around shea butter, an emollient ingredient that isn't what someone struggling with acne needs because it is extremely emollient and greasy and can clog pores. It also contains a potentially effective amount of tea tree oil, but Iredale also included fragrant oils of geranium, ylang-ylang, and lavender, which cause irritation; they don't kill acne-causing bacteria. Meanwhile, the Hide portion shares the same formulary drawbacks. It would be nothing more than a happy accident if you saw any sign of blemish relief using this well-intentioned, but poorly formulated, product.

BLUSH AND BRONZER: ☺ **$$$ So-Bronze** *($41)* is a talc-free, pressed bronzing powder that comes in two shades. The number 1 option is best for fair to light skin and features minimal shine, while number 2 is darker and has a separate, crescent-shaped shiny powder segment that really lays on the sparkles. Both options have a smooth but dry texture and apply evenly (just use them sparingly).

☹ **$$$ Brush-Me Bronze** *($44)*. Housed in a small oval component outfitted with a built-in brush is this loose-powder bronzer. The mica-based, talc-free formula has a soft, dry texture and more opacity than most bronzing powders due to its titanium dioxide and zinc oxide content (note that this product does not come with an SPF rating). The result is color that doesn't enliven skin the way the best powder bronzers do. Instead, skin looks a bit flat, but the mica lends a sheen that makes the finish less drab than it would otherwise be. Two shades are available, and both are acceptable bronze tones for light to medium skin. Overall, this is a messier and definitely pricey way to use bronzing powder!

☹ **$$$ In Touch Cream Blush** *($26)* has a smooth, almost slick texture and comes in a portable, twist-up stick. Each blush shade is sheer and leaves skin with a moist-glow finish. The drawbacks are that this won't last the whole day, you get a surprisingly small amount of product for the money, and the artificial chocolate scent and flavor will be off-putting for many. It does not, as the company states, smell "just like your favorite truffle." Wet 'n' Wild and Avon make better twist-up blush sticks for less money; those looking to spend this amount should consider the options from NARS or Bobbi Brown.

EYESHADOW: ✓ ☺ $$$ **Duo Eye Shadows** *($27)* have the same formula as the Pure-Pressed Eye Shadows, and the same review applies. All of the pairings are well done, but you will need a deeper shade for eye lining.

☺ $$$ **Lid Primer** *($18)* comes with your choice of two cream-to-powder shades, a soft pearlized ivory or a shimmering pink. Both apply easily, have a slight tendency to crease, and offer significant coverage. Despite the shine, these are good choices if you have any discoloration on your eyelid and don't like the look you get using concealer and powder prior to eyeshadow.

☺ **Eye Gloss** *($15)*. Housed in small plastic tubes are various colors of Iredale's lightweight, sheer liquid eyeshadow. Every shade piles on the shine and has enough slip to allow blending to be smooth yet controllable. Once set, this has a tendency to settle into lines and eye creases, so this isn't quite as good as similar eyeshadows from L'Oreal HIP and Clinique.

☺ **Eye Highlighter Pencil** *($15)* is a standard chunky pencil with a pale pink shade on one end and an opalescent white shade on the other. The shine is intense without being glittery, and the only issue is that the creamy texture doesn't last too long around the eye, so some fading and creasing are unavoidable.

☺ $$$ **Triple Eye Shadows** *($27)* suffer from mostly poor or exceedingly shiny color combinations, and most of the colors still use the drier-textured version of Iredale's shadows, which isn't as easy to work with as their newer formula (only available in certain shades, though not clearly identified). The only workable sets are Triple Cognac and Cloud Nine, but two of the three shades in Pink Bliss are good.

EYE AND BROW SHAPER: ✓ ☺ $$$ **PureBrow Colours** *($16)* are soft-tinted brow mascaras that ably enhance the brows. Five superior shades are available, including options for blonde and auburn brows. It does not get sticky or make brows look greasy or too thick, and the brush deposits just the right amount of product (unless your brows are very full or bushy).

☺ $$$ **Liquid Eye Liner** *($20)* goes on slightly wetter than most, but the brush is great, being flexible enough to glide easily along the lash line, yet it lets you maintain control. Dry time is slower than average, but once set the formula stays in place and wears well. I would encourage you to explore the liquid eyeliner options from L'Oreal or Almay first, but this is an option if you want to spend more money.

☺ $$$ **PureBrow Fix & Mascara** *($20)* is a standard, PVP-based, clear brow gel that works as well as those sold at the drugstore. The only advantage of this is that it comes with two brushes, though most will find one preferable.

☹ $$$ **Cream to Powder Eyeliner** *($26)* includes one matte and two shimmer-finish, cream-to-powder shades in a single compact. Each applies smoothly and sets to a relatively solid powder finish, though it isn't impervious to smudging and smearing. All in all, this doesn't compare to the long-wearing, gel-type eyeliners from Bobbi Brown, M.A.C., or Stila.

☹ **Eye Pencils** *($9)* are creamy, run-of-the-mill pencils that apply a bit too thick and smudge easily. Iredale's Cream to Powder Eyeliner lasts longer, as do her powder eyeshadows.

LIPSTICK, LIP GLOSS AND LIPLINER: ☹ $$$ **Lip Crayon Box** *($55)*. Unless the concept of thick, chunky lip crayons and the routine sharpening they need appeals to you, there's no reason to consider this overpriced collection. These chubby pencils have a greasy texture and a glossy finish that doesn't last as long as traditional cream lipsticks.

☹ **Lip Definer** *($9)* has a creamy texture and attractive colors, but is otherwise standard and requires routine sharpening.

⊗ **Just Kissed Lip Plumper** *($24)*. This sheer lipstick has a slick, greasy texture and a glossy finish. The fruit-scented shades are attractive, but it's flavored with spearmint and peppermint oils and, according to the company's description, also contains lemon and tangerine oils. Combined, this definitely will make lips plumper by virtue of irritation, which leads to chapped lips after repeated use.

⊗ **Multi Colour for Lips SPF 18** *($38)*. This lip palette features Iredale's PureMoist LipColours with SPF 18 along with one shade of her PureGloss. The LipColour's sunscreen is pure zinc oxide, which is great. However, each shade also contains peppermint, which makes them too irritating. Meanwhile, the PureGloss contains ginger root oil, which is also way too irritating for routine use on lips.

⊗ **Multi-Gloss for Lips** *($38)*. This palette of Iredale's best-selling PureGloss shades is enticing, and each has an alluring shimmer. However, the formula contains a lot of ginger root oil, which makes them too irritating. There are numerous excellent glosses to consider before this one!

⊗ **PureMoist LipColours SPF 18** *($19)* are one of the few lipsticks with sunscreen that offer UVA protection (Iredale uses zinc oxide), but this plus is sidelined by the irritating peppermint extract that is also included. Granted, these lipsticks don't have the most elegant texture, but the boon of sun protection would have made them worth trying if not for the irritating peppermint.

⊗ **PureMoist LipSheres SPF 18** *($19)* are sheerer versions of the PureMoist LipColours above, and share the same pro (excellent broad-spectrum sunscreen) and con (too much peppermint).

⊗ **PureGloss for Lips** *($19)* has been reformulated and now comes with a flocked sponge-tip applicator. These sheer, minimally sticky glosses are available in some enticing colors, but the inclusion of ginger root oil produces a tingly warm sensation, which means lips are being irritated, not cared for.

MASCARA: ☺ **$$$ Longest Lash Thickening and Lengthening Mascara** *($32)*. I have no idea why this Iredale mascara costs twice as much as her other lash-enhancing options because the results certainly aren't worth the price. (I actually called the company to see if the price was listed correctly—it was, but even the sales rep didn't have a good explanation as to why, and usually a sales person can spin just about anything in the world of cosmetics.) That's not to say this isn't a good mascara, because it most certainly is—lashes are appreciably lengthened, separated without clumps, and left with a soft fringe. Any thickness is hard to come by, so ignore all claims that this brings lashes to their fullest potential. I can think of several mascaras at the drugstore whose all-around performance beats this handily, so there is no reason to spend this kind of money. Longest Lash is available in several colors, including plums, grays, and even a dark blonde shade, which is unusual. These can be a fun departure from classic black or brown, but they don't have a huge impact on enhancing eye color. Besides, if you're interested in trying mascara shades beyond black or brown, Almay has various options for less than $10.

☺ **$$$ PureLash Conditioner** *($16)* is essentially a basic mascara formula without pigment. Used as a primer, it bulks up lashes prior to mascara application, although it's no better than applying two or three coats of a good mascara. This does contain conditioning agents, but lashes don't need conditioning the same way hair does.

☺ **$$$ PureLash Lengthening Mascara** *($16)* builds moderate length with a very clean, clump-free application. Thickness is scarce, and this isn't what I would call dramatic mascara, but it does the job and stays on all day.

☺ **$$$ PureLash Mascara** *($15)* offers decent (but unimpressive) length with a soft curl. This doesn't thicken lashes in the least, but it wears well and removes easily.

FACE AND BODY ILLUMINATING/SHIMMER PRODUCTS: ☺ **$$$ Moonglow** *($46)* comes with four pressed shimmer-powder wedges in one compact. There are no dividers between the colors, but each is big enough to use alone with any number of eyeshadow brushes. Using a blush or powder brush is tricky and will result in one color (a soft golden bronze with a hint of copper—shades having nothing to do with the moon), but the effect is flattering for evening or glamour makeup.

☺ **24-Karat Gold Dust** *($12)* is just mica, iron oxides, and real gold flakes. Combined, they make this simply a shiny loose powder whose glistening effect works nicely for evening glamour.

☺ **$$$ 24-Karat Gold Mine Kit** *($58)* includes six shades of loose shiny powder. The powder has a very silky texture and each shade is infused with obvious gold sparkles that have minimal ability to cling to skin. The brush that's included is workable. The product's description recommends using it on hair, which is a really bad idea unless you want to see it quickly flake onto your clothing, and onto anyone else nearby every time you move your head or touch your hair.

BRUSHES: ☺ **Jane Iredale Brushes** *($9-$39)* are mostly excellent, and the ones to consider for their workable shapes and soft but firm feel are the Chisel Powder, Eye Shader, and Eye Contour; the Eye Liner/Brow and Camouflage Brush are options as well, and both are synthetic. ✓ ☺ **Deluxe Eye Shader** *($21.50)* is one to consider for its workable shape and soft but firm feel. ☺ **$$$ Foundation Brush** *($35.80)* is also worth auditioning if you're curious to see if you prefer this type of brush to a makeup sponge. ☺ **$$$ Handi Brush** *($39)* is recommended for applying Jane Iredale's powder bases. It is cut straight across and applies the powder much like a sponge would, and may be worth a test to see how you like the results. It definitely provides a heavier coverage and matte finish. ☹ **White Fan Brush** *($12)* has little practical purpose and is easily replaced by other brushes.

☹ **$$$ Botanical Brush Cleaner** *($15 for 4 ounces)* is mostly alcohol and witch hazel (which is partially alcohol) along with citrus oils for fragrance. Alcohols function as solvents and will break down makeup on your brushes, but not without the eventual side effect of making the brush bristles feel dry. This is a decent option if you don't want to dampen your brushes with water, but one you should use only intermittently.

Several ☺ **Cosmetic Bags** *($22-$45)* round out Iredale's implement collection, with many including room for brushes and additional compartments, pouches for traveling, or space just to keep your most-used cosmetics organized. You may not find these at salons or spas selling Jane Iredale products, but they are available online.

The ☺ **$$$ One-4-All** *($56)* is meant for serious Jane Iredale fans. Included in one sleek, mirrored compact are three eyeshadows, two cream-to-powder eyeliners, two shades of lip gloss, a cream-to-powder blush, and brow powder. Three palettes are available, with Neutral being the easiest to work with. The Warm and Cool sets contain either blue or green eyeshadow and liner colors, which won't do much to shape and shade the eye. A brush is included as well, and it's a step above what you'll find in similar kits. Although this is rated highly, keep in mind that kits like this are a value only if you know you will use most, if not all, of the colors.

SPECIALTY PRODUCTS: ☺ **$$$ Corrective Colors** *($21)* provides four shades of creamy-bordering-on-greasy color correctors housed in one compact. You get a Yellow, Peach, Beige, and Lilac shade, along with a brief explanation of what color each shade is supposed to cancel or neutralize. The Yellow and Beige shades are acceptable; yellow tones do help cancel red tones (much better than mint green does). The Peach and Lilac shades share the same issue, which is that both look unnatural on skin and replace one coloration problem with another. Regardless of shades, the texture is thick and tends to look heavy and obvious on skin, even with careful blending. Without question, this isn't an essential kit and the fact that half the colors are unusable makes this a tough sell.

JURLIQUE INTERNATIONAL (SKIN CARE ONLY)

JURLIQUE INTERNATIONAL AT-A-GLANCE

Strengths: A handful of good moisturizers whose plant extracts have established benefit for skin; no jar packaging.

Weaknesses: Expensive; only one sunscreen, which does not list active ingredients and contains potent irritants; all of the toners contain alcohol; minimal to no preservatives means the water-based products have a reduced shelf life; irritating lip balm; no products to successfully address the needs of those with acne or blackheads; most of the facial mask formulas will leave skin confused.

For more information about Jurlique International, call (800) 854-1110 or visit www.jurlique.com or www.Beautypedia.com.

JURLIQUE INTERNATIONAL BIODYNAMIC BEAUTY PRODUCTS

☺ **$$$ Biodynamic Beauty Refining Treatment** *($35 for 1.4 ounces)* is a very expensive way to exfoliate skin given that all you're getting is some emollients and ground-up apricot seeds in a very small container. Despite being a natural ingredient, apricot seeds cannot be made perfectly spherical, so you run the risk of abrading your skin. Ironically, such a risk is much lower using synthetic polyethylene beads (composed of plastic) as the abrasive agent, or on the "natural" side, even jojoba beads can be gentler. This is still a good scrub for dry to very dry skin. It contains some problematic plant extracts (especially for those with flower allergies), but they are present in only minimal amounts relative to the helpful emollient ingredients.

☹ **Biodynamic Beauty Eye Cream** *($45 for 0.5 ounce)*. It's a fantasy to think that the plant extracts in this eye cream can have a positive effect on dark circles. Although some of the ingredients have benefit for skin (but not a unique benefit for eye-area skin because they are used in many products for skin anywhere on your body), others are just downright irritating. In particular, the amount of arnica is cause for concern, while the daisy flower can exacerbate allergies (Source: www.naturaldatabase.com). The amount of mica in this emollient eye cream casts a shine that can, to some degree, make dark circles less apparent, but that effect is strictly cosmetic and is easily replaced (and improved upon) by using any good concealer.

☺ **$$$ Biodynamic Beauty Night Lotion** *($55 for 1.3 ounces)* contains so many plant oils and emollients it is suitable only for normal to dry skin, despite this moisturizer being described as "lightweight." This is a mostly good formula that contains an impressive amount of anti-irritant licorice root extract. The litany of plant extracts that follows is a mixed bag of good (Matricaria, calendula) and not-good-but-not-terrible (witch hazel, *Calophyllum tacamahaca*, the latter being less of a problem than usual because of the small amount present). The licorice extract is claimed to be able to fade discolorations, but there is limited research on its use for skin lightening (Sources: *Planta Medica*, August 2005, pages 785-787; and *Journal of Agriculture and*

Food Chemistry, February 2003, pages 1201-1207). It's worth a try, but because concentration protocols haven't been established, you can't be sure you're getting enough licorice root to have a noticeable effect (of course, no skin-lightening product of any kind will work successfully without regular use of a sunscreen). However, this still has merit as a moisturizer.

☹ **Biodynamic Beauty Serum** *($75 for 1 ounce)* should be brimming with state-of-the-art ingredients—considering this serum's price and claims, you'd expect no less. It does contain some interesting ingredients, but in disappointingly low amounts. Plus, the "living energy" claims made for the plant ingredients in this product don't improve the quality of the formulation. (They're hokey because once a plant is harvested, prepared as a skin-care ingredient, preserved, and formulated into a product, it retains little to none of the "energy" it had when it was rooted.) What you're left with is a water- and slip agent–based serum that contains a lot of problematic daisy flower extract. Also known as tansy, daisy flower has a high risk of causing severe contact dermatitis (Source: www.naturaldatabase.com). And black elder flower certainly isn't an antiaging superstar, not any more than watching television is an aerobic activity.

JURLIQUE INTERNATIONAL MAINTAIN BALANCE PRODUCTS

☹ **Balancing Cleansing Lotion** *($40 for 6.7 ounces)* contains some wonderful ingredients to nurture and protect dry to very dry skin. Unfortunately, it also contains several irritating plant extracts along with essential oils of lavender and rosewood. Considering the price and the risk of irritation you encounter with each use, this cleansing lotion just isn't worth it.

☹ **Balancing Foaming Cleanser** *($40 for 6.7 ounces)* contains some very gentle detergent cleansing and foaming agents, yet loses credibility due to its irritating witch hazel base and several fragrant oils, including lemon peel and peppermint. Using this water-soluble cleanser around your eyes or nose is just asking for immediate irritation; as such, it is not recommended. Skin balancing this is not!

☹ **Chamomile-Rose Hydrating Essence** *($38 for 1.6 ounces)* smells divine, but eau de cologne is not smart skin care, regardless of claims. No one needs this "pre-treatment" because it only exposes skin to irritating amounts of alcohol (it's the third ingredient) and fragrance, including several fragrance chemicals known to cause irritation.

☹ **Rosewater Balancing Mist** *($31 for 3.3 ounces)*. Balancing skin isn't in this toner's bag of tricks, but its alcohol content (it's the second ingredient) and several fragrance chemicals will cause irritation and stimulate excess oil production, which is never the goal. Alcohol also causes free-radical damage and dries out skin, and nothing about that is balancing.

☺ $$$ **Balancing Day Care Cream** *($76 for 4.3 ounces)* is a good but not exceptional moisturizer for normal to very dry skin. It is not appropriate for daytime use unless your foundation contains sunscreen rated SPF 15 or greater (or if you're willing to pair this with a separate sunscreen). Several of the plant oils and extracts are great for skin and have antioxidant ability, while the packaging ensures their stability during use. This is not rated better because it lacks skin-identical ingredients and cell-communicating ingredients, and because it contains a small but notable amount of irritating plant extracts and fragrance chemicals.

☺ $$$ **Intense Recovery Mask** *($89 for 4.7 ounces)* is described as a hydrating mask, but the amount of clay in this mask makes that descriptor inaccurate. But is this a good absorbent mask for oily skin? No! Why? Because it contains plant oils and emollients that those with oily skin don't need. So, this rather confusing mask is best for normal skin, but someone with normal skin doesn't really need a mask that's hydrating or absorbing, at least not as part of their skin-care essentials. I would love to hear Jurlique's explanation of how the clay and oils can maintain skin balance—in essence, they cancel each other out.

JURLIQUE INTERNATIONAL REBALANCE DRYNESS PRODUCTS

☹ **Lavender-Lavandin Hydrating Essence** *($38 for 1.6 ounces).* Looking for a sure way to irritate skin? Use this product. A "pre-treatment" without any treatment benefits, it exposes skin to several plant irritants, including lavender oil, horsetail, lemon balm, and various fragrance chemicals. The biggest offenders in this product are lavender oil, which causes skin cell death, and its fragrant component, linalool. When linalool is exposed to air, it oxidizes and forms by-products that are known to cause contact dermatitis (Sources: *Contact Dermatitis,* January 2008, pages 9-14; and *Cell Proliferation,* June 2004, pages 221-229).

☹ **Replenishing Cleansing Lotion** *($40 for 6.7 ounces)* contains some wonderful ingredients to nurture and protect dry to very dry skin. Unfortunately, it also contains several irritating plant extracts along with fragrance chemicals (such as linalool and geraniol) that are known irritants. Considering the price and the risk of irritation you encounter with each use, this cleansing lotion just isn't worth it.

☺ **$$$ Replenishing Foaming Cleanser** *($40 for 6.7 ounces).* What begins as a gentle, soothing cleanser for dry to very dry skin becomes less impressive because of the potentially irritating plant extracts it contains (none of which are skin-replenishing). The fragrance chemicals aren't great for skin, but at least their contact with your skin will be brief. This is an OK (yet overpriced) option and it will remove makeup.

☹ **Lavender Hydrating Mist** *($31 for 3.3 ounces).* As gentle as lavender might sound, this mist lists alcohol as the second ingredient, which makes it completely nonhydrating and very drying, and it also contains irritating fragrance chemicals. This is not skin care! It should be skin caution, because alcohol causes free-radical damage and cell death, and can trigger oil production in the pore lining.

☺ **$$$ Moisture Replenishing Day Cream** *($76 for 4.3 ounces).* What's sad about this emollient moisturizer is that although it contains some very good ingredients to make dry skin look and feel better, some of the plant extracts are potential irritants or have unknown benefits for skin. Plus, the inclusion of several fragrance chemicals isn't the best, either, nor is the price (but size-wise this could be considered a beauty bargain). All told, this water, oil, and wax concoction isn't as elegant as several other moisturizers from the drugstore or department store.

☺ **$$$ Moisture Replenishing Mask** *($80 for 5.2 ounces).* With absorbent kaolin (a type of clay) listed as the second ingredient, you don't want to count on this mask being all that replenishing because clay is an absorbent! Oddly, the clay is followed by several emollients and oils, which will leave oily skin overloaded with what it doesn't need or leave dry skin confused. This mask is best for normal skin, the very skin type few people have and not a skin type that stands to benefit much from a facial mask. By the way, the fragrance chemicals this contains do not qualify this mask as "gentle."

JURLIQUE INTERNATIONAL REBALANCE OILINESS PRODUCTS

☹ **Lemon-Lime Hydrating Essence** *($38 for 1.6 ounces).* Alcohol, lemon and lime peel oils, and several fragrance chemicals conspire to make this a very irritating product for all skin types. Plus alcohol causes free-radical damage and cell death, and can trigger oil production in the pore.

☺ **$$$ Purifying Cleansing Lotion** *($40 for 6.7 ounces).* Sold as being ideal for "rebalancing" oily skin, the formula of emollient triglyceride with alcohol and plant oil will do nothing of the sort. Instead, oily skin will only end up confused and potentially irritated due to several problematic plant extracts in this cleansing lotion. It is a below-average option for normal to dry skin, but Jurlique has better cleansing lotions for those skin types.

☺ **$$$ Purifying Foaming Cleanser** *($40 for 6.7 ounces)* is a good option for normal to oily skin. The mélange of plants is both beneficial and potentially irritating, so in essence the good cancels out the bad. Although this standard water-soluble cleansing gel will remove surface oil, makeup, and impurities, it isn't "rebalancing" any more than any other detergent-based cleanser. And this does contain irritating fragrant extracts.

☹ **Citrus Purifying Mist** *($31 for 3.3 ounces)* lists alcohol as its second ingredient and also contains irritating plant extracts and fragrance chemicals. The claim of essential oils of tangerine and lemon isn't indicated on the ingredient list, but "fragrance" (which these citrus oils qualify as) is. Nothing in this spray-on toner has any documented benefit for oily skin, and alcohol causes free-radical damage and cell death, and can trigger oil production in the pore lining.

☺ **$$$ Clarifying Day Care Lotion** *($76 for 3.3 ounces)* should only be considered if you have normal to slightly dry or dry skin not prone to blemishes and don't mind spending more than you need to for a formula that leaves your skin wanting more. Calendula, chamomile, and daisy cannot rebalance oily skin. This contains some good antioxidant plants (such as green tea and turmeric root), but that's not enough to elevate it to "best" status. If you decide to try this, keep in mind that it is inappropriate for daytime use unless you pair it with a sunscreen rated SPF 15 or greater.

☺ **$$$ Purifying Mask** *($80 for 4.9 ounces)* works well to absorb excess oil, and it doesn't contain the same lineup of skin-confusing ingredients as Jurlique's other masks, but this pricey mask cannot rebalance oily skin. The sesame oil isn't what someone with oily skin needs, but the small amount of it makes it unlikely that it will be problematic. As usual for Jurlique, their selection of plant extracts presents skin with a mix of beneficial and potentially irritating plants, whose effects mostly cancel each other out. This does contain fragrance chemicals that may cause irritation; however, only small amounts are included, which reduces the risk.

JURLIQUE INTERNATIONAL REBALANCE SENSITIVITY PRODUCTS

☹ **Calendula-Lavender Hydrating Essence** *($38 for 1.6 ounces)* is just as problematic for skin as Jurlique's Lavender-Lavandin Hydrating Essence reviewed above, yet it is marketed to those with sensitive skin. How ludicrous! Anyone (truly sensitive skin or not) will find matters worse after applying this cocktail of irritating fragrant ingredients and alcohol.

☺ **$$$ Soothing Cleansing Lotion** *($40 for 6.7 ounces)* would indeed be a soothing cleansing lotion for sensitive skin if it didn't include the fragrance chemicals and peppercorn extract. As is, the fact that this doesn't rinse completely means the peppercorn extract is left on your skin, where it can cause irritation. The gromwell extract has research demonstrating its antioxidant, anti-tumor, and anti-inflammatory actions, particularly on sun-exposed skin. It also has been shown in limited research to enhance skin's barrier function (Sources: *Archives of Dermatological Research*, July 2008, pages 317-323; and *Biological and Pharmaceutical Bulletin*, May 2007, pages 928-934).

☹ **Soothing Foaming Cleanser** *($40 for 6.7 ounces)* is an initially gentle cleanser that contains several ingredients that make it a problematic product for sensitive skin. Any company that adds fragrance, lavender oil, and peppercorn extract to products designed for sensitive skin needs to go back to the drawing board!

☹ **Chamomile Soothing Mist** *($31 for 3.3 ounces)* lists alcohol as the second ingredient, plus has added fragrance and irritating fragrance chemicals, and as such this is about as well-suited for those with sensitive skin as pats of butter are smart snacking for those trying to lose weight. Alcohol causes free-radical damage and cell death, and can trigger oil production in the pore.

☹ **Soothing Herbal Recovery Gel** *($134 for 3.3 ounces)* contains soothing gromwell extract, but this emollient moisturizer's effect is canceled out by the peppercorn and fragrance chemicals. What a shame, because with some slight formulary adjustments this could have been a great option for sensitive skin.

☺ **$$$ Nurturing Mask** *($89 for 5.2 ounces)* is another confusing mask from Jurlique, with their blend of absorbent clay and emollient oils that leaves skin confused more than anything else. The peppercorn, fragrance, and fragrance chemicals (such as limonene and geraniol) make this completely inappropriate for sensitive skin. It's an OK option for normal skin not prone to breakouts, but don't expect much.

OTHER JURLIQUE INTERNATIONAL PRODUCTS

☺ **$$$ Eye Makeup Remover** *($25 for 1.4 ounces)* contains plant oils that will definitely remove eye makeup, but they can leave a greasy film that isn't preferable to the results you can get from a silicone- or detergent-based eye-makeup remover. Making this remover even less of an option are the numerous potentially irritating plant extracts, especially if used in the delicate eye area. Growing plants "biodynamically" may be good for the environment, and perhaps for the plant as well, but not all plants are good for skin, no matter how they're grown.

☺ **$$$ Herbal Recovery Night Mist** *($49 for 1 ounce)* is a mixed bag of ingredients that have soothing and potentially irritating effects on skin. I suspect the soothing agents will prevail because they are present in greater amounts, but if Jurlique hadn't been so plant-happy this would have been a much gentler option for normal to dry skin. The fragrance chemicals and rose essential oil have irritating properties, too; overall, this isn't going to do much for your skin beyond making it smell good, but that's not wise skin care.

☺ **$$$ Daily Exfoliating Cream** *($54 for 4.3 ounces)* contains almonds and oats as the abrasive agents. Natural, yes, but not the gentlest options around, especially for daily use. The amount of alcohol is potentially irritating and drying, which also contributes to this needlessly expensive scrub for normal to slightly dry skin getting a less than good rating. Several scrubs at the drugstore not only cost much less, but also offer better formulas. Or, for even less money, you can use a washcloth with your cleanser instead.

☹ **Arnica Cream** *($36 for 1.4 ounces)* contains too much arnica, which may appeal to fans of natural products, but serves only to make this moisturizer an irritating experience for skin.

☹ **Arnica Lotion** *($27 for 1.6 ounces)* is the lotion version of the Arnica Cream above, and aside from a texture change and the addition of alcohol, the same comments apply: it's an irritating experience for skin.

☺ **Calendula Cream** *($67 for 4.3 ounces)* is a popular Jurlique product that has been reformulated and isn't as good as it once was. The amount of alcohol is cause for concern, especially because its prominence diminishes the effectiveness of the beneficial ingredients that follow. It is an OK moisturizer for normal to dry skin not prone to blemishes, but your skin deserves more than what this provides.

☹ **Calendula Lotion** *($27 for 1.6 ounces)* contains enough witch hazel and alcohol to be considered a problem for all skin types, not to mention that these ingredients undermine the effectiveness of the calendula.

☺ **Elder Cream** *($40 for 1.4 ounces)* contains elderberry extract, a plant whose flavonoid content makes it an antioxidant-rich option for skin. This cream for normal to dry skin also contains stabilized vitamin C and, surprisingly for Jurlique, no other plant extracts besides elderberry and a tiny amount of grapefruit seed (likely included for its mild preservative ability). The amount of alcohol keeps it from earning a happy face rating.

☹ **Herbal Recovery Eye Gel** *($121 for 1 ounce)* is a ridiculously expensive water-based gel containing several plant ingredients that are not recommended for use around the eye area, including arnica, daisy, and violet. Moreover, the amount of alcohol can cause irritation and free-radical damage and this also contains fragrance chemicals, which, you guessed it, should not be applied near the eyes.

☹ **Herbal Recovery Gel** *($134 for 3.3 ounces)*. The evening primrose oil in this product is a plus, but the alcohol that precedes it on the list is a major minus (alcohol causes free-radical damage and cell death), as are the many fragrance chemicals (including irritating eugenol). This absolutely cannot reduce the signs of aging with daily use, but it may cause aging skin to look worse by serving as a daily source of inflammation.

☺ **$$$ Herbal Recovery Neck Serum** *($80 for 1 ounce)* is one of the better formulas from Jurlique, although it's not without its problems. The soy protein, rose hip oil, and avocado oil are helpful for dry skin that needs an antioxidant boost, and the potentially irritating plant extracts Jurlique is fond of using only make a minor appearance in this product. Aside from the fragrance chemicals and the eyebrow-raising price, this is an option for normal to dry skin as long as you keep it away from your eyes, and it holds no special benefit for skin on the neck.

☺ **$$$ Purely Age-Defying Day Cream SPF 15** *($45 for 1.4 ounces)*. Labeling this a revolutionary daily moisturizer is like labeling a grilled cheese sandwich haute cuisine. Yes, it's great that it provides sufficient UVA protection, thanks to titanium dioxide and zinc oxide, and it also has a base formula that's good for dry skin not prone to breakouts. However, the mix of plant oils and plant extracts is, well, a mixed bag. Some benefit skin (e.g., jojoba and licorice root extract), while others are busts causing irritation (such as an unidentified essential-oil fragrance). On balance, this is an acceptable daytime moisturizer with sunscreen, but the cost isn't justified given the formula.

☹ **Skin Balancing Face Oil** *($50 for 1.6 ounces)*. This emollient plant oil mix could have been great for dry skin, but ends up being a mixed bag when all is said and done. First, there's the company's assertion that this product is "rich in the living energy of biodynamic and organic" ingredients; that's mumbo jumbo and has no relevance to taking great care of your skin. Keep in mind that once a plant oil is harvested, extracted, and prepared for use in a cosmetic, its "living energy" is gone. That doesn't mean the plant extract has lost all benefit, but its living energy is effectively cut off once it's uprooted or cut off. Although the blend of oils offers relief for dry skin, this product loses points by including problematic plant extracts and an unidentified essential-oil fragrance blend, which add up to irritation your skin doesn't need. It also contains fragrance chemicals known to cause irritation. You'd be better off blending the nonfragrant oils in this product yourself; all of them are available at health food stores and, used alone or together, can be helpful for dry skin. Plus, they'd be far less expensive than this mixture.

☺ **Soothing Day Care Lotion** *($40 for 1 ounce).* This water- and oil-based moisturizer is anything but soothing due to the numerous problematic ingredients. Witch hazel, peppercorn, and lavender oil are not what sensitive skin needs to look and feel better because they all can cause irritation. Plus, there are synthetic fragrance additives as well.

☺ **$$$ Viola Cream** *($36 for 1.4 ounces)* contains viola extract, also known as heart's ease, a plant with established anti-inflammatory and antioxidant activity. The chickweed and daisy don't add much beyond fragrance, and this would be better without the questionable amount of alcohol, but it's still an option for normal to dry skin.

☺ **$$$ Wrinkle Softening Cream** *($76 for 1.4 ounces)* has an attention-getting name, but also an odd one, because in essence all moisturizers can soften wrinkles, especially wrinkles that result from dryness rather than sun damage. The formula for this moisturizer isn't too different from Jurlique's formulas for other emollient options for dry skin; all will leave skin softer and smoother while supplying it with some plant-based antioxidants. There are some problematic ingredients (including several fragrance chemicals) to be concerned about, particularly the daisy extract, which can cause contact dermatitis (Source: www.naturaldatabase.com).

☹ **Sun Lotion SPF 30+** *($58 for 3.3 ounces)* deserves praise for its in-part titanium dioxide sunscreen, but the price is unreasonable and definitely won't encourage liberal application, an essential element of making sure you're getting the SPF stated on the label. Further, this is impossible to recommend because it contains irritating pine leaf, bitter-orange, lavender, and cypress oils. Note: It is definitely cause for concern that the sunscreen agents in this product are not listed separately as active ingredients.

☹ **Blemish Cream** *($28 for 0.5 ounce)* contains several thickeners that can be a problem for blemishes. Tea tree oil has not been shown to be effective as a topical disinfectant for acne in the amount this product contains. The colloidal sulfur can have disinfecting properties, but is also significantly irritating, and for most acne sufferers the trade-off isn't worth it. The fact that this cream is flesh-toned so it doubles as a concealer for blemishes doesn't change the drawbacks mentioned above.

☹ **Lip Care Balm** *($27 for 0.5 ounce)* is a castor oil–based product containing ingredients that soften and smooth dry, chapped lips. The fragrant ylang-ylang and pepper seed oils will cause inflammation and end up making chapped lips worse.

☹ **Citrus Silk Finishing Powder,** ☹ **Lavender Silk Finishing Powder,** and ☹ **Rose Silk Finishing Powder** *($36 for 0.35 ounce)* are all quite absorbent thanks to their cornstarch and rice starch base coupled with dry-finish silica. Although such ingredients can be a boon for oily skin, these powders' dry texture doesn't look flattering and they contain several plant-based irritants. The natural fragrances used are composed of several fragrance chemicals known to be irritating, which is yet another reason to skip these overpriced, underperforming pressed powders.

KIEHL'S

KIEHL'S AT-A-GLANCE

Strengths: Provides complete ingredient lists on their Web site; Kiehl's staff is generous when it comes to providing samples and product information; some good cleansers; a worthwhile selection of sunscreens with avobenzone for UVA protection; a reliable lip balm; many fragrance-free items.

Weaknesses: Expensive for what you get; the Blue Herbal products are terrible for acne; no products to successfully address skin discolorations; the toners; the self-tanner; jar packaging.

For more information about Kiehl's, owned by L'Oreal, call (800) 543-4572 or visit www. kiehls.com or www.Beautypedia.com.

KIEHL'S SKIN CARE

KIEHL'S ABYSSINE + PRODUCTS

☺ **$$$ Abyssine Cream +** *($42 for 1.7 ounces)* contains a meager amount of exciting ingredients for skin, and what little there is will quickly break down once this jar-packaged cream is opened. At best, this is an extremely average, overpriced moisturizer for normal to dry skin. Like any moisturizer applied to dry skin, it can make superficial lines look better—but your skin deserves a lot more than this can provide.

☹ **Abyssine Cream + SPF 23** *($45 for 1.7 ounces)* provides an in-part avobenzone sunscreen, but otherwise has a formula that's similar to the boring Abyssine Cream + above. Although this provides great broad-spectrum sun protection, the inclusion of several fragrant oils makes it too irritating for all skin types, plus the jar packaging won't keep the tiny amount of antioxidants stable during use.

☺ **$$$ Abyssine Eye Cream +** *($32 for 0.5 ounce)* contains mostly water, glycerin, silicone, several thickeners, and a preservative. The called-out "survival molecule" ingredients, even if they were somehow special and unique, are barely present in this formula and won't remain stable once this jar-packaged eye cream is open. This is a barely passable fragrance-free option for normal to dry skin anywhere on the face.

☺ **Abyssine Lotion + SPF 15** *($42 for 2.5 ounces)* provides an in-part titanium dioxide sunscreen in an incredibly ho-hum base formula for normal to slightly dry or slightly oily skin. There are some good antioxidants and a couple of cell-communicating ingredients are included, but in amounts too small for skin to notice. However, your skin may end up irritated from the small amount of fragrant oils included, and that's not good news.

☹ **Abyssine Serum +** *($44 for 1.7 ounces)* lists alcohol as the second ingredient (alcohol causes free-radical damage and triggers oil production in the pore lining), and that makes this expensive serum a skin-damaging waste of time and money. What a shame, because there are some impressive antioxidants in this formula.

KIEHL'S BLUE HERBAL PRODUCTS

☹ **Blue Herbal Gel Cleanser** *($14.50 for 4.2 ounces)* does contain 1.5% salicylic acid, but in a cleanser this ingredient is wasted because it's not left on the skin long enough to have an effect. The real problem with this cleanser is the inclusion of ginger, cinnamon, menthol, and camphor. If you are using this product, believe me, I feel your pain!

☹ **Blue Astringent Herbal Lotion** *($15 for 8.4 ounces)* has been part of the Kiehl's line since 1964. Considering how much more we know about what skin needs to look and feel its best, it's hardly surprising that this alcohol-based toner is outdated; but with menthol, camphor, and aluminum chlorohydrate (an ingredient in many antiperspirants) as well, this is also incredibly irritating! This isn't a treatment for blemished skin, it's a punishment.

☹ **Blue Herbal Moisturizer** *($22 for 3.4 ounces)* is an ultralight, matte-finish moisturizer for oily skin that contains 0.5% salicylic acid as its active ingredient. Although the pH makes the salicylic acid content minimally effective as an exfoliant, what keeps this from earning a recommendation is the inclusion of menthol and plant irritants such as cinnamon and ginger. Irritation is a problem for all skin types, causing collagen to break down and increase oil production in the pore. This is not preferred to Clinique's Mild Clarifying Lotion or any of the BHA products from Paula's Choice.

☹ **Blue Herbal Spot Treatment** *($15.50 for 0.5 ounce)* lists alcohol as the second ingredient, and further down the list are a slew of other irritants, including menthol, camphor, witch hazel, cinnamon, and ginger. The alcohol causes a host of problems, not the least of which is triggering oil production in the pore. What was Kiehl's thinking?

KIEHL'S BRIGHT PRODUCTS

☹ **Brightening Botanical Cleansing Cream** *($22.50 for 5 ounces)* contains a large amount of the alkaline ingredient potassium hydroxide, which makes this foaming cleanser too drying for all skin types.

☹ **Brightening Botanical Clarifying Toner** *($34.50 for 8.4 ounces)* lists alcohol as the second ingredient, which makes this an expensive burn for skin. It also contains the potent menthol derivative menthoxypropanediol.

☺ **$$$ Brightening Botanical Moisture Fluid** *($40 for 2.5 ounces)* contains a very small amount of plant extracts with limited research concerning their skin-lightening ability (and what research exists studied much higher concentrations than Kiehl's uses). This is just a water- and silicone-based moisturizer with vitamin C. The vitamin C, as ascorbyl glucoside, has limited research pertaining to its skin-lightening ability. The most current study involved pairing an unknown amount of it with niacinamide and using ultrasound technology to enhance penetration, possibilities that don't come with this product (Source: *Skin Research and Technology*, May 2006, pages 105-113).

☺ **Brightening Botanical Hydrating Mask** *($40 for 2.5 ounces)* isn't all that full of botanicals (all of those ingredients are listed after the preservative, so they don't count for much), but I suppose this moisturizing mask for normal to dry skin is a good option if you want to treat your skin to a decent amount of vitamin C. The form of the vitamin C that Kiehl's uses is ascorbyl glucoside, which is good, but there is limited research pertaining to its skin-lightening (or "brightening") ability. Besides, even if this form of vitamin C were the best skin-lightening choice, you'd want to leave it on your skin as long as possible, not rinse it off within minutes as you're directed to do with this mask (which is what you would want to do given the amount of polyacrylamide, a film-forming agent—think hairspray—this product contains).

☺ **$$$ Brightening Botanical Spot Treatment** *($50 for 1 ounce)* stands as great a chance of lightening skin discolorations as typewriters do of making a comeback! The star ingredient (listed, as usual in Kiehl's products, after the preservative—meaning it is a meager amount) is ellagic acid, a polyphenol antioxidant found in many fruits, including pomegranate and strawberry. Although there is research demonstrating its antioxidant potential on human skin cells, there isn't any proof it can lighten skin discolorations. Even if it were a skin-lightening wonder, the amount of it in this needlessly pricey product would likely have minimal to no effect (Sources: *Photochemistry and Photobiology*, January/February 2005, pages 38-45; and www.naturaldatabase.com). At best—and this isn't saying much—this product is an average lightweight moisturizer for normal to oily skin.

KIEHL'S CRYSTE MARINE PRODUCTS

☺ **$$$ Cryste Marine Firming Cream** *($47.50 for 1.7 ounces)* makes a big deal out of the Mediterranean-sourced flower *(Crithmum maritimum,* or rock samphire) extract it contains. Supposedly, this flower can increase the renewal rate of skin cells, but there is no information to support this claim. Even if it had such an effect, the amount in this product is minuscule (there's more preservative than flower extract). That leaves you with a pricey moisturizer that has some respectable qualities (the glycerin, silicone, and squalane base gets things off to a good start), yet this remains an ordinary choice when compared to similarly priced products from other department-store lines, such as Clinique and Estee Lauder. Nothing in this product is capable of firming skin.

☺ **$$$ Cryste Marine Firming Eye Treatment** *($36 for 0.5 ounce)* is incapable of firming skin and the jar packaging will render the tiny amounts of antioxidants ineffective shortly after you open the product. At best, this will make dry skin anywhere on the face feel softer and smoother. For the money, you should expect more.

☹ **Cryste Marine Firming Serum** *($50 for 1.7 ounces)* is primarily water, glycerin, silicone, alcohol, and slip agents. The rice protein cannot firm skin, although it and a few other ingredients in this serum are good water-binding agents. This would be an OK option if it did not contain the irritating menthol derivative menthoxypropanediol.

☺ **$$$ Cryste Marine "Ultra Riche" Lifting and Firming Cream** *($47.50 for 1.7 ounces)* makes a claim that conflicts with basic physics. According to Kiehl's, this rather boring but emollient moisturizer for normal to dry skin contains "Hyaluronic Filling Spheres." The sponge-like absorbency of these spheres is said to trap the skin's own water, causing the molecules to expand, which "immediately" lifts skin. Assuming the spheres work as claimed (although the amount of sodium hyaluronate in this product is next to nothing), the effect would not be to lift skin but rather to stretch it or make it puffy. Of course, when you look at it that way, the appeal pretty much vanishes.

KIEHL'S RARE EARTH PRODUCTS

☺ **$$$ Rare Earth Oatmeal Milk Facial Cleanser #1, for a Normal to Oily Skin Type** *($20.50 for 8.4 ounces)* doesn't contain any earth that is remotely rare, just standard kaolin, better known as clay. But I guess if you want to make something ordinary sound unique, that is one way to do it. All in all, what you're getting in this product is standard detergent cleansing agents and clay. Clay can be slightly tricky to rinse off, but it does leave skin soft and is an option for someone with oily skin.

☹ **Rare Earth Face Masque (Gently Astringent for Oily-Acne Skin)** *($17.50 for 4.2 ounces)* is not preferred to the Rare Earth Facial Cleansing Masque because it lacks the bells and whistles available in many other masks, and adds irritating sulfur, despite an overall claim of being a gentle product.

☺ **$$$ Rare Earth Facial Cleansing Masque, for Normal to Oily and Oily Skin Types** *($20 for 5 ounces)* is a very standard, but effective, clay mask for normal to oily skin. The addition of some soothing plant extracts may be helpful for inflamed or irritated skin.

KIEHL'S ULTRA FACIAL PRODUCTS

✓ ☺ **$$$ Ultra Facial Cleanser, For All Skin Types** *($17.50 for 5 ounces)* is an excellent, fragrance-free water-soluble cleanser for all skin types. Effective yet gentle, this product foams slightly and can remove all but the most tenacious makeup. Now this is how to formulate a cleanser (but please note that you don't have to spend this much to get an equally good cleanser).

☺ $$$ **Ultra Facial Toner, For All Skin Types** *($15 for 8.4 ounces)* has its name all wrong, because if this is the ultra (as in "ultimate") toner for all skin types, then the formulators at Kiehl's haven't updated their notes since, oh, the early 1970s. This toner for normal to dry skin consists primarily of water, slip agents, emollient, and preservatives. The tiny amount of vitamin C and plant oils doesn't compensate for the ho-hum ingredients that precede them.

☺ $$$ **Ultra Facial Cream** *($24.50 for 1.7 ounces)* provides another story about two special ingredients extracted from remote locations, also claimed to be valuable for skin because they can survive in harsh climates (lots of plants can survive harsh climates, but rubbing them on your skin is not going to help you with sun damage or with frigid conditions). It also doesn't help that these miracle plants are present in such tiny amounts, and the jar packaging won't keep any of the token amount of antioxidants stable during use. This is definitely more ordinary than ultra for normal to dry skin.

☺ $$$ **Ultra Facial Moisturizer** *($15.50 for 2.5 ounces)* remains a very popular product for Kiehl's, sort of like the original Dramatically Different Moisturizing Lotion remains a hot seller for Clinique. Both products cover the basic needs of someone with normal to dry skin, but lack anything truly beneficial or state-of-the-art for skin. The tiny amounts of plant oils and vitamins in this moisturizer will have little to no impact, though it is fragrance-free.

☹ **Ultra Facial Moisturizer SPF 15** *($18.50 for 2.5 ounces)* lacks the UVA-protecting ingredients of titanium dioxide, zinc oxide, avobenzone, Tinosorb, or Mexoryl SX, and is not recommended. Even if this had sufficient UVA protection, it is an exceptionally boring moisturizer for the money.

☹ **Ultra Facial Tinted Moisturizer SPF 15** *($24.50 for 2.5 ounces)* comes in three sheer shades and has a much more interesting (though still lackluster) formula than the Ultra Facial Moisturizer SPF 15. However, the absence of sufficient UVA protection makes this a poor choice for daytime.

KIEHL'S YERBA MATE TEA PRODUCTS

☺ $$$ **Yerba Mate Tea Cleanser** *($20.50 for 8.4 ounces)* is a very standard, but good, water-soluble cleanser for normal to oily or slightly dry skin. The amount of black tea ferment is too small to matter, but even if it were present in prodigious amounts it would just be rinsed down the drain before it could exert any antioxidant benefit. This cleanser contains fragrance in the form of lemon fruit extract.

☹ **Yerba Mate Tea Toner** *($24.50 for 8.4 ounces)* is mostly water with slip agents, but loses points for including irritating peppermint and ivy stem. The amount of yerba maté (*Ilex paraguariensis*) is minimal and of little benefit for skin.

☺ $$$ **Yerba Mate Tea Lotion** *($35 for 2.5 ounces)* is infused with yerba maté, but this caffeine-containing plant (most often consumed as tea) has no established benefit for skin. It contains several vitamins and minerals, but not in amounts that would allow the skin to derive much benefit, and its volatile components (including tannins and theobromine) cancel out any potential benefits of the other constituents. In the case of this lotion, the amount of yerba maté is minimal. This is a good moisturizer for normal to slightly oily skin. It has a soft matte finish and provides skin with some effective water-binding agents, a tiny amount of antioxidants, and a cell-communicating ingredient.

OTHER KIEHL'S PRODUCTS

☺ **$$$ Centella Skin-Calming Facial Cleanser** *($28.50 for 8 ounces)* costs a lot of money for what amounts to a standard, gentle, fragrance-free lotion cleanser for normal to dry skin. *Centella asiatica* is a plant extract with wound-healing and antibacterial properties; however, the amount Kiehl's uses is minuscule and the potential benefit is rinsed down the drain. Still, this is a good option for those with sensitive skin, including those with rosacea.

☹ **Foaming Non-Detergent Washable Cleanser, for Combination or Oily Skin** *($17.50 for 8.4 ounces)* is not in the least a nondetergent cleanser because the second ingredient listed is sodium C14-16 olefin sulfate, a detergent cleansing agent (technically called a surfactant) that is present in shampoos and known for stripping hair color. By any dictionary definition, this is a standard detergent cleanser that can be drying and irritating for skin.

☺ **Gentle Foaming Facial Cleanser, for Dry to Normal Skin Types** *($17.50 for 8.4 ounces)* is accurately named. This standard, water-soluble cleanser doesn't have much to it, but it's fragrance-free and does the job for its intended skin types.

☺ **Oil-Based Cleanser and Make-Up Remover** *($20.50 for 8.4 ounces)* ends up being an emollient, somewhat greasy way to remove makeup, but it works for dry to very dry skin not prone to blemishes. The small amount of alcohol is not a cause for concern.

✓☺ **Ultra Moisturizing Cleansing Cream** *($14.50 for 8 ounces)* is a standard, cold cream–style cleanser that is an impressive option for dry, sensitive skin, including those with rosacea, and is fragrance-free. You may still need to use a washcloth to remove all of your makeup, but this cleanser's value for sensitive, dry skin elevates it to Paula's Pick status.

☺ **Washable Cleansing Milk, for Dry, Normal to Dry or Sensitive Skin Types** *($17.50 for 8.4 ounces)* is a lotion cleanser that is an option for normal to dry skin, though it isn't all that washable without the help of a washcloth. The trace amounts of milk and vitamins in this product are barely detectable.

☺ **$$$ Supremely Gentle Eye Make-Up Remover** *($16.50 for 4.2 ounces)* has gentle written all over it, but they should have added "greasy," too, because the amount of oil in this remover leaves a discernible film on skin. This is best for dry skin, and best used before a standard, water-soluble cleanser. It will remove makeup with minimal effort.

☺ **$$$ Epidermal Re-Texturizing Micro-Dermabrasion** *($40 for 2.5 ounces)* is your basic microdermabrasion-in-a-jar topical scrub, with alumina as the abrasive agent. The emollients and silicone in this product help protect skin from the alumina, which can be rough on your skin if not used very gently. Although pricey, this is a good, fragrance-free scrub for normal to dry skin.

☹ **$$$ Milk, Honey and Almond Scrub** *($20.50 for 6 ounces)* is a rather inelegant, from-the-kitchen scrub that contains almond seed meal and grain flours to exfoliate skin. The honey base makes this somewhat sticky while the plant oils impede rinsing, which adds up to a passable but barely worthwhile scrub for normal to dry skin.

☹ **$$$ Pineapple Papaya Facial Scrub, Made with Real Fruit** *($25 for 3.4 ounces)* relies partly on pineapple enzymes to exfoliate skin. Not only are enzymes unreliable exfoliants, but the jar packaging chosen for this product won't keep them stable. The corncob powder is a low-tech exfoliant, but is what saves this scrub for normal to oily skin from being a total waste of time and money.

✓☺ **Ultra Moisturizing Buffing Cream with Scrub Particles** *($14.50 for 4 ounces)* is a very good moisturizing scrub for dry skin. Unlike the other Kiehl's scrubs, this contains rounded polyethylene (plastic) beads as the abrasive agent. It is fragrance-free.

☹ **Calendula Herbal-Extract Toner, Alcohol-Free, for a Normal to Oily Skin Type** *($34.50 for 8.4 ounces)* is such a basic, nearly do-nothing toner that the price is ludicrous. If you're interested in calendula for skin care, buy a bottle of the oil from a health food store or steep the plant in hot water, let it cool, and bottle your own. Either option is an improvement over this product.

☹ **Cucumber Herbal Alcohol-Free Toner, for Dry or Sensitive Skin** *($15 for 8.4 ounces)* contains balm mint, juniper, pine needle, and arnica, making it too irritating for all skin types, especially sensitive skin.

☹ **Herbal Toner with Mixed Berries and Botanical Extracts, for Normal to Oily Skin Types** *($24.50 for 8.4 ounces)* contains berries supposedly placed in each bottle by hand, but aside from looking kind of neat, they have no impact on skin. What will impact skin (negatively) is the peppermint in this poorly formulated toner.

☹ **Rosewater Facial Freshener-Toner, for Normal to Oily Skin** *($15 for 8.4 ounces)* lists alcohol as the second ingredient and contains too little of anything of redeeming value for skin. The alcohol will make oily skin worse by triggering more oil production in the pore lining.

☹ **Tea Tree Oil Toner, for Oily or Normal to Oily Skin Type** *($15.50 for 4.2 ounces)* contains some tea tree oil, but any benefit it has is offset by the irritation caused by the eucalyptus, sage, lavender oil, and other volatile fragrant oils in this toner.

☺ **$$$ Highly Effective Skin Tone Corrector** *($50 for 1 ounce)*. Just how "highly effective" this product is depends on what your expectations are. Kiehl's maintains it is able to reduce the appearance of brown spots and an uneven skin tone, both of which are signs of sun damage. The ingredient that could possibly have some impact on this problem is glycolic acid, and this product's pH of 3.8 means it will function as an exfoliant. The thing is, you don't need to spend this much money (not even close to it) for an effective AHA exfoliant. Besides, the percentage of glycolic acid in this product is likely less than 5%—Kiehl's Customer Service told me that the exact percentage is proprietary, a line we hear over and over again, even though there's no reason to not be forthcoming about this information—so it's actually not as potent as many other well-formulated AHA moisturizers, from Alpha Hydrox, Neutrogena Healthy Skin, and Paula's Choice, among others. Using this fragrance-free product along with a broad-spectrum sunscreen rated SPF 15 or greater will likely improve your skin, but the bottom line is you can achieve better (at least more reliable) results for a lot less money. Those loyal to Kiehl's and wishing to try this product should know it is suitable for all skin types. By the way, there is absolutely nothing natural about this product in any way, shape, or form.

☺ **$$$ Anti-Oxidant Skin Preserver** *($60 for 1.4 ounces)* is an incredibly rich moisturizer for very dry skin, but comes up short with antioxidants, including just a tiny amount of vitamins A, C, and E—none of which will survive for long because of jar packaging.

☺ **Centella Recovery Skin Salve** *($42 for 2.5 ounces)* contains mostly water, silicones, glycerin, slip agents, and preservatives. The tiny amount of plant extracts has negligible benefit for irritated skin, but at least nothing in this fragrance-free moisturizer is likely to cause irritation or bother sensitive skin.

☺ **$$$ Creamy Eye Treatment with Avocado** *($24.50 for 0.5 ounce)* is good for dry skin anywhere on the face, but the amount of antioxidants is tiny and they won't last long once this jar-packaged product is opened.

☺ **Creme D'Elegance Repairateur, Superb Tissue Repairateur Creme** *($49.50 for 4.2 ounces)* is nothing more than an average emollient moisturizer for dry skin. The name is fancy, but the formula is outdated, and the most intriguing ingredients amount to less than a dusting.

The Reviews K

☹ **Eye Alert** *($20.50 for 0.5 ounce)* lists alcohol as the third ingredient, so it's not the "ultimate solution" for improving skin in the eye area because alcohol causes cell death and free-radical damage. All of the potentially helpful, intriguing ingredients are listed after the preservative, so it's too little, too late. The only alert tied to this product is to avoid it at all costs.

☺ $$$ **High-Potency Skin-Firming Concentrate** *($55 for 1.7 ounces)* is a lightweight, serum-type moisturizer with a fairly modern assortment of helpful ingredients for skin. Of course, none of them are capable of addressing "multiple skin firmness concerns," but they can help skin restore a healthy barrier and prevent moisture loss. This is fragrance-free.

☺ **Imperiale Repairateur Moisturizing Eye Balm** *($22.50 for 0.5 ounce)* contains some outstanding ingredients to treat and protect very dry skin, so it's unfortunate that the impressive amount of vitamin E won't remain stable for long due to jar packaging. This still has merit as a balm for dry patches.

☺ $$$ **Line-Reducing Eye-Brightening Concentrate** *($40 for 0.5 ounce)* contains mostly slip agent, silicone, vitamin C (as ascorbic acid, which can be irritating if used around the eyes), glycerin, thickeners, and more silicones. Kiehl's claims the vitamin C content is 10.5%, and it may well be, but there is no research proving this is the magic number needed to reduce wrinkles or under-eye circles. Still, it's a good antioxidant for skin and comes in opaque packaging to keep it stable during use. This isn't a slam-dunk for use around the eyes, but should be OK for use on other areas of the face by all skin types. Fragrance in the form of orange flower extract is one more reason to keep this away from the eye area.

☺ **Panthenol Protein Moisturizing Face Cream, for Normal to Dry and Dry Skin Types** *($25.50 for 4 ounces)* is an OK emollient moisturizer for its intended skin type. Most of the interesting ingredients are listed well after the preservative, so they don't count for much.

☺ $$$ **Powerful Strength Line Reducing Concentrate** *($55 for 1.7 ounces)* is mostly slip agent, silicone, vitamin C, more silicones, film-forming agent, and the cell-communicating ingredient adenosine. Although this is a one-note product, it's an option if you want a stably packaged vitamin C serum.

☺ **Sodium PCA "Oil-Free" Moisturizer** *($17.50 for 2 ounces)* is oil-free but also very boring, offering little for normal to oily skin other than silicone and thickeners. The tiny amount of antioxidants will deteriorate quickly due to jar packaging.

☺ $$$ **Ultra Moisturizing Eye Stick SPF 30** *($20 for 0.18 ounce)* is a rich, balm-like sunscreen stick that contains an in-part avobenzone sunscreen. The amount of synthetic active ingredients may be too high to use around the eyes, but this can be a very good sunscreen for other exposed areas, such as the ears, scalp, or the top of your feet. It is fragrance-free.

☺ **UV Protective Everyday Facial Moisturizing Sunscreen Cream SPF 15** *($29.50 for 3.4 ounces)* is Kiehl's version of similar sunscreens with Mexoryl SX from L'Oreal-owned Lancome, La Roche-Posay, and L'Oreal's own line (recall that L'Oreal holds the patent for Mexoryl, which is why for the time being only their brands contain it). Although each of these companies' options provides sufficient UVA protection via Mexoryl SX (ecamsule) and avobenzone, each has a boring lotion formula that is void of antioxidants or other state-of-the-art ingredients. This is recommended for normal to oily skin needing a lightweight, effective sunscreen, but for the money this should have provided more.

☺ **Acne Blemish Control Daily Skin-Clearing Treatment** *($30 for 1 ounce)*. This anti-acne product contains 1.5% salicylic acid (BHA) as its active ingredient, but unfortunately its pH is too high for exfoliation to occur. You may get minimal results using it, but it doesn't compete favorably with better and far less expensive BHA products from Neutrogena, Bare Escentuals, and the many options from Paula's Choice. If it were formulated within the proper pH range, this lightweight lotion would've been an excellent product to help combat acne and blackheads.

☺ $$$ **Over-Night Biological Peel** *($42 for 1.7 ounces)* is supposed to be as potent as a 10% glycolic acid product, but it contains no alpha hydroxy acids, or beta hydroxy acid for that matter. Instead, this water- and silicone-based fluid contains urea, which is indeed an exfoliant, albeit a far less sexy version than AHAs or BHA because it's derived from urine. Urea definitely has exfoliating and water-binding properties when used on skin, and unlike AHAs and BHA, its efficacy is not pH-dependent. Much as AHAs do, it can cause a stinging sensation on application. Urea can be beneficial for those with dry skin because, although the manner in which it works isn't fully understood, it has proven very effective at reducing moisture loss from the epidermis (Source: *Dry Skin and Moisturizers Chemistry and Function*, Loden & Maibach, 2000, pages 235-236). Kiehl's ingredient list also points to HEPES as an enzyme activator. However, this ingredient (hydroxyethylpiperazine ethane sulfonic acid) functions as a buffering agent, which should help reduce any potential irritation from the urea. Although this peel is pricey and not necessarily superior to an AHA (or BHA) product, it is nevertheless a novel approach to exfoliating skin if you're curious to try something different, or if your skin has not responded favorably to AHA products.

☺ **Soothing Gel Masque** *($18.50 for 2 ounces)* is a lightweight gel mask suitable for normal to oily skin experiencing dry patches. The green tea has soothing benefits, but the jar packaging won't keep it stable for long.

☺ **Drawing Paste** *($16.50 for 0.5 ounce)* is supposed to control surface oiliness and maintain "skin integrity," but it contains several plant oils, wax, shea butter, and lanolin oil, which make it completely inappropriate for oily or blemish-prone skin. There are absorbents in this product, but what they can do is counteracted by the waxes and oils. At least Kiehl's didn't put irritating sulfur in this product.

☹ **Lip Balm SPF 15** *($9.50 for 0.5 ounce)* is an emollient lip balm available in clear or tinted shades, but none of them provide sufficient UVA protection, which leaves lips vulnerable to sun damage.

☺ **Lip Balm #1 SPF 4** *($6.50 for 0.5 ounce)* is a very standard, Vaseline-based lip balm that contains a good blend of emollients to prevent dry, chapped lips. It is fragrance-free.

KIEHL'S SUN & SELF-TANNING PRODUCTS

☺ **All-Sport "Non-Freeze" Face Protector SPF 30** *($18.50 for 1.4 ounces)* features avobenzone for sufficient UVA protection and has a nonaqueous, wax-based formula suitable for very dry skin, particularly in cold climates. This sunscreen is too heavy for day-to-day wear, and is not recommended for use over blemish-prone areas.

☺ $$$ **Creme de Corps Light-Weight Body Lotion with SPF 30 Sunscreen** *($26.50 for 8.4 ounces)* is a good sunscreen for the body if you're looking for a lightweight texture, smooth finish, and UVA protection courtesy of stabilized avobenzone. There are few bells and whistles to speak of, and the price is out of line for what you are buying, but this does provide sun protection without the heavy, sometimes thick feel you get from some sunscreens for the body.

☹ **Sun-Free Self-Tanning Formula** *($22.50 for 5 ounces)* doesn't distinguish itself performance-wise from other self-tanners containing dihydroxyacetone. However, it can be irritating to skin because it contains many volatile fragrant oils and extracts.

☹ **Ultra Protection Water Based Sunscreen Lotion SPF 25** *($27 for 4.2 ounces)* doesn't provide ultra protection because it lacks sufficient UVA-protecting ingredients of titanium dioxide, zinc oxide, avobenzone, Tinosorb, or Mexoryl SX. What a shame, because this has a great lightweight texture.

☺ **UV Protective Suncare Sunscreen Cream, For Face And Body SPF 20** *($32.50 for 3.4 ounces)* is nearly identical to the UV Protective Everyday Facial Moisturizing Sunscreen Cream SPF 15 except this version adds titanium dioxide to gain its higher SPF rating. Otherwise, the same comments apply; UVA protection is definitely assured with this blend of Mexoryl SX, avobenzone, and titanium dioxide.

☺ **Vital Sun Protection Lotion SPF 15** *($18.50 for 5 ounces)* is a very good, in-part avobenzone sunscreen for UVA protection; it is appropriate for someone with normal to slightly oily skin. It contains a film-forming agent that provides water resistance, which Kiehl's advertises on the product label. My only point of contention with this sunscreen is the claim that "minimal chemical ingredients" are used, which I'm sure they've chosen to say to try to imply that their sunscreen is superior to others, and it just isn't true. It contains 18% active ingredients—all of them synthetic sunscreen agents—and synthetic preservatives and film-forming agents. Kiehl's claim of using a "minimal" amount doesn't add up to anything like a genuine definition and is a completely disingenuous statement. This product is fragrance-free and does contain vitamin E for some antioxidant benefit.

☺ **Vital Sun Protection Lotion SPF 30** *($18.50 for 5 ounces)* is similar to the Vital Sun Protection Lotion SPF 15, except this contains a higher concentration of active ingredients to achieve its SPF 30 rating. Otherwise, the same basic comments apply.

☺ **Vital Sun Protection Lotion SPF 40** *($18.50 for 5 ounces)*. Just to be clear, sunscreens with higher SPF ratings do not provide better protection, just the same amount of protection for a longer time (meaning the amount of time you can stay in the sun without getting burned). For example, an SPF 30 and an SPF 40 (as long as they both have UVA-protecting ingredients) both protect skin from the same amount of the sun's rays. Currently, the FDA is considering raising the SPF labeling allowance from the current recommended maximum SPF rating of SPF 30 to SPF 50. However, that still has to do with longer, not better, protection. Regardless of the SPF number, liberal application and regular reapplication are keys to staying protected during prolonged periods of sun exposure. This sunscreen is similar to the Vital Sun Protection SPF 15 and SPF 30 products, except that it contains a higher concentration of active ingredients and a larger amount of film-forming agent for water resistance. Otherwise, the same comments apply regarding formula and skin type.

☺ **Vital Sun Protection Spray SPF 25** *($17.50 for 4.2 ounces)* is a very good, in-part avobenzone sunscreen in a moisturizing, water-resistant spray formula. The intriguing ingredients are listed after the preservative on the ingredient statement, so they don't count for much, but this is a good option for normal to dry skin types, and it is fragrance-free.

KIEHL'S MAKEUP

CONCEALER: ☹ **Concealing Stick for Blemishes** *($18.50 for 0.18 ounce)*. This flesh-toned, slightly peach stick concealer is a huge mistake to use on blemishes. The main ingredient is occlusive zinc oxide, and the formula also contains several thickeners, waxes, and lanolin oil. (I mean, really, lanolin oil in a blemish product?! What were they thinking? That's like trying to put out a fire with gasoline!) Concealing blemishes with a water-based liquid concealer is a much better choice. This product missed the boat completely.

LIP GLOSS: ☺ **Lip Gloss** *($14.50)*. This is a standard tube lip gloss that provides sheer colors (lots of them) and a thick, emollient texture. The glossy finish feels moist and sticky, but at least it doesn't slide off your lips within 30 minutes.

MASCARA: ✓☺ **$$$ Marvelous Mineral Mascara** *($16.50)*. When I first heard that Kiehl's had launched a mascara, I was surprised, because it isn't a line known for makeup. Then I remembered—Kiehl's is owned by L'Oreal. Knowing that L'Oreal mascaras typically are excellent, I wasn't too surprised when Marvelous Mineral Mascara performed beautifully. This is terrific mascara that, quite simply, does everything well and nothing to excess. Outrageously long lashes are its strong point, but it builds a lot of thickness, too, and without clumps or flakes. Consider this a sleeper mascara that I hope gets the attention it deserves. Ignore the mineral claims, however, because they are nothing more than marketing ploys—minerals add little of significance to a mascara.

KINERASE (SKIN CARE ONLY)

KINERASE AT-A-GLANCE

Strengths: Some antioxidant-rich products in stable packaging; every sunscreen offers sufficient UVA protection; mostly fragrance-free products.

Weaknesses: Cleanser; toning mist; some moisturizers and a serum with irritating ingredients; the Clear Skin products; unknowns about topical application of kinetin and zeatin.

For more information about Kinerase, call (800) 826-9755 or visit www.kinerase.com or www.Beautypedia.com.

KINERASE PHOTOFACIALS PRODUCTS

☺ **$$$ PhotoFacials Sun Damage Reversal System Daily Exfoliating Cleanser** *($40 for 5 ounces)*. This cleanser is supposed to be the first step in Kinerase's kit to undo sun damage. The cleanser itself is quite ordinary and, although effective for all skin types except dry, is incredibly overpriced for what you get, which is just a detergent-based cleanser. The plant extracts are included for show; they do not impact exfoliation because they are rinsed down the drain. By the way, cleansers can't undo sun damage in the least though a gentle cleanser is the first step in a sensible skin-care routine.

☺ **$$$ PhotoFacials Sun Damage Reversal System Day Moisturizer with SPF 50** *($88 for 1.7 ounces)*. This daytime moisturizer contains only mineral sunscreen ingredients (titanium dioxide and zinc oxide) and it can protect skin from further sun damage, just as any well-formulated sunscreen can. However, given the large amount of mineral sunscreen agents (about 20%), it has a heavy feel that won't be welcomed by everyone, a definite shortcoming of this type of SPF product.

Labeling this as akin to a PhotoFacial is nothing more than marketing hype. A real PhotoFacial (also known as Intense Pulsed Light or IPL) can help mitigate signs of sun damage such as minor discolorations and redness and can help build some amount of collagen. And, of course, sun protection is the key to maintaining those results. That's where this needlessly expensive product comes in to play, but to think that using this or any part of Kinerase's PhotoFacials system is the same as having the in-office IPL procedure is pure fantasy. The inactive ingredients in this product are listed in alphabetical order, which is an acceptable, albeit confounding, practice for over-the-counter drugs. There are several intriguing ingredients in the base formula (which is best for normal to dry skin not prone to blemishes), but the alphabetical listing makes it impossible to determine how much of the good stuff your skin is getting. This contains fragrance in the form of orange oil.

☹ **PhotoFacials Sun Damage Reversal System Night Moisturizer** *($88 for 1.7 ounces)*. This moisturizer contains the ingredient undecylenoyl phenylalanine, which has limited research pertaining to its skin-lightening benefit, so I wouldn't consider it a reliable choice for improving brown patches. This moisturizer absolutely cannot replicate the benefits of an in-office IPL procedure. That's like thinking you can perform a convincing face-lift at home by doing a handstand and taping loose skin in place. As it turns out, this moisturizer is hardly an exciting formula and it contains several fragrant plant oils (including skin cell-damaging lavender) and unnecessary or useless plant extracts that make it a problem for all skin types, both for the health of your skin and your budget.

KINERASE PRO+ THERAPY PRODUCTS

☺ **$$$ Pro+ Therapy Skin Smoothing Cleanser** *($43 for 5.1 ounces)* is a basic, water-soluble cleanser that is a good, though pricey, option for normal to oily skin. The AHAs in this cleanser cannot exfoliate skin due to their brief contact with it, though the pH is within range.

☺ **$$$ Pro+ Therapy Advanced Radiance Facial Peel** *($89 for 15 packets)* ends up being an expensive way to experience the benefits of the AHA lactic acid. Each packet contains a sponge-tip applicator steeped in this water- and aloe-based solution. The pH of 3.2 allows the approximately 8% lactic acid to exfoliate as you swab this over skin, but it is overall no more effective than considerably less expensive AHA lotions or serums. The only reason to consider this product is if you're intrigued by the combination of lactic acid with zeatin, though there is no research to support their combined use.

☹ **Pro+ Therapy Advanced Repair Serum** *($132 for 0.5 ounce)* lists alcohol as the second ingredient, which makes this a very expensive way to irritate skin, and it just can't repair skin the way they claim it can. In addition to kinetin, this serum contains zeatin, another plant growth hormone responsible for cell differentiation. Suresh I. S. Rattan, the same doctor who published research on kinetin, was responsible for the sole study on zeatin's effects on skin. The study was performed in vitro and had some promising results, including increasing the ability of skin cells to decompose hydrogen peroxide, meaning that zeatin can be considered an antioxidant. Interestingly, Dr. Rattan's study specifically mentions zeatin's ability to help skin cope with ethanol (alcohol) stress (Source: *Rejuvenation Research*, March 2005, pages 46-57). That revelation, however, neither explains nor justifies Kinerase including so much alcohol in this serum, unless they wanted to prove Dr. Rattan right at the expense of irritating their customers' skin!

☹ **Pro+ Therapy C6 Intensive treatment with Kinetin & Zeatin** *($105 for 1 ounce)*. All of the peptides, antioxidants, and cell-communicating ingredients you can pack into a moisturizer don't matter if you're also going to include a potent skin irritant. In the case of this product, the irritant is lime oil, and it instantly makes this a product to ignore. You can read about the pros and cons surrounding topical use of kinetin in my Cosmetic Ingredient Dictionary at www. Beautypedia.com. If you're interested in trying a product that contains it, Kinerase has other options that don't irritate skin. Ironically, the irritation negates a portion of kinetin's benefit when used topically.

☺ **$$$ Pro+ Therapy Daily Defense Cream SPF 30** *($140 for 2.8 ounces)*. A daytime moisturizer with sunscreen at this price point should be brimming with antioxidants and other skin-beneficial goodies. It's great that Kinerase includes avobenzone for UVA protection, but the really interesting ingredients are in short supply. It is doubtful that the meager antioxidant content will impact skin in the slightest, making this product vastly overpriced for its main benefit, which is sun protection. This product is a "Pro" in name only, although it is a good sunscreen. One other point: You have to apply sunscreen generously, and how generously are you going to apply a sunscreen at this price point?

☺ $$$ **Pro+ Therapy Daily Defense Lotion SPF 30** *($140 for 2.8 ounces)* is similar to Kinerase's Pro+ Therapy Daily Defense Cream SPF 30 except it contains greater amounts of antioxidants. UVA protection is assured from avobenzone, and the lotion formula is best for normal to dry skin. It is fragrance-free. Labeling this "non-prescription" is a joke because all sunscreens fall into that category, and there is nothing particularly medicinal about this product. I also disagree with the non-irritating claim, which won't be true for everyone who tries this product because the sunscreen actives it contains have the potential to cause a reaction. That doesn't mean they will, but it does mean it's disingenuous to label such a product "non-irritating." Keep in mind that you must apply sunscreen generously; how generously are you going to apply a sunscreen at this price point?

☹ $$$ **Pro+ Therapy Cream with Kinetin & Zeatin** *($129 for 2.8 ounces)* is sold as "non-prescriptive"—funny because it is strictly a cosmetic, as is every other Kinetin product and every other cosmetic being sold. Perhaps in their attempt to make the cost of this moisturizer for normal to dry skin seem more reasonable to the consumer they're marketing it as somehow associated with medicine. However, you can ignore the medical claims because this is an embarrassingly ordinary moisturizer that, with the exception of kinetin and zeatin, is similar to many moisturizers from Aveeno. The collagen and elastin in this product cannot fuse with or boost these structural components in your skin. As for kinetin and its plant growth hormone "cousin" zeatin, there is only limited research and minimal reason to consider either for aging skin. For details on rarely used zeatin, please refer to the review of Kinerase Pro+ Therapy Advanced Repair Serum above. Detailed information about kinetin can be found in my Cosmetic Ingredient Dictionary, accessible from www.Beautypedia.com.

☹ $$$ **Pro+ Therapy Lotion with Kinetin & Zeatin** *($129 for 2.8 ounces)* is the lotion version of Kinerase's Pro+ Therapy Cream with Kinetin & Zeatin and, other than being preferred for normal to slightly dry skin, the same comments apply.

☹ **Pro+ Therapy Procedure Recovery SPF 30** *($109 for 1.7 ounces)* has rampant problems, although at least the in-part zinc oxide sunscreen is good news. The biggest marks against this daytime moisturizer product are its excessive price (How liberally are you going to apply this moisturizer with sunscreen knowing that every 2-3 months you'd have to buy another one?) and the inexplicable inclusion of several irritating plant oils. There is no reason why rosemary, thyme, sage, and coriander oils need to be in any skin-care product. Yes, each does have antioxidant benefit (especially rosemary), but the flip side is that the oil form of each also contains volatile components that cause skin problems. There are plenty of other antioxidants that offer skin benefits without the risks.

☹ $$$ **Pro+ Therapy Ultra Rich Day Repair** *($149 for 1.7 ounces)* isn't as rich as the name states, but has some emollient properties for dry skin. Jar packaging compromises the effectiveness of most of this product's intriguing ingredients. If you're interested in seeing how the plant growth hormones kinetin and zeatin may affect aging skin, this may be worth a try. However, we don't know at this point if light and air exposure from jar packaging may negatively affect these ingredients too. In theory, I suspect it would at least diminish their antioxidant potential.

✓☺ **$$$ Pro+ Therapy Ultra Rich Eye Repair** *($88 for 0.5 ounce)* is, aside from the unknowns surrounding ongoing use of the plant growth hormones kinetin and zeatin, a very good moisturizer for dry skin anywhere on the face. It contains some great water-binding agents along with cell-communicating ingredients, antioxidants, and ingredients that reinforce skin's support structure. This product is fragrance-free, too.

☺ **$$$ Pro+ Therapy Ultra Rich Night Repair** *($149 for 1.7 ounces)* contains some impressive ingredients for skin, including several ceramides, a peptide, and a significant amount of the antioxidant ergothioneine. How disappointing that jar packaging won't keep these ingredients stable once this emollient, fragrance-free moisturizer for normal to dry skin is opened.

☺ **$$$ Pro+ Therapy Ultra Hydrating Repair Mask** *($89 for 1.7 ounces)* is a lightweight, but hydrating mask for normal to slightly dry skin. It does not contain significant amounts of ingredients known to repair skin, but will feel soothing. The pH, at above 5, prevents the salicylic acid from functioning as an exfoliant.

OTHER KINERASE PRODUCTS

☹ **Gentle Daily Cleanser** *($33 for 6.6 ounces)* lists sodium lauryl sulfate (SLS) as the main detergent cleansing agent, which makes this water-soluble cleanser far from gentle. It is otherwise indistinguishable from countless options at the drugstore (except for the price and inclusion of SLS). Paying this much money for something so standard and ordinary should be illegal.

☹ **Hydrating Antioxidant Mist** *($35 for 6.6 ounces)* has a lot going for it, including glycerin and hyaluronic acid as water-binding agents; antioxidants such as green tea, ergothioneine, and beta-glucan; and an alcohol-free formula. What a shame all this good stuff is degraded by the inclusion of bergamot oil. This citrus oil has photosensitizing and melanogenic (melanin-producing) properties, and should absolutely not be included in skin-care products (Source: *Journal of the American Academy of Dermatology*, September 2001, pages 458-461).

☺ **$$$ Instant Radiance Facial Peel** *($75 for 0.75 ounce)*. Let me preface my review by saying that the happy face rating is merely for the very basic but effective exfoliating formula. It is in no way a recommendation that this is preferred over versions from other companies that are far better and far less expensive. Having said that, what you are wasting your money on are premoistened, individually packaged sponge applicators on a stick. Each sponge is about the size of a quarter and is steeped in a solution of primarily aloe, fruit acids, and lactic acid. Kinerase claims that aloe and fruit acids exfoliate, too, but there's no substantiated proof of that, and the amount of aloe and fruit acid in this peel is insignificant anyway. Although the company would not reveal the percentage of lactic acid, it's likely around 5%, and the pH of 3.2 permits exfoliation to occur. This is an incredibly and unnecessarily expensive way to exfoliate skin, but it's an option. In other words, economically speaking, this is not preferred over numerous AHA lotions, gels, or creams that contain at least 5% or more glycolic or lactic acids, or BHA products that contain 2% salicylic acid. Nevertheless, it is an AHA-containing product with an effective pH. It's a bit like paying $75 for a small bottle of aspirin; the aspirin will work, but at the price, it's just a burn.

☺ **$$$ C6 Peptide Intensive Treatment** *($96 for 1 ounce)* expands on kinetin products by adding vitamin C and peptides to the mix, so it would seem kinetin isn't quite the answer to skin-care woes after all. When bragging about kinetin didn't get much attention from the consumer, Kinerase must have decided to jump on the peptide/vitamin bandwagon by creating this product with acetyl hexapeptide-3, the ingredient used in many products claiming to work "better than Botox." I have discussed this ingredient in the past and it appears that I'll have to keep commenting on it because cosmetics companies keep using it—even though there is no substantiated evidence concerning its effectiveness. For a detailed description of this ingredient, please refer to the Cosmetic Ingredient Dictionary at www.Beautypedia.com. In the end, this product is a good moisturizing lotion that contains antioxidant vitamins C and E, and some standard, but effective, water-binding agents. Whether or not to spend almost $100 to see what kinetin and acetyl hexapeptide-3 might do for your skin is up to you, but I don't recommend it. That $100 could achieve a much more reliable benefit for your skin elsewhere.

☺ $$$ **C8 Peptide Intensive Treatment** (*$98 for 1 ounce*) is a good formula, although this "treatment" moisturizer is one of the more expensive around. The blend of nonfragrant plant oil with fatty acids, cell-communicating ingredients, and antioxidants in stable packaging is nicely done. The effectiveness of applying kinetin topically, however, remains questionable because the studies pertaining to its benefit were paid for by companies selling products with kinetin or by companies selling kinetin as an antiaging ingredient. As it turns out, the amount of kinetin in this product isn't likely going to impact skin anyway, but it's good news that there are other helpful ingredients included. This would be rated a Paula's Pick if it did not contain orange oil for fragrance. The amount is likely too low to be cause for concern, but it's an extraneous ingredient your skin is better off without. One more comment: Labeling this product as "the modern fountain of youth" is stretching its capabilities to the breaking point. This is a beneficial, though overpriced, moisturizer for normal to dry skin that contains ingredients that can help skin function better, but there are a lot of other products that can do the same or better. One more point: there is no question peptides play a significant role in the body and the health of skin, but whether or not they have value in skin-care products has not been proven. Theoretically, it is intriguing, but theory doesn't make it fact. Overall, many peptides clearly play various roles in the aging of skin, but there is no information whether or not peptides included in skin-care products can remain stable, are biologically active, or can affect skin cells. Women want to believe these ingredients can make a difference, but believing doesn't make it true. The potential for peptides playing a role for skin is an interesting and developing field, with most of the ongoing research being conducted within the cosmetics industry (which clearly has exceptional bias and should be looked at with a skeptical eye), but we are not there yet.

☹ $$$ **Clear Skin Moisture Light** (*$75 for 1.7 ounces*) is an insanely overpriced moisturizer with ludicrous claims. Kinerase maintains that this emollient lotion (a triglyceride and thickeners comprise the bulk of the formula) banishes shine upon application while also reducing blemishes. Don't bet on it; in fact, the thickening agents in this moisturizer, which is best for normal to dry skin, may make blemishes worse or prompt new ones. And it absolutely won't leave a shine-free finish. This contains an ineffective amount of salicylic acid, though even if more was used, the pH is above 5, which means it cannot work to exfoliate clogged pores.

☹ $$$ **Daily Defense Cream SPF 30** (*$135 for 2.8 ounces*). For nearly $150, you're getting an in-part avobenzone sunscreen in a moisturizing formula that's so basic the price becomes insulting and offensive. The star ingredients (including kinetin, vitamin C, collagen, and elastin) barely make an impact in this product as there is so little of each. Plus I thought most people knew how ordinary collagen and elastin are in skin care products? Kinetin remains a contro-versial ingredient for skin: its safety is questionable due to the proposed manner in which it is supposed to work on skin, namely keeping cells reproducing possibly for longer than is healthy. It is not recommended for use by pregnant or lactating women (Source: www.naturaldatabase.

com). Given the itty-bitty amount of kinetin in this daytime moisturizer for normal to dry skin, I wouldn't be alarmed. What's most alarming is the price for this mundane formula.

☹ **$$$ Daily Defense Lotion SPF 30** (*$135 for 2.8 ounces*) is the lotion version of Kinerase's Daily Defense Cream SPF 30 (which sells for the same price). Like its cream counterpart, this includes an in-part avobenzone sunscreen for UVA protection, and a basic formula that is so short on significant amounts of exciting ingredients the price is completely unwarranted. The main point of difference for Kinerase is their use of the ingredient kinetin, which remains a controversial ingredient for skin. The controversy is related to the manner in which it works—it potentially keeps skin cells reproducing longer than normal, but perhaps longer than is healthy. Cells that continue to reproduce at an undetermined rate are a recipe for cancer. Kinetin is not recommended for use by pregnant or lactating women (Source: www.naturaldatabase.com). However, given the tiny amount of kinetin in this moisturizer for normal to slightly dry skin, I wouldn't be alarmed. Instead, be alarmed by the price, which isn't likely to encourage the liberal application that's essential for attaining the amount of sun protection stated on the label.

☹ **Extreme Lift Eye** (*$95 for 0.5 ounce*). The only things extreme about this product are the claims and its price! This product is supposed to produce results similar to Botox, "but won't leave you without facial expressions." Keep in mind that these "works like Botox" products can't come even remotely close to the results possible from the real thing. And when done properly, Botox injections won't leave patients expressionless. If they did, most of Hollywood would have immobile faces, and that's certainly not the case. I also find it insulting that a product claiming to include the most advanced ingredients has a formula that consists primarily of water, silicone, alcohol, and pullulan (a polysaccharide related to glucose). Pullulan isn't the antiaging, skin-tightening wonder we've been waiting for. There isn't any research to support its topical use for wrinkled, sagging skin in the eye area or elsewhere, although it likely functions as a water-binding agent, which is good, but hardly significant. The amount of alcohol in this product is very disappointing, and is likely enough to cause eye-area irritation and to negate any benefit the pullulan may have. The potential swelling from the irritation this causes may have a minor impact in lessening the appearance of wrinkles, but in the long run this is absolutely not good for skin; nor is this product "advanced" in any legitimate way.

☹ **Extreme Lift Face** (*$150 for 1 ounce*). Wow! For $150, you're getting a serum that's mostly water and alcohol, two of the least expensive cosmetic ingredients available. The amount of alcohol is irritating and causes free-radical damage, while nothing else in this formula is capable of "instantly" relaxing and filling in wrinkles. The claim that using this totally un-extreme product is similar to in-office procedures is meant to make you think it's topical Botox or a dermal filler, when in reality it is neither. This is about as similar to those procedures as filling out preoperative medical paperwork is to having an actual face-lift! I won't even comment on the kinetin because the amount in this product is too small for your skin to notice.

☹ **HydraBoost Intensive Treatment** (*$75 for 1 ounce*) is a lightweight, gel-type moisturizer that is said to contain 25% hyaluronic acid to help plump skin to a youthful state. Kinerase did not put hyaluronic acid in this "Treatment." Instead, they included sodium hyaluronate, the salt form of the ingredient. Although sodium hyaluronate is in fact a very good water-binding agent, it is not the same as hyaluronic acid, and if you're going to claim that your product contains hyaluronic acid, then that's what it should have in it. Although this product has the potential to hydrate normal to oily skin, the amount of orange flower oil makes it too potentially irritating. Not to mention that the price is insulting for what you get.

☹ **$$$ Intensive Eye Cream** *($62 for 0.7 ounce)* contains a very small amount of kinetin (which is fine, because we don't know how much is needed to exert a benefit) and is otherwise a basic, slightly emollient eye cream comparable to several options at the drugstore, including those from Nivea, Dove, and Neutrogena.

☺ **$$$ Kinerase Cream** *($119 for 2.8 ounces)* combines very standard thickening and emollient ingredients with a soybean-based antioxidant, silicone, preservatives, vitamin C, water-binding agents, and a tiny amount of kinetin (N6-furfuryladenine). There is no reason to choose this over several more elegant formulas loaded with antioxidants and cell-communicating ingredients, unless you think kinetin is the ultimate antiaging ingredient.

☺ **$$$ Kinerase Lotion** *($119 for 2.8 ounces)* is a lighter version of the Kinerase Cream, and is suitable for normal to slightly oily skin. The tiny amount of antioxidants doesn't justify the price, so be aware you're paying a premium to find out if kinetin is the answer for your wrinkles and other aging-skin issues (thus far, research hasn't proven kinetin all that amazing).

☹ **Under Eye Rescue** *($78 for 0.7 ounce)* would be more truthfully labeled "Under Eye Irritation," thanks to menthyl lactate, a derivative of menthol. Although only a tiny amount is included, any amount is problematic in a product designed for application around the eyes. This is otherwise a respectable formula, though not worth its cost, especially when compared with state-of-the-art products like those in the Clinique Repairwear line.

☹ **Ultimate Day Moisturizer** *($125 for 2.8 ounces)* is not the ultimate choice for daytime because it does not contain sunscreen. This slightly emollient moisturizer contains some state-of-the-art ingredients to help dry skin look and feel better. However, the latest research on kinetin hasn't proven it to be an antiwrinkle luminary or even a dim light (Source: *Annals of the New York Academy of Sciences*, May 2006, pages 332-342). Despite some positives, this moisturizer is problematic for all skin types because it contains grapefruit peel oil, which can cause contact dermatitis and a phototoxic reaction due to its volatile components (Source: www.naturaldatabase.com).

☹ **Ultimate Night Moisturizer** *($125 for 2.8 ounces)* is similar to the Ultimate Day Moisturizer, except it contains a higher concentration of irritating grapefruit peel oil. What a shame, because aside from the potential unknowns of topical kinetin, this moisturizer contains some brilliant ingredients for dry skin.

☹ **Brightening Anti-Aging System** *($140)* consists of Kinerase's **Brightening Face Serum** and **Concentrated Spot Treatment**. Both are designed to "enhance and brighten overall skin tone by lightening dark spots and promoting rejuvenation." The Serum is a water- and silicone-based solution that doesn't contain any notable ingredients for lightening pigment discolorations, though it does contain pearl powder, which has a cosmetic brightening effect; but that isn't skin care, that's makeup. The amount of kinetin is impressive, but this plant growth hormone does not have any convincing research pertaining to its ability to affect discolorations on human skin. Kinerase uses two forms of the antiseptic resorcinol, most likely as a preservative because as a lightening agent it would be problematic. It is potentially irritating and doesn't make this Serum any more attractive to use. The Spot Treatment is packaged in a pen-style applicator, and includes many of the same ingredients as the Serum. It contains a smaller amount of kinetin, but that's not such a loss. The main problem is the amount of daisy flower extract. Also known as tansy, this plant is known to cause severe contact dermatitis (Source: www.naturaldatabase. com), and so is not recommended, despite its folklore tie to lightening freckles. This kit doesn't compare to proven skin-lightening products that contain hydroquinone or arbutin. For the money, see your doctor for a prescription for Tri-Luma, which would guarantee far better results and ongoing improvement.

☹ **Clear Skin Blemish Dissolver** *($39 for 0.12 ounce)* lists alcohol as the second ingredient and also contains a high amount of lemon extract, which only serves to create a very irritating product that triggers oil production in the pore.

☹ **Clear Skin Regulating Mask** *($56 for 2.8 ounces)* proves Kinerase should stick with kinetin because they clearly know nothing about what blemish-prone skin needs. If they did, they wouldn't have launched this irritant-laden mask. Lime, basil, and spearmint oils are just a sampling of the offenders in this unhelpful product.

☹ **Clear Skin Treatment Serum** *($79 for 1 ounce)* lists alcohol as the second ingredient, which makes this too drying and irritating for all skin types, not to mention this much alcohol can trigger oil production in the pore lining. The amount of salicylic acid is too small to exfoliate skin, and kinetin has no research proving its anti-acne worth.

☺ **$$$ Lip Treatment** *($38 for 0.35 ounce)* ranks as one of the most expensive lip balms around. But to Kinerase's credit, it's not your typical wax-based formula (although there's nothing wrong with those). More a lip cream than a balm, and designed to be used on and around the lips, it contains an intriguing blend of thickeners usually found in moisturizers, such as non-volatile plant oils, potent antioxidants (present in amounts greater than mere window dressing), soothing plant extracts, water-binding agents, kinetin, and peptides. This product won't make lips plump because it doesn't contain ingredients that cause lips to swell, but it will make dry lips feel smooth and soft, and, as with any moisturizer placed over fine, dry lines, it will make them look better, although the effect is not permanent. Lip Treatment would get a Paula's Pick rating if not for the unknowns surrounding topical use of kinetin.

KORRES NATURAL

KORRES NATURAL AT-A-GLANCE

Strengths: Excellent pressed powders, powder blush, eyeshadow, and lip gloss; some good cleansers and makeup removers; the sunscreens for the body (except for the one that encourages tanning).

Weaknesses: Blatantly dishonest claims; several products contain irritating ingredients, including volatile fragrance chemicals; no products for managing acne or skin discolorations; jar packaging; bar soaps; average moisturizers, including some with disappointing SPF ratings; lackluster masks; the foundation primer contains potent irritants; standard eye pencils; the tinted moisturizer with sunscreen; some of the plant extracts are from endangered species of plants.

For more information about Korres Natural, visit www.korres.com or www.Beautypedia.com.

KORRES NATURAL SKIN CARE

KORRES NATURAL MATERIA HERBA PRODUCTS

☺ **$$$ 3 in 1 Cleansing Emulsion, All Skin Types** *($27 for 5.07 ounces)* is an exceptionally standard cleansing lotion that lists witch hazel extract as the second ingredient, and that is not gentle on skin. As a cleanser this has minimal capacity to clean off makeup, at least not without the help of a washcloth. This is an option for normal to dry skin, but at this price point you're better off leaving it on the shelf.

☹ **Toning Cleansing Foam, All Skin Types** *($27 for 5.07 ounces)* is a lightweight cleanser that contains a couple of very gentle cleansing agents, but their mildness is compromised by the inclusion of several parts of the witch hazel plant, plus alcohol and rosemary oil. Ironic that alcohol passes muster in the world of natural skin care when it kills skin cells, causes free-radical damage, and is drying and irritating for skin. None of this is good news for your skin, and this cleanser is assuredly a problem if used near your eyes, too. *Centaurea cyanus* flower water (which is fragrance, not skin care) is included, and *C. cyanus* is an endangered species.

☺ **$$$ Anti-Ageing Cream, Normal to Dry Skin** *($46 for 1.01 ounces)* is a below-standard emollient moisturizer for dry skin. The emollients (including nonfragrant and fragrant plant oils—fragrance in almost any form is a skin irritant) are fine, but the amount of irritating melissa is hard to ignore. In addition, for the money, this moisturizer is woefully short on notable antioxidants, skin-identical ingredients, cell-communicating ingredients, and, well, other essentials that help skin defend itself against signs of environmental aging. Think of this product as using a horse and buggy instead of a car to get you where you want to go.

☺ **$$$ Anti-Ageing Cream, Oily to Combination Skin** *($46 for 1.01 ounces)*. Those with oily or combination skin won't appreciate the amount of plant oils and fatty acids in this moisturizer because they add emollients to the skin that can clog pores and/or leave it feeling greasier. This is far better for normal to dry skin that doesn't break out, but it isn't a standout formula for that skin type either. The overall formula leaves much to be desired. The amount of bitter-orange flower water is potentially irritating and is there mainly to add fragrance (fragrance is not skin care). What is clearly absent is an appreciable amount of state-of-the-art ingredients like antioxidants, cell-communicating ingredients, and skin-identical ingredients that can combat signs of environmental aging by supplying skin with what has been depleted due to sun damage and irritating skin-care products, among other factors. This ends up being exceedingly overpriced for what you get.

☺ **$$$ Anti-Ageing Eye Cream** *($40 for 0.51 ounce)* is a really basic, overall unimpressive eye cream that isn't worth even half its price. Yes, it will remedy dry skin anywhere on the face, but that's the result of commonplace ingredients, including several that show up in thousands of products from lines that don't make the exotic and misleading claims that Korres does. This contains a tiny amount of plant extract *Pecudanum ostruthium*, also known as masterwort, which is known to cause a reaction when skin is exposed to sunlight, a fact that decreases this product's appeal even further (Source: www.naturaldatabase.com).

☹ **Moisturising Cream, Normal to Dry Skin** *($39 for 1.69 ounces)* lists melissa, which can be a skin irritant, as the second ingredient. Irritating your skin can cause collagen to break down and impair your skin's ability to heal. Several parts of that plant are included, and they contain irritating constituents that your skin is better off without. Like most plants, melissa has antioxidant ability; however, lots of plants provide that benefit without causing irritation, so there's no need to compromise. Even without the problematic plant, this is a shockingly boring formula that contains many of the same emollients (fatty acids) and plant oils present in lots of other products that cost a lot less and without the natural hype.

☹ **Moisturising Cream, Oily to Combination Skin** *($39 for 1.69 ounces)* is a moisturizer (and I use that term very loosely) that lists alcohol as the second ingredient. Alcohol (which is natural) causes free-radical damage, irritation, and dryness, and stimulates oil production in the pore—it has no benefit for skin whatsoever. Also high up on the ingredient list is bitter-orange flower water, and there are several other fragrant plants present, too, all irritating for skin. Think of this as eau de cologne for skin because that's a more accurate description of what you can expect from this moisturizer (eau de cologne is not skin care). This product is not recommended; labeling it as soothing is a joke.

☹ **Moisturising Eye Cream, Anti-Dark Circles** *($36 for 0.51 ounce)*. Considering how ordinary this eye cream is and given its similarity to several other emollient moisturizers in the Korres Natural Materia Herba line, which also make the dark circle–diminishing claims, you shouldn't need this one anyway. So, the question is, why do you need this product? The answer is: probably because you've been convinced that there is something unique in it for your eye area. However, a quick comparative look reveals that this is absolutely not true, and there is no research showing that eye-area skin needs anything different from skin on the rest of your face. Did anybody ever buy a skin-care product claiming to get rid of dark circles that actually did something? If the first product made had worked, then there wouldn't be thousands of others today claiming they are the answer. There is nothing in this product that will smooth puffy eyes or remedy "vascular imperfections" through "an advanced vessel-protecting process." Protecting or not protecting blood vessels isn't why the under-eye area may be dark anyway. What nonsense! If anything, the amount of irritating melissa flower, leaf, and stem extract will make the skin around your eyes look worse. This is an exceedingly ordinary emollient moisturizer with claims that are far more interesting, albeit without merit, than the formula.

OTHER KORRES NATURAL PRODUCTS

☹ **Calendula Softening Soap** *($8.50 for 2.82 ounces)* is a standard-issue bar soap with the plant ingredient calendula thrown in as window dressing. It also contains synthetic coloring agents, which is bizarre for this so-called natural line of products. This has no benefit over Aveeno Moisturizing Bar, which is actually more natural and less irritating than Korres'; in fact, the Aveeno product omits the irritating fragrant extracts. Regardless, this is just a too drying, irritating, and potentially pore-clogging cleanser for all skin types.

☹ **Echinacea Soap for Oily Skin** *($8.50 for 2.82 ounces)* is a standard-issue bar soap with the plant ingredients echinacea and thyme thrown in as window dressing, along with a lot of fragrance. It is too drying and irritating for all skin types.

☺ **$$$ Milk Proteins 3 in 1 Cleansing Toning and Eye Make-Up Removing Emulsion** *($21 for 6.76 ounces)* is an effective, albeit greasy, way to remove makeup and cleanse dry to very dry skin. Its toning properties are questionable and, contrary to claims, you will want to use this with water (and a washcloth) to avoid leaving a greasy residue on your skin. Surprisingly, this is fragrance-free and suitable for sensitive skin. The amount of milk protein (listed as whey protein) is so small your skin won't notice it. In the long run, there is little reason to use this instead of pure sunflower oil or canola oil, which is in essence all you are buying.

☺ **$$$ Milk Proteins Cleansing & Demake Up Wipes** *($12 for 25 wipes)* is a lightweight cleansing solution infused into soft, disposable wipes. They don't remove long-wearing or matte-finish makeup very well, but they're fine for removing lightweight makeup or for refreshing normal to dry skin. For less money, consider using fragrance-free baby wipes. The milk protein in these Korres wipes is listed last on the ingredient list, and clearly is an afterthought, not the emphasis the name implies.

☹ **Milk Soap for Stressed Skin** *($8.50 for 2.82 ounces)* is standard-issue bar soap with milk protein thrown in as window dressing. It is too drying and irritating for all skin types. The amount of fragrance in this soap is not what you want to see in a product sold as being "mild." What is most shocking is that the first ingredient is sodium tallowate, an animal-derived ingredient

☺ **$$$ Orange Blossom Cleansing Emulsion** *($19 for 6.76 ounces)* is an emollient cleansing balm that's suitable for dry to very dry skin. It removes makeup well, but contains enough fragrant plants that its use in the eye area is ill-advised. There are plenty of synthetic ingredients framing the natural ones Korres is supposed to be all about (further proof that the entire premise of this line is marketing hype to the max), but they contribute to this cleanser's texture and skin-softening effect.

☺ **$$$ Pomegranate Cleansing & Make Up Removing Wipes** *($12 for 25 wipes)* are nearly identical to the Korres Milk Proteins Cleansing & Demake Up Wipes above, aside from the tiny amount of pomegranate extract (which your skin won't notice). As such, the same review applies.

☺ **$$$ Thyme and Sage Facial Gel Cleanser** *($21 for 5.07 ounces)* is a very standard, but good, water-soluble cleanser for normal to oily skin. Light, effective, and clean-rinsing, its only drawback is the inclusion of a tiny amount of fragrant plants and, of course, the price. You can find gentler yet still effective gel cleansers at the drugstore for one-fourth the cost of this option.

☹ **Wheat Face Soap** *($8.50 for 2.82 ounces)* is standard-issue bar cleanser, which means it is too drying and irritating for all skin types. The tiny amount of wheat included doesn't change that fact, but the numerous fragrance chemicals do make this soap more irritating than it would be without them.

☺ **$$$ White Tea Facial Fluid Gel Cleanser** *($21 for 6.7 ounces)* is a standard, but good, water-soluble cleanser for all skin types except sensitive. It would be rated a Paula's Pick if it did not contain fragrance chemicals known to cause irritation. White Tea Facial Fluid Gel Cleanser works quite well to remove all but the most stubborn makeup, including waterproof mascara.

☹ **$$$ Jasmine Eye Make-Up Removal Lotion** *($21 for 6.7 ounces)*. First, this eye-makeup remover isn't fragrance-free; it contains jasmine extract, and that is absolutely a fragrant, potentially skin-irritating plant extract. This is a reasonably effective makeup remover in lotion form, but it certainly isn't one of the gentlest formulas around. This is not as effective at removing waterproof mascara as a silicone- or oil-based makeup remover would be.

☹ **$$$ Almond Meal Soft Scrub** *($19.50 for 6.7 ounces)* is not recommended for sensitive skin because this scrub includes almond meal as the abrasive agent. Almond meal, while natural, can actually be more abrasive than synthetic scrub beads, which are engineered to be spherical. As such, that type of synthetic bead glides over skin as it removes built-up dead skin cells. In contrast, almond meal particles have an uneven, possibly jagged shape that can cause tiny tears in skin. This scrub has a cushiony texture that will make the almond meal less abrasive, but it's still not a scrub someone with sensitive skin should use. It is an OK option for normal to dry skin, though it's possible to get better results using a washcloth with your favorite gentle cleanser. The presence of almonds doesn't make this more natural; there are plenty of synthetic ingredients in here as well—in fact, far more than in many other scrubs you can buy.

☹ **$$$ Olive Stones Scrub** *($19.50 for 1.4 ounces)*. Unlike the Almond Meal Soft Scrub from Korres, this version contains ground-up olive pits. Olive or almond, both have an uneven shape, and thus the potential to abrade skin more than gently polish it. Just because a scrub contains a natural ingredient to exfoliate skin doesn't mean it's better for your skin, and let's not forget, a washcloth made from 100% cotton is natural, too. This is an OK scrub for normal to dry skin that is not sensitive. Given the hype and the misleading information this line immerses itself in, this formula isn't natural in the least; it's loaded with synthetic ingredients.

☹ **Hamamelis Face Water** *($21 for 3.4 ounces)* has a first ingredient listed as a concentrated form of witch hazel (which is mostly alcohol), making this too irritating and drying for any skin type. Alcohol also causes free-radical damage and impairs the skin's ability to heal. As such, and despite the inclusion of some good water-binding agents, this is not recommended. There is nothing moisturizing or hydrating about this product in the least.

☹ **Cinnamon and Echinacea Cream Gel** *($25 for 1.35 ounces)* contains several ingredients that are irritating for skin. Although none are present individually in great amounts, their combined total is significant; that plus this product's overall lack of impressive ingredients makes it not worth considering. By the way, this is not at all a good moisturizer for blemish-prone skin; the thickening agents it contains are capable of clogging pores and making blemishes worse. In terms of a natural formula, this contains enough synthetic ingredients to make it completely offensive to anyone thinking they are getting something plant-based for their skin.

☺ **$$$ Evening Primrose Eye Cream SPF 6** *($34 for 1.01 ounces)* is quite similar to Korres' Borage Men's Eye Cream SPF 6 (review available on Beautypedia), except you get half as much product for roughly the same price. (Women are always willing to pay more, something many cosmetics companies count on.) Regardless of the packaging deception, both are underwhelming with their disappointing SPF rating, even though it's pure zinc oxide (SPF 15 is the standard from medical boards worldwide). The base formula is suitable for normal to dry skin, but it is exceedingly ordinary, not particularly natural, and a poor choice for use near the eyes because it contains fragrance.

☺ **$$$ Eyebright Firming Eye Cream** *($38.50 for 1.01 ounces)* is a glycerin-rich moisturizer that has a smooth texture capable of making dry skin anywhere on the face look and feel better. It contains some antioxidants, though some of the plant extracts are problematic due to their fragrant nature. Consider this eye cream a mixed bag; it has potential, but certainly isn't capable of undoing the damage time and stress can cause.

☺ **$$$ Olive and Rye Day Cream** *($38 for 1.35 ounces)* is an ultra-rich, greasy balm–like moisturizer that contains some formidable ingredients for dry skin. Korres maintains this is great for anyone over age 50, essentially classifying that age group and above into one neat little category, even though plenty of people over age 50 don't have dry skin; in fact, some women find they're dealing with acne for the first time as they reach their 50s. Age-related recommendations aside, the antioxidant plant oils in this balm will see their potency reduced thanks to the jar packaging. And if rye extract is as firming and restructuring as Korres maintains, then they're the only company promoting it, and there is no research showing that they've found the answer for skin. But, of course, if they have, then why don't all of their antiwrinkle products contain it?

☺ **$$$ Olive and Rye Eye Cream** *($38.50 for 0.51 ounce)* is a fairly thick moisturizer that isn't well-suited as an eye cream because it contains fragrance. This product offers no special benefit for "mature skin types" and is a far cry from what a modern antiaging moisturizer should be. It contains a few beneficial antioxidants, but any of the moisturizers I rate a Paula's Pick are worth a look before settling for this eye cream.

☺ **$$$ Olive and Rye Night Cream** *($39 for 1.35 ounces)* is nearly identical to the Korres Olive and Rye Day Cream. As such, the same review applies.

☺ **Pomegranate Balancing Moisturiser SPF 6** *($29.50 for 1.4 ounces)*. What is with Korres and their low SPF ratings? SPF 6 is unacceptable in Greece (where Korres is based) or anywhere else in the world—medical boards maintain SPF 15 as the standard and higher is probably better. Titanium dioxide is the active ingredient in this daytime moisturizer with sunscreen for normal to slightly dry skin, and it does contain an impressive amount of the super antioxidant pomegranate, but the SPF number is just deplorable. In addition to the SPF debacle, this is packaged in a jar, so even the antioxidant boost is going to be short-lived. This also contains fragrance chemicals that can cause irritation, and it's another strike against what could've been an exemplary product. In terms of natural, this product is chock-full of unnatural ingredients; Korres seems to enjoy pretending that the line is all natural, when it absolutely is not!

☺ **$$$ Sugar Crystal Cream Multivitamin Skin Shield** *($39.50 for 1.7 ounces)* has slip agents and film-forming agents comprising the bulk of this formula, which don't do much to "shield" skin from drier climates as claimed, and they're anything but natural. The plant oils are the real reason this could be labeled a good moisturizer and there is an OK amount of antioxidants. Glycolic acid also is present, but too little to have any impact on skin in regard to exfoliation. This is an average lightweight moisturizer with retinol for normal to slightly oily skin. It is packaged so the retinol will remain stable during use.

☹ **$$$ Thyme Honey Cream** *($32.50 for 1.35 ounces)*. Thyme honey simply refers to regular honey that has been infused with the herb thyme. Although honey has antioxidant and anti-inflammatory benefits for skin, adding thyme doesn't help matters because it has volatile fragrant components. The good news is that thyme appears nowhere on the ingredient list for this moisturizer. The bad news is that the honey and several emollient plant oils will see their beneficial components squandered due to the jar packaging. At best, this is a decent emollient moisturizer for normal to dry skin. For the money, this doesn't get close to being a smart purchase, and it isn't all natural in the least.

☹ **$$$ Wheat and Honey Intensified Vitamin E Anti-Ageing Cream** *($32.50 for 1.35 ounces)*. There is nothing about this utterly standard moisturizer that's antiaging. Thinking otherwise is like awarding Lubriderm® the grand prize as the one antiaging product everyone needs. That would be silly, and so is claiming that this product can help prevent signs of premature aging. The teeny amount of vitamins thrown in at the end won't help skin fend off anything. At best (and I use that term loosely), this is an average, jar-packaged moisturizer (which means the natural ingredients won't remain stable after opening) for normal to dry skin.

☹ **$$$ Wild Rose 24-hour Moisturiser SPF 6** *($32.50 for 1.4 ounces)*. SPF 6 is an embarrassingly low and harmful SPF rating! Despite titanium dioxide as the sole active ingredient, this isn't a daytime moisturizer I can recommend for sufficient sun protection, and it wouldn't be recommended by any medical board in the world because SPF 15 is considered minimum and higher is better. This does contain some beneficial plant oils and extracts, but much of their potential is diminished due to the jar packaging, which won't keep those ingredients stable. This also contains several fragrance chemicals known to cause irritation, so keep that in mind if you find yourself drawn to this moisturizer's scent.

☹ **Wild Rose Serum** *($38 for 1.01 ounces)*. Irritating, drying witch hazel distillate, which contains alcohol, is the second ingredient in this poorly formulated serum, and alcohol causes free-radical damage and irritation, and impairs the skin's ability to heal. Beneficial plant ingredients and other antioxidants are in short supply, while fragrance chemicals present the risk of further irritation. The form of rose used in this serum is rose hip, which is not the same as traditional rose. Its vitamin C content is well-known, but lots of products contain rose hip or other forms of vitamin C, without adding irritants that your skin doesn't need.

☹ **Yoghurt Cream** *($29.50 for 1.35 ounces)*. Supposedly, this moisturizer is made using full-fat Greek yogurt. If that's true, then your skin will be treated to fats that occur naturally in milk, as well as to protein and other trace nutrients. There is no research anywhere documenting that any type of yogurt is a must for skin, though you'll find plenty of studies pertaining to the potential health benefits of oral consumption. The concern I have with this product is that even if there were research showing that the yogurt and numerous plant oils it contains had superior benefit for skin, they won't last long due to the jar packaging, which won't keep them stable. Think of how long a cup of yogurt would last on your bathroom counter if you opened it once per day and scooped out a small amount. Within a week it would be molding and not smelling too pretty. This cream contains numerous fragrance chemicals that offset any anti-inflammatory benefit you may get from some of the helpful ingredients. Bottom line: Why bother?

☹ **$$$ Chlorophyll Deep Cleansing Face Mask** *($24.50 for 1.35 ounces)* is a very standard clay mask for oily skin that doesn't distinguish itself as cleansing any "deeper" than others of its ilk and it is about as natural as polyester. If anything, it sets itself apart as a less desirable option because it contains several fragrance chemicals known to cause irritation. The clays in this mask cannot regulate sebum (oil) production; that process is controlled by hormones. The only thing that clays can do (regardless of their color, purity, or source) is absorb excess oil on the skin's surface, leaving it temporarily smoother and shine-free.

☹ **$$$ Cinnamon and Natural Clay Mask** *($27 for 2.03 ounces)* is a below-standard clay mask because it contains the potentially irritating plant extracts cinnamon and sage. Anti-irritant willow herb is present, but its benefit will be offset by the problematic ingredients. There are better clay masks for those with oily skin.

☒ **Cinnamon and Thyme Gel for Topical Use** *($16 for 0.51 ounce)*. Cinnamon and thyme may make for a tasty addition to a recipe for dinner, but they have no effect on skin imperfections, at least not without causing more trouble along the way. Besides, alcohol is the second ingredient in this gel, and it's going to have a detrimental effect on skin whether acne is present or not. Alcohol causes free-radical damage, impairs the skin's ability to heal, and causes irritation that includes triggering oil production in the pore lining.

☹ **Thyme Honey Mask** *($27 for 1.35 ounces)*. Despite the name, there is no thyme in this creamy facial mask for normal to dry skin. Its honey content ensures skin will get some benefit from honey's anti-inflammatory properties, but honey has no impact on skin's elasticity. And besides, its potency will be diminished due to the jar packaging, and that goes for the effectiveness of the other plants and vitamins in this mask, too. It's a good mask for normal to dry skin, but the packaging is a letdown.

☺ **$$$ Wild Rose Imperfection-Targeting Oil** *($25 for 0.06 ounce)* is a fragrance-free specialty product that is primarily rose hip oil along with a silicone-like slip agent, vitamin C, and alcohol. The amount of alcohol is probably not cause for concern. Although rose hip oil is a beneficial nonfragrant plant oil for skin, you can use the pure stuff from the health food store and save some money. Those opting for this product should know it is best for dry skin, though its antiwrinkle effect isn't going to be startling, but there is the potential that it can be helpful for skin discolorations.

☹ **Wild Rose Mask Instant Brightening and Illuminating Vitamin C Mask** *($27 for 1.35 ounces)* is a thick, paste-like mask that contains enough titanium dioxide to leave a white cast on skin because this much titanium dioxide isn't easy to rinse off. Perhaps that's where the "brightening and illuminating" comes into play, because it's certainly not from the small amount of vitamin C it contains. Although vitamin C has merit when it comes to reducing skin discolorations, you need to use it daily and you need to leave it on your skin, and that's not what this mask was designed for. And when it comes to natural, this product does not come close to fitting that category.

☺ **Yoghurt Velvety Moisturising Mask** *($27 for 1.35 ounces)* is a fairly good moisturizing mask for normal to dry skin. However, there's no reason you couldn't make this at home and spare your skin the potential irritation from the fragrance chemicals Korres includes in the product. All you'd need is some yogurt and nonfragrant plant oils (such as olive oil or almond oil), blended to whatever consistency you prefer. You won't notice miraculous results with the Korres version or the do-it-yourself version, but at least your skin will be smoother, and with the home version you'll save money.

☺ **Lip Butters** *($9 for 0.21 ounce).* Korres offers several flavors of the same basic emollient lip balm formula. Whether you choose Guava, Quince, Plum, Pomegranate, or Wild Rose, the only difference is the fragrance and a token amount of the namesake plant extract. These lip balms have a thick but smooth consistency and a glossy finish that works well to keep lips moist and protected. The Guava and Quince butters contain fragrance chemicals known to cause irritation, and are not recommended over the others. Note that these lip balms are packaged in jars.

KORRES NATURAL SUN PRODUCTS

☺ **$$$ Sweet Orange Sunscreen Emulsion Face & Body SPF 15** *($23 for 5.07 ounces).* Thankfully, sweet orange is but a small, inconsequential part of this sunscreen's formula because it can be irritating for skin. What is good about this product is that finally Korres has a broad-spectrum protection sunscreen with SPF 15 (not the pathetic SPF 6 of several of their other sunscreens) and the in-part zinc oxide and titanium dioxide base is great. The emollient base formula is suitable for normal to dry skin. The formula lacks a significant amount of antioxidants, which is why it missed a Paula's Pick rating, but all things considered it's a good sunscreen that you can use on face or body. One more comment: contrary to claim, shea butter does not provide sun protection! What a terrible piece of information for a cosmetics company to assert!

☹ **Walnut and Coconut Suntan Oil Face & Body SPF 4** *($20 for 5.07 ounces).* The SPF rating on this product is dangerously low (although it does include avobenzone, listed by its chemical name butyl methoxydibenzoylmethane), but even worse is that this product encourages tanning right on the label. I can't abide by the flawed ethics of a cosmetics company selling so-called antiwrinkle products right alongside products designed to promote tanning. Like cigarettes, this product should come with a warning that it can cause skin cancer and wrinkles. Adding to the pathetic nature of this product is that it contains several fragrance chemicals that can cause a phototoxic reaction when skin is exposed to sun. What an unethical product for any skin-care company to be selling. Korres should be ashamed.

☺ **Watermelon Sunscreen Face Cream SPF 20** *($25 for 1.69 ounces)* is a good sunscreen with the minerals titanium dioxide and zinc oxide as the active ingredients. This also contains synthetic sunscreen ingredients not listed as active, which means this sunscreen isn't a slam-dunk for those with sensitive skin. The amount of watermelon is not enough to impart any benefit, although watermelon doesn't have much to offer skin anyway. This facial sunscreen is best for normal to dry skin.

☺ **Watermelon Sunscreen Face Cream SPF 30** *($28 for 1.69 ounces)* is very similar to Korres' Watermelon Sunscreen Face Cream SPF 20 above. The main difference is that the active ingredients in this one list two additional sunscreen agents that in the SPF 20 version are listed as inactives. Strange, yes, but perhaps it helps them set this higher SPF product apart. In any event, the same review applies.

☹ **Yoghurt Cooling Gel** *($23.50)* provides a cooling sensation that comes from the irritating menthol derivative menthyl lactate. If that weren't disappointment enough, this also contains several fragrance chemicals known to cause irritation. None of these make this gel ideal after sun exposure, unless you want to add insult to skin injury.

KORRES NATURAL MAKEUP

FOUNDATION: ☺ **$$$ Wild Rose Foundation SPF 20** *($28)* is a liquid foundation with a thin, fluid texture that smooths easily over skin, setting to a finish that feels moist but looks matte. It's best for normal to slightly dry or slightly oily skin. The shade range is mostly great, but there are no options for dark skin tones. Avoid WRF6 due to its strong peach cast. Wild Rose Foundation provides sheer to light coverage and has a lingering scent. The sunscreen is in-part titanium dioxide; so, as long as you apply this liberally and evenly, it can serve as your daytime facial sun protection.

☺ **$$$ Ginger and Vitamins Foundation SPF 10** *($28)* has a creamy but lightweight texture that's easy to blend, yet its soft matte finish tends to be slightly chalky. As such, this isn't an all-around attractive foundation for those with normal to dry skin. The sunscreen is pure titanium dioxide, but the SPF rating is disappointing. (Perhaps Korres isn't aware that SPF 15 is the minimum recommended by most major medical organizations.) If you decide to try this foundation anyway, it provides sheer to light coverage and its shade range is best for light to medium skin tones. There are no options for fair or dark skin. Shade LF4 is slightly peach, but workable. In terms of this foundation's vitamin content, it's barely present and not a reason to consider this over countless other better foundations.

☹ **Watermelon Lightweight Tinted Moisturiser SPF 30** *($28)* is a tinted moisturizer with an in-part avobenzone sunscreen that has one of the most unusual finishes I've ever felt. It blends on well enough, but once set it makes skin feel uncomfortably dry and sticky. Most people use tinted moisturizers to create a glow on skin and to add soft color. This provides the soft color (each shade is acceptable), but the glow never happens, not to mention that this just doesn't feel "right" on skin.

CONCEALER: ☺ **$$$ Vitamin Concealer** *($20)* is housed in the same pen-with-brush applicator that Korres uses for their Wild Rose Concealer below. It has a creamier consistency than the Wild Rose Concealer, and its finish on skin tends to look more obvious than concealer should. This is partly due to Vitamin Concealer's less desirable colors and drier finish. I wouldn't choose this over drugstore concealers from L'Oreal, Revlon, or Maybelline New York, all of which cost much less. The vitamins in this product are barely present, so don't believe this is an antioxidant treat for skin.

☺ **$$$ Wild Rose Concealer** *($20)* is housed in a click-pen applicator with a built-in synthetic brush built to dispense this slightly thick yet smooth concealer. It blends well with just enough slip and sets to a satin matte finish that's moderately crease-prone unless set with powder. Compared with similarly packaged concealers, each of its acceptable shades provides average coverage.

POWDER: ✓ ☺ **$$$ Multivitamin Compact Powder** *($28)* has a misleading name, considering vitamins play such a minor role in this pressed powder. Consider this a very silky pressed powder whose formula is best for normal to slightly oily skin. It lays a translucent matte finish on skin without ever looking thick or chalky. The small range of shades caters to those with fair to medium skin tones, and all are recommended.

✓ ☺ $$$ **Rice and Olive Oil Compact Powder** *($28)* is a talc-based pressed powder that is nearly identical to Korres' Wild Rose Compact Powder below. As such, the same review applies: this luxuriously silky talc-based pressed powder foundation is outstanding. It feels and finishes ultralight on skin, providing sheer coverage that lets skin show through yet look beautifully refined. The formula is best for normal to dry skin; those with oily skin will find it doesn't do a formidable job of keeping excess shine in check. The single shade is best for light skin tones.

✓ ☺ $$$ **Wild Rose Compact Powder** *($28)* is an outstanding, luxuriously silky talc-based pressed-powder foundation. It feels and finishes ultralight on skin, providing sheer coverage that lets skin show through yet look beautifully refined. The formula is best for normal to dry skin; those with oily skin will find it doesn't do a formidable job of keeping excess shine in check. Each shade goes on lighter and softer than it appears in the compact and, while all are recommended, each has a soft shine you need to be OK with before purchasing.

BLUSH AND BRONZER: ✓ ☺ $$$ **Blush** *($22)*. The powder blush from Korres is one of the highlights of the makeup line. Although each shade has some degree of shine, the creamy smooth texture and near-seamless application are commendable. Other strong points include the color payoff (a little goes a long way) and the way each shade enlivens cheeks without looking dry or powdery. This is a blush to check out if you don't mind (or simply want) shiny cheeks.

☺ $$$ **Monoi Oil Bronzing Powder** *($28)* is a talc- and aluminum starch–based pressed bronzing powder that has a smooth yet dry texture with a sheer application. As is the case with most bronzers today, the finish is shiny (even though a real tan doesn't glisten). Sunglow Light is the better of the two shades because Sunglow Warm is a bit too peachy to pass as bronzing powder (it's better as a blush).

EYESHADOW: ✓ ☺ $$$ **Eyeshadow** *($16)*. Another high point of the makeup from Korres is their powder eyeshadow. Sold as singles, each shade has the most sublimely silky texture that feels featherlight and blends remarkably well. Pigmentation is excellent, so unless you want a stronger eye design be sure to start sheer and build from there. A few matte shades are available, and these are identified by their raised horizontal-stripe pattern as you survey the colors. The remaining shades have varying degrees of shine, from soft shimmer to a metallic gleam. In every case, unless you really overdo it, the shine clings well. Given the large shade range, there are some blues and greens to watch out for; however, there also are some beautiful browns and earth tones.

EYELINER: ☺ $$$ **Eyeliner Pencil** *($16)*. I want to stress what an ordinary pencil this is, and remind you that spending this much for a pencil that needs sharpening is generally not a good idea. This has a creamy texture that gives way to a smooth, even application. The problem is that the finish stays creamy, and tends to smear and fade unless set with a corresponding shade of powder eyeshadow. You might as well skip the pencil; line your eye with the powder shadow instead. If you're determined to try this, think twice before purchasing the obvious green and bright blue shades.

☺ $$$ **Soft Eyeliner Pencil** *($16)* is a needs-sharpening pencil that has a soft application that seems to glide over skin, even with minimal pressure. That's nice, but it sets to a tacky finish that is prone to smudging and the colors are a mostly odd bunch with very little practical use.

LIPSTICK AND LIP GLOSS: ✓ ☺ $$$ **Cherry Full Color Gloss** *($16)* is packaged with a wand applicator, and appears to be just like countless other glosses. However, it isn't. You'll notice its balm-like texture that keeps lips protected from moisture loss is its main point of difference. It feels substantial without being sticky and leaves a wet shine finish that doesn't immediately slide right off the lips. I disagree that the colors are "full" (as in full coverage) because they aren't; however, Plum 27 is a must-see if you're looking for a stunning plum-red to wear alone or over lipstick.

☺ $$$ **Guava Lipstick** *($22)* is a creamy, lightweight lipstick that feels great and has an attractive satin finish with a hint of gloss. The colors are gorgeous, and provide more pigment than Korres' Mango Butter Lipstick below. As such, they tend to last longer before you need a touch-up.

☺ $$$ **Mango Butter Lipstick SPF 10** *($18)*. I wish this lipstick had a higher SPF rating because its in-part avobenzone sunscreen is terrific. This sheer lipstick has a smooth, moisturizing texture and glossy finish. The colors are well edited, at least if you prefer rose and pink tones. It's worth considering if you want a sheer lipstick with sunscreen; alternatively, you can look to Paula's Choice or Neutrogena for lipsticks that provide more sun protection. The SPF rating is why this lipstick is rated with a neutral face instead of a happy face.

MASCARA: ✓ ☺ $$$ **Abyssinia Oil Volumising/Strengthening Mascara** *($20)* is an outstanding mascara that excels at lengthening lashes while keeping them soft. The formula is slightly different from most mascaras because the standard waxes take a backseat to an olive-based emollient and glycerin. I suspected that may lead to the formula breaking down as the day wore on, but that didn't happen. Instead, lashes stayed perfectly defined and completely free of flakes and smudges. You don't have to spend this much to get a superb mascara (and this isn't all natural), but it is one of the better Korres makeup products to consider. Avoid the Cobalt Blue shade, a shocking blue that harkens back to the early 1980s.

☺ $$$ **Provitamin B5 & Rice Bran Mascara** *($18)*. I wasn't expecting to like this mascara as much as I did. Formula-wise, it's nothing special and many of the ingredients aren't the least bit natural, which is true for most of Korres' products, but the claims are so maddening (forgive me for being repetitive). Still, the brush allows for nimble lash separation and soft definition with appreciable length and no clumps. Thickness isn't much to speak of, but this is worth a try if you want long, defined lashes that look great all day. Note: This product is also known as Deep Colour Mascara. Another Note: There isn't enough Pro-vitamin B5 (panthenol) in this to condition one eyelash.

SPECIALTY MAKEUP PRODUCTS: ☹ **Face Primer** *($28)*. Korres makes a big deal about the fact that this primer is silicone-free, as if silicone were some evil ingredient for skin, which is especially disingenuous for a line whose products are filled with synthetic ingredients. Silicone is not a problem for skin; if anything, research shows it has remarkable healing properties. Whether or not this product is or isn't natural doesn't tell you anything about its benefit for skin. Claims aside, this could have been a worthwhile pre-makeup moisturizer for those with normal to slightly dry skin. Unfortunately, it contains a high amount of melissa, a plant whose various parts are irritating for skin. Melissa has antioxidant benefit, but so do many other plants that don't come with the inherent risk of irritation. This also contains grapefruit peel oil, which also is irritating. The salesperson at Sephora went on and on about how good this primer smells, but that's not a good way to shop for skin care because eau de cologne is not skin care.

L'OCCITANE (SKIN CARE ONLY)

L'OCCITANE AT-A-GLANCE

Strengths: Provides complete ingredient lists for some of its products on company Web site; some very good cleansers, including for sensitive skin; some facial sunscreens provide sufficient UVA protection.

Weaknesses: Expensive; many products are heavily fragranced or contain irritating fragrance chemicals; jar packaging is prevalent, which won't keep ingredients stable; the products are not all natural in the least.

For more information about L'Occitane, call (888) 623-2880 or visit www.loccitane.com or www.Beautypedia.com.

L'OCCITANE IMMORTELLE PRODUCTS

L'Occitane wants you to think that, because the Immortelle flower does not wither or lose its color even after it's been picked, applying its oil to your skin will somehow provide the same benefit and help it resist signs of aging. Whatever prevents the Immortelle flower from withering and fading cannot be transferred to your skin or body, and there is no research proving otherwise. Actually, L'Occitane's claim is not all that unusual; over the years other product lines also have attributed interesting properties to various plant extracts, trying to convince you that they can be passed on to your skin—those were gimmicks, too.

☺ **$$$ Immortelle Brightening Cleansing Foam** *($24 for 5.1 ounces)* is a standard, fairly unnatural, water-soluble cleanser that cannot lighten your complexion, which is its big selling point. The flower and fruits chosen do not have any research showing them to be powerhouse lightening solutions for skin discolorations. Even if they were (which they aren't, not in the slightest), the effect would be severely compromised because this is a rinse-off product and the ingredients are rinsed down the drain. As a cleanser, this foams (for those who like a foaming wash) and is a good, though fragrant, option for normal to slightly dry or slightly oily skin. It is capable of removing makeup, which is always a plus.

☹ **$$$ Immortelle Milk Makeup Remover** *($27 for 6.7 ounces)*, a very basic blend of thickeners and glycerin, is a modified version of cold cream, that works well to remove makeup with or without water (though you'll definitely want to rinse it to avoid leaving a greasy film and to ensure all your makeup is gone). It is an acceptable, though needlessly pricey, option for dry skin. The flower extract in this product is from the daisy family and has a scent reminiscent of curry. There is nothing about this that makes it preferred over many cleansers available at the drugstore, including Pond's Cold Cream.

☺ **$$$ Immortelle Eye Make-Up Remover** *($18 for 4.2 ounces)* Giving a fancy name to floral water (which is primarily eau de cologne) doesn't make this overpriced eye-makeup remover a cut above the rest. The silicone-based formula works swiftly to dissolve all types of makeup, including waterproof formulas and lip paints. One of the plant extracts is anti-inflammatory, while the others are mostly included for fragrance, which isn't the best thing to apply right next to your eyes. Still, this does work as directed. And, like most L'Occitane products, it isn't all natural; it even contains synthetic dye Blue #1.

☺ **$$$ Immortelle Brightening Smoothing Exfoliator** *($36 for 2.5 ounces)* has pumice as the main abrasive agent in this overpriced, ordinary scrub, and it's a good thing it's at least partially buffered by emollient ingredients because it can be rough on skin. The amount of fragrance is cause for concern, while all of the alluded-to plants supposedly "enriching" this product are present in tiny amounts and are rinsed down the drain anyway. This is an OK scrub for normal to dry skin provided that you use very gentle pressure and take care to rinse thoroughly. My strong suggestion, however, is to stick with a washcloth instead and save your money.

☺ **$$$ Immortelle Essential Water for the Face** *($27 for 6.7 ounces).* What a great name to describe a really ordinary, boring toner for normal to dry skin! Some of the plant extracts it contains are beneficial, but the problem is the number of fragrance chemicals that dull the positives and that also pose a risk of irritation. In the end, this toner doesn't deserve consideration. Estee Lauder offers far better toner formulas for those looking to spend in this price range.

☺ **$$$ Immortelle Brightening Toner** *($27 for 6.7 ounces)* is a lighter, less moisturizing version of L'Occitane's Immortelle Essential Water for the Face above, and the same basic review applies. Estee Lauder offers far better toner formulas for those looking to spend in this price range.

☹ **$$$ Immortelle Brightening Renewing Serum** *($52 for 1 ounce).* This water-based serum scrimps on much of what's really helpful for aging skin (like cell-communicating ingredients and skin-identical ingredients), but it does supply some helpful plant extracts and a respectable amount of vitamin C in the form of ascorbyl glucoside. This form of vitamin C isn't the most researched among the many types available, and its skin-lightening ability is not conclusively proven, at least not in terms of concentration protocols for efficacy (Source: *Journal of Separation Science*, February 2008, pages 229-236). This serum would be rated a happy face for all skin types if it did not contain so many fragrance chemicals because there are better fragrance-free options available from Clinique and Olay, among others.

☹ **Immortelle Elixir** *($50 for 1 ounce)* has the same host of problems that plague the rest of this sub-brand, and cannot pass on any of its namesake's "immortal" properties on to your skin.

☹ **Immortelle Eye Balm** *($36 for 0.5 ounce)* is a water- and rose hip–based moisturizer with a light texture and contains enough film-forming agent (a type of ingredient typical in hairsprays) to help make wrinkles look temporarily smoother. But polymethyl methacrylate is about as natural as polyester and it can be an irritant. The plant extracts are mostly ordinary and innocuous, but the inclusion of ivy extract isn't good news. Combine this with a lack of significantly helpful ingredients and jar packaging and this eye balm is best left on the shelf, especially considering that it offers no special benefit for dark circles or puffy eyes.

☹ **$$$ Immortelle Precious Cream** *($53 for 1.7 ounces)* contains several good ingredients (particularly antioxidants), but there is also a generous supply of ingredients that aren't helpful or precious in the least. And when it comes to natural, polyester is looking more like an eco-friendly material than this product. Add to this L'Occitane's choice of jar packaging and you end up with a product that is anything but precious—rather it is an ersatz zirconium. You're left with a standard, emollient moisturizer for normal to dry skin and a product that contains far more fragrance and preservative than the natural ingredients that L'Occitane wants you to focus on.

☹ **$$$ Immortelle Precious Fluid** *($42 for 1 ounce)* is essentially a thinner version of L'Occitane's Immortelle Precious Cream. It feels silkier and is less emollient, and as such is better for normal to slightly oily skin. Aside from the overly hyped nonsense about the Immortelle flower, the synthetic ingredients are abundant, particularly the acrylates (think hairspray), and you're not getting a lot of beneficial ingredients to balance it out. Almost all of the good stuff is listed after the fragrance and preservative.

☺ **$$$ Immortelle Protective Lotion SPF 15** *($46 for 1 ounce)* Broad-spectrum sun protection is assured thanks to this daytime moisturizer's in-part titanium dioxide sunscreen—but that's where the excitement starts and stops (and really, is a sunscreen with the right UVA-protecting ingredients that exciting any more?). Sun protection is critical, but given the many options that provide that key skin-care element along with a sophisticated blend of state-of-the-art ingredients, there is no need to bother with an overpriced product whose formula doesn't surpass average. There is more preservative and fragrance in this moisturizer than good-for-skin ingredients, and some of the plant extracts and fragrance chemicals pose a risk of irritation.

☹ **$$$ Immortelle Very Precious Cream** *($75 for 1.7 ounces)* Apparently, L'Occitane's "regular" Immortelle Precious moisturizers needed a very special counterpart because in and of themselves they weren't quite good enough for your skin and not worth a high price tag. But other than adding some flower extracts (which aren't precious in the least) there is little difference between this product and the others in the Immortelle group to make the price jump worth it. If anything, this moisturizer is a huge disappointment because its jar packaging compromises the stability of the good ingredients that it does contain. Ignore the claims about skin going into repair mode at night; skin needs great ingredients both day and night, and this product isn't going to kick-start skin's repair processes because it barely has what it takes to do so, regardless of what time of day it is.

☺ **$$$ Immortelle Very Precious Eye Serum** *($52 for 0.5 ounce)* is a lightweight, silky serum that is one of the better products in L'Occitane's Immortelle line, but that's not saying much because this still misses the mark compared with superior serums from other brands (lots of other brands, from Olay to Dr. Denese, Clinique, Cosmedicine, Estee Lauder, and on and on). However, it's a relatively good blend of moisturizing ingredients and anti-inflammatory plant extracts along with more antioxidants than L'Occitane typically includes. This does contain a couple of fragrance chemicals, which aren't ideal for eye-area use, but their presence is minor and most likely not a problem.

☹ **$$$ Immortelle Very Precious Fluid SPF 40** *($54 for 1 ounce)* deserves credit for including a pure titanium dioxide sunscreen to ensure broad-spectrum protection, and its fluid, silky texture is nonintrusive and works well under makeup, especially on normal to very oily skin. It would be better if the formula's bells and whistles made more noise, because for the money you're really getting shortchanged! Preservative and fragrance rank higher than the ingredients you're supposedly paying extra for (this is a lot of money for such a small amount of sunscreen), which is never the way to go. As for the Immortelle flower's "immortal" benefits being conveyed to your wrinkles, don't count on it. This product is antiaging because of its sun-protecting ability, not because it contains trace amounts of a legendary flower.

☹ **$$$ Immortelle Cream Mask** *($60 for 4.4 ounces).* "Creamy" is an appropriate word to describe this ultra-moisturizing mask for dry to very dry skin not prone to breakouts. Although it contains some substantial emollients to help dry skin look and feel better, there's also a lot of fragrance, and most of the really intriguing ingredients (such as antioxidant vitamins and nonfragrant plant oils) are barely present. Even if these extras were included in greater amounts, the choice of jar packaging won't keep them stable once this mask is in use.

☹ **$$$ Immortelle Lip Lift** *($24 for 0.5 ounce)* is nothing more than a light-textured lip moisturizer that contains more fragrance than it should to be beneficial for the sensitive, vulnerable skin of the lips, plus several potentially irritating fragrance chemicals. The Immortelle flower, in extract form rather than in oil form as claimed in the marketing material for this product, is not going to make lips look younger or fuller. Those looking to spend this much on a lip balm should consider the options from Estee Lauder or SkinCeuticals before this lackluster lip moisturizer.

L'OCCITANE OLIVE TREE PRODUCTS

☺ **$$$ Olive Tree Cleansing Milk** *($22 for 5.1 ounces)*. This cleansing lotion is a fairly greasy and fragrant option for dry to very dry skin. The amount of alcohol helps cut the oily nature of several other ingredients it contains, but that isn't helpful for skin. Plus you'll still need a washcloth for complete removal and the alcohol poses a slight risk of irritation, especially around the eyes. Olive Tree Cleansing Milk does an OK job of removing makeup, but I wouldn't choose this over CeraVe Hydrating Cleanser, which also costs a lot less.

☹ **Olive Tree Radiance Cleansing Foam** *($22 for 3.4 ounces)*. This would've been an excellent foaming cleanser for normal to oily skin if it didn't contain a problematic amount of irritating spearmint oil, which doesn't balance skin in the least. As such, it is not recommended for any skin type.

☹ **Olive Tree Toning Mist** *($22 for 5.1 ounces)*. This spray-on toner lists spearmint oil as the second ingredient and contains enough alcohol to make it a problem for all skin types. Even if the alcohol posed minimal risk, the amount of spearmint oil is a deal-breaker, because irritation is always damaging for skin.

☺ **$$$ Olive Tree Moisturizing Face Mask** *($36 for 1.7 ounces)*. Because alcohol is the fifth ingredient in this average moisturizing mask, you're not going to see much relief from dryness or surface dehydration. Even without the alcohol, this is an entirely boring formula that isn't worth a fraction of what L'Occitane is charging. Those who want to spend in this range for a moisturizing mask should check out the options from Estee Lauder or Aveda or Paula's Choice instead.

L'OCCITANE RICE PRODUCTS

☺ **$$$ Foaming Rice Cleanser** *($20 for 6.7 ounces)* is an ordinary, unnatural water-soluble cleanser that has an unusual formula because its main cleansing agent is very mild, but there's more acrylate film-forming agent (think hairspray) here than there is in almost any other cleanser. Considering L'Occitane makes such a to-do about being all natural, this is just a really odd misstep. True to its name, this does foam, but that has no bearing on how clean your skin will be when you're done. The inclusion of vinegar and lime peel extract negates the initial gentleness of this cleanser, making it a tough recommendation for any skin type, though I suppose it's an OK option for normal skin as long as you don't use it around your eyes.

☺ **$$$ Exfoliating Rice Powder** *($18 for 1.7 ounces)* is an exfoliating product that is dispensed dry and must be mixed with water prior to use. Once water is added it turns into a decent cleanser/scrub hybrid that polishes skin with polyethylene beads (ground plastic). Polyethylene is a great topical scrub ingredient, but an odd choice for a line that sells itself on how natural it is. If anything, this is further proof of how misused that term really is! Interestingly, L'Occitane included some natural abrasive agents, although their contribution is minor compared with that of the polyethylene. Although this is a novel way to cleanse and exfoliate normal to oily skin, the inclusion of a small amount of lemon peel oil makes it less desirable than many other scrubs. Of course, simply using a washcloth works very well and is considerably more cost-effective.

☹ **Purifying Rice Toner** *($20 for 6.7 ounces)* is a dual-phase toner that contains mattifying silica, but ultimately proves to be a confusing and irritating experience for oily skin. The amount of rice vinegar and lemon peel oil is reason enough to completely avoid this toner because there is no research showing those ingredients to be beneficial for any skin type, especially if your goal is to reduce the inflammation acne causes. What was L'Occitane thinking?

☹ **Rice Ultra-Matte Face Fluid** *($26 for 1 ounce)*. Although this lightweight, silky moisturizer has a suitably matte finish for oily skin, the amount of rice vinegar (which has no benefit for skin) and the lemon peel oil make it too irritating for even occasional use. Mattifying serums from Smashbox, Clinique, and Paula's Choice omit the irritants and supply skin with a shine-free finish and with the ingredients it needs to function in a healthy manner.

☺ **Rice Mattifying Papers** *($12 for 50 sheets)* are blotting papers composed of hemp coated with wood fiber and various absorbents, including clays and rice powder. They work well to absorb excess oil and perspiration, but leave a slight powder finish that can clump in areas if you aren't careful; and that is something to be aware of if you plan to blot first and then touch up with your regular pressed powder.

L'OCCITANE SHEA BUTTER PRODUCTS

☹ **Shea Butter Extra Gentle Cold Cream Soap** *($10 for 5.2 ounces)* is nothing more than standard bar soap beefed up with emollient shea butter and a lot of fragrance. Bar soap is never a good option for facial cleansing because of its drying, alkaline nature and poor rinsability. The cold cream referred to in this soap's name is nothing more than mineral oil—a really bizarre choice from a line that wants you to believe their natural hype—although technically mineral oil is derived from a natural ingredient. It gets its bad rap from the perpetual false information provided by this "natural" sect in the cosmetics industry.

☹ **Shea Butter Gentle Face Buff** *($32 for 1.7 ounces)* is a very expensive, relatively unnatural, ordinary scrub that is a confusing blend of absorbent clay and emollient shea butter, plus a lot of fragrance. This scrub contains more potentially irritating fragrance chemicals than I've ever seen in a single product, and that's not good news for anyone's skin. Moreover, the amount of shea butter in this scrub makes it difficult to rinse, and you don't want to leave the irritants this contains on your skin. Gentle this is not!

☺ **Shea Butter Ultra Moisturizing Fluid SPF 20** *($32 for 1.7 ounces)* isn't a very exciting daytime moisturizer formula, but the sun protection is right on, with pure titanium dioxide, and the texture is silky, with enough emollient heft to satisfy those with normal to dry skin. As is the case with most L'Occitane moisturizers, the intriguing ingredients make up only a small portion of the formula. Still, this doesn't have an offensive price and certainly will protect skin from sun damage. It would be far better if it didn't contain several potentially irritating fragrant ingredients, but they are not overwhelming, and there aren't many emollient sunscreens with just titanium dioxide as the active, which is great for those whose skin is sensitive to synthetic sunscreen ingredients.

☺ **$$$ Shea Butter Ultra Rich Eye Balm** *($32 for 0.5 ounce)* lists coconut oil and shea butter as the main ingredients, so the "ultra rich" name for this eye cream is apropos. Although both ingredients are helpful for dry skin anywhere on the face, the amount of fragrant orange-flower water is cause for concern. Orange-flower water is nothing more than a way to add fragrance to a product, and an eye cream is one skin-care product where fragrance should be omitted, or at least minimized. Believe it or not, the jar packaging isn't a big issue for this product. That's

The Reviews L

because the formula sorely lacks antioxidants, which is the group of ingredients (along with skin-identical ingredients and cell-communicating ingredients) your skin really needs, and that's why this doesn't deserve better than a neutral rating. You can get the same if not better results just using pure shea butter, which you can buy at most drugstores for a fraction of this price.

☺ **Shea Butter Ultra Rich Face Cream** *($38 for 1.7 ounces)* is a decent moisturizer to consider, if you're sold on the benefits of shea butter for dry skin, but it certainly isn't all natural and isn't an improvement over pure shea butter, which you can buy for a fraction of the cost at the drugstore. However, I wouldn't encourage anyone to seek out any one key emollient at the expense of other critical ingredients to help skin look and feel its best, such as antioxidants, cell-communicating ingredients, and skin-identical ingredients. Unfortunately, choosing this product is saying yes to one-note skin care, not to mention that you're exposing your skin to several potentially irritating fragrance chemicals. By the way, assuming this cream really does contain 25% shea butter, the jar packaging will routinely expose this fatty acid–based emollient to oxygen, which will cause it to become rancid over time.

L'OCCITANE ULTRA COMFORTING PRODUCTS

✓☺ **$$$ Ultra Comforting Cleansing Milk** *($22 for 6.7 ounces)*. Wow! Here's a L'Occitane product that does not contain any fragrance or fragrant plants (What a shock!), which makes it a very good option for sensitive skin. This fluid yet milky cleanser feels soothing, removes makeup, and rinses better than expected, though some may find they need to use a washcloth for complete removal. It is fragrance-free and also does not contain preservatives, at least if the ingredient list on the package is accurate. That lack of preservatives is a slight cause for concern because a water-based product like this should have a reliable preservative system, although this is packaged so that the product remains hygienic during use. By the way, if this product that's formulated without fragrance is good for sensitive skin, does that mean that all the other L'Occitane products laden with fragrance are bad for sensitive skin, by L'Occitane's own standards? Just a question to ask yourself if you are considering purchasing from this line.

☺ **$$$ Ultra Comforting Cream** *($38 for 1 ounce)* is a good emollient moisturizer recommended for dry to very dry skin that is also sensitive or affected by rosacea. It certainly isn't the most impressive moisturizer around, but the lack of fragrance and fragrant plant extracts, combined with the skin-comforting emollients, makes it a viable option for reactive skin. This would be rated a Paula's Pick if it contained a larger amount and/or array of anti-irritants and skin-identical ingredients.

☺ **$$$ Ultra Comforting Serum** *($38 for 0.5 ounce)* is billed as the solution for sensitive skin, but that is going w-a-a-a-a-y too far. Yes, this fragrance-free, water-based serum contains some ingredients that help restore and protect skin's barrier function (those with sensitive skin tend to have easily disrupted or malfunctioning barriers, which makes their skin more prone to redness and irritation), but there are other serums that best this one in terms of anti-irritants and other restorative ingredients. Two great alternatives to this serum are the Paula's Choice Super Antioxidant Concentrate and the Elizabeth Arden Ceramide Gold Ultra Restorative Capsules. Both cost more than this option from L'Occitane, but the containers are larger, so you get more product for your money.

☺ **$$$ Ultra Comforting Mask** *($36 for 2.6 ounces)*. Those with dry to very dry and sensitive skin, take note: This emollient mask (which can also be used as a moisturizer or eye cream) is a simple yet very effective formula to ease and help prevent dryness. The fragrance-free formula would have been even better if L'Occitane had increased the anti-irritant content and added more skin-identical ingredients, but this remains one of their better products, especially for sensitive skin (including for those dealing with rosacea).

OTHER L'OCCITANE PRODUCTS

☺ $$$ **Almond Apple Cleansing Oil** *($22 for 6.7 ounces)* is an emollient fluid cleanser that changes into a milky emulsion when mixed with water, and is a suitable, though overly fragrant, cleanser and makeup remover for dry to very dry skin. All in all, it is just too ordinary and unimpressive, other than the cute chemistry experiment when it's mixed with water.

☺ $$$ **Ultra Rich Foaming Cleanser** *($20 for 4.2 ounces)* is a very good, detergent-based, creamy yet water-soluble cleanser for normal to dry skin. Formulated with few extraneous ingredients, this is one of the better choices if you're considering L'Occitane skin-care products. Those not looking to spend in this range should consider the cleansers from CeraVe, Good Skin (available at Kohls), or Boots (available at Target) before this one.

☹ $$$ **Almond Apple Sweet Peel** *($34 for 3.5 ounces)* looks fresh from the French countryside thanks to its homemade packaging, but this scrub contains synthetic polyethylene beads (think plastic) as the abrasive agent. The glycerin-rich formula cushions skin as you scrub, but using this product exposes your skin to a great deal of fragrance, which increases the risk of irritation. Apple cider vinegar and malic acid from apples aren't reliable exfoliating agents anyway, and even if they were, they're rinsed down the drain before they can have an impact on skin. There is no research showing that scrubs can be as effective as well-formulated AHA or BHA products. This scrub may look quaint and decorative on your bathroom shelf, but decorative touches don't make for smart skin care.

☹ $$$ **Olive Face Scrub Mud** *($30 for 3.5 ounces)* is yet another skin-confusing blend of clay with plant oils and emollients, two groups of ingredients with opposing effects. This works OK when used as a clay mask, but only if your skin is slightly oily and not prone to blemishes. Olive seed powder provides some mild abrasion so you can get a scrub-like effect when you're rinsing. For the money, you'd be better off investing in separate products—a clay mask and a scrub—rather than accepting the trade-offs this product presents.

☹ **Almond Apple Toning Cider** *($24 for 6.7 ounces)* lists alcohol as the second ingredient and also contains fragrance chemicals to magnify the irritation the alcohol causes. Alcohol also causes free-radical damage and cell death. This product is not recommended.

☹ **Fresh Face Water** *($20 for 6.7 ounces)* contains some good water-binding agents for all skin types, but it is mostly water and fragrance, which isn't good skin care in the least, any more than eating chocolate cake would be considered a healthy diet. This is a very disappointing toner for the money; any alcohol-free toner at the drugstore would be a better choice.

☺ $$$ **Almond Apple Velvet Concentrate** *($42 for 1.7 ounces)* has some impressive ingredients and it will take care of dry skin in terms of helping it feel smoother and softer. The reason for the neutral rating is the jar packaging, which diminishes the effectiveness of the antioxidants it contains.

☺ $$$ **Olive Express Eye Treatment** *($32 for 0.5 ounce)* is a basic, overwhelmingly synthetic gel moisturizer that contains more film-forming agent (think hairspray—it's the second ingredient) than anything else. That can temporarily smooth superficial lines (meaning really minor wrinkles and for only a few minutes), but at the risk of irritating skin. The bulk of the water-binding agents and the peptide are present in amounts too small for skin to really gain benefit. It almost goes without saying that this product is not a treatment for dark circles or puffy eyes.

L'OCCITANE SUN PRODUCTS

☺ **$$$ After-Sun Balm** *($24 for 5.1 ounces)* is a very emollient balm that is a suitable option for dry skin anywhere on the body, whether it's sun exposed or not. If skin is sunburned, applying a buttery product like this is not advised because its thickness and occlusive nature will trap the heat in, pushing the burn deeper into the skin. (Cool water or aloe gel compresses are better, along with making sure you're vigilant about applying and reapplying sunscreen so you don't get burned again.) Dry, weather-worn skin would do better with a balm that includes more antioxidants and anti-irritants than fragrance, but for the most part L'Occitane seems to be more concerned with scent than with superior skin care.

☺ **$$$ Face Sunshine Veil** *($24 for 1.7 ounces)*. It is completely inaccurate to label this self-tanner "chemical-free" because it absolutely contains chemicals. In fact, this contains dihydroxyacetone, the same self-tanning ingredient in almost every self-tanner. Of course, this product contains lots of other chemicals, too—does L'Occitane think PPG-5 ceteth-20 or hydroxyethyl acrylate/sodium acryloyldimethyl taurate copolymer is a plant species? There is also the issue that everything in skin-care products, even water, is a chemical, so labeling a product "chemical-free" is never correct. Misused words aside, this is a good self-tanner for normal to dry skin not prone to blemishes. It contains caramel coloring, which aids in application because you can instantly see where you've applied the self-tanner and where you haven't. This also contains the slower-acting self-tanning ingredient erythrulose, so you'll get prolonged color after the dihydroxyacetone has developed your tan. Ignore the "veil" portion of the name because a sunless tan doesn't provide any sun protection.

☹ **Sunscreen Cream High Protection SPF 30** *($26)* is not recommended because it does not list any active ingredients. L'Occitane mentions a mineral sunscreen on their Web site, and this does contain an appreciable amount of titanium dioxide, but if it's not listed as active you cannot and should not rely on this for sun protection. This product was manufactured in Brazil, and although sunscreens sold in Brazil are considered cosmetics, that's not the case in the United States, Canada, and Australia. Sunscreens are considered cosmetics throughout Europe too, though they are still beholden to tighter regulations. Given the number of sunscreens available in the world that follow the regulatory standards for sunscreens and list active ingredients, there is no reason to risk your skin's health by choosing one that doesn't comply.

☹ **Sunscreen Milk Medium Protection SPF 15** *($26 for 5.1 ounces)* is similar to the Sunscreen Cream High Protection SPF 30 above, except this has a lighter texture. Otherwise, the same review applies.

☹ **Sunscreen Veil High Protection SPF 30, for Face/Eyes** *($25 for 0.8 ounce)* is not recommended because it does not list active ingredients. Although it contains a high amount of titanium dioxide, unless it is listed as active you should not rely on it for sun protection. Given the number of sunscreens available in the world that do follow the regulatory standards established for sunscreens in most countries and that do list active ingredients, there is no reason to risk your skin's health by choosing one that doesn't comply.

☹ **Sunscreen Veil Low Protection SPF 6** *($26 for 5.1 ounces)*. Not only is the SPF rating of this sunscreen embarrassingly and damagingly low (and this is supposed to be a reputable skin-care line?), but also it does not list any active ingredients. Almost every medical association in the world recommends a minimum SPF 15. This should not be relied on for sun protection from any perspective.

L'OREAL PARIS

L'OREAL PARIS AT-A-GLANCE

Strengths: Inexpensive, quality makeup; some good to outstanding water-soluble cleansers; nice assortment of self-tanning options; one of the best, most comprehensive makeup collections at the drugstore, with superb options in every category except eyeshadow, shimmer products, and specialty products; L'Oreal's mascaras (along with those from sister company Maybelline New York) are a tough act to follow.

Weaknesses: Jar packaging; almost all of the daytime moisturizers with sunscreen lack sufficient UVA protection; terrible adult acne management kits; no product to successfully combat blemishes (at least not without causing more irritation); no skin-lightening options; boring to problematic toners; several foundations with sunscreen still lack sufficient UVA protection; the Lineur Intense Liquid Brush Tip Eyeliner.

For more information about L'Oreal, call (800) 322-2036 or visit www.lorealparisusa.com or www.Beautypedia.com.

L'OREAL PARIS SKIN CARE

L'OREAL PARIS ADVANCED REVITALIFT PRODUCTS

☺ **Advanced Revitalift Radiant Smoothing Cream Cleanser** *($6.99 for 5 ounces)* is a good, though very basic, water soluble cleanser for normal to slightly dry skin. It cannot nourish skin or boost radiance, both strange claims to make for a cleanser because the nourishing part (even if it could do that) would be rinsed down the drain, and the radiance part is just clean skin, something most cleansers can do. The salicylic acid in this cleanser is too low to function as an exfoliant, not to mention you rinse it from skin before it has a chance to work. The fragrance in here is pretty intense, and there is a lot of titanium dioxide, which makes the product look white but also makes it harder to rinse. All in all it's just an OK cleanser with a great price.

☺ **Advanced Revitalift Radiant Smoothing Wet Cleansing Towelettes** *($6.99 for 25 towelettes)* are cloths soaked in a cleaning lotion whose alcohol concentration (as in denatured alcohol, not the benign cetyl or stearyl alcohol fatty acids) is a slight cause for concern. But coupling that with the many fragrance chemicals included makes these towelettes a source of potential irritation if skin is not rinsed afterward. Since part of the convenience of using cleansing cloths is not having to rinse, why bother with these when there are plenty of better options at the drugstore? Even fragrance-free baby wipes would be a better option than this.

☹ **Advanced Revitalift ReNoviste Anti-Aging Glycolic Peel Kit** *($24.75)* consists of three steps, beginning with the **Soft Glycolic Peel**. This liquid solution contains primarily water, alcohol, and 10% glycolic acid. Its pH of 3.6 allows exfoliation to occur, but there is no reason for your skin to tolerate the irritation from the alcohol when effective AHA products *sans* alcohol are available. You're instructed to leave this solution on your face for no more than five minutes, at which time you apply the **Post Peel Neutralizer**. This simple, toner-like formula has a pH of 6.3, enough to neutralize the acidic pH of the Soft Glycolic Peel. Yet because rinsing with plain tap water has the exact same effect (tap water has a pH of 7), the Post Peel Neutralizer is an unnecessary product. Besides, after applying the Neutralizer, the instructions indicate you should rinse the skin anyway, which essentially confirms the "why bother?" premise of this step.

After the peel, you finish with an application of **Rebalancing Moisturizer**. This is a thoughtfully formulated, fragrance-free moisturizer that actually bests many of L'Oreal's stand-alone options. The formula contains mostly water, silicone, glycerin, emollients, mineral oil, water-binding agents, antioxidants, thickeners, petrolatum, plant oils, and preservatives, and is good to use whether or not you go through this two-step rigmarole. Its lightweight texture and silky finish are suitable for normal to slightly dry or slightly oily skin, and the opaque tube packaging will help keep the antioxidants stable. All in all, there's not much reason to consider buying this product. Even though the kit is not much of a financial investment, there are better ways to exfoliate skin, soothe it, and moisturize it. More important, this is absolutely not similar to the type of AHA peel you can get from a dermatologist or at a medical spa. You can find the 10% concentration of glycolic acid in several creams and lotions at department stores, salons, and the drugstore that are much simpler to use. Plus, for most skin types daily use of an AHA product is far better than only once a week. If you want a streamlined approach, consider the 10% glycolic acid products from Alpha Hydrox, Peter Thomas Roth, M.D. Formulations, or my product line, Paula's Choice.

☺ **Advanced Revitalift Anti-Wrinkle Concentrate** (*$16.49 for 1 ounce*). You have every right to expect a brilliant, advanced formula owing to L'Oreal's claim that this product is their most potent antiwrinkle serum ever. But because L'Oreal historically (more often than not) likes making lofty claims without backing them up with superior formulas, all you really end up with is wordplay and a product that is better left on the shelf. This is nothing more than an average water-based serum that possesses a silky texture suitable for normal to slightly dry or slightly oily skin, but that's about it. Antioxidants are in woefully short supply (the retinyl palmitate they use is not the same as retinol, despite their labeling it as "Pro-retinol A"), skin-identical and cell-communicating ingredients are lacking, and the pH of this serum won't permit the salicylic acid to function effectively as an exfoliant. You're getting more shiny mineral pigments than the bells and whistles L'Oreal touts on the packaging. This does contain several fragrance chemicals that pose a risk of irritation. Any of the serums from Olay are distinctly preferred to this far-from-advanced (and incapable of lifting even one skin cell) serum.

☹ **Advanced Revitalift Complete Day Cream SPF 18** (*$15.99 for 1.7 ounces*) does not contain the UVA-protecting ingredients of titanium dioxide, zinc oxide, avobenzone, Tinosorb, or Mexoryl SX, and is not recommended.

☹ **Advanced Revitalift Complete Day Lotion SPF 15** (*$15.99 for 1.7 ounces*) is the lotion version of the Advanced Revitalift Complete Day Cream SPF 15, and the same review applies.

☹ **Advanced Revitalift Complete Day Lotion SPF 15, Fragrance-Free** (*$15.99 for 1.7 ounces*) is indeed fragrance-free, but what it's also lacking is sufficient UVA protection, making it a poor choice for daytime (and it's a really boring moisturizer, too).

☺ **Advanced Revitalift Deep-Set Wrinkle Repair Night Creme** (*$19.99 for 1.7 ounces*) is a moisturizer described and packaged as a luxurious cream with a medical look, and in terms of texture, that's correct. If only silky emollients and thickening agents could thwart expression lines and deep, etched wrinkles! Because they can't, they are good only for temporarily smoothing dry skin; they can't enhance the skin's barrier or protect the skin from free-radical damage. So in this case you're left with an ordinary but decent moisturizer for dry to very dry skin, nothing more. What's particularly disappointing is the preponderance of fragrance chemicals; they're even listed before L'Oreal's touted Pro-Retinol A (retinyl palmitate), which is truly disappointing. Having met L'Oreal's spokesperson Andie McDowell, I can attest to how stunning she is, but it isn't because of L'Oreal, and especially not because of this product.

☹ **Advanced Revitalift Deep-Set Wrinkle Repair SPF 15 Day Lotion** *($19.99 for 1.7 ounces)*. Maddening and disingenuous are the two words that aptly summarize my feelings about this terribly formulated sunscreen. The active ingredients will not provide sufficient UVA protection, a topic L'Oreal is well aware of because they have a patent on a UVA-protecting ingredient. Not only are you putting your skin at risk of UVA damage if you choose this foundation as your only source of sun protection, but also the base formula contains enough alcohol to cause irritation and, potentially, free-radical damage. Sun-exposed skin needs free-radical protection, not an invitation for more damage. I could go on about other deficiencies of this formula, but let's just leave it with me stating that this isn't advanced, it won't do a thing to improve wrinkles, and it's a waste of money.

☺ **Advanced Revitalift Double Eye Lift** *($15.99 for 0.5 ounce)* packages two products in one dual-chambered pump container. You're supposed to apply both products in sequence, because one is designed to reduce wrinkles while the other firms and lifts—an odd instruction given how many individually packaged L'Oreal moisturizers claim to do the same thing at once. Step 1 is the Under Eye Anti-Wrinkle Cream. This emollient, cushy moisturizer with a silky finish will improve the appearance of dry skin (and fine lines caused by it) under the eye. However, the only compelling antioxidant is retinyl palmitate (not retinol, as claimed), so this isn't as exciting as it could have been, though it is fragrance-free. Step 2 is the Upper Eye Lifting Gel, a mix of water, silicone, glycerin, thickener, film-forming agent, vitamin E, and the cell-communicating ingredient adenosine. This won't lift skin but it is a decent lightweight moisturizer. Combined, this duo is more impressive than what L'Oreal usually produces, but that isn't saying much.

☹ **Advanced Revitalift Double Lifting, Intense Re-Tightening Gel & Anti-Wrinkle Treatment** *($15.99 for 1 ounce)* can make skin feel tighter temporarily because of the amount of alcohol and absorbent magnesium sodium silicate it contains, but that's about drying up skin and causing irritation, which is actually wrinkle-inducing. There isn't much else to extol in this gel, and calling it advanced must be L'Oreal's idea of sarcasm.

☺ **Advanced Revitalift Eye Day/Night Cream** *($15.99 for 0.5 ounce)* is a water- and silicone-based moisturizer for normal to dry skin anywhere on the face. It is fragrance-free, as claimed. The tiny amount of vitamin A is the only antioxidant, though jar packaging won't keep it stable. Of course, nothing in this product will lift skin or reduce puffy eyes.

☺ **Advanced Revitalift Face & Neck Day Cream** *($15.99 for 1.7 ounces)* has some emollient properties and a silky texture suitable for normal to dry skin, but it's inappropriate for daytime use unless you pair it with a foundation rated SPF 15 or greater. The soy and vitamin A antioxidants won't last long once this jar-packaged product is opened, and the volatile fragrance components may cause irritation.

☺ **Advanced Revitalift Night Cream** *($16.49 for 1.7 ounces)* doesn't differ significantly from the Advanced Revitalift Face & Neck Day Cream, but it has a thicker texture. Otherwise, the comments for skin type, jar packaging, and fragrance chemicals apply here, too.

☺ **Advanced Revitalift UV, Daily Moisturizing Cream with Sunscreen SPF 15** *($16.49 for 1.7 ounces)* is identical in every respect to Lancome's UV Expert 20, Face & Body Protection Daily Moisturizing Cream SPF 20. Both sunscreens include Mexoryl SX (ecamsule), avobenzone, and titanium dioxide for excellent UVA protection. Neither formula is that moisturizing, while both of them are devoid of antioxidants or any other interesting ingredients. This is a good sunscreen for normal to slightly dry or slightly oily skin, and despite the mundane base, it's still worthy of a happy face rating due to its combination of active ingredients.

☹ **Advanced Revitalift Intense Lift Treatment Mask** *($16.49 for 4 masks)* contains enough alcohol to be irritating to all skin types, and is a completely uninspired, ineffective formula that doesn't stand a chance of lifting skin.

L'OREAL PARIS AGE PERFECT PRODUCTS

☺ **Age Perfect Anti-Fatigue Lotion Cleanser** *($6.99 for 6.7 ounces)* is a standard, mineral oil–based cleanser that is an option for dry skin, but it tends to leave a greasy feel. It's nearly identical to Galatee Confort, Comforting Milky Creme Cleanser, so if you enjoy that Lancome cleanser, there is no reason you won't like this product too, and for a fraction of the cost.

☺ **Age Perfect Rich Restorative Cream Cleanser for Mature Skin** *($6.99 for 5 ounces)*. Let me be perfectly clear: nothing about this cleanser represents a special formula for mature skin. In fact, it isn't a special formula for anyone's skin at any age; it is just a standard lotion-style, water- and oil-based formula that contains a small amount of detergent cleansing agent that would work well for someone with normal to dry skin. (But keep in mind that not everyone with mature skin, whatever that means, has dry skin!) Combined, they do a thorough job of cleansing normal to dry skin and removing makeup. The calcium in here is a gimmicky ingredient that cannot strengthen skin the way drinking calcium-contained beverages (milk) strengthens bones. Skin is not affected by topically applied calcium. All in all, this is a very good cleanser with a great price tag but with really misleading, fabricated claims.

☺ **Age Perfect Rich Restorative Wet Cleansing Towelettes for Mature Skin** *($6.99 for 25 towelettes)* are housed in an emollient formula suitable for normal to dry skin of any age, so ignore the "mature skin" positioning, which is just silly (not everyone with mature skin, whatever that means, has dry skin). These very basic cleansing cloths work well to remove makeup but would be better for skin without the inclusion of fragrance chemicals. Leaving those ingredients on skin isn't the best idea, so if you decide to try these cleansing cloths, make sure you rinse well.

☺ **Age Perfect Anti-Sagging & Ultra-Hydrating Eye Cream** *($16.49 for 0.5 ounce)* is an emollient moisturizer for normal to dry skin that loses points for its jar packaging and the mere dusting of antioxidants. This contains mineral pigments that leave a soft-shine finish on skin, but that won't diminish wrinkles (though it does "brighten").

☹ **Age Perfect Anti-Sagging & Ultra Hydrating Day Cream SPF 15** *($18.99 for 2.5 ounces)* is imperfect for skin of any age because it lacks active sunscreen agents that provide sufficient UVA protection. As you may have guessed, this is not the solution for sagging skin.

☺ **Age Perfect Anti-Sagging & Ultra Hydrating Night Cream** *($17.99 for 2.5 ounces)* is nearly identical to the Advanced Revitalift Face & Neck Day Cream above, except this one contains vitamin E instead of vitamin A. Otherwise, the same review applies.

☺ **Age Perfect Double Action De-Crinkling & Illuminating Treatment** *($18.99 for 1 ounce)* invites you to brighten and "de-crinkle" mature skin in one step, and features a dual-chamber container to keep the two products separate until the pump dispenser mixes them just prior to use. Is any of this necessary? L'Oreal claims that this packaging keeps the vitamin C (ascorbyl glucoside, an antioxidant with minimal research on its effectiveness) stable before each use, but an opaque airless pump component would have worked just as well, assuming the product's pH level would keep the vitamin C stable. L'Oreal also claims this product helps alleviate age spots and discolorations, but it contains nothing that can improve such pigmenta-tion problems. This is just a light-textured moisturizer suitable for normal to dry skin of any age, with an antioxidant content that is meager, at best. That doesn't mean this product should be ignored; rather, its capabilities are limited to smoothing and softening the skin while leav-ing behind a subtle, moist finish. This fragranced product contains salicylic acid, but it is not formulated at the proper pH level to allow exfoliation.

☹ **Age Perfect Re-Cushioning Serum** *($16.99 for 1 ounce)* has a great name that makes it seem as though it can lift and inflate sagging skin to its youthful density, but that's an impossible feat for a skin-care product. Even a well-formulated serum isn't going to do much to fight the signs of aging related to menopause, gravity, and facial movement, and that's how this poorly made serum is marketed. How this blend of water, slip agent, alcohol (I mean really: alcohol!?), silicones, plus plenty of fragrance is supposed to do much of anything beneficial for aging skin is a complete mystery, and in truth it can't. The only way to solve this mystery is to move on to a serum or moisturizer that takes the needs of aging skin seriously by paying attention to current, substantiated research to produce products that truly help skin, which means including antioxidants, skin-identical ingredients, and cell-communicating ingredients. That's something Age Perfect Re-Cushioning Serum is simply incapable of doing; though it will make your skin smell well-perfumed, eau de cologne is not skin care.

☺ **Age Perfect Pro-Calcium Eye & Lip Cream, for Mature, Fragile Skin** *($19.99 for 0.5 ounce)* is a very thick moisturizer for dry to very skin anywhere on the face. The combination of water, thickener, silicone, glycerin, and wax isn't exciting, but it does make dry skin smoother and soften the appearance of wrinkles. The same comments about calcium for the Age Perfect Pro-Calcium SPF 15 Day Cream, for Mature, Fragile Skin (reviewed below) apply here. This is fragrance-free.

☹ **Age Perfect Pro-Calcium Night Cream, for Mature, Fragile Skin** *($19.99 for 1.7 ounces)* promises users will wake up with crease-free skin thanks to L'Oreal's double calcium blend. Calcium isn't an antiwrinkle wonder, and this moisturizer ends up being remarkably similar to several others from L'Oreal and sister company Lancome. Its emollient formula is suitable for dry to very dry skin, but the few antioxidants won't survive long once this jar-packaged product is opened. This also contains potentially irritating fragrance components.

☹ **Age Perfect Pro-Calcium Radiance Perfector Sheer Tint Moisturizer SPF 12** *($19.99 for 1.7 ounces)* is a very sheer tinted moisturizer with an in-part avobenzone sunscreen and is available in two shades, Light and Medium. Both dispense out of the container looking somewhat gray but then transform to a skin tone color (well, the Medium shade veers toward being peachy, which isn't really anyone's skin tone) once blended. The color release is a gimmick to make you think the product is adapting to your skin color, but it isn't. The color is just encapsulated and released when you start blending. Although it's good that L'Oreal included avobenzone in this product, the SPF rating is disappointing for a product meant to be used as a daytime moisturizer (SPF 15 is considered basic by the American Academy of Dermatology and the Skin Cancer Foundation). As for the base formula, it contains a few interesting ingredients but not enough to make it worth considering over tinted moisturizers with sunscreen from Neutrogena, Olay, or Estee Lauder. The calcium in here doesn't have any research showing it is a must-have ingre-dient for aging skin. L'Oreal's anti-age-spot claim is also a bust because the amount of vitamin C (ascorbyl glucoside) they included isn't what the research has shown to be effective for skin lightening (Source: *Journal of Nutritional Science* and *Vitaminology*, 1998, pages 345-359). And the salicylic acid, likely present at or just below 1%, cannot exfoliate skin because this product's pH is too high (it's above 5). That leaves you with a decent tinted moisturizer for normal to dry skin, not a "technological innovation" to rush out and buy.

☹ **Age Perfect Pro-Calcium SPF 15 Day Cream, for Mature, Fragile Skin** *($19.99 for 1.7 ounces)* is yet another antiaging moisturizer from L'Oreal that lacks sufficient UVA-protecting ingredients. This is maddening given that they clearly know about the issue. But what's really disheartening is that women who use such a product are putting their skin at risk for more wrinkles. Adding insult to injury is a pathetic formulation that is about as state-of-the-art as Wonder Bread. And by the way, the calcium in here (in the form of calcium pantethene sulfonate) cannot be absorbed through skin and has no benefit for skin (or bones) when applied topically.

☹ **Age Perfect Pro-Calcium SPF 15 Day Cream, Fragrance Free, for Mature, Fragile Skin** *($19.99 for 1.7 ounces)* is the fragrance-free version of the Age Perfect Pro-Calcium SPF 15 Day Cream, for Mature, Fragile Skin, and the same review applies.

L'OREAL PARIS SKIN GENESIS PRODUCTS

☹ **Skin Genesis Deep Purifying Foaming Cream Cleanser** *($7.99 for 5 ounces)* is a water- and clay-based cleanser, but it isn't creamy, so don't let the name fool you. Most of the major ingredients have absorbent qualities while not being much good for cleansing. This would work best as a mask/scrub hybrid for those with normal to oily skin, but the menthol it contains makes it too irritating to consider.

☺ **Skin Genesis Micro-Smoothing Wet Cleansing Towelettes** *($7.99 for 25 towelettes)* have a textured fabric, which is the best part of these cleansing cloths because it works well to hold onto what you're trying to remove from your face (e.g., makeup, excess oil) rather than simply spreading it around (which would require rinsing) like some cleansing cloths. The formula is best for normal to dry skin not prone to blemishes, and it can remove eye makeup. These would be better without the fragrance, but are still recommended if you're looking to try a new spin on cleansing cloths.

☹ **Skin Genesis Pore Minimizing Gel Cleanser** *($7.99 for 8 ounces).* Describing this as a new-generation gel cleanser is like Sony relaunching the Walkman as a next-generation portable music player! Everything about this cleanser screams standard or problematic, with the latter being attributed to the menthol. As for pore-minimizing, no cleanser can make pores smaller. However, cleansing skin and removing excess oil and debris from pores can keep them as small as they're genetically predisposed to be. It may surprise you to know that's true of any well-formulated cleanser, which this product happens not to be.

☹ **Skin Genesis Multi-Layer Cell Strengthening Daily Moisturizer, SPF 15 Lotion** *($24.99 for 1.7 ounces)* not only leaves skin vulnerable to UVA damage because it lacks the right active sunscreen ingredients, but also lists alcohol as the third ingredient, making this moisturizer about as moisturizing as using vodka as a toner. What a disappointing, skin-detrimental product!

☹ **Skin Genesis Multi-Layer Cell Strengthening Daily Moisturizer, SPF 15 Lotion, Fragrance Free** *($24.99 for 1.7 ounces)* is, save for the omission of fragrance, identical to the Skin Genesis Multi-Layer Cell Strengthening Daily Moisturizer, SPF 15 Lotion above, and registers the same disappointment!

☺ **Skin Genesis Multi-Layer Cell Strengthening Daily Moisturizer, Oil-Free Lotion** *($24.99 for 1.7 ounces)* has a brilliant name, one that implies that this rather ordinary lotion can bring about the rebirth of healthy, glowing, beautifully smooth skin. Skin will be smoother and softer thanks to the silky silicone base and similar ingredients, but that's about it. A more flawless complexion is what's promised, but what's delivered is not as state-of-the-art as the claims. Mineral pigments titanium dioxide and mica are on hand to create a subtle glow, and are present in greater amounts than the couple of antioxidants L'Oreal included. For a moisturizer that purports to work deep within the skin's surface, this formula is pretty superficial stuff.

☺ **Skin Genesis Multi-Layer Cell Strengthening Daily Treatment, Eye Serum** *($19.99 for 0.5 ounce)* doesn't contain anything to make skin cells stronger, whether they're around your eyes or anyplace else. The silicone and isohexadecane leave a silky-smooth finish, but denatured alcohol is present in a greater amount than the sole antioxidant (vitamin E, an established, now unexciting ingredient L'Oreal tends to use consistently), and the alcohol's potential for irritation and free-radical damage cancels out any benefit your skin might have received from this bland serum. Applying this around the eye area will make your skin feel tighter, but the effect is temporary and courtesy of several film-forming agents (think hairspray), and is not due in any degree to stronger skin cells that are more resistant to aging.

☹ **Skin Genesis Multi-Layer Cell Strengthening Daily Treatment, Serum Concentrate** *($24.99 for 1.7 ounces)* lists alcohol as the third ingredient, and this watery product contains nothing of substantial value to the health and appearance of your skin. The couple of potentially worthwhile ingredients in this serum are found in countless others whose formulas (even from those that have been around for years) are a huge improvement over this.

☺ **Skin Genesis Multi-Layer Cell Strengthening Intensive Treatment, Deep Action Night Complex** *($19.99 for 1.7 ounces)* is a serum said to be inspired by the repair process skin goes through with each hour of sleep. Apparently, according to L'Oreal, each hour of sleep improves another layer of skin. (So does that mean someone with pronounced wrinkles can sleep for a few weeks and wake up looking 20 again?) The body as a whole goes through repair processes at night and also throughout the day. Because skin is the body's largest organ, much of this repair work is devoted to keeping skin in good shape (assuming you're not exposing it to a bevy of harmful influences, like sunlight on a daily basis), but skin cannot tell time, so the whole notion of layer-by-layer nighttime repair with each passing hour of sleep just doesn't make sense. L'Oreal could have loaded this serum for normal to oily skin with lots of good-for-skin ingredients, but they neglected those in favor of mostly water, silicone, and alcohol. The tiny amount of spiffy water-binding agents and antioxidant vitamin E is little consolation for a formula that is only state-of-the-art if you believe the claims. The alcohol just weakens skin; it doesn't help anything.

☹ **Skin Genesis Pore Minimizing Skin Re-Smoother** *($19.99 for 1 ounce)* lists alcohol is the second ingredient, making this a worthless serum. How are the hyaluronic spheres L'Oreal brags about supposed to combat the drying, irritating, free-radical-generating effect of so much alcohol? They can't. And the amount of hyaluronic acid (listed as sodium hyaluronate) in this serum is minuscule at best, not enough to help skin in any significant way. Even more problematic is that the alcohol content can stimulate oil production in the pore. This product is not recommended. Clinique, Smashbox, and Cosmedicine offer much better pore size–reducing options, but keep in mind that none of these products have a permanent effect on pore size.

L'OREAL PARIS SUBLIME GLOW PRODUCTS

☺ **Sublime Glow Daily Moisturizer, for Fair Skin Tones** *($10.49 for 8 ounces)* is a lightweight moisturizer for normal to oily skin. The glow comes from the mica, while a relatively small amount of the self-tanning agent dihydroxyacetone provides a hint of tan color.

☺ **Sublime Glow Daily Moisturizer, for Medium Skin Tones** *($10.49 for 8 ounces)* is nearly identical to the Sublime Glow Daily Moisturizer, for Fair Skin Tones, except this one contains more dihydroxyacetone. Otherwise, the same comments apply.

☹ **Sublime Glow for Face Daily Moisturizer SPF 15, for Fair Skin Tones** *($9.99 for 2.5 ounces)* lacks the UVA-protecting ingredients of titanium dioxide, zinc oxide, avobenzone, Tinosorb, or Mexoryl SX, and is not recommended.

☹ **Sublime Glow for Face Daily Moisturizer SPF 15, for Medium Skin Tones** *($9.99 for 2.5 ounces)* lacks the UVA-protecting ingredients of titanium dioxide, zinc oxide, avobenzone, Tinosorb, or Mexoryl SX (ecamsule), and is not recommended.

☹ **Sublime Glow Moisturizing MicroFine Mist, for Medium Skin Tones** *($10.69 for 4.2 ounces)* would be a slam-dunk for all skin types if it did not contain so many volatile fragrance components. The mist facilitates application, but other self-tanners offer this format without the risk of irritation. A great one to try instead is Banana Boat Summer Color Self-Tanning Mist, for All Skin Tones.

L'OREAL PARIS SUBLIME BRONZE PRODUCTS

☺ **Sublime Bronze, Gradual Self-Tanning Lotion** *($10.49 for 6.7 ounces)* is an OK self-tanning lotion that would be better if it didn't contain alcohol and fragrance chemicals known to cause irritation. There are many other self-tanners that work gradually as this one does, but without the potentially troublesome ingredients.

☹ **Sublime Bronze Luminous Bronzer Instant Action Self-Tanning Lotion** *($10.49 for 6.7 ounces)* lists alcohol as the second ingredient, which makes it too drying and irritating for all skin types. There is no reason to tolerate a self-tanner that causes irritation when so many of them don't have this issue.

☺ **Sublime Bronze ProPerfect Airbrush Self-Tanning Mist** *($10.40 for 4.3 ounces)* is an intriguing, fast way to get a self-tan at home. The fine mist dries quickly as claimed, and requires minimal blending and minimal time spent waiting for the mist to dry (though do make sure it is completely dry before getting dressed). The only drawback is the fragrance chemicals, which are known to cause irritation, although the small amount means they are not likely to be much of a concern.

☺ **Sublime Bronze Self-Tanning Gelee, Medium-Deep, for Body** *($9.49 for 5 ounces)* has a smooth, nearly weightless texture and thus is ideal for normal to oily, blemish-prone skin. The tan comes from dihydroxyacetone, while caramel coloring leaves a sheer tint. This can be used on the face, too!

☺ **Sublime Bronze Self-Tanning Gelee, Deep, for Body** *($9.39 for 5 ounces)* is nearly identical to the Sublime Bronze Self-Tanning Gelee, Medium-Deep for Body, except this version contains more dihydroxyacetone for darker skin tones.

☺ **Sublime Bronze Self-Tanning Lotion SPF 15, Deep** *($9.39 for 5 ounces)* includes avobenzone for sufficient UVA protection, and is otherwise a fairly standard self-tanning lotion for normal to oily skin. The amount of alcohol poses a slight risk of irritation. Keep in mind you will need to apply this tanner liberally if it is going to be your only source of sun protection.

☺ **Sublime Bronze Self-Tanning Lotion SPF 15, Light-Medium, for Face/Body** *($9.49 for 5 ounces)* is remarkably similar to the Sublime Bronze Self-Tanning Lotion SPF 15, Deep, yet likely contains a bit less dihydroxyacetone for a tan that's not as dark as the Sublime Bronze Self-Tanning Lotion SPF 15, Deep would provide.

☹ **Sublime Bronze Self-Tanning Towelettes, for Face, Light-Medium** *($9.99 for 6 towelettes)* may seem convenient, but these single-use cloths are an expensive way to self-tan! The cloths are steeped in a solution that contains the self-tanning agent dihydroxyacetone, but the number of volatile fragrance components (and the expense—six uses and you'll have to buy more) makes them not worth considering.

☺ **$$$ Sublime Bronze Self-Tanning Towelettes, for Body, Medium** *($9.99 for 6 towelettes)*. Assuming you don't mind the added expense of self-tanning with disposable towelettes, these are a better option than the Sublime Bronze Self-Tanning Towelettes, for Face, Light-Medium below. That's because they do not contain volatile fragrance components and so are much less likely to cause irritation.

L'OREAL PARIS WRINKLE DE-CREASE PRODUCTS

☹ **Wrinkle De-Crease Collagen Filler, Targeted Wrinkle Reducer** *($19.99 for 1 ounce)* is meant to give the impression that it's a substitute for collagen injections. It isn't. The "technology targeted to wrinkles" sounds new, but it is nothing more than a new spin on the old notion that topically applied collagen can somehow penetrate and supplement your skin's own collagen—it can't. We know collagen damage and depletion lead to wrinkles and other signs of skin aging, but whether it comes in special "bio-spheres" or not, collagen applied in a cosmetic isn't the same substance as the collagen that physicians inject; they have different properties. Even if collagen in a cosmetic could somehow attach to and build up your own collagen, this L'Oreal product contains barely any of it (though you may wonder, if it really worked wouldn't your face change its shape from the buildup of too much collagen?). At best, this is a decent moisturizer for normal to slightly dry skin.

☹ **Wrinkle De-Crease Collagen Filler Eye Illuminator, Targeted Eye Treatment** *($19.99 for 0.5 ounce)* lists alcohol as the third ingredient, which means this "treatment" puts your skin on target for irritation. The amount of collagen and vitamin E is meager, and the collagen can absolutely not work in any way, shape, or form to fill in crow's feet or expression lines.

☺ **Wrinkle De-Crease with Boswelox Advanced Wrinkle Corrector & Dermo Smoother, Day** *($19.99 for 1.7 ounces)* doesn't work to systematically reduce expression lines, but is an OK, slightly emollient moisturizer for normal to dry skin. The jar packaging won't keep the vitamin E stable.

☺ **Wrinkle De-Crease with Boswelox Night** *($19.99 for 1.7 ounces)* functions well as a run-of-the-mill moisturizer for normal to dry skin, but it cannot correct wrinkles or expression lines caused by furrowing one's brow, squinting, or smiling. This product will make dry skin feel smooth and soft, just like most moisturizers, but that's where the benefits start and stop.

☹ **Wrinkle De-Crease with Boswelox Advanced Wrinkle Corrector & Dermo Smoother SPF 15** *($19.99 for 1.7 ounces)* lacks the UVA-protecting ingredients of titanium dioxide, zinc oxide, avobenzone, Tinosorb, or Mexoryl SX (ecamsule), and is not recommended.

☺ **Wrinkle De-Crease with Boswelox Daily Smoothing Serum** *($20.32 for 1 ounce)* is a thinner version of the same basic formula L'Oreal recycles for most of their moisturizers. It is primarily water, silicone, glycerin, thickener, slip agent, film-forming agent, vitamin E, plant extract, preservatives, and fragrance. It will make normal to slightly dry skin smoother, but will not reduce expression lines.

☺ **Wrinkle De-Crease with Boswelox Eye Wrinkle Corrector & Dermo Smoother** *($19.99 for 0.5 ounce)* contains what L'Oreal refers to as a "breakthrough phyto-complex, combining a powerful dose of boswellia extract and manganese," all of which are said to reduce the appearance of lines around the eyes resulting from "facial micro-contractions." This is a simple, but effective, moisturizer for dry skin anywhere on the face. It contains mostly water, silicone, mineral oil, glycerin, thickeners, plant extract, manganese, more thickeners, vitamin E, film-forming agent, and preservatives. It does not contain fragrance, but because *Boswellia serrata* extract is derived from the same family of plants as frankincense, it has a trace of that scent.

OTHER L'OREAL PARIS PRODUCTS

☺ **Hydra Fresh Foaming Face Wash, for Normal to Dry Skin** (*$6.26 for 6.5 ounces*) is a creamy, foaming, water-soluble cleanser whose potassium hydroxide content, while not a deal-breaker, isn't the best for normal to dry skin. This can, however, be an OK cleanser for normal to very oily skin, and the amount of corn oil is unlikely to exacerbate blemishes.

☺ **Nutri-Pure Foaming Cream Cleanser** (*$5.49 for 6.5 ounces*) features myristic and palmitic acids as the main cleansing ingredients, and although they both produce copious foam (something many consumers appreciate), they can be drying and are the wrong choice for use in a cleanser designed for dry skin. This also contains a higher than normal amount of potassium hydroxide, which will further enhance the drying effects of the cleansing agents. This would be an OK cleanser for someone with oily skin, but better options abound from L'Oreal and most other lines.

✓☺ **Clean Artiste Waterproof & Long Wearing Eye Makeup Remover** (*$6.99 for 4 ounces*). This is a very good dual-phase eye-makeup remover that also happens to be exceptionally gentle and fragrance-free. It works quickly and efficiently to remove all types of makeup, including waterproof mascara. The price is great, too!

☺ **Refreshing Eye Makeup Remover, Oil-Free** (*$6.11 for 4 ounces*) is a standard, detergent-based eye-makeup remover that works best before cleansing and removes most types of eye makeup. It is not rated as highly as others because it contains fragrance.

☹ **HydraFresh Toner** (*$6.99 for 8.5 ounces*) lists alcohol as the third ingredient, which isn't terrible, but it's not helpful either. What follows is barely interesting for skin and makes this a toner you should ignore.

☹ **Nutri-Pure Soothing Toner, for Dry Skin** (*$6.29 for 6.7 ounces*) would have been a decent, though boring, toner for normal to dry skin were it not for the inclusion of alcohol (it's the third ingredient). Although the amount of alcohol is likely too small to be a big problem, your skin deserves better. This toner has no other significant redeeming qualities to make it worth auditioning.

☹ **Active Daily Moisture Lotion SPF 15, for All Skin Types** (*$7.99 for 4 ounces*) isn't good for those who are active or even for couch potatoes to use daily because it lacks the UVA-protecting ingredients of titanium dioxide, zinc oxide, avobenzone, Tinosorb, or Mexoryl SX (ecamsule).

☹ **Collagen Remodeler Contouring Moisturizer for Face & Neck SPF 15, Day** (*$19.99 for 1.7 ounces*) makes a big deal about how its Collagen Bio-Activator "infuses volume and shape within skin's surface for smoother, more defined facial features." At the same time, L'Oreal alludes to this product being akin to doctor-administered collagen injections, which it absolutely is not. Believing that would be like believing that sparkling apple cider is on par with Dom Perignon or a toy car can run like a Mercedes! But perhaps what's most frustrating about this sleekly packaged product is that the active ingredients do not include UVA-protecting ingredients. How maddening! It is indisputable and well-known that exposure to UVA rays causes cumulative collagen destruction, yet here we have a daytime moisturizer claiming to restore skin's collagen while at the same time leaving your skin vulnerable to more damage! All I can say is: L'Oreal, what were you thinking?! OK, one more thing: this cannot remodel collagen in skin and if you depend on this for sun protection, it will only serve to deplete collagen.

☺ **Collagen Remodeler Contouring Moisturizer for Face & Neck, Night** *($19.99 for 1.7 ounces)* is said to infuse your sagging skin with volume and shape while you sleep, presumably so you will wake up and cancel that appointment you made for a consultation about cosmetic surgery. It's a good thing L'Oreal states "results not equal to medical procedures," because that's the truth. In fact, all this vial-packaged moisturizer can reliably do is make normal to dry skin feel smoother and softer. The amount of collagen this contains is tiny, but even in greater amounts topically applied collagen cannot remodel the skin's supply. This does contain fragrance components that may cause irritation.

☺ **Eye Defense** *($13.74 for 0.5 ounce)* is a simply formulated, fragrance-free moisturizer for dry skin anywhere on the face. It contains mostly water, glycerin, plant oil, cholesterol, caffeine, thickener, anti-irritant, and preservative.

☹ **Hydra-Renewal Continuous Moisture Cream, for Dry/Sensitive Skin** *($7.99 for 1.7 ounces)* contains the preservatives methylisothiazolinone and methylchloroisothiazolinone, which are contraindicated for use in leave-on products due to their irritation potential. Needless to say, this product is ill-advised for use on all skin types, especially sensitive skin.

☺ **Nutrissime Reactivating Dry Skin Cream** *($10.86 for 2.5 ounces)* doesn't really break any new ground as far as moisturizers go, but it's a decent formula to address the rudimentary needs of normal to dry skin (your skin deserves a more advanced formula, but that doesn't seem to be something L'Oreal can pull off). It is fragrance-free, but the jar packaging will render the vitamin E ineffective shortly after opening. More to the point, it's about time for L'Oreal to start providing more than just vitamin E for antioxidant benefits because one antioxidant isn't ideal for skin and not in the teeny amounts found in this product; not to mention L'Oreal should be providing better packaging.

☺ **Revitalift Deep-Set Wrinkle Repair 24 HR Eye Repair Duo** *($19.99 for 0.4 ounce total)*. This dual-sided product includes an eye cream with sunscreen for A.M. application and an eye cream without sunscreen for use at night. First, before I review the products, I must tell you that there is no research showing that eye-area skin needs anything different from skin elsewhere on the face. Eye creams are a waste of money. A well-formulated face product will work under the eye area as well.

The **A.M. Formula** includes an in-part avobenzone sunscreen, though avobenzone and the other sunscreen actives in this formula aren't the best for use in the immediate eye area (titanium dioxide and/or zinc oxide are preferred). Still, it provides broad-spectrum sun protection. I wish the base formula were at least a little exciting, but it isn't. The amount of alcohol and the lack of truly state-of-the-art ingredients make it a very disappointing eye cream or face cream. It does contain cosmetic pigments that impart a subtle brightening effect.

The **P.M. Formula** is a basic emollient moisturizer suitable for dry skin anywhere on the face. There are some intriguing ingredients in this eye cream, but none of them are present in amounts worth getting excited about. In the end, this is just another lackluster antiwrinkle product from L'Oreal. It cannot repair deep wrinkles and neither product contains a signifi-cant amount of vitamin A. L'Oreal refers to it as Pro-Retinol A, but the actual name is retinyl palmitate, an antioxidant that shows up in hundreds of moisturizers and is hardly the only helpful ingredient for skin.

☹ **Visible Results Eye Skin Renewing Treatment** *($19.84 for 0.42 ounce)* cosmetically diminishes the appearance of dark circles due to the amount of brightening pigments it contains. However, beyond these minimally visible cosmetic results (meaning you won't be impressed with the difference this makes), the lavender oil makes it too irritating, especially for use around the eyes.

☺ **Visible Results Skin Renewing Moisture Treatment SPF 15** *($19.09 for 1.6 ounces)* is one of the only daytime moisturizers with sunscreen from L'Oreal available in the United States that includes a UVA-protecting ingredient (titanium dioxide). Unfortunately, it doesn't add much that's new compared to the many other well-formulated sunscreens that are available from Olay, Dove, or Neutrogena. This contains mostly water, glycerin, silicone, thickeners, shine (in the form of mica), more thickeners, film former, fragrant plant oil, preservatives, and coloring agents. The lack of any significant antioxidants, anti-irritants, skin-identical ingredients, or even a vaguely interesting formulation, makes this disappointingly boring. There are far better ways to take care of your dry skin and get sun protection at the same time.

☺ **Wrinkle Defense** *($12.49 for 1.7 ounces)* is similar to most of the L'Oreal moisturizers, all of which make various antiwrinkle claims that, for one reason or another, cannot be fulfilled. This is a standard mix of water, silicone, thickeners, slip agent, vegetable oil, sunscreen agents, water-binding agents, a tiny amount of vitamin A, fragrance, and preservatives. It's about as exciting as sitting down to do your income tax (my apologies to all of the accountants who get a thrill out of number-crunching).

☹ **Acne Response Daily Adult Acne Regimen** *($23.99)* is a seemingly sensible anti-acne skin-care routine consisting of cleanser, toner, and topical disinfectant. However, for a complete regimen during the day, you would need a separate sunscreen and at night, if needed, a gel- or serum-type moisturizer for dry areas. Going product by product, you begin by washing with **Pore-Clearing Cleanser**. It contains 1% salicylic acid, but any benefit that might bring is lost because you quickly rinse this down the drain. More problematic is the amount of alcohol, and it also contains clay, which adds to the dryness and makes it tricky to rinse. Next up is **Skin-Clarifying Toner**, which contains too much alcohol to make it worth considering, though the amount of glycolic acid and the pH are just sufficient to cause some exfoliation (never mind that glycolic acid isn't nearly as effective against acne as salicylic acid). The only worthwhile product in this kit is the **Blemish-Fighting Lotion** with 2.5% benzoyl peroxide in a nonirritating, fragrance-free lotion base. It is a simple but effective option to kill acne-causing bacteria, but you don't need to spend this much money for such a product or waste your money on the other products in the kit that you shouldn't be using. Instead, consider the benzoyl peroxide–based topical disinfectants from Neutrogena, Stridex, or Paula's Choice.

☹ **Collagen Filler Lip** *($19.99 for 0.4 ounce)*. L'Oreal is partly right with their statement that collagen and hydration are key to keeping lips looking young, but what they produced to address this need is abysmal. The **Lip Plumping Serum** is applied first, but I don't advise applying it at all. That's because it contains lip-irritating menthol and coriander oil. The irritation that results from these ingredients causes collagen to break down, not increase. The tiny amount of the water-binding agent sodium hyaluronate isn't going to plump lips one bit, despite its association with certain lip fillers used by dermatologists. The Lip Plumping Serum is followed by the **Anti-Feathering Creme**, which is designed to keep lipstick from bleeding into lines around the mouth. The texture of this moisturizer works to temporarily fill in lines on the lips (just like most lip balms of this type), but it is too emollient to keep lipstick from traveling into lines around the mouth. Further, the small amount of collagen this contains isn't going to fuse with or shore up your lip's own collagen. You'd be better off getting collagen lip injections, although, yes, you're right, that's costly when compared with products like this—but wouldn't you rather put your money toward something that works?

L'OREAL PARIS MAKEUP

L'OREAL PARIS BARE NATURALE PRODUCTS

FOUNDATION: ☺ **Bare Naturale Powdered Mineral Foundation SPF 19** *($15.25)* is one of the few L'Oreal foundations with sunscreen that contain the right UVA-protecting ingredients. However, the titanium dioxide and zinc oxide in this loose-powder "mineral makeup" conspire to create an opaque, heavy-looking finish, no matter how well you blend. If you're considering this foundation as your sole source of sun protection you'll need to use a generous amount, which only makes your skin look coated and powdery, not bare or the least bit natural. Curiously, although L'Oreal is the first major cosmetics company to venture into the category of mineral makeup, their version, unlike most others, contains talc, which most mineral makeup lines decry as being a problem for skin. (Of course, talc is absolutely a natural earth mineral with a magnificent texture when it is finely milled.) Nonetheless, the natural sunscreen agents zinc oxide and titanium dioxide, and bismuth oxychloride—the more typical ingredient found in "mineral" makeups—are present in high enough concentrations to be comparable to others in this category of makeup, such as the options from Bare Escentuals. What's odd about this type of makeup is that the opacity and the dry feel seem less bothersome than they are because it leaves your skin with a soft glow. Such radiance usually denotes moisture, but not here. If anything, skin feels increasingly dry the longer this type of powder foundation is worn. Still, if you're curious to see how mineral makeup looks on your skin, L'Oreal did produce eight soft, neutral shades for light to tan skin tones, and the brush applicator is soft and dense enough to allow controlled application of the powder.

CONCEALER: ☺ **Bare Naturale Gentle Mineral Concealer SPF 25** *($11.95)* contains 20% titanium dioxide as an active ingredient, which means this loose-powder concealer definitely provides significant sun protection, assuming you apply it evenly and liberally. Surprisingly, this has a beautiful, soft texture that doesn't look thick or chalky on skin. When applied with the cap-attached synthetic brush, you'll get smooth, medium coverage and a satin-matte finish that leaves a soft sheen. The finish feels dry but doesn't look that way on skin. Although someone with oily skin won't like the finish this powder concealer provides, it is a gentle option to use around the eyes if you don't have lines or dry skin in that area, or for concealing minor redness. All five shades are recommended, but note that they go on lighter than they appear in the jar.

POWDER: √ ☺ **Bare Naturale Soft-Focus Mineral Finish** *($15.25)* is a talc-free loose powder available in one shade (Translucent). The mineral part comes from the sodium-calcium-magnesium silicate base, and it lends this sheer finishing powder a soft, nearly weightless texture that perfects without looking dry or flat. This does a great job of making skin look better without making it look made-up, and the color works for most fair to medium skin tones. The built-in brush applicator, though stubby, is better than average. I could see using this for evening makeup or for touching up instead of using regular powder; however, the component doesn't lend itself to being slipped into an evening bag.

☺ **Bare Naturale Gentle Mineral Powder** *($15.25)* is an unusual pressed-powder formula because it is wax-based, so while it still has a very smooth texture, it tends to drag on skin and the final application can make it feel coated. Oddly, you'd expect such a powder to look thick and heavy on skin and it doesn't, unless you purposely overdo it. Applied with a brush, this supplies sheer coverage and has an attractive, skin-like finish; you just might have to get used to the feel. All of the shades are soft and neutral, but there are no options for dark skin tones. This powder is best for normal to dry skin not prone to blemishes or blackheads. Note: the shades tend to apply considerably lighter than they appear in the compact. In order to find the best match, you will need to go a bit darker than your natural skin color.

BLUSH AND BRONZER: ✓ ☺ **Bare Naturale Gentle Mineral Blush** *($15.25)* is a loose-powder blush that is talc-based (remember, talc is a mineral, too—so you can think of this in the mineral makeup category) and has an airy, gossamer texture that looks beautiful and blends superbly. The workable, built-in brush sweeps on a sheer layer of color and imparts a glowing (not sparkling or distracting) finish to perk up the complexion. The shade selection isn't large, but each is worth considering if you don't want a matte-finish blush. Best of all, this formula doesn't feel or make skin look dry or flat, and layers well if you wish to build more color.

☺ **Bare Naturale All-Over Mineral Glow** *($15.25)* has the same formula as the Bare Naturale Soft-Focus Mineral Finish, and the same texture and finish comments apply here as well. The differences are twofold: (1) the small but good selection of shades is best for blushing or bronzing, and (2) the built-in brush has longer, wispier hairs and isn't as dense. As such, it applies the loose powder more sheer, and works for a soft touch of all-over color, as L'Oreal suggests. This loses points because the sparkling particles it contains do not cling well to skin, but it's otherwise a good option for evening makeup.

EYESHADOW: ☹ **Bare Naturale Gentle Mineral Eye Shadow** *($9.95)* is a collection of loose-powder eyeshadows, almost all of which have a noticeable shine, though several neutral colors are available. These have a feather-light texture and very sheer application that imparts more shine than color, so trying to shadow eyes won't do much. This eyeshadow's application isn't nearly as foolproof as that of pressed-powder eyeshadows, and the results are less impressive too, especially because the powder doesn't completely set, making slippage and fading inevitable.

EYE SHAPER: ☺ **Bare Naturale Gentle Mineral Eyeliner** *($9.95)*. Loose powder isn't the best way to line the eyes, regardless of how careful you are. That's what you're getting with this silky-smooth powder liner that comes in a beguiling (yet practical) range of shades, most with glints of shine. Although not preferred to a pressed powder or gel- or liquid-type eyeliner, this loose powder does apply beautifully when used sparingly. The pigment is concentrated, so a little goes a long way. What's especially impressive for this type of eyeliner is that flaking is nearly a non-issue and the formula lasts surprisingly well (it even resists smudging). L'Oreal's packaging includes a built-in brush, and it is a surprisingly workable tool. You may prefer a different type of eyeliner brush, or may want a longer handle, which does make it easier to apply, but the comes-with-it brush isn't bad.

☺ **Bare Naturale Gentle Mineral-Enriched Eyeliner** *($7.99)* is a standard pencil that needs routine sharpening and is no gentler than most other eye pencils. It applies smoothly and remains creamy enough to smudge, so it's best for a smoky eye design rather than a precise, fine line. The color selection features a couple of less common shades, including Olive, which has a taupe/gold undertone that's quite attractive.

LIP GLOSS: ✓ ☺ **Bare Naturale Gentle Lip Conditioner** *($9.95)* is an excellent cross between lip balm and lip gloss. It has a smooth, slightly thick texture that's easy to apply, isn't sticky, provides substantial moisture, and leaves lips looking glossy but not overtly so. The sheer, lip-toned colors are beautiful and workable for a variety of skin tones.

MASCARA: ☺ **Bare Naturale Luminous Lengthening Mascara** *($9.95)*. The mineral makeup trend has expanded to mascara, with L'Oreal adding this good but superfluous lash enhancer to their lineup. The minerals, which are the same cosmetic pigments that show up in many mascaras (mica is the best example) are said to create luminous lashes. You won't notice much luminosity, but this is an easy-to-apply formula that lengthens slightly without a trace of clumps or flaking. It is good for those who want to slightly enhance their lashes rather than wanting to really play them up. The formula keeps lashes soft and is easy to wash off with a water-soluble cleanser.

L'OREAL PARIS H.I.P. MAKEUP

FOUNDATION: ✓ ☺ **H.I.P. Flawless Liquid Makeup SPF 15** *($13)* is nearly identical to L'Oreal's True Match Super Blendable Makeup SPF 17 reviewed below. The same comments for texture, application, finish, and UVA protection apply here, too. The difference is the more varied selection of shades for women of color, and these shades are a bit more intense (less is more, but don't skimp too much if you're relying on this as your sole source of sun protection). The 16 shades present options that favor medium to deep skin tones; there are no suitable shades for fair skin. The following shades are too peach, orange, or copper: Fawn, Terra, and Cappuccino (slightly orange; may work with some tan skin tones). Mahogany is a beautiful shade for darker African-American skin tones. Last, but not least, the sunscreen is pure titanium dioxide.

BLUSH AND BRONZER: ☺ **H.I.P. Blendable Blushing Creme** *($10)* is a somewhat thick-textured cream-to-powder blush. Each of the three shades is strongly pigmented and finishes with a soft metallic shine. Elated is suitable only for dark skin tones, the others are more versatile—but due to the color intensity, these are tricky to apply softly. They do have good staying power, though.

☺ **H.I.P. Vibrant Shimmer Bronzing Powder** *($12)* is a talc-based pressed bronzing powder with a smooth, dry texture and relatively soft application. The shine is a bit obvious and sparkling, but clings decently. Radiant is the most versatile shade among the three; Blesses is more gold than bronze, and works best as a highlighting powder on medium to dark skin tones.

EYESHADOW: ✓ ☺ **H.I.P. Cream Shadow Paint** *($12)* deserves your attention if you're seeking an alternative to powder eyeshadows or are a fan of M.A.C.'s Paint. While the formula isn't identical, the packaging and performance are the same. That means long-wearing, shine-infused cream eyeshadow that has enough slip to be blendable without sliding all over your eye area. Although the H.I.P. line is known for bolder hues, the shade selection of this product doesn't follow suit. There's a shimmering gunmetal gray shade, but the rest are softer, neutral colors that work well as base shades or mixed (and you can use this formula with powder eyeshadows). Whether used alone or with other eyeshadows, Cream Shadow Paint does not crease and is only prone to minimal fading. L'Oreal's packaging for this product includes a case with a reservoir to mix colors, plus a workable synthetic eyeshadow brush. Bravo!

☺ **H.I.P. Color Rich Cream Crayon** *($9.79)* is a wind-up, retractable cream eyeshadow in a pen-style component, with a thick tip. It glides on easily and has a slight slip for controlled blending. Color and shine impact are strong, and most of the shades are better for shock value than for shading or shaping the eye. If that doesn't bother you, this sets to a long-wearing finish and the shine doesn't flake.

☺ **H.I.P. Concentrated Shadow Duo** *($7)* has contrasting, sometimes shocking, colors as its biggest drawback. Most of the duos have more to do with creating colorful rather than artfully shaded eyes. Application-wise, these are very smooth, so blending is effortless. They have a silky texture and moderate pigment saturation (which means that even the darkest shades may need to be layered for more intensity). Every duo has at least one shiny shade, but it clings well. The most workable duos are Shady, Mischief, Dynamic, Foxy, and Saucy.

☺ **H.I.P. Pure Pigment Shadow Stick** *($10)* resembles tiny pieces of chalk and has a talc-based, slightly dry texture that applies better than you'd think. Drag is present but tolerable, and once you "draw" the shadow where you want it, you can blend a bit and soften any hard edges. Speaking of edges, using this stick on its edge allows it to function as a long-wearing powder eyeliner, too. It may also be used wet, which intensifies the effect of each shade. Alluring, Dazzling, and Majestic are the best shades for shadow, while Exquisite is an option for highlighting. The other shades aren't as impressive.

☹ **H.I.P. Bright Shadow Duo** *($7)* is identical to H.I.P.'s Concentrated Shadow Duo above, except these duos feature very colorful, bright combinations, all of which are difficult to work with if your goal is a natural eye design. These are options if you want bold colors that draw attention to themselves rather than to your eyes.

☹ **H.I.P. Metallic Shadow Duo** *($7.99)*. This powder eyeshadow has a smooth but dry texture that blends decently, but tends to flake during application, at least if you use more than a sheer amount. Knowing most women will go for this eyeshadow for its color payoff, which requires more product than you'd think, avoiding the flaking becomes quite the feat. The finish is more iridescent than metallic, and most of the duos are contrasting, which doesn't lend itself to the best look unless you use only one of the colors with another eyeshadow in a complementary shade.

☹ **H.I.P. Shocking Shadow Pigments** *($12)* come packaged in a tiny jar (with a sifter to keep things tidy) and include a small but workable eyeshadow brush for application. The colors and intense shine are way too magnified and noticeable (and not in a good way), making this best for evening makeup when you really want strong shine; in daylight it looks way too obvious and overdone. Tenacious, Intrepid, and Restless are the easiest hues to work with. This would be rated higher if the shine had better cling; the texture is supremely smooth.

EYE SHAPER: ✓ ☺ **H.I.P. Color Truth Cream Eyeliner** *($12)* is L'Oreal's version of the long-wearing gel eyeliners sold by some department-store lines, as well as my Paula's Choice line. Just like all the others, this has a soft, cream-gel texture that must be applied with a brush. A mini angled eyeliner brush is included, and is workable, but most consumers will want something more elegant or capable of drawing a thinner line. Performance-wise, this applies smoothly and sets quickly to an immovable finish. Oddly, color saturation isn't as strong as for other H.I.P. products, so you may need to layer to get more dramatic results. Still, this matches its competitors for long wear without smearing, and requires an oil- or silicone-based remover. All five shades are worth considering, depending on whether you want a classic or trendy look.

☺ **H.I.P. Color Truth Eyeliner** *($8)* needs routine sharpening, but that's the only drawback that keeps this from earning a Paula's Pick rating. It applies easily without skipping and the silicone-enhanced formula sets quickly to a smudgeproof powder finish. Try Black and Brown, but avoid Green and Navy because they are both a bit extreme.

☺ **H.I.P. Color Chrome Eyeliner** *($10)*. This pencil eyeliner requires routine sharpening. If it didn't, it would earn a happy face rating for its super-smooth application (few pencils are this easy to apply) and intense pigmentation. Although this seems too creamy at first, the silicone base sets to a powder finish that resists smearing and fading. The best shade is Black Shock, and it has a sparkling, chrome-like finish. The gold and silver shades are all about personal preference, not fashion.

☺ **H.I.P. Kohl Eyeliner** *($11.99)* has a fine point that makes precise application of these kohl eyeliners a cinch. The powder texture of H.I.P. Kohl Eyeliners also makes them easily blendable, and they work wonderfully to create the ever-popular smoky eye design. Unfortunately, unless used sparingly, the powdery nature of these liners means they flake around the eye area during application, and then need to be cleaned up carefully to avoid smearing and leaving unflattering dark circles around the eye. If you can avoid this mess, and are interested in trying a kohl liner, this may be worth your while. Each of the available shades has some shimmer, making these best reserved for evening wear.

LIPSTICK LIP GLOSS AND LIPLINER: ✓ ☺ **H.I.P. Intensely Moisturizing Lipcolor** *($10)* has a luscious, creamy texture and fully saturated colors. This has a slight tendency to bleed into lines around the mouth, but is otherwise recommended for fans of creamy lipsticks with a plush, moist finish. The shade selection is beautiful, especially if you favor bold colors.

✓ ☺ **H.I.P. Jelly Balm** *($9)*. Don't let the deep, dark colors fool you: this is a sheer, jelly-textured lip balm that smooths over lips and feels decadently soft. The colors, while sheer, are still strong enough to wear on their own, or you can increase the intensity and add a patent-leather gloss shine to any lipstick. Either way, this is another fantastic product from L'Oreal's HIP line.

✓ ☺ **H.I.P. Shine Struck Liquid Lipcolor** *($12)* is an outstanding product to consider if you want the opacity of a traditional lipstick and the finish of a standard lip gloss. This cake-scented liquid lip color feels great, and its pigmentation ensures above-average longevity, though you may want to retouch once the emollient feel wears away. It lacks even a hint of stickiness and has a thinner, non-goopy texture that still feels moisturizing. The shade selection offers a nice mix of nude pinks and riveting reds.

☺ **H.I.P. Color Presso** *($13)*. It's a shame this gloss duo comes in such awkward-to-use packaging because the gloss itself is very good. According to L'Oreal's Web site, the inspired nature of the two-sided plastic packaging means you can use and blend the colors separately or combined, giving you endless color options. In reality, the packaging simply makes dispensing the gloss tedious. Once opened, you need to use your fingertips or a brush to evenly apply the gloss because the wide concave plastic tip makes even application on the lip impossible. All of this work ruins what is otherwise an elegant, non-sticky gloss that comes in a beautiful array of shades. The very good rating is for the gloss itself; the packaging deserves a thumbs-down.

☹ **H.I.P. Brilliant Shine Lip Gloss** *($9.50)* is an average tube lip gloss that has a very thick, unusually sticky texture. This makes it last longer than many other glosses, but that's not too exciting given how uncomfortable it can feel. The shimmer-laced colors are quite pigmented and apply almost the way they look in the tube.

MASCARA: ✓ ☺ **H.I.P. High Drama Volumizing Mascara** *($10)* has a brush that's similar to L'Oreal's Lash Architect 3-D Dramatic Mascara below, and performs about the same. You'll get long, thick, lush lashes with nary a clump, and all in a few strokes. Someone asked me if I was wearing false eyelashes or had lash extensions when I wore this out to dinner—that's how

The Reviews L

dramatic the results are, yet it keeps lashes soft. The Ultimate Blue Black shade isn't noticeably blue; it's just a very deep, inky black.

FACE ILLUMINATING PRODUCTS: ☺ **H.I.P. Illuminating Highlighter** *($10)* presents two complementary shades of a cream-to-powder shimmer in one compact. The shine stays on well and this sets to a finish that tends not to smear. The color saturation isn't anyone's definition of high intensity, but this blends well over foundation, blush, or eyeshadow.

L'OREAL PARIS IDEAL BALANCE PRODUCTS

FOUNDATION: ☺ **Ideal Balance QuickStick Balancing Foundation for Combination Skin SPF 14** *($14.95)* is a slightly revised version of L'Oreal's former stick foundation, with the most notable improvement being the colors, which are now much more neutral. There really aren't any bad options among the 12 shades, primarily because each blends out so well. As stick foundations go, this has a thicker, less silky texture and tends to drag over skin a bit. You can remedy this by applying a light layer of moisturizer first, but that's not a good choice for oily areas, so blend carefully. Coverage goes from sheer to medium, and this foundation builds well without looking too heavy. The sunscreen is all titanium dioxide, and because SPF 14 is so close to the benchmark SPF 15, I opted to rate this with a happy face. By the way, this foundation is not a "fast, smart solution" for both oily and dry areas. The silicone-enriched matte finish exaggerates the slightest amount of dry skin, so be sure to prep any dry areas with moisturizer before applying this.

☺ **Ideal Balance Balancing Foundation for Combination Skin SPF 10** *($14.95)* is another foundation claiming to moisturize dry areas while keeping shine in check over oily ones. Considering the number of people who readily identify with the combination skin profile, it's not surprising that products with promises to reconcile the demands of this skin type keep appearing. Despite the name, this makeup is not capable of balancing anything, though the slightly thick, noticeably silky texture glides on and feels smooth. This has a soft matte finish that won't hold back excess oil for long; you can almost sense the moisture in the formula at war with an army of dry-finish ingredients. Overall, this formula is best for someone with normal to slightly oily skin, because it is matte enough to look unflattering over dry or flaky patches. If you decide to try this, the best almost-neutral shades from the assortment of eight colors are Beige, Caramel, Mocha, and Cappuccino (the last two are excellent for dark skin tones). The remaining colors are unabashedly pink or peach. The SPF 10 is a nice touch and is pure titanium dioxide, but falls short of the minimum SPF 15 recommended by almost all dermatology organizations.

CONCEALER: ☺ **Ideal Balance Stick Concealer for Combination Skin** *($8.99)* is a creamy, twist-up stick concealer that goes on opaque but can be blended to achieve medium coverage. The formula remains creamy on the skin, so this isn't the best choice for use under the eyes (some creasing is inevitable, but not intolerable), or over oil-prone areas and blemishes. The six shades walk the line between acceptable and unattractive peach, which isn't the best tone to use over dark under-eye circles or reddened areas. The best shades are Cream Light, Medium, and Deep. The Corrector shade is too yellow to work for most skin tones, but may be worth a try if you have minor red discoloration or prefer a creamy texture. For best results, set this concealer with powder.

POWDER: ☺ **Ideal Balance Pressed Powder SPF 10** *($10.99)* has a supremely silky, talc-based texture and applies evenly, if quite sheer. The titanium dioxide sunscreen is a nice touch, but the SPF rating is disappointing. Oddly, not all of the four shades include sunscreen, so choose carefully. You're likely wondering whether this powder can balance the skin, keeping dry areas from looking too powdery and oily areas from showing breakthrough shine. As smooth as this no-coverage powder is, meeting two such dissimilar expectations is a dream that won't come true for anyone with combination skin. Even so, this doesn't leave a dry or powdered finish, so although skin won't be balanced, it does fare better over dry areas than many other powders.

L'OREAL PARIS INFALLIBLE PRODUCTS

FOUNDATION: ☺ **Infallible Never Fail Makeup SPF 18** *($13.89)* is a mixed bag. On the pro side, this is one of the few L'Oreal foundations to feature an in-part titanium dioxide sunscreen, plus it feels nearly weightless and undeniably silky on skin. The major con is the way this foundation looks on skin—in a word, heavy. I doubt most women will like the strong, dry-matte finish and full coverage of this foundation. Its silicone technology ensures long wear without fading or streaking, but also demands careful, precise, and efficient blending before it sets. It is best for those with normal to very oily skin who are seeking a long-wearing matte finish and need substantial coverage, even at the expense of looking made-up. Among the 14 shades, 4 are disappointingly pink or peach: avoid Natural Ivory, Buff Beige, True Beige, and Cocoa. The remaining shades include options for fair to dark skin, though the choices aren't as impressive as L'Oreal's True Match Super-Blendable Makeup SPF 17. By the way, not only do the vitamins and minerals not fight signs of facial fatigue (as L'Oreal claims), but also the amount of them in this foundation is inconsequential for providing skin with any level of benefit.

CONCEALER: ☺ **Infallible 16-Hour Concealer** *($9.99)* won't really last for 16 hours without minor signs of fading or creasing (when applied to the under-eye area), but it is still a formidable stick concealer with a slightly creamy texture that doesn't have too much slip. It provides good coverage and sets to a soft powder finish that does a good job of staying in place, plus each of the four shades is worth considering. This type of concealer is not recommended for use over blemishes because of the wax-like thickening agents necessary to keep it in stick form.

POWDER: ☺ **Infallible Never Fail Powder SPF 20** *($12.99)*. L'Oreal promises their new Infallible powder will provide 16 hours of flawless, versatile coverage, but that is the epitome of over-promising. This compact pressed powder does indeed do a good job of controlling shine, but 16 hours just isn't possible unless you never touch your face, don't have any problem with oil, and never use a phone or hug someone. Infallible Never Fail Powder SPF 20 works better dry than wet. Dry it's a reliable, sheer powder that provides a soft matte finish to the skin. When applied wet it goes on heavy and has a cakey appearance on the skin. The included latex sponge is handy for application on the go, but you'll get a finer and more professional application with a powder brush. The number of available shades is small, but the sheerness of this powder means that most skin tones will be able to find a workable option. The SPF 20 is nice, but don't rely on this as your sole source of SPF protection because it doesn't contain sufficient UVA-protecting ingredients.

EYE SHAPER: ☺ **Infallible Never Fail Eyeliner** *($7.99)* is an automatic pencil with a built-in sharpener and sponge tip (to soften the line) that has longevity and a smooth application going for it. However, after an initially seamless application, the pencil never sets to a soft powder finish. Instead, it remains tacky and is prone to fading (the color intensity doesn't hold for 16 hours, as claimed). The liner doesn't smudge or flake once set, but the overall performance isn't on par with Cover Girl's Outlast Smoothwear All-Day Eyeliner or any of the gel eyeliners available from numerous brands, including L'Oreal H.I.P.

LIPSTICK, LIP GLOSS, AND LIPLINER: ✓ ☺ **Infallible Never Fail Lipliner** *($8.99)* is a very good automatic, retractable lip pencil. The base of the pencil's component houses a built-in sharpener for those who want a finer point before lining. The pencil glides on and imparts rich, lasting color, obviously dependent on what your lips are doing. The color selection is versatile enough that most women will find a workable shade, though it lacks any true red tones.

☺ **Infallible Never Fail Lipstick** *($11.99)*. Sixteen-hour wear from a lipstick is a big deal, and this two-step option from L'Oreal almost reaches that goal (as long as you aren't eating anything particularly greasy). As expected, there are some caveats and trade-offs along the way. You begin by applying the lipstick to clean, dry, flake-free lips (any sign of dryness will be magnified, so be sure lips are ultra-smooth), allow it to set for one minute, and then apply the balm-style top coat stick. The second step is a must if you want comfortable wear—the lip color makes lips feel incredibly dry as it sets, but that's part of the transfer-resistant process. Because the top coat is wax-based and less glossy than top coats on products such as Max Factor Lipfinity, it tends to be more tenacious, so you use it less often to touch up—at least that's the theory. In reality, you really need to layer and reapply the top coat to keep lips feeling smooth and comfortable during the day. Once that's done Infallible Never Fail Lipstick wears and wears, with only minimal issues with the lip color "beading" if you wait too long to touch up. L'Oreal's range of shades is impressive, favoring pinks and reds. The Zippo lighter–style packaging is a sleek way to combine both products, and is small enough to fit into any evening bag.

☺ **Infallible Never Fail Lipcolour** *($11.99)* is another lip paint/top coat duo, although this one is packaged to resemble a Zippo lighter (that probably wasn't the intention, but the similarity is impossible to ignore). The problem right off the bat is that although the base color applies sheer, it goes on unevenly, which was a problem with the darker shades. In fact, the darker shades went on so unevenly that I could not get them applied smoothly, and trying to blend it out with the top coat turned the whole thing into a mess, and I had to start all over. Application of the lighter, paler colors was better. The Lipcolour is, as expected, a bit drying and the color wears off unevenly, although a sheer wash of color did adhere to my lips throughout the day while eating and drinking. Reapplication of the top coat solved dryness issues, but it had to be reapplied several times during the day. Also, while the top coat is moisturizing and has a nice sheen, if you want a glossier finish for evening, you'll be disappointed with this. Back to the packaging: Although it is compact and portable, it isn't as convenient as the packaging for the superior long-wearing lip color products from Cover Girl, Max Factor, or Maybelline New York.

☺ **Infallible Never Fail Lip Gloss** *($9.99)* is the lip gloss partner to L'Oreal's Infallible Never Fail Lipcolor. Like its lipstick partner, this gloss presents more problems than solutions. The triangle-shaped applicator would have been helpful in getting a precise application, except for the fact that it's not stiff enough, making it a struggle to achieve an even application. The gloss applies sheer yet feels dry and tacky throughout its wearing time. It does stay on reasonably well through drinking and eating, but certainly does not last the promised six hours. The color starts to bleed into lip lines and wears off unevenly after a couple of hours, requiring reapplication or touch-ups throughout the day. The uncomfortable wear, combined with the need for frequent reapplication, makes this gloss not worth considering over better traditional lip gloss options from L'Oreal as well as from other lines.

☺ **Infallible Plumping Lipgloss** *($7.99)*. This lip gloss has a smooth texture and relatively non-sticky finish. It imparts more color than the average lip gloss, and that aids in longevity. Similar to the long-wearing lip paints, the longer this is on your lips the more uncomfortable it becomes. Unlike lip paints, there's no top coat to apply; if you want to make lips feel moist again, you have to apply more of this gloss. Doing so makes the claim of six-hour wear questionable. After all, any lip gloss will wear that long if you keep reapplying it. In this case, reapplication doesn't do much to help the gloss feel measurably better, so you're left with a pigmented gloss whose strong color deposit is the main reason it outlasts standard lip gloss.

L'OREAL PARIS TRUE MATCH PRODUCTS

FOUNDATION: ✓☺ **True Match Super Blendable Makeup SPF 17** *($10.95)* is L'Oreal's best foundation for normal to very oily skin. The fluid, silky formula feels almost weightless on skin and blends superbly, setting to a natural matte finish that is translucent enough to let your skin show through, while still providing light coverage that diffuses minor flaws and redness. The original version of this foundation did not include sunscreen, but L'Oreal wisely added one with the sole active being titanium dioxide. Now True Match Super Blendable Makeup is an even better choice for those with oily skin. The palette of 24 shades is not only one of the largest shade selections for a single drugstore foundation, but also, for the first time, L'Oreal's shades take a strong cue from Lancome's typically superior selection of neutral colors. Almost all of the shades are excellent, and they cover a wide range of skin tones from porcelain to deep tan. The only shades to avoid are Natural Ivory C2 and Classic Beige C5 (both too pink), and Tawny Beige C6 (too peach). The only drawback to this foundation is its drier finish. Although it does a good job of reducing oily shine and keeping skin looking polished, it tends to emphasize the slightest bit of dry skin, and can also make lines around the eye look more apparent. If you have dry areas or visible lines around the eye, it is imperative that you smooth and hydrate these areas before applying this foundation. An emollient moisturizer lightly applied around the eyes and regular use of an effective topical exfoliant should minimize this problem and make work- ing with this foundation a better experience. Note: This foundation contains subtle shimmer particles that impart a barely perceptible shine to the skin. The particles are so small you have to look very closely to see them in daylight, but it's worth mentioning for those who wish to avoid any type of shimmer in their makeup.

☺ **True Match Super-Blendable Compact Makeup SPF 17 Sunscreen, Oil-Free** *($12.99)* has a creamy texture that blends easily into the skin. The included latex sponge is excellent for application and once blended, this cream-to-powder foundation sets to a soft matte finish that leaves skin looking more natural than made-up. The creaminess of the formulation makes it best for those with normal to dry skin not prone to blemishes. True Match's large shade range is impressive and includes options for fair to dark skin tones. The only shades to consider cau- tiously are C1 and C2, which are likely too pink for most skin tones. Despite these accolades, True Match Super-Blendable Compact Makeup doesn't provide sufficient UVA protection, which keeps it from getting a better rating and means you will need to use another product with it during the day for complete SPF protection. If you're looking for a compact makeup with better UVA protection and that costs less, try the excellent Maybelline New York Instant Age Rewind Custom Face Perfector Cream Compact Foundation SPF 18. The irony is that L'Oreal owns Maybelline New York and managed to get the sunscreen element right with that line, but not with their namesake line.

CONCEALER: ✓☺ **True Match Concealer** *($8.95)* comes with a brush applicator (rather than the standard sponge tip), and is truly a beautiful liquid concealer thanks to its smooth, even-blending texture that feels ultralight, yet provides fairly good coverage. It sets to a natural matte finish and does not crease, though the coverage isn't opaque enough to hide prominent dark circles. Nine shades are available, and six of them are ideal neutral options for light to medium skin tones. Avoid N6-7-8, which tends to turn peach, C1-2-3 (too pink), and C6-7-8 (too orange).

POWDER: ✓☺ **True Match Super-Blendable Powder** *($10.95)* has the distinction of offering the largest palette of shades available at the drugstore. That is to the advantage of almost all skin tones, because this is an outstanding, talc-based pressed powder. Its texture isn't quite as otherworldly as Estee Lauder's AeroMatte Powder, but it's close, and the price difference between the powders should give you pause. True Match Super-Blendable Powder is suitable for all but blemish-prone skin (owing to the inclusion of cornstarch, a food-based ingredient that can feed the bacteria that contribute to blemishes). Among the 24 shades, divided into groups of warm (W), cool (C), and neutral (N), the only ones to avoid are W5 (too peach), N5 and N6 (too orange), C4 (too ash), and C7 (too copper). Shade C2 is great for very fair skin because it is neither too white nor too pink.

BLUSH: ✓☺ **True Match Super-Blendable Blush** *($10.95)* is a collection of silky powder blushes whose sheer colors and seamless application do indeed make them super-blendable. The palette of soft colors is beautiful and is divided into warm, cool, and neutral tones just like L'Oreal's True Match foundation, powder, and concealer. You might find their blush groupings confusing (some of the cool shades go on more golden or peach than befits that description), but if you shop by the color itself rather than by its classification you should be satisfied. Each blush also indicates a coordinating shade of L'Oreal True Match foundation and powder, but blush color and foundation or powder color are unrelated, so you can ignore that matching as well. Aside from those details, this is one of the better powder blushes at the drugstore. (Note: Each shade has a subtle shine, but it gives a soft glow to the cheeks, not distracting sparkles.) Compared to L'Oreal's equally impressive Feel Naturale Light Softening Blush, True Match has a lighter feel and deposits slightly less color on skin.

L'OREAL PARIS VISIBLE LIFT PRODUCTS

FOUNDATION: ☺ **Visible Lift Line-Minimizing & Tone-Enhancing Makeup Normal to Oily Skin SPF 17 Oil-Free** *($14.49)*. Sunscreen is the only antiaging element in this reformulated version of the company's longstanding Visible Lift foundation. A visible lift is not what you'll see from this makeup, regardless of how long you wear it. On the positive side, it does have a nearly weightless, fluid texture that seems to float over skin, setting to a satin matte finish. Sheer to light coverage is possible and this does an impressive job of not readily sinking into lines and large pores. The formula is indeed suitable for its intended skin type. As for the claims of containing a special serum to help make aging skin look better, that's another story. Based on the ads, you'd assume this foundation contains retinol and hyaluronic acid, but in fact, it contains neither. Instead, L'Oreal uses retinyl palmitate and the salt form of hyaluronic acid, sodium hyaluronate—both in the lowest amounts imaginable, so your skin is not going to net a benefit from either ingredient. The foundation itself has a silky serum-like texture and most of the 12 shades are great, except for Natural Ivory, which is too pink, and the peach-tinged True Beige. There are no options for fair or very dark skin tones.

☹ **Visible Lift Line Minimizing & Tone-Enhancing Makeup SPF 17** *($14.49)* is still, without the UVA-protecting ingredients of titanium dioxide, zinc oxide, avobenzone, Tinosorb, or Mexoryl SX, not recommended for sun protection. Without that critical element, forget about any line minimizing! As for the touted Pro-Xylane and Hyaluronic, forget about it. Those ingredients are barely present and have no lifting effect on skin, visible or not. On the plus side, it does have a silky texture that melds with the skin and dries to a soft matte finish. You'll get light to medium coverage and, despite the fact that the target market for this is women with dry skin, the non-emollient formula is best for normal to oily skin. There are ten shades, including a couple of options for very light skin tones. The following shades should be avoided due to overtones of pink and peach: Pale, Buff, Creamy Natural, Golden Beige, and Sand Beige.

CONCEALER: ✓☺ **Visible Lift Line-Minimizing & Tone-Enhancing Under Eye Concealer SPF 20** *($8.99)*. L'Oreal has come up with a very good liquid concealer that includes titanium dioxide as the sole active ingredient. That means it is suitably gentle for use around the eyes and it excels at covering dark circles and other discolorations. It is dispensed from a click-pen applicator onto a built-in synthetic brush and it's easy to blend over spots because it has minimal slip. It sets to a satin finish that you must set with powder to avoid creasing into lines and to enhance longevity. This can look slightly opaque unless carefully blended, but with practice the resulting camouflage is worth it, not to mention the extra bit of sun protection. All four shades are excellent and designed for fair to medium skin tones. It goes without saying that this doesn't lift skin anywhere, but that doesn't change its wonderful concealing ability.

POWDER: ☹ **Visible Lift Line-Minimizing & Tone-Enhancing Powder All Skin Types SPF 12 Sunscreen** *($12.99)*. A pressed powder with sunscreen is a great addition to your makeup routine, because each time you touch up you're reinforcing the sun protection provided by your foundation or daytime moisturizer. However, the issue of sufficient UVA protection is still important, and that's where this L'Oreal powder falters. A broad-spectrum sunscreen with the right UVA-protecting ingredients can minimize lines and help enhance skin tone by preventing sun-induced discolorations, but that's not what you'll get from this smooth-textured powder. It lacks the UVA-protecting ingredients of titanium dioxide, zinc oxide, avobenzone, Tinosorb, or Mexoryl SX, which on the part of L'Oreal is just nonsense, because they absolutely know about the issue of UVA protection (in fact, they have a patent on one of the UVA-protecting ingredients). The talc-based formula glides over skin and provides a seamless, translucent finish that won't make skin look over-powdered and doesn't quickly sink into pronounced wrinkles (though no powder is impervious to eventually magnifying, rather than downplaying, wrinkles). All of the shades are soft and neutral, too, which makes the insufficient sunscreen all the more disappointing.

OTHER L'OREAL PARIS MAKEUP PRODUCTS

FOUNDATION: ☺ **Cashmere Perfect Soft Powdercreme Foundation** *($10.99)* has an accurate name, at least in terms of this nonaqueous foundation's powder attribute. It dispenses as a thick cream but once blended melts into a silky fluid that quickly sets to a smooth, powdered finish. It has so much slip that controlled blending is a challenge, but this can be remedied by carefully applying the makeup to one area of the face at a time. L'Oreal claims the powder finish lasts for 12 hours, a marker I suspect most women who use this foundation won't reach. It is appropriate for normal to very oily skin, provides light to medium coverage, and is available in nine shades, though only five actually look like skin. Classic Ivory is a good pale shade with a slight (not objectionable) pink cast, while Nude Beige, Natural Beige, Buff Beige, and Sand Beige are also recommended. Avoid Natural Ivory, Creamy Natural, Classic Beige, and Honey Beige, which are all too peach or pink to look convincing. Note: Unlike most L'Oreal foundations, Cashmere Perfect has a strong fragrance.

☺ **Age Perfect Skin-Supporting & Hydrating Makeup for Mature Skin SPF 12** *($16.99)* is supposed to be makeup with built-in skin-care benefits, but the most significant benefit is the titanium dioxide sunscreen (though SPF 12 still falls short of the benchmark for daytime protection). This water- and silicone-based, whipped-cream foundation has a phenomenally silky texture that smooths on like a second skin and provides light coverage with a radiant matte finish that looks beautiful. If your mature skin is dry, you'll need to pair this with a moisturizer because it isn't too "skin-supporting" in that regard. The ingredients that are supposed to support the claim of "making skin age perfect" are present in amounts too small to function as anything but window dressing, but the feel of this makeup makes it worth considering if you have normal to slightly dry or slightly oily skin and are willing to pair it with an effective sunscreen rated SPF 15 or greater. More good news: 11 of the 12 shades are suitably neutral! The only shade to avoid due to a noticeable peach cast is True Beige. Interestingly, several of the shades that appear too pink or peach in the jar set to a neutral hue. There are no shades for dark skin tones, an odd oversight given how well L'Oreal did with darker shades for their True Match liquid makeup.

☺ **Feel Naturale Light Softening One-Step Makeup SPF 15** *($12.79)* is a cream-to-powder makeup with a smooth, creamy application and a soft, slightly matte finish. It's an older formula that's not as elegant as today's best cream-to-powder makeups, and the lack of sufficient UVA protection makes it a tougher sell. If you decide to try this anyway, it is best for normal to slightly dry skin. Although the label makes the ubiquitous "oil-free" claim, this does have waxes that will likely aggravate the situation for those prone to breakouts. The 12 shades feature some good neutral choices; the ones to avoid are Sand Beige, Golden Beige, Buff (can be too peach), Soft Ivory (slightly pink), Sun Beige (too peach), and Cocoa (ash).

POWDER: ✓ ☺ **Translucide Naturally Luminous Powder** *($10.59)* is a talc-free loose powder with a marvelous, powdered-sugar texture and a smooth, even finish. It feels like silk on the skin and leaves a subtle radiant finish. The amount of vitamin C is negligible, but the packaging isn't the type to keep it stable anyway. All four sheer shades are excellent. This fragranced powder is perfect for those with normal to dry skin who hate to look powdered but want to look polished.

BLUSH AND BRONZER: ✓ ☺ **Feel Naturale Light Softening Blush** *($11.99)* remains one of the best pressed-powder blushes at the drugstore thanks to its super-silky formula, expert application, and shades with enough pigment to last all day without fading. It is recommended for all skin types, and most of the shades are matte (or nearly so). The following shades are quite shiny, and best for evening, if at all: Charmed Peach, Mauvelous, Mocha Rose, and Plume.

☺ **Blush Delice Sheer Powder Blush** *($9.99)* may be sheer when it comes to color impact, but not when it comes to shine. Wearing any one of the five shades is more about adding iridescence than color, but if that's your goal or you have a disco night planned, this smooth blush won't disappoint.

☺ **Glam Bronze Bronzing Powder** *($12.49)* presents three shades of talc-based pressed bronzing powder. Two have a soft, radiant shine that isn't distracting, while Enchanting Sunrise is ultra-sparkly. Regardless of which shade you choose, this applies evenly and deposits soft color, though it would be nice if the shades leaned more toward tan to bronze rather than peach to copper. You may want to use this as a blush rather than a bronzer, especially if you have fair to light skin.

EYESHADOW: ☺ **Touch-On Colour for Eyes and Cheeks** *($10.19)* imparts minimal color but maximum shine. This soft-textured cream-to-powder product works best to highlight the top of the cheekbone or brow bone, but only if you want intense shine. It blends well without too much slip, and the shine tends to stay put, especially compared to shiny loose powders.

☺ **De-Crease Eye Shadow Base** *($7.99)* has its purpose, but doesn't replace a long-wearing, matte-finish concealer, which is essentially how this product works. It's a powdery liquid that comes in a single pale peach-toned shade. You'll get light coverage and a solid matte finish suitable for powder eyeshadow application. The talc-based formula keeps lids matte, but again, so does a matte-finish concealer, and unlike De-Crease, your matte-finish concealer works elsewhere (such as under the eyes), too.

☺ **Wear Infinite Eyeshadow** *($3.99)* comprises the bulk of L'Oreal's eyeshadow offerings. The colors are divided into Perle (noticeably shiny), Matte (true matte to subtle shine), and Rich (deeper matte and soft-shine colors for contour or lining) finishes, and the color selection presents plenty of classic shades. For example, there are a number of viable options among the quads, although, with the exception of Wood Rose and Subtle Berries, each has at least one shiny shade. The formula is very silky, but also very sheer and almost waxy-feeling. Don't count on anything close to infinite wear from these, but for very soft color and easy application, they'll do. The best matte Singles are Sandy Shores, Brushed Suede, Deep Mocha, Lush Raven, Smooth Latte, and Midnight Sky. From the Duos, only Classic Khakis is matte.

☺ **Wear Infinite Holographic Eyeshadow Single** *($3.89)* has a creamier, thicker texture than the original Wear Infinite Eyeshadows and has a bit more pigment, too, which makes application and building intensity easier. There are only a handful of shades, each with a strong metallic sheen that's best for unwrinkled eyes. The holographic effect is just a way to describe shine that in different lighting or from different angles goes from bronze to plum to dusky pink. That can make coordinating an eye design tricky, but it's fun for special occasions.

EYE AND BROW SHAPER: ✓ ☺ **Lineur Intense Felt Tip Liquid Eyeliner** *($8.29)* used to be known as Line Intensifique, and previously it was a favorite liquid liner. It still is, and one to seriously consider if you're a fan of Lancome's equally impressive but much costlier Artliner Precision Point Eyeliner. The felt-tip applicator makes applying liquid eyeliner easier than ever, and the formula dries quickly and has amazing tenacity, not to mention a resistance to smudging, smearing, or flaking.

✓ ☺ **Voluminous Eyeliner** *($7.49)* has an applicator the company refers to as a "mistake-proof marker," which involves an even, steady flow of liquid color. It works quite well, and allows better precision than you'll get from a standard, thin liquid eyeliner brush. The versatility of the slanted tip is supposed to let you draw a thin or thick line, but I couldn't get the line as thin as L'Oreal's illustration, regardless of how I held the tip or how much pressure I applied (or didn't apply, which I also tried). Still, unless you insist on a thin line, this eyeliner is definitely recommended. Application is easier than most, the formula dries quickly and doesn't smear or flake, and it removes with a water-soluble cleanser.

☺ **Brow Stylist Brow Shaping Duet** *($7.49)* is marketed to women who have a difficult time finding a brow pencil to match their brows. You get two small, standard pencils in lighter and darker variations of classic colors (including options for blondes and redheads). The color pairings are thoughtful, but with the wealth of brow-enhancing options available, it really isn't necessary to use two pencils to get your perfect shade. If anything, it can make an otherwise easy application step awkward and choppy looking. In addition, L'Oreal's formula is a bit too creamy to last and can make brows feel slightly matted.

☺ **Brow Stylist Professional 3-in-1 Brow Tool** *($9.95)* offers a brow pencil, a brow brush, and a mini pair of tweezers in one. The design is quite clever, and many will find the additions useful rather than gimmicky. As for the brow pencil itself, application is sheer and even, and builds well (for more intensity) without clumping. However, because the pencil is oil-based, it is prone to smearing and fading, with fading being the more obvious problem. It is also worth noting that the colors, which are quite good, are imbued with a small amount of shine.

☺ **Extra-Intense Liquid Pencil Eyeliner** *($7.29)* needs sharpening, but it also has the interesting feature of being a pencil that, true to its name, goes on with the intensity of liquid eyeliner. The effect is startling due to its ease of application; indeed, making a mistake with this pencil would be tough. It sets quickly to a long-wearing finish that resists smudging or fading. Note that all of the shades have a sparkling shine. This pencil would be rated a Paula's Pick if it didn't require sharpening.

☺ **Le Kohl Duo Shadow + Liner Smooth Defining Pencil + Powder Eye Shadow** *($9.49)* is a dual-sided pencil that includes a standard, needs-sharpening eyeliner on one end and a pointed sponge tip on the other. The cap for the sponge-tip portion of the pencil houses a tiny disc of powder eyeshadow. Every time you replace the cap, more powder eyeshadow is deposited onto the sponge. Both sides are easy to apply and come in a range of well-coordinated colors. The pencil has a slight tendency to smudge and fade, but this is primarily a problem for those struggling with oily eyelids (in which case one of the long-wearing gel eyeliners is a much better choice). This would rate a happy face if not for the fact that the pencil portion needs routine sharpening.

☺ **Le Kohl Smooth Defining Eyeliner** *($7.49)* is a standard, needs-sharpening pencil reminiscent of Lancome's Le Crayon Kohl ($22). It applies smoothly without being greasy and stays in place quite well. The shade selection has been edited down to just the classics, and all of them have merit.

☺ **MicroLiner Ultra Fine Eyeliner** *($8.29)* is a needs-sharpening pencil that promises "the precision of a liquid liner." Considering how tough it is to be precise with a liquid liner, that's not much of a claim! The advantage of this pencil is its slender tip that allows for a thin, discrete line, or you can build the line for more drama. Because this stays creamy, some smudging is apparent by day's end (much sooner if you have oily eyelids), but it is an option if you prefer pencil and want a very fine line.

☺ **Pencil Perfect Automatic Eye Liner** *($7.49)* isn't what I would call perfect; if anything, it tends to go on creamier than most and that means greater risk of smearing. As a plus, it doesn't need sharpening, but it's nonretractable, so don't wind up more than you need. Avoid green Sage and the self-explanatory Paris Blue.

☺ **Telescopic Precision Liquid Eyeliner** *($7.99)* is outfitted with an excellent slanted-tip brush that makes it relatively easy to draw an even line following the curvature of the eye. The formula takes a bit longer to dry than usual, which can encourage smearing, but what's most disappointing is that the color saturation runs out before you've made it to the end of the lash line, necessitating another application. This stays in place and wears quite well once set, but it turns out to be a liquid eyeliner that demands more patience than many others, including L'Oreal's own Lineur Intense Felt Tip Liquid Eyeliner.

☺ **Wear Infinite Soft Powder Eye Liner** *($7.19)* is a standard pencil with a swift, smooth application and a reliable powder finish. If you prefer pencils and don't mind routine sharpening, this is one to consider because it is less likely to smudge or fade than many others. However, the color selection is mostly shiny, and there are several hues that are inappropriate for lining the eyes, unless you're going for all-out techno-glamour.

☺ **Wear Infinite Waterproof Self-Sharpening Eyeliner** *($7.49)* is an automatic, nonretractable pencil with a thick tip that makes it tricky to draw a thin line. Application is easy due to this pencil's smooth glide, but its finish is somewhat sticky. It is partially waterproof and getting it wet results in some loss of color, but you'll still have some definition.

☹ **Lineur Intense Brush Tip Liquid Eyeliner** *($7.99)* is a surprisingly bad liquid liner. The main problem is the stiff brush that tends to splay and deposit color unevenly. The formula dries quickly, but remains smear-prone longer than it should, which is reason enough to leave this on the shelf.

LIPSTICK, LIP GLOSS AND LIPLINER: ✓ ☺ **Colour Riche Lip Gloss** *($5.49)* is L'Oreal's best lip gloss, period! It has a silky yet moisturizing texture that imparts sheer to medium color (depending on the shade) and leaves lips with a glossy finish free of stickiness. The shades, including the goes-with-anything Rich Pink, are bound to please—and don't be nervous about trying the deeper hues; each goes on softer than it appears.

✓ ☺ **Glam Shine Dazzling Plumping Lipcolour** *($8.99)* makes lips look plump only by virtue of its coverage and shimmery finish. However, do take the "glam" part of this name seriously, because each color (mauve and plum tones dominate) is definitely about putting the spotlight on lips. This lightweight, slightly creamy gloss feels supremely smooth and completely non-sticky, and has longer-than-average staying power.

☺ **Colour Juice Stick** *($9.49)* advertises "sheer, light, luscious" as its selling points, yet this creamy lipstick isn't nearly as lightweight as L'Oreal's Endless Comfortable 8-Hour Lipcolour, nor are the colors that sheer. Rather, this is a moisturizing, light-coverage lipstick with a soft glossy finish and an enticing range of fruit-scented colors. Despite the glossy finish, this isn't too slippery, and lasts a bit longer than standard glossy lipsticks.

☺ **Colour Riche Anti-Feathering Lipliner** *($7.79)* is a standard, twist-up, retractable pencil with a built-in sharpener. The sharpener part isn't really necessary given the finer point that most twist-up pencils like this one already have; plus, after one use the shavings clog the sharpener and that's that. Application is smooth and creamy, and the available colors are versatile. Oh, and it does a great job of preventing lipstick from feathering into lines around the mouth!

☺ **Colour Juice Sheer Juicy Lip Gloss** *($7.79)* is a tube lip gloss that comes in a dazzling array of shades, from sheer cherry to sparkling pale gold and peachy bronze tones. As glosses go this is nothing exceptional, but the deeper shades impart longer-lasting color and the formula provides a minimally sticky, wet-look finish that leaves lips feeling moist rather than slippery. I actually preferred this to Lancome's Juicy Tubes Ultra-Shiny Lip Gloss ($17.50) and encourage you to compare them and walk away with the savings when you notice how much better the L'Oreal version is.

☺ **Colour Riche Nurturing and Protective Lipcolour** *($7.49)* is rich in every way except price, which is a boon for you and your lips! This decadently creamy lipstick offers intense colors that have admirable staying power, although it is creamy enough to slip into lines around the mouth. You'll find this almost identical to Lancome's Rouge Sensation Multi-Sensation Lip-Colour, right down to the fragrance. In terms of being nurturing and protective, it is no more so than many other creamy lipsticks. L'Oreal's in-store displays nicely divide this large collection of lipsticks into color families, making it easy to find the type of shades you like.

☺ **Endless Comfortable 8-Hour Lipcolour** *($9.99)* feels remarkably light and has a minimally creamy finish, yet imparts intense, pulls-no-punches color that really lasts, although not for eight hours. You'll need to touch up after coffee breaks or eating (this isn't a transfer-resistant formula), but for the most part this leaves standard creamy lipsticks behind in the longevity department. The Endless Platinum colors are infused with lots of silver glitter and have a slight metallic finish, but are otherwise identical to the original formula. (The Platinum version is packaged in silver while the other colors come in a gold tube.)

☺ **Endless Kissable ShineWear, The Glossiest Zero-Transfer Lip Duo** *($9.99)* is a two-part system that's somewhat of a spin on long-wearing lip products such as Max Factor's Lipfinity. Lancome fans will recognize this duo as being nearly identical to the company's Juicy Wear Ultra-Lasting Full Colour and Shine Lip Duo ($25.50). The concept is the same: Apply a seemingly regular lipstick, allow one or two minutes for it to set, then (because lips will feel dry and tight) slather your lips with an ultra-shiny, wet-look gloss. The gloss ensures comfortable wear without causing the lipstick color to fade, travel into lines, or smear. If you follow the instructions, this (just like Lancome's version) really does stay put for hours and transfers minimally onto napkins, coffee cups, and significant others. The all-silicone gloss coat feels slick and unlike traditional gloss, but if you find its texture agreeable, it allows for even wear—no balling, chipping, or peeling lipstick. I still prefer Estee Lauder's and M.A.C.'s versions to this, but L'Oreal comes close, the price is right, and the shade range is tempting.

☺ **Colour Riche Anti-Aging Serum Lipstick** *($7.99)*. This very fragrant lipstick includes a clear or tinted (depending on the shade) moisture core that supposedly contains an antiaging serum composed of collagen and L'Oreal's sugar ingredient Pro-Xylane. The sticker on the side of this creamy lipstick advises users that they may feel a slight tingling sensation, and the first several minutes you have this on, that is indeed the case. Perusing the ingredient list, I saw nothing obvious that would cause the tingling I felt or that would prompt L'Oreal to issue that cautionary statement. This lipstick is oil-based and greasy enough to slip into lines around the mouth, but its only unique ingredient is argan oil, and the formula contains only a tiny amount of it. I suspect the tingling came from the fragrance chemicals that are present, or simply from the amount of fragrance itself. In either case, the tingling is a sign that your lips are being irritated, and in no way is this lipstick head and shoulders above many other cream lipsticks. One more thing: The ingredient list does not include collagen or xylane, but that's OK because they have no antiaging effect on lips anyway.

☺ **Endless Kissable Lipcolour** *($8.79)* promises to be a "zero-transfer, extremely long lasting" experience for your lips. I am pleased to report that this lipstick succeeds in staying put and, aside from the occasional trace of color, does not transfer onto objects (think coffee cups) or people (think a friendly "hello" kiss, not a passionate smooch). Its matte-finish formula dries quickly, leaving pigment on your lips without a trace of moisture or gloss, so your lips have color, but no slip or moistness. The instructions state that this product is not to be used with another balm, lip gloss, or lipstick, an advisory I found wise, because adding an emollient product on top of this lipstick definitely cuts its longevity. However, because this lipstick makes lips feel dry, most women will want to pair it with something that feels creamy, as I did, which only minimally affected the staying power. It's worth a try, but it's not in the same league as two-step products such as Max Factor's Lipfinity or M.A.C.'s Pro Longwear Lipcolour.

☺ **Crayon Petite Automatic Lip Liner** *($7.49)*. Crayon Petite Automatic Lip Liner is an automatic, nonretractable lip pencil that is definitely creamier than most and offers some good colors, including a Clear version. Unlike the Colour Riche Anti-Feathering Lipliner, this doesn't stop lipstick from bleeding into lines around the mouth.

☺ **Volume Perfect Re-Shaping Lipcolour** *($9.99)* is a dual-ended lipstick. One side is a colorless lip balm/stick that is supposed to fill in lines and ridges on the lips. This is a "primer" step, and is said to create a uniform surface that allows the lipstick to go on more smoothly, resulting in lips that appear fuller and more youthful. The ads for this lipstick (featuring the unquestionably gorgeous Andie MacDowell) make it look as if her lips have almost no lines at all. Your real-world experience will prove otherwise—the lip primer feels like a silicone and wax mixture, and makes little visible difference when the lipstick is applied over it. Actually, I preferred the way the lipstick looked without the primer underneath. Even though the extra step isn't warranted, this is a decent creamy lipstick whose semi-opaque colors come in a striking palette, though most are infused with large particles of silver shimmer, which tend to stay on (and around) the lips as the color fades—not the best look for the mature woman this product is targeted toward.

MASCARA: ✓ ☺ **Double Extend Lash Extender & Magnifier Mascara** *($10.49)* is a dual-ended mascara, including a lash "Magnifier" (primer) on one end and actual mascara on the other. The Lash Magnifier is just clear mascara, adding extra layers that you can't really see. It's no different from adding extra layers of the black mascara on the other end of the tube, so it's a relatively unnecessary step because this mascara does magnificently well on its own, building incredible length and thickness without clumps or flakes.

✓ ☺ **Lash Architect 3-D Dramatic Mascara** *($8.29)* remains a prime pick if your goal is long, thick, dramatic lashes. With just a few sweeps lashes go from blah to wow, with only minor clumping (and only then if you're overzealous during application). Whether you use the straight or curved brush option you will not be disappointed; either formula also leaves lashes curled in a way the Panoramic Curl Extreme Mascara can't touch.

✓ ☺ **Voluminous Full Definition Volume Building Mascara** *($6.99)* is another stellar mascara from L'Oreal. This formula closely matches, if not mimics, the performance of Lancome's Definicils Mascara *($23)*, meaning it excels at creating long, softly fringed, and separated lashes with some thickness. It keeps lashes soft yet wears all day without smudging or flaking, and comes off easily with a water-soluble cleanser.

✓ ☺ **Voluminous Naturale Natural-Looking Volume & Definition Mascara** *($6.99)* is the first Voluminous mascara to use the new rubber-bristled brush applicator. This style of brush has really caught on, and many women now prefer it to traditional nylon bristles (though there are still many mascaras with nylon brushes that are just as, if not more, impressive). This offering from L'Oreal produces prodigious length and clean definition with just a few strokes. Building thickness takes some effort, but can be done, and without leaving lashes looking heavy or spiky. True to claim, this really is 100% clump-free. It stays on quite well, and removes easily with a water-soluble cleanser. Compared with L'Oreal's original Voluminous Mascara, this version provides greater thickness, but otherwise is very similar, save for the different brushes.

☺ **Double Extend Beauty Tubes Lash Extension Effect Mascara** *($10.99)* is a two-step mascara involving the typical white, wax-based primer followed by mascara. The point of difference is that the mascara forms tubes around each lash, but other than easy removal you won't gain any performance difference by choosing this concept over a traditional mascara formula.

If anything, the tubes (which really do come off with water and slight agitation) can stick to your skin during the rinsing process. That's not a deal-breaker, but something to be aware of if you decide to try this mascara. Overall, the primer adds bulk and separation to lashes while the mascara extends lashes to an impressive length. Although this is recommended, I have to give the price and performance edge to Maybelline's similar (non-tube-forming) XXL Extensions XX-Treme Length Microfiber Mascara. Maybelline's version makes lashes even longer and adds more thickness, too. (Oh, and by the way, Maybelline is owned by L'Oreal.)

☺ **Double Extend Lash Fortifier & Extender Mascara Waterproof** *($10.49)* is a dual-ended mascara with a lash primer/conditioner on one end and mascara on the other. You apply the white "Extender" first and then sweep on the mascara. Supposedly, this pairing should bring about "lush lashes up to 60% longer," but what ends up happening is that the results with the Extender, though assuredly impressive, are the same as applying two or three coats of the mascara alone, which is exactly what I did. When I asked friends if the lashes on one eyelid looked longer, thicker, and more dramatic than the other, no one could tell a difference. Both the Extender and the mascara contain ingredients necessary for a waterproof mascara, and true to claim, this does not budge when lashes are wet, nor does it clump during application or flake during wear. This is another stellar mascara, but one that doesn't need the gimmick of a primer step to sell itself.

☺ **Extra-Volume Collagen Hydra Collagen Plumping Mascara** *($7.99)*. Let me state from the start, just so there are no false notions about this mascara: the amount of collagen this contains is so tiny that even if it could have an impact, there isn't enough for even a minute segment of eyelashes to notice. However, collagen has nothing to do with hair growth or thickness. Collagen is a support structure in skin, it isn't related to the hair. What does plump lashes is the combination of this mascara's brush and the waxes in the formula, just like every other mascara on the market. You'll get lots of length and enhanced volume without clumps, plus near-perfect lash separation with minimal effort. This isn't much for significant thickness, but it leaves lashes softly curled and wears without flaking or smearing. If you're already using and liking one of L'Oreal's other mascaras, there is no reason to jump ship and switch to this one. It's a very good mascara, but other than the laughable collagen-plumping claim, it doesn't distinguish itself from their best.

☺ **Extra-Volume Collagen Waterproof Mascara** *($11.99)* is waterproof as claimed and, after several coats, builds remarkable length and some thickness. There's a bit of clumping along the way and it smears easily while applying, so be extra careful. Otherwise, it's another good mascara from L'Oreal. As for the collagen, it is a minor part of the formula, but in any amount, collagen isn't going to plump lashes from the inside out, no more than a moisturizer with collagen will fill wrinkles.

☺ **FeatherLash Water Resistant Mascara** *($7.49)* is marginally adept at lengthening, but won't build even a hint of thickness. It goes on easily, with no globs or clumps, but be prepared to work for anything more than a subtle effect. What's best about this mascara is that lashes stay soft to the touch and the formula nicely resists water, yet is easily removed with a water-soluble cleanser. Those traits make it worthy of a happy face rating.

☺ **Lash Out Waterproof Lengthening and Separating Mascara** *($7.49)* produces better-than-average length and creates lifted, slightly curled lashes that remain soft. The formula is waterproof, too.

☺ **Panoramic Curl Extreme Curl & Separating Mascara** *($8.49)* disappoints when it comes to curling lashes. It can go on a bit unevenly, but the brush allows for easy comb-through—and once dry, the formula wears and removes well. This is still a worthwhile option for equal parts moderate length and thickness.

☺ **Panoramic Curl Extreme Curl & Separating Waterproof Mascara** *($8.49)* leaves lashes soft while being tenaciously waterproof and allowing you to build long lashes that maintain a slight curl. You'll get a bit of thickness, too, and no clumps or flakes, which make this one of L'Oreal's better waterproof mascaras.

☺ **Telescopic Mascara** *($7.99)* is L'Oreal's version of Lancome's superior Fatale Exceptional Volume Sculpting 3D Comb-Mascara. Lancome's version has the edge due to a better application, but results with either mascara amount to dramatically long, thick lashes. Telescopic uses a multisided comb (rather than brush) applicator and its biggest problem is immediate clumping and a too-heavy appearance. Luckily, the flipside of the comb allows for smoothing things out, but it still takes patience (and perhaps a separate lash comb or brush) to get all the clumps combed through. Although this mascara does not apply in a wink, it wears beautifully all day and keeps lashes soft.

☺ **Volume Shocking Mascara** *($12.99)* is shocking, at least if you're used to average or natural-look mascaras! This two-step mascara includes a **Lash Defining Base Coat** and a **Volume Constructing Top Coat**. The Base Coat is a white "primer" whose formula is similar to that of most mascaras, minus the pigment. It nicely separates and lengthens lashes, but things really get exciting when you apply the Top Coat. It goes on with a comb instead of a brush applicator, and the result is a heavier application of mascara that dramatically lengthens, thickens, and curls with a few strokes. As usual, I applied the primer step on one set of lashes and then used just the mascara on the other. Usually the difference isn't noticeable, but it was this time, albeit marginally. The side with the Base Coat produced fewer clumps when the Top Coat was applied, although some clumping was apparent with or without the Base Coat, as was minor flaking during wear. That's the trade-off if you decide to try this product: magnificently enhanced lashes, but an application process that demands precision and, preferably, a clean brush to comb through lashes so clumps are smoothed out. This is surprisingly easy to remove with a water-soluble cleanser.

☺ **Voluminous Original Volume Building Mascara** *($6.99)* remains a superior lengthening mascara, but falters when it comes to creating noticeably thick, lush lashes. It doesn't clump or smear, however, and it does hold up beautifully throughout the day, making it a good choice if you're not expecting dramatic results as claimed.

☺ **Voluminous Original Volume Building Mascara, Curved Brush** *($6.99)* is nearly identical to the Voluminous Original Volume Building Mascara above, except for its curved brush, which is really personal preference more than performance-related.

☺ **Waterproof Volume Shocking Mascara** *($12.99)* is a waterproof mascara that really did produce shocking results, and I mean that in a good way! Although the lash-enhancing result isn't as prodigious as its non-waterproof partner, you'll still be shocked by how long and thick this two-part mascara makes your lashes. A translucent white primer is applied first, using a standard mascara brush. This is followed by mascara, applied with a serrated comb applicator. It's the applicator that takes lashes from blah to bountiful in seconds, and the more you comb it through your lashes, the longer and thicker they get. However, if you can't restrain yourself, you'll find this produces a too-heavy look that must be smoothed out lest you go all day with thick, spidery-looking lashes. The formula wears well (an overzealous application may produce minor flaking) and takes patience to remove, so be prepared. Otherwise, if you want a false-eyelash effect that holds up to rain and tears, you've found it!

The Reviews L

☺ **Clean Definition Telescopic Clean Definition & Lengthening Mascara** *($7.99)* has a name that contradicts its uneven, too-wet application that tends to stick lashes together for a look that says, "I just got out of the pool and need to take a shower." You can make lashes quite long with only minimal clumping, and the wetter formula allows darker emphasis at lash roots, which can help a bit if you can avoid smearing. With lots of comb-through using a separate, clean brush, the results from this mascara are attractive. However, lots of mascaras do all this without the extra step of comb-through, and in the end this is more trouble than it's worth.

☺ **FeatherLash Softly Sweeping Mascara** *($7.49)* has a clean, slightly wet application, but does little to magnify lashes beyond their natural state. Most women will want more than that, but for those seeking a "natural look" mascara that leaves lashes slightly gelled yet soft, this is an OK option.

☺ **FeatherLash Softly Sweeping Mascara, Curved Brush** *($7.49)* has the same traits as the original FeatherLash, but this time the curved brush makes it easier to apply an even, sheer layer for barely defined lashes.

☺ **Lash Architect Waterproof 3-D Dramatic Mascara** *($8.29)* has the same brush as the non-waterproof Lash Architect, but the results here prove that the best mascaras are an ideal union of brush and formula. Because this waterproof formula is thinner, you get less than half the oomph of the non-waterproof version, making for a less impressive mascara. It lengthens well, doesn't clump, and is waterproof, which may be reason enough for you to give it a try.

☺ **Lash Out Lengthening and Separating Mascara** *($7.49)* doesn't extend lashes as much as the name implies. This is one of the more lackluster mascaras from L'Oreal, but it serves its purpose if all you need is a satisfactory lengthening mascara that provides minimal thickness.

☺ **Voluminous Waterproof Mascara** *($6.99)* won't knock your socks off with prodigious length and thickness, but it does a respectable job in both departments. The main reason to choose this is for its clump-free application and strong waterproof properties.

FACE AND BODY ILLUMINATING/SHIMMER PRODUCTS: ☺ **Glam Bronze All-Over Loose Powder Highlighter** *($12.49)* is a mostly impressive loose powder with shine. Designed for use on face or body, the color goes on quite different from how it looks in the jar container. You get a sheer, rosy bronze tone with a striking gold shimmer and hints of copper. The color works for most skin tones and the shine clings better than expected (loose powders with shine generally have poor cling ability). It's worth auditioning if you prefer your shine to be dusted on in powder form. Note: this contains a tiny amount of fragrance chemicals that pose a slight risk of causing irritation.

BRUSHES: ✓☺ **All Purpose Shadow Brush** *($7.89)* is excellent, a soft, elegantly tapered brush great for applying all-over color or for softly defining the eye's crease. ☺ **All Purpose Powder Brush** *($12.89)* is a workable brush that is nicely shaped and dense enough for controlled application of powder. It isn't luxuriously soft, but does the job at an attractive price. ☺ **Makeup Artiste Travel Brush Set** *($13.89)* comes with four tiny brushes for applying powder, eyeshadow, concealer, and lipstick. They're housed in a thick plastic pouch, and while the small size isn't as elegant as brushes with longer handles, it's a convenient set to toss in your purse or desk drawer for quick touch-ups. ☺ **Precision Concealer Brush** *($7.89)* is also good, though I prefer something that is thinner and has a more pointed tip. This synthetic brush moves across the skin without pulling or dragging, and is worth a look if the shape appeals to you. ☺ **Brow/Lash Brush** *($5.49)* is OK, and the price isn't off-putting—but softer bristles would have been better. ☹ **Lip Brush** *($7.89)* has a decent shape, but the bristles are too soft and sparse for controlled application of lip color.

SPECIALTY PRODUCTS: ☺ **Clean Artiste Makeup Corrector Pen** *($9.49).* Think of this as a makeup remover in pen form and you'll have an idea of how it works. The slanted tip dispenses a mild solution capable of removing minor makeup mistakes such as flaking mascara or a too-heavy application of eyeliner. It is best for corrections in small areas—this isn't a cost-efficient or time-friendly way to remove a full face of makeup or even your eye makeup; it's just for minor repairs! The drawback is that it takes a fair amount of pressure to get this to remove eyeliner mistakes, and pressure isn't what you want in the eye area. Although this works for its intended purpose, you can get even better results with less pressure simply by dipping a cotton swab in your usual makeup remover. Consider Clean Artiste Makeup Corrector Pen as a handy option to keep in your purse for on-the-go makeup fixes.

LA MER

LA MER AT-A-GLANCE

Strengths: Sunscreen provides sufficient UVA protection; effective cleansers; one very good serum, though less expensive options are available from other Lauder-owned lines; mostly good foundations; supremely good powders; the makeup brushes.

Weaknesses: Outlandish claims; ultra-pricey; several products contain irritants, including eucalyptus oil and lime; no AHA or BHA products; an incomplete makeup selection; one of the foundations with sunscreen does not provide sufficient UVA protection.

For more information about La Mer, owned by Estee Lauder, call (866) 850-9400 or visit www.cremedelamer.com or www.Beautypedia.com.

LA MER SKIN CARE

☹ **$$$ The Cleansing Fluid** *($65 for 6.7 ounces)* removes makeup quickly due to its emollient ingredients. However, they're standard to most cleansing lotions and creams for dry skin, while the "extras" in this version (such as tourmaline and pearl powder) have no established benefit for skin. I suppose the algae extracts provide additional hydration, but that still doesn't justify the price.

☺ **$$$ The Cleansing Foam** *($65 for 4.2 ounces)* is a foaming, water-soluble cleanser for normal to oily or normal to slightly dry skin, and it does remove makeup swiftly. But the gemstones do not have a brightening effect on skin, although that's the claim you're paying dearly for; all you're getting is an ordinary cleanser.

☺ **$$$ The Cleansing Gel** *($65 for 6.7 ounces)* is an exceptionally standard, detergent-based, water-soluble cleanser that would be an option for normal to oily skin. But at this price, can anyone's skin really feel better?

☺ **$$$ The Cleansing Lotion** *($65 for 6.7 ounces)* is a milky emulsion that supposedly derives its remarkable cleansing powers from magnetized tourmaline and declustered water, but there is no proof such water makes a cleanser any better. This is a standard, wipe-off cleanser for dry skin that is not all that different from Neutrogena's Extra Gentle Cleanser.

☺ **$$$ Blanc De La Mer The Whitening Lotion** *($75 for 6.7 ounces)* is just a standard toner that contains some good water-binding agents for all skin types, along with a few antioxidants (and packaging that does keep them stable during use). The Whitening Lotion will make skin feel soft and smooth, but any whitening is coincidental. This does contain a small amount of volatile fragrance components that may cause slight irritation.

☺ **$$$ The Hydrating Infusion** (*$95 for 4.2 ounces*) has a lightweight, fluid gel texture that resembles a moisturizer but feels more like a toner; however, given that La Mer doesn't give it a typical name designation you're left guessing. But, based on the directions, which tell you to use it after cleansing but before your moisturizer, you might as well think of it as a toner hybrid. Supposedly, this is another product designed to "enhance" the fabled, near-miraculous benefits of the original Crème de la Mer, but you have to wonder: If that cream was so superior on its own, why does La Mer continue to offer product after (expensive) product to allegedly make it work better? If it's so brilliant (and expensive) on its own, it shouldn't need any enhancement, especially not from products that are essentially watered-down versions of the original. No matter how you look at it, the original Crème de la Mer didn't work as claimed and it is absolutely not the best moisturizer around. Lauder offers dozens of better formulations in their other lines for less money. But back to The Hydrating Infusion. Aside from a potentially irritating amount of lime extract, it is actually chock-full of seaweed-based water-binding agents and plenty of antioxidants and cell-communicating ingredients. Many of the state-of-the-art ingredients in this product are also present in products from other Lauder-owned lines, none of which have the elite price point of La Mer. The major difference between this product and other La Mer products is that they contain declustered water, gemstones, and "hydrating ferments" (whatever those are—you could describe raw sewage the same way) that La Mer claims makes them high-potency treatments. Regardless of what La Mer asserts—the Lauder company asserts myriad miraculous claims about all of their products—there is no published research to support La Mer's "our products have the edge" claims. As a consumer, you're left to decide if you want to go along with the hype or bypass it in favor of less expensive options that are also well-formulated. Those still considering The Hydrating Infusion should know it is best for normal to oily skin; but again, the amount of lime extract is cause for concern, especially if your skin is sensitive.

☹ **The Lifting Intensifier** (*$150 for 0.5 ounce*) is mostly water and alcohol with tiny amounts of plant extracts and a slip agent. The algae and gemstones are barely present, and do not have any miraculous benefits for aging skin. This product is not recommended.

☹ **The Mist** (*$55 for 4.2 ounces*) contains a eucalyptus derivative called eucalyptol, which is a skin irritant. It would have been an OK toner without that irritant, but the price is a joke given the basic ingredients and the small amount of antioxidants.

☹ **The Oil Absorbing Tonic** (*$60 for 6.7 ounces*). Supposedly, the algae extracts La Mer includes not only can turn back time, mend wrinkles, and heal skin, but also can reduce excess oil production for those struggling with acne. There is no research showing that algae can affect oil production. Oil production is controlled by hormones, and regular skin-care products can't affect hormone production. The first ingredient is squalane, a good emollient for dry skin but a problem for oily skin. The acrylates (think hair spray) and salts have some oil-absorbing properties, but the other emollients get in the way of that. I'm not quite sure what this Tonic can do for skin, but it won't absorb oil and it won't keep oily skin matte. It contains lime and eucalyptol (also known as eucalyptus), both of which irritate skin, and as a result may stimulate oil production directly in the pore. In the end, there isn't a valid reason to try this toner unless you enjoy spending way too much money for a product that will leave your skin irritated and confused.

☹ **The Radiant Infusion** (*$95 for 4.2 ounces*) comes with fascinating claims describing its "radical, fluid architecture" that delivers "extraordinary activity on demand," all to set in motion a "continuous wave of radiance-enhancing benefits." Quite honestly, you'd get more radiance from a brisk jog around the block than from applying this toner-like product. Considering the price, it's disheartening (and not the least bit helpful for skin) that the second ingredient is alcohol. Several of the plant extracts have benefit as water-binding agents and/or antioxidants, but the lime extract can be irritating, and nothing in this product will noticeably change skin discolorations. This should be renamed The Radiant Impediment.

☺ **The Tonic** *($60 for 6.7 ounces)* is an alcohol-free toner for normal to dry skin that's standard fare. It contains a minimal amount of ingredients that are beneficial for skin.

☺ **$$$ Blanc De La Mer The Whitening Essence** *($210 for 1 ounce)* is a water- and silicone-based serum that contains some yeast extract and a tiny amount of vitamin C, neither of which is "the ultimate in deep whitening." They're not even good at superficial whitening! Although this serum contains some impressive antioxidants and a few notable skin-identical ingredients, it doesn't best products from the Estee Lauder Perfectionist or Clinique Repairwear lines. At the drugstore, Olay's Definity and Regenerist products stand a much better chance of reducing skin discolorations, because they contain niacinamide. The mica and titanium dioxide in this serum provide a soft glow to skin, but that is strictly a cosmetic effect.

☹ **Creme De La Mer** *($130 for 1 ounce)* is the original product created by Max Huber, as described in the introduction to La Mer (this introduction is available to anyone who visits www.Beautypedia.com). As enticing as this dramatic story sounds, the reality is that this very basic cream doesn't contain anything particularly extraordinary or unique, unless you want to believe that seaweed extract (sort of like seaweed tea) can in some way heal burns and scars. Even if it could, burns and scars don't have much to do with wrinkling, and this product is now being sold as a wrinkle cream. According to Susan Brawley, professor of plant biology at the University of Maine, "Seaweed extract isn't a rare, exotic, or expensive ingredient. Seaweed extract is readily available and [is] used in everything from cosmetics to food products and medical applications." Creme de la Mer contains mostly seaweed extract, mineral oil, Vaseline, glycerin, wax-like thickening agents, lime extract, plant oils, plant seeds, minerals, vitamins, more thickeners, and preservatives. This rather standard moisturizer also contains some good antioxidants, but the jar packaging won't keep them stable during use. This also contains a skin-stressing amount of eucalyptus oil, as well as Kathon CG, a preservative that is recommended for use only in rinse-off products. Consumers who have a "steadfast devotion" to this product are not only wasting their money but also hurting their skin.

☹ **The Concentrate** *($350 for 1.7 ounces)* is, first and foremost, not worth even a fraction of its price. All you're getting is a nonaqueous product containing mostly silicones, seaweed extract, glycerin, film-forming agents, and several plant extracts, some of which (lime, lavender, and basil extracts, and also eucalyptus oil) are irritating to skin. The formula is rounded out by trace amounts of minerals and some additional plant extracts, but none of these, and definitely not in the amounts used here, are particularly helpful for skin, be it wrinkled or not. Seaweed (also known as algae) extract has antioxidant and anti-inflammatory properties, but it is not the magical elixir of youth La Mer makes it out to be, nor is it expensive to include in skin-care products. Bulk liquid seaweed extract costs an average of $1.50 per liter, and the amount used in this product barely amounts to a teaspoon, despite being the second ingredient listed. Like all silicone-based serums, this product will leave skin feeling incredibly smooth and silky. But knowing you can achieve this same feeling with other products that cost $250 less than La Mer's version (and that still have beneficial antioxidants) is a sobering fact, to say the least! The eucalyptus oil makes this too irritating for all skin types, and overall this serum pales in comparison to those from other Lauder-owned lines, all of which cost considerably less.

The Reviews L

unrated **The Essence** *($2,100 for 1.5 ounces).* I wonder sometimes if the cosmetics industry simply has a sardonic sense of humor or whether it's possible they merely don't like women very much. How else can you explain La Mer launching a product that costs $2,100 and whose primary ingredient is seaweed? At least according to the ingredient list it has a lot of seaweed—well, as much as can be present in a 1.5-ounce product—along with a huge list of other ingredients. The primary ingredient in this nonaqueous serum is seaweed extract, but what type of seaweed was used is unknown so there is no way to evaluate its benefit for skin. (There are endless kinds of seaweed extracts, some potentially quite dangerous.) Actually, I wonder how the FDA lets Lauder get around this generalized ingredient identification because it is definitely not according to the regulation. This product also contains silicones, emollients, more seaweed (this time listed by type), ingredients that mimic the structure of skin, an assortment of antioxidants, a tiny amount of niacin (the form of vitamin B that can cause flushing, which is actually a problem for skin), and acetyl hexapeptide-3. The peptide is the ingredient that's supposed to work like Botox, but of course, it can't—even Botox can't work like Botox when applied topically to skin. And just in case you weren't sure the product was doing anything for your skin, they included a few irritating, skin-tingling plant extracts, including eucalyptus, lime, and citronella, to create the impression that it is doing something on your face. For this kind of money it should really be doing something other than irritating skin. Other than that, it's not possible to ascertain any other information because Lauder has no published studies and offers no clinical evidence (other than press releases, which fashion magazines use as if they were factual information) to support the value of the product or the efficacy of the claims. Along with seaweed, The Essence also contains an assortment of yeast extracts: saccharomyces lysate, micrococcus lysate, artemisia extract, and bifida ferment lysate. But whether or not seaweed or yeast in any form can affect wrinkles is still not known. Indeed, that ability is something ingredient manufacturers do claim, but there are no supporting published or substantiated double-blind studies showing this to be true. Research from ingredient manufacturers is interesting, but obviously self-serving; somehow all their ingredients are always miracles. Trying to find independent research about these substances is difficult, and what does exist involves in vitro or animal studies (Sources: *Journal of Burn Care and Rehabilitation*, March-April 1999, pages 155-162; and *Wound Repair and Regeneration*, January 2002, page 38). I could carry on about how these various ingredients are theoretically supposed to affect skin without any research to even rationalize them for skin care, but at some moments in my career I just have to throw my hands up in the air and say, "I give up, the cosmetics industry is just crazy and I have no words left to explain why." I think I'll go get a Starbucks latte.... I don't understand $5 for a cup of coffee either, but at least I know exactly what I'm getting!

☹ **The Eye Balm** *($140 for 0.5 ounce)* is a good moisturizer for normal to dry skin, but the supposed benefits of fish cartilage and malachite? Well, it's up to you to decide, because there is no research showing they're worth this kind of investment for skin. What should give you something to think about is the inclusion of eucalyptus oil (a considerable amount) and mint, which are both unnecessary and very irritating to delicate eye-area skin.

☹ **The Eye Concentrate** *($165 for 0.5 ounce)* contains some incredibly helpful, state-of-the-art ingredients for creating and maintaining healthy skin. What a shame so many of them are subject to reduced potency because of jar packaging! Moreover, how depressing that La Mer included a troubling amount of eucalyptus oil, which only serves to irritate skin. Without that and in better packaging, this really would have been an "ultraluxe eye treatment."

☺ **$$$ The Lifting Face Serum** *($235 for 1 ounce)* is a souped-up version of Lauder's Advanced Night Repair Protective Recovery Complex, with the extras being more antioxidants and algae and a greater complement of skin-identical ingredients. Blue algae are present, but there is no substantiated research anywhere stating that they can lift sagging skin or increase collagen synthesis so skin becomes less wrinkled. However, in terms of providing skin with some state-of-the-art ingredients, this excels, assuming you don't mind the price. Once again, several other Lauder-owned companies offer similar versions of this product at more realistic prices.

☹ **The Moisturizing Gel Cream** *($230 for 2 ounces)* is simply a lighter version of the original Crème De La Mer, and promotes a silkier finish due to the silicone it contains. Despite a light texture, this contains a lot of lime extract and enough eucalyptus to be more irritating than miraculously healing, as claimed.

☹ **The Moisturizing Lotion** *($190 for 1.7 ounces)* would have been a good moisturizer for normal to dry skin, but for the inclusion of lime and eucalyptus extracts, which are potentially irritating and sensitizing for all skin types. And the price is just outrageous!

☹ **The Oil Absorbing Lotion** *($190 for 1.7 ounces)* is the lotion version of the original Crème de la Mer, and it does have a much lighter texture. However, the emollients and the lack of absorbents in this product won't keep oily skin in check. That's forgivable, but the inclusion of a significant amount of eucalyptus oil and lime is not.

☺ **$$$ The SPF 18 Fluid** *($65 for 1.7 ounces)* is a good, in-part avobenzone-based sunscreen in a rather standard emollient base that would be an option for normal to dry skin. Remember, you have to use sunscreen liberally to gain the SPF benefit. How liberally are you going to apply this product given the price? The volatile fragrance components in this sunscreen keep it from earning a higher rating. It is available in various tints, and all of them are acceptable.

☺ **$$$ The SPF 30 UV Protecting Fluid** *($65 for 1.4 ounces)* is a good, though exceedingly overpriced, daytime moisturizer with sunscreen for normal to slightly dry or slightly oily skin. It has a lightweight, silky texture and contains plenty of zinc oxide for UVA protection. Although it does contain some interesting water-binding agents, antioxidants make up only a minor part of the formula, and for the price tag this carries, they should be more prominent. Skin also could do without the fragrance chemicals this contains, but at least those are in short supply, too. One more comment: The sunscreen blend in this product is not unique, at least not in terms of the ingredients themselves, which show up in hundreds of sunscreens for a lot less money.

☹ **The Lip Balm** *($45 for 0.32 ounce)* ranks as one of the most expensive lip balms sold, and the first ingredient is Vaseline. Amazing! The seaweed and plant seeds may make this seem like more than it is, but the amount of eucalyptus oil is not lip-friendly, and it also contains the menthol derivative menthyl PCA.

☹ **The Radiant Facial** *($320)* should leave me speechless, but two words come to mind right away: Don't bother. This kit includes **The Radiant Primer** and **The Radiant Mask**, and both have the same ingredients because the Mask is pre-moistened with the Primer (which basically negates the need to apply the Primer first). The mask is just two pieces of cloth intended to fit over the upper and lower halves of the face. The whole system is as misguided as it gets, so the duplication is just silly. For over $300, you're getting mostly water (it's La Mer's "declustered" water, but simply making water less clustered doesn't translate into outstanding skin care), alcohol, and yeast. These ingredients cannot bring your skin to its utmost clarity, luminosity, and brightness in eight minutes. There are several skin-identical ingredients, plant extracts (most with antioxidant ability), and gemstones in the formula, all claiming to work in biofermented synergy to perform miracles for your skin. None of them will do much for your skin in the presence of this much alcohol, and none of them is capable of lightening skin discolorations and preventing their return. There's no reason at all to consider this occasional-use product over an alcohol-free, antioxidant-laden serum or moisturizer for daily use.

☹ **The Refining Facial** *($75 for 3.4 ounces)* is a relatively standard clay mask. The "sea stuff" is in here, as are tourmaline and diamond powder. If you feel that scrubbing with microscopic amounts of gemstones (and then rinsing them down the drain) is the way to go, that's your decision—but doing so with this product will irritate your skin because of the mint and citrus ingredients. Estee Lauder and Clinique sell less expensive and less offensive versions of this product.

LA MER MAKEUP

FOUNDATION: ☺ **$$$ The Treatment Crème Foundation SPF 15** *($85)* isn't as creamy as the name suggests, but the treatment portion is fairly accurate, at least in terms of all the bells and whistles in this slightly thick but silky foundation. Like The Treatment Fluid Foundation below, this is also a water-in-silicone emulsion, although a few emollients that make it better suited for normal to dry (but not very dry) skin have been added here. It offers medium coverage (and is difficult to sheer out, so be sure you are comfortable with this), and sets to a satin-matte finish that feels slightly moist but doesn't look dewy. The in-part titanium dioxide sunscreen provides broad-spectrum protection, but the nine shades have a few problematic colors. Avoid Golden (too orange), Beige (rosy), and Tan (too peach). Crème and Caramel are slightly peach, but still worth considering. Natural, Buff, Bronze, and Neutral are the best of the bunch. Although this is an elegant foundation with a higher-than-usual amount of antioxidants and other beneficial ingredients, its finish doesn't make wrinkles look less obvious as claimed.

☺ **$$$ The Treatment Fluid Foundation SPF 15** *($85)*. It's a good thing this water- and silicone-based liquid foundation contains an in-part titanium dioxide sunscreen, because that's the least you should expect at this price! This has a fluid, moist texture that goes on slightly silky and sets to a satin finish replete with a glow-y shine. Although the coverage is light, this somehow doesn't look as natural on skin as it should. I've seen more natural-looking foundations from L'Oreal and Maybelline, just to give you an idea of how out of whack this foundation's price is. If you're determined to try it, you'll be pleased to know that most of the shades are impressively neutral. The Natural and Beige shades are slightly peach to peach and should be considered carefully. Consider Linen and Sand carefully, too, because they may be too yellow for some light skin tones.

☺ **$$$ The Treatment Powder Foundation SPF 15** *($95)*. This is a talc- and silicone-based pressed-powder foundation that includes an in-part titanium dioxide sunscreen. For the money, it doesn't rise to the top of the list of powder foundations. It's silky-sheer application feels great and it leaves a soft, slightly dry matte finish. Coverage goes from sheer to medium, as is true for most powder foundations. La Mer's shade range excludes those with dark skin tones, but there are plenty of neutral options for light to medium skin tones. The claims about what this foundation can do for your skin are beyond exaggerated, but there's no denying it is one more good powder foundation to consider. It is best for normal to slightly dry skin.

☹ **The SPF 18 Fluid Tint** *($65)* doesn't have the same array of skin-beneficial ingredients as the two La Mer foundations reviewed, nor does its sunscreen offer sufficient UVA protection. For the money, that's a real burn, and although there are some textural benefits to extol, they're not enough to make this worth considering over the tinted moisturizers with sunscreen available from Bobbi Brown, Aveda, Neutrogena, or Paula's Choice.

POWDER: ✓ ☺ **$$$ The Powder** *($65)* is one of the most expensive loose powders I've reviewed, yet despite the luxurious feel of this talc-based powder, the money doesn't translate into a noticeable difference worth the price. Nonetheless, it does look incredibly skin-like and creates a beautifully natural yet polished finish from each of its four sheer shades. You can find similar loose powders from other Lauder-owned lines (including M.A.C.), but if you're attracted to La Mer's miracles-from-the-sea claims, this one is bound to impress you, especially if you have normal to dry skin.

BRUSHES: ☺ **$$$ The Foundation Brush** *($40)* is composed of synthetic fibers and differs little from almost every other foundation brush available. In fact, the only differences are in the price and La Mer's inflated pedigree. You won't be disappointed with it if you prefer applying foundation with a brush; you just don't need to spend this much to get the same result. ☺ **$$$ The Powder Brush** *($70)* is a very good, retractable powder brush that the company maintains can be used to apply loose or pressed powder. That's hardly unique, and the fact that the bristles of this brush can be "extended" based on your powder preference doesn't make a noticeable difference during application. As a portable powder brush, this is a pricey but good option.

LA PRAIRIE

LA PRAIRIE AT-A-GLANCE

Strengths: All of the facial sunscreens include avobenzone for UVA protection; some very good serums; helpful products to smooth lines around the mouth and on lips; mostly good masks; one well-formulated AHA product; most of the makeup categories present good, though needlessly expensive, options that include foundations with reliable sun protection.

Weaknesses: Very expensive; overreliance on jar packaging; many products contain a potentially irritating amount of astringent horsetail extract; the sun products for the body are a mixed bag; no effective skin-lightening options; poor options for anyone dealing with blemishes (though La Prairie is concerned primarily with selling wrinkle creams anyway); the eyeshadow options are average, as are the pencils.

For more information about La Prairie, owned by Beiersdorf, call (800) 821-5718 or visit www.laprairie.com or www.Beautypedia.com.

LA PRAIRIE SKIN CARE

LA PRAIRIE ADVANCED MARINE BIOLOGY PRODUCTS

☹ **Advanced Marine Biology Tonic** *($95 for 5 ounces)* has an exceptionally long ingredient list, although the lineup begins with alcohol (unbelievably, it is the first listed ingredient), and that instantly makes this toner-like product far from advanced. Alcohol not only causes dryness, irritation, and excess oil production but also generates free-radical damage—none of which stimulates collagen synthesis or improves elasticity. If anything, swabbing alcohol over your skin will help break down these fundamental support elements of your skin. And the sea water and extracts are just gimmicks, meant solely to convince you that they are something special for aging skin, nothing more.

☺ **$$$ Advanced Marine Biology Cream** *($175 for 1.4 ounces)*. What would La Prairie be without lots and lots of antiwrinkle creams, especially very expensive ones? The women who shop this line expect nothing less. The problem is that expensive rarely means better in the cosmetics world, and the same is true for the entire La Prairie line. This cream doesn't raise the bar, but its price should raise your eyebrows, because you're not getting anything substantial for your money. The silicone-enhanced formula leaves skin feeling silky-smooth, but the numerous antioxidants present are performance-handicapped due to the unfortunate choice of jar packaging. This does contain some novel water-binding agents and several cell-communicating ingredients, but these are nestled alongside potentially irritating fragrance ingredients, and that doesn't qualify as advanced care for aging skin. If you decide to try this anyway, it is best for normal to slightly dry skin.

☹ **$$$ Advanced Marine Biology Cream SPF 20** *($175 for 1.7 ounces)*. With a name that sounds more like a high school or college science course than a daytime moisturizer with sunscreen, at least this tremendously overpriced product includes avobenzone for UVA protection. The emollient base formula for dry skin contains a smattering of marine ingredients, but there's no proof (other than from La Prairie's marketing department) that they are stellar antioxidants or have any effect on skin's firmness. What's really frustrating is that none of the plant ingredients will remain potent for long due to the jar packaging. And, of course, you must ask yourself how liberally you'll apply this product knowing that if you apply it correctly to face and neck, you'll be replacing it every couple of months.

☺ **$$$ Advanced Marine Biology Night Solution** *($175 for 1.7 ounces)* is absurdly overpriced, although this water-based serum has the most intriguing formula among La Prairie's Advanced Marine Biology lineup. By the way, I can't be the only one who thinks the name of this sub-brand is more in line with a collegiate course of study than anything related to skin care, can I? But, back to the product: it contains several water-binding agents and cell-communicating ingredients (glycoproteins and peptides among them) along with a lesser amount of antioxidants. The packaging is such that this product should be stored away from direct light to avoid deterioration of the light-sensitive ingredients, but at least it won't let unwanted air in. The amount of horsetail extract in this product is potentially irritating, which keeps this from earning a better rating. Last, the amount of film-forming agent can help make your skin feel tighter temporarily and enhance smoothness, but the effect is strictly cosmetic, and totally unrelated to ocean plants, regardless of how they were harvested.

LA PRAIRIE ANTI-AGING PRODUCTS

☹ **$$$ Anti-Aging Complex** *($220 for 1.7 ounces)* has over a dozen state-of-the-art ingredients for skin, but what precedes them isn't exciting, and the amount of irritating horsetail is larger than the amount of beneficial ingredients. Then, the jar packaging renders the retinol ineffective shortly after you open the product. Considering the price, this is very disappointing!

☹ **$$$ Anti-Aging Day Cream SPF 30** *($200 for 1.7 ounces)*. The obnoxious price for this daytime moisturizer with sunscreen is bound to discourage liberal application, despite the fact that liberal application is essential if you are to get the amount of sun protection stated; that makes this tough to recommend even though its actives list includes avobenzone. This product has a creamy, lush texture that those with dry skin will appreciate, and the formula contains several beneficial ingredients, plus some exotic plants with no known benefit for skin. Unfortunately, none of the plants or antioxidants will remain stable during use thanks to the jar packaging, which makes this product even more a waste of money when compared with countless other daytime moisturizers with sunscreen.

☹ **$$$ Anti-Aging Emulsion SPF 30** *($195 for 1.7 ounces)* contains avobenzone for reliable UVA protection and has a lotion base that those with normal to slightly oily skin will appreciate. My concern, however, is twofold. One, how liberally are you going to apply this each day considering the cost? Two, the horsetail in this product is in a larger amount than the antioxidants and cell-communicating ingredients. Of lesser concern are the volatile fragrance components, but the tiny amount in here is unlikely to cause trouble. Still, this is a tricky product to enthusiastically recommend.

☹ **Anti-Aging Eye Cream SPF 15** *($155 for 0.5 ounce)* is an emollient eye cream with an in-part avobenzone sunscreen that has a lot of potential; however, most of the really helpful ingredients are undermined by jar packaging. The horsetail and balm mint can cause irritation (along with the many volatile fragrance components in this product), making it one to skip.

☹ **$$$ Anti-Aging Longevity Serum** *($225 for 1.7 ounces)* isn't a true serum, but rather a lightweight yet emollient lotion for normal to dry skin. It contains a selection of intriguing ingredients, including several plant-based antioxidants and glycoproteins, which have cell-communicating properties. The disappointment is the amount of horsetail extract, which is irritating to skin. This also contains other plant extracts that have dubious benefits for skin but do have the potential to cause irritation, and that's not going to help skin's natural repair process. I wouldn't bank on this being the antiwrinkle solution any more than I consider a rice cake a satisfying meal. For the money, you're getting a substandard product that absolutely cannot keep dermal tissues from becoming rigid, as claimed. If that were true, given the basic formulation, lots of other less expensive moisturizers would be doing that too. Although La Prairie includes some effective ingredients to help skin look and feel better, pairing them with problematic plants is disappointing.

☹ **$$$ Anti-Aging Night Cream** *($200 for 1.7 ounces)*. Packaged in a jar, so the "special" ingredients you're paying extra for won't remain stable during use, is this rich moisturizer for very dry skin. It feels as luxurious as the image La Prairie strives to maintain, but a luxurious texture doesn't mean much if the formula isn't outstanding or if several key ingredients have their efficacy depleted due to a bad packaging decision. What a shame, because overall this is a really impressive moisturizer, although it isn't worth the price and it doesn't have special antiwrinkle abilities. This contains a small amount of fragrance chemicals known to cause irritation.

☹ **$$$ Anti-Aging Stress Cream** *($195 for 1.7 ounces)* tries to sway consumers with the statement that the natural relaxant valerian root (which is known to have a calming effect when consumed orally) also works via topical application to relax expression lines and promote firmer, lifted skin. Even if we assume that the plant by itself has wondrous properties for wrinkles and stressed skin, La Prairie's choice of jar packaging will quickly degrade its alleged potency. Even more depressing is that there is far more alcohol in this product than there are exciting antiaging ingredients (alcohol causes free radical damage). At its best (which isn't that great) this is nothing more than a standard emollient moisturizer for dry skin. It does contain fragrance in the form of fragrant chemical compounds.

LA PRAIRIE THE CAVIAR COLLECTION PRODUCTS

☹ **$$$ Essence of Skin Caviar Eye Complex** *($120 for 0.5 ounce)* is a lightweight moisturizer that doesn't instantly firm skin, but will hydrate to make superficial lines less apparent. The amount of horsetail extract may cause irritation in the eye area due to its astringent properties, while the caviar extract shows up as the last ingredient on the list.

☺ $$$ **Extrait of Skin Caviar Firming Complex** (*$130 for 1 ounce*) would rate much higher and be worth the splurge if it did not contain problematic plant extracts (including horsetail and sage) along with volatile fragrance components. The amount of sunscreen agent included is odd, given that this product does not advertise an SPF rating. Taking these points into account, this rates as an average option for normal to slightly dry skin.

☹ **Skin Caviar** (*$175 for 1.7 ounces*) is a silicone-based serum whose negatives are strong enough to make it not worth considering. In addition to some irritating plant extracts, this also contains the germicidal agent O-phenylphenol, which research has shown can cause acute skin inflammation and, potentially, ulceration (Sources: *National Toxicology Program Technical Support Series*, March 1986, pages 1-141; and *Critical Reviews in Toxicology*, 2002, pages 551-6250).

☹ **Skin Caviar Crystalline Concentre** (*$375 for 1 ounce*). There are no words fit to print that I can use to describe what a terrible, waste-of-time-and-money product this is. If I were working for La Prairie, I would not be able to sell this catastrophe to a single consumer without feeling like the ultimate snake oil salesperson. The concept and claim behind this serum is to create smoother, firmer skin that has increased elasticity so that wrinkles are filled out and a younger-looking visage emerges. Based on the formula, someone at La Prairie either has a cruel sense of humor or absolutely no concept of what aging skin needs to make it look and feel as good as possible. And the price goes beyond insulting! For nearly $400, you're getting mostly water, slip agents, silicones, thickener, alcohol (the drying, irritating, free-radical-generating kind), and a derivative of resorcinol, which has no proven benefit for skin yet retains resorcinol's irritating properties. The peptides, caviar extract, and diamond powder may attract the cost-is-no-deterrent consumer, but none of these ingredients add up to a brilliant, elite skin-care product that provides even a modicum of antiwrinkle benefit. There are far better (and I mean much, much better) moisturizers than this available for less than $30 at the drugstore.

☺ $$$ **Skin Caviar Intensive Ampoule Treatment** (*$570 for 6 treatments*) consists of six ampoules each of **Solvent** and **Lyophilized Substance**, which you mix together to—what else—guard against accelerated skin aging." Neither product has an SPF rating or contains a UVA-protecting sunscreen, and since that's the only reliable way to prevent accelerated aging with a skin-care product, right away you can tell things are bogus. The Solvent is a lightweight moisturizer that contains some slip agents, emollients, film-forming agent, plant extracts (some are irritating, while most of the others have no established benefit for skin), ceramide, and vitamin E. This also contains volatile fragrance components that may cause irritation. The Lyophilized Substance is a sugar-based powder that contains a salt form of vitamin C along with water, thickener, and the antioxidant superoxide dismutase. There's no reason those ingredients could not have been added to the Solvent, but I suppose the two-step process makes women think the set is somehow more special or customized. In the end, this isn't that exciting, and wouldn't be at even one-fourth the cost.

☹ **Skin Caviar Luxe Cream** (*$390 for 1.7 ounces*) may have a luxe texture, but the ingredients used to create it are commonplace and do not justify the ridiculous price. This jar-packaged moisturizer contains many antioxidants that won't remain stable once you open it, and the pH of this cream is too high for the AHA it contains to exfoliate skin. Topping things off is the inclusion of the irritants sage, arnica, and horsetail, coupled with several volatile fragrance components. Buyer beware!

☺ **$$$ Skin Caviar Luxe Eye Lift Cream** *($295 for 0.68 ounce)* has an incredibly insulting price for what amounts to mostly water, thickeners, Vaseline, and vegetable oil. Many intriguing ingredients are included in this eye cream, but all of them are listed after the pH-adjusting agent, and many won't remain stable once this jar-packaged product is opened. This isn't luxe; it's a bona fide bad beauty investment, at least if you were hoping that the cost would translate to a superior product to vanquish every eye-area woe.

☹ **Skin Caviar Firming Mask** *($145)* might make skin appear firmer temporarily, but that effect results from the extreme irritation this two-step mask causes. The **Penetrating Serum** contains several fragrant oils, including rosemary, rosewood, and sweet marjoram. The **Skin Caviar Firming Complex** lists alcohol as the second ingredient, furthering the irritation from the Penetrating Serum.

OTHER LA PRAIRIE PRODUCTS

☹ **Cellular Cleansing Water Face/Eyes** *($75 for 5.2 ounces)* contains gentle cleansing agents to remove makeup (but not waterproof formulas) and some interesting water-binding agents. However, almost all of the plant extracts can be irritating to skin, especially around the eyes, making this a poor choice at any price.

☺ **$$$ Cellular Comforting Cleansing Emulsion** *($75 for 5.2 ounces)* is a very standard, very overpriced cleansing lotion for normal to dry skin. It does remove makeup but you need to use a washcloth to eliminate any residue. Some of the plant extracts can be a problem for skin if not completely removed.

☺ **$$$ Foam Cleanser** *($75 for 4 ounces)* is a standard, but good, water-soluble cleanser that produces copious soap-like foam. It's an option for normal to slightly dry or slightly oily skin, if the price doesn't make you faint. For the record, several drugstore lines offer similar cleansers for less than $10.

☺ **$$$ Purifying Cream Cleanser** *($75 for 6.8 ounces)* is a cold cream–style cleanser the company states can be rinsed or tissued off, but this requires effort to completely remove it. It's an OK option for very dry skin but is absurdly overpriced.

☺ **$$$ Suisse De-Sensitizing Cleansing Emulsion** *($70 for 5 ounces)* is very similar to the Cellular Comforting Cleansing Emulsion, save for fewer plant extracts, none of which are a particular problem for skin, sensitive or not. Otherwise, the same comments apply.

☹ **Cellular Eye Make-Up Remover** *($60 for 4.2 ounces)* is a water- and silicone-based eye-makeup remover that is less impressive than similar options from Almay or Neutrogena. This version presents problems for eye-area skin because it contains astringent plant extracts and fragrance.

☹ **Age Management Balancer** *($80 for 8.4 ounces)* contains lactic acid and has a pH of 3.6, but the amount of AHA present is too low to exfoliate skin. This toner has some very good ingredients for all skin types, but the amount of horsetail can be irritating, and the lavender extract isn't good news either.

☹ **Cellular Purifying Dual-Phase Toner** *($70 for 8.4 ounces)* lists alcohol as the second ingredient—so, dual-phase or not, this is too irritating for all skin types and won't "nourish" skin as claimed.

☹ **Cellular Refining Lotion** *($80 for 8.4 ounces)* contains irritating horsetail and ivy extracts as well as several volatile fragrance components that won't firm or hydrate skin in the least.

☹ **Cellular Softening and Balancing Lotion** *($140 for 8.4 ounces)* should be brimming with ingredients that put skin in its optimum state, but La Prairie couldn't resist including the irritants horsetail, arnica, witch hazel, and eugenol, among others.

☺ **$$$ Suisse De-Sensitizing Soothing Mist** *($70 for 4.2 ounces)* could have been a very good toner for dry skin, but the balm mint, horsetail, and rose extracts are potential skin irritants, while the other plant extracts and oils are anti-irritants. I suspect that there isn't enough of any of these to make a difference, but at this price and given the claims, it's disappointing.

☺ **$$$ Cellular 3-Minute Peel** *($200 for 1.4 ounces)* justifies its price by claiming to use professional-strength AHAs and BHA, and stating that it works without irritating skin. First, professional-strength hydroxy acids are typically used in concentrations of 20% and up, such as for facial peels. The amount of lactic acid in this product is likely around 5%, which does not distinguish this product from other 5% AHA options available at the drugstore. As far as working without irritating skin, that's not possible. This product has a pH of 2.9, which means the lactic acid will exfoliate skin. The addition of a small amount of glycolic acid and an even smaller amount of salicylic acid likely brings the total amount of exfoliating ingredients to about 7%, which is still not what any dermatologist or aesthetician would consider "professional strength," that is, in the realm of 15% to 30%. Although this product will exfoliate skin, it needs more than three minutes to do a thorough job, and the price is just insulting for what is easily exchanged for far less pricey options that are just as if not more effective.

☹ **Cellular Retexturizing Booster** *($185 for 1 ounce)* is not the way to enjoy the benefits of glycolic and salicylic acid in one product. Although the pH is within range for exfoliation to occur, the amount of alcohol is needlessly irritating and the lavender oil damages otherwise healthy skin cells. It's insulting to the consumer that La Prairie refers to this Booster as non-irritating.

☹ **Cellular Microdermabrasion Cream** *($255 for 4.2 ounces)* is a thick-textured yet surprisingly abrasive scrub that is too rough for most skin types, and irritating for all skin types because of the grapefruit peel oil it contains. Moreover, at this price, you might as well go for professional microdermabrasion treatments, although even those aren't turning out to be all that great.

☺ **$$$ Essential Exfoliator** *($75 for 7 ounces)* is an OK scrub for normal to dry skin, and features apricot seed powder as the abrasive agent. Plant seeds or shells are not preferred to synthetic polyethylene beads because the former typically do not have perfectly smooth surfaces, and therefore can cause tears in the skin and trigger inflammation.

☺ **$$$ Cellular Anti-Spot Brightening Serum** *($185 for 1 ounce)* doesn't contain a high enough concentration of ingredients that research has shown can inhibit melanin production, but it is an excellent serum for normal to dry skin. It contains stabilized vitamin C along with soothing agents, antioxidants, some good water-binding agents, and a couple of cell-communicating ingredients. The inclusion of horsetail extract keeps this from earning a higher rating, but it's nice that this is fragrance-free.

☺ **$$$ Cellular Anti-Wrinkle Firming Serum** *($185 for 1 ounce)* is a very good, antioxidant-rich moisturizer for normal to slightly dry skin. The truly helpful ingredients outnumber the problem-children additions, making this a contender if you prefer to spend in the upper echelon for your skin-care products.

☺ **$$$ Cellular Anti-Wrinkle Sun Cream SPF 30** *($140 for 1.7 ounces)* protects skin from UVA radiation with its in-part avobenzone sunscreen, and has an antioxidant-laden base formula suitable for normal to dry skin. What a shame jar packaging won't keep the numerous antioxidants stable during use. The tiny amount of lavender extract is not likely to be a problem for skin.

☹ **Cellular Cream Platinum Rare** *($650 for 1 ounce)*. Supposedly, real platinum is the justification for the absolutely insane price tag of this moisturizer. If this really contains any discernable amount of platinum, what a waste of a good metal. What you are supposed to believe, and undoubtedly there will be those who do believe it, is that applying platinum and La Prairie's "Exclusive Smart Crystals" (now if that isn't new age mumbo-jumbo lingo, I don't know what is) are said to guard your skin's youthfulness. Next thing you know La Prairie is going to be selling shares of the Brooklyn Bridge at its counters all over the world. I'm tempted to stop here because this doesn't really deserve a second more of my time, and definitely not yours, but just in case someone really wants to understand what kind of formulation this price tag has affixed to it, I'll finish. First, the amount of platinum powder is a mere dusting. However, even in greater amounts, platinum (despite its use in making exquisite jewelry) has no special antiaging or any benefit for skin whatsoever. La Prairie simply chose to use it because they were banking that platinum's jewelry reputation for being prized and expensive would transfer to skin care, thus allowing them to set an extremely high price for what, in many ways, couldn't be a more basic, ordinary moisturizer for dry skin. The only possible association of platinum with skin is how it functions in some chemotherapy medications. It's included in these medications for its cytotoxic (i.e., it kills cells) capabilities when combined with other substances, but that has nothing to do with topical application or with restoring youth (Source: *Journal of Clinical Oncology*, August 2007, pages 3266-3273). That is, it has to do with killing rapidly growing cells to restore equilibrium and to shrink tumors. In all honesty, you'd be better off buying a platinum ring and rubbing that on skin than using this product. The platinum won't be helpful but at least you'll have a beautiful piece of jewelry to wear as compensation! The amount of mica in this moisturizer is enough to cast a shimmering glow on skin, but that effect is strictly cosmetic and has nothing to do with "smart crystals." Actually, it would be much smarter to use a lightweight shimmer lotion to revive the radiance of aging skin than this product! This does contain some beneficial plant extracts and antioxidants, but not nearly as much as it should, especially at this price. And the fact that they chose jar packaging is just maddening, so any beneficial ingredients won't remain stable. Even if you were undeterred by cost and overinflated claims, this product would still not be recommended because it contains silver oxide. Silver oxide is a germicide composed of silver nitrate and an alkaline hydroxide (a metallic compound bound to a metal atom). Silver nitrate is known to be caustic to skin, while silver itself can cause a permanent bluish discoloration on skin (Sources: www.naturaldatabase.com; and *Colloidal Silver: A Literature Review: Medical Uses, Toxicology, and Manufacture*, 2nd Edition, Clear Springs Press, LLC, John Hill).

☹ **$$$ Cellular Day Cream** *($135 for 1 ounce)* is a lot of money for a product that is mostly thickeners, vegetable oil, and Vaseline, but La Prairie was undoubtedly hoping you wouldn't notice. Plus, without a sunscreen it is a definite no-no for daytime. This would be good for dry skin, but doesn't compare with some of the other more interesting products in this line or from many other lines, because it lacks the array of antioxidants, skin-identical ingredients, and anti-irritants the others contain.

☹ **$$$ Cellular De-Sensitizing Serum** *($160 for 1 ounce)* is a poor choice for sensitive skin because of the irritating plant extracts horsetail and balm mint. These irritants are outnumbered by the anti-irritants and several antioxidants, but for this kind of money there shouldn't be any problems; and, at any price, your skin deserves the best ingredients possible.

☹ **$$$ Cellular Eye Contour Cream** *($125 for 0.5 ounce)* cannot help prevent more lines from forming, as claimed, because it does not contain sunscreen. This is a very standard, emollient moisturizer for dry skin anywhere on the face, although the amount of horsetail extract may prove problematic if used in the eye area. Antioxidants are in short supply, but the number of skin-identical ingredients is good.

☺ $$$ **Cellular Eye Moisturizer SPF 15, "The Smart Eye Cream"** *($155 for 0.5 ounce)* has an in-part avobenzone sunscreen, but it isn't inherently smarter than other eye creams, including many that cost much less. The amount of balm mint is likely too small to cause irritation, but why put it in a product meant to be used around the eyes? More disappointing is that jar packaging ensures that the many antioxidants in this product will be less potent shortly after you open it.

☺ $$$ **Cellular Hydrating Serum** *($185 for 1 ounce)* would rate a Paula's Pick if it did not include more horsetail extract than it does several other ingredients that are of value for all skin types. The amount of horsetail is unlikely to be problematic, but without it, this serum would be a slam-dunk recommendation because it is loaded with antioxidants, cell-communicating ingredients, and ingredients that mimic the structure and function of healthy skin. The texture makes this best for normal to slightly dry or slightly oily skin.

☺ $$$ **Cellular Intensive Anti-Wrinkle Anti-Spot Cream** *($205 for 1 ounce)* purports to offer continuous management of "age" spots while you sleep, but that's just making a claim without really saying anything at all. I'd rather get rid of my age spots—which are really sun damage spots—than manage them (do age spots get their own 401(k) portfolio?). Regardless, this product cannot do anything for these dark spots because the potentially effective amount of vitamin C will be compromised once this jar-packaged cream is opened. The citrus and other fruit extracts in this product will not exfoliate or lighten skin, and the volatile fragrance components (present in tiny amounts) are potential troublemakers. Somehow, none of these features is exciting for a product that costs this much money.

☹ **Cellular Moisturizer SPF 15, "The Smart Cream"** *($165 for 1 ounce)* contains a frustrating mix of spectacular and suspect ingredients, complete with an in-part avobenzone sunscreen. The sunscreen is smart, but the decision to package such an antioxidant-rich formula in a jar was not, nor was the inclusion of balm mint and horsetail. Those irritants are present at more than a dusting, and when combined with the many volatile fragrance components ... well, it would be smarter to avoid it.

☺ $$$ **Cellular Night Repair Cream** *($220 for 1.7 ounces)* has jar packaging that will render most of the exciting ingredients ineffective shortly after you begin using the product. Still, the peptides, oil, and silicones will make dry skin look and feel better (though for this much money every last bit of potency should be preserved).

☺ $$$ **Cellular Nurturing Complex** *($255)* is sold as a set, and features a tiny amount of **Balm** and a standard size of **Serum**. The Balm is packaged in a flip-top component that sits atop the bottle that houses the Serum. Formula-wise, the Balm is a very good blend of waxes, nonvolatile plant oils, fatty acids, and a tiny amount of antioxidants. The Serum is silicone-based and contains some good water-binding agents, but the amount of horsetail extract may cause irritation. The anti-irritants in the Serum may seem impressive, but they're barely present, and as such have little to no impact on reducing surface redness. Although this duo has potential for dry to very dry skin, it really isn't worth the expense.

☺ $$$ **Cellular Nurturing Cream** *($205 for 1.7 ounces)* is a standard, slightly emollient moisturizer that contains a minimum amount of soothing agents coupled with some irritating plant extracts, so they cancel each other out. Don't expect this jar-packaged moisturizer to make quick work of facial redness, though it will relieve dryness-related discomfort.

☹ **$$$ Cellular Radiance Concentrate Pure Gold** *($570 for 1 ounce)* sounds like it's the quick-fix solution for those who want to look younger in a hurry. This is said to plump lines and wrinkles within an hour, speed exfoliation, and immediately reduce age spots, but nothing in this formula will make these claims a reality. The formula contains mostly water, silicones, alcohol, solvents, slip agents, thickener, water-binding agents, plant extracts, vitamin C, and several more plant extracts. Yes, it does indeed contain gold (it's the third to last ingredient listed), but that has no established benefit for skin, especially when it comes to turning back the hands of time. (What a waste of good metal!) Most of the plant ingredients in this serum show up in all of the La Prairie moisturizers, so I suppose those can make you look younger in an instant, too. Considering that this formula cannot make good on its claims (not even a little), the price is nothing less than absurd.

☹ **$$$ Cellular Radiance Cream** *($570 for 1.7 ounces)* is a water- and Vaseline-based moisturizer that takes an everything-but-the-kitchen-sink approach to moisturizers by including tiny amounts of dozens of plants along with gemstones and natural ingredients believed to be helpful for women experiencing skin changes due to menopause (though there is little research to support that line of thinking, at least in terms of using tiny amounts of such ingredients topically rather than orally). The price is ridiculous for what amounts to an emollient moisturizer for dry to very dry skin, and jar packaging renders the many antioxidants unstable shortly after you begin using it. The mineral pigments in this moisturizer are what give skin a luminous finish, which is strictly cosmetic, not skin care.

☹ **$$$ Cellular Radiance Eye Cream** *($285 for 0.5 ounce)* contains some good emollients for dry skin, but none that you won't find in hundreds of other moisturizers throughout the price spectrum. There is more mica (a mineral pigment that adds shine to skin) in this eye cream than there are state-of-the-art ingredients, and most of those will be compromised by jar packaging, which doesn't leave you with much for your money.

☺ **$$$ Cellular Resurfacing Cream** *($180 for 1.4 ounces)* has a beautifully emollient texture that addresses the needs of those with dry to very dry skin. However, the formula suffers from the unfortunate choice of jar packaging, which won't keep the light- and air-sensitive ingredients in this product stable during use. The amount of lactic and salicylic acids is likely enough for exfoliation, but the pH is too high for that to happen. Even if the pH were within range, you do not need to spend this much money for a well-formulated AHA or BHA product. Alpha Hydrox, Neutrogena, Olay, and Paula's Choice all have excellent, affordable options (though none of them are as emollient as this cream).

☹ **Cellular Revitalizing Eye Gel** *($155 for 0.5 ounce)* contains a large amount of horsetail extract as well as lesser amounts of chemical components of the plant. Horsetail has research on its ability to relax veins when taken orally, but that does not translate to mean it can reduce puffy eyes and dark circles when applied topically. The volatile components in horsetail (including trace amounts of nicotine) can be irritating to skin. It has potential antioxidant ability, but isn't preferred to other antioxidants that provide a benefit without the potential risk (Source: www.naturaldatabase.com). This product also contains a preservative that is not recommended for use in leave-on products.

☹ **Cellular Serum Platinum Rare** *($650 for 1 ounce)*. As one of the most expensive products La Prairie, or any other cosmetic line for that matter, sells, you might be intrigued if you weren't so shocked by the price. Does it really contain anything that can dramatically change the face of aging skin? Of course not. For all the claims of DNA repair, Smart Crystals, and immediate firming, La Prairie's formula is mostly water, slip agents, and alcohol. This much alcohol in an antiaging product that costs more than $600 per ounce is what should be rare. Alcohol causes cell death and free-radical damage, and that's not something you should be paying even $1 for, let alone $650. Please refer to the review for Cellular Cream Platinum Rare for information on platinum's effect on skin.

☺ $$$ **Cellular Time Release Moisture Lotion SPF 15** *($150 for 1.7 ounces)* is an in-part avobenzone sunscreen in a lotion base suitable for normal to dry skin not prone to blemishes. It contains some good water-binding agents and tiny amounts of antioxidants that will likely be compromised due to the translucent glass bottle that holds them.

☺ $$$ **Cellular Time Release Moisturizer, Intensive** *($150 for 1 ounce)* claims to moisturize for up to 16 hours, and has an oil-rich formula that likely lasts that long. However, time-released or not, many emollient moisturizers can keep skin comfortable all day and prevent moisture loss. This overall unimpressive formula doesn't break new ground and the antioxidants won't last long due to jar packaging.

☹ $$$ **Cellular Treatment Gold Illusion Line Filler** *($150 for 1 ounce)*. This silicone-based product has a silky, spackle-like texture that does to a minor degree fill in superficial wrinkles. How long the effect lasts depends on what else you apply with this product and how expressive you are. La Prairie included a large amount of the shiny mineral pigment mica and potentially irritating horsetail, which may cause irritation. Shine can make wrinkles more noticeable, so tread carefully no matter what your final thoughts about this formula.

This does contain some good antioxidants, but they're joined by alcohol, fragrance, several fragrance chemicals, and pure gold, which is known to cause contact dermatitis on the face and eyelids (Sources: *Inflammation and Allergy Drug Targets*, September 2008, pages 145-162; *Dermatologic Therapy*, volume 17, 2004, pages 321-327; and *Cutis*, May 2000, pages 323-326). There isn't much gold in this product, but there isn't much of anything else helpful for skin either. All told, the concern about the gold still exists and this isn't worth considering over better, less expensive versions of this product without the gold. An example would be Good Skin's Tri-Aktiline Instant Deep Wrinkle Filler, which costs around $40 for the same amount of product.

☹ $$$ **Cellular Wrinkle Cream** *($130 for 1 ounce)* is yet another emollient moisturizer for normal to dry skin that, just like all of the other options from La Prairie, claims to fight wrinkles. The emollients and thickeners can make wrinkles look less apparent, but all told this water-, oil-, and wax-based formula is drastically overpriced.

☺ $$$ **Cellular Protective Body Emulsion SPF 30** *($140 for 5 ounces)* includes an in-part avobenzone sunscreen and has a silky base formula built around silicone and emollients. The formula is also loaded with antioxidants, though all of them are listed after the potentially irritating horsetail extract, which is what keeps this pricey sunscreen for normal to dry skin from earning a Paula's Pick rating.

☹ **Cellular Self Tan For Face and Body SPF 15** *($115 for 3.4 ounces)* does not contain the UVA-protecting ingredients of titanium dioxide, zinc oxide, avobenzone, Tinosorb, or Mexoryl SX, and is not recommended. Self-tanner-wise, dihydroxyacetone shows up in almost every sunless tanning product being sold, and for far less money than this misguided formulation.

☹ **Cellular Balancing Mask** *($135)* is a two-part mask: the **Solvent** consists of water, citric acid, slip agents, and plant extracts, and the **Powdered Substance** is mostly baking soda, clay, silica, and the film-forming agent PVP. The Solvent is acidic while the Powdered Substance is alkaline, so they cancel each other out and haven't a snowball's shot in you-know-where of balancing skin. If anything, these ingredients will leave your skin wondering what you could have possibly been thinking!

☺ **$$$ Cellular Cycle Ampoules for the Face** *($360 for 7 treatments)* is a less expensive, slightly stripped-down version of the Skin Caviar Intensive Ampoule Treatment reviewed above. The ingredients in this version are truly an embarrassment, but not because they're irritating. Rather, they're so ordinary that it's almost funny, although when I think that lots of women are wasting their money on this overpriced mixture, it's actually rather depressing.

☺ **$$$ Cellular Deep Cleansing Mask** *($140 for 1.7 ounces)* is an exceptionally standard clay mask for normal to oily skin that contains token amounts of plant extracts, most of which are beneficial. The AHAs in this product cannot exfoliate skin because the pH is too high.

☹ **Cellular Energizing Mask** *($140 for 1.7 ounces)* contains a solvent that enhances penetration of the other ingredients, but that's not good news for skin because this mask contains irritating amounts of horsetail, lemon peel oil, orange oil, and juniper, and you don't want them penetrating any more than you want them on the surface of your skin.

☺ **$$$ Cellular Hydralift Firming Mask** *($140 for 1.7 ounces)* won't firm skin, but will reinforce its moisture barrier as claimed because of the Vaseline it contains, along with triglycerides and silicone. Several very good antioxidants are included, but their potency will be diminished due to jar packaging.

☹ **Cellular Purifying Blemish Control** *($80 for 0.5 ounce)* contains an unknown amount of salicylic acid as the active ingredient, but the base formula is mostly alcohol, and that's too irritating and drying for all skin types. Further, many of the plant extracts in this product can cause inflammation.

☹ **Cellular Luxe Lip Treatment SPF 15** *($50 for 0.12 ounce)* has deluxe packaging, but leaves lips vulnerable to UVA damage because the sunscreen is *sans* titanium dioxide, zinc oxide, avobenzone, Tinosorb, or Mexoryl SX. The base formula couldn't be more ordinary, and is a further insult at this price.

☺ **$$$ Cellular Lip Renewal Concentrate** *($95 for 0.5 ounce)* is the weakest of La Prairie's three lip products, and makes the odd claim of being able to revive natural lip color (which it cannot do; stick with lipstick for that!). It's essentially a lightweight moisturizer for lips that has more flavor than antioxidants or other helpful ingredients for lips.

✓ ☺ **$$$ Cellular Lip Line Plumper** *($85 for 0.08 ounce)* contains no retinol, but it does contain a blend of silicones and silicone polymers that do a good job of serving as a soft spackle for lip lines. This also contains some very good water-binding agents and cell-communicating ingredients, and omits the irritants typically found in lip-plumping products. It's not as miraculous as the claims imply, but it does work temporarily to fill in lines around the mouth and makes lips look and feel noticeably smoother.

LA PRAIRIE MAKEUP

FOUNDATION: ☺ **$$$ Cellular Treatment Foundation Powder Finish** *($80)* is a talc-based wet/dry powder foundation that has a wonderfully smooth texture and a gorgeous silky finish. It would work best for normal to slightly dry or slightly oily skin types. Companies such as Laura Mercier, Lancome, Chanel, and M.A.C. offer even more impressive powder foundations for much less money, but if you're stuck on La Prairie, this won't disappoint. Four of the six shades are great, but avoid Rose Beige (too rose), and if you have a medium to tan skin tone, consider Soleil Beige carefully.

☺ **$$$ Cellular Treatment Foundation Satin SPF 15** *($70)* provides an in-part titanium dioxide sunscreen, which is the least you should expect from a foundation at this price. It has a fluid yet creamy texture and blends from sheer to medium coverage with a satin finish. The La Prairie salesperson was steering me away from this option, indicating that it uses "older technology" and isn't as advanced as their other foundations. However, getting the sunscreen right (as this one does), along with the comparably lower price point, makes this not only advanced but also the only La Prairie liquid foundation worth considering. Among the nine shades, the four best avoided are 1.0, 3.2, 4.0, and 4.5.

☹ **Cellular Treatment Foundation Cream Finish** *($95)* tries to justify its price by claiming to be a perfect fusion of makeup with state-of-the-art skin care. What's not mentioned is how ordinary most of the ingredients in this cream-to-powder compact foundation are. Yes, it contains some antioxidants, including a few original choices; but the manner in which this is packaged won't help keep them stable during use, and most likely their potency is diminished because of the potential irritation from the many volatile fragrance components present (including eugenol), which is disappointing. This ends up being an unimpressive, overly fragranced foundation whose better attributes (blends easily, offers a smooth-matte finish, and comes in mostly good colors) are offset by the formulary negatives and the shocking price. Estee Lauder's Resilience Lift Extreme Ultra Firming Crème Compact Makeup SPF 15 far surpasses this and is available at one-third the price.

☹ **Anti-Aging Foundation SPF 15** *($100)* is a problem for anyone concerned with antiaging. Not only does it lack sufficient UVA protection (i.e., it doesn't contain avobenzone, titanium dioxide, zinc oxide, Tinosorb, or Mexoryl SX), which isn't antiaging in the least, but also it is pro-aging because it also contains more alcohol than any state-of-the-art ingredients (and this is one long ingredient list!), and alcohol only increases your risk of irritation, dryness, and free-radical damage. The good ingredients in this formula have to fight the alcohol as much as the environment and they are hampered by the lack of UVA protection. What a headache.

CONCEALER: ☺ **$$$ Light Fantastic Cellular Concealing Brightening Eye Treatment** *($70)* has a silky, silicone-enhanced texture and is dispensed onto a synthetic brush via a click-pen component. The product comes with a refill cartridge, which is seemingly generous for La Prairie. In terms of camouflage, this doesn't conceal more than very minor discolorations. It works best as a subtle highlighter. The "powerful" antiaging complex is barely present, and there is no research anywhere to support the claim that glycoproteins and plant extracts, especially in the tiny amounts here, can have an antiwrinkle effect. Although this has an attractive creaseless finish and comes in three good colors, I wouldn't choose it over similar, less expensive highlighters from Estee Lauder or Yves Saint Laurent.

POWDER: ☺ **$$$ Cellular Treatment Loose Powder** *($75)* has an ultra-fine, talc-based texture and a sheer, minimalist finish that leaves skin looking polished and dusted with sparkles. If shiny, expensive powder is your thing, here's a good option, and both shades are translucent.

BLUSH AND BRONZER: ☺ **$$$ Cellular Radiance Cream Blush** *($70)* would be enthusiastically recommended were it not for the ridiculous price. It's a very good, nontraditional cream blush that applies and blends nicely, leaving a soft, transparent wash of color. Skin looks healthy and glowing from each of the four colors, and the shine level is almost on mute. If you're going to indulge in some La Prairie makeup and have dry skin, this would be something to seriously consider, but only for a splurge, because your cheeks won't look like you spent this kind of money on your face.

☺ **$$$ Cellular Treatment Bronzing Powder** *($60)* features two attractive tan colors in one compact, but this pressed bronzing powder's texture is noticeably dry, and although the shine is soft it doesn't cling well, making this a below-average option, especially for the money.

☺ **$$$ Cellular Treatment Powder Blush** *($55)* doesn't impress with its drier-than-usual, slightly grainy texture, though it still applies smoothly. Every shade is shiny, but the effect is closer to a soft glow than sparkles, which is a nice change of pace. Still, countless cosmetic lines offer less expensive powder blushes that have a superior texture and better array of shades.

EYESHADOW: ☺ **$$$ Cellular Treatment Eye Colour Ensemble** *($70)* provides four eyeshadows in one compact, with one shade in each being dark enough to use as eyeliner. These have a smoother, silkier feel and apply better than the Cellular Treatment Eye Colour (below), though still a bit unevenly. Every set has quite a bit of shine, and that's not the best for wrinkled eye-area skin; the least shiny (and most workable) set is called Les Bruns.

☹ **Cellular Eye Colour Effects** *($35)* has a slick, cream-to-powder texture that leaves a silky, very shiny finish. The sheer colors impart much more shine than pigment, which won't deemphasize wrinkles or a drooping eyelid. Given the price and the "mature" positioning of this line, a product like this doesn't make much sense, nor does it last that long without creasing.

☹ **Cellular Treatment Eye Colour** *($45)* is La Prairie's name for their powder eyeshadow singles, and is the most enticing thing about this otherwise unremarkable product. The smooth but dry texture and too-soft pressing lead to a chunky, flake-prone application, and there are far too many pastel tones that do little to shape or shade the eye.

EYE AND BROW SHAPER: ☺ **$$$ Luxe Eye Liner Automatique** *($50)* is an automatic, retractable eye pencil, but the sleek metal component is what you end up paying for. Each color goes on smoothly and leaves a slightly creamy finish that won't be impervious to smearing unless set with a powder eyeshadow. Of course, you could just line with a powder eyeshadow and be done, but this is a decent option for those who prefer pencils. Avoid Lavande, which is way too purple.

☺ **$$$ Luxe Brow Liner Automatique** *($50)* comes in the same type of retractable metal component as the Luxe Eye Liner Automatique, and also features a brow brush on the other end. This is a very good brow pencil that has a smooth but dry application and a soft powder finish that won't budge. The only issue (beyond the price) is that it takes some effort to get the colors to show up.

LIPSTICK, LIP GLOSS, AND LIPLINER: ☺ **$$$ Cellular Lip Colour Effects Luminous Transparent Glaze** *($40)* has an elegantly smooth, not-too-thick texture and a minimally sticky, sparkling finish. Featuring a brush applicator, this gloss does have movement—despite claims to the contrary—so don't expect it to not feather into lines around the mouth, just like most glosses do.

☺ **$$$ Luxe Lip Liner Automatique** *($45)* has a luxurious metal component and above-average brush on the opposite end to soften and blend the line from this automatic, retractable pencil. Because it stays creamy it can't help keep lipstick from migrating into lines around the mouth, so if that's a concern, it's best to skip this one. The Nude shade is a versatile color.

☺ **$$$ Cellular Luxe Lip Colour** *($55)* leans to the greasy side of creamy, which doesn't bode well for those prone to lipstick traveling into lines around the mouth. These light- to medium-coverage shimmer-laden lipsticks leave no stain, so their wear time is relatively brief. All told, there isn't a strong argument to consider these over many other creamy lipsticks, but they're not terrible either.

The Reviews L

☹ **Cellular Luxe Lip Enhancer** *($50)* is a slightly dry, waxy, peach-toned lipstick that claims to prevent every problem you've ever had using a lipstick, but it's just a barely passable concealer that can lightly smooth the lip's surface. Don't bother with this unless you get a thrill out of wasting money.

MASCARA: ☺ $$$ **Cellular Treatment Mascara Instant Curl** *($40)* doesn't do anything instantly, but with patience this extends lashes to fluttering length and leaves them with a soft, fringed curl. Thickness is harder to come by, but the application is clump-free and wearability is uneventful.

☺ $$$ **Cellular Treatment Mascara Instant Build** *($40)* won't clump at all and leaves lashes remarkably soft, but otherwise takes a long time to produce meager lengthening. This isn't any more of a treatment for lashes than most mascaras, and the amount of La Prairie's "Cellular Complex" is minuscule compared to the standard waxes seen in this and most mascaras available today.

BRUSHES: ☺ $$$ **Art of the Brush Collection** *($250)* gets you every brush in a sleek, roll-up case, but a few of these brushes are low quality and don't make this complete set a value. La Prairie's handsome **Brushes** *($28-$65, $125-$250 for collections)* are frustrating because only four of the nine are sold separately. If you want more than that, you have to buy one of the kits. In or out of the kits, most of these brushes are nicely shaped and have comfortable handles, but you will find similarly priced and far more appealing brushes from Trish McEvoy and Stila. The best single brush is the **Professional Concealer Brush** *($30)*, which can double as an eyeshadow brush.

SPECIALTY PRODUCTS: ☺ $$$ **Cellular Treatment Rose Illusion Line Filler** *($115)* supposedly works to make wrinkled skin look smooth and line-free, but don't get your hopes up and don't open your pocketbook. This thick but silky gel-cream is mostly silicone and has an opalescent pink tint to slightly brighten skin. Silicone primers have a softening effect—and that's it; they don't erase lines.

LA ROCHE-POSAY (SKIN CARE ONLY)

LA ROCHE-POSAY AT-A-GLANCE

Strengths: Very good cleansers; well-formulated, stably packaged options for those seeking products with hydroquinone or retinol or stabilized vitamin C; many fragrance-free options; a unique lip moisturizer.

Weaknesses: Some problematic, overly irritating exfoliants; lack of anti-acne products that target blemishes effectively, yet gently; several ho-hum moisturizers and sunscreens.

For more information about La Roche-Posay, owned by L'Oreal, call (888) 577-5226 or visit www.laroche-posay.com or www.Beautypedia.com.

LA ROCHE-POSAY BIOMEDIC PRODUCTS

☺ $$$ **Biomedic AntiBac Acne Wash** *($32 for 6 ounces)* is a very standard, water-soluble cleanser that contains 1.8% salicylic acid as the active ingredient, though its benefit in a cleanser is negligible because it is rinsed from skin before it has a chance to work. This is still a good option for normal to oily skin, provided you keep it away from the eye area.

☹ **Biomedic LHA Cleansing Gel** *($46.50 for 6.76 ounces)*. The LHA in this product's name refers to lipo-hydroxy acid, a term La Roche-Posay made up to make the form of salicylic acid they use (capryloyl salicylic acid) seem more impressive than it is. The only research on this ingredient was done by L'Oreal, La Roche-Posay's owner. Their single study showed that an LHA peel at 5-10% strength was as good as, but tolerated better than, a glycolic acid peel at a concentration range of 20-50%, which can be quite irritating, so the comparison doesn't make sense; it's like comparing apples to lettuce. The take-home message is this quote from the study: "there were no statistically significant differences between the two groups." Clearly, not even L'Oreal believes there is much to be gained from going with LHA peels over AHA peels (Source: *Journal of Cosmetic Dermatology*, December 2008, pages 259-262). Regardless, a medical peel isn't the same as what you buy in a skin-care product. A well-formulated glycolic acid or salicylic acid leave-on skin-care product can help skin feel smooth and look "younger," but when it comes to using LHA or glycolic acid in a cleanser, forget about it because both are just rinsed down the drain. And forget about this overpriced cleanser because it offers no special benefit for skin, but it will cause irritation due to the menthol it contains.

☺ **$$$ Biomedic Purifying Cleanser** *($37.50 for 6 ounces)* is an excellent, water-soluble cleanser for all skin types except very dry. It doesn't purify skin better than similar options, but it's gentle, removes makeup well, and does not contain fragrance. The tiny amount of glycolic acid functions as a water-binding agent, not as an exfoliant.

☹ **Biomedic Micro Exfoliating Scrub** *($36.50 for 6 ounces)* is an overly abrasive scrub that contains almost every irritating volatile oil known, including lemon, lime, and grapefruit. Ouch!

☹ **Biomedic LHA Pre-Peel Solution** *($46.50 for 6.76 ounces)*. This is about as problematic a product as you're likely to find in the name of being an exfoliant. First, it is not a pre-peel product; given the amount of glycolic and salicylic acids, it is an exfoliant. However, alcohol is the second ingredient, which instantly makes it a problem for all skin types (alcohol causes free-radical damage and cell death). As for helping oily, acne-prone skin, alcohol does nothing of the sort. Instead, it stimulates nerve endings in the pore and triggers more oil production. This is a misguided, overpriced product that should absolutely be left on the shelf.

☺ **Biomedic Conditioning Cream** *($44 for 2 ounces)* is a very standard 6% glycolic acid moisturizer best for normal to dry skin. The low pH makes it very effective for exfoliation, but the other ingredients are no different from what you would find in AHA products at the drugstore from Alpha Hydrox or Neutrogena Healthy Skin.

☹ **Biomedic Conditioning Solution** *($37.50 for 6 ounces)* contains a lot of alcohol and also includes irritating eucalyptus oil, neither of which will help the glycolic and salicylic acids increase skin's health or renew skin.

☹ **Biomedic Extra Rich Moisturizer** *($60.50 for 2 ounces)* contains an excellent complement of ingredients for dry, sensitized skin, but the inclusion of sage oil and lavender makes it impossible to recommend. Although sage oil has antioxidant ability, two of its main volatile components (thujone and camphor) are skin irritants.

☺ **$$$ Biomedic Gentle Moisturizing Lotion SPF 15** *($37.50 for 2.5 ounces)* is an exceptionally basic, but effective, daytime moisturizer for normal to minimally dry skin. It features an in-part titanium dioxide sunscreen and is fragrance-free, but that's about it.

☺ **$$$ Biomedic Gentle Soothing Ointment** *($22 for 1.76 ounces)* is, in essence, just a very pricey version of Vaseline because it contains mostly Vaseline, mineral oil, and wax. Yes, it can help very dry skin feel better, but not any better than pure Vaseline. It is incredibly similar to much less expensive products at the drugstore, such as Aquaphor Healing Ointment.

☺ $$$ **Biomedic Hydra-Recovery** (*$44 for 1.35 ounces*). I'm not sure why La Roche-Posay mentions that this moisturizer contains multiple calming agents because it doesn't, at least not in terms of what published research has demonstrated concerning anti-irritants for skin. This is really just a very basic, exceedingly overpriced (and I mean really overpriced) moisturizer for normal to slightly dry skin. The "1% dermobiotic" referred to in the claims is about the company's vitreoscilla ferment ingredient. There is no research proving this ingredient has any benefit for skin, and I am doubtful it's present at 1% given where it appears on the ingredient list. But even if this product contained 10% of the stuff, what benefit does it provide? Your skin would be far better off with a product loaded with anti-irritants, antioxidants, and skin-identical ingredients.

☺ $$$ **Biomedic Hydrating Serum** (*$71.50 for 1 ounce*) is a good, lightweight serum for all skin types that provides a small selection of water-binding agents and antioxidant vitamins. Considering its price, it should contain more bells and whistles than it does, yet it is a suitable option for sensitive skin due to the fragrance-free simplicity of the formula.

☹ **Biomedic Hydro Active Emulsion** (*$42 for 2 ounces*) claims to be antioxidant-rich, but contains only a small amount of vitamin E, which is hardly exciting. This is otherwise an average emollient moisturizer for normal to dry skin. It is fragrance-free.

☹ **Biomedic LHA Serum** (*$68.50 for 1 ounce*). Your skin has nothing to gain but much to lose if you apply this serum because it contains a skin-damaging amount of alcohol. Alcohol causes free-radical damage, dryness, and irritation. Interestingly, glycolic acid is the predominant exfoliant in this serum, again proving that L'Oreal doesn't believe their LHA concept is the best thing going for obtaining smoother, younger looking skin.

☺ $$$ **Biomedic Potent-C 10.5 Concentrate** (*$72.50 for 1 ounce*) contains 10.5% stabilized vitamin C, and comes in packaging that preserves the stability of this antioxidant. There's not much else to say about this product, other than that the glycol base will enhance penetration of the vitamin C, which could pose problems for those with sensitive skin.

☺ $$$ **Biomedic Exfozyme** (*$40 for 1.69 ounces*). I don't know why this mask is labeled "professional-quality" because there isn't anything special or professional about it, and what constitutes a professional designation anyway? Perhaps it's the fact that the product is sold only to aestheticians or physicians? Those decisions and distinctions are all about marketing, not special formulas. This mask is meant to prepare skin for in-office cosmetic procedures such as peels. It contains a high amount of urea, an ingredient that is known as a keratolytic, which means that it softens/weakens dead skin cells to encourage shedding. Applying this pre-peel should net better results because the peel has less surface debris to get through and can have a greater impact on the lower layers of the epidermis, potentially influencing the dermis to produce new collagen. There isn't much else to this mask, and actually you could try using a urea-containing moisturizer from the drugstore before spending so much on this product. Examples of good options are Nutraplus Therapeutic Lotion with 10% Urea and Carmol 10 Total Body Lotion for Dry Skin, both of which are available online at www.drugstore.com.

☺ $$$ **Biomedic Collagenist Powder** (*$43 for 0.5 ounce*) contains three forms of vitamin C. It is designed to be added to any moisturizer to customize it, but doing so will alter the pH of this powder, potentially making the vitamin C ineffective. Moreover, an excess of ascorbic acid can be irritating to skin, and you'd have no way of knowing how much you're adding in terms of potency. It is far better to stay with a serum or moisturizer whose vitamin C content has been calibrated and stabilized within that formula rather than experimenting with this do-it-yourself powder.

☹ **Biomedic Conditioning Gel** *($41 for 2 ounces)* lists 2% hydroquinone as the active ingredient, but this effective, time-proven skin-lightening agent is joined by enough alcohol to make it too irritating and drying for all skin types. The glycolic acid and pH of 3.5 make the alcohol that much more problematic.

☹ **Biomedic Conditioning Gel Plus** *($54 for 2 ounces)* is similar to the Biomedic Conditioning Gel, except this contains more glycolic acid. Otherwise, the same comments apply.

☺ **$$$ Biomedic Retinol Cream 15, 30, & 60** *($52-$57.50 for 1 ounce)* all come in the same lotion base with varying amounts of retinol in what La Roche-Posay refers to as a Customizable Step-Up system. Retinol 15 contains the lowest amount of retinol (0.15%), Retinol 30 contains 0.30%, and, as expected, Retinol 60 contains 0.60%. All are fragrance-free and packaged so the air- and light-sensitive retinol remains stable. Which one you choose isn't of much importance given that there are no formulary standards for retinol concentrations. However, it is a very good antioxidant and cell-communicating ingredient for skin because it helps create better, healthier skin cells and increases the amount of skin-support substances. Keep in mind that retinol should not be the only ingredient you look for in a moisturizer. Skin needs a combination of ingredients to function optimally, including cell-communicating ingredients (of which retinol is one), an array of antioxidants (to reduce free-radical damage), and substances that mimic skin structure. Together, all these various ingredients and elements combine to create a powerful part of any skin-care routine. Biomedic Retinol is best for normal to dry skin.

LA ROCHE-POSAY EFFACLAR PRODUCTS

☺ **$$$ Effaclar Deep Cleansing Foaming Cream** *($19.50 for 4.2 ounces)* produces a foamy lather, but contains a high amount of the alkaline ingredient potassium hydroxide, making this an option only for very oily skin, and even those folks may find this too drying.

☺ **Effaclar Purifying Foaming Gel** *($19.50 for 5.1 ounces)* is similar to the Biomedic Purifying Cleanser above, and aside from producing a more copious lather and containing fragrance, the same comments apply.

☺ **Effaclar Active Matte Moisturizer** *($25 for 1.69 ounces).* This lightweight moisturizer with mattifying properties contains a small amount of dry finish silicones, but the matte finish you'll get is short-lived due to the amount of glycerin and the thickener isocetyl stearate. The amount of alcohol in this product isn't good news, and is borderline for causing irritation. La Roche-Posay maintains that this exfoliates skin with something they refer to as LHA, but nothing on the ingredient list matches that acronym. This contains a form of salicylic acid, but not in an amount considered effective, so don't expect any exfoliation from this merely average product. By the way, given that La Roche-Posay prides itself on being a product line for someone with sensitive skin, the number of potentially risky ingredients is embarrassing, including fragrance, acrylamide/sodium acryloyldimethyltaurate copolymer, and polymethyl methacrylate.

☹ **Effaclar Astringent Lotion Micro-Exfoliant** *($19.50 for 6.76 ounces)* lists alcohol as the second ingredient, and the amount of salicylic acid is too low for exfoliation to occur.

☺ **Effaclar K Acne Treatment Fluid** *($19.90 for 1 ounce)* is a BHA product that contains 1.5% salicylic acid, now listed as an active ingredient. I remain doubtful of that concentration, but even if it is accurate, the pH of 4.4 is not low enough for much, if any, exfoliation to occur.

This is an OK option as a lightweight, very fluid moisturizer for normal to oily skin, but that's it. In Canada, this product is sold under the name Efficlar K Daily Renewal Fluid for Oily Skin; the formulas are identical.

LA ROCHE-POSAY HYDRAPHASE PRODUCTS

☺ **Hydraphase Hydrating Cleansing Milk** *($22 for 6.76 ounces)* is a good cleansing lotion for normal to dry skin. It contains more thickening agents than detergent cleansing agents, but removes makeup well. This may require a washcloth for complete removal, and is not recommended for blemish-prone skin.

☹ **$$$ Hydraphase Hydrating Toner** *($26 for 6.76 ounces)* doesn't do much to impress, but its basic formula will help remove the last traces of makeup and make normal to dry skin feel softer.

☹ **$$$ Hydraphase Eyes** *($26.50 for 0.5 ounce)* is a lightweight, fragrance-free moisturizer for slightly dry skin anywhere on the face. It contains antioxidant vitamin A and soy.

☹ **Hydraphase Light Facial Moisturizer** *($28 for 1.69 ounces)* is a substandard, rather lackluster moisturizer for normal to slightly dry skin. The amount of alcohol is unlikely to cause irritation, but antioxidants are conspicuously absent.

☹ **$$$ Hydraphase Riche Facial Cream** *($28 for 1.7 ounces)*. This is a good, though exceptionally ordinary moisturizer if you want something basic for your skin, although your skin really deserves much more. It provides lubrication from time-honored emollients such as shea butter and mineral oil, plus hydrating ingredients such as urea. Some antioxidants and skin-identical ingredients would have made all the difference in the world.

☺ **Hydraphase UV SPF 30** *($29 for 1.69 ounces)*. The best part about this daytime moisturizer for normal to oily skin is its in-part avobenzone sunscreen. The base formula, while it does have a silky lotion texture, doesn't treat skin to much beyond the basics. Almost all of the antioxidants are listed after the preservative, and as such don't count for much. Still, this provides great broad-spectrum sun protection and works well under makeup. The tiny amount of plant oils is unlikely to be a problem for blemish-prone skin (although those with very oily skin may want to avoid this product). Contrary to claim, the active ingredients plus the inclusion of fragrance do not make this safe for sensitive skin. Those with sensitive skin would do better using a mineral-based (titanium dioxide and/or zinc oxide) sunscreen that is fragrance-free.

LA ROCHE-POSAY MELA-D PRODUCTS

☺ **$$$ Mela-D Bright** *($43 for 1 ounce)* is La Roche-Posay's solution to improving discolorations without using hydroquinone despite the fact that it is the most effective ingredient for that purpose available. The problem with hydroquinone is that it has become controversial and is now banned in many countries (for more information on hydroquinone, please refer to the Cosmetic Ingredient Dictionary at www.Beautypedia.com). Instead of hydroquinone, this light-textured treatment product contains a blend of ascorbic acid (vitamin C) and kojic acid. Both have research proving their effectiveness for lightening hyperpigmentation, although both also have issues of stability and the pure form of vitamin C can be irritating due to its acid component. (Sources: *Biological and Pharmaceutical Bulletin*, August 2002, pages 1045-1048; *Analytical Biochemistry*, June 2002, pages 260-268; *Cellular Signaling*, September 2002, pages 779-785; *American Journal of Clinical Dermatology*, September-October 2000, pages 261-268; *Archives of Pharmacal Research*, August 2001, pages 307-311; and *Dermatologic Surgery*, July

2005, pages 814-817). Although these ingredients do have potential as skin-lightening agents, concentration is directly related to efficacy, and that's where this product is questionable. It is likely that even when combined, the amounts of kojic and ascorbic acids in this product may not be enough to have a significant effect on hyperpigmentation. However, the only way to know for sure (because the company certainly won't divulge the percentages) is to give this product a try (keeping in mind that no skin-lightening product can work without the diligent, daily use of a well-formulated sunscreen). It is best for normal to dry skin.

☺ **Mela-D Dark Spots SPF 15** *($45 for 1 ounce)* includes avobenzone for UVA protection, but the base formula for this daytime moisturizer with sunscreen contains enough alcohol to cause irritation and free-radical damage for all skin types. Moreover, the amount of kojic acid is likely too low to impact skin discolorations. Daily sun protection is a key element of keeping discolorations related to sun damage from recurring or getting worse, but this product isn't a sound way to go about doing that; there are far better options for a lot less money.

☺ **$$$ Mela-D Skin Lightening Daily Lotion** *($45 for 1 ounce)* contains 2% hydroquinone in packaging that will keep it stable during use. Interestingly, the base formula contains several sunscreen agents (including avobenzone), but does not sport an SPF rating, so you should not rely on this for daytime protection. (Note that if you opt to use this product at night, the sunscreens are useless and may cause irritation.) The amount of salicylic acid in this product is too low to exfoliate skin. Still, this is an option for daytime wear if you pair it with another product that is rated at least SPF 15 and includes UVA-protecting ingredients.

LA ROCHE-POSAY NUTRITIC PRODUCTS

☹ **Nutritic Ultra-Fine Cream, Transforming Care For Very Dry Skin** *($27 for 1.35 ounces)* contains an unwelcome amount of coriander oil, making it too irritating for all skin types. The volatile compounds in this oil (mostly linalool) can cause photosensitivity.

☹ **Nutritic Ultra-Fine Emulsion, Transforming Care for Dry Skin** *($27 for 1.35 ounces)* is a more emollient, Vaseline-based version of the Nutritic Ultra-Fine Cream, Transforming Care for Very Dry Skin, and the same review applies.

☹ **Nutritic Lips** *($12.50 for 0.15 ounce)* contains a very good blend of emollients, waxes, and oils to protect and soften lips. Unfortunately, this lip balm in stick form also contains coriander oil, a fragrant oil that can cause contact dermatitis and photosensitivity (Source: www.naturaldatabase.com). Given that this lip balm doesn't contain sunscreen, it is risky to wear during daylight hours, and the potential for irritation is too high to make it worth considering over several other lip moisturizers.

LA ROCHE-POSAY REDERMIC PRODUCTS

☺ **$$$ Redermic Daily Fill-In Anti-Wrinkle Firming Care, Face and Neck, for Dry Skin** *($45.50 for 1.35 ounces)* differs little from La Roche-Posay's Active C, for Dry Skin reviewed below, though this one doesn't ballyhoo its vitamin C content. Otherwise, the same comments apply: The silky, silicone-enhanced base with its nearly matte finish is ideal for normal to oily skin. Just to be clear, vitamin C is a very good, well-established antioxidant for skin, but it isn't the only one to consider, and in that sense you are getting a one-note product by choosing this.

☺ **$$$ Redermic Daily Fill-In Anti-Wrinkle Firming Care, Face and Neck, for Normal to Combination Skin** *($45.50 for 1.35 ounces)* is similar to, but less desirable than, the Active C, for Dry Skin below due to its alcohol content. However, it's still an option if you're curious to try a vitamin C product and you have combination skin.

☺ **$$$ Redermic Eyes, Daily Fill-In Anti-Wrinkle Firming Care** *($36.50 for 1.5 ounces)* is a basic lightweight moisturizer that contains a good amount of vitamin C. The silky, nearly matte finish is suitable only if skin around the eyes is minimally dry. Think of this as a fragrance-free way to supply skin with vitamin C (though it would be better if a variety of antioxidants were included).

☺ **$$$ Redermic UV SPF 15** *($47.50 for 1.35 ounces)*. The supposedly big-deal ingredient in this daytime moisturizer with an in-part avobenzone sunscreen is an extract from the plant *Centella asiatica* that La Roche-Posay refers to as madecassoside. Supposedly, this can tighten loose skin and help heal wrinkles, leading to firmer skin. There is research pertaining to this ingredient's ability to improve sun-damaged skin when combined with vitamin C (as is the case with this product); however, the research was performed by a dermatology lab in France (where the company is based) and La Roche-Posay paid for the study. Still, there is enough animal research on madecassoside to give it a try. It likely has a positive, antioxidant effect on skin, but probably not the lifting, tightening, and line-filling results La Roche-Posay promises (Sources: *Planta Medica*, June 2008, pages 809-815; and *Experimental Dermatology*, May 2008, ePublication). Redermic UV SPF 15 is best for normal to oily skin. It definitely qualifies as a daytime moisturizer with a sufficient quantity of vitamin C, which also plays a role in mitigating sun damage.

LA ROCHE-POSAY TOLERIANE PRODUCTS

✓☺ **$$$ Toleriane Dermo-Cleanser** *($19.50 for 6.76 ounces)* is a very simple, fragrance-free cleansing lotion for dry skin. It poses no risk of irritating skin unless you know you're sensitive to one of the ingredients it contains, and it does a decent job of removing most types of makeup. Its value for dry, sensitive skin earns it a Paula's Pick rating.

☹ **Toleriane Gentle Cleansing Bar** *($8 for 4 ounces)* doesn't contain fragrance, which is good; however, this is standard-issue bar soap and as such it is too drying and irritating for all skin types.

✓☺ **$$$ Toleriane Purifying Foaming Cream** *($21 for 4.22 ounces)* is a very good water-soluble foaming cleanser with a soft cream texture suitable for normal to slightly dry skin, and it removes makeup quickly. The detergent cleansing agents are not bad, but they're also not the best for "intolerant" skin, as La Roche-Posay asserts.

☺ **Toleriane Eye Make-Up Remover** *($22 for 6 ounces)* is a basic, fragrance-free eye-makeup remover packaged in single-use ampoules so it does not need to contain preservatives. Although it's an effective option for sensitive skin around the eyes, the honey in this product (it's the third ingredient) lends a somewhat tacky finish that must be rinsed.

☺ **Toleriane Fluide, Soothing Protective Non-Oily Emulsion** *($24 for 1.35 ounces)* is an average, fragrance-free moisturizer for normal to dry skin not prone to blemishes. Given the simplicity of the formula, this may indeed be a good option for those dealing with rosacea and the sensitivity it entails; it's just so no-frills, I couldn't possibly rate it higher.

☺ **Toleriane Riche, Soothing Protective Cream** *($22 for 1.35 ounces)*. It's interesting to note that the same thickening agent in this product meant for dry skin also contributes significantly to the texture of the company's Effaclar Active Matte Moisturizer, which is designed for oily skin. The truth is that it's much better for dry skin, so in this product it makes sense; it doesn't make sense in the Effaclar. Viewed as a simple fragrance-free formula for sensitive skin, this is worth considering, but overall it is just completely ordinary and not worth the price tag in the least. There isn't one state-of-the-art ingredient and it contains aluminum starch octenylsuccinate, a drying ingredient that isn't the best for sensitive skin. For the money, the company should have at least included one antioxidant or skin-identical ingredient!

☹ **Toleriane Soothing Protective Skincare** *($22 for 1.35 ounces).* Toleriane Soothing Protective Skincare is a very basic, fragrance-free moisturizing lotion for normal to slightly dry skin. It does not contain a single anti-irritant or antioxidant, so it ends up being neither protective nor any more soothing than any other ordinary moisturizer.

OTHER LA ROCHE-POSAY PRODUCTS

☹ **Lipikar Surgras Lipid-Enriched Cleansing Bar, for Severely Dry Skin** *($9 for 5.2 ounces)* has a fancy name and affordable price, but it's still old-fashioned bar soap and can be drying and irritating for all skin types.

✓ ☺ **$$$ Rosaliac Gelee Micellar Make-Up Removal Gel** *($23.50 for 6.76 ounces)* is a gentle, water-based eye-area cleanser that removes most types of eye makeup (though some waterproof mascaras may prove resistant to this formula). It is great for sensitive eyes because fragrance, fragrant plant extracts, and coloring agents are excluded.

☹ **Thermal Spring Water** *($7 for 1.8 ounces)* comes with claims of soothing, toning, refreshing, and providing antioxidant protection to skin, yet all it contains is water and nitrogen. Thermal Spring Water is just water and some extra nitrogen. This product is said to be "rich in selenium, a powerful antioxidant." Whether or not that is true (though obtaining pure selenium as an oral supplement is preferred) is irrelevant because the nitrogen used as a propellant to create a mist of water can generate free-radical damage and cause cell death (Sources: *Cellular and Molecular Biology*, April 15, 2007, pages 1-2; *Mechanisms of Ageing and Development*, April 2002, pages 1007-1019; and *Toxicology and Applied Pharmacology*, July 2002, pages 84-90).

☺ **$$$ Active C Eyes** *($35 for 0.5 ounce)* is a silky, silicone-enriched lightweight moisturizer for slightly dry skin anywhere on the face. It contains a good amount of vitamin C (as ascorbic acid) and contains fragrance in the form of bitter-orange flower extract.

☺ **$$$ Active C, for Dry Skin** *($43.50 for 1 ounce)* would be an outstanding way to see if a 5% stabilized vitamin C product (packaged to ensure stability and potency) improves your skin. The silky, silicone-enhanced base with its nearly matte finish is ideal for normal to oily skin. Just to be clear, vitamin C is a very good, well-established antioxidant for skin, but it isn't the only one to consider, and in that sense you are getting a one-note product by choosing this.

☺ **$$$ Active C, for Normal to Combination Skin** *($43.50 for 1 ounce)* is similar to the Active C, for Dry Skin, and the same review applies.

☺ **Rosaliac Skin Perfecting Anti-Redness Moisturizer** *($32 for 1.35 ounces)* is a product I am asked about fairly often, and the questions come from the product's target audience: women dealing with the redness and sensitivity of rosacea. Rosaliac Skin Perfecting Anti-Redness Moisturizer is said to neutralize redness while calming and soothing inflamed skin. It does have a mint green color, but that has minimal to no effect on reducing or covering facial redness of any kind. A sheer foundation or tinted moisturizer with real skin–tone shades would do a better job of softening skin's reddened appearance. Overall, this is a simply formulated, fragrance-free moisturizer for normal to slightly dry skin. It's just not the solution or even a great option for someone with rosacea. Anyone dealing with rosacea is likely aware that it is wise to avoid topical irritants, especially since many cases of rosacea react to various seemingly benign ingredients with no rhyme or reason. It is therefore best to shop for skin-care products without known irritants or potentially "active" ingredients, particularly when they're intended to be left on the skin. In the case of this product, it does not make sense to include alcohol, caffeine, and niacinamide. Alcohol and caffeine have irritant properties, while niacinamide is derived from niacin, which, although it can be beneficial, has the potential to cause facial flushing—not what someone with reddened skin needs.

☺ **$$$ Substiane** *($49.50 for 1.35 ounces)* makes a big deal about the amount of Pro-Xylane it contains, but what exactly is this Pro-Xylane complex? L'Oreal (La Roche-Posay's owner) includes it in several of their products as well as in their Lancome Absolue line, but not the 5% amount that's being hyped with this product. Suffice it to say, Pro-Xylane is not an essential ingredient for skin, mature or not. It certainly isn't a worthy stand-in for retinoids, which is what it's often compared to! For detailed information about L'Oreal's Pro-Xylane, please refer to the review for Lancome Absolue Eye Premium Bx, Absolute Replenishing Eye Cream. Regarding Substiane, it ends up being little more than a good emollient moisturizer for normal to dry skin not prone to blemishes. It does contain the amino acids serine and arginine as claimed, but not in any amount that's likely to have a specific or noticeable effect on skin.

☹ **$$$ Substiane Eyes** *($39 for 0.5 ounce)* is described in a manner that makes it sound much more scientific than it is. Apparently, it contains 5% Pro-Xylane, an ingredient that L'Oreal (La Roche-Posay's owner) created and includes in its products quite often despite never revealing what it really is or the research for what makes it good for skin. As for it being a "cutaneous substance replenishing ingredient," that description applies to many cosmetic ingredients that replenish substances occurring naturally in skin, which this product woefully lacks. Even more confusing is the presence of cornstarch and silica high up on the ingredient list because both of those ingredients absorb moisture, which makes them a strange addition to any moisturizer meant to hydrate skin. At best, this is a basic emollient moisturizer for slightly dry skin anywhere on the face. It contains very few state-of-the-art ingredients and given the size, this is really outrageously overpriced for what amounts to a poorly conceived product.

✓ ☺ **Ceralip Lip Repair Cream** *($13.50 for 0.5 ounce)* is a sufficiently creamy lip moisturizer that differs from the usual wax-based sticks or oil-based balms. It is definitely an option for dry lips, and is fragrance- and flavor-free.

☺ **Lipolevres Lip Protector** *($12 for 0.1 ounce)* is a standard oil-based lip balm whose ingredients protect lips from dehydration and keep them soft. It isn't quite as elegant as the Ceralip Lip Repair Cream.

LA ROCHE-POSAY SUN PRODUCTS

☺ **Anthelios 15 Sunscreen Cream SPF 15** *($29.95 for 3.4 ounces)* follows many of the other L'Oreal-owned brands by combining an in-part Mexoryl SX (ecamsule) sunscreen in a lightweight, bland moisturizing base suitable for normal to slightly dry or slightly oily skin. Avobenzone is included, too, so without a doubt UVA protection is assured (although Mexoryl SX isn't the only ingredient that provides that benefit). If only the formula included at least one antioxidant and some other state-of-the-art ingredients for skin! Still, it deserves a happy face rating on the basis of its value as a sunscreen.

☺ **Anthelios 40 Sunscreen Cream SPF 40** *($32 for 1.7 ounces)*. The best thing I can say about this incredibly mundane daytime moisturizer with sunscreen is that the UVA range is more than covered because it contains avobenzone and ecamsule, also known as Mexoryl SX. L'Oreal continues to hold the patent on Mexoryl, which is why only their brands (of which La Roche-Posay is one) can use it. The base formula is as bland as all of the company's other sunscreens with Mexoryl SX, but this is an OK option for normal to slightly dry or slightly oily skin.

☺ **Anthelios 60 Melt-In Sunscreen Lotion** *($26 for 1.7 ounces)*. It's interesting that La Roche-Posay's Anthelios 60 sunscreens do not contain Mexoryl SX (ecamsule), the UVA-protecting active ingredient that their parent company, L'Oreal, has the patent on. Instead, Anthelios 60 contains avobenzone for UVA protection. The big thing with this lightweight, matte-finish lotion is the claim that it contains powerful antioxidants. It does contain antioxidants, but only two—vitamin E and *Cassia alata* leaf—and they are barely present; however, they're not all that powerful anyway, so even if there were more of them in this product it wouldn't be a significant improvement. This daytime moisturizer with sunscreen provides broad-spectrum protection and has a texture that those with normal to very oily skin will appreciate, but it doesn't "walk the talk" when it comes to providing a superior antioxidant boost.

☹ **$$$ Anthelios 60 Melt-In Sunscreen Milk** *($32 for 5 ounces)*. It's interesting that La Roche-Posay's Anthelios 60 sunscreens do not contain Mexoryl SX (ecamsule), the UVA-protecting active ingredient patented by their parent company L'Oreal. Instead, Anthelios 60 contains avobenzone for UVA protection. The big thing with this lightweight, matte-finish lotion is the claim that it contains powerful antioxidants. It does contain antioxidants, but only two—vitamin E and *Cassia alata* leaf—and they are barely present so they aren't particularly powerful or potent anyway. This sunscreen provides broad-spectrum protection and has a texture those with normal to very oily skin will appreciate, but it doesn't "walk the talk" when it comes to providing a superior antioxidant boost. Actually, there's more damaging alcohol in here than there are antioxidants, which further dulls what little effectiveness they have, especially given the low amounts.

☺ **Anthelios SX Daily Moisturizing Cream with Sunscreen SPF 15** *($29.95 for 3.4 ounces)* made a big media splash with overblown stories that one of its active ingredients (ecamsule, also known as Mexoryl SX) was a new UVA filter approved by the FDA. What wasn't routinely mentioned was that (at the time of the press release) the FDA approved this active ingredient for only one product, which is the subject of this review. What's noteworthy about this sunscreen is its combination of ecamsule with avobenzone, as stabilized by octocrylene. You can be assured of sufficient UVA protection if you apply this liberally and long enough before venturing outdoors. What's disappointing is that the excitement starts and stops right there. Nothing else about this silicone-enhanced sunscreen is that intriguing, and it doesn't contain even a single antioxidant. For the money and with all the hype this product has generated, you should expect more. Still, it deserves a happy face rating for its sunscreen alone, and the formula is suitable for normal to slightly dry or slightly oily skin. One more thing: Although Mexoryl SX is a good UVA sunscreen, it does not provide the highest level of UVA protection as claimed on the label. Lest we forget, titanium dioxide and zinc oxide can screen UVA rays well beyond their measurable threshold, so Mexoryl SX, while viable, is not intrinsically the best.

☹ **Anthelios 60 Ultra Light Sunscreen Fluid** *($27.50 for 1.7 ounces)*. This has the same active ingredients and percentages as the Anthelios 60 Melt-In Sunscreen Lotion, but the base formula is different. UVA protection is assured from avobenzone, but the amount of alcohol in the base formula is cause for concern (alcohol causes free-radical damage and cell death). The big claim about this daytime moisturizer with sunscreen is how its potent antioxidants provide additional protection for sun-exposed skin. Antioxidants can boost a sunscreen's effectiveness and help skin defend itself better against environmental damage, but not in the paltry amounts present in this product—and not with alcohol being so high up on the ingredient list. How disappointing!

LANCOME

LANCOME AT-A-GLANCE

Strengths: Some good cleansers; well-formulated scrubs; almost all of the sunscreens contain either avobenzone, ecamsule (Mexoryl SX), or titanium dioxide for sufficient UVA protection; an outstanding retinol product; a large selection of self-tanning products; several excellent foundations with beautiful shades for almost every skin color; some great concealers; Lancome is known for their mostly outstanding mascaras; the Absolue powder; the liquid eyeliner; all of the powder eyeshadows; one fantastic lipstick and automatic lipliner.

Weaknesses: Expensive for what amounts to mostly mediocre to below-average skin-care products; no AHA or BHA products; no products to effectively treat blemishes or lighten skin discolorations; average toners; moisturizers that are short on including state-of-the-art ingredients; jar packaging; several foundations with sunscreen do not provide complete UVA protection; the pressed bronzing powder; average powder blush, eye pencils, and long-wearing lip color; none of the lipsticks with sunscreen include adequate UVA protection; relatively unimpressive makeup brushes.

Note: Unless mentioned otherwise, all Lancome products contain fragrance.

For more information about Lancome, owned by L'Oreal, call (800) 526-2663 or visit www.lancome.com or www.Beautypedia.com.

LANCOME SKIN CARE

LANCOME ABSOLUE PREMIUM BX PRODUCTS

☹ **$$$ Absolue Premium Bx Advanced Replenishing Cream Cleanser** *($55 for 6.7 ounces).* Wow! This absurdly expensive, completely ordinary cleansing cream leaves me nearly speechless (well, not completely); it is beyond standard and ends up being a completely antiquated mix of water and mineral oil. Though an option for dry to very dry skin, this is just cold cream, I mean like Pond's Cold Cream. How Lancome has the audacity to claim that it "sets a new standard, in age-targeted skincare" is just obnoxious. First, if this is a new standard then so is paper. Second, even though I've already said this, it needs repeating: this formula is so poor that the price is an insult. Yes, it will remove makeup, but not without leaving a greasy film, just like any cold cream. The amount of wild yam isn't enough to feed a flea at Thanksgiving, and the fragrance chemicals (which will be left on your skin because this cream doesn't rinse easily) can cause irritation.

☹ **$$$ Absolue Eye Premium Bx, Absolute Replenishing Eye Cream** *($85 for 0.5 ounce)* is said to combine two advanced discoveries: Lancome's patented Pro-Xylane and their "intensely replenishing" Bio-Network. According to a report on www.happi.com (the *Household and Personal Products Industry* magazine Web site), Pro-Xylane is derived from xylose, a type of sugar that has water-binding properties for skin. L'Oreal Senior Vice President Alan Meyers reported that in vitro skin tests and testing on human skin showed that their Pro-Xylane complex stimulated the production of glycosaminoglycans in the skin. Glycosaminoglycans are one part of the intricate network that makes up the skin's intercellular matrix. Topical application of substances that mimic what's found in skin's intercellular matrix do help reinforce the skin's barrier function, thus allowing the intercellular matrix to function normally. L'Oreal (Lancome's parent company) may be convinced that Pro-Xylane has some wonderful effect on skin, but lots of other ingredients can do the same thing, and as it turns out, this product doesn't contain all that much Pro-Xylane. Moreover, the tiny amount of Lancome's Bio-Network—consisting of soy, wild yam, sea algae, and barley—won't have the slightest rejuvenating effect on skin, nor counteract changes in skin that result from menopause. As is true for many of Lancome's skin-care products, this is yet another lackluster moisturizer. There's more titanium dioxide, mica, and iron oxides (all mineral pigments that are included in this product to create a radiant glow, which is strictly a cosmetic effect) than anything that could be considered innovative or of "premium" benefit for your skin, and the price for such a mundane formula has everything to do with market positioning, not real, revolutionary results.

☹ **$$$ Absolue Night Premium Bx, Absolute Night Recovery Cream** *($145 for 2.6 ounces)* makes additional claims for the Pro-Xylane discussed in the previous review, such as that it restores essential moisture deep in the structure of the skin's surface. Talk about something that sounds a lot better than it is! Moreover, there are lots of ingredients found in other products that do the same thing. Actually, there's not much of anything substantial in this moisturizer, given that alcohol, wax, and coloring agents are listed well before anything interesting or even remotely worth the money. This is one to leave on the shelf!

☹ **$$$ Absolue Premium Bx, Absolute Replenishing Cream SPF 15** *($120 for 1.7 ounces)* features an in-part avobenzone sunscreen and has a slightly better base formula than the other Absolue Premium Bx products reviewed, but for the money this should be brimming with state-of-the-art ingredients, and it's not. In addition, the effectiveness of the few antioxidants present in this product is diminished by the jar packaging, which is disappointing. Last, if you're considering this for sunscreen (and that's the only claim you can bank on with this product), ask yourself how liberally you'll apply a sunscreen that is this expensive. And if you're still not convinced, at least put yourself in front of the Estee Lauder counter because their moisturizers with sunscreen have formulas that are way ahead of those from Lancome and many of them cost a lot less.

☹ **$$$ Absolue Premium Bx, Absolute Replenishing Lotion SPF 15** *($120 for 2.5 ounces)* has an in-part avobenzone sunscreen, and its opaque, pump-bottle packaging will keep the vitamin E stable (that's the only antioxidant of note in this product). Those are the positives. The bad news is that alcohol is the fourth ingredient. That isn't terrible, but it isn't what you want to see in a costly product meant to combat the visible signs of aging. Despite all the ballyhoo for Pro-Xylane and the Bio-Network (consisting of algae, soy, and wild yam), these ingredients are barely present. The salicylic acid in this product does not function as an exfoliant.

☹ **$$$ Absolue Soleil Premium Bx SPF 30 Sunscreen Absolute Replenishing Sun Protection Face Cream** *($35 for 1.7 ounces)* is an OK option for normal to slightly oily or slightly dry skin. Other than an in-part avobenzone sunscreen, this cream contains more fragrance and alcohol than anything else that could potentially be beneficial for skin.

☹ **$$$ Absolue Ultimate Bx Replenishing and Restructuring Serum** *($130 for 1 ounce)* promises to be a breakthrough for mature skin due to its supposed clarifying power. Those with dull, lackluster skin tones will see radiance returned, but that's due to the mica particles in this product that simply add a soft shine to skin, which is about makeup rather than skin care. Lancome never explains exactly what ingredients comprise their Pro-Xylane complex, but it is supposedly "highly concentrated" in this serum. It could be they're referring to the wild yam, soy, and algae in this product, but these ingredients are barely present (there's much more fragrance than showcased plant extracts), so "highly concentrated" is clearly a marketing concept, not reality. The only potentially helpful ingredient in the product for possibly "clarifying" skin is kojic acid. Lancome doesn't scrimp on this ingredient, and it is indeed known for inhibiting melanin production. However, it is not considered as efficacious as hydroquinone, especially when the latter is combined with tretinoin. Moreover, other research indicates that kojic acid is not as effective as other potential skin-lightening agents (Sources: *Journal of the American Academy of Dermatology*, December 2006, pages 1048-1065; and *The Journal of Biological Chemistry*, May 2002, pages 16340-16344). Kojic acid is also prone to deterioration on exposure to light and air unless it is stably packaged, which is the case with this serum. Although it's rather one-note, this serum has the potential to lighten discolorations. But keep in mind, there are several other options (including prescription TriLuma) that stand a greater chance of producing superior results, and for less money. The overall formula of this serum makes it best for normal to slightly dry skin.

☺ $$$ **Absolue Ultimate Night Bx, Intense Night Recovery and Replenishing Serum** (*$140 for 1 ounce*) has a name that is by far the best thing about it. Lancome just can't seem to get its antiaging act together when it comes to creating a state-of-the-art formula that comes close (even a little) to justifying the cost. This serum contains mostly water, slip agents, thickeners, more slip agent, film-forming agents, plant extract, plant oil, and coloring agents. There are more artificial coloring agents in this product than there are the "bio-network" ingredients Lancome calls out on the label. Completely absent are noteworthy antioxidants, skin-identical ingredients, and anti-irritants. In short, anyone looking to spend in this range for a state-of-the-art serum should know that this product competes with others about as well as a rotary-dial wall phone would compete with an iPhone. Just about every line surrounding Lancome at the department store offers better serums than they do, and that statement also applies to this lackluster entry.

☺ $$$ **Absolue Soleil Premium Bx SPF 30 Sunscreen Absolue Replenishing Sun Protection Body Cream** (*$38 for 5 ounces*). The only, and I mean the only, exciting part of this sunscreen for the body is that it includes avobenzone for UVA protection. Otherwise, the base formula fails to impress even a little, though the claims state otherwise. Alcohol, film-forming agents, and fragrance supersede the special ingredients Lancome touts, making this as far from a "premium" or "replenishing" sunscreen as you can get. It's an OK option for normal to slightly oily or slightly dry skin, but for the money there are far better options to consider.

LANCOME AQUA FUSION PRODUCTS

☺ **Aqua Fusion Cream, Continuous Infusing Moisturizer** (*$37 for 1.7 ounces*) contains more coloring agent than anything exciting for skin, though at least the price isn't too out-of-line. The amino acids and minerals are but a dusting, leaving this as an average, jar-packaged moisturizer for normal to slightly dry skin.

☺ **Aqua Fusion Lotion, Continuous Infusing Moisturizer, for Normal/Combination Skin** (*$37 for 1.7 ounces*) touts the essential minerals it contains as being able to charge skin and keep it hydrated all day. Not only are the minerals not essential for skin (at least not topically; oral consumption as part of a healthy diet is another story), but there is also more artificial color in this moisturizer than ingredients such as calcium or zinc. At best, this is a very standard, lightweight hydrating option for normal to oily skin. You should be aware, however, that this product lacks significant levels of antioxidants or water-binding agents. Glycerin is the second listed ingredient, but alcohol is the third, so the classic ability of glycerin to moisturize skin is compromised. Aqua Fusion Lotion does contain fragrance.

☺ **Aqua Fusion Lotion SPF, Continuous Infusing Moisturizer SPF 15, for Normal/ Combination Skin** *($37 for 1.7 ounces)* is a good, lightweight daytime moisturizer with sunscreen for normal to oily skin. Titanium dioxide is on hand for UVA protection and this contains some good skin-identical ingredients and antioxidant vitamin E.

LANCOME BIENFAIT MULTI-VITAL PRODUCTS

☹ **$$$ Bienfait Multi-Vital Eyes SPF 28** *($36 for 0.5 ounce)* includes titanium dioxide for UVA protection, but the sunscreen ingredient octinoxate is not ideal for use in the eye area, which is where you're directed to apply this product. Even if your eye area can tolerate any sunscreen just fine, there is nothing else of benefit for your skin in here. Like many Lancome skin-care products, the really intriguing ingredients are barely present, while the standard cosmetic ingredients are front and center. The amount of mica is enough to lend a soft shimmer, but you can get that effect with other products that provide more for your money than this average mixture.

☹ **Bienfait Multi-Vital Glow SPF 15** *($46 for 1.7 ounces)*. It's amazing and infuriating that despite L'Oreal's media blitz for their UVA-protecting sunscreen ingredient Mexoryl SX, also called ecamsule, Lancome (L'Oreal owns Lancome) is still launching sunscreens that leave skin vulnerable to UVA damage! That is just shocking! Can you imagine?! A company knows about UVA protection, it advertises in the media how important it is for skin, and then it goes and offers sunscreen products that not only leave out their pivotal ingredient but also do not include any other viable option, such as titanium dioxide, zinc oxide, or avobenzone (the latter also called butyl methoxydibenzoylmethane). There are numerous UVA-protecting products available, including some from Lancome. Really, at this point in the sunscreen game, Lancome should be hanging their heads in shame.

☹ **$$$ Bienfait Multi-Vital SPF 30 Cream** *($43 for 1.7 ounces)* has avobenzone for sufficient UVA protection, but that's the only highlight of this daytime moisturizer for normal to oily skin. Alcohol is the fourth ingredient, which isn't great but is not abysmal, and the antioxidants are subject to deterioration due to jar packaging. What a shame, because this moisturizer has more antioxidants than Lancome typically offers.

☺ **$$$ Bienfait Multi-Vital SPF 30 Lotion** *($43 for 1.7 ounces)* would rate a Paula's Pick if not for the many volatile fragrance components. Although these aren't predominant, they're a potential cause for concern and don't add anything helpful to this in-part avobenzone sunscreen. The base formula is antioxidant-rich and stably packaged, two uncommon traits for a Lancome product. This is still appropriate for normal to oily skin.

☹ **$$$ Bienfait Multi-Vital Night, High Potency Night Moisturizing Cream** *($48 for 1.7 ounces)* makes a big deal out of the vitamins it contains, which are said to help with skin's nightly recovery process. Don't bet on it, because the jar packaging won't keep them stable once this product is in use, and the amount of vitamins is paltry—there's actually more coloring agent. (What would you rather have, a pretty tinted moisturizer or an antioxidant-rich one?) This has the requisite silky, moist texture for normal to dry skin, but that's not enough to justify the price or jibe with the state-of-the-art claims being made for this average moisturizer.

LANCOME BRIGHT EXPERT PRODUCTS

☺ $$$ **Bright Expert Intense Brightening Cleansing Foam** *($32 for 3.4 ounces)* is a creamy, pearlescent foaming cleanser that contains enough potassium hydroxide to make it too drying an option, except possibly for someone with oily skin. None of the many plant extracts in this cleanser have a proven track record for brightening skin, intensely or otherwise, and most of them are listed after the preservatives and fragrance, meaning they can't do much other than look enticing on the label. Besides, even if they could be helpful in some way, they would just be rinsed off the skin before they had a chance to have an effect. This is an OK cleanser for someone with oily skin but the price is unwarranted for what you get, and it's easily replaced by far less expensive and less drying options.

☺ $$$ **Bright Expert Intense Brightening Toner, Hydrating & Conditioning** *($38 for 6.7 ounces)* has an appreciable amount of the vitamin C–derived ingredient ascorbyl glucoside, but there's only limited research indicating this ingredient can improve hyperpigmentation (what Lancome refers to as "dark spots"). Also, the peppermint extract can be a problem for irritation, though there's not a lot of it in this toner. This is an OK option for normal to dry skin as long as you don't expect significant lightening of sun- or hormone-induced skin discolorations.

☺ $$$ **Bright Expert Intense Brightening Moisturizing Night Cream** *($74 for 1.7 ounces)* is a jar-packaged moisturizer that contains mostly water, glycerin, silicone, alcohol, thickener, vitamins, amino acids, and fragrance. It's hardly an exciting or breakthrough formula, and the amount of alcohol keeps it from being too moisturizing, making this an OK, but overpriced, option for someone with normal to slightly dry skin. None of the ingredients in this moisturizer has a lightening effect on skin discolorations, and the jar packaging would not be helpful for the vitamins or amino acids.

☺ $$$ **Bright Expert Intense Brightening Spot Correcting Serum** *($90 for 1 ounce)* ranks as the most expensive product in the Bright Expert lineup, but unless you're convinced ascorbyl glucoside is the skin-lightening answer, there's no reason to consider this water- and silicone-based, alcohol-free serum. Even as a moisturizer this is a fairly boring formulation with minimal beneficial (meaning state-of-the-art) ingredients for skin. The amount of ascorbyl glucoside is sufficient for it to function as an antioxidant and the opaque tube packaging will help keep it stable, but if you know this won't lighten skin discolorations, why choose it over less expensive, better-formulated serums from Olay, Clinique, or Neutrogena?

LANCOME HIGH RESOLUTION PRODUCTS

☺ $$$ **High Resolution Collaser-5X Intense Collagen Anti-Wrinkle Serum** *($65 for 1 ounce)*. The amount of intriguing ingredients in this water-based, silky-textured serum is a pittance, and none of them are capable of pushing wrinkles "up and out" to restore a youthful bounce to aged skin. Lancome tries to impress with claims of ingredients such as coenzyme-R and vitamin C, but much like parent company L'Oreal's overused Pro-Xylane, those are just made-up buzzwords. Wouldn't you rather spend your money on a serum with efficacious amounts of proven ingredients? If so, any of the serums from Olay and Neutrogena, or from MD Skincare by Dr. Dennis Gross are distinctly preferred to this. If you're considering this serum (though I can't imagine why), it's best for normal to slightly oily skin. And, of course, using this product inspired by laser technology doesn't at all equate with actually receiving laser or light-emitting treatments for your skin concerns.

☺ **$$$ High Resolution Eye Collaser-5X Intense Collagen Anti-Wrinkle Eye Serum** *($59 for 0.5 ounce)* doesn't contain a substantial amount of anything that can stimulate collagen production, at least no more so than your average moisturizer. When you protect your skin from sunlight and needless irritants, it is capable of generating new collagen (in a controlled manner) on its own. Lancome's blend of mostly water, silicone, glycerin, plant oil, mineral pigments for shine, and a tiny amount of antioxidant vitamins isn't what I would consider an impressive formulation. Compared to the best serums for the eye area of your face, this water-based serum for all skin types is merely an average option.

☺ **$$$ High Resolution Eye Refill 3X** *($55 for 0.5 ounce)* is supposed to stimulate substances in skin that contribute to its support structure, but this poorly formulated eye cream doesn't even add up to a very good moisturizer. The titanium dioxide and mica it contains lend a soft white shine to the eye area, which is what's responsible for the "luminous" appearance Lancome mentions. This has no more than a cosmetic effect on dark circles (a concealer would net far better results) and nothing in this eye cream will alleviate puffiness because the ingredient list couldn't be more ordinary; there isn't even an ingredient in here that could fake having benefit. Lancome did include a couple of novel peptides, but they're near the end of the ingredient list, which means they are barely detectable in this formula. In fact moisture-absorbing talc and nylon 66 are listed well before any of the interesting ingredients. It is also not good news that this formula includes fragrance chemicals known to cause irritation. Fragrance in any form is a problem for skin anywhere on the body, but especially around the sensitive eye area. In no way, shape, or form is this eye cream akin to dermal fillers that are injected into lines and folds to plump them.

☹ **High Resolution Refill 3x Triple Action Renewal Anti-Wrinkle Cream SPF 15 Sunscreen** *($75 for 1.7 ounces).* Amazing and endlessly frustrating, but true: Lancome is still launching products with sunscreen that leave skin vulnerable to UVA damage because the active ingredients they choose don't protect across the entire UVA spectrum. Lancome knows this all too well; after all, they own the patent on Mexoryl SX, an ingredient that does provide protection across the entire UVA spectrum. How does that make sense? When people ask me why cosmetics companies do what they do, I can often surmise the marketing logic (like jar packaging, because lots of women like using jars), but when it comes to protecting your skin from UVA rays from the sun, which are responsible for serious skin damage and wrinkling, I can't fathom why a company like Lancome, given their ingredient resources, would ignore this. It makes me want to scream (and sometimes I do). As usual for Lancome's daytime moisturizers with sunscreen, the base formula has an elegant silky texture, but it offers skin little in the way of exciting, helpful ingredients. You won't even get single-action antiwrinkle power by using this product.

☺ **$$$ High Resolution Refill 3X Triple Action Renewal Anti-Wrinkle Night Cream** *($90 for 2.6 ounces).* In some small ways, this emollient moisturizer for dry skin is a cut above what Lancome typically offers, but that doesn't say much because generally Lancome and L'Oreal make some of the most disappointing moisturizers and "antiwrinkle" creams available. The notion that this product has anything to do with the effects of a dermal filler or that it contains ingredients that stimulate the production of skin's supportive elements (they probably want you to think of collagen and elastin) is a joke. It won't do that any more than will the thousands of other creams on the market. This actually contains more coloring agents than state-of-the-art ingredients, which is really depressing when you weigh the cost of this moisturizer against its limited benefits. Lancome refers to anisic acid helping to "complete the nightly cellular renewal process." Not only is there no research to support this statement, but it also ignores the fact that lots of ingredients can help skin do that, either by exfoliation (think AHA or BHA) or with antioxidants and cell-communicating ingredients, which skin needs both night and day; it doesn't go into overdrive at night and slow down in the morning. Despite fancy jar packaging and lofty claims, this is nothing more than a moisturizer. Those looking for skin care with antiaging benefits should know that Lancome's offerings consistently come up short.

LANCOME PRIMORDIALE & PRIMORDIALE SKIN RECHARGE PRODUCTS

☺ $$$ **Primordiale Cell Defense Double Performance Cell Defense & Skin Perfecting Serum** *($64 for 1 ounce)* was launched with much ballyhoo about how it is supposed to fight aging by blocking 99% of free radicals in an effort to attain visibly perfect skin, but then Lancome offers no explanation or proof of just how this product goes about blocking nearly all free-radical damage. And logically, given the constant onslaught of the sun, air, pollution, and free radicals generated naturally inside your body there is no way any product or substance can live up to that claim. Moreover, the claims made for this product go beyond any alleged benefit Lancome has previously attributed to the same or similar antioxidants in their products. But what's most maddening is that this isn't even a very good formula! The primary ingredients are water, silicones (which create a silky finish), and alcohol. The amount of alcohol is potentially irritating, while the main antioxidant (ascorbyl glucoside, a form of vitamin C) doesn't play more than a moderate supporting role in a lackluster formula. In fact, coloring agents get more prominence in this serum than the other antioxidants included, so really, how serious is Lancome about this product's prodigious free-radical-scavenging ability? Getting back to the testing Lancome uses to make the free-radical claim, the only details were that it was in vitro and that the free-radical reduction was in response to UVA light exposure. But what about free radicals generated by UVB light, smog, car exhaust, air, heat, and so many other things? UVA light is but one source of damage. In reality, Lancome's test results don't indicate any benefit for skin.

☹ $$$ **Primordiale Eye Skin Recharge Visibly Smoothing & Renewing Eye Treatment** *($50 for 0.5 ounce)* contains mostly water, silicones, glycerin, film-forming agent, plant oils, vitamin E, more film-forming agent, preservatives, and fragrance, truly a boring list if ever there was one. It feels light and silky, but it takes more than vitamin E to treat skin anywhere on the face, and Lancome's choice of jar packaging wasn't wise because vitamin E can deteriorate with routine exposure to light and air. Moreover, as an eye-area moisturizer, this should not contain fragrance or coloring agents. This won't help your skin or reduce wrinkles, and is just a waste of money and effort.

☹ $$$ **Primordiale Night Skin Recharge** *($66 for 1.7 ounces).* Reviewing moisturizers from Lancome has taken on the equivalency of hitting my head against a wall. Try as I might, I'm not going to break through to the other side and the disappointment is never-ending. This product continues the company's pattern of creating antiwrinkle moisturizers whose claims go far beyond what their rudimentary formulas can do. This product claims to recharge skin cells while you sleep, for radiant, healthy skin. It is said to do this with biotin, and, as you may have guessed, the amount of biotin in this product is negligible. Besides, biotin (a B vitamin) isn't capable of recharging skin cells all by itself any more than plain water can remove all types of makeup. Getting past the cellular nonsense, this is just an emollient moisturizer for normal to dry skin. The antioxidant properties of the plant oils and vitamins will be diminished due to jar packaging, while the amount of fragrance trumps the ingredients Lancome claims are doing the amazing anti-wrinkle work.

☹ **Primordiale Skin Recharge Visibly Smoothing & Renewing Moisturizer SPF 15 Sunscreen Cream** *($65 for 1.7 ounces)* lacks the UVA-protecting ingredients of titanium dioxide, zinc oxide, avobenzone, ecamsule (Mexoryl SX), or Tinosorb and is not recommended. This also contains a lot of fragrance, offers few benefits to skin of any age, and is enormously overpriced for what it does (and doesn't) provide.

☹ **Primordiale Skin Recharge Visibly Smoothing & Renewing Moisturizer SPF 15 Sunscreen Lotion** *($65 for 1.7 ounces)* lacks the UVA-protecting ingredients of titanium dioxide, zinc oxide, avobenzone, ecamsule (Mexoryl SX), or Tinosorb and is not recommended. Not only is the lack of sunscreen a huge letdown, but claiming that the ingredients in this product will make pores smaller must be a joke! Regrettably, lots of women will believe the claims only to be disappointed when nothing changes. All told, this is one of the worst daytime moisturizers Lancome has ever launched, and deserves zero consideration unless you like more artificial coloring than antiaging ingredients in your skin-care products.

LANCOME PURE FOCUS PRODUCTS

☹ **Pure Focus Pore Tightening Toner with Matifying Powders** *($24 for 6.8 ounces)* lists alcohol as the second ingredient and contains the potent menthol derivative menthoxypropanediol. The focus is purely on irritation here, and the alcohol will stimulate oil production in the pore.

☺ **$$$ Pure Focus Deep Pore Refining Scrub with Purifying Micro-Beads** *($24 for 3.4 ounces)* is a gel-based scrub that contains polyethylene (plastic) as the abrasive agent. The small amount of detergent cleansing agents makes this a good choice for normal to oily skin.

☹ **Pure Focus Matifying Moisturizing Lotion** *($36 for 1.7 ounces)* barely moisturizes thanks to its alcohol content, and irritates with the menthol derivative menthoxypropanediol. Skin does not need to tingle or be irritated to look matte! The alcohol in this product will make oily skin worse by stimulating oil production in the pore.

☺ **$$$ Pure Focus T-Zone Powder Gel for Instant Shine Control** *($27 for 1 ounce)* is just silicone with fragrance and volatile fragrance components. It provides a silky matte finish, but is not preferred to Clinique's Pore Minimizer Instant Perfector or Paula's Choice Skin Balancing Super Antioxidant Mattifying Concentrate.

LANCOME RENERGIE PRODUCTS

☺ **$$$ Renergie Cream, Anti-Wrinkle and Firming Treatment** *($80 for 1.7 ounces)* remains a perennial favorite of Lancome customers, but it doesn't increase skin's firmness or reduce the appearance of wrinkles better than most emollient moisturizers, which is all this product is. It's a decent option for dry skin, but definitely leaves it wanting more for the money, and the various fragrance components pose a risk of inflammation.

☺ **$$$ Renergie Eye, Anti-Wrinkle and Firming Eye Creme** *($60 for 0.5 ounce)* is a good, fragrance-free, emollient moisturizer for dry skin anywhere on the face. Nothing in it will firm skin, but its rich texture will soften the appearance of wrinkles. Jar packaging doesn't make this an optimum choice if you want to provide skin with antioxidants.

☹ **Renergie Microlift R.A.R.E., Superior Lifting Cream SPF 15 Sunscreen** *($80 for 1.7 ounces)* doesn't deserve consideration because it does not contain the UVA-protecting ingredients

The Reviews L

of titanium dioxide, zinc oxide, avobenzone, Mexoryl SX (ecamsule), or Tinosorb. Lancome knows better (they own the patent on Mexoryl SX and tout the need for UVA protection) and should be ashamed to offer such an inferior product as a means for making collagen-depleted skin look better. By the way, the base formula is as boring as watching paint dry.

☺ $$$ **Renergie Microlift Eye R.A.R.E., Superior Lifting Eye Cream** *($60 for 0.5 ounce)* has aspirations to defy gravity's pull on skin, and is said to be inspired by "the latest vertical surgery techniques" which grant this cream "exceptional lifting power." Such claims may make you think twice about booking a consultation with a cosmetic surgeon, but let me assure you such an appointment would be time well spent compared to using this inferior product. Apparently a "breakthrough" oligopeptide in this product is able to double the synthesis of protein linked to shoring up collagen. If that was true, the result would be smoother, less lined, plumped skin. The only peptide in this product is acetyl tetrapeptide-9, and it is barely present. In fact, there are far more preservatives and volatile fragrance components in this jar-packaged cream than peptide (and the amount of alcohol, while not likely irritating, is still disappointing). Acetyl tetrapeptide-9 is part of a trademarked complex known as Dermican manufactured by Laboratoires Serobiologiques. That company's research shows that this peptide acts on a certain proteoglycan (a sugar molecule that forms the ground substance of connective tissues such as collagen) known as lumican, which is said to play an important role in the synthesis and organization of collagen fibers in skin. The kicker is twofold: the company's research is not substantiated, and the usage level they recommend (1%-3% Dermican) is not even remotely close to what Lancome chose to use. Even if Dermican could work as claimed, you're barely getting any of it in this product, which leaves you with another mundane moisturizer for normal to slightly dry skin. One last note regarding lumican: there is research showing that this proteoglycan's deterioration in skin over time likely plays a role in skin's aged appearance. In addition, animal research suggests that lumican expression is reduced as estrogen levels decrease, such as occurs after menopause (estrogen plays a role in collagen synthesis and organization). (Sources for the above: *Journal of Dermatological Science*, September 2007, pages 217-226; *Molecular and Cellular Biochemistry*, September 2005, pages 63-72; and *Glycoconjugate Journal*, May-June 2002, pages 287-293).

☺ $$$ **Renergie Microlift Neck R.A.R.E., Superior Lifting Neck Cream** *($80 for 1.7 ounces)*. Lancome wants you to believe that this moisturizer is the answer for the "thin, delicate skin" on the neck and chest when these areas begin to show a lack of firmness. To that end, they've developed what they refer to as Bio-Stimulating Technology that, are you ready for this, sends a "dynamic impulse" that spreads throughout the layers of skin. First of all, this product is not a defibrillator for aging skin; second, what exactly is a "dynamic impulse"? A dynamic impulse could be the urge to eat chocolate cake or to drink a glass of water. In this case, "dynamic impulse" is mere marketing chicanery. Most important is the fact that this moisturizer is another in Lancome's endless parade of ordinary formulas with claims that are far more elaborate than the ingredients inside. For as much money as they're charging, it's disheartening to realize you're getting mostly water, slip agents, Vaseline, emollient thickeners, wax, silicone, and coloring agents. The jar packaging won't keep the minimal amount of intriguing ingredients stable during use, and this also contains fragrance chemicals that can cause irritation, especially on "thin, delicate skin." Labeling this product as a superior lift for sagging neck skin is an affront to all cosmetic surgeons, whose skilled handiwork really can make a beautiful difference when skin becomes lax due to a combination of age and sun damage.

☹ **$$$ Renergie Microlift Night R.A.R.E, Superior Firming Night Cream** *($95 for 2.5 ounces)*. Reading the claims for this moisturizer, you can't help but think it is essentially shock therapy for skin that has lost its firmness and youthful contours! But, this is a Lancome moisturizer and, therefore, you shouldn't expect much because Lancome makes some of the most ordinary, poorly formulated moisturizers around. What you end up getting is an average moisturizer with an absurd price tag. The amount of intriguing ingredients pales in comparison to the amount of those that Lancome deems more important for a product's appeal, namely fragrance, coloring agents, and mica, the latter of which lends a soft glow to skin. This is a mundane option for dry to very dry skin, but there is nothing rare, lifting, or superior about it, and your skin truly deserves better.

☹ **$$$ Renergie Night, Night Treatment** *($95 for 2.5 ounces)* claims to accelerate surface cell renewal so that skin is "re-energized" and "looks well-rested." Sounds great, but those benign claims can be made for just about any moisturizer no matter what it contains. All in all, Renergie Night is a very expensive basic moisturizer whose jar packaging won't keep the good ingredients (which there are woefully little of) stable. It contains mostly water, squalane, silicone, glycerin, thickeners, coloring agent, and wax. The formula may be exclusive to Lancome, but no one else would want it anyway.

☹ **$$$ Renergie Oil-Free Lotion, Anti-Wrinkle and Firming Treatment** *($80 for 1.7 ounces)* is a silicone-enhanced lightweight lotion for normal to slightly oily skin. Although the packaging will keep the vitamin E stable, there's barely a drop of it in here.

LANCOME SECRET DE VIE PRODUCTS

☹ **$$$ Secret De Vie Precious Reviving Creme Cleanser** *($55 for 4.2 ounces)* ranks as one of the most expensive cold cream–style cleansers you're likely to find. Although this is an indulgent option for dry to very dry skin and it liquefies with water to a cleansing lotion texture (and it will remove most types of makeup), it does not rinse well without the aid of a washcloth.

☹ **$$$ Secret De Vie Precious Reviving Toner** *($60 for 5 ounces)* ends up being a very boring toner for the money, serving normal to dry skin with mostly water, slip agents, alcohol, and mineral pigments that provide shimmer to this liquid. This does not contain hyaluronic acid as claimed; rather, it contains a teeny-tiny amount of the salt form of this ingredient, which costs significantly less than pure hyaluronic acid and doesn't work quite the same (especially given the cost of this product, they should have used the real thing).

☹ **$$$ Secret De Vie, Ultimate Cellular Reviving Creme** *($240 for 1.7 ounces)*. The major secret here is how utterly ordinary this ultra-pricey moisturizer is. I suppose Lancome didn't want to be left out of the burgeoning group of moisturizers with high-tech claims and staggering price tags. Describing itself as "Lancome's ultimate luxury," Secret De Vie asks you to believe that its key ingredient complex, Extrait de Vie (extract of life), "delivers intense restorative action to six major cell types for instant, visible, exceptional results." Notice that Lancome is trying very hard in this seductive wordplay to attempt to convince consumers that spending this much on a special formula (one that is shockingly similar to almost every other Lancome cream being sold) is somehow worth the extra expense. The company didn't even bother to use stable packaging, instead choosing a futuristic, orb-like jar. Extrait de Vie does sound romantic and exotic, but there is nothing in this product that is in any way unique or even moderately interesting. The majority of the product consists of water, silicones, glycerin, thickener, silicone polymer, aluminum starch, wax, vitamin E, and several plant extracts, including peppermint leaf (though the amount is likely too small to cause irritation). Paying significantly more for this versus almost any of Lancome's other moisturizers, none of which are as impressive as what most other Lauder-owned companies are offering, is not good skin care.

☹ **Secret de Vie, Ultimate Cellular Reviving Life Source Serum** (*$265 for 1 ounce*). There are few words suitable for print that can be used to honestly describe what a poorly formulated, inadequate, and absolutely pathetic water-based serum this is. Calling this an "awesome discovery" for skin is marketing hubris. For the money, you should know up front that the core ingredients in this product are extremely common and mundane. In fact, several L'Oreal products offer similar formulations. However, L'Oreal's status as a mass-market brand means they'd never charge this much money for anything, even when it's almost identical to its expensive counterpart. Because this is a premium product (in price and claims only), Lancome had to devise a story to convince consumers that it's worth the splurge. This time the fabled Extrait de Vie (extract of life) is said to be made super potent because Lancome combines marine ingredients from bodies of water with different temperatures (as in hot and cold). There is no published research anywhere proving these sea extracts (listed as algae and various ferments, the same ingredients that show up in Biotherm products, another L'Oreal-owned company) are capable of prolonging the life of skin cells. Even if they could, merely allowing skin cells to live longer doesn't mean that skin gets firmer or that wrinkles diminish. If the skin cells are damaged (such as from sun exposure) they'll still be damaged, it's just that they'll hang on longer before dying out—and how is that helpful or healthy for skin? It isn't, and it's one of many reasons why this serum is a complete waste of time and money.

☺ $$$ **Secret De Vie Eye, Ultimate Cellular Reviving Eye Creme** (*$140 for 0.5 ounce*) is an emollient moisturizer for dry skin anywhere on the face, but the price is outrageous for what you get. Here, there's no reason to comment on the jar packaging, because there are no light- or air-sensitive ingredients in this far-from-ultimate eye cream.

LANCOME SOLEIL ULTRA EXPERT PRODUCTS

☹ $$$ **Soleil Ultra Expert Sun Care SPF 50 Sunscreen Face and Body Lotion, for Sensitive Skin** (*$34.50 for 5 ounces*) contains too many sunscreen actives to be considered a viable option for sensitive skin, and the propylene glycol can enhance their penetration into skin, another minus for sensitive skin. And why add fragrance? Someone at Lancome must have missed Skin Care 101 if they thought that would be good for sensitive skin! An in-part titanium dioxide sunscreen helps provide broad-spectrum protection, but the base formula is mundane and not worth the expense.

☹ $$$ **Soleil Ultra Expert Sun Care SPF 50 Sunscreen Face Cream, for Sensitive Skin** (*$31.50 for 1.7 ounces*) is a lighter version of the Soleil Ultra Expert Sun Care SPF 50 product. It also features an in-part titanium dioxide sunscreen, and contains fragrance. Another point of contention for those with sensitive skin is the amount of alcohol in this product, not to mention the amount of preservatives, listed well before any type of soothing agent.

· OTHER LANCOME PRODUCTS

☺ $$$ **Ablutia Fraicheur, Purifying Foaming Cleanser** (*$30 for 6.8 ounces*) is a very standard, detergent-based, water-soluble cleanser that can be drying for some skin types, though it is appropriate for someone with normal to oily skin.

☺ **$$$ Clarifiance Oil-Free Gel Cleanser** *($30 for 6.8 ounces)* is an exceptionally basic water-soluble cleanser for normal to slightly oily skin. The price is completely out of whack for what you get, but it is an option if you want to overspend and ignore the better options from L'Oreal or Neutrogena.

☺ **$$$ Creme Mousse Confort, Comforting Creamy Foaming Cleanser** *($24 for 4.2 ounces)*. This is a very good, creamy-feeling foaming cleanser (at least the name is accurate) for normal to dry skin. It works swiftly to completely remove makeup and rinses well without the need for a washcloth. This would be rated a Paula's Pick if it did not contain potentially irritating fragrance chemicals (of which there are many in this rather standard cleanser).

☺ **$$$ Galatee Confort Comforting Milky Creme Cleanser** *($30 for 6.8 ounces)* remains a standard, creamy cleanser for dry to very dry skin. It does not rinse without the aid of a washcloth, and is not for anyone with blemishes, however small. The amount of fragrance components demands complete removal from skin lest you risk irritation.

☹ **Gel Pure Focus, Oil Control Cleansing Gel for Oily Skin** *($24 for 4.2 ounces)*. This water-soluble cleanser has too many strikes against it to make it worth considering over dozens of others, most of which cost considerably less. The alcohol content, the amount of fragrance, and the inclusion of the irritating menthol derivative menthoxypropanediol are all cause for concern and provide ample reasons to ignore this cleanser. It will not tighten or refine pores, nor does it deeply cleanse the skin. A well-formulated, gentle cleanser (which this isn't) will do a great job of removing excess oil and impurities to make pores appear smaller and to reduce surface shine from excess oil, and there are many cleansers that fit this description and for a lot less money, too.

☺ **$$$ Huile Douceur, Remove-All Deep Cleansing Oil Face & Eyes** *($34.50 for 6.8 ounces)*. Lancome plays up the white lotus and Japanese cedar bud in this cleansing oil, but they make up only a minimal part of the formula. It is composed primarily of mineral oil along with corn oil, two ingredients you can purchase for a lot less money and that work just as well to remove makeup. Of course, neither rinses well from skin, but this product doesn't rinse well, either—so plan on using a washcloth. It is recommended only for those with dry to very dry skin. The fragrance and fragrance chemicals make it inappropriate for sensitive skin.

☺ **$$$ Bi-Facil, Double-Action Eye Makeup Remover** *($26 for 4.2 ounces)* is a good water- and silicone-based makeup remover that would be rated higher if it were fragrance-free and left out the questionable preservative quaternium-15. Still, this works well to quickly remove stubborn and waterproof makeup.

☺ **$$$ Effacil, Gentle Eye Makeup Remover** *($26 for 4.2 ounces)* is not gentle due to the amount of detergents and fragrance it contains. It's essentially a watered-down water-soluble cleanser, and not really worth adding to your routine unless you're a soap devotee.

☺ **$$$ Exfoliance Clarte Clarifying Exfoliating Gel** *($24 for 3.4 ounces)* is a cleanser/scrub hybrid that is a good option for normal to oily skin. The exfoliating agent is polyethylene. The amount of papaya is barely worth mentioning, and has no effect on removing dulling impurities.

☺ **$$$ Exfoliance Confort Comforting Exfoliating Cream** *($24 for 3.4 ounces)* is a rich, creamy topical scrub for dry to very dry skin. It contains polyethylene as the abrasive agent, which is great. The only drawback is that the emollients and silicone don't rinse well from skin, so you may need to use this with a washcloth, which exfoliates too (so why use the scrub at all?).

☺ **$$$ Resurface-C Microdermabrasion, Skin Polishing and Radiance Renewing System** *($88)* marks Lancome's contribution to the group of microdermabrasion-at-home kits. The twist they provide here is a vitamin C serum in place of the more standard soothing moisturizer or battery-operated polishing sponge. As it turns out, this serum is the best part of the kit, though it's a surprisingly one-note product, as I'll explain in a moment. Sold as a two-step system, Step 1 is the **Polishing Cream**. It contains aluminum oxide crystals, just like most microdermabrasion-in-a-jar products. Lancome's up-sell is something the company refers to as Physio-Polish Enhancer, which is described as "a safe and gentle exfoliation process that breaks the bonds holding the dead skin cells to the surface." The skin cells then "travel to the top layer so the mechanical exfoliator, Aluminum Oxide Crystals, can sweep them away more effectively." A washcloth can provide the exact same benefit. There is nothing special about the scrub particles that enhance this process. It appears that Lancome's claim is nothing more than marketing nonsense. At its heart the Polishing Cream is merely a mechanical scrub, though the abrasiveness of the aluminum oxide crystals is softened by the emollient base of mineral oil, silicone, glycerin, and shea butter. The mineral oil slightly impedes rinsing, but the instructions do correctly indicate to "rinse thoroughly," so it's a minor issue. After rinsing, you're directed to apply the **Radiance Renewing Vitamin C Serum**. This somewhat thick serum makes skin feel wonderfully silky thanks to its silicone content, and it contains 5% ascorbic acid (vitamin C) in very stable packaging. It would be better, however, if this serum contained an array of antioxidants as well as some cell-communicating ingredients and an anti-irritant or two. As is, it's noteworthy as a vitamin C product, but as beneficial as this ingredient is for skin, it takes more than one good antioxidant (or any other "buzz" ingredient) to take the best care of skin. Of more concern for use following the Polishing Cream is that the acid component of ascorbic acid can irritate skin. That's not the best thing to do immediately following a topical abrasive scrub, though this serum can be used separately if you're curious to see what vitamin C does for your skin. Immediately following the Polishing Cream, you would be wise to apply a soothing moisturizer loaded with antioxidants, such as those from the Clinique Repairwear line.

☺ **$$$ Eau Fraiche Douceur** *($34.50 for 6.8 ounces)*. A fancy French name with scientific claims and a spa personality cannot change the fact that this toner is a great big "why bother?" of a product. For your money, you're getting mostly water, slip agents, fragrance, and preservatives. Any alcohol- and menthol-free toner from the drugstore would beat this product by a long shot, and save you a good deal of money to boot.

☺ **$$$ Tonique Confort, Comforting Rehydrating Toner, for Normal to Dry Skin** *($24 for 6.8 ounces)* is a very good toner for its intended skin type. It contains plenty of water-binding agents, plant oil, and antioxidant vitamin E, all in stable packaging.

☺ **$$$ Tonique Douceur, Alcohol-Free Freshener** *($24 for 6.8 ounces)* is mostly water, glycerin, and rose water. This product is basic and minimally effective for normal to dry skin, unless your only objective is to use a toner to remove the last traces of makeup.

☺ **$$$ Genifique Youth Activating Concentrate** *($78 for 1 ounce)*. How many "firsts" can one cosmetics company have? In the case of Lancome, just like most cosmetics companies, a new "first" launches almost every month, and most consumers never notice that once the fervor subsides, there's another "first" ready to take its place. Without question, Lancome did create fervor for this product. My research assistant witnessed women lined up at the Lancome counter to try this product, and it wasn't even free-gift-with-purchase time! Aside from advertising there is no reason to be excited or even mildly amused by this lackluster formula (lackluster is the standard Lancome has maintained for some time as it's been years since they launched a truly outstanding or even interesting skin-care product). Lancome's claim for this water-based serum is that it boosts the activity of skin's genes, and by doing so, specific proteins tied to youthful skin are expressed, thus leading to younger-looking skin. Before I discuss the lack of science behind that claim, it's critical to note that Lancome couches every cosmeceutical and drug-like claim for this product in cosmetic-lingo disclaimers. For example, they follow their statement "Lancome invents our first skincare that boosts the activity of genes" with a footnote—that tiny superscript number after the statement. In this footnote at the bottom of the ad is another statement in fine print that reads "Activate skin's youthful look." So they aren't really saying anything about your genes (because that would be a medical claim and really get the ire of the FDA). The more obscure, meaningless claim of "activate skin's youthful look" is far safer, but what does that mean? It could mean whatever the company or the consumer wants it to mean. A bland moisturizer could "activate" a youthful look on dry skin by making it look moist, and that claim could appear on any product. Achieving a youthful look has nothing to do with this product or any effect on skin's genes. Back to the science (which is really complicated, but bear with me). It is absolutely true that there are genes in our skin responsible for generating proteins. These proteins create antioxidant pathways that protect skin from intrinsic (internal) and external signs of aging. As we age (actually, as we accumulate more sun damage from years of exposure), these genes become less able to "express" themselves in a healthy manner. That leads to oxidation within the skin and a decreased ability for the gene-generated proteins and enzymes to handle oxidative stress. The result of these deficiencies is damaged collagen, inflammation, and unwanted changes to skin texture, such as roughness, increased sensitivity, and, yes, wrinkles (Sources: *Planta Medica*, October 2008, pages 1548-1559; *Pigment Cell & Melanoma Research*, February 2008, pages 79-88; and *Free Radical Biology & Medicine*, August 2008, pages 385-395). What is Lancome's solution to this issue? A yeast ingredient known as bifida ferment lysate. This same ingredient is the backbone of Estee Lauder's Advanced Night Repair Concentrate Recovery Boosting Treatment, which is overall a significantly better formula. The problem is that there's no research proving that this specific form of yeast has any antiaging or gene-stimulating activity when applied to skin. There is limited research showing that yeast ferment filtrate (a compound different from bifida ferment lysate) does reduce oxidative skin damage in the presence of UV light, but this research also showed that many other antioxidants have a similar effect (Sources: *Archives of Dermatological Research*, April 2008, pages S51-S56; and *Journal of Dermatological Science*, June 2006, pages 249-257). Lancome says this product took 10 years of research, but given the formula they've created, a high school chemistry student could have done this in six days. Outside of the bifida ferment lysate, you're getting a mix of slip agents with alcohol and a tiny amount of water-binding agent. The rest of the formula is mostly preservatives, fragrance, and fragrance chemicals. The fragrance ingredients can cause irritation and inflammation on their own which breaks down collagen and is counterproductive to the claims. Irritation will diminish any youth-giving qualities this formula has (which is to say, zero, but still…). The same is true for the amount of alcohol in this product; while the amount is likely too little to be drying or irritating, it is still capable of causing free-radical damage, something the ideal gene-assisting product should strive to reduce. What's so unfortunate is that countless women will believe the hype and go out and waste their money on this half-baked serum. Lancome could've really hit a home run by formulating this with a different type of yeast ferment and joining that with a potent cocktail of antioxidants and no alcohol. As is, you're left with a lightweight serum that will make skin feel smooth, but that offers precious little additional benefit for all skin types.

☺ $$$ **Hydra Zen, Advanced De-Stressing Moisturizing Cream, for Dry Skin** *($50 for 1.7 ounces)* has a lot more going for it formula-wise than the version for Normal/Combination Skin below. Unfortunately, most of the intriguing ingredients are going to break down shortly after this jar-packaged product is opened. What a shame, because it is otherwise a great option for normal to dry skin.

☺ $$$ **Hydra Zen, Advanced De-Stressing Moisturizing Cream, for Normal/Combination Skin** *($50 for 1.7 ounces)* is supposed to be relaxation in a jar, or at least that's what the name and ad copy suggest. Even if you could apply something to the face to make it calmer, according to Hydra Zen that would only take a moisturizer, because that's all this product is. The only unique thing about Hydra Zen is the name. If mind over matter works, then you will feel calmer, but it probably isn't from applying this good, but rather ordinary, ho-hum, silicone-based, lightweight moisturizer that contains minimal water-binding agents and antioxidants.

☺ $$$ **Nutrix Royal, Intense Lipid Repair Cream, for Dry to Very Dry Skin** *($55 for 1.6 ounces)* contains a terrific blend of emollients to address the needs of its intended skin types. Jar packaging won't keep the tiny amount of antioxidants stable, so this ends up being a fairly expensive moisturizer whose benefits are easily obtained from other products that offer dry skin even more.

☺ $$$ **Nutrix, Soothing Treatment Cream, for Dry to Very Dry/Sensitive Skin** *($45 for 1.9 ounces)*. First launched in 1936, this remains a very good, though basic, moisturizer for very dry skin. The fragrance components (and fragrance itself) are not suitable for sensitive skin. Two forms of lecithin are nice for skin, but skin needs more and, when you think about it, you wouldn't now be using just about anything that was made in 1936, from a washing machine to a typewriter (and TVs and microwaves weren't even invented).

☹ $$$ **Platineum Eye & Lip Hydroxy(a)-Calcium, Restructuring Eye and Lip Treatment** *($85 for 0.5 ounce)* debuts as Lancome's version of L'Oreal's Age Perfect Pro-Calcium Eye Cream. Lancome uses a different base formula and contains insignificant amounts of novel ingredients that L'Oreal left out, but the claims of calcium fortifying aging skin are the same, and they are just as silly because calcium can't fortify skin. As is the case for most Lancome moisturizers, there isn't much to extol. The majority of the formula is standard slip agents and thickeners along with a couple of emollients and wax. The calcium ingredient is hydroxyapatite, and the company claims this is continuously released, working to strengthen fragile skin around the eyes and lips. Hydroxyapatite is the calcium compound found in our bones and teeth. It is also used in dermal fillers such as Radiesse, and for other types of soft tissue augmentation. It's no secret that injecting this substance in a controlled manner can have a positive effect on the appearance of wrinkles, but that is radically different from applying a small amount of it topically when it's blended into a moisturizer. There is no evidence that topically applied hydroxyapatite works even remotely like dermal fillers that contain it, yet Lancome is hoping you won't make that connection. If you're curious to see what calcium can do for your skin, consider L'Oreal's less expensive version or, even better, try adding more calcium-rich foods to your diet and forgo this poorly formulated moisturizer (which would be far better for skin if it contained antioxidants, cell-communicating ingredients, and skin-identical ingredients).

☺ $$$ **Platineum Hydroxy(a)-Calcium Extra Riche, Restructuring and Reinforcing Cream SPF 15** *($120 for 1.7 ounces)* provides an in-part avobenzone sunscreen in a slightly hydrating base. Don't interpret the "Extra Riche" name to mean this is a stellar product for dry to very dry skin; L'Oreal's Age Perfect Pro-Calcium Day Cream SPF 15 is much more emollient and preferred to this one. Although this is an option for those with normal to slightly dry skin seeking a daytime moisturizer, the formula is disappointing for the money. Unless you believe Lancome's claims about calcium restructuring skin (which it absolutely cannot do), you're not getting much from this product beyond light moisture and sun protection. The small amount of antioxidants is disappointing, as is the choice of jar packaging, which won't keep them stable.

☹ **Progres Eye Cream** *($55 for 0.5 ounce)* is an emollient moisturizer for dry skin anywhere on the face. It is not recommended because it contains two preservatives that are contraindicated for use in leave-on products, not to mention that the fragrance is overkill for the delicate eye area.

☹ **Hydra-Intense Masque Hydrating Gel Mask with Botanical Extract** *($28 for 3.4 ounces)* lists alcohol as the second ingredient, which doesn't make this mask the least bit hydrating. This is about as do-nothing (except irritate) as do-nothing products get!

☹ **Pure Empreinte Masque Purifying Mineral Mask with White Clay** *($28 for 3.4 ounces)* has the makings of a very good clay mask for oily skin, but the inclusion of camphor was unwise and makes this not preferred to almost any other clay mask being sold.

☺ **UV Expert 20, Face & Body Protection Daily Moisturizing Cream SPF 20** *($35 for 3.4 ounces)* got a lot of press as L'Oreal blitzed the media with claims that their ecamsule (Mexoryl SX) sunscreen is the preferred active sunscreen for UVA protection. Ecamsule is a very effective, worthwhile UVA sunscreen. However, it is not a must-have. It also doesn't offer the best protection under the sun (titanium dioxide and zinc oxide still provide more protection than ecamsule, especially when you consider that they also provide UVB protection). And it isn't preferred to avobenzone, provided the avobenzone is carefully formulated so it remains stable. This sunscreen lotion contains ecamsule, avobenzone, and titanium dioxide as actives (along with octocrylene, which primarily provides UVB protection and helps to stabilize avobenzone), so the UVA spectrum is definitely covered. What's disappointing is that the base formula is so boring. Not a single antioxidant, elegant water-binding agent, or cell-communicating ingredient shows up. Compare this to the Estee Lauder and Clinique sunscreens that provide broad-spectrum protection and have an array of skin-identical substances plus antioxidants, and honestly, what's all the fuss about?

LANCOME MAKEUP

FOUNDATION: ✓ ☺ **$$$ Absolue BX Makeup Absolute Replenishing Radiant Makeup SPF 18** *($57)* is one of Lancome's most expensive foundations, and thankfully they got the sunscreen part right: it's partly titanium dioxide so the UVA range is covered. Positioned as antiaging makeup for mature skin, the only legitimate antiaging element is the effective sunscreen. The "bio-network" of wild yam, sea algae, and other plant extracts cannot rejuvenate skin or increase its firmness. Even if these plants were the answer to forestalling that face-lift, the amount of them in this foundation is paltry. Taken on its merit of foundation alone, this has an exquisite, fluid texture that glides over skin. It provides almost full coverage and sets to an attractive satin-matte finish that won't make dry skin look dull (that's assuming you've taken pre-makeup steps to smooth over dry patches). Lancome claims this will not settle into lines, and for the most part, that's true. Deep wrinkles will see some settling, but this does a good job of smoothing over superficial to moderate lines. Almost all of the shades are impressive, and there are options for fair to dark (but not very dark) skin tones. Be careful with Absolute Almond 310 and Absolute Almond 320 because both are slightly peach; Absolute Ecru 240 is noticeably peach and should be avoided; and Absolute Caramel 420 has a copper cast that limits its usage, but it may work for some dark skin tones. The Paula's Pick rating has to do with this foundation's attributes, not with its antiaging claims or preferential use for those with mature skin (whatever "mature" means, as not everyone in the mature category has the same needs or preferences).

✓ ☺ **$$$ Dual Finish Fragrance Free Versatile Powder Makeup** *($35.50)* has the same formula as the original Dual Finish Versatile Powder Makeup reviewed below, minus the fragrance. An interesting point is that this version comes in only eight shades, but they're all excellent and correspond exactly with the same-named shades in the fragranced Dual Finish.

✓ ☺ **$$$ Dual Finish Versatile Powder Makeup** *($35.50)* has been part of Lancôme's foundation lineup for years and has deservedly attained classic status. This talc-based wet/dry-powder foundation offers a soft matte finish and a selection of 28 beautiful colors for fair to very dark skin. The application, especially when used dry, is smooth and even with a silky, almost creamy-feeling texture that's best for normal to dry skin. The squalane and mineral oil in the formula are not the best ingredients to temper shine, but they keep this powder from looking too dry or chalky. Using Dual Finish wet is tricky because these types of foundations tend to go on streaky. It is best used dry, and applied with a brush for sheer coverage or a makeup sponge for medium coverage.

✓ ☺ **$$$ Teint Idole Ultra Enduringly Divine and Comfortable Makeup** *($40)* has a near-weightless, silky texture with a fluidity that makes blending a breeze. It sets to a strong matte finish (and still does so faster than other foundations for oily skin), but you have enough play time to get it blended on smoothly and evenly—and if you don't, mistakes can be buffed out. The latest pigment technology allows Lancôme to achieve a long-wearing, oil-absorbing matte finish without creating a flat or masklike appearance. Seventeen medium-to-full-coverage shades are available, and here's where things start to decline a bit. Most of the fair to light shades are excellent, but the deeper shades have an orange to copper cast that even the Lancôme counter makeup artist commented were "bad shades" that "need more work." I love it when cosmetics salespeople openly agree with me; after all these years I still savor those moments. You should be cautious with the following shades: Suede 2, which can turn peach, and Suede 1, and Bisque 8, which are all blatantly peach or copper. Overall, the Buff range of shades (also known as Intensity II) is the most workable for light to medium skin tones. Does this foundation last for 14 hours? Yes, but those with very oily skin will still need to blot and powder before the end of the day.

☺ **$$$ Ageless Minerale Skin-Transforming Mineral Powder Foundation with White Sapphire Complex SPF 21** *($40)* is Lancôme's contribution to the mineral makeup craze, and it's fairly impressive. With titanium dioxide as the sole active ingredient, broad-spectrum protection is assured. This loose-powder foundation has an almost creamy texture that is easy to buff on skin, though it must be done quickly and not over a surface that's too moist or it will grab and change color almost immediately. This provides light to medium coverage with a single application, or can be layered for additional coverage, although doing so can create a too heavy appearance, so use restraint. The sifter comes equipped with a closure to keep mess to a minimum, which is great. This powder's finish on skin is best described as "glowing matte" because the overall effect is matte, but it contains shiny pigments that give skin a dimensional glow, which is not the best for those with oily skin who are trying to suppress shine. By the way, despite the name, this foundation doesn't contain any white sapphire. All told, this mineral-powder foundation is better than what L'Oreal or sister company Maybelline New York did, and is worth a look if you think mineral makeup is the bee's knees. This is best for normal to slightly dry skin. Contrary to claims, it will settle into lines, so it's not a foundation to try if wrinkles are prominent.

☺ $$$ **Bienfait Multi-Vital Teinte High Potency Tinted Moisturizer SPF 30** *($44)* is one of the few tinted moisturizers with a high SPF rating and sufficient UVA protection, thanks to its in-part titanium dioxide sunscreen. Although closer to a light-coverage foundation than a tinted moisturizer (it isn't as sheer as you might think given the name), it has a light lotion texture that blends easily and would be suitable for normal to slightly dry skin. It has a soft, dewy finish and blurs minor flaws nicely. The main issue is that all but one of the four shades lean toward the peachy side, and this isn't sheer enough to accommodate for the color shift. This is definitely one to test at the counter, though if you have a light (not fair) skin tone, Shade 1 is worthwhile. By the way, Lancome's claim that this product is vitamin-enriched makes it sound like it's bursting with antioxidants, and it isn't. They're in here, but not in amounts that will make a discernible difference.

☺ $$$ **Color Ideal Precise Match Skin Perfecting Makeup SPF 15** *($37)* does have impressive UVA protection (titanium dioxide is the sole active ingredient). The big claim is that the pigments in this makeup adapt to your skin tone to provide a perfect match. Although the selection of 19 shades is a mostly neutral lot that includes options for fair to dark skin, it turns out that Lancome's "precision matching" isn't that precise. I tried a couple of shades on my skin, one of which initially matched quite well. Yet the final result revealed that the color lightened noticeably as it dried, making me look unnaturally pale. The darker shade (too dark to match my skin exactly) also lightened a bit, but remained an obvious mismatch. This was very unlike my experience with Cover Girl's TruBlend Make-Up, a foundation that makes similar shade-matching claims that in that case are legitimate. Still, there is much to love about this Lancome foundation. It has a supremely silky, nearly weightless texture that meshes well with skin, setting to a satin-matte finish that does a great job of keeping excess shine in check. Given that, it's not surprising that those with normal to very oily skin will appreciate this foundation the most. Coverage goes from sheer to medium, and building coverage doesn't create a thick or heavy appearance. The following shades are too pink, peach, or copper for most skin tones: I-40C, III-20C, and IV-20C. Shade II-20W may be too yellow for some medium skin tones, while shade IV-40N is a beautiful option for dark skin tones. The bottom line is that this, like all foundations, demands careful evaluation in natural light so you can be sure you're getting the best match. The good news is that most Lancome counters offer trial samples, an option I encourage!

☺ $$$ **Photogenic Lumessence Compact Light-Mastering & Line-Smoothing Makeup SPF 18** *($42)* is a very good, modern cream-to-powder makeup that—big Gasp!—actually provides sufficient UVA protection thanks to its pure titanium dioxide sunscreen. (Gasp! Because Lancome rarely includes UVA-protecting ingredients in any of their products.) This smooths over skin easily and blends to a soft powder finish that leaves a subtle glow. Best for normal to slightly dry skin not prone to breakouts, this foundation provides sheer to medium coverage, although medium coverage requires layering and diminishes this makeup's natural look. It poses a slight risk of creasing into lines around the eye and isn't the best for those with large pores because after a few hours it slips into them and magnifies their appearance. As for the shade selection, it is mostly excellent and includes options for light to dark, but not very dark, skin tones. Be careful with Bisque 6W and Bisque 8N because both can be too peach for their respective skin tones.

☺ **$$$ Renergie Lift Makeup SPF 20** *($40)* is positioned as Lancome's antiaging makeup (which it isn't), but thankfully it does have excellent sun protection and that goes a long way toward reducing the development of wrinkles and skin discolorations when worn daily! All the antiaging claims and statistics in the world don't mean a thing without a sufficient sunscreen in your daily routine, and this in-part titanium dioxide foundation is a great way to get it. This silky liquid foundation is smooth and a pleasure to blend. The finish is natural and slightly moist, and provides medium coverage without creasing into lines. You probably guessed that this won't lift the skin anywhere, but by creating the illusion of smoother, even-toned skin it can make wrinkles (we're talking superficial lines, not pronounced wrinkles) look less apparent; silicone technology comes through again! Of the shades available, the only missteps are the slightly peach Lifting Dore 10, Lifting Clair 30, and slightly orange Lifting Dore 30. If you have normal to dry skin and want to experience a state-of-the-art foundation with effective sun protection, this is highly recommended.

☺ **$$$ Absolue Makeup Absolute Replenishing Cream Makeup SPF 20** *($57)* is Lancome's most expensive foundation. Is it worth it? The disappointing lack of sufficient UVA protection doesn't get this foundation off to a good start. However, its creamy application and silky, slightly moist finish are bound to please those with dry skin. Ironically, for a creamy foundation this isn't an ideal formula for someone with very dry skin. That's because it contains silicone and water-binding agents rather than the oils or emollient ingredients that would provide the extra moisturizing necessary to make very dry skin feel smooth and comfortable. The real reason to consider this foundation is that it provides full coverage without looking heavy or too thick. It conceals without looking too conspicuous, so if you need significant coverage, have dry skin, and are willing to pair this with a broad-spectrum sunscreen, it is an option. The shade selection is smaller than Lancome's typical assortment. With ten colors, you'd hope every one would be a winner, but watch out for Absolute Almond 10 (too pink), and use caution with Absolute Almond 20 (slightly peach, but may be OK for tan skin tones). Absolute Pearl 10 is excellent for fair skin, and the remaining shades are fittingly neutral. One last comment: Lancome's justification for this foundation's high price is its claim that the product's "exclusive bio-network" (featuring wild yam and algae) helps "revitalize and restore skin elasticity." Unfortunately, there's no proof anywhere that those ingredients can do that. Just as their Absolue skin-care products are ineffective for this purpose, so is this foundation that shares the Absolue name and overhyped ingredients. And anyway, there's more fragrance in this makeup than yam or algae.

☺ **$$$ Aqua Fusion Teinte Continuous Infusing Tinted Moisturizer SPF 20** *($37)* lacks the UVA-protecting ingredients of titanium dioxide, zinc oxide, avobenzone, Tinosorb, or Mexoryl SX, which is a shame—because this is otherwise an excellent sheer-to-light-coverage foundation for normal to oily skin. It begins creamy, but dries to a matte finish that remains slightly moist to the touch (it appears matte but feels moist). All four shades are terrific—if only this could be a one-step product for color, coverage, and sufficient sun protection! Since it isn't, this is best for someone with normal to slightly dry skin willing to wear an effective sunscreen underneath, which seems unnecessarily redundant.

☺ **$$$ Color Ideal Hydra Compact Precise Match Skin-Perfecting Cream Makeup SPF 10** *($50; $35 for refills)* is similar to but lighter in texture than traditional cream-to-powder makeup. Although Lancome gets the UVA protection issue right with its all-titanium dioxide sunscreen, the SPF rating is disappointing, at least if you plan to use this as your sole source of facial sun protection. This silicone-in-water foundation applies smoothly and blends over skin well, enhancing it and providing sheer to medium coverage while looking surprisingly natural. The formula contains waxes, which aren't the best for breakout-prone skin, but this is a good option for normal to slightly dry or slightly oily skin without blemish concerns. Among the eight mostly neutral shades are options for fair to tan skin tones. The only shade to consider carefully is the slightly peach Beige Noisette. One note about the packaging: Be sure to close the foundation portion's compact tightly after each use to keep the product from drying out. Color Ideal Hydra Compact makeup does have a lingering fragrance.

☺ **$$$ Photogenic Lumessence Light-Mastering & Line-Smoothing Makeup SPF 15** *($40)*. Lancome has once again created a foundation that has a lot going for it until you realize that it doesn't provide sufficient UVA protection because it doesn't contain avobenzone, titanium dioxide, zinc oxide, Tinosorb, or Mexoryl SX. Lancome knows better because they have the patent on the UVA-protecting ingredient ecamsule, and they have for years. So, the fact that they keep launching foundations whose sunscreens fall short is maddening. If you're willing to pair this foundation with a daytime moisturizer that contains the right UVA-protecting ingredients it is an option, but considering there are lots of foundations that get this aspect of their formula right, why bother with this one? As a foundation this has a fluid, very silky texture that feels amazing and blends easily. It provides light to medium coverage and has a marvelously skin-like finish. The formula is best for normal to slightly dry or slightly oily skin. As usual for Lancome these days, the shade range is excellent, especially for those with fair to light skin tones. The dark shades don't do as well, with Suede 0 and Suede 2 being too orange and copper. What about the light-mastering claims? You won't see any refraction going on, but the pigments in this foundation look quite natural, although it absolutely will not make lines, wrinkles, and pores vanish. Despite the lofty claims, this foundation would be rated a Paula's Pick if not for the deficient sunscreen.

☹ **Imanance Tinted Day Creme SPF 15** *($43 for 1.7 ounces)* has some positives, including an in-part titanium dioxide–based SPF 15 and natural-looking sheer coverage. Yet what outweighs these traits is that almost all of the shades are appalling and the formula contains the preservatives methylisothiazolinone and methylchloroisothiazolinone (also known as Kathon CG), which is not recommended for use in leave-on products, particularly any to be used around the eye area.

CONCEALER: ✓ ☺ **$$$ Maquicomplet et Eclat Eye Brightening Concealer** *($27.50)*. This fluid, smooth brightening concealer is best for highlighting, be it under the eyes, along the bridge of the nose, or elsewhere on the face. It applies smoothly and blends expertly to a finish that is matte in feel but leaves a soft, lit-from-within glow. It is a brilliant choice for subtle highlighting, and all four shades are recommended. Think of this as a full-size version of the highlighting portion of Maybelline New York's Instant Age Rewind Double Face Perfector.

☺ **$$$ Effacernes Waterproof Protective Undereye Concealer** *($27.50)* has a creamy texture that provides significant coverage and allows for smooth blending. The squeeze tube takes some getting used to (it's easy to dispense too much product), but once you acclimate, this concealer is aces, and it doesn't crease! The four shades are mostly neutral, though Porcelaine I is slightly pink. Contrary to the name, this concealer is not waterproof.

☺ **$$$ Flash Retouche Perfecting Brush-On Concealer Radiance & Anti-Fatigue** *($28)* is a slightly creamy liquid concealer housed in a pen-style applicator. A pushbutton at the bottom of the component sends the product onto the built-in synthetic brush. The application is smooth and even, and it dries to a matte finish that has a soft sheen. Coverage isn't significant, so this is best used as a complexion highlighter. Three shades are available, and although Rose Lumiere is slightly pink, the sheerness negates that. As nice as this is for highlighting, Estee Lauder's Ideal Light Brush-On Illuminator is better because it has a larger shade selection and provides enhanced coverage (meaning you can use it as a concealer or highlighter).

☹ **$$$ Maquicomplet Complete Coverage Concealer** *($27.50)* is a smooth, liquidy concealer with excellent, crease-free, medium to full coverage, though each shade suffers from too much shine, and adding shiny particles to a concealer won't distract anyone from what you're trying to hide. What a shame, because most of the shades are impeccably neutral. If you decide to try this, avoid the slightly ash-pink Clair II and use caution with the yellow Correcteur shade.

POWDER: ✓ ☺ **$$$ Absolue Powder Radiant Smoothing Powder** *($52)* carries a price that may make you look anything but radiant, but wait until you feel its ultra-silky, otherworldly texture. This is one of the most elegant loose powders available. Although the talc-based formula isn't too different from many other powders, the milling process does create a slight difference. This has a non-drying sheer finish suitable for normal to dry skin. All of the shades resemble real skin tones, but watch out for the very shiny Absolute Peche and Absolute Golden—both are suitable for nighttime glamour only, unless you want showgirl shine while at the office or out shopping.

✓ ☺ **$$$ Ageless Minerale Perfecting and Setting Mineral Powder with White Sapphire Complex** *($36)* is a loose powder designed to set Lancome's Ageless Minerale Skin-Transforming Mineral Powder Foundation reviewed above. When I learned that was the intent, I asked the salesperson why a person needs a loose powder to set another loose powder. Isn't one powder enough? She explained that the Perfecting and Setting Mineral Powder is designed to give the Mineral Powder Foundation an airbrushed, buffed look. In other words, the Mineral Powder Foundation isn't good enough on its own. Sigh. Overlooking Lancome's reason behind this powder, it's actually a very silky, sheer setting powder that leaves an attractive satin finish on skin. The pale flesh tone is supposed to be translucent, but is too white for tan to dark skin tones. This is very similar to L'Oreal's Bare Naturale Soft-Focus Mineral Finish powder, except that L'Oreal's version is half the price of Lancome's. If you have a light skin tone and normal to dry skin, this is a very good setting powder to consider.

✓ ☺ **$$$ Color Ideal Pressed Powder Precise Match Skin Perfecting Pressed Powder** *($33)* is Lancome's updated version of their former Colour ID Precise Match Weightless Portable Powder. The latter was a talc-free loose powder housed in a component with a built-in brush, while this is a talc-based pressed powder that's much easier to apply. In fact, don't shed a tear over the discontinued powder, because Color Ideal is one of the most exquisite powders you'll find at the department store. It has a beautifully smooth texture and a finish that meshes so well with skin that it just looks better, rather than powdered or starkly matte. My only complaint, and this is primarily for those with oily skin, is that each of the 11 superb shades is laced with sparkles, and adding shine to already shiny skin is counterproductive, although in this case the effect is really subtle. By the way, this is almost identical to, but less expensive than, Giorgio Armani's Luminous Silk Powder. You may recall that L'Oreal owns both companies (and as

L'Oreal often does, will likely launch their own version of this pressed-powder formula at the drugstore soon and, of course, I will let you know when).

☺ **$$$ Photogenic Sheer Loose Powder** *($34)* and **Photogenic Sheer Pressed Powder** *($29)* claim to contain the "Photo-Flex Complex of 2-D reflecting powders and 3-D diffusing powders." That's a great hook for these pricey powders! Admittedly, both powders have a soft, finely milled, sumptuous texture and a smooth, dry finish (the Pressed Powder version is slightly drier), but the special effects are nothing more than subtle shine, plain and simple. Although the shine is barely discernible, those hoping to reduce shine may want to look elsewhere. The loose version offers five shades and the pressed version has four shades. With either powder, almost all of the shades are beautifully soft and neutral.

BLUSH AND BRONZER: ✓☺ **$$$ Color Design Blush Sensational Effects Cream Blush, Smooth Hold** *($27)*. Although this doesn't produce an effect I'd label "sensational," it has a lovely modern cream-to-powder texture that blends on sheer and smooth and, yes, "holds" well, at least for those with normal to dry skin (those with oily skin should avoid this type of blush). Most of the attractive shades have a hint of shine, but it's acceptable for daytime wear. The Freeze Frame and Model Mocha shades have a strong shimmer and are best for evening wear when you want more shine than color. As much as I like this blush, you should know that Maybelline New York's Dream Mousse Blush produces a similar effect for one-fourth the price.

☺ **$$$ Blush Subtil Duo Delicate Oil-Free Powder Blush and Cream Highlighter** *($40)*. Lancome has packaged their popular Blush Subtil (a powder blush that works just fine, but isn't as impressive as several less expensive blushes) with a corresponding shade of creamy highlighter. Most of the pairings are inspired and the highlighter is easy to blend and sets to a soft powder finish (with shimmer, of course). The rose and mauve tones are the most versatile.

☺ **$$$ Tropiques Minerale Mineral Smoothing Loose Bronzer** *($38.50)*. Applying powder bronzer in loose form isn't the tidiest way to fake a tan, but with the right brush, this sheer, soft powder produces an attractive bronze sheen that includes a hint of sparkles. Among the three shades, Natural Ambre is the most convincing. Natural Copper is too orange for most skin tones, so consider it carefully.

☹ **$$$ Blush Subtil Delicate Oil-Free Powder Blush** *($29.50)* has gotten pricier, but its formula hasn't kept pace with the latest and greatest powder blushes from Estee Lauder and, more importantly for the budget-conscious, L'Oreal. The latter's True Match Super-Blendable Blush is superior to Blush Subtil's dry texture and slightly choppy application. If you decide to try this, it includes mostly matte options and each of the colors goes on quite sheer. Miel Glace is shiny.

☹ **$$$ Blush Subtil Shimmer Delicate Oil-Free Powder Blush** *($29.50)* has the same texture as the original Blush Subtil, but each shade is imbued with sparkles (this isn't a low-glow shimmer). The good news is the sparkles cling well and the colors apply softly, but this isn't enough to make it worth choosing over better blushes that cost less.

☹ **$$$ La Rose Liberte Highlighting Bronzer** *($40)*. This is nothing more than a flesh-toned pressed powder that doesn't have a bronze effect, but does enliven skin with a soft gold shine. The smooth, dry texture goes on sheer, and the sparkling shine has OK cling.

☹ **$$$ Star Bronzer Magic Bronzing Brush-Automatic Powder Brush for Face and Body** *($33)* is a soft, tapered powder brush whose handle is a reservoir for a sheer, shiny golden copper powder. A pushbutton at the base of the handle shoots powder into the brush, and from there it can be dusted over the face or body. A clever execution to be sure, but this pricey product has little impact other than the sparkling shine it leaves.

The Reviews L

☻ **Poudre Soleil Sun-Kissed Bronzing Powder** *($36.50)* is a pressed bronzing powder. The Bronze Solaire shade is the best of the colors, but the too-dry texture and flaky shine are disappointing at any price.

EYESHADOW: ✓ ☺ **$$$ Ombre Absolue Duo Radiant Smoothing Eye Shadow Duo 6 Hour Hold** *($35)*. Talk about a beautiful sumptuous texture! This eyeshadow formula is one of the silkiest around, and it applies evenly. Color deposit is smooth and allows for much versatility, unless you want a sheer look. The only downside is that these eyeshadow duos are marketed to older women, and every pairing has shine. The shine itself is understated on some of the duos, but even so shine is not the best for all-over eye-area use once wrinkles and crepey skin are present because shine only accentuates these signs of aging. These duos would work well combined with a matte shade used all over, saving the shiny shades for highlighting under the brow bone. The best duos are Golden Grandeur, Ivory Opulence, and Crystal Rose.

☺ **$$$ Color Design Sensational Effects Eye Shadow Quad Smooth Hold** *($42)*. I am pleased to report that, although this is an expensive way to assemble an eyeshadow collection, every quad has well-coordinated colors that apply smoothly, if a bit soft, and have a suede-smooth texture. At first glance, some of the quads appear contrasting, but the colors blend together well, with most imparting a soft shimmer finish. Among the available sets, Modern Edge is the shiniest and thus not recommended for use on wrinkled or less-than-taut eyelid skin. The effect of any of the quads isn't necessarily sensational, but definitely versatile, and the shine doesn't flake.

☺ **Color Design Sensational Effects Eye Shadow Smooth Hold** *($16.50)* adds to Lancome's impressive roster of powder eyeshadows, and for the first time in a long time the shades are divided by finish on the tester unit, a very helpful concept. The formula (sold as singles) feels quite silky and applies smoothly without flaking or skipping. Medium to deep shades are easy to soften, and overall this eyeshadow takes full advantage of advances in powder technology. The shades and finishes are divided into matte, sheen, shimmer, metallic, and intense. The matte shades are my preference (no surprise there) and the best ones are Daylight, Positive, Faux Pas, Ciel du Soir, and Waif. The sheens have a low-luster finish, appropriate unless your eyelid skin is noticeably wrinkled. Shimmer and Metallic are the shiniest group, while the Intense group is primarily deep shades best for eye lining. Among them, avoid Makeover and Garment, unless you want people to notice your for-shock-value eyeshadow rather than your eyes! As much as I liked this eyeshadow formula, it isn't quite on par with the latest options from Clinique and Estee Lauder.

☹ **$$$ Ombre Perfecteur Perfecting EyeShadow Base** *($23)* is a waterproof concealer for the eyelid area that is also supposed to extend the wear of eyeshadows. The nude, matte color is applied from a pen outfitted with an angled sponge tip. It tends to go on thick, but does blend evenly. It's OK, but not really necessary if you already use a matte-finish concealer.

☻ **Aquatique Waterproof EyeColour Base** *($24)* is still around and that means Lancome is succeeding at convincing some women to use a separate product (beyond foundation or concealer) to even out the skin tone on their eyelids and to prevent eyeshadows from creasing. The opaque, thick formula creases, and what's worse is that the single color is strongly peach, not exactly what all women need or want.

EYE AND BROW SHAPER: ✓ ☺ **$$$ Artliner Precision Point EyeLiner** *($28)* remains one of the best liquid eyeliners around thanks to its easy-to-apply, quick-drying, long-lasting formula and superior brush. For considerably less money, you can get the same results from

L'Oreal's Line Intensifique. Regardless of whether you overspend or save, both liquid liners are top picks.

☺ $$$ **Modele Sourcils Brow Groomer** *($21)* is a brow mascara available in clear or with a tint. The lightweight formula keeps the brow groomed without being sticky, and the densely bristled brush is best for thicker, unruly brows.

☺ $$$ **Le Crayon Kohl** *($23.50)* needs routine sharpening, which is why it is not rated higher; but for those willing to tolerate that drawback this is a very good eye pencil. It applies smoothly and is minimally prone to smudging or smearing. There are some wild colors that do little to emphasize eyes, but the classics are there as well.

☺ $$$ **Le Crayon Poudre Powder Pencil for the Brows** *($23)* is one of the best needs-sharpening brow pencils. It goes on easily, if a bit creamy, and the colors (with options for all but black brows) are matte and soft. There's even a good brush at one end for softening and blending the color. This would be rated better if not for the need to keep it sharpened, which isn't convenient.

☺ $$$ **Le Stylo Waterproof Long Lasting EyeLiner** *($23.50)* is a smooth-textured, automatic, nonretractable eye pencil with mostly shiny colors that all tend to smudge, though no more so than most creamy pencils. This is fine for a smoky look, but it breaks down readily when wet.

☹ **Le Crayon Khol Kajal** *($23.50)*. Don't bother with this needs-sharpening pencil. It's too creamy to last (though it applies smoothly), it smudges easily, and the texture is soft enough that the point routinely breaks, requiring you to sharpen again and again.

LIPSTICK, LIP GLOSS, AND LIPLINER: ✓ ☺ $$$ **Color Design Sensational Effects Lipcolor Smooth Hold** *($22)* has a smooth, creamy texture that hydrates lips without feeling too thick or greasy. Lancome offers a gorgeous range of shades, divided by finish (though all have the same creamy feel). Shimmer shades impart soft shine, Sheens impart a metallic iridescence, Metallics offer a strong metallic finish, and Creams have a soft, semi-gloss finish. Each shade, particularly the reds, has a great stain so these last longer than standard cream lipsticks. Quite simply, this is Lancome's most impressive lipstick, and at this price it should impress!

✓ ☺ $$$ **Le Crayon Lip Contour** *($22)* is an above-average automatic, retractable lip pencil with good colors and a smooth application. This lipliner really stays put and is an ideal choice for those prone to having lipstick feather into lines around the mouth.

☺ $$$ **Color Fever Gloss** *($25)* is billed as a lip gloss, but is closer to a liquid lipstick thanks to its smooth, moist feel and pigment level. A glossy, non-sticky finish is part of the deal, and most of the colors are striking. Paying this much for gloss is definitely not necessary, but at least Lancome provided exquisite packaging and a cleverly angled sponge-tip applicator that lets you apply more color in less time.

☺ $$$ **Color Fever Lipstick** *($25)* has a name that may make you think the shades are richly opaque, yet that's not the case with this lightweight, semi-creamy lipstick. Color saturation is moderate even when layered. This lipstick's appearance is helped considerably by the light-catching shimmer particles in it, which give each shade an alluring glow that doesn't look over-the-top (meaning you won't have pieces of glitter dotting your lips). Contributing to the price is the debut of Lancome's sleekest lipstick component yet, a gunmetal gray mirrored surface flanked on each side by translucent deep-amber panels.

☺ $$$ **Color Fever Shine Sensual Sheer Color Vibrant Lipshine** *($25)*. If you're looking to overspend on a sheer lipstick, here's a good one to consider. It feels smooth and light and most of the sheer colors are infused with a glittering shimmer. The finish is pretty, but won't meet most women's definition of long-lasting.

☺ **$$$ Color Fever Plumper Plumping Vibrant Lip Shine** *($29)* is Lancome's version of Maybelline New York's Lip Plumper XL (Lancome and Maybelline are both owned by L'Oreal). The formulas are nearly identical, and both contain a potent menthol derivative (ethyl menthane carboxamide, to be exact) that makes lips tingle (as claimed) and enlarge slightly, from the resulting irritation. This plumper is too irritating for daily use, but is an OK option for special occasions when you'd like a sheer, sparkling lip gloss that adds a little something extra to lips.

☺ **$$$ Juicy Tubes Jelly Ultra Shiny Lip Gloss** *($18)*. This tube lip gloss has a thick, syrupy texture and each translucent color leaves lips with a wet-look shine and a slightly sticky feel. The shades in this Juicy Tubes product are among Lancome's softest.

☺ **$$$ Juicy Tubes Smoothie Ultra Shiny Lip Gloss** *($18)*. This tube lip gloss offers a creamier feel and stronger color payoff than Lancome's other Juicy Tubes lip glosses. Think of it as a liquid lipstick with a very glossy finish and subdued shimmer. It retains the stickiness of the other Juicy Tubes glosses, which keeps it from earning a Paula's Pick rating.

☹ **$$$ La Laque Fever Lip Shine** *($26)*. The enticing claims for this semi-sheer lip gloss are that it provides high-potency color and shine that lasts for six hours. Don't count on it! Even though this gloss is more pigmented than most, its slick texture tends to fade quickly, necessitating frequent touch-ups. It isn't the least bit goopy or sticky, and the wet-looking, prismatic shine is attractive—but at best you'll get slightly longer wear time than what you get from a standard lip gloss. The applicator for this gloss is unique and won't be to everyone's liking, so be sure to test it before purchasing. (Swatch some gloss on your hand so you get an idea of how the applicator deposits product.)

☹ **$$$ Le Lipstique LipColouring Stick with Brush** *($23)* is a standard pencil with a tapered blending brush at the other end. That's convenient, but not worth the price. This does have some staying power, leaving a slight stain on the lips, and the shade selection is plentiful.

☹ **$$$ Le Rouge Absolu Reshaping & Replenishing LipColour SPF 15** *($26)* not only continues the trend of department-store lipsticks' prices hitting higher and higher price points, but also continues Lancome's pattern of launching makeup products with insufficient UVA protection. I could begin to justify the high price of this lipstick if you were at least getting superior sun protection from it, but since that's not the case you're left with a smooth, standard creamy lipstick that, while indeed pleasant, isn't reason enough to indulge. If you're curious about how the alleged reshaping of lips is supposed to work, it's impossible to say. If you have uneven lips, applying this lipstick won't correct that, and there's nothing in it that can make lips more plump—this isn't a mini collagen injection in the form of a lipstick. Lancome refers to their "plumping polymer," but it's all wordplay without proof.

☹ **L'Absolu Rouge Advanced Replenishing & Reshaping Lipcolor Pro Xylane SPF 12 Sunscreen** *($29)*. Before you seriously consider this lipstick, please know that the sunscreen lacks the right UVA-protecting ingredients to protect lips (which get sun damage too) from the entire UVA spectrum, which is an insult at this price. Labeling this "advanced" is a joke, and the formula doesn't contain anything called Pro Xylane—even Lancome's staff couldn't explain what it was; they simply read from their sales training manual. This cream lipstick does have a unique texture that is light yet substantially moisturizing (it contains a lot of nut oil) and the colors plus the dimensional shimmer most of them have are riveting, as is the magnetic closure of the case. But to go as far as stating this lipstick can reshape lips is a joke. Any shimmer lipstick applied well can make lips look slightly fuller due to its reflective quality, and smoother due to its combination of lip line–filling waxes and polymers. Such technology isn't unique to Lancome, and this lipstick doesn't deserve your attention.

MASCARA: ✓☺ **$$$ Definicils High Definition Mascara** *($24)* is an extraordinary lengthening mascara that builds some thickness with minimal to no chance of clumping. The only drawback, and this is a minor complaint, is it can go on a bit too wet, which increases the chance of it smearing before your lashes dry.

✓☺ **$$$ Definicils Waterproof High Definition Mascara** *($24)* does everything Lancome's regular Definicils mascara does to lengthen, lightly thicken, and separate the lashes, but with a waterproof formula that wears and wears. It is Lancome's premiere waterproof mascara, and the formula now leaves lashes feeling soft (an uncommon trait for waterproof mascaras).

✓☺ **$$$ Fatale Exceptional Volume Sculpting 3D Comb Mascara** *($23)* takes some getting used to, but once you've mastered the tricky application process, you'll be rewarded with unbelievably long, supremely thick lashes that seem too good to be true. Using a three-sided comb rather than a traditional brush, Fatale demands precise application to avoid clumps and a too-heavy appearance. The instructions tell you to rotate the wand so you're using different sides of the comb, which does help. There's no doubt that applying mascara with a brush is faster, but if you're looking to build dramatically long, lush lashes with minimal clumps, this product should be on your short list. In case you're curious, Fatale is very similar to L'Oreal's Volume Shocking Mascara, except that Lancome's version eliminates the lash primer step and offers even more oomph, which is why it is rated higher.

✓☺ **$$$ L'Extreme Instant Extensions Lengthening Mascara** *($24)* is positioned as a lengthening mascara, and it does just that. With a brush similar to mascara hall-of-famer Definicils, L'Extreme quickly elongates lashes with barely a clump. It allows you to create long, fringed lashes with subtle thickness and wears well throughout the day. As impressive as this mascara is, you don't have to spend this much for such results, because other L'Oreal-owned lines have excellent options. Maybelline New York Lash Discovery Mascara and L'Oreal Voluminous Volume Building Mascara are equally adept at lengthening and expertly defining lashes, but that doesn't mean this entry from Lancome is undeserving of a Paula's Pick rating!

☺ **$$$ Cils Booster XL Super-Enhancing Mascara Base** *($21.50)* is a lash primer that really works, and is much better than Lancome's original Cils Booster Mascara Enhancing Base. A pre-mascara, it adds bulk and length to lashes, allowing the actual color-enhancing mascara to cling better and apply evenly. What you'll notice is more thickness and oomph to lashes than using just mascara alone. This type of product isn't for everyone (most women won't want to bother with two steps), but those with short or sparse lashes should give this a try and see for themselves what a difference it makes.

☺ **$$$ Definicils Pro High Definition Curved Brush Mascara** *($24)* has a curved brush with different lengths of bristles on either side. Although not as instantly impressive as original Definicils, this produces long, noticeably thicker lashes after several coats. It also has a slight lifting and curling effect on lashes, and wears all day without flaking or smearing. I agree with Lancome's claim that, compared to regular Definicils, this does create fuller lashes. However, the results aren't so spectacularly better that you should switch to this version, though if it's included in a free gift with purchase, why not give it a try?

☺ **$$$ Hypnose Custom Volume Mascara** *($24)* dares you to go "up to 6 times the volume" for "hypnotic eyes," but real-world testing confirmed this mascara doesn't perform as claimed.

This is far from being a poor mascara because it does do a reasonably good job of separating, lengthening, and slightly thickening lashes without a single clump, leaving lashes soft rather than brittle. It also removes well with a water-soluble cleanser. But if you were expecting impossibly long, voluminous lashes, this isn't the mascara for you, especially if you're currently a fan of Lancome's classic Definicils High Definition Mascara.

☺ **$$$ Oscillation Powerbooster Vibrating Amplifying Primer** ($39). Lancome is on a vibrating mascara spree, and the spree extends to this lash primer, which comes with claims of making lashes stronger, fuller, and longer. The claims are intended to make this sound like several of the expensive lash growth products being sold, including prescription-only Lastisse. However, Lancome words the claims very carefully so that the claims remain cosmetic. After all, "amplifying lashes" could mean several things or nothing at all. As it turns out, this product is little more than an expensive way to add bulk to lashes before applying mascara.

The formula contains standard thickeners and waxes and absolutely nothing that can impact lash growth or thickness, at least nothing beyond a cosmetic effect that will be gone as soon as you remove the product from your lashes. The vibration element is more gimmicky than helpful (it's difficult to keep the button depressed, which is what turns on the vibration), but this primer does add extra oomph to lashes and enhances mascara application. This isn't a necessary product if you're already using a great mascara (Lancome offers several), but this primer does make a difference when used with less impressive mascaras.

☺ **$$$ Oscillation Vibrating Power Mascara** ($34). Just like Estee Lauder, Lancome is in on the power (as in vibrating brush) mascara game. As I reported in my review of Lauder's TurboLash All Effects Motion Mascara, I couldn't get the unit to work as it should have, despite purchasing two of them and following the directions to the letter. Unlike Lauder's "some assembly required" version, Lancome's is ready to go as soon as you pull off a tiny plastic band that keeps the motor inactive. Once that's removed, you can get the wand/brush to vibrate at the push of a button. I wish this was an ingenious, futuristic way to get a better, cleaner application of mascara but it isn't. In the case of Oscillation Vibrating Power Mascara, activating the brush drenched lashes in mascara and caused wet clumps that were tricky to smooth out. Ironically, taking the brush off vibration mode allowed for better smoothing, lash separation, and dramatic length. Lots of mascara gets deposited at lash roots, so the effect when you're done cleaning things up is startling, especially if your lashes are already longer than average. Although I can't recommend this mascara for its special features (and the price is sticker shock given great or even better mascaras that are available for one-third the price), I cannot deny its impressive lengthening ability, either. Note: this mascara has a pervasive rose fragrance and is not recommended for sensitive/teary eyes.

☹ **$$$ High Definicils High Definition Lash by Lash Precision Length Mascara** ($24) is an inferior version of Lancome's sister company Maybelline New York's Define-a-Lash Mascara. Both applicators are variegated rubber bristles on a flexible wand, and both promise optimum length and lash separation. This pricey version from Lancome deposits mascara unevenly and the brush does not allow for easy comb-through without clumping and, if you're not careful, minor smearing. It wins points for how well it separates lashes, but again, the separation comes with some clumps and uneven application. Although not a complete dud, it certainly doesn't impress enough to justify choosing it over Maybelline's option (whose brush is different enough from Lancome's that it avoids the latter's pitfalls).

☺ **$$$ Hypnose Drama Instant Full Body Volume Mascara** *($24.50)*. Lancome normally excels in the mascara department, so it's surprising how disappointing this one is. The problems begin with a very large, unwieldy brush that practically guarantees you'll get mascara where you don't want it, like on the eyelid and the skin along the lower lash line. Application is uneven to the point of being messy, but with patience you can smooth things out and avoid a clumpy, spiked appearance. With proper cleanup (have a clean lash brush or comb handy) the result is very long, dark, and slightly thickened lashes. Lancome's original Hypnose Mascara is preferred, or, for less money, go for L'Oreal's Voluminous or Lash Architect mascaras.

☺ **$$$ Hypnose Waterproof Custom Volume Mascara** *($24)* disappoints compared to its non-waterproof counterpart, but is nevertheless a respectable mascara for length and clean lash separation. Thickness (referred to in the name as "volume") is fairly scarce, but at least this holds up well under water or during a good tear-jerker film.

☺ **$$$ L'Extreme Waterproof Instant Extensions Lengthening Mascara** *($24)* marks one of the few times I have been disappointed by a Lancome mascara. Although this withstands tears and swimming (actually, it's so tenacious that it takes more effort than usual to remove it), it builds minimal length and thickness. At best you'll achieve moderate length and a smidgen of thickness with lots of effort, and for this price (and Lancome's reputation as a mascara leader) that's disappointing. If you insist on using a waterproof mascara from Lancome, try their Definicils Waterproof before this unexciting option.

☺ **$$$ Oscillation Water-Resistant Vibrating Infinite Powermascara** *($34)*. This is another battery-powered mascara from Lancome. The battery causes the wand to vibrate each time you apply the mascara, and it's supposed to improve not only how it's applied but also how much of it is deposited on lashes. In this instance, the vibration makes little difference. I removed the battery to deactivate the special effect and tried it that way, and I tried with the vibration; in both cases this mascara provides impressive thickness and stunted length. Thick, clump-free lashes are this mascara's key selling points, not the vibrating wand. On the downside, once set this breaks down readily with water. In fact, I was able to remove most of it by splashing my face with water, so don't count on the water-resistant claim even a little.

☺ **$$$ Virtuose Black Carat Diving Lasting Curves, Length & Volume Mascara** *($23.50)*. This isn't one of Lancome's better mascaras, but it has novelty appeal for anyone looking to add sparkles to their lashes. The wax-free formula adds no bulk to lashes. Instead, you'll get a smidgen of length and greater emphasis from the pigments than what you'd see without a mascara. The formula dries quickly and the sparkles have only a slight tendency to flake. This is an OK option for special occasions, but avoid the Platinum Carat shade—it's an ugly gray that can make lashes look dingy.

☹ **Courbe Virtuose Divine Lasting Curves Mascara** *($23.50)* comes with beguiling claims, but is a rare letdown from Lancome. I'll even go so far as to say that this is their most disappointing mascara in years. The full, slightly curved brush eventually produces long, curvy lashes, but what a mess to apply! Things are uneven from the start, trying to comb through the clumps only seems to make them worse, and this begins flaking almost as soon as it dries. As for applying this to the lower lashes? Forget about it, unless you want to look like you went to sleep without washing off your mascara!

FACE ILLUMINATING/SHIMMER PRODUCTS: ✓ ☺ **$$$ Color Ideal Illuminateur Sheer Highlighting Pressed Powder** *($31)* is a very silky pressed shimmer powder that casts a subtle yet radiant glow on skin. Color deposit is very sheer, so this is more about adding a hint of shimmer to skin, regardless of which of the three flesh-toned shades you choose. Another impressive trait this powder has is its ability to cling well—flaking is minimal and it can be used over a regular powder blush or bronzing powder if shine is desired.

BRUSHES: ✓☺ **Ageless Minerale Mineral Powder Foundation Brush** *($36)*. This synthetic-hair powder brush is phenomenally soft and perfectly shaped for expert application of loose or pressed powder. It is one of Lancome's better brushes and definitely worth considering for its performance and price.

☺ **$$$ Lancome Brushes** *($24–$56)*. Lancome offers a decent assortment of Brushes, but although many of them are worthwhile, the overall collection is disappointing compared to those from Bobbi Brown, Stila, Laura Mercier, M.A.C., or Paula's Choice. A consistent issue is the overall size of the brush, with an overriding tendency to be either too small or too large for the intended area. Still, there are some winners here, including the **Foundation Brush #2** *($33)*, **Concealer Brush** #8 *($25)*, **Retractable Lip Brush #9** *($24.50)* and **Angle Shadow Brush #13** *($25)*.

SPECIALTY PRODUCTS: ☺ **$$$ Teint Optim'Age Line Blurring Concentrate Face Primer** *($30)*. This primer is nothing more than a blend of silicones, but they work well to help fill in large pores and superficial lines while leaving skin supremely smooth and matte. Test it first to see if the subtle, temporary improvement is what you're looking for. The line-blurring effect works to some extent, but how well and how long it lasts depends on the depth of your wrinkles and on how expressive you are. This is an option for all skin types, and would be rated a Paula's Pick if it contained a few skin-beneficial extras.

☺ **$$$ La Base Pro Perfecting Makeup Primer Smoothing Effect, Oil Free** *($42)*. This "exclusive" formula is nothing more than silicone and a silicone polymer. You'd think for the cost they could have at least added some vitamin E or a soothing agent, though they thankfully omitted fragrance. This clear primer has a thick, slight gel texture that instantly transforms into a weightless silky feel that smooths skin. Applying a sheer layer of dry-finish silicones to skin can help enhance makeup application, but you don't need to seek out a special primer to find these traits. Instead, and for the benefit of your skin, look for an antioxidant-laden silicone serum that also contains some other helpful ingredients. Olay, MD Skincare by Dr. Dennis Gross, Dr. Denese, Paula's Choice, and Smashbox offer such products (all of these companies have added some great bells and whistles Lancome ignored) and they would work equally well pre-makeup. You're simply not getting your money's worth with this no-frills primer from Lancome.

LAURA GELLER

LAURA GELLER AT-A-GLANCE

Strengths: Liquid foundation and concealer; lots of products to add shine to skin; good selection of pressed powders; the cream and liquid blush; enviable lip gloss; the sugar-themed eyeshadows; great brow tint; one remarkable mascara; original Spackle.

Weaknesses: Only one foundation (sold at Sephora; Geller has a hodgepodge of others that come and go on QVC); no foundations, concealers, or powder shades for dark skin tones; contour powder is way too shiny; several average powder eyeshadows; disappointing long-wearing lip paint; incomplete and often not-well-made assortment of brushes; the daytime moisturizer and lip scrub contain needless irritants; claims that products do not contain parabens or mineral oil, but they do.

Note: The Laura Geller products I reviewed are primarily the ones you will find at Sephora stores. These and other Laura Geller products are also sold on QVC, and several of the products have limited runs on the network. Most of the Geller products sold at Sephora are the mainstays of this line.

For more information about Laura Geller, call (800) 625-3874 or visit www.laurageller.com or www.Beautypedia.com.

LAURA GELLER SKIN CARE

☹ **Moisture Compound** *($26.50).* The best and only commendable part of this product is its in-part avobenzone sunscreen. The base formula is ho-hum and more damaging than helpful to skin due to the amount of alcohol and menthol. There is more alcohol in this daytime moisturizer with sunscreen than there are antioxidants—never a good sign. If you're shopping this line at Sephora, they sell dozens of daytime moisturizers with sunscreen that are distinctly preferred to this product.

LAURA GELLER MAKEUP

FOUNDATION: ✓ ☺ **$$$ Barely There Tinted Moisturizer SPF 20** *($30).* This is a superb tinted moisturizer that includes mineral sunscreens titanium dioxide and zinc oxide as active ingredients. It has a silky, lightweight texture that's a pleasure to blend. This sets to a delicate satin-matte finish and provides sheer to light coverage that diffuses minor flaws and redness. The formula contains several antioxidants, but the choice of clear tube packaging means they won't last for long unless you're diligent about keeping this protected from exposure to light. Otherwise, this is recommended for normal to dry or slightly oily skin, and is suitable for sensitive skin provided you're not sensitive to the plant extracts this contains. Those looking for a similar, less expensive product in better packaging should consider Paula's Choice Barely There Sheer Matte Tint SPF 20. If you opt for Geller's version, all of the shades are workable, though Deep is slightly orange and the trickiest to use.

☺ **$$$ Phenomenal Foundation** *($36.50).* Claiming that this liquid foundation is "phenomenal" is pushing things a bit because it automatically implies this is the ultimate foundation—it isn't. I am not, however, saying that it isn't worth considering, because it is in fact a very good option; it's just not the best of the best. Dispensed from a pump, it has a creamy texture that applies light and silky, setting to a satin-matte finish that remains slightly moist. It is best for normal to slightly dry skin (oily areas will show shine in short order). Coverage is in the medium range and this does a reasonably good job of not magnifying pores and lines (it works much better if you apply Geller's Spackle primer first, but there are other foundations that look better on skin and that don't need a primer). Among the small selection of shades, Medium is slightly peach and should be considered carefully. Deep is not that dark and is best for tan skin tones.

CONCEALER: ☺ **$$$ Crease-Less Concealer** *($23.50)* is packaged in a pen-style component that includes a built-in synthetic brush applicator. The fluid, silky texture has an excellent, weightless application that sets to a matte finish with a hint of shine. You'll get moderate coverage, so this is best for minor flaws and slight darkness under the eyes (those with pronounced dark circles will need better camouflage). Two of the three shades are great; avoid Deep, which is too peachy rose to look convincing. This is a very good option for concealing minor blemishes.

☺ **$$$ Caulk Pencil & Sharpener** *($23.50)*. What a name! Who would want to use a concealer with a name reminiscent of that goop that comes in a tube and that you use to seal holes and prevent water damage? Apparently someone does, because this is supposedly one of Geller's better selling items. The good news is that this isn't really caulk. It is a chunky, needs-sharpening pencil outfitted with a sponge tip on one end for blending. The "caulk" end has a silicone-based texture that glides on and blends superbly, while the texture feels lighter than you'd expect. Dotting this on skin provides instant full coverage that can look heavy, but it softens well during blending and winds up being a good option for those who need ample coverage that doesn't appear too opaque. The problem is that among the three shades, two (Medium and Dark) are very peach. The peachiness softens as you blend, but it will still look odd on many skin tones. The best shade to try, if you don't mind sharpening, is Light. It will crease into lines around the eyes unless carefully set with powder, which can make lines look more obvious. So, all in all, there are better concealer options.

☺ **$$$ Hide-N-Shine** *($20.50)* comes in a compact with two colors, one of which is too peach or orange to use regardless of the duo you're considering. Mixing the shades to get a better color is an option, but one that's not really necessary given the plethora of good neutral-toned concealers available in many formats (e.g., liquid or cream). I wish the colors were better because this cream-to-powder concealer applies, blends, and covers beautifully, setting to a soft matte finish with a hint of shine. It is minimally prone to creasing into lines around the eye. All told, this is recommended only if you're OK with mixing two shades for a result that's not as good as it should be.

☺ **$$$ The Real Deal Concealer Serious Coverage** *($20)*. Housed in a flat, small tube, this is a slightly thick, creamy concealer that really does provide serious coverage. It's the type of coverage that can conceal dark circles and pigmented discolorations, including birthmarks (although most port wine stains will need something more for complete camouflage). This is surprisingly easy to blend due to its inherent silky texture, and it's a plus that thinning this out during blending doesn't significantly decrease coverage. What will be a deal-breaker for many people, however, is the fact that this never really sets to a long-wearing finish; it remains moist and slick, and as such is prone to creasing, fading, and smearing unless set with a lot of powder. Of course, setting it with powder can make such opaque coverage more obvious, so it isn't the best look unless you have something major to hide. If you're willing to accept the trade-off, this concealer is an option, but I would definitely test it if possible before buying. Among the four shades, Light and Medium are best. Medium Deep tends to be too orange, and Deep is workable but will be too dark for those with tan to light brown skin.

☺ **$$$ Vanishing Act Duo Concealer** *($20.50)* has a beautifully smooth texture that feels lighter than you would expect, and it sets to a cream finish that will crease unless you set it with powder (and even then you may still get some creasing, and adding powder just makes wrinkles more obvious). There is only one duo available, and both shades are noticeably peach, even when combined. Some people may prefer the peachy tone for concealing dark circles, but in my experience it just doesn't look nearly as good as using a neutral to yellow-toned concealer instead.

POWDER: ☺ **$$$ Balance-N-Brighten** *($29.50)* has a marbled pattern that blends several colors together. The visual appeal of this pressed domed-sculpted powder is nice, but once you swirl a brush over the melange of colors and apply it to your skin, the effect is a sheer beige to sheer peach that works best for fair to light skin tones. The powder has a smooth, dry texture that applies sheer and builds well for additional depth. Its finish is matte (in feel), but it leaves a soft glow on skin. Less expensive versions of this product are readily available from Jane or Physician's Formula, but this is still an option if you're looking to spend more, but not get more for your money (which to my way of thinking is not a good idea).

☺ $$$ **Matte Maker** *($25)* contains a high amount of the very absorbent ingredient calcium carbonate. As such, this sheer, talc-based powder is effective at keeping excess shine in check and is best for oily to very oily skin. The smooth, drier-than-usual powder can be difficult to pick up with a brush, but you don't need much to achieve a mattifying effect. Best for blotting, only one color is available and it applies transparently.

☺ $$$ **Powdered Silk Pressed Powder SPF 8** *($21)*. Despite the embarrassingly low SPF rating, it's good news that this talc-free pressed powder contains titanium dioxide and zinc oxide as the active ingredients. As such, it can be a good adjunct to your sunscreen or foundation with sunscreen, assuming that those are rated SPF 15 or greater to ensure sufficient daytime protection. This powder's slightly thick texture applies smooth and even, while its matte finish looks natural without being chalky. All three shades are recommended. The happy face rating pertains to the powder overall; the low SPF number doesn't deserve more than a neutral face rating.

☺ $$$ **Optilusion Powder SPF 8** *($42.50)* is more about adding a translucent pale-pink sheen with white shimmer to your skin than anything else, and that isn't much of an illusion. The SPF rating is too low for it to provide reliable protection even though the actives are titanium dioxide and zinc oxide. The larger problem is that you'd have to apply a lot of this talc-free loose powder to get even the minimal SPF 8 protection stated on the label, which is why pressed powders with sunscreen are preferred. This does have an extremely soft texture that applies sheer, and the shine clings better than expected. This is not recommended for use as a concealer (the way Geller advertises) because it can look too pale when applied in an amount concentrated enough to achieve concealer-like coverage.

☺ $$$ **Shade-N-Sculpt Contouring Powder with Brush** *($38)*. Housed in one compact without a divider are a muted brown pressed powder and a pale beige-gold highlighting powder. The brown shade is acceptable for contouring medium to tan skin tones, but the effect will be anything but subtle thanks to the large flecks of gold shine that were added. The highlighting powder's shine is subtle and much more workable. Contouring is never about adding shine to skin, and should be a deal-breaker for most professional makeup artists; but of course there are always exceptions to every rule in the world of makeup application. The full-size brush that comes with the kit is an acceptable option, so you don't need to purchase an additional brush.

BLUSH AND BRONZER: ✓ ☺ $$$ **Cheek Sweeps** *($17)* is a very clever, easy way to apply a lightweight cream blush to your cheeks. The stout container houses a domed cream-blush top that fits the curvature of the face and provides a soft wash of translucent color with a satin finish that's not the least bit greasy. There are only few shades available, but if one of them suits you and you have dry skin, this is a blush to check out.

✓ ☺ $$$ **Tint Hint** *($23)* is Geller's version of Benefit's classic BeneTint. Although it's a copycat product, the application method beats that of BeneTint if your primary area of application is the cheeks rather than lips (BeneTint's brush applicator has the edge for use as a lip stain). Geller's sponge-tip applicator has dozens of tiny perforations through which the sheer rose liquid is dispensed. You twist the base until the appropriate amount appears, then simply dab it on your cheeks and blend. This type of blush isn't for someone with an uneven skin texture or large pores, but if that doesn't apply to you and if you prefer liquid blush, this is a very good long-wearing option to explore.

☺ **$$$ Balance-N-Bronze** *($29.50)* has a marbled pattern that blends several colors together. The visual appeal of this pressed domed-sculpted powder is nice, but once you swirl a brush over the melange of colors and apply it to your skin, the effect is a soft rosy tan that looks best on fair to medium skin tones. The powder has a smooth, dry texture that applies sheer and builds well for additional depth. Its finish is matte (in feel), but it leaves a soft glow on skin. Less expensive versions of this product are readily available from Jane or Physician's Formula, but this is still an option if you're looking to spend more but not get more for your money (which to my way of thinking is not a good idea).

☺ **$$$ Blush-N-Brighten** *($29.50)*. This marbled pressed powder presents a blend of colors in one compact. Swirling a brush over the tablet blends the hues together to create one shade that enlivens cheeks with color and a strong shimmer finish. The texture is smooth yet dry and application is sheer and even. You don't have to spend this much money for shiny blush, but it is an option, and all of the colors are workable.

☺ **$$$ Bronze-N-Brighten** *($29.50)* has a marbled pattern that blends several colors together. The visual appeal of this pressed domed-sculpted powder is nice, but once you swirl a brush over the melange of colors and apply it to your skin, the effect is a muted bronze with rose undertones that looks best on light to medium skin tones. The powder has a smooth, dry texture that applies sheer and builds well for additional depth. Its finish is matte (in feel), but it leaves a soft glow on skin. Less expensive versions of this product are readily available from Jane or Physician's Formula, but this is still an option if you're looking to spend more, but not get more for your money (which to my way of thinking is not a good idea).

EYESHADOW: ☺ **$$$ Marble Cakes Baked Eyeshadow & Liner Duo** *($26)*. This circular 2-in-1 baked powder compact offers a cake eyeliner and shimmery coordinating powder shadow, and comes with a dual-ended synthetic brush for blending and lining. Available in only two shade options (Blue or Brown), the eyeliner is exceptional, with a rich, lasting color deposit that performs best when applied wet and that won't budge once dry. The shadow is too shimmery for wide appeal or real versatility, but it does complement the liner nicely, and could work in addition to a more deeply pigmented contour shadow. The real star here is the multi-functional full-size brush, which has the density to capture and distribute powder nicely, while the angled liner end delivers precision results.

☺ **$$$ Sugar Free Matte Baked Eyeshadow Duo** *($22)* is a standard, but good, powder eyeshadow whose name makes it sound like something to snack on if you're concerned about carbs. The "baked" concept refers to the fact that these eyeshadows begin in liquid form and then are cooked at high heat in terracotta pots until they solidify. There's really no benefit to making eyeshadows this way (though it sounds good in marketing materials), and in the case of this product, the result is the same smooth texture and even application of many good eyeshadows. The duos are nearly matte—only a soft shine is visible—and the shades work well together.

☺ **$$$ Sugared Baked Pearl Eyeshadow** *($23)* is just a shiny powder eyeshadow with a very smooth texture and even, flake-free application (unless you overdo it). The small selection of shades has a strong shimmer and works best for highlighting the brow bone.

☺ **$$$ Wonder Wand** *($18.50)*. I wish Geller would parlay this loose-powder eyeshadow into a pressed eyeshadow because it has an otherworldly smooth texture that clings like a second skin and imparts sheer, buildable color with an attractive, though none-too-subtle, shimmer. As a loose powder, however, it's hard to blend on as eyeshadow. At least the packaging minimizes mess and the pointed sponge-tip applicator (while not preferred to a good eyeshadow brush) allows for greater versatility than standard sponge applicators. If used sparingly, this is a very good way to highlight the brow bone or under-eye area for evening glamour.

☺ **$$$ Baked Marble Eyeshadow** *($23)*. Although the marbled pattern is eye-catching, this powder eyeshadow isn't quite as good as Geller's other "Baked" shadows (but then there is no advantage to the formula being baked). The large particles of shine not only distract from the result once applied, but also give this eyeshadow a slight grainy feel. Color deposit is good and the shine clings decently, so this is still an OK option if you want impact accompanied by large flecks of shine for your eyeshadow look.

☺ **$$$ Eye Rimz Baked Wet/Dry Eye Accents** *($26)* is marbleized and flecked with two colors in one compact. As described, the dominant color is pitch black and you swirl it with another color to achieve a dimensional, metallic effect. This comes with a good brush and applies smoothly, but you have to be careful to not pick up too much on the brush or it will flake. As with most powder eyeshadows, this may be used wet or dry. Eye Rimz works best to line the eyes or create a smoky eye design for evening makeup. Note that the emollients in this powder lead to some fading and smearing after several hours of wear.

☺ **$$$ Eye Spackle** *($23)*. Sold as a prep product to apply to the eyelid and under-brow area pre-eyeshadow, this is nothing more than a cream concealer whose opaque and whitish finish brightens the eye area but also leaves an unattractive heavy look unless applied sparingly. The creamy finish is crease-prone, and this is not preferred to numerous matte-finish concealers that work beautifully as a base for eyeshadows.

☺ **$$$ Eye Stay Duo** *($17.50)* is a dual-sided liquid eyeshadow that presents two complementary colors (one for highlighting, the other for shading) in one sleek package. Although the formula has a silky texture that applies evenly, blending takes more time than it should because the colors are slow to set. Even when you think they've set you'll still get some slippage and movement, so these aren't the best if you want hours of fail-safe wear. Some fading occurs and anyone with oily eyelids will find creasing a problem. In the end, despite some innovative elements by Geller, Revlon and Clinique offer more intriguing alternatives to powder eyeshadow.

☺ **Eye Shadow** *($15)*. There isn't much to say about this collection of eyeshadow singles except that they are run-of-the-mill in every respect. That doesn't make them poor performers, just ordinary (and every shade has moderate to strong shine).

EYE AND BROW SHAPER: ✓ ☺ **$$$ Eyebrow Tint & Tamer** *($21.50)*. Housed in one dual-sided package are a clear brow gel and a brow tint. Both are applied with built-in mascara brushes, and each has a clean, smooth application that sets unruly brows without feeling tacky or gummy. The brow tint is sheer yet does its part to define, and there are three good colors (there are no options for black or auburn/red brows).

☺ **$$$ Baby Cakes Baked Eyeliner Palette** *($34)*. A flip-top palette houses four shades of super-smooth powder eyeliner made for wet or dry application, the former being preferable because it yields more intense and lasting results, with no flaking. The included synthetic eyeliner brush is tiny and unsuitable for dry application, but when wet it creates a beautiful and exact pencil-thin line that lasts. The major drawback is the shades, all of which contain noticeable shine, with Blue Sugar wearing far more like a stripe of glitter than an eyeliner. Dutch Chocolate is vibrant and gorgeous, but as a whole the palette is hardly worth the price for one or two viable shades. Consider cherry-picking shades you'll actually use, as Laura Geller offers larger sizes of this product in workable duos of colors for nearly half the price—and with a larger brush to boot!

☺ **$$$ Baked Cake Eyeliner Duo** *($23)*. Housed in a flip-top compact are two shades of pressed-powder eyeliner designed to be applied wet or dry. Dry application is sheer and slightly flake-prone, even when used sparingly. Wet application is preferred because the immediate result is an intense line that works well to define the eyes without any mess or flaking. The included synthetic eyeliner brush is ideal for creating either a thin or thick line. Both shades (one is distinctively dark and the other is a colorful, medium tone) contain noticeable shine, so this isn't for anyone who wants a matte-finish eyeliner. Those hoping for longevity won't be disappointed, but should know that gel eyeliners last even longer and aren't prone to fading.

☺ **$$$ Brow Marker Long-Lasting Brow Color** *($22)* is a liquid brow color housed in a felt-tip pen-style applicator. The thin, precision brush allows you to get in between brow hairs to create the illusion of a fuller brow, and it's surprisingly easy to apply. The problem is that the amount of alcohol in this formula and the film-forming agent can make brow hairs feel dry and slightly sticky at the same time. Although the application and concept are admirable, the formula itself needs work. If you overdo this even a little you'll notice some flaking color at some point during the day. It isn't terrible, but with some slight tweaks this could be a formidable option to color and shape the brows (speaking of colors, Geller needs to expand its options beyond just those for brunette brows).

☺ **Brow Pencil** *($12.50)* is another pencil from Laura Geller that would be rated a Paula's Pick if it did not require routine sharpening (which is a waste of time and readily uses up more pencil in the process). If that doesn't bother you, this is an excellent brow pencil and all three shades are recommended (there are no shades for black or auburn/red brows). It has a super-smooth texture that glides easily between brow hairs and sets to a soft powder finish. The cap includes a mini brow brush that works in a pinch to get the job done.

☺ **$$$ I-Care Waterproof Eyeliner Duo** *($25)*. This retractable eyeliner pencil, available in classic black or brown, glides on nicely, requires no sharpening, and is definitely waterproof. Due to the product's quick grab and blunt tip, it's difficult to achieve a thin line or to smudge it out; sadly, the rubber smudger tool on the other end of the pencil doesn't do the trick and pulls on eyelids more than it blends the color. The eyeliner performs well until it gets wet, and even though it resists smearing, the line tends to separate on exposure to moisture, and then it appears flaky and dry. All in all, if you need waterproof eyeliner and prefer a thicker line, this is an OK, albeit pricey, option.

☺ **Powder Pencil Eyeliner** *($15.50)* would be rated a Paula's Pick, with its smooth application and powder finish, were it not for the fact that it needs routine sharpening. Once set, this is minimally prone to smudging and wears beautifully. Application, while smooth, is sheer, so you must layer it to truly define your eyes. The silver and green shades have shine, and are alternatives only for special occasion makeup.

☹ **Double Eye Appeal & Sharpener** *($19.50)*. The appeal of this needs-sharpening pencil sounds good on paper, but in practice you'll be left wondering why you wasted your money. Designed to highlight and clarify skin with its dual-sided nude cream and pale gold colors, the texture of this pencil is too thick and creamy to last, so the minor results are short-lived and look sloppy in short order. Besides, the promises this pencil makes are a better bet (and more easily attainable) from liquid or powder shine products than from a pencil.

LIPSTICK, LIP GLOSS, AND LIPLINER: ✓☺ **Creme Couture Soft Touch Matte Lipstick** *($15.50)*. Much more unique than Geller's regular Lipstick, Creme Couture Soft Touch Matte Lipstick feels creamy and light at the same time, and it has a rich cream finish with a low shine that helps spotlight this lipstick's bold opacity. It is recommended for fans of semi-matte lipstick, and the formula allows it to wear longer than standard cream lipsticks. If only Sephora offered more colors!

✓☺ **$$$ Lip Shiner** *($16)*. Excellent lip glosses aren't exactly hard to find, but there are proportionately fewer of them than there are average to poor lip glosses. Lip Shiner is one of the former: An excellent, non-sticky lip gloss that feels great on and that is available in a beautiful range of shades, including Clear. The best part is that this gloss lasts longer than many others, so you won't feel constantly compelled to add more.

☺ **$$$ Lipstick** *($15.50)* is a standard, lightweight cream lipstick with a creamy finish plus shimmer. It provides moderate coverage and comes in an acceptable range of shades, though non-shimmer and darker colors are lacking.

☺ **Lip Liner** *($12)*. There's not much to say about this standard, needs-sharpening pencil. It is typical in every respect, right down to the range of safe yet versatile nude and pink-brown colors. The finish is creamy, but it stays in place reasonably well.

☺ **Lip Parfaits** *($16)* may be visually appealing in its container due to the swirled, intertwining colors, but in the end it's just a standard lip gloss with a moderately thick texture and slightly sticky but glossy finish. It's not the type of lip gloss worth mail ordering because you can find much better lip gloss formulas at the drugstore for half the price (plus QVC's shipping charges quickly mount up because they charge per item, not per order).

☺ **Lip Stay** *($14.50)* is a dual-sided lip color product that is Geller's contribution to the type of long-wearing lip paint first made famous by Max Factor's Lipfinity. Geller's begins well, with a silky-textured coat of color that applies evenly and allows for full coverage. It sets in 30 seconds, and then you can apply the glossy top coat. Actually, you need to apply this top coat, because without it the lip paint makes your lips feel progressively drier. After less than an hour of wearing this and with one gloss touch-up, I began to notice problems. The color was peeling and fading toward the center of my mouth, the smooth gloss feeling was wearing off too soon, and the gloss itself was, if you can believe it, difficult to apply. Let's chalk this up to "nice try but no cigar," and stick with companies that offer better versions of such products, including Max Factor, Cover Girl, M.A.C., Estee Lauder, and Maybelline New York.

☹ **Lip Heal & Seal Lip Gloss** *($18)*. Packaged in one tube are two separate products for lips. The **Lip Heal** portion is housed in a separate inner tube (a tube within a tube) and dispenses with the **Lip Seal** portion of the product. Although this has a great smooth feel and glossy finish, it is not recommended because it contains the irritating menthol derivatives menthyl lactate and menthoxypropanediol—neither of which is the least bit healing for lips.

MASCARA: ✓☺ **$$$ Creamy Mascara** *($15.50)*. Naming a mascara "Creamy" isn't the smartest way to assure your customers that the formula won't smear or smudge and is long-wearing. As it turns out, you can forget the negative connotation of the name. This is an impressive lengthening mascara that allows you to make lashes incrementally longer and more defined without a trace of clumping or uneven application. If you're not concerned about building thickness, this is highly recommended. It removes easily with a water-soluble cleanser.

☺ **$$$ Mighty Mascara & Fortifier** *($21.50)* features a regular mascara on one end and a lash primer on the other of its dual ends. Both products have the same ingredient list, and there is nothing fortifying about it. Including a tiny amount of panthenol and elastin in a lash product isn't going to produce stronger lashes. The **Mascara** builds equal parts length and thickness without clumping or smearing (but be sure to let it dry completely before blinking too much), while the **Fortifier**, if applied before the mascara, allows you to add a bit more thickness at the expense of some clumping and a less even application. Used alone or together, this duo is workable, but L'Oreal and Maybelline New York sell similar products that perform better at one-third the price.

FACE AND BODY ILLUMINATING/SHIMMER PRODUCTS: ☺ $$$ **Baked Body Frosting** *($40)*. Given this product's name, you may be envisioning a whipped cream–textured product. However, the "frost" refers to the shine of this pressed shimmer powder. This mica- and talc-based formula goes on smooth and dry and isn't too powdery, and it finishes to a satin shine that works best for fair to medium skin tones. Dusted on with a brush or applied with a sponge, this is an attractive way to highlight skin from the neck down (though it can certainly be used on the face, too). Caution: The shine and some color will come off on clothing.

☹ $$$ **Ethereal Rose Baked Powder** *($29.50)* is designed to give skin a "fresh luminosity" and does so via its very soft (and, unfortunately, fleeting) shine. The pale pink powder has a silky yet dry texture that provides minimal color deposit and that doesn't cling to skin as well as it should. The sole shade is best for fair skin, though it almost goes without saying that there are better versions of this product available at the drugstore.

☺ **Liquid Candlelight Face & Body Glow** *($23.50)* imparts sheer shine. Its application has a lot of slip, which makes blending this liquid shimmer over large areas easier, though it does take time to set. The problem is that the shine is mostly from obvious gold particles rather than from finely milled shimmer pigment. Therefore, the effect is showy instead of "glow-y," and not something to consider if your objective is to re-create the soft, alluring glow that real candlelight has on skin; Lorac, Chanel, and Stila have better options in that regard.

BRUSHES: ☺ **Camouflage Brush** *($17)* is a standard, synthetic concealer brush that works as well as many others to apply and blend liquid- or cream-based products. It is well-shaped to fit into tiny corners, such as the inner portion of the under-eye area or the side of the nostrils. ☺ **Eyeshadow Double-Ended Brush** *($15)* features two eye-shading options in one, allowing you to apply shadow to your eyelid and crease area with ease. Both ends are soft and well-shaped for their intended purpose. ☹ **Contour Highlights Brush** *($16)* is another Geller dual-sided brush. One end is for contouring and the other is a domed, dense eyeshadow brush that works well for shaping and shading the eye. Although the eyeshadow end of the brush is good, the contour side should've been angled rather than rounded off for better application. ☹ **Duo Brush** *($19)* features a large sponge tip on one end and an oversized eyeshadow brush on the other. The flocked sponge has minimal practical usage, while the eyeshadow brush is too large for most eye shapes, making this one brush whose two sides have extremely limited appeal.

☹ **Professional Brush Collection** *($68)*. This seven-piece brush set has an attractive price and even comes with its own brush holder (not a brush roll or bag; instead it's a cup like what you'd use to store pencils on your desk). The set turns out to be not as much of a value as it could've been because half of the brushes are either not needed or are poorly made. The worthwhile brushes in this set include the Angled Powder Brush, Eyeshadow Brush, and Eyeliner/Eyebrow Brush. The others just don't pass muster for professional makeup tools, and the flat, fan-like Blush and Highlighter Brush is no substitute for a traditional domed powder-blush brush.

SPECIALTY PRODUCTS: ☺ $$$ **Line & Define** *($20)*. Sold as "a careful pairing of color-coordinated eyeliner and mascara," this duo is a good option if you don't mind shiny eyeliner. The mascara lengthens and separates lashes quickly without clumping, but doesn't do much to build thickness. The liquid liner's thin brush applies color well and it goes on evenly and dries fast, which is a plus. Liquid liner wearability is generally good, save for some minor fading (but no flaking).

☺ **Spackle Under Make-Up Primer** *($23)*. By far this is Geller's most popular product and the one from her line I am asked about most often. And it's no wonder: This pump-dispensed primer is sold as the ideal undercoat to perfect skin's texture. Most primers contain a lot of silicone to smooth skin and provide a silky canvas for foundation (and, to some extent, help to temporarily fill in large pores and superficial lines). Spackle is mostly water and film-forming agent with lesser amounts of silicone. It feels very light and has a smooth finish that is ever-so-slightly tacky at dry-down. This is easy to apply, sets quickly, and contains shiny pigments to lend a subtle glow to skin (this glow may be why so many women feel their skin looks better with this product; if you have a dull complexion, applying any slightly shimmery product will help, but it's more effective to deal with dullness during your skin-care routine than with makeup effects). I sampled Spackle both with and without Geller's foundation, and found that the Spackle did enhance the effect of the foundation. It was easier to apply and it looked better because it didn't show signs of sinking into pores and lines. Does that mean Spackle is a must-have? Absolutely not. There's nothing wrong with adding this product to your routine, but your skin would be better off using a weightless matte- or satin-finish serum loaded with beneficial ingredients (the botanicals in Spackle don't quite cut it, and some, such as witch hazel, are irritating). Moreover, almost all of today's best foundations (those I rate Paula's Pick) can make skin look smooth and even without the need for a primer. If your foundation isn't making your skin look the way you want it to, consider trying a new foundation before trying a primer. Those who remain intrigued by this product should know it is suitable for all skin types except sensitive.

☺ $$$ **Spackle Tinted Under Make-Up Primer** *($23 for 2 ounces)* is nearly identical to Laura Geller's original Spackle Under Make-Up Primer, except for its sheer bronze tint that leaves skin with a subtle radiant glow. The product feels silky and light, and helps enliven dull or sallow skin tones, whether worn alone or under a sheer- to medium-coverage foundation.

☺ $$$ **Welcome Matte Skin Enhancer** *($23.50)*. I'm surprised this product isn't named Spackle, like others from Laura Geller, because this nonaqueous silicone-based gel really does have a spackle-like texture. It feels very silky and works to a minor extent to temporarily fill in large pores and smooth superficial lines. The weightless finish is ideal for oily skin and facilitates makeup application. Because this isn't super-absorbent, those with very oily skin should explore Smashbox's Anti-Shine before this.

☹ $$$ **Face Folio** *($23.50)*. Geller offers two variations for her Face Folio sets, each housed in a faux leather case. The **Face and Eye Palette** includes pressed powder, cream concealer, several powder eyeshadows, and mini applicators (none of which are that impressive). The **Lip and Cheek Palette** includes powder bronzer, powder blush, cream lip colors, an eye pencil, mascara, and mini applicators that are not a good substitute for professional brushes. The products in each set range from good to average, which makes the price a bit steep for what you get. If you're new to makeup and want several colors to experiment with, the Face Folio may be worth it. However, I'm fairly certain most women would get better results by shopping around for makeup or assembling their own palette from brands such as M.A.C., Stila, Trish McEvoy, or Bobbi Brown.

☹ $$$ **Lip Spackle** *($23)* is sold as a base for lipstick and for filling in lines on lips for smoother application of lipstick and gloss. It feels light and has a soft, sheer powder finish that doesn't impede lipstick application. Lipstick appearance is another thing: unless you apply your lipstick very carefully and don't push lips together to blend (as many women do), this product can make lipstick look oddly colored and uneven. It is definitely not recommended for use with sheer lipsticks or glosses. If you're curious to try this cream-to-powder product, it functions best with opaque matte or semi-matte lipsticks.

☺ **$$$ Mascara Sealer** *($15)* can be applied over regular mascara without disrupting it, but it goes on very wet and heavy, so some cleanup is needed. Because the main ingredient in the Sealer is a solvent that's present in many waterproof mascaras, it does indeed work to make a regular mascara impervious to water. For the money, you're better off purchasing a good waterproof mascara for those times when you need such a product. Note that even with makeup remover, the Mascara Sealer is very difficult to remove.

☺ **$$$ Spackle Trio** *($31.50).* This cleverly packaged set provides all of Geller's Spackle products in one unit. The original Spackle (used as a foundation primer) is an option, but the Lip and Eye Spackle products are average at best and easily replaced by better products. If you're interested in the original Spackle, I advise you to purchase the full-size version rather than get a reduced amount coupled with two other products that you likely won't find all that great to use.

☺ **Lip & Eye Spackle** *($23)* combines Geller's Lip Spackle and Eye Spackle in one compact, and neither is anything to get excited about. Please refer to the individual reviews for each product for details. Suffice it to say, the Lip Spackle isn't necessary and the Eye Spackle is easily replaced (and improved upon) by numerous matte-finish concealers.

☹ **Lip Strip Cooling Sugar Scrub** *($16)* contains sugar granules as the abrasive agent. Although sugar can be rough for lips, the formula's oil and emollient content helps offset this, allowing for smooth exfoliation. Although this will eliminate immediate signs of dry, flaky lips, the irritating oils of peppermint and spearmint along with menthol can make perpetually chapped lips worse. Exfoliating your lips doesn't require a cooling sensation, and your lips deserve better than this misguided product.

LAURA MERCIER

LAURA MERCIER AT-A-GLANCE

Strengths: Many fragrance-free products; top-notch water-soluble cleansers; very good eye-makeup remover; the serum and serum-type moisturizers are worth a look; some extraordinary foundation and powder products; great powder blush, cream blush, and powder eyeshadows; one impressive mascara; mostly great shimmer products; the makeup brushes; the Bronzing Gel.

Weaknesses: Expensive; some of the products with sunscreen lack sufficient UVA-protecting ingredients; no product to treat acne or lighten skin discolorations; jar packaging; none of the makeup products with sunscreen contain the right UVA-protecting actives; the various Primers are merely OK; average eye pencil, brow-enhancing, and lip pencil options.

For more information about Laura Mercier, call (888) 637-2437 or visit www.lauramercier. com or www.Beautypedia.com.

LAURA MERCIER SKIN CARE

LAURA MERCIER FLAWLESS SKIN PRODUCTS

☺ **$$$ Flawless Skin Creme, Anti-Aging Treatment** *($95 for 1.7 ounces)* has a great name—is there any doubt what this product promises? Yet the miracle ingredient is "deep sea water." Regardless of depth, water of any kind is not the key to flawless skin. The majority of ingredients in this product appear in hundreds of other moisturizers, which is all this "treatment" really is: a basic moisturizer. What's particularly dismaying is that the many antioxidants and cell-communicating ingredients won't stay potent for long because of jar packaging. Spending this much for what amounts to a letdown isn't advised, but it still has potential for normal to dry skin.

☺ **$$$ Flawless Skin Day Creme SPF 15** *($95 for 1.7 ounces)*. It would be incredibly convenient if all it took to attain flawless skin was one product with sunscreen, but Mercier is simply capitalizing on a name that has worked well for her makeup line (not to mention that as a makeup artist Mercier is known for creating "the flawless face"). There are no active ingredients listed, so this isn't a reliable daytime moisturizer with sunscreen. Oddly, this contains two sunscreen agents (including a tiny amount of avobenzone, listed by its chemical name butyl methoxydibenzoylmethane), but they don't count because they're not listed as active. Beyond the sunscreens, the base formula is quite good, even assuming that you know the powerful Deep Sea Water claim is just plain hokey. What's not so good is that several state-of-the-art ingredients in this daytime moisturizer are going to lose potency due to the jar packaging, which is really unsettling given how much this product costs. It you're up for throwing money away on a product whose main benefit is sun protection (something that indeed is needed, but that is readily available at a much fairer price), this day cream is best for normal to slightly dry skin.

☺ **$$$ Flawless Skin Day Lotion SPF 15** *($95 for 1.7 ounces)* is nearly identical to the Flawless Skin Day Creme SPF 15 above, except this has a thinner lotion texture. Otherwise, the same review applies.

☹ **Flawless Skin Eye Creme, Anti-Aging Eye Creme** *($75 for 0.7 ounce)* mentions that it contains deep sea water, and describes this as a "key ingredient that enhances metabolic reaction within the skin and helps cell renewal." That must mean scuba divers can cross "worry about wrinkles" off their list! Getting back to reality, there is no proof anywhere that water alone, whether from a shallow pool or from fathoms deep, can affect skin cell renewal. If anything, quite the opposite is true: too much water is bad for skin, leading to an impaired barrier and inflammation as the skin cells take on more water than they can handle. I'd say forget the water claim and concentrate on the plethora of excellent ingredients in this eye cream for normal to dry skin; but there are drawbacks. Jar packaging won't keep the antioxidants and plant oils stable during use, some of the plants (geranium, arnica) are present in amounts that can cause irritation, and arnica in any amount is never a good idea for skin around the eye. With the elimination of a handful of undesirable ingredients and better packaging, this would have easily rated a Paula's Pick.

☹ **Flawless Skin Eye Serum, Rejuvenating Eye Concentrate** *($80 for 0.63 ounce)* is a water-based serum that lists most of its really intriguing ingredients after the mineral pigment mica, which lends a shimmer finish to the eye area. How disappointing, but the deal-breaker is the inclusion of geranium and arnica in amounts bound to be troublesome for the skin around the eyes or anywhere on the face for that matter. Please see the review for Laura Mercier's Flawless Skin Eye Creme, Anti-Aging Eye Creme for a discussion of the company's claims about deep sea water.

OTHER LAURA MERCIER SKIN-CARE PRODUCTS

✓ ☺ **$$$ Foaming One-Step Cleaner** *($35 for 5 ounces)* is a liquid-to-foam, water-soluble cleanser that's an excellent option for normal to dry skin. It removes makeup and rinses easily, and is fragrance-free. The tiny amount of witch hazel is not a cause for concern.

✓ ☺ **$$$ Oil-Free Gel Cleanser** *($35 for 8 ounces)* is pricey, but is nevertheless an outstanding gentle cleanser for normal to oily skin. The fragrance-free formula contains over a dozen water-binding agents and also some very good soothing agents, though their brief contact with skin doesn't allow them to do much. However, such additives are much better than the exotic and/or potentially irritating plant extracts that most cosmetics include!

✓ ☺ **$$$ One-Step Cleanser** *($35 for 8 ounces)* is nearly identical to the Foaming One-Step Cleanser above, except this one doesn't have the liquid-to-foam dispensing system. Which one you use is a matter of personal preference, but you get more cleanser for your money here, and the consistency makes this one easier to stretch, which helps offset the expense.

☹ **$$$ Purifying Oil - Light** *($40 for 6.7 ounces)* is an oil-based cleanser and makeup remover for dry to very dry skin. The main ingredients are not "light," and this should not be used by anyone with oily skin. Mercier claims this "leaves less oil molecules on the surface of skin," but that's impossible. The mineral oil-base doesn't rinse easily without a washcloth, and no matter how you slice it, more oil molecules will be left on your skin than when you began.

☹ **$$$ Purifying Oil - Rich** *($40 for 6.7 ounces)* is more oily than the Purifying Oil - Light, and is appropriate only for dry to very dry skin. This removes makeup easily, just like most oil-based cleansers, but leaves a greasy film. It contains fragrant plant extracts.

☹ **Gentle Eye Makeup Remover** *($20 for 4 ounces)* is a below-standard, detergent-based eye-makeup remover that is not gentle because it contains comfrey extract and methylisothiazolinone, a preservative not recommended for use in leave-on products.

✓ ☺ **$$$ Waterproof Eye Makeup Remover** *($20 for 4 ounces)* is a very good, water- and silicone-based eye-makeup remover. The fragrance-free formula is ideal for all skin types, and not a single irritating ingredient was used. You'll find similar options from Almay and Neutrogena for less money, but this is still a winner.

☺ **$$$ Face Polish** *($30 for 3.5 ounces)* is a standard but good topical scrub for normal to slightly oily or slightly dry skin not prone to blemishes. The tiny amounts of irritating plant extracts are not likely to be a problem.

☺ **$$$ Perfecting Water - Light** *($38 for 6.7 ounces)* claims to temporarily "over-hydrate" skin, which isn't a benefit. Too much water isn't healthy for skin, but the reality is that this toner is a fairly basic option for normal to slightly dry skin. The amount of alcohol is not likely to cause irritation, but this fragrance-free toner would be better without it.

☺ **$$$ Perfecting Water - Rich** *($38 for 6.7 ounces)* is a better option than the Perfecting Water - Light. The alcohol- and fragrance-free formula contains some good skin-identical ingredients and soothing agents for normal to dry skin.

☺ **$$$ Eyedration Firming Eye Cream** *($40 for 0.5 ounce)* features an absolutely huge ingredient list—but the "meat" of this product is mostly water, emollient, thickener, glycerin, several more thickeners, silicone, and film-forming agents. Barely weighing in for a supporting role are several plant extracts (mostly nonirritating) and antioxidants, along with a few water-binding agents. Had these ingredients been included in greater amounts (and not in jar packaging), this would have been a more impressive formula. It does contain fragrant plant extracts, and nothing in it will significantly firm the skin or reduce puffiness.

☺ **$$$ Illuminating Brightener** *($70 for 1 ounce)* purports to work on sun spots (brown skin discolorations) while improving skin's clarity. It contains a small amount of sodium ascorbyl phosphate, a stable form of vitamin C—but unlike other forms of vitamin C, this one doesn't have any research proving its skin-lightening ability (though it does function as an antioxidant). In fact, none of the ingredients in this product can act on skin discolorations. It's just a lightweight moisturizer with some good water-binding agents and antioxidants. This would be appropriate for normal to slightly oily or slightly dry skin.

☺ **$$$ Mega Moisturizer Cream with SPF 15** *($45 for 2 ounces)* is a silky moisturizer that features an in-part avobenzone sunscreen. The silicones are suitable for normal to oily skin, but the emu oil and wax are not for anyone prone to breakouts. Unfortunately, jar packaging undermines the effectiveness of the antioxidant vitamins this contains.

☺ **$$$ Moisturizer Cream with SPF 15** *($45 for 2 ounces)* includes avobenzone for UVA protection, and wraps it in a decently emollient base for normal to dry skin. The vitamins will be subject to deterioration shortly after this jar-packaged product is opened.

☺ **$$$ Multi-Vitamin Serum** *($65 for 1.2 ounces)* is a two-part product consisting of water-based **Phase 1** and silicone-based **Phase 2**. Both contain ingredients that will smooth and hydrate skin, and both contain several antioxidants, although Phase 2 has slightly more. From a formulary standpoint, there was no need for this product to be split into two phases. The explanation I was given by a Mercier salesperson was that the water in Phase 1 doesn't mix with the plant oils in Phase 2, but that is an issue that any cosmetics chemist could overcome by choosing the correct ingredients to keep them blended together. I suppose Mercier simply wanted her serum to seem different and more scientific, and so consumers are directed to mix several drops from both phases before applying it to the skin. If the mixing step doesn't bother you, this is a very well-formulated, antioxidant-rich serum that is recommended for all but blemish-prone skin. Its packaging ensures the antioxidants will remain stable during use. The firming sensation you get from this product comes from the film-forming agent in Phase 1, which can temporarily make skin feel tauter and look smoother. This product does not contain fragrance, but does contain a small amount of orange oil, which imparts a scent (and may cause irritation, the only misstep in an otherwise superb product).

☺ **$$$ Night Nutrition Renewal Creme, for Normal to Dry Skin** *($55 for 1.7 ounces)* is an OK, rather standard moisturizer for someone with normal to dry skin. The tiny amounts of antioxidants and water-binding agents make the price a bit of a burn. For this amount of money, you should expect much more and it should be in packaging that keeps the antioxidants stable.

☺ **$$$ Night Nutrition Renewal Creme, for Very Dry and Dehydrated Skin** *($55 for 1.7 ounces)* is similar to the Night Nutrition Renewal Cream, for Normal to Dry Skin, except this contains slightly more emollients, including canola oil. As such, it is preferred for very dry skin, although the shortage of state-of-the-art ingredients, coupled with the steep price, makes it a less-than-satisfactory choice.

☺ **$$$ Night Nutrition Renewal Eye Creme** *($45 for 0.5 ounce)* is a more emollient version of the Eyedration Firming Eye Cream, and would work well for dry to very dry skin anywhere on the face. The same comments made for Eyedration about the antioxidants, skin-identical ingredients, and jar packaging apply here as well.

☹ **Oil Free Moisturizer SPF 15** *($45 for 4 ounces)* lacks sufficient UVA-protecting ingredients and contains enough lavender extract to make it potentially irritating, which isn't good news for any skin type.

☺ **$$$ Renewal Serum** *($80 for 1.5 ounces)* claims to stimulate skin-cell turnover, but it doesn't contain ingredients capable of doing that. It's a water-based serum for all skin types that does contain an impressive amount of green tea. Yet all by itself green tea is a one-note song and not nearly as interesting for skin as healthy amounts of other antioxidants, skin-identical ingredients, and cell-communicating ingredients. This is fragrance-free and an option, just not an exciting one.

☺ **$$$ Secret Finish** *($27 for 1 ounce)*. The real secret is that this ordinary, overpriced, lightweight moisturizer will not make a discernible difference in how your makeup wears. It is merely water, slip agent, thickener, rice starch (for a soft matte finish), plant extracts (including witch hazel, an irritant), vitamins, preservatives, more silicone, fragrance, and coloring agents. If anything, this formula isn't nearly as modern or effective as the less pricey handful of silicone-based mattifiers sold by M.A.C., Smashbox, and Paula's Choice.

☹ **Deep Cleansing Clay Mask** *($32 for 3.7 ounces)* contains a significant amount of irritants, including arnica, balm mint, and orange oil. The clay is joined by emollients, making this both confusing and irritating for all skin types.

☹ **Hydra Soothing Gel Mask** *($32 for 3.7 ounces)* contains lavender oil, which isn't soothing due to its negative effect on skin cells. Without it, this would be a recommended mask for normal to slightly dry skin.

☺ **$$$ Intensive Moisture Mask** *($32 for 3.7 ounces)* promises immediate firming, but doesn't deliver. However, what this does do brilliantly is make dry to very dry skin look and feel replenished. More than just a moisturizing mask, the formula contains some very good antioxidants, plant oils, and soothing agents.

☺ **$$$ HydraTint SPF 15** *($20)*. This emollient tinted lip balm has a smooth, cushiony texture and provides a soft gloss finish. The sheer colors are beautiful, so all things considered, it's a shame that the sunscreen doesn't provide sufficient UVA protection.

☹ **Lip Balm SPF 15** *($20 for 0.12 ounce)* does not contain the UVA-protecting ingredients of titanium dioxide, zinc oxide, avobenzone, Tinosorb, or Mexoryl SX, and is not recommended. What a shame, because this is otherwise a stellar lip balm.

☺ **$$$ Lip Silk** *($20 for 0.4 ounce)* is a very good, Vaseline-based lip balm that contains silicone for a silky finish and lighter texture. This also contains vitamin E and a cell-communicating ingredient. The glycolic and salicylic acids do not function as exfoliants.

☺ **$$$ Lip Treatment Kit** *($28 for 0.61 ounce total)* contains a lip scrub and a lip balm, a nicely formulated duo that helps exfoliate and protect. The **Lip Polish** is a gentle, gel-textured scrub that exfoliates lips with bamboo powder and polyethylene beads. This is followed by the **Lip Conditioner**, which is a standard, but good lip balm. The Lip Conditioner contains a couple of fragrance chemicals known to be irritating, but the small amount is not likely a cause for concern.

LAURA MERCIER MAKEUP

LAURA MERCIER MINERAL MAKEUP

✓ ☺ **$$$ Mineral Powder SPF 15** *($35 for 0.34 ounce)* is the first loose-powder mineral makeup from a makeup artist–based line, and right out of the gate Mercier's option trounces the competition. The drawbacks of mineral makeup (potential discoloring over oily areas, making dry skin or dry areas look and feel even drier, messy application—after all, it is loose powder) do apply here to some extent. However, this product's overall excellent attributes balance those negatives and make this a mineral makeup worth exploring. The broad-spectrum sunscreen is provided by 20% zinc oxide, an amount that also lends this powder its opacity and ability to provide nearly full coverage and an absorbent finish. The zinc oxide is joined by pearl powder and lesser amounts of other ingredients common to mineral makeup, including mica and bismuth oxychloride. Together they create a silky, dry texture that blends better on skin than any other mineral makeup I've tested (and I've tested them all!). Its finish is matte in feel, but the pearl powder lends an attractive, non-sparkling, dimensional glow to skin that keeps it from looking too dull or flat. Eight shades are available (with no options for tan to dark skin tones), but they demand careful testing because they apply either lighter or darker than they appear in the container. Speaking of the container, the sifter has a clever closure that keeps the powder from spilling out during travel, a thoughtful touch. Applying this with a brush nets the most natural results; applying it with a sponge provides a noticeably opaque finish.

☺ **$$$ Mineral Primer** *($30)* is a silky loose powder with a natural affinity for skin. Although the color is pure white, it applies sheer and creates a slight brightening effect without looking chalky or too shiny. Despite this, it's not for everyone and is definitely something you'll want to test before purchasing. This mica-based powder is said to boost the effectiveness of the sunscreen(s) in other mineral formulas, but it cannot do that. In fact, that's a sketchy claim to make since this powder does not sport an SPF rating or active sunscreen ingredients.

☺ **$$$ Mineral Cheek Powder** *($22)*. If you want the shiniest cheeks around and if you want to be shimmering, look no further than this loose-powder blush. It has a sublime texture and silky application that clings well and adds concentrated color to your cheeks. All three shades are workable, though predominantly warm-toned (you're out of luck if you want a soft pink or pastel rose shade). Again, the shine each powder leaves is intense, even if applied softly. Such a look is best for evening makeup or special occasions.

☹ **$$$ Mineral Eye Powder** *($20)* is a loose powder packaged in a pot with a sifter to control how much is dispensed. The sifter consists of one hole in the center, which keeps this from being too messy, but it still dispenses too much powder at once, and this is concentrated, pigment-rich stuff! The shine is intense and clings reasonably well, though it is way too much for aging eyelids or use near wrinkles. If that's not a problem for you, this is worth a look.

☹ **$$$ Mineral Illuminating Powder** *($32)* creates a multidimensional shine from its pearl and diamond powders. Unfortunately, the shine clings poorly. You'll get illumination from this silky, weightless mica- and talc-based loose powder, but there are other ways to get there that don't involve the mess and that don't leave you with short-lived results. A great example would be Mercier's Illuminating Tinted Moisturizer SPF 20 with sunscreen below.

☹ **Mineral Finishing Powder** *($32)*. This loose powder is designed to "set" other mineral powders, which is a ridiculous notion—on a par with stating you need to set your liquid foundation with another liquid foundation because somehow your usual foundation just isn't setting well on its own. As it turns out, this sheer powder has a very dry texture that feels scratchy and effectively dulls the complexion. This is a must to avoid and one of Mercier's only resounding disappointments.

OTHER LAURA MERCIER MAKEUP

FOUNDATION: ✓ ☺ **$$$ Flawless Face Silk Creme Foundation** *($42 for 1.18 ounces)* has a name that not only makes you want to try it immediately (Flawless? Silk? Yes, please!), but also happens to be 100% accurate. One of the hallmarks of Mercier's foundations is how well they mesh with skin. Her formulas, even this one that provides significant coverage, somehow manage to look very skinlike, primarily because they don't settle into lines, pores, and minor crevices. Flawless Face Silk Creme Foundation's silicone base blends expertly and sets to a silky matte finish. It is one of the few almost-full-coverage foundations that don't look too thick or dull down healthy skin's natural luminosity. Granted, as exceptional as these qualities are, this foundation still looks like makeup—no one will believe you're sporting a sheer look—but if that's the kind of coverage you're looking for, this deserves serious consideration by those with normal to oily skin. Each of the shades is impeccable, but there are no options for someone with dark skin.

✓ ☺ **$$$ Foundation Powder** *($40)* is a superlative powder foundation that comes in seven gorgeous shades, including options for light and dark (but not very dark) skin tones. This talc-based powder offers a suede-smooth texture, even application, and light to medium coverage when used dry. If you use it wet it provides fuller coverage, but you also run the risk of streaking if you're not careful. If the price isn't too off-putting and you have normal to oily skin, this is a must-try and it's on the very short list of today's best pressed-powder foundations. One caution: Each shade has a hint of shine. While the shine isn't distracting, you should be aware of it if you're looking for a completely matte finish.

✓ ☺ **$$$ Illuminating Tinted Moisturizer SPF 20** *($42 for 1.7 ounces).* I'll get right to the point: This is an awesome tinted moisturizer if you have normal to dry skin and want an attractive glow finish that is sophisticated without being sparkly. Unlike Mercier's other tinted moisturizers, this one gets the UVA issue right by including avobenzone. The silicone-enhanced formula contains several antioxidants, is fragrance-free, and comes in three versatile sheer shades ideal for fair to medium skin tones. Unless your skin is sensitive to synthetic sunscreen actives or you want more coverage, there is every reason to consider this formidable tinted moisturizer. You also can blend it with a foundation if you need more coverage, but keep in mind that doing so will diminish the amount of sun protection you get (unless your foundation also includes sunscreen).

✓ ☺ **$$$ Moisturizing Foundation** *($42 for 1 ounce)* would be suitable for normal to dry skin seeking medium to almost full coverage. The texture is elegantly light and creamy, leaving a beautiful, slightly dewy finish. Six of the seven colors are excellent, although shades for darker skin tones are absent. Avoid Shell Beige, which is too pink.

☺ **$$$ Oil-Free Foundation** *($42)* still has a lot going for it, but as foundation technology has improved this product has stayed the same, so it is no longer the "top dog," so to speak. But it is definitely worthy of consideration by anyone with normal to oily skin. The fluid, densely pigmented texture blends out to a seamless, soft matte finish with medium coverage that can appear thick unless you blend it meticulously. Twelve shades are on hand, with options for very light but not for very dark skin tones. The only shades to consider avoiding are Shell Beige (slightly pink) and Suntan Beige (slightly peach). Porcelain Ivory is a very good shade for fair skin.

☹ **$$$ Stick Foundation SPF 15** *($40 for 0.33 ounce)* shares the same drawback present in most of Mercier's foundations with sunscreen: a lack of sufficient UVA-protecting ingredients. That's always disappointing, but even more so here because this is an otherwise fantastic stick foundation. Its silicone base smooths over skin easily and blends to a natural-looking finish that is skinlike, while still providing light to medium coverage. The formula is perfect for those with normal to dry skin not prone to blemishes (the high wax content that keeps this foundation in stick form is the culprit). As usual, Mercier's shade range is nearly flawless. Among the eight options (no colors for darker skin tones), the only slightly suspect shade is Tawny, but it's still worth testing. If you'd prefer a stick foundation that does provide sufficient sun protection, consider Shiseido Stick Foundation SPF 15 instead.

☒ **Tinted Moisturizer Oil-Free SPF 20** *($42 for 1.7 ounces)* is oil-free but is also unfortunately free of the UVA-protecting ingredients of titanium dioxide, zinc oxide, avobenzone, Tinosorb, or Mexoryl SX, and is not recommended.

☒ **Tinted Moisturizer SPF 20** *($42 for 1.5 ounce)* isn't worth considering, despite its light, creamy texture and its easy-blending application, because the SPF lacks UVA-protecting ingredients and because many of the colors, while sheer, tend to be too pink or peach. Until Mercier gets the sunscreen right, look to Bobbi Brown, Aveda, or Stila for superior tinted moisturizers.

CONCEALER: ☺ **$$$ Secret Concealer** *($22)* is meant for the eye area and is far more user-friendly than Mercier's Secret Camouflage concealer reviewed below. It comes in a small pot and offers three decent shades, each with a very creamy-smooth, petrolatum-based texture. It covers well but does tend to crease during the day. Give this a test run before you decide to purchase, and be sure to set it with powder.

☺ **$$$ Undercover Pot** *($34 for 0.2 ounce)* combines two of Mercier's concealers and her Loose Setting Powder reviewed below in one stacked package. The concealers are in a flip-top compact while the loose powder rests in a jar underneath. I'm not sure how to rate this trio because the Secret Camouflage received a neutral rating on its own, the Secret Concealer earned a happy face, and the loose powder remains a Paula's Pick for its many wonderful attributes. If you're not familiar with Mercier's products, please access the individual reviews for the products in this set. The Secret Concealer and Loose Setting Powder combination is great; the Secret Camouflage is a heavy duty, thick-textured concealer that can be mixed with Secret Concealer to aid application or soften the coverage a bit. There are four pairs of shades offered, all of which can be mixed to work for light to medium skin tones. The loose powder is the same translucent shade regardless of which set you choose. Be sure to test this at the counter before purchasing; blending your own concealer shades isn't the easiest way to go, and some will find the texture of both too much.

☹ **$$$ Flawless Fix Pencil** *($20)* needs routine sharpening (hence the neutral face rating because there are so many great pencils that don't take work to use) and isn't my favorite format for a concealer, but its texture is creamy without being slick, so it stays in place better than similar options and manages to provide medium to full coverage without looking thick. This type of concealer is a no-no for use over blemishes, but is ideal for camouflaging red spots or minor, sun-induced skin discolorations. All four shades are neutral and best for fair to medium skin tones.

☹ **$$$ Secret Camouflage** *($28)* is a two-sided compact concealer with a thick, dry texture and truly opaque camouflage coverage. All of the duos have yellow to beige or peach to copper colors that can work if mixed in the right proportions, but why would you want to do that when there are so many excellent one-step concealers available? Secret Camouflage was designed as a cover-up for facial blemishes, dark circles, or birthmarks, and if all else has failed, it is an option because of the high level of coverage you'll get. SC4 and SC6 are too peach or copper to recommend; SC3 is the most neutral duo.

☹ **$$$ Secret Brightener** *($30)* is a creamy highlighting pen with a brush-tip applicator. It goes on so sheer you're left wondering if you've really applied anything, but you will see a subtle shimmer finish. When used correctly, this product can create extremely subtle highlights under the eyes, on the brow bone, down the bridge of the nose, or on the collarbone. Both shades are suitable for their intended purpose.

POWDER: ✓ ☺ **Pressed Setting Powder** *($30)* has many of the same qualities as the Loose Setting Powder (below), minus the cornstarch. The texture is smooth and dry but the sole Translucent shade is recommended only for fair to medium skin tones.

✓ ☺ $$$ **Loose Setting Powder** *($34)* has an out-of-this-world silky texture that blends beautifully over the skin and leaves a satiny-smooth, dry finish. All of the shades are workable and have a subtle yellow undertone. The formula is talc-based and also includes a small amount of cornstarch, but likely not enough to be problematic for blemish-prone skin. All three shades are beautiful.

☺ $$$ **Pressed Powders** *($32)* are either bronze, shimmery, or both. They have a silky, non-flaky texture and apply evenly, imparting a soft shimmer finish and healthy color. Matte Bronze Light has the least amount of shine, while the intense shine of Matte Bronze is best for evening glamour only.

☺ $$$ **Secret Brightening Powder** *($22)* is a weightless, talc-based loose powder that is meant for (and does a great job of) highlighting skin, especially under the eyes—but again, the effect is subtle. There is no reason a similar effect cannot be created by the artful use of a standard concealer and powder, but for those inclined to experiment (and especially for makeup artists) this product, though pricey, may be worth experimenting with.

BLUSH AND BRONZER: ✓ ☺ $$$ **Creme Cheek Colour** *($22)* ranks as an outstanding cream blush for normal to dry skin. It's creamy without being greasy, has enough slip to blend evenly, and offers a smooth satin finish from each of its three sheer colors. Those who find this type of blush appealing may wish there were more shades available, but each one is excellent.

✓ ☺ $$$ **Second Skin Cheek Colour** *($24)* is an amazingly good powder blush. It feels beautifully smooth and application is soft with even results. Best of all, the finish is almost matte and the amount of shine is completely suitable for daytime wear. The attractive range of shades is tailored to those with fair to medium skin tones. The company claims this blush makes skin look "naturally blushed" and, thanks to this product's affinity for skin and seamless application, it does!

☺ $$$ **Bronzing Duo** *($32)* combines a pressed bronzing powder and powder blush in one compact. The colors are not separated by a divider, so it's best to swirl your brush over both. Doing so results in a soft bronze color with a hint of pink, peach, or muted rose, depending on which duo you choose. The texture is soft and slightly powdery and application is good. You'll get a strong color payoff and the finish is laced with shine, but it's soft.

☺ $$$ **Bronzing Gel** *($32 for 1.69 ounces)* is a standard, sheer gel bronzer that's infused with particles of shine that call attention only to themselves in daylight. If you're a fan of shine you'll find this a tempting option, and the color is utterly believable, even on fair skin tones. It has just enough copper-red pigment to closely mimic a natural tan, but the consistency makes it best for use over bare or lightly moisturized skin rather than blended over foundation (especially matte-finish foundation, which causes the gel to grab and look dotted on the skin).

EYESHADOW: ✓ ☺ $$$ **Eye Colour Trio** *($38)* are similar to Mercier's other powder eyeshadows, but these have a greater color deposit from all the shades (Mercier's other shadows tend to be softer, except for the darkest shades). The texture and the enhanced pigmentation are superb. Each shade is easy to blend and melds with skin rather than looking like powder sitting on top of it. Mauve Sunset and Midnight Sun are the most workable trios. The Blue Hour trio suffers from the darkest shade being too blue, especially for use as a crease color.

✓ ☺ **$$$ Luster Eye Colour** *($22)* is a smooth-textured, highly blendable eyeshadow that goes on soft and requires layering for shading and detail. The "luster" part of the name refers to this powder eyeshadow's satin sheen. Avoid the green Sherazade shade. If you insist on blue eyeshadow, Celestial is tolerable because it goes on more as a muted bluish gray.

✓ ☺ **$$$ Matte Eye Colour** *($22)*. Once again, Mercier has crafted a powder eyeshadow with an unbelievably smooth texture and near-perfect application, even for the darkest shades. The finish on each shade isn't true matte, but it comes very close, with only a hint of sparkle. The shade range is good, but would be better if it had more mid-toned shades. There are plenty of options for those seeking lighter colors.

☺ **$$$ Eye Basics** *($24)* are liquid eyeshadows that come in a tube with a sponge-tip applicator. Each neutral yet shiny shade has a lightly creamy, sheer texture that blends easily and dries to a natural matte (in feel) finish. This works almost as well as a matte-finish concealer over the eyelids.

☺ **$$$ Sateen Eye Colour** *($22)* has a supremely smooth texture that blends with ease. Each shade of this high-shine powder eyeshadow applies softer than it appears (by about 50%), so layering is required for a notable color payoff. Still, there are some excellent colors if you want sparkling shine. Avoid St. Germain, which is too green to look anything but overly colorful. Note that Sateen Eye Colour's formula is different from that of Mercier's Luster Eye Colour; the latter is smoother and has a more sophisticated shine.

☺ **$$$ Metallic Creme Eye Colour** *($22)* is the one to choose if you want strong colors with a metallic finish but don't want to get it from a powder eyeshadow. This silky cream blends seamlessly, with just the right amount of slip. Its powdery (in feel) finish doesn't hold up all day, so expect some movement and a bit of creasing, though blending it with a powder eyeshadow all but eliminates this side effect.

☺ **$$$ Satinee Creme Eye Colour** *($22)* is tenacious. The shimmer factor is pretty high, so if you have any lines or less-than-taut skin around the eye area, these pearlescent cream shadows are not for you. However, if you don't have those issues, these cream shadows have a lot going for them. The available shades range from sheer to strong; with each, a little goes a long way. These shadows layer well and blend easily (though you have to be quick), allowing you to customize the shade and depth you want. Once on, these shadows wear for hours with minimal fading or creasing.

EYE AND BROW SHAPER: ☺ **$$$ Eye Brow Gel** *($19)* is a basic, efficient, clear brow gel. It's a great way to keep unruly brows in place, but there is no reason to spend this much when there are equally good options available from several drugstore lines.

☹ **$$$ Brilliant Eye Liner** *($22)*. With this product Mercier adds her own contribution to the crop of gel eyeliners, but it doesn't rise above them the way a latecomer should. Packaged to resemble a small bottle of nail polish, application requires you to dip a brush into the container, so it's nearly impossible to gauge how much product you're getting on the brush—until you pull it out. If you overload the brush, it's difficult to put product back in, and actually can be quite messy. Once you have the right amount on whichever brush you prefer (a brush is not included with the product), application is even and slightly wet. This remains smudge- and smear-prone for several seconds, but stays in place once it sets. All of the colors, even black, are imbued with shine, and each applies sheer, so you'll need successive layers for impact. If you want this type of eyeliner and crave shine, try M.A.C.'s Fluidline or Bobbi Brown Long Wear Gel Eyeliner instead. Both cost less and are easier to use.

☺ **$$$ Caviar Eye Liner** *($22)* is sort of like a soft-textured kohl pencil in compact form. It begins slightly creamy and sets to a dry finish. Application is smooth but sheer, so you'll need to layer for the best definition. A matte powder eyeshadow or one of the cream-gel eyeliners produces longer-lasting results with less effort.

☺ **$$$ Eye Brow Pencil** and **Eye Pencil** *($19)* are utterly standard, with traditional colors, and are not worth more than a fraction of this price. Mercier apparently developed "an exact texture" for these, but there isn't any difference between these and most other pencils. Each has a dry, stiff texture that isn't the easiest to work with, but the finish stays in place so smearing is much less likely. Avoid the Bleu Eye Pencil shade because it is too intensely blue and will compete with your eye color.

☺ **$$$ Eye Liner** *($22)* is a standard powder-cake liner that must be used wet with an eyeliner brush. The texture is the same as most cake liners, except that these all have a bit of sparkle to them and the shiny particles can flake off and get in your eye, which is annoying to say the least.

☺ **$$$ Kohl Eye Pencil** *($19)* has a creamy, soft texture and must be applied gently or the pencil tip will break. The creamy finish is meant to be smudged for a smoky look, but you can get similar results from many other pencils that don't require sharpening.

☺ **$$$ Brow Definer** *($20)* is sold in tiny glass pots and is accurately described as a wax/gel formula. The wax content lends a stiff texture to this product and also makes for a less-than-smooth application. However, with a good brush and some patience, this is an option to fill in, groom, and define brows with soft color and a non-sticky finish. All three shades are recommended but are best for brunettes.

☺ **$$$ Brow Powder Duo** *($24)* features two dry-textured brow powders in one compact. The color combinations are quite good, and there are suitable options for redheads and blondes, along with traditional options for brunettes—but all the colors are sparkly. Why the eyebrows need to shine is beyond me, but if this appeals to you, these brow powders do apply and blend well.

LIPSTICK, LIP GLOSS, AND LIPLINER: ✓ ☺ **$$$ Lip Velvet** *($22)*. Wow! Talk about color payoff! Mercier has done it again with this creamy lipstick, which applies like a gloss and really does feel like velvet on the lips. The colors are matte and apply thickly to the lips, so be careful. Wear time is commendable and Lip Velvet is so heavily pigmented that it will stain the lips a bit, so you can go longer between applications. This is a creamy product, so I encourage those prone to lip color bleeding into lines around the mouth to use a lipliner before applying. Ignore the antiaging claim for this product; it's without merit and completely hype due to the paucity of any ingredient that could be considered antiaging.

✓ ☺ **$$$ Liquid Crystal Lip Glace** *($22)* provides a striking, unique finish, all in a silky-feeling, non-sticky gloss. The shade selection is limited, but this deserves an audition because it is something fresh in the overcrowded, extremely repetitive lip gloss category.

☺ **$$$ Lip Colour Creme** *($22)* is pricey for a standard cream lipstick with a slightly glossy finish. However, the colors are beautiful and it isn't slippery or greasy, so it's unlikely to migrate into lines around the mouth (and even less likely if you use an anti-feather lipliner with it).

☺ **$$$ Lip Colour Sheer** *($20)* is exactly that, a sheer lip color with a glossy finish and marvelous, versatile colors that all have a slight stain.

☺ **$$$ Lip Colour Shimmer** *($22)* has the same formula as the Lip Colour Creme, though each shade has a soft to moderate shimmer finish and the colors aren't as rich. Otherwise, the same review applies.

☺ **$$$ Lip Colour StickGloss** *($20)* is aptly named! This is truly a lip gloss in lipstick form, and it provides a very glossy, non-sticky finish from each of its sheer but juicy colors.

☺ **$$$ Lip Stain** *($20)* is said to provide the visual effect of a stain along with the comfort and sheen of a gloss. A pot-packaged lip gloss is what this is; the stain effect is minimal yet the sheer colors are great and bound to please those looking for a softer lip color to wear alone or over lipstick. It has a slightly sticky yet glossy finish.

☺ **$$$ Lip Glace** *($22)* costs too much to make it worth strong consideration over many other standard lip glosses, but if you decide to indulge, this is a moderately sticky, sparkling wet gloss applied with a sponge tip.

☹ **Lip Kisses SPF 15** *($20)* lacks sufficient UVA protection, and the colors are too sheer to provide the opacity necessary to shield lips from sun damage. What a shame, because the colors are lovely.

☺ **$$$ Lip Pencil** *($19)* has a standard creamy texture and a dry finish. The expansive color range includes options that coordinate well with the lipsticks. Less expensive pencils abound, but these work well if you don't mind routine sharpening.

☺ **$$$ Lip Sheer Pencil** *($19)* is meant to be used with sheer lipsticks or lip glosses because it imparts softer (fleeting) color. The creamy texture is comfortable to apply, but don't expect much longevity from this needs-sharpening pencil.

☺ **$$$ Long Wear Lip Pencil** *($19)* is an automatic, retractable lip pencil. This has a smooth, silicone-enhanced application and feels slightly creamy, but otherwise is no different from many other automatic lip pencils, and Mercier's shade selection is not extensive.

☺ **$$$ Lip Plumpers** *($30)* contain a flavoring agent that works with other ingredients in the gloss to build a progressive cooling sensation. Within several minutes of applying this lip gloss–like product (which comes in a small but pleasing range of sheer to clear shades), your lips will be tingling like church bells on Sunday and may be a bit plumper as a result. Of course, that tingling and any increased fullness is the result of irritation, and that's not the best thing to do to lips on a routine basis. For occasional use (or applied over lipstick, which blocks most of the active minty flavor from causing irritation) this is an option, and it does have a rich, glossy finish that feels smooth and surprisingly light, though the subtle difference isn't really worth the money.

MASCARA: ✓☺ **$$$ Thickening and Building Mascara** *($20)* is a pleasure to apply, and it builds impressively long, lifted lashes with a fair amount of thickness. Lashes look full, soft, and fringed—all without clumping or smearing.

☺ **$$$ Waterproof Mascara** *($20)* has a formula that is easy to apply, makes it through the day without flaking, and really is waterproof (though you may notice slight smearing). It takes some effort to build long, thick lashes, but the result is worth it and your lashes aren't left feeling stiff or brittle.

☺ **$$$ Mascara** *($20)* creates subdued definition and average length. Thickness is a foreign concept to this mascara, and overall the payoff isn't worth the price.

FACE AND BODY ILLUMINATING/SHIMMER PRODUCTS: ✓☺ **$$$ Shimmer Bloc** *($38)* deserves consideration if you're looking for a shiny pressed powder to highlight or add a glow to your skin. You get four colors in one compact, and the tightly pressed formula is not flyaway, which makes application that much easier. Even better, the prismatic shine clings well and tends to not flake. Very well done!

☺ **$$$ Illuminating Powder** *($35)* presents four squares of color in one compact, without dividers between them. The result from either of the two quads is akin to a shimmery blush, with the shine level being moderate and best for evening. This has a silkier, more refined texture than Mercier's powder blush, and applies smoothly.

☺ **$$$ Illuminating Stick** *($25)* offers a lot more than a healthy glow, because this is one intensely shiny (almost metallic) finish! Application of this cream-to-powder stick is quite good, although the colors are intense and require careful blending. Illuminating Stick is best for normal to very dry skin.

☹ **$$$ Loose Shimmer Powders** *($34)* comprise the long-standing Star Dust and Sun Dust powders, each with a sheer, silky texture and sparkling, dimensional finish. The formula doesn't cling as well as it should, so you'll get some flaking, but if you're going for all-over shine, that's not such a big deal.

BRUSHES: ☺ **$$$ Laura Mercier Brushes** *($10-$250)*. Mercier has done her homework when it comes to brushes. Most of these are masterfully shaped and are dense enough to hold and deposit color evenly on the skin. Almost every brush is available with a long or short handle, which is an attractive option. The best among this collection of either natural or synthetic hairs are the **Powder Brush** *($52)*; the synthetic-hair **Camouflage Powder Brush** *($28)*, which is more appropriate for eyeshadows; **Bronzer Brush** *($45)*; and the **Cheek Colour Brush** *($45)*. Almost all of the **Eyeshadow Brushes** *($24 to $30)* are worth a closer look, particularly the **Eye Crease Brush** *($29)*, **Smudge Brush** *($24)*, and **Corner Eye Colour Brush** *($25)*. The Brush Sets are pricey, and the **Micro Mini Brush Set** *($50)* isn't much for the money, so make sure you're going to use every brush in these sets regularly.

SPECIALTY PRODUCTS: ☹ **$$$ Foundation Primer** *($30 for 1.7 ounces)* is a thin, lightweight cream-gel that contains some antioxidants whose effects are counteracted by too many fragrant extracts. It's supposed to contain light-reflecting ingredients that protect the skin, but it doesn't (unless you consider the emollient shine from the finish protecting). It is a good, simple, matte-finish moisturizer for someone with slightly oily skin, but that's about it. It does not, as claimed, "act as a buffer to outside elements," especially when you consider that the major outside element is sunlight.

☹ **$$$ Foundation Primer - Hydrating** *($30 for 1.7 ounces)* contains a minimal amount of hydrating ingredients and more witch hazel than should be applied to normal to dry skin, though overall the amount is unlikely to cause irritation. All of the antioxidants and other intriguing ingredients are listed well after the preservatives. At best, this water- and silicone-based lotion will create a silky-smooth surface for makeup application, but so will many other serums and moisturizers that, while not officially sold as primers, will perform the same function while providing greater benefit.

☹ **$$$ Foundation Primer - Mineral** *($30)*. Mercier didn't need another primer in her line, but because all things labeled "mineral" get the consumer's attention I suppose her marketing team couldn't help themselves. This is a silky, lightweight lotion whose main mineral is absorbent silica. It leaves a radiant finish that doesn't feel the least bit greasy, likely because alcohol is the fifth ingredient. Even if you have oily skin and want a matte-finish primer, there are better options than this.

☺ **$$$ Foundation Primer Oil-Free** *($30 for 1.7 ounces)* has a thinner, less silky texture than the original Foundation Primer, and the formula is less exciting, too. It is oil-free, but it lacks absorbent ingredients and contains too many thickeners to make someone with oily skin happy. It is best viewed as an ordinary, lightweight moisturizer to remedy slightly dry skin.

LORAC

LORAC AT-A-GLANCE

Strengths: Mostly great foundations in a neutral shade range; beautiful pressed powder and bronzing powder; several super blush and lipstick options; one superior lip gloss; awesome collection of shimmer products.

Weaknesses: Limited, average skin-care options; average to problematic concealers; unimpressive eyelining and brow-enhancing options; the Lotsa Lip products; the mascaras are a mixed bag with mostly disappointing results; no brushes.

For more information about Lorac, call (800) 845-0705 or visit www.loraccosmetics.com or www.Beautypedia.com.

LORAC SKIN CARE

☺ **$$$ MakeupPREP Gentle Skin Resurfacer** *($32 for 3.7 ounces)* is an at-home microdermabrasion topical scrub product that contains aluminum oxide as the main abrasive agent. This gritty-feeling scrub is formulated in a creamy base to help cushion your skin as you apply it. Even so, it should be used very gently because you can easily go overboard with this type of harsh scrub. Rinsing is a bit difficult due to the oil in the formula. Aluminum oxide is not a "gentle" scrub ingredient, so the name is misleading, and it doesn't work any better than (and is definitely not as gentle as) a washcloth.

☺ **$$$ Vitamin E Stick** *($16)* is available in tinted or untinted versions. The former isn't really tinted, it's just an emollient lipstick that's loaded with white iridescence. Used alone, this can make lips look ghostly. The untinted version is a standard, emollient lip balm. Both versions contain a meager amount of vitamin E.

LORAC MAKEUP

FOUNDATION: ✓ ☺ **$$$ Natural Performance Foundation** *($35 for 1 ounce)* comes in a nice range of colors to suit very fair to dark skin tones. The satin finish on this medium-coverage foundation is more semi-matte than dewy and best for normal to slightly dry or slightly oily skin. It blends beautifully and wears well, though over oily areas you will definitely need to set it with a loose or pressed powder. Note: Those with sensitive skin may also find this a good option because it is fragrance free.

✓ ☺ **$$$ Oil-Free Wet/Dry Powder Makeup** *($36)* is fantastic. This ultra-smooth, almost creamy, talc-based pressed-powder foundation is a joy to apply. It blends imperceptibly over the skin and creates a sheer, polished finish. All five shades are superior, with options for light to tan skin. Few pressed-powder foundations look this beautiful on skin, and wet application is a step above the rest, too (but be careful to avoid streaking).

☹ **Breakthrough Performance Foundation SPF 14** *($38 for 1 ounce)* is meant to be Lorac's answer to combining high-tech skin care with makeup, but it's not a merger that translates to gorgeous, healthy skin in any way shape or form. This creamy liquid foundation contains what the company refers to as "SMS Complex," which they claim will stimulate cell turnover, stimulate collagen production, and create a better support system for skin. Of course none of that is legitimate, because not a single ingredient in this foundation is capable of such feats, at least not in the teeny amounts Lorac included (the amount of tripeptide is nearly zero). The only truly antiaging element in this foundation is its in-part titanium dioxide sunscreen—but at this point, its inclusion is more a nice me-too than breakthrough! Still, this definitely provides broad-spectrum sun protection. Outside the claims, you'll find the best part of Breakthrough Performance is its smooth application and blending. It sets to a satin finish that feels moist, and it's best for normal to dry skin. The problem is that this foundation tends to emphasize pores and lines, be they superficial or deep. At first the finish looks beautiful, but within minutes it sinks into the slightest depression in skin, calling attention to it in an unflattering way, and this is true for each of the seven shades. For that reason alone, I cannot recommend this foundation over several others.

☹ **ProtecTINT SPF 30 Oil-Free Tinted Moisturizer** *($32)* has a water-fresh, moist texture with lots of slip and a dewy finish suitable for normal to dry skin. The five shades are very sheer and workable for all but very dark skin tones, but this is not recommended because it lacks sufficient UVA-protecting ingredients. With so many tinted moisturizers with sunscreen that get this fundamental element right, why choose one that puts skin at risk for more sun damage?

CONCEALER: ☺ **$$$ Double Feature Concealer/Highlighter** *($24)* combines a twist-up creamy stick concealer with a liquid shimmer highlighter and roller ball for blending, all in a unique package. The stick concealer provides ample coverage, but is crease-prone and definitely not for use on blemishes. Using the roller-ball blender helps soften edges and reduces the amount of coverage, if that's what you need. While clever, this isn't an essential addition because it doesn't do anything more than what a clean fingertip or concealer brush can do, and if not used carefully, it can roll off enough concealer so that flaws show through. You apply the highlighter part with an angled sponge-tip applicator and it sets to a very shiny finish that has more longevity than the concealer. Three shades are available: the first and second shades (DF1 and DF2) are acceptable, although some with light skin will find them too yellow, and DF3 is for medium to tan skin, but will be too orange for most. Maybelline's Age Rewind Double Face Perfector is a better choice, and the price makes it a steal compared to Lorac's version. Still, when used carefully and if you set the concealer with powder, this is an option to consider.

☺ **Coverup** *($18)* comes in a pot and offers great emollient coverage, but it also tends to crease almost immediately and keeps on creasing. If creasing isn't a concern for you, the range of shades (which apply less yellow than they appear) is quite good.

POWDER: ✓ ☺ **$$$ Translucent Touch Up Powder** *($32)* is a talc-based pressed powder that has a smooth-as-silk texture and three very good colors, each with a slight amount of shine. It provides a bit more coverage than traditional pressed powder, and blends on easily.

BLUSH AND BRONZER: ✓ ☺ **$$$ Blush** *($19)* offers a small, but very good, palette of colors. Plum, Rose, Soul, and Peach are particularly great. Avoid Desire and Crimson unless the goal is extreme shimmer on your cheeks. The texture and application are beautiful, and the color begins sheer but builds well.

✓ ☺ **$$$ Sheer Wash** *($20)* is comparable to but slightly better than Benefit's BeneTint. Sheer Wash comes in two beautiful colors suitable for a wide range of skin tones. As is true for all liquid stains, this dries almost immediately and tends to work best on smooth, flawless skin. If you can master the application quirks inherent to this type of product, it lasts all day without fading.

☺ **$$$ Baked Matte Satin Blush** *($24)*. Ignore the "matte" in this product's name because this powder blush is heavy on shine. The shine clings decently, but adding this much shine to cheeks is best reserved for evening makeup. This blush has a strong color payoff, so a little goes a long way.

☺ **$$$ Bronzer** *($28)* comes as a pressed powder and is available in two attractive, shine-infused shades. A natural tan doesn't add shine to skin, but at least this silky powder applies evenly and lasts, plus the shine stays put.

☺ **$$$ Cheek Duo** *($28.50)* offers a pressed-powder blush and bronzer in one compact, and the pairings are well done. Both colors have noticeable shine, but can work for evening glamour or to highlight younger skin.

☺ **$$$ TANtalizer Baked Bronzer** *($30)* downplays talc (only a small amount is included) in favor of a triglyceride base. That makes this creamy pressed bronzing powder a good option for normal to dry skin. It has a smooth, non-powdery application with a natural affinity for skin. If you want a bronzer with tan overtones and a soft shimmer, this is one to check out!

☹ **$$$ TANtalizer SPF 15 Baked Matte Satin Bronzer** *($30)* may seem like a boon to your regular sun protection, but the active ingredients in this shiny, mica-based pressed bronzing powder don't provide sufficient UVA protection. As a bronzer, this has a very smooth texture and applies evenly, but the color is a strange peachy yellow tone that doesn't resemble a real suntan.

EYESHADOW: ☺ **$$$ Baked Matte Satin Eye Shadow** *($22)*. Ignore the "matte" in this product's name because these powder eyeshadows are heavy on shine. The texture is very silky and pigmentation is strong, so you can get dramatic results with ease. And there's more good news: the shine stays in place well. This isn't the eyeshadow to choose if you have wrinkles or a less-than-taut eyelid area, but it's an option for all others. Avoid Insider; it's too blue.

☹ **$$$ On Screen Duo** *($24)* combines a powder highlighter and cream eyeshadow/eyeliner in one component, the idea being to provide a brown-toned shade for shadowing and creating shape, and a pale flesh tone for adding highlights. The powder is smooth and imparts sheer color with a soft shine that clings. Unfortunately, the cream eyeshadow/eyeliner portion is too thick and waxy to work well as an eyeshadow and too creamy to last long as eyeliner. For less money, better application, and much longer wear consider L'Oreal HIP Cream Shadow Paint instead.

☹ **$$$ Starry-Eyed Baked Eyeshadow Trios** *($24)*. These are strongly pigmented powder shadows that apply smoothly and wear and wear for hours without flaking. Unfortunately, all of the color options are so shiny that it will look like you've applied glitter directly to your eyelids. None of these trios will work for understated or professional daytime makeup, and unless you're headed out to the disco, circa 1976, or want the focus to be on your glitter instead of your eyes, they're not a slam-dunk for evening wear either. The application is commendable, but it's hard to recommend an eyeshadow whose intense shine has limited appeal.

EYE AND BROW SHAPER: ✓ ☺ **$$$ Front of the Line PRO** *($22)* is a felt-tip marker-style liquid eyeliner. The best part is that it really works, and so there's very little, if any, skip or drag when drawing even the finest lines. The formula dries almost instantly and then doesn't budge, making this a good choice for those whose eyeliner (be it pencil or powder) tends to fade during the day.

✓ ☺ **$$$ Front of the Line Waterproof Eyeliner** *($20)* is a liquid eyeliner with a felt-tip marker-style applicator that makes drawing a line easy. The formula dries almost instantly and then doesn't budge, making this a good choice for those whose eyeliner (be it pencil or powder) tends to fade during the day. Among the three shades, Black is classic while Brown is actually a teak-like red and Green is an olive-brown shade some may find appealing. As the name states, this is waterproof—though it does fade slightly if worn when you're immersed in water (as in going for a swim). This requires an oil- or silicone-based product for removal.

☺ $$$ **Take A Brow** *($22)* contains two brow powders, a mini brow brush, and a clear brow wax in one slim compact. The brow powders have a silky-smooth texture and are easy to work with, though each has a slight shine. The various sets present shade options for blondes, redheads, and brunettes, whether you want to use one or blend two to best match your brow color. As for the clear wax, it is unusually gummy (likely due to the mix of castor oil with cornstarch) and not preferred over setting your brows with a clear gel or a touch of hairspray. The included brush is functional despite its small size, but is still best for touch-ups.

☺ $$$ **Creamy Brow Pencil** *($19)* has a texture that's more thick than creamy, though it does leave a moist finish. This needs-sharpening pencil comes in four excellent shades that with practice can be feathered through brows to create a natural, defined appearance. Application can drag a bit if the pencil is not kept consistently sharp, while the mascara-type brush on the opposite end helps complete the brow-enhancing result.

☺ **Eye Pencils** *($16)* are standard fare and more or less available to appease pencil lovers. You can find comparable pencils that don't need routine sharpening at the drugstore.

☹ **Eye Shadow/Liner** *($16)* needs sharpening and, although that may be tolerable, you likely won't want to put up with this chunky pencil's too-creamy application and the fact that the large particles of glitter built into each color flake.

LIPSTICK, LIP GLOSS, AND LIPLINER: ✓ ☺ $$$ **Co-Stars** *($19)* are a late entry into the ring of long-wearing, two-part lip colors—but it was worth the wait, because Co-Stars is one of the best to come along since M.A.C.'s equally impressive Pro Longwear Lipcolour. The color coat feels creamier than most when first applied, and imparts rich, nearly opaque color. It feels remarkably less creamy as it sets, which is why the glossy top coat is necessary for comfortable wear. Staying power is where this product excels. Lorac pledges eight-hour wear, and this delivers. Aside from reapplying the glossy top coat, the color stays on through eating, drinking, smooching—anything that causes traditional lipstick to transfer or come off. Removing this requires an oil-based product, because silicone makeup removers do not work well. The shade selection is smaller than that offered by other lines, but if you find one you like (and there are some very good nude pink and rose tones), this is something to check out!

☺ $$$ **Couture Shine Liquid Lipstick** *($22).* Think of this smooth-textured, brush-on lip product as a cross between a lipstick and lip gloss. You get more color than you do from most lip glosses, but definitely not as much as you get from traditional lipsticks. In typical Lorac fashion (at least when it comes to lip products) the shade range is well edited. Every shade has shimmer, and they make a big deal about it coming from mother of pearl, but mother of pearl is just a mineral (primarily calcium carbonate) that isn't nearly as shimmery as mica, which is also present in this liquid lipstick. The bottom line is that each shade provides a beguiling sheen to lips while being minimally sticky.

☺ $$$ **Cream Lipstick** *($19)* is a light, decadently creamy lipstick with a slightly greasy finish that goes on smoothly and imparts rich color. The large selection of shades is stunning, although most of the celebrity-inspired shades have disappeared.

☺ **$$$ Matte Lips** *($19)* are not matte, but these do have a less creamy texture than the Cream Lipstick, and offer more intense colors that last without feeling dry or cakey on the lips. Although the color selection is limited to only three shades, Explore is one of the best red hues you'll find.

☺ **$$$ Sheer Lipstick** *($19)* is the exact same formula as the Cream Lipstick, but with less pigment, so these tend to fade quickly. The soft colors work for a variety of skin tones.

☹ **$$$ Breakthrough Performance Lipstick SPF 15** *($22)*. This creamy lipstick claims to go beyond ordinary lipsticks by doing such things as stimulating collagen production and providing a slew of antiaging ingredients, including sunscreen. Things don't get off to a good start because the sole active ingredient (octinoxate) does not provide sufficient UVA protection. As for unique elements of the formula, they are absent, so this lipstick isn't much different from almost every other good creamy lipstick being sold. It has a smooth texture, soft cream finish, and great color payoff. The creaminess doesn't last for long, but the color definitely does—and this doesn't easily slide into lines around the mouth. I suppose one could consider those attributes enough of a breakthrough performance, but the insufficient sunscreen keeps this from earning a better rating.

☹ **$$$ Mocktail** *($18)* is a series of lip glosses named after and flavored to taste like various cocktails. I don't quite get the association of lip gloss and cocktails, never mind that flavored lip glosses tend to encourage the wearer to lick her lips, which promotes dryness and means you have to reapply the gloss more often. This is an OK gloss with a moderately thick texture and slightly sticky feel. For the money, it's not worth choosing over numerous drugstore lip glosses. If the novelty of flavored gloss speaks to you, Jane and Bonne Bell have copious options available.

☹ **Lip Pencil** *($16)* is just a standard pencil with a great color selection that coordinates nicely with the majority of Lorac's lipsticks. The application is creamy but these have a drier finish, which keeps them in place longer, though you still have to sharpen them.

☹ **Lotsa Lip Plumping Lip Gloss** *($18.50)* has much more pigment than the Lotsa Lip Plumping Lipstick below, as well as a smooth, non-sticky texture and sexy gloss finish. The problem is it contains capsicum extract. This ingredient, typically extracted from peppers, is a counterirritant when used in topically applied arthritis treatments. It works by confusing the pain receptors (creating inflammation on the skin, which "tricks" the nerves around the joints), but in a lip gloss it's just a potent irritant (Source: www.naturaldatabase.com). While it can temporarily swell lips, the long-term results are not pretty (irritation is bad for skin).

☹ **Lotsa Lip Plumping Lipstick** *($18.50)* is disappointing. Lorac's other lipsticks are quite lovely, with elegant textures and enticing colors, but not so here. This sheer, slick lipstick is infused with large glitter particles that look silly, not seductive, and they actually claim that this provides "long-lasting color." Don't believe it for a second—this slips off before you know it, leaving behind noticeable pieces of glitter. Does this lipstick have a plumping effect to offset its inadequacies? Lorac uses Maxi-Lip, an ingredient mixture from Croda (a large supplier of raw materials to the cosmetics industry). Maxi-Lip is a blend of standard thickeners and emollients along with palmitoyl oligopeptide, which is said to reduce lines, add moisture, and increase the lip's volume. There is no substantiated research showing that Maxi-Lip has a legitimate plumping effect on lips. The only supportive information is from Croda, and that's hardly impartial. Peptides can help bind moisture to skin (and lips), but for now we have no idea whether or not they can affect collagen in any way, and for certain this product can neither duplicate nor come close to the results you get from lip injections of collagen or hyaluronic acid.

MASCARA: ✓ ☺ **\$\$\$ Visual Effects Curling, Separating, and Lengthening Mascara** *(\$19.50)* has an oddly shaped brush, but if you're feeling experimental, the reward is tremendously long, dramatically defined lashes. It's a breeze to build thickness where you need it most (at the lash roots) and you'll get noticeable lift, soft separation, and a touch of curl. The drawbacks, both of which are minor, include a slower-than-average drying time (so be careful or you may end up with some smearing) and slight clumping that is combed through easily. The Midnight Blue shade looks off-putting in the tube, but its effect on lashes is a silver-tinged smoky gray. (I prefer the Jet Black, but Midnight Blue is an interesting alternative shade that isn't brown.)

☺ **\$\$\$ Lorac Lashes** *(\$19)* is a good lengthening mascara that applies cleanly and wears all day without flaking or smudging. This is Lorac's original mascara, and it's down to one color, Brown, which is fine for lighter eyelashes or when you want a softer look.

☺ **\$\$\$ Special Effects Conditioning Primer and Defining & Lengthening Mascara** *(\$22)*. Here we have another dual-sided mascara (in ultra-sleek packaging) where one end is a lash primer and the other a mascara. Both sides feature rubber-bristled brushes to deposit product on your lashes. The primer goes on too wet, but if smoothed out it does add noticeable bulk to lashes when paired with the mascara. Apply the mascara carefully over the primer because imprecise application can lead to a gloppy look that's not easy to comb through. Used on its own, the mascara provides clean definition and length with a hint of thickness. It's nothing special, but the pair works quite well to produce voluminous lashes. It's up to you whether to engage in a two-part process or just spend less money on a mascara that provides length, separation, and ample thickness in one tube.

☺ **\$\$\$ Publicity Stunt Lashes** *(\$19)* is billed as a breakthrough formula because it lasts for days and is gymproof, cryproof, and waterproof. The formula eschews standard waxes in favor of the film-forming agent polyester-3, which is what ensures long wear and makes this mascara impervious to water and water-soluble cleansers. It's not much different from standard waterproof mascaras, except that when you use an oil- or silicone-based remover, it comes off in flakes and chunks. That's messy, and this mascara's performance isn't good enough to make the odd removal tolerable. You'll get longer, separated lashes (the built-in lash comb is a nice but unnecessary touch), but the real publicity stunt is in convincing consumers that this mascara really is a breakthrough and that it is OK to keep mascara on for days!

☹ **Lotsa Lash Fiber Mascara** *(\$19.50)* has one of the largest mascara brushes I've ever seen, and it doesn't make for better application. If anything, it demands extra vigilance because it's too easy to get excess mascara on the skin around your lashes, and it makes it nearly impossible to reach the lashes at the inner corners of your eyes (at least not without some risk of hurting yourself). This formula does contain fibers, which Lorac claims "cling to lashes like mini lash extensions" for "baby doll-like lashes." It turns out this mascara is lotsa talk and very little action because it takes longer than usual to build mediocre length and minimal thickness. The fibers don't create baby-doll lashes, nor do they have a curling effect. Instead, they make lashes feel brittle and the fibers tend to flake off, which is a problem for eyes in general, and especially for those who wear contact lenses.

☹ **Waterproof Lashes Waterproof Mascara** *(\$18.50)* is waterproof, but it smears with little provocation (even after lashes have dried) and tends to flake, making it an expensive mistake. Even without those surprising setbacks, the application is uneven, looking too heavy in one place and too sparse in others. In short, this is a mess of a mascara!

FACE AND BODY ILLUMINATING/SHIMMER PRODUCTS: ✓ ☺ $$$ **Oil Free Luminizer** *($28)* is a sheer liquid shimmer product that has a silky, lightweight texture and very smooth application. This leaves a shiny finish that is noticeable without being distracting, perfect for dressing up evening makeup with hints of sparkle and a soft radiance. Perhaps best of all, this stays put without flaking and doesn't feel slick or greasy. The sole shade, L1 (sheer white with pale pink and gold undertones), is versatile, especially for lighter skin tones. One caveat: This product is packaged in a pump bottle that dispenses more product than you're likely to need. A little of this stuff goes a long way and too much can look too obvious—so dispense carefully.

✓ ☺ $$$ **Perfectly Lit Oil-Free Luminizing Powder** *($32)* is a talc-free, mica-based pressed shimmer powder that has an amazingly smooth texture and applies beautifully. This is an outstanding way to highlight skin or specific features with a soft glow, and the shine stays in place. Each of the three shades is versatile and flattering.

✓ ☺ $$$ **TANtalizer Body Bronzing Luminizer** *($30)* basically takes the concept of the Oil-Free Luminizer and parlays it into a bronze-toned body lotion laced with radiant shimmer. This sheer-tinted lotion feels silky and light, and its finish on skin (especially medium to tan skin) is gorgeous. This is sure to be a summertime favorite, especially for evening. One caution: The lotion comes off on clothing, so apply carefully.

☹ **TANtalizer Award-Show Glow** *($32)* claims to be a body-firming bronzing mousse, but although the bronzing part definitely happens, the firming won't—not with drying, irritating alcohol as the second ingredient. The color is concentrated and ends up being a soft bronze with a rosy undertone and silvery shimmer. Although it dries down to soft matte (in feel), this is not long-wearing as claimed. It comes off readily on clothing or simply a swipe of your finger, so don't count on it for worry-free wear on hot summer nights. Actually, I wouldn't count on this at all given the alcohol content.

SPECIALTY PRODUCTS: ☺ $$$ **Greatest Hits CDs** *($48)* feature four eyeshadows, one blush, one lip/cheek tint, and a lip gloss. Not bad, considering that purchasing these items singly (instead of as an "album") would cost over twice as much. CD1 showcases warm colors, while CD2 spotlights cool tones. Depending on your preferences, both are worthwhile.

☺ $$$ **aquaPRIME Oil-Free Makeup Primer** *($30)* departs from the typical silicone-based, nonaqueous foundation primer with its simple formula of water, acrylate film-forming agent, water-binding agent, and preservative. It has a super-light gel texture and is oil-free, yet can make skin feel slightly tacky, and this much acrylate can cause irritation.

☺ $$$ **Oil-Free Neutralizer** *($30 for 0.9 ounce)* is supposed to even out any blue or red discolorations. It works to some extent because of its semi-opaque coverage and whitening effect (the green tinge has been minimized), but the same results can be achieved with a single foundation—though not with Lorac's liquid foundations, which are too sheer to conceal bothersome redness.

LUSH (SKIN CARE ONLY)

LUSH AT-A-GLANCE

Strengths: OK, they do offer complete ingredient lists in their newspaper-like catalog.

Weaknesses: Almost every product contains at least one potent skin irritant; no sunscreens to be found, nor are they recommended by the company; no products to address common skin conditions such as acne, hyperpigmentation, or eczema; jar packaging.

For more information about Lush, call (888) 733-5874 or visit www.lush.com or www.Beautypedia.com.

☹ **Angels on Bare Skin** *($9.95 for 3.5-ounce bar)* contains lavender and patchouli oils, and is not recommended. This recipe claims to be from the Middle Ages, which to my way of thinking is not a positive selling point! Back in those days, life expectancy was drastically short and bloodletting was the pinnacle of medicine!

☹ **Aquamarina** *($9.75 for 3.5-ounce bar)* contains irritating calamine powder as well as orange and patchouli oils. This is not something you should use if your face has caught too much sun.

☹ **Baby Face** *($9.35 for 1.2 ounces)* is a very fragranced bar cleanser that irritates skin with tangerine oil and concentrated narcissus fragrance.

☹ **Coalface** *($10.95 for 3.5 ounces)* assaults skin with sandalwood and rosewood oils plus sodium lauryl sulfate and genuine coal powder. Washing your face in the fireplace would be preferred to this product.

☹ **Dark Angels** *($10.95 for 3.5 ounces)*. This cleanser is mostly mud mixed with oil and charcoal. It's a mess to use, is difficult to rinse, and irritates skin with the fragrant oils of sandalwood and rosewood. Nothing about this cleanser is specific to the needs of darker skin; that claim is just bizarre. There is no research showing different skin tones require different skin-care ingredients. The black sugar in this product is not effective for any skin type or skin color.

☹ **Fresh Farmacy** *($8.95 for 3.5-ounce bar)* is based around calamine powder and irritates skin with lavender oil and sodium lauryl sulfate (and how often do you see that growing on the farm?).

☹ **Sweet Japanese Girl** *($10.25 for 1.2-ounce bar)* is a rich, buttery soap that irritates skin with lemon and juniper oils.

☹ **Ultra Bland** *($14.45 for 1.5 ounces)* is indeed bland, yet it's also irritating to skin due to the iris, rose absolute, and benzoin it contains.

☹ **Herbalism** *($10.75 for 3.5 ounces)*. This very abrasive scrub contains ground almonds to exfoliate skin, but the amount of clay makes it difficult to move over skin. This isn't nearly as elegant as many other scrubs, the almonds can scratch skin, and almost all of the plant extracts and oils it contains do nothing but irritate skin. This is a natural product, but it clearly proves the point that natural does not automatically, or even frequently, equal great skin care.

☹ **Ocean Salt** *($18.55 for 4.2 ounces)* rubs salt in the wound (figuratively speaking), thanks to lemon and lime additives. This would be a great way to break down skin's protective barrier and create dull skin.

☹ **Breath of Fresh Air** *($17.45 for 8.4 ounces)* is better dabbed on as perfume given the amount of volatile (and irritating) fragrant oils it contains. You've been warned!

☹ **Eau Roma Water** *($17.45 for 8.4 ounces)* is an unexceptional toner that's mostly perfumed lavender and rose water. It is not beneficial for any skin type.

☹ **Tea Tree Water** *($17.45 for 8.4 ounces)* has tea tree oil in it, which is fine. But the grapefruit and juniper turn what was fine into irritation, and that's not helpful for "troublesome teenage problems."

☹ **Tea Tree Toner Tab** *($1.50 for one 0.28-ounce tab)*. This is one way to get a single use of tea tree oil, but you're better off buying a small bottle of the pure stuff. That's because the main ingredient in this toner-like product is citric acid, which, in this amount, can be exceedingly irritating (Source: *International Journal of Toxicology*, 2001 Supplement, pages 47-55).

Citric acid is recommended for use in cosmetics only in small amounts, as a pH adjuster or an antioxidant.

☺ **Vitamin C Toner Tab** *($1.50 for one 0.28-ounce tab)*. This single-use toner's main ingredient is citric acid, which is exceedingly irritating for skin in this amount (Source: *International Journal of Toxicology*, 2001 Supplement, pages 47-55). Citric acid is recommended for use in cosmetics only in small amounts, as a pH adjuster or antioxidant. This also contains fragrant oils that will cause further irritation.

☺ **Vitamin E Toner Tab** *($1.50 for one 0.28-ounce tab)*. This single-use toner's main ingredient is citric acid, which is exceedingly irritating in this amount (Source: *International Journal of Toxicology*, 2001 Supplement, pages 47-55). Citric acid is only recommended for use in cosmetics in small amounts as a pH adjuster and antioxidant. This also contains fragrant oils that will cause further irritation.

☺ **Celestial** *($21.35 for 1.5 ounces)*. Finally a product in the Lush lineup with minimal fragrance! Though it still contains vanilla water and orchid extract, I imagine that it contains the least amount of fragrance of all the Lush products. But while this may contain the least amount for Lush, it isn't little enough to make this a good moisturizer because it doesn't contain one water-binding agent, antioxidant (vanilla water doesn't count), or anti-irritant.

☹ **Cosmetic Lad** *($20.45 for 1.5 ounces)* isn't a good choice for lads or lasses because it's based around lavender and also contains irritating sandalwood and tangerine oils.

☹ **Enchanted Eye Cream** *($22.35 for 1.5 ounces)* would be an OK emollient eye cream for dry skin if it weren't based on lavender, but that makes it is too potentially irritating for all skin types.

☹ **Enzymion** *($35.95 for 1.5 ounces)* contains enzymes naturally present in papaya juice to exfoliate skin, but those aren't reliable (not when compared to a well-formulated AHA or BHA product) and the jar packaging makes these unstable ingredients even less active. That's not good news, and things only get worse because Lush added lemon juice and lime oil.

☹ **Gorgeous** *($85.45 for 1.5 ounces)* claims to leave a matte feeling, but the olive and evening primrose oil base doesn't allow that. The lemon juice, orange flower, neroli, and myrrh resin are all fragrant and problems for skin, at least if you want yours to be described as "gorgeous."

☹ **Imperialis** *($21.35 for 1.5 ounces)* contains too many problematic plants and fragrant extracts to make it the "imperial majesty of moisturizers." Of particular concern is St. John's wort, which can cause a phototoxic reaction when skin is exposed to sunlight.

☹ **Mirror Mirror** *($21.45 for 1.7 ounces)* won't make you the fairest of them all, but will cause irritation thanks to sandalwood oil and other volatile fragrant extracts. Lush actually sells this for use either as a moisturizer or a fragrance!

☹ **Paradise Regained** *($46.95 for 1.7 ounces)*. This product claims to provide natural sun protection, but it contains two synthetic sunscreen ingredients (ethylhexyl methoxycinnamate and avobenzone, listed as butyl methoxydibenzoylmethane) that aren't listed as active, but they are present nonetheless. That fact and the lack of an SPF rating means this moisturizer cannot be relied on for sun protection. I wouldn't rely on it for anything else either, especially not for bringing skin to a state of paradise; it contains several fragrant oils and fragrance chemicals that cause pronounced irritation and hurt skin's ability to heal. Interestingly, this is one of the only Lush products containing preservatives.

☹ **Skin Drink** *($18.55 for 1.5 ounces)* contains neroli and rose absolute oils, which makes it too irritating for all skin types. Plain aloe vera gel and sesame oil (the main ingredients in this product) would be much better, though still far from what skin needs to function optimally.

☺ **$$$ Skin Nanny** *(46.95 for 1.7 ounces)*. Skin Nanny isn't a great way to keep a watchful eye on your complexion. This moisturizer has an emollient base that can be beneficial for dry skin (it's borderline greasy), but, like every Lush product, it contains irritating fragrant oils that make it a less desirable option. It is worth noting that this product isn't as fragranced as most other Lush products, but that's not saying much. It contains two synthetic sunscreen ingredients not listed as active, and this product does not have an SPF rating. It shouldn't be relied on for daytime protection.

☺ **Skin's Shangri La** *($45.95 for 1.5 ounces)* is an extremely emollient moisturizer for dry skin that contains some good plant oils and a tiny amount of antioxidants. The fragrance is a bit much, but not terrible.

☹ **Ultralight** *($13.95 for 3.3 ounces)* contains the sunscreen agent octyl methoxycinnamate, but does not have an SPF rating (nor is the sunscreen listed as "active"), so it cannot be relied on for daytime protection. The sandalwood and lavender oils plus myrrh resin in this emollient moisturizer make it unsuitable for all skin types.

☹ **Vanishing Cream** *($35.95 for 1.7 ounces)*. This moisturizer is recommended as "perfect" for those with acne, but the risk of causing more blemishes and making skin redder is obvious when you look at the ingredient list. The plant oils will make skin greasy and keep skin cells from shedding and the shea butter has the potential to clog pores. The overly fragrant base is closer to eau de cologne than skin care. Vanishing Cream also contains potent skin irritants such as lavender oil, tincture of benzoin, and fragrance chemicals. Lush says you don't have to have problem skin to use this, but there is a strong probability that using this will cause problem skin. At the very least, the problem will be irritation, which is a bigger issue than most people realize.

☹ **A Crash Course in Skincare** *($7.95 for 2.6 ounces)*. This facial mask for dry skin is a crash course only in irritation for your skin and the risk of potential bacteria contamination due to the lack of preservatives. This product must be kept refrigerated and most likely will spoil within days of being opened, as will any mix of plants you keep in your refrigerator; think about how long a head of lettuce lasts when refrigerated. This also irritates skin with a host of ingredients that include lemon juice (ouch!) and lavender oil. Maybe if the chemists at Lush took a crash course in skin care they'd see how incapable most of their products are of keeping skin in optimum condition.

☹ **Ayesha** *($7.95 for 2.6 ounces)*. This mask contains absorbent fuller's earth along with a floral blend, some food ingredients, and irritating fragrant oils of rosemary and patchouli. The drying nature of the fuller's earth makes skin feel temporarily tighter, but that temporary benefit is negated by the irritating, skin-damaging plant extracts.

☹ **BB Seaweed** *($7.95 for 2.6 ounces)*. Nothing about this mask, which must be refrigerated because it lacks preservatives, is deep cleaning or the least bit beneficial for skin. It contains some good ingredients, but they're trumped by the number of irritating ones, including the too-abrasive amount of ground almonds. That type of exfoliant tears the skin, damaging the outer barrier, and the fragrant oils are irritating, not hydrating. The scent of this mask will knock your socks off!

☹ **Brazened Honey** *($7.95 for 2.6 ounces)*. This mask contains fresh lime juice, which is exceedingly irritating for skin—and that's just the beginning of its many problems. Sage, rosemary, and juniper add their irritating kick as well, and ground almond shells give this mask a scratchy scrub quality that can damage skin. Ouch, ouch, ouch! That's what your skin would scream if it could talk and you applied this mask.

☹ **Catastrophic Cosmetic** *($7.95 for 2.6 ounces)*. I love the name for this mask because it aptly describes how much of a problem it is for your skin. Calamine powder (the main ingredient) is a counter-irritant. That means the irritation it causes is stronger than the irritation (such as itchiness) that it is meant to reduce. It definitely stops itchy skin, but it's suitable only for short-term use. This is just a very strange formulation that doesn't deserve consideration unless you're actively seeking to confuse your skin.

☹ **Cosmetic Warrior** *($7.95 for 2.6 ounces)*. The ingredient list for this mask reads more like a food recipe than an effective skin-care product. There is no research showing what free-range eggs are supposed to do for skin, although they are natural. The garlic in this mask is bound to be irritating due to its chemical constituents—you're better off eating garlic than smearing it on your face. The texture of this clay-based mask makes it difficult to apply and rinse, not to mention that all the fragrance it contains is just irritating and, therefore, skin damaging.

☹ **Cupcake** *($7.95 for 2.6 ounces)*. Cupcake contains fresh lemon juice and several fragrant oils that only cause irritation and offer your skin zero benefits. Please skip this product and eat a frosted cupcake instead. Your hips won't benefit, but at least you won't be damaging your skin!

☹ **Love Lettuce** *($7.95 for 2.6 ounces)*. This clay-based mask contains oil, which works against the absorbent properties of the clay and Fuller's earth. It also irritates skin and causes cell death with lavender oil, and the ground almonds can scratch and tear at the skin as this is being rinsed. Who comes up with these terrible concoctions for Lush?

☹ **Mask of Magnaminty** *($11.55 for 4.4 ounces)* contains peppermint oil and African marigold oil, which can cause contact dermatitis (Source: *Encyclopedia of Common Natural Ingredients Used in Food, Drugs and Cosmetics*, 2nd Edition, John Wiley & Sons, 1996).

☹ **The Sacred Truth** *($7.95 for 2.6 ounces)*. Forget about whether it's sacred or not, the real truth is that using this mask is an invitation for skin to become irritated and potentially break out in a rash, which to me would be unholy rather than sacred. The papaya can be very irritating and your skin is bound to be 100% confused by this odd mix of absorbents (clay, talc) with emollients and oils (shea butter, lanolin—and lanolin is an animal by-product). The biggest offenders are the numerous fragrant oils and fragrance chemicals.

☹ **Lip Balms** *($8.75 for 0.3 ounce)*. **Chocolate Whipstick Lip Balm, Dream Time Temple Balm, Flying Fox Temple Balm, Honey Trap Lip Balm, Lip Lime Lip Balm, Lip Service Lip Balm, Lite Lip Balm, Party On Temple Balm, T Tree Simplex Lip Balm,** and **Whoosh Balm Temple Balm** are emollient balms meant for the lips or, as the name states, temple area (for pressure-point massage). All of them contain one or more irritating essential oils, including peppermint, lavender, rosemary, lime, lemon, ginger, palmarosa, and jasmine. Expect them to cause redness and make dry, chapped lips look and feel worse.

M.A.C.

M.A.C. AT-A-GLANCE

Strengths: A Lauder-owned company, with some impressive moisturizers; all the daytime moisturizers with sunscreen include sufficient UVA protection; excellent lip balm and toner; excellent foundations (some whose sunscreen includes the right UVA-protecting ingredients) in a mostly gorgeous range of shades; great concealers; the Select Sheer and Mineralized powders; the Sheertone Blush and traditional cream blush; wide selection of powder eyeshadows in various finishes; Fluidline and Technakohl Liner; dizzying array of lipstick shades in mostly sumptuous formulas; Lipgelee; all of the Pro Longwear Lipcolour options; several very good mascaras (regular and waterproof); the makeup brushes; most of the Prep + Prime products work as claimed.

Weaknesses: A few products with uncomfortably high levels of known or potential skin irritants; no AHA or BHA products; no anti-blemish products; the Lightful products can't affect sun-induced skin discolorations; some of the foundations were downgraded because their sunscreen did not offer sufficient UVA protection; several average pressed and loose powders; the pencil concealer; Cream Colour Base; the Lustre and Velvet eyeshadows; the traditional eye pencils (that need sharpening); Brow Set and Brow Finisher; Lipglass and Plushglass; the Brush Cleanser.

For more information about M.A.C., owned by Estee Lauder, call (800) 588-0070 or visit www.maccosmetics.com or www.Beautypedia.com.

M.A.C. SKIN CARE

M.A.C. LIGHTFUL PRODUCTS

☺ **$$$ Lightful Foaming Cleanser** *($24 for 3.4 ounces)* underwent some minor formulary changes that change its original review. This foaming cleanser now deserves a happy face rating due to its gentler yet still effective formula. It remains preferred for normal to oily skin; those with dry skin may still find this facial wash doesn't leave their skin feeling as comfortable as they'd like. It removes makeup easily and contains some plant extracts with research pertaining to their skin lightening ability; however, in a cleanser these ingredients are rinsed down the drain before they can affect discolorations.

☺ **$$$ Lightful Active Softening Lotion** *($30 for 5 ounces)* has been reformulated and isn't as impressive a toner as it originally was. This is still a good option for normal to dry skin, though the cost is more of an issue since the formula isn't as well-rounded as it used to be. Despite this slight disappointment, it remains one of the better toners available at the department store.

☺ **$$$ Lightful Charged Essence** *($40 for 1 ounce)*. Lightful Charged Essence is a decent vitamin C serum, but the form of vitamin C (ascorbyl glucoside) doesn't have nearly as much substantiated research on its side as other forms, including magnesium ascorbyl phosphate or L-ascorbic acid. Still, this is hardly a one-note product, and it's good news that M.A.C. removed the problematic plant extracts this used to contain. It offers skin an impressive mix of antioxidants and water-binding agents. This is a good serum option for oily skin.

☺ **$$$ Lightful Ultramoisture Creme** *($36 for 1.7 ounces)* is a lightweight but substantially hydrating moisturizer for normal to slightly dry or dry skin, and it is jam-packed with cell-communicating ingredients, antioxidants, and beneficial plant extracts. How frustrating that all of these ingredients will quickly become less effective due to jar packaging that doesn't keep these air-sensitive ingredients stable.

OTHER M.A.C. SKIN-CARE PRODUCTS

☹ **Cleanse Off Oil** *($21 for 5 ounces)* isn't any better than removing makeup with a gentle cleansing lotion or even plain olive oil because it contains irritating bitter-orange and lavender oils. This is not recommended for any skin type, and would be a problem for eye-area use.

☺ **$$$ Cremewash** *($19.50 for 3.4 ounces)* is a water-soluble cleanser that produces copious foam. The main cleansing agent is the soap constituent potassium myristate, which means this cleanser can be drying for some skin types, rather than "super-hydrating" as claimed. It is an OK option for normal to oily skin, and removes makeup easily. Cremewash is similar to but better formulated than Clinique's Rinse-Off Foaming Cleanser ($17.50 for 5 ounces).

☺ $$$ **Green Gel Cleanser** *($19.50 for 5 ounces)* is an OK, water-soluble cleanser for normal to very oily skin. The drying TEA-lauryl sulfate cleanser is third on the ingredient list, which doesn't make this preferred to several other (less expensive) gel cleansers.

✓ ☺ $$$ **Wipes** *($17 for 45 sheets)* are a favorite at the M.A.C counter and it's not hard to see why: these sturdy yet soft cloths easily and quickly remove all types of makeup, including long-wearing lip stains and waterproof mascara. The formula combines gentle cleansing agents with a solvent and silicones to accomplish this, and most will find it a soothing experience. Wipes are convenient, but keep in mind that a water-soluble cleanser with a washcloth is just as effective (and costs less per use).

☺ $$$ **Cleansing Tips** *($12.50 for 30 swabs)* are cotton swabs whose hollowed-out center is filled with a gentle cleansing fluid, similar to most nonsilicone eye-makeup removers. One end is pointed for quick cleanup around the lash line, while the other end is rounded for cleaning up larger areas such as the eyelid. These work well and can be convenient, but they're not a cost-effective way to remove makeup, especially when you can just purchase a bottle of eye-makeup remover and a large box of pointed cotton swabs for roughly half the price. If you love the concept of pre-filled cotton swabs for makeup removal, check out the equally effective Swabplus Liquid Filled Cotton Swabs ($3.79 for 72 swabs) available online at www.drugstore.com.

☺ $$$ **Gently Off Eye and Lip Makeup Remover** *($18 for 3.4 ounces)* is a standard, but effective, dual-phase makeup remover with silicone. The plant extracts are a mix of fragrant rose and soothing cucumber, with rose extract not being the best for use around the eyes. Although this works very well, it doesn't best less expensive options from Almay or Neutrogena that are available at the drugstore.

☺ $$$ **Pro Eye Makeup Remover** *($18 for 3.4 ounces)* is a standard, detergent-based eye-makeup remover that works as well as any, and is fragrance-free. The formula claims to be pro-quality, but isn't different from what most other lines offer for less money.

☹ $$$ **Fix +** *($17 for 3.4 ounces)* is a standard, but good, alcohol-free toner for normal to dry or slightly oily skin. The mist application is convenient, but don't mist this over your makeup—nothing in the formula will "finish" it or prolong wear. Quite the opposite is true!

☹ $$$ **Microfine Refinisher** *($26.50 for 3.4 ounces)* contains "microfine crystals" of alumina to polish skin, so it's a good thing this scrub is blended with oil to cushion your skin because it can be fairly abrasive. And keep in mind, a washcloth works far better than almost any scrub.

☹ $$$ **Fast Response Eye Cream** *($28.50 for 0.5 ounce)* is a silicone-based moisturizer that contains several antioxidants, but also enough caffeine to make it problematic for use around the eyes due to its irritant potential. This contains fragrance in the form of methyldihydrojasmonate.

☺ $$$ **Oil Control Lotion** *($29.50 for 1.7 ounces)* doesn't control oil as much as it just leaves a smooth matte finish. This is a good moisturizer for oily skin types with dry patches. It contains a few antioxidants and cell-communicating ingredients in stable packaging.

☺ **Prep + Prime Skin Refined Zone Treatment** *($17.50 for 0.5 ounce)* is a good, light-weight mattifier for oily to very oily skin. It may be applied under or over makeup (pat it on oily areas to touch up and be careful not to rub) and helps keep skin shine-free. This does not contain ingredients capable of exfoliating skin, so that part of the claim is inaccurate. Sodium salicylate cannot exfoliate like salicylic acid does, and the pH of this product isn't within range for exfoliation anyway.

✓☺ $$$ **Studio Moisture Fix SPF 15** *($29.50 for 1.7 ounces)* has an in-part zinc oxide sunscreen with a beautiful silky texture, provides a soft matte finish, and is loaded with anti-oxidants, skin-identical substances, and anti-irritants. It is a brilliant option for normal to oily skin, although the amount of zinc oxide (and its slight whitening effect) may prove tricky to work with on darker skin tones. This product does contain fragrance.

✓☺ $$$ **Strobe Cream** *($29.50 for 1.7 ounces)* contains mineral pigments to optically "brighten" skin, which basically means particles of shine to make skin look radiant rather than dull. Looking beyond the light show reveals a well-formulated moisturizer brimming with the essential elements that normal to dry skin needs to look and feel its best. Almost all of the anti-oxidants included have considerable research documenting their topical benefit for skin.

☺ **Strobe Liquid** *($29.50 for 1.7 ounces)* is the fluid version of M.A.C.'s popular Strobe Cream. Strobe Cream is one of the better moisturizers M.A.C. offers, and Strobe Liquid follows suit by treating normal to oily skin to an impressive mix of antioxidants and water-binding agents. Although not as well-rounded as Strobe Cream, this is still worth considering as long as you're OK with the obvious opalescent pink shimmer that it leaves. Strobe Cream's shimmer is subtle, giving your skin a well-rested glow, while Strobe Liquid tosses subtlety out the door and turns the shine dial to "loud," which won't please someone with oily skin.

☹ **Studio Moisture Cream** *($31 for 1.7 ounces)* contains a large amount of *Aleurites moluccana* oil. Also known as tung seed oil, it is known to cause sweating on contact and can cause acute contact dermatitis. It is also a good source of linolenic and linoleic acids, but so is evening primrose oil, without the negatives (Source: www.naturaldatabase.com).

☹ $$$ **Studio Moisture Fix** *($29.50 for 1.7 ounces)* is a slightly more emollient version of the Strobe Cream, but doesn't contain the same impressive array of antioxidants. This is still a good moisturizer for normal to dry skin, and works well under makeup (assuming your foundation is rated SPF 15 or greater).

☺ $$$ **Blot Film** *($12.50 for 30 sheets)* is a set of 30 uncoated sheets of thin plastic material with absorbent properties. They work well to soak up excess shine and perspiration. Whether you choose them over tissue paper–style blotting papers comes down to personal preference.

✓☺ $$$ **Lip Conditioner** *($12.50 for 0.5 ounce)* is an exemplary, stably packaged lip balm that's based around Vaseline, but contains appreciable amounts of several antioxidants and skin-identical substances. It is highly recommended for dry, chapped lips, and the tube applicator is convenient when you're on the go.

☹ **Lip Conditioner SPF 15** *($13.50 for 0.5 ounce)* leaves lips vulnerable to UVA damage because it does not contain titanium dioxide, zinc oxide, avobenzone, Tinosorb, or Mexoryl SX (ecamsule). Its formula is also not nearly as elegant as that of the regular Lip Conditioner.

☺ $$$ **Lip Conditioner Stick SPF 15** *($13.50)* contains 1% titanium dioxide, which is decent, but not great, UVA protection. A higher percentage would be far better for your lips. The balm itself is basic and will shield your lips against moisture loss while providing a smooth finish.

✓☺ **Prep + Prime Lip** *($14.50)* is a base that is applied before lipstick to facilitate application and prevent it from feathering into lines around the mouth. Guess what? It works! The silicone- and wax-based stick forms a great barrier to keep color in place, in a way similar to long-discontinued products such as The Body Shop's No Wander and Coty's Stop It! As good as this product is, keep in mind that it won't prevent greasy, slippery lip glosses from migrating into lines around the mouth. It works best with moderately creamy or satin matte lipstick formulas, of which M.A.C. has plenty!

☢ **Tinted Lip Conditioner SPF 15** *($14.50)* is an emollient tinted lip balm whose petrolatum and castor oil base will make dry, chapped lips feel better. If only the sunscreen included sufficient UVA-protecting ingredients, this would be recommended. As is, the colors are too sheer to provide any natural protection.

M.A.C. MAKEUP

M.A.C. MINERALIZE MAKEUP

FOUNDATION: ☺ **$$$ Mineralize SPF 15 Foundation Loose** *($29)*. I had to stifle a chuckle as I watched the M.A.C. salesperson bring out the testers for this loose-powder "mineral" foundation. They were in a black plastic bag, which was dusty with powder. As she removed each shade, even though all were capped, powder was everywhere. Therein is one of my major gripes about this type of makeup: it is incredibly messy unless it comes in a component that minimizes powder spill. M.A.C.'s packaging doesn't quite cut it, but I've seen worse. In terms of performance, this wins points for its all-titanium dioxide sunscreen and feather-light, mica-based texture. Although this provides light to barely medium coverage, it feels like you're wearing nothing at all. Shine is there, but definitely on the subtle side. This has a dry matte finish but still casts a soft glow on skin. Among the nine shades, Light, Light Medium, and Medium are excellent. The middle range of colors—Medium Plus, Medium Deep, and Dark—tends to be slightly peach to orange, and should be considered carefully. The Deeper Dark shade is a very good bronze tone for those who want a loose bronzing powder without a rosy cast. The cap for this foundation features a sponge for applying the makeup. It works decently, but a larger sponge or full (meaning dense) powder brush is preferred. All told, this is a fairly impressive entry into the ever-expanding category of mineral makeup. However, at the department store, the mineral foundation champ remains Laura Mercier.

☹ **$$$ Mineralize Satinfinish SPF 15** *($28)* has so much going for it, yet the sunscreen lacks sufficient UVA protection. Surprisingly for this mineral-themed foundation, M.A.C. did not opt to use titanium dioxide or zinc oxide for the sunscreen, a typical standard in this category of makeup. This fluid foundation dispenses from a pump and has a beautifully smooth texture and soft matte finish that gives a good dimensional (rather than flat) quality to skin. Achieving medium coverage is easy; in fact, this is difficult to make sheer. It has a hint of shine and is available in 18 shades, of which the following should be considered carefully due to their peachy casts: NW30, NW35 (way too peach for most), NW43 (also quite peach), and NW45. This is a product to consider if you have normal to slightly dry or slightly oily skin and are willing to pair it with a separate product during the day that contains the UVA-protecting ingredients of zinc oxide, titanium dioxide, avobenzone, Tinosorb, or Mexoryl SX.

POWDER: ✓ ☺ **$$$ Mineralize Skinfinish** *($26.50)* is a sheer, talc-based pressed powder that looks wonderfully natural on skin. It's almost impossible to make this powder look heavy, thick, or dry. Those with normal to dry skin will appreciate the slight sheen this leaves behind (and remember, talc is a mineral, too, so M.A.C.'s name for this product is accurate). All four shades are neutral and highly recommended, but there are no options for very dark skin tones.

BLUSH: ☺ **$$$ Mineralize Blush** *($21)* is a shine-infused pressed-powder blush that has a silky, slightly dry texture and reliable application with an even color deposit. The marbleized pattern of each shade is infused with sparkles that give this blush its shiny finish, and they tend to cling well. This is a very good blush for those looking to color and add shine to their cheeks.

EYESHADOW: ☹ **$$$ Mineralize Eye Shadow Trio** *($17.50)* is truly an eyeshadow addition the M.A.C. line did not need. The color combinations are either shocking or just plain odd, and the domed strips of powder shadow have no dividers, which makes using them with almost any size eyeshadow brush especially tricky. The colors on either side of the trio apply smoothly and deposit color well, but the center strip is garishly shiny and applies sheer, and the shine flakes in short order (and in this case, we're talking large flecks of glitter on cheeks and lashes). When you consider that the "minerals" in this shadow aren't contributing to it in a good way, the concept becomes silly and unattractive.

M.A.C. PRO MAKEUP

FOUNDATION: ☹ **$$$ Full Coverage Foundation** *($28)* is a creamy, thick compact makeup whose level of coverage is indeed full and more akin to a concealer than a traditional foundation. The concentrated formula blends out well, leaving a cream finish. It no longer includes sunscreen, and is best for normal to dry skin that needs serious camouflage. M.A.C. offers 18 shades for fair to dark skin tones, and most are quite good. The only troublesome colors are the peachy NW25 and pink NW30. Shade C35 is excellent for concealing dark circles on light skin tones.

☹ **$$$ Hyper Real SPF 15 Foundation** *($28)* lacks the UVA-protecting ingredients of titanium dioxide, zinc oxide, avobenzone, Tinosorb, or Mexoryl SX, and so is not to be relied on for daytime protection. This is otherwise a very good foundation whose slightly thick, lotion-like texture blends to a smooth matte (in feel) finish that has enough soft shine to make skin look radiant rather than glittery. Coverage runs from light to medium and the formula is best for normal to oily skin. The range of 15 shades offers many beautiful options for fair to dark skin tones. The only shades to view cautiously are NC500 and NW500 (both are slightly peach). NW700 is a beautiful non-ashy shade for dark skin tones, while Bronze Reflections has a soft, peachy gold shimmer that's attractive on medium to tan skin.

POWDER: ☺ **$$$ Hyper Real Pressed Powder** *($23)* is talc-based powder with a soft shimmer finish. Available exclusively in M.A.C. Pro stores, the six shades are best for highlighting areas of skin rather than for dusting all over. Half the shades fall into the category of color correctors, but the sheer application has minimal corrective impact (which in this case is good). The flesh-toned shades to consider include Extra Light, Light, and Medium.

☹ **$$$ Blot Powder Loose** *($21)* is identical to M.A.C.'s Set Powder (reviewed below) but is more widely available and comes in four classic shades for medium to dark skin tones. It leaves a soft, sheer matte finish and is absorbent enough to help manage oily areas. Still, neither this nor the Set Powder is in the same league as the Select Sheer powders.

OTHER M.A.C. MAKEUP

FOUNDATION: ✓ ☺ **$$$ Select SPF 15 Moistureblend** *($29)* gets everything right, from its elegantly creamy texture (those of you with dry to very dry skin, take note!) and soft glow finish to its brilliant, in-part zinc oxide sunscreen. Not a cream-to-powder makeup, but instead a plant oil–based creamy compact makeup, this blends superbly and is neither too greasy nor too slick. Coverage stays in the medium range (this isn't an easy foundation to make sheer), but the finish keeps skin looking fresh and dimensional. The range of 23 shades is remarkably good, and includes options for all skin tones. The only shades to consider carefully are the slightly pink-to-peach NW30 and the obviously peach NW25.

✓☺ **$$$ Studio Sculpt SPF 15 Foundation** *($28)* is a creamy liquid foundation with an in-part titanium dioxide sunscreen that doesn't offer the user any greater sculpting abilities than any other foundation. Besides, it isn't foundation that plays a large role in sculpting the face via makeup; that type of detailing is done with contouring, blush, and eyeshadow placement (plus proper blending). Aside from the name, as a foundation with sunscreen, this is a workable option for those with normal to slightly dry or oily skin. It dispenses somewhat thick at first, but softens as it warms to skin temperature. Application is smooth and even, and this provides no less than medium coverage (you can get nearly full coverage if needed). It finishes satin-matte with a powdery feel, and does a reasonable job of keeping shine in check. Another attribute of this foundation is its long-wearing, tenacious nature. It holds up really well if you perspire (those in humid climates, take note) and requires more than a water-soluble cleanser when you're ready to remove it. As usual, M.A.C's shade range is extensive and mostly impeccable; there are equally good options for fair to dark skin tones. The shades to avoid due to overtones of orange, peach, or copper are NC45, NW30, NW35, and NW45. The NC35 shade is slightly peach but workable for medium skin tones. Studio Sculpt SPF 15 Foundation deserves a Paula's Pick for its sunscreen, long-wearing nature, and blending ease. The formula also contains some antioxidants, but it isn't packaged to keep them stable during use unless you keep the translucent tube away from light.

✓☺ **$$$ Studio Stick Foundation SPF 15** *($29)* is a stick foundation that includes an in-part titanium dioxide sunscreen for UVA protection. It has a silky, initially creamy texture that allows ample play time before it sets, providing light to medium coverage. This layers well for additional coverage over more obvious imperfections; it also can be sheered out, but keep in mind that doing so will reduce the amount of sun protection. As usual, M.A.C.'s shade selection is mostly top-notch; among the 18 options to consider only two shades should be avoided—NC40 and NC45 can be too peach for most skin tones. As with all foundations of this type, the ingredients that keep the product in stick form can be potentially problematic for blemish-prone or very oily skin. Studio Stick Foundation is ideal for normal to slightly dry or slightly oily skin. Just make sure any dry areas are smoothed before applying, because this foundation's somewhat powdery finish will not be kind to them.

✓☺ **Studio Fix Powder Plus Foundation** *($26)* remains one of the top pressed-powder foundations available, despite several impressive entries from other companies. It has an exceptionally silky, talc-based texture that applies and blends like a dream. As usual, wet or dry application is possible, but using this wet poses the risk of streaking. Dry application provides light to medium-full coverage. If you prefer this type of foundation and have normal to slightly dry or slightly oily skin, it is highly recommended. Almost all of the 37 colors are impressive (albeit repetitive) for a broad range of skin tones, but the following shades are best avoided due to pink, orange, or peach overtones: C6, NC42, NW25, NW30, NW40, and NC40.

☺ **$$$ Studio Tech Foundation** *($29)* is a next-generation cream-to-powder foundation that offers a lighter, almost weightless texture, smooth application, and a soft satin finish that tends not to grab onto dry areas. It combines the super-light feel of a water-to-powder makeup with the slip and smoothness of silicone-based cream-to-powder makeups. Studio Tech applies easily and provides light to medium coverage. A staggering range of 27 shades is available, with suitable options for very light (NC15, NW15) and darker (NW50, NW55) skin tones. Although the majority of the shades lean toward neutral, six of them are too orange or peach for their intended skin tones: NC40, NC45, NC55, NW25, NW30, and NW40. This formula is best for normal to slightly dry and dry skin—the non-matte, non-powdery finish won't do much to temper shine, and even though this is not traditional cream-to-powder makeup, enough waxes and thickeners are present to make it problematic for those battling blemishes. If your skin fills the bill for this makeup, it's certainly worth checking out.

☺ **$$$ Face and Body Foundation** *($32)* comes in a 4-ounce bottle and is very liquidy and sheer. It takes some patience to blend on because it tends to slide around a lot before drying. This can be layered for more coverage (as can most foundations) and is reasonably waterproof. For body makeup it can be a problem, however, because it can come off on clothes, and it's not a great choice for major flaws you want to fully conceal. There are 11 shades, and most are neutral and workable. The deeper shades can be sketchy because most of them have a slight peach-to-red cast that won't work for many skin tones. This also contains grapefruit oil, though likely not enough to cause irritation.

☺ **$$$ Select SPF 15** *($26)* has a formula very similar to the Studio Fix Fluid SPF 15 below, and is another M.A.C. foundation whose sunscreen lacks sufficient UVA-protecting ingredients. If you're already using a separate sunscreen rated SPF 15 or higher and want to give this a try, it has a fluid, lightweight texture that blends easily and sets to a silky matte finish. This offers slightly less coverage than the Studio Fix Fluid and is preferred for normal to slightly dry or slightly oily skin. Among the 21 mostly excellent shades are a few duds: NC45 is slightly orange, NW25 slightly peach, NW35 very peach, NW45 a bit too coppery, and NW50 slightly ash.

☺ **$$$ Studio Fix Fluid SPF 15** *($26)* has so much going for it, but it doesn't come out a winner because it lacks UVA-protecting ingredients. If you're willing to wear an effective sunscreen underneath, this has a beautifully silky texture and ultra-smooth application that sets to a natural matte finish. Best for normal to oily skin, Studio Fix Fluid provides medium coverage and comes in 23 shades, of which only 4 are poor contenders: NC55 is too ash, NW30 and NW35 too peach, and NW45 has a copper overtone that makes it a tough match for darker skin tones. NW50 and NW55 are ideal shades for dark skin, and there are options for very light skin, too.

CONCEALER: ✓ ☺ **Select Cover-Up** *($15.50)* is a great concealer. Lightly creamy with a natural matte finish, this liquid concealer provides good camouflage with minimal risk of creasing. Fifteen mostly neutral shades are available, plus four color correctors, of which Colour Corrector Peach is an OK option. Colour Corrector Pink may work for some porcelain skin tones, though it has an opalescent finish. Of the regular shades, the ones to be cautious with are NC45, NW35, and NW45.

☺ **Select Moisturecover** *($15.50)* is another great liquid concealer, though this definitely has a creamy feel. Easy to control during application and providing medium to full coverage, this sets to a smooth finish that's minimally prone to creasing. The palette of 15 shades is practically a case study in neutral to yellow tones for fair to dark skin, and the only color to consider carefully is the slightly peach NW30.

☺ **Studio Finish Concealer SPF 35** *($15.50)* has a formidable sunscreen that's in-part titanium dioxide, and the creamy texture is smoother and thus easier to blend. This is still a full-coverage concealer, and it takes practice to achieve the level of coverage you want without using too much product. It is excellent for concealing redness, dark circles, and other discolorations, but too emollient to use over blemishes. A wide range of shades is available, and almost all of them are exceptional. NC42 is too yellow for most skin tones, while NC45, NW35, and NW40 suffer from peach overtones. NW45 is too coppery for most dark skin tones, but the deeper NW50 is ideal. Fair to light skin tones will find more than one suitable shade, so be sure to test this at the counter before making a purchase.

☺ **Studio Stick Concealer** *($15.50)* is the partner product to M.A.C.'s Studio Stick Foundation, and this creamy, full-coverage concealer nicely complements it. Smooth, even coverage is obtainable with one stroke, and this concealer blends exceptionally well considering its opacity. It's a superb option for concealing dark circles and other discolorations, but has a slight tendency to crease before the end of the day when used under the eyes. There are 15 shades and, given the number of shades, there are some to avoid, including NC45 (too orange), NW15 (too white but may be an option for porcelain skin), and NW25, NW30, and NW40 (all three of which are too peach).

☹ **$$$ Studio Sculpt Concealer** *($16.50)* is a thick, creamy concealer with just enough slip to make blending a non-issue, but it remains creamy and is crease-prone unless set with powder. Even when you use powder, this concealer's finish doesn't hold up nearly as well as its partner product, Studio Sculpt SPF 15 Foundation. Still, it provides good coverage without looking heavy and the shade range is impressive. You'll find colors for fair to dark skin tones and only a few to avoid. Those to avoid are the peachy NW30 and the orange-ish NC50, and consider NC42 carefully. One other comment: This concealer is packaged in a heavy glass jar that some will find cumbersome, especially for travel.

POWDER: ✓ ☺ **$$$ Prep + Prime Transparent Finishing Powder** *($21)* is described as "an invisible way to set makeup." It has a finely milled cornstarch-based texture that feels weightless and, despite its pure white color, actually does go on transparent. I asked a M.A.C. makeup artist with a darker skin tone to show me how this powder looked on her hand, and sure enough, it didn't appear whitish or ashen. This finishes matte with just a hint of shine, and is a good choice for oily skin that needs extra absorbency. This is not recommended for blemish-prone skin because cornstarch can "feed" the bacteria that contribute to acne. This loose powder can be used over most shades of foundation without affecting the color.

✓ ☺ **$$$ Select Sheer Loose Powder** *($21)* sets a new powder precedent by offering an ultralight texture that seems to disappear into the skin, yet provides a smooth, dimensional, polished finish. The talc-based formula has an understated shine that is visible, but that doesn't detract from this powder's incredibly light texture and fine finish. The 14 shades are typically M.A.C., meaning there are many noteworthy neutral tones. Each shade goes on very sheer and imparts just a hint of color, so getting an exact match isn't essential, and the choices are plentiful. NW35 is a beautiful option for bronzing powder, and shade NC5 is for the most porcelain skin tone.

✓ ☺ **$$$ Select Sheer Pressed Powder** *($21)* is basically a pressed version of the Select Sheer Loose Powder, except that this powder does not have any shine and, as is true for most pressed powders when compared to loose powders, it offers more coverage. Most of the 17 shades are exceptional, although NW43 may be a touch too copper for some dark skin tones and NW50 is slightly ash. Shade NC55 makes an excellent bronzing powder color. Overall, this is a wonderful pressed powder, especially if you want a finished look but aren't a fan of traditional powders. Those with oily skin may find this not absorbent enough, but it's still worth auditioning.

☹ **$$$ Blot Powder Pressed** *($21)* has been reformulated and is now a talc-free, silicone-based powder that feels silky yet looks a bit chalky and dry on skin. It is best for taming oily skin, and all five shades are worth considering—but check the finish in natural light to make sure you like it.

☺ **$$$ Iridescent Powder Loose** *($21)* comes in a tub, and this talc-free powder is appropriately named. The two sheer colors do well in terms of providing high shine, but the shine doesn't cling as well as the Iridescent Powder Pressed, so the effect doesn't last as long.

☺ **$$$ Iridescent Powder Pressed** *($21)* has a dry, slightly grainy, talc-based texture and is available in two pale, iridescent shades that impart noticeable shine and cling moderately well.

☹ **$$$ Set Powder** *($24)* is a talc-based loose powder that contains silica and film-forming agent to create a waterproof finish. Sold exclusively at M.A.C. Pro stores (which, confusingly, are not the same as "regular" M.A.C. stores), it comes in several shades, many of which are color correctors. However, because this goes on so sheer and isn't much for pigment, any correction is very subtle. It does help waterproof your complexion, but so will many other powders that contain similar ingredients.

BLUSH AND BRONZER: ✓ ☺ **$$$ Bronzing Powder** *($21)* is a talc-based, pressed-powder bronzer with an extremely smooth texture and dry finish. It comes in five believable tan shades, three of which have a very shiny finish. Matte Bronze is truly matte and Bronze is almost matte. Looking to spend less money for similar results? Try Wet 'n' Wild's Bronzer ($2.99).

☺ **$$$ Blushcreme** *($18)* brings back the old-fashioned (in a good way) true cream blush. Those with dry to very dry skin, take note: The emollient, oil-based feel and dewy finish of this blush make skin look radiant and healthy. The colors are all classics, with an equal representation of warm (peach) and cool (pink/rose) tones. The moist texture takes some getting used to during blending, so be sure to use less than you think you need and blend purposefully for best results. This does not work for those with normal to oily skin or if you have enlarged pores over the cheek area.

☺ **$$$ Powder Blush - Satins** *($18)* presents almost 50 shades, from the palest pinks and peaches to the deepest browns and plums. The vast palette is divided into five finishes and two formulas. The Satins feel silkier than the Mattes or Frosts and have good pigmentation with less of a tendency to grab.

☺ **$$$ Powder Blush - Sheertone/Sheertone Shimmer** *($18)*. Best among the powder blushes are the Sheertone and Sheertone Shimmer shades. Although both lack the pigmentation of the other M.A.C. blushes, they apply extremely well and have a super-silky texture, and the regular Sheertone comes in a beautiful range of true matte colors. The Sheertone Shimmer version is just that, sheer colors with a soft shimmer finish. They work well for evening makeup, but most have too much shine for daytime, at least if you work in a professional environment. Both Sheertone formulas have limited options for darker skin tones, but fair to medium skin tones are well served.

☹ **$$$ Powder Blush - Frosts** *($18)* have the same dry texture and application as the Mattes below, but each shade has a soft to medium shimmer finish.

☹ **$$$ Powder Blush - Mattes** *($18)* are a standard, pressed-powder blush with a reasonably smooth application and dry texture that causes the colors (especially the deeper shades) to grab a bit.

☹ **$$$ Cream Colour Base** *($16.50)* has been around for years, and the color collection keeps expanding, so there must be a lot of people buying these somewhat slick, crease-prone (when used as eyeshadow) colors. The shade range offers options for eyes, lips, and cheeks, and their intensity varies, so this is definitely a product to test at the counter before purchasing. The creamy base is ill-advised for blemish-prone skin, but normal to dry skin looking to add a soft, radiant (or iridescent, depending on the shade) glow may want to give this a try.

EYESHADOW: ✓ ☺ **Eye Shadows - Veluxe** *($14.50)*. Veluxe shades (don't ask me what Veluxe means; I assume it's a combination of velvet and luxurious) have the most beautifully silky texture and even application. I wish there were more shades, but the following shades are excellent: Dovefeather, Llama, Samoa Silk, Mink Pink, and Brown Down.

✓ ☺ **Matte2 Eye Shadow** *($14.50)* marks the resurgence of eyeshadows that have a true matte finish (other trend-driven lines, such as Urban Decay, are following suit), which is great! This time around the emphasis is on creating a dimensional rather than a flat matte finish, courtesy of improved pigment technology. The result is definitely matte, but more skin-like than the many chalky matte eyeshadows from years ago. However, there have always been exemplary matte eyeshadows to be found; it was just difficult to locate them in a sea of shiny eyeshadows (which have also come a long way over the years). M.A.C. has produced a pressed-powder eyeshadow with a luxuriously smooth, almost creamy-feeling texture that, as expected, blends easily. That fact is a plus because all of the shades (including some odd ones, mentioned below) are pigment-rich. You'll get excellent coverage with these shadows, and they have a silky-smooth finish with staying power. Among the mostly workable selection of shades, avoid Post Haste, Clarity, and Newly Minted, which are all very strong, bright colors that are difficult to work with and do nothing to shape or shade the eye.

✓ ☺ **$$$ Paint Pot** *($16.50)* comes in, you guessed it, a pot. Basically a newfangled version of a cream-to-powder eyeshadow, Paint Pots have a soft, buttery texture that leads to a smooth, even application, whether applied with a natural-hair or synthetic brush (the synthetic brush produces a stronger color, while natural-hair brushes net a softer color deposit). These set quickly to a long-wearing, waterproof powder finish, so be sure blending is quick and precise. Once set, these absolutely do not crease, fade, or smudge, which is very impressive. All of the colors are workable, though some are a bit too colorful. The only matte option (and also a great base color for the eyelid) is Painterly. The others have a soft to brazen shine. Because of Paint Pot's finish, you can apply other shadows or pencil liner over it without disruption.

☺ **Eye Shadows - Matte and Satin** *($14.50)*. The Eye Shadows maintain the same almost-smooth, dry texture they've had for the past several years. The only real difference this time around is that many of the colors go on softer and sheerer. You'll notice less of this with the medium to dark shades, which tend to go on grainier and deeper than they look and don't blend as evenly as the best eyeshadows, but there is minimal flaking. These are not the smoothest shadows in town, but they do the job. Although the shades are labeled Satin, Frost, Lustre, Matte, Velvet, Veluxe, and Veluxe Pearl, they are arranged by color, not formula or finish, on the tester unit. The large number of Matte (most of the shades are indeed matte) and Satin shades apply much better, though the darker Matte shades drag a bit, so blending must be precise.

☺ **$$$ Paint** *($16.50)* is essentially a cleverly named and packaged cream-to-powder eye-shadow. Dispensed from a tube (don't apply too much pressure because you'll end up wasting product), the concentrated formula blends very well and has a natural opacity that can almost take the place of your foundation or concealer as a means for evening-out skin on the eyelid and under-brow area. Most of the 20 colors are neutral and workable yet supply intense shine. There are a few softer shades that can work for a mildly shiny look. Paints can be used alone or mixed with other products, and they sheer out well if you prefer a subtle wash of color. Regardless of color or shine intensity, these tend not to crease and last all day without fading or smearing.

☺ **Prep + Prime Eye** *($16)* works well as a cream-to-powder concealer for the eye area as well as for other discolorations. Its creamy texture quickly morphs into a silky, weightless matte finish that is minimally prone to creasing. The finish can look slightly powdery, but the effect is canceled once eyeshadow is blended over it. The five shades present options for light to dark skin tones, but nothing for someone with porcelain to fair skin. But that's OK, because although this product has its purpose, it is easily replaced by a matte-finish concealer, such as M.A.C. Select Cover-Up.

☺ **Eye Shadows - Veluxe Pearl** *($14.50)* have a drier texture and slightly flaky application, and the colors have a strong metallic finish. Not bad, but a couple of steps down from the regular Veluxe.

☹ **$$$ Shadestick** *($16.50)* is a twist-up, retractable eyeshadow stick whose texture is neither creamy nor too dry. Unfortunately, it is still dry enough to make using it as eyeshadow a problem because it tends to drag and pull over eyelid skin, though it creases surprisingly little. This works best to emphasize the lower lash line, or to dot across the upper lash line and blend with a brush or your fingertip for a smoky, deliberately smudged look. Each shade is shine-laden, a finish that is not kind if you have moderate wrinkles. For the most versatility, I still prefer M.A.C's powder eyeshadows, used wet or dry with all manner of eyeshadow and eye-lining brushes.

☹ **Eye Shadows - Lustre and Velvet** *($14.50)*. Among the various finishes and formulas, the most problematic are Lustre and Velvet due to their grainy, difficult-to-blend texture and flaky shine.

EYE AND BROW SHAPER: ✓ ☺ **Eye Brow Pencils** *($14.50)* are automatic, nonretractable, ultra-sleek pencils that apply easily and impart soft color without being greasy or smudging. The colors are brow-perfect, but don't ask me to explain the sexually charged names such as Stud, Lingering, and Fling!

✓ ☺ **Fluidline** *($15 for 0.1 ounce)* is nearly identical to Bobbi Brown's Long-Wear Gel Eyeliner, a once-unique product of which I am a fan because of its remarkably easy application and tenacious wear. Long Wear Gel Eyeliner, M.A.C. Fluidline, and Stila's Smudge Pots are the only eyeliners that can stand up to oily eyelids without fading, smearing, or running. All of these have a slightly moist application that sets to a long-wearing matte finish. Fluidline is every bit as tenacious as Brown's Long-Wear Gel Eyeliner, but the colors are mostly … well, they're odd. Yes, classic browns and black are available, but the majority of the shades are not meant to define the eye so much as to add a shock of color. Peacock blue and bright purple are indeed eye-catching, but neither fulfills the main purpose of eyeliner, which is to define and accent the eye and enhance the depth of eyelashes. Not surprisingly, the M.A.C. counters and stores I visited while doing research were consistently sold out of the black and brown shades, but had plenty of the Halloween-appropriate tones! Rich Ground, Dipdown, and Blacktrack are the most versatile choices.

✓ ☺ **$$$ Penultimate Eyeliner** *($16.50)*. What a great name for a liquid eyeliner! The precision brush allows one to draw an extremely thin line that can be easily thickened with a successive coat. Application is even, it dries fast (which is desirable because it minimizes the chance of smearing), and, once set, it lasts quite well. Those with moderately oily to oily eyelids will find this a bit smudge-prone and not preferred to silicone-enhanced gel liners (such as M.A.C. Fluidline). If oily eyelids aren't a concern and you prefer liquid liners, this is a terrific choice. It is available only in Rapidblack, which is rich and dramatic.

✓ ☺ **Technakohl Liner** *($14.50 for 0.01 ounce)* is the eyeliner pencil to choose if you want a smooth application that doesn't drag or skip while imparting rich color. Initially creamy, this automatic, retractable pencil's formula sets to a soft powder finish that remains smudge-resistant. All but one of the shades are laced with shine, so if that's not on your must list, stick with Brownborder. And unless your eye-lining goal is to draw attention to the liner rather than to your eyes, skip Jade Way, Auto-de-blu, and Smoothblue.

☺ **$$$ Liquid Eye Liner** *($16.50)* is fairly straightforward, applying nicely with a thicker, firmer brush than the Liquidlast Liner, yet with a faster dry time. You're unlikely to experience flaking or smearing.

☺ **$$$ Liquidlast Liner** *($16.50)* has a thin, flexible brush to ensure even application (assuming you have a steady hand). Dry time is average, so this isn't a liquid liner for anyone who flinches easily. Once set, it wears quite well, fading only slightly, and without smearing or flaking. Coco Bar and Point Black are the classic colors for a variety of eye-makeup designs. The remaining shades have a strong shimmer or metallic finish that is best for evening makeup and not appropriate for wrinkled eyelids.

☺ **Brow Set** *($13.50)*. Brow Set is a basic brow gel formula that comes with a very good brush and has a minimally sticky finish. The Clear option is best; the others imbue brows or lashes with noticeable shimmer and have a tacky finish that can feel strange.

☺ **Eye Kohl** *($14.50)* is another group of pencils that are an unnecessary addition, but here's one more twist on the creamy, standard pencil formula. The chance of smearing is slightly less than for the Eye Pencils, but don't bet on them not smearing, despite their powdery finish.

☺ **Eye Pencils** *($13)* are utterly standard (right down to the commonplace colors) and comparable to most of the other pencils out there. For lining the eyes, M.A.C.'s matte eyeshadows or Fluidline shades are a better alternative.

☺ **Powerpoint Eye Pencil** *($14.50)* glides on with no tugging or skipping, but smears easily before it sets. Allow a minute or two for this to set, and you will be treated to several hours of fail-safe wear. As usual, M.A.C.'s shade selection is a mix of classic (brown and black) shades with trendy and unusual shades (jade green) meant to satisfy a wide variety of tastes. The soft, creamy texture of this pencil means it is difficult to create a fine, thin line, but it works great for thicker or smokier lines. The only other drawback? It needs to be sharpened, which keeps it from earning a happy face rating.

☹ **Brow Finisher** *($15)* is a twist-up, waxy, tinted stick that's packaged like a brow pencil. The texture is so waxy that application is difficult and it tends to stick brow hairs together, not to mention the waxy smell (all of the testers I played with had an "off" odor). This also feels tacky on brows and isn't something most women would want to tolerate given the variety of other options (including clear and tinted brow gels) that groom and define while being almost imperceptible.

LIPSTICK, LIP GLOSS, AND LIPLINER: M.A.C.'s **Lipsticks** are a standout attraction of this line. The majority of the formulas provide lush textures and feel comfortable, and the color range is nearly unparalleled. The ✓ ☺**Amplified Cremes** *($14)* are excellent and among the best cream lipsticks anywhere. They're similar to the Satin Lipsticks, but these offer enhanced opaqueness and a touch more gloss. The ✓ ☺ **Mattes** *($14)* are not true mattes, but come pretty close with their deeply pigmented, full-coverage colors and non-glossy finish. ✓ ☺ **Satins** *($14)* are softly creamy with a rich, opaque texture and moist finish, and offer the best compromise of long wear and desirable creaminess. ☺ **Frosts** *($14)* are creamy lipsticks with medium coverage and a soft-shimmer to true-frost finish, available in over 30 colors; ☺ **Glazes** *($14)* were the predecessors to Lustre Lipsticks and present a much smaller shade selection. The colors are sheerer and less glossy than the Lustres. ☺ **Lustres** *($14)* are M.A.C.'s largest collection of sheer lipsticks, each with a glossy finish and enough slip to easily make its way into any lines around the mouth. If that's not an issue for you, these are worth checking out.

✓ ☺ **$$$ Cremesheen Glass** *($18)* is, believe it or not, a unique lip gloss. Think of it as a cross between a standard brush-on gloss and a lip balm and you'll have a good idea of how it feels and looks on lips. In a word, the effect is beautiful. The texture is very smooth and it leaves lips with a balm-like sheen that fills in superficial lip lines. The shade range is pleasing, and tends to favor sheer pastels and brighter tones.

✓ ☺ **Lipgelee** *($14)* is a far cry from the thick, sticky feel of M.A.C.'s Lipglass or Tinted Lipglass reviewed below. Packaged in a tube with an angled plastic applicator, Lipgelee is wonderfully smooth, completely non-sticky, and provides a high-shine finish. The shades appear much bolder than they look on the lips, so if you're looking for a sheer gloss, this should be on your short list.

✓ ☺ **$$$ Pro Longwear Lipcolour** *($20)* is M.A.C.'s version of Max Factor's Lipfinity. It is a dual-sided product, one end holding the lip color and the other a brush-on, glossy top coat. Although the concept is the same as Lipfinity, Outlast from Cover Girl, and all the other imitators, M.A.C.'s version excels because the colors go on so easily and evenly with a single application and, more important, because the top coat feels better than those of competing products. It actually goes a long way, not only in keeping lips glossy, but also in preventing the color beneath from chipping or peeling as the top coat wears off. As a result, you get amazingly long-lasting lip color combined with a superior top coat that keeps up appearances, and that makes this option from M.A.C. a must-try. You could argue that M.A.C. has attempted to mimic the technology Procter & Gamble developed for their Max Factor and Cover Girl long-wearing lipsticks, but the way I see it, M.A.C. took a good thing and made it even better—improvement is the new sincerest form of flattery!

✓ ☺ **$$$ Pro Longwear Lustre Lipcolour** *($21)* is a departure from the original Pro Longwear in two ways: the colors (they're less opaque, though not sheer) and the accompanying top coat, called Mirror (which is infused with multi-colored glitter rather than being clear and glossy). The application process and impressive wear time are the same, but I am not a fan of the glittery top coat because it limits the use of the striking but soft colors of the Pro Longwear Lustre Lipcolour. The good news is you can purchase one of M.A.C.'s other top coats to accompany the Lustre shade you like—the bad news is it must be purchased separately (it screws onto the color-base component so you can alternate top coats as needed). See if you like the glittery top coat before committing to this. Otherwise, this product is highly recommended.

☺ **$$$ Dazzleglass Lipcolour** *($16.50)* was once a limited-edition gloss, but has become a stable part of M.A.C.'s line due to its popularity. The sheer- to light-coverage shades are infused with crystalline-like sparkles that cast a sultry multi-dimensional shine to lips. Unlike many sparkle-infused lip glosses, the sparkle particles are very tiny, so they look sophisticated rather than showy, and they don't feel grainy as the moisturizing feel of the gloss wears away. The slightly thick texture isn't as uncomfortably sticky as M.A.C.'s Lipglass, but it isn't as smooth as that of their outstanding Lipgelee, either. Consider this a middle-of-the-road option whose main selling point (beyond the shade selection) is its, to borrow from the product's name, dazzling shine.

☺ **Lip Treatment** *($14)* is a standard, colorless lipstick designed to work as a lip balm. It does just that, but no better than any of M.A.C.'s other lipsticks.

☺ **Lustreglass** *($14)* has the same wet-look shine as M.A.C.'s original Lipglass (below), but the Lustre version kicks up the color, so this is more of a lipstick/gloss hybrid than standard gloss. The brush applicator helps the gloss glide on, and considering this gloss' thicker texture, it is comparably non-sticky. The shimmer-infused shades feature mostly conservative (meaning softer and less intense) choices that should please most gloss fans, especially if they plan to apply this over a regular lipstick.

☺ **Pro Longwear Gloss Coat** *($14)* is described in the review for Pro Longwear Lipcolour above, and is available in five finishes to be purchased separately. Whichever one you choose, each fits the component for either of M.A.C.'s Pro Longwear formulas. Mirror adds a sparkling shine with multicolored glitter; and Clear is the original top coat, which adds a wet-look shine without shimmer or glitter.

☺ **Slimshine Lipstick** *($14.50)* is for women who prefer sheer, glossy colors. That's exactly what this smooth, lightweight lipstick provides, and the color range is a smart blend of the trendy along with the tried-and-true. These slim lipsticks have a very glossy finish but aren't the least bit sticky. They're not much for longevity (and not for anyone prone to lipstick bleeding into lines around the mouth), but if those concerns don't apply to you, this is another sheer lipstick to consider.

☺ **Cremestick Liner** *($14.50)* is an automatic, retractable lip pencil that comes in an enticing range of neutral, versatile shades, but that's the best compliment I can offer. This pencil is too creamy for its own good. The creaminess enhances application, but because it stays creamy, you'll find it fades and is definitely capable of traveling into lines around the mouth. One other point: This applies sheer, so if you want to define your mouth you need to layer quite a bit, which only makes the creamy finish more fleeting.

☺ **Lip Pencils** *($13)* have a superior color selection, but that's the only thing that separates these standard, needs-sharpening pencils from nearly identical pencils found in almost every other line.

☹ **Lipglass, Clear and Tinted** *($14)* are very thick, tenacious glosses whose heavy, syrupy texture is not for everyone. The tinted version has a slightly thinner texture and comes in a tube with a wand applicator; original Lipglass is packaged in a squeeze tube. The extensive shade range for Tinted Lipglass goes from sheer to dramatic.

☹ **Plushglass** *($17.50)* is similar to Clinique's Full Potential Lips Plump and Shine, but omits the peppermint oil. Still around to irritate lips into a plump state are ginger root and capsicum (pepper) oils, neither of which are great to use consistently. This is otherwise a standard sheer lip gloss with a smooth feel and minimally sticky finish (it does feel nicer than Clinique's version). Compared to Clinique's plumping option, the omission of peppermint oil makes this the lesser of two evils, though it's still difficult to recommend for anything but occasional use.

MASCARA: ✓ ☺ **Pro Lash Mascara** *($12)* is in a league all its own! This home-run mascara builds dramatic thickness and length, while being only slightly difficult to control. It's almost too easy to over-apply this mascara, so be sure to exercise restraint to avoid a heavy, clumped appearance. Otherwise, you will be impressed at how quickly this revs up your lashes!

✓ ☺ **Zoom Lash Mascara** *($12)* can go on a bit too heavily (especially if you're too zealous while applying it), but it builds impressive thickness with minimal effort and does so without bothersome clumps or smudges. This is also supposed to curl lashes, but the effect is subtle; you'll still need your eyelash curler (assuming you ordinarily use one). This mascara is best for those who want lash drama, not demureness.

☺ **Plush Lash** *($12)* doesn't, despite its name, leave lashes feeling or looking all that plush. The oversized brush is difficult to work with, but with practice, the results can be evenly defined, long, and slightly curled lashes. Thickness doesn't come easily to this mascara, even with successive coats—though you can apply a lot of this without a hint of clumping. Although this has its strong points, it is not preferred to M.A.C.'s Zoom Lash or Pro Lash mascaras, both of which produce results that wow and leave lashes feeling plush.

☺ **Pro Longlash Mascara** *($12)* is touted as extreme lengthening mascara, and it does lengthen—just not that well or that fast. It adds no thickness and finishes lashes with a soft curl. But for all the promises, it just doesn't have the "wow" factor of the Pro Lash Mascara.

☺ **Splashproof Lash Waterproof Mascara** *($12)* allows you to create lasting thickness and length with minimal effort, though it can clump slightly as it builds. This is also tenaciously waterproof, and a bit difficult to remove (have a silicone- or oil-based makeup remover handy). This mascara competes nicely with the top choices from drugstore lines Maybelline New York, L'Oreal, and Jane, and is only a bit more expensive.

☺ **$$$ Dazzle Lash** *($12)* is supposed to create the effect of a starburst pattern of lashes. It certainly makes lashes longer and the brush tends to bunch lashes together with minimal clumping for an elongated, stylized look that leaves lashes looking slightly wet and with a subtle shimmer. The result is flattering, but definitely not for everyone, which may be why the M.A.C. salesperson kept trying to get me to consider one of their other mascaras instead. (It's not often I go to purchase a mascara and the salesperson says, "Are you sure?") After wearing this for a day, I found out why—the fibers, which add bulk to the lashes, tend to flake and get into the eye. I was finding traces of this mascara around my eye even after washing it off, which is not a good sign. This is not crowd-pleasing mascara, but I understand why some will find its effect alluring.

☺ **Fibre Rich Lash Mascara** *($12)* does contain tiny, hair-like fibers, but unlike similar mascaras from a decade or more ago, these fibers tend to stay on the lashes rather than flake off (and into your eyes) throughout the day. Why M.A.C. needed this mascara is a question worth asking because, aside from the fibers, it doesn't distinguish itself from their Pro Lash or Pro Longlash Mascaras. It does just an OK job and doesn't impress with its lengthening ability.

☺ **Mascara X** *($12.50)* is said to deliver dramatically longer, thicker lashes, but it isn't nearly as impressive as M.A.C.'s newer mascaras, not to mention that several L'Oreal and Maybelline New York mascaras outperform this one at half the cost.

☺ **Prep + Prime Lash** *($13.50)* is meant to smooth and condition lashes, but doesn't do much better in this regard than most mascaras—there is nothing in this product that is all that conditioning for lashes, though it does make them feel soft. It is also supposed to intensify "the build and lengthening quality of all [mascara] formulas," but that didn't happen. Side-by-side testing confirmed what is true of almost all lash primers: they tend to make mascara trickier to apply and don't help lengthen or thicken lashes any more than simply applying two or three coats of regular mascara. I suppose this is an OK option if you're using a lackluster mascara, but the bigger question is why you're not using a superior mascara, given how many there are! This does make a noticeable difference with average mascaras.

FACE ILLUMINATING/SHIMMER PRODUCTS: ☺ **$$$ Pigment** *($19.50)* comes in small jars of shiny loose powder, available in almost every color imaginable and with a shininess scale that goes from sheer to POW! Most of the colors cling surprisingly well and allow you to create an array of effects. The shades labeled Glitter cling terribly and flake everywhere. Although Pigments can be messy to use, they add some kick to evening or special-occasion makeup. The best colors include Naked, Dark Soul, Melon, Tan, Vanilla, and Chocolate Brown.

BRUSHES: ✓☺ **M.A.C. Brushes** *($11-$71)* are one of the best selections of brushes you'll find anywhere (over 40 different brushes). The big brushes are a little pricey, but they last forever if you take care of them. Though there are indeed good, inexpensive brushes to be found, if you're going to splurge, this is one area where the extra expense won't be wasted. Be sure to check out M.A.C.'s variety of eyeshadow brushes, particularly the **#275 Medium Angled Shading Brush** *($24.50)*, an excellent, versatile eyeshadow brush. Also, test the **#217 Blending Brush** *($22.50)*. Other top choices include the **#168 Large Angled Contour Brush** *($32)*, **#192 Cheek/Face Brush** *($32)*, **#194 Concealer Brush** *($18.50)*, **#208 Small Angled Brow Brush** *($19)*, **#219 Pencil Brush** *($23)*, **#239 Eye Shading Brush** *($24.50)*, **#242 Shader Brush** *($23)*, **#249 Large Shader Brush** *($27)*, and all of the various **Angled Shader Brushes** *($17-$24.50)*. Avoid the **#202 Replaceable Sponge Tip Applicator***($18.50)*, which comes free in most eyeshadow kits, as well as the **#204 Lash Brush** *($11)*, which is easily duplicated by washing off an old mascara wand. The freestanding M.A.C. stores sell pricier brushes known as M.A.C. Pro brushes, and these are definitely worth a look, especially if you're a working makeup artist with a generous budget. In particular, **Brush #136** *($62)* and **Brush #174** *($71)* are softer, more refined versions of M.A.C.'s regular loose-powder brushes. ☺ **Brush Cleanser** *($11)* is an alcohol-based solution that does remove makeup and excess oil from brushes, but will eventually make natural hair dry and stiff. Although it's OK for occasional quick cleanups, washing your brushes with a gentle shampoo and water is preferred.

☺ **$$$ Carry All Case** *($225)* is a sturdy, multi-compartment makeup case for die-hard makeup artists only, and even they may find it lacking. It excels in durability and overall quality—you could toss this down a flight of stairs and it wouldn't register a dent—but I would have preferred more organizational versatility. You get one deep central compartment with two smaller top-storage compartments that swivel out on sturdy hinges. Some drawers or a secret compartment or two would have gone a long way toward making this a must-have accessory to house your color and brushes. The case can be locked and also comes with a removable shoulder strap for travel, features professional makeup artists will appreciate.

SPECIALTY PRODUCTS: ✓☺ **Prep + Prime Line Filler** *($19.50 for 0.5 ounce)*. Now this is what I mean by a well-formulated primer! Rather than just being a mix of silicones and fragrance, this combines a dry-finish silicone polymer with emollients, film-forming agents, and copious antioxidants to help smooth skin, temporarily fill in superficial lines, and create an even canvas for foundation. It is similar to any well-formulated serum because it leaves skin feeling silky while imparting lots of beneficial extras that go beyond just prepping skin for makeup. The line-filling ability of this Prep + Prime product is minor and short-lived, but it will make a subtle difference. The matte finish of this product makes it suitable for all skin types, but those of you who tend to break out may want to choose a serum that doesn't contain emollients. The good news is there are plenty of serums that meet that description.

☺ **$$$ Prep + Prime Face Protect SPF 50** *($28 for 1 ounce)* is disappointing given the price tag and the shortage of antioxidants. It is otherwise a very good in-part zinc oxide sunscreen in a silicone-enriched base that is ideal for use under makeup. The amount of zinc oxide leaves a slight white cast, but this is a non-issue if you're going to follow with foundation. Unless you are prone to breakouts from zinc oxide, this is an excellent, fragrance-free daytime moisturizer (or primer, if you prefer) for normal to very oily skin.

☺ **$$$ Prep + Prime Skin** *($23)* is an ultralight, fragrance-free lotion meant to be applied to skin before foundation. This product doesn't necessarily prime skin better than similar products labeled as moisturizers, gels, or serums, but it does indeed create a silky-smooth, non-greasy surface that facilitates makeup application. Whether it's for you depends strictly on whether your skin needs help in this regard. Compared with other products sold as primers, this formula goes a bit further by being more than a mixture of silicones and water. Prep + Prime Skin contains appreciable amounts of plant extracts that serve as antioxidants and anti-inflammatory agents. It is a suitable formulation for normal to slightly dry or slightly oily skin, but has one potential drawback: shine. This M.A.C. product's shine is more obvious and more glittery than shimmery. If you don't mind added shine under your makeup (or on bare skin), this won't be an obstacle. All others are encouraged to sample this product with foundation to make sure the amount of shine is not objectionable.

☺ **$$$ Matte** *($18)* is a thick, but silky, silicone-based gel that creates a smooth skin texture and has a long-wearing matte finish. It isn't as absorbent as other products in this category (Smashbox's Anti-Shine trumps this one), but is nevertheless worth a try.

☹ **Clear Gloss** *($17.50)* is a thick, clear gloss meant to add "polish, shine and highlights to bare or made-up skin." It certainly adds shine, but why anyone would want to tolerate this product's sticky finish is a good question, especially when there are so many smooth, non-sticky shine alternatives. Applying this over makeup will ruin any careful blending, and if you have long hair, expect it to get stuck in this gloss.

MAKE UP FOR EVER

MAKE UP FOR EVER AT-A-GLANCE

Strengths: A couple of good cleansers and makeup removers; one good lip balm; the newer foundations have many wonderful qualities; impressive options (and shade ranges) for powders, powder blush, and powder eyeshadow; some extraordinary lip glosses and lipstick/lip color options (and again, the shade ranges are remarkable); a few formidable mascaras; good shimmer options; the huge selection of makeup brushes.

Weaknesses: Expensive; a few products suffer from needlessly irritating ingredients; average toner; the foundations and concealers that have been in this line longest are behind the times; mostly average eye and lip pencils; the Transparent Mascara; the Diamond Powder; mostly lackluster specialty products.

For more information on Make Up For Ever, call (877) 757-5175 or visit www.makeupforever.com or www.Beautypedia.com.

MAKE UP FOR EVER SKIN CARE

☹ **Extreme Cleanser, Balancing Cleansing Dry Oil** *($30 for 6.76 ounces)* is a lotion-textured creamy cleanser that contains a dry skin–compatible amount of oil, which also helps dissolve makeup. Despite this, it is not recommended for any skin type because it contains rosemary oil, pepper extract, and volatile fragrance components that can cause irritation.

☺ **$$$ Gentle Milk, Moisturizing Cleansing Milk** *($23 for 6.76 ounces)* omits most of the irritants found in the Extreme Cleanser, and is an OK option for normal to slightly dry skin not prone to blemishes. The milky cleanser removes makeup easily and leaves minimal residue. It would be better without the volatile fragrance components, but their presence is minor.

☺ **$$$ Pure Water, Moisturizing Cleansing Water** *($23 for 6.76 ounces)* is a basic liquid cleanser that combines slip agents with gentle detergent cleansing agents. It's an option for normal to slightly dry or slightly oily skin when minimal makeup is used, or as a morning cleanser.

☺ **$$$ So Divine, Moisturizing Cleansing Cream** *($27 for 4.4 ounces)* is a cold cream–style cleanser for very dry skin, and requires a washcloth for complete removal. The tiny amount of plant extracts either have a soothing quality or impart subtle fragrance.

☺ **$$$ Sens'Eyes, Waterproof Sensitive Eye Cleanser** *($23 for 3.38 ounces)* works well to remove waterproof eye makeup, but isn't preferred for sensitive eyes over similar but less expensive options from Almay, Neutrogena, or Clinique. This product is fragrance-free.

☹ **$$$ Cool Lotion, Moisturizing Soothing Lotion** *($23 for 6.76 ounces)* costs a lot for what amounts to an average toner that's primarily water, grape water, solvent, and slip agent. It's a mediocre option for normal to dry skin.

☹ **$$$ Mist & Fix** *($27 for 4.22 ounces)* is supposed to be used not only to touch up makeup but also to protect skin against external damage. This spray-on product consists primarily of water, slip agent (methylpropanediol, which absolutely won't refresh makeup), and film-forming agent, similar to what's used in hairsprays. This has a slightly sticky finish that can feel odd, but I suppose it does provide some protection from makeup fading and slipping. Overall, this is a gimmicky product that's a poor solution for those looking to reinforce or touch up makeup on the go. A good oil-blotting paper and quick dusting of pressed powder (and lipstick touch-up, of course) are much better.

☹ **$$$ HD Elixir** *($38 for 0.40 ounce)* is a lightweight moisturizer with a toner-like consistency. Its main ingredients are as ordinary and mundane as it gets: water, glycerin, slip agents, and a couple of emollient thickeners. Marketing this as a "breakthrough formula" is just silly; it's akin to suggesting a skateboard is a breakthrough vehicle. This contains a smattering of impressive ingredients, but the amounts are too small for your skin to notice. As for the hydration boost claim—"520% increase after 15 minutes"—it's just an overhyped and trivial skin effect. For example, simply sitting in the bathtub for several minutes can boost skin's hydration (water content) that much and more, but that's not good for skin. Too much water can disrupt skin's barrier function, leading to a loss of the critical substances skin needs to stay intact and healthy. In the end, you don't want this product to work as claimed—thankfully, it doesn't.

☺ **$$$ Stop Shining +** *($16)* is a thick, nonaqueous, silicone gel with absorbent properties meant for use over oily areas. It doesn't hold up all day, nor is it as effective as similar products from Clinique and Smashbox that combine silicones with absorbent magnesium, but it may be worth a try if your oily areas aren't too out of control.

☺ **$$$ Moisturizing Lip Balm** *($18)* is a colorless, emollient, glossy lip balm that works well to remedy and prevent dry, chapped lips. It does not contain any irritants and it does not feel too thick or waxy.

MAKE UP FOR EVER MAKEUP

FOUNDATION: ✓ ☺ **$$$ Duo Mat Powder Foundation** *($32)* provides everything a pressed-powder foundation should, and excels in each area. The talc- and silicone-based formula feels buttery smooth and blends on like a second skin. The slightly dry, non-chalky matte finish is ideal for normal to very oily skin, and this provides light to medium coverage that doesn't mask skin, but does make it look refined and polished. The selection of 11 shades is first-rate; the only questionable colors are the slightly orange 209 Warm Beige and the slightly peach 214 Dark Beige. Shades 216 Caramel and 218 Chocolate are beautiful for darker skin tones or used as matte bronzing powders. Shade 200 Beige Opalescent has a soft shine that will magnify oily areas. This powder foundation does contain fragrance.

✓☺ **$$$ HD Invisible Cover Foundation** *($40)*. This water- and silicone-based liquid foundation is among the best of the best, assuming your preferences mesh with what it provides. The creamy, fluid texture has great slip, but not so much that blending is a problem. It sets to a natural matte finish that looks incredibly skin-like, while offering medium to almost full coverage. The pigment technology behind this makeup, like many of today's best foundations, allows it to blur imperfections and improve skin tone without feeling or looking like a mask. The selection of no less than 25 shades is staggering, and staggeringly good, too. The range offers options for fair to very dark skin tones, and the pump-bottle packaging is sleek and easy to use. As is often the case when a product has more than two dozen shades, not all of them are slam dunks. The following shades are not recommended because they are too rose, pink, orange, or peach: 135 Vanilla, 145 Neutral, 150 Pink Beige, 160 Golden Beige, 170 Caramel, and 165 Honey Beige. The shades 177 Cognac, 178 Chestnut, and 180 Brown are beautiful dark tones; 125 Sand is slightly peach, but still worth considering; and 130 Warm Ivory is slightly pink, but may work for some light skin tones. Whether you choose this for day-to-day or on-camera use, its skin-perfecting qualities are exemplary. The formula makes it best for normal to very oily skin.

✓☺ **$$$ Mat Velvet + Mattifying Foundation** *($34 for 1.01 ounces)* has a thin, fluid texture with enough slip to allow smooth blending before setting to a strong matte finish. Coverage goes from medium to almost full, and this foundation camouflages diffuse redness on skin quite well. The absorbent formula is ideal for oily to very oily skin, with the only caveat being the prominence of cornstarch and its potential for feeding the bacteria responsible for blemishes. Sixteen mostly impressive shades are available. The ones to avoid due to obvious peach or orange tones are Sand, Neutral Beige, and Golden Beige. Soft Beige and Honey Beige may be too peach for some skin tones, but are worth a look. Alabaster is a superb shade for very fair skin, while the Brown and Chocolate shades are gorgeous, non-ashy shades for ebony skin tones.

✓☺ **$$$ Powder Foundation** *($40)* is talc-based and has an outstanding, finely milled texture that sweeps over skin, providing a flawless, soft powder finish with sheer coverage. All four shades are exemplary. Note: Some shades list SPF 8, but the ingredient list does not indicate any sunscreens, so don't rely on this powder foundation for any amount of sun protection. This is recommended for all skin types except very dry.

☺ **$$$ Face and Body Liquid Makeup** *($38)* is a liquidy, water-based foundation that also contains a blend of silicone and mineral oil, so this has a good amount of slip on the skin, yet blends readily to a natural matte finish. Coverage can go from sheer to medium, and allows you to build coverage without it looking thick. The collection of ten shades is deceiving, because many of them look too peach or pink in the bottle, yet almost all of them end up being soft and neutral on the skin—plus there are equally good options for light and dark skin tones. Test Natural 3 and Bronzed Beige 26 carefully, as both finish slightly peach. This can be used on the body if desired, but it isn't as tenacious or clingy as products like DermaBlend, so the results can be mixed. This lightweight formula works best for normal to slightly dry or slightly oily skin.

☹ **$$$ Liquid Lift Foundation** *($41)* is overpriced for what amounts to a very basic formula that absolutely cannot lift skin or impart a tightening effect. It has a fluid, silky texture and nice slip, which makes blending easy. Coverage is medium and it leaves a slightly dewy finish suitable for someone with normal to dry skin. Among the six shades (best for fair to medium skin) only Golden Beige 5 stands out as too peach.

☹ **$$$ Pan Stick** *($30)* has a thick, petrolatum- and wax-based creamy texture that's not too far removed from traditional theatrical makeup. Unless you need full coverage and are willing to trade that for a makeup that doesn't look natural no matter how well it's blended, this has limited appeal. Considering the ingredients, it doesn't feel or look as oily as you'd think. Five shades are offered, and only Caramel 5W is slightly peach. The others, while heavy, are surprisingly neutral.

CONCEALER: ✓ ☺ **$$$ Full Cover Concealer** *($30).* Take the name for this concealer seriously, because Make Up For Ever certainly did! This fairly thick concealer softens on contact with skin and provides superior coverage for all manner of discolorations and flaws. It has minimal slip, so is best dotted on small areas and blended quickly. It sets to a long-wearing matte finish that resists creasing, but the texture and drier finish of the product is capable of exacerbating lines around the eye, which is true for concealers in general. Most of the shades are remarkable and there are options for fair to dark skin tones. Beige 8 and Dark Beige 12 are slightly peach, but still worth considering; avoid Fawn 14, which is decidedly orange. Ebony 20 is very dark and has a slight ash finish, so consider it carefully if your skin tone is dark enough to warrant using this color. Full Cover Concealer is excellent to use over blemishes and to cover the pink to red marks that linger after a blemish has healed.

☺ **$$$ Lift Concealer** *($22)* begins liquidy, but dries quickly to a long-lasting, powdery matte finish. It provides good coverage that you can build to move up from light to medium coverage. This water-, talc-, and silicone-based formula comes in a tube and is best for oily skin or for use over oily areas. Five shades are available, with the best ones being Medium Beige 2, Neutral Beige 3, and Matte Beige 4. By the way, this won't lift skin in the least, so don't bank on that benefit.

☹ **$$$ 5-Camouflage Cream Palette** *($36)* comes in a palette with four flesh-toned colors that veer slightly to the peachy side, along with a green color corrector. You can blend the shades together to create a custom match, but unless you need significant coverage and are willing to put up with this difficult texture, this is easy to pass up. The waxes in this concealer are a poor choice for use over blemishes, but do lend an opacity that helps conceal red marks, dark circles, or flat scars.

☹ **$$$ Camouflage Cream** *($18)* is a range of cream concealers that are identical to those in Make Up For Ever's Camouflage Cream Palette above. The palettes hold five shades, and the most popular shade in each palette is now sold separately exclusively at Sephora. Each has a thick, creamy texture that applies decently and offers full coverage (those with stubborn dark circles, take note). The formula makes this not the easiest to work with, but it's still an option if you need significant coverage. Avoid all of the color-correcting shades because they look nothing like real skin and they are so pigmented you'll need another product to cover the obvious, "wrong" shade you've just applied. The shades to avoid include Yellow Green 16, Green 17, Mauve 18, Pink 19, and Orange 20.

☹ **Concealer Pencil** *($18)* is a dual-sided pencil that comes in two different skin tones, one for lighter skin and one for medium skin. It's greasy, looks heavy, and is unsuitable for use over blemishes.

POWDER: ✓ ☺ **$$$ Super Matte Loose Powder** *($24)* has a super fine, ultralight texture and a soft, dry finish that's ideal for oily skin. This talc- and silica-based loose powder looks beautiful on skin, and all of the three translucent shades are great.

☺ **$$$ Compact Powder** *($30)* is talc-based and has a silky, dry texture and sheer finish that doesn't look chalky or too powdery on skin. The three shades are all decent, but this isn't quite as good as the Super Matte Loose Powder.

☺ **$$$ Velvet Finish Compact Powder** *($29)* has a talc- and kaolin (clay)-based texture that feels slightly thick and dry, but it applies smoothly, leaving a velvety matte finish. Failing to blend carefully or brushing on too much of this powder results in a chalky appearance, so use restraint. Each of the eight shades applies lighter than it appears in the compact, but all of them are very good. Caramel and Chocolate are great for dark skin tones or for use as bronzing powder on medium to tan skin tones.

☹ **$$$ High Definition Microfinish Powder** *($30)* has a sole ingredient of silica in this one-shade-fits-all loose powder. This dry-finish mineral is engineered to have a very unusual texture in this powder, which it does. A simple touch and you'll know that it is truly unusual. It has a strange sensation of movement and feels unbelievably and immeasurably silky. So while touching it may feel good, wearing it is an entirely different issue, and one you won't find as interesting. Although this is designed to be "universally flattering," it wouldn't be flattering on anyone. The silica will exaggerate even the slightest amount of dry skin, while the whiteness of this powder can make even fair skin tones look artificially pale. Moreover, this is simply too sheer to completely even out all skin tones as claimed. High definition may be akin to high-tech, but this powder doesn't give you a visage that will have you ready for an extreme close-up.

BLUSH AND BRONZER: ✓ ☺ **$$$ Sculpting Blush Powder Blush** *($24)* ranks as Make Up For Ever's best lineup of powder blush in the last ten years. The talc- and clay-based formula feels gossamer smooth and applies evenly. Almost all of the colors are matte but still beautifully enliven skin, and the pigmentation is strong (so begin with a sheer application and build color as needed). Shade #2 Matte Blue Pink has the faintest hint of pink and won't show up as "blush," even on someone with very fair skin (but it's OK as a highlighting powder). Shades #24 Matte Fawn, #26 Matte Sienna, and #28 Brown Brick are workable, warm-toned hues for women of color.

☺ **$$$ Mat Bronze** *($30)* is a good talc-based bronzing powder whose smooth texture prompts a noticeable color payoff and even application. All of the shades are matte, which is a real find in this age of shimmering bronzing powders. I just wish the shade range were more bronze-like. As is, the best shade is Earth 6. Dark Bronze 4 is good, too, but for some reason tends to grab on skin more than the other colors. Light Bronze 0 and Medium Bronze 2 are too fleshy or peachy to approximate a tan.

☺ **$$$ Powder Blush** *($19)* comes in a bountiful array of shades, from the pinkest pinks to the most understated neutrals. These are strongly pigmented shades, and without careful, sheer application they tend to grab on the skin, which is a side effect of this blush's drier texture. Use restraint and you likely will be pleased with the results and the long wear. Several shiny shades are also available, and the good news is the shine clings well and applies evenly.

EYESHADOW: ☺ **$$$ Aqua Black Waterproof Cream Eye Shadow** *($22)* is a pure-black cream eyeshadow and meant to be your secret weapon for creating the ultimate smoky eye. Applied with the brush of your choice, this glides on easily and sets to a soft matte finish that resists smearing. The formula allows enough time before drying for you to "smoke out" the effect, and then layer for added intensity. It is waterproof, as claimed. Although pure black is a severe way to go about creating a smoky eye, this product serves its purpose and, used carefully and artfully, works well.

☺ **$$$ Eyeshadow** *($19)* has a texture, application, and intensity that are nearly identical to those of the Powder Blush. The range of shades is staggering (125 in all, though most Sephora boutiques only stock a fraction of them), with some of the most imaginative (and largely unnecessary) shades right next to the earth and neutral tones that are universally flattering. These apply evenly, and most of the shades provide opaque coverage, which lets them last without creasing or fading.

☺ **$$$ Diamond Shadow** *($20)* is positioned as a long-wearing iridescent eyeshadow, but the large particles of holographic glitter don't cling well—you'll notice them on cheeks and clothing shortly after application. Although these shadows have a dry, almost grainy texture, and they blend smoothly, which is a positive, the shade range presents mostly unworkable options unless you want strong, contrasting colors to make more of a statement than your eyes do.

☺ **$$$ Pearly Waterproof Eyeshadow Pencil** *($18)* is a standard chubby pencil with a creamy texture that glides over the skin and imparts sheer, shimmering color. This pencil is not preferred to the Eyeshadow, but some will undoubtedly find it intriguing, and the formula is waterproof.

EYE AND BROW SHAPER: ☺ **$$$ Aqua Creamliner** *($20 for 0.14 ounce)* is similar to the many long-wearing gel eyeliners being sold at department stores. Make Up For Ever's point of difference is a creamier formula that contains some oil, so don't expect this to last as long as the competition. Still, application is swift and pigmented and it sets quickly and won't budge, at least not for several hours. Those with oily eyelids may find this breaks down before they'd like; others without that problem may want to give this an audition.

☺ **$$$ Color Liner** *($19)* is a good liquid eyeliner that features a soft but firm-textured brush and a formula that applies easily and dries quickly. All of the colors have a strong iridescent finish, making them best for evening makeup on unwrinkled eyelids. Best of all, once dry, the formula holds up remarkably well.

☺ **$$$ Waterproof Eyebrow Corrector** *($19)* is a creamy liquid eyebrow tint packaged in a squeeze tube. The idea is to dispense a small amount on your brow brush and then fill in and shade the brows. It's an intriguing way to experiment with brow color and, with practice, you can create defined brows that look natural. All of the shades are workable and best for dark blonde to dark brown brows. If you need your brow color to be waterproof, this fills the bill, and once set, it doesn't smudge or smear.

☺ **$$$ Aqua Eyes Waterproof Eyeliner Pencil** *($17)* needs sharpening and has an unusual base of cottonseed and jojoba oils, neither of which is as waterproof as silicone-based pencils, though it does hold up to minimal water exposure (think crying versus swimming). Although the application is creamy, this sets to a tacky finish that stays put. All of the shades are laced with shine, so choose carefully. Turquoise 7L is recommended only if you're a performer in Cirque de Soleil.

☺ **$$$ Eyebrow Pencil** *($18)* has to be sharpened, which is a pain, but it applies very smooth and has a lightweight, non-waxy texture and a soft powder finish that won't smear or smudge. All of the colors are workable (and matte), making this an easy recommendation if you don't mind sharpening.

☺ **$$$ Waterproof Eyeliner** *($22)* has an ultra-thin brush that applies the slow-drying liquid liner well. It is reasonably waterproof once set, but has a tendency to fade, making it an average choice and not really worth its price.

☺ **$$$ Eye Pencil** *($16)* needs routine sharpening and has a slightly stiff, fine-tipped application that finishes slightly creamy. It's OK, but rather basic for the money. Avoid Dark Blue 11 and Bright Blue 31.

☹ **Kohl Eye Pencil** *($17)* is a substandard pencil that applies too thick, flakes a bit, and is very prone to smearing. Avoid it unless you like eye makeup that demands constant upkeep!

LIPSTICK, LIP GLOSS, AND LIPLINER: ✓☺ $$$ **Fascinating Lip Gloss** *($18)* is applied with a sponge tip and is just as smooth and refreshingly non-sticky as the Super Lip Gloss. It has a slightly lighter texture and all of the sheer colors are infused with glitter, but it doesn't feel grainy on the lips.

✓☺ $$$ **Liquid Lip Color** *($20)* remains a favorite, but the shade selection has been streamlined since the previous review. The ultra-smooth texture imparts intense, opaque color and a completely non-sticky, high-gloss finish. This lipstick/gloss hybrid comes in a tube with a brush applicator, and the opening of the tube is large enough to prevent the brush from splaying—a major plus. Consider this a must-try if you like the opacity of lipstick with the finish of a lip gloss.

✓☺ $$$ **Super Lip Gloss** *($16)* is a favorite of Make Up For Ever fans, and it's not hard to see why. This is one of the smoothest, least sticky glosses you're likely to find. It comes in a tube and is silicone-based, so it can feel slippery (and can encourage lipstick feathering if you're prone to that), but women who have a problem with bleeding lipstick should stay away from glosses in the first place. The available shades are beautiful and include some unconventional (but sheer) options.

☺ $$$ **Lipstick** *($19)* is the general name for Make Up For Ever's newest lipstick option, available in four finishes, each with the same basic formula (what differs is the level of pigment). The **Lacquered Creams** *($19)* are shades numbered in the 200s, and are lightweight yet sufficiently creamy, with medium coverage and a slight gloss finish. **Pearly** *($19)* are shades numbered in the 300s, and are identical to the Lacquered Creams, but with a soft, pearlescent finish. **Lacquered Transparent** *($18)* are shades numbered in the 400s, and offer sheer to light coverage and a gorgeous selection of colors, each with a soft glossy finish and minimally greasy texture. The **Mattes** *($19)* are shades numbered in the 500s and provide opaque coverage and opulent colors, but do not have a true matte finish—it's definitely creamy—but these last the longest due to the high level of pigment. The red shades in this range are stunning!

☺ $$$ **Aqua Lip Waterproof Lipliner Pencil** *($17)* is a standard, needs-sharpening lip pencil that glides on swiftly for quick application, but remains creamy until it has set (which takes a few minutes); after it sets, it feels a bit tacky. This is waterproof, yet comes off easily with a water- and detergent-based makeup remover. The shade range is quite good, with no oddities and plenty of pink-brown and red tones. As you may know, most lip pencils are waterproof to some extent simply because of the silicones and waxes used to create them. This pricier option is OK, but doesn't distinguish itself in any positive way from less expensive pencils.

☺ $$$ **Lip Pencil** *($16)* is a standard pencil with a good creamy application and some unique but wearable shades among a few standbys. It's longer than most, so keep in mind that that makes it a tough fit for small makeup bags.

☺ $$$ **Matte Lip** *($20)* is designed to be used over lipstick to minimize a glossy or creamy finish. It's somewhat odd given that you can achieve this finish by simply choosing a demi-matte or regular matte lipstick. Dabbing this colorless, cornstarch-based cream over lipstick can be a messy task, but it does mattify and is an option if applied very carefully.

☹ **Glossy Full** *($20)* adds a striking vinyl sheen to lips when applied over any lipstick. Essentially a colorless lip gloss, this product loses points for its undeniable mint flavor and for containing fragrance components that can be irritating to lips. The amount of pentapeptide won't plump lips even a little.

MASCARA: ✓☺ $$$ **Lengthening Mascara** *($19)* has a small brush that provides big results, and quickly. This is a fantastic lengthening mascara that just doesn't know when to stop, making lashes impossibly long, all without clumps. Thickness is incidental, but for lash-fluttering length that wears all day, this excels!

✓ ☺ $$$ **Lengthening Waterproof Mascara** *($20)* has been improved and is an excellent lengthening mascara that is indeed waterproof. The tiny, tailored brush allows easy access to every lash, extending them beautifully, but building little in the way of thickness. Clumps are absent though, so if length and waterproofing are what you're after, this works beautifully.

☹ $$$ **Smoky Lash Extra Black Mascara** *($22)* is a very black mascara that makes eyes noticeably more dramatic, especially if you have fair to light skin and light-colored eyes. It goes on a bit heavy, but builds considerable length and separates lashes well. Unless you wipe down the wand before applying, you will notice some slight flaking, which is not great news for any mascara, especially one in this price range. However, the flaking doesn't occur throughout the day, so if you're craving very dark, long lashes, this may be worth auditioning.

☹ $$$ **Volume Mascara** *($19)* comes off easily with a water-soluble cleanser, but is otherwise very boring and doesn't live up to its enticing name, at least if your expectation is thick, voluminous lashes.

☹ **Aqua Smoky Lash Waterproof Extra Black Mascara** *($22)*. It has been a long time since I've been so disappointed by a mascara. This extra-black formula definitely makes lashes dramatically dark, but its messy, uneven application smears from the beginning and doesn't let up. Within moments I noticed flaking and by midday my entire upper lash line was splotched with smeary mascara. All this for average length and a formula that is moderately waterproof. Even though much of it comes off before you want it to, removing the rest of it is no easy feat—the ultimate irony for one of the worst waterproof mascaras in recent memory.

☹ **Transparent Mascara** *($18)*. Transparent Mascara is basically a styling-gel formula in mascara form. The small brush works for lashes and brows, but the clear gel is too sticky for either. Considering the number of inexpensive non-sticky and minimally sticky brow gels, this isn't worth the bother.

FACE AND BODY ILLUMINATING/SHIMMER PRODUCTS: ☺ $$$ **Compact Shine On** *($29)* is a smooth-textured, talc-based pressed powder with a shine that has elements of subtle glow (finely milled shimmer pigments) and visible sparkles (which, while visible, aren't gaudy). The shine clings better than you'd expect, and all three shades are soft, sheer options for highlighting areas of the face or body.

☺ $$$ **Diamond Cream** *($36)* presents shimmer in lotion form and it's another concentrated product, so apply sparingly until you get the desired effect. It does have a slightly tacky finish, but the shine doesn't flake. It actually works best mixed with a standard body lotion for a soft glow.

☺ $$$ **Shine-On Powder** *($26)* has an honest name, as most powders with shine also claim to keep skin matte while concurrently adding sparkles to the skin. This talc-based loose powder has a pleasant texture and its finely milled shiny shades work well for a low-key evening look.

☺ $$$ **Star Powder** *($18)* is simply a very shiny loose powder that comes in a wide variety of shades, from gold and silver to lots of pastel hues, as well as finishes ranging from soft shimmer to metallic. They're versatile and include several deeper colors for dramatic effects, and they cling reasonably well. Be forewarned, however, a little goes a long way and even tiny amounts can be messy to use, so build slowly.

☹ **Diamond Powder** *($24)* offers truly diamond-like shine in the form of another messy loose powder. Unfortunately, although the effect is very cool, the powder flakes endlessly and feels slightly grainy.

BRUSHES: ✓ ☺ **$$$ HD Kabuki Brush** *($39)* is a short, squatty powder brush that is composed of exquisitely soft, dense bristles, which work beautifully to deposit powder on skin. Unless you simply can't get used to the stubby handle, this is an excellent powder brush to consider. It comes with its own zippered case for storage or travel.

✓ ☺ **Make Up For Ever Brushes** *($13-$54)* have something to offer everyone, whether you're a makeup brush neophyte or connoisseur. The brushes include both natural and synthetic hair options, and the majority are expertly shaped and sized appropriately for their intended purpose. There are some superfluous ones to consider carefully, but that chiefly depends on what your needs are. All in all, the choices are plentiful and the prices are comparatively reasonable. The only unfortunate element is that most Sephora stores sell only a small portion of this company's brushes. To view the entire collection, you need to find a Make Up For Ever counter in a department store or visit their flagship store in New York.

SPECIALTY PRODUCTS: ☺ **$$$ HD Microperfecting Primer** *($32)*. As a makeup primer this works fine, but the inclusion of color-correcting pigments (something almost all other primers exclude) is a twist worth ignoring. The biggest offenders in this group are the Green and Mauve shades, both of which, though sheer, add an odd tone to skin that doesn't mesh well with foundation and that definitely don't fly on their own. The Blue color is barely blue (which is good) and applies like an ethereal white. As such, it is an acceptable option for very fair skin tones with a pink cast that needs neutralizing. The Neutral shade adds a soft luminescence to skin, while Caramel and Yellow (which isn't pure yellow, rather more of a neutral putty color) also are workable options. The silky, lightweight texture of this primer helps smooth and enhance skin texture while adding a subtle shine that can boost dull or sallow complexions. The "nourishing" ingredients mentioned in the claims for this primer are present in such tiny amounts that your skin won't notice, so this isn't preferred to prepping your skin with a silky serum that contains beneficial ingredients. Still, this is worth a try if you need to brighten your complexion or tone down (in a subtle manner) an uneven skin tone. Be sure to test this in natural light before purchasing—something Sephora stores (where this product is exclusive) readily allow.

☺ **$$$ UV Prime SPF 50/PA +++** *($30)* straddles the line between a primer (which usually is silicone based and nearly weightless) and a lightweight moisturizer with sunscreen. The sun protection is plentiful and powered by titanium dioxide for sufficient UVA protection. The formula lends it a silky texture and a finish that gets progressively matte as it sets. However, it doesn't make skin look flat or dull, although it does leave a soft white cast. You get what can only be described as a matte glow. This works great under makeup, especially for those with normal to oily skin. It would be rated a Paula's Pick if the formula contained a more substantial amount or range of antioxidants and it was formulated without potentially irritating fragrance chemicals.

☺ **Aquarelle** *($18)* is a specialty makeup item that Make Up For Ever recommends using for detail work on the face or body. (Think theatrical or Halloween costume makeup for drawing tattoo-like designs on your skin.) Aquarelle is a liquid body paint available in several colors, from soft pastels with shimmer to rich primary colors. It's easy to work with, dries quickly (the formula has quite a bit of alcohol in it), and lasts until you remove it. This is an option if your makeup needs require such a product.

☺ **$$$ Lip Palettes** *($39)* feature the new lipstick formula in its various versions packaged in a slim palette with a workable brush. The mix of shades is complementary, allowing you to blend two or three together for an attractive custom color.

☺ **Eyelashes Individual** *($15)* are sold in a kit that includes several smaller bunches of natural lashes without going overboard. The individual pieces can be cut to size, but before you attempt that, make sure you have the hang of the application and removal process.

☺ **Eyelashes Strip** *($15)* consists of just what the name states: strips of reusable false eyelashes. They're sold in a variety of styles, from subtle strips meant to be affixed to corner lashes to full-on theatrical sets that don't work for daily makeup unless your makeup icon is RuPaul or your profession is being a drag queen. Note that these lashes are not sold with glue, so you need to purchase that separately.

☹ **$$$ Eye Seal** *($20)* is meant to turn any powder-based eye makeup into a waterproof formula. The alcohol-free liquid formula contains quick-drying solvents and film-forming agents that are water-resistant, but application is an issue. For example, when you use a brush to apply Eye Seal over, say, a powder eyeshadow, the fluid removes the makeup. I couldn't figure out a way around this, but the Sephora salesperson had a solution: apply the powder product to your hand, then add a drop of Eye Seal and mix it together with the brush. That worked better, but it's messy and the results can still be uneven. In short, the formula contains ingredients typically seen in eye-makeup removers, although it's intended to enhance the longevity of makeup. I'd advise you to leave this on the shelf and use almost any other way to line your eyes.

☹ **$$$ All Mat, Face Matifying Primer** *($45 for 1.01 ounces)* creates a smooth matte finish thanks to its formula of silicone, slip agent, silicone polymers, and mineral-based absorbents. It is an option for normal to very oily skin looking to prolong a matte finish, but what a shame this pricey product lacks truly helpful ingredients for skin. If anything, the fragrance chemicals in this primer put skin at risk for irritation.

☹ **$$$ Flash Color** *($18)* comes in a theatrical range of colors, including several shades rarely seen in everyday makeup (bright yellow, kelly green, and day-glo orange among them). Meant for use on eyes, cheeks, or lips, this potted cream product has a texture that works best on lips. It is workable as a cream blush if your skin is dry to very dry; used as eyeshadow, this will crease almost immediately and few of the shades are usable for shaping and shading the eyes. As lip color, the red, purple, and burgundy hues have a good stain, though this isn't as fast or convenient to apply as a standard lipstick.

☺ **Pure Pigments** *($13)* is exactly as the name states: pure cosmetic pigments ready for a variety of uses. Sold in a tiny jar with a built-in sifter, each color is presented in powder form. The pigmentation is intense, but can be blended on sheer if you're careful. Although this can be mixed with almost any makeup product, from eyeshadow to blush or lip gloss, the colors aren't what anyone would consider understated. Most are vivid hues that have no practical place in day-to-day makeup. However, a theatrical or special effects makeup artist would find this product quite useful. Note that when used by itself, Pure Pigments tends to have a dry finish and uneven application.

☺ **Star Glitter** *($13)*. If you want flecks of multi-colored loose glitter shaped like five-sided stars, this is the product for you. Although it's more arts-and-crafts project than sophisticated, easy-to-work-with makeup, this is an OK option for special occasions if you're in the mood to confetti yourself before others throw some your way.

☹ **Glitter** *($13)*. Glitter is glitter, and in this case, just like in kindergarten art class, these tiny pots spread sparkles anywhere you want them to go as well as places where you don't want them. The problem is with the product's extremely poor cling factor. It gets everywhere without staying where you originally placed it.

MARCELLE (CANADA ONLY)

MARCELLE AT-A-GLANCE

Strengths: Inexpensive; Marcelle provides complete ingredient lists on its Web site; drugstores that retail this brand provide testers, including makeup testers; almost every product is fragrance-free; some good cleansers and makeup removers; impressive eyeshadows; great lipsticks and lip glosses.

Weaknesses: The hypoallergenic claims are bogus, as is this brand positioning itself as being a smart choice for those with sensitive skin; formaldehyde-releasing preservatives, not recommended for those with sensitive skin; the anti-acne products are mostly alcohol, which is damaging to skin and can increase oil production, making acne worse; dated moisturizer formulas; some greasy cleansers; a general lack of state-of-the-art ingredients; foundations with sunscreen do not provide sufficient UVA protection; average to poor mineral makeup; no shades for those with tan or darker complexions; mostly lackluster mascaras.

For more information about Marcelle, call (800) 387-7710 or visit www.marcelle.com or www.beautypedia.com.

Note: All prices are in Canadian dollars.

MARCELLE SKIN CARE

MARCELLE AC-SOLUTION PRODUCTS

☹ **AC-Solution Anti-Imperfections Purifying Foaming Cleanser** *($13.50 for 5.07 ounces)* contains sodium C14-C16 olefin sulfonate as the main cleansing agent, which means it is too drying and irritating for all skin types. The salicylic acid isn't helpful for acne-prone skin because it must be left on the skin to provide any benefit, and cleansers must be rinsed from the skin because if they're left on, they damage the skin.

☹ **AC-Solution Anti-Imperfections Clarifying Lotion** *($13.50 for 6.76 ounces)* lists alcohol as the second ingredient, which isn't what you want to see. Alcohol causes irritation and free-radical damage, and stimulates oil production in the pore. I am also concerned that the amount of pH-adjusting agent, sodium hydroxide (lye), is high enough (the fourth ingredient) that it will cause further dryness and irritation.

☹ **AC-Solution Anti-Imperfections Oil-Free Moisturizing Regulating Lotion** *($19.95 for 1.7 ounces)* is nothing this problematic BHA product can regulate, at least not in a good way. The amount of alcohol it contains will only help skin become more irritated, red, and dry. This absolutely cannot keep drier areas "superbly hydrated," and the alcohol, due to the irritation it generates, will stimulate oil production in the pore, which may lead to more breakouts and inflammation of existing acne lesions. With some minor formulary adjustments, this could have been an effective BHA product for blemished skin.

☹ **AC-Solution Blemish Control** *($9.95 for 0.2 ounce)*. Alcohol is the first ingredient in this seriously problematic anti-acne product. Actually, it would be more accurate to call this pro-acne. The blend of glycolic and salicylic acids would make it capable of exfoliating skin, but the alcohol-caused irritation and inflammation, surface dryness, and enhanced oil production in the pore lining are not what skin affected by acne needs.

MARCELLE ESSENTIALS PRODUCTS

☺ **2 in 1 Face & Eye Cleanser** *($13.50 for 5.6 ounces).* Labeling this "the most practical product ever designed" is a dubious assertion. Practical for whom, I ask? Certainly not for the consumer, and that's for sure! This tube-packaged makeup remover has a lotion texture and an exceedingly simple formula. It removes makeup, but it's not as adept at removing waterproof formulas as a silicone- or oil-based product. This is not rated with a happy face because it contains plant extracts that shouldn't be used around the eyes.

☺ **$$$ Cleansing Cloths** *($11.50 for 25 cloths)* is a very basic, relatively ordinary cleansing lotion steeped into disposable cloths. The formula is fragrance-free and does a decent job of removing most types of makeup. The amount of benzyl alcohol is potentially irritating and keeps these cloths from earning a happy face rating. Products like this from Olay and Dove are far better formulated and far less pricey.

☺ **Cleansing Cream** *($14.95 for 7.3 ounces)* is a very basic, very old-fashioned oil- and wax-based cleanser. Similar to standard cold cream, it removes makeup easily, but definitely leaves a greasy film. It also contains sodium lauryl sulfate, a detergent cleansing agent that is too sensitizing for all skin types though the relative amount of it in this cleanser coupled with the oil and wax is unlikely to be a problem.

☹ **Cleansing Milk, Combination Skin** *($13.50 for 8.1 ounces)* is a very basic cleansing lotion that contains enough witch hazel to make it a potential problem for all skin types because witch hazel contains alcohol. The main thickening agent is ill-suited for use on oily areas, and this doesn't begin to compare favorably with a water-soluble cleanser.

☺ **Cleansing Milk, Normal to Dry Skin** *($13.50 for 8.1 ounces).* This cleansing lotion is nearly identical to Marcelle's Cleansing Milk, Combination Skin. The difference is that this version omits the potentially irritating witch hazel. It is a minimally effective cleanser for dry skin, but wiping off makeup is not the preferred way to daily clean your skin because it pulls on the skin, causing sagging. A gentle water-soluble cleanser is far better.

☺ **Gentle Foaming Wash** *($13.50 for 6.2 ounces)* is an effective water-soluble formula that works great for normal to oily skin. It is fragrance-free and capable of removing makeup without leaving a residue. The tiny amount of sodium lauryl sulfate, thankfully for Marcelle, is not cause for concern.

☺ **Eye Makeup Remover Cloths** *($11.50 for 2 packs of 15 cloths; 30 cloths total)* is nearly identical to Marcelle's regular Cleansing Cloths above. As such, the same review applies.

☺ **Oil-Free Eye Makeup Remover Lotion** *($11.50 for 4 ounces)* is a basic, detergent-based eye-makeup remover that's suitable for all skin types. It is fragrance-free and requires rinsing from skin, so it's best to use this before you use your regular water-soluble cleanser.

☺ **Soothing Eye Makeup Remover Gel** *($11.50 for 3.5 ounces)* is a very good, soothing eye-makeup remover in gel form. The fragrance-free formula is mild and suitable for all skin types. The only caveat is that it isn't strong enough to remove long-wearing or waterproof makeup. However, if you don't routinely use such formulas, this is an option. The formaldehyde-releasing preservative diazolidinyl urea makes it inappropriate for sensitive skin.

☺ **Waterproof Gentle Makeup Remover for Sensitive Eyes** *($13.50 for 5 ounces)* is a standard silicone- and oil-based makeup remover that dissolves all types of makeup. However, for some inexplicable reason (I couldn't get an answer from the company) it contains hydrochloric acid, a highly corrosive ingredient that I have never seen in a cosmetic formula before, and that's really saying something given the thousands of products I've reviewed over the years!

The small amount of hydrochloric acid in this product likely isn't cause for concern, but it shouldn't be in here at all.

☹ **Tonifying Lotion, Combination Skin** *($13.50 for 8.1 ounces)* lists alcohol as the second ingredient, and also contains several forms of the witch hazel plant. It is not recommended. The alcohol will stimulate oil production in the pore due to the irritation it generates, which is not something those with combination skin need; plus, it kills skin cells and generates free-radical damage.

☺ **Tonifying Lotion, Normal to Dry Skin** *($13.50 for 8.1 ounces)* is an exceptionally basic toner that's an OK option for normal to dry skin, but any skin type deserves much more than this boring concoction.

☹ **1st Wrinkles Eye Contour Cream** *($27.50 for 0.5 ounce).* Almost all of the intriguing ingredients are listed after the preservative in this poorly textured eye cream. The amount of absorbent aluminum starch (third ingredient) lends a powdery matte finish that is a problem for dry skin anywhere on the body, not to mention that it prevents the olive oil and other emollients from being as hydrating as they naturally are. It cannot reduce puffiness or dark circles; if anything, the amount of aluminum starch can irritate skin and make the eye area look puffier, nor does it have any antiwrinkle prowess.

☺ **Anti-Wrinkle Cream** *($18.95 for 1.3 ounces)* is a very basic moisturizer for normal to dry skin. Between the lackluster formula and the jar packaging, this seriously shortchanges your skin. One more comment: Applying collagen and elastin topically does not stimulate or shore up these substances in the lower layers of your skin; they do not fight wrinkles in any way.

☺ **Aqua-Matte Hydrating Fluid** *($18.50 for 4 ounces)* is a very basic, minimally beneficial, lightweight moisturizer that's a below-average option for normal to oily skin. Marcelle claims it is fragrance-free, but it definitely isn't because two of the main ingredients in this formula—farnesol and farnesyl acetate—are forms of fragrance.

☺ **Moisture Cream** *($16.95 for 2 ounces).* Unless you're OK with giving your dry skin the bare minimum to keep it smooth and soft, there's no reason to consider this incredibly dated, mineral oil-based moisturizer. The jar packaging in this case isn't an issue because there isn't anything that matters for skin that would deteriorate on exposure to light and air.

☺ **Moisture Lotion** *($18.95 for 4 ounces)* is nearly identical to Marcelle's Moisture Cream above, but with a lotion texture, and the same review applies.

☹ **Multi-Defense Cream SPF 15** *($18.95 for 2 ounces)* lacks the UVA-protecting ingredients of titanium dioxide, zinc oxide, avobenzone (also known as butyl methoxydibenzoylmethane), Tinosorb, or Mexoryl SX and is not recommended. Even if better UVA protection were provided, the overall formula leaves much to be desired, although it is fragrance-free.

☺ **Night Cream** *($14.25 for 1.3 ounces).* This exceptionally dated, mineral oil-based moisturizer is only a minimally effective option if your goal is to provide dry skin with an array of ingredients it needs to function optimally and resist signs of aging, such as antioxidants, skin-identical ingredients, and cell-communicating ingredients. For any skin type, this is a waste of money. The jar packaging for this product doesn't matter because there is nothing in here worth keeping stable.

☹ **Oil-Free Multi-Defense Lotion SPF 15** *($18.95 for 4 ounces)* lacks the UVA-protecting ingredients of titanium dioxide, zinc oxide, avobenzone (also known as butyl methoxydibenzoylmethane), Tinosorb, or Mexoryl SX and is not recommended. Even if better UVA protection were provided, the overall formula leaves much to be desired, although it is fragrance-free.

☹ **Clay Mask** *($13.50 for 3.7 ounces)* doesn't deserve consideration because several forms of the witch hazel plant are listed as the second ingredient, and witch hazel naturally contains alcohol and astringent constituents that irritate skin. It's a very basic clay mask that would be better for oily skin without the irritating, astringent witch hazel.

☺ **Lip Balm** *($6.95 for 0.1 ounce)* has an emollient, oil-based formula that does a great job of protecting lips from moisture loss and chapping. This is fragrance-free and contains a small amount of antioxidant vitamins E and A, but those are merely window dressing; there isn't enough of them to have a positive impact on skin.

MARCELLE HYDRA-C COMPLEXE PRODUCTS

☺ **Hydra-C ComplexE Facial Cleansing Gel** *($13.50 for 6.4 ounces)* is a standard water-soluble, detergent-based cleanser that contains fragrance in the form of fennel seed extract. The vitamins and antioxidants in this cleanser don't have a brightening effect because they are rinsed down the drain before they can have any benefit.

✓☺ **Hydra-C ComplexE Gentle Self-Foaming Cleanser** *($13.50 for 5.5 ounces)* is an excellent, fragrance-free, water-soluble cleanser suitable for all skin types except very dry. It removes makeup easily and rinses cleanly. Ignore the claims about the vitamins in this cleanser being able to invigorate skin, however, because vitamins don't have that effect. Even if they did, their presence in a cleanser provides negligible benefit because they are just rinsed down the drain.

✓☺ **Hydra-C ComplexE Facial Exfoliating Gel** *($13.50 for 3.4 ounces)* is a very good, fragrance-free cleanser that also functions as a scrub. The abrasive agent is polyethylene (plastic beads), which are preferred to natural abrasive agents (such as ground-up nut shells and fruit pits) because they are spherical in shape. This rinses cleanly and is suitable for all skin types.

☹ **Hydra-C ComplexE Tonifying Lotion** *($13.50 for 8.1 ounces)*. This toner is short on vitamins; instead, it contains more witch hazel plant extract, which can irritate skin. There isn't much else to say, except leave this on the shelf.

☺ **Hydra-C ComplexE 24H Hydrating Fluid** *($22.95 for 1.6 ounces)* doesn't have an SPF rating despite the fact that it contains several sunscreen ingredients. The second-listed ingredient (not active) is ethylhexyl methoxycinnamate, and the formula also contains avobenzone (listed by its chemical name butyl methoxydibenzoylmethane). The lack of an SPF rating on the package and the lack of an actual percentage of active ingredients means you cannot rely on this for sun protection. The overall formula is very basic and contains emollients that those with oily skin (to whom this is marketed) should avoid. The touted ingredient Fillagryl is a made-up word Marcelle uses to make the truly do-nothing contents sound more interesting—it doesn't. Marketing claims aside, the few helpful ingredients are barely present.

☹ **Hydra-C ComplexE Eye Contour Gel-Cream** *($20.95 for 0.51 ounce)* has a lightweight, silky texture but is an ordinary formula with a silicone and Vaseline base that also contains several plant extracts (including various forms of witch hazel) that are a problem for irritation. The inclusion of aluminum starch makes it not the best for the eye area because it is drying and absorbent, which doesn't help hydrate, but rather soaks up the moisture in your skin. The silicones help to temporarily fill in superficial lines, but this effect is attainable from other products with better, irritant-free formulas.

☹ **Hydra-C ComplexE 24H Moisturizing Gel-Cream** *($22.95 for 1.7 ounces)*. This moisturizer is nearly identical to Marcelle's Hydra-C ComplexE 24H Hydrating Fluid above, and the same review applies.

☹ **Hydra-C ComplexE 24H Moisturizing Gel-Cream, Dry Skin** *($22.95 for 1.8 ounces)* is nearly identical to Marcelle's Hydra-C ComplexE 24H Hydrating Fluid reviewed above, and the same review applies.

☹ **Hydra-C ComplexE Moisturizing Gel-Cream** *($22.95 for 1.7 ounces)* is mostly water, thickener, film-forming agent, and a form of wax, which is about as exciting as watching grass grow. This dated, do-nothing formula shortchanges your skin of a state-of-the-art formula with ingredients that truly could help make your skin function like younger skin. The amount of vitamin C it contains is trivial and it won't remain potent for long thanks to this product's jar packaging.

MARCELLE NEW•AGE PRODUCTS

✓ ☺ **$$$ New•Age Comforting Foaming Cleanser** *($14.25 for 5.8 ounces)*. If this cleanser is the "ultimate" for skin as Marcelle claims, then they should stop selling all of their other cleansers and direct their customers to this ultimate option—Right? "Ultimate" is just an adjective, used frequently in marketing, but in this case, as it turns out, this product is one of Marcelle's several excellent cleansers, and one to consider. The fragrance-free formula is a water-soluble, detergent-based cleansing lotion that's ideal for normal to dry skin. You'll find the lightly foaming texture works great to remove makeup and leaves skin silky-smooth. I wouldn't consider it a "new age" of cleansing, but it's still a great fragrance-free cleanser worth checking out.

☺ **New•Age Soothing Hydrating Tonifying Lotion** *($14.25 for 8.1 ounces)* has a lot going for it, but hits a couple of snags that keep it from earning a better rating. The first snag is that it would be a more well-rounded formula if it contained a broader range of antioxidants. That's not a deal-breaker, but the inclusion of witch hazel (the second snag) isn't going to benefit your skin. The amount of witch hazel isn't enough to discount this toner altogether, but what a shame it was included at all because it can be a skin irritant, and irritation is never the goal because it damages skin!

☺ **New•Age Anti-Wrinkle + Firming Cream** *($27.50 for 1.7 ounces)*. There is nothing about this emollient moisturizer that makes it preferred for women over age 35, as claimed. Age is not a skin type. In the case of this product, someone over the age of 35 with oily skin will find it too greasy, and what about someone who's 29 and struggling with dry skin? Are they out of luck because their skin isn't "mature" enough for this moisturizer? As it turns out, this is one of Marcelle's only impressive moisturizers, and it would be recommended for dry skin of any age if not for the jar packaging, which means this fragrance-free formula's most elegant ingredients won't remain stable because of repeated exposure to light and air. What a shame! One more comment: Ignore the claim about caffeine stimulating lymphatic drainage. If that were possible, simply chugging a cup of Starbucks coffee would go a longer way toward slimming skin than applying the minute amount of caffeine in this product.

☺ **$$$ New•Age Anti-Wrinkle + Firming Eye & Lip Contour Cream** *($27.50 for 0.49 ounce)* is an OK fragrance-free moisturizer but it has problems that keep it from being suitable for any skin type anywhere on the face, especially around the eye area. The amount of aluminum starch keeps this from being moisturizing because that is an extremely absorbent ingredient. There are the tiniest amounts of antioxidant, peptides, and skin-identical ingredients, but that's about it. Marcelle's touted NOVA-CELL complex is as made up as their Fillagryl complex in their other products. This isn't a terrible product, but when it comes to skin, there is no reason it should get shortchanged, especially when this product is so pricey.

☺ **New•Age Anti-Wrinkle + Firming Night Cream** *($27.50 for 1.6 ounces)*. It's unfortunate Marcelle selected jar packaging for this moisturizer because in most respects it is one of Marcelle's better formulas, although that's not saying much. As is, most of the state-of-the-art ingredients won't remain effective with repeated exposure to light and air. This also contains a blend of plant extracts with irritating properties; although none of them are present in a troublesome amount, any amount is a waste of time and a risk for your skin. Needless to say, it's 100% false that this moisturizer allows your skin to defy the effects of time. That's just wishful thinking at its best!

MARCELLE MAKEUP

FOUNDATION: ✓ ☺ **Satin Matte Mousse Make-Up** *($16.95)*. This nonaqueous, silicone-based foundation housed in a glass jar is Marcelle's best. Its sponge-like texture gives way to a silky-smooth blending experience that sets to a beautifully natural matte finish. Skin looks polished and minor imperfections are nicely blurred thanks to this makeup's sheer to light coverage. The shade range is attractive and best for light to medium skin tones. Note that each color goes on lighter than it appears in the jar. Satin Matte Mousse Make-Up is best for normal to very oily skin. Its finish is not the best for those with dry skin or dry patches, however, because it tends to magnify rather than downplay dry areas.

☺ **True Radiance Radiant Complexion Make-Up SPF 15** *($14.50)* has a fluid, sheer texture that slips easily over skin and sets to a lightweight matte finish. Sheer to light coverage is possible, but this isn't a slam-dunk recommendation for normal to oily skin because its sunscreen does not provide sufficient UVA protection. What a shame, because the shade range is neutral and well-suited to those with fair to medium skin tones.

☺ **Moisture Rich Moisturizing Make-Up** *($14.50)* is a very standard, somewhat dated, water- and oil-based foundation. Its fluid, moist texture blends well and sets to a satin finish suitable for normal to dry skin. Light to medium coverage is possible and the shade selection, while neutral, favors light to medium skin tones only.

☺ **Matte Finish Make-Up** *($14.50)* has a soft matte finish that's suitable for normal to oily skin, but feels a bit old-fashioned when compared with today's best matte-finish makeup. It has a decent slip and provides medium coverage, but again, it simply isn't one of the better foundations. If you decide to give this a go, the shade range is limited to those with light to medium skin tones. Avoid Mocha, which is too peach.

☺ **Sheer Tint Fluid Moisturizer SPF 15** *($14.50)*. What a shame this lightweight tinted moisturizer doesn't provide sufficient UVA protection. It has a very smooth, mousse-like texture that's easy to blend and it sets to a slightly moist finish. With proper UVA protection, this would be an easy recommendation for those with normal to dry skin. As is, you're losing one of the conveniences that a tinted moisturizer with sunscreen can provide. If you decide to try this anyway, avoid the darker shades (Mocha Beige, Café Au Lait, and Bronze Soleil) because all of them have a noticeable peach tinge.

☹ **Marcelle Minerals Powder Make-Up** *($17.95)*. Marcelle's foray into mineral makeup isn't all that successful. This loose-powder makeup is packaged in a cylindrical container outfitted with a brush applicator. The brush is OK, but really too small to use for application over the entire face. Moreover, the midsection of the component loosens easily, which leads to powder spilling everywhere. (I'm still trying to get mineral powder out of the white grout on my bathroom counter.) Even in better packaging, this bismuth oxychloride-based powder has a very dry, thick texture that manages to make skin look ashen and shiny at the same time. It feels increasingly drier the longer it's on your skin, making even the oily areas feel and look dehydrated. That is not attractive; this is a mineral makeup you can and should ignore.

CONCEALER: ☹ **Concealer Palette** *($15.95)* is a very creamy, thick formula that offers four shades in one compact. The included synthetic brush is a thoughtful touch, but it's too small for practical use. Regardless of whether you use one shade or blend several to create a custom match, this concealer applies and looks heavy, even when blended out sheer. You get almost full coverage, but with the trade-off of makeup that is needlessly apparent.

POWDER: ✓☺ **Face Powder** *($13.50)*. Housed in a generous-size tub is this talc- and mineral oil-based loose powder. It has a silky, almost creamy texture that makes skin look polished and satiny rather than flat and powdered. If one of the two translucent shades works for you, this is a great, affordable loose powder for those with normal to dry skin.

☺ **Pressed Powder** *($13.50)* is a very standard, talc-based pressed powder. It has a sheer, dry texture that feels slightly silky and provides a soft, translucent matte finish. Both shades are fine, but reserved for those with fair to light skin tones. The formula is best for normal to slightly dry or slightly oily skin.

☺ **Pressed Powder Bronzer** *($13.50)* is nearly identical to Marcelle's Pressed Powder, except the shades are best for creating a soft tanned appearance. Suntan is the preferred color; Natural Bronze is OK, but tends to go on a bit orange, so it's less convincing.

BLUSH AND BRONZER: ☺ **Cream Blusher** *($10.25)* is a traditional oil-based cream blush that's best for dry skin not prone to blemishes. It applies smoothly and leaves a moist finish that doesn't slip-slide all over the face. Both shades are bright and leave a subtle shine.

☺ **Marcelle Minerals Powder Blush** *($15.95)* is a loose-powder blush housed in a slim component outfitted with a brush applicator. The mica-based formula isn't nearly as drying as Marcelle Minerals Powder Make-Up, and is much easier to blend. Both shades are sheer pastel and leave a soft-shine finish. Ideally, this is best dusted on to highlight cheeks after you apply a regular powder blush, at least if your objective is to add color to the cheeks.

☺ **Velvety Powder Blush** *($10.25)*. Despite the touted Grand Prix of Beauty award this product won from *Elle* magazine, it's as ordinary as it gets for a pressed-powder blush. The texture is smooth, dry, and slightly waxen, while application is sheer, providing soft color that most skin tones will need to layer. Among the four shades, only Blushing Bronze has noticeable shine.

☹ **Marcelle Minerals Bronzing Powder** *($15.95)*. This loose-powder bronzer is terrible. It has a dry texture and barely-there colors plus a finish that tends to make skin look shiny and ashen at the same time. Why anyone would choose this to bronze skin over several better options at the drugstore is beyond me.

EYESHADOW: ✓☺ **Wet & Dry Eyeshadow Quad** *($13.95)* is Marcelle's best powder eyeshadow due to its silky texture and superior blendability. It has an extra silkiness that their single and duo eyeshadows lack, though both of those are still recommended. All of the quads are shiny, but it's understated. Still, this isn't the best if your eyelid area is wrinkled or sagging. The most attractive sets are Bohemian and Goddess.

☺ **Wet & Dry Eyeshadow** *($8.50)* has a soft, dry texture that could be silkier, but it applies fairly well, with each shade providing impressive color payoff. Every shade has some amount of shine, but most merely leave a subtle shimmer. Avoid the green Amazone and the blue Electric Dream. Choco Chic and Cabaret are excellent crease colors.

☺ **Wet & Dry Eyeshadow Duo** *($10.50)* has a formula that's identical to Marcelle's single Wet & Dry Eyeshadow above, and the same review applies.

☹ **Marcelle Minerals Eye Shadow** *($10.95)*. This loose-powder eyeshadow is messy to apply, and even if you get it in place without any flaking, it's difficult to blend, despite feeling smooth. It tends to grab the skin and the colors have a slight ashen look most will find intolerable. Definitely a tough sell on all counts!

EYE AND BROW SHAPER: ☺ **Kohl Eyeliner** *($8.95)*. This needs-sharpening pencil has a thick, creamy texture made for smudging. It applies imprecisely, so you'll want to smudge this for a softer look. Once set, this wears decently and has minimal tendency to smear or fade.

☺ **Powder Eyeliner** *($9.50)*. This pencil's best attribute is its nearly effortless application and soft-powder (in feel; most of the shades finish with a shine) dry-down. It requires routine sharpening, but if that doesn't bother you, this pencil lasts longer than its creamy brethren.

☺ **Waterproof Eyeliner** *($9.50)* needs regular sharpening. Its silicone base is waterproof, but leaves a tacky finish that can interfere with eyeshadow application, assuming you want to blend shadow over the pencil. Application-wise, this glides on easily and imparts rich color. Avoid the Indigo shade.

☺ **Accent Eyebrow Crayon** *($9.50)* is a very good eyebrow-enhancing option for fans of brow pencils, though it requires sharpening. It applies smoothly and slightly dry, setting to a soft powder finish. Each color goes on soft and builds well without balling up or flaking. Blondine is an excellent shade for medium blonde brows.

LIPSTICK, LIP GLOSS, AND LIPLINER: ✓☺ **Vita-Lip Plumping Gloss** *($10.95)* comes packaged in a squeeze tube and is easy to apply. It has a wonderfully silky texture and soft, sheer colors that leave a markedly pearlescent finish. It is 100% non-sticky, yet isn't so slick that you'll be reapplying every few minutes; unfortunately, however, like all glosses with movement, this isn't for those with lines around the mouth. The small shade range is versatile and the pearlescent finish is very attractive.

☺ **Rouge Vitality Lipstick** *($10.25)* is a standard, but good, cream lipstick. The shade selection is impressive, and most of the shades go on opaque and provide a moderate to strong shimmer finish that feels comfortably smooth.

☺ **Lux Gloss** *($10.95)* is nothing more than a standard, slightly thick-textured lip gloss with moderate color payoff and a minimally sticky finish that adds lots of shine to lips.

☺ **Lux Gloss Sheer** *($10.95)* is identical to the Lux Gloss above, except the shades are softer and more versatile, which means you can pair this with a lipstick if you like. Otherwise, the same review applies.

☺ **Rouge Reflex Lipstick** *($10.25)* has a slick texture that glides over lips but feels heavy. The shades impart minimal color, but leave lips softly glossed. It's best described as a tinted lip balm in stick form.

☺ **Waterproof Lip Definition Crayon** *($9.50)* requires routine sharpening and, true to its name, it is waterproof. The texture is creamy and each shade is more pigmented than you might expect. Caution: The Nude shade is actually a rosy mauve that doesn't approximate what most women would consider a "nude" shade.

MASCARA: ☺ **Ultimate Lash Mascara** *($9.95)* ranks as Marcelle's best mascara, though none of them are the cream of the crop when compared with the best mascaras from Maybelline New York, L'Oreal, Revlon, and Cover Girl. Ultimate Lash is a good choice if you want cleanly separated lashes with moderate length and minimal thickness. The formula doesn't clump and it wears without flaking or smearing.

☺ **Lash Extreme Mascara** *($9.95)* is one of the most do-nothing mascaras available. Even with considerable effort, the best this manages is average length and good lash separation. Talk about a real snoozer!

☺ **Healthy Lash Mascara** *($9.95)*. This mascara, which isn't healthier than any other, is an OK option if you need subtle length without clumps and without even a hint of thickness. It has a slight tendency to flake throughout the day, but that may be because I applied too much in the hope that this would amount to more than it did. It's worth a shot if you prefer modest lash enhancement.

☹ **Volume Precision Mascara** *($11.95)* has a rubber-bristle brush that feels unusually scratchy along the lash line and even as you comb through lashes, feeling almost as if it's snagging in your lashes. Successive coats produce average length and no thickness. Although this doesn't clump, it tends to smear shortly after application.

MARY KAY

MARY KAY AT-A-GLANCE

Strengths: Most of the products are fragrance-free; some noteworthy cleansers, serums, and sunscreens; every sunscreen offers sufficient UVA protection; packaging that keeps light- and air-sensitive ingredients stable during use; very good eye-makeup remover and topical disinfectant with benzoyl peroxide; two good foundations; the Concealer; the eyeliner pencils; the Lip Gloss; the Brush Set (individual brushes are sold separately, but these are a mixed bag).

Weaknesses: The overall collection is a mixed bag of exciting and disappointing products; several outdated moisturizers and greasy cleansers; no AHA or acceptable BHA products; no products that can successfully address skin discolorations; unexceptional topical scrub; irritating lip balms; average powder blush; the Medium Coverage Foundation; the Waterproof Mascara; the Eye Primer isn't necessary.

For more information about Mary Kay, call (800) 627-9529 or visit www.marykay.com or www.Beautypedia.com.

MARY KAY SKIN CARE

MARY KAY TIMEWISE PRODUCTS

☹ **TimeWise 3-In-1 Cleanser, for Combination to Oily Skin** *($18 for 4.5 ounces)* lists the drying detergent cleansing agent TEA-lauryl sulfate as the second ingredient and also contains a couple of irritating plant extracts, making this expensive cleanser a poor choice for anyone.

☺ **$$$ TimeWise 3-in-1 Cleanser, for Normal to Dry Skin** *($18 for 4.5 ounces)* is a very standard and somewhat greasy cleansing lotion for dry to very dry skin. The mineral oil, Vaseline, and clay make this difficult to remove with a washcloth, and this should be avoided if you have dry skin with blemishes.

☹ **TimeWise 3-in-1 Cleansing Bar** *($18 for 5-ounce bar)* is a standard, drying bar soap that does not contain a single ingredient capable of exfoliating skin as claimed. On that same note, this soap cannot "reduce the visible signs of aging." What a ridiculous claim for a product that's basically a bar of Dove Soap!

☺ $$$ **TimeWise Microdermabrasion Set** *($55)* is Mary Kay's contribution to the growing number of at-home microdermabrasion kits. Just like its numerous competitors, this two-part product features a topical scrub and post-treatment moisturizer. **Step 1: Refine** *($30 for 2 ounces; may be purchased separately)* contains alumina crystals as the abrasive agent, and yes, this is the same ingredient used in professionally administered microdermabrasion treatments. But there's a difference between massaging a scrub on your skin and how the microdermabrasion machine works (and the way it's operated). Further, recent research has shown that microdermabrasion doesn't appear to have a cumulative benefit. Either way, products like this (when used gently) are indeed viable topical scrubs. What I like is that Mary Kay's version is free of added irritants and that it rinses easily (many microdermabrasion scrubs are difficult to remove with water). **Step 2: Replenish** *($25 for 1 ounce; may be purchased separately)* is to be applied after Step #1: Refine, though I can think of many other serum-type moisturizers that have formulas superior to this, including those from Aveda, Clinique, Estee Lauder, Olay, and Paula's Choice. Rather than create a product brimming with antioxidants, anti-irritants, and cell-communicating ingredients, Mary Kay created a functional, but ordinary, product that is just an OK option for normal to slightly oily skin. It's being marketed for dry or oily skin, but if you have dry skin, Replenish will leave your skin wanting more, and for oily skin it may prove too emollient. It has some good antioxidants and the packaging will keep them stable, but the amounts are likely too small to bring much benefit to your skin. Overall, there is nothing about the scrub in this kit that can't be replaced by a washcloth, and there are better moisturizers than this. But if you're still interested in trying a microdermabrasion-at-home product, consider Neutrogena's Advanced Solutions At-Home Microdermabrasion System, which costs less and comes with a rotating brush applicator and cleanser.

☺ $$$ **TimeWise Age-Fighting Eye Cream** *($26 for 0.65 ounce)* is a decent, lightweight moisturizer for slightly dry skin anywhere on the face. The lack of antioxidants and skin-identical ingredients is disappointing, but this contains peptides, which theoretically function as cell-communicating ingredients.

☺ **TimeWise Age-Fighting Moisturizer, for Combination/Oily Skin** *($22 for 3.3 ounces)* has a fluid texture and silky feel. It's a suitably light moisturizer for its intended skin types, and leaves a soft matte finish. Regrettably, it lacks a good selection of antioxidants and ingredients that mimic the structure of healthy skin. And, of course, without a sunscreen, this product cannot fight aging any more than an ant can drive a car.

☺ **TimeWise Age-Fighting Moisturizer, for Normal/Dry Skin** *($22 for 3.3 ounces)* has a creamy but light texture and contains some helpful ingredients for normal to dry skin, but most of the impressive ingredients are listed after the preservatives, so they're barely functional. Moreover, antioxidants are in very short supply.

☺ **TimeWise Age-Fighting Moisturizer Sunscreen SPF 15** *($22 for 3 ounces)* deserves kudos for its in-part zinc oxide sunscreen, but the base formula for normal to slightly dry skin is rather boring, with insignificant amounts of antioxidants and water-binding agents.

✓ ☺ **TimeWise Day Solution Sunscreen SPF 25** *($30 for 1 ounce)* is the most impressive daytime moisturizer in the TimeWise collection. The in-part zinc oxide sunscreen provides sufficient UVA protection, while the fluid but creamy formula contains a great selection of antioxidants, skin-identical ingredients, and lightweight emollients for normal to dry skin. This also has a silky finish that wears beautifully under makeup.

☺ **$$$ TimeWise Firming Eye Cream** *($30 for 0.5 ounce)* is a very emollient, Vaseline-based moisturizer for dry to very dry skin anywhere on the face. Lots of thickening agents combine with smaller amounts of peptides and a few antioxidants to round out the skin-beneficial traits of this product (but, regrettably, it won't firm skin).

☹ **TimeWise Night Solution** *($30 for 1 ounce)* is a clear, slightly tacky serum that's loaded with antioxidants and peptides. The unhappy face rating is because these ingredients are joined by several fragrant plant extracts that cause irritation, including geranium, wild mint, rose, orange, and jasmine. The tingling sensation this causes is not good news for aging skin.

☹ **TimeWise Targeted-Action Eye Revitalizer** *($35 for 0.34 ounce)* asks you to "imagine a product so powerful, it can reduce the appearance of both dark circles and under-eye puffiness in just two weeks." That's something many people would love to achieve given how common these eye-area skin conditions are. But can this product and its roller-ball applicator produce such results? Sadly, it cannot. The water- and film-forming agent–based fluid contains some state-of-the-art ingredients, but neither they nor the numerous plant extracts (some of which are irritating) have been proven to lighten dark circles and make puffiness recede. This is actually more of a problem for skin around the eyes because it contains the irritating menthol derivative menthyl lactate (for the cooling sensation mentioned in the claims).

✓ ☺ **$$$ TimeWise Targeted-Action Line Reducer** *($40 for 0.13 ounce)* deserves a Paula's Pick rating for its elegant formula laced with several antioxidants, soothing agent, and a cell-communicating ingredient. The antiwrinkle claims for this product are farfetched because this click pen–dispensed product works poorly and doesn't really act like spackle, especially if you smile. This will not fill in deep, etched lines like those that occur along the nasolabial folds. Wrinkles aside, the formula as a whole is very good for normal to dry skin, whether around the eyes or on other areas that need temporary smoothing. And thank you, Mary Kay, for not implying in the least that this product is better than Botox or dermal injections!

✓ ☺ **$$$ TimeWise Age-Fighting Lip Primer** *($22 for 0.5 ounce)* is a silicone- and wax-based spackle for filling in lines on the lips and around the mouth. It works to a minor extent, but the effect is temporary and diminishes faster if you wear greasy or overly glossy lipsticks. What's particularly impressive is the amount of antioxidants and cell-communicating ingredients this contains. Those help skin repair itself while reducing inflammation, and earn this product a Paula's Pick. By the way, this is worth considering over Lauder's more expensive Perfectionist Correcting Concentrate for Lip Lines ($35 for 0.08 ounce).

✓ ☺ **$$$ TimeWise Even Complexion Essence** *($35 for 1 ounce)* promises to restore a natural, even tone to skin while helping to reverse skin discolorations. Eschewing the established skin-lightening agent hydroquinone, this water-based serum contains niacinamide and ascorbyl glucoside instead. There is some research showing that niacinamide can interrupt the transfer of melanocytes (pigmented skin cells) to keratinocytes (regular skin cells that make the protein keratin), which would essentially cut the discoloration process off at the pass. However, these studies were done in vitro (test tube) rather than on human skin. Moreover, while the researchers pointed out that a positive outcome was dose-dependent, the dosage was not revealed (Source: *Experimental Dermatology*, July 2005, pages 498-508). A smaller study, which was done on human skin, revealed that a 5% concentration of niacinamide produced a noticeable effect on discolorations after four weeks of use (Source: *British Journal of Dermatology*, July 2002, pages 20-31). It should be noted that this study was done on only 18 women, and was from Procter & Gamble, whose Olay and SK-II lines are big on the use of niacinamide. There is no substantiated research concerning the ability of the vitamin C derivative ascorbyl glucoside to lighten skin, although vitamin C in other forms has shown potential. So what we have here is a potentially good alternative skin-lightening product, though Mary Kay is definitely not using 5% niacinamide. Nonetheless, this product is worth considering by all skin types as a lightweight serum that contains several vitamin- and plant-based antioxidants as well as water-binding agents, including peptides.

MARY KAY SUN CARE PRODUCTS

☺ **After-Sun Replenishing Gel** *($12 for 6.5 ounces)* is a lightweight, soothing gel that contains mostly water, slip agent, glycerin, silicone, green tea and other antioxidants, thickener, preservatives, fragrance, and coloring agents. It is recommended for normal to slightly dry skin, and the green tea may help skin repair itself to some extent from sun exposure—though it's far better not to let sun-exposed skin get to a point where a "repair" product is needed.

✓ ☺ **SPF 30 Sunscreen** *($14 for 4 ounces)* is a water-resistant sunscreen for normal to oily skin. It includes avobenzone for UVA protection and contains a nice selection of vitamin-based antioxidants (plus green tea) known to help skin defend itself better from sun exposure. This is an outstanding sunscreen formulation that's priced right; it does contain fragrance.

✓ ☺ **Lip Protector Sunscreen SPF 15** *($7.50 for 0.16 ounce)* combines an in-part zinc oxide sunscreen with petrolatum and other lip-smoothing emollients and antioxidant soybean oil along with vitamin E. This smart lip balm is a beautiful option for keeping lips smooth and protected year-round. The addition of yellow coloring agents helps offset the slight white cast from the zinc oxide, a thoughtful touch.

☺ **Subtle Tanning Lotion** *($16 for 4 ounces)* is labeled a "subtle" self-tanner because it contains less dihydroxyacetone, the ingredient that turns skin a tan color. That's nice, but nothing special that cannot be found at the drugstore from lines such as Dove, Neutrogena, and Jergens for less money. If you're considering this product, it's best for normal to dry skin, but it contains too much fragrance to be suitable for sensitive skin.

✓ ☺ **Tinted Lip Balm Sunscreen SPF 15** *($13)* is a superior tinted lip balm with sunscreen. UVA protection is assured from zinc oxide, and it's accompanied by other sunscreen actives (based on the percentage of actives alone, this likely could've earned a much higher SPF rating). The smooth, emollient texture has a slight waxy feel and imparts sheer color with a soft gloss finish. Speaking of the shades, all of them are great! This is highly recommended for those looking to combine sun protection and color for lips.

OTHER MARY KAY PRODUCTS

☺ **Creamy Cleanser Formula 2** *($12 for 6.5 ounces)* is an exceedingly standard water- and mineral oil-based cleanser for normal to dry skin not prone to blemishes. It requires a washcloth for complete removal.

✓ ☺ **$$$ Deep Cleanser Formula 3** *($12 for 6.5 ounces)* is a very good water-soluble cleansing lotion for normal to slightly oily skin. It rinses cleanly, removes makeup, and does not contain fragrance.

✓ ☺ **$$$ Facial Cleansing Cloths** *($15 for 30 cloths)*. These cleansing cloths are a convenient way to refresh your face on the go. The mild formula is fragrance-free and it contains soothing plant extracts that don't pose even a slight risk of irritation (that is, unless you're allergic to them). The cloths don't work well to remove most types of makeup, including waterproof mascara, but they're great for freshening up post-workout or while traveling.

☺ **Gentle Cleansing Cream Formula 1** *($12 for 4 ounces)* is a cold cream–style cleanser for dry to very dry skin. It removes makeup easily but you need a washcloth to make sure you don't leave a greasy residue.

☹ **Velocity Facial Cleanser** *($10 for 5 ounces)* uses TEA-lauryl sulfate as the main detergent cleansing agent, which makes this too drying and irritating for all skin types. In addition, several of the plant extracts are irritants, and the fragrance is not needed.

✓ ☺ **Oil-Free Eye Makeup Remover** *($14 for 3.75 ounces)* works quickly and beautifully to remove all types of makeup. The silicone-enhanced formula may be used before or after cleansing and, unlike many makeup removers, this one omits the fragrance.

☹ **Blemish Control Toner Formula 3** *($13 for 6.5 ounces)* won't control blemishes, but will instead cause irritation and redness due to the alcohol, eucalyptus oil, and menthol it contains.

☹ **Hydrating Freshener Formula 1** *($13 for 6.5 ounces)* consists primarily of water, slip agent, and preservatives, but the menthol makes it not worth considering over dozens of other toners.

☹ **Purifying Freshener Formula 2** *($13 for 6.5 ounces)* lists alcohol as the second ingredient, making this too drying and irritating for all skin types.

☹ **Advanced Moisture Renewal Treatment Cream** *($19 for 2.5 ounces)* covers the basics for replenishing dry to very dry skin, but is an overall lackluster (not advanced) moisturizer whose token amounts of antioxidants and the cell-communicating ingredient lecithin are a too little, too late approach.

☺ **Balancing Moisturizer Formula 2** *($18 for 4 ounces)* is similar to Clinique's original Dramatically Different Moisturizing Lotion, and just as boring. It is an outdated, inadequate option for normal to dry skin.

☺ **Enriched Moisturizer Formula 1** *($18 for 4 ounces)* is a thicker, more emollient version of the Balancing Moisturizer Formula 2, and the same comments apply, except that this is suitable for dry to very dry skin.

☹ **Extra Emollient Night Cream** *($11 for 2.1 ounces)* is basically Vaseline and mineral oil along with several waxes. Yes, it will make dry skin feel smooth and lubricated, but the inclusion of menthol is a burn.

☹ **Indulge Soothing Eye Gel** *($15 for 0.4 ounce)* contains a frustrating mix of helpful and skin-hindering ingredients, with the negatives (comfrey, witch hazel, and eyebright) outweighing the positives and making this more a problem than an indulgence for skin.

☺ **Intense Moisturizing Cream** *($30 for 1.8 ounces)* is a very standard, humdrum moisturizer that is primarily water, mineral oil, Vaseline, and waxes with little to no antioxidants or water-binding agents. In the end, this is an OK moisturizer for dry to very dry skin. However, in this price range, far better options are readily available.

☺ **Oil Control Lotion Formula 3** *($18 for 4 ounces)* doesn't carry a high price, which it shouldn't, because this is a very ordinary mix of water, silicone, slip agent, thickener, and film-forming agent. It is a substandard option for normal to oily skin, and does not do a remarkable job at keeping skin shine-free.

☺ **Oil-Free Hydrating Gel** *($30 for 1.8 ounces)* is considerably more modern than the Intense Moisturizing Cream, and has a wonderfully silky, lightweight texture for normal to oily or combination skin. The drawback is jar packaging, which won't keep the antioxidants in this product stable once it's opened.

☺ **Oil Mattifier** *($15 for 0.6 ounce)* is much better at curtailing surface shine (oiliness) than the Oil Control Lotion Formula 3. The tiny amount of alcohol isn't cause for concern. The solvent isododecane and the silicones help promote and maintain a lightweight matte finish. It would have earned a higher rating had it included antioxidants, cell-communicating ingredients, or skin-identical ingredients, something all skin types can benefit from immensely.

☺ **Tinted Moisturizer with Sunscreen SPF 20** *($18)* has a fluid, beautifully smooth texture that blends easily, providing sheer to light coverage and a satin matte finish. The in-part zinc oxide sunscreen makes this a smart choice for daytime use by those with normal to slightly dry or slightly oily skin. The six shades could have been more neutral (for a newer product, the overtones of pink and peach are odd), but the good news is that this is sheer enough so that the lesser shades (which would be Beige 1 and Bronze 1) are still options should one of the other colors not work for you.

☹ **Velocity Lightweight Moisturizer** *($12 for 4 ounces)* offers minimal benefit for skin and contains enough alcohol to be potentially irritating. It also contains several irritating plant extracts, including cinnamon and sandalwood.

✓ ☺ **Acne Treatment Gel** *($7 for 1 ounce)* lists 5% benzoyl peroxide as the active ingredient, and is a very good, gel-based topical disinfectant for those battling blemishes.

☺ **Beauty Blotters Oil-Absorbing Tissues** *($5 for 75 sheets)* are non-powdered thin sheets of linen-type material that do their job to absorb excess oil and perspiration. The price is good, too.

☺ **Clarifying Mask Formula 3** *($14 for 4 ounces)* is a standard clay mask that is an OK option for oily to very oily skin, but contains potentially problematic lavender along with a tiny amount of TEA-lauryl sulfate. It's not terrible, but better clay masks abound.

☹ **Moisture Rich Mask Formula 1** *($14 for 4 ounces)* is below standard because it lacks state-of-the-art ingredients for dry skin and contains menthol, which serves no purpose other than to cause irritation and convince you the product is "working."

☺ **Revitalizing Mask Formula 2** *($14 for 4 ounces)* may cause your skin to be confused due to its contrasting mix of absorbent clay with moisturizing agents, waxes, and exfoliating walnut shell powder. I don't know whom to recommend this mask for; it's too drying for normal to dry skin and too emollient for oily skin.

☹ **Satin Lips Lip Balm** *($9.50 for 0.3 ounce)*. Your lips will thank you if you skip this menthol-laced balm in favor of plain Vaseline, which is the main ingredient in this pricey product.

☹ **Satin Lips Lip Mask** *($9.50 for 0.3 ounce)* isn't satiny in the least and lips don't need a clay mask with the kind of aggressive exfoliation this causes when massaged over the mouth. Furthermore, the menthol in here isn't the least bit helpful, and may make chapped lips worse.

MARY KAY MAKEUP

MARY KAY MINERAL MAKEUP

FOUNDATION: ✓ ☺ **Mineral Powder Foundation** *($18)* is technically not on a par with "standard" mineral makeup because the main ingredient is talc. The irony is that talc is a mineral, yet that doesn't stop most mineral makeup brands from avoiding its use due to unfounded health concerns. Mary Kay has crafted a loose-powder foundation with a superior smooth texture that feels almost creamy and blends beautifully. What you will get with this foundation is an initially sheer application with light to medium coverage (depending on how you layer it) that's not nearly as heavy as that from several other mineral foundations. It also won't give your face that "glow" or sparkling shine that mineral foundations are well known for (which may not be the best for someone with oily skin who might want a more a matte appearance from their powder application). The application brush (sold separately) does a respectable job, although the bristles are a bit stiff and I suspect many women will prefer a softer powder brush, which works far better for applying foundations like this one. The six shades are mostly impressive, neutral options. Bronze 1 will be too peach for most medium to tan skin tones, but Bronze 2 is a winner. If you're curious to try a mineral foundation and don't mind the mess they can cause (it is loose powder, after all, and Mary Kay doesn't offer a tidy component), this is highly recommended as one of the best available, most notably for how great it looks on skin. As is the case with all mineral-type foundations, it can make dry skin or dry spots look worse unless they're sufficiently prepped with moisturizer (and you must allow the moisturizer to absorb, or the powder will grab in spots and look uneven).

POWDER: ☺ **Mineral Highlighting Powder** *($12)* has a different formula from Mary Kay's Mineral Bronzing Powder, and is similar to the company's Mineral Cheek Color (both reviewed below). That means you get a smooth, dry texture that offers a soft, even color deposit. Both the shimmer and matte options are attractive and best for highlighting fair to light skin tones (and the highlighting will be subtle, which is what you want for artfully applied makeup). Purchased individually, the powder tablet arrives enclosed in a handy plastic case. If you opt to purchase the Mary Kay Compact, it can house two Mineral Highlighting Powders.

BLUSH AND BRONZER: ☺ **Mineral Cheek Color** *($10)* is a talc-based blush (remember, talc is a mineral) that isn't as beautifully silky as Mary Kay's Mineral Eye Color below, but still acquits itself nicely for those seeking a smooth, sheer, dry pressed-powder blush. The matte shades include Berry Brown, Cinnamon Stick, and Pink Petals. If you prefer a subtle shine, consider Cherry Blossom, Shy Blush, Strawberry Cream, or Sparkling Cider. The remaining shades are noticeably shiny and really too much for daytime wear (plus the colors are the least appealing even if they didn't have shine). Mineral Cheek Color is suitable for all skin types; it is fragrance-free. Purchased individually, these powder tablets arrive enclosed in a handy plastic case. If you opt to purchase the Mary Kay Compact, it can house two blushes.

☺ **Mineral Bronzing Powder** *($12)* is a creamy-smooth pressed-powder bronzer whose main mineral is talc, which is fine because talc is a mineral, despite being maligned by many mineral makeup-only companies. Although Mary Kay offers matte and shimmer duos (each featuring a tan to bronze tone alongside a complementary lighter shade), the color deposit is minimal even if you intentionally try to apply a lot of it. The shimmer options impart more shine than color, while the matte options may leave you wondering why you bothered. This just goes to show that a sublime texture is not enough if it doesn't apply and build well. Still, this is worth considering if you want really sheer color or hints of shimmer. Purchased individually, the powder tablet arrives enclosed in a handy plastic case. If you opt to purchase the Mary Kay Compact, it can house two Mineral Bronzing Powders.

EYESHADOW: ✓ ☺ **Mineral Eye Color** *($6.50)* lists talc as its main mineral ingredient in these sold-singly powder eyeshadows. Talc is not a bad thing—quite the contrary—most other minerals have a drier texture that hinders smooth application, and that's not the case here. Their previous powder eyeshadows (which this is very similar to) were also enviably silky. The matte shades include Sweet Pink, Hazelnut, Silky Caramel, Coal, Espresso, Cinnabar, and Raisin; soft-shine shades include Spun Silk and Ivy Garden. The remaining shades are very shiny, though the shine does cling well. Avoid the too-purple Iris and too-blue Denim Frost, and watch out for the very shiny shades if your eyelid is wrinkled. Purchased individually, these powder tablets arrive enclosed in a handy plastic case. If you opt to purchase the Mary Kay Compact, it can house up to six eyeshadows.

BRUSHES: ☺ **Mineral Powder Brush** *($10)* was created to apply Mary Kay's Mineral Powder Foundation. It does work for that purpose, but it is neither as soft nor as dense as it should be. However, for the money it's not a bad choice if you need a powder brush for travel.

MARY KAY SIGNATURE MAKEUP PRODUCTS

FOUNDATION: ☺ $$$ **Creme-to-Powder Foundation** *($14)* is smooth without feeling greasy or too thick, and provides medium coverage with an effect that's not too powdery or too creamy. This is more akin to traditional cream-to-powder foundation, which means it is best for normal to slightly oily skin without dry patches—which this foundation's finish exaggerates. Ten shades are available; among them, Ivory 2, Beige 2, Bronze 1, and Bronze 2 are best avoided due to overtones of rose or orange.

☺ **Full Coverage Foundation** *($14)* has a smooth, emollient formula that is suitable for those with normal to dry skin. It provides medium to full coverage and is relatively easy to blend, but it can look masklike on the skin, though the overall effect is more attractive than that of the Medium Coverage Foundation below. This is an option if you need significant coverage, but the trade-off is a finish that makes skin look covered rather than enhanced. Twenty shades are offered, with options for very light to dark skin. The following shades are too pink, peach, or rose for most skin tones: Beige 304, Beige 404, Bronze 500, Bronze 507, and Bronze 607. Due to this makeup's high talc content, the darkest shade, Bronze 808, can look slightly ash, but this effect can be minimized by mixing the foundation with a dab of moisturizer.

☹ **Medium Coverage Foundation** *($14)* feels (and looks) like a giant step backward compared to the marvelous foundations from the Lauder companies, L'Oreal, Cover Girl, and many others. It is a fairly smooth liquid foundation, but it doesn't blend all that well and ends up having a dry, slightly chalky, flat finish that can look artificial and masklike on skin. Rather than floating over or merging with the skin, the pigments in this foundation tend to creep into every crevice, which magnifies dry areas and can make skin look tired and older than it is. Twenty shades are available; although most of them are just fine, the overall look of this foundation isn't one I'd encourage you to explore.

CONCEALER: ✓ ☺ **Concealer** *($10)* comes in a squeeze tube and is very concentrated. This has an excellent, silicone-enhanced texture that blends without slip-sliding all over your face. It provides almost full coverage without looking thick or creasing, so it's a top choice if you have very dark circles. The six colors are fairly good, with the best ones being Light Ivory, Ivory, and Beige. The Yellow shade is too yellow for just about everyone.

POWDER: ☺ **Loose Powder** *($14)* is a talc-based powder with a soft, dry consistency and sheer finish. Five of the six colors are quite good—only Bronze 1 can be too peach for most skin tones.

EYESHADOW: ☺ **Eyesicles Eye Color** *($10)* comes in a tube and is available only in two colors (soft vanilla and coppery bronze). This cream-to-powder eyeshadow has enough slip to make controlled blending a problem, though once set it doesn't crease and it is waterproof as claimed. Mary Kay states that Eyesicles have a soft matte finish, but that's only true in terms of how this product feels once it sets. Rather, the look is very shiny and not for wrinkled eyes.

☺ **Eye Primer** *($12)* is a slightly thick, water- and talc-based white cream meant to prevent eyeshadows from creasing or smudging. Despite the prominence of talc, this remains slightly moist and doesn't work as well for its intended purpose as a flesh-toned matte-finish concealer. It's OK, but not suitable for anyone who has trouble getting eyeshadows to stay put.

EYE AND BROW SHAPER: ☺ **Eyeliner** *($10)* is an automatic, retractable pencil that has a smooth application, a smear-proof finish, and a reasonable price. There are some attractive soft colors available along with classic brown and black. This requires an oil- or silicone-based makeup remover.

☺ **Liquid Eyeliner** *($11)* has been improved and now sports a brush that's easier to control and a formula that dries faster and lasts. This liner is water-resistant as claimed, but note that if you swim with this and then rub your eye, it comes off immediately.

☹ **Brow Definer Pencil** *($10)* is a standard brow pencil that needs routine sharpening, but if you're OK with that, the results are great, as is the soft powder finish. Application and color deposit are good, and in fact the shades themselves are impressive, with options for blondes and redheads. This would get a happy face rating if sharpening wasn't a requirement.

☹ **Classic Blonde Brow Definer Pencil (wood)** *($10)* is a standard pencil that is a bit stiff yet has a long-lasting powder finish. The blonde shade is suitable for blonde eyebrows, and the color goes on sheer but builds if you need more intensity.

LIPSTICK, LIP GLOSS, AND LIPLINER: ✓☺ **Creme Lipstick** *($13)* replaced the MK Signature Cream lipstick, and it is a welcome improvement. Whereas the previous formula leaned toward the greasy side of creamy, this version feels creamy without a hint of greasiness, and imparts rich, riveting color that really lasts. As before, the range of shades is divided into color groups, and it's a logical system that makes it easy to focus on the types of shades you prefer. This offers a soft gloss finish without feeling slick, and doesn't fade into lines around the mouth as quickly as many creamy lipsticks do. We have a winner!

☺ **Lip Liner** *($10)* is recommended as a good, automatic, retractable lip pencil whose shade selection has been attractively expanded. The packaging is nicely color-coded, too, and this would be a Paula's Pick if it were more adept at keeping lipstick from feathering into lines around the mouth.

☺ **Nourishine Lip Gloss** *($13)* isn't as impressive as the original MK Signature Lip Gloss, but this replacement formula offers colors that are much more sheer, while keeping the formula smooth (though it has become thicker and now finishes with a slight stickiness) and the shimmer intact. A few of the colors work well over any shade of lipstick.

MASCARA: ☺ **Lash Lengthening Mascara** *($10)* does just what the name says, and accomplishes its task without clumping, flaking, or smearing. You won't notice any thickness, but if longer lashes are all you're after, this is one to try.

☺ **Ultimate Mascara** *($15)* doesn't reach the status of being worthy of its "ultimate" name, but it's nevertheless a good mascara that builds length and thickness quickly and in equal measure. Subsequent applications yield diminishing returns, which is why this isn't the one to choose if your objective is "ultimate" lashes.

☹ **MK Signature Waterproof Mascara** *($10)* works just as most waterproof mascaras do, meaning it lengthens lashes, doesn't do much to thicken, yet holds up when lashes get wet. The average aspect of this mascara is that it takes longer than it should to provide any noticeable difference in your lashes.

FACE ILLUMINATING PRODUCTS: ☹ **$$$ Facial Highlighting Pen** *($18)* is housed in a pen-style component with a built-in synthetic brush applicator. Although labeled a highlighter, its finish and coverage on skin are closer to that of a true concealer, as are the four shades.

Among those, shades 1 and 3 have a peach cast that's tricky to soften. Estee Lauder's Ideal Light Brush-On Illuminator costs slightly more, but is an overall much better product if your goal is to highlight skin and reflect light to make shadowy areas brighter.

BRUSHES: ☺ **Brush Set** *($48)* includes five brushes in a well-constructed synthetic leather case that includes extra pouches so you can add more brushes in the future. The **Powder Brush** and **Blush Brush** are quite soft and appropriately dense, though the **Blush Brush** would work better if its head were larger. The **Eye Definer Brush** and **Eye Crease Brush** don't fare as well, but aren't terrible, while the dual-sided **Eyeliner/Eyebrow Brush** is practical and functional (though the **Eyebrow Brush** is a bit too stiff). It's an overall worthwhile brush set that is priced fairly for what you get.

☹ **Cheek Color Brush** *($2.50)* is a compact-size blush brush similar to many prepackaged powder-blush brushes. It's not recommended over a regular, full blush brush.

☺ **Compact** *($18)* is Mary Kay's sleek solution for combining eyeshadows, blush, bronzing, and highlighting powders in one compact. Though not all of the aforementioned products will fit at once, you can mix and match whatever combination of Mary Kay pressed-powder items you'd like. The mirrored compact is sturdy, includes room for mini brushes (which is thoughtful, although the mini brushes the company offers are not on par with their full-size versions), and has a slot for a lipstick or lip gloss. And if you decide to forgo the compact and still want to order some Mary Kay eyeshadows or blushes, you'll find these items come packaged in their own resealable plastic cases.

☺ **Compact Pro** *($35)* is a larger version of Mary Kay's Compact. It includes enough room for 18 eyeshadows or a lesser combination of shadows (four would be plenty) along with powder blush, bronzer, highlighter, or an eyeshadow used for filling in brows or eyelining. The large compact also houses up to four pencils and has room for two lipsticks or a lipstick and lip gloss. Finally, there is room for Mary Kay's small brushes which, as mentioned in the review of their regular Compact, are not as good as their full-sized brushes (those do not fit in Compact Pro). If you're a fan of Mary Kay's powder-based makeup and want the option to store many shades in one case, this is a compact worth considering!

MAYBELLINE NEW YORK (MAKEUP ONLY)

MAYBELLINE NEW YORK AT-A-GLANCE

Strengths: The line earned Paula's Pick ratings for products in almost every category; many excellent foundations; superior mascaras; inexpensive makeup brushes; some terrific concealers, powders, blush, eyeshadow, eyeliner, lipstick, and bronzer options.

Weaknesses: The makeup removers; the foundations with sunscreen lack the right UVA-protecting ingredients; disappointing lipliners; average lip gloss; the loose-powder eyeshadow; Great Lash mascaras.

For more information about Maybelline New York, owned by L'Oreal, call (800) 944-0730 or visit their interactive Web site at www.maybelline.com or visit www.Beautypedia.com.

MAYBELLINE MINERAL POWER PRODUCTS

FOUNDATION: ☺ **Mineral Power Natural Perfecting Powder Foundation** *($8.29)* is Maybelline's answer to the mineral makeup craze, and they're promoting their entire Mineral Power line in a big way. This refined loose powder is based around zinc oxide, so it has a dry finish and provides adequate coverage for minor flaws or redness. It blends on smoothly, but it's unfortunate that Maybelline didn't take the extra step to evaluate this powder's sun-protection value (it seems to contain enough zinc to warrant the effort). But the big question is, should you try this mineral makeup? In no way does it distinguish itself from the competition, other than costing less and imparting minimal shine. The claim that the minerals are "triple-refined" means an improved texture, but mineral makeup options from L'Oreal, Laura Mercier, and Revlon among others have comparable textures. Application can still be a messy proposition, and the included "kabuki" brush is too small to be practical, not to mention it should be softer. For those who think loose-powder foundation is the way to go, this lends a dry matte finish that will do a good job of controlling oil, but the finish will look and feel too dry for anyone with dry areas. As with most mineral makeups, you may notice some deepening of the shade over oily areas (this tends to happen after several hours of wear). Maybelline offers eight shades, most of which go on more neutral than they appear in the container. The only one to consider carefully is the slightly rose Creamy Natural; avoid Sandy Beige, as this is too peach for most medium skin tones. The happy face rating pertains to this product's value for those seeking mineral makeup. I maintain that a liquid or compact foundation bests such makeup in most respects, and is easier to work with.

☺ **Mineral Power Natural Perfecting Foundation SPF 18** *($8.29)* disappoints in name and for its sunscreen's lack of sufficient UVA-protecting ingredients. This isn't a mineral foundation in the true sense of the word because none of the traditional mineral-type ingredients are in this liquid foundation. Although it could be argued that the silicones are derived from the mineral silica, they don't resemble this mineral by the time the finished ingredient (such as dimethicone) is added to the product. Despite the misleading name, this foundation has many good qualities. Of course, that makes it all the more disheartening that the sunscreen comes up short. This silky foundation that provides medium coverage and a smooth matte finish would have been ideal for normal to oily skin. Its finish is beautiful and doesn't feel the least bit thick or make skin look pasty. The range of 16 shades is one of the best Maybelline has ever produced; only Creamy Natural suffers from being more than slightly peach. There are suitable shades for fair and dark skin, too, so if you're willing to pair this with a broad-spectrum sunscreen with UVA-protecting ingredients, it's worth auditioning.

CONCEALER: ☺ **Mineral Power Liquid Concealer** *($6.49)* beckons you to replace artificial colorants with mineral pigments for natural coverage. Such a claim may make you think this concealer is different from the norm, but it isn't. The minerals in question (iron oxides, mica, and titanium dioxide) are present in almost every foundation or concealer being sold today. Besides, what good are mineral pigments if what they're mixed with doesn't create a pleasing texture and long-wearing finish? Luckily, Maybelline succeeded with that task. This concealer has a smooth, lightweight texture, and just enough slip. It provides good coverage and a solid matte finish with a hint of shine. Creasing should not be an issue, but this concealer's finish can magnify the look of wrinkles around the eye. Each of the six shades is worth considering, particularly the lighter colors. Beige Medium may be too peach for some medium skin tones, but isn't terrible.

POWDER: ☺ **Mineral Power Finishing Veil Pressed Powder** *($7.49)* is a mica-based powder that comes in three very good shades. It leaves a touch of shine on skin, but the effect is more radiant glow than glittery. It has a silky, sheer texture that is best for making normal to dry skin look polished. Those using powder to control shine (oil) will want something more absorbent.

BLUSH AND BRONZER: ☺ **Mineral Power Finishing Veil Bronzing Powder** *($8.99)* has a different formula and thicker texture than Maybelline's Mineral Power Finishing Veil Pressed Powder. The texture can result in a too-heavy application, especially if you use the enclosed sponge. However, this works great for medium to tan skin tones when dusted on with a large powder brush. The finish is matte in feel yet softly radiant in appearance. This is a good compromise between a shimmering and matte-finish bronzing powder.

☺ **Mineral Power Naturally Luminous Blush** *($7.49)* is a loose-powder blush, so right off the bat you're dealing with a product that is tricky to apply without overdoing it, not to mention inherently messy. The concentrated, surprisingly bright colors impart a lit-from-within glow, and the dry finish tends to hold up well over normal to oily skin. Those with dry skin will find this blush a mixed bag: the glow is nice, but the finish will likely feel too drying. I don't know why anyone would want to bother with this instead of using a pressed-powder blush, but for those so inclined, this is a decent choice.

LIPSTICK: ☺ **Mineral Power Lipstick** *($5.99)* is by far the weakest (or should I say least "power"ful?) entry in Maybelline's Mineral Power sub-brand, because this sheer, slick lipstick has nothing to do with minerals and everything to do with colors that are so fleeting you'll wonder why you bothered. Yes, this does feel ultralight and many of the colors have an enticing shimmer, but this practically slides right off your lips! It doesn't deserve an unhappy face rating, but at the same time it isn't a lipstick I would recommend to anyone unless they want sheer colors and short-lived results. Almost any lip gloss outperforms this one.

OTHER MAYBELLINE MAKEUP

FOUNDATION: ✓☺ **Dream Liquid Mousse Airbrush Finish** *($8.79)* has a name that makes this foundation seem as though flawless skin is within your reach, and guess what? That's not too far from the truth! This liquid foundation is dispensed via an elegant pump and has a luxuriously silky texture that meshes so well with skin it looks like a second skin. In that sense, and because this offers light to medium coverage, it's not going to conceal moderate to glaring flaws. However, it will blur minor flaws and discolorations and leave your skin with a luminous matte finish that's very attractive. The formula is best for normal to oily skin, but those with dry areas will do fine with this foundation as long as they prep their skin with a moisturizer (preferably one that contains sunscreen). The range of 12 shades is commendable and includes options for fair to dark (but not very dark) skin tones. Avoid Honey Beige and Pure Beige because both lean toward being too peach for medium skin tones. All told, this is another winner from Maybelline New York!

✓☺ **Instant Age Rewind Custom Face Perfector Cream Compact Foundation SPF 18** *($7.99)*. This cream-to-powder foundation is one of the best at the drugstore. The sunscreen is pure titanium dioxide, which is great news not only for sun protection but also for those with sensitive skin. The silky, initially creamy texture is a pleasure to blend and sets to a soft, natural matte finish that enlivens skin. Despite my enthusiasm, there was a compromise made to ensure such a beautifully smooth application. This foundation has so much slip that even once it sets it keeps slipping, and that includes slipping into wrinkles and creasing on the eyelids, even when set with powder. This drawback will be most apparent to those with oily skin or oily areas, which makes this foundation best for normal to dry skin (the finish does not exaggerate dry spots in the least). In fact, the Paula's Pick rating is only for those with normal to dry skin considering this foundation. Coverage varies depending on which side of the included sponge you use. The white side of the sponge produces nearly full coverage and does a good job of keeping the foundation out of lines and large pores. The pink side produces sheer coverage and tends to exaggerate lines and pores, so it is not preferred. Actually, a flat, round latex sponge is the best way to apply this foundation, but you can also use a foundation brush if that's your preference. Whichever you choose, there's no denying this is a brilliant cream-to-powder foundation with sunscreen that is highly recommended for normal to dry skin not prone to blemishes (the waxes this contains can contribute to clogged pores). Among the eight shades are mostly neutral options suitable for light to tan skin tones. Pure Beige will be too peach for most medium skin tones, and Tan has the same issue but is still worth considering.

☺ **Dream Matte Mousse Foundation** *($8.79)* has a smooth, whipped texture that feels wonderfully light on the skin and blends impeccably, setting to a slightly powdery matte finish. Coverage can go from sheer to medium, and this foundation layers well for additional coverage without a heavy or caked appearance. The nonaqueous silicone formula's main drawback is that it exaggerates any degree of dry skin. Therefore, either exfoliate your skin before using it or make sure your skin is prepped by applying a moisturizing sunscreen. Of course, applying a moisturizer negates this matte makeup's benefit for oily skin, but someone with very oily skin (who is unlikely to have any dry patches) can skip this step. Twelve shades are available, with options for light and dark (but not very dark) skin tones. The only shades to steer clear of due to strong overtones of pink or peach are Creamy Natural, Pure Beige, Medium Beige, and Tan. Porcelain Ivory is a good shade for fair skin tones, while Cocoa is a deep brown shade that doesn't turn ashy on skin, always a plus! Classic Ivory may be too peach for some light skin tones.

☺ **Pure.Makeup** *($4.99)* is a simply formulated, lightweight liquid foundation that smooths beautifully over skin and sets to a soft matte finish. The level of coverage is light but can be built up to medium if needed. The formula and finish are ideal for someone with normal to oily skin. Twelve shades are available; the lightest and darkest hues are the best options. Among the mid-tones, Light 3 and Medium 2 are slightly peach; Light 5, Medium 3, and Medium 4 are strongly peach; and Dark 1 is too rosy. By the way, despite the "won't clog pores" claim, this foundation contains enough titanium dioxide so that this is not a worry-free choice for the blemish-prone.

☺ **Superstay Makeup 24HR** *($10.49)*. This liquid foundation boasts of its 24-hour wear time, but that begs the question of why you'd want to wear your makeup for that long. At some point during the day you should remove your makeup (and whatever was applied underneath) to treat your skin to other products that don't involve color or camouflage. That said, Superstay Makeup has a formula that all but guarantees long wear. It has a smooth, semi-fluid texture that blends well and sets to a strong matte finish that feels and looks powdery. I wish this foundation looked better on skin, but as is, it casts a somewhat dull finish that isn't as good as, say, L'Oreal's True Match Super Blendable Makeup, or, for oily skin, Clinique's Superfit Makeup. The finish isn't a deal-breaker, but many of the shades look neutral in the bottle and then set to an unattractive peach, rose, or pink tone. Avoid any shades ending in "Beige" (e.g., Pure Beige, Honey Beige) and consider the medium tones carefully. The lightest and darkest shades are best. Back to wearability, this foundation stays on so well it practically stains the skin. A water-soluble cleanser won't work; you need an oil- or silicone-based makeup remover or plain cold cream to take this off. This foundation is best for oily skin in humid climates; it is not recommended for dry skin or skin with signs of dryness.

☺ **Instant Age Rewind Cream Foundation SPF 18** *($9.49)* is remarkably similar to the original Instant Age Rewind Foundation below, right down to its insufficient amount of UVA protection. This has a slightly thicker texture and slightly moist finish, but isn't what most people (especially those with dry skin) would consider creamy. This version also has the same noticeable sparkles as its predecessor, and they're very obvious in daylight. Among the 12 mostly good shades, the problematic colors include Medium Beige, Creamy Natural, and Honey Beige. This foundation is best for normal to slightly dry skin and must be paired with a sunscreen that provides sufficient UVA protection.

☺ **PureStay Powder Plus Foundation SPF 15** *($8.99)* is a talc-based pressed powder with slightly heavier coverage so it can double as a foundation. It has a superior, smooth texture, an even application, and a soft matte finish that can go from sheer to medium coverage. What a shame the sunscreen lacks significant UVA-protecting ingredients! Still, if you're already using a well-formulated sunscreen rated SPF 15 or higher, this is worth considering by those with normal to very oily skin. Most of the eight shades are excellent neutrals; the ones to avoid due to pink or peach overtones are Soft Cameo, Golden, and Sand.

☺ **Instant Age Rewind Foundation SPF 18** *($6.59)* has a great name! Maybelline even included the classic VCR "rewind" symbol as part of this product's logo. But clever names and logos don't relate to fact: no one's skin will be any firmer or "look younger instantly" with this water- and silicone-based foundation. And any age-rewinding credibility this foundation hoped to have is lost in advance because its sunscreen does not provide sufficient UVA protection. That lack of protection is disappointing, because this foundation's texture and application are beautiful. It provides medium coverage and sets to a smooth matte finish that is laced with shiny particles. The shine isn't as subtle as that of similar products from Revlon or M.A.C., so consider this factor carefully. The selection of 12 shades includes some excellent options for fair to light and tan to dark skin tones, including Porcelain Ivory, Classic Ivory, Tan, Caramel, and Cocoa. Those with medium skin tones will be disappointed, however, because those shades (Creamy Natural, Honey Beige, Sandy Beige, and Pure Beige) all lean toward or are blatantly peach. In summary, this foundation has more pros than cons, and is an option for normal to slightly dry or slightly oily skin if you're willing to pair it with a sunscreen that provides better UVA protection.

☺ **Superstay Silky Foundation SPF 12** *($10.99)* is a two-part foundation that combines a primer and foundation with a pure titanium dioxide sunscreen and a too-low (but not terrible) SPF rating (SPF 15 would have been best). The first time you use this, the primer is dispensed before the foundation, which is wasteful. But when the foundation joins the primer (each is packaged in its own chamber, visible through the plastic component) they mesh together well—until you notice the colors. Almost all of them are noticeably pink, peach, orange, rose, or copper. What you see in the bottle is very close to what you get on your skin once this foundation sets to its silky matte finish. It has a very good, lightweight texture that allows plenty of time to blend, and the finish holds up quite well, providing medium coverage and a slightly too-opaque look. But among the 12 colors, the only recommended shades are Light 2, Light 4, and Medium 1—and even these aren't as stellar as what you'll find at L'Oreal.

CONCEALER: ✓ ☺ **Instant Age Rewind Double Face Perfector** *($7.09)* provides a liquid concealer and coordinated highlighter in one sleek, dual-sided package. The concealer has a supremely lightweight texture that is easy to apply, but blending must be quick because it sets to a creaseless matte finish in short order. Coverage-wise, this really excels. It's meant to camouflage "adult imperfections" such as discolorations from the sun or broken capillaries, and does so without calling attention to itself. The highlighter has a thinner texture, more slip (so you have more time to blend), and offers a sheer finish with a hint of shine. It is ideal for highlighting small areas and may be used around the eyes. Among the four shade duos, only Medium falls short because it's borderline peach. This remarkable duo is otherwise highly recommended.

☺ **Pure.Concealer** *($5.79)* is an automatic, nonretractable pencil concealer, the type that makes pinpoint application to red spots and blemishes a cinch. The silicone-based formula applies smoothly and provides sufficient, non-cakey coverage, but it does contain waxes and wax-like ingredients that aren't the best for routine use on blemishes. This contains 2% salicylic acid (BHA), but a pH cannot be established in a waterless medium, so there's no way the BHA will exfoliate. Pure.Concealer comes in three very good shades (for light to medium skin) and is an option to spot-conceal redness or minor discolorations.

☺ **True Illusion Undetectable Concealer SPF 10** *($5.79)* has no UVA-protecting ingredients and the SPF 10 is too low for all-day protection, so it is unreliable for sunscreen; but it is a very good concealer with a smooth texture and a semi-opaque, natural-matte finish. It blends easily and does not crease. True Ivory and True Beige are both great options for light skin tones.

☹ **Coverstick Corrector Concealer** *($5.49)* is a dated, oil- and wax-based formula that is too greasy to stay put for long, and it creases easily. It also tends to look too thick and heavy on skin, even when blended thoroughly. Maybelline claims this is their #1-selling concealer, and while that may be true in volume, it is not so in performance, especially when compared to their other concealers.

☹ **Superstay Concealer 24HR** *($7.59)*. This liquid concealer promises to wear for 24 hours without transferring. It contains an ingredient that can definitely go the distance in terms of long wear, but the bigger concern is why you'd be wearing makeup for 24 hours straight. This certainly won't hold up well if you sleep in it, and at some point in the day, makeup needs to be removed so that your skin can be treated with other products. I have no complaints about the minimal slip of this concealer, plus it covers well and sets to a matte finish. One problem is that this absolutely cannot be blended once it sets, so you have to get it right the first time. That can be accomplished with practice, but it doesn't take away the bigger issue, which is with the shades. Maybelline really regressed here and for whatever reason created five shades that go on much more pink, rose, or peach than you'd expect. The Fair shade is the only acceptable option, and that's being generous.

POWDER: ✓ ☺ **Dream Matte Face Powder** *($6.49)* has a silky-smooth yet dry texture, allowing it to make good on its claim of providing an air-soft matte finish. It is a very good pressed powder for normal to very oily skin. Application is sheer, and applying more doesn't lend a thick, powdery look (though it can make skin look dull, so do use some restraint). Eight shades are available, all of which are beautiful, including options for very fair to tan skin tones. Well done!

☺ **Shine Free Oil-Control Loose Powder** *($5.99)* is a talc- and clay (kaolin)-based powder that comes in two translucent colors and has a soft texture and sheer matte finish. It isn't quite as elegant as L'Oreal's Translucide Naturally Luminous Powder, but for half the price you may not mind! This powder is suitable for normal to very oily skin.

☺ **Shine Free Translucent Pressed Powder** *($5.99)* can't control shine any more than most powders, but it is a suitably soft, dry-finish powder that applies smooth and sheer and is indeed oil-free. The talc-based formula is available in four colors. Natural Beige 04 is too pink, especially for those battling excess oil, but the other three shades are fine.

BLUSH AND BRONZER: ✓ ☺ **Dream Mousse Blush** *($5.99)* is accurately described as "air-whipped." It has a soft, spongy texture that gives way to a superior application for what's essentially a modified cream-to-powder blush. Each shimmer-infused shade blends on soft and sheers out quickly, so you can experiment without imparting too much color. Those who want to add more color will find this product layers well. Even better, this really stays in place after it sets, and you'll experience only minimal fading. It is a fun-yet-functional departure from powder blush, and is best for normal to slightly dry or slightly oily skin (provided you don't mind having shiny cheeks).

✓ ☺ **Dream Mousse Bronzer** *($5.99)* has the same formula and thus deserves the same accolades as the Dream Mousse Blush, only here you get two shiny bronze tones. Glistening Sun is preferred for fair to light skin, while Sun Glow is ideal for medium skin tones. This is one to try if you don't mind a tan with noticeable shine.

☺ **Expertwear Blush** *($5.49)* doesn't deserve its "silky-smooth" description because this pressed-powder blush is a bit too dry and thus tends to apply a bit unevenly. The less-than-ideal application isn't a deal-breaker because each shine-infused shade goes on sheer, but I wouldn't choose this over L'Oreal's True Match Super-Blendable Blush. Maybelline's shade selection does not offer deeper hues for women of color.

☺ **Expertwear Blush Duo** *($4.49)* has the same formula and application issues as the Expertwear Blush, but here you get a slightly shiny powder blush paired with a shinier highlighting powder. The Two to Glow duo is an option as a bronzing powder for someone with fair skin.

☺ **Expertwear Blush Bronzer** *($5.49)* also has the same formula as the Expertwear Blush, except that the two shades are meant to be used as bronzing powder. The Salsa Sun shade is matte and can work as a bronzer or for contouring.

EYESHADOW: ☺ **Cool Effect Cooling Shadow/Liner** *($4.69)* feels cool due to the water and glycol base, and although this glides on easily, it sets quickly. That means using any of the shine-infused shades as eyeshadow or highlighter (there are lots of pale colors) requires quick, precise blending. You'll find that as eyeliner these last all day without smearing, though the amount of shine is too strong for someone with wrinkled or drooping eyelids. The following shades are either too contrasting or odd for an attractive eye makeup design: Cool as a Cucumber, Frosty Pink, Sugar Plum Ice, and Midnight Chill.

☺ **Expert Eyes Designer Selections Shadow** *($7.39)* provides eight powder eyeshadows in one compact, though you get just a small amount of each. Four of the shades are matte and four are shiny. These apply and feel just like Maybelline's Expertwear Eye Shadow, which means they're good but not great. If you decide to try this, the best set is Sunbaked Neutrals.

☺ **Expertwear Eye Shadow** *($2.99)* is a notable improvement over previous versions of Maybelline powder eyeshadows, though it doesn't surpass the top picks in this category. What's missing from these shadows is that lush, almost suede-like smoothness and impeccable blending found in superior options. Expertwear Eye Shadow does have a nice silkiness, but also has a waxy feel that prevents smooth, even blending. Pigmentation has improved, as has these eyeshadows' ability to cling to skin. You won't get as much color payoff as you will with eyeshadows from M.A.C. or Stila, but the sheerness is bound to please those looking for softer eyeshadow shades. There appear to be some matte options among the singles, but closer inspection reveals that even these have some shine, so avoid them if matte is your goal. The almost-matte single shades include Vanilla, Earthly Taupe, Champagne Fizz, and Creme de Cocoa. All of the duos have a soft shine, but if that doesn't bother you, the best pairings are Indian Summer, Browntones, and Grey Matters. Two of the three shades in each trio set are shiny, but again, there are some attractive combinations, including Almond Truffles, Chocolate Mousse, and Impeccable Greys. Among the quads, most sets have at least one matte shade, and at least one shade is suitable for use as powder eyeliner. The most workable quads include Mocha Motion, Designer Chocolates, Sunlit Bronze, and Time for Wine.

☹ **Shadow Stylist Loose Powder** *($5.19)* is packaged like the inkwell-style liquid eyeliners, but this is loose-powder eyeshadow that's applied with a synthetic, pointed sponge tip. Although the powder's texture is smooth and blendable, the application method causes way too much flaking, even if you dab off excess product. Given that the results are comparable to what you can achieve with a powder eyeshadow that doesn't flake, there is no reason to consider this.

EYE AND BROW SHAPER: ✓☺ **Define-A-Brow Eyebrow Pencil** *($5.49)* is an ultra-thin, automatic, nonretractable brow pencil that comes in a terrific range of shades, including two options for blonde brows. Even better, this does everything a stellar brow pencil should, while offering an exemplary texture and long wear. The component includes a useful brow comb for tidying the results. This is definitely one of the better brow pencils at the drugstore!

✓☺ **Expertwear Defining Liner** *($5.79)* used to go by the name Expert Eyes Defining Liner, and it remains a great automatic, retractable eye pencil whose dry finish isn't as smudge-prone as most eye pencils, though it's not quite as worry-free as lining with a matte-powder eyeshadow. It's definitely worth a look for pencil lovers, and the smudge-tip concealer has a built-in sharpener for those desiring a finer point.

✓☺ **Line Stiletto Ultimate Precision Liquid Eyeliner** *($6.99)*. This liquid liner contains a flexible felt-tip brush meant to create "slender lines," which it absolutely does. Rich color is deposited evenly and the formula dries quickly to a patent-leather shine. The formula has impressive wear time and doesn't flake, though anyone with oily eyelids will likely find that this doesn't go the distance as well as the gel-type eyeliners.

✓☺ **Line Stylist Eyeliner** *($5.79)* is another excellent automatic pencil, though this one isn't retractable. However, the wind-up is calibrated, so there's little chance you'll break the pencil tip. The tip allows you to draw a thin or thicker line, and application is smooth and even. Once set, this feels powdery and stays in place all day. Most of the shades have shimmer or sparkle, but those looking for classic colors will appreciate Onyx and Espresso. Note: This tenacious product is difficult to take off without an oil- or silicone-based remover.

✓☺ **Unstoppable Smudge-Proof Waterproof Eyeliner** *($7.29)* is an automatic, retractable pencil that applies swiftly without skipping and really doesn't smudge, even with provocation. It's waterproof, too, yet removes easily. The only drawback is its slightly tacky finish. That's a minor issue for such an outstanding pencil, and with the exception of Jade, the color selection is reliable.

☺ **Brow Styling Gel** *($5.69)* is a standard brow gel that is very easy to apply and feels light and non-sticky. There are two sheer colors, which would work for dark blondes and brunettes, as well as a clear shade for just holding unruly brows in place. It's a good, inexpensive option if you're looking to tame your brows or add a soft sheen.

☺ **Define-A-Brow Brow Gel** *($4.99)* doesn't set a new pace for clear brow gels, but instead uses a standard gel formula that works well to neaten brows and hold them in place throughout the day. The finish is minimally sticky, and brows are left soft with a natural, non-glossy appearance.

☺ **Define-A-Line Eye Liner** *($6.29)* is supposed to glide on smoothly, and it does. This automatic, retractable pencil needs no sharpening, but includes a built-in sharpener (housed under the sponge-tip smudger) if you desire a finer point. Because this pencil's finish is quite smudge-prone on its own, it is best for creating a smoky eye effect. The shade range offers several variations on brown along with gray and black. Khaki Green is an intriguing departure: a shiny golden olive that can look alluring blended with (or over) a black or deep brown eyeliner (or powder eyeshadow).

☺ **Expertwear Brow and Eyeliner** *($4.49)* is an automatic, retractable pencil that can be sharpened to a finer tip than most (the sharpener is built into the pencil). This pencil has a dry texture, which means less smudging. The sheer application and drier finish are well-suited to brows.

☺ **Ultra Brow Brush-On Brow Color** *($4.99)* is a standard, matte brow powder that comes packaged with the standard hard brush that you should toss away and replace with a good soft professional brush. There are two shades, which is limited to say the least, but what's available works if it matches your brow color.

☺ **Ultra Liner Waterproof Eyeliner** *($6.29)* is a liquid liner with a brush that only allows you to draw an intense, thick line. It takes a bit longer to dry than it should, but once it does it won't move, even under water. If you're going swimming and want thickly lined, dramatic eyes, here's your solution!

☺ **Waterproof Liquid Eyeliner** *($6.99)* has a finer tip and thus allows for a more versatile application (you can easily go from thin to thick) than the Ultra Liner Waterproof Eyeliner. Another plus is that this formula dries almost instantly, which reduces the chance of smearing. It stays on well, too, and is waterproof. The only issue is that it tends to apply unevenly, so you have to smooth out the line before it sets. It would otherwise be rated a Paula's Pick.

☺ **Expert Eye Twin Brow and Eye Pencil** *($2.99)* has been part of the Maybelline line for decades, and it's still a standard small pencil whose dry, stiff texture is somewhat workable for brows. However, it would still net you a dated look, and you don't want to use this for eye-lining because it is so dry that it would actually hurt as you tried to move it along the skin. There are ample colors for all brow colors, from blonde to black, and the dry finish really stays put. If you don't mind sharpening and you prefer pencil to powder, this is one to consider.

☺ **Expertwear Softlining Pencil** *($4.79)* is a standard "sharpen me again" pencil that goes on creamy but doesn't smudge or smear as readily as it once did. It isn't exceptional, but is worth considering if you don't mind routine sharpening.

☺ **Line Express Eyeliner** *($4.69)* needs routine sharpening, so right off the bat it isn't worth considering over automatic pencils. The pencil comes with a pointed sponge tip at one end that is designed for smudging the line. You'll want to do that before this creamy formula (which applies smoothly) smudges on its own. The colors are described as intense, and though they do apply darker than some pencils, the difference isn't enough to make this a must-have for sultry, smoky eyes.

LIPSTICK, LIP GLOSS, LIPLINER: ✓☺ **Color Sensational Lipcolor** *($7.19)*. This cream lipstick is excellent. It has a smooth, emollient texture that glides on without being too slick and makes lips feel indulgently moist with a soft cream finish. The 48 shades (yes, 48 shades!) are divided into color families of Pinks, Plums, Reds, and Naturals (tan to brown tones) and each group has a color-coordinated cap that makes it easy to figure out which group you're looking at. With this many shades to choose from, you can have a field day in the drugstore.

Most of the shades have some degree of shimmer finish. Note that you need several layers of this to build what Maybelline describes as "rich, stunning color." This lipstick is prone to feathering into lines around the mouth, but if that's not an issue for you, it is highly recommended.

✓ ☺ **Color Sensational Lip Gloss** *($6.19)* appears to be another standard lip gloss, but it rises above much of the competition with its supremely smooth texture, luxurious feel on lips, and attractive colors that go on moderately strong and impart a glossy sheen. The shade range is excellent and this isn't the least bit sticky. It's a great option to wear alone because the color deposit approaches that of many lipsticks, although it wears off faster.

✓ ☺ **Superstay Lipcolor** *($9.19)* bests Max Factor's original Lipfinity because it wears more evenly. The now-familiar two-step application process involves applying the color coat, then waiting two minutes for it to set (it feels very sticky as it dries, unlike most of the other long-wearing lip paints out there). Next you apply a glossy top coat to ensure a shiny finish and, more important, comfortable wear. Whereas Lipfinity, like Cover Girl's identical Outlast Lipcolor, tends to wear off at the inner portion of the lips, Superstay Lipcolor stays and stays. There's just one caveat: This is not a liquid lipstick that makes it through a meal, although it's fine with just drinks. This is partially because Maybelline's shade range is so soft. Most of the colors, even those that appear intense, apply sheer, and layering doesn't build significantly more color. Removing this product requires mineral oil, Vaseline, or an oil-based cleanser. The top coat is in stick form, and feels similar to the top coats that accompany Lipfinity and Outlast. Although I disagree with Maybelline's claim that Superstay Lipcolor lasts 16 hours (only if you hold perfectly still, don't talk, and don't eat anything), it is another terrific alternative to traditional lipstick. Maybelline also deserves kudos for packaging the two steps in one component, similar to what M.A.C. and Estee Lauder have done with their competing products.

☺ **Shine Seduction Glossy Lipcolor** *($6.49)* takes a standard sheer lip gloss and packages it in a sleek tube with a click-dial that feeds product onto an angled applicator. The high-shine gloss has a moderately thick texture and a wet, slightly sticky finish with fair tenacity. Seduction-wise, this is easily kissed off, but it will look alluring, and that may be all it takes!

☺ **Superstay Gloss** *($8.99)* claims to deliver "double-duty beauty" because one end is a sheer liquid lip color and the other is a clear, patent leather–shiny gloss. This Max Factor Lipfinity–like product is applied in two steps. You paint on the lip color, let it dry for two minutes, then brush on the thick, clear gloss. This is an option if you're looking for long-wearing sheer colors and want a super glossy finish; however, it is not preferred to Maybelline's original Superstay Lipcolor because the Gloss version's top coat is sticky and doesn't do a great job of making the liquid lip color increasingly comfortable. Great colors, though, including "your lips, but better" shades. Wear time is definitely longer than a traditional gloss, which is the main reason to consider this product.

☺ **Superstay Topcoat** *($3.99)* is the same product that's paired with Maybelline's outstanding Superstay Lipcolor. It's a smooth, colorless lip balm in stick form that may be used over the company's long-wearing lip color or on its own (should you just want moisture and a soft gloss finish). This is recommended if you use one of Maybelline's Superstay products and find that you go through the top coat faster than the lip paint portion of these dual-sided products. This top coat is available in Clear or with a golden shimmer.

☺ **Color Sensational Lipliner** *($6.19)*. Although this lip pencil requires routine sharpening, it's a very good option for those who don't mind the chore. It applies evenly and sets to a slightly powdery finish that resists smudging and doesn't fade (at least for the first few hours it's worn). I wish the shade selection were larger, but what's available is great. This would earn a Paula's Pick rating if not for the need to sharpen.

☺ **Line Stylist Lip Liner** *($5.19)* is an automatic, very thin-tipped, nonretractable lip pencil with a smooth but dry application that goes on a bit unevenly. It finishes dry rather than creamy, and although that helps it last longer, the shades are pigment-shy and tend to fade sooner than they should. There are better lip pencils at the drugstore from L'Oreal, Cover Girl, and others.

☺ **$$$ Lip Gloss/Lip Stain** *($28)* offers a dual-sided product: one end is a silicone-based, deeply pigmented lip stain, the other a sheer, standard lip gloss. The stain goes on more like a liquid lipstick, imparting rich, opaque color without a trace of heaviness. The gloss makes things more comfortable, but the problem is it wrecks the stain beneath it, meaning that you have to blend the two together, which diminishes longevity. This lip paint/top coat product is an OK option, but should have been much better this late in the game, especially given the competition from Lorac Co-Stars and M.A.C. Pro Longwear Lipcolour.

☺ **Lip Polish Hi-Shine Color** *($4.69)* provides a somewhat creamy, but also powdery, texture that spreads sheer, colored glitter over the lips. It isn't as greasy or messy as some glosses, but it also isn't as smooth—it just has lots of sparkle.

☹ **Moisture Extreme Lipcolor SPF 15** *($5.59)* provides lips with lots of emollient moisture, but disappoints with a sunscreen that fails to deliver sufficient UVA protection. This creamy-bordering-on-greasy lipstick feels almost like a slick balm when applied to lips, and leaves a glossy finish. The shade selection is plentiful (almost 40 colors), but none has much staying power, especially if you're prone to lipstick feathering into lines around the mouth.

☺ **Moisture Extreme Lipliner** *($4.69)* needs sharpening and is creamy enough to be worthy of its name. The application is ultra-smooth, but the downside is this pencil is too creamy to last as long as many others, and it puts up little resistance when your lipstick starts migrating into lines around the mouth.

☺ **VolumeXL Seduction Xtreme Lip Plumper** *($8.99)* contains a potent menthol derivative (ethyl menthane carboxamide, to be exact) that makes lips tingle (as claimed) and enlarge slightly from the resulting irritation. The plumping effect won't cause people who know you to do a double-take over your inflated mouth, but this is an inexpensive option for occasional use because irritating lips like this daily can cause chapped lips. Maybelline offers a clear shade along with several sheer colors (they look much darker in the container than they apply). The texture of each is akin to traditional lip gloss, meaning slightly thick and sticky with a glossy finish. All in all, this is an OK option for special occasions and the dispensing method from the sleek component is better than that of many other lip plumpers.

☹ **Shiny-Licious** *($5.79)* has a smooth application and a glossy finish that isn't too slick or slippery, but the formula has mint in it, as evidenced by the tingling feel after it's applied. There is little question that this gloss irritates lips, making it not worth choosing over dozens and dozens of others that don't have this problem.

MASCARA: ✓ ☺ **Define-a-Lash Volume Mascara** *($6.29)* has the same type of hourglass-shaped rubber-bristled brush as the original Define-a-Lash Mascara, but Maybelline made some minor tweaks that produce major (positive) results! The promises of "zero clumps, clean definition, and voluptuous volume" come true with just a few swipes of the wand, though some may find the slightly wetter-than-usual application a bit dismaying. The application can initially make lashes look stuck together, but the brush allows for nimble comb-through, so you can soften the result, making lashes look fringed while building considerable thickness and length. As a final plus, lashes remain very soft, there's no flaking or smearing, and removal is complete with just a water-soluble cleanser.

✓☺ **Define-A-Lash Waterproof Lengthening Mascara** *($6.29)* is a superior waterproof mascara that makes lashes impressively longer and well-defined with minimal effort. True to claim, the rubber-bristled brush applies product without a trace of clumping, and allows you to reach every lash. Get lashes as wet as you'd like: This isn't budging! It took several attempts with a silicone-based makeup remover to completely remove this tenacious mascara!

✓☺ **Define-A-Lash Volume Waterproof Mascara** *($6.99)* is aces if you're looking for more length than thickness, with beautifully clean lash separation and soft definition. The formula is waterproof and applies easily with its rubber-bristled brush. You will need an oil- or silicone-based makeup remover when you're ready to take this off. True to the company's claim, this mascara doesn't clump.

✓☺ **Full 'n Soft Mascara** *($6.59)* ranks as Maybelline's best mascara for those desiring equal parts impressive length and thickness. The balanced application sweeps on without clumps, separates lashes evenly, and wears all day. Marvelous!

✓☺ **Intense XXL Volume + Length Microfiber Mascara** *($6.79)* is similar to L'Oreal's Volume Shocking Mascara *($12.95)*, but (despite the name) this is less intense. It involves a two-step process of base plus top coat, although—just like Maybelline's other XXL mascaras— the base coat makes little difference, assuming you're willing to apply two or three coats of the mascara itself. The best news is that whether or not you use the base coat, you'll get beautifully long, nicely separated, and moderately thickened lashes with absolutely no clumps. The formula wears well and removes easily, making for hassle-free work all around.

✓☺ **Lash Discovery Mascara** *($6.59)* has a very small brush that initially made me skeptical. Yet this tiny, short-bristled brush let me be adept not only at getting to each and every lash, but also at expertly lengthening, separating, and providing appreciable thickness without clumping or smearing.

✓☺ **Lash Discovery Waterproof Mascara** *($5.99)* lacks the noticeable thickness of its non-waterproof counterpart, but this is otherwise an extraordinary mascara that lifts, lengthens, and leaves lashes with a soft, fringed curl. It's also waterproof and the tiny brush makes application to the lower lashes a cinch.

✓☺ **Sky High Curves Extreme Length and Curl Mascara** *($6.49)* almost lives up to its lofty name. This is a thoroughly impressive mascara! The easy-to-wield brush allows for ample (not extreme) lengthening and almost instant, high-impact thickness that just keeps getting better the longer you apply it. Perhaps the best news is that for all this lash-building, clumping is barely a problem.

✓☺ **Sky High Curves Extreme Length and Curl Mascara Waterproof** *($6.49)* isn't much for creating curled lashes, but wow, does this make lashes incredibly long, and quickly, too! The smearproof formula holds up beautifully to water exposure, yet isn't overly difficult to remove. It is one of the better lengthening waterproof mascaras at the drugstore.

✓☺ **The Colossal Volum' Express Waterproof Mascara** *($6.99)* became an instant favorite of mine for its ample lash-magnifying results that look great, so I had high hopes for the waterproof version. I wasn't let down. Although this version doesn't leave lashes as thick and lush as its non-waterproof counterpart, the worry-free, easy application still leaves most other waterproof mascaras in the dust. Unless you want ultra-thick lashes, you'll be impressed by the results from this Colossal, and it is waterproof as claimed. You will need more than a water-soluble cleanser to remove it.

✓ ☺ **The Colossal Volum' Express Colossal Mascara** *($5.99)* has a huge rubber-bristled brush that allows you to be surprisingly nimble as you elongate and thicken every lash. The volumizing results are evident almost immediately, though not without some clumping that needs to be smoothed out. Make no mistake, this mascara is not for the lash-timid. It produces Texas-size lashes that keep getting bigger the more you apply (though layering this tends to worsen the clumps and cause slight flaking). This goes slightly beyond the outstanding results from rival Cover Girl's Lash Blast Mascara, but with Lash Blast, clumps and a too-heavy appearance are rarely an issue. Either way, both are excellent mascaras to consider.

✓ ☺ **Volum' Express Mascara 3X** *($6.69)* isn't the best thickening mascara in Maybelline's lineup anymore, but it still excels at creating long, thick lashes without clumps. Results are noticeable immediately, and layering makes lashes slightly more dramatic.

✓ ☺ **Volum' Express Mascara 3X, Curved Brush** *($6.69)* isn't the best thickening mascara in Maybelline's lineup anymore, but it still excels at creating long, thick lashes without clumps. Results are noticeable immediately, and layering makes lashes slightly more dramatic. The curved-brush version produces even faster results than the traditional brush style and makes lashes look slightly more lifted.

✓ ☺ **Volum' Express Turbo Boost Mascara 7X** *($7.79)* advertises that users will achieve seven times the volume in one stroke, and guess what? It works! This is certainly one of Maybelline's most impressive thickening mascaras, with an application that's quick and clump-free and a lash look that's only for those who covet long, impossibly thick lashes.

✓ ☺ **XXL Curl Power Volume + Length Microfiber Mascara** *($6.79)* is another two-step mascara whose results are excellent whether you apply the base coat or just the mascara alone. I used the base coat with two coats of mascara on one side, then applied two coats of mascara to the other side. In both cases the result was long, slightly thickened, clump-free lashes upswept to a soft curl. The only drawback is that the inclusion of the non-value-added base coat means you get less mascara, and that's the part that really delivers. Still, for those who like the novelty of such mascara pairings, this is a prime choice.

✓ ☺ **XXL Extensions XX-Treme Length Microfiber Mascara** *($7.59)*. Fans of DiorShow mascaras take note: here is your drugstore double. This two-step mascara will give your lashes the kind of prodigious length that will get your eyes noticed. Step one is the base coat, which applies cleanly and separates lashes, preparing them for step two, the mascara. The large brushes mean that applying it to smaller lashes can be tricky, but other than that this mascara applies very easily with no clumping. It also wears beautifully throughout the day without smearing or flaking. XXL Extensions does create more length than thickness, but it will still give you va-va-voom lashes that are gorgeous and perfectly separated. Removal is a cinch with any eye-makeup remover.

✓ ☺ **XXL Volume + Length Microfiber Mascara** *($7.59)* is similar to L'Oreal's excellent DoubleExtend Lash Extender & Magnifier Mascara *($9.99)*. Both are dual-ended mascaras: one end contains a lash primer and the other a mascara. Just as I did with L'Oreal's version, I applied the "microfiber base coat" to my left eyelashes and followed with the mascara. Results were impressive. On my right lashes I applied two coats of the mascara only. As expected, both sides looked nearly the same, with the slight length and thickness edge going to the mascara-only lashes. The bottom line is that Maybelline's XXL Microfiber Mascara (which, by the way, doesn't contain any fibers) is an outstanding lengthening/thickening mascara all by itself. The base coat is no more effective than applying two coats of regular mascara, and, if anything, including the base coat wastes space that could be filled with mascara instead! Whether you use this product's two steps or just apply the mascara, you're not likely to be disappointed.

☺ **Define-A-Lash Mascara** *($7.95)*. Promising zero clumps with stunning definition and length, this mascara really delivers! It isn't much for creating thicker lashes, but each stroke makes them longer without any mishaps. The brush doesn't take as much getting used to as does the fact that the wand is too flexible. Sweeping this through lashes causes the wand to bend more than it should, which can affect application, but for the most part it wears without a hitch, keeping lashes exceptionally soft.

☺ **Full 'n Soft Waterproof Mascara** *($5.99)* is said to build "full, soft thick lashes." It does a decent job of fulfilling that claim, albeit with less thickness than you may be expecting. Still, it bests several other waterproof mascaras that make thicker-lashes claims, and this one won't come off in the pool or inclement weather.

☺ **Great Lash Clear Mascara** *($4.79)* is a multi-purpose clear mascara that adds a touch of length and a glossy finish to lashes while also grooming unruly brows. The standard formula is similar to that of most other clear mascaras and brow gels, but it does its job without flaking or feeling sticky. It does take a bit longer than usual to dry, but that's a minor quibble for this versatile, affordable product.

☺ **Lash Stiletto Ultimate Length Mascara** *($7.49)* claims to do for your lashes what stiletto heels do for your legs. That could mean any number of things, but what this fairly average mascara will do is lengthen well with minimal clumping. Lash Stiletto doesn't build much thickness, but it does wear well through the day with no flaking or smearing. The long brush takes some getting used to, but the tapered end makes it easy to reach smaller lashes. Lash Stiletto does not give your lashes a shiny patent finish as claimed; the color deposit is the same as that of any other good mascara.

☺ **Pulse Perfection by Define-A-Lash Vibrating Mascara** *($14.99)* is Maybelline's version of Lancome's Oscillation Mascara. Although Maybelline's version is at the top of the price scale for expensive drugstore mascaras, it's still less than half the price of Lancome's version (remember, L'Oreal is the parent company of both brands). Whether you choose to spend more on Lancome or a lot less on Maybelline, does the concept of a vibrating mascara have merit? Yes, but not nearly as much as the ads and claims for such mascaras would have you believe. Pulse Perfection offers very good length and thickness and all-day wear without flaking or smearing. The vibration makes a subtle difference, mostly in terms of a clump-free deposit of mascara at the base of the eyelashes. To enable the vibration feature you must keep the tiny button on the cap of the mascara wand depressed. Unfortunately, it requires a lot of pressure, which makes maneuvering the brush through your lashes more difficult than it should be. The results with the vibration off are good enough that I wasn't willing to tolerate the awkwardness that came with having to keep the button depressed during application. This mascara is easy to remove with a water-soluble cleanser.

☺ **Pulse Perfection by Define-A-Lash Vibrating Mascara Waterproof** *($14.99)* is Maybelline's version of Lancome's Oscillation Water-Resistant Mascara. Although Maybelline's version is at the top of the price scale for expensive drugstore mascaras, it's still less than half the cost of Lancome's version (remember, L'Oreal is the parent company of both brands). Whether you choose to spend more on Lancome or a lot less on Maybelline, does the concept of a vibrating mascara have merit? Yes, but not nearly as much as the ads and claims for such mascaras would have you believe. In this case, you'll find the vibrating brush deposits extra mascara at the base and outward along the lashes, but not so much that you couldn't do the same thing by simply applying another coat or two. Enabling the vibration feature requires you to keep the tiny button on the cap of the mascara wand depressed. Unfortunately, it requires a lot of pressure and that makes maneuvering the brush through lashes more difficult than it should be. The results were negligible enough that I preferred to use this mascara without the vibration. You'll get beautifully elongated lashes and some thickness with ample definition and the formula is waterproof. This would be rated a Paula's Pick if not for its minor tendency to smear.

☺ **Volum' Express Waterproof Mascara 3X** *($6.69)* builds quickly and makes lashes moderately longer and noticeably thicker without clumps. It is waterproof.

☺ **XXL Volume + Length Waterproof Microfiber Mascara** *($6.79)* is indeed a tenaciously waterproof version of the XXL Microfiber Mascara. One end of this dual-sided product is a lash primer and the other a lengthening mascara. I applied the primer and mascara combination to one set of my eyelashes and used just the mascara on the other. The mascara alone produced copious length and beautifully defined, clump-free lashes. However, if you apply mascara immediately after using the primer, you'll notice slightly more length than with the mascara alone. It's not enough of a difference to justify two steps, but at least it's something.

☹ **Great Lash Big Mascara** *($4.99)*. Maybelline's Great Lash Mascara has never been among their best, despite its continued popularity. Adding to the folly of that poorly performing product, they've now launched this version with a different, much larger brush. I wish the new brush made a big improvement, but it's only marginally better than the original Great Lash Mascara. You won't get any thickness and its lengthening abilities are average. The best I can say is that this darkens and separates lashes well, but you'll notice slight flaking during wear.

☹ **Lash Stiletto Ultimate Length Waterproof Mascara** *($6.99)*. It takes several coats to build merely average length with this mascara. The formula is waterproof and applies without clumping, but it flakes a bit during wear. It isn't one of Maybelline's best waterproof mascaras, but it's an OK option for occasional use if you don't need much more than modest length.

☹ **Volum' Express Turbo Boost Mascara Waterproof 5X** *($7.79)* is said to make lashes five times thicker in one stroke. Its turbo effect is more akin to a standard 4-cylinder engine because it takes its time to get going, and you will be dealing with clumps and uneven application along the way. It builds reasonable length, but is really more for thickening lashes, an area where it does not perform as well as Maybelline's other Volum' Express mascaras. The best reason to consider this is because it's tenaciously waterproof. It requires a silicone- or oil-based makeup remover; a water-soluble cleanser (even those with some oil) won't do the job.

☹ **Great Lash Mascara** *($4.99)* builds some length, though it takes a good deal of effort to get anywhere, and pales in comparison to most of Maybelline's other mascaras. Great Lash does not build any thickness and it has a tendency to smear. The curved-brush version does little to make an unimpressive mascara any better. It may (shockingly) be the #1-selling mascara, but that doesn't mean it's the best.

☹ **Great Lash Waterproof Mascara** *($4.99)* is an utterly boring mascara that takes lots of effort for an "Is that all there is?" result. It stays on in the rain or pool, but so do Maybelline's other waterproof mascaras—all of which are preferred to this.

☹ **Lash Stylist Mascara** *($6.99)* is another brushless mascara that, instead of a brush, uses tiny, comblike teeth arranged in a V-pattern, which is said to lift and lengthen lashes. It definitely does that, and dramatically so. You'll quickly achieve long, lightly curled lashes that have impact—this isn't a mascara for a natural look. So why the unhappy face rating? Because, despite the impressive application, it consistently flakes and smears easily. What a shame, because it is otherwise a premier option. For a similarly dramatic effect without the problems, try L'Oreal's Volume Shocking Mascara ($12.95).

☹ **Lash Stylist Waterproof Mascara** *($6.99)* has the same comb applicator as the regular Lash Stylist Mascara, but it deposits too much product on lashes, leaving them looking too heavy and wet. This takes longer than it should to dry, and also tends to smear, making it not recommended despite the fact that once it sets, it holds up well under water.

BRUSHES: ☺ **Blush Brush** *($4.49)* is extremely soft, but firm, and it works decently well. ☺ **Expert Eyes Brush 'n Comb** *($4.49)* is a standard, feasible brow and lash comb that's afford-ably priced. ☺ **Expert Tools Eyelash Curler** *($4.49)* is a very standard, but workable, eyelash curler. The price is right and the classic curved shape is suitable for quickly curly lashes, unless you have small eyes, in which case the shape of this kind of curler can be trickier to work with. ☺ **Eye Contour Brush** *($4.99)* is a synthetic brush option for brows or eyelining, but not for eyeshadow. ☺ **Eyeshadow Brush** *($3.99)* is extremely soft, but firm, and it works decently well. ☺ **Retractable Lip Brush** *($6.99)* is a standard lip brush that travels well, though it could be firmer. Less impressive is the ☹ **Face Brush** *($8.49)* which feels soft but is too floppy for con-trolled application of powder, though some women may prefer a "looser" powder brush.

MAKEUP REMOVERS: ☺ **Expert Eyes Eye Makeup Remover Towelettes** *($5.49 for 50 towelettes)* are small cloths packaged in a resealable pouch. The simple, gentle formula works well to remove makeup unless the formula is long-wearing or waterproof, in which case too much "elbow grease" is needed, and that's not great for skin around the eyes. The tiny amount of lavender extract is not cause for concern.

☺ **Superaway Lipcolor Remover** *($4.99)* is a tube of makeup remover with an angled tip that's meant to take off long-wearing lip color, either from Maybelline or any other company. The silicone-enriched formula feels silky and, as long as you let it sit on lips for a moment after application, it works great to remove tenacious color while leaving a smooth finish.

☹ **Expert Touch Moisturizing Mascara Remover** *($4.79 for 2.23 ounces)* is an incred-ibly simple concoction of mineral oil, emollient thickener, lanolin oil, and preservative. This greasy liquid will indeed remove mascara and most other makeup as well—but the greasy film it leaves

☹ **Expert Eyes 100% Oil-Free Eye Makeup Remover** *($4.59 for 2.3 ounces)* is an anti-quated eye-makeup remover with too much boric acid and isopropyl alcohol to use it around the eyes. It is not recommended.

MD FORMULATIONS (SKIN CARE ONLY)

MD FORMULATIONS AT-A-GLANCE

Strengths: The entire line is fragrance-free; some well-formulated AHA products featuring glycolic acid and ammonium glycolate; a selection of very good cleansers; some extraordinary moisturizers and serums; very good toner; an oil-rich lip balm with broad-spectrum sunscreen; a skin-lightening product with retinol and arbutin.

Weaknesses: Some AHA products that include alcohol and other irritants; jar packaging; sunscreens without sufficient UVA protection; the at-home peel kit is an irritation waiting to happen; adhering to a routine of several MD Formulations products may expose skin to an excessive amount of exfoliation; incomplete routine(s) for blemish-prone skin.

For more information about MD Formulations, call (800) 451-3940 or visit www.mdformulations.com or www.Beautypedia.com

MD FORMULATIONS CONTINUOUS RENEWAL PRODUCTS

☺ **$$$ Continuous Renewal Complex** *($35 for 1 ounce)* is a basic, fragrance-free, pH-correct AHA moisturizer for normal to dry skin. Bells and whistles are absent, but it does the job to exfoliate skin and renew its texture. Between the glycolic acid and ammonium glycolate, the AHA content is at least 10%.

☹ **$$$ Continuous Renewal Complex, Sensitive Skin Formula** *($35 for 1 ounce)* contains enough AHAs to exfoliate, but the pH of 4.4 doesn't allow that to occur; AHAs do best at a pH of 3 to 4. So this product really isn't worth considering for any skin type (Source: *Cosmetic Dermatology*, October 2001, pages 15-18).

☺ **$$$ Continuous Renewal Serum** *($53 for 2 ounces)* claims to deliver the same benefits of glycolic acid without the irritating side effects. However, this doesn't contain anything too different from the other products in this line that contain glycolic acid. Despite the contradictory claim, this is an effective (meaning pH-correct), no-frills AHA product for all skin types. It contains approximately 12% AHA.

☹ **$$$ Continuous Renewal Serum, Sensitive Skin Formula** *($53 for 2 ounces)* has a more elegant formula than the Continuous Renewal Serum, but the pH of 4.4 reduces the potential for the AHAs it contains to exfoliate skin.

MD FORMULATIONS MOISTURE DEFENSE PRODUCTS

✓☺ **Moisture Defense Antioxidant Spray** *($28 for 8.3 ounces)* is pricey, but in this case you're getting a well-done spray-on toner. It supplies skin with very good skin-identical ingredients, antioxidants, and a couple of notable soothing agents, all without any irritants or fragrance.

☹ **$$$ Moisture Defense Antioxidant Comfort Creme** *($45 for 1 ounce)* is a basic moisturizer for normal to dry skin. The meager amount of antioxidants will become less effective once this jar-packaged product is opened.

☹ **$$$ Moisture Defense Antioxidant Creme** *($55 for 1.7 ounces)* contains a selection of ingredients capable of reinforcing skin and rebuilding its protective barrier as claimed, and that's excellent. What's not so great is that the jar packaging will render the many antioxidants ineffective shortly after you begin using this cream. In better packaging, this would be a slam-dunk recommendation for normal to slightly dry skin.

☹ **$$$ Moisture Defense Antioxidant Eye Creme** *($35 for 0.5 ounce)* contains too few impressive ingredients and earns its stripes primarily via cosmetics trickery. The amount of titanium dioxide and iron oxides creates a whitening, slightly pearlescent finish that helps mask the appearance of dark circles. It's not as effective as a concealer, and overall not worth considering over many other eye creams.

✓☺ **$$$ Moisture Defense Antioxidant Hydrating Gel** *($45 for 1 ounce)* contains effective, state-of-the-art water-binding agents, antioxidants, and cell-communicating ingredients in an ultralight base suitable for all skin types (or for very oily skin seeking an antioxidant-laden gel). This would also be worthwhile for someone with rosacea.

✓☺ **$$$ Moisture Defense Antioxidant Lotion** *($50 for 1 ounce)* lists urea as the fourth ingredient, and thus has some exfoliating properties; it is also a very good moisturizing agent for dry skin. A lesser amount of lactic acid (likely 2%) boosts the exfoliation potential, and the pH of 3.8 is within range. Even better, this lotion for normal to dry skin is loaded with antioxidants and ingredients that reinforce skin's healthy functioning. A beautiful formulation that's packaged right, too!

✓☺ **Moisture Defense Antioxidant Moisturizer SPF 20** *($36 for 1.7 ounces)*. Now this is how to formulate a great daytime moisturizer with sunscreen! UVA protection is assured thanks to zinc oxide, and the silky lotion formula feels great and works beautifully for normal to dry skin. Antioxidants are plentiful, the formula includes some good water-binding agents, and it is fragrance-free. "Moisture and protection without a greasy look and feel" is a fairly accurate way to describe this product. Those with slightly oily skin will find this doesn't hold back shine, but those with normal to dry skin will find it leaves a natural matte finish that is comfortable under makeup. Well done, MD Formulations!

☺ **$$$ Moisture Defense Antioxidant Treatment Masque** *($26 for 2.5 ounces)* contains approximately 8% AHAs, but the pH of 4.4 reduces the potential for effective exfoliation. This is otherwise a thick, creamy mask for dry skin that contains some good antioxidants and soothing agents. These ingredients are best left on skin rather than rinsed off.

MD FORMULATIONS THE TEMPS PRODUCTS

☹ **The Temps Brighten & Tighten Eye Serum** *($36 for 0.16 ounce)* comes packaged with a roller-ball applicator that allows this water-based solution to glide onto the under-eye area. Contrary to claims, this product doesn't contain any ingredients that can vanquish dark circles or puffiness. Actually, it's a problem for use around the eye area because it contains arnica extract, which can cause contact dermatitis and be very irritating to mucous membranes (Source: www.naturaldatabase.com). By the way, this also contains PVP/polycarbamyl polyglycol ester (a hairspray-type ingredient) that can also be a skin irritant.

☹ **The Temps Lip Plumping Treatment** *($28 for 0.27 ounce)* is an emollient lip balm that contains some excellent moisturizing ingredients for dry, chapped lips. Unfortunately, the plumping comes from the irritating, potent menthol derivative menthoxypropanediol. The inflammation this causes will make lips swell a little, but causing such inflammation daily isn't a good idea for the health of your lips.

☺ **$$$ The Temps: Oil Control Pore Refiner** *($28 for 0.5 ounce)* is a good silicone-based serum with retinol for normal to oily skin. The blend of silicones leaves a smooth matte finish and this also contains another form of vitamin A (retinyl palmitate) plus tea tree oil, though not in an amount that would be effective against acne-causing bacteria. This can help control oily shine on skin's surface, but cannot control oil production because that is regulated by hormones. This contains fragrance in the form of farnesol. One more comment: This would work well as a retinol-based primer to wear under makeup.

☺ **$$$ The Temps Wrinkle Filler & Deep Crease Relaxer** *($36 for 0.06 ounce)* is basically positioned as a "Botox-on-the-go" product that is packaged in a pen-style applicator. This nonaqueous blend of silicones feels great on skin, but the peptides in this product won't relax expression lines, although it is reasonable to expect them to attract moisture to skin and, therefore, make lines look less apparent by virtue of hydration. Unlike the ill-advised The Temps Brighten & Tighten Eye Serum, this product is gentle enough to use on wrinkles around the eye area.

MD Formulations Vit-A-Plus Products

☺ $$$ **Vit-A-Plus Anti-Aging Serum** *($55 for 1 ounce)* is a heavier (but not occlusive) version of the Vit-A-Plus Anti-Aging Eye Complex, with an improved selection of helpful ingredients for normal to dry skin. The pH is too high for the 10% concentration of AHAs to exfoliate, but the vitamin A (as retinyl palmitate) content is good.

☺ $$$ **Vit-A-Plus Anti-Aging Eye Complex** *($53 for 0.5 ounce)* contains 10% AHAs, but the pH of 4.4 limits their exfoliating properties, though they will serve as water-binding agents. This lightweight moisturizer is an option for slightly dry skin. Vitamins A and E are the only antioxidants on board, but the packaging will keep them stable during use.

✓☺ $$$ **Vit-A-Plus Illuminating Serum** *($65 for 1 ounce)* combines the benefits of AHAs (15%) at a pH of 4 with retinol and other cell-communicating ingredients, plus a good complement of antioxidants, all in packaging that keeps them stable during use. This is highly recommended for normal to dry skin not prone to breakouts (the plant oil and wax may prove problematic for blemishes). The AHA content is likely to be problematic for those with sensitive skin.

☺ $$$ **Vit-A-Plus Intensive Anti-Aging Serum** *($55 for 1 ounce)* is similar to the Vit-A-Plus Anti-Aging Serum, except it has a higher concentration (20%) of AHAs. Once again, the pH does not permit optimal exfoliation; however, the amount of retinyl palmitate is good.

✓☺ $$$ **Vit-A-Plus Night Recovery** *($50 for 1 ounce)* is a combination AHA/BHA product with 8% glycolic compound (consisting of ammonium glycolate and glycolic acid) and 2% salicylic acid. The pH of 4 is borderline for exfoliation, but you should net some results. The lightweight texture and reduced amount of thickening agents are preferred for normal to slightly oily skin, but this can be used by all skin types. The amount of antioxidants and water-binding agents isn't expansive, but the concentrations of each are above average.

☹ **Vit-A-Plus Clearing Complex** *($39 for 1 ounce)* lists alcohol as the second ingredient. Without it, the blend of AHAs and salicylic acid plus retinol in this product would have been great for battling blemishes.

☺ $$$ **Vit-A-Plus Clearing Complex Masque** *($30 for 2.5 ounces)* contains lactic acid and sodium lactate at a pH of 3.6, so some exfoliation will occur. This is first and foremost a clay mask for oily skin, and the amount of exfoliation won't be great because you'll want to rinse this off after several minutes. The small amount of rosemary oil may cause irritation.

☺ $$$ **Vit-A-Plus Firming Treatment Masque** *($36 for 2.5 ounces)* contains a small amount of vitamin A and not enough AHA or BHA to function as an exfoliant. This is otherwise an OK clay mask for normal to oily skin not prone to blemishes (the amount of ceresin, a wax-like thickening agent, isn't the best for blemish-prone skin).

☹ **Vit-A-Plus Illuminating Masque** *($42 for 2.5 ounces)* contains 5% AHAs at a pH of 4, so some exfoliation will occur. However, this moisturizing mask for normal to dry skin is not recommended because it contains irritating lavender oil.

Other MD Formulations Products

☺ $$$ **Facial Cleanser** *($32 for 8.3 ounces)* is a basic, slightly creamy but water-soluble cleanser that contains 12% glycolic acid at a pH of 3.8. That's nice, but it's all for naught because the benefit is rinsed from your skin, when in fact it should be left on (though you wouldn't want to do that with a cleanser). It's an option for normal to oily skin, provided you avoid the eye area.

✓☺ **$$$ Facial Cleanser, Sensitive Skin Formula** *($32 for 8.3 ounces)* includes a tiny amount of glycolic acid and some soothing agents. The glycolic acid isn't helpful in a cleanser and is an odd choice in a product meant for sensitive skin. Still, this is a gentle, effective cleanser for normal to dry skin, and it's fragrance-free.

☺ **$$$ Facial Cleansing Gel** *($32 for 8.3 ounces)*. This basic, fragrance-free, water-soluble cleanser works well but the amount of glycolic acid may prove too irritating for use around the eyes. The glycolic acid won't exfoliate skin due to its brief contact with it, and you don't want to leave a cleanser on your face for longer than is needed to cleanse.

☹ **Daily Peel Pads** *($30 for 40 pads)* would be recommended as pH-correct glycolic and salicylic acid pads if the formula did not include several irritants, including alcohol, juniper oil, lavender oil, and witch hazel.

☹ **Glycare Acne Gel** *($30 for 2.5 ounces)* lists alcohol as the second ingredient, which makes it too drying and irritating for all skin types. Alcohol can stimulate oil production in the pore lining, too.

☺ **$$$ Face and Body Scrub** *($35 for 8.3 ounces)* is a standard, detergent-based scrub that contains plastic beads as the abrasive agent. The inclusion of 15% glycolic acid (in a base with a pH of 3.8) guarantees exfoliation only if this is left on skin for a prolonged period—much longer than a product like this should be left on. There's nothing about this product that isn't easily replaced by a washcloth.

✓☺ **$$$ Critical Care Calming Gel** *($39 for 1 ounce)* is designed to minimize redness and irritation, and contains impressive levels of ingredients research has shown do just that because of their anti-inflammatory properties. This is an outstanding, fragrance-free gel moisturizer for all skin types that contains lots of antioxidants and a cell-communicating ingredient.

☺ **$$$ Critical Care Shielding Creme** *($85 for 1 ounce)* has a beautifully silky texture built around silicones, and also includes some well-researched antioxidants and ingredients that reinforce skin's structure. Yet, for the money it ends up being a disappointment because of the jar packaging, which won't allow the antioxidants to stimulate skin's healing process.

☺ **$$$ Critical Care Skin Repair Complex** *($100 for 1 ounce)* promises to restore the smooth, beautiful skin you were born with, but it cannot replace what time and years of sun damage take away. It's just a lightweight, silky-textured moisturizer in which the effectiveness of the antioxidants is diminished due to jar packaging. MD Formulations should have taken "care" to get this "critical" aspect right!

☹ **Glycare Lotion** *($40 for 2 ounces)* contains too much alcohol and causes further irritation due to eucalyptus oil. This is not the way to control excess oil or reduce the appearance of large pores. If anything, the alcohol will make oily skin oilier by stimulating oil production in the pore lining.

☹ **Sun Protector 30 Spray, SPF 30** *($24 for 4 ounces)* lacks the UVA-protecting ingredients of titanium dioxide, zinc oxide, avobenzone, Tinosorb, or Mexoryl SX (ecamsule), and is not recommended. Even if it had the right UVA protection, this would be a problem for all skin types because it contains cedarwood bark and lavender oils.

☺ **Total Protector 30** *($22 for 2.5 ounces)* is a good, but basic, sunscreen that provides UVA protection via its in-part zinc oxide sunscreen. It isn't nearly as state-of-the-art as many other daytime moisturizers with sunscreen, but is workable for normal to dry skin not prone to blemishes.

☺ **Benzoyl Peroxide 10** *($20 for 2 ounces)* works swiftly to kill acne-causing bacteria with its 10% concentration of benzoyl peroxide. You shouldn't start with such a high concentration, but it may be worth stepping up to if your blemishes don't respond to 2.5% or 5% concentrations.

☺ **$$$ Lip Balm SPF 20** *($12 for 0.33 ounce)* contains an in-part titanium dioxide sunscreen, but the amount (0.8%) is on the low side in terms of providing superior UVA protection. This is still worth considering as a unique lip balm that contains some very good emollients and oils to stop chapped lips.

☹ **My Personal Peel System** *($85)* consists of five separate products meant to be customized according to your skin's needs; however, all of them contain at least one irritating ingredient. The **Power Peel Pads** contain 20% AHAs, but irritate the skin with alcohol, witch hazel, lavender oil, and juniper oil. The **Firming Anti-Wrinkle Booster** only boosts skin inflammation because it contains the menthol derivative menthoxypropanediol. The **Extra Clear Booster** contains irritating grapefruit oil (which won't promote clear skin, but can cause a phototoxic reaction). The **Brightening Booster** contains menthoxypropanediol and lavender oil. And the **Post-Peel Restorer** contains strawberry oil, which can cause contact dermatitis and has no established soothing benefit for skin, particularly if it's as irritated as it will be after proceeding through the steps of this at-home peel.

MD SKINCARE BY DR. DENNIS GROSS (SKIN CARE ONLY)

MD SKINCARE BY DR. DENNIS GROSS AT-A-GLANCE

Strengths: Almost all of the products are fragrance-free; several serums and moisturizers contain a brilliant assortment of beneficial skin-care ingredients; all of the sunscreens contain sufficient UVA protection; almost all of the antioxidant-rich products are packaged to ensure stability and potency.

Weaknesses: Expensive; no effective AHA or BHA products (including the at-home peel the line is "known" for); problematic toner; incomplete selection of products to treat acne, and what's available is more irritating than helpful; a few "why bother?" products.

For more information about MD Skincare by Dr. Dennis Gross, call (888) 830-7546 or visit the Web site at www.mdskincare.com or www.Beautypedia.com.

☺ **$$$ All-In-One Cleansing Foam** *($36 for 5 ounces)* is a good water-soluble cleanser for normal to oily skin, but would be rated higher if it did not contain witch hazel bark, leaf, and twig extract. The amount is not likely cause for concern, but why include it at all?

☺ **$$$ All-in-One Facial Cleanser with Toner** *($38 for 8 ounces)* is an exceptionally standard, detergent-based cleanser that is an option for someone with normal to oily skin. The teeny amount of emu oil provides no emollient benefit for skin, but the witch hazel base is potentially irritating.

☹ **Botanical Bar with Tea Tree & Aloe** *($24 for 7 ounces).* The presence of botanicals doesn't keep this bar from being a problem for all skin types. The cleansing agents are drying and irritating and the irritation is made worse by the inclusion of rosemary and orange oils. This isn't good medicine for anyone.

☺ **$$$ EZ4U 4-In-1 Facial Treatment, for Dry/Normal Skin** *($35 for 30 towelettes).* Those looking to cleanse, tone, moisturize, and fight wrinkles all at the same time are supposed to have found what they need in this product, at least according to the claims. These individually wrapped, water-based towelettes (right, just ordinary towelettes) are said to be your do-it-all option (though sun protection was left out, so right away you know this isn't an all-in-one solution for keeping skin healthy). All these really do is minimally cleanse skin and provide it with a smattering of antioxidants. Most of the intriguing ingredients are listed after the preservative (caprylyl glycol) and as such don't count for much. The realistic way to view this product is as a slightly moisturizing toner you wipe over skin after a workout or long day outdoors if you're not wearing makeup. That's the "EZ" part, but you'll still need a real cleanser and the rest of your skin-care routine because this is only the beginning, and a poor beginning at that.

☺ **$$$ EZ4U 4-In-1 Facial Treatment, for Normal/Oily Skin** *($35 for 30 towelettes)* is similar to the EZ4U 4-In-1 Facial Treatment, for Dry/Normal Skin above, and the same basic comments apply. The realistic way to view this product is as a soothing, oil-absorbing toner whose alkaline nature (from the sodium bicarbonate) may cause slight dryness, while the witch hazel and fragrant citrus extracts can cause irritation. There is nothing "easy" about this product because you'll still need a real cleanser and the rest of your skin-care routine because this is only the beginning, and an average beginning at that.

☺ **$$$ EZ4U to Go, Facial Towelette** *($10 for 7 towelettes).* My goodness! The physician namesake of this line has no shame, or is so disconnected from reality that it's scary. The claim is that in 20 seconds after wiping these over the skin you "will effectively cleanse, repair, firm, and moisturize skin." That isn't even remotely true. These individually wrapped, water-based towelettes are said to replace four different skin-care products, including your "wrinkle fighter," although there is no sun protection, so right away you know this isn't an all-in-one solution for keeping skin healthy. But that's just the half of it. The only thing these glorified towelettes can do is cleanse skin and provide it with a dusting of antioxidants. The realistic way to view this product is as an ordinary toner with way too much sodium bicarbonate, making it too alkaline for all skin types. There is nothing "easy" about this product because you'll still need a real cleanser and the rest of your skin-care routine because this barely makes it as a cleanser. Did you notice that these price out to be more than $1 per towelette? Now that's a pricey way to get average results!

☹ **Hydra-Pure Mist** *($32 for 5 ounces)* has a lot going for it, including some very effective water-binding agents and a few antioxidants. But the inclusion of comfrey extract makes this problematic for all skin types. Please refer to my online Cosmetic Ingredient Dictionary for an explanation of comfrey's negative impact on skin.

☹ **Antioxidant Enzyme Buff with Berry Seeds & Dead Sea Salt** *($57 for 14.1 ounces)* is a standard scrub that is mostly table salt and plant oil along with lots of fragrance. Though absurdly overpriced (you could pull the salt out of your cupboard and use it in the bath with a cleanser and do far better than this formula), it could have been a good scrub for skin from the neck down, but it is not recommended because it contains enough irritating plant extracts to make it not worth the effort. Plus, the jar packaging makes this a mess of a product to use, and repeatedly sticking wet fingers into a jar is not the most sanitary way to access skin-care products of any kind.

☹ **Creamy Cleansing Polish** *($38 for 5.2 ounces).* This glycerin-rich cleansing scrub could have been a brilliant option for normal to dry skin. However, the formula contains several potent irritants, including clove and lime oils. As such, it is not recommended. Sad to think that this product, merely because of the product line's name, is associated with having anything to do with the medical care of skin.

☹ **Alpha Beta Daily Face Peel Two-Step System** *($78)* is the system that made Dr. Gross famous, or so the company says. Step 1 involves the salicylic, glycolic, and lactic acid-infused **Alpha Beta Peel Refining**. The amount of AHAs pales next to the BHA content, but none of these exfoliants function as expected because the pH of the pads is 4.4. Step 2, the **Neutralizing System**, has been improved, but it's still superfluous (plain tap water can neutralize a peel). This is basically a good toner formula in pad form, and includes several antioxidants and retinol, but the jar packaging won't keep them stable during the lifespan of this product. In the end, this is a great big "why bother?"

☺ **$$$ All-In-One Tinted Moisturizer Sunscreen SPF 15** *($44 for 1.7 ounces)* contains an in-part avobenzone sunscreen in a silicone-enhanced moisturizing base for normal to dry skin. The six sheer shades are all worth trying, each providing a hint of color but no meaningful coverage. A higher amount of antioxidants would have netted this tinted moisturizer a Paula's Pick rating.

☺ **$$$ Auto-Balancing Moisture Sunscreen SPF 10** *($42 for 1.7 ounces)*. A dermatologist selling a sunscreen with an SPF 10 is very disappointing. This sunscreen does contain avobenzone, but the gold standard for sunscreens today is SPF 15 (Source: American Academy of Dermatology, www.aad.org). The base formula is appropriate for normal to dry skin, though it doesn't automatically balance skin.

✓☺ **$$$ Continuous Eye Hydration Advanced Technology** *($45 for 0.5 ounce)* has what it takes to address the needs of slightly dry to dry skin anywhere on the face. The formula includes effective emollients along with several antioxidants, water-binding agents, and a cell-communicating ingredient. The claims that this can reduce puffy eyes with caffeine and cucumber are unfounded, and this also cannot lighten dark circles (though the mica cosmetically "brightens" shadowed areas). Still, there's no denying that this is a well-formulated, stably packaged product.

✓☺ **$$$ Hydra-Pure Antioxidant Firming Serum** *($95 for 1 ounce)* has a texture that's more lotion than serum, and it contains a brilliant assortment of ingredients to help normal to dry skin look and feel its best. The amount of lactic acid is impressive, but the pH of 4.7 significantly reduces any potential for exfoliation. The lactic acid still has merit as a water-binding agent, however, and the formula contains appreciable amounts of several well-researched antioxidants, plus retinol and other cell-communicating ingredients. One more thing: Dimethyl sulfone is the fourth listed ingredient. Also known as methylsulfonylmethane (MSM), there is limited research supporting its benefit for skin. The only published study was a single case report of a man with a rare skin disorder (ichthyosis) who responded well to topical treatment with a moisturizer that contained, among several other ingredients, MSM. The case report did not elucidate if it was the MSM or another ingredient (or a synergistic combination) that provided relief (Source: *Ostomy/Wound Management*, April 2006, pages 82-86).

☹ **Hydra-Pure Firming Eye Cream** *($90 for 0.5 ounce)* contains some incredibly helpful, state-of-the-art ingredients for all skin types, but the jar packaging won't keep them stable, and lavender oil (of which there is a significant amount) only wreaks havoc on skin cells, not to mention being problematic for use around the eyes. What was Dr. Gross thinking?

☹ **Hydra-Pure Intense Moisture Cream** *($125 for 1.7 ounces)* shares the attractive points and drawbacks of the Hydra-Pure Firming Eye Cream, and the same comments apply.

✓☺ **$$$ Hydra-Pure Oil-Free Moisture** *($78 for 1 ounce)* is said to be a best-seller for the brand, but it also makes the claim that it removes unwanted heavy metals left on skin from tap water. How it goes about doing that isn't explained, other than that it works via the company's Chelating Complex. Chelating agents prevent metals from binding to other substances, but the amount of metals in tap water (and their potential subsequent effect on skin) isn't cause for concern. In the end, this is a very good moisturizer for normal to slightly dry skin. It contains a nice array of antioxidants, cell-communicating ingredients, and a tiny amount of water-binding agents.

✓ ☺ $$$ **Hydra-Pure Radiance Renewal Serum** *($95 for 1 ounce)* is designed to address skin discolorations from sun damage, and handles this task beautifully. This water-based serum has a silky texture and contains arbutin and uva ursi leaf extract in amounts that are likely to have an effect on hyperpigmentation (assuming your routine includes daily application of sunscreen rated SPF 15 or greater). The formula also contains numerous antioxidants and the cell-communicating ingredients creatinine and retinol, and it's fragrance-free. This is suitable for all skin types.

✓ ☺ $$$ **Hydra-Pure Redness Soothing Serum** *($85 for 1 ounce)* contains efficacious amounts of several well-researched soothing agents, including bisabolol, green tea, and licorice root extract. This fragrance-free, water-based serum's only misstep is the inclusion of witch hazel, though the amount is most likely too small to be of concern for irritation. This is recommended for any skin type dealing with redness or irritation, and would indeed be suitable for post-laser treatment or after other cosmetic procedures, such as peels or waxing.

✓ ☺ $$$ **Hydra-Pure Vitamin C Serum** *($95 for 1 ounce)* has a beautifully smooth silicone base and contains an impressive amount of vitamin C (as ascorbic acid, whose acid component can be a skin irritant). Two other stabilized forms of vitamin C are also in the formula, along with the antioxidants quercetin, vitamin E, willow bark, and kudzu. Gross also added cell-communicating ingredients and salicylic acid, but the amount of the latter is too low (and the pH of this product too high) for exfoliation to occur. All in all, this is a well-formulated antioxidant serum that is packaged to ensure potency. It is a great way to see how vitamin C works for you while also exposing skin to other beneficial ingredients.

☹ **Lift & Lighten Eye Cream Advanced Technology** *($60 for 0.5 ounce)* is one of the least impressive MD Skincare products because it contains far more fragrance than it does the bells and whistles that Dr. Gross wisely added to most of the other moisturizers and serums in this line. This also contains arnica, which is a problem for all skin types, and even more so in a product meant for application to the eye area.

☺ $$$ **Maximum Moisture Treatment** *($54 for 1.7 ounces)* is an effective but comparably basic moisturizer for normal to dry skin not prone to blemishes. It does not contain the same amount or selection of antioxidants or other goodies present in other MD Skincare moisturizers.

✓ ☺ $$$ **Powerful Sun Protection SPF 30 Sunscreen Lotion** *($42 for 5 ounces)* claims it is the only sunscreen that addresses the increased risk of sun damage caused by iron that's left on your skin from tap water. Of course, this statement isn't backed up by any research on Dr. Gross' Web site, so we're left to take his word for it. This product does contain chelating agents, which can possibly prevent iron from damaging skin in the presence of sunlight. Chelating agents are compounds that bind with a metal (such as iron) and change its function by affecting its molecular makeup. Chelating agents are often used in laundry detergents to prevent trace metals in the water from binding to clothing. Left on clothing, these trace metals can react with perspiration and cause clothing to discolor, so in that context preventing this is a good thing and chelating agents are helpful. The chelating agents in Dr. Gross' product are tetrasodium

EDTA and disodium EDTA, common chelating agents found in hundreds of products, from shampoos to moisturizers. They are not unique to his product and there is no reason to choose this over another well-formulated sunscreen because of its allegedly special protective ability. Dr. Gross focuses on chelating agents to keep iron from damaging your skin, although it's likely the amount of iron left on your skin (if any) from tap water is completely insignificant. What he doesn't mention is that there is research showing that the antioxidants present in skin-care products do a great job of keeping the iron in our skin from converting to reactive oxygen species (ROS) and causing free-radical damage in the presence of sunlight (Source: *Free Radical Biology and Medicine*, October 2006, pages 1197-1204). In addition, although there is research showing that specific iron chelators added to a sunscreen increase its ability to protect skin from sun damage, Dr. Gross didn't use either of the above compounds in this product (Source: *The Journal of Investigative Dermatology*, October 2006, pages 2287-2295). That said, if you ignore the "one-of-a-kind" claims, this is a very good, fragrance-free, in-part avobenzone sunscreen that comes in a lightweight lotion base and contains several potent antioxidants. It's expensive, but is nevertheless an excellent option for normal to slightly dry skin.

✓ ☺ **$$$ Powerful Sun Protection SPF 30 Sunscreen Packettes** *($42 for 60 packettes)* makes the same iron-squashing claims as the Powerful Sun Protection SPF 30 Sunscreen Lotion above, and is also the same product, just packaged in single-use, take-along packets. Although pricey, it's a good way to pack extra sunscreen for unanticipated long days outdoors or for use after washing your hands when you're away from home.

✓ ☺ **$$$ Powerful Sun Protection SPF 45 Sunscreen Cream** *($42 for 4.2 ounces)* is a very good sunscreen that includes zinc oxide for sufficient UVA protection (among other sunscreen actives). The iron-encapsulating chelating claims made for the product are discussed in detail in the review of this brand's Powerful Sun Protection SPF 30 Sunscreen Lotion, but suffice it to say, this isn't a special feature worth seeking out (though it's certainly not harmful, either). This water-resistant sunscreen is great for normal to dry skin not prone to blemishes, and contains some unique antioxidants to help boost skin's environmental defenses, and it's fragrance-free.

☹ **Alpha-Beta Body Peel** *($78 for 30 applications)*. This two-step product doesn't come close to living up to the claim of being an "effective way to solve every skincare concern that you may have on your body." It doesn't solve anything, although one of the steps in this routine can cause skin problems, and the price will hurt your pocketbook.

The pads in Step 1 contain 2% salicylic acid as the active ingredient, but also contain alcohol and witch hazel, which isn't good news because they are drying and cause free-radical damage and irritation, which is not good for skin anywhere on the body. The pads in Step 2 are meant to be applied after the solution from Step 1 has been on skin for 2 minutes. The Step 2 pads are steeped in a water-based serum containing several antioxidants and retinol. Although the Step 2 pads contain many helpful ingredients for all skin types, the jar packaging means they won't remain stable for long after opening, so you're losing benefits with each use rather than building on them. Interestingly, the directions for this peel tell you not to apply any products with alcohol afterward—how ironically pathetic. Clearly, Dr. Gross knows alcohol is a problem for skin, but then he went ahead and included it in Step 1 of this duo!

☺ **$$$ Intense Hydra Mask** *($62 for 6 treatments)* is not intense in the least. And what is it with dermatologist lines and their two-step kits? And why, almost without exception, do these kits feature products that are either inferior to or the equivalent of other products in the line (yet the products in the kit claim to do something completely different or better)? Gripes aside,

Step 1 of this duo is the **Hyaluronic Gel**, which purports to plump skin and fill in wrinkles. Its name (and the claims) implies hyaluronic acid, which is the ingredient used in dermal fillers such as Restylane, so you'll think it will work the same. However, it actually contains sodium hyaluronate, the less expensive salt form of this ingredient, which doesn't work even vaguely in any way, shape, or form like Restylane. It does contain a good selection of antioxidants with this skin-identical ingredient, but it's still nothing that isn't found in most of the other MD Skincare moisturizers and serums. Once you've brushed the Gel on (a brush is included in the kit), you apply the **Self-Heating Mask**. This is simply a mixture of slip agent, mineral, thickener, and antioxidants. The sodium silicoaluminate reacts with water and causes a warming sensation, though it has little effect on skin other than feeling pleasant. I suppose that is intended to re-inforce the treatment angle for which this kit is striving. Both steps contain helpful ingredients for all skin types, but if you're using one or more of MD Skincare's best products, this kit isn't a must-have.

☹ **Correct & Perfect Spot Treatment** *($28 for 0.5 ounce)* will irritate and aggravate thanks to the 3.25% concentration of the potent disinfectant sulfur and the inclusion of menthol. Sulfur can be helpful for blemish-prone skin, but its side effects and irritation potential are more problematic than beneficial.

☹ **All-Over Blemish Solution** *($84 for 1.7 ounces)* has a jaw-droppingly ridiculous price that's even more insulting when you find out that the pH is above 5, so the 2% salicylic acid won't function as an exfoliant. Want more bad news? The menthol will cause irritation and possibly worsen the appearance of reddened, blemished skin.

✓☺ **$$$ Powerful Sun Protection SPF 25 Lip Balm** *($18 for 0.25 ounce)* provides UVA protection via its in-part avobenzone sunscreen, and is a brilliantly formulated, antioxidant-rich lip balm in a tube. The oil-based formula does its job to keep lips from chapping, while the sunscreen provides protection for long days outdoors (be sure to take this with you for reapplication). Ignore the claim that iron residue left on your skin from tap water requires the chelating agents in this formula to help prevent skin cancer. That's a bogus claim with no research indicating that it's true. Dr. Gross should have left that claim in the "discard" pile of marketing ideas.

☺ **$$$ Serious Lip Treatment** *($58 for 0.54 ounce)* claims to be a two-step process for plumping lips, but it ends up being two steps too many and a waste of money. **Step 1** consists mostly of water, glycerin, honey, and preservative; **Step 2** is mostly water, a plant oil copolymer, thickener, silicones, honey, film-forming agent, and several nonvolatile plant oils. The ingredients in both tubes can smooth and soften lips, but that's about it. Honey appears to be the link between the two, but it has no plumping or antiaging effect on lips; it's merely a good water-binding agent and likely contributes the flavor to both products. The only serious thing about this product is its name, although its benign, ho-hum formula doesn't deserve an unhappy face rating. But the price did make me bite my lip!

MURAD (SKIN CARE ONLY)

MURAD AT-A-GLANCE

Strengths: A few good water-soluble cleansers; a selection of well-formulated AHA products centered on glycolic acid; most of Murad's top-rated products are fragrance-free; the sunscreens go beyond the basics and include several antioxidants for enhanced protection.

Weaknesses: Expensive; no other dermatologist-designed line has more problem products than Murad; irritating ingredients are peppered throughout the selection of products, keeping several of them from earning a recommendation.

For more information about Murad, call (888) 996-8723 or visit www.murad.com or www. Beautypedia.com.

MURAD PROFESSIONAL PRODUCTS

☹ **Activating Cleansing Emulsion** *($65 for 3.4 ounces)* claims to be oxygen-activated, but that doesn't convey any special benefit to skin. If you think about it, all cleansers used with water are oxygen-activated because water is partly oxygen molecules—so big deal. Aside from its hyper, overly absurd price, this cleanser is not recommended because it contains orange, eucalyptus, cedarwood, and Siberian fir oils, all of which are irritating. As a physician, Dr. Murad should be ashamed: both for creating such a problematic cleanser and for price-gouging his customers, who believe that as a physician he has their best interests at heart.

☺ **$$$ Daily Eye Lift** *($89 for 0.5 ounce)*. This overpriced eye-area moisturizer's formula isn't very exciting and there is nothing about it that makes it better for the eye area, or any area of the face for that matter. It's problematic in that one of the main ingredients is sodium polystyrene sulfonate, a polymer that's known to be unstable and potentially irritating to skin, especially around the eyes. Some good water-binding agents and soothing plant extracts are included, but this also contains plant extracts that cause irritation (e.g., comfrey and myrtle), making it confusing for your skin. If you want to spend in this range and insist on eye creams even though they don't differ from facial moisturizers, your skin will thank you for considering the options from Cosmedicine or Dr. Denese New York.

☹ **Daily Moisture Charge SPF 30** *($100 for 1.7 ounces)* lacks the UVA-protecting ingredients of titanium dioxide, zinc oxide, avobenzone, Tinosorb, or Mexoryl SX, and is not recommended. Even if it did have the right UVA active ingredients, the fragrant oils in this daytime moisturizer would present problems of their own.

☹ **Immuno-Skin Age Inhibitor** *($150 for 1 ounce)* lists polyvinyl alcohol as the third ingredient, which makes this water-based product too drying for all skin types (and not the least bit age-inhibiting, though polyvinyl alcohol can have a plasticizing, temporary tightening effect on skin). For inexplicable reasons, this fraudulent antiaging product also contains irritating eucalyptus, cedarwood, and orange oils, all in amounts greater than what's typically seen in skin-care products.

☺ **$$$ Nightly Hydro-Lock** *($120 for 1.7 ounces)* has the potential to be an excellent moisturizer for normal to dry skin. It contains an elegant blend of silicones, triglycerides, antioxidant plant oil, and vitamins. What's not so great is the inclusion of balm mint (*melissa*) along with oils of eucalyptus, cedarwood, and orange. None of these are present in prodigious amounts, but they're not helpful for skin regardless of how little is used. As such, this moisturizer isn't worth considering over many less expensive options that omit the potential irritants.

MURAD RESURGENCE PRODUCTS

☹ **Renewing Cleansing Cream** *($35 for 6.75 ounces)* isn't that creamy and will cause irritation because it contains lime, orange, tangerine, rosewood, and buchu oils (the buchu oil includes camphor).

The Reviews M

☹ **Age-Balancing Night Cream** *($82 for 1.7 ounces).* Age balancing? At what age does age become imbalanced? And, more to the point, can a moisturizer do anything to balance one's age? Of course not. This is another moisturizer with wild yam extract, directed toward those with peri-menopausal and menopausal skin. You might as well use the wild yams for your Thanksgiving feast because they have not been demonstrated to have any effectiveness when used on skin. Murad also puts the spotlight on chaparral extract, stating that it is clinically proven to slow down the growth of facial hair. Chaparral is extracted from a desert plant whose leaves (like those of most plants) contain antioxidant compounds. Topical application of chaparral is known to cause contact dermatitis (Source: www.naturaldatabase.com), and it's the fourth ingredient listed in this product. There's not a shred of published research on chaparral's alleged ability to slow facial-hair growth, though according to Murad it can reduce hair growth by 22%. Even if that were true, is a 22% reduction what you would consider significant? This moisturizer is also a perplexing mix of good-for-skin and bad-for-skin ingredients, including several antioxidants and retinol as well as several irritating essential oils. There is no logical reason to consider this product.

☹ **Age-Diffusing Serum** *($72 for 1 ounce)* does have a lot going for it when you consider this water-based AHA serum's level of silicones, range of antioxidants, and several water-binding agents. Yet, like so many Murad products, too many irritating ingredients that have no benefit for skin corrupt its good start. Clove flower and iris extracts are the prime offenders, and further down on the ingredient list orange, lime, tangerine, and rosewood oils are joined by buchu leaf oil, which contains camphor as a major constituent. How disappointing!

☺ **$$$ Renewing Eye Cream** *($73 for 0.5 ounce)* includes some good moisturizing agents for normal to dry skin, though none of them are capable of firming skin or diminishing puffiness. The amount of iris and clover extracts is potentially irritating, while the amount of the most intriguing ingredients isn't as impressive as it could have been.

☹ **Sheer Lustre Day Moisture SPF 15** *($68 for 1.7 ounces)* is an in-part avobenzone sunscreen that contains far too many problematic, and often photosensitizing, ingredients to make it a smart choice for daytime wear. Putting lemon and tangerine oils in a sunscreen is just asking for trouble. Price notwithstanding, this would have been highly recommended if it did not contain so many irritants.

☺ **$$$ Resurgence Renewal Home Facial Treatment** *($75 for 4 treatments)* is supposed to be an antiaging hero that mitigates wrinkles and signs of hormonal aging. That overblown-sounding claim can easily be asserted by any moisturizer because when you lose estrogen as you go through menopause, skin can become drier if it also has been sun damaged. Don't let the seductive claim waylay you because there is nothing in this product worth the expense.

This kit includes **Firming Facial Mask Treatment Powder**, a product you mix with something the company calls **Treatment Activator**, which is mostly water. You apply the moistened mixture to your face and follow with the **Firming Facial Treatment Gel** and **Hydrating & Firming Gel Eye Mask** over key areas. This trio is left on for 10 minutes and then rinsed, just like a regular mask. The Treatment Powder is mostly potato starch with enzymes and vitamin C; it's doubtful the enzymes remain stable enough to exfoliate skin after they've been mixed, but you may notice a slight benefit. The Treatment Gel contains too many fragrant irritants to be worthwhile for any skin type and the wild yam it contains isn't going to deliver progesterone to your skin. The Hydrating & Firming Gel Eye Mask is a decent blend of lightweight moisturizing ingredients and film-forming agents that make skin look temporarily smoother. All told, this is far from an ideal at-home treatment and, as mentioned, it won't do a thing to reduce signs of hormonal aging, which by the way includes bone loss, but who knows what hormonal aging this product was supposed to deal with in the first place?

OTHER MURAD PRODUCTS

☺ **$$$ AHA/BHA Exfoliating Cleanser** *($35 for 6.75 ounces)* can be a good cleanser for normal to dry skin, but the amount of jojoba oil makes it slightly difficult to rinse without the aid of a washcloth. This contains dissolving beads which exfoliate skin; the AHAs and BHA will not exfoliate because this cleanser is rinsed from the skin before they can be of much benefit.

☹ **Clarifying Cleanser** *($26 for 6.75 ounces)* contains essential oils that have antibacterial properties, but they're also very irritating. In addition to the lemon, bitter-orange, and lime oils, this irritation-waiting-to-happen cleanser contains menthol.

☹ **Energizing Pomegranate Cleanser** *($26 for 5.1 ounces)* irritates rather than energizes because this liquid-to-foam cleanser lists alcohol as the second ingredient. Further, it doesn't even do a good job at cleansing!

☹ **Essential-C Cleanser** *($35 for 6.75 ounces)* states it is designed to soothe environmentally stressed skin, but the orange, basil, and grapefruit peel oils do just the opposite, making this a nonessential cleanser.

☺ **$$$ Moisture Rich Cleanser** *($29.50 for 6.75 ounces)* is one of the only Murad cleansers not containing one or more problematic ingredients. This is a slightly creamy but water-soluble cleanser for normal to dry skin not prone to blemishes. The rosemary and grapefruit extracts aren't the best additives, but they're not going to bother skin the way they would if they were used in their essential oil form.

☺ **$$$ Refreshing Cleanser** *($29.50 for 6.75 ounces)* is a very standard, but good, water-soluble cleanser for normal to oily skin. It does not contain fragrance, but does include fragrant plant extracts. The amount of glycolic acid will not function as an exfoliant.

☹ **Soothing Gel Cleanser** *($25 for 6.75 ounces)* irritates rather than soothes due to the number of volatile fragrant oils, along with the potent menthol derivative menthoxypropanediol. Murad sells this as their redness-relieving cleanser, which is unbelievable.

☹ **Clarifying Toner** *($22 for 6 ounces)* lists witch hazel as the second ingredient and also contains menthol and its derivative, menthoxypropanediol. The citronella oil doesn't help matters, and certainly isn't clarifying.

☹ **Essential-C Toner** *($30 for 6 ounces)* contains a lot of witch hazel and lesser, but still problematic, amounts of citrus and basil oils. This will not balance stressed skin!

☺ **$$$ Hydrating Toner** *($24 for 6 ounces)* offers skin some helpful water-binding agents, but the amount of witch hazel is potentially problematic and keeps this otherwise well-done toner for normal to dry skin from earning a higher rating.

☹ **Cityskin Night Treatment** *($140 for 1 ounce)* has the ability to exfoliate skin thanks to its AHA concentration (glycolic acid is the second ingredient) and pH value, but like so many other Murad products, the good-for-skin ingredients are joined by those that cause needless irritation and, therefore, collagen breakdown. Cityskin Night Treatment contains some problematic plant extracts along with the fragrant oils of juniper, clove, sage, lemon, clary, and rosewood, among others. They may make this product smell lovely, but they assuredly aren't doing your skin any favors. The epidermal growth factor this treatment contains is potentially risky because growth factors can trigger skin cells to overproduce out of control.

The Reviews M

☺ **$$$ Intensive Resurfacing Peel** *($165 for 2.04 ounces)*. You're not getting much product for your money, but housed in each of these tiny vials is a water-based exfoliant serum whose blend of glycolic and salicylic acid is, according to a representative from Murad, between 3% and 5%. Given the pH of 2.8, it definitely will exfoliate skin. The issue I have is that the 4% glycolic acid (AHA) and the approximately 1% salicylic acid this peel contains aren't "intensive" in the least. A 10% concentration of glycolic acid would have been more "intensive." In addition, a pH of 3.5 would have been adequate (and is within the pH range recommended for AHA products by the FDA), and without the extra irritation that results from a product with a pH of less than 3. Either way, the amount of AHA and BHA Murad used isn't akin to what they use in an in-office AHA peel (where concentrations of glycolic acid typically range from 20% to 40%). The bamboo extract in this product provides mild mechanical exfoliation as you wash this product away, but you could easily get the same mechanical exfoliation using a washcloth. This ends up being an effective AHA option that is needlessly expensive and not a substitute for the peels a doctor can perform. For a lot less money and beautiful results, without the need to wait and then rinse the product off, check out the various AHA options from Alpha Hydrox, Neutrogena Healthy Skin, and NeoStrata.

☺ **$$$ Intensive Wrinkle Reducer** *($150 for 1 ounce)* may be one of the most expensive AHA products around, though it's definitely an effective one, containing at least 10% glycolic acid in a gel base with a pH of 3.2. The formula also contains several outstanding water-binding agents and plenty of antioxidants along with some good anti-irritants. It's a suitable option for all skin types, but you don't need to spend this much money to enjoy the benefits of AHAs. This product did not rate a Paula's Pick because it contains cinnamon bark extract and fragrance components that can be irritating to skin. Cinnamon has antioxidant ability, but its irritation potential when applied topically doesn't help move this product to the top of the must-have list.

☺ **$$$ Intensive Wrinkle Reducer for Eyes** *($90 for 0.5 ounce)* is a viable option if you're looking for a pH-correct AHA product with approximately 3-5% glycolic acid. There isn't anything about this formula that makes it a specialized treatment for eye-area skin; it's suitable for normal to dry skin anywhere on the face. What's disappointing, especially for this amount of money, is that other than the glycolic acid (which can be found in dozens of products that cost much less), the other state-of-the-art ingredients are barely present—and there are a lot of them. I suppose the tiny amounts of each antioxidant and cell-communicating ingredient might add up to provide some benefit for skin, but at this price you should expect a lot more. Apparently, this product is supposed to be worth it because it contains Dr. Murad's antiaging Durian Cell Reform, which they claim reverses signs of aging. Durian is a tropical fruit that research has shown to be a potent antioxidant when consumed orally. It contains high levels of antioxidants such as caffeic acid and quercetin, and likely has topical benefit as well, though this hasn't been proven (Sources: *Food and Chemical Toxicology*, February 2008, pages 581-589; and *Journal of Agricultural and Food Chemistry*, July 2007, pages 5842-5849). However, there isn't a shred of published research (including from Dr. Murad himself) that demonstrates durian fruit has a pronounced effect on skin wrinkles or firmness. Plus, there are other products that contain the active ingredients in durian and that would be far more effective in protecting skin. Intensive Wrinkle Reducer for Eyes is just another way for Dr. Murad to market his latest antiwrinkle products as superior; basically this is just a good AHA moisturizer barely worth your attention, especially at this price. Still, it deserves a happy face rating due to its effectiveness as an exfoliant.

✓ ☺ **$$$ Night Reform Glycolic Treatment** *($66 for 1 ounce)* is an outstanding fragrance-free AHA product for all skin types, but the texture is best for normal to very oily skin. Approximately 10% glycolic acid and a pH of 3.5 help create smoother, softer, even-toned skin, while the numerous antioxidants and anti-irritants provide further benefit. The cost is the only drawback, but at least you're getting more for your money than just another functional AHA product.

☺ **$$$ Optimal Skin Health Treatment** *($70 for 1 ounce)*. I would love to see the research or study that led Dr. Murad to conclude that this product could increase skin's firmness by 41% in 10 minutes. Does this mean that in half an hour skin will be over 100% firmer, and maintain it? And if you keep reapplying it do you consistently get firmer until your skin is firm like a tabletop? Talk about speedy antiaging! If this claim is true, which I doubt, then it would mean that any well-formulated AHA product with glycolic acid would have similar results because that is all you're getting in this overpriced, overhyped product. We know that's not the case based on copious research, but without question ongoing use of a well-formulated AHA product like this can gradually increase your skin's firmness because it stimulates collagen production and improves skin's texture along with its moisture-binding ability. But that doesn't happen in 10 minutes, nor would you want it to. Doing so would mean too much irritation at one time, and that isn't a good skin-care tactic to follow daily. Optimal Skin Health Treatment contains approximately 8-10% glycolic acid at a pH that allows exfoliation to occur. It is best for normal to slightly dry skin, although the wasabi root extract has the potential to cause irritation. There are lots of intriguing ingredients in this product, but most of them are listed after the pH-adjusting agent sodium hydroxide, which means you're not getting much of the good stuff for your money. However, that doesn't change the fact that this is another AHA option to consider.

☹ **T-Zone Pore Refining Gel** *($40 for 2 ounces)* lists alcohol as the second ingredient, which makes this gel too drying and irritating for all skin types. How disappointing, because this otherwise contains the makings of a very good AHA/BHA product for oily skin.

☹ **Pomegranate Exfoliating Mask** *($22.50 for 3.25 ounces)*. Murad has repackaged and renamed this enzyme mask, perhaps in an effort to keep the enzymes (bromelain and papain, the latter being from papaya fruit) stable prior to use. The packaging change helps to some extent, but the stability of these enzymes is still questionable and doesn't make this exfoliating mask preferred to a well-formulated AHA or BHA product. Even if enzymes were the equal of other exfoliants, this mask contains the irritating menthol derivative menthoxypropanediol and is not recommended.

☹ **Active Radiance Serum** *($89 for 1 ounce)*. The claims for this product are as disingenuous and as obnoxious as it gets. It is supposed to "Undo sun damage and erase a lifetime of summers," which it absolutely cannot do in any way, shape, or form. Ignoring the exaggeration and façade, this is merely a serum with a helpful amount of glycolic acid. Although research on that ingredient has shown it can help improve sun-damaged skin, it's hardly a panacea for a lifetime's worth of sun damage, any more than eating broccoli is a cure for a lifetime's worth of smoking.

As it turns out, the pH of this product is too high for the glycolic acid to exfoliate, which means you're pinning your hopes on Dr. Murad's vitamin C technology, said to deliver "50 times the free radical neutralizing power of prior generations." What prior generations is he referring to? Could it be his own products that contain vitamin C, which means they are no longer worthwhile for skin and he should stop selling them?

Either way, there are no substantiated data proving the claims are true and, in fact, there isn't much vitamin C in this serum anyway, so it is an empty message for your skin. There also are other antioxidants in this product, which is good because there is no single antioxidant that is the best for skin. Where this serum really comes up short is in including two forms of menthol along with fragrance chemicals known to cause irritation, and that is skin damaging, not healing.

☹ **Correcting Moisturizer SPF 15** *($37 for 1.7 ounces)* provides broad-spectrum sun protection via its in-part zinc oxide sunscreen. The base formula isn't too exciting, and this is a poor option for all skin types because of the peppermint extract and lemon peel oil.

☹ **Day Reform Treatment** *($66 for 1 ounce)* is a silky, silicone-based serum with retinol and tiny amounts of a few other antioxidants. It is not recommended over other retinol serums because it contains too much tannic acid. According to www.naturaldatabase.com, "Tannic acid has astringent effects. It dehydrates tissue, internally reducing secretions, and externally forming a protective layer of harder, constricted cells." That's not what you want from a product that pledges to reverse the damage caused by environmental elements.

☺ **Energizing Pomegranate Moisturizer SPF 15** *($33 for 2 ounces)* contains an in-part avobenzone sunscreen in a lightweight lotion formula suitable for normal to slightly oily skin. Pomegranate is a very good antioxidant; it's a shame there isn't more of it in here. Still, this is one of the few Murad products not waylaid by needless irritants, and it contains some effective soothing agents. It does contain fragrance.

☹ **Essential-C Daily Renewal Complex** *($92 for 1 ounce)* is another formula that should make you question Dr. Murad's formulary expertise. This silicone-based moisturizer contains several light- and air-sensitive ingredients (including retinol), yet it's packaged in a jar. The orange, grapefruit peel, basil, and galbanum oils included here may smell nice, but they also may cause skin irritation.

☹ **Essential-C Eye Cream SPF 15** *($67 for 0.5 ounce)* lacks the UVA-protecting ingredients of titanium dioxide, zinc oxide, avobenzone, Tinosorb, or Mexoryl SX (ecamsule), and is not recommended.

☺ **$$$ Essential-C Moisture SPF 30** *($60 for 1.7 ounces)*. This daytime moisturizer with an in-part titanium dioxide sunscreen is a very good option for normal to dry skin. Although not as impressive as some less expensive options from department-store brands, this sits nicely in the happy face column thanks to its lightweight lotion formula that contains several antioxidants and some good skin-identical ingredients. It is not rated a Paula's Pick because it contains a small amount of fragrance chemicals known to cause irritation.

☹ **Essential-C Night Moisture** *($60 for 1.7 ounces)* isn't the least bit essential despite containing some proven antioxidants for skin. The pros are just overwhelmed by the cons, which include irritation from the inclusion of several fragrant oils, including lavender, thyme, and grapefruit.

☺ **$$$ Eye Treatment Complex SPF 8** *($59 for 0.5 ounce)* includes an in-part titanium dioxide sunscreen, but an SPF rating that's embarrassingly low, especially from a dermatologist-developed line. The pH of 4 is borderline but still allows the approximately 8% concentration of glycolic acid to exfoliate. The SPF rating is the only weak spot in an otherwise well-formulated, antioxidant-rich, fragrance-free product for normal to dry skin.

☹ **Moisture Silk Eye Gel** *($49.50 for 0.5 ounce)* has many excellent, skin-friendly ingredients such as silicones, water-binding agents, and an anti-irritant, all in a silky gel-based formula.

Yet all of this is for naught because Murad couldn't resist adding cassia, grapefruit peel, orange, and bitter-orange oils—all potent skin irritants that should not be used near the eye area. This also contains a greater amount of caffeine than many products, which won't wake up the eye, but will increase the potential for irritation.

☺ **$$$ Oil-Control Mattifier SPF 15** *($39.50 for 1.7 ounces)* would rate a Paula's Pick, were it not for a small amount of potentially irritating cinnamon bark extract. The in-part zinc oxide sun protection is broad-spectrum and the matte-finish base formula is excellent for oily to very oily skin. What's more, the formula contains several antioxidants, including pomegranate, which is known to boost the efficacy of sunscreen actives. A small amount of cell-communicating niacinamide is included along with some anti-irritants, making this an overall well-rounded product that works beautifully under makeup.

☹ **Perfecting Day Cream SPF 30** *($47 for 1.7 ounces)* contains hydrogen peroxide and lavender oil, two ingredients capable of causing skin-cell death and free-radical damage. There are plenty of well-formulated sunscreens with avobenzone that omit problematic ingredients, so choosing this option would just be an expensive mistake.

☺ **$$$ Perfecting Night Cream** *($49 for 1.7 ounces)* is a very good, fragrance-free moisturizer for normal to dry skin. It would be rated a Paula's Pick if it contained more antioxidants. However, this contains some outstanding plant oils and a few good water-binding agents.

☺ **$$$ Perfecting Serum** *($62 for 1 ounce)* provides normal to very dry skin types with many of the ingredients needed to ensure a healthy barrier and allow skin to repair itself. It's a shame the clear glass bottle will compromise the effectiveness of the vitamin A and antioxidant-rich plant oils. However, the ceramides and lipids will make dry skin look and feel better.

☹ **Recovery Treatment Gel** *($52 for 1.7 ounces)* is supposed to fortify delicate, sensitive skin and make it feel comfortable, but that's not going to happen when you add peppermint, lemon peel oil, and hydrogen peroxide to the mix.

☺ **$$$ Sensitive Skin Soothing Serum** *($49.50 for 1 ounce)* has a formula that surprised me. Dr. Murad is notorious for infusing even his so-called gentle products with appreciable amounts of irritating ingredients. As a dermatologist, he should know better, but that hasn't proven itself to be true over the years. This water-based serum almost makes it to a Paula's Pick. It contains some very good soothing agents, water-binding agents, and antioxidants. It misses the mark only due to the inclusion of ivy extract, arnica flower, and pellitory. None of these plant extracts are what is needed for sensitive skin or for decreasing irritation. They're not present in large amounts, but including them at all wasn't a wise choice. Although this is a risky proposition for someone with irritated, sensitive skin, its texture is suitable for normal to oily or breakout-prone skin.

☹ **Skin Perfecting Lotion** *($33 for 1.7 ounces)* would be a much better moisturizer with retinol if it did not contain so much arnica extract. Arnica does not reduce redness or clogged pores, as claimed. It can cause irritation due to its volatile components and the amount of data compiled for this ingredient isn't sufficient to support its use or efficacy (Source: 2007 *CIR Compendium*).

☹ **Sleep Reform Serum** *($97 for 1 ounce)*. Because skin cannot tell what time it is and because its daily repair needs and function are occurring all the time, how is this product supposed to enhance skin's sleep cycle? Is it going to send a signal to cell receptors that the person is asleep now, so let's put the little skin-saving elves to work before the alarm clock buzzes? No, that's not going to happen. In fact, about the only things that will occur from using this serum is that your skin will feel smoother and perhaps a bit tighter (due to the amount of film-forming agent—similar to putting hairspray on the skin). But for long-term benefit of your skin the downside is the potential for irritation because this serum contains lavender oil, which can cause skin-cell death and serves as a pro-oxidant (Sources: *Contact Dermatitis*, September 2008, pages 143-150; and *Cell Proliferation*, June 2004, pages 221-229) along with other irritating fragrant ingredients. It also contains synthetic coloring agents, which is sad to see in a product supposedly from a dermatologist. Sleep Reform Serum also contains the hormone ingredient melatonin, but the only research pertaining to its effect on skin (as opposed to oral consumption) demonstrates it has a protective effect when skin is exposed to sunlight (Source: www.naturaldatabase.com). Given that this product is meant for nighttime use, including melatonin seems to be a marketing maneuver, not a skin-care essential. Another ingredient worth explaining is human oligopeptide-1. This is a type of epidermal growth factor whose benefits, if any, and the risk of long-term use on healthy, intact skin are unknown. We do know that such growth factors play a role in wound healing and reducing inflammation, but wrinkles are not wounds and there are many anti-inflammatory ingredients that have stronger safety profiles than epidermal growth factors. One potential negative of topical application of growth factors is the potential to cause cells to overproliferate. That's not what aging skin needs, and the possible side effects include cellular changes that could prove unhealthy or cosmetically undesirable (e.g., psoriasis is a skin disorder that involves overproliferation of skin cells). In short, topical application of growth factors isn't worth the potential risks to your skin, especially given that growth factors do not have any firmly established benefit as an antiaging wonder.

☺ **$$$ Firming Bronzer SPF 15, for Face and Body** (*$48 for 3.4 ounces*) is a good, though pricey, sunscreen for normal to dry skin, and its cost means you probably won't apply it liberally, which in turn means that you won't be getting sufficient sun protection. Avobenzone is on hand for sufficient UVA protection, and cosmetic and mineral pigments are included for a sheer bronze tint and shimmery finish. (The color is fairly natural, but it can be too peachy for very fair skin.) This sunscreen does not contain a self-tanning ingredient, just cosmetic pigments for color. Dr. Murad claims this increases skin's firmness by 32% in just 15 minutes, but because none of the ingredients in this product make skin firmer, you'll be waiting a lot longer than that for no improvement. However, keeping skin protected from sunlight will discourage the breakdown of collagen and elastin, and that helps prevent skin from sagging.

☹ **Oil-Free Sunblock SPF 15 Sheer Tint** (*$26 for 1.7 ounces*) has much going for it, including a pure titanium dioxide sunscreen, soft tint, and copious antioxidants to keep skin protected from inflammation, so it doesn't make a shred of sense that several irritating ingredients were included, too. Grapefruit, lavender, thyme, and orange oils all have their share of problems for skin, and make this sunscreen impossible to recommend.

☹ **Oil-Free Sunblock SPF 30** (*$30 for 1.7 ounces*) is built around synthetic sunscreen ingredients, including avobenzone for UVA protection. However, the roster of irritants is the same as for the Oil-Free Sunblock SPF 15 Sheer Tint above; therefore, this is not recommended.

☹ **Waterproof Sunblock SPF 30 for Face and Body** (*$31 for 4.3 ounces*) is similar to the Oil-Free Sunblock SPF 30, except it is water-resistant. The irritants still make this an ill-advised product for all skin types.

☹ **Acne Treatment Concealer** (*$21*) is not the kind of formula that's good for use on blemishes. Although the 2% salicylic acid gives it anti-acne potential, the nonaqueous formula makes it impossible to establish an acidic pH, which means the salicylic acid won't be effective as an exfoliant. Although this wind-up stick concealer covers well without looking thick, and all three shades are workable, the sage oil it contains causes irritation. You may think the immediate tingle means that the product is working to heal your blemishes, but the tingle is irritation, and that is actually an impediment to your skin's healing process. Camphor is a natural component of sage oil, and is not an ingredient proven to be helpful for blemishes.

☹ **Acne Spot Treatment** *($17.50 for 0.5 ounce)* lists 3% sulfur as the active ingredient, which makes this spot treatment an irritating, drying experience for skin (though sulfur can kill acne-causing bacteria). This has merit as a pH-correct AHA product, but it isn't worth considering over other AHA products that don't contain additional irritants.

☹ **Age Spot and Pigment Lightening Gel** *($60 for 1 ounce)* is a very expensive skin-lightening product that contains 2% hydroquinone. The problem is the alcohol base, which makes this gel too irritating for all skin types. Paula's Choice Clearly Remarkable Skin Lightening Gel contains the same amount of active ingredient along with salicylic acid to help exfoliate, and no needlessly irritating ingredients.

☹ **Clarifying Mask** *($37 for 2.65 ounces)* lists 4% sulfur as the active ingredient, which makes this an incredibly drying, irritating mask for acne-prone skin, or for any skin. Sulfur is joined by camphor and lavender oil, which are as appropriate for blemishes as using bacon grease to absorb excess facial oil.

☹ **Exfoliating Acne Treatment Gel** *($54 for 3.4 ounces)* features 1% salicylic acid as the active ingredient, but it's in a base that's mostly water and alcohol, and the arnica extract isn't helpful for any skin type. The anti-irritants in this gel can't compete with the problematic ingredients.

☹ **Firm and Tone Serum** *($77 for 6.75 ounces)* features an ingredient list with a "who's who" of skin-beneficial and skin-detrimental additives. Firm and Tone Serum claims to minimize body imperfections ranging from cellulite to stretch marks and sagging skin, leaving you "proud to show off." I wouldn't bank on this water- and alcohol-based concoction for any amount of body perfection, especially when you consider the amount of irritation your skin will experience from the peppermint, menthol, and several fragrant, volatile oils that have no established benefit for skin. Last, but not least, this product also contains esculin, a component of horse chestnut, which is considered toxic and is not recommended for topical application (Source: *Ellenhorn's Medical Toxicology: Diagnoses and Treatment of Human Poisoning*, 2nd Edition, Baltimore, MD: Williams & Wilkins, 1997).

☹ **Hydrating Gel Mask** *($30 for 2.65 ounces)*. This gel mask is not recommended because it contains ivy and arnica extracts as well as lavender oil. Even a small amount of lavender oil can cause skin cell death and enhance oxidative damage (Sources: *Contact Dermatitis*, September 2008, pages 143-150; and *Cell Proliferation*, June 2004, pages 221-229).

☹ **Lighten and Brighten Eye Treatment** *($75 for 0.5 ounce)* contains 1.5% hydroquinone as the active ingredient. Hydroquinone is adept at lightening melanin-based skin discolorations, whether they result from sun exposure or hormonal influence. However, this product is positioned as being able to lighten dark circles under the eyes, and hydroquinone cannot do that. Some people may have darkness under the eyes that results from excess pigmentation, but most cases of dark circles result from microscopic blood vessels showing through the very thin skin under the eyes. There's also the fact that this area is naturally shadowed just because of the way our skulls are shaped, as well as the fact that the infraorbital fat pads thin over time, which creates a sunken, hollow appearance. None of this is affected by topical application of hydroquinone. Not only is that disappointing in regard to this product, but also the inclusion of several irritating oils is completely wrong for use anywhere on skin, especially near the eyes.

☹ **Post-Acne Spot Lightening Gel** *($60 for 1 ounce)* could have been an effective option for treating hyperpigmentation because it contains 2% hydroquinone along with a good amount of glycolic acid. However, the amount of alcohol makes this too irritating for all skin types. If you're keen on spa or salon lines, the skin-lightening products from Peter Thomas Roth are much better formulations.

☺ **$$$ Vitamin C Infusion Home Facial Kit** *($70 for 4 treatments)* could have been an interesting, if somewhat gimmicky and overpriced, way to experiment with vitamin C for your skin, but the overall formulation has more problems than benefits.

You begin by mixing the **Vitamin C Infusion Treatment Powder**, which is just ascorbic acid and tapioca starch, with the **Vitamin C Infusion Treatment Gel**, which contains mostly glycerin, film-forming agent (think hairspray), vitamins, and the irritating plant extract *Ranunculus ficaria* (Source: www.naturaldatabase.com). After leaving this concoction on your skin for several minutes, you rinse, and are instructed to follow with the **Sensitive Skin Soothing Serum**, but this serum isn't recommended for anyone's skin because it contains problematic ivy and arnica extracts. Those plants mar an otherwise well-formulated serum, which is a shame, because in kits like this every product should be beneficial for your skin. Given the price and the inclusion of irritants that don't offer a benefit for skin, this kit really isn't worth the time or expense.

☹ **Energizing Pomegranate Lip Therapy SPF 15** *($17 for 0.5 ounce)* lacks the UVA-protecting ingredients of titanium dioxide, zinc oxide, avobenzone, Tinosorb, or Mexoryl SX (ecamsule), and is not recommended.

☹ **Soothing Skin and Lip Therapy** *($15 for 0.5 ounce)* lists benzyl cinnamate as the second ingredient. This is the chief fragrant component of balsam peru, and can be very irritating to skin and lips.

MYCHELLE DERMACEUTICALS

MYCHELLE DERMACEUTICALS AT-A-GLANCE

Strengths: MyChelle provides complete ingredient lists on their Web site; one good sunscreen for sensitive skin; sheer coverage stick foundation for dry skin.

Weaknesses: A natural product line that overemphasizes what their products don't contain, yet offers no conclusive proof that their list of allegedly bad ingredients is harmful; almost every product contains one or more irritating ingredients (most notably lavender oil); ineffective routines for improving acne and skin discolorations; only one sunscreen and no facial sunscreen is recommended for any of the daytime routines; no pH-correct AHA or BHA products; jar packaging; most of the makeup is difficult to blend due to its high wax and oil content; no makeup options for oily or blemish-prone skin.

For more information about MyChelle Dermaceuticals, call (800) 447-2076 or visit www.mychelle.com or www.Beautypedia.com.

MYCHELLE DERMACEUTICALS SKIN CARE

MYCHELLE DERMACEUTICALS APPLE BRIGHTENING PRODUCTS

☺ **$$$ Apple Brightening Cleanser** *($13.34 for 2.1 ounces)*. This water-soluble cleansing gel contains ingredients known to inhibit melanin production (at least in vitro), but they're of little use for skin discolorations when formulated in a cleanser because they are mostly rinsed down the drain. Although this could have been a very good cleanser for normal to oily skin, it contains citrus oils that may cause irritation and are definitely a problem if used in the eye area. Do I need to mention that this is *not* an all-natural cleanser and that the size is ridiculously small for the price?

☹ **Apple Brightening Mist** *($16.68 for 2.1 ounces)* lists witch-hazel water as the second ingredient. This ingredient often contains alcohol, but it's hard to tell from the ingredient list, so it may not be a problem. However, it also contains several plant irritants, including daisy flower, grapefruit oil, and two forms of orange oil, and contains fragrance chemicals that compound the irritation from the other problematic plants. Frustratingly, this formula contains some very good antioxidants and would have been a great toner for all skin types if it didn't contain the needless irritants.

☹ **Apple Brightening Peel** *($31.70 for 1.2 ounces)*. Apple isn't much of an exfoliant, which is apparent to MyChelle because this product also includes 5% lactic acid. Although it contains a potentially effective amount of AHA, the pH is really too high for effective exfoliation to occur. Even if the pH were within range, this peel wouldn't be recommended due to the many irritating fragrant oils it contains. All of the helpful ingredients in this product will be fighting the inflammation and other skin problems that the plant irritants will cause, and that doesn't equate to smart skin care. What a disappointment, because there really is a wonderful array of good ingredients in this product. This is much like a diet where you're eating chocolate cake with a healthy fresh salad, which isn't the way to take care of your diet. Leaving out the bad is as important as putting in the good.

☹ **Apple Brightening Serum** *($44.22 for 1 ounce)*. Witch-hazel water (which may contain enough alcohol to cause irritation and, likely, free-radical damage) is the main ingredient in this serum. It also contains a trio of irritating fragrant oils, including lavender. The lavender oil causes skin cell-death and promotes oxidative damage (Sources: *Contact Dermatitis*, September 2008, pages 143-150; and *Cell Proliferation*, June 2004, pages 221-229). This contains some potentially effective skin-lightening ingredients, but the irritants prevent a recommendation.

MYCHELLE DERMACEUTICALS CLEAR SKIN PRODUCTS

☹ **Clear Skin Cleanser** *($9.95 for 2.1 ounces)* offers no special benefit to acne-prone skin. It cleanses and removes makeup proficiently, but contains too many fragrant plant oils to make it worth considering over many other cleansers. The only ingredient with antibacterial activity is totarol, which is extracted from the heartwood of the Totara tree, as well as from plants such as rosemary and juniper. The research about this ingredient as it pertains to acne-causing bacteria is scant; the only study I found involved one person (a 14-year-old male), and even the study's author admitted he wasn't sure if the totarol produced the results or something else. He went on to state "This case provides anecdotal evidence of improvement in acne with the use of topical totarol; however to establish a casual relationship, large controlled clinical trials are needed." Moreover, the study involved using totarol in a leave-on product, not in a cleanser like this, which is quickly rinsed from skin (Source: www.natureshopnz.com/assets/Totarol_Case_Study.pdf).

☹ **Clear Skin Clarifying Pads** *($9.95 for 30 pads)* contain witch-hazel water as the main ingredient and may contain alcohol, which would be damaging to skin. They also contain the fragrant oils of lavender, grapefruit, and lemongrass, which are too drying and irritating for all skin types, and the irritation will make redness from acne worse. Of course, nothing in these pads provides control over oil production. If anything, irritating your skin increases oil production in the pore.

☹ **Clear Skin Balancing Cream** *($24.95 for 1 ounce)* contains several thickening agents that can potentially clog pores, which is something someone struggling with blemishes doesn't need, at least if the goal is clear skin. It contains some anti-inflammatory plant ingredients, but also contains irritating fragrant oils, so don't expect this moisturizer to reduce redness from acne or to have a calming effect on skin. One ingredient (totarol) deserves some explanation: Totarol is extracted from the heartwood of the Totara tree, as well as from plants such as rosemary and juniper. The research about this ingredient as it pertains to acne-causing bacteria is scant; the only study I found involved one person (a 14-year-old male) and even the study's author admitted he wasn't sure if the totarol produced the results or something else. He went on to state "This case provides anecdotal evidence of improvement in acne with the use of topical totarol; however to establish a casual relationship, large controlled clinical trials are needed" (Source: www.natureshopnz.com/assets/Totarol_Case_Study.pdf). I wouldn't pin my hopes for clear skin on totarol, definitely not when the product in question contains needless irritants.

☹ **Clear Skin Serum** *($31.70 for 1 ounce)* lists witch-hazel water as the main ingredient, followed by alcohol. Between the pure alcohol and the possible alcohol content of the witch-hazel water, you can expect dryness, irritation, free-radical damage, and increased oil production in the pore lining. These effects are compounded by the handful of fragrant plant oils. Clear Skin Serum does have some potentially helpful ingredients, but nothing that you can't find in other anti-acne products that treat your skin gently and that don't have unnecessary irritants.

☹ **Clear Skin Spot Treatment** *($14.95 for 0.5 ounce)*. The only thing this spot treatment for acne will do is induce on-the-spot irritation from the sulfur, zinc sulfate, and fragrant plant oils. While sulfur does have research showing it can have benefit for reducing blemishes, the dryness and irritation it can cause don't make it the first step in finding what will work to clear up your skin. There are many other products offering skin benefits that you should try first before trying one with irritants. Please refer to the review of the Clear Skin Balancing Cream above for an explanation of the totarol ingredient this contains.

OTHER MYCHELLE DERMACEUTICALS PRODUCTS

☹ **Creamy Pumpkin Cleanser** *($9.66 for 2.1 ounces)*. This cleansing lotion with a small amount of detergent cleansing agent is not recommended because it contains several incredibly irritating fragrant oils. Clove, cinnamon, nutmeg, and lime are great for cooking, but applied topically, the only thing they cook up is problems for your skin.

☺ **$$$ Fruit Enzyme Cleanser** *($9.66 for 2.1 ounces)*. This water-soluble cleanser does contain a small amount of fragrant plant oils, but not enough to be a deal-breaker; however, that doesn't make this cleanser worth considering over several other less expensive options ($9.66 is a strange price if I've ever seen one; for 2.1 ounces, it makes this a fairly pricey cleanser, coming in at just about $30 for 6.3 ounces). The pectin in here doesn't exfoliate skin and neither does the teeny amount of glycolic acid.

☺ **Honeydew Cleanser, Unscented** *($9.66 for 2.1 ounces)*. Technically, this cleanser is not unscented because it contains fragrant melon fruit extract derived from the honeydew melon, although the fragrance isn't as potent as that in other MyChelle products. Plus, this cleansing lotion for normal to dry skin omits the irritating plants the company is so fond of using. In addition, it's reasonably adept at removing most types of makeup, and rinses without the need for a washcloth.

☺ **White Cranberry Cleanser** *($9.66 for 2.1 ounces)* is nearly identical to MyChelle's Apple Brightening Cleanser, except for a change in plant extracts, which have no effect on this product's ability to cleanse skin or remove makeup. This contains fragrant oils that aren't the best, making this a problem for use around the eyes, but they're not present in an amount that warrants an unhappy face rating.

☺ **$$$ Fruit Enzyme Scrub** *($17.10 for 2.3 ounces)* is a creamy scrub and an OK option for normal to dry skin. The abrasive agents are a blend of jojoba beads and bamboo powder; it's not the fruit enzymes that are exfoliating skin, at least not to any noticeable degree. This is less desirable than several other scrubs (or just using a washcloth with your favorite cleanser) because it contains fragrant lemongrass oil.

☹ **Tropical Skin Smoother** *($31.70 for 1.2 ounces)*. The claim about this product tantalizing your olfactory (nose) senses says it all: this scrub contains citrus peel and oil that make it too irritating for all skin types. Choosing this for its citrus scent isn't a wise way to take the best care of your skin. By the way, the jar packaging won't keep the fragile enzymes stable during use.

☹ **Fruit Enzyme Mist** *($14.18 for 2.1 ounces)* contains an irritating amount of witch-hazel water and contains lesser, but still potentially problematic, amounts of alcohol, lavender oil, and grapefruit peel oil. There are some intriguing ingredients, too, but they're of little use to skin in the presence of so many irritants.

☹ **Pumpkin Hydrating Mist** *($39.95 for 2.1 ounces)*. Pumpkin and poppy extract are not rejuvenating for skin. You might think this is a do-nothing product, but the fragrant oils it contains do something—they irritate your skin.

☹ **Fruit Fiesta Peel** *($28.36 for 1.2 ounces)* is supposed to "romance your skin to a more radiant, youthful glow." You will be far better off with a dozen roses than you will be if you use this product. This peel contains a blend of AHAs but is formulated at a pH level that limits effective exfoliation. The pure fruits it contains can be irritating, while the fragrant citrus oils and synthetic fragrant components aren't helpful for skin in the least. All told, this formula has more in common with a fruit smoothie than skin care!

☹ **Capillary Calming Serum** *($42.21 for 1 ounce)*. Although this water-based serum contains an impressive amount of the plant soothing-agent willow herb, among other really interesting ingredients, the third ingredient is alcohol, which doesn't calm skin in the least. Alcohol causes free-radical damage, cell death, and irritation. This serum also contains several fragrant plant oils that someone with sensitive skin should steer clear of at all costs. The claims this serum can remove toxins is sheer myth; there is no proof there are toxins in skin in the first place, and certainly no evidence that they could be coaxed out by a skin-care product.

☺ **Deep Repair Cream** *($28.36 for 1.2 ounces)* is far more ordinary than reparative, although it does contain some emollient ingredients that are helpful for dry skin and several of the plant extracts have antioxidant ability. Unfortunately, other components keep this moisturizer from doing much that's positive for skin. The jar packaging won't keep the good antioxidants stable during use, the inclusion of epidermal growth factor is a potential risk for skin due to the unknowns associated with daily application, and this contains fragrant oils and fragrance chemicals that are known irritants.

☺ **Deep Repair Cream, Unscented** *($28.36 for 1 ounce)* is nearly identical to MyChelle's regular Deep Repair Cream above, and the same review applies. It definitely contains fragrance in the form of plant oil (neroli), so the unscented claim is bogus.

☹ **Fabulous Eye Cream** *($28.36 for 0.5 ounce)*. The name for this eye cream would ring true if it did not contain several irritating fragrant oils. These oils are a problem for use on skin anywhere on the body, but even more so for use around the eyes. What a shame, because this does contain some very impressive ingredients that skin really needs. By the way, there isn't any research showing that eye-area skin needs anything different from skin elsewhere on the face; that is, if you have dry skin on your face and are using a brilliant moisturizer for that area, and you have dry skin in the eye area, you should use the same moisturizer for that area.

☹ **Fresh Eyes** *($41.71 for 1.2 ounces)* has the same problem as MyChelle's Fabulous Eye Cream above: a preponderance of fragrant plant oils that are irritating for use anywhere on the face, but especially near the eyes. Fresh Eyes is the worse of the two because one of its main ingredients is witch-hazel water, a plant that constricts skin and whose potential alcohol content can be a problem. Again, what a shame, because this product also contains several beneficial ingredients, although the jar packaging won't keep them stable because they deteriorate in the presence of air.

☹ **G2 Instant Firming Serum** *($59.95 for 1 ounce)*. You're supposed to believe that the goji berry fruit in this serum instantly lifts skin and offers long-term prevention of lines and wrinkles. It's all bogus, but if it were true, why doesn't MyChelle include it in all their antiaging products? The truth is that this serum has a few too many negatives over the positives. Witch-hazel water is a major ingredient that can potentially contain a good deal of alcohol, which isn't firming but instead rather irritating. This also contains fragrant oils, including lavender, which kills healthy skin cells and promotes oxidative damage (Sources: *Contact Dermatitis*, September 2008, pages 143-150; and *Cell Proliferation*, June 2004, pages 221-229).

☹ **Magnolia Fresh Eyes** *($38.95 for 0.5 ounce)*. Magnolia as a skin-care ingredient has no research pertaining to its benefit for skin in the eye area, whether the concern is dark circles or anything else. This also contains daisy extract, a plant that can cause severe contact dermatitis (Source: www.naturaldatabase.com). Add to that the fact that the witch-hazel water usually contains alcohol, making this something not to use around the eye or anywhere on the face.

☹ **NoTox Anti-Wrinkle Serum** *($54.95 for 1 ounce)*. Just like most cosmetics companies that espouse their products' natural content, MyChelle has to offer products that claim to work like Botox (oddly Botox is indeed natural, as it is derived from a bacteria, and bacteria is surely natural). The peptides in this water-based serum cannot replicate in any way what Botox can do for wrinkles and expression lines. At best, the peptides in here serve as water-binding agents and theoretically as cell-communicating ingredients, but none of them can prevent wrinkles. It is very disappointing that witch-hazel water (which almost always contains alcohol, and that's damaging for skin) is a main ingredient in this product, and it also contains fragrant oils. Epidermal growth factors are on board, too, and that's a risky ingredient to apply daily due to the unknown effect of using it on otherwise healthy, normal skin.

☹ **Oil Free Grapefruit Cream** *($29.95 for 1 ounce)*. The emollients that comprise the bulk of this product can make skin feel greasier and potentially clog pores. Salicylic acid is included, but the amount is borderline for being effective for oily skin, not to mention the fact that the pH of this moisturizer is too high for effective exfoliation to occur. Also, there is more alcohol in this moisturizer than beneficial ingredients for oily skin, and it contains several fragrant plant oils that can irritate skin, causing it to increase oil production rather than decrease it.

☹ **Pumpkin Renew Cream** *($25.86 for 1.2 ounces)* contains several fragrant oils (including clove and cinnamon) that make it very irritating for all skin types. It also contains antioxidants, but they are sensitive to air and won't remain stable in the jar packaging. The fragrance is quite potent, but scent isn't the key to taking great care of your skin. It also contains epidermal growth factor, an ingredient whose impact on healthy skin is unknown. Adding to the confusion is the 0.5% glycolic acid, which is too little for it to have any effect as an exfoliant. Plus, the showcased pumpkin has no research showing it to be of benefit for skin. This also contains totarol, an ingredient with no real research showing it can benefit someone with oily skin. The claim that this works for all skin types is like suggesting one-size-fits-all pantyhose was a realistic concept.

☹ **Pumpkin Renew Cream, Unscented** *($25.86 for 1.2 ounces)* is identical to MyChelle's Pumpkin Renew Cream above and the same review applies. This contains fragrance.

☹ **Revitalizing Night Cream** *($38.38 for 1.2 ounces)* is an emollient moisturizer for dry skin that contains a handful of uncommon plant extracts, but none of them are known to provide benefits for skin. It also contains a bevy of star ingredients, from antioxidants to cell-communicating ingredients. The problem is that most of them are air-sensitive and, therefore, won't stay stable in the jar packaging. Add to that the inclusion of fragrant plant oils (including cell-damaging, oxidative lavender oil) and this isn't your nighttime ticket for healthier skin.

☺ **$$$ Revitalizing Night Cream, Unscented** *($38.38 for 1.2 ounces)* is similar to MyChelle's regular Revitalizing Night Cream above, except it omits the fragrant oils. That's an improvement, and something they should do for all their products, but it's still disappointing that the numerous antioxidants and other air-sensitive ingredients (retinol among them) will lose their potency because of the jar packaging. What a foolish oversight for what would have otherwise been an excellent product.

☹ **Serious Hyaluronic Firming Serum** *($42.21 for 1 ounce)*. Not much about what MyChelle offers for skin is serious, at least not in terms of what published research has shown skin needs. Mostly, they offer what skin doesn't need to reach its optimum potential, and this serum is no exception. It lists witch-hazel water as the second ingredient, which most likely includes alcohol, and that's a problem for skin. It also contains skin cell-damaging lavender oil. Several impressive ingredients are on board, but you don't have to tolerate irritants to get these essential ingredients into your skin-care routine.

☹ **Supreme Polypeptide Cream** *($53.39 for 1.2 ounces)*. If this is MyChelle's supreme moisturizer, then why do they sell so many others with varying degrees of antiwrinkle claims? This is described as an "unsurpassed wrinkle defense nourishing cream," so wouldn't you think the company should stop selling all of their other antiwrinkle products, or at least put a disclaimer on them that says "These don't work as well as our Supreme one?" As it turns out, this isn't supreme in the least. This moisturizer is quite similar to the many other emollient options MyChelle offers. It contains several antioxidants and a cell-communicating ingredient, but these air-sensitive ingredients won't remain stable in the jar packaging. By the way, the claim that this product contains "dermaceutical-grade" ingredients is sheer nonsense. This is a made-up marketing term that has no counterpart in the world when it comes to ingredient regulations. Supreme Polypeptide Cream earns its unhappy face rating due to the presence of several irritating fragrant oils.

☹ **Supreme Polypeptide Cream, Unscented** *($53.39 for 1.2 ounces)* is identical to the regular Supreme Polypeptide Cream above, and the same review applies. The only difference is that this product is scented!

☹ **The Perfect C** *($41.71 for 1 ounce)* is hardly the perfect choice for anyone's skin because it contains several irritating ingredients, including citrus oils that can cause a phototoxic reaction when skin is exposed to sunlight. This contains vitamin C (ascorbic acid) along with retinol and some good antioxidants, but the irritants are too potent to ignore. Several other brands offer well-formulated vitamin C products without including the extraneous irritants. The glycolic acid in here can have exfoliating properties, but there are many products that contain that ingredient in a gentler base.

☺ **$$$ Ultra Hyaluronic Hydrating Serum** *($42.21 for 1 ounce)*. This water-based serum is one of the few well-formulated MyChelle products. Fragrant geranium oil is the only real problem, but the amount is probably not enough to be of concern. It does contain some very good skin-identical and cell-communicating ingredients, but it's short on significant antioxidants. Regrettably, the formula leaves out many of the state-of-the-art ingredients that show up in other MyChelle products, which is disappointing because this could have been a great formula instead of just good.

☹ **X-zema Balm** *($15.01 for 0.5 ounce)*. This wax-based balm contains several plant ingredients, most of which are helpful for skin either as antioxidants or as soothing agents. The wax and plant oils form a protective barrier that helps dry skin improve, but what's missing are key structural components of skin. Including them would have made this a much better product. As is, it's not recommended because it contains lavender oil. Research has shown that even a small amount of this plant oil can kill healthy skin cells (Source: *Cell Proliferation*, June 2004, pages 221-229).

☹ **Del Sol Bronzing System** *($13.34 for 2.3 ounces)*. There are no toxic chemicals in other self-tanners, so you can ignore MyChelle's misguided claim that theirs is the only safe self-tanner, not to mention that this self-tanner is *not* all natural. If anything, this self-tanner ends up being the unsafe option because it contains several citrus oils that can cause a phototoxic reaction when skin is exposed to sunlight (Source: www.naturaldatabase.com). Because this self-tanner includes the same ingredients to turn skin color that countless other self-tanners contain, there's no reason to risk irritation and other problems for skin or to spend this much money.

☺ **$$$ Sun Shield SPF 28** *($19.19 for 2.3 ounces)* is a very good, very basic, fragrance-free mineral sunscreen suitable for normal to dry or sensitive skin. It contains a couple of antioxidants and omits the fragrant plant oils found in most of MyChelle's other skin-care products, which is really a welcome relief for your skin.

☹ **Cranberry Mud Mask** *($25.03 for 1.2 ounces)* is a below-standard clay mask that irritates and dries skin with its alcohol content and several skin-irritating fragrant oils, including rosemary and lavender. The antibacterial agent totarol has only minimal research behind its anti-acne prowess. Nothing in this mask can detoxify skin because the skin has no toxins in it that can be coaxed out by a skin-care product.

☹ **Guava Cactus Mask** *($31.70 for 1.2 ounces)*. None of the chief plant extracts in this moisturizing mask are all that helpful for skin, but they do support MyChelle's natural angle. What also supports this angle, though assuredly not to skin's benefit, is the inclusion of several fragrant oils, including lavender, which causes skin cell death and oxidative damage (Sources: *Contact Dermatitis*, September 2008, pages 143-150; and *Cell Proliferation*, June 2004, pages 221-229). This mask is not recommended.

☹ **Incredible Pumpkin Peel** *($26.69 for 1.2 ounces)*. Pumpkin wine is the main ingredient in this specialty peel, but there's no legitimate research anywhere proving it is preferred to established ingredients for exfoliation such as AHAs and BHA. Plus, wine has a high alcohol content and that causes irritation, which is a problem for all skin types. This peel also contains several potent irritants that no one's skin needs. This product smells like a dessert, but that won't help your skin. The claim it can detoxify skin is bogus; there are no ingredients that can coax toxins out of the skin, and the claim it can aid in "tissue respiration" is meaningless. This product has little potential to absorb (which is good news because you don't want the irritants this product contains causing more problems than they already do), but the surface skin cells are dead and can't breathe.

☺ **$$$ Lip Plumping Treatment** *($26.69 for 0.5 ounce)* is available in either a Pina Colada or Mint flavor. The Pina Colada version is recommended as a good emollient lip balm; the Mint version is not recommended. The Mint version has a formula similar to that of the Pina Colada version, bit it irritates lips with spearmint and peppermint oils plus menthol. Of course, the Mint version is the more "plumping" of the two balms (because of the irritation it causes), but neither will replace "up to 40% of lost volume" after less than one month's use. There is nothing in either of these products that restores lip content. The Maxi-Lip ingredient complex doesn't have a shred of substantiated research proving it increases lip fullness.

☺ **Love Your Lips** *($12.01 for 0.5 ounce)* lists titanium dioxide as its active ingredient, but it doesn't have an SPF rating. The company told my research assistant that they haven't yet tested this product via FDA protocols, so they didn't attach an SPF rating or go on record stating one. That's a strange answer, but the packaging information doesn't meet FDA regulations for sunscreens and, therefore, you can't rely on this for sun protection. Regardless of the flavor you choose, this balm won't love your lips as much as it should, especially if they're exposed to sunlight.

MYCHELLE DERMACEUTICALS MAKEUP

☺ **$$$ Cream Foundation** *($25.86)* is a stick foundation that is decidedly more waxy than creamy. Its oil base makes it best for dry to very dry skin, although it's not very easy to blend. It also tends to drag over skin, but with patience, you can achieve a natural-looking finish that feels moist and provides sheer coverage. All of the shades are workable and include options for dark (but not very dark) skin tones. The mica in this foundation casts a subtle shine.

☺ **Concealer** *($12.93)* has a formula that's nearly identical to MyChelle's Cream Foundation, except it provides noticeably more coverage. Because the formula is oil- and wax-based, the increased coverage tends to look heavy on skin (the Cream Foundation's sheerness negates this issue) and it definitely creases into lines around the eyes. This is not recommended for use over blemishes. Each of the three shades is acceptable.

☺ **$$$ Blush Stick** *($20.85)* is a twist-up stick blush with a thick, waxy texture that glides poorly over skin, which makes blending a challenge. The formula is only for those with normal skin; with patience you can produce a sheer wash of soft color with a moist finish. All of the shades are attractive and most add a soft shimmer to skin.

☹ **Eye Shimmer** *($12.93)*. All of the shades in this twist-up eyeshadow stick have shimmer, but so what? Eyeshadows with shimmer are a dime a dozen, and you shouldn't have to put up with this one's drawbacks. It has a sheer, waxy texture that makes skin look dotted with color, and the cream finish doesn't last. Trying to blend this just makes it look choppy, and I can't imagine women putting up with this given the number of superior eyeshadows available.

☺ **$$$ Lip Gloss** *($26.69)* is a very expensive lip gloss with an oil-based formula that makes it feel quite slick and protective on lips. Packaged in a squeeze tube with an angled applicator, it glides on and imparts surprisingly rich color with a glassy finish. This product is also known as Lip Plumping Gloss, but it doesn't contain ingredients proven to make lips bigger. Instead, you get the optical illusion of fuller lips due to this product's reflective finish. You can get the same result from most lip glosses.

☹ **Little Kisses** *($10.42)* are just tiny tubes of lipstick. The texture is similar to that of MyChelle's Eye Shimmer, which means it is thick and waxy and has an uneven application. This may very well be one of the most difficult lipsticks to apply because the color deposit and the finish are uneven and chunky.

NARS

NARS AT-A-GLANCE

Strengths: One good cleanser and lip balm; great range of foundation shades; the powder blush; the lipsticks, including a sheer option with broad-spectrum sunscreen; some of the makeup brushes are excellent.

Weaknesses: Expensive; jar packaging; drying cleansers and irritating toners and mask; no exfoliants; no sunscreens; ineffective skin-lightening products; average to poor pencils; the liquid liner; single eyeshadows; mascaras that are not impressive given their cost.

For more information about NARS, owned by Shiseido, call (888) 903-6277 or visit www.narscosmetics.com or www.Beautypedia.com.

NARS SKIN CARE

☺ **$$$ Balancing Foam Cleanser** *($35 for 4.4 ounces)* is a standard, detergent-based cleanser that can be more drying than most due to the amount of potassium hydroxide. The orange oil prevents this cleanser from being a safe bet for use around the eyes. It's an OK option for normal to oily skin.

☺ **$$$ Gentle Cream Cleanser** *($35 for 4.4 ounces)* is gentle in name only. This water-soluble cleanser is quite similar to the Balancing Foam Cleanser above, except it contains some additional thickening agents. Otherwise, the same comments apply.

☹ **Purifying Soap** *($22 for 7 ounce bar)* is a standard, detergent- and tallow-based, highly alkaline soap that can be drying and irritating for most skin types.

☺ **$$$ Softening Milk Cleanser** *($36 for 4.4 ounces)* is the best among NARS' cleansers, but that isn't saying much. This basic, cold cream–style milky cleanser removes makeup with mineral oil and other emollients, and contains a small amount of detergent cleansing agents. A washcloth may be needed for complete removal, but this is an option for normal to dry skin.

☺ **$$$ Eye Makeup Remover** *($25 for 3 ounces)* is a very standard, but effective, water- and silicone-based fluid that removes most types of makeup. The inclusion of fragrant plant extracts isn't the best, and the price is extraordinary for what amounts to ordinary. This is easily replaced with better formulas for far less money.

☹ **Balancing Toning Lotion** *($36 for 6.7 ounces)* lists alcohol as the second ingredient and contains isopropyl alcohol, too, for a double whammy, plus camphor and eucalyptus oil. Ouch!

☹ **Hydrating Freshening Lotion** *($36 for 6.7 ounces)* omits the camphor and eucalyptus oil in the Balancing Toning Lotion, but contains too much alcohol to be even a little hydrating. This is just irritating and the alcohol will trigger excess oil production in the pore lining.

☹ **Balancing Moisture Lotion** *($55 for 2.5 ounces)* contains more alcohol and potassium hydroxide than it does any beneficial ingredients. The antioxidants are present in such teeny amounts that they are meaningless for skin.

☺ **$$$ Brightening Serum** *($61 for 2.5 ounces)* contains enough talc to leave a slight white cast on skin, which is what "visibly brightens skin after one application." This is otherwise a standard, overpriced, silicone-based moisturizer that lacks truly beneficial ingredients for skin.

☹ **Essential Vitamin Serum** *($75 for 2.5 ounces)* irritates skin with alcohol and contains more film-forming agents (the same kind used in hairstyling products) than vitamins or anything else beneficial for skin. This is just an overpriced waste of time.

☺ **$$$ Hydrating Moisture Cream** *($72 for 3.4 ounces)* is an OK emollient moisturizer for normal to dry skin. The jar packaging won't keep the tiny amount of antioxidant vitamins stable.

☺ **$$$ Nourishing Eye Cream** *($76 for 0.5 ounce)* is an average, jar-packaged moisturizer for normal to slightly dry skin anywhere on the face. The iron oxides (a cosmetic pigment) are what create the "radiant luminosity" the company brags about.

☺ **$$$ Aqua Gel Hydrator** *($76 for 3.6 ounces)* is a water- and silicone-based moisturizer with many of the same problems as the other moisturizers in this line, including jar packaging (a true disappointment with this product, as it contains more antioxidants than other NARS moisturizers). The claim that it contains 87% water is basically letting you know that there isn't much of anything else in here. Plus your skin doesn't need water (healthy skin is only 10% water, and too much water destroys the skin's structure). Rather, the skin needs ingredients that support and enhance its structure, antioxidants to reduce free-radical damage, and sunscreen to prevent sun damage—something this line almost completely ignores.

☺ **$$$ Lightening Cream** *($98 for 3.5 ounces)* does not contain any ingredients capable of lightening skin discolorations. Even the form of vitamin C used (ascorbyl glucoside) has minimal research proving its worth for pigmentation issues, and the jar packaging won't keep it stable during use. That leaves you with a very expensive silicone-based moisturizer for normal to slightly dry skin.

☹ **Mud Mask** *($45 for 3.4 ounces)* is an exceptionally standard clay mask whose alcohol content makes it even more drying, while the eucalyptus oil causes irritation. The Masada Mud from the Dead Sea may sound impressive, but your skin wouldn't know the difference between mud from that part of the world and mud from Lake Michigan.

☺ **$$$ Rain Lip Treatment** *($23 for 0.14 ounce)* is essentially a colorless emollient lipstick NARS sells as a lip moisturizer. It contains oils and waxes to ensure smooth, flake-free lips, has a nice selection of antioxidants, and is fragrance-free.

☺ **$$$ Sabrina Lip Balm** *($23 for 0.14 ounce)* claims an SPF 20 but because it doesn't list active ingredients you can't rely on it for sun protection. It is otherwise very similar to the Rain Lip Treatment, and the same basic comments apply. The neutral face rating is for this balm's misleading claim of sun protection.

NARS MAKEUP

FOUNDATION: ☺ **$$$ Firming Foundation** *($50)*. You can ignore the firming claims for this creamy liquid foundation; the amount of beneficial ingredients is practically an afterthought, and they're not particularly stable in this formula. Moreover, none of them can firm skin, no matter the amount or the type of packaging. Despite that disappointment and this foundation's absurd price tag, it is worth considering if the wasted money doesn't bother you and if your skin is normal to slightly dry. The slightly thick texture means that it takes a little more time than usual to set while blending, with the result being a soft matte finish and medium to almost full coverage. This doesn't look quite as skin-like as similar foundations from Laura Mercier, but NARS is getting better. Among the many shades are some notable options for fair and very dark skin tones. The darker shades actually look more natural than the lighter shades, some of which appear slightly chalky after they set. Consider the Stromboli shade carefully. Avoid Cadiz—whose skin is this orange?—and if it is, why aren't they asking a doctor what's wrong with them?

☺ $$$ **Powder Foundation SPF 12** *($45)* has a silky texture and seamless application that is far more advanced than either of NARS other liquid foundations reviewed. Even better, the talc-free formula's sunscreen is in-part zinc oxide, though SPF 15 is preferred for minimum daytime protection. Still, this deserves a happy face rating for those seeking a pressed-powder foundation to wear over a regular sunscreen or over a foundation with sunscreen. It provides sheer to light coverage and leaves a soft matte finish with a hint of shine. The range of ten shades is mostly gorgeous and suitable for a wide range of skin tones; only Jamaica pulls a bit too copper for its intended dark skin.

CONCEALER: ☺ $$$ **Eyebrightener** *($22)*. Although positioned as a specialty product, this is really just a good liquid concealer with a light, sheer texture and a soft matte finish. Paired with it is a soft, off-white highlighter that can be used on its own or blended with the flesh-toned concealer shade. This duo covers minor imperfections reasonably well, but isn't what you want if hiding blemishes or dark circles is the goal. Six shades are available (the highlighter shade is the same for each) and four are great. Praline is too peach and Toffee is slightly gold, but still worth testing.

☺ $$$ **Concealer** *($22)* provides creamy, opaque coverage that can look heavy, as though it's just sitting on skin rather than melding with it. NARS claims this is crease-resistant, but it can indeed slip into the lines around the eyes. If you prefer creamy, lipstick-style concealers, there are some decent colors, but avoid Honey and Praline (both too peachy pink). Toffee is an OK option for darker skin, but may turn slightly copper.

POWDER: ☺ $$$ **Loose Powder** *($34)* remains one of the messier loose powders to use due to its awkward, oversized packaging and lack of a sifter. This is otherwise a gorgeous talc- and cornstarch-based powder that looks beautifully natural on the skin, with only a trace of shine. The six shades are exemplary—Snow is ideal for very fair skin, but watch out for Mountain, which can be too ash on dark skin (though applied sheer this becomes a non-issue).

☺ $$$ **Pressed Powder** *($30)* has been improved and as a result has been given a higher rating. The talc-based formula shares most of the attributes of the Loose Powder version, including a sheer finish that looks natural rather than powdered. The texture is drier than the Loose Powder, too, but that doesn't affect how nice this looks on skin. All eight shades are superb, though Mountain is tricky due to its stronger yellow tone.

BLUSH AND BRONZER: ✓☺ $$$ **Blush** *($25)* is definitely the star attraction of this line and it's easy to see why. These have a splendid texture and apply beautifully with a sheer initial application that builds to any depth of color you want because most of the colors have strong pigment (a plus for women with dark skin). The following shades are almost matte and highly recommended: Amour, Desire, Exhibit A, Gina, Gilda, and Mata Hari. The very shiny shades, which you should consider carefully, include Angelika, Crazed, Lovejoy, Mounia, Outlaw, and Torrid. The remaining palette features shiny shades that aren't the best for daytime makeup, but are great for a sultry evening look.

✓ ☺ **Color Wash** *($25)* is the NARS version of Benefit's BeneTint liquid blush, but NARS bests Benefit by offering more color choices, and each is suitable for a natural, flushed appearance or subtle lip stain.

☺ **$$$ Bronzing Powder** *($30)* shares the same positive traits as the Pressed Powder above, and is also talc-based. Two shades are available, each with moderate shine. Laguna is best for fair to light skin, while Casino meshes well with medium to tan skin colors. Although a real tan doesn't sparkle, at least the shine in this bronzer adheres well to skin.

☺ **$$$ Creme Blush** *($25)* is definitely creamy but not too thick or greasy. It smooths over skin, delivering sheer color and a radiant finish. Although the colors look way too intense in their compacts, each goes on translucent and layers well if you want a bit more color. You will find that this works best on dry to very dry skin.

EYESHADOW: ☺ **$$$ Cream Eye Shadow** *($21)* is quite shiny but has a smooth texture and just enough slip to make application and blending easy. However, because the finish stays moist, it won't stay in place and it will fade and crease slightly. If creamy eyeshadows are what you're after but you want longevity, look to Revlon or M.A.C. first.

☺ **$$$ Duo Cream Eyeshadow** *($32)* has the same pros and cons as M.A.C.'s Cream Eye Shadow above.

☹ **$$$ Single Eye Shadow** *($22)* has a dry but smooth texture, but a somewhat choppy application. Part of the application issue has to do with how deeply pigmented and chalky these shadows are. Stronger colors aren't inherently a problem and can be easily blended if the silkiness and slip is there. Regrettably, that is exactly what is absent here.

☺ **$$$ Duo Eye Shadow** *($32)* has an improved texture and formula that is different from (and preferred to) the Single Eye Shadow. What that lacks in silkiness, the duo Eye Shadow more than compensates for, and each duo applies color-true. The number of duos, all of which have some shine, is a bit overwhelming, though the majority of them feature pairings that are too contrasting or just too colorful for day-to-day makeup. The most attractive, versatile duos include All About Eve (great name, even better film), Bellissima, Charade, Key Largo, Madrague, Pacifica, and Tokyo.

EYE AND BROW SHAPER: ☹ **$$$ Eyebrow Pencil** *($20)* needs sharpening, but if you're OK with that, all of these have a suitably dry texture and smooth-powder finish that stays in place. The three shades present options for blondes and brunettes, but nothing for redheads or those with raven brows.

☹ **Eye Liner Pencils** *($20)* have a too creamy application that is very prone to fading and smearing, and the colors are too unnatural or too clownish to take seriously, at least for most women.

☹ **Glitter Pencil** *($24)* is a fairly creamy, thick pencil infused with flecks of glitter. The glitter tends to separate from the pencil's base formula and chip off onto your face.

☹ **Liquid Liner** *($27.50)* is absurdly priced given the number of superior liquid liners available for less than $10. The NARS version comes in a nail-polish bottle and features an OK brush (which must be assembled prior to use) and mostly wild colors that go on too sheer. Repeated applications are necessary to build intensity, and that increases the odds against precise, even application. Why anyone would bother with this is beyond me—if you want to spend this kind of money on liquid liner, I suggest Lancome's fantastic Artliner, but there are less expensive options at the drugstore from L'Oreal and Maybelline.

LIPSTICK, LIP GLOSS, AND LIPLINER: ✓ ☺ **$$$ Semi-Mattes** *($24)* are the real standouts here; they have an opaque, slightly creamy finish and a good stain. Creamy lipsticks don't get much better than this, and this formula is available in over 20 colors, including some of the best reds available.

☺ **$$$ Lip Lacquer** *($24)* isn't the easiest to use due to its glass jar packaging, but its thick, lanolin oil–based texture leaves lips heavily moisturized and beaming, although with a slightly sticky finish that won't be to everyone's liking. The large color palette includes both sheer and strongly pigmented colors, making this one to test before purchasing (the shade names are no help in determining this—what does "Chelsea Girls" tell you about opacity or color shade?).

☺ **$$$ Lip Stain Gloss** *($24)* is for those who love the opacity of traditional lipstick but also want the shiny finish of a lip gloss. This two-in-one product has a slick, silicone-based texture without a trace of stickiness and provides a high-gloss shine. The intense colors leave a good stain, but are not for the timid. Think glam to the max and you'll love this!

☺ **$$$ Satins** *($24)* are creamy, bordering on greasy, and are fairly opaque yet have a soft gloss finish.

☺ **$$$ Sheers** *($24)* finish glossy, aren't too slick, and offer coverage that is light rather than genuinely sheer. The colors are great.

☹ **$$$ Lip Gloss** *($24)* features several bold colors in a sticky, thick formula whose price is unwarranted for what you get, which is just a gloss, and a rather tacky-feeling one at that. If you're going to indulge in a NARS gloss, go for the Lip Lacquer.

☹ **$$$ Lipliner Pencil** *($20)* claims it won't bleed or feather, and although that won't hold true for everyone, this does have a drier finish that should keep those problems in check at for least a few hours. The color selection has been expanded and coordinates well with the many lipsticks (and glosses) this line offers. This would rate a Paula's Pick if it didn't require routine sharpening.

☹ **$$$ Velvet Matte Lip Pencil** *($24)* has a beautifully smooth texture that goes on silky and feels light, and has enough creaminess to look soft and still wear comfortably. It isn't a true matte, but velvet matte is a fairly accurate description of this pencil's finish. The shade selection is nicely varied. This pencil's creaminess is enough to pose a slight problem for those prone to lipstick bleeding into lines around the mouth, and the sharpening and resharpening is just not fun, hence the neutral face rating.

MASCARA: ☹ **$$$ Mascara** *($23)* just doesn't impress enough, at least not for what it costs. You'll be able to build decent length, but this mascara takes time to show its stuff and can be slightly clumpy. There are at least a dozen or more mascaras at the drugstore that significantly outperform this one.

☹ **Waterproof Mascara** *($23)* has characteristics similar to the Mascara, only this one tends to stick the lashes together and creates a spiky look. This is hardly waterproof either, which is a real letdown given the price.

FACE AND BODY ILLUMINATING/SHIMMER PRODUCTS: ☹ **$$$ Body Glow** *($59)* comes in a heavy glass bottle and is just coconut oil with golden bronze shimmer and potent fragrance. It adds a sexy, though oily-feeling, sheen to bare skin and will definitely complement a tan (which hopefully came from a bottle and not from the sun). Be careful, this will rub off on clothing.

☺ **$$$ Sparkling Loose Powder** *($35)* is identical to the NARS Loose Powder, only the single shade is infused with a subtle but sparkling shine. It clings OK, but isn't really worth the money given the number of shiny powders available at the drugstore that work far better.

☺ **$$$ Monoi Body Glow II** *($59)* was launched because presumably the original Body Glow needed a sequel. Unlike the original, this version has a different scent (it's still very perfume-y) and is colorless. It retains the original's coconut oil base and is a workable, though pricey, body oil option for dry skin.

☺ **$$$ Sparkling Pressed Powder** *($31)* doesn't do much to impress other than adding sparkling shine to skin. It has a smooth but dry texture and a shine that tends to apply unevenly and not stay in place for long. It's an option, but only if you're willing to pay more for fewer positives. As a plus, the three shades are versatile and sheer.

☺ **$$$ The Multiple** *($37)* is a chunky wind-up stick with a creamy yet lightweight texture and soft, sheer colors that would work for cheeks, eyes, and, in some cases, lips. Although all of the colors have varying degrees of shine (and go on softer than they appear in the stick), these are an option for a fun evening look, though the price is extraordinary for what amounts to a soft wash of glow-y color. Sonia Kashuk's namesake line at Target uses the same concept for her Illuminating Color Stick, which is just as worthwhile and sells for one-fourth the price.

BRUSHES: ✓ ☺ **$$$ NARS Brushes** *($21-$75)* almost all have a lovely, soft feel and are appropriately shaped for a variety of application techniques. The best brushes are the synthetic **Flat Concealer Brush 07** *($25)*, the pricey but luxurious **Eye Shader Brush 03** *($55)*, and the **Liquid Eyeliner Brush 09** *($21)*. ☺ **$$$ Push Eyeliner Brush 02** *($26)* is identical to those found in many other lines, except that NARS charges more. ☺ **$$$ Smudge Brush 15** *($25.50)* has a unique cut and shape that work for smudging or other eyeshadow detail work. It's worth testing if you're in the mood for something different. ☺ **$$$ Loose Powder Brush 01** *($50)* should have better-quality hair for the money. Steer clear of the ☹ **Retractable Lip Brush 11** *($25)*, which is really too small for most women's lips.

SPECIALTY PRODUCTS: ☺ **$$$ Makeup Primer with SPF 20** *($33)* contains an in-part titanium dioxide sunscreen and as such can protect your skin from UVA rays whether worn alone or under a foundation. Because this is a primer, most women will use it under foundation, so the question of whether or not this product "primes" the skin needs to be addressed. The water-in-silicone base formula will leave skin feeling silky-smooth, which will facilitate foundation application and, depending on your skin type and condition, potentially improve wear time. However, many other lightweight moisturizers (with or without sunscreen) do this, too, as such combinations of silicone and lightweight hydrating ingredients are becoming increasingly common. For example, a less expensive option that provides the same feel and finish (minus sunscreen) is Olay's Regenerist Perfecting Cream. This NARS product might have been worth the splurge if it contained an array of antioxidants and other bells and whistles to help skin, but they're in short supply. The orange oil has a slight potential to cause irritation, but is included mostly for fragrance. If you want to audition this, the formula is best for normal to slightly dry or slightly oily skin.

☺ **$$$ Makeup Primer** *($33)* is just an ultralight moisturizer that supposedly "primes" the skin for foundation. As a moisturizer, it lacks any state-of-the-art water-binding agents or antioxidants and isn't worth considering over the state-of-the art gel-creams and serums offered by many other lines, from Olay to Estee Lauder.

NEOSTRATA (INCLUDING EXUVIANCE)

NEOSTRATA (INCLUDING EXUVIANCE) AT-A-GLANCE

Strengths: Huge assortment of AHA and PHA products, all with correct pH to exfoliate; sunscreens that include AHA and/or PHA at right pH and provide reliable broad-spectrum sun protection; good cleansers; some excellent serums and lightweight moisturizers; the Exuviance makeup products are worth a try if you need full coverage with sufficient sun protection.

Weaknesses: No BHA products (better for blemish-prone skin or for those who can't tolerate AHAs or PHA); no topical disinfectants (a basic for those with acne); all hydroquinone products have at least one major negative; irritating toners; jar packaging; potentially problematic self-tanning products; lip balms contain irritating spearmint oil; most NeoCeuticals products are terrible.

For more information about NeoStrata, call (800) 225-9411 or visit www.neostrata.com or www.Beautypedia.com.

NEOSTRATA SKIN CARE

NEOSTRATA EXUVIANCE PRODUCTS

☺ **$$$ Gentle Cleansing Creme** *($25 for 6.8 ounces)* a standard, lightweight cleansing lotion that does not contain detergent cleansing agents. It removes makeup and is best for normal to slightly dry skin. It would be even gentler without the fragrance.

☹ **$$$ Purifying Cleansing Gel** *($25 for 6.8 ounces)* is a good water-soluble cleanser for normal to very oily skin. The amount of gluconolactone and glycolic acid will be rinsed away, so their inclusion isn't helpful for skin, plus it's a potential problem for the eyes.

☹ **Moisture Balance Toner** *($25 for 6.8 ounces)* lists alcohol as the second ingredient, which makes this neither moisturizing nor balancing for skin. The pH of 4.1 keeps the AHA and PHA from performing optimal exfoliation.

☹ **SkinRise Bionic Tonic** *($40 for 30 pads)* are pads (also sold in packette form) that serve only to irritate skin because of the amount of peppermint oil. Other irritants include eucalyptus, grapefruit, and menthyl lactate. Barbara Green, NeoStrata Vice President of Technical and Consumer Affairs, wrote to me that this product is "a very soothing, non-irritating formulation" and supported this point by referring to the Repeat Insult Patch Testing (RIPT) results. This test is performed by many cosmetics companies (including mine) to purportedly gauge the potential for irritation and skin reactions. However, the protocols for this test involve putting a dab of product on the arm or back of volunteers, and keeping it semi-occluded. The site is then routinely checked for signs of irritation. If minimal to no reactions are noted, the product is considered non-irritating. The problems? This test doesn't correlate with how consumers use the product on their faces, and a substance applied on the arm for a few days doesn't have anything to do with using it on the face day after day. Even more to the point, there's the issue that irritation can occur without visible proof, such as redness or flaking (think of the silent damage UVA rays from the sun cause). RIPT testing may make regulatory boards happy, but it has limited relevance for the consumer.

☹ **$$$ Soothing Toning Lotion** *($25 for 6.8 ounces)* contains a good amount of the PHA gluconolactone, but the pH of 4.7 reduces its effectiveness as an exfoliant. This is otherwise a fairly standard toner for normal to dry skin. It would be better for sensitive skin if it did not contain fragrance or coloring agents.

☺ **$$$ Skin Healthy Home Resurfacing Peel System** *($65)* is a four-step system that consists of smaller sizes of two products sold separately from the kit (the **Purifying Cleansing Gel** and **Evening Restorative Complex**). The first step is the **Activator Pads**, which combine AHAs and the PHA gluconolactone at a combined concentration of 25% and pH of 3.6. You're directed to leave this solution on skin for no more than ten minutes (and at this concentration that seems like a long time to me), at which point you apply the Neutralizing Solution to stop the peel's exfoliating action. This step isn't essential considering you can net the same result by simply rinsing the solution with tap water, but I suppose it makes the kit seem more "clinical." The amount of AHAs and PHA is indeed on par with the type of peels performed in a doctor's office or by an aesthetician. In that sense, this kit bests similar options available from drugstore lines. However, I'd caution you to use this only occasionally if you routinely use another AHA or BHA product. The skin can only handle so much exfoliation before it starts reacting negatively, so pay attention to its response and remember that the amount of exfoliants in this kit can cause noticeable irritation (and don't forget to protect your skin with an effective, broad-spectrum sunscreen).

☺ **$$$ Essential Daily Defense Creme SPF 15** *($28 for 1.75 ounces)* works beautifully to provide sun protection (it contains an in-part titanium dioxide sunscreen) and exfoliates skin with 8% glycolic acid in a pH of 3.8. The moisturizing base is suitable for normal to dry skin. Unfortunately, jar packaging renders the plant-based antioxidants ineffective shortly after you begin using it. However, this still has merit as a dual-purpose daytime moisturizer, so a happy face rating applies.

☺ **$$$ Essential Daily Defense Fluid SPF 15** *($28 for 1.75 ounces)* is similar to but has a slightly lighter texture than the Essential Daily Defense Creme SPF 15, and the same basic comments apply, except that this one is preferred for normal to slightly dry skin. Although not packaged in a jar, the translucent glass bottle means that the antioxidants will be exposed to light, and that's not the way to keep them stable and potent.

☺ **Evening Restorative Complex** *($38 for 1.75 ounces)* is a boon for normal to dry skin due to the amount of gluconolactone, the pH of 3.8 promises exfoliation, and the antioxidant-rich base formula (now in stable, non-jar packaging). This also contains some good cell-communicating ingredients, and is definitely worth considering as an exfoliant/night moisturizer.

☹ **$$$ Hydrating Eye Complex** *($30 for 0.5 ounce)* contains 3% gluconolactone and 1% lactobionic acid at a pH of 3.6. The amount of PHA won't prompt much exfoliation, but that's not such a bad thing for a product to be used around the eye. The fragrance-free base is silky and slightly emollient, but what a shame the numerous antioxidants will be compromised due to jar packaging.

☺ **$$$ Multi-Protective Day Creme SPF 15** *($28 for 1.75 ounces)* is preferred for sensitive skin because its PHA content is 5%, and the pH of 3.4 is effective for exfoliation. For those with sensitive skin, any AHA or PHA may prove too irritating, and the synthetic sunscreen agent in here can do the same. This does contain titanium dioxide for sufficient UVA protection.

☺ **$$$ Multi-Protective Day Fluid SPF 15** *($28 for 1.75 ounces)* is a good daytime moisturizer for normal to dry skin. It has a lotion texture and includes an in-part titanium dioxide sunscreen. This has a pH of 4, which still allows the PHAs to be effective exfoliants while being potentially less irritating for sensitive skin.

☺ $$$ **Vespera Bionic Serum** *($55 for 1 ounce)* is a good lightweight gel moisturizer for normal to slightly dry or slightly oily skin that contains small amounts of some good antioxidants along with water-binding agents and effective PHAs for exfoliation. The packaging will keep the antioxidants stable during use. This product also contains mandelic acid, but this AHA is not as effective as others.

☹ $$$ **Skin Healthy Sunless Tanning Facial Pads** *($15 for 12 packettes)* are difficult to recommend because the amount of gluconolactone and the pH of 3.2, which allows for effective exfoliation, are not what you want while you're waiting for your self-tan to develop (the pads contain dihydroxyacetone to turn skin color). Exfoliating before self-tanning is an important step, but combining the two at the same time can result in an uneven, blotchy color.

☹ $$$ **Skin Healthy Sunless Tanning Mousse** *($24 for 3.4 ounces)* has the same drawbacks as the Skin Healthy Sunless Tanning Facial Pads above, and the lower pH of 2.9 makes the PHA that much more effective (though also potentially too irritating).

☹ **Blemish Treatment Gel** *($18 for 0.5 ounce)* has a pH above 5, which prevents the 2% salicylic acid from functioning as an exfoliant. The amount of alcohol makes this gel too drying and irritating for all skin types, plus the alcohol stimulates excess oil production in the pore lining.

☹ **Purifying Clay Masque** *($30 for 1.7 ounces)* tried to go beyond standard by including NeoStrata's AHA alternatives, gluconolactone and glucohepatanolactone. However, neither will offer much of an exfoliating benefit because this mask's pH is borderline for them to be effective. Although this clay mask for oily skin has good oil-absorbing potential, inclusion of the irritating menthol derivative menthyl lactate makes it impossible to recommend.

☹ **Rejuvenating Treatment Masque** *($26 for 2.5 ounces)* only treats skin to irritation due to its blend of alcohol and polyvinyl alcohol (a common ingredient in hairspray and peel-off masks). The alcohol is joined by some problematic plant extracts and the pH of 4.4 prevents the AHA and PHA from exfoliating.

☹ **Essential Multi-Protective Lip Balm SPF 15** *($10 for 0.14 ounce)* would be a brilliant lip balm with sunscreen if it did not contain irritating spearmint oil. The titanium dioxide and zinc oxide (along with other actives) ensure UVA protection, but such protection shouldn't come with the trade-off of irritated lips.

NEOSTRATA EXUVIANCE PROFESSIONAL PRODUCTS

☺ $$$ **Moisturizing Antibacterial Facial Cleanser** *($25 for 6.8 ounces)* is a standard, water-soluble gel cleanser for normal to oily skin; the triclosan and other additives don't make this a "professional" option any more than renaming a Big Mac "Filet Mignon Sandwich" would change the fact that it is still just a Big Mac. Still, the triclosan is likely a helpful first step toward reducing acne-causing bacteria on skin.

☹ **Clarifying Solution** *($20 for 3.4 ounces)* is an alcohol-based toner that contains 8% glycolic acid at a pH that allows it to exfoliate. Many other products have the same AHA positive without the negative that this much alcohol presents.

✓ ☺ $$$ **Rejuvenating Complex** *($45 for 1 ounce)* exfoliates skin with 12% gluconolactone and a pH of 3.2, all in an emollient base suitable for dry to very dry skin. The "Pro-Retinol" in this stably packaged product isn't actually retinol. It's retinyl acetate, which is the ester of retinol and acetic acid (an ester is an organic compound formed from the reaction of an acid and an alcohol). Despite the different name, it's still a retinoid, but it doesn't work as well as pure retinol. Overall, this is an excellent exfoliant that provides the additional benefit of antioxidants.

☺ **$$$ Ultra Restorative Creme** *($45 for 1.75 ounces)* is similar to the Exuviance Evening Restorative Complex reviewed above, except this contains more PHAs (12% versus 8%). Otherwise, the same review applies. The amount of sodium hyaluronate in this product isn't worthy of the company's "moisture sponge" claim.

☹ **Intense Lightening Complex** *($42 for 1 ounce)* contains too much alcohol to make it a worthwhile hydroquinone product. Additionally, this contains oxalic acid, which is corrosive to skin and nails. Maybe that's what they mean by "intense"?

NEOSTRATA NEOCEUTICALS PRODUCTS

☺ **$$$ NeoCeuticals Antibacterial Facial Cleanser, PHA 4** *($22 for 6 ounces)* is nearly identical to the Exuviance Professional Moisturizing Antibacterial Facial Cleanser above, and the same review applies.

☹ **NeoCeuticals Oil Control Gel** *($23 for 1 ounce)* won't control oil as much as it will irritate skin given the amount of alcohol it contains. NeoStrata recommends this as an ideal after-shave product for men—talk about a painful ending!

☹ **NeoCeuticals PDS Treatment Regular Strength Cream** *($30 for 3.4 ounces)* is a very emollient AHA moisturizer that contains glycolic acid and gluconolactone as the main exfoliating ingredients. Although this can exfoliate skin, it irritates it with spearmint oil, so it is not worth considering.

☹ **NeoCeuticals Problem Dry Skin Gel** *($24 for 4 ounces)* contains 20% urea as the active ingredient, an amount known to cause skin inflammation and promote moisture loss from skin. Urea can be an outstanding moisturizing agent for all types of dry skin, but concentrations of 10% or less are preferred, and there is extensive research to support the therapeutic benefits of this amount (Sources: *Dry Skin and Moisturizers: Chemistry and Function*, Maibach and Loden, CRC Press, 2000, pages 243-250; and *CIR Compendium*, 2007, pages 314-315). This product will likely cause, not mitigate, problem dry skin, and it can cause stinging on contact.

☹ **NeoCeuticals Skin Brightening Gel** *($38 for 1 ounce)* contains many remarkable ingredients in this hydroquinone-free, skin-lightening gel, including an effective blend of the polyhydroxy acid gluconolactone and the alpha hydroxy acid glycolic acid. The formula also includes kojic acid to lighten hyperpigmentation. However, all of these potentially helpful ingredients are a wash because alcohol is a major ingredient. Peter Thomas Roth and my line (Paula's Choice) offer effective skin-lightening gels with hydroquinone that do not include extraneous irritants.

☹ **NeoCeuticals Acne Spot Treatment Gel** *($15.50 for 0.5 ounce)* is identical to the Blemish Treatment Gel above, and the same comments apply.

☹ **NeoCeuticals Acne Treatment Solution Pads** *($16.50 for 40 pads)* are alcohol-based pads that include 2% salicylic acid at a pH that's too high for exfoliation. Two words: Don't bother.

OTHER NEOSTRATA PRODUCTS

☺ **$$$ Facial Cleanser, PHA 4** *($24 for 6 ounces)* is a standard, detergent-based, water-soluble cleanser with 4% PHA (polyhydroxy acid). Even though this doesn't contain much AHA, it is still of concern in a cleanser that may get into the eye area.

☹ **Foaming Glycolic Wash, AHA 20** *($25 for 3.4 ounces)* contains a lot of glycolic acid, but that's not helpful in a cleanser because it is rinsed down the drain before it can go to work. Additional problems include the amount of alcohol and the drying detergent cleansing agent sodium C14-16 olefin sulfonate.

✓ ☺ **$$$ Brightening Bionic Eye Cream** *($42 for 0.5 ounce)* provides exfoliation with 4% gluconolactone in a pH of 3.5, which may be too irritating for some when used around the eye. Considering that gluconolactone has some antioxidant capacity and that this product also contains other antioxidants, it is worth considering if you have normal to dry skin. The vitamin K in here does not impact dark circles; nothing in this product will, but it has other benefits.

✓ ☺ **Daytime Protection Cream SPF 15, PHA 10** *($33 for 1.75 ounces)* is a very good fragrance-free daytime moisturizer with sunscreen (titanium dioxide is one of the active ingredients). It also contains 8% PHA at a pH that allows exfoliation to occur in a standard emollient base, and is an option for normal to dry skin.

☺ **Face Cream Plus, AHA 15** *($29 for 1.75 ounces)* contains 15% glycolic acid at an effective pH range. The simple moisturizing base is suitable for normal to very dry skin, and is fragrance-free. One caution: Daily use of products containing more than 10% glycolic acid is of concern to the FDA, but the research isn't there to support the long-term effects of such usage, for better or worse.

☹ **Gel Plus, AHA 15** *($33 for 3.4 ounces)* lists alcohol as the second ingredient, which makes this 15% glycolic acid gel too irritating for all skin types. The alcohol will also stimulate oil production in the pore lining.

☺ **$$$ High Potency Cream, AHA 20** *($40 for 1 ounce)* contains 20% glycolic acid at a pH of 3.5. This will exfoliate skin, but the kickback from irritation due to such a high concentration of AHA may not be worth the risk, at least not for daily use. There isn't any research on this issue to help point you in a safe direction. This product is only recommended if your physician advises you that such potency is necessary.

☺ **Lotion Plus, AHA 15** *($28 for 6.8 ounces)* is similar to but less emollient than the Face Cream Plus, AHA 15 above, and the same concerns apply.

☹ **Oily Skin Solution, AHA 8** *($23 for 3.4 ounces)* lists alcohol as the second ingredient, and is not recommended over other products with 8% glycolic acid that exfoliate without unnecessary irritants. The alcohol will stimulate oil production in the pore lining.

✓ ☺ **$$$ Renewal Cream, PHA 12** *($43 for 1.05 ounces)* is very similar to the Exuviance Professional Rejuvenating Complex reviewed above, right down to its 12% concentration of gluconolactone and inclusion of retinyl acetate.

☺ **Ultra Smoothing Cream, AHA 10** *($23 for 1.75 ounces)* combines 8% glycolic acid and 2% citric acid, for a total 10% AHA product, although citric acid is not nearly as effective as glycolic acid. Still, the pH of 3.5 means this will exfoliate, and it is a good, basic, fragrance-free AHA moisturizer for normal to dry skin.

☺ **Ultra Smoothing Lotion, AHA 10** *($27 for 6.8 ounces)* is the lotion version of the Ultra Smoothing Cream, AHA 10 and, other than being preferred for normal to slightly dry or slightly oily skin, the same review applies.

☺ **Bio-Hydrating Cream, PHA 15** *($32 for 1.75 ounces)* contains 15% PHA (using gluconolactone). Since this exfoliant works in a manner similar to glycolic acid, the same concerns about using concentrations above 10% apply. This is an OK option for intermittent use by those with normal to dry skin.

✓ ☺ **$$$ Bionic Eye Cream, PHA4** *($50 for 0.5 ounce)* provides exfoliation with 4% gluconolactone in a pH of 3.5, which may be too irritating for some when used around the eye. Considering that gluconolactone has some antioxidant capacity and that this product also contains other antioxidants, it is worth considering if you have normal to dry skin. The vitamin K in here does not impact dark circles; nothing in this product will, but it does have other benefits.

☺ **$$$ Bionic Face Cream, PHA 12** *($47 for 1.75 ounces)* contains 12% PHA (polyhydroxy acid) in a silicone-based moisturizer that also contains some good plant oils and small amounts of water-binding agents, which make it good for normal to dry skin. However, there is concern about using such a high concentration of AHA (over 10%) given its unknown long-term effects on skin, but this is a reliable option for normal to slightly dry or slightly oily skin.

☺ **$$$ Bionic Face Serum, PHA 10** *($47 for 1 ounce)* contains only the PHA lactobionic acid, and there is no substantiated research proving this exfoliates skin, so it's not necessarily a slam-dunk if you're hoping for that benefit. This ends up being a well-packaged, water-based, fragrance-free antioxidant serum for all skin types. For that reason, it certainly deserves consideration.

☺ **$$$ Bionic Lotion, PHA 15** *($25.50 for 3.4 ounces)* exfoliates skin with the PHA gluconolactone at a concentration of 12% and a pH of 3.8. The bland moisturizing base is suitable for normal to dry skin. Given the high concentration of PHA, this product may provide the best results when alternated with another AHA product with a lower acid concentration.

☺ **$$$ Eye Cream, PHA 4** *($26 for 0.5 ounce)* includes 4% gluconolactone with a pH of 3.2 to prompt exfoliation. The eye area may not be able to tolerate this product, but it's fine for use elsewhere on the face where skin is dry. The antioxidants and antioxidant plant oils are a nice touch, but they're not a prominent part of the formula.

✓ ☺ **Oil Free Lotion SPF 15, PHA 4** *($30 for 1.75 ounces)* is very similar to the Daytime Protection Cream SPF 15, PHA 10 reviewed above, except with a 4% concentration of gluconolactone. Otherwise, the same comments apply.

☺ **Ultra Daytime Smoothing Cream SPF 15, AHA 10** *($30 for 1.75 ounces)* exfoliates skin with 10% glycolic acid in a pH of 3.2, while an in-part titanium dioxide sunscreen shields skin from UVA rays. The base formula for normal to dry skin isn't terribly exciting, but this is highly recommended if you're looking for a combination AHA sunscreen product.

☺ **$$$ Ultra Moisturizing Face Cream, PHA 10** *($28 for 1.75 ounces)* is an effective, though basic, PHA moisturizer that includes 10% gluconolactone formulated at a pH of 3.5, so exfoliation will occur. The fragrance-free formula is best for normal to dry skin; what a shame the jar packaging won't keep the selection of antioxidants stable during use.

☹ **Bionic Skin Lightening Cream SPF 15, PHA 10** *($28 for 1 ounce)* contains 2% hydroquinone, but the sunscreen actives do not provide sufficient UVA protection, making this an almost-there product that doesn't deserve a purchase.

☹ **Lip Conditioner SPF 15** *($6.50 for 0.14 ounce)* is identical to the Exuviance Essential Multi-Protective Lip Balm SPF 15, and the same (unfortunate) comments apply. Spearmint oil can cause contact dermatitis on the lips (Source: *Contact Dermatitis*, October 2000, pages 216-222).

NEOSTRATA EXUVIANCE MAKEUP

FOUNDATION: ☺ **$$$ CoverBlend Concealing Treatment Makeup SPF 20** *($22.50)* is a remarkable full-coverage foundation that effectively conceals minor and major discolorations without feeling thick and greasy on the skin. Since this is a rather opaque makeup, I don't agree with Exuviance's claim that it provides "natural" coverage. But the effect, while perceptible, is certainly more attractive on the skin and easier to work with than DermaBlend or most other heavy-duty foundations you may have tried. The silicone-based formula features an excellent titanium dioxide– and zinc oxide–based sunscreen, and although it appears thick in the jar, it has a soft, light texture that is surprisingly easy to blend. Concealing Treatment Makeup dries to a solid matte finish, which may not be to everyone's liking, but you will certainly get more longevity out of it than you will with traditional creamy or greasepaint-type foundations. Those with normal to dry skin will definitely need to apply moisturizer before using this makeup, and you're not likely to need any setting powder, unless you want to further enhance the matte effect (which can be a mistake). Almost complete coverage is achieved with one application, and it layers well for areas that need more camouflage. There are 14 shades, but not all of them are praiseworthy. The following colors are too pink, peach, or rose for most skin tones: Neutral Beige, True Beige, Blush Beige, Honey Sand, and Palest Mahogany. Bisque and Ivory are slightly peachy pink, but may work for some fair skin tones because the dry-down result is lighter than the color you see in the container. True Mahogany, Blush Mahogany, and Deep Mahogany are beautiful for dark skin tones, although the titanium dioxide and zinc oxide sunscreen can result in a slightly ashen finish.

☺ $$$ **CoverBlend Skin Caring Foundation SPF 15** (*$30 for 1 ounce*) has a titanium dioxide sunscreen and a strong silicone base that starts out feeling light and silky but blends down to an ultra-matte, dry finish that only those with very oily skin will appreciate. Coverage is sheer to light and it does maintain its solid matte finish for most of the day. As with most ultra-matte foundations, it will exaggerate dry spots, however minor. There are 14 shades available, and though some of them appear too pink, peach, or rose in the bottle, most dry down to a soft, semi-sheer color. The following colors are noticeably peach, pink, or rose on the skin: True Beige, Neutral Beige, Palest Mahogany, Honey Sand, and Blush Mahogany.

☹ **CoverBlend Corrective Leg & Body Makeup SPF 18** (*$18*) is more akin to traditional full-coverage makeup when compared to the CoverBlend Concealing Treatment Makeup above. Although this silicone- and talc-based makeup with a titanium dioxide– and zinc oxide–based sunscreen does indeed provide substantial, water-resistant coverage, three of the four shades are simply too peach or pink to look convincing on most skin tones. If you're going to wear opaque makeup on the body (presumably concealing a large area of skin), you don't want to use colors that stand out against the skin and draw attention to what you're trying to hide. If you have dark skin and need this type of camouflage makeup, Mahogany is a worthwhile deep tan shade to consider.

CONCEALER: ☺ $$$ **CoverBlend Multi-Function Concealer SPF 15** (*$16.50*) is a slightly creamy, full-coverage concealer that includes a titanium dioxide– and zinc oxide–based sunscreen. This applies quite well, and has only a slight tendency to crease—though the complete coverage may be of interest only to those with severe dark circles or other skin flaws that are not effectively covered by traditional concealers. If you need serious coverage and don't mind the trade-off of a less-than-natural finish, this is worth a try. There are four shades available; the following two are problematic: Mahogany has strong peachy gold overtones that don't mesh well with most dark skin tones, while Sand dries to an ashy rose color that doesn't do anything to enhance the complexion.

POWDER: ☺ $$$ **CoverBlend Anti-Aging Finishing Powder** (*$18*) is a fine-textured, satin-finish loose powder that contains only talc, gluconolactone, pigments, and preservatives. The gluconolactone is supposed to provide a moisturizing benefit, but don't count on significant hydration from an absorbent powder containing this ingredient. This simple formula works well with the CoverBlend foundations, and the two shades are equally good options, each imparting a sheer wash of color.

NEUTROGENA

NEUTROGENA AT-A-GLANCE

Strengths: Inexpensive; some superior water-soluble cleansers; good topical scrubs; effective AHA and BHA products; several retinol options, all in stable packaging; vast selection of sunscreens, most of which offer excellent UVA protection; good variety of self-tanning products; several fragrance-free options; most Healthy Skin products are state-of-the-art; almost all of the foundations with sunscreen provide sufficient UVA protection; the Moistureshine Gloss; a tinted lip balm with broad-spectrum sunscreen; the Shimmer Sheers; enticing mineral makeup with sunscreen.

Weaknesses: An overabundance of antiaging products that is perennially confusing for consumers; bar soap; most toners are irritating or boring; a handful of bland moisturizers and eye creams; some sunscreens lack sufficient UVA protection or contain too much alcohol; Advanced Solutions products are advanced in name only; most of the Deep Clean products are terrible; no effective skin-lightening products; jar packaging; mostly disappointing concealers and eyeshadows; most of the lip balms with sunscreen provide inadequate UVA protection; poor mascaras.

For more information about Neutrogena, owned by Johnson & Johnson, call (800) 582-4048 or visit www.neutrogena.com or www.Beautypedia.com.

NEUTROGENA SKIN CARE

NEUTROGENA ADVANCED SOLUTIONS PRODUCTS

☺ $$$ **Advanced Solutions At Home MicroDermabrasion System** *($39.99)* is an all-in-one kit for those who want to try a microdermabrasion treatment at home before making a far more expensive, one-time appointment for the real-deal procedure with an aesthetician or dermatologist. Included is a battery-powered, hand-held device (batteries included) with two speeds, two sponge heads, a unit for storing the device between uses, and the **Micro-Oxide Crystallized Cream**. The cream product contains the same ingredient (aluminum oxide) used in professionally administered microdermabrasion treatments and, thankfully, does not contain unnecessary irritants such as menthol. You're instructed to use the sponge tip (with the device turned off) to dot the exfoliant cream on key areas of your face, then switch the device on, which causes the attached sponge head to vibrate. After moving the device over your entire face to enhance the mechanical skin-scrubbing action, you're instructed to rinse the product. That's where things got tricky for me. Massaging the Micro-Oxide Crystallized Cream into my skin wasn't difficult, though it did feel a bit gritty, almost as if I were stroking my skin with soft sandpaper. However, rinsing the cream off proved a lengthy process, and hours later I was still feeling traces of the crystals on my face. Not the best. Because this is an effective topical scrub, there is no question your skin will feel softer and smoother after a treatment (mine had a noticeable glow). However, I am concerned that the aluminum oxide crystals may cause problems in the long run if people overdo this, because irritation is a concern. When microdermabrasion is performed with a professionally guided machine, the crystals are suctioned off the skin during treatment, which drastically minimizes their potential for causing post-treatment problems. With at-home systems like Neutrogena's, the likelihood of problems increases. Of course, it all

The Reviews N

depends on how zealous consumers are about it, but it's easy to get carried away while running the device over your face. Neutrogena does have research, which they paid for, showing that their At Home MicroDermabrasion System works as well as microdermabrasion performed in an office setting (Source: *The Rose Sheet*, March 7, 2005, page 3). Their comparison is impressive; 60 women received in-office microdermabrasion treatments or used the At Home MicroDermabrasion System. The two groups felt equally happy with their results! Keep in mind the study did not examine whether either treatment was as effective as a topical scrub (including just using a washcloth) paired with regular use of an effective AHA or BHA product, which has the potential to net better results for your skin (and recent research suggests that repeated microdermabrasion treatments may yield diminishing returns). Plus, published research indicates that salon/doctor-performed microdermabrasion treatments may have either marginal benefit or diminishing results. That means that if Neutrogena's works as well as the professional version, that might not be good news (Sources: *Dermatologic Surgery*, June 2006, pages 809-814, and March 2006, pages 376-379; and *Journal Watch Dermatology*, May 2004).

☹ **Advanced Solutions Acne Mark Fading Peel** *($15 for 1.4 ounces)* is designed to fade post-inflammatory hyperpigmentation from acne—those telltale marks left on skin long after a blemish has healed. On lighter skin tones, the marks are traditionally pink or red, while darker skin tones typically have brown to almost black marks. These marks are the remnants of your skin's healing response to blemishes, and usually fade within 12 to 18 months—an eternity when they are staring you in the face each morning. Will this Neutrogena product be the "Advanced Solution" you've been looking for? Probably not, but the 2% salicylic acid in a base with a pH of 3.8 means you can get beneficial exfoliation, and that can help the discolorations. However, the product's directions indicate that you can use it as many as three times per week and you should leave it on for periods of 5 to 10 minutes, which means you rinse it off before it really has a chance to work. The inclusion of irritating menthol makes it inherently problematic for healing. To gain maximum benefit from salicylic acid, it is best to leave it on the skin. The anti-inflammatory effect of the salicylic acid in this product is negated when paired with menthol, which has absolutely no fading or peeling abilities. Exfoliation with glycolic or salicylic acids can indeed speed the fading of post-inflammatory hyperpigmentation, as can receiving doctor-supervised facial peels or laser treatments, but using this product in the hopes that its "Celluzyme" technology will diminish these discolorations is nothing more than wishful thinking.

☹ $$$ **Advanced Solutions Complete Acne Therapy System** *($24.99)* features a cleansing scrub, daytime moisturizer with sunscreen, and topical disinfectant (labeled as a nighttime product, but it can certainly be used as part of your daytime routine, too). The **Skin Polishing Acne Cleanser** contains 0.5% salicylic acid, an amount really too small to provide much exfoliation, not to mention that the pH is really too high for that to occur anyway. However, this cleanser also includes polyethylene (plastic) beads, which provide manual exfoliation. The cleansing base is fairly gentle. Skin Polishing Acne Cleanser works best as a topical scrub rather than as a daily cleanser. Use caution and avoid scrubbing over raised blemishes or reddened areas. The **Sun Shield Day Lotion with SPF 15** is a standard sunscreen lotion with an in-part zinc oxide sunscreen. Although zinc oxide is a great broad-spectrum sunscreen, it is not the best for use over blemished skin because its occlusive nature can contribute further to clogged pores. This means you have to experiment to see if that's true for your skin. Its base formula isn't anything special or interesting, and a couple of fragrant extracts may cause irritation, but broad-spectrum sun protection is assured. Last up is the **Overnight Acne Control Lotion**, a

2.5% benzoyl peroxide product that is as straightforward as it gets. This works well to disinfect the skin, but would have been better if Neutrogena had added some soothing agents or anti-irritants. Still, it is an option as a topical disinfectant and does not contain needless irritants. Given that the three-piece kit above lacks a leave-on, pH-correct salicylic acid exfoliant and features a sunscreen with an active ingredient that can be problematic for someone with acne, you might ask, how is this an advanced solution? In short, this collection of products, though attractively packaged, is not necessarily one-stop shopping for blemished or blemish-prone skin. A one-size-fits-all approach to treating blemishes may seem convenient, but it takes systematic experimentation to find the best combination of products for you. If Neutrogena's offerings in this kit were a bit more sensible, it would have received a higher recommendation.

☺ **$$$ Advanced Solutions Facial Peel** *($25.99 for 1.7 ounces)* is an interesting product, mainly because its "peeling" comes from the directions on the package to manually rub the skin, which in essence exfoliates the skin. Advanced Solutions Facial Peel does not contain an AHA or BHA. What it does contain is *Mucor miehei* extract, which Neutrogena refers to as "mushroom protein." From what I could find out about this ingredient, it is an acid protease (protease is an enzyme that breaks down protein—which would break down the substances that hold the cells on the surface of skin together) derived from a type of fungus. As you might suspect, the next question is whether this ingredient can exfoliate (peel) skin or have any benefit whatsoever. In this scenario you've got to take Neutrogena's word for it, because there is no research pointing the way on this one (at least not in the concentration used in this product). I suspect this product's skin-smoothing ability comes from the exfoliating beads it contains, not from a "breakthrough" ingredient capable of providing "dramatic, skin-revitalizing benefits." If you decide to try this product as a topical scrub, be forewarned that it has a lot of fragrance.

NEUTROGENA AGELESS ESSENTIALS PRODUCTS

☺ **Ageless Essentials Continuous Hydration Cream Cleanser** *($7.99 for 5.1 ounces)* is a good, water-soluble cleansing lotion for normal to dry skin not prone to blemishes. It removes makeup easily and rinses surprisingly well without the need for a washcloth. The amount of feverfew extract is not likely cause for concern. One more point: although this cleanser doesn't strip skin or leave it feeling dry, it isn't capable of providing continuous hydration. You will notice almost immediately that this cleanser doesn't replace the need for a good toner or moisturizer if your skin is dry.

☹ **Ageless Essentials Continuous Hydration Eye Cream** *($14.99 for 0.5 ounce)*. The only reason to consider this silky-textured lightweight eye cream is if you believe that dimethyl MEA (also known as dimethylaminoethanol [DMAE]) is an antiaging essential. Despite the lack of evidence supporting any claim that DMAE has any effect on skin, there are hundreds of Web sites claiming that it does. While it is possible that DMAE can help protect the cell membrane and keep cells intact, that is only conjecture, and is not supported in the scientific literature. If anything, a study published in *The British Journal of Dermatology* (May 2007) has shown contrary evidence that it may actually pose risks for the skin. In vitro tests of the pure substance, as well as tests of creams that contain DMAE, demonstrated a fairly fast and significant increase in protective elements around the skin cell. However, a short time later the researchers observed a significant decrease in cell growth and, in some cases, they found that it had halted cell growth altogether. In short, DMAE's benefits are questionable and it appears there are risks. It isn't an antiaging ingredient that should be on anyone's short list. Lastly, Neutrogena should know better than to formulate an eye cream with fragrance! Even if DMAE could protect cells, the fragrance hurts cells and ends up causing problems that even the DMAE couldn't fix.

☹ **Ageless Essentials Continuous Hydration Moisture SPF 25** *($14.99 for 1.7 ounces)* is not recommended because it contains the preservative methylisothiazolinone, which is a known sensitizer and generally not recommended for use in leave-on products (Sources: *Contact Dermatitis*, November 2001, pages 257-264; and *European Journal of Dermatology*, March 1999, pages 144-160). Add to this the absence of any exciting antiaging ingredients and it's apparent how non-essential this daytime moisturizer with sunscreen really is in comparison to other options in this price range from Olay or even Neutrogena.

☺ **Ageless Essentials Continuous Hydration SPF 25 with Helioplex** *($14.99 for 1.7 ounces)*. For the most part, Neutrogena does sunscreens right, and that's the case here. This in-part avobenzone sunscreen is formulated in a lightweight cream suitable for normal to dry skin. That's the good news. The bad news is that (especially considering the "Ageless Essentials" name), other than the sunscreen actives, there are no notable antiaging ingredients in this daytime moisturizer. It contains a preservative that is a known sensitizer and not recommended for use in leave-on products, and the feverfew extract has the potential to be irritating. Neither fact is good news. In fact, both make this a tough sell, especially given that Neutrogena offers better options in their enormous range.

☺ **Ageless Essentials Continuous Hydration Time Released Moisturizer, Night** *($14.99 for 1.7 ounces)* is a basic, lightly emollient moisturizer for normal to slightly dry skin. There is nothing particularly exciting about the formula, so calling it "Ageless Essentials" is a bit like serving a plain baloney sandwich and calling it fine dining. I am concerned about the amount of *Chrysanthemum parthenium* (feverfew) extract in this product. However, it appears that Neutrogena's owner Johnson & Johnson is aware of the irritants in this plant, and so has developed and is using a form of feverfew that does not contain the suspect chemicals (Sources: *Inflammopharmacology*, February 2009, pages 42-49; and *Archives of Dermatological Research*, February 2008, pages 69-80). What's uncertain is whether they're using the irritant-free form of this ingredient in their products (research is one thing, but it's meaningless if it's not carried through to the formulary stage). Either way, it isn't a miracle ingredient and there is more alcohol in this product than any interesting ingredients anyway.

NEUTROGENA AGELESS INTENSIVES PRODUCTS

☺ **Ageless Intensives Tone Correcting Peel** *($21.99 for 1.4 ounces)* is a scrub that contains nothing intensive, ageless, or correcting. The name for this product is far more interesting than what you get. As far as the "peeling" goes, you will only get that from the manual scrubbing/massaging you're directed to perform while you have this so-called unique ingredient on your skin. Ageless Intensives Tone Correcting Peel does not contain an AHA or BHA, nor does it have a pH level that approximates that of the acid peels performed by dermatologists. What it does contain is *Mucor miehei* extract, which Neutrogena refers to as a "brightening enzyme." From what I could find out about this ingredient, it is an acid protease (protease is an enzyme that breaks down protein—which would break down skin cells) derived from a type of fungus. The question is whether this ingredient can stay stable in a formula (enzymes are notorious for breaking down in a skin-care product) especially in a rinse-off product. In the long run this is nothing more than an overpriced topical scrub. This product's skin-smoothing ability, for all intents and purposes, comes from the exfoliating beads it contains, not from a "concentrated" ingredient capable of providing dramatic, skin-revitalizing benefits.

☺ **Ageless Intensives Deep Wrinkle Anti-Wrinkle Eye Cream** *($21.99 for 0.5 ounce)* is a decent lightweight moisturizing cream for use around the eyes or anywhere your skin is experiencing mild dryness. It contains a standard array of thickeners and emollients along with silicones, glycerin, several antioxidants (which is good, because none of them are present in any significant amount), an anti-irritant, retinol, film-forming agent, and preservatives. It is fragrance-free and packaged so the retinol will remain stable during use. This eye cream will (like almost any moisturizer) reduce the appearance of fine, dry lines and wrinkles. However, contrary to Neutrogena's claim, it won't reduce the appearance of dark circles or fill in deep wrinkles. The only reason to consider this product is if you want to try an eye-area moisturizer with retinol.

☹ **Ageless Intensives Deep Wrinkle Anti-Wrinkle Moisture, Night** *($21.99 for 1.4 ounces)*. Am I the only consumer utterly baffled by Neutrogena's spiraling-out-of-control range of antiwrinkle moisturizers? They have their Ageless Intensives brand along with several others, including Ageless Essentials, Ageless Restoratives, Healthy Skin Anti-Wrinkle, and Visibly Firm—with seemingly more antiwrinkle products launching every couple of months. If any of these worked as claimed, who would still have wrinkles? The fact is, none of these products work as claimed, and Neutrogena doesn't believe this either. If they did believe their own hype, why would they keep launching new ones with the same claim? Personal preference counts, but come on—as of this writing they have 42 antiwrinkle moisturizers on their Web site! All this Ageless product ends up being is an unnecessary addition. It has a decent formula with some antioxidants and a skin-identical ingredient with stable packaging but for the money, Neutrogena offers more impressive moisturizer formulas, as does their competitor Olay.

Note: This product was previously named "Healthy Skin Anti Wrinkle Intensive Night Cream"($17.99 for 1.4 ounces) and the formulation has not changed. It was originally rated Paula's Pick in error.

☺ **Ageless Intensives Deep Wrinkle Anti-Wrinkle Moisture SPF 20** *($21.99 for 1.4 ounces)* provides a convenient, elegant way for you to experience an in-part avobenzone sunscreen in a lightly moisturizing base with retinol and a tiny amount of water-binding agents. This isn't at the same level of formulary excellence as Neutrogena's tinted Healthy Skin Enhancer SPF 20 reviewed below, but it's worth a try if you have normal to slightly oily skin. This product will not fill in the look of deep wrinkles within two weeks. That's wishful thinking! Neutrogena should have settled for what works and left the other claim to less reputable cosmetics companies.

☹ **Ageless Intensives Deep Wrinkle Anti-Wrinkle Serum** *($21.99 for 1 ounce)* has a silky, gel-cream texture rather than that of a true serum, and includes a blend of silicones, film-forming agents, anti-irritants, and retinol. The variety of antioxidants found in the two Healthy Skin Anti-Wrinkle products reviewed below is absent here, making this more of a one-note product, with retinol as the star ingredient. However, the amount of retinol appears to be the same in the three different products (several calls to Neutrogena asking about whether this serum indeed contained more retinol didn't help answer that question). The decision about which one to use comes down to formula, and because the amount of film-forming agents in here is potentially problematic the other two are better options. Nonetheless, it is fragrance-free and comes in packaging that will definitely keep the retinol stable.

☺ **Ageless Intensives Firming Moisture SPF 20** *($21.99 for 1.7 ounces)* deserves praise for its in-part zinc oxide sunscreen, but the base formula for normal to slightly oily skin is bland, with the antioxidants and copper listed after the preservative. For the money, this doesn't measure up against any of Olay's Regenerist or Total Effects products with sunscreen, but is still an option.

☺ **$$$ Ageless Intensives Lifting Treatment, Eye** *($21.99 for 0.43 ounce).* The only unique ingredient in this otherwise lackluster eye moisturizer is sodium methylesculetin acetate. This ingredient is supposed to reduce capillary leakage and improve circulation, which, as you may have guessed, is tied to reducing dark circles. This ingredient does not have any notable anti-wrinkle properties. In fact, the only information about it comes from the companies that sell it, which is about as reliable as casino owners telling you they're in business to make sure you make money, not the other way around. This product cannot lift skin anywhere and its strengthening ability is not evidenced by its average formula.

☺ **Ageless Intensives Lifting Treatment, Night** *($21.99 for 1.6 ounces).* This lightweight moisturizer for normal to oily skin has so little going for it that the price is ridiculous. Even the called-out "fortifying minerals" are nothing more than very standard cosmetic pigments.

☺ **Ageless Intensives Tone Correcting Moisture SPF 30** *($19.99 for 1 ounce).* Although this daytime moisturizer with sunscreen doesn't contain a significant amount of ingredients known to lighten skin discolorations (other than what every sunscreen offers skin in that regard), it is a very good option for those with normal to oily skin. The silky formula includes avobenzone for sufficient UVA protection and also includes several antioxidants, cell-communicating ingredients (including retinol), and a tiny amount of anti-irritants. The consistency of this moisturizer with sunscreen allows it to work well under makeup, too.

☺ **Ageless Intensives Tone Correcting Concentrated Serum Night** *($21.99 for 1 ounce).* I don't know how consumers are supposed to decide between all of Neutrogena's "Ageless" products. If the Ageless range is "essential," then why offer another range that's labeled "intensive" and yet another labeled "restorative"? And what do they mean by ageless anyway? More to the point, why do so many of them have such ordinary, boring, antiquated formulas? Maybe it's because Neutrogena is trying to please everyone by offering dozens of options, when all they're really doing is creating confusion and shortchanging their consumer with really mediocre products. This water-based product is closer to a moisturizer than a serum, and it contains nothing known to correct skin tone, unless your only complaint is minor dryness (but usually, skin tone refers to overall color, not to moisture content). This contains salicylic acid, an ingredient that can exfoliate skin and improve signs of sun damage, but it won't work here because this product's pH is too high. Retinol is a great cell-communicating ingredient for skin and it can help improve skin's overall appearance, but there are better products that contain this vitamin A ingredient, including some from Neutrogena itself and from sister company RoC. All told, this is an average moisturizer for slightly dry skin, not at all an "intensive" corrective product to address multiple signs of aging.

☹ **Ageless Intensives Lip Plumping Treatment SPF 20** *($21.99 for 0.33 ounce)* does not contain the UVA-protecting ingredients of titanium dioxide, zinc oxide, Mexoryl SX (ecamsule), avobenzone, or Tinosorb and is not recommended for daytime protection. The lip balm itself leaves much to be desired, and isn't as good as the other lip options from Neutrogena.

NEUTROGENA AGELESS RESTORATIVES PRODUCTS

☺ **Ageless Restoratives Energy Renewal Cleanser** *($7.99 for 5.1 ounces)* is a standard water-soluble foaming cleanser that contains a small amount of polyethylene beads for a mild scrub action. It doesn't energize or renew skin better than any other cleanser used with a washcloth (and there are certainly scrubs from Neutrogena that have a more invigorating effect), but this is a good option for normal to oily skin. It removes makeup and rinses easily, but the scrub particles aren't the best way to remove makeup; so this is best used as your morning cleanser.

☺ **Ageless Restoratives 5 Minute Facial** *($21.99 for 1.7 ounces)*. I imagine lots of people will be drawn to this product's claim of being able to provide a professional peel at home, and within five minutes, too! The results are said to equal those of a 20-35% strength glycolic acid peel—they can't, not even remotely. What you need to know is that in no way is this product comparable to a professional peel, any more than roller skates are comparable to a limousine. For the most part, this is just a glorified scrub that's suitable for all skin types. The ingredient Neutrogena maintains has an AHA peel benefit "without the irritation" is *Mucor miehei* extract. This ingredient is an acid protease derived from a type of fungus. (A protease is an enzyme that breaks down protein, which would break down the substances that hold the cells on the surface of the skin together.) Whether or not that ingredient can exfoliate skin in any manner is something you have to take Neutrogena's word for, because there is no research pointing the way on this one, at least not at the small concentration in this product. This is just one more scrub to consider with the same overblown claims, though in this case the jar packaging isn't a sanitary way to use such a product and would allow the *Mucor miehi* extract to break down anyway.

☺ **Ageless Restoratives 3-in-1 Skin Enhancer SPF 30** *($19.99 for 1.7 ounces)* is a standard daytime moisturizer with an in-part avobenzone sunscreen. It has a sheer tint that adds a bit of color to skin, but the effect is subtle so this works for various skin tones. Neutrogena's Celluzyme technology is supposed to invigorate and refresh the look of dull skin, but there's no proof the plant extracts in this Celluzyme complex do that. The claim itself is wide open to interpretation because lots of products (and cosmetic ingredients) can make skin look more refreshed or "awake." Any foundation, concealer, or moisturizer (with or without a tint) could make the same boast, so Celluzyme is mostly just a cool name, not a skin-care must-have. Actually, this formula ends up shortchanging your skin of many of the ingredients it needs, such as antioxidants, skin-identical ingredients, and cell-communicating ingredients, though it does provide adequate sun protection. It is suitable for normal to slightly dry skin.

☺ **Ageless Restoratives Anti-Oxidant Booster Serum** *($19.99 for 1 ounce)*. Considering the name of this product, the overall formula for this serum is really a disappointment. The small amount of antioxidants included is less than stellar. Other than that, it is just too mundane and ordinary for it to be considered a boost for any skin type.

☹ **Ageless Restoratives Anti-Oxidant Eye** *($19.99 for 0.5 ounce)*. Although several aspects of this formula are quite impressive, this eye cream is a problem for all skin types because it contains a high amount of the sensitizing preservative methylisothiazolinone. The titanium dioxide and mica are what provide a brightening effect, but this is strictly cosmetic.

☹ **Ageless Restoratives Energy Renewal Day Lotion SPF 15** *($18.99 for 1.7 ounces)* may appeal to the environmentally aware consumer concerned with aging, given its emphasis on "energy renewal," but this daytime moisturizer with an in-part avobenzone sunscreen has too many drawbacks to make it worth considering over several other options in this price range. The amount of antioxidant soybean is impressive, but the feverfew extract contains chemical components that can be irritating. Often touted as an anti-inflammatory, feverfew has that effect, but it also can irritate, so in essence the anti-inflammatory benefit is canceled out. This product also contains the sensitizing preservative methylisothiazolinone, which is not recommended for use in leave-on products. Neutrogena is including this preservative in more and more of their sunscreens, despite the research proving that it's a problem (Sources: *Regulatory Toxicology and Pharmacology*, December 2003, pages 269-290; and *Toxicology and Applied Pharmacology*, August 2002, pages 226-233). Neutrogena makes better sunscreens and better makeup with sunscreen to consider than this one.

☺ **Ageless Restoratives Energy Renewal Eye Cream** *($18.99 for 0.5 ounce)* has a silky texture and lightweight finish that work well under makeup, and other than that, there is little to extol in this eye cream. It doesn't wake up tired eyes, and the energizing effect (if you want to call it that) comes from the mineral pigments it contains, which brighten and add a soft shine (but that's a cosmetic effect, not a skin-care benefit). The amount of the preservative BHT is cause for concern due to its carcinogenic potential (Sources: *Mechanisms of Ageing and Development*, May 2002, pages 1203-1210; and *Free Radical Biology and Medicine*, February 2000, pages 330-336). BHT's appearance on the ingredient list before most of the other ingredients (including anti-irritants) is worrisome, and given the overall lack of bells and whistles in this eye cream, it is one you can leave on the shelf.

☹ **Ageless Restoratives Anti-Oxidant Moisture Night** *($18.99 for 1.7 ounces)* contains the same problematic ingredients as the Anti-Oxidant Age Reverse Day Lotion SPF 20 reviewed below, and the same concerns apply. This formula differs little from the Ageless Restoratives Anti-Oxidant Eye above, except that the more state-of-the-art ingredients are given less prominence. All the Age Reverse products contain soy as the star antioxidant; if that's of interest to you then consider the Positively Ageless products from Aveeno; they omit the irritants Neutrogena includes.

☺ **Ageless Restoratives Energy Renewal Hydrating Night Cream** *($18.99 for 1.7 ounces)*. The same concerns expressed for the amount of preservative BHT in Neutrogena's Ageless Restoratives Energy Renewal Eye Cream above apply here, too. BHT is a potential carcinogen and in this amount may pose risks for skin (Sources: *Mechanisms of Ageing and Development*, May 2002, pages 1203-1210; and *Free Radical Biology and Medicine*, February 2000, pages 330-336). Given that this nighttime moisturizer's only exciting ingredient is the cell-communicating ingredient carnitine, it isn't worth considering over many other moisturizers that do not contain BHT or that at least include a much smaller amount of BHT (0.1% or less is considered safe). Moreover, the jar packaging will compromise the stability of several ingredients in this moisturizer for normal to slightly dry skin, which makes it even less appealing. Neutrogena needs to rethink the speed at which they launch new products and spend more time in the lab working out the problematic kinks before launching.

☺ **Ageless Restoratives Instant Eye Reviver** *($19.99 for 0.5 ounce)* is an average, extremely ordinary lightweight eye cream that is not specially formulated for the eye area, but rather is suitable for slightly dry skin anywhere on the face. It is fragrance-free and contains a smattering of minerals, though none of these or any other ingredient in this product can noticeably diminish puffy eyes or dark circles. The *Saccharomyces lysate* extract is a yeast extract with no published research showing it to be of benefit for skin, though it may have antioxidant properties.

☺ **Ageless Restoratives Skin Renewal Moisture SPF 30** *($19.99 for 1.7 ounces)*. Despite the name and the healthy, vibrant skin claims, the most you can expect from this daytime moisturizer with sunscreen is broad-spectrum sun protection. Avobenzone is on hand for reliable UVA protection, and it's stabilized with Neutrogena's Helioplex complex. The plant extracts that comprise the company's Celluzyme technology are barely present, but that's not such a loss when you consider they have only negligible benefit for skin. This is best (although in no way is it the ideal daytime product) for normal to slightly dry skin.

☺ **$$$ Ageless Restoratives Total Skin Renewal** *($27.99 for Starter Kit with Applicator and 12 Puffs)* is a two-part system that includes a battery-powered, hand-held cleansing device similar to Neutrogena's Wave Power-Cleanser product (reviewed below) coupled with disposable cleansing pads attached to the device. The pads are steeped in a cleansing solution that is activated on contact with water. It ends up being just a standard water-soluble cleanser that, coupled with the textured pads and the battery-powered device, functions as a sort of supercharged washcloth for your face. This provides cleansing with exfoliation, but you must use the device with care so you don't overdo it, and do not use it in the eye area. Unlike the cleansing pads sold with Neutrogena's Wave system, these do not contain irritating menthol.

NEUTROGENA DEEP CLEAN PRODUCTS

☹ **Deep Clean Cream Cleanser** *($6.99 for 7 ounces)* contains menthol and is not recommended. The minty sensation has nothing do with skin being deeply cleansed.

☹ **Deep Clean Facial Cleanser, for Normal to Oily Skin** *($6.89 for 6.7 ounces)* leaves out the menthol in the Deep Clean Cream Cleanser above, but is based around the drying detergent cleansing agent sodium C14-16 olefin sulfonate.

☹ **Deep Clean Invigorating Daily Cleanser** *($7.99 for 6.7 ounces)* had the potential to be an excellent water-soluble cleanser for normal to dry or sensitive skin, but the inclusion of menthol (quite a bit of it) makes this a no-go for all skin types.

☹ **Deep Clean Invigorating Ultra-Foam Cleanser** *($6.99 for 6 ounces)* has every element of a brilliantly formulated liquid-to-foam cleanser until you get to the menthol, which is just irritating, literally and figuratively.

☺ **Deep Clean Relaxing Nightly Cleanser** *($7.49 for 6.7 ounces)* is too mild to remove any amount of makeup and would be unsuitable for oily skin. Plus, no cleanser can go deeper than the skin's surface layers, so ignore the name. Still, this gentle water-soluble cleanser is a good option for normal to dry skin if full-face makeup removal isn't needed. Ironically, despite the name, this would also make a good A.M. cleanser! The aroma this product releases as you wash is its main selling point, but that is not helpful for skin in the least. The chemistry trick of encapsulating fragrance to be released when water is added doesn't change its negative impact on skin.

☹ **Deep Clean Invigorating Dual Action Toner** *($6.79 for 6.7 ounces)* promises to give pores a tighter feel to "seal in the tingly sensation," which is a roundabout way of telling you that this alcohol-laden toner with menthol causes lingering irritation and will stimulate oil production in the pore lining.

☺ **Deep Clean Gentle Scrub** *($6.49 for 4.2 ounces)* is indeed gentle, and makes a very good cleanser/scrub hybrid product for normal to oily skin. The salicylic acid isn't doing the exfoliating; the polyethylene (plastic) beads do that when massaged over the skin.

☹ **Deep Clean Invigorating Foaming Scrub** *($7.59 for 4.2 ounces)* is not preferred to the Deep Clean Gentle Scrub above because it contains menthol.

☺ **Deep Clean Relaxing Nightly Scrub** *($7.49 for 4.2 ounces)* releases fragrance as you wash, a neat trick for a chemist but utterly useless for your skin. Fragrance has a negative impact on skin; it is only helpful for your sense of smell. This version contains synthetic scrub particles that can gently exfoliate skin. Although this is a good scrub for normal to slightly dry or slightly oily skin, it's an extraneous, gimmicky addition to Neutrogena's overcrowded product selection.

NEUTROGENA HEALTHY SKIN PRODUCTS

☺ **Healthy Skin Anti-Wrinkle Anti-Blemish Cleanser** *($7.69 for 5.1 ounces)* contains 0.5% salicylic acid, which is too low a percentage to have much of an effect on blemishes, especially when included in a cleanser that is rinsed off shortly after it's applied. This also contains glycolic acid, but the pH of 4.5 is too high for effective exfoliation, and again, it will be rinsed off before it has a chance to work. What's best about this softly fragranced cleanser is the gentle cleansing agents it contains, which are effective for makeup removal and excellent for all but the driest skin types. The product name is a tongue twister (and has no effect on either wrinkles or blemishes), but this is a good cleanser and that's great all by itself.

☺ **Healthy Skin Visibly Even Foaming Cleanser** *($7.99 for 5.1 ounces)* has a slightly richer texture than the Healthy Skin Anti-Wrinkle Anti-Blemish Scrub below and omits the salicylic and glycolic acids, but is otherwise a comparable product and good choice for normal to dry skin.

☺ **Healthy Skin Anti-Wrinkle Anti-Blemish Scrub** *($7.99 for 4 ounces)* contains 0.5% salicylic acid as an active ingredient and also includes 2% glycolic acid. Neither will exfoliate, because of their brief contact with the skin before being rinsed down the drain. However, this is worth considering as a cleansing scrub for all skin types except very dry. It is more abrasive than several other scrubs that also contain polyethylene beads, but if used gently can be a helpful addition to your routine.

☺ **Healthy Skin Anti-Wrinkle Anti-Blemish Clear Skin Cream** *($12.99 for 1 ounce)* sounds like a treat for consumers battling wrinkles and breakouts, an all-too-common frustration. However, the 2% salicylic acid cannot exfoliate very effectively because the pH is too high. This is worth considering as an antioxidant-rich moisturizer that also contains additional antioxidants (and not just a dusting, either). It is suitable for normal to dry skin but is not rated a Paula's Pick because it contains kawa extract, which can cause dermatitis and be sensitizing (Sources: *Alternative Medicine Review*, December 1998, pages 458-460; and *Clinical Experimental Pharmacology and Physiology*, July 1990, pages 495-507). The amount of kawa extract is likely too low for it to be problematic, but it's a needless inclusion.

✓ ☺ **Healthy Skin Anti-Wrinkle Cream, Original Formula** *($13.99 for 1.4 ounces)* is a good, fragrance-free moisturizer with retinol for normal to dry skin. The retinol is packaged to keep it stable, the amount of green tea is impressive, and the formula contains tiny amounts of two forms of Vitamin E. It is definitely one of the better retinol products at the drugstore.

☹ **Healthy Skin Anti-Wrinkle Cream, Original Formula SPF 15** *($13.99 for 1.4 ounces)* disappoints because it lacks the UVA-protecting ingredients of titanium dioxide, zinc oxide, avobenzone, Mexoryl SX (ecamsule), or Tinosorb and is not recommended.

✓ ☺ **Healthy Skin Enhancer SPF 20** *($11.99 for 1 ounce)* combines an in-part titanium dioxide sunscreen with retinol and a hint of color, all of which enhance skin due to their respective qualities. Moreover, there is more than just a dusting of retinol in this product, which makes it unique! It has a light, creamy texture and a satin finish appropriate for those with normal to dry skin. If an oily T-zone is an issue, this product should be set with powder to reduce the sheen it leaves on skin. The six sheer shades are great and include options for fair (but not very fair) to tan skin tones. In addition—and this is again unusual for a foundation—plenty of antioxidants are included. This product proves that Neutrogena is capable of setting new makeup benchmarks for their drugstore contemporaries to strive for, rather than just keeping up with their competitors.

☺ **Healthy Skin Eye Cream** *($12.29 for 0.5 ounce)* does not contain glycolic acid, at least according to the ingredient list on the package. Calls to Neutrogena received the nonsensical answer that just because the company states that the product contains an AHA on the packaging doesn't mean they have to list it on the ingredient statement (What nonsense!). With or without an AHA (and make no mistake, it absolutely must be listed if the product contains it), this generic eye cream has a pH of 5.5, so no exfoliation will take place. It's an OK option for normal to dry skin and contains a few vitamin-based antioxidants.

☹ **Healthy Skin Face Lotion SPF 15** *($12.59 for 2.5 ounces)* leaves skin vulnerable to UVA damage because it lacks sunscreen agents capable of shielding skin from the entire spectrum of UVA light. What a shame, because the 8% glycolic acid and pH of 3.3 allow exfoliation to occur, which would have made this a convenient, dual-purpose product.

✓ ☺ **Healthy Skin Glow Sheers SPF 30** *($12.79 for 1.1 ounces)* is a very sheer, tinted moisturizer that's ideal for normal to slightly oily skin. It has a feather-light texture that glides over skin and sets to a soft matte (in feel) finish. Left behind is almost translucent color and a soft, natural-looking glow. Of course, the glow makes oily areas appear oilier, but if that's not a cause for concern (or if you have slightly dry skin) this will be perfect. The base has several antioxidants to help the in-part titanium dioxide sunscreen keep skin protected. One caution: The Bronze Glow shade does not contain any UVA-protecting ingredients (meaning titanium dioxide, zinc oxide, or avobenzone) and should be avoided. The other five shades are all recommended, but consider Light carefully because it is slightly peach, though it's likely too sheer to matter.

✓ ☺ **Healthy Skin Visibly Even Daily SPF 15 Moisturizer** *($13.09 for 1.7 ounces)* includes an in-part avobenzone sunscreen in a lightweight lotion formula enriched with the antioxidant soy. Although the pH of 4 is within range for the salicylic acid to function as an exfoliant, there isn't enough of it in here. Still, this is highly recommended as an antioxidant-rich daytime moisturizer for normal to slightly dry or slightly oily skin.

☺ **$$$ Healthy Skin Rejuvenator, the Anti-Aging Power Treatment** *($38.99)* contains "power" that comes from the supplied batteries that power this hand-held scrub device. This is Neutrogena's second attempt to woo customers interested in the concept of giving themselves some incarnation of microdermabrasion treatments at home. Now they offer this seemingly simpler yet supposedly more effective option. The kit includes a device whose top portion is outfitted with a Velcro-like material that holds the cleansing pads in place. The textured pads are steeped in a mild cleanser, so this lathers slightly as you use it. After putting the pad in place, you wet the sponge, turn the device on, and massage over each area of your face for 1 to 2 minutes. The result, not surprisingly, is smoother, softer skin. This type of exfoliation is similar to using a powered washcloth, but this has greater potential to be irritating, so be careful; after one minute of "gently" massaging this over my face, it was visibly red. Neutrogena's spin on this irritation is that the device is stimulating circulation to improve oxygen flow, but that's not the way to get that benefit. That's like saying that when you fall down and cut yourself it promotes skin healing; it's true that your skin will heal after being cut, but you don't want to encourage healing by hurting yourself. And in this case, it would be better to stimulate your body's circulation with exercise or with a very gentle massage than by irritation. The benefit you get from mechanical exfoliation is just that—exfoliation—period. Neutrogena has all manner of convincing claims, including graphs, charts, and statistics to convince you this is the key to younger, firmer skin, but the truth is that the only thing this will unlock is smoother skin, and you don't need to spend this much money or go through the routine this device involves to get it. Still, for those impressed by the novelty, this is an effective scrub device if used gently (and preferably not for as long as Neutrogena advises). As for the wrinkle reduction you may see, it's due to the fact that this device causes inflammation, which makes your skin swell, and the effect is only temporary. However, just in case you might be convinced this is an antiwrinkle wonder—let me assure you, it isn't.

NEUTROGENA OIL-FREE ACNE PRODUCTS

☹ **Oil-Free Acne Stress Control Night Cleansing Pads** *($6.29 for 60 pads)*. These cleansing pads aren't anti-acne stress control for anyone's skin, but they will stress your skin because of the amount of alcohol. Alcohol not only causes dryness and irritation, but also can trigger oil production in the pore because the irritation triggers the release of androgens, the hormone responsible for causing oily skin. What a shame, because without the alcohol this would've been an effective cleanser with salicylic acid, and the fact that you don't rinse skin afterward means that the salicylic acid would have a chance to get into the pore and work.

☹ **Oil-Free Acne Stress Control Power-Cream Wash** *($7.99 for 6 ounces)* may make you think this is an ideal cleanser for normal to dry skin that's blemish-prone, given its combination of 2% salicylic acid along with approximately the same amount of glycolic acid and a creamy base. Alas, it isn't for two reasons: the AHA and BHA ingredients aren't in contact with skin long enough for them to function effectively as exfoliants, and leaving this on skin for any longer than what's necessary to clean the face will only increase the irritation from the menthol and cleansing agents. Neutrogena knows menthol is a problem for skin, but they consistently use it in most of their anti-acne products because so many consumers love that "refreshing tingle." If the tingle were somehow conveying an anti-acne benefit, I could concede to the sensation, but that's not the case.

☺ **Oil-Free Acne Stress Control Power-Foam Wash** *($8.79 for 6 ounces)* contains 0.5% salicylic acid, but it's a useless ingredient in a cleanser because it is rinsed down the drain before it has a chance to work. This is otherwise a standard, water-soluble cleanser that's suitable for normal to oily skin. It removes makeup easily and does contain fragrance.

☹ **Oil-Free Acne Wash** *($6.89 for 6 ounces)* purports to be the #1 cleanser recommended by dermatologists for their patients with acne. If that's true, then lots of dermatologists are swayed by advertising and not up to speed on skin-care formulas. A dermatologist should know better than to endorse a cleanser that contains the drying, irritating detergent cleansing agent sodium C14-16 olefin sulfonate as a major ingredient, not to mention the fact that salicylic acid is wasted in a cleanser because it is just rinsed down the drain before it can be effective.

☺ **Oil-Free Acne Wash Cleansing Cloths** *($6.99 for 30 cloths)* are a better option than the Oil-Free Acne Wash because the problematic detergent cleansing agent is a much smaller proportion of the formula. These cloths are a good option for normal to oily skin, but don't forget to rinse the solution from your skin.

☹ **Oil-Free Acne Wash Cream Cleanser** *($6.99 for 6.7 ounces)* has a slightly creamy texture, but that's not enough to keep the main detergent cleansing agent (sodium C14-16 olefin sulfonate) from drying skin. In no way is this a "gentle treatment" for acne; the 2% salicylic acid is rinsed away before it has a chance to work.

☺ **Oil-Free Acne Wash Foam Cleanser** *($6.99 for 5.1 ounces)* contains 2% salicylic acid, but that won't help acne in a cleanser because it is rinsed down the drain before it can go to work. This is still a good water-soluble cleanser for normal to oily skin.

☹ **Oil-Free Acne Wash Pink Grapefruit Facial Cleanser** *($7.99 for 6 ounces)* is nearly identical to Neutrogena's Oil-Free Acne Wash above, except this version contains grapefruit extract and a grapefruit fragrance. This product is an unnecessary addition to an already overcrowded line; it's sort of equivalent to launching a new Barbie doll whose only difference from last year's doll is a new, though thoroughly unattractive, pink hat. Big deal! Neither this nor the original Oil-Free Acne Wash is recommended due to their drying detergent cleansing agent and the fact that the 2% salicylic acid is rinsed from skin before it can penetrate to have any positive effect against built-up, pore-clogging dead skin cells.

☹ **Oil-Free Acne Wash, Redness Soothing Cream Cleanser** *($7.99 for 6 ounces)*. This creamy cleanser contains 2% salicylic acid as its active ingredient and also contains a fair amount of glycolic acid, which could have been helpful, but in a cleanser these ingredients are rinsed down the drain before they have a chance to do much good, so they're essentially worthless in this formula. Labeling this cleanser "soothing" is a mistake because Neutrogena included menthol, which is one of the least soothing ingredients around, not to mention that it has zero benefit for acne.

☺ **Oil-Free Acne Wash, Redness Soothing Facial Cleanser** *($7.99 for 6 ounces)* is a very good water-soluble cleanser for normal to slightly dry skin. The cleansing agents are mild enough that those with oily skin will likely want a more thorough cleansing, but using a washcloth could help in that regard. This contains anti-irritants capable of reducing redness, but in a cleanser they are rinsed off the skin too quickly to impart that benefit. The same issue applies to this cleanser's active ingredient of 2% salicylic acid; you need to leave this on the skin to get maximum benefit, but leaving a cleanser on skin is too irritating and damaging for any skin type.

☹ **Oil-Free Acne Stress Control Triple-Action Toner** *($7.49 for 8 ounces)* causes stress (and stimulates more oil production) thanks to its irritating, drying alcohol content—a far cry from being able to control skin stress! The pH of this product is just low enough to allow the 2% salicylic acid to function as an exfoliant, but that comes at the cost of subjecting your skin to the free-radical damage of the alcohol. Not good, and not recommended considering that there are BHA exfoliants available that work against acne and that soothe and even skin without also causing undue irritation.

☹ **Oil-Free Acne Stress Control Power-Clear Scrub** *($8.49 for 4.2 ounces)* contains menthol, which makes it too irritating for all skin types. The 2% salicylic acid isn't going to benefit blemish-prone skin when used in a topical scrub because it is basically rinsed down the drain right after it's applied and doesn't have time to absorb into the skin.

☹ **Oil-Free Acne Wash Daily Scrub** *($6.99 for 4.2 ounces)* is nearly identical to the Oil-Free Acne Stress Control Power-Clear Scrub above, and the same review applies.

☺ **Oil-Free Acne Wash Pink Grapefruit Foaming Scrub** *($7.99 for 4.2 ounces)* should only be considered if you like the scent of pink grapefruit. It's an OK option if you have normal to oily skin and it isn't nearly as harsh on your skin as Neutrogena's Oil-Free Acne Wash Pink Grapefruit Facial Cleanser, but the fact remains that the 2% salicylic acid is wasted due to this scrub's brief contact with skin. Besides, the pH of this scrub is too high for the salicylic acid to function as intended anyway. At least this doesn't contain menthol or its derivatives, and it includes grapefruit extract, rather than grapefruit oil, to make good on the product's fruity name.

☹ **Oil-Free Acne Wash, Redness Soothing Gentle Scrub** *($7.99 for 4.2 ounces)*. This creamy scrub for normal to dry skin doesn't do a great job of soothing skin, mostly because it contains the potent irritant menthol. It does include 2% salicylic acid for additional exfoliation, but in a cleanser it's just rinsed down the drain before it can impart that benefit to skin.

✓ ☺ **Oil-Free Acne Stress Control 3-In-1 Hydrating Acne Treatment** *($7.99 for 2 ounces)* got Neutrogena back into the BHA game, and it was about time! Most of their previous BHA products either contained irritating ingredients (particularly alcohol and menthol) or had a pH that was too high for effective exfoliation to take place. This version contains 2% salicylic acid at a pH of 3.4, and comes in a nearly weightless silicone base that includes antioxidants and anti-irritants. Although the inclusion of fragrance and coloring agents is a slight disappointment, it's a relief that Neutrogena omitted menthol or its derivatives, making this an all-around ideal BHA lotion for skin of any type battling blemishes.

NEUTROGENA RAPID CLEAR PRODUCTS

☹ **Rapid Clear Oil-Control Foaming Cleanser** *($8.49 for 6 ounces)* is a simply formulated cleanser that contains the strongly alkaline ingredient potassium stearate as the main cleansing agent. That means this cleanser is about as drying to skin as most bar soaps, and as a result is not recommended.

☹ **Rapid Clear 2-in-1 Fight & Fade Gel** *($8.99 for 0.5 ounce)* is yet another potentially effective anti-acne product from Neutrogena that could have been a great option for skin if it didn't contain alcohol (which is drying, irritating, causes free-radical damage, and stimulates oil production in the pore lining) and witch hazel water (which is mostly alcohol). Neither of these ingredients is effective at helping to fade marks from acne faster. If anything, the irritation and damage it can cause can disturb the skin's healing process and immune response, which means the marks you're trying to fade may actually last longer.

☺ **Rapid Clear Acne Defense Face Lotion** *($8.49 for 1.7 ounces)* is an effective BHA product option in the battle against blemishes. With 2% salicylic acid and a pH of 3.6, this can indeed exfoliate skin and help dislodge blackheads. The product features a lightweight moisturizing base that is best for normal to slightly dry skin dealing with blemishes. The only issue I have is with the irritating fragrant extracts it contains (cinnamon and cedar), though they are present in amounts that are likely too low to cause irritation. Still, they are unnecessary additives and prevent this BHA product from earning a Paula's Pick rating.

☹ **Rapid Clear Acne Eliminating Spot Gel** *($8.49 for 0.5 ounce)* is another product that means well by the inclusion of the proven blemish fighter salicylic acid (in a 2% concentration), but it falters with the pointless inclusion of almost 40% alcohol along with witch hazel extract, cedarwood, and cinnamon. Even without the irritants, the pH of this product is too high for optimal exfoliation to occur.

☹ **Rapid Clear Treatment Pads** *($8.49 for 60 pads)* will rapidly irritate due to the amount of alcohol, an ingredient that also stimulates oil production in the pore lining. The 2% salicylic acid is nice and potentially effective, but this is not a BHA shining star for Neutrogena.

OTHER NEUTROGENA PRODUCTS

☺ **Anti-Oxidant Age Reverse Cleanser** *($8.99 for 5.1 ounces)* is a very good water-soluble cleanser for all skin types. It produces a cushiony lather that removes makeup and rinses completely. This would be rated a Paula's Pick if it didn't contain so much fragrance. Although this is a very good cleanser to consider, keep in mind that it cannot work with Neutrogena's other Anti-Oxidant Age Reverse products to "neutralize 99% of free radicals." Given the nature of free radicals plus our endless and unrelenting exposure to them, this is one claim that's simply too good to be true.

☹ **Blackhead Eliminating 2-in-1 Foaming Pads** *($7.99 for 28 pads)* won't eliminate a single blackhead, but will cause irritation due to the menthol in these pads, and will cause dryness because of the detergent cleansing agent chosen. Textured pads have nothing to do with remedying blackheads.

✓ ☺ **Extra Gentle Cleanser** *($7.99 for 6.7 ounces)* remains one of Neutrogena's standout cleansers. It is an excellent option for those with normal to dry or sensitive skin, including those with eczema or rosacea. The fragrance-free, lotion-textured formula contains mild cleansing agents and some good anti-irritants, but these aren't as effective in a cleanser as they are when they are left on the skin.

✓ ☺ **Fresh Foaming Cleanser** *($6.59 for 6.7 ounces)* is a superb water-soluble cleanser for normal to oily or combination skin. It removes makeup easily and rinses without a trace. This does contain fragrance.

☺ **Liquid Neutrogena Facial Cleansing Formula, Original** *($8.79)* is an option as a fragrance-free, water-soluble cleanser for oily skin, but its combination of detergent cleansing agents is potentially drying. As a result this is not preferred to the Fresh Foaming Cleanser or Neutrogena's One Step Gentle Cleanser below.

✓ ☺ **Make-Up Remover Cleansing Towelettes** *($8.99 for 25 towelettes)* are cleansing cloths whose specialty is makeup removal, and they do an excellent job of breaking up and dissolving foundation, lipstick, and mascara (including waterproof types). These soft-textured cloths do not contain any needlessly irritating ingredients (such as menthol or arnica), making them safe for use around the eyes.

✓ ☺ **One Step Gentle Cleanser** *($7.49 for 5.2 ounces)* removes makeup and leaves skin feeling clean and smooth, all in one gentle step. This water-soluble cleanser feels great on skin, lathers slightly, and rinses easily. It also contains milder cleansing agents than many other cleansers. It is highly recommended for all but very dry skin types. It does contain fragrance. Note: For some reason, most stores that stock this cleanser are stocking it with Neutrogena's makeup rather than with their other cleansers, so it can be a bit tricky to find.

☹ **The Transparent Facial Bar, Acne-Prone Skin Formula** *($3.19 for 3.5-ounce bar)* is a variation on the same standard bar soap based on the drying, irritating cleansing agent TEA-stearate and traditional soap ingredients (such as tallow, which can clog pores). This bar cleanser is not recommended for any skin type.

☹ **The Transparent Facial Bar, Original Formula** *($3.29 for 3.5-ounce bar)* is a variation on the same standard bar soap based on the drying, irritating cleansing agent TEA-stearate and traditional soap ingredients (such as tallow, which can clog pores). This bar cleanser is not recommended for any skin type.

☹ **The Transparent Facial Bar, Original Formula, Fragrance-Free** *($3.29 for 3.5 ounce bar)* is a variation on the same standard bar soap based on the drying, irritating cleansing agent TEA-stearate and traditional soap ingredients (such as tallow that can clog pores). This bar cleanser is not recommended for any skin type.

☺ **Extra Gentle Eye Makeup Remover Pads** *($7.69 for 30 pads)* is akin to a silicone-based makeup remover steeped in plush, slightly textured pads. Although pricier than using a liquid makeup remover on a separate cotton pad, there's no denying that the formula works quickly to dissolve makeup, including waterproof formulas. These pads do contain fragrance.

✓ ☺ **Oil-Free Eye Makeup Remover** *($7.99 for 5.5 ounces)* is a gentle, fragrance-free, silicone-based dual-phase remover that works well to dissolve eye makeup, including waterproof formulas. Removers such as this may be used before or after cleansing.

The Reviews N

☺ **Ultra-Soft Eye Makeup Remover Pads** *($6.69 for 30 pads)* are indeed very soft pads that work to gently remove eye makeup. The formula is very similar to the Extra Gentle Eye Makeup Remover Pads above, and the same review applies.

☹ **Wave Power-Cleanser, and Deep Clean Foaming Pads** *($15.99 for the kit)*. The Wave is a battery-powered hand-held device to which you attach dry cleansing pads, wet the pads, and then massage over skin. This is Neutrogena's attempt to compete with pricey facial cleansing devices such as the Clarisonic. Although the device is just fine for those who want a more thorough cleansing (with the pad attached and the device switched on, this is sort of like a powered washcloth for your face), the pads themselves are a problem. The Deep Clean Foaming Pads are a bit abrasive and the cleansing solution the pads are steeped in contains menthol, so you'll feel the tingle long after you're done using this as instructed. That tingle is your skin telling you it's been irritated, and irritation damages skin and can trigger excess oil production.

☹ **Wave Deep Clean Gentle Exfoliating Pads (Refills)** *($7.99 for 30 pads)*. These refill pads for Neutrogena's Wave device contain menthol, a skin irritant, and are not recommended. If you want to use the Wave device, try doing so with the cleansing pads or pillows from Dove instead.

☺ **Alcohol-Free Toner** *($7.99 for 8.5 ounces)* is an average toner at best because it lacks significant water-binding agents or ingredients that support skin's structure. The formula is OK for normal to slightly dry or slightly oily skin.

☹ **Clear Pore Oil-Eliminating Astringent** *($5.69 for 8 ounces)* contains 45% alcohol followed by witch hazel (which just adds more alcohol), and together these make this astringent too irritating to consider, not to mention the alcohol stimulates oil production in the pore lining. The pH of this product prevents the 2% salicylic acid from functioning effectively as an exfoliant.

☹ **Pore Refining Toner** *($7.99 for 8.5 ounces)* lists alcohol as the second ingredient, and also contains witch hazel. It is even more irritating than usual because it also contains peppermint and eucalyptus. The alcohol will stimulate oil production in the pore lining, which isn't the least bit refining.

☺ **$$$ 14 Day Skin Rescue** *($25.99)* is a kit with a concept to give skin a jump start toward a healthier appearance. The set includes a cleanser, a daytime moisturizer with sunscreen, and a nighttime moisturizer. I suppose if your skin-care routine were dreadful then these products could make a noticeable difference in 14 days, but overall these just aren't exciting products. The **14 Day Skin Rescue Cleanser** *(2 ounces)* is a standard, overly fragranced cleanser containing a small amount of polyethylene beads that provide a mild scrubbing effect and rinse clean. It's a suitable cleanser for normal to oily skin, but very similar to several others Neutrogena offers. Next up is **14 Day Skin Rescue Day SPF 30** *(0.5 ounce)*. This creamy but lightweight sunscreen contains avobenzone for UVA protection and mica for a soft-shine finish. The texture and finish make it best for normal to dry skin, which confuses things because, as mentioned, the cleanser in this kit is preferred for oilier skin. Reserved for evening use is **14 Day Skin Rescue Night Cream** *(0.5 ounce)*. This silky moisturizer has a lightweight feel and smooth finish suitable for normal to slightly dry or slightly oily skin. The formula contains some good antioxidants, though most are present in meager amounts. Retinol is also on hand, just as it is in dozens of other Neutrogena products. Again, nothing in this kit is groundbreaking or exciting. It's basically Neutrogena's attempt to package a pre-selected group of their products in a three-step skin-care routine into one box, something they could've done with many of their existing products rather than creating tiny-sized new ones. As is, once you're done with this two-week kit, you're supposed to move on to other Neutrogena products. The question is, why not just begin your routine with those products I rated with a happy face from the get-go?

☹ **Blackhead Eliminating Daily Scrub** *($6.99 for 4.2 ounces)* contains menthol and is not recommended. As a reminder, using a topical scrub over blackheads removes only the top portion of them. That means that the "root" of the blackhead is still inside the pore, so the effect from the scrub is minimal at best, and for that benefit a washcloth would prove just as effective (without the irritation from the menthol).

✓ ☺ **Fresh Foaming Scrub** *($5.99 for 4.2 ounces)* is a very good cleansing scrub for normal to oily skin, though the amount of salicylic acid isn't enough to exfoliate. The polyethylene beads do that job, and do it well while rinsing cleanly.

✓ ☺ **Pore Refining Cleanser** *($7.99 for 6.7 ounces)* is positioned as a cleanser, but is really a cleanser/scrub hybrid. It's less abrasive than many of the other Neutrogena scrubs, and it's the polyethylene beads doing the exfoliating, not the glycolic or salicylic acids. The gentle cleansing base is appropriate for normal to slightly dry or dry skin.

☹ **Anti-Oxidant Age Reverse Day Lotion SPF 20** *($19.50 for 1.7 ounces)* claims to neutralize 90% of free radicals, but there's no supporting evidence to validate this. Besides, under what conditions was this tested? And what free radicals? Free radicals generated from sun exposure? From breathing? Exposure to secondhand smoke? The only antioxidant of note in this in-part avobenzone sunscreen is soy, and that's hardly the most powerful option (we still don't know which antioxidant, if any, will emerge with this title). Although the sunscreen element can forestall further signs of environmental aging, this product contains methylisothiazolinone, which is not recommended for use in leave-on products due to its sensitizing potential. The inclusion of feverfew extract is also a problem because it can also be sensitizing, though it appears Neutrogena knows how to treat this ingredient so its sensitizing chemicals are removed.

☺ **Healthy Defense SPF 30 Daily Moisturizer** *($14.99 for 1.7 ounces)* is an average daytime moisturizer with sunscreen for those with normal to dry skin. The in-part zinc oxide sunscreen is great, but the lightweight base formula doesn't go the distance.

☹ **Healthy Defense SPF 45 Daily Moisturizer** *($14.99 for 1.7 ounces)* shortchanges skin on antioxidants, but does provide an in-part avobenzone sunscreen. What's problematic is the choice of the sensitizing preservative methylisothiazolinone, which is not recommended for use in leave-on products.

☺ **Illuminating Eye Reviver** *($12.99 for 0.5 ounce)* has a great silicone-enhanced texture and silky finish, but tactile positives aren't enough to make this jar-packaged moisturizer worth considering over many others. Mica adds a soft shine to skin, but it cannot illuminate the eye area in the same way a deftly applied highlighter or concealer can.

☹ **Intensified Day Moisture SPF 15** *($12.99 for 2.25 ounces)* lacks the UVA-protecting ingredients of titanium dioxide, zinc oxide, avobenzone, Mexoryl SX (ecamsule), or Tinosorb and is not recommended. The base formula is also really boring.

☺ **Light Night Cream** *($12.99 for 2.25 ounces)* remains in the Neutrogena lineup, and is still a basic, emollient moisturizer for normal to dry skin. It contains a tiny amount of soy fatty acid, but is otherwise devoid of state-of-the-art ingredients.

☹ **Oil-Free Anti-Acne Moisturizer** *($7.29 for 1.7 ounces)* contains the irritating menthol derivative menthyl lactate, and is not recommended. The amount of salicylic acid is too low to provide much exfoliation or to alleviate acne/blackheads.

☺ **Oil-Free Fresh Moisture, Ultra-Light Moisturizer** *($11.99 for 3 ounces)* is a good, inexpensive, lightweight moisturizer for normal to slightly dry skin. The lack of silicones and the relatively large amount of glycerin and glycol don't translate to ultralight, and a couple of the thickening agents may cause problems for breakout-prone skin. Neutrogena included some vitamin-based antioxidants and the opaque tube packaging will help keep them stable during use.

☺ **Oil-Free Moisture, for Combination Skin** *($12.99 for 4 ounces)* provides lightweight, skin-silkening moisture for its intended skin type, and doesn't contain fragrance. However, your skin deserves more than this basic formula provides.

✓ ☺ **Oil-Free Moisture, for Sensitive Skin** *($12.99 for 4 ounces)* is suitable for dry, sensitive skin (and for those with rosacea) because it contains some good emollients and a small amount of water-binding agents. This is also fragrance-free, but that's where the excitement starts and stops. Still, the other attributes make it worthy of a Paula's Pick status, assuming your skin is sensitive and you want to take a less-is-more approach with your moisturizer.

☹ **Oil-Free Moisture SPF 15** *($12.99 for 4 ounces)* doesn't contain oil, but also doesn't provide sufficient UVA-protecting ingredients. Given Neutrogena's sun-savvy marketing campaigns and its roster of impressive broad-spectrum sunscreens, this product should be discontinued—it's not doing anyone's skin any favors, that's for sure.

☺ **$$$ Retinol NX Concentrated Retinol Serum** *($65 for 1 ounce)*. Johnson & Johnson–owned Neutrogena has decided to enter the home shopping market via QVC, and the result is this serum with retinol. Sales of skin-care products on home shopping channels like QVC continue to climb, so it's not too surprising that the more mainstream lines are dipping their toes into this potentially lucrative pool of business. First, let me say that there is nothing medical or dermatological about this product in any way, shape, or form. There isn't even anything special or unique about the formula when compared with the formulas of other retinol products being sold by Neutrogena at the drugstore. And the same is true for RoC's retinol products, also owned by the same parent company that owns Neutrogena. Claims on infomercials always sound outstanding, and retinol is certainly an advantageous ingredient for sun-damaged, wrinkled skin, but Neutrogena and RoC make similar claims for their less expensive retinol products. J&J is not telling the truth somewhere. In reality, for the money and given the exclusive marketing of this retinol serum, the formula is a letdown given the price and all the associated hoopla (though it still deserves a happy face rating). If this version from Neutrogena is really better than what they are selling at the drugstore, then why don't they stop selling those versions and admit that this pricey retinol serum is the real deal and that what they sell at the drugstore is inferior? What Neutrogena could have done for this pricier, "exclusive" product to make it worthy of the claims is load it with ingredients that strongly differentiate it from their other options with retinol, such as antioxidants, skin-identical ingredients, and other cell-communicating ingredients, like so many other cosmetic companies do. Because they didn't, there's no compelling reason to purchase Retinol NX Concentrated Retinol Serum. Taken on its own merit as a stably packaged serum with an efficacious amount of retinol, it is recommended for all skin types. But when compared with retinol products from other J&J-owned brands, it isn't superior. Think of it as moving from one three-bedroom home to another on the same block with the same interior, but with a different exterior paint job, and the house costs three times as much. I mean really, why would you move? For less money and overall better formulas that offer skin more than retinol, consider Neutrogena Healthy Skin Anti-Wrinkle Cream, Night Formula or RoC Multi-Correxion Night Treatment.

☺ **Visibly Even Daily Moisturizer SPF 30** *($12.99 for 1.7 ounces)* isn't a daytime moisturizer with a bounty of antioxidants to help defend skin, although it does provide sufficient UVA protection with avobenzone and contains Neutrogena's heavily hyped Helioplex technology, which is said to stabilize it. (Helioplex is not the only option to stabilize avobenzone or other sunscreen actives, so don't be fooled into thinking Neutrogena has the edge here.) The somewhat creamy lotion texture is suitable for normal to dry skin and includes soybean seed extract as the main antioxidant. All of the other bells and whistles (of which there are few) are present in amounts likely too small to benefit skin. This is still worth considering as a daytime moisturizer with sunscreen, but it falls short of joining the top brass in this category.

☹ **Visibly Firm Eye Cream, Active Copper** *($18.99 for 0.5 ounce)* won't firm skin, but it's still an OK moisturizer for normal to dry skin anywhere on the face. The amount of antioxidants is paltry, and the jar packaging won't keep them (and likely the copper peptide) stable during use.

☺ **Visibly Firm Night Cream, Active Copper** *($18.99 for 1.7 ounces)* contains some good antioxidants, but once again jar packaging will be their undoing once you begin using this. Reformulated in mid-2007, this remains an OK moisturizer for normal to dry skin, but copper isn't the antiwrinkle, skin-firming answer. If it were, why is Neutrogena selling so many other products without copper, and also making antiwrinkle claims about them?

☹ **Clear Pore Cleanser/Mask** *($7.99 for 4.2 ounces)* can disinfect skin because it contains 3.5% benzoyl peroxide, but the clay base makes this too potentially drying, and the menthol only causes irritation. A well-formulated leave-on benzoyl peroxide product would be far better for treating blemishes.

☺ **On-the-Spot Acne Treatment** *($6.99 for 0.75 ounce)* contains 2.5% benzoyl peroxide as the active ingredient, which is helpful for blemish-prone skin. The formula's clay and wax base is a confusing mix for skin; the clay can exacerbate the drying effect of benzoyl peroxide, while the wax may make blemishes worse. Still, I suppose this is an OK option for spot-treating a blemish (which you should do only if you rarely break out—regular breakouts require treating the entire face).

☺ **Shine-Control Blotting Sheets** *($6.99 for 60 sheets)* are thin polypropylene plastic sheets. They do absorb excess oil and perspiration, but the addition of mineral oil won't keep skin as shine-free as other options.

☹ **Lip Boost Intense Moisture Therapy** *($7.55 for 0.3 ounce)* is a water- and Vaseline-based lip balm that contains several good-for-lips ingredients. However, that's all for naught because they are coupled with menthol and peppermint, two irritants that make this intensely irritating, not therapeutic.

☹ **Lip Moisturizer SPF 15** *($3.89 for 0.15 ounce)* is advertised as being PABA-free, which is nice (PABA is a sunscreen active that's rarely used because it tends to be irritating), but Neutrogena forgot to include sufficient UVA protection, so this isn't a lip balm with sunscreen that anyone should rely on.

☺ **Lip Nutrition Balm** *($8.50 for 0.18 ounce)* is a berry-flavored lip moisturizer that comes in a pot. The emollient formula is good for keeping lips smooth and preventing chapping, though generally speaking unflavored balms are better because they don't encourage licking your lips, which results in needing to reapply the lip balm more frequently.

NEUTROGENA SUNSCREEN PRODUCTS

☹ **Age Shield Face Sunblock Lotion SPF 90+** *($11.99 for 3 ounces).* SPF 90! Really? Before I discuss this sunscreen I'd like to point out that nowhere in the world is there enough daylight to warrant applying this level of sun protection. Remember, SPF is a rating about the length of time you can stay in the sun without burning. It is a time-related number, not quality. Even someone whose skin turns pink after 5 minutes of unprotected sun exposure would get 450 minutes (7.5 hours) of sun protection. Now that's an extreme example for someone with very white skin; most people would get four times that amount of protection, which translates to 30 hours in the sun, and given there are only 24 hours in a day, you start to understand how silly this is. Companies know that consumers think a higher SPF number means "better" protection, but it only means longer protection. You get the same quality of protection from an SPF 90 as you do from an SPF 30. The only reason to consider such a high level of SPF protection is if you know you routinely underapply and if you aren't apt to reapply when needed. A higher SPF means you would be applying more sunscreen ingredients on skin. However, the risk is that with a larger amount of active ingredients your skin is more likely to have a reaction. This sunscreen contains stabilized avobenzone in a lightweight yet slightly waxy base. Unfortunately, like so many other Neutrogena sunscreens, it contains methylisothiazolinone, a sensitizing preservative not recommended for use in leave-on products (Sources: *Contact Dermatitis*, November 2001, pages 257-264; and *European Journal of Dermatology*, March 1999, pages 144-160). Combine this with fragrance and the high amount of sunscreen agents needed to reach SPF 90 and this is very likely to cause needless irritation.

✓ ☺ **Age Shield Face Sunblock SPF 55** *($10.99 for 4 ounces).* Neutrogena has other Age Shield sunscreens with lower SPF ratings, and all of them have similar formulas that provide UVA protection courtesy of avobenzone. The SPF 55 version offers longer protection among the Age Shield options with lower SPF ratings, but as with any sunscreen, reapplication is necessary when you'll be spending many hours outside or have been perspiring heavily. This is a very good sunscreen with antioxidants for all skin types except sensitive. It is suitable for use on the face, but if facial skin is dry, you may want to apply a moisturizer first.

☹ **Age Shield Face Sunblock SPF 70** *($10.99 for 4 ounces).* The combination of active ingredients includes avobenzone for UVA protection, but adds up to a sunscreen that has strong potential to irritate skin. This irritation is compounded by the inclusion of the sensitizing preservative methylisothiazolinone, which is not recommended for use in leave-on products. Lastly, although this sunscreen doesn't deserve to be downgraded because of its SPF rating, it must be said that SPF 70 is nearing overkill for anyone's skin. There just isn't that much daylight in most parts of the world to warrant exposing skin to the concentration of sunscreen actives needed to reach such a high SPF rating.

✓ ☺ **Age Shield Sunblock SPF 30** *($10.69 for 4 ounces)* has a great name, and honestly describes what a well-formulated sunscreen does for your skin. This fragrance-free, in-part avobenzone sunscreen definitely has the UVA range covered, and includes several antioxidants in stable packaging. The initially creamy application dries to a soft matte finish without a hint of greasiness. It's a texture that someone with normal to very oily skin will love, and is suitable for use under makeup. Now to address the claims. Neutrogena maintains that this product is a breakthrough in UVA protection for the United States because of their patented Helioplex technology. Helioplex is composed of avobenzone, oxybenzone, and the solvent 2-6-diethylhexyl naphthalate, a solvent that is believed to make the avobenzone more stable, and avobenzone stability has indeed been a concern. According to Neutrogena, Helioplex "blocks more UVA rays than the leading sunscreen available in the U.S. today, to give you the best antiaging protection around." Yet, without knowing which "leading sunscreen" they are referring to (best-selling products change daily), there is no way to know what they are comparing it to. What if that sunscreen didn't even contain UVA-protecting ingredients? If it is an issue of avobenzone remaining stable, there is substantial research showing that it can be stable without the addition of the naphthalate (Sources: *Journal of Photochemistry and Photobiology*, March 2006, pages 204-213; and *British Journal of Dermatology*, December 2004, pages 1234-1244). Neutrogena is touting this and their other sunscreens with Helioplex as a breakthrough when, in fact, it really isn't anything new under the sun. What is perplexing is that all the ballyhoo about Helioplex and avobenzone completely ignores the UVA screening ability of titanium dioxide and zinc oxide. Both of these mineral sunscreens block light beyond the UVA light range of 320-400 nanometers, screening all the way up to 700 nanometers (Source: *Skin Therapy Letter*, Table 1, 1997), and Neutrogena also sells sunscreens with these two active ingredients. Marketing claims aside, in the end what really counts is that this remains a well-formulated, broad-spectrum sunscreen that deserves consideration when shopping for water-resistant SPF 30 products.

✓ ☺ **Age Shield Sunblock SPF 45** *($10.69 for 4 ounces)* is nearly identical to the Age Shield Sunblock SPF 30 above, and the same review applies.

☹ **Fresh Cooling Body Mist Sunblock SPF 30** *($10.69 for 5 ounces)* comes in a pressurized can and propels a fine-mist formula that includes an in-part avobenzone sunscreen. Unfortunately, the spray is loaded with alcohol (it makes up 67% of the formula) and also includes a menthol derivative; combining the menthol derivative and the alcohol will indeed make your skin feel cool, but not in a good way. The broad-spectrum sun protection and ultralight feel are great, but the irritants are a significant problem for skin, even more so when it is going to be subjected to long-term sun exposure—such as during a day at the beach or on a tropical vacation.

☹ **Fresh Cooling Body Mist Sunblock SPF 45** *($10.69 for 5 ounces)* has a higher SPF rating than the Fresh Cooling Body Mist Sunblock SPF 30, but that's about the only difference

☹ **Fresh Cooling Body Mist Sunblock SPF 70** *($10.99 for 5 ounces)* has a cooling effect due to the amount of skin-drying, irritating alcohol this spray-on sunscreen contains, along with the menthol derivative menthyl PCA. Mist-and-go sunscreens are great, but you don't have to settle for one that exposes skin to alcohol and other irritants. Paula's Choice, Banana Boat, Kinesys (not reviewed in this book), and other lines sell spray-on sunscreens that do not contain needless irritants.

☺ **Healthy Defense Oil-Free Sunblock Lotion SPF 45** *($10.29 for 4 ounces)* is a good basic sunscreen for normal to oily skin, and includes avobenzone for UVA protection. However, I am concerned that the amount of methylpropanediol (a penetration enhancer) may make this more irritating to skin than other sunscreens. After all, 26.5% active ingredients is a lot for anyone's skin to handle. This is worth trying, but is recommended with caution.

☺ **Healthy Defense Oil-Free Sunblock Stick SPF 30** *($7.99 for 0.47 ounce)* brings portable protection for oft-forgotten areas of skin, though the wax base is not the best for blemish-prone areas. UVA protection is assured with avobenzone, and this contains small amounts of vitamin-based antioxidants.

☹ **Pure & Free Baby Sunblock Lotion SPF 60+ with PureScreen** *($10.99 for 3 ounces)* has a lot going for it, especially for babies or those with sensitive skin. It's fragrance-free and contains anti-irritants, and its active ingredients (titanium dioxide and zinc oxide) are as gentle as it gets in the world of sunscreens. Neutrogena even includes some antioxidants, though it's difficult to ascertain their concentration because the inactive ingredients are listed in alphabetical order rather than in descending order of content, which in this case is permissible because sunscreens are over-the-counter drug products. Unfortunately, Neutrogena chose methylisothiazolinone, a preservative that is contraindicated for use in leave-on products due to its sensitizing potential. (Sources: *Actas Dermo-Sifiliograficas*, January-February 2009, pages 53-60; *Archives of Dermatological Research*, February 2007, pages 427-437; and *Contact Dermatitis*, October 2005, pages 226-233). For that reason alone, I am unable to recommend this otherwise beautifully formulated sunscreen.

✓ ☺ **Pure & Free Baby Sunblock Stick SPF 60+ with PureScreen** *($8.99 for 0.47 ounce)* is rated a Paula's Pick because of its value for those with sensitive, reactive skin. The gentle actives consist of titanium dioxide and zinc oxide, while the base formula is fragrance-free and works well over dry areas due to the protective qualities of the waxes that keep this product in stick form. It is ideal for use on children or adults but can feel heavy and sticky.

☹ **Sensitive Skin Sunblock Lotion SPF 60+ with PureScreen** *($10.99 for 3 ounces)* is identical to Neutrogena's Pure & Free Baby Sunblock Lotion SPF 60+ with PureScreen above. As such, the same review applies.

☺ **Summer Glow Daily Moisturizer SPF 20** *($8.99 for 6.7 ounces)* provides sun protection with its in-part avobenzone sunscreen and comes in a lightweight lotion base that includes a bit of dihydroxyacetone, the ingredient in most sunless tanning products. It is suitable for all skin types, but best for normal to oily skin.

☹ **Ultimate Sport Sunblock Lotion SPF 55** *($10.99 for 4 ounces)* makes odd claims because it certainly isn't the first from Neutrogena to include their Helioplex technology to stabilize the avobenzone. (Didn't anyone at the company recall their previous sunscreens they launched with this technology and marketing campaigns?) The company also claims that this replenishes electrolytes to "nourish and restore skin balance," but the electrolytes we lose through our skin from perspiration (such as occurs with sports) are best replenished with fluids we drink. You can't replenish them topically, and especially not from your sunscreen, which is designed to stay on top of your skin to protect it. Although this sunscreen applies smoothly and is tenacious when it comes to staying put, I cannot recommend it because it contains the preservative methylisothiazolinone, which is contraindicated for use in leave-on products due to its sensitizing potential (Sources: *Actas Dermo-Sifiliograficas*, January-February 2009, pages 53-60; *Archives of Dermatological Research*, February 2007, pages 427-437; and *Contact Dermatitis*, October 2005, pages 226-233). The active ingredients in this sunscreen can be sensitizing on their own, so you don't want anything else in the formula adding to that potential.

☹ **Ultimate Sport Sunblock Lotion SPF 70+** *($10.99 for 4 ounces)* is, save for a higher SPF rating, nearly identical to the Ultimate Sport Sunblock Lotion SPF 55 above, and the same review applies.

☹ **Ultimate Sport Sunblock Spray SPF 55** *($10.99 for 5 ounces)* has a wonderfully light feel, in addition to an in-part avobenzone sunscreen (with the avobenzone stabilized by Neutrogena's Helioplex technology). Regrettably, the lightness is due to the amount of drying, irritating alcohol in this spray-on sunscreen. If silicone or a non-drying solvent had been chosen instead, this would definitely have been a sunscreen for active people to try.

☹ **Ultimate Sport Sunblock Spray SPF 70+** *($10.99 for 5 ounces)* contains stabilized avobenzone for UVA protection, which is a good thing for skin, but the base formula of this aerosol spray-on sunscreen is bad for skin because it's mostly alcohol. That means skin is subject to needless irritation and excess free-radical damage, which isn't what sun protection is all about. Coppertone and Paula's Choice offer spray-on sunscreens without such irritants, and you don't have to compromise on broad-spectrum protection.

☹ **Ultra Sheer Body Mist Sunblock SPF 30** *($9.99 for 5 ounces)* features 3% avobenzone for sufficient UVA protection, but the base formula is mostly alcohol, and that makes it too drying and irritating for all skin types. Oddly, this product still leaves a fairly greasy, slick finish.

☹ **Ultra Sheer Body Mist Sunblock SPF 45** *($9.99 for 5 ounces)* is nearly identical to the Ultra Sheer Body Mist Sunblock SPF 30 above, except it contains a higher percentage of active ingredients to achieve its higher SPF rating. Otherwise, the same comments apply.

✓ ☺ **Ultra Sheer Dry-Touch Sunblock SPF 30** *($10.69 for 3 ounces)* really does have a dry finish, and is an outstanding in-part avobenzone sunscreen that begins creamy but quickly dries down to a weightless matte (in feel) finish. The high levels of active ingredients required to net an SPF 30 rating do leave a very slight sheen on the skin, but it's hardly worth complaining about, especially if you are dealing with oily to very oily skin and have been unable to find a stand-alone sunscreen that doesn't feel heavy or greasy. Those with normal to dry skin will likely find this sunscreen too drying, but it's a winning option for oily skin, and it does contain antioxidants.

✓ ☺ **Ultra Sheer Dry-Touch Sunblock SPF 45** *($10.69 for 3 ounces)* is identical to the Ultra Sheer Dry-Touch Sunblock SPF 30 above, but with increased levels of active ingredients to reach SPF 45.

☺ **Ultra Sheer Dry-Touch Sunblock SPF 55** *($10.69 for 3 ounces)* contains the same Helioplex ingredient mixture as the Age Shield Sunblock SPF 30 above, so UVA bases are well-covered. Although this sunscreen is fairly lightweight, it isn't as sheer and it definitely is more apparent on the skin than either of the Age Shield Sunblocks. The formulas are similar, but this Ultra Sheer version lacks a single antioxidant and contains fragrance, which keep it from earning a Paula's Pick rating and also make it not worth considering over Neutrogena's Age Shield Sunblocks.

☹ **Ultra Sheer Dry-Touch Sunblock SPF 70** *($11.29 for 3 ounces)* achieves its ultra-high SPF number because it contains over 25% active ingredients, including avobenzone for UVA protection. The lotion texture has a smooth feel and a dry, almost weightless finish. However, this product has some problems. First, it lacks antioxidants; second, it contains the preservative methylisothiazolinone, which is not recommended for use in leave-on products due to its sensitizing potential (Source: *Archives of Dermatological Research*, February 2007, pages 227-237); and third, its SPF 70 rating means there are an awful lot of sunscreen ingredients for skin to handle. Also, considering that an SPF 70 product provides about 24 hours of daylight protection (assuming you don't perspire or wash your hands), there just isn't enough daylight to warrant this kind of formulation, except in Alaska or Antarctica during their long summer days. The FDA's recent sunscreen proposal to allow SPF ratings only up to 50 may mean products like this will be disallowed, which wouldn't necessarily be a bad thing, for reasons stated above.

☹ **Ultra Sheer Dry-Touch Sunblock SPF 85** *($10.99 for 3 ounces)*. I'm torn about how to review this sunscreen because it certainly provides sufficient UVA protection with its in-part avobenzone sunscreen. It also has a lightweight feel and a soft matte finish not often found in sunscreens with high SPF ratings, but that's part of the dilemma—SPF 85? Really, whose skin sees that much daylight? If someone with very fair skin that burns instantly were to apply this, or even someone whose skin turns pink in ten minutes, they could stay in the sun for 850 minutes (14 hours) without burning, and there simply isn't that much daylight in most parts of the world. Someone with a medium skin tone that tans could stay in the sun for 28 hours! In addition, I am concerned that someone using this product would think they don't need to reapply because, hey, it's SPF 85, so they're covered all day, right? Nope. Higher SPF ratings don't mean better protection, just longer protection—and that does not negate the need to reapply after swimming, toweling off, or perspiring. Lastly, and this is the deal-breaker, the presence of the preservative methylisothiazolinone and the amount of active ingredients (33.5%) likely make this too irritating for most skin types. The aforementioned preservative is recommended for use only in rinse-off products; even small concentrations are known to be sensitizing (Source: *Contact Dermatitis*, May 1998, pages 261-265).

☺ **Ultra Sheer Dry Touch Sunblock SPF 100+** *($10.99 for 3 ounces).* Despite the impressive ultra-high SPF rating, the extra synthetic sunscreen ingredients don't net much added benefit. You will still need to reapply this if you perspire or swim for more than 80 minutes.

SPF 100 is well past the boundaries of how much sun protection anyone needs. Even if your skin turns pink in the sun after 10 minutes (typical of those with very white, fair skin), you'd be protected for 1,000 minutes or 16 hours. There isn't enough daylight in most parts of the world to warrant such protection. The only reason very high SPF ratings have merit is for those who tend to skimp on application. If you're not one to apply sunscreen liberally, you may well be getting SPF 50 instead of the SPF 100 rating, so there is that consideration. However, this sunscreen is difficult to recommend for two reasons: the amount of active ingredients (39% of the formula) increases the risk of a sensitized skin reaction and it contains a preservative (methylisothiazolinone) that is not recommended for use in leave-on products. This does work well as a sunscreen with avobenzone for UVA protection.

☹ **Waterguard Kids Sunblock Mist Spray SPF 70+** *($10.99 for 5 ounces)* may sound like a boon for kids who spend hours outdoors and can't be bothered to stop their activities to have Mom or Dad reapply; but it isn't, at least not without an important caveat. It does include avobenzone for sufficient UVA protection and has a very light texture and non-greasy finish, but because Neutrogena included a sensitizing preservative in the formula, this isn't a sunscreen I recommend. The preservative in question—methylisothiazolinone—is known as one of the most sensitizing preservatives around, which is why it's best reserved for use in rinse-off products (Sources: *Actas Dermo-Sifiliograficas*, January-February 2009, pages 53-60; *Archives of Dermatological Research*, February 2007, pages 427-437; and *Contact Dermatitis*, October 2005, pages 226-233). By the way, on the label for this product Neutrogena is still using the term "waterproof" even though no sunscreen meets that standard (that's why "water-resistant" is the term regulated by the FDA), so you still need to reapply this after swimming, sweating, or toweling off after about two hours.

NEUTROGENA SUNLESS TANNING PRODUCTS

☺ **Build-A-Tan Gradual Sunless Tanning** *($10.69 for 6.7 ounces)* is a very standard, but good, self-tanning lotion for normal to oily skin. It tans skin with dihydroxyacetone, the same ingredient found in most self-tanners.

☺ **Build-A-Tan Gradual Sunless Tanning Face SPF 15** *($10.69 for 2.5 ounces)* is a dihydroxyacetone-based self-tanning lotion that includes an in-part avobenzone sunscreen. It's an option for daytime use, assuming you apply it liberally (not always the best idea for self-tanners because the color can come out too dark or blotchy).

☹ **MicroMist Tanning Sunless Spray, Medium** *($11.99 for 5.3 ounces)* contains too much witch hazel to make it a good choice, especially given the huge number of self-tanning products that work without irritating skin.

☹ **MicroMist Tanning Sunless Spray, Deep** *($11.99 for 5.3 ounces)* has the same irritancy potential as the MicroMist Tanning Sunless Spray, Medium, and the same review applies.

☺ **Sheer Body Tint** *($10.69 for 4 ounces)* is not a self-tanner but rather a cosmetic bronzer in mousse form. The lightweight formula smooths on easily and dries quickly while imparting sheer, buildable color that washes off with any cleanser. It is available in versions for fair to light and medium to dark skin tones. Both versions contain film-forming agents that help keep this on skin, not all over your clothes. However, I wouldn't recommend wearing this under your tennis whites!

☹ **Sun Fresh Sheer Summer Color Sunless Foam** *($9.99 for 4 ounces)* is a lightweight, liquid-to-foam sunless tanner that is available for fair to medium and medium to deep skin tones, with the only difference between them being the amount of dihydroxyacetone (the ingredient that turns skin a tan color). That's good, but things take an irritating turn for the worse with the amount of witch hazel. Neutrogena includes several parts of the plant, and that's not good news. There are plenty of self-tanners available that work beautifully without exposing your skin to irritants, so these should be ignored.

☹ **Sun Fresh Sheer Summer Color Sunless Lotion** *($9.99 for 4 ounces)* is a substandard self-tanning lotion because no matter whether you choose the Fair/Medium or the Medium/Deep option, your skin will be exposed to an irritating amount of witch hazel extract.

NEUTROGENA MAKEUP

NEUTROGENA HEALTHY SKIN PRODUCTS

FOUNDATION: ☺ **Healthy Skin Liquid Makeup SPF 20** *($13.99)* is a reformulation of Neutrogena's longstanding liquid foundation of the same name. There wasn't much need to improve the previous version of this product, but this entry maintains the silky texture, even application, and natural-looking, soft matte finish of its predecessor. Sun protection remains strong with an all titanium dioxide sunscreen, which lends to the finish and opacity of Healthy Skin Liquid Makeup. The range of shades is much better than in Neutrogena's SkinClearing Oil-Free Makeup, which is good news for those with normal to slightly dry and oily skin, but bad news for those with blemish-prone skin. Among the shades for Healthy Skin Liquid Makeup, only Soft Beige stands out as being slightly peach on medium skin tones. As for Neutrogena's touted antioxidant blend, antioxidants are barely present and the clear-glass bottle packaging won't keep them protected from light anyway. One caution: Although it is only one of several preservatives in this foundation, consumers should know that Neutrogena added methylisothiazolinone, which has a history of causing sensitized reactions and is not recommended for use in leave-on products. I suspect the amount present won't be an issue, but it's enough to keep this from earning a Paula's Pick rating.

☹ **Healthy Skin Cream Powder Makeup SPF 20** *($12.19 for 0.4 ounce)* is an outdated cream-to-powder compact makeup with an unpleasant texture that (surprisingly for Neutrogena) lacks sufficient UVA-protecting ingredients. Each of the four shades is glaringly peach or pink, making this one of the most unappealing foundations at the drugstore.

CONCEALER: ☺ **Healthy Skin Smoothing Stick Treatment Concealer** *($7.59 for 0.1 ounce)* wins points for providing nearly opaque coverage with one swipe, but this lipstick-style concealer also looks heavy and creases into lines around the eye. It's an OK option for camouflaging small areas of redness, and three of the four shades are decent (Medium is too peach), but the concealers from L'Oreal and Revlon have much more to offer.

POWDER: ☺ **Healthy Skin Blends Translucent Oil-Control Powder** *($12.79 for 0.2 ounce)* features various color "squares" of powder in one compact, the idea being that swirling the brush over these multiple colors nets you one translucent color on skin. It does apply that way, but I completely disagree with Neutrogena's claim that this product can be used by multiple skin tones. The powder is best for fair to medium skin tones, although some medium skin tones will find it too light. The talc-based formula has a smooth texture and an even, non-powdery application, but those dealing with blemishes should avoid these products because they contain cornstarch.

☺ **Healthy Skin Loose Powder** *($12.19 for 0.7 ounce)* has three shades, suitable for fair to light/medium skin. Its formula is talc-based, with a soft, silky finish. The colors are actually quite attractive, but you have to pry open the boxes to get a glimpse of them (don't tell anyone I said this).

☺ **Healthy Skin Pressed Powder** *($11.87 for 0.35 ounce)* has three shades, suitable for fair to light/medium skin. Its formula is talc-based, with a soft, silky finish. The colors are actually quite attractive, but you have to pry open the boxes to get a glimpse of them (don't tell anyone I said this). The Pressed Powder offers a bit more coverage and has a slightly silkier feel, courtesy of the silicone it contains, than the Healthy Skin Loose Powder.

BLUSH AND BRONZER: ☺ **Healthy Skin Blends Natural Radiance Bronzer** *($12.79 for 0.2 ounce)* is identical in concept, texture, and application to the Healthy Skin Blends Translucent Oil-Control Powder above, except this comes in bronze tones with a hint of shine. The effect on skin is a soft tan that's best for fair to light skin.

☺ **Healthy Skin Blends Sheer Highlighting Blush** *($12.88 for 0.2 ounce)* is identical to the Healthy Skin Blends Translucent Oil-Control Powder, except with this product you get pale to medium pink squares in one pressed-powder compact. The result is akin to a soft pink blush with a hint of shine, and it's best for fair to light skin.

NEUTROGENA MINERAL SHEERS MAKEUP

FOUNDATION: ✓☺ **Mineral Sheers Powder Foundation SPF 20** *($12.99 for 0.34 ounce)* provides light to medium coverage, a soft matte finish, and impressive mineral sun protection (from titanium dioxide) in one sleek mirrored compact. This pressed-powder foundation has a smoother, more elegant texture than Neutrogena's former Healthy Defense Protective Powder SPF 30. Mineral Sheer also looks more natural on skin (though it still looks like makeup). Coverage, even when you apply it with a sponge, is more sheer than what you get with standard pressed-powder foundations. However, this is an excellent way to boost the protection of your foundation or daytime moisturizer with sunscreen. Among the eight mostly excellent shades are options for fair to tan skin tones. Honey Beige 70 is best avoided due to its overt orange tone.

☺ **Mineral Sheers Liquid Makeup SPF 20** *($14.49)* contains only one mineral of note in this liquid-to-powder foundation: silica. One of the most abundant minerals on earth, silica has strong absorbent qualities and contributes to this foundation's dry finish. The company isn't kidding about the sheer part: You get almost no coverage, so even minor flaws stand out unless you pair this with a concealer. The sunscreen benefit is definitely recommended due to the in-part titanium dioxide blend, but if you're going for the mineral claim, why not use titanium dioxide all by itself or paired with zinc oxide, and forgo the synthetic sunscreen agents? Some may enjoy the brush applicator Neutrogena provides (you rotate the top portion of the bottle until foundation is dispensed onto the brush), but I found it was not as good as a synthetic sponge because it tended to produce streaky-looking results. The streaks aren't readily apparent as you brush it on, but after it sets, you'll see streaking unless the shade you choose matches your skin exactly. Therein lies another issue: The colors for this foundation are mostly pink, peach, or orange toned. If this foundation were not so sheer, many of the colors would be unacceptable. As is, there really aren't any to avoid—but you may want to skip this foundation altogether unless you are more interested in sun protection than in coverage or you want SPF with only a hint of a tint (and I mean a really tiny hint).

☺ **Mineral Sheers Mineral Powder Foundation** *($11.99 for 0.18 ounce)*. Housed in a self-contained unit is a loose powder with a built-in applicator brush. You shake the powder into a concealed sifter piece, which then dispenses it onto the brush, ready for you to dust it on. This powder foundation's main weak spot is the brush itself; it just isn't as soft as it should be given the way you are supposed to use it. If you want meaningful coverage, you need to buff this product over your skin using the head of the brush, which feels scratchy. Sweeping the powder over your skin is an option that feels better, but you'll get sheer to no coverage, since the powder is dispensed onto the head (not the sides) of the brush. Application issues aside, this isn't too different from most mineral makeups, with the main ingredients being mica and bismuth oxychloride. The mica adds a subtle glow to the skin while the bismuth oxychloride adds bulk, opacity, and an extremely drying matte finish that tends to get drier as the day goes by. The finish is admittedly attractive at first, but I was less enamored by late afternoon, when I noticed my oily areas looking dull and somewhat flaky. By nighttime, with only one touch-up I was unusually shine-free, but my skin had a flat, drawn appearance that wasn't nearly as nice as the finish you get from some of today's best liquid foundations. I understand the appeal of mineral makeup, yet my comments about this type of makeup remain the same: It may look good at the onset, but the drying, absorbent bismuth oxychloride exaggerates even minor areas of dry skin, and on oily areas it can thicken and look very much like makeup. To Neutrogena's credit, their powder formula is lighter than many others, and its drawbacks take longer to appear. If you're curious to try this, the five available shades are all worthwhile, though the Sheer Bronzer shade leaves noticeable gold sparkles on your skin.

CONCEALER: ☹ **Mineral Sheers Concealer Kit SPF 20** *($14.49)*. I'll get right to the point: Don't bother with this terrible concealer kit! The creamy concealer has a soft, frosting-like texture that makes it very easy to overapply. Even when you're careful about how much you're using, the formula remains creamy (almost greasy) and creases endlessly. Setting it with the accompanying powder (which is cleverly hidden in a jar underneath the concealer) enhances longevity, but actually makes the concealer look worse on your skin. The sunscreen is pure titanium dioxide, but the amount of this active (over 20%) is a major contributor to why it looks so unnatural and chalky on skin. This is not the way to enjoy mineral makeup! The shades are mostly good, but so what—this is one of the worst concealers at the drugstore.

BLUSH: ☺ **Mineral Sheers Blush** *($12.99 for 0.1 ounce)* is a talc-free sheer loose blush that's packaged with a built-in brush applicator. The brush could be softer and tapered better, but it does the job. The problem is the way the powder is dispensed (it tends to be too dusty), and the application is so sheer you really need to pile this on to get color to show. Color takes a backseat to shine, as each shade has rather large crystalline particles that don't cling to skin as well as they should. L'Oreal did much better with their Bare Naturale Gentle Mineral Blush.

EYESHADOW: ☺ **Mineral Sheers for Eyes** *($7.99 for 0.12 ounce)* capitalize on the mineral makeup trend, yet the formula is talc-based just like most powder eyeshadows. Of course, talc is a mineral but most mineral makeup lines eschew it in favor of alternatives. In any case, these eyeshadow duos have a smooth but dry texture that applies and blends fairly well. The dryness causes some flaking unless you dust these on sheer. However, sheerness is the theme here, and you'll notice most of the shades offer more in the way of shine than color. If you're curious to try this and want a duo to shade and highlight, the only ones to really consider are Shell and Clay. The others go on too lightly to shade or shape the eye.

OTHER NEUTROGENA MAKEUP PRODUCTS

FOUNDATION: ☺ **SkinClearing Oil-Free Makeup Microclear Technology** *($13.99)* is an updated version of the company's longstanding SkinClearing Oil-Free Makeup. Both the original and this version contain 0.5% salicylic acid as the active ingredient. Just like before, the salicylic acid won't exfoliate skin because the product's pH is well above 4. The salicylic acid may have a slight antibacterial action, but it would be more effective in that respect if the amount were increased to at least 1%. Outside of the active ingredient letdown, this is a very good, lightweight liquid makeup. It smooths easily over skin, provides light to medium coverage, and sets to a soft matte finish that looks more natural than the original version. The shade range appears questionable at first glance—many appear too orange or too peach in the bottle—but these overtones are neutralized once blended on skin. Still, consider Buff, Warm Beige, and Soft Beige carefully. This is best for normal to oily skin; the wax content makes it questionable for acne-prone skin, unless your blemishes are mild and not an issue over your entire face.

☹ **Skin Clearing Oil-Free Compact Foundation** *($11.99 for 0.4 ounce)* is a thick-textured cream-to-powder makeup that contains absorbent aluminum starch as its main ingredient, which increases the odds that it will irritate skin. The thickening agents that follow aren't the best for oily skin—and that's precisely the skin type this is being marketed to. Although it does have a rather dry matte finish that would please someone with oiliness, almost all of the shades are too peach, pink, or orange to recommend, especially without any testers at the store to see if they can blend unseen into your skin tone. The color swatch on the box barely resembles the actual shade, and with no testers in sight, choosing the wrong color is all but inevitable. The minimal amount of salicylic acid (BHA) comes without a pH (you cannot establish a pH in a waterless product) and, therefore, has no effect on breakouts.

CONCEALER: ☺ **Skin Clearing Oil-Free Concealer** *($8.24 for 0.05 ounce)* is packaged in a click-pen that feeds this lightweight concealer onto an angled sponge tip. It blends very well (and fast) to a matte finish, and provides excellent coverage. The light, silicone- and clay-based formula is fine for use over blemishes—just don't expect the tiny amount (0.5%) of salicylic acid at this high pH to clear things up. There are four shades, three of which are beautifully neutral. Avoid Correcting Green because green does not hide red on the skin, it only adds a Kermit the Frog shade to your face.

☺ **3-in-1 Concealer for Eyes SPF 20** *($9.99)* is positioned as another multipurpose product, this time combining concealer, eye cream, and sunscreen in one convenient package. As a concealer, this provides smooth, even coverage that looks natural and has a satin finish slightly prone to creasing. Both shades are worthwhile. The sunscreen is almost 10% titanium dioxide, which also helps enhance coverage. Where it falls short is the eye-cream claim. This product isn't too creamy (not with talc as the third ingredient) and the amount of fragrance is disappointing. There are better concealers with sunscreen from Revlon, but this is still an option.

☹ **Skin Soothing Undereye Corrector** *($9.59 for 0.05 ounce)* is a sheer highlighter available in two peachy pink shades that are dispensed onto a brush from the click-pen component. Each has a strong matte finish that does little to cast a radiant glow, but the bigger problem is the menthyl lactate, a menthol derivative and an irritant that should not be used on skin, especially around the eyes.

POWDER: ☺ **Skin Clearing Oil-Free Pressed Powder** *($12.08 for 0.35 ounce)* has a dry, smooth texture and an almost-too-powdery finish that is an option only for someone with oily to very oily skin. The inclusion of salicylic acid in a powder is never effective, as the very ingredients that compose a powder have too high a pH to allow the BHA to work as an exfoliant. Three shades are available, and although they appear too peach in the compact, each goes on softly.

BLUSH: ☺ **Soft Color Blush** *($10.33 for 0.16 ounce)* has a smooth but unusually dry texture that makes application spotty. Most of the shades are soft, matte, and muted, but the swatch on the box is not an accurate representation. Although this is an OK blush, it isn't worth considering over powder blushes from L'Oreal, Almay, or Jane.

EYESHADOW: ☺ **Nourishing Eye Duo** *($8.49)* debuts as a powder eyeshadow with alleged skin-conditioning benefits. There is a negligible amount of vitamins present, and a slightly greater amount of silk powder (which doesn't so much condition skin as enhance this eyeshadow's texture and application). Conditioning benefits are not happening, but the formula applies beautifully, blends well, and has a good color payoff. Eight duos are available, all with a slight amount of shine that has moderate shimmer once applied. Most of the pairings are sensible and attractive (though not ideal for dark skin tones).

☺ **Nourishing Eye Quad SPF 15** *($9.99)*. How exciting—Neutrogena is one of the few companies to offer an eyeshadow with built-in sun protection. In this case, the active ingredient is 5% titanium dioxide, which definitely supports this product's SPF rating. How are the eyeshadows themselves? You get one large base shade, with a matte finish, which is the only one of the four that has sunscreen. The three other shades are labeled as highlighter, crease, and accent colors, and each has a soft to moderate shimmer. For the most part, the designations make sense as you survey the available quads (avoid Garden Party, it's too green). Other than the base shade, which tends to go on more opaque, the other shades in each quad, while silky and easy to apply, impart no more than sheer color with shine. You'll have to layer this extensively to get adequate shaping and shading, but if a softer, diffused look is what you're after, these work great and the shine doesn't flake. By the way, despite the name, this powder eyeshadow isn't nourishing (though the sun protection the base shade provides is a nice touch).

☹ **Skin Soothing Eye Tints** *($9.45 for 0.18 ounce)* is sold as a jack-of-all-trades product for use on the eyelids. According to Neutrogena, this product can function as an eyeshadow base, an eye brightener, a puffiness reducer, and an aid to prevent your eyeshadows from creasing. Both shades have a hint of shimmer, and a somewhat dry texture that is a bit tricky to blend. They dry to a matte finish that can help prevent eyeshadows from creasing, but the cooling sensation you feel is from the menthyl lactate, a form of menthol that can be very irritating to the eyelids.

The Reviews N

EYE SHAPER: ☺ **Nourishing Eyeliner** *($7.99)* is a silicone-based automatic, retractable eye pencil that contains only a tiny amount of vitamins, which aren't going to nourish the skin along your lash line or stay stable, so forget that claim. What you should keep in mind when considering this pencil is its smooth application and soft cream finish that won't smudge once set (though it still feels creamy, which is surprising). The other end of this great eye pencil includes a precision sponge tip for softening the line and a built-in sharpener you can use to refine the pencil's tip. The shades are mostly classic options, but be careful with Twilight Blue, a deep navy hue that is attractive but not for everyone (it looks best with dark-colored eyes).

LIPSTICK AND LIP GLOSS: ✓ ☺ **MoistureShine Gloss** *($7.65 for 0.22 ounce)* has all the best attributes of a lip gloss: it comes with a hygienic wand applicator, has a smooth, non-sticky texture that feels moisturizing but not goopy, and leaves lips looking evenly glossed rather than overly wet. The selection of shades (most are shimmer-enriched) is beautiful and each goes on sheerer than it appears. Sweet Nothing is a colorless shade without shimmer.

✓ ☺ **MoistureShine Lipstick with SPF 20** *($9.49)* is a comfortably creamy lipstick that deserves strong consideration if you want to combine opaque lip color and sunscreen in one. The sunscreen includes titanium dioxide for UVA protection, while the pigmented shades have impressive staying power (and a range of attractive, "safe" colors). This is definitely a step forward for Neutrogena, and they made good on the moisture and shine portion of this lipstick's name!

☹ **MoistureShine Soothing Lip Sheers SPF 20** *($8.99 for 0.06 ounce)* are sheer, minimally slick glossy lipsticks with an in-part titanium dioxide sunscreen. These would be a slam-dunk (and the shades are attractive) except that the formula includes the irritating menthol derivative menthyl lactate. The tingle may seem refreshing, but it's persistent (there's not just a dusting of this ingredient in here) and not good news.

☹ **MoistureShine Lip Soother Cooling Hydragel SPF 20** *($7.44 for 0.35 ounce)* has a unique balm/lip gloss texture and each of the sheer, juicy colors leaves lips very shiny, but the sunscreen element lacks sufficient UVA-protecting ingredients and the menthol in this product won't do your lips any favors.

MASCARA: ☺ **Healthy Volume Mascara** *($7.99 for 0.21 ounce)* includes a large mascara brush that takes practice and patience to achieve the best results. Once accustomed to it, you'll find this builds impressive length and decent thickness quite fast. Clumping is minimal, and what occurs is easy to neaten without a separate brush. This also keeps lashes very soft, yet doesn't flake or smear, and it removes easily with a water-soluble cleanser. The only drawbacks are the claims, because this standard mascara formula doesn't contain ingredients that plump lashes from the inside. If it did, you could forgo mascara after a week or so because your lashes wouldn't need any more plumping from the mascara, and that just doesn't happen! Not to mention the fact that mascara can't be absorbed into lashes.

☺ **Weightless Volume Mascara** *($7.67 for 0.28 ounce)* is a wax-free mascara that promises full, weightless lashes with no clumps or smudges. It fulfills the latter part of that promise, but is otherwise one of the most do-nothing mascaras available. The fact that this is wax-free is fine if you're bothered by waxes. If not, waxes are an essential problem-free component of most mascaras, as they add fullness and pliability, and help keep mascara on the lashes.

☺ **Healthy Volume Waterproof Mascara** *($8.99)* is supposed to build lashes from the inside out thanks to olive oil. There's no research to support that claim and, thankfully, there's only a minute amount of olive oil present, because oil in mascara can make for short-lived, smear-prone, flaky results. Application-wise, this mascara's large brush is an impediment to getting fast, clean results. If you're careful and take it slow, you can build decent length and thickness with minimal clumping and a soft curl. The formula is "waterproof," and requires an oil- or silicone-based remover when you're ready for it to come off.

☹ **Clean Lash Tint** *($7.99 for 0.09 ounce)* is sold as a gentle tint for eyelashes, and its advertising recommends using it with Acuvue contact lens solution. (Acuvue and Neutrogena are owned by Johnson & Johnson, so this endorsement is hardly impartial.) However, it does absolutely nothing to lengthen or thicken lashes; all you'll get is slightly darker lashes. That would be fine for those blessed with naturally long lashes, but for some inexplicable reason Neutrogena added grapefruit oil to this product.

NIVEA (SKIN CARE ONLY)

NIVEA AT-A-GLANCE

Strengths: Inexpensive.

Weaknesses: Boring formulas; no products to treat breakouts or lighten skin discolorations; limited options for normal to oily skin; anticellulite products are a joke; jar packaging.

Note: Nivea confirmed that they discontinued U.S. sales of their Visage line, which was composed of facial-care products. The body-care products and some lip balms remain the only points of interest for U.S. consumers, though the line continues to offer facial-care products in many other countries (where Nivea has a stronger following).

For more information about Nivea, owned by Beiersdorf, call (800) 227-4703 or visit www. nivea.com or www.Beautypedia.com.

☹ **Nivea Creme** *($7.49 for 6.8 ounces)* remains one of the star products for this line, and Nivea describes it as "the mother of all modern creams." First made available in 1911, the jar-packaged formula with its familiar scent is an exceptionally basic blend of mineral oil, Vaseline, glycerin, and wax. All of these standbys can make dry skin look and feel better, but there are many more ingredients that have significant benefit for skin—ingredients that weren't even close to being options when Nivea Creme launched. Far from "unmatched," there are dozens upon dozens of moisturizers that offer skin more than this cream does, and without the inclusion of sensitizing preservatives methylisothiazolinone and methylchloroisothiazolinone.

☺ **A Kiss of Flavor Cherry Tinted Lip Care** *($2.49 for 0.17 ounce)* is a basic, wax-based, tinted lip balm that does a good job of taking care of dry lips. It is housed in a convenient Chapstick-style container. Interestingly, this contains a couple of sunscreen agents, including avobenzone (listed by its chemical name butyl methoxydibenzoylmethane). However, because these are not listed as active, they shouldn't be relied on for sun protection. The ingredient neo-hesperidin dihydrochalcone is an artificial sweetener that contributes to this lip balm's flavor.

☺ **A Kiss of Flavor Passion Fruit Tinted Lip Care** *($2.49 for 0.17 ounce)* is a basic, wax-based tinted lip balm that does a good job of taking care of dry lips. It is housed in a convenient Chapstick-style container. The ingredient neohesperidin dihydrochalcone is an artificial sweetener that contributes to this lip balm's flavor.

☺ **A Kiss of Moisture Essential Lip Care** *($2.49 for 0.17 ounce)* is a basic, wax-based lip balm that does a good job of taking care of dry lips. It is housed in a convenient Chapstick-style container. It is irritant-free and a reliable, inexpensive option.

The Reviews N

☺ **A Kiss of Moisture Hydrating Lip Care SPF 4** *($2.49 for 0.17 ounce)*. A cosmetics company that develops an SPF 4 product is either ignorant or foolish; either way, the formulators should know better when formulating products for skin care. You're better off not including sunscreen in your lip balm than bothering to formulate one with a measly SPF value of 4 and misleading people to think they are protecting their lips from sun damage. This does include avobenzone for UVA protection, but SPF 15 is the minimum number you should be looking for. This is otherwise a basic, soft-textured lip balm that works to keep lips smooth. The SPF rating is why it isn't rated with a happy face.

☺ **A Kiss of Protection Sun Protection Lip Care SPF 30** *($2.49 for 0.17 ounce)* is a standard wax-based lip balm that also contains an in-part titanium dioxide sunscreen. As such, it's an excellent (and affordable) daytime option to keep lips smooth and protected from environmental damage. With SPF 30, you're getting more than a kiss of protection, and that's good!

☺ **A Kiss of Rejuvenation Q10+ Anti-Aging Lip Care SPF 4** *($3.29 for 0.35 ounce)*. Nivea added coenzyme Q10 to this lip balm with sunscreen, but don't expect it to have much antiwrinkle benefit because it has an embarrassingly low SPF rating. Yes, avobenzone is on hand for UVA protection, but SPF 4 is cheating sun-exposed lips for no good reason. A cosmetics company offering this pathetic level of sun protection should be strung up by their claims. This lip balm with a shimmer finish is not recommended for daytime use, but is an OK option once the sun sets.

☺ **A Kiss of Shimmer Pearly Shimmer Lip Care** *($2.49 for 0.17 ounce)* is a standard waxy lip balm that contains a lot of mica to add shimmer to the lips, just like you'd get from numerous lip glosses, many of which feel better on lips than this product. Interestingly, this contains a couple of sunscreen agents, including avobenzone (listed by its chemical name butyl methoxydibenzoylmethane). However, because these are not listed as active, they shouldn't be relied on for sun protection.

☺ **A Kiss of Shine Natural Glossy Lip Care** *($3.29 for 0.35 ounce)* is a glossy lip balm with a very sheer tint that is a good option for preventing chapped lips while adding an alluring shine without stickiness. Interestingly, this contains a couple of sunscreen agents, including avobenzone (listed by its chemical name butyl methoxydibenzoylmethane). However, because these are not listed as active, they shouldn't be relied on for sun protection.

☺ **A Kiss of Shine Pink Glossy Lip Care** *($3.29 for 0.35 ounce)*. Except for its sheer pink tint, this glossy lip balm is identical to Nivea's A Kiss of Shine Natural Glossy Lip Care. Therefore, the same review applies. This has an alluring shine without stickiness.

☺ **A Kiss of Shine Red Glossy Lip Care** *($3.29 for 0.35 ounce)*. Except for its sheer red tint, this glossy lip balm is identical to Nivea's A Kiss of Shine Natural Glossy Lip Care. Therefore, the same review applies.

☹ **Good-bye Cellulite Patches** *($12.99 for 6 patches)* are gimmicky adhesive patches meant to fit over the thighs, buttocks, or stomach. The adhesive agents can be irritating to skin, there is no research anywhere proving cartinine has a cellulite-diminishing effect, and this patch system isn't preferred over just rubbing the Good-bye Cellulite, Smoothing Cellulite Gel-Cream into your skin. So don't bother to even say hello to this product, unless you're willing to say goodbye to your money and get nothing of value in return.

☹ **Good-bye Cellulite, Smoothing Cellulite Gel-Cream** *($12.99 for 6.7 ounces)* purports to reduce cellulite because it contains L-cartinine. Also known as carboxylic acid, this ingredient is naturally present in our bodies and may be obtained from dietary sources such as red meat. It has unsubstantiated claims of being able to affect fat metabolism when consumed orally. There is no research pertaining to its anticellulite benefit when applied topically, although it likely functions as an antioxidant (Source: www.naturaldatabase.com). This product won't do a thing to improve cellulite, but its alcohol content will irritate your skin and cause inflammation.

☺ **Sun-Kissed Beautiful Legs Shave Minimizing Gradual Tan Moisturizer** (*$9.99 for 6.7 ounces*) is supposed to provide a sun-kissed tan glow to legs while minimizing the need to shave frequently. This lightweight lotion contains nothing that will slow the growth of hair, and the amount of self-tanning ingredient dihydroxyacetone is at best only enough for a subtle tan. What's problematic compared with many better self-tanning products is the amount of alcohol included. It's likely not enough to cause significant irritation, but why take the chance given there are so many self-tanners that omit this ingredient?

☹ **Sun-Kissed Firming Moisturizer** (*$7.49 for 8.4 ounces*) is another round of moisturizers with a small amount of the self-tanning ingredient dihydroxyacetone built in for a bit of color over several days. Nivea's version (available in Light to Medium or Medium to Dark versions) is not preferred to those from Dove or Olay because alcohol is the third ingredient, which makes Nivea's too potentially irritating (but none of these are firming in the least).

NOXZEMA (SKIN CARE ONLY)

NOXZEMA AT-A-GLANCE

Strengths: None.

Weaknesses: Almost all products reviewed contain a blend of camphor, menthol, and eucalyptus oil; none of the anti-acne or anti-blackhead products work as claimed; no topical disinfectant for acne-prone skin; no sunscreens; no moisturizers.

For more information about Noxzema, call (800) 436-4361 or visit www.noxzema.com or www.Beautypedia.com.

NOXZEMA TRIPLE CLEAN PRODUCTS

☺ **Anti-Bacterial Lathering Cleanser** (*$4.99 for 6.5 ounces*) contains 0.3% triclosan, which is a good antibacterial agent that can be a helpful start toward reducing acne-causing bacteria. However, the amount of potassium hydroxide in this cleanser makes it more drying than most, and there are better cleansers with triclosan. This is still an OK option for those with very oily skin who prefer a foaming cleanser.

☺ **Blackhead Cleanser** (*$4.39 for 5 ounces*) contains 2% salicylic acid, but it won't dislodge blackheads because it is rinsed from the skin before it can exert that benefit. This is otherwise a decent water-soluble cleanser for normal to slightly oily skin, and includes scrubbing beads of polyethylene. The small amount of sodium lauryl sulfate is not cause for concern.

☹ **Anti-Blemish Astringent** (*$4.59 for 8 ounces*) serves only to hurt skin with alcohol, peppermint oil, and menthol, which is triple irritation that won't ban one blemish. None of these ingredients offers a positive outcome for blemish-prone skin and the alcohol can trigger more oil production.

☹ **Anti-Blemish Pads** (*$4.49 for 65 pads*) may seem to be a bargain, but severely irritate skin thanks to the potent combination of alcohol, camphor, eucalyptus, and menthol. The alcohol will trigger oil production that may lead to more blemishes.

OTHER NOXZEMA PRODUCTS

☹ **Daily Cream Cleanser** *($5.49 for 7 ounces)* contains camphor, menthol, and eucalyptus oil and is not recommended for any skin type.

☹ **Deep Cleansing Cloths** *($5.96 for 30 cloths)* are similar to the cleansing cloths offered by Olay (Olay and Noxzema are both owned by Procter & Gamble), but are not recommended because they contain menthol.

☹ **Deep Lathering Cleanser** *($4.79 for 7 ounces)* is an alkaline cleanser that, in addition to drying skin, irritates it with menthol, camphor, and eucalyptus oil.

☹ **Long Lasting Microbead Cleanser** *($4.84 for 6 ounces)* contains menthol and is not recommended for any skin type.

☹ **Original Deep Cleansing Cream, Jar** *($4.52 for 10.75 ounces)* is a slightly modified version of the formula that started it all, when this product was launched in 1914 with its "signature scent" of menthol, camphor, and eucalyptus oil. Those irritants are still present, but at least the phenol and lye aren't included anymore. However, that doesn't bring me any closer to recommending this product.

☹ **Original Deep Cleansing Cream, Pump** *($4.89 for 10.5 ounces)* has a slightly different base formula than the Original Deep Cleansing Cream, Jar, but contains the same irritants and is not recommended.

☹ **Plus Moisturizers Deep Cleansing Cream** *($4.49 for 10.75 ounces)* contains camphor, menthol, and eucalyptus oil and is not recommended for any skin type.

☹ **Plus Moisturizers Deep Cleansing Cream, Pump** *($4.89 for 10.5 ounces)* contains camphor, menthol, and eucalyptus oil and is not recommended for any skin type.

☹ **Wet Cleansing Cloths** *($5.96 for 25 cloths)* get skin wet and irritated because the cloths are steeped in menthol, camphor, and eucalyptus oil. Noxzema advises using these to remove mascara, but that's just begging for severe eye (and eyelid) irritation.

☹ **Daily Exfoliating Cleanser** *($4.49 for 6 ounces)* is primarily a scrub, but one that irritates skin because it contains camphor, menthol, and eucalyptus oil.

☹ **Long Lasting Citrus Scrub** *($4.84 for 5 ounces)* contains menthol and is not recommended. Much better topical scrubs are available from Neutrogena, Olay, and L'Oreal.

NU SKIN

NU SKIN AT-A-GLANCE

Strengths: Workable AHA and BHA products; some state-of-the-art moisturizers and serums; several products are fragrance-free; almost all sunscreens include sufficient UVA protection, and most have impressive levels of antioxidants; good lip gloss, sheer powder blush, and makeup brushes.

Weaknesses: Expensive; drying cleansers; irritating toners; Tri-Phasic White products do not noticeably improve skin discolorations; unimpressive masks and "spa-at-home" products; claims are too far from reality; several categories of Nu Skin's makeup are resounding disappointments, including foundation, concealer, and eyeshadows; the brow pencil; the Eyelash Treatment product; average lipsticks.

For more information about Nu Skin, call (800) 487-1000 or visit www.nuskin.com or www.Beautypedia.com.

NU SKIN SKIN CARE

NU SKIN 180° PRODUCTS

☺ **$$$ 180° Face Wash** *($37.05 for 4.2 ounces)* is an overpriced, standard, detergent-based cleanser that contains sodium C14-16 olefin sulfate as the cleansing agent, making it potentially too drying and irritating for skin. There are plant oils in it that can cushion some of the dryness, but why use any irritants whatsoever? The vitamin C it contains will be washed away before it has a chance to have any benefit for skin.

☺ **$$$ 180° Skin Mist** *($30.88 for 3.4 ounces)* is a good but fairly basic toner in mist form for normal to dry skin. It is fragrance-free.

☺ **$$$ 180° AHA Facial Peel** *($57)* is an expensive but effective way to exfoliate skin. The first part of this two-step kit is the **AHA Facial Peel**. This provides 18 pads, each steeped in a water-based solution of 10% lactic acid. The pH of 3.5 ensures exfoliation, and no needless irritants are included. You swipe the pad over your skin and let it sit for at least 10 minutes, at which point you use the **AHA Facial Peel Neutralizer**, which consists of pads soaked with a water-based toner that contains some very good soothing agents. The pH of the Neutralizer stops the peel action, but so would rinsing your skin with plain tap water. At least Nu Skin made these pads better than most companies that sell at-home peel kits. Although this kit will exfoliate skin, you're better off spending less money and using leave-on AHA products that contain between 8% and 10% glycolic or lactic acids, which you leave on your skin, and there are plenty of these products available. Both products in this set are fragrance-free.

☺ **$$$ 180° Cell Renewal Fluid** *($77.43 for 1 ounce)* exfoliates skin with the polyhydroxy acid (PHA) gluconolactone at a 15% concentration and at a pH of 3.2. This is a good alternative to AHA or BHA products, but research has not shown gluconolactone to be a preferred or a gentler option (at least not in a significant way), and a 15% concentration is high and can be irritating for some skin types. This fluid also contains salicylic acid, but the amount is likely too low to boost exfoliation from the gluconolactone. By the way, if you're curious to try a product with gluconolactone, those from NeoStrata are just as effective for a lot less money.

✓ ☺ **$$$ 180° Night Complex** *($66.50 for 1 ounce)* is a brilliant serum for normal to dry skin because it combines ingredients that restore a healthy look and feel to skin while supporting its structural integrity and supplying it with plenty of antioxidants and cell-communicating ingredients. Well done, though why couldn't this be fragrance-free like the other 180° products?

☺ **$$$ 180° UV Block Hydrator SPF 18** *($56.05 for 1 ounce)* is a great in-part zinc oxide sunscreen for normal to dry skin not prone to blemishes. For the money, this should be brimming with state-of-the-art ingredients, which it's not, but at least broad-spectrum sun protection is assured and fragrance is excluded.

NU SKIN CLEAR ACTION ACNE MEDICATION SYSTEM

☺ **$$$ Clear Action Acne Medication Foaming Cleanser** *($23.28 for 3.4 ounces)* is a medicated liquid-to-foam cleanser that contains 0.5% salicylic acid, which in a cleanser isn't on your skin long enough to exert a benefit. Although this is a good cleanser for normal to dry skin, its oil content is not the best for anyone battling blemishes, and makes it somewhat difficult to rinse completely.

☺ **$$$ Clear Action Acne Medication Toner** *($20.43 for 5 ounces)* is a fragrance-free, pH-correct BHA toner; however, the 0.5% concentration of salicylic acid is too low to significantly impact blemishes and blackheads. This toner is fragrance-free and contains soothing agents.

☺ **$$$ Clear Action Acne Medication Day Treatment** *($38 for 1 ounce)* contains 0.5% salicylic acid at a pH of 3.5, and although that allows exfoliation to occur, it would be better if there were more salicylic acid. Still, the amount of AHA lactic acid is likely around 5%, which provides additional exfoliation, and the base formula contains some good anti-irritants.

✓ ☺ **$$$ Clear Action Acne Medication Night Treatment** *($38 for 1 ounce)* is worth considering as an antioxidant serum but not as an anti-acne treatment. That's because the amount of salicylic acid is too low (0.5%) and the pH too high for exfoliation to occur. Antioxidants include green tea, alpha lipoic acid, and vitamin E. This also contains cell-communicating ingredients (including retinol) and anti-irritants.

NU SKIN EPOCH PRODUCTS

☹ **Epoch Cleansing Bar** *($10.74 for 3.4-ounce bar)* is a detergent-based bar cleanser that is similar to Dove's original Beauty Bar. Although more gentle than true soap, it is still drying for all skin types and the ingredients that keep it in bar form can clog pores.

☺ **$$$ Epoch Calming Touch Soothing Skin Cream** *($38 for 1.7 ounces)* is a good lightweight moisturizer for normal to slightly dry skin. Nu Skin positions this as a product meant to reduce redness and scaly skin from eczema or rosacea, but the ingredients they chose show up in hundreds of moisturizers for the face and body. That doesn't mean they're not effective at reducing dry, scaly skin; rather, it's just that they're not unique to this moisturizer. Oddly, this contains the flavoring agent homoanisaldehyde, likely used to impart fragrance.

☹ **Epoch Blemish Treatment** *($12.35 for 0.5 ounce)* contains 2% salicylic acid as an active ingredient, but the pH of 4.1 prevents it from functioning optimally as an exfoliant. This is an ineffective option for blemishes, and is irritating for all skin types due to the fragrant oils it contains.

✓ ☺ **$$$ Epoch Glacial Marine Mud** *($24.70 for 7 ounces)* is a mud mask whose mud is said to be mineral-rich, but minerals aren't a cure for skin problems in the least, nor are they nurturing (especially when delivered in dirt—imagine adding that to your diet). Still, this can be a good absorbent mask for normal to oily skin, and it's fragrance-free.

NU SKIN NUTRICENTIALS PRODUCTS

✓ ☺ **Creamy Cleansing Lotion, for Normal to Dry Skin** *($17.10 for 5 ounces)* is an outstanding cleanser for its intended skin type. Emollients and plant oils combine with a gentle detergent cleansing agent to remove impurities and makeup without leaving a greasy film. Fans of cleansing lotions, take note!

☺ **Pure Cleansing Gel, for Combination to Oily Skin** *($15.20 for 5 ounces)* is a standard, detergent-based, water-soluble cleanser for its intended skin type, but one that's not highly recommended because of the amount of fragrant plant extracts it contains.

☹ **pH Balance Mattefying Toner, for Combination to Oily Skin** *($13.30 for 5 ounces)* lists witch hazel as the second ingredient and also contains some problematic plant extracts, making this toner (which doesn't set to a matte finish) too irritating for all skin types.

☹ **pH Balance Toner, for Normal to Dry Skin** *($13.30 for 5 ounces)* contains witch hazel and camphor, making this a problem toner for any skin type, and it won't restore skin's optimal pH level (our skin is quite adept at doing so on its own anyway), but the irritation this can cause will make dry skin worse.

☹ **Celltrex Ultra Recovery Fluid** *($36.10 for 0.5 ounce)* has a lot going for it, but ends up being a problem for all skin types because it contains orange and lavender oils. Lavender oil doesn't help skin cells recover, it causes cell death and oxidative damage.

☺ **Moisture Restore Day Protective Lotion SPF 15, for Combination to Oily Skin** *($32.30 for 1.7 ounces)* is similar to the Nu Skin 180° UV Block Hydrator SPF 18 reviewed above, except this contains a greater amount of the antioxidant vitamin E. It loses points for including a tiny amount of St. John's wort, which can make skin more sun-sensitive.

☺ **Moisture Restore Day Protective Lotion SPF 15, for Normal to Dry Skin** *($32.30 for 1.7 ounces)* would rate a Paula's Pick if not for the needless inclusion of St. John's wort, which can cause a skin reaction in the presence of sunlight. The fact that this product contains sunscreen (in-part zinc oxide) helps offset this, but not enough to make it a slam-dunk recommendation for normal to dry skin.

☺ **Night Supply Nourishing Cream, for Normal to Dry Skin** *($37.05 for 1.7 ounces)* features some very good ingredients for dry skin, but the jar packaging won't keep the antioxidants and plant oils stable during use; plus the inclusion of St. John's wort wasn't wise. This is an OK option that could've been a lot better.

☺ **Night Supply Nourishing Lotion, for Combination to Oily Skin** *($37.05 for 1.7 ounces)* is a basic, lightweight moisturizer for its intended skin type. It contains mostly water, silicone, glycerin, soothing agent, emollient thickeners, a cell-communicating ingredient, vitamin E, more thickeners, fragrance, and preservatives.

NU SKIN TRI-PHASIC WHITE SYSTEM

☺ **$$$ Tri-Phasic White Cleanser** *($29.93 for 1 ounce)* costs a lot for what amounts to a standard water-soluble foaming cleanser for normal to oily skin. Not a single ingredient in this pricey cleanser can "inhibit the expression of discoloration on the surface of skin." Even if it contained effective skin-lightening agents, they'd be of no use because they'd be rinsed down the drain before they had a chance to work.

☹ **Tri-Phasic White Toner** *($35.63 for 4.2 ounces)* lists witch hazel as the second ingredient, making this too irritating for all skin types. This cannot exfoliate away dark spots, as claimed.

☺ **Tri-Phasic White Day Milk Lotion SPF 15** *($48.93 for 2.5 ounces)* includes avobenzone for UVA protection and wraps it in a silky lotion base for normal to slightly oily or slightly dry skin. A greater array of antioxidants and a cell-communicating ingredient would have netted this daytime moisturizer a higher rating.

☺ **$$$ Tri-Phasic White Night Cream** *($48.93 for 1 ounce)* is a lightweight, jar-packaged moisturizer formulated with the ingredient diacetyl boldine, which Nu Skin claims works to disrupt the activation phase of skin pigmentation, when melanin (skin pigment) is created. Diacetyl boldine appears to have antioxidant ability but, as this book goes to print, there is still no independent, peer-reviewed research supporting its claim of being able to suppress melanin production. Therefore, I wouldn't count on this otherwise OK moisturizer for slightly dry skin to do anything other than make skin feel softer and smoother.

☺ **$$$ Tri-Phasic White Radiance Mask** *($70.78 for 8 masks)* provides a collection of individually packaged, fragrance-free, pre-moistened masks that contain a good blend of water-binding agents and antioxidants. None of the ingredients in these masks has substantiated research supporting Nu Skin's claims of inhibiting any phase of hyperpigmentation, but they can make skin look and feel better.

The Reviews N

☹ **Tri-Phasic White Essence** *($59.85 for 1 ounce)* contains a good deal of lemon peel extract, whose volatile components can cause irritation. This isn't helped by the lesser amount of peppermint extract, and to top it off, not a single ingredient in this misguided product can have even a slight impact on skin discolorations. Animal testing has shown that lemon peel can cause a phototoxic reaction on skin in as little as three minutes, even when sunscreen is worn (Source: *Photodermatology, Photoimmunology, and Photomedicine*, December 2005, pages 318-321), and it is known to cause contact dermatitis in people, making it something to avoid.

NU SKIN TRU FACE PRODUCTS

☹ **Tru Face Priming Solution** *($35.63 for 4.2 ounces)* contains some helpful, amino acid-based water-binding agents for skin, but the amount of witch hazel makes this toner too irritating for all skin types. A product like this isn't essential to "prepare" skin for the benefits of other Tru Face products.

☺ **$$$ Tru Face Essence** *($140.60 for 60 capsules)* includes mostly silicone, thickeners, plant oils, and antioxidants packaged in tiny capsules meant for single use. The packaging is a good way to keep the antioxidants stable, though it would be better if they were more prominent in this product. For the money, these aren't as elegant as the Ceramide capsules from Elizabeth Arden, which cost half as much for the same amount of product.

✓ ☺ **$$$ Tru Face IdealEyes Eye Refining Cream** *($43.70 for 0.5 ounce)* was designed to send under-eye bags packing, but this fragrance-free eye cream cannot accomplish what genetics, time, sun damage, and an aging face create. What it can do is moisturize and smooth, while supplying skin with a good amount of stabilized vitamin C and lesser, but still potentially effective, amounts of other antioxidants and cell-communicating ingredients.

☹ **$$$ Tru Face Instant Line Corrector** *($67.93 for 0.5 ounce)* is Nu Skin's "works like Botox" product, claiming to relax forehead wrinkles and expression lines. The company's literature for this product mentions the "heavy risks" associated with Botox injections, but the only convincing "risk" they could come up with was the ongoing expense (I admit, Botox isn't a value-driven procedure). Formula-wise, this silicone-enriched moisturizer contains aminobutyric acid, also known as GABA. However, GABA does not inhibit muscle contractions that lead to expression lines. For a detailed explanation of this ingredient, please refer to the *Cosmetic Ingredient Dictionary* on www.Beautypedia.com. This product can make skin feel silky-smooth and, to a small, temporary extent, fill in superficial lines on the face. It actually could have been a lot more impressive than it is if a broader range of state-of-the-art ingredients had been included.

☹ **$$$ Tru Face Line Corrector** *($45.60 for 1 ounce)* is a basic, lightweight, silicone-based moisturizer that contains palmitoyl-pentapeptide-3. In theory, this and other peptides are cell-communicating ingredients that also function as water-binding agents. The antiwrinkle claims come from studies that were funded by the companies that sell these peptides to the cosmetics industry, so they're hardly impartial. This is still a good, basic moisturizer for normal to slightly oily or slightly dry skin.

☹ **$$$ Tru Face Revealing Gel** *($45.13 for 1 ounce)* is similar to the Nu Skin 180° Cell Renewal Fluid reviewed above, except this version contains less gluconolactone (the company did not reveal the percentage difference, but this product appears to have less than a 5% concentration). It is an OK lightweight gel moisturizer for oily skin, but isn't likely to have a noticeable impact on pores—at least not to the extent that dry-finish silicone serums can.

☺ **$$$ Tru Face Skin Perfecting Gel** *($51.78 for 1 ounce)* is a water-based serum that contains a blend of skin-identical ingredients and a small amount of antioxidants. Don't believe the claims that this can stave off the first signs of aging and restructure your skin's collagen, because it absolutely can't do that; do believe, however, that it's a good serum for normal to oily skin, and will work well under makeup.

OTHER NU SKIN PRODUCTS

☺ **Nu Colour Eye Makeup Remover** *($9.50 for 1.76 ounces)* is a silicone-in-water fluid that includes a wax-based ingredient and plant oils to thoroughly remove all types of makeup. The oils contribute a slightly greasy film, making this a product that you should use before your regular cleanser. It is fragrance-free.

☺ **Exfoliant Scrub Extra Gentle** *($13.78 for 3.4 ounces)* contains mostly water, aloe, thickener, seashells (as an abrasive), and vitamins. The seashells can be rough on the skin, so calling this product gentle is a stretch, but it is a good exfoliant for most skin types, even though a washcloth would work as well if not better.

☺ **Facial Scrub** *($13.78 for 3.4 ounces)* is gentler than the Exfoliant Scrub Extra Gentle, despite the name difference. This one contains finely milled walnut-shell powder and husk, which work as a scrub, and it can be good for someone with normal to dry skin.

☹ **$$$ Polishing Peel Skin Refinisher** *($27.55 for 1.7 ounces)* is a clay- and cornstarch-based scrub that isn't as elegant or as rinsable as the two Nu Skin scrubs. The pumpkin enzymes are too unstable to provide extra exfoliation. This is not similar to a microdermabrasion procedure any more than an efficiency apartment is similar to a mansion.

✓ ☺ **NaPCA Moisture Mist** *($10.93 for 8.4 ounces)* is an above-average fragrance-free, spray-on toner for all skin types. The alcohol-free formula contains several skin-identical ingredients and the cell-communicating ingredient niacinamide.

✓ ☺ **$$$ Celltrex CoQ10 Complete** *($48.45 for 0.5 ounce)* supplies skin with a healthy dose of several antioxidants, including ubiquinone (coenzyme Q10). It also contains a cell-communicating ingredient, water-binding agents, and anti-irritants. In short, this fragrance-free, water-based serum is highly recommended for all skin types.

☺ **Enhancer Skin Conditioning Gel** *($13.30 for 4 ounces)* is an OK basic ultralight, gel-based moisturizer for oily skin. It lacks antioxidants but contains several water-binding agents. As claimed, this can be a soothing after-shave product for men.

☹ **Face Lift, Original Formula** *($34.96)* includes the **Face Lift Powder** and the **Face Lift Activator**. These two formulas are meant to be mixed together and then applied to your skin. The Lift Powder contains egg white, cornstarch, and some water-binding agents. The Activator contains water, aloe, some water-binding agents, and preservatives. This won't lift skin anywhere, and the egg white and cornstarch can be skin irritants. In addition, the cornstarch can promote bacterial growth, which isn't good news for blemish-prone skin.

☹ **Face Lift, Sensitive Formula** *($35.63)* is similar to the Face Lift, Original Formula above, except the egg white is replaced by a gum-based thickener and the Activator portion is just a water- and aloe-based toner. This isn't preferred for sensitive skin because the cornstarch can be a problem, and none of this will lift skin one bit.

☺ **$$$ HPX Hydrating Gel** *($50.35 for 1.7 ounces)* contains some intriguing ingredients, but I can't imagine most consumers being impressed by the fact that this contains human placental protein, at least I hope not. Plus, there is nothing about human placental protein that has any unique benefit for skin. Beyond that gimmick, this fragrance-free blend of oil, vitamin E, fatty acids, and preservatives is a good moisturizer for dry skin.

☺ **$$$ Intensive Eye Complex** *($38.95 for 0.5 ounce)* is a decent lightweight moisturizer for slightly dry skin anywhere on the face. It's disappointing that the really intriguing ingredients barely make a showing, though this product is fragrance-free.

☺ **Moisture Restore Intense Moisturizer** *($30.40 for 2.5 ounces)* offers those with dry to very dry skin some helpful ingredients to restore moisture and radiance, but the jar packaging means the antioxidants (of which there's very little) won't remain stable during use.

☺ **NaPCA Moisturizer** *($25.65 for 2.5 ounces)* is an option for normal to dry skin, but what a shame the many antioxidants are subject to breaking down once this jar-packaged product is opened.

☺ **Rejuvenating Cream** *($32.30 for 2.5 ounces)* is very similar to the Moisture Restore Intense Moisturizer above, and the same review applies.

☺ **Clay Pack** *($13.78 for 3.4 ounces)* is a standard clay mask with small amounts of water-binding agents and antioxidants. This is an option for normal to oily skin.

☹ **Creamy Hydrating Masque** *($19 for 3.4 ounces)* ends up being more irritating than indulgent for skin because it contains lavender and sage oils along with pinecone extract. None of these help protect dry skin from harsh environmental conditions.

☹ **Galvanic Spa** *($36.10 for 4 treatments)* is a gimmicky "treatment" system consisting of **Galvanic Spa Pre-Treatment Gel**, which is mostly water, slip agent, film-forming agent, and several plant extracts, and **Galvanic Spa Treatment Gel**, which has a similar formula but also contains an ingredient that has a warming effect on skin, along with fragrant plant extracts that can be irritating. The warming effect can stimulate circulation and cause reddened skin, but this effect is more detrimental than helpful due to the manner in which it is caused, via irritation. It would be much more beneficial to stimulate circulation by exercising rather than wasting time and money on this mostly do-nothing duo.

☹ **Sunright Lip Balm SPF 15** *($7.13 for 0.15 ounce)* lacks the UVA-protecting ingredients of titanium dioxide, zinc oxide, avobenzone, Mexoryl SX (ecamsule), or Tinosorb and is not recommended.

NU SKIN SUN & SELF-TANNING PRODUCTS

☹ **Sunless Tanner** *($21.90 for 3.4 ounces)* lists witch hazel as the second ingredient, which makes this otherwise well-formulated but standard self-tanner too irritating for all skin types.

✓ ☺ **Sunright Body Block SPF 15** *($15.20 for 3.4 ounces)* is nearly identical to the Sunright Body Block SPF 30, except this contains a lower total concentration of active ingredients, resulting in its reduced SPF rating. Otherwise, the same comments apply.

✓ ☺ **Sunright Body Block SPF 30** *($15.20 for 3.4 ounces)* is an excellent, in-part avobenzone water-resistant sunscreen for normal to dry skin. It not only provides broad-spectrum sun protection but also boosts the skin's defenses with antioxidants and soothing agents. Another bonus: the price isn't so high that it's going to discourage liberal application

NU SKIN MAKEUP

FOUNDATION: ☹ **Nu Colour MoisturShade Liquid Finish SPF 15** *($22.80)*, which lacks reliable UVA protection, is a moist-finish, light-coverage foundation that comes in ten noticeably peach, pink, rose, or orange tones. Who thought any of these shades would look convincing on real skin tones? It's a shame these two major faults overwhelm an otherwise well-formulated product, but there you have it.

☹ **Nu Colour Skin Beneficial Tinted Moisturizer SPF 15** *($26.60)* lacks significant UVA protection, which is odd given that Nu Skin's sunscreens do a good job of protecting in that range. That's unfortunate, because this has a light, elegant application that blends superbly to a dry matte finish. The five colors tend to get peachier the darker you go, but this is sheer enough that the peachiness is not an issue. What is an issue (beyond the lack of good UVA protection) is that the base formula lists the irritant witch hazel as the first ingredient, which makes this not worth considering over tinted moisturizers with sunscreen from Bobbi Brown, Aveda, or Neutrogena.

CONCEALER: ☹ **Nu Colour Skin Beneficial Concealer** *($19)* is a cream concealer with a greasy consistency and far too much slip to cover evenly and stay in place. The colors are uniformly unflattering, but even more troublesome is the inclusion of ylang-ylang and sandalwood oils, which have no business being around the eyes (or anywhere on skin for that matter).

POWDER: ☺ **$$$ Nu Colour Custom Colour MoisturShade Wet/Dry Pressed Powder** *($19)* feels very soft, almost creamy, and blends nicely to a dry, light-coverage finish. However, this mica-based powder has shine despite Nu Skin's claim of it being matte. Four of the six shades have an unattractive peach, pink, or rose cast that's strong enough to matter, especially in daylight. The only possible contenders are Buffed Ivory and Creamy Ivory.

☺ **$$$ Finishing Powder** *($23.28)* is a talc-free, rice starch–based powder, so this has a drier texture that can feel a bit grainy. It comes in one shade, and while Nu Skin claims that it's translucent, this will look too white or ashen on all but fair skin, sort of like using plain baby powder to set your makeup.

BLUSH AND BRONZER: ☺ **$$$ Subtle Effects Blush** *($15.20)* is indeed subtle, as each of the six sheer colors attests. It takes some effort to build noticeable color, but the application is smooth and even with just a hint of shine. If you're looking for sheer blush, this is one to consider.

☺ **$$$ Nu Colour Bronzing Pearls** *($35.63)* are bronze-colored powder beads that you sweep a brush over and dust on to complete your sheer, shiny tan. The Body Shop has had this type of product for years, and if the concept appeals to you, check out their less expensive Brush-On Bronze.

EYESHADOW: ☹ **Custom Colour Desired Effects Eye Shadow** *($10.93)* is sold as eyeshadow singles and all have a silky, silicone-based texture, but the shine (present in all of the shades, often to a sparkling degree) flakes regardless of how careful or sheer your application is. Given the number of shiny eyeshadows that don't have this problem, why would you want to consider this?

EYE AND BROW SHAPER: ☺ **Defining Effects Smooth Eye Liner** *($11.40)* is a standard, creamy eye pencil that needs sharpening. It's easy to apply, but like most creamy pencils is prone to smudging and fading before the day is done. If you're curious to try this, avoid the Sapphire and Blue Smoke shades.

☹ **Nu Colour Defining Effects Brow Liner** *($11.40)* needs to be sharpened and you'll be doing a lot of that if you choose this creamy pencil. The colors go on strong, so achieving a softly defined, natural brow is almost impossible; plus this will smudge before the end of the day, which is hardly a strong selling point.

LIPSTICK, LIP GLOSS, AND LIPLINER: ☺ **$$$ Nu Colour Contouring Lip Gloss** *($16.63)* doesn't contour the lips; it is just a shimmer-infused, semi-thick gloss dispensed from a tube that is minimally sticky and yet tenacious enough to not require a touch-up within an hour. The oligopeptide in this product is said to make lips fuller, but there is no proof of that, and even if there were, the amount of it in this product is minuscule.

☺ **$$$ Nu Colour Replenishing Lipstick** *($16.63)* contains more than enough emollient oils to replenish dry lips, but it's too much of a good thing if you were hoping for a creamy lipstick that stays in place and lasts until lunch. This does neither, as it migrates into any lines around the mouth shortly after application. Most of the medium- to full-coverage colors are very attractive, but this is one greasy lipstick!

☺ **Nu Colour Defining Effects Smooth Lipliner** *($11.40)* is nothing unique as far as pencils are concerned, but this sharpen-me tool has a smooth application and a small, but respectable, color collection.

MASCARA: ☺ **$$$ Defining Effects Mascara** *($18.05)* remains an average contender, offering only modest lash enhancement even with considerable effort. It keeps lashes soft and doesn't flake or smear, but is only worth the investment if you aren't expecting much as far as length or thickness is concerned.

☹ **Nu Colour Nutriol Eyelash Treatment** *($26.13)* is a clear mascara that is supposed to be a conditioning treatment for lashes, complete with a swanky European pedigree. Ingredients like PVP (a film-forming agent typically used in hair gels), butylene glycol, and witch hazel are not conditioning in the least, and these are the backbone of this waste-of-time-and-money product.

BRUSHES: ☺ **$$$ Cosmetic Brush Collection** *($59.50)* comes in a cloth case that would be better suited to housing bathroom grooming accessories (think nail clippers, disposable razors, and cuticle nippers) than the seven elegant, well-made brushes it holds. The **Powder** and **Blush** brushes are well-shaped and suitably soft while the two **Eyeshadow** brushes cover the basics for a classic eye design. The **Eyeliner** brush can double as a brow brush, and the rubber smudge tip at the opposite end is an option for creating soft, smoky eyes. If only the case were better, this set would have warranted a Paula's Pick rating. All of the brushes are also sold separately, ranging in price from $8 to $15.

NYX COSMETICS (MAKEUP ONLY)

NYX COSMETICS AT-A-GLANCE

Strengths: NYX provides complete ingredient lists on its Web site; inexpensive for such quality makeup; superior eyeshadows; the non-waterproof mascaras are terrific.

Weaknesses: The complete line, which is huge, is available only from the company's Web site, which means you can't see or test the colors in person (and the company doesn't offer samples); the waterproof mascara isn't waterproof, not even a little.

NYX Cosmetics customer service number is (866) 699-1004 or you can visit www.nyxcosmetics.com or beautypedia.com.

MAKEUP REMOVER: ☺ **Eye & Lip Makeup Remover** *($6 for 4 ounces)* is a very standard but good liquid makeup remover that contains silicone and solvents. It quickly removes even the most stubborn or waterproof makeup. This would be rated a Paula's Pick if it didn't contain fragrance and fragrant orange extract, two ingredients you should be wary of using so close to the eyes.

EYESHADOW: The powder ✓ ☺ **Eyeshadow** *($4.99)* is marvelous and definitely a must-see if you're interested in NYX Cosmetics. It has a velvety-smooth texture that applies and blends superbly (no flaking), even though most of the colors don't skimp on pigment. The company sells an overwhelming collection of 160 shades, of which Ulta stores (the primary retail source for NYX in the United States) stock a couple dozen. There are plenty of matte shades in classic neutral to brown tones, and these work beautifully as powder eyeliner or for defining and filling in eyebrows. You'll also find shades with a metallic, shimmer, sheer, and glitter finish, with the glitter finish being the least desirable. Given the vast number of shades, there are plenty to avoid, including several pink, red, green, vivid blue, bright yellow, and orange hues, none of which work to create sexy, sophisticated eye shaping and shading. Note that the darker shades tend to grab a bit and require more skill to blend, but they certainly hold up well.

☺ **Triple Shadows for Sexy Babe's Eyes Only!** *($7.99)*. You don't have to be a sexy babe to use these eyeshadow trios, but without question you can create all kinds of eye designs with the 45 different trios available. These shadows have a very smooth, slightly dry texture that's not quite as elegant as NYX's single eyeshadows, but is still worth strong consideration. Application is even and color payoff is strong, so a little goes a long way unless you want a dramatic effect. The best trios are Honeycomb, White/Gray/Black, Nude/Taupe/Dark Brown, Highlight/Brown/Suede, Aloha/Mink Brown/Deep Bronze, Sahara/Suede/Chocolate, Very Delight, Rock & Roll, In the Woods, and Copacabana. Unless you want a deliberately colorful eye design that doesn't shape or shade the eye, avoid the many trios with combinations of blue, green, bright pink, orange, and turquoise.

☺ **Jumbo Eyeshadow Pencil** *($3.99)* is a chunky pencil that requires routine sharpening. It has a soft tip that will smush down if you apply more than a light pressure, which doesn't make it any more appealing. Otherwise, this has a creamy texture and smooth application that impart rich color and a shimmer finish that borders on metallic. The creaminess sets to a slightly moist finish that won't resist creasing, making this product not preferred to NYX's powder eyeshadows.

EYE AND BROW SHAPER: ☺ **Felt Tip Liner** *($7.99)* is an excellent liquid eyeliner whose felt-tip pen applicator enables you to create a line that's as thin or thick as you wish. It smooths on beautifully and deposits color evenly. Dry time is quick and once set this doesn't budge, though you may notice slight fading before the end of the day. This would be rated a Paula's Pick if it did not contain fragrant rosemary extract, a plant that may cause irritation along the lash line.

☺ **Eye/Eyebrow Pencil** *($2.99)* is a very standard, slightly creamy eye pencil that is also workable for filling in brows. It glides on and sets to a slightly moist finish that won't make brow hairs look greasy or matted. This pencil needs routine sharpening, but if that doesn't bother you, the price is right and all the classic (and some not-so-classic) shades are available.

LIPSTICK, LIP GLOSS, AND Lipliner: ✓ ☺ **Goddess of the Night Lip Gloss with Mega Shine** *($4.99)* is a very good lip gloss that includes a longer sponge-tip applicator that comes to a rounded point. It takes some getting used to, but this type of applicator makes it easier to apply gloss precisely. The very smooth texture feels emollient, isn't the least bit sticky, and has the expected glossy shine. The shade range is enormous, offering a colorless shade and everything beyond that, from hot pink to rich reds and dark browns. Several of the shades have a much stronger color deposit than standard gloss, so this isn't a gloss to consider if your operative word is "sheer."

☺ **Lip Smacking Fun Colors** *($3.99)* is a standard, but good, cream lipstick that's available in a dizzying array of over 140 shades. Honestly, if you can't find a color you like from this selection, you probably shouldn't be wearing lipstick! Ulta stores (where NYX cosmetics are primarily sold in the United States) stock perhaps 10% of what's available online. Note: This product is listed on the NYX Cosmetics Web site as **Round Lipstick**—Why? Who knows? Their customer service people didn't return our phone calls.

☺ **Lip Liner Pencil** *($2.99)* is an average lip pencil that needs routine sharpening. It's unremarkable in every respect except for the shades, which include many unusual options. This is worth a look if you can't find a lip pencil to match an atypical shade of lipstick. Note: This is listed on the company's Web site as **Slim Pencil Eye & Lip**.

☺ **Jumbo Lip Pencil** *($2.99)* is a chunky, needs-sharpening pencil whose high wax content is inelegant and makes it feel slightly greasy even after it's applied. It quickly creeps into lines around the mouth and the shade selection (at least what Ulta stores stock) is unusually dark (think Goth colors). You can find a broader shade range on the NYX Cosmetics Web site, but I wouldn't encourage you to try this unless you prefer lipstick in pencil form and don't have lines around the mouth.

MASCARA: ✓ ☺ **Doll Eye Mascara Volume** *($10.99)* excels at quickly creating long lashes you'll want to go out and flutter. The name is apropos because with a few coats you'll have beautifully long lashes resembling those on a doll. This builds slight thickness and doesn't clump, smear, or flake.

✓ ☺ **Doll Eye Mascara Longlash** *($10.99)* sells itself as a lengthening option, but it actually builds equal parts length and thickness. If really long lashes are what you want, NYX's Doll Eye Mascara Volume is the one to choose. But this Longlash version is an excellent all-purpose mascara that wears without a hitch and is easy to remove with a water-soluble cleanser.

☺ **Doll Eye Mascara Waterproof** *($10.99)*. What a shame this mascara isn't the least bit waterproof! It dissolves (actually, it begins running right down your cheeks) with a mere splash of water. Application-wise, this produces impressive length and slight thickness, but it can go on a bit unevenly.

FACE AND BODY ILLUMINATING/SHIMMER PRODUCTS: ☺ **Glitter Cream Palette** *($6.39)* is simply large, very shiny particles of glitter mixed in a base of waxes, oil, and lanolin. The waxy base allows the glitter to cling to skin much better than it would if you just dusted on loose glitter, but application is wildly uneven no matter whether you use a brush or your fingertip. This is best for costume or special effects makeup, not for creating alluring gleam for evening makeup.

OLAY (SKIN CARE ONLY)

OLAY AT-A-GLANCE

Strengths: Inexpensive (mostly); several outstanding water-soluble cleansers and scrubs; all sunscreens include UVA-protecting ingredients; some good BHA options (but the low pH is a concern); bountiful selection of state-of-the-art serums and some excellent moisturizers; some of the best products offer fragrance-free versions.

Weaknesses: Bar cleansers; no AHA products; no topical disinfectant for blemishes; random products contain menthol; more than a handful of dated moisturizers; jar packaging; several moisturizers with sunscreen don't offer skin much beyond basic sun protection; repetitive formulas make this line confusing and tricky to shop.

For more information about Olay, owned by Procter & Gamble, call (800) 285-5170 or visit www.olay.com or www.Beautypedia.com.

OLAY AGE DEFYING PRODUCTS

☺ **Age Defying Daily Renewal Cleanser** *($5.99 for 6.78 ounces)* is a good cleansing lotion/scrub for normal to dry skin, though the beta hydroxy complex will not exfoliate skin due to its brief contact and the too high pH. What will exfoliate mildly are the polyethylene beads this cleanser contains.

☺ **Age Defying Anti-Wrinkle Daily SPF 15 Lotion** *($14.99 for 3.4 ounces)* is a lightweight, water- and glycerin-based daytime moisturizer that includes an in-part avobenzone sunscreen. Olay draws attention to this product's pro-retinol and beta hydroxy acid content, but the formula contains neither retinol nor salicylic acid. What it does contain is a small amount of retinyl propionate. Similar to the more commonly used retinyl palmitate, retinyl propionate is a retinoid ester that must be converted to a more active form by enzymes in the skin. Retinyl propionate is apparently more stable and less irritating than retinol, yet offers a similar benefit to skin. However, research on this retinol alternative is scant. And with the most current information coming from dermatologist Dr. Zoe Diana Draelos, who is a consultant to Procter & Gamble (Olay's parent company), it's not exactly impartial. Assuming that retinyl propionate is more stable than retinol (and that's only an assumption because there is no substantiated proof) doesn't fully explain why Olay chose to package this moisturizer in a translucent bottle, which doesn't help keep ingredients stable. Still, it's a good option for someone with normal to slightly oily skin. And, as with most of Olay's latest moisturizers, it includes plenty of skin-beneficial niacinamide.

☺ **Age Defying Anti-Wrinkle Eye Cream** *($14.99 for 0.5 ounce)* is a light-textured, silky moisturizer for slightly dry skin anywhere on the face that contains many commendable ingredients. The problem is that most of the beneficial ingredients will degrade soon after you start using the product because of the jar packaging (something Olay is typically good about avoiding). This product also contains an unusually high number of preservatives, including dmdm hydantoin, which can be a problem for skin, especially in the sensitive eye area.

☺ **Age Defying Anti-Wrinkle Replenishing Night Cream** *($14.99 for 2 ounces)* is similar to the Age Defying Anti-Wrinkle Daily SPF 15 Lotion, minus the sunscreen. It is not rated as highly because the jar packaging will not help keep the antioxidant vitamins stable during use.

☺ **Age Defying Daily Renewal Cream** *($10.99 for 2 ounces)* is an option as a BHA product due to its salicylic acid content (approximately 2%), but the pH of 2.3 is unusually low and may prove too irritating for daily use, so proceed with caution. The base formula is best for normal to slightly dry or slightly oily skin.

☺ **Age Defying Intensive Nourishing Night Cream** *($11.49 for 2 ounces)* is similar to the Age Defying Daily Renewal Cream, and the same review applies.

☺ **Age Defying Protective Renewal Lotion SPF 15** *($10.99 for 4 ounces)* contains an in-part zinc oxide sunscreen, but that's the only exciting element in this rather bland moisturizer for normal to slightly dry skin. The moisturizers with sunscreen in Olay's Regenerist, Total Effects, and Definity lines are more exciting.

☹ **Age Defying Revitalizing Eye Gel** *($10.99 for 0.5 ounce)* lists witch hazel distillate as the second ingredient, which makes this gel too irritating for all skin types.

The Reviews O

OLAY COMPLETE PRODUCTS

☺ **Complete Ageless Rejuvenating Lathering Cleanser** *($8.49 for 6.5 ounces)* is a standard water-soluble cleanser that contains gentle scrubbing beads for enhanced cleansing. It doesn't guarantee ageless skin and the antioxidants will be rinsed down the drain before they can impact skin, but it's suitable for all skin types.

☺ **Complete Lathering Cleanser** *($7.99 for 6 ounces)* is a standard but good water-soluble cleanser for normal to oily skin. It rinses completely and is capable of removing all but the most tenacious or waterproof makeup formulas.

☺ **Complete Ageless Eye Brightening Cream** *($24.99 for 0.5 ounce)* has a lush, silky texture and contains some beneficial antioxidants. What a shame jar packaging will render them ineffective shortly after you begin using it. The amount of niacinamide is impressive and this B vitamin doesn't break down in the presence of light and air, so that's helpful. Although this is an option for slightly dry skin anywhere on the face, Olay offers better moisturizers (including those labeled as special for the eye area).

✓ ☺ **Complete Ageless Skin Renewing UV Lotion SPF 20** *($24.99 for 2.5 ounces)* is an excellent daytime moisturizer for normal to slightly dry or slightly oily skin. UVA protection is assured from avobenzone, and this has a beautifully silky texture that feels great and works well under makeup. Best of all, skin is treated to a bevy of helpful ingredients, including niacinamide and efficacious levels of antioxidants. The amount of vitamin C is too small to matter and this contains fragrance, but that's not enough to keep it from earning my highest recommendation.

☺ **Complete All Day Moisture Cream SPF 15, for Combination/Oily Skin** *($7.99 for 2 ounces)* is a slightly more emollient version of Olay's Age Defying Protective Renewal Lotion SPF 15 reviewed above, and the same review applies.

☺ **Complete All Day Moisture Cream SPF 15, for Normal Skin** *($8.49 for 2 ounces)* is nearly identical to the Complete All Day Moisture Cream SPF 15, for Combination/Oily Skin, and the same comments apply.

☺ **Complete All Day Moisture Cream SPF 15, for Sensitive Skin** *($7.99 for 2 ounces)* is nearly identical to the Complete All Day Moisture Cream SPF 15, for Combination/Oily Skin, except this version omits the fragrance. Otherwise, the same comments apply.

☺ **Complete All Day Moisture Lotion SPF 15, for Combination/Oily Skin** *($10.99 for 6 ounces)* features an in-part zinc oxide sunscreen in a lightweight lotion base suitable for its intended skin type. Aside from broad-spectrum sun protection and a silky texture, skin will be left wanting more, though this works well under makeup.

☺ **Complete All Day Moisture Lotion SPF 15, for Normal Skin** *($10.99 for 6 ounces)* is nearly identical to the Complete All Day Moisture Lotion SPF 15, for Combination/Oily Skin, and the same comments apply.

☺ **Complete All Day Moisture Lotion SPF 15, for Sensitive Skin** *($10.99 for 6 ounces)* is nearly identical to the Complete All Day Moisture Lotion SPF 15, for Combination/Oily Skin, minus fragrance. Otherwise, the same comments apply.

☺ **Complete Defense Daily UV Moisturizer SPF 30** *($14.99 for 2.5 ounces)* is a great, in-part avobenzone sunscreen in a lightweight moisturizing base that is a fine option for normal to dry skin. The base formula isn't too exciting, but Olay did include an appreciable amount of their favorite vitamin, niacinamide, which can help skin retain moisture and may help skin cells function better. The other vitamins, antioxidants, and soothing plant extracts are barely present and don't amount to much for skin. This product does contain fragrance.

☺ **Complete Defense Daily UV Moisturizer SPF 30, for Sensitive Skin** (*$14.99 for 2.5 ounces*) has a lighter moisturizing base than the Complete Defense Daily UV Moisturizer SPF 30 above, but includes 6% zinc oxide. Although zinc oxide provides excellent broad-spectrum protection, it can also leave a whitish cast on the skin when used in this amount. Because Olay included other synthetic sunscreen active ingredients, this is not a slam-dunk choice for sensitive skin (zinc oxide or titanium dioxide are the most gentle choices for this skin type). This fragrance-free daily sunscreen would be best for normal to slightly dry skin not prone to blemishes. It contains a less impressive amount of niacinamide than the Complete Defense Daily UV Moisturizer SPF 30.

☺ **Complete Night Fortifying Cream** (*$14.99 for 2 ounces*) is a lightweight moisturizer for normal to dry skin, but regrettably the antioxidants it contains will deteriorate due to the jar packaging. Several other Olay products have better formulations in packaging that will keep the air- and light-sensitive ingredients well protected.

☺ **Complete Plus Ultra-Rich Day Cream SPF 15, for Extra Dry Skin** (*$12.99 for 2 ounces*) is not ultra-rich in the least. In fact, this is very similar to Olay's Complete All Day Moisture Cream SPF 15, for Combination/Oily Skin, and the same comments apply.

☺ **Complete Plus Ultra-Rich Moisture Lotion SPF 15, for Extra Dry Skin** (*$10.59 for 4 ounces*) has a base formula that's way too light for someone with extra-dry skin. However, this can be an OK, in-part zinc oxide sunscreen for normal to oily skin. The tiny amount of vegetable oil won't make skin oilier and certainly won't provide "intense moisture."

☺ **Complete Plus Ultra-Rich Night Firming Cream, for Extra Dry Skin** (*$12.49 for 2 ounces*) contains some helpful ingredients for dry skin, but someone with extra-dry skin will likely find this formula lacking. The jar packaging won't keep the vitamin E and other antioxidants stable during use.

☺ **Complete Plus Ultra-Rich Tinted Moisturizer, for Extra Dry Skin** (*$11.49 for 1.7 ounces*) is a sheer tinted moisturizer that isn't all that moisturizing, especially as it lists alcohol as the fourth ingredient. There are some ingredients present that are good for dry skin, but the alcohol automatically makes this a lighter product. Olay missed an opportunity to give women an all-in-one option by not including any sunscreen—a strange oversight given how many of the Complete products have very good sunscreens. There are better tinted moisturizer options available at similar prices from Neutrogena and Revlon.

☺ **Complete Touch of Sun Daily UV Facial Moisturizer SPF 15** (*$14.99 for 2.5 ounces*) combines the self-tanning agent dihydroxyacetone (DHA) with an in-part avobenzone sunscreen for color with protection. Not a bad idea, assuming you'll still apply this liberally. Although labeled to imply a sheer hint of color, the amount of DHA in both the Light/Medium and Medium/ Darker versions is similar to what you'd see in a standard self-tanner, so do expect more color.

OLAY DAILY FACIALS PRODUCTS

☹ **Daily Facials Deep Cleansing Cloths, for Combination/Oily Skin** (*$6.49 for 30 cloths*) contains menthol and is not recommended for any skin type.

☺ **Daily Facials Express Wet Cleansing Cloths, for Sensitive Skin** (*$5.99 for 30 cloths*) are an admirable cleansing option for sensitive skin, eschewing fragrance and drying cleansing agents in favor of glycerin, slip agents, and silicones. This combination does not cleanse skin or remove makeup very well, but is fine for a refresher between normal face washings with a regular cleanser. The only ingredient caution for this product is for sensitive skin because it contains dmdm hydantoin, a formaldehyde-releasing preservative. There is nothing about this product that can't be replaced by a gentle cleanser and a washcloth.

☺ **Daily Facials Express Wet Cleansing Cloths, for All Skin Types** (*$5.99 for 30 cloths*) are identical to the Daily Facial Express Wet Cleansing Cloths, for Sensitive Skin, except that these contain fragrance. If that's important to you (it isn't important for good skin care), these are the cloths to choose. There is nothing about this product that isn't replaced by a gentle cleanser and a washcloth.

☺ **Daily Facials Hydrating Cleansing Cloths, for Normal to Dry Skin** (*$7.49 for 30 cloths*) have a gentle formula that can be a very good option for their intended skin types, though the lather they produce requires thorough rinsing to avoid a slightly greasy film. The amount of salicylic acid is too little to exfoliate.

✓☺ **Daily Facials Skin Soothing Cleansing Cloths, for Sensitive Skin** (*$5.99 for 30 cloths*) are wonderfully soothing and a good, disposable cleansing option for someone with dry, sensitive skin. The fragrance-free, emollient formula is exceptionally gentle, yet thoroughly removes makeup. There is nothing about this product that you can't achieve by using a gentle cleanser and a washcloth.

OLAY DEFINITY PRODUCTS

☺ **Definity Illuminating Cream Cleanser** (*$10.99 for 5 ounces*) is said to penetrate deep into the skin's surface for an illuminating cleansing, but the skin's surface isn't that deep and the major ingredients in this cleanser (isopropyl palmitate and petrolatum) do not penetrate skin. This is recommended as a partially water-soluble rich cleanser for dry to very dry skin. You will need a washcloth for complete removal of "the smallest traces of dirt and makeup" and of the cleanser itself, as it doesn't rinse too well.

☺ **Definity Penetrating Mousse Cleanser** (*$9.99 for 5.2 ounces*) includes the water-binding agent acetyl glucosamine. The amount included is a pittance, and it certainly won't have any effect on skin tone (even if it was present in a greater concentration, remember, this is a cleanser and it is just rinsed down the drain). This propellant-based mousse cleanser is an option for normal to oily skin, but in this case there's no need to spend more for the Definity brand.

✓☺ **Definity Pore Redefining Scrub** (*$10.49 for 5 ounces*) has more cleansing ability than exfoliating ability, because the amount of polyethylene beads that do the exfoliating is meager. Meanwhile, the salicylic acid won't work as intended because this product's pH is too high and because it is rinsed off and so has only brief contact with skin. This is still a good, easy-to-rinse cleanser with a mild scrub action for normal to oily skin.

☺ **Definity Color Recapture Anti-Aging UV Moisturizer + Sheer Illuminating Coverage SPF 15** (*$26.99 for 1.7 ounces*). Debuting as one of the most expensive Olay products ever (at least until their Pro-X line hit store shelves), it is good news that this single product offers skin an in-part avobenzone sunscreen, a touch of color, soft matte finish, and a base formula that includes cell-communicating ingredient niacinamide along with antioxidant vitamin E. The matte finish doesn't help make good on Olay's claim of youthful luminosity, but does make this an attractive formula for normal to oily or blemish-prone skin. As for the color portion, whether you choose Fair/Light, Light/Medium, or Medium/Dark, the results are very sheer and workable for a wide range of skin tones. If you have a dark to very dark skin tone, you'll likely find the darkest option here to look grayish, but Olay's sister company Cover Girl offers some good foundations with sunscreens in dark shades.

☺ **Definity Correcting Protective Lotion with SPF 15** *($29.99 for 1.7 ounces)* is a very good daily sunscreen that provides sufficient UVA protection from avobenzone. The base formula consists of several skin-friendly ingredients, including glycerin, niacinamide, acetyl glucosamine, panthenol, and safflower seed oil. It's a worthwhile, if not quite state-of-the-art, formula (a wider array of antioxidants would have been preferred, especially given the price) for normal to dry skin. The mineral pigments provide a radiant finish that's best described as a subtle glow that works fine for daytime.

☺ **$$$ Definity Deep Penetrating Foaming Moisturizer** *($29.99 for 1.7 ounces)* foams because it is pressurized with isobutene and propane gases, but that feature is more a novelty than a particularly effective delivery system because those substances have a negative impact on the stability of the beneficial ingredients. This light-textured moisturizer contains mostly water, silicone, glycerin, niacinamide, acetyl glucosamine, thickener, film-forming agent, slip agents, preservatives, aloe, plant oil, and fragrance. Mineral pigments are included for a glowy finish, but if you're using this in the evening before you go to bed, that cosmetic effect isn't really necessary. This does contain other antioxidants, but the amount is insignificant.

☺ **Definity Deep Penetrating Foaming Moisturizer, Fragrance-Free** *($29.99 for 1.7 ounces)* is identical to Olay's Definity Deep Penetrating Foaming Moisturizer, except this omits the fragrance. Otherwise, the same review applies.

☺ **$$$ Definity Deep Penetrating Foaming Moisturizer SPF 15, Fragrance Free** *($28.99 for 1.7 ounces)* has a unique foam texture, but that won't enhance penetration, nor would you want it to because the active ingredients necessary for sun protection are meant to stay on the skin's surface. The sunscreen includes avobenzone for UVA protection while the base formula is the now-standard Olay blend of glycerin, niacinamide, and silicone. As with the other Definity moisturizer, mineral pigments provide a slight glow to skin, but don't mistake this cosmetic effect for a permanent change in skin's luminosity. This is best for normal to dry skin. The propellant can cause the beneficial ingredients to be unstable.

☺ **Definity Eye Illuminator, Illuminating Eye Treatment** *($29.99 for 0.5 ounce)* combines the key ingredients in the Definity moisturizers, but at higher concentrations. This fragrance-free formula provides a silky texture and finish while also being a good source of cell-communicating ingredients and antioxidant vitamin E. More antioxidants would have catapulted this to a Paula's Pick, but it is still a good consideration for slightly dry skin, and it works well under makeup. The mineral pigments add an "illuminating" shine to skin.

☺ **Definity Intense Hydrating Cream** *($29.99 for 1.7 ounces)* is the richest of the Definity moisturizers, but its formula is most similar to the Definity Deep Penetrating Foaming Moisturizer, minus the propellants. Since niacinamide is the chief beneficial ingredient in this product and it's not affected by exposure to light or air, the jar packaging is appropriate. Other than that, the same comments made previously for the Definity Deep Penetrating Foaming Moisturizer apply here as well.

☺ **Definity Night Restorative Sleep Cream** *($29.99 for 1.7 ounces)* is a standard, silky-textured moisturizer for normal to dry skin, but the choice of jar packaging will render the cell-communicating ingredients and token amount of antioxidants ineffective shortly after you begin using it. The mineral pigments add a soft shine to skin (what Olay refers to as a "luminous surface"), and this cream will make your skin feel great, but the packaging is a problem.

☺ **Definity Self Repair Serum** *($29.99 for 1.7 ounces)* has some of the impressive attributes seen in other Olay serums, including a high concentration of niacinamide and a hydrating mix of silicone and glycerin. However, it pales slightly in comparison because the amount of antioxidants is paltry and it contains a lot of dmdm hydantoin, a formaldehyde-releasing preservative that isn't as gentle as other preservatives (including the parabens, which are not in this serum). The mineral pigments provide a cosmetic glow to skin, but otherwise there's not much of interest here to improve skin tone and create healthier cells.

☺ $$$ **Definity 14 Day Skin Rehabilitation** *($33.99)* is a three-step kit designed to reduce skin discolorations and wrinkles in two weeks. To some extent, it can do that—just not to the point where you'll look like you've had a youth-reviving overhaul or anything approaching a rehabilitation. Despite the claims, how can this product produce any results? Each of the three phases contains one or more state-of-the- art ingredients, in efficacious amounts. These ingredients work to exfoliate skin, repair a damaged barrier, and serve as a starting point to reduce sun-induced skin discolorations. I wrote "starting point" because no skin-lightening ingredient is going to show great results after just two weeks, and certainly not without religious use of a sunscreen on a daily basis. Instead, you'll want to use such a product daily for at least three months. And in most cases, ongoing use is recommended. Olay wisely recommends using one of their Definity sunscreens with this routine. Let's examine each phase. **Phase 1** is to be used for the first week. It is a beta hydroxy acid (BHA, or salicylic acid) lotion that has a silky texture and minimally moist finish. The amount of salicylic acid is at least 1%, and with this product's pH of 2.5, exfoliation will occur. Although the pH is within the range to allow exfoliation, it is also low enough that this BHA lotion may be needlessly irritating, so be cautious. For long-term use, a gentler BHA product (such as those from Neutrogena or Paula's Choice) is advised. **Phase 2** is a very silky serum that contains an impressive amount of niacinamide (which has some research demonstrating skin-lightening ability) and acetyl glucosamine, though there's no substantiated in vivo evidence that the latter works to exfoliate skin. In terms of acetyl glucosamine's impact on skin discolorations, the existing research was performed either by Procter & Gamble (Olay's parent company) or by those on P&G's payroll, such as Dr. Zoe Diana Draelos (Sources: www.pgbeautyscience.com/zoe-diana-draelos-md.html; *Dermatologic Therapy*, September-October 2007, pages 308-313; and *Journal of Cosmetic Dermatology*, December 2006, pages 309-313). Still, acetyl glucosamine is a potentially effective ingredient for skin and most certainly has water-binding properties, which will help improve skin barrier function. You use Phase 2 for six days. By day 14, you're ready for **Phase 3**, which is the Revival Treatment. This is merely a pre-moistened cloth mask that you stretch and form to fit your face. You leave it on for 15 minutes, remove it, discard the cloth, and massage the remaining product into your skin. There is nothing special or essential about this cloth mask. The key ingredients are used to much greater benefit in Phases 1 and 2, so, if anything, Phase 3 is just a pampering experience to end your 14-day skin rehab on a relaxing note. I have to admit, Phases 1 and 2 are interesting formulas with some proven ingredients when it comes to creating the skin you want. However, what counts far more than any "intensive" at-home treatment is what you do to take care of your skin on a daily basis. In that sense, kits like this, while potentially effective to a modest degree, don't replace your daily routine. Olay offers plenty of products from which consumers can assemble a formidable daily skin-care routine, which makes this treatment trio a superfluous addition.

☺ $$$ **Definity Night Anti-Spot Treatment** *($29.99 for 0.17 ounce)* is meant to be a targeted specialty treatment for stubborn brown spots and other discolorations, although its formula isn't much different from Olay's other Definity serums and moisturizers. If you're us-

Olay 901

ing one of those with good results, adding this spot treatment isn't going to up the ante in any noticeable way. The only different ingredient in this product is undecylenoyl phenylalanine. This ingredient was the subject of Procter & Gamble's (Olay's owner) Beauty Breakthroughs newsletter in 2007. According to the company, "Undecylenoyl phenylalanine works as an MSH (melanin stimulating hormone) antagonist, meaning it prevents the melanin synthesis from starting…." "In vitro testing shows that the combination of undecylenoyl phenylalanine, N-acetyl glucosamine, and niacinamide demonstrate an additive effect in reducing melanin production without damaging skin cultures". That sounds promising, but we only have P&G's research to go on, and what's possible on cultured cells in a petri dish may not translate to the same or any level of effectiveness on skin. There is no independent, substantiated research about undecylenoyl phenylalanine, nor did P&G disclose how much of the ingredient was used in their in vitro testing to produce melanin-disrupting results. This product, like all those in the Definity line, also contains niacinamide and acetyl glucosamine. Niacinamide has been shown to lighten and prevent skin discolorations, but again, this research also comes from P&G, and likely was conducted only to justify the claims made for their Definity, Total Effects, and Regenerist products, all of which contain niacinamide (Sources: www.pgbeautyscience.com/breakthroughs-xiii.html; *Journal of Cosmetic Dermatology*, March 2007, pages 20-26; and *The British Journal of Dermatology*, July 2002, pages 20-31). The bottom line is that this product will likely have some effect on skin discolorations, but the lightening agents used are not as well researched as the gold standard, hydroquinone. For the money, I wouldn't invest in this product over other Olay Definity products just because it contains undecylenoyl phenylalanine, or over a well-formulated hydroquinone product. Given all that, the formula itself is worth a happy face rating.

OLAY PRO-X PRODUCTS

☺ **Pro-X Age Repair Lotion with SPF 30** (*$47 for 2.5 ounces*) is a daytime moisturizer with sunscreen with a lotion-like texture that slips easily over skin and sets to a lightweight hydrating finish suitable for normal to slightly dry or slightly oily skin. UVA protection is provided by avobenzone, just as it is for almost every daytime moisturizer with sunscreen that Olay offers. The rest of the formula contains cell-communicating niacinamide along with peptides, vitamin E, and glycerin. Glycerin is a good moisturizing agent that's present in hundreds, if not thousands, of moisturizers. Pro-X Repair Lotion with SPF 30 isn't any more reparative than other well-formulated sunscreens, and would've been even better if Olay had included some potent antioxidants (there isn't that much vitamin E in here, and many dermatologists feel a cocktail of antioxidants is best for skin) for extra environmental defense. Still, this is recommended and its cosmetically elegant texture works beautifully under makeup. As with all Pro-X products, this is fragrance-free. Note: This is not rated with a $$$ because size-wise, Olay provides more product than many competing brands (the standard size is 1.7 ounces).

✓ ☺ **$$$ Pro-X Deep Wrinkle Treatment** (*$47 for 1 ounce*). You might think that this product is another of the spackle-type moisturizers that have been showing up at cosmetic counters with a thicker texture meant to temporarily fill in lines and minor wrinkles. It isn't. Instead, this is akin to a lightweight moisturizer, which is being marketed as a specialty treatment by Olay. This doesn't contain a single ingredient that distinguishes it in any meaningful way from other Olay products, but it's worth considering for its blend of cell-communicating ingredients and antioxidants, all in a silky, thin lotion texture that pairs well with other products.

Olay's packaging helps keep the vitamin A in this product stable, which is a very good thing. The form of retinol included is retinyl propionate, which also appears in Olay's Age Defying line, though jar packaging prevails for most of that line, which makes those products useless. Retinyl propionate is also found in Olay's Regenerist Targeted Tone Enhancer and Total Effects Intensive Restoration Treatment, both of which sell for less than half this product's price. All told, Pro-X Deep Wrinkle Treatment has the better formula compared with Olay's other products with retinol, but its price should give you pause. If retinol is what you're after, keep in mind that RoC and Neutrogena have compelling options in that category for less money.

✓ ☺ **$$$ Pro-X Eye Restoration Complex** (*$47 for 0.5 ounce*). I disagree with Olay's marketing claims that this is a specialized treatment for the eye area because the ingredients also show up in their facial moisturizers. However, it cannot be denied that this fragrance-free formula is outstanding in many respects. It feels lightweight yet substantial, makes skin feel incredibly smooth, and treats it to several cell-communicating ingredients as well as a respectable amount of antioxidants, but the caffeine it contains won't brighten or wake up your eyes. As with most eye creams, the claims of diminishing dark circles and puffiness are dubious at best. By the way, this product is very similar to Olay's Regenerist Eye Lifting Serum, which sells for less than $20 for the same amount of product.

☺ **$$$ Pro-X Hydra Firming Cream** (*$47 for 1.7 ounces*). The cosmeceutical-sounding claims for this moisturizer are tempting, but for the most part, this silky-textured moisturizer for normal to dry skin doesn't distinguish itself from several less expensive Olay moisturizers. It contains some peptides and vitamin E, but all of these state-of-the-art ingredients will see their efficacy diminish due to the jar packaging. There are reasons to consider this fragrance-free moisturizer, but it's not one I recommend with enthusiasm because of the packaging issue. A similar Olay moisturizer in better packaging (and for a lot less money) is Regenerist Deep Hydration Regenerating Cream.

☺ **$$$ Pro-X Wrinkle Smoothing Cream** (*$47 for 1.7 ounces*) has a slightly heavier texture than the Olay Pro-X Hydra Firming Cream, and because of that, those with dry to very dry skin will likely enjoy this product's performance best, but don't take that to mean this is the antiwrinkle moisturizer you've been waiting for. To Olay's credit, their claims for this moisturizer are accurate: It smooths the appearance of lines and wrinkles while improving skin's texture. Those benefits are the beginning of any well-formulated moisturizer, and this one certainly qualifies. What holds it back from a better rating is the jar packaging. When you're loading your moisturizer with peptides and also including antioxidants, you should know that consistent exposure to light and air isn't going to keep these fragile ingredients around for long. A less expensive version of this product that comes in better packaging is Olay Regenerist Reversal Treatment Foam.

☺ **$$$ Pro-X Discoloration Fighting Concentrate** (*$47 for 0.4 ounce*) is packaged in a medicinal-looking tube and its pointed applicator speaks to its spot-treatment nature. Spot-treating discolorations can work, but chances are good that you've got more discolorations that haven't become visible yet. In that sense, you're better off treating the entire face with a skin-lightening product—but if you choose to do so with this lightweight Pro-X lotion option, you'll be replacing it frequently because this is a very small amount of product. The pigmentation-fighting ingredients included in this product are niacinamide, acetyl glucosamine (a blend found in all of the less expensive Olay Definity products, which also make discoloration-fighting claims), and an Olay-developed skin-lightening agent known as undecylenoyl phenylalanine.

Olay's parent company Procter & Gamble are the only ones with research on the latter ingredient, so the research is not exactly unbiased, but it does appear promising. The same is true for the limited but promising research on acetyl glucosamine (a favorite ingredient of Estee Lauder, too). More bankable is the research on the melanin-inhibiting effects of niacinamide (Sources: *Journal of Drugs in Dermatology*, July 2008, pages S2-S6; and *The British Journal of Dermatology*, July 2002, pages 20-31). It's worth noting, however, that the majority of research connecting niacinamide to skin lightening has, you guessed it, been conducted and published by Procter & Gamble. That doesn't make it worthless information, but I eagerly await their positive results being duplicated in larger studies done outside of P&G's control. By the way, the Definity product that is comparable to this Pro-X item is the Night Anti-Spot Treatment. As it turns out, the price per ounce is the same; you pay twice as much for the Pro-X Discoloration Fighting Concentrate but you get twice as much product.

OLAY REGENERIST PRODUCTS

☺ **Regenerist Deep Hydrating Mousse Cleanser** *($9.99 for 6.1 ounces)*. Other than this cleanser being dispensed as cushiony foam, there isn't much to get excited about. The formula is suitable for cleansing and makeup removal for normal to very dry skin, and it rinses better than expected considering its Vaseline and mineral oil content. This product is supposed to be based on Olay's Aquacurrent science, which is their interpretation of the science behind aquaporins. Aquaporins are membrane water channels present in bacteria, plants, and animals, including humans, that help to maintain the water content of cells, including skin cells (Source: www. ks.uiuc.edu/Research/aquaporins/). As fancy as that sounds, it doesn't take much to facilitate that system—research shows that ingredients as simple as glycerin handle this quite nicely.

☺ **Regenerist Micro-Derm Cleansing Cloths** *($9.99 for 30 cloths)* are Vaseline-based cleansing cloths whose texture allows for manual exfoliation, much like using a washcloth. These cloths do remove makeup, but for eye makeup it takes more effort than you might like to expend. They are best for normal to very dry skin, and the solution should be rinsed from your skin because of the detergent cleansing agents in it.

☺ **Regenerist Eye Makeup Remover** *($9.99 for 6.7 ounces)* is a very standard, but effective, eye-makeup remover lotion for normal to very dry skin. The emollients and oils work swiftly to remove all types of makeup, including waterproof formulas, though it's not as easy to rinse from skin as liquid eye-makeup removers. I have no idea what Olay means by their "aminopeptide" ingredient, because it is not evident in this product's formula, which really couldn't be more ordinary unless you used plain mineral oil or Vaseline to remove makeup.

☺ **Regenerist Daily Regenerating Cleanser** *($7.49 for 5 ounces)* is a cleanser/scrub hybrid, and the lotion base allows the polyethylene beads to exfoliate without being too abrasive. It's an OK cleansing scrub for normal to dry skin, but no product can detoxify skin (exactly what toxins are we talking about anyway? and how is this measured?), especially one that is rinsed off shortly after application.

☺ **Regenerist Daily Thermal Mini-Peel** *($18.99 for 6 ounces)* is a topical, nonaqueous scrub that lists magnesium sulfate (commonly known as Epsom salt) as the second ingredient. Massaging it over wet skin (as directed) causes an exothermic (heat-releasing) reaction. While you will feel an intense warming sensation that gets stronger as you continue to massage the product over your skin, the heat doesn't benefit your skin in any way. If anything, heat can be a problem for skin, causing capillaries to break and surface, creating red veining on your face.

The polyethylene beads will exfoliate skin, but the glycolic acid is useless because the magnesium sulfate keeps this product too alkaline, and AHAs need an acidic pH to exfoliate, though in a cleanser they would just be rinsed away, so all around, the AHA is wasted in this product.

☺ **Regenerist Detoxifying Pore Scrub** *($9.99 for 6.5 ounces)*. Forget the pore detoxifying talk surrounding this scrub, because there aren't any toxins lurking in pores that need to be scrubbed away. This is a standard cleanser/scrub hybrid whose benefit is more as a cleanser than as a scrub due to the large amount of detergent cleansing agents relative to the amount of polyethylene beads (that's what has the scrub effect). The salicylic acid has no effect on skin because it is rinsed away before it has a chance to work. This rinses cleanly, removes makeup, and is an acceptable option for normal to oily skin.

☹ **$$$ Regenerist Microdermabrasion & Peel System** *($27.99 for 4.2 ounces)* is a two-part system that includes a **Microdermabrasion Treatment** and **Peel Activator Serum**. The Microdermabrasion Treatment does not contain the usual aluminum oxide crystals. Instead, this bright orange, gel-based scrub contains baking soda (sodium bicarbonate) and silica. You're instructed to apply the exfoliating gel to dry skin and massage for a minute or so. Next, you apply the Peel Activator Serum to fingertips and massage a thick layer over the exfoliating gel. Since the baking soda in the exfoliant gel is alkaline and the serum is acidic, two things happen: a mild, fizzy, foaming action occurs, and there's a slight warming sensation. This happens whenever alkaline and acidic products are mixed together. As the skin's pH acclimates to this change, the warming sensation subsides. After another minute of massaging the mixture over skin, you rinse it off. The abrasiveness of the baking soda makes the skin quite smooth, which is where the bulk of this duo's benefit lies. Although the Peel Activator Serum contains lactic acid and has a pH of 3.6, it is not left on the skin long enough to cause a peeling effect. All of this amounts to a somewhat convoluted way to exfoliate skin with a fairly good risk of irritation given the "salt" scrub followed so closely by the lactic acid. In Olay's attempt to be innovative, they simply combined the benefits of manual exfoliation with chemical exfoliation. I wouldn't suggest using this scrub, but rather just a washcloth with a gentle cleanser that you rinse off—and then apply an AHA or BHA product that you leave on the skin.

☹ **Regenerist Micro-Exfoliating Wet Cleansing Cloths** *($7.99 for 30 cloths)* do not contain cleansing agents or anything capable of exfoliating skin, although the mechanical action of massaging these cloths over skin (similar to using a washcloth) will remove some dead skin cells. The glycol and silicone can help dislodge makeup, but I wouldn't choose these cloths to remove waterproof mascara (Olay claims they do this, but that's debatable). I suppose these are an OK option for normal to dry skin if you wear minimal to no makeup.

☹ **$$$ Regenerist 14 Day Skin Intervention** *($29.99 for 0.7 ounce)* promises a skin turnaround in two weeks, all without surgical intervention. You get 14 tiny tubes of product, divided into phases. **Phase 1** is applied nightly for the first week, and is said to "ignite cellular regeneration beneath the skin's surface." It's a water- and silicone-based serum that contains niacinamide, just like all of the Regenerist, Total Effects, and Definity products Olay sells. However, this also contains lavender (several parts of the plant) along with arnica, and both are troublesome for skin. Other than the gimmick of using this for a week before moving on to **Phase 2**, there is no reason to consider this serum over others from Olay that contain just as much niacinamide and omit the irritants. Phase 2 is silicone-based, and as such has a thicker, spackle-like texture. It won't make your skin look lifted as claimed, but will definitely make it look and feel better, all while supplying your skin with some potent cell-communicating ingredients plus the antioxidants vitamin E and green tea. Phase 2 is also fragrance-free. In summation, Phase 1 is not worth considering over Olay's better serums; Phase 2, on the other hand, is a state-of-the-art serum that stands an excellent chance of strengthening skin's barrier function and allowing it to create healthier new cells. It's up to you to decide if half of this 14-day regimen is worth the expense; I'd recommend you consider one of Olay's Regenerist serums instead.

✓ ☺ **Regenerist Advanced Anti-Aging DNA Superstructure UV Cream SPF 25** *($29.99 for 1.7 ounces)*. Olay is heavily advertising this sleekly packaged daytime moisturizer with an in-part avobenzone sunscreen. The claim of blocking DNA damage sounds impressive, but in fact that's what any well-formulated sunscreen (which this certainly qualifies as) does. Daily use of an effective sunscreen rated SPF 15 or greater protects skin from the pernicious, cumulative DNA damage that sun exposure causes as well as protecting collagen from breaking down. Therefore, this moisturizer with sunscreen isn't the only game in town, nor do you need to spend this much to get an effective sunscreen. That said, there's no denying that once again Olay has crafted a sophisticated formula that is suitable for all skin types except sensitive (because of the nonmineral sunscreen actives) and oily. The intriguing ingredients are mostly the same ones that show up in other Regenerist moisturizers (and serums) so Olay isn't breaking new ground here. But taken together, they do their part to protect and enhance skin so it is better able to repair itself and, as a result, become healthier.

☹ $$$ **Regenerist Advanced Anti-Aging Eye Roller** *($22.99 for 0.2 ounce)*. The trio of metal ball rollers on this product is designed to be massaged around the eye area to reduce puffiness. Unfortunately, puffiness cannot be massaged away, especially if it is from aging (when the fat pads beneath the eye weaken and droop beneath the eye area). Therefore, this pen-style component and its roller-ball applicator mechanism is more gimmicky than useful, though it does a good job of depositing product. The product inside is a water-based serum that isn't nearly as elegant as several other Regenerist formulas, though it does contain a small amount of peptide and omits fragrance.

✓ ☺ **Regenerist Daily Regenerating Serum** *($19.49 for 1.7 ounces)* is a silky, silicone-based serum that contains a nice complement of water-binding agents and antioxidants. It contains approximately 2% to 3% niacinamide, and, in this amount, it can increase the skin's ceramide and fatty acid content as well as have anti-inflammatory action (Source: *Journal of Cosmetic Dermatology,* April 2004, pages 88-93). When it comes to niacinamide being able to affect aging (wrinkled) or sun-damaged (also discolored) skin, research points to a concentration of 5% as necessary to notice any improvement in skin texture and color that's consistent with what is typically seen in young skin (Source: D. L. Bissett, J. E. Oblong, A. Saud, and M. Levine, "Topical niacinamide provides improvements in aging human facial skin," presented at the 60th Annual Meeting of the American Academy of Dermatology, 2002).Olay claims the palmitoyl pentapeptide-3 this contains can regenerate and intensely hydrate skin. However, palmitoyl pentapeptide-3 (also known as Matrixyl) is present in this product at less than 1%, and its value for skin is documented only by Sederma, the company that sells it. As it turns out, Sederma makes lots of peptides, and makes increasingly exaggerated claims about curing every skin-care woe imaginable. Of course, none of this is published research, but that doesn't stop Sederma or any of the numerous cosmetics companies from using their ingredients. In reality, it's the various types of silicones that really give this product its elegant texture and make skin feel unbelievably silky. Regenerist Daily Regenerating Serum won't give aging skin a new lease on life, but it would be a very good serum-type moisturizer for normal to slightly oily skin. This does contain fragrance.

✓☺ **Regenerist Daily Regenerating Serum, Fragrance-Free** *($19.49 for 1.7 ounces)* is identical to the Regenerist Daily Regenerating Serum, except this option excludes fragrance, which is even better for the health of your skin, regardless of age.

☺ **Regenerist Deep Hydration Regenerating Cream** *($19.99 for 1.7 ounces)* contains ingredients capable of hydrating skin (including glycerin and niacinamide), but has a texture that those with dry to very dry skin may find too light. Overall this is a good formula whose only shortcoming is the somewhat disappointing amount of antioxidants.

☺ **Regenerist Eye Derma-Pod** *($17.99 for 24 pods)* not only capitalizes on the name of the popular iPod digital music player, but also takes a cue from its packaging. However, the Olay Derma-Pod has nothing to do with music. It is supposed to resurface, fill in lines, and decongest puffiness around the eyes. Each pod is a tiny packet filled with a silicone-based lotion. Squeezing the pod dispenses the product onto the built-in sponge pad, and you're directed to gently dab the product all around the eye, then use the sponge to massage the area in a circular motion for one minute. The sponge and massage action provides a very mild exfoliation for eye-area skin, while the silicone feels smooth and silky. Olay maintains that the massage action is what helps "remove excess under-eye fluids," but the effect is minimal at best, not to mention that puffiness from fluid buildup is usually temporary and related to diet (high in sodium), allergies, or sinus issues, and the latter two are easily remedied by over-the-counter antihistamines or decongestants. Plus you could just massage the area without the little pads and get the exact same results. The solution dispensed onto the sponge differs little from the other serums in Olay's Regenerist line. It contains a significant amount of niacinamide and lesser amounts of peptides, along with a couple of antioxidants. These pods aren't a necessary add-on to your skin-care routine, but if you're curious to try them the formula itself is definitely beneficial for skin, either around the eyes or elsewhere, and the massage action is best done carefully because massaging too vigorously can pull delicate skin.

✓☺ **Regenerist Eye Lifting Serum** *($18.99 for 0.5 ounce)* is every bit as state-of-the-art as Olay's other Regenerist products. In fact, Eye Lifting Serum differs little from Olay's Regenerist Daily Regenerating Serum, Fragrance-Free, which provides three times as much product for the same price. Both of these products contain silicones, glycerin, niacinamide (which can increase skin's ceramide and free fatty acid content, among other benefits), several water-binding agents, antioxidants, and anti-irritants. You really can't go wrong with most of the Regenerist serums or moisturizers as long as you keep your expectations realistic. In other words, Olay's claim that these products are able to provide "dramatically younger-looking skin without surgery" is stretching the truth—plastic surgeons have not seen a decrease in new patients since the Regenerist line came on the beauty scene. But the fact remains that this fragrance-free moisturizer is an excellent option for use around the eyes or anywhere on the face. In contrast to Olay's Regenerist Daily Regenerating Serum, Fragrance Free, this product contains mineral pigments (including mica) that impart a soft, reflective shimmer to skin. To a slight degree, this can help make dark circles under the eye look less obvious, but the effect is strictly cosmetic.

✓☺ **Regenerist Touch of Concealer Eye Regenerating Cream** *($21.99 for 0.5 ounce)* is a very good moisturizer that Olay is positioning as a tinted eye cream. Its concealing ability comes from the amount of titanium dioxide it contains (which provides soft coverage) along with standard cosmetic pigments. The base formula is lightweight and very silky, and treats skin anywhere on the face to some exceptional ingredients. Niacinamide, peptides, antioxidants, and skin-conditioning agents combine to make this tinted eye cream a top consideration, though the single shade won't work for everyone's skin tone (it is best for light to medium skin tones).

☺ **Regenerist Filling & Sealing Wrinkle Treatment** *($19.99 for 1 ounce)* comes in a medicinal-looking tube and is meant, as the name states, to fill wrinkles and seal in moisture. The silicone and the plastic-based thickening agent that comprise the bulk of this product will function as minor fillers for wrinkles, but the best results will be seen for superficial lines, not deep, etched wrinkles, and the effect is best described as temporary. However, someone in their late 20s or 30s with the first signs of lines around the eyes or mouth may find this works beautifully (if temporarily) to reduce these signs of aging. Olay omits the niacinamide and instead includes an impressive amount of a cell-communicating peptide and antioxidant vitamin E. This line-filling serum is fragrance-free and includes a mineral pigment to help reflect light away from the skin, which can further improve the appearance of superficial lines.

☺ **Regenerist Micro-Sculpting Cream** *($26.99 for 1.7 ounces)* purports to be the result of 50 years of Olay research, so you'd expect this to be a breathtakingly unique formula. It's not, and in fact it's very similar to all of the other Regenerist moisturizers and serums (I can't imagine what Olay was doing for 50 years, because if this is all they came up with, that would not be something to brag about). Increasing hydration can make skin cells plump, but that doesn't restore volume to a face that is sagging due to the complex process of aging. In other words, despite the name, this is not a face-lift in a jar. Actually, the jar packaging does a disservice to the range of antioxidants in this product (it does contain more antioxidants than many Olay products). That leaves you with a decent lightweight moisturizer for normal to slightly dry skin.

☹ **Regenerist Night Recovery Moisturizing Treatment** *($19.49 for 1.7 ounces)* comes in a jar, so the potency of the interesting ingredients such as niacinamide, vitamin E, and green tea is compromised. This also contains lavender and arnica extracts, which won't provide a "mini-lift" to skin, but do have the potential to cause irritation. This has a less impressive formulation than most of Olay's Regenerist products, and if you're already using one or more of those, there is no reason to add this product, especially when there are more state-of-the-art formulas in better packaging available from companies such as Clinique, Neutrogena, and Paula's Choice.

☺ **Regenerist Reversal Treatment Foam** *($29.99 for 1.7 ounces).* What this propellant-based foaming moisturizer is supposed to reverse is merely the appearance of lines and wrinkles, a claim that can be made for almost any moisturizer. With the exception of the fact that this pressurized product foams, its formula differs little from that of all of the other Regenerist moisturizers. If the foaming effect had some positive action on skin this would be worth the splurge, but no such luck, it's just a novel way to dispense a moisturizer. Don't get me wrong—this is a respectable moisturizer for normal to slightly dry or slightly oily skin (it's heads and shoulders above anything L'Oreal or Nivea offers)—it just wasn't a necessary or revolutionary addition to Olay's burgeoning Regenerist lineup. The tin oxide and mica cast a subtle shine on skin that has nothing to do with it being regenerated layer by layer, it is merely a cosmetic sheen. This product is supposed to be based on Olay's Aquacurrent science, which is their interpretation of the science behind aquaporins. Aquaporins are membrane water channels present in bacteria, plants, and animals, including humans, that help to maintain the water content of cells, including skin cells (Source: www.ks.uiuc.edu/Research/aquaporins/). As fancy as that sounds it doesn't take much to facilitate that system—research shows that ingredients as simple as glycerin handle this quite nicely.

✓ ☺ **Regenerist Touch of Foundation UV Defense Regenerating Moisturizer SPF 15** *($19.99 for 1.7 ounces)* is a very good tinted moisturizer with an in-part avobenzone sunscreen. Olay's descriptor of "a touch of foundation" is just a new angle on what this product really is: a tinted moisturizer. It comes in one shade that provides sheer coverage and is workable for light to medium skin tones (those with fair skin will find this goes on too dark). The formula contains some state-of-the-art ingredients just like those found in most of the Olay Regenerist serums and moisturizers. It is best for normal to slightly dry or slightly oily skin.

☺ **Regenerist Touch Of Sun UV Defense Regenerating Lotion SPF 15** *($19.99 for 2.5 ounces)* protects skin with an in-part avobenzone sunscreen and has a silky, moisturizing base that contains a small amount of the self-tanning agent dihydroxyacetone. This provides gradual color (not as much as a standard self-tanner would) and is a good option for daytime use if you have normal to slightly dry skin and are willing to apply it liberally enough to ensure sun protection. Niacinamide, present in most of the leave-on Regenerist products, is absent here.

✓ ☺ **Regenerist UV Defense Regenerating Lotion SPF 15** *($19.99 for 2.5 ounces)* has a lightweight base that is suitable for those with normal to slightly dry or slightly oily skin, while avobenzone is on hand for UVA protection. The formula is loaded with beneficial extras for skin, including a peptide complex, antioxidants, and soothing agents. This does contain fragrance, but is otherwise highly recommended!

✓ ☺ **Regenerist UV Defense Regenerating Lotion SPF 50** *($29.99 for 1.7 ounces)*. I have to hand it to Olay. According to the press release we received for this product, their goal was to create a daytime moisturizer with a high level of sun protection that felt like a silky lightweight moisturizer rather than a heavy, occlusive sunscreen. They succeeded brilliantly. This in-part avobenzone sunscreen feels wonderfully light yet makes skin feel smooth, moisturized, and protected. Yes, there are lighter products out there that carry lower SPF ratings, and many of those are excellent, too. However, people who desire or need a high SPF rating should check this product out. It contains an impressive blend of cell-communicating ingredients and antioxidants and works beautifully under makeup. It really does set quickly and won't leave skin feeling greasy. I hope Olay launches a fragrance-free version, too; it would make an already great product that much better.

☺ **Regenerist Targeted Tone Enhancer** *($18.99 for 1 ounce)* is meant to combine the benefits of niacinamide with what Olay refers to as pro-retinol. However, the form of vitamin A they chose, retinyl propionate, doesn't have anywhere close to the amount of research on pure retinol, so choosing it instead is somewhat of a gamble. This is otherwise a good lightweight moisturizer with niacinamide for normal to slightly dry skin.

☺ **$$$ Regenerist Anti-Aging Lip Treatment** *($19.99 for 0.06 ounce)*, packaged in a pen-style component, is an emollient, shimmery balm that can't change the lines around your mouth. The niacinamide and lecithin are a nice touch, and add to the moisturizing effect of this product, but it won't change the age of your lips by even one day.

OLAY TOTAL EFFECTS PRODUCTS

☹ **Total Effects Age Defying Cleansing Cloths** *($8.99 for 30 cloths)* are pre-moistened cleansing cloths that contain menthol, which makes them too irritating for all skin types.

☺ **Total Effects Nourishing Cream Cleanser** *($9.99 for 6.5 ounces)* is a standard emollient cleansing cream for dry to very dry skin. It requires a washcloth to avoid leaving a greasy film on skin. This fragranced cleansing cream removes makeup easily.

☺ **Total Effects Revitalizing Foaming Cleanser** *($9.99 for 6.5 ounces)* is a great water-soluble cleanser for normal to oily skin. You'll find it builds a soft lather and is capable of removing makeup and rinsing cleanly. It contains fragrance and isn't more revitalizing than similar products, but it certainly cleanses thoroughly.

☺ **Total Effects Age Defying Wet Cleansing Cloths** *($8.99 for 30 cloths)* do not contain cleansing agents or anything capable of exfoliating skin, although the mechanical action of massaging these cloths over skin (similar to using a washcloth) will remove some dead skin cells. The glycol and silicone can help dislodge makeup, but I wouldn't choose these cloths to remove waterproof mascara (Olay claims they do this, but that's debatable). I suppose these are an OK option for normal to dry skin if you wear minimal to no makeup.

☺ **Total Effects Anti-Aging Anti-Blemish Daily Cleanser** *($7.59 for 5 ounces)* contains 2% salicylic acid in a base with a pH below 4, but these positive traits are wasted in a cleanser because it is rinsed from the skin before the BHA has a chance to work, not to mention that salicylic acid should not be used near the eyes or mucous membranes. This is an OK option as a scrub cleanser (a small amount of polyethylene beads is included for manual exfoliation) for oily skin.

☺ **Total Effects 7-in-1 Anti-Aging Booster Eye Cream + Concealer** *($19.99 for 0.5 ounce)* is nearly identical to Olay's Regenerist Eye Touch of Concealer Eye Regenerating Cream, though the latter has a slight formulary edge that earns a Paula's Pick rating. Best viewed as a lightweight silky eye cream rather than a concealer, this has a soufflé-like texture that sets to a smooth matte finish. Coverage is sheer, so this won't hide dark circles, but it also doesn't crease into lines around the eyes or interfere with your usual concealer. The ingredient list definitely contains more state-of-the-art extras not seen in standard concealers, which is why this is worth considering.

☺ **Total Effects 7-in-1 Anti-Aging Moisturizer** *($18.99 for 1.7 ounces)* is a lightweight moisturizer that contains a good amount of niacinamide and silicones for a silky finish. While overall not as state-of-the-art as similar options from Olay's Regenerist collection, this is still a good option for normal to oily skin.

☺ **Total Effects 7-in-1 Anti-Aging Moisturizer, Fragrance Free** *($18.99 for 1.7 ounces)* is identical to the Total Effects 7-in-1 Anti-Aging Moisturizer above, minus the fragrance, which is always a plus for your skin. Otherwise, the same review applies.

✓☺ **Total Effects 7-In-1 Anti-Aging Moisturizer, Mature Skin Therapy** *($19.38 for 1.7 ounces)* is Olay's answer to the needs of women whose skin is suffering from the changes it endures during and after menopause. The seven benefits in one product claim to intensely moisturize skin, reduce wrinkles, enhance skin tone and color, minimize pores, provide free-radical defense, and lift skin. Wow, all this for under $20? Sarcasm aside, this moisturizer for normal to dry skin contains several state-of-the-art ingredients that can improve the appearance and healthy functioning of skin at any age, but without a sunscreen a major necessary benefit is missing! Antioxidant-wise, this bests all of the other Total Effects products, propelling this to the top of the list. Much of the skin-appearance enhancement has to do with visual trickery— the mineral pigments add a subtle soft-focus, brightening effect to dull skin, while niacinamide encourages ceramide production for a smoother surface, which reflects light better. This isn't one-stop shopping for menopausal skin because most of the claims are at best farfetched, but it definitely has many strong points.

☺ **Total Effects 7-in-1 Anti-Aging Moisturizer, SPF 15** *($18.99 for 1.7 ounces)* keeps skin shielded from the sun with its in-part avobenzone sunscreen, but other than that the only exciting element in this lightweight daytime moisturizer for normal to slightly oily skin is niacinamide. The other bells and whistles aren't present in impressive amounts.

☺ **Total Effects 7-In-1 Anti-Aging UV Moisturizer Plus SPF 15, Fragrance-Free** *($19.98 for 1.7 ounces)*. As is typical for Olay's latest sunscreens, reliable UVA protection is provided by avobenzone. Also typical for Olay moisturizers is the inclusion of the cell-communicating ingredient niacinamide, present in this product at what is most certainly an efficacious amount. Other than a silky texture and fragrance-free formula, that's where the excitement stops. All of the other antioxidants and intriguing ingredients are listed after the pH adjuster (triethanolamine), so they don't amount to much. Still, this is a good daytime moisturizer for normal to oily skin that is prone to blemishes.

☺ **Total Effects 7-in-1 Anti-Aging UV Moisturizer Plus Touch of Foundation SPF 15** *($19.99 for 1.7 ounces).* Is this a brilliant way to combine sunscreen, a touch of color, and lots of bells and whistles for skin in one apply-and-get-out-the-door product? The answer is a confusing yes and no. The in-part avobenzone sunscreen is a plus, as is the silky texture laced with an efficacious amount of the cell-communicating ingredient niacinamide. It also applies smoothly, blends well, and sets to a soft matte finish. The problem is that the single shade available won't work for all skin tones (it's best for those with light to medium skin tones that are not overly pink), and although it's sheer, if the color isn't right for you, the difference will be obvious. Olay would have been better off launching this in three or four shades for various skin tones (and they clearly know how to do that given the impressive improvements seen in Cover Girl's foundations; remember, both Cover Girl and Olay are owned by Procter & Gamble). As it turns out, this is a brilliant option only if the single shade matches your skin well enough to look convincing. If that's the case, the formula, which is good but could've ramped up the antioxidants a bit, is best for normal to slightly oily or slightly dry skin. Neutrogena's Healthy Skin Tone Enhancer SPF 20 is a comparable product with a better formula and several shades.

☹ **Total Effects Daily Moisturizer + Blemish Control** *($18.99 for 1.7 ounces)* is an effective beta hydroxy acid option at the drugstore, though the product's pH of 2.3 is lower than usual and definitely poses a risk of causing irritation. The 1.5% salicylic acid will penetrate the pore's follicle lining, exfoliating and helping to dislodge blackheads while smoothing skin and treating inflammatory acne. The fragranced base formula is nothing to write home about, but it has a silky, light texture that won't be bothersome for normal to slightly dry or slightly oily skin. What a shame the low pH makes this a gamble for irritation. It also keeps this BHA product from earning a happy face rating.

☹ **Total Effects Eye Transforming Cream** *($18.99 for 0.5 ounce)* has a formula similar to Olay's other Total Effects products, meaning you get a blend of such ingredients as glycerin, niacinamide, silicone, emollients, and antioxidants. It features a dry-finish ingredient known as isohexadecane, which prevents it from being too creamy. If you prefer a luxurious-feeling eye cream, this is not the one to choose. Another reason to reconsider before buying this: The formulation is similar to Olay's other Total Effects products, but in this case you're getting less product for your money and it's in translucent jar packaging, which compromises the effectiveness of the antioxidants even before you open it.

☺ **Total Effects Instant Smoothing Serum** *($19.99 for 1.7 ounces)* must have been created so that Olay's Total Effects line has a state-of-the-art product similar to their Regenerist line, but Total Effects is far removed from having anything total for skin. Just like Regenerist's Daily Regenerating Serum, this Total Effects silicone-based product contains niacinamide, along with an elegant blend of water-binding agents, silicone, film-forming agents, and antioxidants. The only glaring omission is the palmitoyl pentapeptide-3 (trade name: Matrixyl) that's present in the Regenerist product. Peptides are potentially beneficial ingredients for skin (although the hype over their antiaging prowess is overblown) and so, considering that the two Olay serums

(Regenerist and Total Effects) are nearly identical formulations at the same price and size, why not buy the Regenerist Serum for the "icing on the cake" addition of peptides?

☺ **Total Effects Intensive Restoration Treatment** *($18.99 for 1.01 ounces)* claims to fight past damage in your most "aging-prone zones," yet its formula is remarkably similar to that of all the other Total Effects moisturizers, save for the addition of a few thickeners (none of which can turn back the hands of time). This does contain a tiny amount of retinyl propionate, Olay's version of retinol, but the research isn't there to support its use over pure retinol. However, this is still a good moisturizer for normal to dry skin, and the amount of niacinamide is beneficial.

☹ **Total Effects Night Firming Cream, Face & Neck** *($19.49 for 1.7 ounces)* is a lightweight moisturizer for normal to slightly dry skin, but one whose jar packaging won't keep the antioxidant ingredients stable during use. Niacinamide is on board as usual, but despite the positive research available for this ingredient, it cannot firm skin.

☹ **Total Effects Touch Of Sun, Daily Anti-Aging Moisturizer** *($17.49 for 1.7 ounces)* tries to combine two steps—self-tanning and exfoliation—in one product. While the concept is nice and it sounds like a time-saver, it is probably far better for your skin to apply them separately. The self-tanning process is enhanced when you exfoliate before you apply the self-tanner, not during. Applying them at the same time can be counterproductive. Perhaps more problematic for skin is this product's fairly low pH of 2.3, which, while ensuring exfoliation, is potentially irritating to skin. Overall, the result (or lack thereof) isn't worth it.

OTHER OLAY PRODUCTS

☺ **Deep Cleansing Face Wash, for Combination/Oily Skin** *($5.89 for 7 ounces)* is a very standard but good water-soluble foaming cleanser for its intended skin type, and one that removes makeup easily.

☺ **Dual Action Cleanser + Pore Scrub** *($7.49 for 5 ounces)* is nearly identical to Olay's Complete Ageless Rejuvenating Lathering Cleanser and the same review applies.

☹ **Dual Action Cleanser + Toner** *($6.99 for 6.7 ounces)* contains menthol, which makes it too irritating for all skin types, especially when used to remove makeup around the eyes.

☺ **Foaming Face Wash, for All Skin Types** *($4.90 for 6.78 ounces)* is a great water-soluble cleanser for all skin types except very dry. It removes makeup easily and leaves no residue. This would be rated a Paula's Pick if it did not contain fragrance.

✓ ☺ **Foaming Face Wash, for Sensitive Skin** *($4.49 for 6.78 ounces)* is preferred to Olay's Foaming Face Wash, for All Skin Types, because it has the same formula but without the fragrance. Considering the aesthetics and performance of this cleanser, it is one of the best values at the drugstore, and is ideal for sensitive or rosacea-affected skin.

✓ ☺ **Gentle Foaming Face Wash, for Sensitive Skin** *($5.99 for 7 ounces)* is very similar to the Foaming Face Wash, for Sensitive Skin, and the same review applies. Both are very good water-soluble cleansers for all skin types, particularly those with sensitive skin or rosacea.

☺ **Hydrate & Cleanse Micro-Bead Cleansing Serum** *($8.49 for 6.7 ounces)* contains sodium lauryl sulfate, which can be problematic, but the small amount present coupled with the moisturizing ingredients that precede it in the ingredient list make it no cause for concern. This rinses better than the formula suggests, though you may still prefer to use it with a washcloth to avoid a residue. It is best for normal to dry skin.

☺ **Moisture Balancing Foaming Face Wash, for All Skin Types** *($6.49 for 7 ounces)* is nearly identical to the Foaming Face Wash, for All Skin Types above, and the same review applies.

☺ **Purifying Mud Lathering Cleanser** *($6.99 for 5 ounces)*. This foaming cleanser doesn't contain any mud, just a tiny amount of clay that's not going to have much effect on oily skin. What makes this an option for normal to oily (especially oily) skin is its effective blend of detergent cleansing agents coupled with a lack of ingredients that leave a residue.

☺ **Mascara + Make-Up Remover** *($7.99 for 4.5 ounces)*. This water-based, emollient (and I mean really emollient) makeup remover is a slightly modified version of standard cold cream. As such, it works well to dissolve mascara and other makeup. The problem, however, is that this formula doesn't rinse well from skin on its own, so you'll want to follow with a regular cleanser to avoid build-up around the eye area. Olay thoughtfully omitted fragrance from this makeup remover.

☹ **Refreshing Toner** *($4.29 for 7.2 ounces)* lists alcohol as the second ingredient and witch hazel distillate (which just adds more alcohol) as the third. Menthyl lactate completes the package of ingredients primed to irritate, not refresh, skin.

☺ **Active Hydrating Beauty Fluid, Original** *($11.99 for 4 ounces)* contains mostly water, thickener, glycerin, oil, Vaseline, and more thickeners, plus fragrance and coloring agents to make it smell and look pretty. This is definitely a case where the original isn't the best. Instead, it's uninspiring and minimally helpful for dry skin.

☺ **Active Hydrating Cream, Original** *($8.99 for 2 ounces)* is active in name only, and is one of Olay's most boring, do-nothing moisturizers. It's an average option for dry skin, nothing more.

☺ **Anti-Wrinkle Nutrients Daily SPF 15 Lotion** *($12.99 for 3.4 ounces)* comes in a generous size for facial application, and includes avobenzone for reliable UVA protection. The base formula is the familiar Olay blend of water, glycerin, niacinamide, and silicone, and it's suitable for normal to slightly oily or slightly dry skin. Antioxidants are in short supply, but this does provide an opalescent glow to skin thanks to the titanium dioxide and mica it contains. You may or may not like this effect (it can make oily areas look oilier), but it can be an attractive, subtle boost for dull skin. This daytime moisturizer does contain fragrance.

☺ **Anti-Wrinkle Nutrients Night Renewal Cream** *($12.99 for 2 ounces)* actually contains more antioxidants than the Anti-Wrinkle Nutrients Daily SPF 15 Lotion, which is why the choice of jar packaging wasn't smart. Knowing these skin-defending ingredients won't last long once you begin using this moisturizer leaves you with a fairly basic formula that's an OK option for normal to slightly oily or slightly dry skin.

☺ **Smooth Skin Cream Scrub** *($6.79 for 6 ounces)* is a fairly gentle scrub that contains more salicylic acid than abrasive agent. The salicylic acid won't exfoliate skin due to this product's pH and its brief contact with skin, but it's a good option if you have normal to dry skin and want to try a lotion-like cleansing scrub. The amount of sodium lauryl sulfate is not cause for concern.

☺ **Night of Olay Firming Cream** *($6.99 for 2 ounces)* is sort of a stripped-down version of the moisturizers from Olay Regenerist, Total Effects, or Definity, without all of the intriguing ingredients. That leaves just an average moisturizer for dry skin.

☺ **Sensitive Moisture Therapy Cream, for Sensitive Skin** *($7.79 for 2 ounces)* is sold as an exceptionally mild cream meant to prevent irritation. This lightweight water- and glycerin-based cream is fragrance- and colorant-free. It contains a high amount of niacinamide, which can help reinforce the skin's own structure to keep skin protected from moisture loss (Source: *British Journal of Dermatology*, September 2000, pages 524-531). Niacinamide may also help skin cells function normally (Sources: *British Journal of Dermatology*, July 2002, pages 20-31; *Biomedical and Environmental Sciences*, September 1999, pages 177-187; and *Nutrition and Cancer*, 1997, volume 29, issue 2, pages 157-162). But aside from the niacinamide, all the other antioxidants (and the sole skin-soothing agent) are barely present and will likely have no impact on skin, especially since jar packaging was chosen. This can be a good moisturizer for normal to slightly dry skin, but aside from not containing fragrance, it isn't that different from most of Olay's other moisturizers.

☺ **Sensitive Moisture Therapy Lotion, for Sensitive Skin** *($8.99 for 4 ounces)* is nearly identical to the Sensitive Moisture Therapy Cream above, except with fewer thickeners, which is what gives it a lotion texture. This version is not packaged in a jar. Otherwise, the same comments apply.

☺ **Quench Touch of Sun Body Lotion** *($8.79 for 6.7 ounces)* is a standard self-tanning lotion suitable for normal to dry skin. It turns skin color with a combination of the self-tanning ingredients dihydroxyacetone and the slower-acting erythrulose. The texture and finish of this won't leave skin feeling greasy. By the way, although they're not reviewed in this book due to space concerns, Olay's Quench body moisturizers are among the best at the drugstore (and you can find complete reviews at www.Beautypedia.com).

ORIGINS

ORIGINS AT-A-GLANCE

Strengths: Almost none for the skin-care products, save for a couple of average eye-makeup removers; makeup fares better, with several great options, including liquid concealer, powder foundation, loose and pressed powders, liquid blush, bronzing options, brow enhancer, and automatic lip and eye pencils; very good makeup brushes composed of synthetic hair.

Weaknesses: Almost every skin-care product contains potent irritating ingredients that have no established benefit for skin, though they are natural; no products to address needs of those with acne or skin discolorations; no AHA or BHA products; although sunscreens provide the right UVA-protecting ingredients, they also contain irritating ingredients, some of which are phototoxic; the foundations contain irritating ingredients, as do most of the lip color products; average specialty products.

For more information about Origins, owned by Estee Lauder, call (800) 674-4467 or visit www.origins.com or www.Beautypedia.com.

ORIGINS SKIN CARE

ORIGINS A PERFECT WORLD PRODUCTS

☹ **A Perfect World Deep Cleanser with White Tea** *($20 for 5 ounces)*. It's not even close to a perfect world for your skin when your cleanser contains irritants such as bergamot, spearmint, and lemon peel oils. All of these and many more plant ingredients in this water-soluble cleanser are problematic for skin, and are a must to keep away from the eye area. As for Origins' rarefied silver-tipped white tea, it is barely present. Even if the white tea was a major ingredient in this cleanser, its positive benefit is negated by the litany of irritants present and the fact that it would be rinsed down the drain before it could have a benefit.

☹ **A Perfect World, Liquid Moisture with White Tea** *($21 for 5 ounces)* contains several essential oils (meaning fragrant oils, because essential oils should only be those that are good for your skin) that are extremely irritating to skin, making this product impossible to recommend and far from skin's fountain of youth!

☹ **A Perfect World, Antioxidant Moisturizer with White Tea** *($36 for 1.7 ounces)* starts out strong and, at first glance, has all the elements of what other Lauder companies (of which Origins is one) know is necessary to create a great moisturizer to ease dryness and restore skin to a healthier state. What a shame Origins had to include such unnecessary and irritating ingredients as bergamot, lemon, orange, spearmint, and vetiver oils (among others). Among all of the Lauder-owned companies, there are plenty of other excellent moisturizers whose best qualities compare favorably to this one from Origins, and those thankfully omit the problematic ingredients that create anything but a perfect world for your complexion.

☹ **A Perfect World For Eyes, Firming Moisture Treatment with White Tea** *($32 for 0.5 ounce)* is the eye-area counterpart to the A Perfect World, Antioxidant Moisturizer with White Tea. The formulas for both are similar, but the designated eye-area version contains a hefty amount of peppermint, which you will notice causes a tingling sensation as soon as you apply it to your skin. Peppermint is a potent irritant and is not only an unnecessary ingredient but also should never be used around the eyes. This product also contains several fragrant plant and flower oils that will make someone with allergies miserable, not to mention further the irritation from the peppermint.

☹ **A Perfect World, White Tea Skin Guardian** *($33.50 for 1 ounce)* is a silicone- and water-based serum that contains some good antioxidants (and in stable packaging), but ultimately just irritates skin due to the bergamot, lemon peel, spearmint, and rosewood oils it contains. Your face will smell great, but that has nothing to do with taking the best possible care of skin.

ORIGINS BY DR. ANDREW WEIL PRODUCTS

☹ **Plantidote Mega-Mushroom Face Cleanser** *($26 for 5 ounces)* had potential for being a good cleansing lotion for normal to dry skin, but it includes too many irritating essential oils to earn a recommendation. The various mushrooms have antioxidant ability, but even if that translated to topical application, those benefits are just rinsed down the drain.

☺ **$$$ Plantidote Mega-Mushroom Eye Makeup Remover Pads** *($21 for 60 pads)* are not as gentle and soothing as described, but they are definitely less irritating than all of the other Plantidote products from Origins. These pads are infused with a mild cleansing solution, but hit some speed bumps on the road to recommendation due to inclusion of potentially irritating ginger root and holy basil. Neither ingredient is preferred for use around the eyes, plus there are plenty of eye-makeup removers available without them, making this pricier option a tough sell.

☹ **Plantidote Mega-Mushroom Eye Serum** *($45 for 0.5 ounce)* lists myrtle leaf water as the second ingredient, which is not recommended for contact with skin due to volatile compounds, including 1,8-cineole, the constituent responsible for this plant's toxicity (Sources: *Journal of Natural Products*, March 2002, pages 334-338; and www.naturaldatabase.com). Even without the myrtle, this serum contains several fragrant oils that are troublesome for skin, including patchouli, orange, and lavender oils.

☹ **Plantidote Mega-Mushroom Face Cream** *($61 for 1.7 ounces)* is the cream version of the Plantidote Mega-Mushroom Face Serum below, sharing many of the same ingredients, but it omits the emollients and thickeners needed to create a creamy texture. Assuming the irritating ingredients mentioned in the review of the Plantidote Mega-Mushroom Face Serum are not present, the many antioxidants in this moisturizer for normal to dry skin are compromised by this product's jar packaging, because antioxidants are not stable in packaging that isn't airtight. As it is, this well-intentioned product has too many negatives to make it a calming, age-fighting experience for skin.

☹ **Plantidote Mega-Mushroom Face Lotion** ($61 for 1.7 ounces) contains some novel and potentially effective antioxidants, but it's laced with irritants, including a tea of orange and myrtle and fragrant oils of lavender, patchouli, olibanum, and orange.

☹ **Plantidote Mega-Mushroom Face Serum** ($66 for 1.7 ounces) is a water-based serum that contains a large number of skin-beneficial ingredients, including efficacious plant oils (the kind that aren't fragrant and protect skin), glycerin, lecithin, and many antioxidants, including olive oil, turmeric, and several species of mushrooms. Things go awry then because Origins just couldn't resist adding irritating fragrant oils to the Plantidote products. Lavender, orange, patchouli, geranium, and mandarin oils all have volatile compounds that counter the soothing, anti-inflammatory effects of the ingredients that precede them. Dr. Weil could have easily found this out from a number of sources, including the medical-journal search engine at www. pubmed.com (the National Institutes of Health Web site), www.naturaldatabase.com, and other resources. The oils assuredly make this serum smell wonderful, which is great for your nose, but they aren't helpful to skin in the least, and prevent this product from being recommended. Without these questionable, problematic fragrant extras, this could have been one of the more intelligently formulated antioxidant serums available.

☹ **Plantidote Mega-Mushroom Treatment Lotion** ($30 for 6.7 ounces) contains too many irritating ingredients to make it a smart choice for any skin type, even though several impressive antioxidants are also included. The basil is a problem, as are the lavender, patchouli, orange, geranium, and frankincense oils. If these ingredients are necessary to "address problems that get in the way of skin's healthy appearance," as claimed, how come the other Lauder brands don't also contain them?

☹ **Night Health Bedtime Face Cream** ($55 for 1.7 ounces) is a lush-textured moisturizer for normal to dry skin that's supposed to relieve "tense-looking skin and visible lines" during deep sleep. Just what is tense-looking skin anyway? How is skin tense? Frowning is one issue, but you're probably not frowning when you're sleeping; even if you were, how does a product like this stop you from doing that? Trying to make this logical is making me tense … oh, no, my skin is wrinkling! OK, forget the claims; they are just nonsense because under any circumstance or any time of day or night this product is not capable of "releasing" wrinkles. As usual for Origins products, this is laced with several fragrant oils that serve to irritate skin and, in the case of lavender oil, cause skin-cell death and increase oxidative damage (Sources: *Cell Proliferation*, June 2004, pages 221-229; and *Contact Dermatitis*, September 2008, pages 143-150). This is in no way a healthy means of achieving a better complexion, at any time of day or night.

☹ **Plantidote Mega-Mushroom Skin-Calming Face Mask** ($35 for 3.4 ounces). I find it so hard to accept that Dr. Weil believes mushrooms are the best ingredient for skin. There is no research substantiating any superior benefit, and Weil is a research-oriented kind of guy. Here is one more product in Weil's Plantidote group for Origins that contains various species of mushrooms, just like the other products in the group. Unfortunately, this moisturizing mask for normal to dry skin continues this line's problematic tradition of including several irritating ingredients for skin. The mushrooms are a novel and potentially effective inclusion, and this contains emollient safflower oil and some soothing agents, but that's little consolation when you consider the abundance of fragrant irritants. Both Estee Lauder and Aveda offer non-irritating, wonderfully soothing facial masks packed with ingredients that skin really needs, and without the disingenuous skin-calming claims. One more comment: Weil positions this mask for those with sensitive, reddened skin. Irritants aside, anyone dealing with sensitive skin should be suspicious of a skin-care product that has a lengthy ingredient list like this one, which goes on and on and on. The more ingredients in a product, the greater the chance that your skin will react to one of them. When it comes to choosing products for sensitive skin, fewer ingredients per product is best.

☹ **Conditioning Lip Balm with Turmeric** *($15 for 0.14 ounce)* is a substandard castor oil–based lip balm that leaves lips irritated due to its lime and ginger oils. The lime oil is dangerous to put on your lips if you are going to expose them to sunlight because a phototoxic reaction can occur that can lead to discolorations (Source: www.naturaldatabase.com).

ORIGINS ORGANICS PRODUCTS

☹ **Organics Foaming Face Wash** *($25 for 3.4 ounces)* would have been a great cleanser for normal to dry skin, but the amount of clove, thyme, grapefruit, and patchouli oils makes this an irritating experience for skin, and a distinct problem if it gets near the eyes.

☹ **Organics Purifying Tonic** *($25 for 5 ounces)* lists alcohol as the second ingredient, and also contains vinegar and lavender oil. None of these are helpful for skin, and the calming willow bark extract doesn't stand a chance of soothing skin in the presence of these potent irritants.

☹ **Organics Nourishing Face Lotion** *($42.50 for 1 ounce)* contains too many irritating fragrant oils to list, along with several fragrant components. The amount of alcohol is also a potential cause for concern, and one more factor that causes this moisturizer to pale in comparison with several others from the Lauder stable.

☺ **$$$ Organics Soothing Lip Balm** *($15 for 0.15 ounce)* is a very good emollient lip balm that is based around cocoa butter. It is irritant-free (What a pleasant surprise!) and works as claimed to prevent moisture loss and restore softness to dry, chapped lips.

ORIGINS YOUTHTOPIA PRODUCTS

☹ **Youthtopia Age-Correcting Serum with Rhodiola** *($50 for 1 ounce)* is more accurately described as a perfume than as a state-of-the-art serum for prolonging skin's "youthspan" (another buzzword Origins uses to sell their products). But what is youthspan anyway, other than an obscure marketing term to make you think this product will make you look younger, when it can't. Not even one second younger. The backbone of this water-based serum is fragrant, irritating sage and orange leaf waters. Although the water form of these ingredients has less irritation potential than the oil form, this serum contains several fragrant oils known to be irritating when applied on skin. It also contains several irritating fragrance chemicals, including eugenol, cinnamyl alcohol, and citronellol. It is telling also that all of these skin-damaging ingredients are listed before the intriguing ingredients that stand a good chance of improving skin when it's not being exposed to multiple irritants.

☺ **$$$ Youthtopia, Firming Eye Cream with Rhodiola** *($39.50 for 0.5 ounce)* promises a more youthful-looking eye area "with none of the potential wrinkles," which means, I think, that the ingredients that are present in other eye creams should make you think twice about using them. Well, I'd think twice about using this product because it is based around myrtle and bitter-orange water, neither of which is helpful for skin. These water (tea) infusions aren't as potent as the pure oils or extracts, but they're still not warranted. Although this eye cream isn't likely to cause irritation, it's a shame that jar packaging was chosen, because the rest of the formula is chock-full of outstanding ingredients. Antioxidants are abundant, and this contains some notable cell-communicating ingredients and skin-identical substances, too. It's best for normal to dry skin, but in better packaging and without the myrtle and bitter-orange it would have been an eye cream superior to most others.

☹ **Youthtopia, Skin Firming Cream with Rhodiola** ($48.50 for 1.7 ounces). I have to hand it to Origins for coming up with some of the most clever product names around, because they convey a sense of cuteness. I wish what was inside the jars was just as clever, because—despite some very good ingredients—Origins' penchant for potent, skin-sensitizing essential oils makes almost all of their products too irritating for skin, as is the case with this moisturizer. It contains sandalwood, geranium, orange, patchouli, cinnamon, nutmeg, and thyme oils, all of which present problems for skin and won't do a thing to help it regain its youthful appearance.

☹ **Youthtopia, Skin Firming Lotion with Rhodiola** ($48.50 for 1.7 ounces) is the lotion version of the Youthtopia, Skin Firming Cream, and the same basic review applies. By the way, if you're wondering what rhodiola is, it's a flowering plant that's known as an adaptogen, a term referring to an ingredient that, when consumed orally, helps the body deal with stressors such as intense exercise or a compromised immune system. Although there is a small amount of research pertaining to rhodiola's benefit when consumed orally, information about its effect as a topical application is scant, though components of this plant do have antioxidant properties (Source: www.naturaldatabase.com). Origins uses the active (root) portion of this plant, but its benefit on skin, if any, is diminished by the inclusion of so many irritating essential oils.

OTHER ORIGINS SKIN CARE PRODUCTS

☹ **Checks and Balances, Frothy Face Wash** ($18.50 for 5 ounces) is a very drying, alkaline cleanser that's made even more troublesome because it contains spearmint, lavender, and geranium oils.

☹ **Clean Energy, Gentle Cleansing Oil** ($18.50 for 6.7 ounces) begins with several non-volatile, gentle oils suitable for dry to very dry skin, but quickly turns from mild to irritating due to several fragrant oils, including lavender, lemon, patchouli, and cedarwood.

☹ **Mint Wash, Cooling Gel That Lathers Clean** ($18.50 for 6.7 ounces) has a name that can't possibly translate to a good rating, and it doesn't because of the numerous irritating fragrant oils this cleanser contains.

☹ **Never A Dull Moment, Skin-Brightening Face Cleanser with Fruit Extracts** ($18.50 for 5 ounces). The only thing that isn't dull about this cleanser is the irritating plant extracts—pine, eucalyptus, grapefruit, and mint oils—which will make your face glow with inflammation.

☹ **Pure Cream, Rinseable Cleanser You Can Also Tissue Off** ($18.50 for 5 ounces). Regardless of how you decide to remove this cleanser, it's best not to use it in the first place because of the peppermint, tangerine, lime, and spruce oils. Ouch!

☺ **Well Off, Fast and Gentle Eye Makeup Remover** ($16.50 for 3.4 ounces) is a simply formulated, rosewater-based eye-makeup remover (which is more eau de cologne than skin care) that is only slightly less of a problem than all the other Origins products that are loaded with unfriendly skin ingredients.

☹ **Modern Friction, Nature's Gentle Dermabrasion** *($37 for 4 ounces)* is Origins' take on the group of at-home scrub products that purport to mimic the effect of microdermabrasion treatments. Unlike other microdermabrasion scrubs, which contain aluminum oxide crystals, Modern Friction contains rice starch. Rice starch is considerably less abrasive, but before you get too excited, keep in mind that this is an Origins product. That means you can expect irritation, delivered here by a bevy of essential oils: lemon, bergamot, peppermint, and camphor. These oils are not present in meager amounts either, and you will feel a deep-down tingle (irritation) as you massage this scrub over your skin. Without these additives, this would be a great scrub for normal to dry or sensitive skin types. As is, I do not recommend it.

☹ **Never A Dull Moment, Skin-Brightening Face Polisher With Fruit Enzymes** *($25 for 4.4 ounces)* contains eucalyptus, pine, and mint oils, and is absolutely not recommended.

☹ **Oil Refiner, Skin Purifying Tonic** *($19.50 for 5 ounces)* contains many more irritants than helpful ingredients for skin, and is not recommended.

☹ **Eye Doctor, Moisture Care for Skin Around Eyes** *($30 for 0.5 ounce)* is not what the doctor ordered! This moisturizer contains wintergreen, mint, and lemon oils, all of which are a problem for skin and increasingly so when used around the eyes.

☹ **Have a Nice Day, Super-Charged Moisture Cream SPF 15** *($35 for 1.7 ounces)* contains an in-part titanium dioxide sunscreen, but at only 1%, so I wouldn't bank on it for UVA protection. Beyond that issue, you won't have a nice day because this daytime moisturizer irritates skin with its peppermint base and blend of volatile citrus and mint oils.

☹ **Have a Nice Day, Super-Charged Moisture Lotion SPF 15** *($35 for 1.7 ounces)* is the lotion version of the Have a Nice Day, Super-Charged Moisture Cream above, and the same comments apply (though this contains slightly more titanium dioxide).

☹ **High Potency Night-A-Mins, Mineral-Enriched Eye Cream** *($30 for 0.5 ounce)* has an emollient, silky formula, but it has no business being used around the sensitive eye area due to the many fragrant oils it contains. Without them (and in better packaging), this would have been a Paula's Pick as an outstanding, thoughtfully formulated moisturizer for dry to very dry skin.

☹ **High Potency Night-A-Mins, Mineral-Enriched Moisture Cream** *($35 for 1.7 ounces)*. What significantly hurts this product (and, in the long run, your skin) is the prevalence of several fragrant oils, including orange and neroli. All of these are on hand in greater amounts than the vitamins or the many other skin-beneficial ingredients such as linoleic acid and cholesterol. This product is not recommended.

☹ **High Potency Night-A-Mins, Mineral-Enriched Moisture Lotion** *($35 for 1.7 ounces)* has a lighter texture than the High Potency Night-A-Mins, Mineral-Enriched Moisture Cream above, but the same negative comments apply here, making this product one to avoid.

☹ **Make A Difference, Skin Rejuvenating Treatment** *($36 for 1.7 ounces)* has a silky texture that can translate to smoother skin, but the main difference this product makes is by causing skin irritation with essential oils of citrus, spearmint, and vetiver. The redeeming ingredients can't compete with these irritants, and won't last long due to jar packaging.

☹ **Make a Difference Skin Rejuvenation Treatment Lotion** *($21 for 5 ounces)*. The only difference this will make in anyone's skin is one of irritation, not rejuvenation. Surprisingly short on truly beneficial ingredients, your skin instead is treated to plant irritant after plant irritant, all in the guise of natural ingredients being better for skin. While it's true that many natural ingredients are quite helpful for skin, here's a clear example of several that are not, and skin suffers as a result. How does Origins justify including spearmint and camphor oils (among others) in a product meant to help skin "rebound from dramatic dehydration"? There is no proof anywhere that these irritants serve skin for the better, especially in comparison with plant extracts that do reduce irritation or do have antioxidant properties.

⊗ **Make a Difference Ultra-Rich Rejuvenating Cream** *($36 for 1.7 ounces)* has a reasonably rich texture (without a doubt, the Lauder companies know how to create elegant moisturizer textures), but that's not enough to offset the irritation and resulting cascade of cellular damage from ingredients such as lemon, spearmint, lavender, and bergamot oils. This moisturizer is mostly void of helpful ingredients and the few that are present won't last long due to the jar packaging. If you really want to make a difference for your skin, be sure to avoid this product.

⊗ **Matte Scientist, Oil Controlling Lotion** *($25 for 1.7 ounces)* doesn't contain enough salicylic acid to help skin, and the amount of irritants is considerable, making this a product all skin types should ignore. Those with very oily skin will do much better keeping shine at bay with one of the Pore Minimizing products from Clinique or with Smashbox's Anti-Shine options.

⊗ **Out Smart, Daily SPF 25 Naturally Protective Sunscreen** *($21 for 1.7 ounces)* includes pure titanium dioxide for sun protection, but is not recommended due to the irritation the many essential oils included can cause. Using this product is not smart, not when there are so many sunscreens that shield skin without causing needless irritation.

⊗ **Make A Difference, Skin Rejuvenating Sheet Mask** *($36 for 6 masks)* is a set of cotton masks said to restore a youthful look to skin, whether the damage was done decades or mere days ago. Don't count on it, primarily because each mask contains a lot of problematic ingredients, including lavender, bergamot, and lemon oils.

⊗ **Drink Up, 10 Minute Mask to Quench Skin's Thirst** *($21 for 3.4 ounces)* offers dry skin some relief, but at the expense of causing irritation because this mask contains bitter-orange and camphor oils.

⊗ **Clear Improvement, Active Charcoal Mask to Clear Pores** *($21 for 3.4 ounces)* is a clay and charcoal mask that would have been a good option for oily to very oily skin if it did not contain so much horsetail extract, which can constrict skin and cause irritation.

⊗ **Modern Fusion, Skin Transforming Catalyst** *($37 for 1 ounce)* wants to transform your skin with its rice-based refinishing complex, but this product will only transform skin from healthy to irritated due to the number of sensitizing ingredients it contains. Bergamot, orange, galbanum, field mint, lemon, and tangerine oils are indeed natural, but they are far from what is needed to enhance skin's glow and clarity, or to make pores vanish as claimed. Bergamot and the citrus oils can cause serious problems for skin if it is exposed to sunlight without adequate protection.

⊗ **No Puffery, Cooling Mask for Puffy Eyes** *($21 for 1 ounce)* contains several fragrant oils that shouldn't get anywhere near the eyes (puffy or not), and as such this rosewater–based product (rose water is mostly fragrance anyway) is not recommended.

⊗ **Out of Trouble, 10 Minute Mask to Rescue Problem Skin** *($21 for 3.4 ounces)* gets skin into trouble because it contains camphor. That won't rescue anyone's skin, and those with blemish-prone skin are potentially setting themselves up for more breakouts because of the high amount of zinc oxide in this mask.

⊗ **Spot Remover, Acne Blemish Treatment Gel** *($12 for 0.3 ounce)* is basically a laundry list of irritants, none of which are helpful at making blemishes go away. Alcohol heads the list, but skin is also assaulted with oregano oil and witch hazel.

⊗ **Cover Your Mouth, Lip Protector with SPF 8** *($8.50 for 0.15 ounce)* not only features an embarrassingly low SPF rating, but also irritates lips with peppermint oil, which is present in a significant amount that definitely makes this a lip balm to keep away from.

☹ **Lip Remedy** *($12 for 0.17 ounce)* contains a lot of peppermint oil, which is the opposite of being any sort of lip remedy.

☹ **Zero Oil, Instant Matte Finish for Shiny Places** *($12 for 0.64 ounce)* lists witch hazel as the second ingredient and also contains camphor oil, making this instantly irritating for all skin types.

ORIGINS SUN & SELF-TANNING PRODUCTS

☹ **Faux Glow, Radiant Self-Tanner For Face** *($18.50 for 1.7 ounces)* lists peppermint (ouch!) as the second ingredient, and that makes this otherwise standard self-tanner extremely irritating. And that's before you even get to the orange, spearmint, and rosemary oils—all of them irritants—that are present, too. Instead of this problematic mix, try an irritant-free self-tanner (most of them are, from Coppertone to Neutrogena), and purchase peppermint oil to inhale while waiting for the self-tanner to dry!

☹ **Sunshine State, SPF 20 Sunscreen with Natural Minerals for Face and Body** *($23.50 for 5 ounces)* will leave your skin in an irritated state due to the atypically large amount of peppermint present in this titanium dioxide–based sunscreen. The rather standard base formula contains more irritants than skin-friendly antioxidants or soothing agents, and, given the price, that's insulting.

☹ **The Great Pretender, Shimmery Self-Tanner for Body** *($18.50 for 5 ounces)* is almost identical to the Faux Glow facial self-tanner, and the same comments apply. Without the unnecessary irritants, both of these self-tanners would have been excellent nongreasy options.

ORIGINS MAKEUP

FOUNDATION: ☺ **Silk Screen Refining Powder Makeup** *($24.50)* is the best and only foundation I recommend from Origins. This talc-free pressed-powder foundation does not contain any of the irritating essential oils that plague other options. It has an awesome silky texture and a smooth, dry finish that provides light coverage. There are 15 shades available, including options for fair to dark skin, and there's not a poor one in the lot. This is recommended for normal to oily skin, though it's not quite on par with similar pressed-powder foundations from Estee Lauder, M.A.C., and Lancome.

☹ **Nude and Improved Bare-Face Makeup SPF 15** *($18.50)* has a lot going for it, from its titanium dioxide sunscreen to its mostly neutral colors and natural finish. How unfortunate that Origins chose to add problematic lemon, spearmint, and grapefruit essential oils. Among those, lemon and grapefruit oils are known to be phototoxic, which means this makeup should not be applied to skin about to be exposed to sunlight (Sources: *Archives of Dermatological Research*, 1985, issue 278, pages 31-36; and www.naturaldatabase.com).

☹ **Stay Tuned Balancing Face Makeup** *($18.50)* has a lot in common with sister company Estee Lauder's Equalizer Makeup SPF 10, except the Origins version contains irritating spearmint, geranium, and lavender oils. All of these present their share of problems for skin and yet have no balancing effect whatsoever. What a shame, because the shade range is beautiful and this foundation costs significantly less than Lauder's version (but with theirs you're getting an irritant-free product).

CONCEALER: ✓☺ **Quick, Hide! Easy Blend Concealer** *($14.50)* is Origins' only concealer, but it's an outstanding version whose only plant ingredients are the soothing varieties, a welcome change of pace. This lightweight, water- and silicone-based concealer provides substantial coverage without looking thick or heavy. It sets quickly to a natural matte finish, so blending must be swift—but it stays in place really well and won't crease into lines under the eye. There are seven mostly excellent shades—Dark is too peach for most skin tones and Neutralizer will be too yellow for lighter skin tones, but is still worth considering. Lightest is suitable for very fair skin, while Very Dark is good but misnamed (it's too light for very dark skin).

POWDER: ☺ **$$$ All and Nothing Sheer Finishing Powder** *($24.50)* is a talc-free loose powder whose light, airy texture feels and looks amazing on skin. Origins decided to make only one shade, which works for most light to medium skin tones; on darker skin, it can look too ashy. This powder does contain mica, which adds a subtle shine, but not enough to avoid wearing during daylight hours. If the one-shade-fits-all prospect doesn't work for you, consider M.A.C's Select Sheer Loose Powder, available in several shades. The synthetic-hair brush Origins includes with this powder, though tiny, is remarkably soft and easy to use. Even better, it rests neatly inside the powder's cap, a convenient addition to a great powder.

☺ **$$$ All and Nothing Sheer Pressed Powder** *($24.50)* is, like the loose version, also talc-free and available in only one shade. It applies sheer, but will still look too light on tan or darker skin tones. It has a smooth texture and sheer, dry finish that works best for normal to oily skin.

BLUSH AND BRONZER: ☺ **$$$ Sunny Disposition Liquid Bronzer** *($20)* has a sheer, non-sparkling, pink-bronze tint that would work well on warm or sallow skin tones that want a tanned appearance. Its matte finish makes it preferred for normal to oily or combination skin.

☺ **$$$ Sunny Disposition Powder Bronzer** *($20)* ranks as a very good pressed-powder bronzer that comes in two believable shades. They'd be more convincing without the shine, but it is comparatively subtle. A little of this goes a long way, so apply sparingly and build from there if a darker result is desired.

☺ **$$$ Sunny Disposition Bronzing Stick for Eyes, Cheeks, and Lips** *($20)* has a smoother-than-silk texture that is easy to apply and imparts a soft, golden bronze color. The single shade is loaded with iridescence so it looks distracting, rather than beguiling, in daylight. However, it is appropriate for evening glamour, and looks particularly attractive when used over self-tanned legs, collarbone, and brow bone. The finish of this product does not feel great on lips, unless you're mixing it with a gloss or balm. For evening use, this is an excellent shimmer product that blends nicely and (best of all) tends to stay put. It is irritant-free.

☺ **Pinch Your Cheeks** *($11)* is a liquid cheek stain that blends nicely once you get the hang of it (expect to have to practice), and offers a transparent matte finish. This works best on normal, small-pored, even-textured skin. The original shade is now labeled Raspberry, and two additional shades are also available.

☹ **$$$ Brush-On Color** *($18.50)* is a powder blush with an unusually dry texture yet smooth, even application. Almost all of the shades are laden with shine, which makes them a questionable choice for daytime makeup. The least shiny shades include Crimson and Clover, Pink Petal, and Rose Dust.

EYESHADOW: Origins' powder ☺ **Eyeshadow** *($14)* includes over 20 shiny selections ranging from subtle to striking. These have a buttery-smooth texture and very nice application that is neither too sheer nor too intense. There are no suitable options for lining the eyes or filling in brows, but at least the shine tends to remain flake-free. Be warned that applying shine over the eyelid can make any amount of wrinkles in that area more noticeable.

☹ **Underwear for Lids** *($14.50)* is a creamy eyeshadow base that comes in twist-up-stick packaging. Why Origins thought this slightly greasy, crease-prone concealer hybrid would make a good eyeshadow base is a mystery. This does not come close to the long-lasting effect you can achieve using a good matte-finish concealer, including Origins' own Quick, Hide! Easy Blend Concealer.

EYE AND BROW SHAPER: ✓ ☺ **Fill in the Blanks Eyebrow Enhancer** *($15)* is a prime pick if you prefer filling in and defining brows with pencil rather than powder. This skinny, automatic, nonretractable pencil applies with ease, isn't the least bit greasy or smear-prone, and has a soft powder finish. The two shades (one for blondes, one for brunettes) are limiting, but everything else about this brow pencil is terrific.

☺ **Automagically Eye Lining Pencil** *($14.50)* is an automatic, nonretractable pencil with one of the smoothest applications you're likely to come across. No tugging or dragging here! The pencil's soft texture makes it tricky to draw a thin line, but thicker lines are a cinch and although you'll notice some fading as the day passes, it stays in place very well. Avoid the Jade and Navy shades.

☺ **Eye Brightening Color Stick** *($14)* is a chubby, stout pencil that comes in one shade—a pale, shimmery silver-blue that is intended to line the inner rims of the eye, a technique that is more theatrical than practical. Also, repeated daily applications put your eyes at risk, as cosmetic coloring agents just don't belong next to the cornea. Yes, it can look striking in photographs, but it's not worth doing on a regular (or even infrequent) basis.

☺ **Just Browsing** *($13)* is a lightweight, softly tinted brow gel with an OK brush that adds natural color and definition to the eyebrow. The number of shades now stands at two (one for blondes, one for brunettes), and overall, I'd recommend Bobbi Brown's Natural Brow Shaper over this because it has a better brush and a wider selection of shades.

LIPSTICK, LIP GLOSS, AND LIPLINER: ✓ ☺ **Automagically Lip Lining Pencil** *($14.50)* deserves consideration if you're looking for an automatic, nonretractable lip pencil whose soft and sheer colors have a drier application but enough stain and silicone-enhanced tenacity to stay on for hours. This is an excellent option for those prone to lipstick bleeding into lines around the mouth. However, just like any anti-feathering lipliner, it won't keep slick glosses or greasy lipsticks from straying past the mouth's border.

☺ **Matte, Sheer,** and **Shimmer Sticks** *($13)* are the original "chubby sticks" that Origins has offered for years, and they're about the only cosmetics company that still does. Why these ever caught on is anyone's guess, because they need constant sharpening, and most are too soft to get a controlled lip line. They're all akin to standard, creamy lipsticks in pencil form. The Matte Stick is not matte in the least, and is actually rather greasy. The Sheer Stick is even greasier than the Matte version, but has less pigment. The Shimmer Stick is creamy without being greasy and has a soft metallic finish. This one stands the best chance of lasting beyond your mid-morning break.

☺ **Underwear for Lips** *($14.50)* is not really necessary if you have a traditional matte-finish concealer handy. This comes in a tube with a wand applicator, and is designed to smooth the surface of the lips and make it easier to apply lipstick. Although this does have a soft matte finish, the peachy hue is not for everyone, and this works only marginally well. Depending on how matte or greasy your lipstick is, this will barely enhance application and will leave you wondering why you bothered. However, unlike most Origins lip products, this one is irritant-free.

☹ **Flower Fusion Hydrating Lip Color** *($16)* does contain several plant and flower waxes, and while those are harmless and contribute to this lipstick's creamy but thick texture, the jasmine, tangerine, lavender, and other citrus oils make this way too irritating to use on lips.

☹ **Liquid Lip Color** *($14.50)* presents lip gloss with a bit more pigment than usual, which means you'll get a semi-opaque, glossy finish. What a shame the mint flavoring is so powerful and irritating, because the selection of colors is enticing.

☹ **Liquid Lip Shimmer** *($14.50)* contains enough mint to make lips tingle and, depending on how much or how often you apply this, burn. The irritation is not worth it when many other glitter-infused glosses are so widely available.

☹ **Once Upon a Shine Sheer Lip Gloss** *($14.50)* could just as easily be called "once upon an irritation" because that's what your lips are up against once they come into contact with this peppermint oil–infused gloss.

☹ **Rain and Shine Liptint with SPF 15 Sunscreen** *($14.50)* lacks adequate UVA-protecting ingredients and loses even more points due to the strong presence of peppermint oil. Plenty of sheer, glossy lipsticks are available that don't run the risk of irritating your lips.

☹ **Smileage Plus Liptint** *($11)* is a sheer, glossy tinted lip balm that comes in some enticing, wearable colors and contains several lip-smoothing emollients. What a shame this ends up being irritating for lips due to its essential oils of lime and tangerine. The lime oil is especially problematic for lips exposed to sunlight, as it can cause a phototoxic reaction (Source: *Archives of Dermatological Research*, 1985, volume 278, pages 31-36).

MASCARA: ☺ **Fringe Benefits Lash-Loving Mascara** *($13.50)* remains a commendable but not extraordinary lengthening mascara that applies without clumps and leaves lashes soft and separated. It's best for those looking for natural rather than dramatic lashes.

☺ **Full Story Lush-Lash Mascara** *($13.50)* is more like a novella than a full story, at least when it comes to making the most of your lashes. You're in for a letdown if you expect this to perform as claimed because it's one of the most unexciting mascaras around. Repeated coats will provide some length, but no thickness whatsoever. In fact, trying to build anything impressive with this mascara is akin to reading the same chapter in a book over and over while expecting the story to progress.

☺ **Underwear for Lashes** *($14.50)* is described as a "little lash builder" and is nothing more than a colorless mascara that adds length and bulk to lashes prior to applying a regular mascara. Its formula is nearly identical to that of the Fringe Benefits Lash-Loving Mascara, and two or three coats of that (or an even better mascara) produce the same results as using this before applying the real mascara.

FACE AND BODY ILLUMINATING/SHIMMER PRODUCTS: ☹ **Halo Effect Instant Illuminator for Face** *($17 for 0.5 ounce)* works as a versatile shine-enhancing lotion that has a gorgeous shimmer effect on skin, whether used alone or mixed with foundation. The problem? A plethora of irritating essential oils, including peppermint, orange, and lemon. These make Halo Effect impossible to recommend for any skin type.

BRUSHES: ✓ ☺ **$$$ Origins Brushes** *($16-$33.50)* have always been made of synthetic hair, a boon for animal rights activists (or just for animal lovers). The latest incarnations are better than ever—you have to feel these to believe how amazingly soft and luxurious synthetic hair can be. Every brush has a renewed softness and the hairs are cut more precisely to facilitate a professional makeup application. Even the handles are top-notch, making the entire collection worth looking at. **The Eye Lining Brush** *($16)* could stand to be a bit firmer, but some may appreciate its greater flexibility. **The Lip Brush** *($16)* is standard fare but the price isn't out of line, and it comes with a cap.

SPECIALTY PRODUCTS: ☺ **Brush Cleaner** *($11 for 3.4 ounces)* is a spray-on, solvent-based brush cleaner that is scented with plant extracts so it won't leave brushes smelling medicinal. It works well and dries quickly; however, this type of product is best for makeup artists who may be using the same brushes on multiple faces. If you're the only one using your brushes, an occasional cleaning with a basic shampoo or liquid soap will suffice, and in the long run will be less drying on the brush bristles.

OXY (SKIN CARE ONLY)

OXY AT-A-GLANCE

Strengths: Inexpensive; selection of fragrance-free topical disinfectants with benzoyl peroxide.

Weaknesses: Everything that's a problem for acne! Most products won't help acne, but will irritate skin with alcohol and menthol; BHA products not formulated at correct pH range to exfoliate, and also contain needless irritants.

For more information about Oxy, call (800) 688-7660 or visit www.oxynation.com or www. Beautypedia.com.

OXY ACNE-FIGHTING FORMULA PRODUCTS

☹ **Face Wash Acne-Fighting Formula** *($6.99 for 6 ounces)* may appeal to the male teens for whom it's marketed because it contains dragon's blood *(Croton lecheri)* extract, but this ingredient has nothing to do with fighting acne. In fact, there is no research supporting its use for any skin type. Reverting to what's all too common and unfortunate about anti-acne products, for either gender, this cleanser contains menthol and a drying detergent cleansing agent that those struggling with oily skin and acne don't need.

☹ **Spot Treatment Acne Fighting Gel Formula** *($6.99 for 0.5 ounce)* irritates skin with 25% alcohol plus menthol, while the dragon's blood extract *(Croton lecheri)* does not reduce redness or soothe skin. If soothing is the goal, then this should have been a radically different formula! The 1% salicylic acid has merit, but not against the other irritants. Note: This product is only available in Canada.

☹ **Shave Cream Acne-Fighting Formula** *($6.99 for 5.2 ounces)* offers hope for blemishes in the beard area because it contains 2.5% benzoyl peroxide, but the emollients and coconut oil make it a potential problem for blemish-prone skin (this doesn't rinse nearly as well as a shaving gel). Although the benzoyl peroxide stands a slight chance of disinfecting skin during the shaving process (though it really doesn't stay in contact with skin long enough), the addition of menthol makes this too irritating to consider.

☹ **Post-Shave Lotion Acne-Fighting Formula** *($6.99 for 1.7 ounces)* contains a low amount of salicylic acid, yet any amount in this product wouldn't help fight acne because the pH is too high for exfoliation to occur. This is not recommended at any stage of a male's shaving routine because it contains a mint extract and the irritating menthol derivative menthyl lactate.

OTHER OXY PRODUCTS

☹ **Chill Factor Daily Cleansing Pads** *($6.59 for 90 pads)* contain mostly alcohol and menthol, and are not recommended for any skin type.

☹ **Chill Factor Daily Wash** *($6.59 for 6 ounces)* is a water-soluble cleanser that contains 10% benzoyl peroxide, but any benefit is rinsed down the drain. The chill comes from the menthol added to this daily wash, making it too irritating for all skin types.

☹ **Daily Cleansing Pads, Focus: Blackheads** *($5.69 for 90 pads)* are nearly identical to the Chill Factor Daily Cleansing Pads, minus the menthol. The low amount of salicylic acid and improper pH range means these pads won't help remove blackheads.

☹ **Daily Cleansing Pads, Maximum** *($5.69 for 90 pads)* contain a potentially helpful amount of salicylic acid, but the pH is too high for it to function as an exfoliant, and the almost 50% alcohol base is too drying and irritating.

☺ **Daily Wash, Maximum Strength** *($5.69 for 6 ounces)* is identical to the Chill Factor Daily Wash, except this version omits the menthol, making it a better choice for normal to oily skin seeking a water-soluble cleanser. The 10% benzoyl peroxide will have minimal, if any, impact on acne due to its brief contact with skin.

☹ **Chill Factor Face Scrub** *($6.49 for 5 ounces)* contains menthol, sodium C14-16 olefin sulfonate, and aluminum powder, all of which make this scrub too irritating and drying for all skin types.

☺ **Face Scrub Acne Treatment, Maximum** *($5.59 for 5 ounces)* is a medicated scrub that contains 2% salicylic acid, but the pH is too high for it to exfoliate, not to mention that it is rinsed from skin before it could penetrate into the pore. The detergent cleansing base can be drying unless you have very oily skin; better scrubs are available at the drugstore.

☺ **Daily Moisturizer Oil-Free SPF 15 Formula** *($6.99 for 1.7 ounces)*. This is a lightweight, oil-free daytime moisturizer suitable for normal to slightly oily skin. The active ingredients include avobenzone for UVA protection, although the salicylic acid cannot function as an exfoliant because the pH is too high. This has a semi-matte finish and a masculine scent, which may encourage young men to start using sunscreen on a daily basis.

✓ ☺ **Oxy Spot Treatment** *($5.49 for 0.65 ounce)* is a topical disinfectant lotion that contains 10% benzoyl peroxide as the active ingredient. It comes in two versions: Clear and Light, each fragrance-free. The Light version provides subtle camouflage and a matte finish, but you'll still need a liquid concealer to cover redness from blemishes. This is a great option for battling acne, but keep in mind that 10% benzoyl peroxide can be too potent for many. This amount is not advised unless you have found using a lower-strength benzoyl peroxide product to be ineffective. Even then, you may want to consult your dermatologist about topical prescription products before trying 10% benzoyl peroxide.

PATRICIA WEXLER, M.D. (SKIN CARE ONLY)

PATRICIA WEXLER M.D. AT-A-GLANCE

Strengths: Good selection of well-formulated moisturizers and serums; two highly recommended cleansers; good topical disinfectant with benzoyl peroxide.

Weaknesses: Moderately expensive; at-home AHA peel provides more irritation than help for skin; all lip products contain potent irritants; one sunscreen lacks UVA-protecting ingredients; no non-irritating salicylic acid products for acne-prone skin; skin-lightening product is alcohol-based; jar packaging.

For additional information about Patricia Wexler M.D., call (888) 939-5376 or visit www.patriciawexlermd.com or www.Beautypedia.com.

PATRICIA WEXLER, M.D. ACNESCRIPTION PRODUCTS

☹ **Exfoliating Cleanser with Acnostat** *($16 for 5.1 ounces)* makes claims that would be more genuine if this were a leave-on product. Because it's a cleanser, the 2% salicylic acid won't exfoliate skin and the MMPi ingredients advertised on the label are rinsed from skin before they can exert any benefit. Most bothersome is the inclusion of cypress oil. Although not much is known about this oil, its volatile compounds can be irritating and its safety and effectiveness (if any) are unknown (Source: www.naturaldatabase.com).

☹ **MMPi•20 Anti-Aging Acne Serum with Acnostat** *($45 for 1 ounce)* lists alcohol as the second ingredient, followed by ethoxydiglycol, a penetration-enhancing ingredient that only makes the alcohol that much more irritating and drying. What an expensive way to irritate skin, not to mention the alcohol will trigger oil production in the pore lining.

☹ **Oil Free Hydrator SPF 30+** *($39.50 for 1.7 ounces)*. I am just stunned at this product, and it is absolutely not recommended because it lacks the UVA-protecting ingredients of titanium dioxide, zinc oxide, avobenzone, Mexoryl SX (ecamsule), or Tinosorb. Without these you leave your face vulnerable to a sizable range of damaging sunlight. Elaborate claims and scientific mumbo jumbo can't replace the need for a well-formulated sunscreen. I'm not sure how this was overlooked, as the research about sunscreen formulations shows up in more dermatological journals than you can imagine.

☺ **$$$ Acne Spot Treatment With Acnostat** *($15 for 0.5 ounce)* is a very good, absorbent cream with 10% benzoyl peroxide as the active ingredient. The addition of soothing plant extracts helps calm redness from blemishes, but that effect is counteracted somewhat by the inclusion of cinnamon bark extract, which keeps this anti-acne product from earning a Paula's Pick rating. The amount of salicylic acid is inconsequential for skin.

☹ **Exfoliating Glyco Peel System** *($60)*. Step 1, **10% Glycolic Peel Pads**, do contain 10% glycolic acid, as the label states. That could have made this Peel very effective for exfoliation, but the pH of 4.4 makes it far less effective than it would be with a lower pH, and for this kind of money it should be very effective indeed. This Peel also contains several irritating plant extracts and oils, including lemon, mandarin, and tangerine, which serve no purpose other than to add fragrance and cause irritation. There are better 10% AHA products on the market with an appropriate pH so they will actually facilitate exfoliation, and without the irritating additives. Step 2, **Skin Neutralizer**, is completely unnecessary. A neutralizer is needed only after application of an extremely potent AHA (over 20%) in a base with an effective pH, neither of which applies to the Peel part of this system. In addition, this Neutralizer has a pH of 8, and there is research showing that products with a pH over 7 can increase the bacteria content in skin. Complicating matters further are several problematic plant extracts that can potentially cause irritation. From almost every perspective this is not a good idea. Step 3, **Intensive Hydrator**, is by far the best product in this kit. It contains several state-of-the-art ingredients, but also includes cypress oil, and that is just a mistake for skin. This mistake might have been overlooked, but not when added to the other problems in this group of products.

☹ **Overnight Acne Repair Lotion with Acnostat** *($20 for 1 ounce)*. Day or night, the 1.25% concentration of salicylic acid in a pH of about 3.5 found here can be extremely helpful for combating acne, acting as both an exfoliant and a disinfectant (to kill acne-causing bacteria at the source). But this product ends up being a complete disappointment because alcohol is the second listed ingredient. To claim that this product reduces irritation, when it contains alcohol in such a prominent position, is just wrong. The alcohol can make oily skin worse by triggering oil production in the pore lining.

PATRICIA WEXLER, M.D. FASTSCRIPTION PRODUCTS

✓ ☺ **$$$ Advanced No-Injection Wrinkle Smoother** *($29.50 for 0.5 ounce)* won't replace the need for Botox or dermal filler injections, but if it really could have this effect then wouldn't it put Wexler's medical practice, which includes injections of Botox and dermal fillers, out of business? Shouldn't she just be handing out this product instead of charging her patients $600 for Botox and even more for dermal injections? Despite the disingenuous claim, this is an exceptionally well-formulated serum-type moisturizer that contains several cell-communicating ingredients and proven water-binding agents. This fragrance-free product is recommended for all skin types, but not for those who are dealing with rosacea because the amount of myristyl nicotinate has a chance of triggering facial flushing if the product is not carefully formulated to avoid the release of free nicotinic acid (Source: *Journal of Pharmaceutical and Biomedical Analysis*, February 2007, pages 893-899).

☹ **Instant De-Puff Eye Gel** *($19.50 for 0.5 ounce)* won't deflate puffy eyes instantly or even after a week of diligent use. The formula contains a high amount of an acrylate-based film-forming agent and adds caffeine to the mix (though there is no research proving caffeine wakes up tired, puffy eyes). It is disappointing that Wexler added irritating cinnamon bark extract to this gel, and it also contains the menthol derivative menthone glycerin acetal. What a shame, because these irritants are commingled with some state-of-the-art ingredients, though none of the peptides can deflate puffy eyes. Overall, this is just too potentially irritating for the eye area.

☺ **$$$ No-Injection Instant Line Filler for Lips & Eyes** *($17.50 for 0.5 ounce)* contains fewer exciting ingredients than the Advanced No-Injection Wrinkle Smoother above, yet its nonaqueous silicone base is considerably silkier. Used around the eyes or on the lips, the concentrated silicone functions as a soft spackle for superficial lines. It's a bit of a letdown that most of the cell-communicating ingredients are listed after the preservative. And, of course, this doesn't have a snowball's shot in you-know-where of replacing what dermal injections do for the lips.

☹ **Advanced No Injection Lip Plumper** *($17.50 for 0.16 ounce)*. How does this make lips plump? Not with hyaluronic acid spheres as claimed. Rather, the menthol derivative menthyl lactate slightly swells lips by irritating them. This is not in any way comparable to what dermal injections can achieve for the lips (procedures Wexler performs in her medical practice because she isn't selling this product to her patients as a way to avoid injections).

☺ **$$$ Instant Airbrush Line Smoothing SuperConcealer** *($19.50)* is made to sound like an instant fix in a tube, claiming to relax wrinkles, treat dark circles, and improve skin tone, all while camouflaging flaws. The ingredients in this water- and silicone-based formula cannot relax lines (the GABA complex it includes has never been shown to be effective for this purpose, and there isn't much of it in here anyway), and the tiny amounts of plant extracts that are natural sources of arbutin won't affect skin discolorations (including dark circles) in the least. I would assume that as a dermatologist Wexler knows all this, because this kind of information has been reported on extensively in every dermatologic medical journal I've read. Wexler's concealer has a lightweight, silky texture that covers moderately well and won't crease into lines under the eye, though its strong matte finish can accentuate these lines. It can be used over blemishes, and is a good alternative to creamy or stick-based concealers for that purpose. Both shades are very good, but are limited to those with fair to light skin tones. Last, it's a boon for skin that this brush-on, pen-style concealer contains a nice array of antioxidants and cell-communicating ingredients, all in packaging that will keep them stable.

OTHER PATRICIA WEXLER, M.D. PRODUCTS

✓ ☺ **$$$ Dual Action Foaming Cleanser** *($16 for 5.1 ounces)* is an excellent, fragrance-free, liquid-to-foam cleanser for normal to oily or slightly dry skin. The water-light formula cleans and removes makeup well without leaving a residue or drying skin. The smattering of plant extracts is more for show than effect.

☺ **$$$ Universal Anti-Aging Cleanser** *($16 for 5.1 ounces)* is a standard, but very good, cleanser for normal to dry skin. It's reminiscent of Neutrogena's Extra Gentle Cleanser, except for the price, of course, which is about twice that of Neutrogena's. While nothing in this product has anything to do with fighting aging, the claim will get the attention of many. For removing makeup, you will need to use a washcloth to be sure you've gotten everything off. It does contain fragrance. By the way, if by "universal" Wexler means "all skin types" that's a mistake, because someone with oily to very oily skin won't be happy with this product. This contains fragrance in the form of methyldihydrojasmonate.

☹ **$$$ Resurfacing Microbrasion System** *($60)* is a two-step system. Step 1 is the **Skin Resurfacing Cream with MMPi**, which is nothing more than a scrub in an emollient base with alumina as the abrasive agent. It can be gritty, so use it carefully. As far as scrubs go, this is OK, but the claim that it can inhibit collagen breakdown is wishful thinking because the ingredients are washed away before they can be of much use to the skin. Step 2 is the **Intensive Hydrator with MMPi**, a well-formulated moisturizer with ingredients that mimic the structure of skin, cell-communicating ingredients, and some unique antioxidants. The combination of these two products doesn't hold any special benefit and more to the point, there are better, less expensive scrubs available, and there are other Wexler moisturizers more interesting than this one. Note: A reappraisal of published literature concerning multiple professional microdermabrasion treatments indicates that its overall level of improvement is marginal, at best (Source: *Dermatologic Surgery*, June 2006, pages 809-814).

☹ **$$$ Deep Wrinkle Eye Repair with MMPi** *($29.50 for 0.5 ounce)* is a fairly state-of-the-art formulation, but the jar packaging leaves much to be desired because none of the exciting ingredients fare well when routinely exposed to air.

☻ **Intensive 3-in-1 Eye Cream** *($32.50 for 0.5 ounce).* The blend of glycerin and shea butter in this eye moisturizer makes it intensive for smoothing and softening dry skin, but I am concerned about the amount of cinnamon bark extract and the cypress oil because they both have the potential for irritation, especially if used around the eye area—it's just not worth the risk. Wexler added some intriguing peptides and cell-communicating ingredients to this product, but like many of the products in this doctor's line, this one comes in jar packaging, which compromises the stability of the good ingredients. Wexler may be a wiz at administering dermal fillers and Botox, but outstanding skin-care formularies aren't one of her more notable specialties.

☹ **$$$ Intensive Night Reversal and Repair Cream** *($42.50 for 1.7 ounces)* features a state-of-the-art formula, but much of what makes it an exciting option for normal to dry skin will be lost once this jar-packaged product is opened. The amount of cypress oil is potentially cause for concern; although not much is known about this plant, two of its components are camphor and d-pinene, both of which can irritate skin.

☹ **$$$ MMPi Skin Regenerating Serum** *($55 for 1 ounce)* does have a wonderful silky-smooth texture, but it lacks the impressive state-of-the-art ingredients in Wexler's other products, plus the jar packaging won't help keep the few good ingredients in here stable.

☹ **$$$ Skin Brightening Daily Moisturizer SPF 30+** *($39.50 for 1.7 ounces)* has what the Oil Free Hydrator SPF 30+ sunscreen reviewed above lacks, thanks to its in-part avobenzone sunscreen and some very interesting state-of-the-art ingredients. How foolish to package it in a jar, which leaves the efficacious antioxidants subject to deterioration on exposure to air and light.

☺ **$$$ Under-Eye Brightening Cream** *($29.50 for 0.5 ounce)* is an impressive blend of antioxidants, cell-communicating ingredients, anti-irritants, and ingredients that mimic the structure of skin, and it has a silky, emollient texture. This would be great for any part of the face—under eye, cheek, jaw—because there's nothing about the formulation that makes it specific for the eye area. As state-of-the-art as this formulation is, to hope that it can improve dark circles under the eye is little more than wishful thinking, though the mica (shine particles) and the whitening effect of the titanium dioxide will cosmetically give the skin a light glow. But that's makeup trickery, not a skin-care breakthrough. It does contain *Uva ursi* (bearberry) leaf extract, which in large amounts can have melanin-inhibiting properties, but at this low concentration, it will barely be noticed by your skin.

☺ **$$$ Universal Anti-Aging Moisturizer PM with MMPi** *($39.50 for 1.7 ounces)* is an emollient moisturizer for normal to dry skin. You can be assured you'll get antioxidants, cell-communicating ingredients, and ingredients that mimic the structure of skin, which is good. Unfortunately, this formula also gives you more fragrance (methyldihydrojasmonate) than any of the more fascinating components. It is still a desirable option, but there could have been more of the good stuff up front (meaning higher up on the ingredient list).

☺ **$$$ Universal Anti-Aging Moisturizer SPF 30 with MMPi** *($39.50 for 1.7 ounces)* contains avobenzone, so this nicely covers the UVA spectrum for good sun protection. While the sunscreen ingredients will remain stable in the jar packaging, the plant extracts, peptides, antioxidants, and retinol certainly won't. That's truly disappointing, because every other aspect of this formulation excels, and it would have been worth the investment for those with normal to slightly dry skin.

PAULA'S CHOICE

As I have done for previous editions of this book, I decided to once again ask for help with the following introduction to my own product line Paula's Choice. I felt one of my customers could describe my products far better then I could and far more objectively. I sent out a request in my free email Beauty Bulletin (available at www.cosmeticscop.com) for comments from women who felt they had a strong sense of what my mission is and what my products do, and asked them to submit their thoughts in writing. The responses were incredibly humbling and I'd like to express a special thanks to everyone who took the time to write an entry. After going through all of the submissions with my team, the winner was Sujaan M. Grimson, L.A.c. (Licensed Acupuncturist), from New York City. This is what Sujaan had to say about my mission and products:

"I am a holistic health care practitioner and my patients often ask me about my personal skin care regimen, probably assuming that I buy everything only from health food stores. In fact, that assumption is incorrect. After reading Paula's advice and learning about natural ingredients— those that are healthy and those that are irritating—not to mention that all ingredients are technically chemical from a scientific point of view, I have a wealth of information to help myself and my patients. I refer all of my interested patients and friends to Paula's books, Web site, and

Paula's Choice skin care line. With thousands of new products on the market every year I can honestly say I would never buy a skin-care product of any kind without first checking with Paula. She covers almost every product on the market and not only reviews it but explains why the product is lacking or wonderful, so it becomes a tutorial as well as useful advice.

"Paula has saved me thousands of dollars by clueing me in to which less expensive products equal or better their pricier rivals. And not buying eye cream alone has saved me hundreds more! As an herbalist I was fooled into believing that herbal ingredients would make a product better, but an herb that might be extremely helpful taken internally can be quite damaging externally, especially when used on the delicate skin of the face. Of course, I must admit, after so many years reading her reviews the best products I have found are her own! I love Paula's Choice products. She makes it so easy by designing routines for different skin types. The prices, ingredients, and packaging all comply with what she has been teaching us for so many years. With Paula's Choice, I don't have to think about it; I just order what she tells me is right for my skin. Simple and inexpensive and I get compliments on my 46-year-old skin all the time … people think I'm in my 30s!

"Thank you, Paula, for all the money you've saved me and even better, for how great my skin looks! I have learned so much from you over the years and will continue to be your devoted reader and customer for years to come."

PAULA'S CHOICE AT-A-GLANCE

Strengths: All products are fragrance-free; all products formulated based on published research on ingredients and their functions/benefits for skin; pH-correct AHA and BHA products; effective skin-lightening options; gentle cleansers; toners that go beyond the norm; all sunscreens provide UVA protection; effective topical disinfectants for acne; antioxidant-rich serums and moisturizers with elegant textures; every foundation provides sun protection and comes in a range of neutral colors; pressed powder and lipstick contain effective sunscreens.

Weaknesses: Limited self-tanning options; limited makeup shades for darker skin tones; no longer a complete selection of makeup products (I'm focusing all my energy on skin care because it is my passion).

For more information about Paula's Choice, call (800) 831-4088 or visit www.paulaschoice.com or www.Beautypedia.com.

PAULA'S CHOICE SKIN CARE

PAULA'S CHOICE CLEAR PRODUCTS

✓☺ **CLEAR Normalizing Cleanser Pore Clarifying Gel for All Skin Types** *($10.95 for 6 ounces)* is a water-soluble gel cleanser that feels refreshing and offers thorough yet gentle cleansing for blemish-prone skin. It is formulated with an antibacterial agent designed to begin the process of killing acne-causing bacteria. This cleanser removes makeup and doesn't leave a trace of residue.

✓☺ **CLEAR Targeted Acne Relief Toner with 2% Salicylic Acid, All Skin Types** *($18.95 for 4 ounces)* is an anti-acne toner whose active ingredient is 2% salicylic acid. It exfoliates skin's surface as well as inside the pore lining to dislodge blackheads, prevent acne from recurring, and reduce redness and inflammation. This toner provides a measurable improvement in skin tone and clarity while feeling water-light and refreshing.

✓☺ **CLEAR Extra Strength Targeted Acne Relief Toner with 2% Salicylic Acid, All Skin Types** *($18.95 for 4 ounces)* is similar to my regular CLEAR Targeted Acne Relief Toner except this contains an ingredient that enhances the penetration of 2% salicylic acid into the pores. It is recommended for those with stubborn acne and blackheads. This product is identical to the 2% Beta Hydroxy Acid Liquid for All Skin Types (below), which has remained a best-seller since it launched.

✓☺ **CLEAR Acne Fighting Treatment 2.5% Benzoyl Peroxide, All Skin Types** *($16.95 for 2.25 ounces)* contains benzoyl peroxide as its active ingredient, and it is the gold standard when it comes to over-the-counter ingredients for acne-prone skin. I've formulated this in a lightweight lotion base that sets to a soft matte finish. It contains soothing anti-irritants so it remains effective against acne-causing bacteria while being gentle on skin.

✓☺ **CLEAR Extra Strength Acne Fighting Treatment 5% Benzoyl Peroxide, All Skin Types** *($17.95 for 2.25 ounces)* is nearly identical to the CLEAR Acne Fighting Treatment above, except this version contains double the amount of benzoyl peroxide. It is recommended for those with stubborn acne, and the formulary attributes remain the same as those for the regular strength version.

PAULA'S CHOICE SKIN BALANCING PRODUCTS

✓☺ **Skin Balancing Cleanser, for Normal to Oily/Combination Skin** *($15.95 for 8 ounces)* has a pearlescent, cushiony texture that leaves skin perfectly cleansed and free of makeup. This is the cleanser to consider if you prefer lots of foam (though the foam itself has no effect on cleansing ability).

✓☺ **Skin Balancing Toner, for Normal to Oily/Combination Skin** *($15.95 for 6 ounces)* is based around the cell-communicating ingredients niacinamide and adenosine triphosphate, both of which improve skin and restore balance while also improving hydration. This toner helps eliminate mild dryness and flaking skin while leaving it feeling smooth. It has been incredibly popular since it was launched.

✓☺ **Skin Balancing Daily Mattifying Lotion with SPF 15, for Normal to Oily/Combination Skin** *($20.95 for 2 ounces)* has a weightless texture someone with oily skin will love, yet it provides sun protection and supplies skin with potent antioxidants and cell-communicating ingredients, while leaving a matte finish. UVA protection is assured by stabilized avobenzone.

✓☺ **Skin Balancing Moisture Gel, for Normal to Oily/Combination Skin** *($18.95 for 2 ounces)* leaves skin feeling remarkably silky, while imparting necessary ingredients that maintain and generate healthy skin. It is ideal under makeup, assuming your foundation provides broad-spectrum sun protection.

✓☺ **Skin Balancing Super Antioxidant Mattifying Concentrate Serum, for Normal to Very Oily Skin** *($24.95 for 1 ounce)* is a weightless combination of beneficial antioxidants, cell-communicating ingredients (including retinol), skin-identical ingredients, and soothing agents. It helps to normalize skin-cell function while keeping excess oil in check thanks to its long-lasting matte finish (which also allows this to work as a "primer" under foundation). It has a silky-smooth finish that feels elegant and makes skin look supple and smooth.

✓☺ **Skin Balancing Carbon Mask, for Normal to Oily/Combination Skin** *($14.95 for 4 ounces)* is a unique treatment mask that absorbs excess oil with clay and super-absorbent carbon. This rinses easily, and the drawing action of the mask also helps to dislodge blackheads.

PAULA'S CHOICE SKIN RECOVERY PRODUCTS

✓ ☺ **Skin Recovery Cleanser, for Normal to Very Dry Skin** *($15.95 for 8 ounces)* feels rich and soothing, and its creamy texture cleanses skin while leaving it feeling smooth and supple. It does not leave a greasy residue, nor does it require a washcloth for complete removal.

✓ ☺ **Skin Recovery Toner, for Normal to Very Dry Skin** *($15.95 for 6 ounces)* is truly a moisturizing toner and is ideal for restoring essential elements to environmentally compromised or sensitized skin. It contains antioxidants, anti-irritants, and essential lipids while being a perfect starting point before applying moisturizer, serum, or sunscreen.

✓ ☺ **Skin Recovery Daily Moisturizing Lotion with SPF 15 and Antioxidants, for Normal to Very Dry Skin** *($20.95 for 2 ounces)* combines extra gentle titanium dioxide and zinc oxide for daytime sun protection while pampering skin with a blend of emollients, silicones, lots of antioxidants, and cell-communicating peptides. Surprisingly moisturizing for being so lightweight, it is designed to work well under foundation. It is suitable for sensitive skins, including those dealing with rosacea.

✓ ☺ **Skin Recovery Moisturizer, for Normal to Very Dry Skin** *($18.95 for 2 ounces)* restores vital moisture to its intended skin types and has an elegantly creamy texture. Skin is fortified with emollients, peptides, antioxidants, and skin-identical ingredients, all of which combine to deliver soft, smooth, healthy skin.

✓ ☺ **Skin Recovery Super Antioxidant Concentrate Serum, for Normal to Very Dry Skin** *($24.95 for 1 ounce)* revitalizes dry skin with a team of antioxidants, cell-communicating ingredients (including retinol), and beneficial plant oils. This is a great way to improve the appearance and healthy functioning of sun-damaged skin.

✓ ☺ **Skin Recovery Hydrating Treatment Mask, for Normal to Very Dry Skin** *($14.95 for 4 ounces)* drenches skin in moisture while helping to restore a healthy barrier function and reduce inflammation. Skin is left feeling soft and looking radiant; you can leave this mask on as long as necessary.

OTHER PAULA'S CHOICE PRODUCTS

✓ ☺ **Moisture Boost One Step Face Cleanser, for Normal to Dry Skin** *($15.95 for 8 ounces)* is a water-soluble cleanser with a milky texture and low lather. It works beautifully to remove all types of makeup.

✓ ☺ **Hydralight One Step Face Cleanser, for Normal to Oily/Combination Skin** *($15.95 for 8 ounces)* is a water-soluble gel cleanser that feels silky and rinses cleanly. Skin is left smooth and refreshed, and this cleanser removes most types of makeup.

✓ ☺ **Gentle Touch Makeup Remover** *($12.95 for 4 ounces)* is a water- and silicone-based, dual-phase liquid that quickly removes all types of makeup, from long-wearing foundations to waterproof mascaras and lip stains. It contains soothing agents and is safe for use around the eyes.

✓ ☺ **Healthy Skin Refreshing Toner, for Normal to Oily/Combination Skin** *($15.95 for 6 ounces)* is one of four truly state-of-the-art toners I have formulated, something sorely missing in many product lines. Each goes above and beyond the benefits of a typical toner, all without the common irritants many toners contain such as citrus, alcohol, or menthol. Healthy Skin Refreshing Toner contains ingredients that improve skin function while reducing cellular damage, leaving skin feeling refreshed with a nearly imperceptible finish, and it also removes the last traces of makeup. Note: this product's name will be changing to Hydralight Skin Refreshing Toner.

✓☺ **Moisture Boost Hydrating Toner, for Normal to Dry Skin** *($15.95 for 6 ounces)* helps normalize and optimize skin to function normally. It contains antioxidants, cell-communicating ingredients, and skin-softening agents that leave a satin-smooth finish while also removing the last traces of makeup.

✓☺ **1% Beta Hydroxy Acid Gel, for All Skin Types** *($18.95 for 4 ounces)* features 1% salicylic acid in a pH-correct formula whose gel texture feels silky-smooth. This is ideal for exfoliating the skin's surface and inside the pore to improve its texture and appearance, while minimizing blemishes and blackheads.

✓☺ **1% Beta Hydroxy Acid Lotion, for All Skin Types** *($18.95 for 4 ounces)* contains 1% salicylic acid in a pH-correct lotion formula that contains soothing agents. It exfoliates and improves skin's texture while providing lightweight moisture.

✓☺ **2% Beta Hydroxy Acid Gel, for All Skin Types** *($18.95 for 4 ounces)* is similar to the 1% Beta Hydroxy Acid Gel, but has twice the concentration of salicylic acid for those with stubborn blemishes or blackheads. This is suitable for all skin types, but best for normal to oily skin.

✓☺ **2% Beta Hydroxy Acid Liquid, for All Skin Types** *($18.95 for 4 ounces)* is one of my most popular products and one I personally have used religiously since I created it for my line. I am proud to say that this product's success is because it works efficiently and quickly to remedy breakouts and dislodge blackheads, smooth the surface of skin while imparting no irritation and improving skin tone (due to the gentle but functional exfoliation it offers). This product also can calm pre-existing irritation. You can apply this toner-like solution with fingertips or a cotton pad.

✓☺ **2% Beta Hydroxy Acid Lotion, for All Skin Types** *($18.95 for 4 ounces)* combines 2% salicylic acid in a pH-correct lotion that soothes and softens skin with its combination of water-binding agents and anti-inflammatory ingredients. It is ideal for those with normal to dry skin prone to breakouts.

✓☺ **8% Alpha Hydroxy Acid Gel, for All Skin Types** *($18.95 for 4 ounces)* pairs an effective amount of glycolic acid in a pH-correct, silky gel. It exfoliates and smooths sun-damaged skin and improves signs of unevenness and minor discolorations.

✓☺ **Hydralight Moisture-Infusing Lotion, for Normal to Oily/Combination Skin** *($18.95 for 2 ounces)* is one of my lightest moisturizers, yet its antioxidant-rich formula provides a powerhouse of helpful ingredients skin needs to look radiant and healthy. Skin is left feeling fresh and looking matte; this works great under makeup, too.

✓☺ **Moisture Boost Hydrating Treatment Cream, for Normal to Dry Skin** *($18.95 for 2 ounces)* makes skin feel luxuriously soft with its combination of skin-identical ingredients, plant oil, cell-communicating ingredients, and emollients. The texture and results make this one of my favorite products to use around the eyes when they're showing signs of dryness.

✓☺ **RESIST Barrier Repair Moisturizer, Skin Remodeling Complex** *($22.95 for 1.7 ounces)* is an advanced moisturizer that's formulated to provide skin with key ingredients it needs to resist environmental damage that causes wrinkles and skin aging. Its luxurious, restorative blend of emollients, antioxidants, skin-identical substances, and cell-communicating ingredients works to remodel and significantly improve skin, bringing it to a new level of health and restoration. The state-of-the-art ingredients selected for this moisturizer are proven to generate healthy collagen production, reduce inflammation, and allow skin to repair itself.

✓☺ **RESIST Super Antioxidant Concentrate Serum, for All Skin Types** *($24.95 for 1 ounce)* is my original Antioxidant Concentrate, which was offered in a new, improved formula in early 2009. It remains an excellent all-purpose option that supplies skin with stabilized vitamin C, cell-communicating ingredients, and other potent antioxidants in a base formula that's neither matte nor emollient. It is suitable for sensitive skin because it does not contain retinol.

✓ ☺ **RESIST Clearly Remarkable Skin Lightening Gel, for All Skin Types** *($18.95 for 2 ounces)* packs a one-two punch for discolored areas with its combination of 2% hydroquinone and 2% salicylic acid. (The latter speeds the results from the hydroquinone.) The gel texture feels refreshingly light, and the special packaging is designed to keep the hydroquinone stable during use. Hydroquinone has considerable research showing it to be the most effective skin lightening ingredient available.

✓ ☺ **Remarkable Skin Lightening Lotion, for All Skin Types** *($18.95 for 2 ounces)* lightens sun- or hormone-induced skin discolorations with its blend of 2% hydroquinone and 7.4% glycolic acid. This smooth-textured lotion may be used alone or layered with other products as needed.

Note: As this book goes to print, this product is transitioning to new packaging and will be renamed RESIST Clearly Remarkable Skin Lightening Gel, for All Skin Types.

✓ ☺ **Skin Relief Treatment, for All Skin Types** *($15.95 for 4 ounces)* is a unique toner-like product that contains stabilized aspirin and vitamin C to soothe skin and calm irritation. It does not contain any of the problematic ingredients found in almost all men's products. This is ideal as an after-shave product for both men and women.

✓ ☺ **Lip Recovery Balm** *($7.95 for 0.19 ounce)* is the lip balm that most of my staff says they wouldn't be caught without and that's true for me, too. Supremely emollient, it contains protective oils, waxes, and emollients that prevent moisture loss and restore dry, chapped skin to a normal state. Applying this at night and during the day if you aren't wearing lipstick guarantees you will never have chapped lips again.

✓ ☺ **Moisturizing Lipscreen SPF 15** *($8.95 for 0.16 ounce)* is an in-part titanium dioxide–based lip balm in a twist-up, ChapStick-style container. Lips are protected from the sun while maintaining a glossy, balm-like finish.

✓ ☺ **Oil-Blotting Papers** *($7.95 for 100 sheets; $3.95 for refill pack of 50 sheets)* are thin tissue paper–style sheets that quickly soak up excess oil and perspiration without leaving a powdery residue.

PAULA'S CHOICE SUN PRODUCTS

✓ ☺ **Almost the Real Thing Self-Tanning Gel, for All Skin Types** *($12.95 for 5 ounces)* is a water-based self-tanner that contains dihydroxyacetone to turn skin color. The formula is tinted so you can instantly see where it has been applied, and it dries quickly. It is suitable for all skin colors. It builds color with each application to prevent streaking or a patchy appearance. Instead, you get a natural–looking tan.

✓ ☺ **Essential Non-Greasy Sunscreen SPF 15, for Normal to Oily/Combination Skin** *($14.95 for 5 ounces)* is my classic sunscreen for normal to oily skin types. It contains avobenzone for UVA protection and leaves skin feeling fresh, smooth, and lightly hydrated. It is ideal for use anywhere on the body, and is designed to not pose problems for blemish-prone skin.

✓ ☺ **Extra Care Moisturizing Sunscreen SPF 30+, for Normal to Dry Skin** *($14.95 for 5 ounces)* has a smooth, creamy texture that feels elegant yet provides water-resistant sun protection and includes titanium dioxide and zinc oxide, among other actives, plus antioxidants.

✓ ☺ **Extra Care Non-Greasy Sunscreen SPF 45, for Normal to Oily/Combination Skin** *($14.95 for 5 ounces)* has a lightweight lotion texture that smooths easily over skin and provides a soft matte finish. It has a much more elegant feel than many other high-SPF products, and provides sufficient UVA protection thanks to stabilized avobenzone. The formula contains antioxidants to boost skin's environmental defenses and is very water-resistant. Ideal for active people or anyone spending several hours outdoors. This sunscreen is suitable for normal to oily or blemish-prone skin but can be enjoyed by all skin types.

✓ ☺ **Pure Mineral Sunscreen SPF 15, for Normal to Very Dry Skin** *($15.95 for 6 ounces)* is my favorite sunscreen to use in sunny climates when I'm going to be outside for a long day. This gentle formula contains only titanium dioxide and zinc oxide and has a silky texture that applies easily and feels light. Green tea is the chief antioxidant, and that coupled with the nonsensitizing actives makes this a great choice for those dealing with rosacea or sensitive skin, or for use on children.

✓ ☺ **Ultralight Weightless Finish SPF 30 Sunscreen Spray, for All Skin Types** *($15.95 for 4 ounces)* is a nonaqueous spray that includes avobenzone for sufficient UVA protection and potent antioxidants to help boost skin's environmental defenses. This protects skin beautifully yet feels like you're wearing nothing at all.

PAULA'S CHOICE HAIR CARE AND BODY PRODUCTS

☺ **All Over Hair & Body Shampoo, for All Skin & Hair Types** *($12.95 for 16 ounces)* functions as a shampoo for all hair types (including chemically treated) and works just as well as a body wash. The formula rinses cleanly and does not contain any ingredients that may be irritating to skin or scalp. Unlike most every shampoo this is truly fragrance-free and extremely gentle, making it excellent for use on babies and children, too.

☺ **Smooth Finish Conditioner, for All Hair Types** *($14.95 for 16 ounces)* moisturizes, detangles, and adds shine to hair, all without making it look or feel limp or greasy. This is one of the only fragrance-free conditioners available, and my goal was to make it every bit as elegant as any others I have reviewed. It works for all hair types, which means you only need to change the amount you use (i.e., more for thick, dry hair, less for fine or thin hair) to achieve the desired results of smooth, silky, combable hair.

✓ ☺ **Beautiful Body Butter, for Dry to Extra Dry Skin** *($16.95 for 4 ounces)* is a decadently rich moisturizer that forms a protective barrier on skin. Cocoa and shea butters dramatically improve the appearance of dry, cracked skin while preventing further moisture loss. This works perfectly on heels, elbows, hands, and other severely dry areas of the body.

✓ ☺ **Close Comfort Shave Gel, for All Skin Types** *($8.95 for 6 ounces)* is a cushiony, soothing shave gel for men or women. The concentrated formula does not foam or lather, yet rinses easily from the razor blade while also protecting your skin from nicks and cuts.

✓ ☺ **Cuticle & Nail Treatment** *($10.95 for 0.06 ounce)* comes in a portable package making it an on-the-go, emollient blend of oils and conditioning agents dispensed from a pen-style applicator with a built-in synthetic brush tip. The applicator makes it ideal for targeted use to keep nails looking great.

✓ ☺ **Skin Revealing Body Lotion with 10% Alpha Hydroxy Acid, for All Skin Types** *($19.95 for 7 ounces)* is an extremely effective exfoliant containing 10% glycolic acid in a pH-correct base formula that supplies skin with an array of ingredients it needs to look and feel its best. This is ideal for rough, dry, sun-damaged skin.

✓☺ **Slip Into Silk Body Lotion, for All Skin Types** *($16.95 for 7 ounces)* contains state-of-the-art ingredients that go above and beyond what typical body moisturizers contain. This lotion leaves skin feeling unbelievably smooth while supplying it with antioxidants, cell-communicating ingredients, and proven water-binding agents.

PAULA'S CHOICE MAKEUP

FOUNDATION: ✓☺ **All Bases Covered Foundation SPF 15** *($14.95)* has a light, creamy-smooth texture and is ideal for normal to dry skin. It has a soft matte finish and offers light to medium coverage with excellent blendability in five neutral shades for fair to medium/tan skin tones. It protects skin from sun damage with a pure titanium dioxide SPF 15 sunscreen.

✓☺ **Best Face Forward Foundation SPF 15** *($14.95)* is designed especially for normal to very oily or combination skin. It has a fluid, ultralight texture that blends beautifully and sets to a long-wearing matte finish that doesn't look thick or feel heavy. An in-part titanium dioxide sunscreen provides broad-spectrum protection from the sun, eliminating the need for a separate sunscreen (provided you apply the foundation evenly over your entire face). Available in four neutral shades for fair to medium/tan skin, this foundation offers sheer to medium buildable coverage.

✓☺ **Barely There Sheer Matte Tint SPF 20** *($14.95)* has a creamy but light texture that slips flawlessly over skin and provides a smooth, satin-matte finish. Its sheer-coverage formula provides a hint of color to even out your complexion while still allowing your natural skin tone to show through. The broad-spectrum titanium dioxide and zinc oxide sunscreen included will help shield your skin from harmful UV rays, making this an ideal all-in-one option for broad-spectrum sun protection and light moisturizing, plus soft color that enhances your skin. It comes in four neutral shades for fair to medium/tan skin tones.

POWDER: ✓☺ **Healthy Finish Pressed Powder SPF 15** *($14.95)* offers the option of shine control and additional sun protection, with a titanium dioxide– and zinc oxide–based sunscreen. This has a velvety feel and goes on evenly and smoothly without looking chalky or dry. You'll find this provides light to medium coverage and has a soft matte finish. It can be used as a pressed-powder foundation (best for normal to slightly dry or slightly oily skin) or simply used with a powder brush to set makeup or touch up your sun protection (over sunscreen or foundation with sunscreen) without redoing your makeup. Please keep in mind that I don't recommend relying on any SPF-rated pressed powder as your sole source of sun protection because it is unlikely anyone will layer it thickly enough to achieve optimal sun protection. It is best to use an SPF 15 powder in conjunction with a moisturizer or foundation with an SPF 15 or greater and that contains UVA-protecting ingredients. Three neutral shades are available plus Healthy Tan, which has a soft bronze tone.

CONCEALER: ✓☺ **Soft Cream Concealer** *($9.95)* features everything I want in a cream concealer: it has a smooth texture that blends easily, it covers well without looking thick or cakey, it has a natural satin finish that resembles skin rather than makeup, and it remains creaseless for hours. I created two neutral shades to complement fair to medium skin tones, whether used alone or with foundation and powder.

EYE AND BROW SHAPER: ✓☺ **Brow/Hair Tint** *($9.95)* defines eyebrows with natural-looking color. The brush-on formula is lightweight and flakeproof, and the three shades can also be used to touch up gray hair at the roots between colorings. (This is the one product I keep in my purse, briefcase, car, and desk—if I see gray hair, I quickly cover it up and no one is the wiser.)

✓ ☺ **Constant Color Gel Eyeliner** *($12.95)* is one of my personal favorites. This long-wearing, water-resistant gel-cream eyeliner has a smooth, quick-drying formula with the texture of a cream lipstick. It glides easily over the lid when applied with your favorite eyeliner brush. You get the look of liquid eyeliner and the smooth application of powder liner. Best of all, it won't smudge, fade, smear, or tear off once it has set. It's ideal for those whose regular eyeliner doesn't make it through the day.

LIPSTICK AND LIPLINER: ✓ ☺ **Long-Lasting Anti-Feather Lipliner, Clear** *($7.95)* is an automatic and retractable colorless lipliner that has a smooth application but isn't greasy, and can help prevent feathering (just like most pencils that have this kind of texture). It works beautifully to keep lipstick from bleeding into lines around the mouth.

✓ ☺ **Sheer Cream Lipstick SPF 15** *($10.95)* offers a beautiful palette of sheer, shimmering colors and includes an in-part avobenzone sunscreen to protect lips from the sun. This lipstick has a modern, lightweight texture that feels comfortably creamy while providing a soft, glossy finish. A colorless version (Invisible) is available to use alone or over your favorite lipstick when you want sun protection.

MASCARA: ✓ ☺ **Great Big Lashes Mascara** *($9.95)* has an agile brush whose dense bristles provide instant thickening and considerable length with just a few strokes. The flake-free formula goes on smoothly, defining each lash for maximum impact. It also keeps lashes soft and is easy to remove with a water-soluble cleanser or your favorite makeup remover.

✓ ☺ **Lush Mascara** *($9.95)* quickly creates long, thick lashes without clumping, flaking, or smearing, and it will last all day. It's water-soluble for easy removal.

BRUSHES: ✓ ☺ **Paula's Choice Brushes** *($9.95-$20.95)* are very soft and dense, are precisely cut for their intended purpose, and hold their shape and place color evenly with minimal to no flaking of powder. All of them are short-handled so they fit nicely and conveniently in any makeup bag. **The Powder Brush** *($20.95)*, **Blush Brush** *($16.95)*, two **Eyeshadow Brushes**, **Small** and **Large** *($11.95 each)*, **Wedge/ Brow Brush** *($10.95)*, **Eyeliner Brush** *($9.95)*, **Lipstick Brush with Cap** *($9.95)*, **Shadow Softening Brush** *($12.95)*, **Crease Defining Brush** *($12.95)*, **Precision Shadow Brush** *($12.95)*, and **Concealer Brush** *($12.95)* are all professional-style brushes to help you apply makeup using the same tools on which most makeup artists rely. Additional brushes you might wish to consider based on your needs are the **Soft Blending Brush** *($12.95)*, **Angled Shadow Brush** *($11.95)*, **Precision Liner Brush** *($11.95)*, **Retractable Powder Brush** *($16.95)*, and **Brow/Lash Brush** *($11.95)*.

✓ ☺ **Makeup Application Sponges** *($5.95 for 10 sponges)* are latex-free, and designed for applying foundation and for blending the edges of makeup, an essential step that's all too often overlooked.

✓ ☺ **Pro Basics Brush Set** *($99.95)* provides seven essential brushes tucked in a synthetic-leather carrying case.

✓ ☺ **Mini Brush Set** *($38.95)* includes small yet perfectly functional versions of my Powder, Blush, Large and Small Eyeshadow, Wedge/Brow, and Eyeliner brushes inside a nylon pouch with a Velcro closure. It's great as a secondary brush set for office or travel.

✓ ☺ **Brush Carrying Case** *($12.95)* allows you to carry, store, and protect up to 12 brushes, enough to stock daily essentials and extra, occasional-use brushes. Made of synthetic leather, this soft, flexible case comes in black and features a durable snap to keep your brushes secure. Spot-clean with a gentle liquid soap or shampoo and a damp washcloth.

✓ ☺ **Bags and Cases** *($7.95-$12.95)* for makeup and skin-care products are also available.

PETER THOMAS ROTH (SKIN CARE ONLY)

PETER THOMAS ROTH AT-A-GLANCE

Strengths: Provides complete ingredient lists on Web site; most products are fragrance-free; very good AHA products; wide selection of water-soluble cleansers and scrubs; some excellent sunscreens, skin-lightening products, and benzoyl peroxide products; many antioxidant-rich formulas.

Weaknesses: Expensive; mostly lackluster toners; mostly boring to potentially irritating masks; no BHA products that do not include at least one needless irritant; jar packaging.

For more information about Peter Thomas Roth, call (800) PTR-SKIN or visit www.peter-thomasroth.com or www.Beautypedia.com.

PETER THOMAS ROTH TO DIE FOR PRODUCTS

✓ ☺ **$$$ Lashes to Die For** *($125 for 0.2 ounce)*. I knew it wouldn't be too long before other cosmetics companies jumped on Jan Marini's lash-enhancing bandwagon, and here's Peter Thomas Roth's (PTR) contribution. You can check out the claims for yourself, but the message is loud and clear: use this and your lashes will be longer and thicker, no mascara required. The water-based, brush-on formula contains several vitamins (which won't nourish lashes, but they look good on the label) as well as several water-binding agents. The latter help keep lashes soft and pliable, but they won't impact their growth or thickness. So is there anything in this product that works to make lashes magnificent? Yes. It seems that the folks at Peter Thomas Roth have found another prostaglandin analogue (listed as 17-phenyl trinor Pge2-Sa) that is behind the results, and this ingredient isn't in trouble with the FDA, at least not yet. You may recall that Jan Marini Skin Research's original Age Intervention Lash products each contained prostaglandin analogues (cloaked in their original formula as "eyelash growth factor" and subsequently relabeled to identify the ingredient as required by the FDA). The original formula was removed from the market by the FDA for various reasons, and her second attempt infringed on a patent issued by Botox king Allergan, so Marini discontinued that product instead of facing an uphill legal battle. It turns out Allergan was working on their own lash-growth product based on their ophthalmic drug Lumigan, which contains the prostaglandin analogue bimatoprost. Unlike Marini, Allergan went through the proper channels to seek FDA approval before bringing the product (Latisse) to market. Of course, this begs the question of how can companies like PTR get away with using prostaglandin analogues in their products, while Jan Marini gets admonished for it? PTR makes no claims of using a prostaglandin analogue, nor did Marini, so why pick on her? I don't have an answer to that other than to suppose that the FDA is selective on which companies they choose to confront about this issue. Getting back to Lashes to Die For, it's a lightweight, brush-on gel that contains antioxidants and some good water-binding agents. Research on the 17-phenyl trinor Pge2-Sa ingredient it contains hasn't proven directly that it stimulates eyelash growth and darkening, but we know it's one of many prostaglandin analogues used to treat glaucoma and that a side effect of such drugs is eyelash growth and darkening (Sources: *Progress in Retinal and Eye Research*, July 2000, pages 459-496; and www.caymanchem.com/app/template/Product.vm/catalog/10004238/a/z). The tiny amount of radish root and alcohol is likely not enough to cause irritation, but it is something to be aware of if you choose to use this product and notice signs of irritation or increased sensitivity.

☹ **Lips to Die For** *($25 for 0.3 ounce)* won't make strangers fall at your feet due to your inflated mouth, but it will irritate your lips because there is so much menthol-like menthone glycerin acetyl in here. The special massaging applicator only causes further agitation that temporarily swells lips, but none of this is an equitable substitute for professional lip injections.

☹ **Lips to Die For Pink Bombshell Lip Balm** *($20 for 0.4 ounce)* is a sheer, pale pink lip balm that has an attractive opalescent shimmer and feels very silky on lips. The texture and softening qualities of the emollients are remarkable, but this balm contains the menthol derivative menthone glycerin acetal. You'll feel the cool tingling sensation almost instantly, and it intensifies the longer this balm is on lips. That's not good news and as a result, Lips to Die For Pink Bombshell Lip Balm is not recommended.

PETER THOMAS ROTH UN-WRINKLE PRODUCTS

☺ **$$$ Un-Wrinkle Peel Pads, for All Skin Types** *($45 for 60 pads)* are alcohol-free pads that contain 20% glycolic acid, a level that is close to peel strength, but before you get too excited, know that the pH of the solution is almost a 6, which is well beyond the level needed for the acid to exfoliate skin. There is no reason to consider these pricey pads (though they're certainly not a problem for skin); the many antioxidants and retinol will not remain stable due to jar packaging.

☺ **$$$ Un-Wrinkle, for All Skin Types** *($120 for 1 ounce)* is a serum loaded with peptides in a proportion that the company claims tops out at 23%, therefore enabling this product to prompt up to a 52% reduction in wrinkles after a month of use, or so goes the claim. Yet there is no research showing that higher concentrations of peptides can have such an effect. There are some intriguing (if somewhat scary) assertions made about these peptides, such as the peptide called SYNr-AKE (technically dipeptide diaminobutyroyl benzylamide diacetate), which mimics the activity of snake venom. (This is Roth's claim, not mine.) The effect of real snake venom on skin can range from swelling and redness all the way to severe infection and necrotic (dead) tissue. Why on earth would a company advertise a peptide as being akin to snake venom? Good question, and it's telling that Roth's Web site mentions the correlation to snake venom, while the same product sold on Sephora's Web site leaves this chilling comparison out. Clearly Sephora was as shocked as I was. SYNr-AKE comes from Pentapharm, whose Web site describes it as a "peptide with an Age Killing Effect. Mimics the neuromuscular blocking properties of Waglerin 1, a polypeptide found in the venom of the snake Tropidolaemus wagleri." This snake is a type of viper, and Waglerin-1 is a peptide (composed of 22 amino acids) that is derived and purified from the venom. There is information on how this peptide performs on neurons in the brain and on its relation to GABA (gamma aminobutyric acid), a common ingredient in products claiming to work like Botox. However, information on how this ingredient works when blended into cosmetic products is lacking and I'm not sure anyone should be a guinea pig for a substance like SYNr-AKE. Waglerin-1 is said to be another blocker of the neurotransmitter acetylcholine, which triggers muscle contractions. But if it worked as claimed, when applied topically it would relax muscles in your fingers, too, and what would happen if you used too much at once or accidentally got it too near the area around your eyes or mouth? (Sources: *Journal of Pharmacology and Experimental Therapeutics*, July 1997, pages 74-80; and *Brain Research*, August 1999, pages 29-37).This product also contains a peptide referred to as SNAP-8, which Roth claims targets the "wrinkle formation mechanism" in the same manner as Botox injections. Although there is no substantiated research to support that, keep in mind that not even Botox works like Botox when it's applied topically. Fear the needle or not, if you want Botox to work it must be injected into, not dabbed on, your skin. SNAP-8 (technically acetyl glutamyl heptapeptide-1) is the trade name for an ingredient manufactured by Centerchem. Yet this ingredient is not listed for Un-Wrinkle, for All Skin Types, making an already bogus antiwrinkle product even more suspect. Of course, the only efficacy studies performed for this peptide were conducted by the manufacturer, and done in vitro rather than on human skin (Source: www.centerchem.com/PDFs/SNAP-8%20Tech%20Lit%20Aug05. pdf). The best reason to consider using this water-based serum is not for its litany of peptides or antiwrinkle prowess (which it is most certainly lacking), but for its antioxidants and water-binding agents, all in stable packaging. This is a costly way to get those ingredients, but they nevertheless are the most substantiated, useful ingredients in this product.

☺ $$$ **Un-Wrinkle Day SPF 20** *($90 for 1.35 ounces).* This daytime moisturizer with sunscreen includes titanium dioxide for UVA protection, but suffers from being overly fragrant. The ginger and lemon extracts aren't the best ingredients for skin, and they're present in a greater amount than Roth's blend of "wrinkle relaxing and antiaging peptides and neuropeptides." By the way, none of the peptides in this product have substantiated research proving they have even a slight effect on wrinkles or expression lines. The only research about these peptides (which are sold as named blends that Roth uses to make their products seem more enticing) comes from the companies selling them to brands such as Peter Thomas Roth. Peptides have their place in skin-care products, but they're not the antiwrinkle miracle we've been waiting for. This is still a good option for normal to slightly dry skin, provided you don't expect your expression lines to go away.

☺ $$$ **Un-Wrinkle Eye** *($100 for 0.5 ounce)* makes the same "look years younger" claim as other Un-Wrinkle products, but doesn't have nearly as interesting a formula, at least not if you're looking for a peptide-rich product (there's no pressing need to do that, but peptides do get a lot of buzz). This has purpose as a lightweight moisturizer for slightly dry skin anywhere on the face, and it contains some good antioxidants in packaging that will keep them stable during use. However, this will not lead to lineless eyes.

☹ **Un-Wrinkle Neck** *($100 for 1.7 ounces)* has claims that read a bit like a science project, what with all the talk of complexes such as Syn-Coll, Trylagen, and Pepha+-Tight and their accompanying percentages. All of these complexes are merely the trade names Roth makes up for his ingredient blends, the same blends he claims will treat deep wrinkles on the neck. Most of the claims are tied to the peptides in this product, yet there is no independent, peer-reviewed research anywhere proving the peptides in Un-Wrinkle Neck will reverse signs of aging (or are even that powerful). What we do know is that because the second ingredient in this serum is alcohol your skin will be exposed to needless irritation and free-radical damage. That's probably not what you were expecting for $100, but it's reality nonetheless. There are some intriguing ingredients in this serum-like product, but they're all trumped by the amount of alcohol.

☺ $$$ **Un-Wrinkle Night, for Normal to Dry Skin Types** *($110 for 1 ounce)* sounds like a science project in a jar! It contains several peptides and claims to firm skin, improve its tone, minimize pores, reduce wrinkles, repair damage, and prompt collagen production. All of a sudden the price seems not so bad, until you realize that there isn't any research proving that the multiple peptides in this moisturizer can reach any of the goals mentioned in the claims. Another disappointment is that the jar packaging won't keep the retinol and antioxidants stable during use. And the "mega dose" of glycolic acid amounts to a mere dusting, not to mention that this product's pH won't permit exfoliation. As a moisturizer, this is suitable for normal to dry skin and it doesn't contain fragrance. Otherwise, this is really pricey for what you get, and a letdown when you consider the jar packaging. By the way, the manner in which most of the peptides in this product are said to work is by interrupting the chemical pathways that occur beneath the skin and that allow us to make facial expressions—this isn't possible. However, assuming these "100% active" peptides could do that, the results would be potentially frightening (as in you wouldn't be able to smile, chew, or keep your eyes completely open).

☺ **$$$ Un-Wrinkle Instant Mineral SPF 30** *($35)*. The "instant mineral" portion of this loose powder with sunscreen has to do with the titanium dioxide and zinc oxide actives. These provide great sun protection, but as with any powder, you shouldn't rely on it as your sole source of sun protection unless you apply it liberally. Liberal application with this powder is a problem because of its occlusive, absorbent nature and because its dry matte finish doesn't look particularly natural on skin. This is best used as a supplement to your moisturizer or foundation with sunscreen. When dusted on normal to oily skin, it adds to your sun protection while helping to temper shine. As for the antiwrinkle claims, you'll have to take the company's word for it that their peptide blend is the solution for instant youth. I wouldn't bet on it, and, in fact, I'm curious as to how they keep the peptides stable and viable in a powder medium based on absorbent minerals. From all the research I've seen about the fragile nature of peptides, they wouldn't remain stable. However, according to the raw material suppliers that manufacture some of the peptides in this product, many of them are available in powder form. Either way, what is 100% certain is that there is no substantiated research proving these peptides work like Botox or have any noticeable benefit for skin. If they did work like Botox, the results from a product like this would be disastrous. Think about it like this: if you dust this all over your face for even coverage and sun protection, and if the peptides prevent contractions of the muscles that lead to expression lines, then they'd also be affecting muscles all over your face. Doing so would affect things we take for granted, like the ability to—oh, I don't know—blink, chew food…! Consider this for its convenient sun protection benefit, not for its alleged antiwrinkle prowess.

☹ **$$$ Un-Wrinkle Lip** *($30 for 0.25 ounce)*. Talk about high tech! This water-based lip moisturizer contains several peptides the company refers to as "100% active," while the Maxilip complex is made to sound like a topical way to reproduce the results of collagen lip injections. Don't count on either class of ingredient coming close to what's possible with lip injections. Assuming that the peptides remain stable (active) as they penetrate the lips and surrounding skin, there's no proof that any peptide blend stimulates collagen production to the extent that lips will be noticeably fuller or less lined. The silicones and waxes in this product can help to temporarily fill in superficial lip lines and lines around the mouth, but nothing magical is taking place, it's just fleeting cosmetics trickery, which is helpful but doesn't change anything. Peptides aren't throwaway ingredients for skin (they have water-binding properties and, theoretically, cell-communicating ability), but to think they can restore what time, smoking, and sun damage depletes (or what was never there in the first place, as in taking thin lips to a full-on pout) is fantasy. The peppermint extract in this product poses a slight risk of irritation, and the resulting inflammation may make lips ever-so-slightly larger for a small amount of time.

OTHER PETER THOMAS ROTH PRODUCTS

☺ **$$$ Anti-Aging Cleansing Gel** *($35 for 8 ounces)* purports to contain natural ingredients that boast antiwrinkle technology, but this is nothing more than a standard water-soluble cleanser for normal to oily skin. The amount of glycolic and salicylic acids is too low for ideal exfoliation (though they would be rinsed away before they could have an effect), and the citrus extracts aren't the best for use around the eyes. Although this is an OK cleanser, the price is way out of line for what you get.

☹ **$$$ Beta Hydroxy Acid 2% Acne Wash** *($35 for 8 ounces)* lists 2% salicylic acid as an active ingredient, but this is rinsed from the skin before it can have an effect. This is otherwise a very simple fragrance-free cleanser for all skin types except very dry.

☺ **$$$ Chamomile Cleansing Lotion with Natural Herbal Extract for All Skin Types** *($32 for 8 ounces)* would be a great water-soluble cleanser for any skin type, but because it contains fragrance those with rosacea or sensitive skin should consider it carefully. This will remove makeup well and contains soothing plant extracts.

✓☺ **$$$ Gentle Foaming Cleanser** *($32 for 6.7 ounces)*. I have nothing but praise for this well-formulated water-soluble cleanser. It is indeed gentle, has a mild foaming action many consumers will appreciate, and works beautifully to remove makeup. Best for normal to oily skin, this fragrance-free cleanser is highly recommended, although you don't need to spend this much money for a good fragrance-free cleanser.

☹ **$$$ Glycolic Acid 3% Facial Wash** *($32 for 8 ounces)* may contain 3% glycolic acid, but without the right pH and given this cleanser's brief contact time with skin, it doesn't matter. It is otherwise a very standard, fragrance-free water-soluble cleanser for normal to oily skin.

☺ **AHA/BHA Face & Body Polish** *($35 for 8 ounces)* contains only a tiny amount of AHA and BHA, so the exfoliant duties fall to synthetic polyethylene beads (the third ingredient). This is a good scrub for normal to very oily skin, and it is fragrance-free.

☹ **$$$ Anti-Aging Buffing Beads** *($36 for 8.5 ounces)*. This product is made to sound like an advanced scrub capable of polishing away wrinkles but the company uses the term "fine lines," which aren't true wrinkles but the lines occurring from dryness. Using a scrub over dry skin and following with a moisturizer can eliminate fine lines, but won't help wrinkles. What's iffy about this jojoba bead scrub (an abrasive agent that is quite gentle) is the inclusion of the drying detergent cleansing agent sodium C14-16 olefin sulfonate as a main ingredient. The glycolic and salicylic acids are present in amounts too small to exfoliate skin. This is an OK, needlessly pricey scrub for normal to oily skin.

☹ **$$$ Blemish Buffing Beads** *($36 for 8.5 ounces)*. The fact that jojoba oil is the second ingredient in this body scrub makes it unsuitable for blemish-prone skin. However, the oil keeps the detergent cleansing agent sodium C14-16 olefin sulfonate from being as drying as it typically is. This is otherwise a very basic scrub whose cinnamon bark content isn't going to do your skin any favors. Overall, it is a problematic formula that fights against itself, putting your skin in the boxing ring as well.

☺ **$$$ Botanical Buffing Beads** *($36 for 8 ounces)* is a scrub that contains jojoba beads as the abrasive agent. They're quite gentle and a good option for normal to dry skin. However, they cannot open clogged pores and emulsify sebum (oil) as claimed. In contrast, because jojoba oil's molecular structure is so similar to our skin's oil, it is much more likely to contribute to rather than remedy clogged pores.

☺ **$$$ Aloe Tonic Mist** *($32 for 8 ounces)* is a very basic, alcohol-free spray-on toner that contains mostly water, aloe (which is primarily water), soothing agents, and a dusting of antioxidants. It is fragrance-free, and suitable for all skin types.

☹ **Conditioning Multi-Tasking After Shave Tonic** *($20 for 8 ounces)* contains several irritants, including witch hazel, lauryl leaf oil, menthol, and citrus peel oils. This would be a terrible product to apply to just-shaved skin!

☺ **$$$ Conditioning Tonic** *($32 for 8 ounces)* is an exceptionally basic toner whose salicylic acid content is too low to be effective, even though the pH is within range. Countless other less expensive toners offer your skin more than this.

☺ **$$$ Glycolic Acid Clarifying Tonic** *($32 for 8 ounces)* is a substandard toner that contains a frustrating mix of helpful and irritating ingredients, plus the pH is too high for the glycolic acid to function as an exfoliant. Let me clarify by saying that there are numerous other tonics that provide your skin with more than this.

☺ **$$$ Glycolic Acid 10% Hydrating Gel** *($48 for 2 ounces)* is an excellent fragrance-free AHA product for all skin types, and the pH of 3.6 ensures efficacy. The amount of antioxidants and other beneficial extras isn't enough to keep this product at its former Paula's Pick rating.

✓ ☺ **$$$ Glycolic Acid 10% Moisturizer** *($45 for 2 ounces)* is an ideal AHA moisturizer for normal to dry skin. Glycolic acid at a pH of 3.8 ensures exfoliation, while emollients and antioxidants help dry skin look and feel better, all without added fragrance.

☺ **$$$ Anti-Aging Cellular Eye Repair Gel** *($42 for 0.76 ounce)* is sold as a revolutionary eye treatment whose benefits for wrinkles go beyond retinol. The company's Firme-CELL-4 technology is allegedly responsible for this feat. It combines four peptides (including the works-like-Botox argireline, also known as acetyl hexapeptide-3) said to have a synergistic effect on reducing deep lines and wrinkles. Before you get too excited, there is no substantiated research to support this claim. Peptides have theoretical cell-communicating ability and likely play a role in encouraging healthy skin functioning, but whether or not they can affect wrinkles is unknown; they probably can't. In contrast, retinol has mounds of research pertaining to its ability to improve skin's appearance and stimulate collagen production. Besides, beyond the peptides, this gel is mostly slip agent, film-forming agent (a hairspray-type ingredient), and preservatives, which are hardly worth opening up your pocketbook for.

☹ **Eye Overhaul Duo** *($58 for 0.25 ounce).* This eye-area moisturizer includes two products in one jar. The **Day** eye cream offers SPF 30 and provides UVA protection with avobenzone. That active ingredient isn't the best for use in the immediate eye area (titanium dioxide and zinc oxide are by far preferred for that area) due to its sensitizing potential. The base formula contains several beneficial ingredients, but most of them will lose their potency due to the jar packaging. Cosmetic pigments are included to give the eye area a subtle brightened look.

The **Night** eye cream is supposed to reduce under-eye puffiness and repair skin while you sleep. Will you wake up with lineless, puff-free eyes? Absolutely not, because the ingredients in this product, while helpful for skin in general, do not have the ability to eliminate puffy eyes caused by aging or allergies. It's a shame the many beneficial ingredients (most notably antioxidants) in this eye cream won't last for long because of the jar packaging. This Duo won't overhaul your eye area, but in better packaging it could've gone a long way toward strengthening skin's barrier and encouraging healthy collagen production.

☺ **$$$ Max All Day Moisture Defense Cream with SPF 30** *($42 for 1.7 ounces)* is a good daytime moisturizer for normal to dry skin. The in-part titanium dioxide sunscreen provides sufficient UVA protection, and the formula includes antioxidants (though they should have been given more prominence).

☺ $$$ **Max Anti-Shine Mattifying Gel** *($35 for 1 ounce)* is merely a blend of silicones and a dry-finish solvent. It produces a matte finish, although without absorbent ingredients that offer more absorbency, don't expect shine-free longevity. Also, for the money, the company could have included at least one antioxidant and a single skin-identical ingredient.

☺ $$$ **Max Sheer All Day Moisture Defense Lotion with SPF 30** *($42 for 1.7 ounces)* isn't that sheer, but it's a good daytime moisturizer with an in-part avobenzone sunscreen suitable for normal to dry skin. This product is fragrance-free.

☹ $$$ **Mega Rich Intensive Anti-Aging Cellular Creme** *($85 for 1.7 ounces)* uses the same Firma-CELL-4 technology described for the Anti-Aging Cellular Eye Repair Gel above. This time the base is creamy and only two of the four peptides are present in notable amounts. However, none of the peptides can affect deep wrinkles or expression lines. At best, this moisturizer will make normal to dry skin feel better, but the many antioxidants are subject to deterioration because of jar packaging, making this a mega waste of money.

☹ $$$ **Mega Rich Intensive Anti-Aging Cellular Eye Creme** *($65 for 0.76 ounce)* lists most of the bells and whistles after the preservatives, and the jar packaging leaves all the ingredients vulnerable to the deteriorating effects of exposure to air.

✓ ☺ $$$ **Moisturizing Multi-Tasking After Shave Balm** *($24 for 3.4 ounces)* is a brilliant choice for a moisturizer to use after shaving (or anytime, anywhere skin is dry). The fragrance-free balm contains significant amounts of antioxidants, cell-communicating ingredients, and ingredients that reinforce skin's healthy barrier function. And the price is realistic, too!

☹ $$$ **Oil-Free Moisturizer** *($42 for 1.7 ounces)* remains one of Roth's more basic moisturizers, though it is indeed oil-free. This would be an OK option for normal to slightly oily or slightly dry skin. It does contain fragrance.

☹ **Oxygen Eye Relief** *($52 for 0.75 ounce)* contains hydrogen peroxide, a potent generator of free radicals and a completely inappropriate ingredient for skin care. Although the jar packaging won't keep the peroxide (or antioxidants) stable for long, the entire concept of oxygenating skin to improve wrinkles is just bonkers!

☹ **Power K Eye Rescue** *($100 for 0.5 ounce)* includes several antioxidants front and center, but none of them will do much good for your skin because of the jar packaging. In addition, vitamin K cannot affect dark circles or brighten skin when applied topically, and although arnica has a history of being used for bruising, it is ill-suited for use around the eye, not to mention that very few cases of dark circles are actual bruises.

☹ **Power Rescue Facial Firming Lift** *($150 for 1.7 ounces)* contains a lot of film-forming agent, and also has the same formula pitfalls as the Power K Eye Rescue—making this not worth the investment or the potential irritation to skin.

☹ **Radiance Oxygenating Serum** *($65 for 1 ounce)* is a classic example of cosmetics double-talk because it claims to provide oxygen to skin, while also supplying antioxidants. Given that these two actions are diametrically opposed, how can anyone's skin possibly benefit? The answer is it can't, and it may actually make matters worse. Although this water-based serum doesn't contain pure oxygen, it contains fluorocarbons (chemically inert compounds), which increase the oxygen content in liquids. As an aside, fluorocarbons are also responsible for much of the ozone depletion that occurs in the atmosphere. Peter Thomas Roth's theory and claim is that by increasing the oxygen content of this serum users will be giving skin a potent dose of oxygen with each application. If that's their claim, then one must surmise that no one at the company has taken note of any of the research indicating that oxygen isn't going to help your skin resist wrinkles or look younger. Exposing skin to more oxygen than it is already exposed to will simply generate more free-radical damage (Sources: *International Journal of Cosmetic Science*, October 2008, pages 313-322; and *Human and Experimental Toxicology*, February 2002, pages 61-62). In contrast, applying antioxidants to skin (and consuming them as part of a healthy diet) is supposed to reduce the very damage oxygen exposure causes. See what I mean about opposite actions? Even if increasing the oxygen that is delivered to skin was somehow beneficial, this serum would not be recommended because it contains the irritating menthol derivative menthyl lactate along with peppermint extract. Without question, neither of those ingredients are helpful for skin, regardless of age or concern.

✓ ☺ **$$$ Retinol Fusion PM** *($65 for 1 ounce)* is a very good nonaqueous, silicone-based serum with retinol. It also includes antioxidant vitamins C and E along with a cell-communicating ingredient and anti-irritant. The fragrance-free formula is best for normal to dry skin. The amount of alcohol is so small as to not be cause for concern; likely it's present to make an ingredient in this serum more soluble.

☹ **$$$ Ultra-Lite Anti-Aging Cellular Repair** *($52 for 1.5 ounces)* makes the same anti-wrinkle, our-peptides-pack-a-punch claims as the Anti-Aging Cellular Eye Repair Gel above. Peptides are brimming in this product, but there is no proof they can affect collagen and elastin production or improve the appearance of wrinkles and expression lines. This is an OK option for normal to dry skin, but the smattering of antioxidants is not helped by jar packaging.

☹ **Ultra-Lite Multi-Tasking After Shave Balm** *($24 for 3.4 ounces)* lists witch hazel distillate (which is mostly alcohol) as the second ingredient, and is not recommended.

☺ **$$$ Viz-1000** *($65 for 1 ounce)*. If you believe the claim that this product is super-concentrated with 75% hyaluronic acid, you're in for a surprise. This product doesn't even contain hyaluronic acid (the natural substance used in some dermal fillers to plump wrinkles and facial skin folds). Rather, it contains the salt form (sodium hyaluronate), which, while effective as a water-binding agent, isn't the same thing as the more potent (and expensive) hyaluronic acid. Despite that letdown, this serum contains plenty of water-binding agents that hydrate skin and improve its smoothness while preventing moisture loss. Viz-1000 (whatever that name means) is suitable for all skin types. However, there are many serums at and below this price range that offer skin a more well-rounded formula. And just to be clear, using any form of hyaluronic acid topically on your skin doesn't net the same results, in any way, shape, or form, as dermal injections of hyaluronic acid (such as the dermal filler Restylane). You can't just rub a dermal filler on your skin and expect to get a drop of benefit; it has to be injected.

☹ **Acne Spot And Area Treatment** *($32 for 1 ounce)* lists 5% sulfur as its active ingredient. Although sulfur is a potent disinfectant, it is very drying and irritating for most skin types. For that reason, it is not preferred to benzoyl peroxide or even tea tree oil. The pH of 3.1 serves only to make the sulfur more irritating, but it does allow the blend of glycolic and salicylic acids to exfoliate.

☹ **AHA/BHA Acne Clearing Gel** *($45 for 2 ounces)* contains 2% salicylic acid in the correct pH range for exfoliation to occur, but the amount of alcohol makes this too potentially drying and irritating for acne-prone skin.

☺ **$$$ Aloe-Cort Cream** *($30 for 2 ounces)* is a very standard lotion that contains 1% hydrocortisone as the active ingredient. It's an option for occasional use on minor skin irritations and itching, but for the money you'll get just as much efficacy from less expensive hydrocortisone creams at the drugstore. Aloe alone doesn't justify the price.

☺ **$$$ Cucumber Gel Masque** *($45 for 5.3 ounces)* is an overpriced water-based mask that contains a mixture of irritating and non-irritating plant extracts. It should not be considered calming or capable of reducing under-eye puffiness, at least not any better than using a cold compress to relieve swelling.

☹ **Gentle Complexion Correction Pads** *($36 for 60 pads)* contain an unimpressive amount of salicylic acid, but would have merit as an AHA product if the base did not contain so much alcohol.

☹ **Max Complexion Correction Pads** *($36 for 60 pads)* share the core problems of many anti-acne pads: an alcohol-based solution and a pH too high for salicylic acid to exfoliate, which won't help blemished skin in the least. This is absolutely not recommended.

✓☺ **$$$ Mega Rich Intensive Anti-Aging Cellular Moisture Masque** *($60 for 3.4 ounces)* doesn't have a "mega-rich texture" for those with very dry, dehydrated skin, but those with normal to dry skin looking for an indulgent mask should consider this state-of-the-art formula. The company's comments about the peptides in this product helping to improve skin's texture are legitimate and surprisingly low key. Assuming the peptides can penetrate skin and not be destroyed by enzymes en route, they stand a good chance of improving cellular functioning, which in turn improves skin's texture and appearance. For that reason and because this mask contains impressive levels of well-researched antioxidants, it is best left on skin overnight rather than rinsed after several minutes. There is no reason why you couldn't use this as a nightly moisturizer; it would be a shame to treat skin only intermittently to such an impressive, fragrance-free formula.

☺ **$$$ Pumpkin Enzyme Peel, For All Skin Types** *($44 for 3.3 ounces)* is a simply formulated, non-irritating product that banks on pumpkin enzymes to provide "deep exfoliation" for skin. Most enzymes used in skin-care products are unstable, and this is no exception (and jar packaging doesn't encourage stability). It's very likely the only benefits you'll receive from this non-peeling peel are softer skin (from glycerin) and, if this appeals to you, a pumpkin scent.

☹ **Radiance Oxygenating Masque** *($50 for 3.4 ounces)* is very similar to Peter Thomas Roth's Radiance Oxygenating Serum above and the same claims are asserted: you're supposed to believe that this mask supplies oxygen to skin while also defending against oxidative damage with the antioxidants it contains. Please refer to the Radiance Oxygenating Serum review for a full explanation of how and why these claims are contradictory.

☹ **Sulfur Cooling Masque** *($40 for 5 ounces)* severely irritates skin due to its 10% concentration of sulfur along with eucalyptus oil. This mask is not recommended.

☹ **Hands That Lie SPF 15** *($25 for 2.5 ounces)*. This hand cream with sunscreen lacks the UVA-protecting ingredients of titanium dioxide, zinc oxide, avobenzone, Tinosorb, or Mexoryl SX and, therefore, is not recommended. It also contains several plant irritants that can make skin more sun-sensitive. By the way, although the base formula contains avobenzone (listed as butyl methoxydibenzoylmethane), it doesn't count for sun protection if it's not listed as an active.

☺ **Matte Lip Balm** *($12 for 0.25 ounce)* is a blend of silicones with antioxidant plant extracts, two of which (rosemary and ginger) can be irritating. The silicone has a protective action on your lips while feeling feather-light, and does set to a matte finish.

PETER THOMAS ROTH SUN & SELF-TANNING PRODUCTS

☹ **Continuous Sunscreen Mist SPF 30** *($28 for 6 ounces)* is a spray-on sunscreen that owes its nearly weightless texture to the inclusion of lots of alcohol. Unfortunately, that's bad news for the health of your skin. This provides UVA protection with avobenzone, but for the money, Roth could have had a much better product using silicone instead of skin-damaging alcohol, and the tiny amount of vitamin E is too little, too late.

☺ **$$$ Instant Mineral SPF 30** *($30 for 0.32 ounce)* provides sun protection with titanium dioxide and zinc oxide, and is a mica-based loose powder packaged in a self-contained applicator with a built-in brush. Powder application is sheer, but the brush is merely OK. You'd have to apply this liberally to ensure SPF 30 protection, and doing so is difficult due to the application method. That makes Instant Mineral SPF 30 best as an adjunct to a separate sunscreen or foundation with sunscreen. The product imparts very sheer color and a subtle shine, and has an absorbent finish.

☺ **$$$ Instant Mineral SPF 45** *($30)*. You may think this is simply a more protective version of Roth's Instant Mineral SPF 30 above, but it is different in some key areas. First, the amount of sunscreen actives titanium dioxide and zinc oxide is nearly double (this likely provides more than SPF 45, but as with any powder you'd really have to apply a lot to get the stated amount of protection) while the base formula has a lighter, smoother, and drier texture without an obvious shine. This sheer powder is dispensed from a cylindrical component onto a built-in powder brush. The brush isn't the softest, but works to apply this loose powder evenly. The powder goes on sheer and translucent, and does a good job of keeping oily shine at bay. Those with oily, sensitive skin, take note: this is a great way to add to your daily sun protection.

☺ **$$$ Natural Looking Self-Tanner** *($28 for 4 ounces)* is a good self-tanning lotion for normal to dry skin. Like most self-tanners, it's dihydroxyacetone that turns skin color. This contains fragrance in the form of rose oil.

✓☺ **$$$ Oil-Free Sunblock SPF 30** *($26 for 4.2 ounces)* is a very good in-part avobenzone sunscreen whose antioxidant-rich formula is suitable for normal to slightly dry skin. This is also fragrance-free and while it does not contain any oil, some of the thickening agents may be problematic for blemish-prone skin.

☺ **$$$ Oily Problem Skin Instant Mineral SPF 30** *($30)*. The mineral sunscreens in this tinted loose powder are a great way to get broad-spectrum protection, plus they have the secondary benefit of providing coverage to help even out the complexion. The downside is that the amount of titanium dioxide and zinc oxide is likely to contribute to rather than help clogged pores, but that's always a risk with these two ingredients. This loose powder is housed in a cylindrical applicator with a built-in brush. It has a dry texture and absorbent finish that are ideal for oily skin, but again, if blemishes are a concern the amount of mineral actives may prove problematic. This contains a potentially effective amount of salicylic acid, but the pH is not within range for exfoliation to occur. Although the company positions this product as being perfect for acne-prone skin, it is preferred for oily skin not struggling with blemishes (or dealing with occasional breakouts). By the way, the main ingredient in the base formula is a mineral known as illite, which has a clay-like texture and a luminosity similar to that of mica. Despite that, the mineral actives in this powder keep it from being noticeably shiny. This would be a worthwhile sunscreen addition for someone with oily skin and rosacea.

✓☺ **Uber-Dry Sunscreen Cream SPF 30** *($26 for 4.2 ounces)* has a name that fits, because the base formula of this in-part avobenzone sunscreen feels nearly weightless and provides a silky-matte finish that's sure to please those who dislike the often thick, tacky texture of many high-SPF sunscreens. This earns its stripes not only for providing broad-spectrum sun protection, but also for being fragrance-free and treating skin to antioxidant vitamins and phospholipids. It is an excellent sunscreen option for all skin types, particularly normal to oily skin (and there is no reason this cannot be used on facial skin).

✓ ☺ **$$$ Ultra-Lite Oil-Free Sunblock SPF 30** *($26 for 4.2 ounces)* is similar to but slightly heavier than the Oil-Free Sunblock SPF 30, and the same review applies.

☹ **Ultra-Lite Oil-Free Sunscreen Mist SPF 15** *($28 for 8 ounces)* does not contain the UVA-protecting ingredients of titanium dioxide, zinc oxide, avobenzone, Mexoryl SX (ecamsule), or Tinosorb and is not recommended. Even with sufficient UVA protection, this is a really no-frills formula that is completely devoid of antioxidants or other skin-beneficial ingredients. What a disappointment!

PHILOSOPHY

PHILOSOPHY AT-A-GLANCE

Strengths: Relatively inexpensive; some of the best products are fragrance-free; very good retinol products; selection of state-of-the-art moisturizers; skin-lightening option that includes sunscreen; great lip balms, including those with a tint; impressive specialty makeup products.

Weaknesses: Irritating and/or drying cleansers; average to problematic scrubs for face and lips; at-home peel kits far more gimmicky than helpful; most sunscreens contain lavender oil; several products include irritating essential oils; insufficient options to manage breakouts; the majority of makeup items do not rise above average status.

For more information about philosophy, call (800) 568-3151 or visit www.philosophy.com or www.Beautypedia.com. Note: philosophy opts to use lowercase letters for every product they sell, so the listings below are simply following suit.

PHILOSOPHY SKIN CARE

☹ **never let them see you shine cleanser** *($20 for 5.5 ounces)* is not recommended because this foaming, creamy, water-soluble cleanser contains the irritating menthol derivative menthyl lactate along with skin-unfriendly lavender oil. Neither ingredient has any effect on reducing skin's output of oil, nor can they prolong the time it takes for cleansed skin to show signs of shine.

☹ **purity made simple high foaming cleanser** *($21.50 for 6 ounces)* produces copious foam, thanks to the main detergent cleansing agents in this product (along with supporting lather agents), but that's not what is getting your skin clean. Regardless, some people love cleansers that foam and others can do without it. If you're a foam fan, this cleanser isn't the way to go because it contains several irritating fragrant oils along with irritating citrus and pepper extracts (none of which are capable of calming and refining skin as claimed).

☹ **never let them see you shine scrub** *($20 for 4 ounces)* is not recommended because it contains the irritating menthol derivative menthyl lactate along with skin-unfriendly lavender oil. Also, the abrasive agent is essentially composed of tiny crushed skeletal pieces from sea creatures. Not too appealing, is it?

☺ **$$$ the great mystery** *($25 for 5 ounces)* is basically glycerin, water, sea salt, and thickeners, along with some token marine plant extracts and a tiny amount of lavender oil. Salt can be a problem for the skin due to its high pH and irritation potential, though it does work as a scrub, but for that purpose a simple washcloth will work even better. The only mystery is why more people don't do that instead of bothering with all these scrub particles scraping and abrading their faces.

☺ $$$ **the microdelivery exfoliating wash** *($25 for 8 ounces)* contains a gentle detergent cleansing agent, but the clay it contains can be a bit drying for all but oily skin. The apple amino acids may sound farm fresh, but they have no ability to exfoliate skin, especially not in a product that is quickly rinsed away.

☺ $$$ **the microdelivery peel** *($65)* is a two-step at-home peel kit that ends up being more trouble than it's worth. Step 1 involves the **Vitamin C/Peptide Resurfacing Crystals**. This is essentially a baking soda scrub that contains silica for additional exfoliation and antioxidant vitamins, none of which will remain stable once this jar-packaged scrub is opened. You massage the Resurfacing Crystals over your skin for up to one minute, then apply Step 2, the **Lactic/Salicylic Acid Reactivating Gel**. This gel contains mostly water and lactic acid, and its pH of 2 interacts with the alkaline pH of the baking soda in the Resurfacing Crystals, which is what provides the immediate sensation of warmth. The warm feel doesn't mean the vitamin C and peptides are suddenly active, as philosophy claims; it's merely a chemical reaction. Not surprisingly, it leaves your skin very smooth after rinsing, just as it would be if you used a standard scrub with a washcloth. The lactic acid functions as an AHA product (with a pH that's definitely irritating), but its contact with skin is too brief to do much, so this is essentially a very expensive, potentially irritating baking soda scrub.

☺ **the afterglow** *($20 for 4 ounces)* contains an efficacious amount of the AHA lactic acid at a functional pH of 3.5, all in a supremely lightweight, fragrance-free base. This would be even better with some anti-irritants or more sophisticated water-binding agents, but it's definitely worthwhile as an AHA product for all skin types.

☹ **the microdelivery mini peel pads** *($35 for 60 pads)* contain eucalyptus, tangerine, lemon, lavender, and orange oils, which make these AHA pads (lactic acid is on hand for exfoliation) too irritating for all skin types. If you want an effective AHA product that is free of needless irritants, consider the less expensive options from Alpha Hydrox, Avon, Neutrogena, or Paula's Choice.

☹ **the microdelivery multi-use peel pads** *($55 for 100 pads)* may have multiple uses, but skin will be irritated and sensitized wherever these pads are stroked. The same problematic ingredients mentioned in the microdelivery mini peel pads are present here, too.

☺ $$$ **booster caps retinol capsules** *($50 for 60 capsules)* each contain a blend of silicones with a plant sugar, the algae chlorella (water-binding agents), film-forming agent, retinol, and fragrance. The capsule system is a good way to keep the retinol stable until you use it, and the contents have an extremely silky texture that is suitable for all skin types. Still, this product contains no more retinol than its competitors, and the lack of other antioxidants is short-sighted. Retinol does have research showing it has antiwrinkle benefits for skin (Sources: *Skin Pharmacology and Physiology*, March/April 2005, pages 81-87; and *Radiation Research*, March 2005, pages 296-306), but research also shows that its benefit for skin is further enhanced when antioxidants and ingredients that mimic the skin's intercellular matrix are included. None of this makes this product not worth trying, but given its one-note nature, there are more interesting retinol products available.

☺ $$$ **booster serum** *($60 for 1 ounce)* was created to "give your skin the ultimate antiaging treatment," but it seems no one at philosophy stopped to consider what that should entail because this is one of the most lackluster serums around. It contains more fragrance than antioxidants (much less the talked-up peptides), and is modestly successful at being an OK moisturizer for normal to slightly dry skin.

☺ **$$$ dark shadows** *($33 for 0.5 ounce)* is a good lightweight moisturizer for normal to slightly dry skin anywhere on the face. It contains a couple of unique antioxidants and peptides, which may have cell-communicating ability. What this cannot do is eliminate dark circles or discolorations above the upper lip. It contains fragrance in the form of hibiscus flower.

✓ ☺ **$$$ eye believe** *($30 for 0.5 ounce)* is a thick, silicone-based gel that contains a couple of antioxidants along with retinol and peptides. It's an elegant formula that can smooth the appearance of superficial lines (those related to dryness, not permanent wrinkles), but more important, it provides all skin types with some very helpful ingredients, and does so without fragrance.

☺ **$$$ help me** *($45 for 1 ounce)* is a good retinol product for normal to very dry skin not prone to blemishes (the amount of wax can aggravate breakouts). Content-wise, retinol isn't given more prominence here than it is in several drugstore lines, but it is stably packaged, fragrance-free, and certainly an option.

☹ **hope in a bottle** *($38 for 2 ounces)* contains an unspecified amount of salicylic acid, but regardless of the amount, the pH of this moisturizer is too high for preferred levels of exfoliation to occur. It is not recommended because it contains lavender oil and lacks any significant amounts of beneficial ingredients.

☹ **hope in a jar, for dry, sensitive skin** *($38 for 2 ounces)* is completely inappropriate for any skin type because it contains lavender and sage oils, both of which have components that are irritating to skin and destructive to cells.

☺ **$$$ hope in a jar, original formula** *($28 for 1 ounce)* is sold as philosophy's world-famous therapeutic moisturizer, but it's a rather ordinary formula that does not contain lactic acid as claimed. Instead, this has lauryl lactate, which is the ester of lauric and lactic acids. Although the product has a pH of 3.2, lauryl lactate does not have exfoliating abilities; rather it functions as an emulsifier and enhances the spreadability of creams. Jar packaging won't keep the antioxidants in this product stable, and it's really not deserving of its alleged worldwide fame.

☹ **hope in a jar SPF 20** *($45 for 2 ounces)*. There's hope for protecting your skin from the sun thanks to this daytime moisturizer's in-part avobenzone sunscreen. However, some hope is dashed because the jar packaging exposes the few antioxidants it contains to degrading light and air. In addition, the lavender oil won't do the same favor for your skin as it might for your nose. Applied to skin, lavender oil can cause cell death (Source: *Cell Proliferation*, June 2004, pages 221-229). One of the main ingredients in this product is lauryl lactate, which is the ester of lauryl alcohol and lactic acid. However, the high pH of this product coupled with the non-acidic nature of the ingredient means you cannot rely on Hope in a Jar SPF 20's claims to exfoliate skin. Using pure lactic acid at the right pH would have been better, along with omitting the lavender oil.

☺ **$$$ hope in a tube** *($33 for 0.5 ounce)* is a thick, emollient-rich, fragrance-free cream that will take excellent care of dry, dehydrated skin anywhere on the body, but it won't firm skin one iota. Of course, given the small amount of product, this is best reserved for use on the face, and would work well around the eyes if that area is dry. Classic moisturizing standbys such as glycerin, petrolatum, and mineral oil comprise the bulk of the formula, and philosophy included a few antioxidants, too.

☺ **$$$ on a clear day retinol clarifying lotion** *($40 for 0.75 ounce)*. Before I get into a discussion about the claims philosophy makes for this product, I need to state that this is a very good fragrance-free moisturizer with retinol for normal to dry skin. It is also packaged so that the retinol and antioxidants will remain stable during use, which is exactly what you want to see. The issue with this product is the claims it makes for abating acne, clogged pores, and post-acne scarring. None of that is true, most notably because the base formula contains a lot of triglyceride and wax (yes, wax), both of which are the opposite of what someone with clogged pores or acne needs if their goal is to improve matters. There is also nothing in this product that can stop the growth of bacteria that cause blemishes. As for acne scarring, the company should've been more specific. Retinol and antioxidants bring multiple benefits to skin, but the only type of acne "scarring" they may help improve are not technically scars. Rather, the correct term is "post-inflammatory hyperpigmentation," which refers to the discolorations that linger long after a blemish has gone. Nothing in this product is going to plump up depressed or pitted acne scars. The antioxidants in here can reinforce healthy cells and reduce inflammation, which can help improve the red marks that occur once a blemish has gone away, fading them faster than they would on their own. But this product isn't going to do a better job than many others. Despite the fact that this product isn't an all-in-one solution to a cadre of skin woes, it is, as mentioned, a contender if you have normal to dry skin and want a well-formulated moisturizer with retinol along with other beneficial ingredients.

☺ **$$$ save me** *($60 for 1 ounce)* is first and foremost a vitamin C serum. It contains magnesium ascorbyl phosphate, a stable form of this antioxidant, and there is plenty of it present (it's the second ingredient listed). The other showcased ingredients (peptides, retinol, and additional antioxidants) make a less impressive appearance, but they are present. The opaque, airless pump bottle will help keep the vitamin C stable, but don't expect this product to lift and firm skin as claimed. This is suitable for all skin types and is worth trying if you're curious to see what a vitamin C serum does for your complexion.

☹ **shelter, tinted SPF 30** *($20 for 2 ounces)* contains lavender oil, an ingredient that is toxic to skin cells and increase oxidative damage (Sources: *Contact Dermatitis*, September 2008, pages 143-150; and *Cell Proliferation*, June 2004, pages 221-229).

☹ **shelter, untinted SPF 30** *($25 for 4 ounces)* would rate a Paula's Pick for sun protection if it did not contain lavender oil. The in-part titanium dioxide sunscreen and silky lotion base with plentiful antioxidants could have been a great option for those with normal to dry skin.

☹ **the present** *($25 for 2 ounces)* is supposed to serve as a "second skin," but the lavender oil in this product can cause skin-cell death, which means your "first skin" will be put at risk by using it.

☹ **when hope is not enough, age defense spf 20** *($38 for 2 ounces)* is a pricey sunscreen that doesn't have much going for it, other than including avobenzone for UVA protection. The base formula lacks a blend of antioxidants in appreciable amounts, something that might have made the price tag more reasonable. Lavender oil is added for fragrance, but there is concern that this ingredient, even in concentrations as low as 0.25% (which may be applicable to this product) is toxic to cells (Source: *Cell Proliferation*, June 2004, pages 221-229). It is best to avoid any product, effective sunscreen or not, that features lavender oil, just as you would avoid any other expensive sunscreen—because its price might discourage liberal application.

☺ **$$$ when hope is not enough facial firming and lifting serum** *($38 for 1 ounce)* contains mostly water, film-forming agent, slip agents, glycerin, water-binding agents, antioxidants, anti-irritant, pH adjuster, fragrance, and preservatives. It is a worthwhile, serum-type moisturizer for normal to slightly oily skin because it supplies hydrating agents, antioxidants, and cell-communicating ingredients without thickeners, oils, or oil-like ingredients. This product won't lift skin, and it won't help minimize facial hair growth as claimed, because it contains no ingredients with proven ability to do that.

☺ $$$ **when hope is not enough hyaluronic acid/peptide capsules** *($50 for 60 capsules).* Ever since hyaluronic acid became a popular ingredient in medically injected dermal fillers, it has become a popular cosmetic ingredient claiming to work the same way as the medical version to reduce wrinkles and other age-related lines in skin. Of course, these "alternative to cosmetic corrective procedure injections" don't work in any way, shape, or form as dermal fillers do, but the name association is often all it takes to get consumers to pay attention. This philosophy product is no different, although they went the individual-capsule "dosage" route rather than packaging this serum-type product the standard way. Either way it is just a waste of money. What's frustrating is that the product label mentions "hyaluronic acid," but the ingredient list (the only part of the product that has to tell the truth) indicates sodium hyaluronate, which is the salt form of this ingredient. Sodium hyaluronate is a great water-binding agent for skin, but it's not the same as the considerably more expensive hyaluronic acid. Regarding these capsules, the amount of water-binding sodium hyaluronate and "cutting edge" peptides is almost too small to matter anyway. If you like the idea of single-use capsules for dispensing a serum, Elizabeth Arden's Ceramide capsules have a better formula.

☺ $$$ **when hope is not enough omega 3-6-9 replenishing serum** *($45 for 0.85 ounce).* What's most bothersome about this nonaqueous serum is the amount of fragrance. A product's scent shouldn't take precedence over truly beneficial ingredients, yet almost all of the interesting antioxidants in this serum take a backseat to the fragrance. This serum does contain some helpful, non-irritating plant oils for dry to very dry skin (and they do supply skin with various omega fatty acids, as claimed), but if you want the benefits of these fatty acids, you should use a more advanced serum and mix it with a small amount of the plant oils present in this philosophy product. Note: Depending on the Web site you visit, this serum is also known as When Hope is Not Enough Omega 3-6-9 Replenishing Oil and as When Hope is Not Enough Essential Fatty Acid Replenishing Treatment. We used the name that philosophy printed on the bottle.

☺ $$$ **when hope is not enough replenishing cream** *($48 for 2 ounces)* is an emollient moisturizer whose best, price-justifying ingredients will break down once this jar-packaged product is opened. This will help dry skin look and feel better, but so will many less expensive moisturizers.

✓☺ **a pigment of your imagination SPF 18** *($30 for 2 ounces)* is one of philosophy's most unique products because it combines an effective, in-part avobenzone sunscreen with ingredients that can improve hyperpigmentation. The main ingredient responsible for lightening skin discolorations is arbutin, and that's due to its hydroquinone content. Although the research describing arbutin's effectiveness is persuasive (even if almost all of the research has been done on animals or in vitro), concentration protocols have not been established. That means we just don't know how much arbutin it takes to have an effect in lightening the skin. Related information suggests that a newer compound known as deoxyarbutin also has merit as a skin-lightening agent, though this research was also done in vitro on cultured human skin cells (Sources: *Journal of Cosmetic Science,* July/August 2006, pages 291-308; and *Experimental Dermatology,* August 2005, pages 601-608). A pigment of your imagination is fragrance-free and best for normal to dry skin. It is comparable to but actually a better formulation than Shiseido's Whitess Intensive Skin Brightener.

☺ **$$$ the microdelivery peel, hydrating mask** *($25 for 1.3 ounces)* has lots of potential as a moisturizing mask for normal to dry skin, but the lavender oil it contains is a problem for all skin types. There isn't much of it in here, and this is ideally meant to be rinsed from the skin after a brief period, so the rating is more lenient.

☹ **the oxygen peel kit** *($50)* is a two-step kit that contains **oxygen foam** and **catalase enzyme capsules**. The foam portion contains a good deal of hydrogen peroxide, which is not recommended for anyone, while the capsules contain the enzyme catalase, which is responsible for the elimination of peroxide. Taken together, this is a do-nothing duo that is not akin to any type of in-office professional peel.

☺ **$$$ turbo booster c powder** *($35 for 0.25 ounce)* consists of a bottle of vitamin C powder that contains other antioxidants, amino acids, and a couple of water-binding agents. The powder is designed to be used alone or added to a moisturizer or serum to create "a state-of-the-art vitamin C formula." There are lots of top-notch vitamin C products available that don't involve a messy powder or mixing with another product. This is a viable option if you're curious to see what a vitamin C product will do for your skin; the only issue is that the form chosen (ascorbic acid) can be irritating, while other, more stable forms of vitamin C don't have this drawback.

☹ **kiss me exfoliating lip scrub and facial** *($15 for 0.5 ounce)* is an emollient sugar-based scrub for lips that works to remove dry, flaky skin and leave it smooth. The problem? Peppermint oil, which only causes irritation. You're better off mixing a bit of table sugar with a nonvolatile plant oil or mineral oil and massaging that mix over dry lips.

☺ **$$$ the supernatural oil-control blotting tissues** *($10 for 100 sheets)* are standard, non-powdered oil-blotting papers with a tissue-thin texture. They do soak up excess shine or perspiration, and the dispensing method is unique.

PHILOSOPHY MAKEUP

FOUNDATION: ☺ **$$$ the supernatural powder airbrushed canvas SPF 15** *($35)* deserves credit for its pure zinc oxide sunscreen, but this is otherwise a standard loose-powder mineral makeup that comes packaged with a built-in (and removable, if you want to clean or replace it) sponge applicator. The powder shakes onto the sponge to minimize mess, and you buff it over your skin. Like most mineral makeup, the main ingredient is bismuth oxychloride. Despite a lightweight texture, this can make skin feel increasingly dry during wear, and the strong matte finish is offset by noticeable sparkles. Coverage goes from sheer to medium, but you really have to pile this on to get to that level, which increases the dryness later on. Although the range of nine shades is mostly neutral, if mineral makeup intrigues you, consider the silkier-feeling options from bare escentuals before this.

CONCEALER: ☺ **$$$ the supernatural airbrushed color corrector** *($25)* gets you three creamy concealers in one compact, complete with a synthetic brush. The brush's square tip isn't as easy to work with as those with a rounded or tapered tip, and although the concealer applies smoothly and covers well, it creases unless carefully set with powder. Three palettes are available. Light is the best assortment, Medium is OK but two of the shades pull toward peach, and the shades in the Dark palette are too disparate to work together. This concealer would have been better if it was sold as a single color with a slightly tweaked formula and a less creamy finish.

LIPSTICK, LIP GLOSS, AND LIPLINER: ✓ ☺ **kiss me clear tube** *($12)* is the original, colorless kiss me product and remains an excellent choice for those seeking a lip balm with a non-sticky texture and glossy finish. This lanolin-based balm is a great choice for treating dry, chapped lips and, thankfully, is irritant-free.

☺ **$$$ the supernatural lip gloss** *($15)* is a standard lip gloss with a wand applicator that has a slightly thick, sticky feel and shimmer-infused finish from each of the sheer colors. This is flavored with mint, but it's subtle and the product does not contain direct peppermint oil so the risk of irritation is slim.

☺ **$$$ the supernatural lip pencil** *($12.50)* needs sharpening and is all-around standard except for the fact that the slightly dry application doesn't smear. Otherwise, the few shades are versatile enough to coordinate with several shades of lipstick.

☺ **$$$ think big big mouth lip primer** *($25)* is a semi-matte, colorless lipstick that is supposed to fill in lines on the lips and make them smoother pre-lipstick. It does this to a minor extent, but despite plumping claims, the formula doesn't contain anything that makes lips bigger, even temporarily. This is a pricey, superfluous product whose smoothing benefit you can get from many lipsticks.

☺ **lip shine** *($12)* is a philosophy lip gloss that's exclusive to Sephora stores. It comes in several tempting flavors, including cinnamon buns and mimosa. These thick, sticky glosses are loaded with shimmer and each imparts more sparkle and shine than color. Avoid the empowermint lip shine because it contains peppermint oil.

☹ **kiss me pink tube** *($12)* is a very sheer pink gloss with a slick, emollient texture—too bad it is loaded with peppermint oil, so lips get a potent dose of irritation along with a glossy finish.

☹ **kiss me very emollient SPF 20 lip balm clear** *($14 for 0.5 ounce)* has a sunscreen whose actives do not provide sufficient UVA protection, plus it contains irritating peppermint oil. This is a step in the wrong direction, philosophy!

☹ **kiss me very emollient SPF 20 lip balm red** *($14 for 0.5 ounce)* is identical to the kiss me very emollient SPF 20 lip balm clear above, except this has a sheer red tint. Otherwise, the same comments apply.

MASCARA: ☺ **$$$ the supernatural mascara** *($22)* has been reformulated so it's less of a do-nothing-but-darken-lashes mascara, but it still fails to wow, at least if your goal is to build length or thickness. Truly a natural-look mascara, the unconventional formula coats lashes minimally, basically creating minor improvements all around. It's an option if you're 90% satisfied with the lashes you have, but anything less will leave you disappointed, especially at this price, and you have to be careful that the wetter formula doesn't smear before it dries.

☺ **$$$ think big big gorgeous eyes mascara** *($22)* has an enticing name, but the only thing "big" about this mascara is the box it comes in (which is an unreasonable waste of packaging material). If anything, applying this mascara will be a big disappointment. No matter how many times you stroke the brush through your lashes or dip it into the container hoping more product will produce "gorgeous" results, they won't appear. Minimal length and almost no thickness are all you'll achieve. If you are only interested in modest results, this will work well enough. It doesn't smear or flake during the day and washes off easily, but that is hardly worth the price.

BRUSHES: ☺ **$$$ the supernatural brush** *($25)* is a dense, synthetic powder brush whose head is cut straight across. That makes it a workable choice to apply loose-powder foundation (such as the one philosophy sells) or blush. Whereas philosophy used to sell several brushes (usually in sets), they now have decided that you need only one brush for all your makeup needs. That's not possible, any more than a blouse is all you need to wear to go outside and to the office.

SPECIALTY PRODUCTS: ☺ **$$$ the supernatural poreless flawless tinted SPF 15** *($30 for 1.6 ounces)* is a nonaqueous, silicone-based primer with an in-part titanium dioxide sunscreen. It has the requisite silky texture and smooth matte finish, but is marred by a strange, though sheer, peach tint. This is best for light to medium skin tones (the peachy tinge won't make someone with fair skin happy), and as primers go, this does contain some great antioxidants.

☹ **never let them see you shine primer** *($20 for 1 ounce)*. The silicones in this water-based product can help temper oily skin, but the slip agents and water-binding agents attract moisture to skin, which can make it appear oily. How confusing! This also contains several natural ingredients that can irritate skin, including a bark extract, ginger, and lavender oil. There are better primer-type products that go the distance in terms of keeping shine in check without needlessly irritating skin. Clinique, Smashbox, and Laura Mercier's options are all recommended over this disappointment.

PHYSICIANS FORMULA

PHYSICIANS FORMULA AT-A-GLANCE

Strengths: Inexpensive; almost all products fragrance-free; outstanding cleansers; one worthwhile toner; pressed powder with broad-spectrum sunscreen; several bronzing powder options (primarily for fair to light skin tones); one of the only lines at the drugstore selling matte-finish eyeshadows; the loose powder; most of the blushes; good liquid liner; excellent automatic brow pencil.

Weaknesses: Dated moisturizer formulas; several sunscreens lack sufficient UVA protection; jar packaging; several of the makeup products epitomize wasteful packaging; the shade selection for almost all the foundations and concealers is awful; tons of gimmicky products that don't perform as well as you'd think but are eye-catching in their compacts; bad eyelining options; the lip color and lip plumper; mostly average to disappointing mascaras; the Organic Wear products either have undesirable textures or contain irritating ingredients.

For more information about Physicians Formula, call (800) 227-0333 or www.physicians-formula.com or www.Beautypedia.com.

PHYSICIANS FORMULA SKIN CARE

PHYSICIANS FORMULA ORGANIC WEAR 100% NATURAL ORIGIN PRODUCTS

☹ **Organic Wear 100% Natural Origin Eye Makeup Remover Liquid** *($9.95 for 4 ounces)*. The plant extracts in this liquid makeup remover may be organic, but that doesn't inherently make them better for your skin. The orange fruit–water base coupled with radish root extract and lavender oil is not what you want to apply near the eyes. Ouch!

☹ **Organic Wear 100% Natural Origin Facial Makeup Remover Lotion** *($9.95 for 5 ounces)* would be a good option if not for the amount of orange fruit water it contains and the inclusion of lavender oil. You'd be better off removing your makeup with pure jojoba, safflower, or olive oil—all of which are natural.

☹ **Organic Wear 100% Natural Origin Eye Makeup Remover Pads** *($9.95 for 60 pads)* contain fragrant orange fruit water as a main ingredient and also contain the potent irritants lemon peel and lavender oils. They are a mistake to use anywhere near the eyes, and, organic or not, lavender causes skin-cell death while increasing oxidative damage.

☹ **Organic Wear® 100% Natural Origin Facial Makeup Remover Towelettes** *($9.95 for 25 towelettes)* contain far too many natural irritants to make them a wise choice for makeup removal. Using an organic, nonfragrant plant oil would be a much better solution.

OTHER PHYSICIANS FORMULA SKIN CARE PRODUCTS

✓☺ **Gentle Cleansing Lotion, for Normal to Dry Skin** *($7.25 for 8 ounces)* is a very standard, but also very good, fragrance-free cleansing lotion for its intended skin type. It is also recommended for those with sensitive skin who cannot tolerate detergent cleansing agents. You will need a washcloth for complete removal.

✓☺ **Eye Makeup Remover Lotion, for Normal to Dry Skin** *($4.75 for 2 ounces)* has a formula that's remarkably similar to the Gentle Cleansing Lotion, for Normal to Dry Skin, except this version is marketed as a makeup remover. It works in that capacity, even removing waterproof mascara, but if you're already using or considering the Gentle Cleansing Lotion, you don't need this as well.

☺ **Eye Makeup Remover Pads, for Normal to Dry Skin** *($5.75 for 60 pads)* are an effective but greasy way to remove eye makeup, including waterproof mascara. These pads are best used before washing your face, because the residue they leave behind isn't something you want to go to bed with on your face. By the way, a cheaper version of this product that would work just as well given the ingredient list would be plain mineral oil.

☹ **Oil Free Eye Makeup Remover Pads, for Normal to Oily Skin** *($5.75 for 60 pads)* contain only a tiny amount of cleansing agents capable of removing makeup, and are mostly fragrant rose water and irritating witch hazel. That's eau de cologne, not skin care!

☺ **Vital Lash Oil Free Eye Makeup Remover Lotion, for Normal to Oily Skin** *($4.75 for 2 ounces)* isn't vital to anyone's eyelashes. It's just a standard, detergent-based makeup remover that is effective and that you'll need, particularly around the eyes, if you wear a good amount of makeup, to make sure you're getting everything off.

☺ **Gentle Refreshing Toner, for Dry to Very Dry Skin** *($6.95 for 8 ounces)* is a standard, but OK, alcohol-free toner for normal to dry skin. It is fragrance-free.

☹ **Pore Refining Skin Freshener, for Normal to Dry Skin** *($6.95 for 8 ounces)* is mostly water and alcohol, and as such is an undesirable option, especially for dry skin.

☺ **Collagen Cream Concentrate, for Dry to Very Dry Skin** *($8.95 for 2 ounces)* contains a tiny amount of collagen, but no amount applied topically can impact your skin's own collagen. This is otherwise an average, jar-packaged, fragrance-free moisturizer that's mostly water, plant oil, and lots of thickeners. It's OK for its intended skin types.

☺ **Deep Moisture Cream, for Normal to Dry Skin** *($8.50 for 4 ounces)* is a very basic, fragrance-free moisturizer for dry skin. Although this is inexpensive, it's also short on anything remotely state-of-the-art.

☺ **Elastin/Collagen Moisture Lotion, for Normal to Dry Skin** *($8.50 for 4 ounces)* is similar to and earns the same review above as the Deep Moisture Cream, for Normal to Dry Skin.

☺ **Enriched Dry Skin Concentrate, for Dry to Very Dry Skin** *($8.50 for 4 ounces)* is a blend of plant oils with Vaseline, lanolin, slip agent, preservatives, and fragrance. Nothing too exciting here, but most of these ingredients are appropriate, though exceptionally basic and passé, for dry to very dry skin (though the plant oil's potential will be lost because of jar packaging).

☺ **Extra Rich Rehydrating Moisturizer, for Normal to Dry Skin** *($8.50 for 4 ounces)* is an exceptionally basic, dated moisturizer that's an OK option for dry skin, assuming you're willing to settle for less than what skin deserves.

☺ **Luxury Eye Cream, for Normal to Dry Skin** *($5.95 for 0.5 ounce)* contains some emollient ingredients with a rich texture, but overall is a basic formula that you could easily replace just by using plain Vaseline, or even better by using a plant oil such as olive oil, around the eye area to treat very dry skin.

☺ **Nourishing Night Cream, for Dry to Very Dry Skin** *($5.95 for 1 ounce)* is an oil-based moisturizer for very dry skin, but the formula itself is quite dated and the greasy texture isn't all that appealing.

☺ **Oil Control Oil-Free Moisturizer, for Normal to Oily Skin** *($8.50 for 4 ounces)* contains a minimal amount of absorbent ingredients, and the thickeners that precede them on the ingredient list won't do a thing to keep excess oil in check. This is an average moisturizer for normal to dry skin, but is not appropriate for any degree of oily skin.

☹ **Self Defense Color Corrective Moisturizing Lotion SPF 15** *($7.50 for 2 ounces)* lacks the UVA-protecting ingredients of titanium dioxide, zinc oxide, avobenzone, Tinosorb, or Mexoryl SX (ecamsule), and is not recommended.

☹ **Sun Shield Lip Care SPF 15** *($2 for 0.15 ounce)* lacks the UVA-protecting ingredients of titanium dioxide, zinc oxide, avobenzone, Tinosorb, or Mexoryl SX (ecamsule), and is not recommended.

✓☺ **Sun Shield For Faces Extra Sensitive Skin SPF 25** *($8.95 for 4 ounces)* is a good, gentle sunscreen for someone with sensitive skin that is normal to dry, including rosacea-affected skin. The Paula's Pick rating pertains to this sunscreen's value for sensitive skin. Other skin types should consider a sunscreen that is loaded with antioxidants, which this formula is lacking. Clinique Super City Block Sheer contains SPF 25, mineral sunscreens, and antioxidants, so that would give someone with sensitive skin an even better product than this (but ounce for ounce Physician's Formula's option costs a lot less).

☹ **Sun Shield Sunless Tanning Lotion SPF 20** *($9.95 for 6 ounces)* lacks the UVA-protecting ingredients of titanium dioxide, zinc oxide, avobenzone, Tinosorb, or Mexoryl SX (ecamsule), and is not recommended.

PHYSICIANS FORMULA MAKEUP

PHYSICIANS FORMULA MINERAL WEAR PRODUCTS

FOUNDATION: ☺ **Mineral Wear Mineral Tinted Moisturizer SPF 15** *($12.95)* contains a mineral sunscreen (titanium dioxide) as the sole active ingredient. Its initially fluid texture blends well and sets to a moist finish suitable for normal to dry skin. Worth noting is that this tinted moisturizer feels heavier than many others. All four shades are worthwhile and all go on sheer, and there are options for light to tan skin tones. The very small amount of lavender oil is not likely a cause for concern.

☺ **Mineral Wear Talc-Free Mineral Liquid Foundation** *($11.95)* has an odd name not only because most liquid foundations are talc-free, but also because talc is a mineral! This water- and silicone-based foundation is dispensed from its tube onto an attached sponge. The sponge is a bit small for application to the entire face, but it smooths the product well. Despite an initially attractive texture, this sets to a strong matte finish that appears chalky and tends to just sit on the skin rather than mesh with it, which is not good. Out of the available shades, the only real-skin shades are Classic Ivory and Natural Beige. Although not a total loss, this is only worth considering by those with very oily skin who desire medium coverage.

CONCEALER: ☹ **Mineral Wear Talc-Free Mineral Concealer Stick SPF 15** *($8.95).* With 26% titanium dioxide, sun protection is assured—but I was also anticipating an opaque, dry texture and chalky finish and sadly, my suspicions were confirmed. Overall this looks too obvious and heavy on skin, especially if you need extra coverage on trouble spots. The shade range only compounds the less-than-desirable finish this concealer has.

☹ **Mineral Wear Talc-Free Mineral Cream Concealer SPF 10** *($7.65)* provides sun protection via 15% titanium dioxide, but that amount also gives this liquid concealer an unusually opaque finish, which doesn't make the four awful shades look any better.

POWDER: ✓☺ **Mineral Wear Talc-Free Mineral Face Powder** *($12.95).* When Physicians Formula wants to create an outstanding pressed powder, they pull out all the stops! This talc-free, mica-based pressed powder protects skin from sun damage with its titanium dioxide and zinc oxide sunscreens, which is great. The texture feels wonderfully creamy for a powder, and becomes almost like a second skin after application. I was surprised that this can get powdery (dusty, if you will) as you swirl the brush over the compact, but I suspect this is because the powder isn't pressed as tightly as others. This fragrance-free powder comes in a neutral range of shades best for fair to medium skin tones. It is a brilliant way to add to the sun protection you're getting from your daytime moisturizer or foundation with sunscreen, and is highly recommended. Fans of mineral makeup won't be let down because this product's formula definitely qualifies.

☺ **Mineral Wear Perfecting Mineral Concentrate 3-in-1 Concealer Foundation Powder** *($9.95).* This loose powder tried to be all things to make enhancing your complexion easier, but it doesn't do any of them very well. It is housed in a pen-style component outfitted with a small, firm brush that's about the size of a standard eyeshadow brush. You depress a button at the opposite end of the component to shoot powder onto the brush and apply. The mica-based formula manages to look shiny and dry at the same time, and the colors tend to go on more yellow or peach than they appear in the container. If layered, this provides fairly good coverage, but it can look heavy and cakey on skin unless blended on sheer. Because of that, it's best to use this as a finishing powder, but then you have to contend with a brush that's too small for applying powder to the entire face.

☺ **Mineral Wear Talc-Free Matte Finishing Veil** *($12.95)* is a loose powder packaged in a container that is attached to a sifter which feeds the powder onto the built-in brush. The corn- and aluminum starch–based powder feels weightless and has a very dry texture and finish that is only suitable for very oily skin not prone to blemishes. Further limiting its appeal, the sole shade is only suitable for those with fair skin.

☺ **Mineral Wear Talc-Free Mineral Loose Powder** *($10.95)* contains mica and zinc oxide instead of talc, which adds up to a mineral-based loose powder (but talc is a mineral, so almost all powders meet the criteria). The zinc oxide causes this light-textured powder to feel dry and look somewhat thick and pasty on skin, but that effect is offset to some extent by the mica's shine. Among the available shades, three are too peach to consider, including Creamy Natural, Natural Beige, and Sand Beige. The dry finish of this powder is best for oily skin, but you'll have to be OK with the shine it leaves behind, which kind of defeats the purpose of using powder.

BLUSH AND BRONZER: ☺ **Mineral Wear Talc-Free Mineral Blush** *($11.95)* is a mica-based pressed-powder blush that has a beautifully silky texture and smooth application. The color payoff is great, while the radiant (rather than sparkling) finish is attractive. The Nude Glow shade is closer to overall skin color than what you'd want from a blush, but the other shades are soft and well-suited for application to cheeks.

☺ **Mineral Wear Talc-Free Mineral Loose Blush** *($10.95).* Not only is this not the best way to use powder blush, but also the built-in brush is too small and not nearly as soft as it should be for even, seamless application. However, the powder itself (whose only mineral of note is mica, but hey, that counts) has a gossamer-light texture that imparts very sheer color and noticeable shimmer (the effect is more of a glow than an all-out shine). Most of the colors are pastel, and don't show up well; Warming Glow is a good sheer bronze option, while Classic Glow is a failsafe nude pink suitable for most light skin tones. This is worth a try if you're willing to unscrew the cap and carefully dispense some powder onto a full-sized blush brush rather than deal with the application method Physicians Formula devised.

☺ **Mineral Wear 100% Mineral BronzeBrightener** *($13.95).* This clay-based pressed powder is identical to Physicians Formula's Mineral Wear 100% Mineral FaceBrightener below, except it comes in a range of sheer bronze tones. It's not easy to work with, the texture is very dry, and the shine flakes. All this, and minimal color payoff, too!

☹ **Mineral Wear 100% Mineral FaceBrightener** *($13.95).* This clay-based pressed powder with shine has a very dry texture and sheer color deposit. It isn't pleasurable to work with and the shine flakes almost immediately. The colors are suitable only for fair to light skin tones, but it's not really worth the effort or expense.

☹ **Mineral Wear Talc-Free Bronzing Veil** *($12.95)* has the same formula and packaging as the Mineral Wear Talc-Free Matte Finishing Veil above but comes in a slightly orange/bronze shade that is an OK option for medium skin tones, but not for all-over use.

EYESHADOW: ☺ **Mineral Wear Talc-Free Mineral Fluid Powder Eye Shadow** *($6.95)* has a name that's long, confusing, and inaccurate because minerals comprise a very small portion of this loose-powder eyeshadow. It comes with a pointed sponge-tip applicator, and between that and the initially "wet" feel, this tends to drag over skin and not blend well. It becomes silky once it sets and does not flake or smear, which is a plus especially because the shine from each shade is intense (and slightly metallic). This is an intriguing option if you want something novel for eyeshadow and are willing to apply this with a brush.

☹ **Mineral Wear Talc-Free Eye Shadow Quad** *($8.95)* comes packaged in a compact with no dividers between the colors, though most of the sets are coordinated well and include three matte shades and one shiny shade. The issue is primarily texture: although these feel silky, the formula is very dry, goes on too sheer (so lots of layering is required if you want the color to show), and the dryness causes flaking and shortens wear time.

☹ **Mineral Wear Talc-Free Mineral Eyeshadow Duo** *($6.95)* is talc-free, but the mica base is a bit too dry for smooth, even application. The low-commitment colors are very sheer and the shine is almost nonexistent, but there are better powder eyeshadows at the drugstore.

EYELINER: ☹ **Mineral Wear Talc-Free Mineral Eye Liner Pencil** *($6.95)* contains a couple of minerals, but the very same ones show up in almost every eye pencil being sold (because they help create the color or add texture to the pencil). This is not a unique option; it's just another standard, creamy eye pencil that needs routine sharpening. It is good that this is minimally prone to smearing or fading once it has set.

LIP GLOSS: ☺ **Mineral Wear Mineral Lip Sheen** *($7.95)* is a very standard lip gloss whose main point of distinction is not minerals, but rather gemstones. Ruby, sapphire, and amethyst powders are joined by tourmaline and they give this sheer gloss a fresh, dimensional shimmer that looks crystalline. The gloss finishes and remains somewhat sticky, but that helps it last a bit longer, too. Minerals are present in this gloss, but they're the same cosmetic mineral pigments seen in many lip glosses that don't advertise their mineral content.

MASCARA: ☹ **Mineral Wear Talc-Free Mineral Mascara** *($7.95)* makes a strange claim, because mascaras are never made with talc (and it's not a harmful ingredient for eyelashes anyway). The mineral component comes from the mineral water, which is the main ingredient in this mascara. The product applies heavily from the get-go, and quite wet. It takes several minutes to dry, in which time you run the risk of smearing, making this a poor contender among other mascaras. Another downer is how difficult this is to remove. A water-soluble cleanser and two rounds of a silicone-based eye-makeup remover weren't enough (though the formula does wear well once it finally sets).

PHYSICIANS FORMULA ORGANIC WEAR 100% NATURAL ORIGIN PRODUCTS

FOUNDATION: ☹ **Organic Wear 100% Natural Origin Tinted Moisturizer SPF 15** *($11.95)*. Yes, this tinted moisturizer has all manner of organic certification and contains lots of organically sourced ingredients, something that will appeal to many consumers. It even has a titanium dioxide sunscreen, which is great. The problem is that, organic or not, the overall formula is terrible. Alcohol is the second ingredient (which causes free-radical damage, dryness, and irritation), and that is followed by lavender oil (which causes cell death), adding up to a natural disaster for all skin types. Despite the claims, this contains a few synthetic ingredients, so don't be fooled. However, as stated, there is no way I would recommend anyone try this product. The texture isn't pleasant to deal with, it is very fragrant (even though Physicians Formula labels it fragrance-free—if lavender oil isn't fragrance, I don't know what is) and most of the four shades are too pink or rose to look convincing.

☹ **Organic Wear 100% Natural Origin Liquid Foundation SPF 15** *($13.95)*. This fragrant foundation may be certified organic, but that doesn't mean it's not without considerable problems. The titanium dioxide sunscreen is fine, but the base formula feels and looks heavy on skin. It has been a long time since I've tested a foundation whose texture and finish make skin look worse instead of better, but this one does. Even more distressing, it contains the potent irritants lemon and lavender oils as well as colloidal silver, which can cause a permanent bluish discoloration on skin. This is absolutely not recommended, nor is it the least bit comfortable or natural-looking on skin.

CONCEALER: ☹ **Organic Wear 100% Natural Origin Concealer Stick** *($6.95)*. Prepare to be very disappointed if you purchase this lipstick-style concealer. It contains mostly natural ingredients to support the claims, but the olive oil- and beeswax-based formula has a dreadful texture that drags over skin, feels and looks thick, and yet somehow manages to provide spotty coverage. None of the four shades are workable enough to look convincing, either, and this will readily crease into lines around the eyes. If this is what organic cosmetics means, I'll gladly take synthetic makeup any day!

POWDER: ☺ **Organic Wear 100% Natural Origin Pressed Powder** *($13.95)* is a talc-free, mica-based pressed powder with a formula that's different from (and better than) that of Physicians Formula Organic Wear bronzing powder and powder blush, reviewed below. Although still on the dry side, it feels silkier, is easier to apply and blend, and doesn't leave skin looking overly powdered or matte. The range of nine shades is superb due to the neutral tones of each, and there are options for fair to tan skin tones. This powder is best for normal to oily skin, and provides a touch more coverage than standard pressed powders.

☺ **Organic Wear 100% Natural Origin Loose Powder** *($13.95)*. What's odd about this mica-based loose powder is that it isn't difficult to create a powder composed of entirely natural ingredients—lots of lines offer this, but Physicians Formula, for all their 100% natural origin posturing, didn't! Their claim is misleading to say the least, but what about the powder itself? It has an initially grainy, powdery texture that transforms to a silky-smooth feel that applies evenly. Due to the absorbent nature of the minerals and clay, this leaves skin looking a bit too powdered and matte, almost as if it has a grayish cast. Another oddity is that almost all of the six shades are interchangeable, so there are no options for medium to dark skin tones. Unless you're willing to tolerate the inadequacies this powder has in exchange for getting some organic ingredients, you're better off considering the superior loose powders from Almay, Jane, or L'Oreal before this.

BLUSH AND BRONZER: ☺ **Organic Wear 100% Natural Origin Blush** *($11.95)*. This powder blush has plenty of natural ingredients, but it ends up being difficult to apply due to its dry, powdery texture. Moreover, its flat matte finish on skin isn't attractive, even for those shades with a noticeable shimmer. The overall effect is a blush that tends to sit on top of skin rather than mesh with it, which is what the best powder blushes do. The brush that's included in the paper-wrapped compact is not sufficient for a smooth application.

☺ **Organic Wear 100% Natural Origin Bronzer** *($13.95)* looks pretty and will appeal to natural enthusiasts due to its formula and "from the earth" packaging. However, as far as pressed bronzing powders go, this doesn't come close to benchmark status. Smooth and dry, it is difficult to pick up a sufficient amount of powder with a brush, and as such this applies sheer and uneven. With patience you can get satisfactory results and a soft glow finish, but lots of other bronzing powders do this quickly and seamlessly. I wish this was a better product, because the shade range is gorgeous, with options for fair to medium skin.

☺ **Organic Wear 100% Natural Origin Face Sculpting Trio 3-in-1 Highlighter, Face Powder, Bronzer** *($13.95)*. Housed in an eco-friendly cardboard compact are a talc-based pressed powder, powder bronzer, and powder highlighter. There are no dividers between the products and the crescent shape of each makes it difficult to hone in on one unless you're using a small brush, which isn't that practical for applying powder or bronzer. More important, the color payoff of this product is minimal, especially for the bronzer, so forget about sculpting your features. Each product has the same formula, and the texture is best described as overall smooth with an underlying graininess that hinders application. Buying organic is one thing, but whether you do so or not, you shouldn't be left wondering why you bothered.

☹ **Organic Wear 100% Natural Origin 2-in-1 Bronzer Blush** *($13.95)* includes a pressed bronzer and blush that can be used independently or swirled together for a sheer glow. The brush is too small for practical use, but the real deal-breaker is the strong odor of the powder itself, likely from the plant oils going rancid due to the packaging.

☹ **Organic Wear 100% Natural Origin Liquid Bronzer** *($10.95)* is a liquid bronzer that comes in a range of attractive shades, but shares the same drawbacks as Physicians Formula Organic Wear 100% Natural Origin Tinted Moisturizer SPF 15 above: a formula with way too much alcohol (which causes free-radical damage) and lavender oil (which causes cell death) to be a good option for anyone's skin. What difference does it make if these ingredients are organic if they're not beneficial to skin? Using natural products shouldn't have to involve harming skin, or smelling like a lavender flower all day long (which you will from this unctuously fragranced product).

EYESHADOW: ☺ **Organic Wear 100% Natural Origin Eye Shadow Duo** *($7.95)*. Notice how the wording in the name of this organic product is "100% natural origin" instead of "100% natural." That's how Physician's Formula gets around the fact that not every ingredient in this powder eyeshadow is natural. (Have you ever seen glyceryl caprylate at your local farmer's market?) It's a bit deceptive because I am sure the average consumer interprets the wording in the name as meaning that this product is 100% natural, but it isn't. That said, although the shade selection is limited, these shadow duos have a smooth-but-dry texture that applies well. Color intensity is sheer, but these layer well for more intensity, although you won't be able to create a deep, dark smoky-eye look. Among the duos, the best are Brown Eyes Organics and Hazel Eyes Organics. The other duos are too blue or green to recommend. Each duo has a soft shine that clings well and is suitable for daytime wear. One caution: This product contains a tiny amount of the fragrance chemical cinnamic acid, which may cause allergic contact dermatitis (Source: *American Journal of Contact Dermatitis*, June 2001, pages 93-102).

EYELINER: ☺ **Organic Wear 100% Natural Origin Eyeliner** *($7.95)*. Notice how the wording in the name of this organic product is "100% natural origin" instead of "100% natural." That's how Physician's Formula gets around the fact that not every ingredient in this eye pencil is actually natural, but it makes it sound like it is anyway. The main ingredients in this pencil show up in many other eye pencils that don't make organic certification claims, so unless you're gung-ho on your makeup being approved by the Ecocert group, there's no need to choose this pencil. It needs routine sharpening and remains creamy enough to smudge and smear. It's OK if you want a smoky-eye design or are willing to pair it with a powder eyeshadow, but why not just line your eyes with the longer-lasting powder eyeshadow and skip the pencil?

LIPSTICK AND LIP GLOSS: ☺ **Organic Wear 100% Natural Origin Superfruit Lip Gloss** *($7.95)*. This fruit-scented lip gloss provides moderate color payoff and a non-sticky gloss finish. It's a very good lip gloss that contains several very good natural ingredients, though its main ingredient, bis-diglyceryl polyacyladipate-2, is a synthetic derivative of vegetable oil.

☹ **Organic Wear 100% Natural Origin Lip Veil** *($7.95)*. All of the natural ingredients and organic certification claims in the world can't change the fact that this is a terrible lipstick. It has an uncomfortably dry texture that impedes application, deposits minimal color with an almost tacky finish, and contains two potent lip irritants. Peppermint and lemon peel oils are natural, but that doesn't make them a safe choice for anyone's lips!

MASCARA: ☺ **Organic Wear 100% Natural Origin Mascara** *($9.95)* has a thin application but builds decent length without clumps. Thickness is scant and this is prone to minor flaking. It is unusually fragrant due to its orange fruit–water base. The natural waxes it contains are found in numerous mascaras, yet they're not used to impressive effect here.

OTHER PHYSICIANS FORMULA MAKEUP

FOUNDATION: ☹ **Beauty Spiral Brightening Compact Foundation** *($9.95)* is a cream-to-powder makeup that "spirals" two colors together. It's eye-catching, but that's all this substandard foundation has going for it. The thick texture offers sheer coverage and a dry, powdery finish that just doesn't feel or look great on the skin. The three colors are passable, but there are far more elegant cream-to-powder foundations from Cover Girl or Revlon, and their options include sun protection.

☹ **Beauty Spiral Skin Brightening Liquid Foundation** *($9.95)* is a sheer, light-textured foundation that has an uneven, slightly pasty-looking finish due to the high amount of titanium dioxide. The two shades are passable, but nothing this chalky can have any sort of brightening effect.

☹ **CoverToxTen50 Wrinkle Therapy Foundation** *($12.95)* is one of a few foundations claiming to work like Botox, without painful injections. One of the main ingredients is GABA (gamma amino butyric acid). Please refer to the *Cosmetic Ingredient Dictionary* for an in-depth discussion of this ingredient. Suffice it to say, GABA does not work to smooth wrinkles; not even Botox works for this purpose if it is applied topically rather than injected. Another antiaging ingredient touted on the package is vitamin C (as tetrahexyldecyl ascorbate) but there is so little in this foundation, your skin won't even notice it. Although it is clever and convenient that this initially creamy liquid foundation is dispensed onto a built-in brush, it does little to enhance application. It also doesn't change the fact that no matter how much blending you do, this foundation always looks heavy and somewhat opaque, with a flat, slightly chalky finish. It is not the answer to camouflaging wrinkles; in fact, its finish tends to emphasize them and most of the colors go on too peach or pink to recommend.

☹ **Le Velvet Film Makeup SPF 15** *($5.25)* is an old-fashioned cream-to-powder foundation that goes on surprisingly moist and creamy and can be blended out fairly sheer. The SPF is part titanium dioxide, which is great, but the finish is somewhat chalky and none of the colors resemble real skin tones, making this one to avoid.

☹ **Sun Shield Liquid Makeup SPF 15** *($5.95)*. Insufficient UVA protection, a dated formula, and some incredibly poor colors add up to a foundation that is a must-avoid.

CONCEALER: ☺ **Line Erase Rx Wrinkle-Filling Firming Lifting Concealer** *($9.95)* is closer to a soft spackle for lines than a concealer. Its silicone-based texture is silky-smooth and, when gently tapped into superficial wrinkles, can make them look less apparent for a short period of time. The effect is subtle, and this absolutely doesn't lift the skin or fill in deep wrinkles (the before and after photos on the back of the box are retouched), but if you're willing to settle for a slight difference, this is worth looking into. Note that this provides light coverage that's not akin to what most concealers hide; all of the shades are good, but they're best for fair to light skin tones.

☺ **Blemish Rx Blemish-Healing Concealer** *($8.95)*. Talk about cheesy! Physicians Formula plays the medicinal angle of this liquid concealer to the hilt by packaging it in a component that resembles a syringe, right down to the dosage markers on the side and a needle-like tip. It is "medicated" with 1.7% salicylic acid, but the pH is not low enough to permit exfoliation, a major way salicylic acid helps banish blemishes. This must be shaken before use (the formula tends to separate) and it then dispenses as a thin liquid that supplies modest coverage and a soft matte finish. Although nothing in this formula is likely to aggravate blemishes (there's a tiny amount of cinnamon bark extract, likely not enough to be a problem) most people will want more coverage than this provides. Other than the Green and Yellow shades, it is an OK option for those with oily skin whose blemishes aren't such that serious camouflage is needed.

☺ **Gentle Cover Concealer Stick** *($6)* is a thick, lipstick-style concealer that provides moderate coverage with a heavy-looking, crease-prone finish. Two of the four colors are marginally acceptable, but this is only recommended for those who refuse to consider the many superior concealers at the drugstore.

☺ **Wanderful Wand Brightening Concealer** *($6.95)* is a liquid concealer housed in a pen-style applicator with a built-in synthetic brush. It has good slip and is easy to blend, but coverage is disappointingly sheer and its flat finish doesn't put skin in its best light, so to speak. The Yellow and Green shades are terrible; Light is OK, but not enough to elevate this to a happy face rating.

☹ **Circle Rx Circle Control Concealer** *($8.95)* is only "just what the doctor ordered" if your doctor is in favor of runny concealers that dispense too heavily and look opaque and chalky on skin. Yes, this conceals dark circles but so do many other concealers whose finish doesn't call attention to itself (and also comes in much better colors). By the way, the plastic syringe packaging is corny to the max!

☹ **Conceal Rx Physicians Strength Concealer** *($8.75)* has a ridiculous name, because there is no such thing as a physician's strength concealer. They claim this liquid concealer is the prescription for "any and all imperfections" due to its coverage capability. This does provide full coverage that can camouflage dark circles, redness, or bruising but the result is heavy and chalky, while none of the colors resemble real skin tones in the least.

☹ **Concealer 101 Perfecting Concealer Duo** *($7.25)* doesn't make the grade as an introduction to concealers, at least not if one of your prerequisites is shades that resemble skin. The texture, coverage, and finish of this concealer are quite nice, but that doesn't mean a thing when the unnatural skin colors scream "obvious" over whatever you're trying to hide.

☹ **Concealer Palette 4-in-1 Concealing Palette** *($7.95)* provides three shades of concealer and a pressed powder, each tiny squares in one compact whose top revolves to allow access to one shade at a time. A brush is included, but it's too small for practical use. Even if the brush were better, the creamy concealers have a dry, powdery finish that looks obvious on skin, the powder is waxy, and the whole product is more gimmicky than useful.

☹ **Concealer Twins Cream Concealer 2-in-1 Correct and Cover SPF 10** *($7.65)* has an admirable (though not quite high enough) titanium dioxide sunscreen, but an otherwise lackluster creamy texture. You get a flesh-toned color on one end and a yellow or green hue on the other, but both leave much to be desired.

☹ **CoverToxTen50 Wrinkle Therapy Concealer** *($8.95)* has the most unbelievable claims for a concealer I've ever seen, and that's saying a lot! Billed as serious care for your wrinkles, it promises to not only reduce their appearance, but also to reduce dark circles by 77%, relieve puffy eyes, and enhance collagen synthesis—all with "no prescription needed." There isn't anything remotely drug-like in this product. The wrinkle-erasing claim is tied to GABA (gamma aminobutyric acid), a neurotransmitter inhibitor whose proponents say that it works like topical Botox. Without rehashing all of the details of this ingredient (it's discussed many times elsewhere and in the our online *Cosmetic Ingredient Dictionary*), it doesn't work—not even Botox works like Botox when applied topically rather than injected. This liquid concealer comes in a tube with a built-in synthetic brush applicator. Although quite silky thanks to the high amount of silicone, coverage is sparse and the matte finish manages to creep into every crevice, line, or large pore on the skin. Couple this with mostly peachy pink colors and misleading claims and it's easy to see why this is not recommended.

☹ **Gentle Cover Cream Concealer SPF 10** *($5.45)* is a mineral oil– and wax-based concealer with a wand applicator and a titanium dioxide sunscreen. This formula will easily crease into any lines around the eye. The Yellow and Green shades are horrid, while Light is barely passable.

⊗ **Powder Finish Concealer Stick SPF 15** *($5.45)* is a creamy stick concealer with titanium dioxide as one of the active ingredients for sun protection. This is nice, but the only flesh-toned shade (Light) is too pink to look natural (especially with this concealer's thick texture), and the powder finish is minimal—it tends to stay creamy and creases easily.

POWDER: ✓ ☺ **Loose-to-Go Multi-Colored Loose Powder** *($11.95)* is a pressed powder in a loose-powder tub. The component includes a "shaver" that, with a twist, dispenses a small amount of loose powder out of the slits in the sifter. It is clever, but at times too much powder is shaved off, and the excess remains in the top, making things just as messy as most loose powders. Packaging aside, this talc-based powder has a superior smooth texture and satin finish that leave skin with a soft glow (well, except for the Loose Bronzer, which is very shiny). As with most Physicians Formula powders, multiple colors merge into one on skin, and this follows suit. The formula and finish are best for normal to dry skin.

☺ **CoverToxTen50 Wrinkle Therapy Face Powder** *($12.95)* is a talc-based pressed powder with GABA, which is said to work like Botox to reduce wrinkles and expression lines. It doesn't work as claimed but this sheer, creamy-feeling powder is a very good option for normal to dry skin. The three shades appear slightly pink in the compact, but go on soft enough so as not to be a concern. There are no shades for medium to dark skin tones. Just to be clear: although this is recommended, it does not do a better job of reducing the appearance of wrinkles than any other recommended powder (and, generally speaking, powdering isn't the way to make wrinkles less apparent).

☺ **Magic Mosaic Multi-Colored Custom Pressed Powder** *($13.95)* is a tightly pressed, talc-based powder that features overlapping circles of tone-on-tone colors. Applying this to skin produces a uniform color that is quite sheer and nonintrusive, though it does have a dry texture. The Light Bronzer/Bronzer and Ivory/Creamy Natural shades have noticeable shine, while the other options have a very subtle shine that's suitable for daytime.

☺ **Powder Palette Multi-Colored Face Powder** *($13.95)* is a kaleidoscopic arrangement of different colors that all come off as the same color on the skin, as it should be. The range of shades has improved; although some look a bit odd in the compact, they blend on neutral and leave a soft, translucent finish. The Light Bronzer option is matte, while Peach-to-Glow is better as blush than an allover powder. Avoid the Highlighter shade because of its contrasting colors, and avoid Green for obvious reasons.

☺ **Pearls of Perfection Multi-Colored Powder Pearls** *($12.95)* are large pots of colored, talc-based powder beads, available in bronze, flesh, and shiny highlighting shades. They're fun in concept, but the execution is messy and not worth the effort. Still, if you're a fan of Guerlain's Meteorites Powder for the Face, this is quite similar and only one-fourth the price. Note that the Guerlain line is not reviewed in this book but is reviewed on www.Beautypedia.com.

BLUSH AND BRONZER: ☺ **Baked Bronzer Bronzing & Shimmery Face Powder** *($11.95)* is similar to the Baked Pyramid Matte Bronzer below, except this version is imbued with large flecks of gold shine, whether used wet or dry. The shine clings well either way, and wet application intensifies the color and won't streak, assuming you blend it carefully.

☺ **Baked Pyramid Matte Bronzer** *($11.95)* is a good pressed-powder bronzer that comes in two semi-matte colors. Dry application produces sheer color and an almost matte finish that can be layered for more intensity. Wet application reveals stronger color and a shimmer finish, though you have to blend carefully to avoid streaking (this isn't a problem once the powder dries).

☺ **Bronze Booster Glow-Boosting Pressed Bronzer** *($14.95)* is a good, talc- and mica-based pressed bronzing powder. Its texture is smooth and dry, application is decent, and the color payoff is softer than you might expect, yet workable for lighter skin tones. The Fair to Light shade is too flesh-toned to work as bronzer; the other shades are better and impart a subtle shine.

☺ **Cheek Palette Cream-to-Powder Blush** *($7.95)* doesn't have a powder finish, so ignore the inaccurate name. This is actually a very good, sheer cream blush that blends smoothly, doesn't streak, and leaves a soft cream finish. You get three colors in one compact, but despite looking different, they all appear similar on skin. This blush is best for normal to dry skin that is not prone to blemishes.

☺ **Powder Palette Multi-Colored Blush** *($10.95)* combines several blush shades in a mosaic pattern that is eye-catching, but the fact is the colors come off as one unified shade on skin, just like a standard powder blush. This has a smooth, impressively silky texture and dry finish laced with sparkles. The sparkly effect is subtle, which explains why each shade looks matte in the package. Blushing Mocha is suitable as a powder bronzer—as if this line needs more options in that regard!

☺ **Solar Powder SPF 20 Face Powder** *($12.95)* is a talc-based, pressed bronzing powder that includes an impressive titanium dioxide–based sunscreen. The two shades go on sheer, and each has three colors, representing a picture of the sun setting over a beach (it sounds odd, but it fits the theme). Swirling a powder brush over the entire powder cake results in one uniform color with a tiny amount of shine. Although it would be nice if a greater range of skin-tone shades were available, this pressed powder with sunscreen is one to consider, especially if you want to pair it with a foundation that contains sunscreen for a touch of bronze color without the sun damage.

☺ **Baked Blush Wet/Dry Blush** *($10.95)* is a domed pressed-powder blush whose three shades are all noticeably shiny. The fact that this powder is "baked" doesn't make it better or preferred over other options. If anything, it tends to crumble easily despite applying smoothly (though it's pigment-rich, so apply sparingly unless you want stronger color). Wet application is tricky because of streaking, but if you're careful (and want intense shine) it works.

☺ **Baked Bronzer** *($11.49)*. This talc-based pressed bronzing powder comes in two suitable shades, both with a shiny finish. It has a dry texture (maybe it was baked too long?) but manages to apply smoothly, imparting a soft tan color. The shine detracts from the finish because its gold particles tend to flake easily. Otherwise, this is one more bronzing powder to consider. As usual with pressed powders, wet application produces more coverage and stronger color impact, but you must blend carefully to avoid streaks.

☹ **Bronze Booster Glow-Boosting Loose Bronzing Veil** *($14.95)*. This loose, talc-based bronzing powder is more trouble than it's worth. A small amount of powder is housed in the center of a cylindrical component with a built-in brush. You open the cap and turn the bottom of the component to the desired number on the center dial. This determines how much powder is dispensed onto the brush. After you've dialed in the amount, simply brush on wherever you want a hint of bronze color. Sounds easy, right? Mostly it is; the problems lie in the dry texture of the powder coupled with its sheerness and the harsh quality of the brush. This is not a comfortable product to apply, and you need to keep brushing it on to see any color, a process that becomes painful. Why someone would choose this over a standard bronzing powder is beyond me—it isn't worth the gimmick.

☺ **Magic Mosaic Multi-Colored Custom Blush** *($10.95)* looks pretty and pillowy in its pressed-powder compact, but this blush is so sheer and so difficult to pick up on the brush that you'll be left wondering why you bothered unless your goal is the faintest hint of blush. Even the Soft Mocha/Mocha shade (for bronzing) goes on so soft no one will believe you've been kissed by the sun. Still, this does have a matte finish.

☺ **Planet Blush Powder & Blush 2-in-1** *($10.95)* features a split compact with a shiny pressed highlighting powder on one side and a softly shiny blush tone on the other. The domed top is there to allow a tiny blush brush to stand upright in the center of the compact, but its rough texture and extremely short handle make it impractical to use. This is another gimmicky product that will take up more room in your makeup bag than it should.

☹ **Les Botaniques Botanical Face Powder Bronzer** *($11.95)* is a talc-based pressed-powder bronzer embossed with cutesy designs of flowers and the blazing sun. It contains a few botanicals, but in very small amounts, meaning they're mere window dressing. This has a dry, almost stiff texture that applies unevenly, and both shades impart more of a yellow-orange than tan color to skin, which only makes matters worse.

☹ **Pearls of Perfection Multi-Colored Blush** *($9.95)* looks cute if the idea of pressed spheres of powder blush appeals to you. Application, however, is another issue because it's difficult to pick up enough powder on your brush so that it will show on skin, and all you end up getting is noticeable shine. From concept to execution, this isn't any match for a standard pressed-powder blush.

EYESHADOW: ✓☺ **Bright Collection Shimmery Quads Eye Shadow** *($6.75)* is identical to the Matte Collection Quad Eye Shadow below, except with these sets all four shades have shine (which tends to stay in place, making these highly recommended if you prefer shiny eyeshadows). Otherwise, the same basic comments apply.

✓☺ **Matte Collection Quad Eye Shadow** *($6.75)* has some of the best neutral color combinations around, with a welcome silky texture and a matte finish that applies and blends beautifully. There are only four quads available, but each is excellent, though all of them do not have a suitable shade for eyelining.

✓☺ **Shimmer Strips Custom Eye Enhancing Shadow & Liner** *($10.95)*. The only issue I have with these strips of powder eyeshadows (each one provides nine shades in arrangements of three sets of tone-on-tone colors) is the mistaken notion that blue eyes need blue eyeshadow, green eyes need green eyeshadow, and so on. I've said it before, and I'll say it again: Matching your eyeshadow to your eye color is not the way to showcase your eyes. All it does is put two similar colors in proximity, drawing attention away from what you're using eyeshadow to emphasize. Enough said about that. In every other respect, unless you don't want shine, these eyeshadows have a remarkably smooth texture and an even, flake-free application (unless you overdo it when using them wet). Physician's Formula typically produces outstanding powder eyeshadows, and Shimmer Strips continues the tradition. The offerings for Hazel and Brown eyes feature the best color combinations. The Green group is good if you ignore or downplay the green shades, while Blue is the trickiest because blending blues and peaches with gray tends to produce a muddy yet pastel-looking result. Each set includes one shade dark enough to work as powder eyeliner, making these convenient, all-in-one options to shape and shade the eye.

☺ **Baked Collection Wet/Dry Eye Shadow** *($7.95)* offers three well-coordinated, shiny eyeshadows (what the company refers to a "luminous matte") in one compact. Most of the trios have one darker shade to use as eyeliner, and these have smooth, dry textures that blend nicely and last, plus the shine doesn't flake. True to the name, these may be applied wet or dry (most powder eyeshadows have this feature) with wet application intensifying the color and shiny finish. Watch out for Baked Spices—the orange tones aren't the easiest to work with. Baked Sweets has the same issue with its colors.

☺ **Baked Collection Wet/Dry Eye Shadow Luminous Matte** *($7.95)*. Luminous matte is an oxymoron if I've heard of one. How can something be luminous and matte at the same time? Basically, this powder eyeshadow trio has a matte finish with a hint of sheen, so that's where the luminous part comes in, but the sheen will still make wrinkles around the eye area more noticeable. Although all of the trios are workable with their respective light, medium, and dark shades, each has a dry texture that's not as elegant or easy to blend as today's best eyeshadows. This is still an eyeshadow worth considering, especially if you want a mostly matte finish and don't want to worry about whether the colors in each set work well together.

☺ **Bronze Gems Matte & Bright Bronzer, Highlighter, and Eye Shadow** *($12.95)* combines a bronzing powder with soft shine along with three smaller "sections" of complementary shades of shimmer powder. Whether blended together or used separately (such as bronzing powder on cheeks and highlighting powder as eyeshadow), the result is sheer color and shine that tends to flake. All told, this looks much better in the compact than it does on skin.

☹ **Eyebrightener Multi-Colored Eyelighter** *($7.95)* is definitely eye-catching. Unfortunately, this variegated display of colors ends up placing a sweep of intense shine and is powdery enough to flake endlessly during application, making it more of a bother than it's worth.

EYE AND BROW SHAPER: ✓ ☺ **Brow Definer Automatic Brow Pencil** *($5.95)* ranks as one of the best brow pencils at any price, and the shade selection includes options for all but red or auburn brows. It applies smoothly and allows you to build color in sheer layers, which makes for natural-looking brows. The slightly thick powder finish lasts without smearing, while the brow comb (built into the cap) finishes things with precision.

✓ ☺ **Eye Definer Felt-Tip Eye Marker** *($6.95)* looks like a fine-tipped marker and applies like a liquid eyeliner. The felt tip is firm yet comfortable, making it easy to draw a continuous thick or thin line. You'll find this dries almost immediately and wears all day without chipping, smearing, or fading. Bravo, Physicians Formula!

☺ **Eye Definer Flat Automatic Eyeliner Pencil** *($5.95)* is a twist-up, retractable pencil with an angled, flat, wide tip. The unique shape allows you to draw an unusually thick or traditional thin line, though the formula is creamy enough to smear and fade before the day is done.

☺ **Fineline Brow Pencil** *($4.25)* needs sharpening and comes in two decent shades. It has a standard, dry texture. If you don't mind routine sharpening, this is one of the least expensive reliable brow pencils.

☹ **Brow-Tweez 3-in-1 Tweezer-Brow Pencil-Shaper** *($7.95)*. I'm still unclear about what the third benefit of this pencil is supposed to be, but regardless, it needs routine sharpening and has a stiff, dry texture that can hurt to apply—and you still get sheer color (so successive coats are required). The pencil has tiny tweezers at the end—a seemingly clever touch but they're no match for a standard pair of tweezers, especially for removing tiny brow hairs.

☹ **Eyebrightener Brightening Liquid Eyeliner** *($6.50)* is infused with glitter particles and applies too sheer and choppy. This also takes too long to dry and smears easily, making it an eyeliner to avoid.

☹ **Eye Definer Automatic Eye Pencil** *($5.50)* is a twist-up, retractable eye pencil that is greasier than most, which means it can smear and smudge easily, and it does.

☹ **Wonderful Brow Automatic Brow Wax Stick** *($5.95)* is billed as an all-in-one product for the brows, but remains a below-standard automatic, retractable pencil that doesn't apply as easily as most automatic brow pencils, and remains tacky, which can cause brow hairs to mat. What a shame, because the colors are attractive and don't apply too strongly.

LIPSTICK AND LIP GLOSS: ☹ **Plump Palette Plumping Lip Color** *($7.95)* features four sheer-to-moderate coverage lip colors in one mirrored compact complete with brush. The lipstick texture is subpar, feeling too waxy and looking not the least bit glossy. What's most problematic is the inclusion of cinnamon, ginger, and menthane carboxamide (a potent, synthetically derived form of menthol), which plump lips (minimally) via irritation.

☹ **Plump Potion Needle-Free Lip Plumping Cocktail** *($9.75)* is packaged to resemble a syringe (so much for allaying fear of the needle!) and only provides lips with a cocktail of irritants, including menthol and menthyl nicotinate. These ingredients cause inflammation and increase blood flow to the lips, resulting in a slight increase in fullness—but such irritation is not the key to younger-looking, smoother lips.

☹ **Plump Potion Needle-Free Plumping Lipstick** *($9.95)*. This creamy, smooth-textured lipstick plumps lips with three potent irritants: menthol, benzyl nicotinate, and the menthol derivative ethyl menthane carboxamide. It actually hurts to wear this; I'd rather have a needle injection of collagen or another filler substance because at least the injection sites are numbed before such procedures! Without the trio of irritants, this would be a very good cream lipstick with beautiful, full coverage colors.

MASCARA: ☺ **F.L.A.T. Fabulously Long and Thick Mascara** *($6.95)* makes lashes long and thick in a wink, and the drama continues with each successive quote. This mascara would rate a Paula's Pick were it not for the intermittent flaking experienced throughout the day. If you use restraint during application, the flaking becomes a non-issue—but it's a shame those who go for the gusto must tolerate this side effect.

☺ **PlentiFull Thickening Mascara** *($5.20)* has improved from the last time I reviewed it because it is now a credible mascara to consider if you need primarily a lengthening mascara that, with several coats, builds moderate thickness without clumps or smearing. The tiny amount of botanicals (aloe and chamomile) has no impact on lashes.

☺ **Plump Potion Lash Plumping and Stimulating Mascara** *($9.75)* makes wallflower lashes the talk of the party in no time thanks to its dense brush that deposits a lot of mascara to quickly thicken lashes. You'll get some minor clumps along the way, but they can be smoothed out without a separate brush. Unless you absolutely don't want dramatic lashes in an instant, the only downside of note is that if this gets on your skin (such as the eyelid or lash line) it is very difficult to correct without the help of a makeup remover. Most mascara smudges can be remedied with a cotton swab, but this one won't budge. By the way, none of the ingredients the company uses in an effort to stimulate lashes actually have that effect. Even if they did, the amount of said ingredients in this mascara is insignificant.

☺ **To Any Lengths Lash Extending Mascara** *($5.20)* is excellent for substantial but not excessive length and clean, clump-free definition. Don't expect any thickness from this, but as a lengthening formula this wins high marks, and it wears all day without smearing or flaking.

☺ **AquaWear Waterproof Mascara** *($5.20)* will build some length, but no thickness, and is fairly waterproof. Contrary to the claim here, no waterproof mascara can condition lashes, nor do lashes need conditioning. However, this does make lashes feel softer than a typical waterproof mascara.

☹ **Lash-in-a-Tube Full Coverage Cream Mascara** *($5.95)* promises a false-eyelashes effect without the stiffness, yet all it delivers is appreciable length with minor clumps and some smearing along the way. If you're meticulous during application, this can be an OK lengthening mascara, and it does keep lashes soft.

☹ **Eyebrightener Brightening & Curling Mascara** *($6.95)* is blah all the way around, doing little of anything except making lashes feel especially brittle. This does not curl lashes or make eyes look any brighter.

FACE AND BODY ILLUMINATING/SHIMMER PRODUCTS: ☺ **Shimmer Strips Custom Blush & Highlighter** *($11.95)*. This smooth, dry-textured striped blush is a good way to get shiny cheeks. The highlighting portion of the product's name is from the shine, but it's intense enough so as to make truly subtle highlighting impossible. As mentioned, you get stripes of color in one compact. When swirled together with a brush, the color reads as one soft shade on skin, with the color impact taking a backseat to the high degree of shine. The gleaming finish wears well without flaking.

☺ **Summer Eclipse Bronzing and Shimmery Face Powder** *($12.95)* casts an equal amount of shimmer and sun-kissed bronze tint on the skin. The tightly pressed, talc-based powder applies sheer and even, and the shine clings better than you might think. It's best for evening glamour when you want shine without overdoing it.

☺ **Virtual Face Powder Multi-Reflective Face Powder** *($10.95)* is a talc-based pressed powder that attempts to minimize lines and wrinkles by diffusing light. It doesn't work in that manner, however, because it is so shiny that any flaw or wrinkle it's applied over is magnified. However, this is perfect if you have smooth, unlined skin and want a shiny powder that has a dimensional effect and clings very well. All four shades are enticing if strong shine is your thing.

☺ **Jungle Fever Bronzing & Shimmery Face Powder** *($11.95)* is a shimmering pressed powder that comes in your choice of a tiger or leopard pattern. What that has to do with improving powder application is anyone's guess, but it nicely coincides with the clever jungle name. Each shade mixes light and bronze tones for a sheer tan effect on the skin, but the shine is most prominent—and doesn't stay in place well, making this a lesser option from Physicians Formula.

☺ **Retro Glow Illuminating Face Powder** *($10.95)* is supposed to be a return to the heritage of Physicians Formula. This talc-based powder contains aluminum starch as its second ingredient, so the finish is dry and absorbent though replete with shine. The shine is described as "imperceptible," but that isn't true in the least. Although the two shades are neutral and sheer, the shine doesn't cling well, but this is still an OK option for oily skin that's fair to light.

☹ **Shimmer Strips Custom Bronzer, Blush, & Eye Shadow** *($12.95)* tries to compete with Bobbi Brown's popular Shimmer Brick Compacts, but fails due to its dry, thick texture that applies unevenly. The shimmer tends to sit (and look piled) on the skin no matter how little you use, whereas Brown's option meshes with and uses shimmer to highlight skin.

SPECIALTY PRODUCTS: ☹ **Bronze Booster Self-Tanning Bronzing Veil** *($14.95)*. This butterscotch-scented product is a liquid bronzer with shimmer that also has self-tanning action, courtesy of dihydroxyacetone and erythrulose. Combined, you get instant color and shimmer from the cosmetic pigments plus a sunless tan that develops in a few hours and continues to darken over the next couple of days. It sounds wonderfully convenient, but unless you apply this all over the face and neck, the results once the self-tanner develops will look blotchy and uneven. Rather than combining these products, Physician's Formula should recommend using a self-tanner first (perhaps in the evening) and, once it has developed, augmenting the tan with a liquid bronzer with soft shine. As is, this Bronzing Veil is tricky to get right and the built-in brush applicator doesn't do a thing to promote even, streak-free application. If you decide to try this anyway, it's available in three shades suitable for fair to medium skin tones.

☺ **Custom Eye Enhancing Eyeliner Eye Shadow Highlighter** *($5.37)* is a dual-sided product meant to line, shadow, and highlight the eyes. One end features a pointed sponge tip for lining and crease work, while the other has a larger, rounded sponge tip for applying the highlighter color. The cap for both ends is outfitted with a disc of pressed powder that the sponge tip contacts when the product's caps are on. More powder is deposited on the sponge tip each time you replace the cap. Both powders go on smoothly, but they are a bit difficult to blend. The colors have noticeable shine and are meant to play up one's eye color, but not every pairing is successful. If anything, the color pairings tend to be too extreme, offering a ghostly pale highlighter and a dark liner color.

PROACTIV SOLUTION

PROACTIV SOLUTION AT-A-GLANCE

Strengths: Effective, elegant-textured AHA, BHA, and skin-lightening options; all sunscreens provide sufficient UVA protection; good options for controlling excess oil breakthrough, including a colorless pressed powder.

Weaknesses: Several products contain irritating ingredients that do not help acne-prone skin; some gimmicky products that no dermatologist-created line should be selling (they should know better); mostly substandard to poor makeup options, including a sulfur-based concealer.

For more information about ProActiv, call (800) 876-9717 or visit www.proactiv.com or www.Beautypedia.com.

PROACTIV SKIN CARE

☹ **Clear Zone Body Pads** *($21.75 for 75 pads)* are dual-textured pads medicated with 2% salicylic acid. Although the pH of the solution in which the pads are soaked allows exfoliation to occur, the amount of alcohol and the inclusion of witch hazel do not make these a must-have option for blemished skin.

☹ **Makeup Removing Cloths** *($16.75 for 45 towelettes)* are not adept at removing makeup thoroughly because they lack cleansing agents or solvents, and they contain enough lavender to cause problems for skin. The cleansing cloths from Olay, Pond's, or Dove are preferred to and less expensive than this.

☹ **Deep Cleansing Wash** *($20 for 8 ounces)* cannot help unclog pores as claimed because its 2% salicylic acid is washed down the drain before it can go to work inside the pore lining. More of an issue is that this cleansing scrub contains menthol, which won't help anyone have clearer skin.

☺ **$$$ Renewing Cleanser** *($16 for 4 ounces)* is a water-soluble cleansing lotion that uses 2.5% benzoyl peroxide as the active ingredient. A benzoyl peroxide wash may sound convenient, but it's a problem if used around the eyes, plus in a cleanser, it's in contact with the skin only briefly, which makes it not nearly as potent as when it is used in a leave-on product.

☺ **$$$ Revitalizing Toner** *($16 for 4 ounces)* is a good 6% AHA liquid. However, when it comes to most kinds of breakouts, research indicates that BHA (salicylic acid) rather than AHA is the best way to exfoliate for breakout prevention. Salicylic acid can exfoliate within the pore as well as on the surface of the skin because it is lipid soluble (meaning it can penetrate oil). AHAs exfoliate primarily on the surface of the skin because they are water soluble and can't work beneath the surface. The amount of witch hazel is unlikely to be irritating, but it keeps this from earning a higher rating.

✓ ☺ **Clarifying Night Cream** *($28.75 for 1 ounce)* is a well-formulated BHA lotion that includes 1% salicylic acid at an effective pH of 3.6. As further enticement, the formula also includes retinol and several antioxidants, all in stable packaging. This is highly recommended for normal to dry skin battling blackheads and blemishes. Clarifying Night Cream does contain fragrance.

☹ **Daily Oil Control** *($20 for 1.7 ounces)* lists alcohol as the second ingredient and although that can de-grease skin, it is also very irritating and can cause free-radical damage.

☺ **Daily Protection Plus Sunscreen SPF 15** *($17.25 for 4 ounces)* is a good in-part avobenzone sunscreen for normal to oily skin. It provides a lightweight matte finish and contains some helpful absorbent ingredients. What's missing are antioxidants (the only one of note is a tiny amount of vitamin C). The amount of salicylic acid is too low to affect blemish-prone skin, although the pH is within the ideal range.

☹ **Green Tea Moisturizer** *($24.50 for 1 ounce)* contains a lot of green tea and vitamin A, two antioxidants with considerable value for all skin types. The problem is that the amount of iris root extract (also known as orris root) can cause allergic or sensitizing skin reactions and there is no research showing it to be beneficial for skin (Source: *Botanical Dermatology Database*, http://bodd.cf.ac.uk/BotDermFolder/BotDermC/CACT.html). What a shame, because this is otherwise a great moisturizer for normal to dry skin.

☺ **Nourishing Eye Cream** *($23.25 for 0.5 ounce)* is a good, lightweight, fragrance-free moisturizer for slightly dry skin around the eyes or anywhere on the face. It contains several antioxidants, which is good because none of them are present in a significant amount.

☹ **Oil Free Moisture with SPF 15** *($27 for 1.7 ounces)* is a basic, fragrance-free sunscreen for normal to oily skin. The in-part zinc oxide sunscreen may be a problem for someone struggling with blemishes, but it does contribute to this product's matte finish and UVA protection. It is unfortunate that I am no longer able to recommend this daytime moisturizer with sunscreen because ProActiv changed the preservatives. The formula now contains methylisothiazolinone, which is not recommended for use in leave-on products. Methylisothiazolinone is known for causing contact dermatitis (Source: *Contact Dermatitis*, August 2007, pages 97-99).

☺ **Replenishing Eye Serum** *($23.25 for 0.5 ounce)* lists a film-forming agent as the main ingredient, and at that concentration users may experience some irritation (and it definitely creates a firming, tightening sensation, though the effect is strictly cosmetic). The silicone-enhanced formula contains some impressive water-binding agents and antioxidants, but the potential for irritation makes this a risky consideration.

☺ **Sheer Finish Mattifying Gel** *($18 for 1 ounce)* definitely helps keep skin matte due to its combination of dry-finish silicones and clay. The inclusion of green tea and the omission of fragrance also make this a decent contender for those with oily skin who need shine control. However, it would have achieved a higher rating if it included a complement of antioxidants, skin-identical ingredients, and cell-communicating ingredients. Leaving those out shortchanges any skin type. Note: This product is available exclusively through ProActiv; you will not be able to purchase through QVC.

☹ **Advanced Blemish Treatment** *($17 for 0.33 ounce)* is a 6% benzoyl peroxide solution. However, the fourth ingredient is alcohol, which makes this unnecessarily drying and irritating. There are far more gentle 5% and 10% benzoyl peroxide products at the drugstore for a fraction of this price.

☹ **Clear Purifying Mask** *($18 for 1 ounce)* lists 6% sulfur as its active ingredient. Although sulfur is a potent disinfectant for acne-prone skin, its side effects are pronounced and in most cases it does more harm than good for skin. This mask also contains a potentially troublesome amount of alcohol along with irritating plant extracts.

☹ **Medicated Pore Cleaning System** *($16.50)* is further proof that the dermatologists behind this line are frustratingly endorsing both helpful and harmful products for those with acne. This two-step system includes **Pore Strips** and a **Pore Cleansing Solution**. The Pore Strips are like Scotch tape for skin, and include alcohol, peppermint oil, and menthol to further irritate and inflame skin. The Pore Cleansing Solution doesn't fare much better because it contains a lot of alcohol and irritating arnica extract. This is a mistake from any angle. There is nothing medicated about alcohol, menthol, or peppermint.

☹ **Mild Exfoliating Peel** *($18 for 1 ounce)* is mild to the point of being ineffective because the 0.5% salicylic acid won't work efficiently at this product's pH level. Further, with alcohol and witch hazel heading up the ingredient list, this peel is far from "calming"; rather it is irritating and drying.

☹ **Refining Mask** *($20 for 2.5 ounces)* is a standard clay mask that also contains 6% pure sulfur. Sulfur can be a good antibacterial agent, but its irritant properties outweigh its benefit for most people. There are better ways to disinfect skin than this.

✓☺ **Repairing Lotion** *($21.75 for 2 ounces)* is a very good topical disinfectant for acne. The active ingredient is 2.5% benzoyl peroxide and it is blended in a silky lotion base that contains an anti-irritant. It's pricey for what you get, but is definitely worth considering as part of a battle plan for blemishes. This does contain fragrance.

✓☺ **Skin Lightening Lotion** *($21.75 for 1 ounce)* combines 2% hydroquinone with approximately 4% glycolic acid at an effective pH of 3.3. This is an outstanding option to fade sun- or hormone-induced brown skin discolorations, while also improving skin's texture and reducing inflammation with antioxidants. The opaque packaging ensures the hydroquinone will remain stable during use.

☺ **$$$ Oil Blotter Sheets** *($16.50 for 130 sheets)* are standard, powder-free pieces of paper that work quickly to absorb excess oil and perspiration. They're on the pricey side, but at least you get an abundance of papers.

PROACTIV MAKEUP

FOUNDATION: ☺ **$$$ Sheer Finish Compact Foundation** *($26.25)* is sheer as the name states, but that won't help this cream-to-powder compact foundation provide the coverage those struggling with acne typically desire. Another unhelpful element is that this foundation's finish is more creamy than powdery, so any oily areas become slick and greasy-looking shortly after application. The base formula contains thickeners and waxes that further contribute to clogged pores. As for the salicylic acid, it cannot be effective in this nonaqueous product because water is required to establish a pH. This is most appropriate for those with normal to dry skin not struggling with acne.

☻ **Sheer Tint Moisturizer with SPF 15** *($24.50 for 1.7 ounces)* is quite standard except for the fact that it lacks sufficient UVA protection because it does not contain avobenzone, titanium dioxide, zinc oxide, Mexoryl SX, or Tinosorb. This fragrance-free tinted moisturizer is not recommended over several other tinted moisturizers with sunscreen that get the critical issue of sufficient UVA protection right.

CONCEALER: ☻ **Concealer Plus Sulfur Acne Treatment** *($17.75)* is a terrible liquid concealer in almost every respect. It contains 8% sulfur as its active ingredient, and that makes it incredibly drying and irritating for all skin types. Although sulfur is a viable anti-acne ingredient, its irritant properties outweigh its benefit for those with acne. The sulfur lends this fluid concealer a dry, almost grainy finish that flakes easily, which draws more attention to what you're trying to conceal, as do the mostly peachy or pink colors.

POWDER: ✓ ☺ $$$ **Sheer Finish Pressed Powder** *($26.25)* is a colorless (well, it appears alabaster in the compact but goes on translucent) pressed powder that's quite a find for those with very oily skin. The talc-based formula applies smoothly and evenly, and works beautifully to keep excess shine to a minimum without looking chalky. Wearing this alone is fine unless you need coverage, because this is too sheer to provide any. It is best brushed on or you can use the enclosed sponge to lightly dab powder over shine-prone areas. The formula is suitable for those with acne.

☺ $$$ **Sheer Finish Loose Powder** *($23.25)* is a needlessly expensive loose powder that comes in a very small container. It has a silky, dry texture and contains absorbents to minimize shine, but the powder also has a shiny finish which defeats the purpose of using a powder to temper shine. The Light and Medium shades are fine, but the Dark shade is too ash to recommend. If you have oily skin, think twice before using this powder.

REVLON (MAKEUP ONLY)

REVLON AT-A-GLANCE

Strengths: Superior foundations with sunscreen and all of them provide sufficient UVA protection (though one has a disappointing SPF 6); several outstanding concealers and powders; one of the best cream blushes around; great cream eyeshadow and liquid eyeliner; a beautiful selection of elegant lipsticks, lip gloss, and lipliner; some worthwhile specialty products.

Weaknesses: Average eye and brow pencils; several lipsticks with sunscreen lack the right UVA-protecting ingredients; inaccurate claims surrounding their Botafirm complex; mostly average to disappointing mascaras.

For more information about Revlon, call (800) 473-8566 or visit www.revlon.com or www. Beautypedia.com.

REVLON AGE DEFYING PRODUCTS

FOUNDATION: ✓ ☺ **Age Defying Makeup with Botafirm SPF 15** *($13.99)* comes in two formulas, one for dry skin and one for normal/combination skin. Confusingly, the dry-skin formula lists talc as one of the main ingredients, though it provides a soft matte finish. In contrast, the normal/combination skin formula is more emollient, with a finish that's almost matte. Both foundations provide broad-spectrum sun protection; the dry-skin formula has an in-part titanium dioxide sunscreen, while the normal/combination formula contains titanium dioxide and zinc oxide. Texture- and application-wise, both formulas are equally wonderful.

Which one you choose depends on the type of finish you prefer, because both provide seamless medium coverage without a heavy feel. Each foundation features 12 shades, and they tend to go on lighter than they appear in the bottle. The best news: With the exception of the too-peach Honey Beige (both formulas), there's not a bad shade in the bunch, and there are options for light to dark (but not very fair or very dark) skin tones. Whether you choose the dry or the normal/combination skin formula, both of these foundations are best for normal to slightly dry or slightly oily skin, but neither firms skin nor reduces the look of expression lines.

☺ **Age Defying Spa Foundation SPF 18** *($13.99).* You've probably seen the ads for this foundation with Elle McPherson looking all dewy-skinned and beautiful thanks to how this product from Revlon makes her skin look. Who could resist wanting the same beautiful appearance as Elle? First, to be very clear, Miss McPherson's gorgeous appearance in the ads has nothing to do with this foundation. Talented makeup artists, strategic lighting, digital photo retouching software, and McPherson's natural beauty are responsible. She looked beautiful long before she got this spokesperson role with Revlon, right? Nonetheless, this liquid foundation in a brush-tipped tube does provide medium coverage and a dewy, satin finish to the skin. The brush-tip applicator, which this product would be just as good without, is soft enough to apply the foundation on the skin, but you still need to use your fingers or a sponge for complete blending and to avoid streaks. This formulation also provides excellent broad-spectrum sun protection and is recommended for those with normal to dry skin. Note: The shade selection tends to run darker than you'd think and there are no testers. Therefore, I recommend you select a color one shade lighter than you normally wear. Avoid 005 Light Medium/Medium altogether because it turns orange on the skin. This foundation missed being rated a Paula's Pick because some of the plant ingredients it contains are potentially irritating and because Revlon included a lot of fragrance, in the form of meythldihydrojasmonate.

CONCEALER: ☺ **Age Defying Spa Concealer** *($10.50)* comes packaged with a brush-tipped applicator—I suppose to make it match the brush-tipped packaging of Revlon's Age Defying Spa Foundation SPF 18. While this type of packaging seems to be more common lately, it's more of a novelty and is seldom really helpful or useful for application and blending purposes. Such is the case here. Once this cream concealer is dispensed through the brush, you still need to blend it with your fingertips or a sponge. Once blended, this medium-coverage concealer sets to a matte finish and wears well without sinking into fine lines. The color range is small, but the shades are neutral enough that most light to medium skin tones will be able to find a usable shade. The packaging is the only negative keeping this concealer from earning a Paula's Pick.

SPECIALTY PRODUCTS: ✓☺ **Age Defying Instant Firming Face Primer for Dry Skin** *($13.99)* has a texture that's best for normal to slightly dry skin. Those with dry to very dry skin will need something more emollient than this water- and silicone-based lotion, but it's loaded with antioxidants and performs well under makeup, even if your foundation of choice is rich and dewy.

✓☺ **Age Defying Instant Firming Face Primer for Normal/Combination Skin** *($13.99)* has a lotion texture and leaves a slightly moist finish that casts a sheen on skin. It works beautifully under makeup and is fine for its intended skin types. What propels this to Paula's Pick status are the many antioxidants Revlon added, all in impressive amounts. Consider this an elegant, lightweight moisturizer that rivals the best of the best, but keep in mind that you get only 1 ounce of product.

☺ **Age Defying Precise Wrinkle Eraser with Botafirm** *($13.99)* doesn't really erase wrinkles—but you knew that, right? Instead, the silicones this primer-type product contains help temporarily fill in and reduce the appearance of superficial lines. That's helpful, especially under makeup (even the best foundations tend to accentuate rather than downplay wrinkles), but the product name is definitely misleading. Revlon claims their botanicals and peptide work to inhibit lines, but there is no solid science to support that notion. At best, the botanical ingredients offer antioxidant and anti-inflammatory benefit to skin, and their inclusion allows this to go beyond the basic formulas most primers have.

REVLON BEYOND NATURAL PRODUCTS

FOUNDATION: ✓ ☺ **Beyond Natural Skin Matching Makeup SPF 15** *($12.99)* is the Revlon version of Almay's Smart Shade Makeup (Revlon owns Almay). The product dispenses from the tube as white with dark speckles, but quickly turns into a flesh-toned color as it is applied to skin. The gimmicky notion of a cosmetic changing to match your skin tone aside, this is an excellent tinted moisturizer makeup that provides light to medium coverage (you can definitely get more coverage from this than from many tinted moisturizers). Zinc oxide and titanium dioxide are on hand for broad-spectrum sun protection, and they also contribute to this makeup's matte finish and shine-absorbing quality. There are five shades available, and all of them are great, although Medium will be too peachy yellow for some skin tones. This is a wonderful all-in-one daytime product that will work beautifully for those with normal to oily or even slightly dry skin. If you are prone to dry patches, applying a light moisturizer underneath will ensure a smooth application. Nice work, Revlon!

CONCEALER: ☹ **Beyond Natural Concealer & Highlighter** *($9.99)* applies smoothly and is easy to blend, but has enough slip that coverage can be spotty, and creasing under the eyes is evident shortly after application. True to its name, this creamy concealer with coordinated shimmer highlighter looks natural on skin, but natural needn't mean short-lived wear or a concealer that does only a marginal job of camouflaging dark circles or redness. The selection of four shades is fairly impressive, with only Light being questionable due to its pink tone. This is an OK option if you want a concealer with light coverage and are willing to set it with powder to prolong wear and minimize creasing. As for the highlighter, it works well for its intended purpose, but the formula is best for normal to dry skin not prone to blemishes.

BLUSH AND BRONZER: ☹ **Beyond Natural Blush & Bronzer** *($11.99)* sweeps on incredibly sheer, almost to the point where even those with porcelain skin tones can go overboard during application of this pressed-powder blush and bronzer and not have it look noticeable. Anyone with a medium to tan skin tone will likely wonder why they bothered. It's called cheek color, not cheek un-color! This imparts a soft glow to cheeks, and that's how it is best used: Apply your regular blush or bronzer first, then top with a dusting of this powder—assuming you want to bother with it. All four duos are recommended, and which one you choose is of little consequence because of the "beyond natural" sheerness!

EYESHADOW: ☺ **Beyond Natural Cream to Powder Eye Shadow** *($7.99)* has a smooth texture and soft, well-coordinated colors, and it blends well to a low-glow cream finish. What's not to like? The main drawback is the fact that these crease and tend to fade within a couple of hours after application. Blending the shades together so you get a gradation of color and/or are able to shape and shade the eye (which is the purpose of eyeshadow) is tricky. Even if your blending is precise, the formula tends to cause the colors to migrate into one. If you're looking for cream or cream-to-powder eyeshadows, you'll find better, long-wearing, crease-resistant options from M.A.C., L'Oreal H.I.P., and even Revlon (their Illuminance Creme Shadow is excellent).

EYELINER: ☹ **Beyond Natural Defining Eye Pencil** *($7.99)* is a needs-sharpening pencil that glides along the lash line with the greatest of ease—no pulling or tugging required. Unfortunately, the creamy texture stays that way, and within a short time you'll find this eyeliner fades, although smearing is kept to a minimum (well, unless you rub your eyes). The shades are infused with a touch of sparkle, but that's not enough to warrant a purchase—lots of eyeliners feature varying degrees of shine but last longer than this one.

LIPSTICK AND LIP GLOSS: ✓ ☺ **Beyond Natural Cream Lip Gloss** *($7.99)* comes in a small, but satisfying, group of colors that basically translate to mean "your lip color, only better." Adding heightened, translucent color and a soft, non-sticky gloss finish make this lip gloss even more appealing. The Beyond Natural name is appropriate, and I suspect if this sub-brand doesn't succeed in its entirety, this tube gloss will remain in the line because it certainly stands on its own and serves as a good, sheer alternative to Revlon's other lip glosses.

☹ **Beyond Natural Protective Liptint SPF 15** *($7.99)*. What a shame this sheer lip balm in lipstick form lacks the UVA-protecting ingredients of titanium dioxide, zinc oxide, avobenzone (also known as butyl methoxydibenzoylmethane), ecamsule (Mexoryl SX), or Tinosorb. If one of these actives were included, this would be a brilliant way to provide lips with moisture, a soft cream finish, and adequate sun protection.

MASCARA: ✓ ☺ **Beyond Natural Defining Mascara Waterproof** *($7.99)* is an excellent lengthening mascara that applies evenly, doesn't clump, and provides beautiful lash separation. This is well worth considering if you don't want any thickness, but do want to make lashes impressively long with a waterproof formula that lasts. It requires an oil- or silicone-based remover.

☺ **Beyond Natural Defining Mascara** *($7.99)* isn't the one to choose if you're looking for dramatic, traffic-stopping mascara. However, if you want defined, perfectly separated lashes with moderate length and zero clumps, this is well worth trying! The rubber-bristled, dual-sided brush contains short, thick bristles on one side and long, thin bristles on the other. Using both sides, you can achieve impressive results. No one will think your lashes are natural, but you won't be accused of overdoing it either! This wears well and comes off easily with a water-soluble cleanser.

SPECIALTY PRODUCTS: ☺ **Beyond Natural Smoothing Primer** *($12.99 for 0.85 ounce)* leaves skin feeling very silky with a slightly moist finish, but only because this gel-textured primer is composed mostly of silicones. It can facilitate makeup application, but so do many serums and, yes, many moisturizers, due to the fact that silicones are so widely used. For those who prefer a pre-makeup product labeled a primer (which is more a marketing term than anything else), this is a good option. It is suitable for all skin types except sensitive due to the strong, lingering fragrance. Because of the fragrance, some may find this a problem to use near the eyes. It certainly was for me: I had low-grade stinging and minor eye irritation that lasted all day.

REVLON COLORSTAY PRODUCTS

FOUNDATION: ✓ ☺ **ColorStay Active Light Makeup SPF 25** *($12.99)* has properties similar to Revlon's former ColorStay Light Makeup SPF 15. It's a worthy successor to that formidable foundation, except in one area: coverage. ColorStay Active Light Makeup SPF 25 offers sheer to medium coverage, and medium coverage is obtainable only if you layer the product.

Otherwise, there are more similarities (and improvements) than differences. This version has a slightly fluid texture that applies smoothly, offering enough play time to blend it evenly. As for wearability, ColorStay Active Light Makeup just won't quit. It maintains its finish and appearance on skin almost all day, which is great news for those with oily skin. The trade-off for such long wear is that this foundation is difficult to remove, so be sure to use a soft washcloth with a gentle, water-soluble cleanser to get it all off. Despite this drawback, it remains an excellent foundation with reliable sunscreen (the actives include in-part titanium dioxide and zinc oxide) for someone with oily to very oily skin. The eight shades do not include options for those with very fair or dark skin; however, those with light to medium skin tones are well served. Avoid the darkest shade, Toast, which is noticeably orange.

✓ ☺ **ColorStay Makeup with Softflex for Normal to Dry Skin SPF 15** *($12.99)* contains zinc oxide and titanium dioxide for broad-spectrum sun protection, and although it's not emollient enough to please those with dry skin, it has a beautiful satin-matte finish that feels slightly moist and provides medium to nearly full coverage (if layered). Those with dry skin looking for a long-wearing foundation with sunscreen will find that this pairs well with a moisturizer. This isn't nearly as difficult to remove as the original ColorStay Makeup was, and it's much easier to blend because it is forgiving of any mistakes rather than setting and refusing to budge. There are 12 shades, and nearly all are praiseworthy. The only shades to avoid are the too-pink Fresh Beige and the slightly orange Cappuccino.

☺ **ColorStay Makeup with Softflex for Combination/Oily Skin SPF 6** *($12.99)* is downgraded from the get-go because of its unusually low SPF rating. This is an area where Revlon typically excels, and the fact that this is a reformulation makes the SPF 6 even more frustrating. Still more perplexing is the fact that this version of ColorStay Makeup has a higher percentage of active ingredients than the Normal to Dry Skin version. I thought the SPF 6 (all titanium dioxide) was a mistake, but calls to Revlon confirmed that wasn't the case. If you're willing to pair this with an effective sunscreen rated SPF 15 or higher, it has a superb texture that blends effortlessly and allows enough time to do so before setting to a solid, but not flat-looking, matte finish. It's tricky to get less than medium coverage from this, so if you want something sheer, consider the ColorStay Active Light Makeup SPF 25. In comparison to Revlon's original ColorStay, the improvements found are all around. This version allows you to buff away any blending mistakes, it wears beautifully, and it removes with a water-soluble cleanser. If the sunscreen were rated SPF 15 or higher this would have been a slam-dunk recommendation for normal to very oily skin. Twenty shades are available for fair to dark skin tones, almost all of which are wonderful. Avoid Natural Beige and Golden Caramel. Note: Caramel, Toast, Rich Ginger, Cappuccino, Mahogany, and Mocha shades do not offer any sun protection.

CONCEALER: ☺ **ColorStay Under Eye Concealer SPF 15** *($9.99)* nets its excellent sun protection from a combination of titanium dioxide and zinc oxide, two gentle active ingredients well-suited for use around the eyes. This click-pen concealer has a built-in angled sponge-tip applicator that dispenses a slightly thick but blendable concealer. It smooths over skin, provides decent coverage (this isn't the best choice for very dark circles), and has a satin finish. Overall, this is a great option for normal to dry skin. It poses minimal risk of creasing into lines under the eye, and five of the six shades are superbly neutral. Avoid Light/Medium, which has a peachy cast that doesn't soften enough to look natural.

☺ **ColorStay Blemish Concealer** *($9.99)* contains 0.5% salicylic acid, which is on the low side for handling blemishes, but the pH of this concealer prevents it from working as an exfoliant anyway. This revamped version of the original ColorStay Concealer isn't as winning as its predecessor. It provides uneven, often insufficient, coverage (especially for blemishes), and it never sets to a true matte finish, so slippage and fading will be issues, not to mention that it looks slightly chalky on skin. The six shades are nearly perfect (though Light/Medium is a bit pink), but that's not enough to make this liquid concealer an easy recommendation.

POWDER: ✓☺ **ColorStay Pressed Powder** *($9.99)* claims to wear for 16 hours over makeup, and, yes, it can stay that long (assuming you keep your hands off your face and you're not perspiring), but your oily areas will undoubtedly need a touch-up at some point during the day well before 16 hours. This adds up to a wonderful, talc-based powder for normal to very oily skin. The jet-milled powder has a superfine texture that provides a matte finish that doesn't look cakey or chalky, and of the six shades, only Light/Medium and Deep are too peach for their intended skin tones.

EYESHADOW: ☺ **ColorStay 12 Hour Eye Shadow Quad** *($6.99)* is an impressive eyeshadow whose smooth, slightly thick, but non-powdery texture applies evenly and softly. The color application is on the sheer side, but layering produces more dramatic shading and shaping. Does it last 12 hours without fading or creasing? That's hard to quantify, because so much depends on application, how oily your eyelids are, whether or not you use moisturizer on your eyelids, and what other makeup products you use, such as a matte concealer, foundation, or powder over the eye. The best news is that most of the quads are well coordinated, though all have some degree of shine. Some of the superior quads are Coffee Bean, In the Buff, and Copper Spice. Sandstorm is attractive as well, but the shine is more obvious and not the best for wrinkled eyelids because it will make them more pronounced. Avoid Stonewash Denim and Azure Mist, which are overwhelmingly blue.

EYE AND BROW SHAPER: ✓☺ **ColorStay Liquid Eye Pen** *($8.99)* should be seriously considered by anyone desiring the look of liquid eyeliner. Its pointed, flexible felt-tip applicator makes this a breeze to put on, even if you don't have a very steady hand. The formula dispenses evenly and sets quickly to an immovable finish. Smearing, smudging, and fading simply don't happen with this eyeliner. The only drawback is that the color intensity isn't as strong as that of standard liquid eyeliners. That means the initial application is a bit softer, but if you're adept, you can lay down a second coat for additional emphasis. All of the shades Revlon created are recommended.

✓☺ **ColorStay Liquid Liner** *($7.49)* has an improved brush that enables you to paint a thin or thick line with precision and ease. The formula dries in a flash, so get this on correctly right from the start because once it sets it won't budge all day. This is assuredly worth a look for those who prefer liquid eyeliner or who have trouble getting pencil eyeliners to last. The Black Shimmer shade is infused with obvious silver glitter that doesn't flake, so it's a consideration for evening makeup.

☺ **ColorStay Brow Enhancer** *($8.99)* provides a tinted wax and brow-bone highlighter in one component. The wax is essentially a twist-up brow pencil housed in a retractable base. It definitely has a waxy texture and unless applied sparingly can make brow hairs look and feel coated. Unlike the best brow pencils, the finish of this one remains slightly tacky. The highlighter is simply a twist-up cream-to-powder eyeshadow that leaves a gleaming finish wherever it is used. It applies smoothly and is minimally crease- and fade-prone. You can get better results using a brow powder or any of the brow pencils I recommend (Maybelline has some good ones) plus a standard powder eyeshadow. If you opt for this Revlon product, all of the shades are workable, including the Blonde tone.

☺ **ColorStay Eyeliner** (*$7.49*) is a twist-up, retractable pencil that has almost too much slip and a tip that's soft enough to smush with moderate pressure. Once this sets in place though, it does stay quite well without feeling tacky. If you're willing to acclimate to this pencil's quirks, it is one to consider.

LIPSTICK, LIP GLOSS, AND LIPLINER: ✓ ☺ **ColorStay Lip Liner** (*$7.99*) is a retractable, twist-up pencil that really holds up against greasy lipsticks and, true to its name, stays put. The 16 shades do a formidable job of keeping lipstick anchored in place, making this a must-try if you're prone to feathering.

☺ **Colorstay Overtime Lipcolor** (*$9.99*) competes nicely with Cover Girl's Outlast Lipcolor. The basic application steps and "rules" are the same: you apply a base coat of opaque color using a sponge-tip wand applicator, and wait about one minute for the color to set. Once it has dried (which doesn't feel comfortable, but is integral to the long-wearing part) you can apply the clear, glossy top coat. Unlike Outlast, Revlon's clever packaging houses both base color and clear topcoat in a single unit. I prefer the fact that Revlon's topcoat comes with a brush applicator rather than a solid, swivel-up stick. Also Revlon's top coat also feels thicker and provides a glossier finish. It's more tenacious, too—I reapplied the top coat only a few times throughout the day, whereas similar products require more frequent applications of the top coat to prevent dry lips. Over time, Lipcolor loses points (and a Paula's Pick rating) for not wearing as well as Outlast. It does stay on, but after testing both formulas over the course of several days, I experienced more flaking and color chipping with Revlon's Overtime Lipcolor. It also tended to feel grainy on the lips after a few hours, and reapplying the top coat did not ease this feeling. Still, this definitely has its strong points (such as being easy to take off with an oil- or silicone-based remover) and it's certainly worth a test run if you're curious.

☺ **ColorStay Soft & Smooth Lipcolor** (*$9.99*) initially feels very smooth and creamy, but lightweight. The lightweight texture remains, but the creaminess dissipates quickly, leaving a slightly moist, semi-matte finish that has notable staying power. Although a far cry from the dry, parched feeling of the original ColorStay lipstick, this isn't for someone who likes their lips to remain emollient and look glossy. In fact, applying a lip gloss on top of this shortens its wear time, although not drastically so. Overall, this is a nice update and good compromise between the dryness of traditional ultra-matte lipsticks and the smoothness of today's best creamy lipsticks. Six of the shades are labeled as ColorStay Sheer, and they are indeed softer colors that can be layered for more opacity, but initial application is more translucent. The Sheer formula does not wear as long as the original, but it's impressive compared to many other sheer, glossy lipsticks.

☺ **ColorStay Overtime Sheer Lipcolor** (*$10.29*) is Revlon's version of Lipfinity EverLites and Cover Girl Outlast Smoothwear. It has the same two-phase concept, with color application followed by a top coat to ensure comfortable wear. Revlon's shades do go on sheer, but their formula tends to dry out too soon, even with regular application of the glitter-infused top coat (which has a thicker, stickier feel than those from competing products and is not the same formula as the top coat in Revlon's ColorStay Overtime Lipcolor). As such, you don't really get to enjoy the best feature of products like this—namely, long wear without fading, chipping, or leaving telltale marks.

☹ **ColorStay Ultimate Lipcolor** (*$9.99*). The big to-do with this lip product is that it's supposed to be a lip paint and top coat in one, thus negating the need to use the numerous two-step long-wearing lip products first made famous by Max Factor Lipfinity. That's an admirable goal, but Revlon failed miserably. This liquid lipstick applies smoothly and feels like a lightweight gloss, but within minutes after it dries, your lips literally feel like the moisture is being sucked right out of them. I applied more product, thinking that because the top coat was built in I would get some relief from the parched feeling. That didn't happen. Instead, my lips continued to feel dry. Still, I persevered. About an hour later, this began flaking and looking all-around unattractive. Revlon maintains this wears for 12 hours, but I suspect most women won't tolerate the way it feels for longer than 12 minutes, so their long-wearing claim won't be put to the test. What a shame, because the concept is exciting and the shade range is beautiful.

COLORSTAY MINERAL PRODUCTS

FOUNDATION: ✓ ☺ **ColorStay Mineral Mousse Makeup SPF 20** *($13.99)* has sunscreen actives that are mineral-based, which is typical of Revlon, even in their foundations not labeled as "mineral." This ends up being a very silky, easy-to-blend foundation with a lasting matte finish that's ideal for oily skin. It provides sheer to light coverage and has a silky-smooth, natural affinity for skin. True to its name, it has a mousse-like texture, but not the foamy kind you may equate with standard hairstyling mousse; this is more like a soft pudding. All of the shades are recommended; even the questionable ones for medium skin tones go on softer and more neutral than you might expect. There are no options for very fair or dark skin tones.

☺ **ColorStay Mineral Foundation SPF 10** *($13.99)* This loose-powder foundation is talc-based, yet offers more coverage than a standard loose powder (remember, talc is a mineral). The sunscreen rating is disappointing, although Revlon's on-product information describes it honestly as "secondary sun protection," which is a good idea (and what keeps this from earning a neutral face rating due to its lower SPF rating). The sole active is titanium dioxide, making this suitable for sensitive skin. The packaging for this powder houses a brush that's built into the twist-off cap. Turning the top portion of the cap lowers the brush onto the sifter, where it picks up powder. You need to raise the brush back into the cap to close the component. Although the brush concept is clever, the brush is smaller and the hairs are not as soft as they should be. A regular powder brush is preferred, though Revlon's component deserves credit for reducing the mess loose powders can make. Once applied, this leaves a soft-glow finish and can provide sheer to almost medium coverage. The 16-hour wear claim sounds great, but those with oily areas will find touch-ups are needed, not to mention that the coverage tends to fade over the course of a day. However, this is an overall impressive powder, and the eight shades are almost all neutral, plus there are options for fair to dark skin tones. Shade 080 Deep will be too copper for some dark skin tones, but is still worth considering.

POWDER: ☹ **ColorStay Mineral Finishing Powder** *($11.99)* is pretty to look at in the compact, but terrible in every other respect. It is nearly impossible to pick up any color using a brush; even wiping at this with a fingertip proves futile—product comes off on your finger, but you can't transfer it to facial skin, at least not without it looking streaky (that goes for brush application, too). It's the oddest thing, but you literally cannot do much of anything with this finishing powder; except, of course, refuse to purchase it, which I highly recommend.

BLUSH AND BRONZER: ☹ **ColorStay Mineral Blush/Bronzer** *($13.99)* is a terribly dry, powdery blush (or bronzer, as the product comes in two shades for bronzing) that doesn't last anywhere near its claim of 16 hours. That's because the color payoff is so small; you may find yourself humming Peggy Lee's song "Is That All There Is?" in frustration. Even if wear was exemplary, this blush's texture and application make it one of the worst options at the drugstore. It really is that bad!

EYESHADOW: ☺ **ColorStay Mineral Eye Shadow** *($8.99)* shares a formula that's nearly identical to Revlon's problematic ColorStay Mineral Blush/Bronzer above. That doesn't bode well for application or long wear, but at least with these shiny shadows the pigmentation is improved. That doesn't make them worth considering over most other powder eyeshadows (including Revlon's original ColorStay shadows), but they're not the same letdown the ColorStay Mineral Blush/Bronzer is.

LIP GLOSS: ☺ **ColorStay Mineral Lipglaze** *($8.99).* Never mind the fact that the only minerals in this gloss are mica and iron oxides, the same cosmetic pigments that show up in thousands of lipsticks and glosses—what about Revlon's claim of 8-hour wear from a lip gloss? Well, due to the high amount of (very synthetic) film-forming copolymer, that claim is basically true. This wand-applied lip gloss wears and wears (though the top layer will come off on coffee cups or anything else your lips touch). The problem is that this long wear and lingering color come with the trade-off that your lips constantly feel slightly tacky. This isn't a silky, slick gloss with a wet-looking shine; it's a tenacious gloss with a shimmering finish that doesn't feel as good as it should. That makes ColorStay Mineral Lipglaze a tough sell, but if you're willing to tolerate the drawbacks, it may be worth a try (it certainly wears longer than standard lip gloss).

OTHER REVLON PRODUCTS

MAKEUP REMOVERS: ☺ **Makeup Eraser Pen** *($8.49 for 0.06 ounce)* is a pencil designed for "portable perfection and touch-ups on the go." The solvent- and silicone-based formula is dispensed through a felt-tip marker, and does dissolve eyeliner, mascara, or lipstick mistakes. This is convenient for minor mistakes, but you will need a tissue or cotton swab to completely remove signs of the mistake. I was impressed that this works on stubborn makeup, too, and is fragrance-free. Based on the design, this is best for removing or correcting eyeliner or lipliner mistakes, but it doesn't work any better than a cotton swab with makeup remover dabbed on the tip.

☺ **Makeup Remover Towelettes with Pomegranate and Chamomile** *($6.49 for 30 tow-elettes)* contain a lotion-based cleanser that works fairly well to remove lightweight makeup. Ironically, these don't do a complete job (at least not without a lot of pressure and rubbing, which isn't good for skin) of removing Revlon's ColorStay foundations that contain silicone. Perhaps the strangest part is the really unusual scent of these cloths. I couldn't tell if it was intentional or was just beginning to go bad, but it wasn't pleasant. These cloths are best for normal to dry skin when minimal makeup is used.

FOUNDATION: ✓☺ **New Complexion One Step Compact Makeup SPF 15** *($12.99)* ranks as the best cream-to-powder foundation at the drugstore, hands down, and it includes titanium dioxide as the only sunscreen active. It applies superbly; has a light, silky texture; and sets to a soft, natural-looking powder finish that is best for normal to slightly oily or slightly dry skin. (Just keep in mind that moisturizer must be applied over any dry spots or this foundation will exaggerate them.) Coverage goes from sheer to medium. This is a must-try if you prefer cream-to-powder foundation. Revlon's 12 shades have been improved, and are a mostly neutral lot. Avoid Natural Beige, Cool Beige, and Warm Beige. Tender Peach is fairly true to its name, but may work for some light skin tones. Regrettably, there are no shades for very light or very dark skin tones.

☺ **Custom Creations SPF 15 Foundation** *($13.99 for 1 ounce).* This innovative foundation not only contains titanium dioxide and zinc oxide for superior sun protection, but also is the only foundation that allows the user to customize the shade by adjusting the dual-chambered component. Each of the six base color shades (from Fair/Light to Deep) allows you to create unique shades, depending on where you set the dial. Once the pump is primed, you're free to turn the dial to find your best shade. This can be very convenient if, for example, you're dealing with a paler skin tone in winter months or you occasionally use a self-tanner. The interior of the component is set up to dispense a proportionate amount of the shade you've "dialed in" along with the base color. The differences among the five possible shades are subtle, but this fine-tuning does allow for a more precise match than simply purchasing a single shade. So why doesn't this foundation get a better rating? The drawback is in how it appears on the skin. Once you get the hang of how to control the pump so you're not dispensing too much product, this blends on very well, but the powdery matte finish tends to make skin look dry and pasty. Even when I tried using the darkest possible shade from my bottle (which was definitely too dark to look convincing), my skin still looked washed-out and flat. Considering the number of superior foundations whose finish has an enviable skin-like quality, that's disappointing. This is worth a look for its novelty and customization, but keep in mind that the range of foundation shades available to consumers today provides more than enough selections for all skin tones. There are better foundation options at the drugstore, many by Revlon. One more note: This can become quite messy because the foundation tends to keep oozing out of the dispenser, which means you have to tidy up the component before you replace the cap.

☺ **New Complexion Makeup** *($11.99)* isn't so new anymore—it's actually Revlon's oldest foundation despite a packaging update. Although it isn't a terrible choice, it doesn't have the same great qualities of their more recent additions. This remains a very lightweight option for normal to slightly oily skin. It slips nicely over the skin and sets to a natural matte finish that provides light to medium coverage. Its look on skin isn't as seamless as it could be, and you may notice it sinks into lines and large pores, especially in oil-prone areas. Of the nine shades, the only good options are Sand Beige, Medium Beige, and Sun Beige. The rest are too pink, orange, or peach.

BLUSH AND BRONZER: ✓ ☺ **Cream Blush** *($9.79)* is misnamed because this is really a cream-to-powder blush. However, if you're looking for a smooth alternative to powder blush and have normal to slightly dry or slightly oily skin (that is, not oily in the cheek area) this is an outstanding option. The color selection is small but well edited, meaning every shade is a winner, though each shade has a touch of shimmer (but it's light enough so it's not distracting). Note that all the shades go on softer than they appear. This blends so easily that it is easy for the color to go "out of bounds" as you apply it, so you may need to practice before you get it to go just where you want it to be. It is best to apply this as a series of dots along the cheekbone and onto the apple of the cheek, then carefully blend each dot together to form one smooth wash of color. The compact features a cleverly concealed mirror that pops out at the touch of a button. Very sleek, and the mirror is just big enough for quick lipstick touch-ups or to check for mascara smudges.

☺ **Bronzer Blush** *($9.79)* has a different and silkier formula than the Powder Blush below, and also imparts more color from both soft tan shades (OK, Natural Bronze is a peachy tan). The shine is discreet and the compact's pop-out mirror is an added convenience. Toss the too-tiny brush Revlon included, unless you want a striped effect.

☺ **Matte Powder Blush** *($9.99)* is a very good sheer powder blush with a genuine matte finish. Revlon took the matte name literally and delivered a beautiful yet small range of pastel-ish colors best for fair to light skin tones. The texture is silky and you'll need to layer this if you want more than a soft wash of color, but it's worth considering if you've been dismayed by the lack of good matte blushes and want a soft hint of color.

☺ **Powder Blush** *($9.79)* doesn't impart much color, even with successive applications. It has a silky texture with results that are so soft it's almost like wearing no blush at all, though you are left with sparkles. The sparkles aren't readily visible as you're eyeing the shade in the compact, but don't be fooled—they're part of each shade. This blush is only recommended if you want a hint of color and don't mind sparkly cheeks.

EYESHADOW: ✓☺ **Illuminance Creme Eyeshadow** *($6.50)* offers four shades of cream-to-powder eyeshadow in a sleek compact. Most cream eyeshadows tend to crease and can be troublesome to blend with other colors, but these hold up quite well and go on softly. Your choices are limited if you prefer neutral tones, but those who enjoy cream eyeshadows should strongly consider these. The best sets are Not Just Nudes, Pink Petals, Seashells, Twilight, Va Va Va Bloom, Skinlights, and Wild Orchids. Powder eyeshadows may be applied before or after for different effects, and to give the cream shadow greater staying power.

☺ **Matte Powder Eyeshadow** *($4.99)*. Other than Physician's Formula, Prestige Cosmetics, Jane, and some random shades from L'Oreal, finding a good matte-powder eyeshadow isn't easy when you're shopping at the drugstore. Revlon is now part of this mix. They've crafted a reasonably good powder eyeshadow in a small range of shades, all with a matte finish. The silky, slightly dusty texture applies evenly and builds well for intensity, plus it blends seamlessly with other shades rather than "sticking" where you first touch brush to eye-area skin. I wish more of the colors were workable; as is, there are blues and greens to avoid. The shades to consider are Vintage Lace, Peach Sorbet, Pink Innocence, Aubergine, and Rich Sable.

EYE AND BROW SHAPER: ☺ **Brow Fantasy Pencil & Gel** *($7.49)* combines a standard brow pencil with a sheer brow gel in one component. The pencil needs sharpening; you get a very small amount (it's roughly a quarter of the length of a standard brow pencil); and the brow gel, while completely non-sticky, imparts almost zero color and does not contain the type of ingredients that keep unruly hairs in place. This is more a blah product than a fantasy, unless your imagination is limited to dreaming in shades of gray!

☺ **Luxurious Color Eyeliner** *($9.99)* is a relatively standard eye pencil that needs routine sharpening. The color intensity is strong (Revlon compares it, accurately, to that of a liquid eyeliner), yet the color can be smudged and softened for a smoky effect. It is mildly prone to smearing and some fading, but the rich colors last, making this an option for those who prefer pencils and don't mind sharpening.

☺ **Matte Luxurious Color Kohl Eyeliner** *($9.99)* is a fairly standard pencil that applies smoothly, needs sharpening, and has a tendency to smudge after it has set. Each shade finishes matte, and if you don't mind the sharpening and are trying for a smoky eye design, check this out. Avoid the purple Very Violet and consider Pure White carefully—using white liner around the eyes is a theatrical makeup technique that rarely looks convincing up close in natural light.

LIPSTICK AND LIP GLOSS: ✓☺ **Matte Lipstick** *($7.99)*. I am always searching for matte lipsticks, and have been since I was very young. Glossy, creamy, or even slightly creamy lipsticks have always bled into the lines around my mouth. Matte lipsticks are the only answer for this problem if you're going to wear lip color, but they're hard to find. Over the years that I've been reviewing makeup products, I have come across very few truly matte lipsticks. Even when a lipstick was labeled as being matte, it was still creamy (often even greasy) and so was useless for preventing movement. This product, however, did not disappoint me. It is indeed matte and you can wear it with little risk of having it move into lines. It definitely has a matte finish and a slightly dry texture, but if you are tempted to put a gloss on, it will bleed if you share my problem. If not, take a look at the 10 shades Revlon has to offer. The colors tend to be bold reds and burgundy hues, which are without question limiting. Mauve It Over is the most versatile shade, while Nude Attitude tends to make lips look washed out.

✓ ☺ **Super Lustrous Lipstick** *($7.99)* is a moderately creamy lipstick that feels comfortable without being too slick or greasy and has better-than-average staying power. Revlon claims this is America's #1-selling lipstick, and backs this up with year-long figures from AC Nielsen Scantrak. However, best-selling doesn't mean you should jump on the bandwagon (I can think of a lot of popular items people buy that are not a good idea). In this case, best-seller or not, this is a very good creamy lipstick with a staggering range of 72 shades. If you can't find a color you like, perhaps lipstick just isn't for you!

☺ **Super Lustrous Lipgloss** *($7.69)* is a standard lip gloss with an angled, sponge-tip applicator and smooth application that finishes glossy and feels slightly sticky. The beguiling shade selection offers sheer and dramatic hues that can be worn alone or to add pizzazz to a lipstick. This reasonably priced gloss competes nicely with more costly options from luxury lines such as Chanel and Yves Saint Laurent.

☺ **Creme Gloss** *($9.99)* is a gloss/lipstick hybrid that has a lot going for it; unfortunately, it also has a lot going against it. First, the assets: the creamy texture provides more coverage and you get slightly more wear time than you get from a typical gloss. Now, the drawbacks: the brush-tipped applicator overdispenses the gloss through the middle of the brush, making even application difficult, and it's likely you will need to repeatedly blot excess gloss. Also, the thicker formulation applies sloppily and easily gets on the teeth (yuck)! Considering these negatives, this gloss is recommended only to fans of Dior's Creme de Gloss, which has a similar formulation but better applicator, yet costs considerably less than this option from Revlon.

☺ **Moon Drops Lipstick** *($8.99)* has been around for decades, and even the bright green packaging hasn't changed. Although this is a good, traditional cream lipstick, its fragrance is knock-your-socks-off strong and that also affects how this tastes, which is to say not pleasant. The selection of nearly 30 shades favors bright, bold hues (fans of orange lipstick, take note) rather than the more contemporary palette found in Revlon's Super Lustrous range.

☹ **Moon Drops Lip Conditioner SPF 6** *($8.99)* is a lip balm with sunscreen with an antiquated formula whose sole active ingredient is one that's rarely used anymore due to its tendency to be sensitizing. It only provides UVB protection, so lips are left vulnerable to UVA damage. Moon Drops Lip Conditioner has a smooth, emollient texture but is downgraded because of its cloying fragrance and unpleasant flavor. It contains several fragrance chemicals that can cause irritation.

MASCARA: ✓ ☺ **3D Extreme Mascara** *($13.99)* promises lashes that are curvier, fuller, and longer, and it really delivers! 3D Extreme Mascara has a patented brush in which two-thirds of the bristles are short and densely packed, and the other third are longer and wider spaced. The result is immediate thickness and lengthening that goes on and on, and, yes, a curvy finish that can get quite dramatic with subsequent coats. The formula wears well and removes easily with a water-soluble cleanser. Watch out, L'Oreal!

✓ ☺ **Fabulash Mascara** *($6.99* promises fuller, clump-free lashes, and it delivers—big-time! You'll get a clean application that defines each lash while lengthening and thickening in the right proportions to produce dramatic but not over-the-top lashes. Add to this the fact that lashes stay soft without flaking or smearing, and Fabulash deserves an enthusiastic round of applause!

☺ **3D Extreme Mascara Waterproof** *($9.99)* isn't quite as impressive as the original 3D Extreme Mascara, but is definitely worth considering if you're looking for a waterproof mascara that provides even length and thickness while lasting all day. This applies with slight clumps that must be combed through for best results, but once it sets you won't see a flake or smear.

☺ **Lash Fantasy Total Definition Primer & Mascara** *($8.99)* doesn't reach the same peaks of performance as the Fabulash Mascara, but this two-step mascara is still worth considering. The Primer step is essentially a colorless mascara that's applied first, followed by a regular mascara. Using the Primer versus not using it makes a subtle difference, but whether you do both steps or just apply the mascara, you'll enjoy substantial length and thickness in nearly equal measure. Lashes are perfectly defined without a clump in sight, and this wears beautifully all day.

☺ **Lash Fantasy Total Definition Waterproof Primer & Mascara** *($8.99)* owes its successful results to the lash primer, just as with Revlon's non-waterproof Lash Fantasy Total Definition Primer & Mascara above. Sweeping the primer through lashes and immediately following with mascara produces prodigiously long, appreciably thick lashes. You'll need a lash comb handy unless you want a heavier, dramatic look. Clumping is kept to a minimum, but you may notice some minor flaking if application is overzealous. The mascara applied alone is a snooze; all you get is patchy definition and mediocre length without much thickness, even with successive coats. Whether you use the lash primer with or without the mascara, the formulas are waterproof and require more than a water-soluble cleanser for complete removal.

☹ **Double Twist Mascara** *($8.99)* features short-cut densely packed bristles in the central portion and longer, variegated rubber bristles on the outer portion of this flashy mascara's double-helix brush. The result is incredibly thick, dramatic lashes that become impossibly longer with each coat, although adding more than a couple coats is really overdoing it and leads to flaking and a heavy look. After all that praise, why isn't this mascara rated a Paula's Pick? The formula falls apart shortly after opening. We tried a few tubes of this mascara, being sure to purchase a different color each time. In every case, after a few uses, the mascara softened in the tube and formed thick, creamy globs on the brush. It was impossible to use due to the absurd amount of product "caught" on the brush. What a shame, and what poor quality control, Revlon!

☹ **Fabulash Mascara Waterproof** *($6.99)* has the same type of brush as Revlon's original (and amazingly good) Fabulash Mascara, but that's where the similarities start and stop. The waterproof version does hold up when lashes get wet, but the application and wear leave much to be desired. Although this mascara lengthens and provides decent thickness, it clumps as it is applied, goes on unevenly, and flakes throughout the day, not to mention it makes your lashes feel dry and crispy. Almay (owned by Revlon) produces much more reliable waterproof mascaras, particularly their One Coat Nourishing Mascara Triple Effect Waterproof Mascara. Almay, you should tell Revlon what they're doing wrong!

RIMMEL (MAKEUP ONLY)

RIMMEL AT-A-GLANCE

Strengths: Inexpensive; the pressed bronzing powder; some of the best mascaras at the drugstore; respectable powder blush, cream blush, and powder eyeshadows; excellent automatic eye pencil; Lasting Finish Lipstick and Vinyl Lip are must-sees.

Weaknesses: Packaging that isn't very user-friendly; average concealers; several lackluster eyeshadow options; none of the Extra Super Lash mascaras earn their impressive-sounding names; potentially problematic eye-makeup remover.

For more information about Rimmel, visit www.rimmellondon.com or www.Beauty-pedia.com.

Note: Many Rimmel products featured on their Web site are not available in the United States; they are exclusive to United Kingdom drugstores. The products reviewed below are those that are consistently found at U.S. stores nationwide, specifically Target, Walgreens, and Walmart.

MAKEUP REMOVER: ☺ **Gentle Eye Makeup Remover** *($7.29 for 4.2 ounces)* is a relatively standard, nonsilicone-based eye-makeup remover whose formula is hindered a bit by the inclusion of sodium lauryl sulfate, a cleansing agent known for being a potent skin irritant. There isn't a lot of it in the product, but this strong detergent cleansing agent is best kept away from the sensitive eye area, so this isn't worth considering over gentler options from Neutrogena, Almay, or L'Oreal.

FOUNDATION: ☺ **Lasting Finish Mineral Enriched Foundation** *($7.49)*. Sigh—more mineral makeup. And just like so many others bearing the mineral name, the smattering of mineral-based ingredients aren't unique or present in quantities great enough to qualify as genuine mineral makeup. But, it's a growing trend, and trends sell. In terms of a lasting finish, this liquid foundation delivers, thanks to its silicone-enhanced formula and silky matte finish. This has a beautiful texture suitable for normal to oily skin, and does an above-average job of looking more skin-like than flat. This is especially impressive when you consider the amount of coverage it provides. Although it can be blended on sheer, the standard amount provides nearly full coverage, yet it doesn't look heavy. The best shades include Ivory, Soft Beige, and True Ivory. The options for medium skin tones are not worth considering because of their obvious pink or peach tones.

☺ **Lasting Finish Mineral Powder Foundation** *($8.49)*. This loose-powder foundation is housed in a jar with a built-in sifter and a removable (and washable) sponge applicator. Given the smooth, nearly weightless texture, I suspect the formula is talc-based, and talc is indeed a mineral. Also, compared with many other mineral makeups, this provides sheer coverage that doesn't build well, so don't count on it for coverage or camouflage of any kind. That's not an issue if you want it sheer, but if not, this isn't the "mineral" powder makeup to buy. Each of the five shades leaves a sheen on your skin, which can magnify oily areas, so this foundation is best for those with normal to dry skin. All of the shades are recommended (the range only offers options for light to medium skin tones) except Classic Beige, which is too orange when blended on skin.

☺ **Stay Matte + Skinpure Complex Clarifying Matte Foundation** *($7)* is a great liquid foundation option for those with normal to oily skin looking to control shine. It also applies sheer, leaving the skin with a semi-matte finish that lasts well through the day. Rimmel brags about the "Skinpure Complex" in this foundation, but they're simply referring to the small amount of salicylic acid, which is not enough to help exfoliate or reduce blemishes. The shade selection is small, but the options are sheer enough that most skin tones will be able to find a workable option. The small amount of radish root extract is not likely to be a problem for skin.

☺ **Renew & Lift Foundation + Time Release Complex** *($9.69)* promises younger-looking skin in 12 days, thanks to its complex of ceramides and peptides. Ignoring the look-younger claims, this liquid foundation has a pervasive fragrance and a slightly creamy texture that makes it best for normal to dry skin. It provides medium coverage that is difficult to soften, and so it can look somewhat mask-like if the shade you pick doesn't match exactly. In addition, the shades are a mixed bag; among the six choices, Porcelain, Sand, and Classic Beige are too peachy pink to recommend. The other three options are best for fair to light skin tones. Interestingly, the United Kingdom version of this foundation comes with SPF 15, an asset that goes a lot further to protect skin from aging than any peptide!

☺ **Stay Matte Foundation** *($5.39)* is recommended for normal to oily skin, but the moist texture and slightly creamy finish would be more suitable for normal to dry skin, plus it contains enough oil to make its matte finish short-lived. This comes in a tube, provides light to medium coverage, and blends evenly. There are six shades, three of which—Sand, Soft Beige, and Warm Honey—are too pink or peach for most skin tones. Porcelain is slightly pink, but may work for lighter skin tones.

CONCEALER: ☹ **Hide the Blemish Concealer** *($5.19)* is a very greasy, lipstick-style concealer that doesn't cover that well, though it does come in three very good colors. An emollient, wax-based concealer like this is the last thing you want to place over blemishes, at least if the goal is to not make them worse! If you prefer this type of concealer, it would be OK over unblemished areas, but if you're using it under the eye, creasing is inevitable.

☹ **Clear Complexion Coverstick** *($4.99)* is nearly identical to the Hide the Blemish Concealer above, and the same basic comments apply. This does not contain any ingredients known to promote clear skin, but several of the waxes and the lanolin oil make it a distinct problem for those battling blemishes.

POWDER: ☹ **Stay Matte Pressed Powder** *($4.99)* has a smooth texture and non-powdery, but dry, matte finish laced with a tiny amount of shine. Those with oily skin will find this doesn't stay matte for long, but it doesn't look thick or cakey, either. While not the most elegant-feeling powder, it's a good, inexpensive option for normal to slightly oily or slightly dry skin. There are three shades, with no options for medium to dark skin tones. This contains a small amount of fragrance chemicals known to cause irritation, which is what keeps this from earning a happy face.

BLUSH AND BRONZER: ✓ ☺ **Natural Bronzer** *($5.49)* is a talc-based pressed-powder bronzer that has a beautifully smooth texture and application. Shine from each of the three shades is so subtle as to be almost nonexistent, making this a fine choice for daytime wear (though if you have oily skin it probably isn't the best option; those with oily skin need less shine, not more). Speaking of the shades, all have potential, but the orange tinge of Sun Light makes it trickier for fair to light skin tones to pull off, and it's too light for medium skin tones.

☺ **Blush** *($3.49)* is a pressed powder that comes in a small compact and features predominantly sheer, warm-toned shades, all with a softly shiny finish. If only these were matte, they would be a steal, as the texture and application are wonderful.

☺ **Soft Cream Blush** *($2.24)* has a luscious texture, though it's definitely cream-to-powder rather than a true cream blush. Still, this is worth a look if you prefer this type of blush and don't mind shine. The sheer colors apply well and fade minimally (unless your skin is very oily, in which case you shouldn't be using this type of blush anyway).

EYESHADOW: ☺ **Infinite Waterproof Cream Shadow** *($4.37)* is a cream-to-powder eyeshadow applied with a sponge-tip applicator that's affixed to a wand. Blending is tricky because this has a lot of slip, but with practice it imparts strong, shiny color that stays put and is waterproof (yet removes easily with a water-soluble cleanser).

☺ **Special Eyes Mono Eyeshadow** *($2.69)* has a silky, slightly powdery but easy-to-blend texture, and offers mostly shiny to soft shimmer colors. The only matte shades are Matte White (which has limited appeal) and Romance. If you want shiny eyeshadows, this is a good, affordable option.

☺ **Special Eyes Duo Eyeshadow** *($4.29)* has the same formula as the Special Eyes Mono Eyeshadow below, and a surprising number of well-coordinated pairs, each with one matte shade. Take a look at Walnut Pearls and Orchid (both are matte), Metallic Pearls, Desert, Cream Caramel, Biscuit Box, and Spice, where both shades are matte.

☺ **Special Eyes Trio Eye Shadow** *($5.19)* also shares the same formula and application traits as the Special Eyes Mono Eyeshadow, but unlike the plethora of Duos, the selection of Trios is small. Lynx and Orion are worth considering, though two of the three shades in each are shiny.

☺ **All Over Pencil** *($4.37)* is a chunky, needs-sharpening pencil with colors that are best-suited for eyes rather than cheeks or lips. The application is silky-smooth and the formula sets to a relatively long-lasting finish, putting it a step above the standard creamy pencils that are the norm. This is worth considering if you don't mind routine sharpening, but note that every shade is shiny.

☺ **Cool Touch Shadow** *($5.99)* is a liquid-to-powder eyeshadow whose metallic shades go on much sheerer than they appear in the tube, though the shine is intense. Each shade sets to a matte (in feel) finish, but they don't hold up well. They aren't prone to creasing but they tend to fade, wear unevenly, and aren't tenacious (you can remove the product with just water, and they definitely come off when you're perspiring). Better, longer-lasting examples of this type of product are M.A.C. Paint and Maybelline New York's Dream Mousse Shadow.

☺ **Metallic Eye Gloss** *($2.97)* comes in two formulas, though they perform identically. One is mineral oil–based while the other is petrolatum-based, meaning these are creamy and leave a moist, crease-prone finish. Shinier than they are metallic, they're an OK option if they're strategically placed and your eye area is perfectly taut, but you can still count on this smearing and slipping fairly quickly.

☹ **Smokin'! Kohl Shadow** *($6.99)* is a loose-powder eyeshadow packaged in a tiny, vial-like container that includes a pointed sponge-tip applicator. The mess is surprisingly minimal, but this is difficult to apply evenly and has little movement on skin, so it's difficult to blend and soften the stripe of color that's deposited. The medium to darker shades are options if you use this for soft definition on the upper lash line. As long as you don't overload the applicator, the powder itself doesn't flake.

☹ **Stars Glitter Eye Shadow Pencil** *($3.99)* is a needs-sharpening, slightly chunky pencil that imparts minimal, fade-prone color and lots of glitter. What's unusual for pencils like this is that the glitter tends to stay in place quite well. You'll notice some flaking, but much less than with comparable, pricier pencils from NARS or Hard Candy.

☹ **Eye Twist Automatic Duo Liner & Shadow** *($4.37)* is a dual-ended, automatic, retractable pencil with a creamy eyeliner on one end and a shiny cream eyeshadow on the other. Although both apply well, they're too creamy to last, and some smearing is inevitable.

EYE AND BROW SHAPER: ✓ ☺ **Exaggerate Full Colour Eye Definer** *($6.29)* is a superior automatic eye pencil that's also retractable, and includes a built-in sharpener if you desire a finer tip. This applies well, but it takes a few strokes to build intensity. It sets to a soft powder finish that has a low risk of smudging or smearing. The colored tip on the pencil's package is a good indicator of how the color will look on the skin. Avoid the blue and green hues unless you're wearing eyeliner for notice value.

☺ **Professional Eyebrow Pencil** *($3.49)* has a drier, stiffer texture than most standard brow pencils, but its finish really lasts and application is soft and even. This includes a brush built into the cap, which can come in handy.

☺ **Soft Kohl Kajal Eye Pencil** *($3.49)* needs sharpening but is a better pencil in every respect than the Special Eyes Eye Liner Pencil below. Although it is creamy, it has a longer-lasting finish that's less prone to smudging and it glides on with minimal effort. Among the ten shades, Loveable Lilac, Silver, and Jungle Green are shiny. Avoid the latter as well as Cool Blue and Denim Blue. Chianti is an attractive option if you want to move beyond basic brown, black, or gray.

☹ **Professional Liquid Eye Liner** *($5.99)* is a standard liquid liner that comes with a long, skinny brush that can be hard to control over the lash line. Although some may prefer this type of brush, this formula takes too long to dry (even when applied lightly) and it smears easily.

☹ **Special Eyes Eye Liner Pencil** *($3.49)* is a poor eye pencil choice even if the prospect of sharpening thrills you. It's way too creamy and smears with minimal provocation. Even without provocation you'll notice fading way too soon.

LIPSTICK, LIP GLOSS, AND LIPLINER: ✓ ☺ **Lasting Finish Intense Wear Lipstick** *($5.19)* promises 8-hour wear, and almost makes it to that mark. Color intensity is strong, which lends staying power, but this is still a cream lipstick that comes off on coffee cups and other objects (and it certainly won't last through a meal without a touch-up). That said, you'll find this to be one of the better (and least expensive) elegant cream lipsticks available at the drugstore. It feels supremely smooth and light, yet leaves lips comfortably moisturized with a soft gloss finish (or shimmer, depending on the shade chosen). I'd put this up against any department-store lipstick selling for $20 and up, that's for sure!

✓ ☺ **Lasting Finish Kiss & Stay Lipgloss** *($7.99)* does indeed last and stay. The dual-sided wand features a deeply pigmented gloss on one end and a coordinating shimmery top coat on the other. The colors are darker than they appear in the packaging. Surprisingly, while the shiny top coat has the same amount of wear time as any other standard gloss and needs to be reapplied often, the base color is tenacious and lasts extraordinarily well through drinking and eating. Those who have found long-wearing lipsticks too drying will be pleasantly surprised by how comfortable this product feels on the lips. I needed to use makeup remover at day's end to take this off. All in all, this is impressive, and it's a great price, too!

✓ ☺ **Lasting Finish Lipstick** *($4.99)* is, in short, one of the best creamy lipsticks at the drugstore. It feels wonderful and glides on with a soft, creamy texture and slightly glossy finish, and the color range, while not enormous, is still impressive, each providing a good stain. Check out Ballistic if you are a fan of red lipstick that's neither too blue nor too orange.

✓ ☺ **Vinyl Lip** *($5.79)* is an extremely smooth, decadent-feeling lip gloss that is completely non-sticky and very comfortable to wear. The shade selection is bountiful (a Clear option is available too) and this rates as another gem from Rimmel.

☺ **Cool Shine Lipstick** *($6.25)* adds a lot of sparkling glitter to lips that clings tenaciously but doesn't feel grainy. This is otherwise a light-textured, glossy lipstick with a slightly creamy feel and soft colors revved up by an overdose of sparkles (meaning, be sure you like this effect before purchasing).

☺ **Exaggerate Full Colour Lip Liner** *($5.99)* is an automatic, retractable lip pencil that is creamy without veering into greasiness. It stays on quite well, and the colors are rich with pigment. It doesn't apply as smoothly as others (you have to apply a fair amount of pressure to get the color to show up), but for the money, this is a safe bet.

☺ **Jelly Gloss Sheer Lipgloss** *($5.50)* comes in a tube and offers smooth-textured, non-sticky results with a wet-look glossy shine. You have to tolerate the fruity scents and flavors, but if you're a fan of Lancome's Juicy Tubes Ultra Shiny Lip Gloss this is comparable, and with the benefit of not being the least bit goopy. The color impact is more ultra-sheer with minimal to no color saturation.

☺ **Shock Gloss 3D Magnifying Lipgloss** *($5.79)* doesn't really have a 3-D effect on lips, nor does it make lips appear larger than any other sheer gloss. It has a slightly thick, syrupy texture that feels surprisingly smooth and is minimally sticky. It leaves your lips with a wet-looking shine from a range of juicy colors. The only potential drawback is the flat spatula applicator. This is an awkward way to apply gloss, depositing more product than you may want, and the spatula isn't the best way to evenly blend the excess.

☺ **Vinyl Gloss Mirror Shine Lipgloss** *($2.99)*. Without question, the name of this gloss conjures up images of what we want gloss to do when we wear it. Regrettably, this Rimmel lip gloss doesn't deliver results that come close to the product name. It's a good option for basic lip gloss with a soft shine and sheer colors, and it isn't sticky, but that's as scintillating as it gets!

☺ **Volume Booster Lip Colour** *($6.79)* is a smooth-textured, sheer lip gloss applied with a built-in brush applicator. This feels substantially moist without being sticky or goopy, and leaves a wet, glossy sheen on lips. As with most glosses, this will make a beeline into lines around the mouth. I suspect the tingle is a menthol derivative, but the point is that it is nonintrusive and, therefore, likely not cause for concern. As for collagen, whether it is in here or not (the label states "with collagen"), you cannot plump lips with topically applied collagen. That said, the collection of sheer to light coverage colors is pleasing, and there's a Clear option, too.

☺ **1000 Kisses Stay On Lip Liner Pencil** *($3.49)* is a standard, needs-sharpening pencil. It has a smooth and comfortably creamy texture and stays on as well as most other pencils, which is to say, well but not well enough to withstand even one kiss, much less a thousand!

☺ **Rich Moisture Cream Lipstick** *($5.79)* has a smooth but overly waxy feel reminiscent of traditional ChapStick. That's not so bad, but what really keeps this lipstick from earning a higher rating are its potent fragrance and greasier-than-it-should-be finish.

☺ **Twist & Shine Lip Polish** *($4.37)* is a cross between a liquid lipstick and a lip gloss, and is housed in a click pen with an angled sponge-tip applicator. It's an OK option that leaves lips looking colored and glossed.

☺ **Twist & Shine Sheers Lip Polish** *($4.37)* has the same packaging and basic qualities as the regular Twist & Shine Lip Polish above, except the colors are translucent and the finish slightly glossier.

☺ **Vinyl Jelly Gloss Lip Liner** *($3.99)* combines the sheerness and fleeting quality of standard lip gloss with a needs-sharpening pencil format. The soft, sheer colors are sure to please, but this product isn't for anyone expecting a long-lasting, defined lip line. What this can be used for is lip gloss. It's almost as shiny and definitely sheer, and all you'd need to do is line and fill in lips with the color of your choice (and take it along, because touch-ups will be frequent). Ultimately, this doesn't substitute for far-easier-to-use glosses in standard gloss containers.

☹ **Volume Boost Liquid Lipcolour** *($6.49)* comes in a brilliant array of ten sheer, glossy colors and has a beautifully smooth application and minimally sticky feel. Why the unhappy face rating, then? This liquid lipstick contains a menthol derivative known as ethyl menthane carboxamide that is ten times cooler than menthol itself (Source: www.leffingwell.com/cooler_than_menthol.htm), which means it also is that much more irritating.

MASCARA: ✓ ☺ **Eye Magnifier Exact Definition Clean Definition Lengthening Mascara** *($6.99)* produces long, slightly thick, and dramatically defined lashes with just a few sweeps with the rubber-bristled brush. You may experience some minor clumping that requires smoothing out, but the brush allows for this without making matters worse. This stays on quite well yet removes easily with a water-soluble cleanser.

✓ ☺ **Eye Magnifier Eye Opening Mascara** *($6.99)* is said to "lift lashes vertically by 70%" thanks to its Verti-lift brush, but who wants lashes that go vertical when the most attractive look is a panoramic sweep of softly fringed lashes? Luckily this mascara gets very close to that goal and quickly, too. Working the rubber-bristled brush through lashes produces minor clumping, but that's the trade-off for the dramatic results you get from this mascara. The clumps smooth out quickly and further strokes separate lashes nicely while increasing thickness and, to a lesser extent, length.

✓ ☺ **Lash Maxxx 3X Lash Multiplying Effect Mascara** *($7.49)* replaces the familiar round-brush applicator with a serrated comb whose variegated teeth allow for creating tremendously long lashes without clumps. Successive coats build some thickness and you can really get to the lash roots for emphasis there, but this is mostly about making lashes very defined and long. Lashes stay soft, the formula doesn't flake, and it comes off easily with a water-soluble cleanser.

✓ ☺ **Volume Flash Instant Thickening Mascara** *($7.49)* ranks as a formidable thickening mascara. It lengthens, too, but is best for creating beautifully separated, really thick lashes. You won't find the thickness is instant, but with some effort (and no clumps) your lashes will be captivatingly dramatic! An added bonus: Lashes stay soft, and this removes easily with a water-soluble cleanser.

✓ ☺ **Volume Flash Mousse Air-Whipped Volumizing Mascara** *($6.99)* begins with a slightly messy application that deposits a lot of mascara on lashes, but the result is dramatic with copious thickness. This is one of those mascaras that quickly make the most of lashes, leaving them full, defined, and softly fringed. You may need a separate lash comb to smooth things out, but those looking to make a bold lash statement should give this mousse-like mascara strong consideration!

☺ **Glam'Eyes Lash Flirt Mascara** *($4.49)* isn't one of Rimmel's best though this one does have its strong points. The VolumeFlex brush has spiky bristles spaced farther apart than usual, so the result is uneven length, a slightly heavier application, and subtle thickness after several coats. This earns its stripes as lengthening mascara and the deep black pigments the company uses do add extra impact, but that's about it.

☺ **Volume Flash Instant Thickening Waterproof Mascara** *($7.49)* doesn't have the same wow factor as its non-waterproof counterpart, but it is a slightly thickening waterproof mascara. Application is quick and clean, and unlike the results with many waterproof formulas, lashes aren't left feeling dry and brittle.

☺ **Extra Super Lash Curved Brush Mascara** *($3.49)* performs just as well as the straight brush version, but is the one to choose if you want a more defined curl.

☹ **Extra Super Lash Mascara** *($3.49)* is a reliable lengthening mascara that applies clump-free and tends to not flake or chip, but thickness is harder to come by.

☹ **Extra Super Lash Waterproof Mascara** *($6.49)* won't knock your socks off with its lengthening or thickening abilities, but is a very respectable, long-wearing waterproof mascara for those who want slightly longer, separated, and fuller lashes.

☺ **Extreme Definition Ultimate Lash-Separating Mascara** *($6.99)* is a brushless mascara—meaning that it has a miniature comb to sweep on mascara. It does an impressive job of instantly creating long, slightly thick lashes that I wouldn't consider "ultimate," but that are still definitely above average. This can be a time-saving option because lashes are enhanced and separated after just a few strokes. It is prone to minor flaking throughout the day, which is not the best, especially when there are other options that don't flake even a little.

☺ **Glam'Eyes Mascara** *($7.49)* isn't one of Rimmel's best mascaras because its application is too heavy, which results in clumps that must be smoothed out. However, if you're willing to be patient, you can end up with long lashes and an average amount of thickness for greater glamour. Because this goes on heavy, some flaking may occur by the end of the day. I didn't find it objectionable, though, and this is easy to remove with a water-soluble cleanser. Note: the brush can be unusually scratchy as you apply mascara to the base of the lashes, so use extra caution.

☺ **Lycra Lash Extender Mascara** *($7.49)* makes a big deal out of the fact that it contains the synthetic, amazingly stretchable fiber Lycra. Used in mascara, it is supposed to increase lash length by 60% and curl by 50%, all while helping lashes hold their shape for 14 hours. It sounds impressive, but isn't value added because, for all its ballyhoo, Lycra Lash Extender Mascara doesn't produce results anyone would consider "instant" or "dramatic." With several coats you can elongate lashes, and it sets to a soft, eye-opening curl. But thickness is scant, some clumping occurs along the way, and the performance plateaus far too soon to make good on the claims. It's still a valid option if you want a reasonable (but definitely not dramatic) lengthening mascara. Lashes stay soft and the formula is easy to remove.

☺ **Sexy Curves Mascara** *($7.50)* is another mascara with a rubber-bristled brush, this time one that is wavy to set it apart from the others. Rimmel calls it a "Triple Plump Brush," which is likely to entice those with skimpy lashes. The problem is that the excessively curvy brush makes it unnecessarily difficult to get an even application of mascara onto your lashes. If you're willing to put in the work and layers, you'll be rewarded with longer and slightly thicker lashes. You won't get, as Rimmel claims, lashes that are 70% curlier, because Sexy Curves does little to help curl the lashes. All told, Rimmel has much better options that are easier to work with.

☹ **Sexy Curves Waterproof Mascara** *($7.50)* This mascara has a very scratchy brush that is among the most painful I've encountered in the past decade. Getting this too close to the base of your lashes (where you definitely want to deposit mascara) hurts, and you need several coats to produce average length and no thickness. This doesn't clump, but neither do lots of other mascaras that outperform this one. As for the waterproof claim, it isn't one you can rely on for failsafe results; at best, this is slightly waterproof.

☹ **Eye Magnifier Eye Opening Waterproof Mascara** *($7.49)*. Although this mascara goes on with slight clumping, it allows you to build satisfactory length and minor thickness. However, the reason you're likely considering this is because it is sold as being waterproof—and it isn't. This begins to run and smear with minor exposure to water; take a swim in this and you'll be leaving a trail of black in the water! Because this fails miserably as a waterproof mascara, it is not recommended.

☹ **Lash Maxxx 3X Lash Multiplying Effect Waterproof Mascara** *($7.49)*. This mascara is a rare misfire from Rimmel, and it is terrible in every respect. It isn't waterproof, it goes on too heavy, it tends to clump, and the clumps only get worse the more you try to fix them. The result is spiky, messy-looking lashes and a formula that doesn't resist even a little water.

☺ **Volum'Eyes 5X Volume Comb Mascara** *($6.49)* promises copious volume in one stroke, all without clumping or clogging—and fails miserably. This comb mascara is a mess from the get-go, depositing way too much product and instantly making lashes look clumped and spiky. Trying to smooth things out just causes smearing, and makes this the one Rimmel mascara to absolutely avoid.

SPECIALTY PRODUCTS: ☺ **Fix & Perfect Foundation Primer** *($7.79)* is a silky, lightweight primer that imparts a sheer peach tint that dissipates quickly once applied. The powder-assisted matte finish it provides helps keep excess oil in check and creates a smooth surface to apply makeup. Best for normal to oily skin, this is a good, inexpensive product to consider if you've been curious about whether a primer would be helpful or whether it would be a needless addition to your makeup routine.

ROC (SKIN CARE ONLY)

ROC AT-A-GLANCE

Strengths: Some well-packaged products with retinol; one good cleanser; all the sunscreens provide sufficient UVA protection.

Weaknesses: Mediocrity reigns supreme; none of the formulas are particularly exciting; antiwrinkle claims tend to go too far; jar packaging.

For more information about RoC, call (800) 762-1964 or visit www.rocskincare.com or www.Beautypedia.com. And for a better selection of state-of-the-art retinol products from RoC, see the reviews for RoC Canada.

ROC AGE DIMINISHING PRODUCTS

☺ **Age Diminishing Facial Cleanser** *($7.99 for 5.1 ounces)* won't make you look younger, but you can count on this gentle, water-soluble formula to leave normal to slightly dry or slightly oily skin clean and refreshed.

☹ **Age Diminishing Daily Moisturizer SPF 15** *($14.79 for 3 ounces)* contains an in-part avobenzone sunscreen, and that can definitely help diminish the appearance of aging. This is otherwise a really boring daytime moisturizer unless you want to ignore current skin-care research and put all your eggs in one basket by betting that soy extract will be the antiaging miracle. Substantiated research has many positive things to say about soy, and it is a good antioxidant. But the hope that its topical use can diminish wrinkles and discolorations or boost skin's firmness has not yet appeared on the list of proven accomplishments. Regrettably, other than the sunscreen, soy (albeit only a dusting) is the only ingredient of interest here. The mica and titanium dioxide lend a soft shine finish to skin, but that is a cosmetic attribute, not a skin-care benefit.

☹ **Age Diminishing Moisturizing Night Cream** *($14.99 for 1.7 ounces)* contains an impressive amount of antioxidant soybean seed extract, but its potency will be compromised once this jar-packaged moisturizer for normal to dry skin is opened (though even in airtight packaging, soy isn't going to take even one hour off your age). All told, this isn't worth considering over several other options at the drugstore.

ROC COMPLETE LIFT PRODUCTS

☹ **Complete Lift Daily Moisturizer SPF 30** *($17.50 for 1.3 ounces)* is an incredibly basic, lightweight daytime moisturizer with an in-part avobenzone sunscreen. Broad-spectrum sun protection is assured, but skin is cheated of many other helpful ingredients, not to mention this is completely incapable of lifting or transforming skin in as little as four weeks. This is an average option for normal to dry skin.

☺ **Complete Lift Eye Cream** *($22.99 for 0.5 ounce)* is a lightweight eye cream that won't lift skin anywhere on the face, but you probably already knew that. I wish I could report that even though your wrinkles won't be lifted away you would at least be getting a brilliant, well-formulated moisturizer, but I can't. It simply is not well-formulated in the least—not even close. Although suitable for normal to slightly dry skin, the formula is so mundane and the really intriguing ingredients are so barely present that it really isn't worth considering this over better products from Olay and Neutrogena (the latter also owned by Johnson & Johnson, just like RoC).

☺ **Complete Lift Eye Pen** *($18.99 for 1 ounce)* comes housed in a pen-style component with a special angled-tip applicator and is touted as RoC's solution for lifting sagging skin in the eye area while also reducing under-eye puffiness. Is this the ingenious product lots of us have been waiting for? Sadly, no. Although this has a lightweight texture and starch-based thickener that can give the perception of tighter skin (an effect that's cosmetic and fleeting), you won't see sagging skin firm up or under-eye bags get lost. Such age-related changes to skin around the eye can be remedied only via cosmetic surgery. That's because the underlying causes of wrinkles, sagging, and puffiness (including shifting of fat pads beneath the skin, muscle movement, bone loss, gravity) cannot be addressed by skin-care products or even by prescription topical products. Complete Lift Eye Pen may reduce minor puffiness brought on by allergies or late nights, but you'd likely get even better results by taking an antihistamine. At best, this is an average moisturizer for slightly dry skin anywhere on the face.

☺ **Complete Lift Night Cream** *($22.99 for 1.7 ounces)* has a slight edge over similar products from Neutrogena (also owned by Johnson & Johnson), but in this instance that's not saying much. The ho-hum formula barely passes muster for acceptability, and the glycolic acid won't be effective because this product's pH is 5. Whatever "Protient" is, as claimed in the description for this product, there is no substantiated research anywhere proving it to be a "high performance tightening agent," or even that it exists. So please don't bank on any alleged lifting abilities; your skin isn't going anywhere with this product. I suspect the Protient is tied to the minerals and soy in this moisturizer for normal to slightly dry skin, but even when combined they amount to no more than a dusting, and your skin could get so much more from a better formulated moisturizer.

☺ **Complete Lift Serum** *($22.99 for 1.3 ounces)* claims it's nothing short of a face-lift in a bottle. Worried about sagging skin? After reading the claims, you will certainly want to believe your worries are over, and that all you have to do is apply this product. And if you did believe the claims, you'd assume you could cancel your consultation with the plastic surgeon. Well, don't be fooled, nothing could be further from the truth. In all seriousness this serum couldn't be less impressive. The formula is mostly water, starch-based thickener, wheat protein, and a chelating agent, none of which can restore lost elasticity or facial contours that are drooping from the effects of time and sun damage; it isn't even a very good moisturizer. The starch and wheat protein have a slight tightening effect, but that is temporary and strictly cosmetic (and drying, for that matter). You could bathe day and night in this serum and not see one sagging skin cell spring back to its youthful state. I'm not dismissing serums used for antiaging benefits, because there are many outstanding formulas that treat skin to a range of truly beneficial ingredients that can help reduce wrinkles and other signs of aging. The issue is that this isn't one of them—not even close!

RoC MULTI-CORREXION PRODUCTS

☺ **Multi-Correxion Exfoliating Cleanser** (*$9.99 for 5 ounces*) is a very good cleanser that contains polyethylene beads for gentle exfoliation. The small amounts of soy, vitamin C, and vitamin E make them of little consequence for skin, not to mention the fact that any potential benefit from these meager amounts is rinsed down the drain. This cleansing scrub is best for normal to oily skin.

☺ **Multi-Correxion Eye Treatment** (*$24.99 for 0.5 ounce*) contains a lot to like in this lightweight, silky-textured eye cream, but its treatment benefits don't extend to diminishing dark circles and puffiness (so much for the multi-correction claim). What this will do is provide a light dose of moisture along with the antioxidant benefit of vitamin C, vitamin E, and soy protein. Also on hand is an impressive amount of the cell-communicating ingredient retinol, and this product's packaging will keep it stable during use. So there's much to like about this product because its combination of ingredients can help skin look better, and that includes improving the appearance of wrinkles. This would be rated a Paula's Pick if it did not contain fragrance. I can concede to fragrance in an otherwise well-formulated facial moisturizer, but not in a product meant for use in the eye area. This is suitable for normal to slightly dry skin.

✓ ☺ **Multi-Correxion Night Treatment** (*$24.99 for 1 ounce*) is, with few exceptions, nearly identical to RoC's Multi-Correxion Eye Treatment above. This nighttime version has a serum-like texture and contains a greater amount of vitamin C (as ascorbic acid) than the Eye Treatment. Both also contain additional antioxidants and retinol, all packaged to ensure ingredient stability. RoC's other retinol products aren't as multi-faceted as this one, which begs the question of why they're still around, but I suppose it gives them more presence in stores to offer numerous "treatment" products. This moisturizer with retinol is suitable for normal to slightly dry skin.

RoC RETINOL CORREXION PRODUCTS

☺ **Retinol Correxion Deep Wrinkle Daily Moisturizer SPF 30** (*$21.99 for 1 ounce*) should be considered by those with normal to dry skin looking for a daytime moisturizer with retinol. The in-part avobenzone sunscreen (using Neutrogena's Helioplex technology, though RoC doesn't advertise this; both companies are owned by Johnson & Johnson) has a smooth texture and satin finish. The pH is above 4.5, which means the glycolic acid won't function as an exfoliant. But this does contain retinol and comes in packaging that keeps it stable. Although this should have a better blend of antioxidants and cell-communicating ingredients, it deserves praise for the aforementioned positive traits.

☺ **Retinol Correxion Deep Wrinkle Filler** (*$21.99 for 1 ounce*). RoC has lots of products they describe as "breakthrough formulas," yet it's simply talk. The ingredient list doesn't make this a breakthrough anymore than reverting to rotary dial telephones would be a step forward! The formula is mostly water, thickeners, sunscreen agent (though no SPF rating is listed, so this cannot be relied on for sun protection), silicones, emollient, retinol, hyaluronic acid, and preservatives. It's a good option if you're looking for a standard moisturizer with retinol but more bells and whistles are needed to elevate this to Paula's Pick status. This is best for normal to slightly dry skin.

☺ **Retinol Correxion Deep Wrinkle Night Cream** (*$21.99 for 1 ounce*) makes the same claims as the Retinol Correxion Deep Wrinkle Daily Moisturizer SPF 30, only without the sunscreen. This product contains nothing special to fend off or reduce wrinkles, and is quite a standard moisturizer containing mostly water, silicone, slip agent, several thickeners, pH adjusters, glycolic acid (functioning as a water-binding agent in this amount, not an exfoliant), preservative, film-forming agents, emollients, fragrance, retinol, and antioxidants. For the money and the tiny amount of product, you should expect at least more retinol and antioxidants, but with RoC that appears to be just wishful thinking. This is an OK moisturizer for normal to dry skin, but one that's not nearly as impressive as the nighttime options from Dove, Neutrogena, and Olay, most of which cost less than this product.

☺ **Retinol Correxion Deep Wrinkle Serum** *($21.99 for 1 ounce)* has a silky, silicone-enhanced texture that's suitable for all skin types. It contains an impressive amount of vitamin E, but there's still more fragrance in here than there should be. You can find better retinol products from other drugstore lines (like Alpha Hydrox) and from department store lines.

☺ **Retinol Correxion Eye Cream** *($21.99 for 0.5 ounce)* contains only a tiny amount of retinol (it's listed after the preservatives) and as such this isn't a top choice if retinol is what you're after. This is otherwise a standard lightweight but hydrating eye cream for slightly dry skin. It does not contain fragrance.

ROC CANADA (SKIN CARE ONLY)

ROC CANADA AT-A-GLANCE

Strengths: Some excellent cleansers; many fragrance-free options; several state-of-the-art moisturizers with retinol, including a sunscreen with retinol; lip balm with sunscreen; packaging that helps keep light- and air-sensitive ingredients stable during use; sunscreens with the UVA-protecting ingredient Tinosorb.

Weaknesses: Anti-acne products are irritating and not the least bit helpful for blemish-prone skin; ordinary toners; mostly mediocre moisturizers; no skin-lightening products; pricey for a drugstore line.

For more information about RoC Canada call (877) 223-9807 or visit www.rocskincare.ca or www.Beautypedia.com.

Note: All prices listed are in Canadian currency. The following RoC products are available only in Canada, while other RoC products are available in both U.S. and Canadian markets. Be sure to check the other RoC product reviews (listed simply as "RoC") if unable to find a specific product.

ROC CANADA CALMANCE PRODUCTS

☺ **Calmance Soothing Cleansing Fluid** *($16 for 200 ml)* is a water- and silicone-based makeup remover that works quickly and easily, but is best used before cleansing to avoid a greasy-feeling residue. The amount of feverfew extract is unlikely to cause irritation.

☹ **Calmance Soothing Intolerance Repairing Cream** *($20 for 40 ml)* is a very standard, but good, emollient moisturizer for normal to dry skin. It is designed to soothe skin after laser treatment, but contains only a minor amount of ingredients that can do that, while the feverfew extract can be sensitizing if its irritating chemical constituents haven't been removed.

☺ **Calmance Soothing Moisturiser** *($20 for 40 ml)* is similar to the Calmance Soothing Intolerance Repairing Cream above, except this option contains less feverfew extract and isn't quite as emollient (but that's basically a texture preference). Otherwise, the same review applies.

☺ **Calmance Soothing Regenerating Mask** *($20 for 30 ml)* is a standard moisturizing mask for dry to very dry skin. For a product claiming to soothe redness and irritation, it is surprisingly lacking in ingredients that can do that.

ROC CANADA COMPLETELIFT PRODUCTS

☹ **$$$ CompleteLift Day Lifting and Firming Moisturiser** *($39.88 for 50 ml)* is a very standard lightweight moisturizer whose handful of antioxidants won't remain potent for long due to jar packaging. This absolutely cannot lift or firm skin and isn't an "advanced formula" designed for women aged 50 or older. If anything, a woman in her 50s who uses this product is shortchanging her skin of several key ingredients it needs to look younger longer.

☹ **$$$ CompleteLift Eye Contour Gel** *($33.99 for 15 ml)* is such a boring, do-nothing eye gel that I don't even want to write about it. The wheat polymer and plant extracts this contains may exhibit a slight tightening effect on skin but it's temporary and strictly cosmetic. Your eyes won't experience a complete lift nor will dark circles go away. At best, this is marginally acceptable for slightly dry skin anywhere on the face.

☺ **CompleteLift Eye Pen** *($33.90 for 1.5 ml)* is similar to the Complete Lift Eye Pen offered in RoC's main line that's sold in the United States. This product is reviewed above, and the same review applies.

☺ **CompleteLift Night Lifting and Firming Cream** *($39.88 for 50 ml)* will only completely lift money from your pocketbook or bank account, so you can forget the tempting claims. This moisturizer is primarily a blend of water with glycerin, several thickeners, silicone, emollient, and film-forming agent. The moisturizing ingredients can smooth wrinkles made worse from dry skin, but so can hundreds of other products, many with more interesting formularies than this average option.

☹ **$$$ CompleteLift Immediate Lift Serum** *($44.86 for 40 ml)* is very similar to the Complete Lift Serum that Roc sells in their main line. It is reviewed above under the RoC header, and the same review applies here, too.

ROC CANADA DEMAQUILLAGE PRODUCTS

☺ **Demaquillage Actif Cleansing Lotion, for Dry Skin** *($16 for 200 ml)* is a rich, somewhat greasy cleansing lotion that is an OK option for dry to very dry skin, as long as you don't mind using this with a washcloth.

☺ **Demaquillage Actif Cleansing Lotion, for Normal or Combination Skin** *($16 for 200 ml)* is a much lighter but still effective cleansing lotion compared to the Demaquillage Actif Cleansing Lotion, for Dry Skin. It's a simple option for quick makeup removal from normal to dry skin; someone who has combination skin with oily areas will likely prefer a water-soluble cleanser.

✓ ☺ **Demaquillage Actif Foaming Facial Wash** *($16 for 150 ml)* is a very good, fragrance-free cleanser for normal to oily skin, and it removes makeup easily.

☺ **Demaquillage Actif Eye Makeup Remover Extra Gentle** *($16 for 125 ml)* is a very standard, liquid eye-makeup remover that can be used by all skin types. It is indeed gentle, but would be better without the coloring agents.

☺ **Demaquillage Actif Skin Toner, for Dry Skin** *($16 for 200 ml)* is a basic toner whose dated formula is an OK option for normal to dry skin that needs hydration. It is fragrance-free.

☹ **Demaquillage Actif Skin Toner, for Normal or Combination Skin** *($16 for 200 ml)* contains a lot of alcohol, which makes it too drying and irritating for all skin types (the alcohol will trigger more oil production, among its many detriments). It also contains a film-forming agent commonly found in hairstyling gels, which is an odd addition to an already problematic toner.

✓ ☺ **Demaquillage Actif Gentle Exfoliating Cream** *($16 for 40 ml)* is a great scrub for dry to very dry or sensitive skin because it contains mild cellulose for exfoliation (cushioned by mineral oil), and is also fragrance-free.

ROC CANADA ENYDRIAL PRODUCTS

✓ ☺ **Enydrial Anti-Drying Cleansing Gel** *($16 for 200 ml)* is a well-formulated, fragrance-free, water-soluble cleanser for normal to oily skin. It removes all but waterproof makeup and rinses completely. The only issue is the targeted skin type; someone with very dry skin will likely find this cleanser too strong.

☺ **Enydrial Dermo-Cleansing Lotion** *($16 for 200 ml)* is a good detergent- and fragrance-free cleansing option for someone with dry skin. Ideally you should use it with a washcloth to ensure complete removal.

☺ **Enydrial Extra-Emollient Cream, for Very Dry and Atopic Skin** *($20 for 40 ml)* contains several emollients that are great for very dry skin, and borage has anti-inflammatory properties. Although lacking considerable antioxidants, this moisturizer contains some good anti-irritants. By the way, the ingredient "olus" in this product is the technical name for vegetable oil.

☺ **Enydrial Repairing Lip Care** *($7 for 4.8 grams)* is a good, fragrance-free lip gloss-like lip balm that will prevent lips from ending up in a dry, chapped state.

ROC CANADA HYDRA+ PRODUCTS

☺ **Hydra+ 3 in 1 Cleansing Care** *($17 for 200 ml)* is supposed to function as a cleanser, toner, and moisturizer in one, but this is just a standard, fragrance-free cleansing lotion for normal to dry skin not prone to breakouts. It doesn't eliminate the need for a toner and moisturizer.

☹ **Hydra+ Bio-Active Moisturizing Cream for Combination Skin SPF 15** *($29.99 for 40 ml)* provides sufficient UVA protection with avobenzone but that's the only star attraction of this daytime moisturizer with sunscreen for normal to slightly dry skin. The silica produces a slight matte finish but also serves to blunt the moisturizing ingredients RoC included. The inclusion of feverfew isn't the best news because this plant has constituents that can be irritating unless they're removed before the plant is used. As a consumer you wouldn't know this unless the company confirmed it, which RoC Canada didn't do.

☹ **Hydra+ Bio-Active Moisturizing Cream for Dry Skin SPF 15** *($29.99 for 40 ml)* is a more emollient version of the Hydra+ Bio-Active Moisturizing Cream for Combination Skin SPF 15 above, and as such is preferred for dry skin. Other than this not having a slight matte finish, the same sunscreen and formula comments apply here, too.

☹ **Hydra+ Bio-Active Moisturizing Cream for Normal Skin SPF 15** *($29.99 for 40 ml)* has a texture that's not as creamy as RoC Canada's Hydra+ Bio-Active Moisturizing Cream for Dry Skin SPF 15 but not as lightweight as the company's Hydra+ Bio-Active Moisturizing Cream for Combination Skin SPF 15. The only "bio active" feature is this product's in-part avobenzone sunscreen. It is otherwise an OK daytime moisturizer with sunscreen for normal to slightly dry or slightly oily skin. The comment about feverfew extract made for the other Hydra+ moisturizers with sunscreen applies here, too.

☺ **Hydra+ Destressant Daily Moisturising Care, Day** *($30 for 40 ml)* is a mediocre fragrance-free moisturizer for normal to slightly dry skin. It's not suitable for daytime use unless you pair it with a product rated SPF 15 or greater. This contains a smattering of antioxidants and a cell-communicating ingredient.

ROC CANADA PURIF-AC PRODUCTS

☹ **Purif-AC Purifying Cleanser** *($16 for 150 ml)* contains the drying, irritating detergent cleansing agent sodium C14-16 olefin sulfonate, and is not recommended. Even if the cleansing agent were gentle, the cinnamon and cedar bark extracts can be irritating.

☹ **Purif-AC Exfoliating Lotion** *($16 for 200 ml)* is an irritating, drying toner because of its alcohol content and the presence of cinnamon and cedar extracts.

☹ **Purif-AC Blemish Correcting Emulsion** *($20 for 40 ml)* fails to impress because the pH is too high for the 1% salicylic acid to work well as an exfoliant, and it contains an appreciable amount of irritating cinnamon and cedar.

☹ **Purif-AC Fast Action Gel** *($20 for 15 ml)*. The only thing fast about this product is how quickly it will irritate your skin with the witch hazel, alcohol, and fragrant plant extracts it contains. This concoction will not make blemishes retreat.

ROC CANADA RETIN-OL PRODUCTS

✓ ☺ **$$$ Retin-OL Correxion Intensive Nourishing Anti-Wrinkle Care, for Dry Skin** *($44 for 30 ml)* has a formula that adds up to an outstanding moisturizer with retinol for normal to slightly dry skin. It actually contains much more vitamin C than retinol, but the amount of retinol is comparable to that in most competing products. The addition of anti-irritants is icing on the cake!

✓ ☺ **$$$ Retin-OL Multi-Correxion Multi-Corrective Anti-Ageing Moisturiser, Day/Night** *($42 for 30 ml)* is interchangeable with the Retin-OL Correxion Intensive Nourishing Anti-Wrinkle Care, for Dry Skin, and the same review applies.

✓ ☺ **$$$ Retin-OL Multi-Correxion Multi-Corrective Eye Cream** *($32 for 15 ml)* contains less vitamin C than the other RoC Retin-OL Multi-Correxion products, but its overall formula is very similar. It would have been better if it didn't contain fragrance.

ROC CANADA RETIN-OL+ PRODUCTS

✓ ☺ **$$$ Retin-OL+ Day SPF 30** *($48.99 for 30 ml)* is a brilliant daytime moisturizer that provides a high SPF rating fueled by stabilized avobenzone for UVA protection. Beyond the sun protection you're treating skin to several antioxidants and the cell-communicating ingredient retinol. This has a silky, lightweight lotion texture that's best for normal to oily skin. Ideally it shouldn't contain fragrance and the wrinkle-filling claims won't come true in the cumulative manner described, but this is still a formidable daytime moisturizer with sunscreen (and retinol) to consider.

☺ **$$$ Retin-OL+ Eyes, Intensive Eye Anti-Wrinkle Care** *($34 for 15 ml)* is similar to RoC's U.S.-sold Retinol Correxion Eye Cream, but this version is superior because it contains a more generous amount of retinol. It is fragrance-free.

☺ **$$$ Retin-OL+ Dry Skin, Intensive Anti-Wrinkle Moisturiser** *($44 for 30 ml)* is a lightweight moisturizer with retinol that's best suited for normal to slightly dry skin. The amount of glycolic acid is too low for it to function as an exfoliant.

☺ **$$$ Retin-OL+ Max, Intensive Anti-Wrinkle Serum** *($50 for 30 ml)* is similar to RoC's U.S.-sold Retinol Correxion Deep Wrinkle Serum, except this contains notably more retinol and less fragrance, which makes it the preferred option (especially for those living in Canada). It would be rated a Paula's Pick if not for the potential risk of using products with DMAE (dimethyl MEA).

☺ **$$$ Retin-OL+ Night, Intensive Anti-Wrinkle Care** *($44 for 30 ml)* is similar to RoC's U.S.-sold Retinol Correxion Deep Wrinkle Night Cream, except this version is the better choice because it contains more retinol and a lower concentration of preservatives. The pH is still too high for the glycolic acid to exfoliate skin, but this is still an option for those with normal to dry skin seeking a retinol product.

ROC CANADA MINESOL SUN PRODUCTS

☹ **Minesol Protect Application Express Multi-Position Atomizer SPF 30** *($23.95 for 114 g)* is not recommended even though it contains an in-part avobenzone sunscreen. The reason is because the base formula is mostly alcohol, which makes this too drying and irritating for all skin types (even more so when you consider the amount of sunscreen actives in this product can cause skin irritation on their own).

☹ **Minesol Protect Application Express Multi-Position Atomizer SPF 45** *($23.95 for 114 g)* is nearly identical to RoC Canada's Minesol Protect Application Express Multi-Position Atomizer SPF 30 above, except this contains a higher amount of active ingredients to reach its SPF rating. Otherwise, the same comments apply.

☺ **Minesol Protect Ultra High Protection Suncare Spray SPF 60** *($23.95 for 200 ml)* provides excellent UVA protection thanks to titanium dioxide and two forms of the sunscreen active Tinosorb. The lightweight, water-resistant lotion lacks an appreciable amount of beneficial extras and contains enough film-forming agent to feel a bit tacky on skin, but it's certainly recommended for its sun protection abilities. This is fragrance-free and best for normal to slightly oily skin.

☺ **Minesol Protect Very High Protection Suncare Spray SPF 30** *($23.95 for 200 ml)* is similar to the Minesol Protect Ultra High Protection Suncare Spray SPF 60 above, except it contains a lower amount of active ingredients and omits the titanium dioxide. Tinosorb is still on hand for reliable UVA protection, and this is a good water-resistant, fragrance-free sunscreen lotion for normal to slightly oily skin.

☺ **Minesol After Sun Prolonging Lotion** *($19 for 200 ml)* is a very basic body moisturizer meant to be used after sun exposure to prolong your tan and prevent peeling. Any product that encourages tanning is unethical; ironically, this option doesn't help skin in any way even if it wasn't exposed to the sun.

☺ **Minesol Bronze Express Drying Self Tanning Foam** *($23.94 for 125 ml or 4.2 ounces)* is a good, fragrance-free self-tanner that dispenses as a foam. The novelty of foam may appeal to you, but this isn't any easier to apply than a gel or lightweight lotion with the same self-tanning ingredient this product has, dihydroxyacetone. It is suitable for all skin types.

✓ ☺ **Minesol High Protection Lipstick SPF 20** *($10 for 3 grams)* is a good, glossy-finish lip balm with sunscreen that features avobenzone (listed by its chemical name of butyl methoxydibenzoylmethane) for sufficient UVA protection.

The Reviews R

SALLY HANSEN NATURAL BEAUTY INSPIRED BY CARMINDY (MAKEUP ONLY)

SALLY HANSEN NATURAL BEAUTY INSPIRED BY CARMINDY AT-A-GLANCE

Strengths: Inexpensive; excellent foundation, pressed powder, and bronzers; good cream concealer; well-coordinated eyeshadow trios; enticing shade range for lipstick and lip gloss.

Weaknesses: No testers available; only one type of liquid foundation and it's not suitable for all skin types; overly fragrant, potentially irritating loose powder; messy mascara; foundation primer that stays slick, thus hindering makeup application.

For more information about Sally Hansen Natural Beauty Inspired by Carmindy, call (800) 953-5080 or visit www.sallyhansennaturalbeauty.com or www.Beautypedia.com.

FOUNDATION: ✓ ☺ **Your Skin Makeup** *($12.99)*. The big claim for Carmindy's only liquid foundation is that it adjusts to suit your skin type. That's a bogus claim if ever there was one because no foundation, serum, or moisturizer is capable of self-adjusting to meet the disparate needs of dry and oily skin. (How would the ingredients know what to do?) Although you can ignore the claims, if you have normal to oily skin, this is an excellent option! It dispenses smoothly from the pump applicator, and slips over skin easily, which makes blending a pleasure. This sets to a smooth matte finish that feels a bit more absorbent and dry to the touch than most foundations of this type. Coverage goes from light to medium and, assuming you choose the right shade, it can look surprisingly natural on skin. There are a dozen shades available, with some beautiful shades for fair to light skin. True Beige is slightly peach and should be considered with caution, while Mocha is slightly ash. Avoid Warm Beige entirely—it's noticeably peach. The only drawback for those with oily skin is this foundation's lack of sunscreen. Sunscreen in foundation isn't required, but for those who have oily skin, it is always better to use fewer products, and not having to wear an extra sunscreen product under your makeup can prevent problems.

☺ **Airbrush Spray Makeup** *($13.99)*. The directions for this aerosol foundation tell you to spray it on your hands and then apply it to your face, so it isn't one-step complexion perfection in a can; it doesn't create an airbrushed look at all, unless your hand is where you wanted to wear your makeup. When you follow these directions, the pressurized foundation blasts onto your fingers and can quickly make a mess if you're not very careful. You can also spray a foundation sponge, but again, overdoing it is an issue and the sponge tends to soak up a lot of this foundation due to the force of the mist. Once on skin, this is relatively easy to blend and the finish is smooth and natural-looking. It provides sheer to light coverage and has a strong matte finish that feels nearly weightless. The fair to light shades are very good, but the darkest shades (Medium to Deep and Deep) tend to be too yellowish orange, although they may work for some skin tones. Overall, the application is too problematic and wastes too much makeup, plus, as nice as it may look on skin, you can achieve the same effect from any well-formulated liquid foundation.

CONCEALER: ☺ **Fast Fix Concealer** *($8.99)* comes in a slim flip-top component and has a beautifully smooth texture and application. Although I wouldn't use this cream concealer for areas that need serious camouflage, it does a very good job concealing minor to moderate dark circles, red spots, and other minor discolorations. It isn't prone to smearing once set, but because the finish remains slightly moist, you will notice some creasing and fading unless you set it with powder. The only problems with this concealer, which seriously limit its appeal, are the colors. The All Over Neutralizer is too yellow for most skin tones; Brightener is lavender and doesn't look good on anyone; and Dark is strongly peach. That leaves you with Light, Medium, and Medium Deep as choices, and the latter is sketchy due to its tendency to turn peach. Still, if one of the limited recommended shades works for you, this is worth a look.

POWDER: ✓ ☺ **Luminous Matte Pressed Powder** *($11.99)* is a superior choice for those with normal to dry skin. This talc-based pressed powder has a silky, cashmere-soft texture that meshes with skin to leave a polished satin finish. Beautifully sheer, this is ideal to set makeup without making skin look dull or dry or exaggerating flaky areas. Some of the shades appear iffy when viewed in the compact, but they apply so sheer that it doesn't really matter. But just in case, consider the peach-tinged Medium Deep and orange-tinged Dark carefully. The Light shade is excellent for fair skin. One more comment: Unlike Carmindy's Truly Translucent Loose Powder (below), this pressed powder is fragrance-free.

☹ **Truly Translucent Loose Powder** *($12.99)* has a dry, airy texture that remains true to its translucent name as it appears on skin, regardless of the shade. This talc-free loose powder lays down a sheer layer of absorbency yet leaves skin with a polished soft sheen that's quite becoming. Unfortunately, despite all of these positive traits, this is not a loose powder I can recommend. Why? It contains an unusually high amount of fragrance (you'll be smelling this on your face all day) and, unlike just about any other loose face powder I can think of, this also contains several potentially irritating fragrance ingredients. Although I don't normally comment on my personal experience with powders, this one actually made my face sting. That has never happened to me from a face powder! What is more important is that eau de cologne is never good for skin.

BLUSH AND BRONZER: ✓ ☺ **Sun Glow Powder Bronzer** *($12.99)* is a talc-based pressed bronzing powder that has a wonderfully smooth texture and soft, sheer application. Skin is enlivened with subtle tones of bronze, tan, and soft pink from the Spring shade or with tones of bronze, gold, and soft peach from the Summer shade. Either is great for fair to light skin. Those with medium to dark skin will have difficulty getting this bronzer to show up unless you apply a lot of it. The finish is subtle radiance with a hint of translucent sparkle. The sparkles don't last too long, but the overall radiant/sheer color effect tends to go the distance.

☺ **Sheerest Cream Bronzer** *($11.99)* isn't the sheerest cream bronzer out there, but it does apply softly. You can layer for additional depth and intensity, but the overall effect remains translucent. The silicone-rich texture is cream-to-powder with a satin finish that highlights the complexion with a very subtle shine. This is easy to blend and a good option for normal to dry skin not prone to blemishes. Among the shades, Miami Glow will be too orange-y for light skin tones. Havana Glow and Rio Glow are easier to work with. Sheerest Cream Bronzer does contain fragrance.

☺ **Natural Beauty Powder Blush** *($10.99)*. It seems Carmindy thinks shine is a big part of being a natural beauty, because each shade of this blush is replete with it. Unfortunately, it's not the low-glow shimmer that gives you that attractive luminous look; instead, it's large particles of glitter. The shine tends to cling better than expected, but it's not a look I'd encourage for daytime professional or casual makeup. Beyond the shine, this is a fairly standard smooth but dry-textured blush in a small range of vibrant-looking shades that apply sheer.

☺ **Sheerest Cream Blush** *($8.99)* has a formula completely different from that of Carmindy's Sheerest Cream Bronzer. The silky silicones of the bronzer are replaced by emollient, wax, and cornstarch in this cream version. The result is a very sheer, true cream blush that feels lighter than you might expect but that leaves skin with a sheen that borders on greasy. This is not for anyone with any degree of oiliness in the cheek area and is best for dry skin not prone to blemishes. The available shades don't offer much choice, but all are attractive and wearable.

EYESHADOW: ☺ **Instant Definition Eye Shadow Palette** *($7.99)*. Carmindy skipped right past eyeshadow singles and duos and instead launched these trios, each packaged in a pressed powder-sized compact. The result is a well-coordinated selection of powder eyeshadows designed to shape, shade, and highlight the eye area, and it doesn't flake. Although every trio is shiny, most of them have a moderate shimmer that's wearable only if your eye area isn't wrinkled or crepey. I am most impressed with the color combinations, almost all of which are excellent and truly what a makeup artist would use for many eye designs. None of the darkest shades in any of the trios are well suited for use as eyeliner unless you want a softer effect. Otherwise, the formula applies smoothly, blends well, and allows for sheer to moderate coverage. The only trio to avoid is Ocean due to its blue tones. This group of products would have received a Paula's Pick rating had it offered just one or two matte options.

☺ **Fast Fix Eyeshadow Base** *($7.99)* is a silicone-enhanced product meant to improve the look and wear of eyeshadow. Initially creamy and slick, this glides over the eyelid and quickly sets to a sheer powder finish. The thickening agents it contains won't keep eyeshadows from creasing; plus there is nothing special about it in terms of extending the wear time of your eye makeup, at least not any better than a well-formulated concealer would, that's for sure. Some women may find this type of product useful; however, for the most part, you'll get better results from a matte-finish liquid concealer and, unlike Fast Fix Eyeshadow Base, you can also use that on other areas of the face. Without question this product will not help those who have oily eyelids or who use makeup that doesn't last.

EYELINER: ☺ **Forever Stay Eye Pencil** *($6.99)*. This creamy eye pencil needs routine sharpening, but if that doesn't bother you, it has a smooth, slightly thick application that sets to a soft powder finish. This doesn't stay on forever, but it will get you through the day unless you have oily eyelids, in which case the gel-type cream eyeliners are without peer for longevity.

LIPSTICK AND LIP GLOSS: ☺ **Color Comfort Lip Color** *($9.99)*. There isn't much to say about this cream lipstick other than it applies smoothly, imparts rich color, has a soft cream finish, and comes in an enticing range of shades that's bound to please most women.

☺ **Ultra Soothing Lip Tint** *($4.99)* is just a standard lip gloss that feels smooth, is non-sticky, and comes in an array of soft colors that go on translucent. Some may appreciate the jelly-like texture, but the glossy finish is similar to what you'd end up with from most lip glosses. There is nothing "ultra soothing" about the formula.

☺ **Natural Shine Lip Gloss** *($7.99)* has a strong fragrance that many will find off-putting. Still, this brush-on lip gloss does the job to give lips sheer, shimmery color and a wet-looking finish that's slightly sticky. The shade range consists of modestly bright hues along with can't-go-wrong colors, including Clear Shimmer, which will work with any lipstick. This isn't one of the best lip glosses we've tested, and the amount of fragrance on your lips, where the skin is especially sensitive, is not the best idea, but it's not worth avoiding 100% either.

MASCARA: ☺ **Lift & Define Mascara** *($7.99)*. Some mascaras apply wet and deposit too much mascara during the first few strokes. That's exactly how Lift & Define Mascara starts out, but unlike mascaras with those beginnings, this remains a messy proposition from start to finish. Although the result is remarkably long lashes with a touch of thickness, you will need to comb through lashes for a neatened effect. This is also prone to minor flaking, another blemish that keeps it from earning a happy face rating.

SPECIALTY PRODUCTS: ☺ **Luminizing Face Primer** *($9.99)* contains a blend of silicones that differs from that of many primers because it contains enough mica (a mineral) to leave a sparkling sheen on skin. That may or may not be what you want under makeup, but it's an unavoidable fact if you use this product. One other point of difference is that this remains slick-feeling on skin. It isn't easy to apply foundation over this primer because it has so much slip, and it doesn't ever set to a powdery finish the way many others do. Luminizing Face Primer is a tricky product with limited appeal. It is best for those who want to add shine to skin and not bother with foundation or concealer.

☺ **Natural Highlighter** *($7.99).* There isn't anything natural about the finish this has on skin. The cream-to-powder texture applies smoothly and quickly sets to a powdery dry finish that leaves skin laced with sparkles. This isn't a subtle way to highlight skin, but is an OK option for evening glamour. The particles of shine have minimal ability to cling to skin, and the colors go on much softer than they look in the compact.

SEPHORA

SEPHORA AT-A-GLANCE

Strengths: Inexpensive; some good cleansers and makeup removers; the Blotting Papers; good powder foundation; the Light Touch Highlighter; Impressive blush and shiny eyeshadow options; great metallic-finish eyeliner; awesome brow kit; bountiful selection of lipsticks and lip glosses; a couple of very good mascaras; several outstanding makeup brushes; testers are available in-store for each product, and sales pressure is practically nonexistent.

Weaknesses: Mostly average to below-average toners, moisturizers, and sunscreens; no options for those dealing with acne or skin discolorations; some SPF-rated products (including foundations) lack sufficient UVA-protecting actives; the lip plumper is too irritating; too many disappointing eye-makeup products, including several disappointing eyeliners and brow pencils; unappealing shimmer powders.

For more information about Sephora, call (877) 737-4672 or visit www.sephora.com or www.Beautypedia.com.

SEPHORA SKIN CARE

SEPHORA FACE PRODUCTS

☹ **FACE 25 Makeup Removing Wipes, for Face, Eyes & Lips** *($8 for 25 wipes)* are not only expensive for the number of cloths you get, they also don't do a great job of removing makeup, plus the formula contains fragrance components that will be irritating when used around the eyes.

☺ **FACE Eye Makeup Remover** *($8 for 4.22 ounces)* has a combination of slip agents and a solvent that do a fairly good job removing most types of makeup, but I wouldn't choose this over silicone-in-water formulas because they do a more thorough job and glide more smoothly over the eye area.

✓☺ **FACE Waterproof Eye Makeup Remover** (*$10 for 4.22 ounces*) is a very good water- and silicone-based dual-phase makeup remover, and it effectively takes off all types of eye makeup, including waterproof mascara. The formula is fragrance-free, too.

☺ **FACE Refreshing Toner** (*$10 for 6.76 ounces*). If you're looking for a basic toner simply to remove the last traces of makeup you might have missed when washing your face, this qualifies. It's not a particularly beneficial or even mildly interesting formula, but then again, that describes 98% of the toners sold today! It is suitable for all skin types except sensitive, but mostly you are buying water, glycerin, and preservatives.

☺ **FACE Soothing Toner** (*$5 for 6.76 ounces*) is very similar to Sephora's FACE Refreshing Toner above and the same review applies.

☺ **FACE Age Prevention Moisturizer SPF 15, for Combination to Oily Skin** (*$20 for 1.69 ounces*) is a below-standard daytime moisturizer whose only redeeming quality is its in-part titanium dioxide sunscreen. The silicone-enhanced base formula is suitable for normal to oily skin, but there are far more fragrance and preservatives present than anything exciting for skin. Furthermore, the really, really tiny amount of antioxidants will suffer upon opening due to the jar packaging.

☺ **FACE Age Prevention Moisturizer SPF 15, for Dry Skin** (*$20 for 1.69 ounces*) is the emollient version of Sephora's FACE Age Prevention Moisturizer SPF 15, for Combination to Oily Skin. That means this one is preferred for normal to dry skin, but you're still getting little in return other than an in-part titanium dioxide sunscreen and lots of fragrance.

☺ **FACE Age Prevention Moisturizer SPF 15, for Normal Skin** (*$20 for 1.69 ounces*) offers a slightly more interesting formula than Sephora's FACE Age Prevention Moisturizer SPF 15, for Combination to Oily Skin, but that's not saying much. Titanium dioxide is on hand for UVA protection, but the amount of fragrance and preservative trumps the antioxidants, and the choice of jar packaging means these antioxidants won't remain stable once you begin using this daytime moisturizer for normal to slightly dry skin.

☺ **FACE Hydrating Balancing Cream, for Combination to Oily Skin** (*$18 for 1.69 ounces*) doesn't offer skin anything special, but its silky texture sets to a matte finish thanks to the clays it contains. It is a suitable option for oily skin or oily areas, and works well under makeup; it's unfortunate that greater amounts of beneficial ingredients weren't included.

☺ **FACE Moisturizing Cream, for Dry Skin** (*$18 for 1.69 ounces*) is an average moisturizer whose blend of glycerin and several thickeners can make dry skin look and feel better. The tiny amount of vitamin E does not make this a "vitamin-enriched moisturizer."

☺ **FACE Moisturizing Gel Cream, for Normal Skin** (*$18 for 1.69 ounces*) is a boring moisturizer that will do a moderately effective job of keeping normal skin hydrated; however, without any additional benefits, such as antioxidants (which are barely present), there is no reason to consider this an option. Another shortcoming is that the amount of cornstarch can be a problem for those with blemish-prone skin.

☹ **FACE Peel Off Purifying Mask, for Combination to Oily Skin** (*$12 for 1.69 ounces*) is a standard, irritating peel-off mask that contains polyvinyl alcohol and regular denatured alcohol as major ingredients. The alcohol will trigger oil production in the pore lining, which isn't what oily skin needs.

☺ **FACE Concealing Blemish Pen, for Combination to Oily Skin** (*$14 for 0.09 ounce*) dispenses a thin, tinted fluid from a pen-style component with a brush applicator. The neutral shade is fine for light to almost-medium skin tones, but don't count on the salicylic acid to help heal blemishes because the amount is likely too low, while the alcohol that precedes it on the list is potentially drying.

SEPHORA POWER MASK PRODUCTS

☹ **Power Mask Fusio-Fiber Face Mask** *($12 for 1 mask)* is a great example of a gimmicky, do-nothing product masquerading as a specialty treatment. This cloth mask, pre-cut to fit over your face, is supposed to be a groundbreaking treatment. The thing is, formula-wise, Sephora didn't even crack the dirt. It's mostly water, slip agents, skin-damaging alcohol, and preservative. This is far removed from a "super-soothing face mask," though they did include a token amount of notable anti-irritants. Considering the benefits that you won't see from this single-use mask, the price is a burn.

☺ **Power Mask Hydrogel Eye Mask** *($8 for 1 mask)* is a cloth-like gel mask designed to fit evenly over your eyes as you lie back and let the refreshment begin. The only real perk you'll get from applying this mask is the downtime while you're waiting patiently until you remove it, because the formula itself is a ho-hum concoction. You're getting mostly water, slip agent, and film-forming agents. Expect a bit of a sticky finish that requires you to rinse any remaining solution from your skin when done relaxing, which may just leave you wondering why you bothered.

☺ **Power Mask Hydrogel Face Mask** *($10 for 1 mask)* is a two-piece cloth mask designed to be used on the upper and lower areas of your face, and is said to dramatically refresh skin for "super-moisturizing renewal." That sounds great—too bad the formula is mostly disappointing and mostly void of moisturizing ingredients (glycerin is on board, but it's in so many other products with better formulas that its inclusion here isn't really a plus). At best, the main benefit you'll get from this mask is the time you take to relax while you wait for it to "work." As long as you don't expect noticeable results, that may be worth the price of admission.

SEPHORA TRICKS OF THE TRADE SKIN CARE PRODUCTS

☺ **Tricks of the Trade Radiance Mist** *($12)* is a basic, spray-on toner that's mostly water, slip agents, fragrant plants, and preservatives, which is little more than eau de cologne for skin, and it doesn't do a thing to make skin look radiant or to set makeup. Misting your face after makeup application is not a trick I'd encourage anyone to try, unless you're looking to reduce wear time and possibly cause streaking and smearing. This is an OK toner for normal to dry skin, but use it before, not after, applying your makeup.

☹ **Tricks of the Trade Complete Lip Balm** *($8)*. Although it's Vaseline-based like many others, it has a wonderfully silky texture and a smooth finish that's a cross between a balm and a lip gloss. It pains me to write that Sephora couldn't resist tainting this otherwise top-notch balm with menthol. Drat! And it's such a good price, too! Those looking for a tenacious lip balm with an elegant texture should consider my own Lip & Body Treatment Balm.

☺ **Tricks of the Trade Lip Peel** *($12)* is essentially a peel-off gel mask for lips. I couldn't locate an ingredient list for the product, but I suspect it contains polyvinyl alcohol to form a film on your lips. Then you peel away the film and it takes dry, dead skin cells with it, leaving your lips smooth and ready for moisture. This is an OK product for occasional use, but there are gentler ways to exfoliate lips, including lightly massaging them with a baby toothbrush and water.

OTHER SEPHORA SKIN CARE PRODUCTS

☹ **Professional Radiance Flash Spray** ($12 for 1.6 ounces) is a so-so toner that contains mostly water, slip agents, and preservative. The small amount of glycolic acid likely has no benefit at all, and definitely not as an exfoliant. This also contains a number of fragrance components that don't make it worth considering over many other toners.

☺ **Super Shield Skin Saver SPF 15** ($10 for 6 ounces) is a lightweight sunscreen that includes avobenzone for UVA protection. I am concerned that one of the main ingredients is a known penetration enhancer that may cause the sunscreen actives to be needlessly irritating. The amount of fragrance this contains only makes the potential for irritation stronger.

☺ **Matte Blotting Film** ($10 for 50 sheets) consists of blotting papers of a synthetic material coated with mineral oil and a polymer blend. They do an average job of absorbing excess oil, but are not as efficient as tissue-paper blotters.

✓ ☺ **Natural Matte Blotting Papers** ($8 for 100 sheets) work very well to soak up excess shine and perspiration.

SEPHORA MAKEUP

SEPHORA TRICKS OF THE TRADE MAKEUP

LIP GLOSS: ☺ **Tricks of the Trade Instant Lip Plumper** ($14) is a brush-on, gelatinous clear lip gloss that has a lightweight texture that leaves lips looking slick and glossy. It does little to plump your lips beyond the illusion of fuller lips that any lip gloss can provide, so consider this a basic gloss rather than a sure way to make lips bigger.

SPECIALTY PRODUCTS: ☺ **Tricks of the Trade Eye Primer** ($12). Sephora recommends using this beige-toned eye primer to extend the staying powder of your eyeshadow. It does indeed work for that purpose; however, so would your foundation or concealer. Tricks of the Trade Eye Primer dispenses from its brush-tipped applicator thickly and needs to be thinned and blended with a sponge or fingertip to keep it from being too cakey on the eye area. Once set, apply your shadow on top and it will last and last with no creasing.

☺ **Tricks of the Trade Eyeshadow Transformer** ($14). The purpose of this product is to turn any powder eyeshadow into a liquid liner. You apply the clear fluid (like eyeliner) over your powder eyeshadow, which deepens the color and forms a long-wearing finish that keeps the color from fading or smearing. It's easier to use than liquid liner, and worth checking out if you're curious to see the effect and/or need help getting your powder eyeliner to last.

☺ **Tricks of the Trade Perfection Primer** ($18) has a much better application and finish than the company's Tricks of the Trade Anti-Shine Primer below. The fluid texture applies sheer and helps subtly brighten skin tone with its pale-pink opalescent shimmer. It is light enough to use under any makeup and is suitable for all skin types. You're not getting any beneficial extras with this product (as you would with an antioxidant-rich lightweight serum applied pre-makeup), but it serves its purpose for those looking to cast a subtle glow or to softly highlight features.

☺ **Tricks of the Trade Immediate Wrinkle Filler** ($20 for 0.42 ounce) is a thick, nonaqueous cream based on silicones and talc. It feels very silky, and goes on lighter than you might expect. The silicones have a soft spackle effect on minor lines and wrinkles, temporarily smoothing their appearance. This also reduces the appearance of large pores, though how long that effect lasts depends on what other products you apply and how oily your skin is. This is comparable to the more expensive Instant Smooth Perfecting Touch from Clarins.

☺ **Tricks of the Trade Eye Brightener** *($14)* is a standard, chunky pencil, which needs routine sharpening to maintain a workable tip, is creamy, is tinted a pale pink, and has a soft shine finish. It is meant to highlight the inner corners of the eyes or along the lash line, but it doesn't last as long as it should. You can get better results using a powder eyeshadow or liquid highlighter with soft shine.

☺ **$$$ Tricks of the Trade Mineral Matte Setting Powder** *($18)* is a translucent loose powder whose mica and silica base combine to produce a texture that's airy and dry and a finish that offers absorbent properties but adds a hint of shine. The shine means that those with oily skin won't find this the ideal powder. As sheer as this powder is, I was surprised that it still manages to leave a noticeable white cast on skin. Even when lightly brushed on, those with skin tones darker than fair will be buffing away a residual white cast.

☹ **Tricks of the Trade Anti-Shine Primer** *($18)* isn't one you'll want to add to your makeup routine. Generally speaking, a primer isn't essential and certainly not preferred to using an antioxidant-rich serum, many of which have silky, primer-like finishes and as such perform double duty. The trick is on you if you choose this Sephora product, because the formula contains enough alcohol to cause irritation and the finish of this gel-textured primer remains tacky. Any of the primers from Smashbox (a brand Sephora sells in many of their stores) are preferred to this.

☹ **Tricks of the Trade Eyeliner Last** *($14)* is a clear fluid that comes equipped with a brush-on applicator, just like many liquid eyeliners. It is meant to prevent your eyeliner from creasing or fading, but the amount of alcohol in the formula is bound to be irritating. Given the number of superior long-wearing eyeliner options available, this potentially irritating product is completely unnecessary.

☹ **Tricks of the Trade Lip Last** *($14)* is a clear lip sealant meant to be applied after lipstick, with the goal being to keep the color from fading or smearing for hours, if not all day. Well, don't count on this working, not even marginally. The formula contains a lot of alcohol (you'll feel the sting, even through your lipstick) and it tends to make a mess of carefully applied lipstick (alcohol is a solvent and can remove makeup). Why bother with this when there are so many excellent, long-wearing lip paint/top coat products to consider?

☹ **Tricks of the Trade Lip Primer** *($12)* is a chunky, flesh-toned pencil that's Sephora's version of Benefit's D'Finer D'Liner, except that Benefit's product doesn't contain lip-irritating menthol, which is the "natural plumping ingredient" referred to in the claims for this primer. The oil-based formula is greasy and does little to fill in lines on the lips or to help the color last longer.

OTHER SEPHORA MAKEUP PRODUCTS

FOUNDATION: ✓ ☺ **Matifying Compact Foundation** *($20)* is an outstanding talc-based pressed-powder foundation for those with normal to oily skin. It has a silky application and sheer matte finish that looks practically seamless on skin. True to claim, this really does make your complexion "look like sheer perfection," assuming that you don't have any discolorations or blemishes, in which case you should use this foundation with the appropriate concealer. Sephora provides a huge range of shades with options for fair to dark skin tones. Given the number of shades, I expected some of them to be duds, and I was right. Consider the following shades carefully due to slight overtones of rose, copper, peach, or gold: R30, D32, D33, R33, D40, and R55. On the other hand, avoid D34, R40, and R50 because they don't resemble real skin tones. Shade D65 is an impressive non-ashen dark tone.

The Reviews S

☺ **Base Primer** *($18)* is a primer with shine, and it comes in two soft, flesh-toned shades that work well under foundation. Although primers make foundation go on better, they don't offer skin the beneficial, essential ingredients found in many other silicone-based serums. The wax content of this primer helps temporarily fill large pores and superficial lines, but it's not the best for blemish-prone skin.

☺ **Double Compact Mineral SPF 10** *($22)* lists 20% titanium dioxide as its sole active ingredient, so the SPF rating is likely quite conservative. That amount of titanium dioxide could easily net SPF 50 in the right formula! This talc-free, mica-based pressed-powder foundation for normal to very oily skin has a thick, dry texture that blends surprisingly well. It leaves a silky matte finish that doesn't look chalky, and provides light to medium coverage. The formula is fragrance-free and most of the shades are good. R30 Cool Beige is slightly pink, but still worth considering, while R40 Cool Cognac is rosy ash and best avoided. This deserves a happy face rating because it is an excellent way to touch up your sunscreen during the day, or to pair with a liquid foundation that contains sunscreen.

☺ **Hydrating & Smoothing Foundation SPF 10** *($20)* includes avobenzone for UVA protection, but the SPF rating is below the benchmark for daytime protection. If you're willing to pair this foundation with a sunscreen rated SPF 15 or greater, it is recommended for dry skin. The creamy-smooth texture blends well and leaves a fresh, radiant finish that keeps skin hydrated. Medium coverage is the norm with this foundation; it's difficult to make it sheer due to the opacity of the pigments. The selection of shades includes some great neutral colors for fair skin and plenty of options for medium to tan skin tones. Shade D28 Warm Golden Natural is slightly gold, but still worth considering; avoid R35 Cool Tan because it is too rosy and be careful with R40 Cool Cognac, as this will be too rosy copper for some dark skin tones. This would earn a happy face rating if the SPF rating were better.

☹ **Tinted Moisturizer SPF 15** *($18)* does not contain the UVA-protecting ingredients of titanium dioxide, zinc oxide, avobenzone, Mexoryl SX, or Tinosorb, and is not recommended. Otherwise, this is a very standard, emollient, tinted moisturizer that provides just a hint of color. Given that tinted moisturizers with sunscreen should be a convenient all-in-one product, this misses the mark and should be avoided.

CONCEALER: ☺ **Light Touch Highlighter** *($12)* is aptly named, because this brush-on concealer functions best as a highlighter due to its sheer to light coverage. It has a very smooth texture, just the right amount of slip to make blending easy, and five of the six shades are great. Watch out for Apricot, which is slightly peach, although passable.

☹ **Buildable Cover Concealer** *($16)* is interesting. Viewed in its compact, it appears to have a pressed-powder texture. However, it's actually a cream texture with a soft-powder finish. There's something slightly off about the texture, which makes blending tricky; it tends to sit on top of the skin rather than mesh with it, and the result (plus its powdery finish) is unflattering. It is slightly crease-prone. You can build coverage, but that's true for almost any concealer, including many that outdo this one.

☺ **$$$ Concealer Palette** *($20)* presents four creamy concealers in a compact, and comes with a brush that's too small to use unless you like a challenge. This applies well and provides nearly opaque coverage, which results in a heavy look. The creaminess means this is prone to creasing, but setting it with powder minimizes this effect. The flesh-toned palette is neutral, but the color-correcting palette is not. All told, this is an OK option only for those seeking full coverage.

☺ **Cooling Cover Stick** *($12)* is a twist-up concealer that feels cool and slightly wet when applied, but it dries quickly to a matte finish laced with sparkles. Coverage is a bit on the sheer side, and given the lack of slip, blending must be swift. This doesn't feel or look as good on skin as many other concealers, but two of the three shades are suitably neutral.

POWDER: ☺ **$$$ Powder in a Brush** *($22)* brings portability to loose powder. Housed in a self-contained unit, it contains a small amount of sheer, whitish pink, talc-based powder. The powder shakes through a sifter onto a built-in brush (the brush is nicer than expected), allowing for quick touch-ups. The single shade goes on practically colorless and leaves a sheer matte finish, but this is best for fair to medium skin tones.

☹ **$$$ Sculpting Disk** *($24)* consists of three stripes of pressed powder separated by a plastic divide, housed in one giant compact slightly larger than a CD. The center stripe, the largest, is a regular, flesh-toned pressed powder. To the left is a peachy tan bronzing powder; to the right is a pale peach highlighting powder. All three have a decently smooth, dry texture and soft application. Those with light skin tones can use these shades to "sculpt" the face, but doing so is tricky and the color combinations aren't going to work for all light skin tones.

BLUSH AND BRONZER: ☺ **Blush Me Twice** *($8)* is a standard pressed-powder blush/bronzer in one compact. You can apply the blush or the bronzer separately because the products are separated by a divider, or you can pick up a little of both with your blush brush. Not much to get excited about, but the price is attractive and it applies evenly. Note that this leaves a soft shine on skin.

☺ **Bronzer Powder SPF 15** *($16)*. If the bronze tones of this pressed bronzing powder were better, it would be easier to recommend. It's great that the sunscreen is in-part titanium dioxide, and the talc-based formula applies well and has a minimally shiny finish. Bora Bora is the shade to consider if you want a bronze effect; Bahamas works great for contouring; but Riviera is too peachy to pass as bronze or tan.

☺ **Cheek Stain** *($12)* is meant for those with normal to dry skin because its moist application and finish will likely prove too intrusive for any other skin type (or anyone with large pores). Those searching for a sheer, balm-like blush whose color impact is akin to the many liquid cheek stains available should check this out. Each translucent color is beautiful and easy to blend, leaving a fresh, dewy finish.

☺ **Sun Disk** *($20)* is a pressed-powder bronzer that is as large as a compact disc. While it won't fit into most makeup bags, the talc-based formula applies smoothly and imparts sheer, buildable peachy tan color that is best for fair to light skin tones. The shine is toned down, making this a suitable bronzing powder for daytime. And given the amount of product you get in this huge compact, I suspect you'll have it around for years!

☹ **Blush Me Mono** *($12)* comes in a tempting range of matte and shimmer finish colors. The texture is standard-issue smooth, but this blush's problem becomes apparent as soon as you apply it: the color payoff is almost zero. This powder blush tends to go on very sheer yet spotty, and you can layer it from morning till night and not build more than a hint of color. Unless your intent when you apply blush is make it look like you didn't apply blush, don't bother.

☹ **$$$ Duo Bronzer** *($16)* is a creamy-feeling pressed bronzing powder along with a coordinating shade of highlighter powder. There is no divider between the colors, but there's enough space to place your brush on either shade and apply as usual. Unfortunately, color payoff is minor compared to the flood of golden to copper sparkles this lays on your skin—and the sparkles cling poorly.

☺ **Harmony Trio Bronzer** *($16)* is an average version of the Shimmer Brick-type shiny pressed powders made popular by Bobbi Brown. Sephora's bronzer costs half what Brown's does, but its texture and application aren't as smooth, plus the shine is more showy than glowing. This bronzer with shine is housed in a compact without dividers between the trio of colors, but they end up looking uniform when swirled on skin. The Bronze Trio is the only option if you want a tanned effect; the other trios work best as blush with lots of shine.

EYESHADOW: ✓ ☺ **Colorful Mono Eyeshadow** *($12)*. This powder eyeshadow collection replaces all of Sephora's other eyeshadow singles. The huge assortment of shades comes in three finishes: matte, metallic, and glittering. Among them, the mattes (which really are matte!) and metallic (most of which produce a subtle shine that doesn't look metallic at all) are the best. Avoid the glittering shades at all costs; not only is the glitter blatantly obvious and overdone, but also the formula has a dry, grainy texture that clings poorly, so the glitter flakes immediately. The matte and metallic shades have a smooth, non-powdery texture that applies evenly and deposits soft color. You'll need to layer for more than nuanced shading and shaping, but I suspect most women will prefer how softly these apply at first. Those interested in matte powder eyeshadows should not miss this collection.

☺ **$$$ Colorful 9 Eyeshadow Palette** *($28)*. This collection of nine powder eyeshadows in one compact gives you tiny dots of each shade, so although nine seems impressive, you're not getting a lot of product for the money. Each shade has a smooth, dry texture that lends itself to a decent application. Color payoff is good, but more than half the shades are tricky to work with, so watch out for going overboard with clashing colors.

☺ **$$$ Colorful Eye Shadow Palette** *($24)* is a collection of powder eyeshadow quads that are talc-based and have a smooth, dry texture. The dryness hinders application a bit, but the shadows are still workable if applied in sheer layers. The formula for this powder eyeshadow is different from that of Sephora's Colorful Pro Eyeshadow Palette (below), and the difference is enough to earn it a happy face rating. The most versatile quads are: Kiss From ___ (you're supposed to fill in the blank), Abricot Pulp, Camel Leon, and Taupe Model.

☺ **Eye Primer Pot** *($8)* is a tiny pot of wax and emollients that goes on colorless and is meant to enhance the cling and wear time of loose-powder shimmer and glitter products, including those sold in Sephora's own brand. Although this has a lingering tacky finish, it certainly keeps loose shine, which would otherwise flake mercilessly, in place. This is best used after concealer, powder, and eyeshadow are applied to the eye area.

☺ **Colorful Duo Eyeshadow** *($16)* includes two eyeshadows in one compact, and there's a divider between the shades. The texture is smooth, but powdery enough to make flaking during application an issue unless you blend in sheer layers. The shade range is hit-or-miss; roughly half are too odd or contrasting to work for an attractive eye design. Duo No. 05 and Duo No. 06 are matte, while Duo No. 07 is the best one if you want a smart pairing of shades with shine. Shades labeled "shimmer" have a more obvious, glitzy shine than those labeled "metallic."

☺ **$$$ Colorful Pro Eyeshadow Palette** *($26)* is available in options for brown, blue, and green eyes. Each compact is filled with six strips of pressed-powder eyeshadow, and at least one color in each set has a strong glitter finish. The glitter flakes quickly, but the non-glittery shades apply surprisingly well considering their drier texture. The palettes for green and brown eyes are the best. The one for blue eyes offers, what else, blue eyeshadow. The result is your sparkling blue eyes get lost next to shadows that are close to the same hue.

☺ **$$$ Smoky Eyes Palette** *($38)*. This kit is packaged as a small hardcover book. Inside are four shades of powder eyeshadow, a mini eye pencil and mascara, and a dual-sided applicator that is so small that you'd have to have the world's tiniest fingers to wield it effectively and create an attractive eye design. The powder shadows are labeled base, contour, lid, and light, and Sephora includes step-by-step instructions for creating a smoky eye. There's no reason you cannot create the classic smoky eye with this palette, and the instructions are great, but the products themselves don't move past ho-hum. The eyeshadows have a waxy feel and deposit color too softly for much drama, unless you want to apply several layers of color—even the black shade goes on a tad soft. The pencil is standard fare and the mascara thickens lashes to complete the look. The concept and packaging are commendable, but you're better off creating a smoky eye with other products.

EYE AND BROW SHAPER: ✓ ☺ **$$$ Arch It Brow Kit** *($35)* is just about one of the cutest and most practical brow kits I've ever seen. Packaged in a chic leather case about the size of a change purse are a compact that houses brow powder, brow wax, two synthetic brushes, a mini clear brow gel, a full-size pair of tweezers, brow stencils, instructions, and a larger (but too scratchy) brow brush. The brow powder is matte, and although the accompanying wax looks too dark to coordinate with the powder, it applies sheer. The instructions indicate how to use the stencils (three shapes are included) to perfect your brows, and although they're brief they're also accurate. If you are new to the practice of brow tweezing and shaping, this kit will get you off to a great start and is highly recommended!

✓ ☺ **Long Lasting Metallic Eyeliner** *($10)* is Sephora's best liquid eyeliner thanks to its easy-to-use tapered brush that allows for precise, even application of this fast-drying formula. Once set, this wears and wears. The only limitation is that all of the colors have a sparkling metallic finish. If you want a dramatic, shiny effect, this is highly recommended.

☺ **Brow Tint** *($12)* is sort of a non-permanent marker pen for brows. Rather than a pencil or powder, it's a liquid housed in a pen-style component with a synthetic brush applicator affixed. The fine-tipped brush allows you to place color between brow hairs for emphasis and definition. This is a fast-drying formula that supplies sheer, buildable color that lasts. I'd consider this an ingenious alternative to standard brow makeup if only the two shades were better. Both brunette-themed shades have a reddish-orange cast that limits their appeal. But, if one of these shades works for you, this is definitely worth considering.

☺ **Nano Eyeliner** *($5)*. This pencil needs routine sharpening and the "nano" in the name refers to how small it is (about half the size of a regular eye pencil); it's got nothing to do with the formula. This has a minimally creamy texture and smooth application, though it goes on a bit thick. Because the finish stays creamy, this is best used for smoky eyes when you intend to smudge the line. The colors feature mostly glittery or shimmer finishes.

☺ **Lash & Eyebrow Mascara** *($8)* comes in two shades, but only the Clear version is worth considering. The other shade is metallic, which looks artificial on brows. The dual-sided brush works well and the formula remains non-sticky, though you can find clear brow gels for less money at the drugstore.

☺ **Long Lasting Eye Liner** *($10)* has a very thin brush that can be tough to control, resulting in sketchy application. This also takes longer than it should to dry and, despite the name, its wear time doesn't match that of the prime picks in this category.

☺ **$$$ Retractable Waterproof Eyeliner** *($12)*. The trade-off for this automatic, retractable eye pencil's waterproof finish is that it remains tacky to the touch. That's not a big deal because you shouldn't be touching your eyes anyway if you want your eye makeup to last, but those who draw a thick line may notice the tacky feeling during wear, especially if you have deep-set eyes and small eyelids. This pencil applies easily and most of the shades provide an intense, metallic shine, plus there are some truly odd colors that do little to emphasize the eye. Still, classic black is available and some of the metallic shades can be fun for evening makeup.

☺ **Slim Pencil-Eye** *($5)* comes in a dizzying array of colors, which is really the only reason to consider this otherwise very standard, creamy pencil. At this price, you can afford to experiment with several shades, but I encourage you to look past the many blue, green, and purple choices.

☹ **Cream Eyeliner Palette** *($15)* may tempt you with its striking, metallic-tinged colors, but be aware that this cream eyeliner is way too emollient and applies unevenly, balling up and smearing as you attempt to smooth things out and build intensity (the colors look rich, but apply sheer), and its wear time is brief and fraught with problems.

☹ **Eyebrow Palette** *($12)* is a good concept with poor execution. Housed in a round compact are two brow powders, a clear brow wax, and a tiny (mostly useless) applicator. The shades of matte brow powder are too sheer and don't correspond well to their intended brow colors, while the wax keeps things in place, but with an unpleasant feel. For brows, you are far better off with the Arch It Brow Kit.

☹ **Eyebrow Pencil** *($10)* comes in two good colors, but this needs-sharpening pencil has a creamy application that is too thick and leads to a smear-prone finish. Almost any brow pencil at the drugstore (or department store) outperforms this one.

☹ **Jumbo Pencil-Eye** *($6)* needs sharpening and applies smoothly, but the texture is too creamy and it stays that way, leading to smearing and fading too soon.

☹ **Kohl Pencil** *($8)* is a below-standard pencil that drags and tugs during application yet has a creamy finish that won't stay in place for long.

LIPSTICK, LIP GLOSS, AND LIPLINER: ☺ **Lip Attitude Glamour** *($12)* is a good creamy lipstick with a glossy finish and an attractive group of sheer to light coverage colors. The longevity of each shade is brief at best, but that tends to be the norm with sheer lipsticks anyway, so it doesn't make this less worthy of consideration.

☺ **Lip Attitude Star** *($12)* has an elegantly smooth, creamy feel that moisturizes lips without feeling thick. Each shade leaves a soft to moderate shimmer, but has minimal stain, so frequent touch-ups will be necessary. Still, this is a very good modern cream lipstick with a shade range that's bound to please.

☺ **Lush Flush Wine Lip & Cheek Stain** *($10)*. Meant for use on lips or cheeks, this standard gel formula comes in packaging that makes it preferred for use on lips. The sponge-tip applicator is great for quickly staining the lips with sheer yet vivid color. Used as a gel blush, this demands lightning-fast blending to avoid a streaked or spotted look, and mistakes aren't easily wiped away. The sole shade is a boysenberry-plum that looks better on lips than it does on cheeks.

☺ **Maniac Long-Wearing Lipstick** *($12)* promises "the satiny radiance of a second skin," and although it doesn't feel quite that light, for a creamy lipstick this is not nearly as thick-textured as many. It applies smoothly and imparts nearly opaque color with a satin finish. The shade selection is well-rounded, but small by Sephora standards, offering mostly shimmer- or glitter-infused colors. As for the long-wearing claims, this doesn't fade within an hour, but it also doesn't make it past lunch without a touch-up either, making it a decent lipstick.

☺ **Shimmer Harmony Gloss Palette** *($14)*. Can't decide on a lip gloss shade? You could go with this sleek palette, which contains six shades of soft, creamy lip gloss. The drawback is that the shades deposit almost no color, so you're basically left with a translucent sheen that's not the least bit sticky.

☺ **Ultra Shine Lip Gloss** *($15)* does leave lips ultra-shiny as well as glittery. This showy gloss isn't for the demure, and its slightly thick application feels a bit sticky, but that contributes to its high-gloss finish. Give this a sniff before purchasing to make sure the fruit scent appeals to you.

☹ **Lip Attitude Chic** *($12)* claims its vitamin E protects lips from premature aging, which isn't true in the least (and, let me tell you: they do use the least amount of vitamin E in this lipstick). Ignore the antiaging claims because this is merely a standard cream lipstick whose emollient texture feels lighter on lips than expected. This finishes creamy with a slight gloss, and provides medium coverage. The shade range features several colors that are so pale or beige they make lips look dull, almost as if they have vanished. Sephora's Lip Attitude Star has a more pleasing palette.

☺ **Maniac Mat Long-Wearing Matte Lipstick** *($12)* is a true matte lipstick and I wish I liked it more than I do. Application is smooth and even and it imparts pure, rich color with a soft matte finish. The problem is that within minutes this lipstick becomes uncomfortably tacky. Lips feel slightly stuck together, which reminded me of how the old ultra-matte lipstick felt. This does a good job of not cracking or balling up and it wears longer than a cream lipstick, but it's definitely one to test before purchasing.

☺ **Nano Lip Liner** *($5)*. The name of this standard, needs-sharpening pencil has to do with its tiny size. I imagine it will be used up or barely usable within a month or so. That's especially true because this pencil is too creamy and the colors have minimal stain, so they don't last long on lips. Knowing this, the price isn't such a value!

☺ **Nectar Shine Hydrating Lipgloss SPF 8** *($14)*. Not only does this lip gloss with sunscreen leave lips vulnerable to UVA damage, but its SPF rating is paltry. This brush-on gloss has a thick, moist texture and the requisite glossy finish that leaves lips feeling a bit sticky. The sheer, shimmer-infused colors are pretty, but given the inadequacy of the sunscreen this isn't a gloss worth considering.

☺ **Slim Pencil-Lip** *($5)* is similar to the Slim Pencil-Eye, and, just like it, the best reason to explore this pencil is the vast shade selection. The creamy formula applies well but doesn't do much to keep lipstick from feathering into lines around the mouth. If that's not an issue, this is a reliable, basic pencil.

☹ **Fresh Gloss** *($7)* contains and is flavored by mint, which makes it not worth considering over countless other tube lip glosses, including several sold by Sephora.

☹ **Professional Flash Lip Plumper** *($6)* contains a blend of menthol and pepper to plump lips in a flash, but the resulting irritation isn't worth the minor results.

MASCARA: ✓ ☺ **Atomic Volume Mascara** *($16)* has a misleading name because it doesn't produce lots of volume (i.e., thickness). What it does do easily and copiously is make lashes wonderfully long and beautifully defined, especially if you want a soft, fringed look without clumps. Some comb-through is needed to avoid a slightly spiked look, but otherwise this works well and wears without a hitch. It leaves lashes noticeably soft and removes easily with a water-soluble cleanser.

✓ ☺ **$$$ Lash Plumper** *($16)* pledges to "fatten your flutter" (meaning lashes) and does so quickly! This is an awesome mascara if your goal is length and volume without clumps. The brush is a bit larger than standard, but once you adapt it isn't too tricky to reach even the shortest lashes. This wears all day without a hitch and comes off easily with a water-soluble cleanser.

✓☺ **Lengthening Mascara** *($10)* does just that and quickly, too! It builds beautifully, creating long, fringed lashes without any clumps. This has much more curling impact than other Sephora mascaras, and lashes stay soft.

☺ $$$ **Lash Plumper Waterproof** *($16)* isn't nearly as impressive as its non-waterproof counterpart. The full, plump-bristled brush allows you to build ample length and definition with some thickness. Clumps are absent, but this has the uncommon tendency to dry with tiny balls of product at the very tip of your lashes. It's not a deal-breaker, but it doesn't make for the cleanest look. This is waterproof, and removing it requires something with oil, where you'll find it tends to come off in pieces and flecks rather than just a smear of dissolved color.

☺ **Lash Stretcher Mascara** *($16)* is supposed to be like false lashes in a tube, but it isn't. The formula adds bulk and drama to lashes with tiny fibers, but for all the good they may do appearance-wise, they end up being a nuisance. That's because they tend to flake as the day wears on, depositing themselves in your eye or on your cheek. As you can imagine, that gets annoying pretty quickly, and doesn't make the enhanced results (which are messier than what you can achieve with false eyelashes) worth it.

☺ **Professional Clear Natural Mascara** *($10)* is a very standard, colorless gel mascara that has minimal impact on lashes beyond slightly darkening them and creating a minimal groomed look. This actually works better as a brow gel, but isn't worth the splurge over similar products from Cover Girl or Maybelline New York.

☺ **Triple Action Mascara** *($14)*. If this does three things for lashes, it doesn't do any of them very well! This Sephora-described "best of both worlds" mascara is merely average in all departments, though it is easy to remove with a water-soluble cleanser.

FACE AND BODY ILLUMINATING/SHIMMER PRODUCTS: ✓☺ **Luminizer** *($18)* is a silicone-in-water shimmer lotion housed in a glass bottle with a pump applicator. It has a silky application and a dry finish that leaves skin softly glowing. This is an excellent way to subtly highlight skin, and it mixes well with moisturizer or foundation. All three shades are very good.

☺ **Luminous Trio** *($15)* is a less expensive copy of Bobbi Brown's popular Shimmer Brick Compact, except that in this instance you get just three stripes of shimmering pressed powder. It feels very smooth and applies well, if a bit heavy. The shine is intense, making this best for highlighting small areas rather than for dusting all over. Both trios are attractive.

☺ **Glitter Pot** *($8)*. What you get with this product is just what the name states: A pot of glitter. Loose glitter may be fun for party or Halloween makeup, but little else. Glitter Pot is large flecks of glitter, like what you'd buy at an arts-and-crafts store. The difference is that this clings to skin decently, so flaking isn't a major problem. This is special-occasion fun makeup, and only for when you really want pure glitter as part of your cosmetic adornment.

☺ **Highlighting Compact Powder** *($15)* is an average pressed powder with shine. It has a dry texture and sheer application that imparts more shine than is warranted, at least for daytime makeup. The shine clings marginally well, but Sephora sells better versions of this type of product from brands such as Benefit, Stila, and Dior.

☺ **Shimmer Pot** *($8)*. Similar to Sephora's Glitter Pot in terms of packaging and dispensing via a sifter, Shimmer Pot offers a smooth, pigmented loose powder with lots of shine, but the effect isn't glittery or garish. This clings OK, but applying shimmer with a loose powder is not preferred to adding it with a product in pressed or liquid form because both of the latter versions are easier to control and tend to last longer.

BRUSHES: ✓☺ **Sephora Brushes** *($5-$58)* present some prime choices, especially for applying eyeshadow and powder eyeliner. Over 50 brushes are available, with the best ones being the **Professional Foundation Brush** *($25)*, **Bronzer Brush** *($26)*, **Professional Natural All Over Shadow Brush** *($23)*, **Professional Angle Brush** *($14)*, **Slanted Contour Eyeshadow Brush** *($22)*, and **Eyeshadow Brush** *($15)*.

✓☺ **Professional Platinum Air Brush #55** *($34)* is a top-notch powder brush composed of soft yet densely packed synthetic bristles. Sephora sells this as a way to apply foundation, but it works best with powder products, including pressed-powder foundations. The price is a bit steep, but given you only have to purchase a brush once, this well-made brush may be worth the splurge.

SPECIALTY PRODUCTS: ☺ **Deluxe Lash Kit** *($18)* is available in classic black or glitter lashes, which have a shiny strip at the base of the lashes. Included are a pair of pre-cut false eyelashes, adhesive, a lash curler, and a storage case. This is worth checking out if you like the look of these lashes and want to experiment, or if you just want to add some drama to your natural lashes for a special occasion.

☺ **Flirt-It Lash Duo** *($8)* is a kit with pre-cut strips of false eyelashes and adhesive. It's well priced and a basic kit for beginners interested in experimenting with this type of product. The second version features rhinestones at the lash base for a sparkling effect.

☺ **Makeup Bags** *($5-$50)*. You will not be disappointed by Sephora's vast selection of Makeup Bags. The variety is astounding. The selection tends to vary by store, so if you want to see everything that's available, check out the Sephora Web site.

☺ **Makeup Eraser Pen** *($12)* does come in handy when you need a fast makeup fix for flaking mascara or smeared lipstick. This pen has a wax- and silicone-enriched tip that allows precise application to the trouble spot. Just dab on, blend a bit, and then use a tissue or cotton swab to remove. While not an essential, you may want to consider adding this to your stash of office or evening makeup.

☹ **Correcting Smoothing Primer** *($18)* is nearly identical to Sephora's Base Primer, except it offers the "correcting" of a sheer green tint. Green color correctors are very difficult to work with—they often make matters worse when it comes to neutralizing redness and they add yet another layer of makeup to skin. However, this silicone-enriched primer's green tint is so sheer it becomes a non-issue, and, therefore, a waste of time.

☹ **$$$ PURE Natural 7-Color Palette** *($36)*. Sephora's PURE line is their attempt to offer natural and organic products, ostensibly to compete with the other natural product brands they sell. This palette, housed in a recyclable wood compact with a built-in mirror, contains six powder eyeshadows and one powder blush. All have a smooth, powdery texture and sheer application that leaves skin gleaming with shine. The blush is less shiny than the eyeshadows, and the eyeshadows present some workable shade combinations, but avoid the blue and green hues. As for the ingredients, most of them in each formula are, in fact, natural, but none of them are unique to this palette.

☹ **$$$ PURE Natural Island Sunset Palette** *($30)* is nearly identical to the PURE Natural 7-Color Palette above, save for a change of shades that favors bright hues. Otherwise, the same review applies.

SERIOUS SKIN CARE (SKIN CARE ONLY)

SERIOUS SKIN CARE AT-A-GLANCE

Strengths: Provides complete ingredient lists on Web site; several good cleansers; some impressive serums (with and without retinol) and primers; the A-Stick balm; one good scrub; one effective BHA (salicylic acid) product; effective AHA (glycolic acid) pads; effective 5% benzoyl peroxide product; the lip line–filling products (though the effect is not akin to dermal fillers as claimed).

Weaknesses: Too many products, which makes determining what to buy incredibly confusing; several good formulas hampered with needless irritants; no effective skin-lightening options; incomplete lineup for managing acne; jar packaging for many moisturizers, which allows the important, but unstable, ingredients to degrade; average masks; the at-home peels are terrible; too many gimmicky products; very small assortment of sunscreens, especially considering all of the antiaging products; the Beauty Treatment patches are gimmicky and useless; the Glucosamine and Calstrum sub-brands are mediocre; an irritating lip plumper.

For more information about Serious Skin Care, call (800) 540-8662 or visit www.seriousskincare.com or www.Beautypedia.com.

SERIOUS SKIN CARE A-DEFIANCE PRODUCTS

☺ **$$$ A-Wash, Vitamin A Gel to Foam Cleanser** *($19.95 for 4 ounces)* is expensive for what you get, but it is an effective, fairly gentle option for normal to slightly dry or slightly oily skin. The inclusion of retinol and other antioxidant vitamins looks good on the label, but their benefit is nil given that this product is designed to be rinsed from your skin, so the ingredients just end up down the drain, not on your face. And why on earth does this product require a synthetic blue dye and lemon peel extract, which are completely unnecessary and problematic, especially for a skin-care line labeling themselves as serious?

☺ **$$$ A-Wash, Vitamin A Gel to Foam Cleanser with Triple Peptides** *($21.95 for 4 ounces)* is very similar to Serious Skin Care's A-Wash Vitamin A Gel to Foam Cleanser above. The differences are that this version contains peptides and some skin-identical ingredients. In a cleanser, these peptides are rinsed from the skin before they can penetrate (which is what you want peptides to do to obtain results), but the skin-identical ingredients help make this cleanser more conditioning than a standard, detergent-based cleanser. It is a good, though pricey, option for normal to slightly dry to slightly oily skin. And why does this product require a synthetic blue dye and lemon peel extract, which are completely unnecessary and problematic, especially for a skin-care line labeling themselves as serious?

☹ **A-Cream XR** *($34.95 for 2 ounces).* This product is incredibly misguided and not recommended. It does not list any active sunscreen ingredients or include an SPF rating, so forget about it for sun protection. Almost as bad is the inclusion of several fragrant plant oils, all of which are irritating to skin and make this a retinol product that, nanoencapsulated or not, pales in comparison to several other retinol products rated Paula's Pick. Examples of brands with very good retinol products include Skinceuticals, Peter Thomas Roth, RoC, and Dr. Denese New York. When all is said and done, this is just an ordinary badly formulated moisturizer. As for the 2 Million International Units of vitamin A, that sounds wholly impressive, but ends up accounting for only 0.02 ounce of the product's contents!

☹ **A-Cream XR, SPF 30** *($34.95 for 2 ounces)*. Never mind the potentially controversial claims about nanotechnology for this daytime moisturizer with an in-part avobenzone sunscreen, and the fact that they exaggerate the amount of retinyl palmitate (retinyl palmitate is derived from vitamin A) by referring to the amount of International Units it contains (a measurement that makes it sound like there must be an awful lot in here, when there really isn't; 2 million IUs works out to 600 milligrams in the entire product, which is equivalent to 0.02 ounce—hardly an impressive amount of vitamin A!). This product is absolutely not recommended because it contains too many potent irritating plant oils. Geranium, ylang-ylang, jasmine, rosewood, grapefruit, and especially lemon oil have no business in any well-formulated skin-care product, especially one meant to protect skin from sunlight.

☺ **A-Eye XR** *($21 for 0.5 ounce)*. This lightweight eye-area moisturizer contains a good amount of retinol and comes in packaging that will keep it stable during use. It is not rated a Paula's Pick because, despite the fact that it contains beneficial ingredients in addition to the retinol, it contains potential irritants such as horsetail, witch hazel, and elderflower, all of which have an astringent or constricting effect on skin. The amounts are small enough that they aren't likely to be a problem, but they're worth calling out because this product is designed to be used near the eye, and retinol as an active ingredient can cause problems by itself on the skin, so staying away from any additional risk is best.

✓ ☺ **A-Force XR, Retinol Serum** *($15.75 for 1 ounce)*. This water-based serum contains an impressive amount of vitamin A (mostly as retinyl palmitate), along with a smaller but still efficacious amount of retinol. The formula also contains a good anti-irritant as well as antioxidants, including vitamin C and green tea. Although glycolic acid is present, the amount is too low for it to function as an exfoliant; however, it has water-binding properties for skin, and that's helpful. This serum is best for normal to dry skin; the castor oil will be a problem for those with oily or breakout-prone skin. The only slight drawback is that it contains fragrance.

☹ **A-Good Nite, Beta Carotene Night Cream** *($26.50 for 2 ounces)*. The amount of vitamin A in this product paltry, and the jar packaging will compromise the stability of it and the other antioxidants it contains. Even more of an issue is the amount of fragrant rosewood oil, which is an irritant and serves no useful purpose for skin.

✓ ☺ **A-Stick, Vitamin A Moisturizer Stick** *($8 for 0.17 ounce)* is a balm-like, oil-based moisturizer in lipstick form and it is not Chapstick (meaning you won't have to reapply every few minutes). It works very well to smooth and soften dry lips, or can be spot-applied to very dry areas of the face or anywhere on the body where dryness is a problem. The wax-heavy formula adheres well, which is just what lips need to protect from moisture loss and climate extremes, while containing a healthy assortment of emollient plant oils. It is also fragrance-free. Your lips will be happy with this exceptionally done product.

☺ **DNA Eye Beauty Treatment Cream** *($22.50 for 0.5 ounce)*. This water- and oil-based moisturizer is suitable for dry skin anywhere on the face. The formula includes some good water-binding agents along with antioxidants. It also contains a tiny amount of the controversial growth hormone prasterone, also known as DHEA. Please refer to the *Cosmetic Ingredient Dictionary* on www.Beautypedia.com for detailed information about DHEA. As for the DNA, it won't have any impact on your skin, but then you wouldn't want it to, either!

☺ **$$$ DNA Facial Beauty Treatment** *($34.50 for 1 ounce)* is nearly identical to Serious Skin Care's DNA Eye Beauty Treatment Cream, but it is less emollient because it contains less plant oil. This is merely a good moisturizer for dry skin anywhere on the face.

☹ **InstA-Tox Temporary Facial Firming Wrinkle Smoothing Serum** *($28.50 for 0.75 ounce)* is the company's works-like-Botox product (something numerous cosmetics companies have added to their product lines over the past few years). Serious Skin Care does state that the effect of their serum isn't as dramatic as the effect you get from the actual medical procedure, but they also state that the results are still "remarkable." What a joke! It isn't dramatic, remarkable, or anything resembling good skin care. The alkaline pH of this mineral-heavy serum can cause skin irritation, resulting in inflammation that will temporarily reduce the appearance of wrinkles. This product does not provide moisture—on the contrary—it can draw moisture from the skin due to sodium silicate's irritating, astringent quality (Source: *American Journal of Contact Dermatitis*, September 2002, pages 133-139). Believe me, just about any serum or moisturizer is preferred over this mistaken concoction.

☺ **A-Facial, Meringue Exfoliating Mask** *($22.50 for 2 ounces)*. The formula for this meringue-textured product is that of an absorbent cleanser, not an exfoliant or a mask. Used as a mask, the sodium laureth sulfate (a detergent cleansing agent listed second on the label) can be extremely irritating and drying when left on the face for a period of time, as you are supposed to do with masks. The plant oils won't do much moisturizing due to the amount of clay this contains, which makes it OK as a cleanser for oily skin, but overall truly a product to be ignored. What was this company thinking?

☹ **A-Peel, Derma Peel Kit** *($13.25 for 2 ounces)*. This two-part at-home peel is a waste of time and a detriment to skin. The **A-Peel** contains a lot of alcohol and a grand total of approximately 3% AHAs and BHA, minimally worthwhile for skin, and the fragrant orange oil only compounds the irritation from the alcohol. The **A-Neutralize** is just baking soda with slip agent, aloe, and some vitamins. Given that the A-Peel isn't pH-adjusted to remain acidic, neutralizing it is a useless step. Besides, even if this were an effective peel, you could use plain tap water to stop the process and not send your skin's pH into the alkaline range, which is what applying baking soda does.

☺ **A-Primer, Vitamin A Line Filler** *($22.50 for 1 ounce)* serves as a soft spackle for lines, and can temporarily fill in superficial wrinkles. The mica adds a bit of shine, but the amount of vitamin A is nothing to write home about. This can help makeup go on smoother and give skin a polished, luminous look, as claimed, but given the number of serums that perform this function and add other beneficial ingredients to their formulas, this is just too ordinary to consider. Your skin deserves better.

☺ **$$$ Slice of Life Cucumber Slices** *($11.25 for 24 pads)* is nothing more than pads saturated with a water- and glycerin-based toner. It contains some helpful ingredients for skin, but the jar packaging won't keep the antioxidants stable. The inclusion of *Sophora japonica* (pagoda tree) is odd because there is no research demonstrating its topical benefit, and consumed orally it can be fatal (Source: www.naturaldatabase.com). I wouldn't worry about its presence in this product, but I can't imagine why Serious Skin Care included it!

SERIOUS SKIN CARE CAPOMINERALE PRODUCTS

☺ **$$$ Capominerale Mineral Rich Foaming Cleanser** *($36.50 for 4 ounces)* is a very expensive water-soluble cleansing scrub dressed up with several natural abrasive agents, including pumice. The abrasive agents make up only a small portion of the formula, but you still should use extra care with this scrub to avoid irritating your skin. Those with normal to oily skin will fare best with this product, but please keep in mind that a washcloth used with your regular cleanser is a better and less costly option.

☺ **$$$ Capominerale Mineral Rich Eye Creme** *($32.50 for 0.5 ounce).* Serious Skin Care seemingly has a moisturizer or eye cream for any and every ingredient trend going, so why not add one enriched with minerals? It doesn't matter that minerals applied topically offer no benefit to skin around the eyes; minerals are the "it" category so let's create more products with them while we also carry on about our other products with olive oil, vitamin A, vitamin C, and on and on. Can't they make up their mind about what ingredients really work? Getting back to this eye cream: you're getting mostly watered-down minerals with silicone and wax (by the way, the molecular size of minerals makes them too large to penetrate skin anyway). There are a few antioxidants and a couple of the plant extracts (iris and arnica) are troublemakers for skin, though likely not in the amounts used here. If you're planning to spend in this range for an eye cream or facial moisturizer, this isn't the one to pick.

☺ **$$$ Capominerale Mineral Rich Facial Creme** *($44.50 for 1.7 ounces).* Despite the claim that this is densely packed with minerals, which it isn't because they are barely present, the minerals that it does contain—malachite and hematite—can't penetrate skin and there is no research showing they have any benefit anyway. Aside from the outlandish promise of minerals being the skin-care answer for your wrinkles or other concerns (what a sad joke), this moisturizer is identical to Serious Skin Care's Capominerale Mineral Rich Eye Creme. There is no reason you can't use this moisturizer in the eye area, and as usual, you get a lot more (almost three times as much) face cream product for your money than you do eye cream product. It is also good news that this Capominerale product does not contain the potentially irritating plant extracts that are in their eye cream version. This moisturizer doesn't qualify as state-of-the-art, but it's an OK option for normal to dry skin not prone to blemishes.

SERIOUS SKIN CARE C-NO WRINKLE PRODUCTS

☺ **$$$ C-Clean, Vitamin C Ester Facial Cleanser** *($21.95 for 4 ounces).* Positioning this cleanser as being for skin over age 40 is a marketing decision, because there is nothing about the formula that is unique for skin of a particular age range. This is suitable for normal to oily skin. There are a lot more plant extracts and multiple forms of vitamin C in this cleanser than is needed because this antioxidant/collagen-stimulating vitamin is of little use in a cleanser because any benefits are just rinsed down the drain. Some of the citrus extracts pose a risk of skin and eye irritation, so careful use is advised.

☺ **$$$ C-Scrub Vitamin C Facial Polish** *($22.50 for 2 ounces).* There are stabilized forms of vitamin C in this scrub, but they're of little use for skin because they are quickly rinsed down the drain. This ends up being a standard scrub for normal to dry skin not prone to blemishes. Polyethylene beads are the abrasive agent, and they're buffered by safflower oil. This scrub also has a mild cleansing action, so it can serve you well as a morning cleanser/scrub product, but it's awfully pricey for the amount of product.

☺ **C-Cream SPF 30, Vitamin C Ester Protective Daytime Moisturizer** *($26.50 for 2 ounces).* The numerous citrus fruit extracts in this product put a damper on an otherwise brilliantly formulated daytime moisturizer for normal to dry skin. Avobenzone is on hand for sufficient UVA protection and the amount of vitamin C (known to help protect skin from sun damage) is appreciable. Unfortunately, citrus extracts are plentiful as well, making this sunscreen a potential problem, especially for sensitive skin. Parts of this product's formula are worthy of a Paula's Pick rating, but taken as a whole, a neutral face and a caution are warranted.

☹ **C-Eye, Vitamin C Ester Eye Beauty Treatment** *($21.50 for 0.5 ounce)* contains an amount of irritating citrus extracts that is too great to ignore, and none of them have any notable benefit for wrinkles or eye-area skin. Without the citrus extracts, this would be an impressive lightweight vitamin C moisturizer for normal to slightly dry skin.

☺ **C-Repair, Vitamin C Ester Moisturizing Night Cream** *($24.50 for 2 ounces)* will see its vitamin C content squandered as a result of the jar packaging. Furthermore, the amount of citrus extracts (all listed before the really beneficial ingredients for skin) makes this a potentially irritating waste of your time and money for all skin types. Although the price is attractive, you're not getting much for your money beyond softer skin and potential irritation.

☹ **C-Serum, Vitamin C Ester Skin Conditioner** *($28.50 for 1 ounce)* contains far too many irritating citrus extracts to make it worthwhile for any skin type. Lots of companies offer much better vitamin C formulations, including Perricone, MD Skincare by Dr. Dennis Gross, Jan Marini, and Skinceuticals. Those brands' products cost more, but at least you're getting the goods without several extraneous irritants taking precedence over the beneficial ingredients.

☺ **$$$ C-Appeal System, Vitamin C Micro-Peel Spa Quality Facial Regime** *($26.50 for 3 ounces)* is meant to help you achieve an immaculate complexion in only seven days. Don't count on it. The best you can expect from this product is wasting your time and money. Step 1 is the **Exfoliating Serum**, which contains approximately 5% lactic acid along with lesser amounts of other AHA ingredients in a gel base that also contains vitamin C and some good water-binding agents. The pH of 3.2 allows for effective exfoliation to occur, assuming you leave this on for longer than directed (the two minutes advised isn't going to provide much exfoliation). You're then supposed to use Step 2, the **Neutralizing Solution**, to stop the peel action. This solution is mostly water, baking soda, and slip agents. The alkaline pH of the baking soda will stop the action of the peel, but so will rinsing with plain tap water, so Step 2 is superfluous. Step 3, applying the **Moisturizing Serum**, completes the process. The serum is primarily a blend of water with slip agents, water-binding agents, vitamin C, and plant extracts (including arnica, which can be irritating). The only worthwhile product in this trio is the Exfoliating Serum, and it is best left on skin for several minutes or overnight for best results. There are better moisturizing serums to consider, while the Neutralizing Solution is a waste and potentially problematic because of the alkaline direction it pushes skin toward.

☺ **$$$ C-Extreme Results** *($44.50 for 2 ounces)* begins with the application of **C-Resurface**. This is a baking soda–based gel scrub that contains vitamin C and fragrant citrus oil. The vitamin C is wasted in a rinse-off product and the baking soda creates a pH that is too high and not the best for skin. After rinsing, you apply the **C-Potion**, which is a lactic acid–based exfoliant whose pH is too high for exfoliation to occur. This is a very expensive way to scrub skin and treat it to a vitamin C "potion," which isn't nearly as impressive as it should be. If you're anxious to try it, those with normal to slightly dry skin will fare best—but don't expect extreme results, or really any real results of any kind.

☺ **C-Mask, Vitamin C Conditioning Mask** *($21 for 3 ounces)*. Vitamin C takes a backseat to the clay and silt (sedimentary soil) in this absorbent mask that is best for oily skin. Most of the plant extracts have soothing benefits, which add to this mask's appeal. As long as you're not expecting vitamin C to be the star performer, this is a worthwhile, though basic, clay mask.

☺ **$$$ C-Radiance, Self Tanning Facial Care** *($26.50 for 1 ounce)*. This lightweight, silky-textured product is a very expensive way to try a self-tanner. The amount of alcohol is potentially irritating, while the vitamin C isn't all that plentiful. There are much better self-tanners available from the drugstore for a lot less money (keep in mind that 99% of all self-tanners contain the same ingredient [dihydroxyacetone] to turn skin a brown shade, and this one is the same as all of those).

☹ **C-Zone Anti-Wrinkle Vitamin C Infused Hydrogel Treatment Patch, Eyes** *($24.50 for 4 patches)*. Vitamin C gets short shrift in these stick-on eye patches that contain enough acrylate-based film-forming agent to cause irritation. The plant extracts are but a dusting, and these patches are about as far from being "antiaging elixirs" as you can imagine. What you are getting mostly in this product is hairspray, mineral oil, lye, and thickening agents. This is one of the worst product formulations I've run into in quite some time. The claims for this product are nothing short of offensive.

☹ **C-Zone Anti-Wrinkle Vitamin C Infused Hydrogel Treatment Patch, Forehead** *($26.50 for 4 patches)*. These patches are nearly identical to Serious Skin Care's C-Zone Anti-Wrinkle Vitamin C Infused Hydrogel Treatment Patch, Eyes, except this version adds a teeny-tiny amount of a peptide. Otherwise, you're getting the same embarrassing formulation.

☹ **C-Zone Anti-Wrinkle Vitamin C Infused Hydrogel Treatment Patch, Neck** *($29.50 for 4 patches)*. Offering no special benefit for skin on the neck, these sticky patches are identical to Serious Skin Care's C-Zone Anti-Wrinkle Vitamin C Infused Hydrogel Beauty Treatment Patch, Forehead. As such, the same review and sense of genuine dismay apply.

SERIOUS SKIN CARE CONTINUOUSLY CLEAR PRODUCTS

☹ **Clear Wash, Acne Medicated Targeted Cleanser** *($16.50 for 4.2 ounces)* is medicated with 1% salicylic acid, which is an effective anti-acne ingredient but whose contact with skin as a cleanser will be too brief for it to work as intended. Even if you left this on your skin for several minutes, the pH is too high for exfoliation to occur, plus the peppermint oil causes instant irritation.

☺ **$$$ Daily Ritual, Acne Medication Cleanser** *($21 for 4 ounces)*. Although this omits the irritating peppermint oil found in Serious Skin Care's Clear Wash, Acne Medicated Targeted Cleanser, the 2% salicylic acid isn't going to be effective in a product that is quickly rinsed from skin. This is otherwise a good water-soluble cleanser for normal to dry skin. The tiny amount of jojoba wax beads provides a mild abrasive action. Because of the salicylic acid and the exfoliant beads, you should not use this cleanser in the eye area.

☺ **Clarify, Acne Medication Clarifying Treatment** *($17.50 for 2 ounces)* contains 2% salicylic acid at a pH of 4.1, so some exfoliation will occur. There are more effective BHA products available, but this lightweight, simply formulated anti-acne product is an option.

☹ **Continuously Clear, Acne Medication Moisture Replenishing Cream** *($26.50 for 2 ounces)* contains 0.5% salicylic acid and is formulated at an effective pH. So why the unhappy face rating, you ask? The high amount of paraffin can contribute to clogged pores and the rosemary oil is needlessly irritating.

☺ **Repairz-It, Youth Formula Oil Free Skin Hydrator Acne Medication** *($26.50 for 2 ounces)*. Although this isn't a bad product, it is not effective for its intended purpose due to a low amount of salicylic acid and a pH of 4.5, so exfoliation is only minimally able to take place. There isn't any other reason to consider this product unless you're OK with using an average moisturizer that may contribute to the clogged pores you're trying to diminish due to the amount of wax it contains.

The Reviews S

☹ **Clear Pads, Acne Medicated Pre-Soaked Wipes** *($19.95 for 45 wipes)*. The 2% salicylic acid steeped onto these cleansing pads would be much better for skin if it weren't formulated in a base of strong alcohol. As such, these are too irritating and drying for all skin types (plus alcohol generates free-radical damage) and the formula's pH is too high for the salicylic acid to function as an exfoliant.

✓ ☺ $$$ **Clearz-It Acne Medication** *($17.50 for 2 ounces)* is the only topical disinfectant I know of that combines an effective amount of benzoyl peroxide (in this case, 5%) with a high amount of tea tree oil, also known to have disinfecting properties for skin. The lightweight lotion formula is suitable for all skin types experiencing acne, and it's fragrance-free. This is definitely one of the better products from Serious Skin Care.

☹ **Dry-Lo, Acne Medication Spot Treatment** *($22.50 for 1 ounce)*. If you're looking for a quick way to irritate and dry out your skin, check out this skin-disrupting blend of 10% sulfur, rubbing alcohol, and camphor. Sulfur is a potent disinfectant for acne, but in this amount (and compared to benzoyl peroxide) and with the other unfriendly skin-care ingredients, it is exceedingly irritating to skin.

☹ $$$ **Unmasked, Acne Medication Sulfur Mask** *($22 for 2.5 ounces)*. Ignore the sulfur portion of the name because, at least if the company-supplied ingredient list is correct, this clay mask doesn't contain any. It would work well to absorb excess oil and rinse cleanly from the skin, but it's a shame the effect of the anti-irritant licorice is canceled out by irritating cinnamon bark extract. The tea tree oil could be helpful as a disinfectant, but the jar packaging wouldn't help keep it or any of the other potentially helpful plant extracts in this mask stable.

SERIOUS SKIN CARE FIRST PRESSED PRODUCTS

☺ $$$ **Olive Oil Emulsifying Cleanser** *($39.95 for 12 ounces)* is an oil-based cleanser that contains an emulsifier which turns it into a softly foaming cleanser when mixed with water. It is a good cleanser and makeup remover option for those with dry to very dry skin, but likely will require use of a washcloth for complete removal. The price is over the top for what ends up being a fairly ordinary emollient cleanser.

☹ **Olive Oil Face Polish** *($22.50 for 2 ounces)*. This emollient face scrub tries to appeal to those seeking natural ingredients by advertising that it contains finely ground olive pits as the exfoliating ingredient. It does contain them, but even when they are finely ground olive pits can still have rough edges that may scrape or abrade your skin. The fact that they're cushioned in olive oil helps, but that feature also makes this scrub difficult to rinse completely. Add to that the irritation potential from the rosemary oil and this ends up being better as a condiment than as a face scrub (though obviously you wouldn't want to eat it).

☺ $$$ **O3 Mega Omega 3 Restoring Beauty Therapy** *($32.50 for 1 ounce)*. Trying to be more than a one-note product, this olive oil–based moisturizer (which isn't in the least therapeutic) also contains glycerin along with a cell-communicating ingredient and some silicones. There are omega fatty acid oils in the product, which is good for skin, but they are hardly unique to this product. When this simple ingredient list is added up you end up with a decent moisturizer for dry skin, but from a therapy point of view you would not be getting your money's worth.

☺ **Olive Oil Moisture Cream for Face and Neck** *($26.50 for 2 ounces)*. First-pressed or not, the antioxidant benefits and stability of the olive oil in this moisturizer for dry to very dry skin will be compromised because of jar packaging. That's unfortunate, because otherwise this is an exceptionally emollient formula that contains some good antioxidants and a cell-communicating ingredient.

☺ **Olive Oil Moisture Replenishing Eye Balm** *($19.50 for 0.5 ounce)* is based on a blend of a nonfragrant plant oil and cornstarch, which helps keep things from getting too greasy and likely enhances spreadability. Rather than use this product (the rosemary oil is irritating), however, you can treat areas of very dry skin to plain olive or canola oil from your kitchen cupboard. As is, this product should not be used routinely around the eyes because of the fragrant rosemary oil and because this is just a really boring, ordinary group of ingredients that leave skin wanting so much more.

☺ **$$$ Olive Oil Deep Facial Peel** *($26 for 4 ounces)*. I don't know what to say about this product other than don't bother. This oil-based product is an exceedingly odd combination of ingredients that offer little benefit for skin, and if anything, would end up confusing it. The peeling is supposed to come from the enzyme papain, but papain is an unstable ingredient that definitely won't remain active in this jar packaging. The canola oil and cornstarch base is a strange mixture, the oil being greasy and the cornstarch drying. Those with dry skin would be better off exfoliating with a well-formulated AHA moisturizer and applying plain olive oil to dry areas afterward. Hmmm … I guess I did know what to say about this product after all!

☹ **Olive Oil Hydration Mask** *($24.50 for 2 ounces)*. A facial mask designed for dry skin shouldn't contain clay (bentonite) as a main ingredient, followed by another absorbent ingredient, as this product does. If you're thinking that it must be good for oily skin, you'd be fooled again because the thickeners and plant oils in here aren't going to do that skin type any favors either. Ironically, this ends up being ideal for normal skin, but if your skin is truly normal (meaning no discernible oily or dry areas) you don't need a mask!

☺ **Olive Oil Hydrating Skin Primer** *($24.50 for 1 ounce)* is a good, lightweight moisturizer for normal to dry skin not prone to blemishes. It doesn't feel like most primers designed to be used under makeup (and with other products), but it stands well on its own and in fact does work well under makeup, provided you don't apply too much. Unlike most primers, this contains antioxidants and a cell-communicating ingredient—good news for anyone's skin!

☹ **Olive Oil Replenishing Oil** *($26.50 for 1 ounce)*. Consisting mostly of olive oil, this product also contains skin-irritating rosemary oil. Because of that and the price-per-ounce issue, you're much better off applying plain extra virgin olive oil (or any nonfragrant plant oil) to areas of very dry skin as needed.

SERIOUS SKIN CARE SENSITIVE PRODUCTS

☹ **Glucosamine Skin Resurfacing Cleanser** *($21 for 5 ounces)*. The big deal with this cleanser is that it is supposed to be an acid-free way for those with sensitive skin to exfoliate. That may sound intriguing, but the ingredient in here that is meant to have exfoliating properties, acetyl glucosamine, doesn't have research supporting that benefit, and definitely would not have that benefit in a cleanser where it is rinsed off before it can have an effect. Moreover, the amount of acetyl glucosamine in this cleanser is tiny, so even if it did work as claimed this wouldn't be the product to test out. This cleansing lotion is also not the best option for sensitive skin because it contains sodium lauryl sulfate, a well-known skin irritant. So, not only are the claims over the top, but the formulation is notoriously unacceptable.

☺ **$$$ Glucosamine Phyto-Pumpkin Scrub** *($21 for 2 ounces)*. The acetyl glucosamine in this oil-based topical scrub for dry to very dry skin isn't doing the exfoliating. It does not have this ability, but in a leave-on product it does have water-binding properties for skin. Instead, the sucrose (sugar) is the granular abrasive agent, and it is buffered by several oils. The oils help cushion skin, but they impede rinsing, so you may need to follow with a washcloth (which can also be used in place of any scrub, especially in place of this overpriced mixture).

☺ $$$ **Glucosamine Hydrating Facial Mist** *($18 for 4 ounces)*. Because acetyl glucosamine does not function as an exfoliant, this isn't the toner to choose if your goal is to dissolve dead skin cells. However, it does function as a good water-binding agent, and as such this is a good, though basic, one-note toner for all skin types. Skin needs more than this single ingredient to function optimally.

☹ **Glucosamine Acid-Free Eye Firming Gel** *($19.50 for 0.5 ounce)*. This lightweight, water-based gel is acid-free as claimed, but acetyl glucosamine isn't a reliable stand-in for ingredients like glycolic or salicylic acids. The third ingredient in this jar-packaged gel is *Ceratonia siliqua*, more commonly known as carob. This plant's tannin content is part of what helps it have a tightening (read: firming) effect around the eye, while the mica adds shine for a reflective effect. The tightening from carob is temporary and its tannin content can make it problematic for use around the sensitive eye area, plus it's not good news that this product also contains fragrance.

☺ **Glucosamine Acid-Free Skin Resurfacing Moisturizer** *($22 for 4 ounces)*. Given that this moisturizer for normal to dry skin doesn't contain any exfoliating ingredients, the resurfacing claim is farfetched. This can deliver "immediate hydration," but so can any moisturizer when applied to dry skin, so the urgency behind that claim is not tied to anything unique about this product. Most of the antioxidants are present in amounts too small to matter, though at least it's better than nothing.

☺ **Glucosamine Skin Refining Eye Cream** *($19.50 for 0.5 ounce)*. There is little to get excited about in this moisturizer for normal to dry skin anywhere on the face. The amounts of the mineral pigments mica and titanium dioxide lend a slightly opaque shiny appearance to this cream, and this is what causes the "brightening" effect. The intriguing ingredients don't amount to much, so at best this is a below-average fragrance-free moisturizer.

☺ **Glucosamine Skin Resurfacing Serum** *($26.50 for 1 ounce)*. Even though acetyl glucosamine is the second ingredient in this water-based serum, it cannot resurface skin—at least not in the same manner as using a well-formulated AHA or BHA product. Acetyl glucosamine is similar to the skin-identical ingredient glycosaminoglycans, so it functions as a water-binding agent and can help hold moisture in skin. The pore- and redness-reducing claims aren't in acetyl glucosamine's bag of tricks, but the antioxidants can exert an anti-inflammatory benefit. In the end, this isn't as impressive as serums from Olay or Garnier Nutritioniste, two brands that not only offer better formulas but also cost less.

OTHER SERIOUS SKIN CARE PRODUCTS

☺ $$$ **Glycolic Cleanser** *($21.95 for 4 ounces)* contains a hefty amount of glycolic acid and has a pH low enough to allow exfoliation. However, you're not going to get that benefit unless you leave this on your skin for several minutes. Doing so poses a serious problem for your skin because you never want to leave detergent cleansing agents on your skin for any longer than you have to; ideally, that should be just a few seconds because they can be extremely drying if left on skin longer than necessary. As is, this cleanser is a good option for normal to oily skin, but only if you take care to completely avoid the eye area (due to the low pH and the potential for glycolic acid to get into the eye).

☹ **Buff Polish, Facial Exfoliation Treatment** *($21 for 4 ounces).* This cleanser/scrub hybrid contains several irritating ingredients, including lemon, balm mint, and jasmine oils. It is not recommended.

☹ **Quick Lift, Firming Facial Mist with Argifirm** *($21 for 2 ounces).* The only thing you'll reverse by using this mess of a toner is the care you've taken to not irritate your skin or cause undue inflammation. Coupled with several questionable and gimmicky ingredients are irritating fragrant oils along with sodium polystyrene sulfonate, which is rarely seen in skin-care products (it can be drying and is more typical in firm-hold hairsprays). The locust bean gum is what has a tightening effect on wrinkles, but the effect is temporary and strictly cosmetics trickery, not a "lift" that lasts.

☺ **$$$ Unplugged, Pore Purifying Spray** *($22.50 for 2 ounces)* is a very basic toner that contains a tiny amount of one unusual ingredient, sodium scymnol sulfate. As it turns out, this ingredient is a salt that makes up a portion of the bile excreted by the liver of sharks. Also known as isolutrol, this substance has limited research demonstrating it to be almost as effective as 5% benzoyl peroxide for reducing acne. The comparative study noted that benzoyl peroxide was more effective at reducing non-inflamed acne lesions than isolutrol (Source: *The Australasian Journal of Dermatology*, February 1995, pages 13-15). Although the research isn't extensive, this deserves consideration if you're someone who cannot tolerate benzoyl peroxide yet need a topical disinfectant for acne.

☺ **$$$ Serious Firming Facial Pads** *($32.50 for 60 pads)* contain approximately 8% to 10% glycolic acid at an effective pH to ensure exfoliation. The inclusion of witch hazel rather high on the ingredient list doesn't make this as gentle as many competing AHA products in gel or lotion form, but the potential irritation from it is likely countered by the soothing agents in the formula. The minuscule amounts of amino acids have no effect on skin.

☺ **A-Copper Oil Control Cream with Copper Peptides** *($13 for 2 ounces).* Serious Skin Care offers some of the buzz ingredients the cosmetics industry likes to tout, yet they never combine them in one product. Instead they offer several sub-brands with dozens of formulas, which basically amount to one-note products that are some of the least interesting for skin I've seen in a long time. That's the case with this moisturizer and its copper sulfate, which still has no research proving its benefit for use in skin-care products; however, even if it did have such research to back up the claims, your skin needs lots more state-of-the-art ingredients to keep it healthy. As for the oil control claims, no way! The thickening agents in this moisturizer for normal to dry skin are not capable of controlling oil, but they will make oily skin feel and look oilier. The jar packaging won't help keep the small amount of antioxidants in this product stable during use.

☺ **A-Copper Oil Control Serum with Copper Peptides** *($28.50 for 1 ounce).* This water-based, somewhat sticky-feeling serum contains two forms of copper, yet the lack of research attesting to copper's antiwrinkle prowess means this isn't a serum anyone should choose over others that contain proven ingredients, such as a wide range of antioxidants, skin-identical ingredients, exfoliants, sunscreens, and on and on. Moreover, the inclusion of sodium polystyrene sulfonate (an ingredient found in firm-hold hairspray products) may cause irritation and doesn't have a pleasant after-feel on skin. The remaining ingredients include some novel antioxidants (meaning versions with minimal supporting research), but they don't make up for copper's lack of efficacy or the problematic ingredient. If you still wish to try this serum, it is best for normal to oily skin.

☺ **B-Glow, Vitamin B Moisturizing Complexion Enhancer** *($22.50 for 2 ounces)* is a decent option for normal to dry skin that's looking dull. I'd suggest a tinted moisturizer with sunscreen instead of this product, including one with shine, such as Laura Mercier Illuminating Tinted Moisturizer SPF 20. That's because despite some formulary positives, the jar packaging won't keep the retinol and antioxidant plant oils stable once this is opened. By the way, the B-complex referred to in the claims amounts to only one form of vitamin B (pyridoxine), which is OK, but not worthy of being showcased in the product's name.

☹ **B-Surge** *($12.25 for 1 ounce)*. The invigorating sensation from this water-based serum comes from menthol, and that makes it too irritating for all skin types. What a shame, because this is otherwise an interesting serum for normal to oily skin.

☺ **Calstrum La Creme, Moisture Cream** *($34.50 for 2.6 ounces)*. Serious Skin Care wants women with mature skin (whatever that means—in the case of this product, it translates to dry skin) to believe that calcium and colostrum whey (a protein-based substance secreted by a cow's mammary gland before milk is produced) are what their skin needs. Although colostrum is loaded with nutrients and growth factors, there is no research anywhere proving it makes skin look "younger and more vibrant." (For more information about colostrum please refer to the *Cosmetic Ingredient Dictionary* at www.Beautypedia.com.) The calcium gluconate in this cream does have research showing it to be helpful in healing burns, which makes it a good skin-care adjunct, but it won't make your skin look younger. This moisturizer would be more enticing if it were not packaged in a jar. Because of that, the various antioxidants (none present in a really impressive amount) will break down shortly after you open the jar.

☺ **Calstrum La Creme, Moisture Eye Cream** *($24.50 for 0.5 ounce)*. This eye cream has a silky texture and contains several cell-communicating ingredients, but their stability will likely be compromised because of the jar packaging. Otherwise, the same comments made for the Calstrum La Creme, Moisture Cream above apply here, too.

☺ **Calstrum Intense, Hydrating Restoration and Support Serum** *($28.50 for 1 ounce)*. Those with mature skin, be it dry or oily, should know that there is nothing intense or restorative about this water-based serum. The olive oil provides antioxidant benefit, but only if you take care to keep this translucent-packaged product away from light, which will cause any oil to become rancid over time. The amounts of calcium and colostrum are insignificant, but that's OK because neither is capable of making older skin younger in any way. The most intriguing ingredients in this serum are but a dusting.

☹ **COQ10, Around the Clock Antioxidant Beauty Treatment** *($39.50 for 1.4 ounces)*. The entire concept of this kit is to provide 24-hour antioxidant protection to skin. However, whether you use the **Daytime** or **Nighttime** version, both expose your skin to a damaging amount of alcohol (listed as ethanol in the nighttime version). Talk about counterproductive! Alcohol generates free-radical damage! How foolish is that? Furthermore, in both products, the only antioxidant of note is ubiquinone (coenzyme Q10). If you assume that round-the-clock antioxidant protection is possible, it would take more than one antioxidant to do the job. Also worth mentioning is the skin cell–damaging lavender oil present in the Nighttime version and the fact that the Daytime version doesn't contain sunscreen. This kit is an antiaging joke, with ingredients that cause more problems than they help.

☹ **Correc-Chin, Firming Beauty Cream** *($24 for 1 ounce)*. This moisturizer claims to be the solution for a sagging jawline or less-than-taut profile, thanks to a French anticellulite ingredient. Getting past the nonsense, if this product worked, that would have to mean that cellulite and sagging skin are related, and they aren't. Women with perfectly firm skin and good muscle tone still have cellulite. More to the point, there is nothing in this product that can improve the look of a sagging face or thigh. And the French don't have the answer to cellulite, no one does. Plus this product lists alcohol pretty high up on the ingredient list, and alcohol generates free-radical damage. In truth, a cosmetic corrective procedure or, in pronounced cases, cosmetic surgery, is the only way to treat sagging skin that results from aging. This cream is nothing more than a sham treatment that doesn't deserve your attention.

☺ **C-Primer, Vitamin C Line Filler** *($22.50 for 1 ounce).* If vitamin C is your thing and you want a stabilized serum whose silicone base makes skin feel very silky and helps makeup glide on smoothly, this is recommended. The formula includes skin-identical ceramide as well as a cell-communicating ingredient. Though it could be more interesting with a more diversified formula, as a vitamin C serum at this price point you're definitely getting your money's worth!

☺ **Eye Help, Daily Moisture Eye Cream** *($19.95 for 0.5 ounce).* Other than having a silky-smooth texture, this ordinary, boring eye cream for normal to slightly dry skin doesn't offer much for your skin. The effectiveness of the plant extracts and their antioxidant ability will be squandered once this jar-packaged product is in use. None of the ingredients in this eye cream will promote firmer skin. It is fragrance-free.

☹ **Glyco-Youth Eye Conditioner, SPF 15** *($21 for 0.5 ounce).* This sounds like a convenient product for those looking to combine moisture, sun protection, and exfoliation from AHAs in one product. Sun protection is assured thanks to the pure titanium dioxide active ingredient, but the small amount of glycolic acid and the pH of 4.4 do not permit exfoliation to occur. Consider this a decent daytime moisturizer for normal to slightly dry or slightly oily skin. Most of the bells and whistles are listed after the preservative, and as such don't count for much.

☹ **Glyco-Youth Serum** *($26.50 for 1 ounce).* With some key omissions, this would be a very good AHA serum for all skin types. The pH is within range for exfoliation to occur, but the inclusion of rose and balm mint oils, along with sage extract, makes this too irritating for all skin types. Adding needless irritants to a product certainly isn't the way to help skin look youthful.

☺ **$$$ Hi-Bright with Haloxyl** *($32.50 for 1 ounce)* is merely a good lightweight moisturizer for slightly dry skin anywhere on the face, not an answer for under-eye bags or dark circles. This product's supposedly special ability to treat the eye area is tied to the Haloxyl complex, the trade name for a mixture of ingredients from raw material supplier Sederma. According to Sederma, Haloxyl is supposed to be able to minimize hemoglobin by-products that accumulate in the skin and lead to dark circles. Hemoglobin is the oxygen-carrying pigment in red blood cells. If only it were that simple. The reality, however, is that numerous factors contribute to dark circles, including heredity, allergies, problem veins, skin thickness, sun damage, and inflammation (Source: www.emedicine.com). Hemoglobin by-products aren't much of a factor by comparison, and outside of Sederma's own in vitro studies (meaning the studies weren't done on people), there is no evidence that Haloxyl complex is the fix that those with dark circles have been waiting for. Although this isn't going to lighten dark circles or send under-eye bags packing, it is still a decent moisturizer, and it is fragrance-free. The mica adds a soft shine to skin.

☺ **$$$ Ice Age Wrinkle Cream** *($34.50 for 1 ounce)* is not going to do anything special for wrinkles, frown lines, dark circles, or discolored skin. If it really were that wondrous, why would Serious Skin Care need to sell so many other antiwrinkle products? It is discouraging, but also empowering, to realize this is just a standard moisturizer for normal to dry skin. It contains several antioxidants, but their efficacy will begin to degrade once this jar-packaged product is opened. The fragrance chemical eugenol poses a slight risk of irritation.

☺ **Line Redefine Correcting Concentrate for Lip Lines** *($17.50 for 0.33 ounce)*. There is no really line-correcting activity taking place with this faux line-filling product. Estee Lauder, M.A.C., and Good Skin (sold at Kohl's) offer similar products with better formulas, at least in terms of giving your skin more than just thick-textured but lightweight, powder-finish silicones.

☺ **$$$ Nanofill Topical Collagen** *($27 for 0.5 ounce)* is supposed to be the answer to getting collagen into skin because Serious Skin Care claims to have made the collagen molecule very small via nanotechnology. OK, so let's assume they're right and that the hydrolyzed collagen molecules in this product really are able to penetrate the skin. Does that mean they'll seek out and attach to your skin's own supply of collagen? No, of course not; but there are lots of consumers who will likely make that association. In contrast, the purified, highly concentrated collagen (whether animal sourced or bioengineered) used for injections is a relatively thick gel that is injected just under the wrinkle, filling it out. Over time, this collagen breaks down, and then you must have another injection. So, even if nanosized collagen were being used in this product (which it isn't), it won't bind to the collagen in your skin; even the collagen fillers don't do that. And keep in mind how small nanosized particles are—if Serious Skin Care is really using such small particles of collagen, there's not much to stop them from penetrating where you don't want them to go (which is one of the reasons nanotechnology in cosmetics is controversial). By the way, the ingredient *Pseudoalternomonas* ferment extract is a form of bacterium sold by cosmetic ingredient supplier Lipotec. According to the company, this bacterium has an amazing ability to increase skin's collagen production. If that were true, then presumably Serious Skin Care wouldn't need to tout their nanosized collagen molecules because the bacteria would go to work and super-stimulate skin to produce more collagen to fill lines. Of course, there is no published, peer-reviewed research supporting the claims for *Pseudoalteromonas* ferment, just Lipotec's unduplicated studies (as you might expect, Lipotec's study of its own product will show results that are nothing short of miraculous). In the end, this is a good fragrance-free moisturizer for normal to slightly dry skin not prone to blemishes, and it can be used around the eyes.

☹ **No. 8 By SSC, Facial Beauty Serum** *($21 for 1 ounce)* is supposed to be all about antiaging antioxidants, but it contains so few of them that the hype for the product is almost laughable. What you do get is some good water-binding agents and cell-communicating ingredients, but those looking for an antioxidant boost will be disappointed. As a reminder, peptides can be helpful ingredients for skin (though there is no conclusive research about this yet, plus it is very difficult for peptides to remain stable as they penetrate the layers of skin), but they're neither youth-restoring nor wrinkle-preventing as often claimed.

☹ **Reverse Lift, Firming Facial Cream with Argifirm** *($29.95 for 2 ounces)*. This jar-packaged moisturizer for normal to dry skin contains the works-like-Botox ingredient argiline. Please refer to the *Cosmetic Ingredient Dictionary* on the Home page of www.Beautypedia.com for details on this ingredient. Suffice it to say, argiline does not work like Botox or have remarkable wrinkle-reducing ability. This product is not recommended because it contains menthol, which is irritating for skin.

☹ **Reverse Serum, Firming Facial Serum with Argifirm** *($26.50 for 1 ounce)*. Incapable of lifting or firming skin, this serum will cause irritation due to some problematic plant extracts along with camphor, menthol, and the potent menthol derivative menthoxypropanediol. The redeeming ingredients are so few and far between, it's impossible to recommend this serum.

☹ **Rulinea-FX Topical Aging Skin Regenerating Cream** *($32.50 for 2 ounces)*. The power of penetrating botanicals is said to be at the heart of this moisturizer's formula, but although it does contain several helpful plant ingredients with documented evidence of their benefit for skin, the inclusion of peppermint oil (which doesn't have a regenerating effect on skin) is a major strike against it. Without the peppermint oil, this would've been one of Serious Skin Care's better moisturizing formulas.

☺ **Rulinea-FX Topical Intensive Wrinkle Serum** *($29.50 for 1 ounce)* is a very good anti-oxidant serum for all skin types. It contains an impressive amount of the cell-communicating ingredient niacinamide, which offers multiple benefits to skin, including barrier repair. It is not rated a Paula's Pick because several of the good-for-skin ingredients are listed after the preservative; for a product at this price point, you want to see as much of the good stuff up front as possible. The skin tightener referred to in the claims is likely the film-forming agent glyceryl polymethacrylate, which is included in many serums and moisturizers for its smoothing ability.

☺ **Rulinea-FX Topical Regenerating Eye Cream for Aging Skin** *($21.25 for 0.65 ounce)* is yet another eye cream from a line that already has too many eye-area options. If any of them worked as claimed, why would they keep offering more, all with similar line-diminishing claims? Overall, this product's formula is very similar to the company's Rulinea-FX Topical Aging Skin Regenerating Cream above, except with this version you get less product and it does not contain peppermint oil. Overall, this is an impressive moisturizer for dry skin anywhere on the face. Some of the plant extracts pose a slight risk of irritation, but the amounts of these potential irritants are likely too small to matter.

☹ **$$$ Skincandescence, Illuminating Skin Serum** *($44.50 for 1 ounce)*. This water- and olive oil-based moisturizer contains a small amount of arbutin, a plant ingredient whose hydroquinone content has skin-lightening ability, though likely not when present in such a small amount as in this product. Another ingredient, diacetyl boldine, is said to disrupt the activation phase of the melanin production process (remember, melanin is the pigment that darkens skin cells). Diacetyl boldine appears to have antioxidant ability, but there is no independent, peer-reviewed research supporting the claim that it can suppress melanin production. Although you shouldn't rely on this serum for lightening skin imperfections, it is an OK option as a moisturizer for dry skin. The inclusion of BHT as an antioxidant preservative is not cause for concern, not only because only a small amount is present but also because BHT's link to being a carcinogen has to do with oral consumption (it is used in many foods to prevent spoilage) rather than with topical application.

☺ **Squalane 99, 99% Pure Olive Squalane** *($29.50 for 1 ounce)* is almost 100% squalane, an emollient derived from olives or sharks (in this case, it appears to be from olives). The sea buckthorn oil offers antioxidant benefit, while the fragrance is extraneous. Squalane is a good ingredient for dry to very dry skin, but not one you want to use to the exclusion of others or of more well-rounded products that offer skin a variety of benefits. If you do want a single-note product, pure extra virgin olive oil from the grocery would work as well, and for far less money.

☺ **$$$ Super Creamerum** *($55 for 0.5 ounce)*. No question that this product is designed to be a cross between a cream and a serum, but how does the formula stack up? For the most part, quite well. The glycol-based product (which has a more serum-like texture than moisturizer texture) applies smoothly and treats your skin to an impressive amount of alpha lipoic acid (listed as thioctic acid) and lesser amounts of other antioxidants along with some cell-communicating ingredients. The amount of glycolic acid is too low for it to function as an exfoliant, but it will function as a water-binding agent. I wouldn't be concerned about the amount of alcohol in this product either, though I would have preferred to see it even lower on the ingredient list. This is a suitable, yet pricey, serum option for normal to oily skin.

☺ $$$ **Super Eye Creamerum** *($44.50 for 0.5 ounce)* isn't as impressive as Serious Skin Care's Super Creamerum and there is no reason you can't use that product around the eyes. Almost all of the really intriguing ingredients are listed after the preservative, though you are getting some peptides that theoretically have cell-communicating ability. The bismuth oxychloride functions as a thickening and opacifying agent, while also lending a subtle brightening effect to the eye area (the effect is strictly cosmetic). Normal to dry skin will do best with this product, though again, it isn't as impressive or as "super" as it could have been.

☺ **SuperMel C, An Antioxidant Rich Beauty Cream** *($39.50 for 1.7 ounces)*. You can forget about getting much antioxidant benefit from using this product because the jar packaging will routinely expose it to degrading light and air. The meager amounts of antioxidant included in this product make it all the more disheartening. By the way, just because the antioxidants in this product are encapsulated does not mean they are impervious to light and air. Most ingredient encapsulations use a lipid (fat) membrane, and the lipids are prone to oxidation, too.

☺ **SuperMel C, An Antioxidant Rich Eye Cream** *($24.50 for 0.5 ounce)* is nearly identical to the SuperMel C, An Antioxidant Rich Beauty Cream above, and the same comments apply. The melon extract, present in an extremely small amount, contains superoxide dismutase as one of its constituents, but in this small amount, so what?

☺ **SuperMel C, An Antioxidant Skin Beauty Cocktail** *($18.25 for 1 ounce)* is a product that is supposed to be an antioxidant powerhouse, but ends up falling a bit flat. The olive and sunflower seed oils have antioxidant ability and the packaging will keep these oils stable during use; however, this product does not contain superoxide dismutase as claimed. Even if it is encapsulated, as the label states, it would still have to be listed on the ingredient statement, and it isn't. Despite this omission, it is worth noting that a constituent of the melon extract in this product is superoxide dismutase (Source: *Journal of Agricultural and Food Chemistry*, May 2008, pages 3694-3698), but the amount of melon extract is next to nothing, which makes its ability to impart the beneficial component to skin at best remote. This is a relatively unexciting overly hyped moisturizer for dry skin.

☹ **Total Youth Recall, All Over Facial Firmer** *($44.50 for 1.7 ounces)* is primarily a blend of water with acrylate-based film-forming agents (think hairspray) along with drying, irritating, free-radical-generating alcohol. There is no redeeming quality to this product whatsoever.

☹ **Bi-Layer Facial Lift** *($44.50)*. The **Serum** is a very good, fragrance-free, silky-finish option for all skin types, including sensitive. You're supposed to apply this to clean skin, allow it to dry, and follow with a layer of the **Sealing Mask**. The mask is a standard, alcohol-based peel-off mask that will do nothing but irritate your skin. You're directed to let the mask dry, then peel it off, taking the remnants of the serum with it. So, in summary, one product in this pair is recommended, while the other is not (using a peel-off mask isn't going to lift sagging facial skin any more than using Scotch tape to prevent expression lines from forming is the same as getting Botox injections). You may think the relatively low cost would merit purchasing just to use the serum, except that you can find similar (and better) serums from Olay for half the cost of this kit.

☹ **Ice Age Full Lip Service** *($22.50 for 0.2 ounce)*. This viscous, sticky lip gloss is sold as having line-filling and lip-plumping abilities, yet the only plumping that occurs comes from the irritating menthol in this product. So much for this being a treat for lips! Other than containing a peptide with no proven lip-enhancing traits, this isn't too far removed from standard lip gloss with menthol, so the price is approaching ridiculous.

☺ **Glycolic 3, Cleansing, Exfoliating and Tightening Mask** *($19.50 for 5 ounces)*. The tiny amount of glycolic acid in this mask isn't going to exfoliate skin, so this mask is best as a standard absorbent product for oily skin. It contains some good plant soothing agents, though the witch hazel distillate can make this more drying than other clay masks because witch hazel is mostly alcohol.

☺ **Reverse Facial, Five Minute Firming Mask** *($22.50 for 2 ounces)*. It would be great if this standard clay mask could firm and lift skin, but it absolutely cannot. All you can expect is oil absorption and a slight tight feeling after rinsing (but that isn't related to skin being firmed or lifted in any way). The aluminum chlorohydrate (the main ingredient in most deodorants) makes this clay mask extra-drying, and it is advised only for oily to very oily skin.

☺ **Reverse HD, High Definition Diffuser with Argifirm** *($24.50 for 1 ounce)* is a silicone-heavy serum that contains shimmer pigments to add a glow to skin. The effect isn't necessarily soft-focus, but this can be considered a good primer-type product to use pre-makeup. It contains a few bells and whistles for skin, but nothing that elevates it to must-have status, particularly because there are other antioxidant-rich serums available that have a finish similar to the finish of this product, so they also work well under makeup.

☹ **Serious Conceal Acne Treatment Pen** *($19.50 for 0.05 ounce)* contains 10% sulfur, a potent amount of this antibacterial agent. There is definitely research showing sulfur has a positive effect on acne, but not in comparison to benzoyl peroxide. Plus, sulfur can be irritating, especially at this concentration. In addition, research indicates that sulfur works better when paired with salicylic acid (BHA) (Source: *Journal of Drugs in Dermatology*, July-August 2004, pages 427-431). What is most problematic about this formula is the amount of thickeners, titanium dioxide, and zinc oxide it contains, which could potentially clog pores. There are far better options to consider than this product.

SHEER COVER

SHEER COVER AT-A-GLANCE

Strengths: One well-formulated toner; the mineral foundations (particularly the pressed version) are a cut above most others; surprisingly good powder eyeshadow set; Guthy-Renker has an excellent return policy.

Weaknesses: Mostly unimpressive skin care, including a sunscreen that leaves skin vulnerable to UVA damage; poor concealer; average mascara.

For more information about Sheer Cover, call (800) 506-6281 or visit www.sheercover.com or www.Beautypedia.com.

SHEER COVER SKIN CARE

☺ **$$$ Conditioning Cleanser** *($23.95 for 4 ounces)* is a water-soluble cleansing lotion that's best for normal to dry skin not prone to blemishes. It produces a slight lather and leaves skin feeling very smooth. This would be rated a Paula's Pick if it did not contain fragrance chemicals that pose a risk of irritation.

☺ **$$$ Purifying Cleanser** *($20.95 for 4 ounces)* is a lightweight, water-soluble cleansing lotion that contains a tiny amount of detergent cleansing agent. The main issue with this cleanser is that it doesn't remove the Sheer Cover Mineral Foundation (reviewed below) very well. This fragrance-free cleanser is best for someone with normal to dry skin who wears minimal to no makeup.

☺ **$$$ Refreshing Face Mist** *($22.95 for 2 ounces)* is a spray-on, alcohol-free toner that is suitable for normal to dry skin. It contains several good water-binding agents and also has some vitamin-based antioxidants, but the clear bottle packaging won't keep them stable for long. This does contain fragrance. The instructional DVD and how-to guide for Sheer Cover recommends misting this toner over your Mineral Foundation, but doing so encourages streaking and can make the color look a bit blotchy, necessitating more blending.

☺ **$$$ Soothing Mineral Toner** *($22.95 for 4 ounces)* does contain minerals, but none of them have substantiated proof that they can encourage collagen production to create firmer skin. Beyond the water and minerals in this toner, there are a few plant extracts and soothing agents, as well as minuscule amounts of witch hazel and alcohol. You're not getting a lot of bang for your buck here, but this fragranced toner is an OK option for all skin types.

☹ **Nourishing Moisturizer SPF 15** *($30.95 for 2 ounces)* does not contain the UVA-protecting ingredients of titanium dioxide, zinc oxide, avobenzone, Mexoryl SX, or Tinosorb, and has a boring water- and wax-based formula, making it a poor choice all around.

SHEER COVER MAKEUP

FOUNDATION: ☺ **$$$ Mineral Foundation SPF 15** *($29.95)* is the core product of the Sheer Cover line. It's a fragrance-free loose powder whose primary ingredient is zinc oxide, which lends opacity and allows a small amount of product to provide sufficient coverage, not to mention providing broad-spectrum sun protection (though if you brush a sheer layer on skin you won't be getting the amount of sun protection advertised, which is why foundations like this are best paired with a daytime moisturizer rated SPF 15 or greater).

The good news is that, texture-wise, this is one of the most finely milled mineral foundations I've reviewed. That makes it look more natural on skin, though it can still look a bit thick and opaque unless applied sheer.

The bad news (though it may not be bad, depending on your preference) is the amount of shine each shade leaves behind. Unlike other mineral makeups whose shine casts an all-over radiant glow, Sheer Cover's version makes skin look sparkly, which is distracting for daytime wear and definitely calls attention to the fact that you're wearing makeup. Eight shades are available and segmented into four kits (Light, Medium, Tan, and Dark). The idea is to blend the shades in each kit to achieve a perfect match, though this won't work for everyone and the process is anything but tidy. The Almond shade in the Dark kit tends to turn peach over oily areas, while the Nude shade in the Light kit tends to go on too pink (Bisque is much better).

In summary, the Mineral Foundation from Sheer Cover has the same basic traits as most mineral makeup. It can provide full coverage (which will conceal redness from rosacea) and leaves a slightly thick, dry matte finish that is laced with shine. It wears quite well except over very oily areas. Unless the oil-prone areas are set with powder (a step Sheer Cover recommends), you'll notice the color getting darker as the day goes on, or the foundation pooling in pores, neither of which is attractive. Sheer Cover's point of distinction (and the reason to consider it if you can tolerate the clingy sparkles) is a finer texture that blends very well and lends itself to a more natural look—about as natural as this type of foundation can appear on skin, which is a step in the right direction!

As for the antioxidants this contains, they won't remain stable thanks to this product's clear jar packaging. I wouldn't rely on the antioxidants in this loose powder makeup to keep my skin looking younger, that's for sure! Still, this simple formula can be helpful for those with sensitive or rosacea-affected skin.

☺ $$$ **Pressed Mineral Foundation SPF 12** *($29.95)* is a smoother, neater way to experiment with mineral makeup, though the composition of this talc-free, pressed-powder foundation is not akin to traditional mineral makeup. This has a beautiful soft, dry texture that blends very well and leaves skin with a subtle glow, courtesy of mica and boron nitride, a texture enhancer. Coverage goes from sheer (if applied with a brush) to medium (if used with a sponge) and does not look too thick, powdery, or heavy on skin, though like most powder foundations it will magnify dry areas. All five shades are excellent, and there are options for light to dark (but not very dark) skin tones. The sunscreen is pure zinc oxide, though an SPF 15 rating would've been better (and it's what keeps this from earning a Paula's Pick). Unless you need significant camouflage, consider spending your Sheer Cover dollars on this product instead of their loose Mineral Foundation.

CONCEALER: ☺ $$$ **Conceal and Brighten Trio** *($31.95)* provides two cream concealers and a creamy highlighter (to "brighten" skin) in one sleek compact. Each has a smooth texture and blends quite well while providing moderate coverage. Because the finish stays creamy, these are prone to creasing unless set with powder. Although the finish isn't as skin-like as today's best concealers, this is an option if you need to mix shades and want the addition of a highlighter for key areas.

☹ **Duo Concealer** *($24.95)* has a creamy-slick texture that slips over skin easily, but it just keeps slipping. Because this surprisingly lightweight concealer never sets, creasing and fading are inevitable, even when set with powder. It also doesn't provide much coverage, as is evidenced by watching the women in the Sheer Cover how-to DVD apply it. Most of the shades are quite good (and blend well together), but the aforementioned drawbacks still make this a concealer to ignore.

POWDER: ☺ **Finishing Powder** *($23.95)* is a talc-free loose powder with a weightless texture and a soft, dry finish. This product is included in the Sheer Cover Intro Kit, and is recommended for use after applying the Mineral Foundation (I know, it's odd that you need to set a powder with another powder, but whether this works for you is a personal preference, not a must-have). Three shades are available, all of which apply very sheer, leaving skin matte but dusted with a fine layer of sparkles.

BLUSH AND BRONZER: ✓ ☺ $$$ **Mousse Blush** *($24.95)* is an outstanding cream-to-powder blush that has a whipped mousse texture. Just a dab provides a soft wash of color with a shimmer finish that's great for evening or "beach-y" makeup. This looks beautiful dabbed over a bronzing powder for added color and dimension. Both shades are beautiful and best for fair to medium skin tones. Maybelline and Rimmel sell less expensive versions of this product, but Sheer Cover devotees won't be disappointed.

☺ $$$ **Lip-to-Lid Highlighter** *($22.95)* is a mica-based, shiny loose powder available in a pink shade for blush or a tan shade for bronzing, contouring, or use as eyeshadow. Both shades leave skin quite shiny, but not ultra-sparkling, making this a good choice for evening glamour. The shine clings well and the effect from either shade is pretty if applied sparingly. Using this on the lips is another story, however, because you have to combine it with a lip balm so it feels comfortable, and doing so isn't as easy or nice looking as just using a regular lipstick or lip gloss.

☺ **$$$ Pressed Mineral Blush Duo** *($31.95)* is an expensive powder blush that includes two tone-on-tone colors in one compact without a divider between the shades. Best swirled together with your brush, this Duo goes on sheer and provides equal parts color and soft shine. The main ingredients are minerals (well, at least partially) but the irony is the texture isn't as smooth and seamless as powder blushes made with talc. Talc is also a mineral but one most mineral makeup lines characterize (unjustly) as a problem for skin. Both shades in this duo are also sold separately as **Pressed Mineral Blush** for the same price as the Duo.

EYESHADOW: ☺ **$$$ Eye Collection** *($39.95)* provides six pressed-powder eyeshadows in one compact. Each shade has a soft to moderate shimmer, but they apply smoothly, don't flake, and impart soft color that can build to a deeper hue. Only one medium shade is included, leaving you with five colors best for lids or under-brow. With a slightly more thoughtful shade assortment this would have been a Paula's Pick.

☺ **$$$ Single Eyeshadow** *($19.95)* shares the same characteristics as the powder eyeshadows in Sheer Cover's Eye Collection above, which is good news. All of the shades are worthwhile, though you have to be OK with each having some degree of shine.

EYE AND BROW SHAPER: ☹ **$$$ Defining Mineral Eye Liner** *($21.95)* is a standard eye pencil that needs routine sharpening and comes equipped with a pointed sponge tip to smudge or soften the line. You'll want to use the smudge tip before this pencil smudges on its own, which will happen due to the soft cream finish. The color range is attractive.

☹ **$$$ Eye Enhancer Pencil** *($24.95)* is a dual-sided chunky pencil that requires sharpening to maintain a usable tip. One end is a very pale lavender eyeliner that is meant to give eyes a wide-awake look but ends up looking eerie instead. The other end is very pale gold shade with shimmer, and it's designed to be used to highlight the brow bone. This is more gimmicky than helpful, though the pale gold shade works OK to highlight the under-brow area (a powder eyeshadow lasts longer).

☹ **$$$ Cream Eyeliner** *($16.95)* comes in a pot and suffers from an application that's too sheer and creamy. This takes longer to set than most other the cream-gel eyeliners, and once it does the finish is still prone to minor smearing and fading. This just isn't in the same league as the long-wearing eyeliners from L'Oreal, Bobbi Brown, M.A.C., and several others.

☹ **$$$ Cream Eyeliner Quad** *($45.95)* offers four shades of Sheer Cover's Cream Eyeliner in one large compact. Although the laced-with-shine colors are pretty to look at, the performance of these liners isn't on par with today's best long-wearing gel-cream eyeliners.

LIP GLOSS AND LIPLINER: ☺ **$$$ Lip Collection** *($31.95)* comes complete with six sheer, sparkling lip glosses in one compact. The tiny brush applicator isn't helpful and should be discarded. Otherwise, as far as lip gloss goes, each shade has a smooth texture and a wet shine finish, and is minimally sticky. This is pricey for what you get, but if you're looking to splurge on sheer lip gloss it won't disappoint.

☹ **$$$ Defining Lip Liner** *($21.95)* needs sharpening and is priced outlandishly, but it happens to be a good, slightly creamy lip pencil that applies well and stays in place. Only two shades are available, but they work with a variety of lipstick colors.

☹ **Lip Gloss Pot** *($13.95)* is a sheer lip gloss that feels smooth and emollient, and doesn't leave a trace of stickiness. It is rated with a neutral face because of the waxy smell and taste. Hundreds of lip glosses don't suffer from this trait, so there's no need to seriously consider this one, plus it leaves a residual minty tingle that isn't good news for lips.

☹ **Lipgloss Collection** *($31.95)* provides six shades of lip gloss and a lip brush in one mirrored compact. Unfortunately the gloss is the same formula as Sheer Cover's Lip Gloss Pot above, which means you have to tolerate a waxy smell and taste, plus the peppermint kick, which causes irritation.

MASCARA: ☺ **$$$ Extra Length Mascara** *($19.95)* is a minimalist mascara that does nothing but make lashes look darker and a bit more separated. Yes, it is misnamed, but this may be worth a try if you're pleased with your lashes in their natural state and just want to darken them.

BRUSHES: Sheer Cover's ☺ **Brushes** *($17.95–$39.95)* are a mostly average assortment of tools that don't measure up to brushes from department-store lines, particularly those fronted by makeup artists. The shapes and density are mostly good, but the brush hair quality isn't as silky-soft as it should be. As a result, several brushes, such as the ☺ **Kabuki Brush** *($25.95)* and ☺ **On-The-Go-Brush** *($25.95)* just aren't that pleasant to use. Believe me, if you used high-quality brushes (and there are several in this price range), the difference is obvious. The best brushes to consider are the dual-sided options, which include ☺ **Dual-End Eyeshadow/ Eyeliner Brush** *($27.95)*, ☺ **Double End Eyeliner Brush** *($27.95)*, and ☺ **Dual-End Shadow Brush** *($27.95)*.

☺ **$$$ Deluxe Mini Brush Set** *($59.95)* includes four dual-sided brushes, so you're essentially getting the capability of eight brushes, all packaged in a black carrying case. The brushes are mostly for eyeshadow design, filling in brows, and eyelining, but all are workable. This is on the pricey side for what you get, but is still worth considering if you already have good powder and blush brushes but need better eyeshadow brushes.

☹ **$$$ Travel Brush Set** *($59.95)* is way overpriced for the average brushes it contains. Even at the Sheer Cover Member price, these are still not recommended over most other brush sets. The Sponge Applicator brush is a terrible way to apply eyeshadows, and the other brushes in this set simply aren't the epitome professional (and at this price, they should be).

FACE AND BODY SHIMMER/ILLUMINATING PRODUCTS: ☺ **$$$ Highlighting Corrector Pen** *($25)* is too sheer to correct anything, but this liquid highlighter, which is dispensed onto a brush applicator, is a very good way to add long-lasting sheer shimmer to skin. The nearly translucent result casts a pale golden peach glow to skin. This is way too sheer to cover dark circles, but can be dabbed over your regular concealer to brighten the under-eye area further.

☺ **Cream Highlighter** *($13.95)* feels (and smells) more waxy than creamy, and doesn't have much slip on skin. The low slip factor could be viewed as a plus when you want to highlight key areas. As for the finish, it also feels waxy and the shine is of the sparkling variety rather than being a radiant glow.

☺ **Cream Highlighter Trio** *($13.95)* offers three smaller versions of the Cream Highlighter above, packaged in one sleek compact. The shades are identical to what's sold singly, and the same comments made above apply here, too.

SPECIALTY PRODUCTS: ☺ **$$$ Base Perfector** *($29.95 for 0.5 ounce)* is a mixed bag of positives and negatives. This nonaqueous, silicone-based gel leaves skin feeling very smooth, and it feels nearly weightless. Green tea, vitamin E, and vitamin A are on hand as antioxidants, but the fragrance and fragrant extracts basically cancel out their benefit. This is a decent option if you're looking for a foundation primer, but it is not as matte as many others, so isn't ideal for very oily skin.

☺ **$$$ Sheer Cover Intro Kit** *($29.95)*. Most customers who order Sheer Cover take advantage of the Sheer Cover Intro Kit, which allows you to sign up for an automatic replenishment program that bills your credit card the same amount each month. I wouldn't recommend doing that until you're sure you like the products (based on the small sizes, you would need to replenish most of the products monthly anyway). Included in the kit are two shades of the **Mineral Foundation**, **Duo Concealer**, **Finishing Powder**, a sponge applicator, two brushes, and smaller sizes of the **Conditioning Cleanser** and **Nourishing Moisturizer SPF 15**. Aside from the skin-care products, the color items in this kit are reviewed because they are also sold separately, and the kit's overall neutral face rating was based on the mixed-bag nature of the products it contains.

SHISEIDO

SHISEIDO AT-A-GLANCE

Strengths: Most of the sunscreens provide sufficient UVA protection and present a variety of options, whether you're looking for titanium dioxide, zinc oxide, or avobenzone; a handful of good (but not great) moisturizers; an excellent sunscreen for lips; worthwhile oil-blotting papers; every foundation with sunscreen provides sufficient UVA protection (and there are some wonderful foundations here); pressed powder with sunscreen for oily skin; the unique Hydro Powder Eye Shadow; Perfecting Lipstick is one of the best creamy lipsticks at the department store; mostly good mascaras; all of the Veil products are worth considering.

Weaknesses: Expensive; several drying cleansers; boring toners; a few sunscreens offer insufficient UVA protection; no AHA or BHA products; no products to effectively manage acne; no reliable skin-lightening options despite a preponderance of products claiming to do just that; irritating self-tanners; gimmicky masks; jar packaging; uneven assortment of concealers (and some terrible colors); the eyeshadow quads; average to disappointing eye and brow shapers; average makeup brushes.

For more information about Shiseido visit www.sca.shiseido.com or www.Beautypedia.com.

SHISEIDO SKIN CARE

SHISEIDO BENEFIANCE PRODUCTS

☺ **$$$ Benefiance Creamy Cleansing Emulsion** *($34 for 6.7 ounces)* is a very standard, water- and oil-based cleansing cream for dry to very dry skin. This is essentially glorified cold cream, and although it removes makeup in a flash, you'll need a washcloth to avoid the greasy residue it leaves behind.

☹ **$$$ Benefiance Creamy Cleansing Foam** *($34 for 4.4 ounces)* is a foaming, creamy-textured, water-soluble cleanser that contains alkaline cleansing agents capable of causing dryness for most skin types.

☺ **$$$ Benefiance Balancing Softener** *($42 for 5 ounces)* won't balance anything and is nothing more than a basic, alcohol-free toner for normal to dry skin. It contains mostly water, glycerin, slip agents, thickeners, a water-binding agent, preservatives, fragrance, a cell-communicating ingredient, and coloring agents.

☹ **$$$ Benefiance Enriched Balancing Softener** *($42 for 5 ounces)* is similar to the Benefiance Balancing Softener above, but is less interesting because most of the helpful ingredients are listed after the preservative. That's really disappointing considering this toner's cost.

☺ **$$$ Benefiance Concentrated Neck Contour Treatment** *($50 for 1.8 ounces)* is primarily a blend of water, silicones, and slip agents along with film-forming agents and some antioxidants, none of which are specific to the neck area. This serum-like product also contains potentially irritating ingredients, although the small amounts means they are likely inconsequential. This product has no hope of making lines on the neck a thing of the past, and there are products from other lines that are better formulated than this gaffe.

☹ **$$$ Benefiance NutriPerfect Eye Serum** *($75 for 0.5 ounce)* claims to counteract hormonal changes that cause skin to look aged, but the infusion of nutrients in this serum absolutely cannot do that. Hormonal changes that take their toll on skin must be addressed medically, not with cosmetics. It is very disappointing that this product contains not only fragrance but also several fragrance chemicals known to cause skin irritation, which causes collagen to breakdown. What are those doing in a product meant to be used around the eyes?! The sole intriguing ingredient in this serum is carnosine, an amino acid that has anti-inflammatory and antioxidant properties, but these potentially positive effects are muted by the inclusion of denatured alcohol. For the money, this serum should've been significantly better, and it definitely won't make good on its claims to restore youthful vitality to aging eye-area skin.

☹ **$$$ Benefiance Concentrated Anti-Wrinkle Eye Cream** *($50 for 0.51 ounce)* has a thick, lush texture tailor-made for dry skin anywhere on the face, and contains some tried-and-true emollients. A nice selection of antioxidants is on hand, too, but the jar packaging won't keep them stable during use, which knocks this product's rating down.

☹ **Benefiance Daytime Protective Cream SPF 15** *($46 for 1.3 ounces)* not only leaves skin vulnerable to UVA damage because its sole active ingredient does not cover the full spectrum of UVA light, but the base formula is terribly boring for the money. Plus it is packaged in a jar, so the few antioxidants it does contain won't be around for long.

☹ **Benefiance Daytime Protective Emulsion SPF 15** *($46 for 2.5 ounces)* is an even worse formula compared to the Benefiance Daytime Protective Cream SPF 15 above, and does not deserve even a second's worth of thought.

☹ **Benefiance Energizing Essence** *($55 for 1 ounce)* cannot energize skin, but it contains enough alcohol to cause irritation. Another concern is the inclusion of tranexamic acid. This synthetic ingredient is a drug used to control bleeding during surgical procedures, and it has no purpose or business being in a skin-care product (Sources: www.drugs.com; and *The Journal of Thoracic and Cardiovascular Surgery*, September 2000, pages 520-527).

☹ **Benefiance NutriPerfect Day Cream SPF 15 Sunscreen** *($88 for 1.7 ounces)* lacks the UVA-protecting ingredients of titanium dioxide, zinc oxide, avobenzone, Tinosorb, or Mexoryl SX and is not recommended. The cell-communicating ingredient carnosine and the few antioxidants in this formula will soon become useless due to the jar packaging, making this product an expensive mistake for its target audience of women age 50 and older.

☺ **$$$ Benefiance NutriPerfect Night Cream** *($92 for 1.7 ounces)* is Shiseido's answer for women dealing with skin changes that occur during and after menopause. With claims talking about restoring skin's density, renewing its vitality, and strengthening skin weakened by hormonal shifts, this is truly a disappointing and vastly overpriced moisturizer. Other than the addition of carnosine, this differs little from the dozens of other emollient moisturizers for normal to dry skin Shiseido sells. Carnosine is composed of amino acids and has benefit as an antiaging ingredient for skin because of its antiglycation properties, but it is not a superior ingredient to address the many skin changes that occur during and after menopause. For example, it cannot stop skin sagging from loss of estrogen, cannot stimulate collagen production, and cannot correct decreased oil gland functioning that leads to dry skin (Sources: *Pathologie Biologie*, September 2006, pages 396-404; and *Life Sciences*, March 2002, pages 1789-1799). The amount of fragrance, relaxing or not, is greater than the amount of vitamin-based antioxidants, but those won't last long once the product is opened because the jar packaging won't keep them stable.

☺ **$$$ Benefiance Revitalizing Cream** *($49 for 1.3 ounces)* is a relatively standard moisturizer for normal to dry skin, and is definitely overpriced for what you get. The tiny amount of antioxidants will break down shortly after this jar-packaged product is opened.

☺ **$$$ Benefiance Revitalizing Emulsion** *($49 for 2.5 ounces)* is similar to the Benefiance Revitalizing Cream above, but in better packaging and with a greater amount of antioxidants. It is recommended for normal to dry skin.

☺ **$$$ Benefiance Wrinkle Lifting Concentrate** *($63 for 1 ounce)* is sold with the promise of, what else, lifting wrinkles. But Shiseido goes on to claim that this product allows skin to resist future wrinkles, something that's not possible without an effective sunscreen, which is absent here. The showcased ingredient in this product is chlorella extract. According to Shiseido, this reinforces the presence of a protein in skin that's critical to halting the wrinkling process. But none of that is substantiated, and even if it were, there's so little chlorella that your wrinkles wouldn't even notice. Chlorella is an algae and, like almost all species of algae, can act as a water-binding agent and antioxidant on skin. A good question for Shiseido: If this ingredient is that important for stopping wrinkles, why isn't it in every "antiwrinkle" product this line sells? This product is chiefly a lightweight moisturizer that contains more alcohol than it does beneficial ingredients for skin. Several antioxidants appear, but they're of little use when combined with the potentially drying and irritating effect of the alcohol and the lack of sunscreen. At best, this is a substandard moisturizer for slightly dry skin that has no positive effect on wrinkles—either past, present, or future.

☺ **$$$ Benefiance Eye Treatment Mask** *($39 for 10 pairs)* seems like a specially targeted product, but it isn't. Although it contains some helpful ingredients for skin, the exciting ones are but a dusting, while the amount of acrylate-based film-forming agent may cause irritation around the eyes. Nothing in this mask solution can treat dark circles.

☹ **Benefiance Firming Massage Mask** *($45 for 1.9 ounces)* contains tranexamic acid, a synthetic drug that has no proven purpose in a skin-care product. One study that involved applying a 2%-3% concentration of the drug to guinea pig skin indicated severely reduced melanin formation resulting from concentrated UV exposure (Source: *Journal of Photochemistry and Photobiology*, December 1998, pages 136-141). In contrast, another study showed that topical applications of vitamin E (as alpha tocopherol) and ferulic acid (another antioxidant) were more effective at inhibiting melanin production than a higher dose of tranexamic acid, and did so while having an added, potent antioxidant benefit (Source: *Anticancer Research*, September/October 1999, pages 3769-3774). Given the precautions and side effects associated with oral administration of tranexamic acid and the unknowns of topical application, it is an ingredient that is best avoided.

☹ **Benefiance Full Correction Lip Treatment** *($35 for 0.5 ounce)* irritates lips with menthol and has only a scant amount of antioxidants. The waxlike thickeners in this product can help temporarily fill in vertical lip lines, but so can similar products from Olay, for less money and with a much better formula.

☺ $$$ **Benefiance Pure Retinol Intensive Revitalizing Face Mask** *($62 for 4 masks)* has a formula very similar to the Benefiance Pure Retinol Instant Treatment Eye Mask below, but this option includes pre-cut mask sheets for the upper and lower eye area. It is not intensive if you are looking for a potent dose of retinol, and won't do much beyond providing mild hydration for slightly dry skin.

☺ $$$ **Benefiance Pure Retinol Instant Treatment Eye Mask** *($62 for 12 pairs)* is basically a gimmicky mask that has a very tiny amount of retinol. The bulk of this formula is water, slip agents, silicone, and alcohol, making it an average option that costs far more than it should.

SHISEIDO BIO-PERFORMANCE PRODUCTS

☺ $$$ **Bio-Performance Super Exfoliating Discs** *($65 for 8 discs)* are said to work like microdermabrasion, and manually exfoliate skin due to their texture and a mixture of talc and rice bran. These discs differ little from those sold in many drugstore lines, including Olay, Neutrogena, and Dove.

☺ $$$ **Bio-Performance Advanced Super Revitalizer (Cream)** *($71 for 1.7 ounces)* isn't advanced when compared to today's state-of-the-art moisturizers, but it does contain several ingredients (including glycerin, squalane, fatty acids, and silicone) that are helpful for dry skin. The tiny amounts of antioxidants will suffer from the jar packaging. The iron oxides produce a slight glow on skin, but don't mistake that for skin being revitalized.

☺ $$$ **Bio-Performance Advanced Super Revitalizer (Cream) Whitening Formula** *($98 for 1.7 ounces)* is similar to the Bio-Performance Advanced Super Revitalizer (Cream) above, except this pricier option contains a selection of plant extracts and vitamin C (as ascorbyl glucoside), which have some research showing them to be effective for skin lightening. However, due to jar packaging, none of these potentially efficacious ingredients will remain stable during use.

✓ ☺ $$$ **Bio-Performance Super Eye Contour Cream** *($55 for 0.53 ounce)* is an excellent emollient moisturizer suitable for dry to very dry skin anywhere on the face. It is stably packaged, to the benefit of the many vitamin- and plant-based antioxidants it contains.

☹ **Bio-Performance Super Refining Essence** *($76 for 1.8 ounces)* is a water- and glycerin-based serum that contains some good water-binding agents and small amounts of vitamins E and C. The problem is that it also contains numerous fragrance components, which can cause irritation, and that isn't what should be applied to freshly scrubbed skin.

☺ $$$ **Bio-Performance Super Lifting Formula** *($74 for 1 ounce)* is similar to the Benefiance Concentrated Neck Contour Treatment above, and the same basic comments apply. The addition of a few more water-binding agents in this product doesn't change the fact that it cannot lift skin.

☺ $$$ **Bio-Performance Super Restoring Cream** *($98 for 1.7 ounces)* is sold as an unparalleled age-defying cream, which doesn't explain why Shiseido sells dozens of other moisturizers with this same claim. After all, if this is the one, why bother with the rest of them? As it turns out, this is a very good moisturizer for dry skin. Yet it ends up being disappointing because of jar packaging, which hinders the effectiveness of the impressive amount of antioxidants in this product.

☺ **$$$ Bio-Performance Intensive Skin Corrective Program** *($300)* has an eyebrow-raising price accompanied by claims that make this combination of products sound like a NASA project for aging skin. Something Shiseido refers to as "Bio-Recharger MC" is said to strengthen skin by "optimizing the calcium-magnesium ion distribution," the result of which is allegedly smoother, firmer skin. Shiseido talks about ion exchange in relation to this product. Briefly, an ion is any atom that has either lost or gained an electron. When an ion loses an electron, it becomes positively charged and is called a cation. When an ion gains an electron, it becomes negatively charged, and is called an anion. Ion exchange is a natural process that occurs in many different substances. Skin can act as an ion exchange medium due to its water content, and cosmetics chemists the world over know that various cosmetic ingredients, used alone or in combination, can make a product positively or negatively charged. Shiseido's idea seems to be that aging skin needs an infusion of calcium and magnesium ions in order to regain its youthful appearance. In reality, these minerals play a minor role (at best) in skin function and appearance; they certainly are not critical ingredients to look for in the quest for the ultimate antiwrinkle product because they cannot be absorbed into the skin. This kit consists of two products, neither of which is impressive or worth even one-fourth the cost. The **Serum Essence** is the portion that contains the calcium and magnesium, very tiny amounts of both. It is mostly a blend of water and slip agents with alcohol, a humectant, and preservative. Talk about boring, and the alcohol, while not likely to cause irritation, is a letdown. The **Balm** is a nonaqueous blend of silicone with Vaseline, film-forming agents, and wax. It can function as a spackle for wrinkles, but the effect is temporary—plus the amount of fragrance components in this product is likely to cause irritation. All told, this set is an utter disappointment, with a price tag that is over the top for what you get by any standard. Consumers looking to spend this much on an antiwrinkle product would do better with the various options from DDF, M.D. Skincare by Dr. Dennis Gross, or even the products from Dr. Perricone. All of them have overinflated claims, too, but at least many of the formulas approach or surpass the current state-of-the-art, which this Shiseido duo absolutely does not.

SHISEIDO ELIXIR PRODUCTS

☺ **$$$ Elixir Superieur Cleansing Foam with Collagen Extract I, for Normal/Oily Skin** *($27 for 4.5 ounces)* promises lifted skin as you wash, thanks to the collagen extract it contains. It's a bogus claim because collagen applied topically cannot do a thing to correct sagging. Besides, this is a rather drying cleanser because it contains a high amount of potassium hydroxide. It is only an option for very oily skin, and even for that skin type it's not a very good option.

☺ **$$$ Elixir Superieur Cleansing Foam with Collagen Extract II, for Normal to Dry Skin** *($27 for 5.1 ounces)* is a foaming cleanser that's too drying for its intended skin types. It's an OK option for oily skin, but adding a tiny amount of collagen to a cleanser isn't going to lift skin anywhere.

☹ **Elixir Superieur Makeup Cleansing Cream** *($30 for 4.9 ounces)* costs a lot of money for what amounts to mostly mineral oil, water, and emollient thickeners. Although this will remove all types of makeup and contains several ingredients helpful for those with very dry skin, the inclusion of menthol makes it a problem and impossible to recommend.

☹ **Elixir Superieur Makeup Cleansing Gel** *($30 for 4.9 ounces)* is an average, overpriced liquid makeup remover that loses points for including alcohol (in an amount not too likely to cause irritation, but still, it shouldn't be in such a product) and fragrance. While the alcohol is likely not problematic, the menthol assuredly is. This cleanser is not recommended.

☹ **Elixir Superieur Makeup Cleansing Oil** *($30 for 5.7 ounces)* is just mineral oil with thickeners, silicone, emollient, water, preservative, and fragrance. Mineral oil removes makeup quickly and easily, but why spend this much when plain mineral oil costs mere pennies by comparison? Besides, this product contains menthol which only serves to irritate skin and, ironically, break down collagen (which this cleanser is supposed to supply).

☹ **Elixir Superieur Lifting CE Lotion I** *($34 for 5 ounces)* lists alcohol as the third ingredient and also contains menthol, both of which make it too drying and irritating for all skin types, not to mention the free-radical damage the alcohol will cause.

☹ **Elixir Superieur Lifting CE Lotion II** *($35 for 5 ounces)* contains menthol, which makes it too irritating for all skin types. Even without the menthol, this is hardly an exciting toner formulation, nor is it worth its price.

☹ **Elixir Superieur Lifting CE Lotion III** *($35 for 5.7 ounces)* isn't much different from the other Elixir Superieur toners. It contains menthol, which makes it too irritating for all skin types and the formula quite underwhelming for the money.

☹ **Elixir Superieur Toning Lotion** *($34 for 5.7 ounces)* removes surface oil and "stickiness" due to its alcohol content, but degreasing your skin in this manner is irritating and triggers excess oil production in the pore lining. The inclusion of menthol makes this even more irritating and a must to avoid. The only thing this product can lift is the money from your pocketbook.

☺ **Elixir Lifting Daytime Protector SPF 25 PA++** *($38 for 1.6 ounces)* includes an in-part titanium dioxide sunscreen, but the base formula is mostly water, silicone, and alcohol, which doesn't make it worth considering over several superior sunscreen options. It goes without saying that nothing in this product can lift sagging skin.

☺ **$$$ Elixir Eye Radiance (Eye Cream)** *($56 for 0.7 ounce)* shortchanges skin of antioxidants and other intriguing ingredients, and instead provides it with an average blend of moisturizing agents and thickeners. This is an OK option for dry skin, but it's not worth the price.

☺ **$$$ Elixir Lifting Eye Treatment EX** *($55 for 0.53 ounce)* is a decent moisturizer for dry skin, but a product meant for use around the eyes should be fragrance-free, and this isn't. Still, it contains some good antioxidants and plant oils, and if you're going to devote your cosmetics dollars to Shiseido, this is one of their better products.

☹ **Elixir Superieur Lasting Lift Essence** *($56 for 1.6 ounces)* does contain collagen, but soluble or not, it cannot lift skin to reduce signs of sagging. If anything, because alcohol is the third ingredient, this gel may prove too irritating for most, and that cancels out any positive impact the antioxidants in here could have had. It is quite possible the amount of alcohol in this product will trigger free-radical damage, and the menthol Shiseido added will definitely cause irritation.

☹ **Elixir Superieur Lifting CE Emulsion I, for Normal/Oily Skin** *($38 for 4.3 ounces)* is a formulary embarrassment that offers not a shred of hope for aging skin. Alcohol is the second ingredient, and it will cause irritation, exacerbate dryness, and trigger free-radical damage. This also contains menthol for further irritation, while the collagen has zero effect on wrinkles.

☹ **Elixir Superieur Lifting CE Emulsion II, for Normal Skin** *($38 for 4.3 ounces).* This lightweight moisturizer contains some good ingredients to make slightly dry skin feel smooth and healthy, but like all of the Elixir products, it contains menthol, so it's too irritating for all skin types. Your skin deserves much more than this provides.

☹ **Elixir Superieur Lifting CE Emulsion III, for Normal/ Dry Skin** *($38 for 1.5 ounces)* is an incredibly standard, jar-packaged moisturizer for its intended skin types. It is interesting to notice that while this has a lower price, it contains many of the same ingredients Shiseido uses in their most expensive moisturizers. However, this one isn't recommended because it contains menthol, which only serves to irritate, not lift, your skin.

☹ **Elixir Superieur Lifting Night Cream** *($50 for 1.4 ounces)* is a below-standard moisturizer for normal to slightly dry skin. The tiny amount of antioxidants won't hold up due to jar packaging, while the menthol is irritating and has no place in a moisturizer.

☹ **Elixir Superieur Vitalizing Massage Cream** *($37 for 3.5 ounces)* contains some of the most common emollient ingredients ever, and in many ways is a dated formula whose greasy texture is only suitable for very dry skin. Unfortunately, it is not recommended for anyone's skin because it contains menthol. Menthol only serves to cause irritation, and massaging it into skin only makes that irritation worse.

☺ **$$$ Elixir Superieur Pore Care Essence** *($38 for 0.52 ounce)* consists primarily of water, silicones (including those that have a dry finish), and alcohol. The handful of interesting ingredients are barely present, and that doesn't make this serum worth considering over others that have a lasting matte finish and supply skin with a better range of ingredients. If you're stuck on Shiseido, they offer better options in their Pureness line, or you can forget Shiseido and look to the mattifying products from Clinique, Smashbox, or Cosmedicine.

☹ **Elixir Superieur Clarifying Moisture Recharge Mask** *($32 for 6 masks)* contains a potentially irritating amount of alcohol and offers skin precious little in the way of moisturizing ingredients. This is a gimmicky way to minimally moisturize skin, and it pales in comparison to the moisturizing masks from most other department-store lines.

☹ **Elixir Treatment Mask** *($40 for 3.6 ounces)* is a standard, peel-off mask that lists polyvinyl alcohol as its second ingredient, which makes it too irritating for all skin types.

SHISEIDO PURENESS PRODUCTS

☹ **Pureness Deep Cleansing Foam** *($21 for 3.6 ounces)* contains potentially drying cleansing agents and irritates skin with menthol, making this a cleanser to avoid.

☹ **Pureness Foaming Cleansing Fluid** *($21 for 5 ounces)* contains potassium myristate as its main cleansing agent. A constituent of soap, it can be drying for most skin types.

☺ **$$$ Pureness Refreshing Cleansing Sheets, Oil-Free, Alcohol-Free** *($17 for 30 sheets)* are cleansing wipes suitable for all skin types, but their cleansing ability isn't such that makeup removal is swift. The *Palo azul* wood extract in this product has no documented benefit for skin.

☺ **$$$ Pureness Refreshing Cleansing Water, Oil-Free, Alcohol-Free** *($21 for 5 ounces)* is basically the same formula as the Pureness Refreshing Cleansing Sheets above, only not steeped onto cloths. As such, the same review applies.

☺ **$$$ Pureness Pore Purifying Warming Scrub** *($23 for 1.7 ounces)* doesn't make much sense as a scrub product designed for someone with oily skin and clogged pores because its main ingredient is mineral oil, followed closely by petrolatum (Vaseline). Although neither of these ingredients poses a risk of clogging pores, both have a thick, greasy texture that won't make someone with oily skin happy. This scrub is actually very good for someone with dry skin. The polyethylene beads (standard for most scrubs) are buffered by the mineral oil base, leaving skin with a soft, smooth feel along with some residual moistness. The warming effect is in the name only, because this scrub contains nothing to warm the skin (although the mechanical action of scrubbing can create a slight sense of warmth). This product does contain fragrance.

☹ **Pureness Anti-Shine Refreshing Lotion** (*$23 for 5 ounces*) contains a low amount of salicylic acid and has a pH that prevents it from functioning effectively as an exfoliant. This also contains enough alcohol to cause dryness, yet also stimulate oil production in the pore and cause irritation, all of which won't help treat acne in the least.

☺ $$$ **Pureness Balancing Softener, Alcohol Free** (*$23 for 5 ounces*) is an OK toner for normal to oily skin, but it absolutely cannot create stronger skin that resists adult acne, as claimed.

☺ **Pureness Matifying Moisturizer, Oil Free** (*$32 for 1.6 ounces*) is a nearly weightless lotion for normal to oily skin, though its alcohol content may cause problems. Still, this is an option for those who need a bit of hydration with a matte finish.

☺ **Pureness Moisturizing Gel-Cream** (*$32 for 1.4 ounces*) provides a hint of moisture along with a tiny amount of water-binding agent. It is an average option for normal to oily skin.

☹ **Pureness Blemish Clearing Gel** (*$19 for 0.5 ounce*) contains a barely effective amount of salicylic acid and the pH of this gel is too high for it to function as an exfoliant. Further, the amount of alcohol this contains makes it too irritating and drying for all skin types.

☺ $$$ **Pureness Matifying Stick, Oil Free** (*$25 for 0.14 ounce*) is a silicone-based stick that contains the absorbent ingredient silica, so it does provide a matte finish. However, the waxes that keep this in stick form should not be applied over blemish-prone areas.

☹ **Pureness Pore Minimizing Cooling Essence** (*$27 for 1 ounce*) lists alcohol as the second ingredient, and that, coupled with the menthol in this product, produces its "cooling essence" on skin. These two ingredients cause needless irritation and won't do a thing to benefit blemish-prone skin, nor will they reduce the appearance of pores as Shiseido (incorrectly) claims. Instead, the alcohol will trigger oil production in the pore lining.

☺ $$$ **Pureness Oil-Control Blotting Paper** (*$17 for 100 sheets*) consists of blotting papers laced with clay to provide oil absorption and a lasting matte finish. The rosemary extract isn't the best, but without question these work to keep excess shine in check.

SHISEIDO THE SKINCARE PRODUCTS

☺ $$$ **The Skincare Extra Gentle Cleansing Foam** (*$29 for 4.7 ounces*) is a standard, glycerin-based foaming cleanser that is an option for all skin types except very dry. It removes makeup completely and rinses well. Shiseido mentions that this is formulated with patent-pending yuzu (*Citrus junos*) seed extract, but it is nowhere to be found on the ingredient list.

☹ **The Skincare Purifying Cleansing Foam** (*$29 for 4.6 ounces*) contains the drying, alkaline cleansing agent potassium myristate, which makes this cleanser/scrub hybrid a problem for all skin types.

☺ $$$ **The Skincare Rinse-Off Cleansing Gel** (*$29 for 6.7 ounces*) doesn't rinse completely due to its silicone content, but this is a new twist on standard, water-soluble cleansers and is a consideration for normal to oily skin. The tiny amount of alcohol is not likely to be a problem for skin. This is capable of removing all but the most stubborn types of makeup.

☺ $$$ **The Skincare Instant Eye and Lip Makeup Remover** (*$26 for 4.2 ounces*) is a water- and silicone-based makeup remover that is below standard due to its alcohol content. Several other companies offer a better version of this type of makeup remover for a lot less money, including Almay, Neutrogena, and Paula's Choice.

☺ $$$ **The Skincare Hydro-Balancing Softener, Alcohol-Free** (*$34 for 5 ounces*) is an OK toner for all skin types. It provides water-binding agents, but that's it, so it's up to you to decide if spending this much for such a basic formula is worthwhile.

☹ **The Skincare Hydro-Nourishing Softener** *($34 for 5 ounces)* costs a lot of money for what amounts to mostly water, slip agent, alcohol, and glycerin. There's enough alcohol to make this a non-softening problem for all skin types, and the peppermint extract only makes matters worse.

☹ **The Skincare Day Moisture Protection SPF 15 PA+, Regular** *($39 for 2.5 ounces)* lacks sufficient UVA-protecting ingredients, which makes this new daytime moisturizer—especially with its lackluster base formula—a resounding disappointment. What is extremely detrimental is that the PA+ is supposed to represent Japan's standard for some level of UVA protection. This system applies only to sunscreens manufactured in Japan, and does not imply superiority, as clearly evidenced here.

☹ **The Skincare Day Moisture Protection SPF 15 PA+, Enriched** *($39 for 1.8 ounces)* is a slightly more emollient version of The Skincare Day Moisture Protection SPF 15 PA+, Regular, but other than that the same review applies.

☹ **The Skincare Eye Moisture Recharge** *($40 for 0.54 ounce)*. Talk about disappointing! This lightweight eye-area moisturizer for slightly dry skin has a substandard formula that subjects skin to more alcohol than state-of-the-art ingredients. It also contains fragrance, which isn't what you want in a product meant for use around the eyes, and peppermint, another problem. Last, almost all of the really intriguing ingredients (including the thiotaurine Shiseido spotlights) are listed after the fragrance and preservative. This is a "why bother?" product if ever there was one!

☺ $$$ **The Skincare Eye Revitalizer** *($40 for 0.53 ounce)* is a rather boring moisturizer for dry skin anywhere on the face. The bells and whistles barely make a sound because they are present in such paltry amounts. Meanwhile, the wild thyme extract may cause irritation.

☹ **The Skincare Eye Soother** *($40 for 0.54 ounce)* contains too much alcohol (three forms of the drying, irritating kind) to be soothing, and what precedes the alcohol is as common as a cloudy day in Seattle.

☺ **The Skincare Multi-Energizing Cream** *($43 for 1.7 ounces)* is far from an intensive treatment for dull, dehydrated skin, but is an OK jar-packaged moisturizer for normal to dry skin.

☺ **The Skincare Night Moisture Recharge, Light** *($41 for 2.5 ounces)* contains mostly water, glycerin, silicone, and alcohol. The few intriguing ingredients are listed after the preservative, making this yet another disappointing, boring fluid moisturizer.

☺ **The Skincare Night Moisture Recharge, Regular** *($41 for 2.5 ounces)* is a lightweight moisturizer that's an average option for normal to slightly dry skin. Shiseido maintains that the yuzu seed extract (present in a next-to-nothing amount in this product) is a "breakthrough ingredient" that encourages the skin to produce more hyaluronic acid. There is no research anywhere to support this claim, but yuzu is a popular citrus fruit in Japan and Korea, and the peel does have considerable antioxidants. However, that's all related to eating the fruit and its skin, not putting it on your skin (Source: The *Journal of Agricultural and Food Chemistry*, September 2004, pages 5907-5913).

☺ $$$ **The Skincare Night Moisture Recharge, Enriched** *($41 for 1.8 ounces)* contains more thickening agents than The Skincare Night Moisture Recharge, Regular, but is otherwise an equally uninspired moisturizer with a very small amount of the star ingredient, yuzu seed extract.

☺ $$$ **The Skincare Renewing Serum** *($46 for 1 ounce)* makes skin of any age feel silky-smooth due to its silicone content, but it lacks state-of-the-art ingredients and may prove irritating due to the peppermint and wild thyme extracts.

☺ **$$$ The Skincare Tinted Moisture Protection SPF 20** *($37 for 1.7 ounces)* has a rather lackluster ingredient mix, at least when it comes to replenishing "generous moisture" as claimed. The slightly creamy texture blends well and sets to a soft matte finish courtesy of the silicone and talc in the formula (neither are particularly moisturizing on their own). True to its name, coverage amounts to a sheer tint. The shade range is small, and what's available tends to be a bit too yellow or peach, but they're sheer enough to be workable for light to medium skin tones (there are no shades for fair or dark skin). This is a good daytime moisturizer with sunscreen for normal to slightly dry or slightly oily skin. The in-part titanium dioxide sunscreen is excellent, while the formula itself contains more water-binding agents than anything else considered "moisturizing."

☹ **The Skincare Visible Luminizer Serum, Anti-Dullness** *($46 for 1.6 ounces)* lists alcohol as the second ingredient and also contains peppermint, making this serum (which actually has a lotion texture) too irritating for all skin types. Even without so much alcohol, this is not an impressive formula, and it is incapable of leaving skin energized or taking care of enlarged pores.

☺ **The Skincare Moisture Relaxing Mask** *($33 for 1.7 ounces)* contains many of the same ingredients Shiseido uses in all of its moisturizers, which means those would be appropriate for masking, too. This version supplies dry skin with an OK selection of emollients and some water-binding agents, but is a more or less superfluous product.

☹ **The Skincare Protective Lip Conditioner SPF 10** *($22.50 for 0.14 ounce)* lacks the UVA-protecting ingredients of titanium dioxide, zinc oxide, avobenzone, Mexoryl SX (ecamsule), or Tinosorb, and is not recommended.

☹ **The Skincare Purifying Mask** *($29 for 3.2 ounces)* has clay to absorb excess oil, but so do many other masks for oily skin, and most of those don't contain irritating eucalyptus oil.

SHISEIDO WHITE LUCENT PRODUCTS

☺ **$$$ White Lucent Brightening Cleansing Foam** *($34 for 4.7 ounces)* is a standard, water-soluble foaming cleanser whose detergent cleansing agents can be slightly drying. This is a decent option for oily skin.

☺ **$$$ White Lucent Brightening Refining Softener, Enriched** *($46 for 5 ounces)*. I don't know what they've "enriched" this misguided toner with, but it has nothing of value for skin. The amount of alcohol poses a slight risk of irritation and likely counteracts the anti-irritant properties of the licorice extract. The inclusion of St. John's wort means this toner should never be applied to skin that's about to be exposed to sunlight.

☹ **White Lucent Brightening Refining Softener, Light** *($46 for 5 ounces)* lists alcohol as the second ingredient, making this overpriced toner too drying and irritating for all skin types, not to mention the alcohol will trigger oil production in the pore lining.

☹ **White Lucent Brightening Toning Lotion, Cool** *($46 for 5 ounces)* is even more irritating than the White Lucent Brightening Refining Softener, Light, because it adds menthol to the mix.

☹ **White Lucent Brightening Eye Treatment** *($50 for 0.5 ounce)* contains too much alcohol and not enough of what eye-area skin in need of help requires. The amount of titanium dioxide in this poorly formulated eye cream creates a brightening effect due to the white coloration it imparts to skin (this would be most noticeable on Asian skin tones, which tend to be strongly yellow), while mica adds shine. Big deal! This also contains several fragrance ingredients that can compound the irritation from the alcohol, and nothing in this product can address the poor circulation issues that lead to dark circles.

☹ **White Lucent Brightening Massage Cream** *($52 for 2.8 ounces)* is a basic, unimpressive moisturizer that contains more alcohol than ingredients with potential skin-lightening ability (and jar packaging won't keep these ingredients stable anyway). Chalk this up to a huge waste of time and money.

☺ **$$$ White Lucent Brightening Moisturizing Cream** *($54 for 1.4 ounces)* is similar to the White Lucent Brightening Massage Cream above, only with a more emollient base formula. The concern about the alcohol remains, but the emollient helps offset the irritation potential. Still, this is a lot of money for a really basic, jar-packaged moisturizer that cannot lighten discolorations.

☺ **White Lucent Brightening Moisturizing Emulsion** *($54 for 3.3 ounces)* is an OK lightweight lotion for normal to slightly dry or slightly oily skin, but it cannot lighten discolorations, not even a little. The sleek packaging will keep the antioxidants stable during use, but they would be more potent without the alcohol that precedes them on the list.

☹ **White Lucent Brightening Moisturizing Gel** *($54 for 1.4 ounces)* contains enough alcohol to cause dryness and irritation, and there's more salt in here than any potentially helpful skin-lightening agents.

☹ **White Lucent Brightening Protective Moisturizer SPF 16 PA++** *($52 for 2.5 ounces)* offers skin an in-part avobenzone sunscreen, but its lotion base contains enough alcohol to cause irritation and undermine the effectiveness of the antioxidants it contains.

☺ **$$$ White Lucent Concentrated Brightening Serum** *($120 for 1 ounce)* is mostly water, slip agents, alcohol, and silicone. It contains vitamin C as ascorbic acid, but not in an amount that can impact skin discolorations. The same goes for the numerous exotic-sounding plant extracts in this product. I imagine most of them were added to make this pricey serum seem unique, but they do not lighten discolorations.

☺ **$$$ White Lucent Brightening Mask** *($68 for 6 masks)* contains a handful of intriguing ingredients, but none of them are present in impressive amounts. That means, for example, that the ascorbic acid (vitamin C) won't fade discolorations or even provide much antioxidant benefit. You're getting mostly water, slip agents, alcohol, and the water-binding sugar xylitol. None of this is brightening or whitening and some of the plant extracts can be irritating, although it's not likely given the small amounts found in this mask. Nevertheless, for this kind of money you should be getting only skin-beneficial ingredients, not this do-nothing mixture.

OTHER SHISEIDO SKIN CARE PRODUCTS

☺ **Ultimate Cleansing Oil, for Face & Body** *($23 for 5 ounces)* is marketed as a cleanser that will remove long-wearing makeup and water-resistant sunscreens, and although it can do that, the formula is mostly mineral oil, which you can buy for less than a few dollars at any pharmacy around the world.

☹ **Eudermine Revitalizing Essence** *($56 for 4.2 ounces)* is outrageously priced for what amounts to mostly water, slip agent, and alcohol. It contains a few good water-binding agents, but in amounts too small for skin to notice, especially with the alcohol involved.

☺ **Extra Smooth Sun Protection Cream SPF 36 PA+++, for Face** *($28 for 1.9 ounces)* deserves a bit of explanation because of its PA+++ designation. This rating system was developed in Japan (where Shiseido is based) as a means to quantify the level of UVA protection a sunscreen can provide. "PA" stands for Protection-Grade of UVA. A PA+ rating signifies some UVA protection (which would apply to most sunscreens today), while a PA++ means moderate

UVA protection, and PA+++ symbolizes high UVA protection. Because this particular sunscreen contains over 9% zinc oxide, it qualifies for its PA+++ rating. (This system is not recognized in the United States, Canada, or Australia.) The base formula is suitable for normal to oily skin not prone to blemishes. This would be rated higher if it included greater amounts of antioxidants and did not contain a potentially problematic plant extract.

☺ $$$ **Future Solution Eye and Lip Contour Cream** *($125 for 0.7 ounce)* comes packaged in a luxurious jar, but no matter how beautiful the container, it can only serve to sabotage the effectiveness of the few antioxidants in this otherwise standard moisturizer. Nothing in this product is exclusive for the eye or lip area, while a couple of the plant extracts can be irritating. A natural constituent of *Ononis spinosa* root (also known as spiny restharrow) is menthol and that makes it potentially irritating (Source: *PDR for Herbal Medicines*, 1st Edition, Montvale, NJ: Medical Economics Company, 1998). Other Japanese plant extracts in this moisturizer have no established benefit for skin, and there is only sketchy research on their benefits when consumed orally.

☺ $$$ **Future Solution Total Revitalizing Cream** *($230 for 1.8 ounces)* is said to work on every aspect of skin to alleviate all signs of aging, from wrinkles to sagging. But, without a sunscreen, don't bet on this for any future protection against wrinkles and loss of resilience. For the money, this should be brimming with a who's who of today's top ingredients for helping skin function at its best, but it isn't. Even if some of those were included, they'd suffer from the unfortunate choice of (pretty) jar packaging. At best, this is an acceptable moisturizer for normal to dry skin; some of the plant extracts can be irritating, as described above in the review for Future Solution Eye and Lip Contour Cream.

☺ $$$ **Revitalizing Cream** *($140 for 1.4 ounces)* is an incredibly basic, shockingly priced moisturizer for dry to very dry skin. Not a single ingredient in this emollient product is justified by the cost, and jar packaging won't keep the two forms of vitamin E stable during use.

☺ $$$ **Sun Protection Eye Cream SPF 32 PA+++** *($31 for 0.6 ounce)* deserves kudos for its in-part zinc oxide sunscreen and silky-cream texture, but it sorely lacks sufficient amounts of state-of-the-art ingredients for skin, and given the price that's an insult. Although the sunscreen is very good, this doesn't compete favorably with similar products from the Lauder-owned lines at the department store (including their relatively inexpensive Good Skin line, which is sold at Kohl's). Still, it would work as a good sunscreen.

✓ ☺ $$$ **Sun Protection Lip Treatment SPF 36 PA++** *($20 for 0.14 ounce)* is a very good, in-part titanium dioxide lip sunscreen that includes emollients to keep lips soft and smooth. The added bonus of an antioxidant and anti-irritant make this even better.

☺ **The Makeup Pre-Makeup Cream SPF 15** *($29.50 for 1 ounce)* contains an in-part titanium dioxide sunscreen, but that's the only exciting element in this pre-makeup moisturizer for normal to dry skin. The mineral pigments give a slight glow to skin, but that will be concealed after you apply makeup.

☺ $$$ **Ultimate Sun Protection Cream SPF 55 PA+++, for Face** *($34 for 2 ounces)* is an in-part zinc oxide sunscreen for normal to slightly dry skin that definitely covers the broad-spectrum bases and has a silky texture. It's a shame antioxidants are scarce here, because in a sunscreen that costs this much they should be plentiful.

☺ $$$ **Whitess Intensive Skin Brightener** *($130 for 1.4 ounces)* is an absurdly overpriced skin-lightening product that contains a high concentration of arbutin to inhibit melanin production. Arbutin is a constituent of cranberries, bearberries, and blueberries, among other fruits. Although arbutin has been shown to have the same skin-lightening capability as hydroquinone, that fact has been established only in animal, human skin model, and in vitro studies, rather than on intact skin (Sources: *Biological and Pharmaceutical Bulletin*, April 2004, pages 510-514; and *Pigment Cell Research*, August 1998, pages 206-212). It is interesting to note that arbutin degrades to become hydroquinone, a change that is related to its efficacy (Source: *Journal of Chemical Ecology*, May 2004, 1067-1082). Still, it might be worth the price to see if this amount of arbutin, as an alternative to hydroquinone, can have an effect on skin. (Actually, arbutin ends up having more in common with hydroquinone than its natural association would indicate.) The amount of alcohol in this product isn't terribly bad, but keeps it from earning a happy face rating.

SHISEIDO SUN & SELF-TANNING PRODUCTS

☹ **Brilliant Bronze Quick Self-Tanning Gel, for Face/Body** *($29 for 5.2 ounces)* lists alcohol as the second ingredient and isn't really worth the irritation given the number of less expensive self-tanners at the drugstore that have no irritating ingredients.

☺ **$$$ Brilliant Bronze Self-Tanning Emulsion, for Face/Body** *($26 for 3.5 ounces)* is a lightweight face and body lotion that works the same as any self-tanner.

☹ **Brilliant Bronze Tinted Self-Tanning Gel, for Face/Body** *($29 for 5.4 ounces)* is available in a light or medium tan shade, but both versions list alcohol as the third ingredient, making this tinted self-tanning gel an irritation waiting to happen.

☺ **$$$ Daily Bronze Moisturizing Emulsion, for Face/Body** *($36 for 5 ounces)* is a self-tanning lotion that works the same way as any self-tanner with dihydroxyacetone. Considering the volatile fragrance components in this product, you're better off trying one of the subtle self-tanners from Jergens, Dove, or Olay available at the drugstore.

☺ **Extra Smooth Sun Protection Lotion SPF 33 PA++, for Face/Body** *($29 for 3.3 ounces)* is preferred to the Extra Smooth Sun Protection Cream SPF 36 PA+++, for Face above because it omits a questionable plant extract and because it provides more product for the same price. It would be rated a Paula's Pick if it contained more than one antioxidant.

☹ **Refreshing Sun Protection Spray SPF 16 PA+, for Body/Hair** *($28 for 5 ounces)* includes avobenzone for UVA protection, but is an alcohol-based product, which makes it a problem for all skin types, as does the orange oil that is present.

☺ **Sun Protection Lotion SPF 18 PA+, for Face/Body** *($26 for 5 ounces)* is a standard, in-part titanium dioxide sunscreen suitable for normal to oily skin. Talc contributes to this sunscreen's smooth matte finish. For the money, this should contain more bells and whistles than it does.

☺ **$$$ Ultimate Sun Protection Lotion SPF 55 PA+++, for Face/Body** *($38 for 3.3 ounces)*. This silky sunscreen includes an in-part zinc oxide sunscreen for sufficient UVA protection. It is a very good option for normal to oily skin and would be rated a Paula's Pick if Shiseido had included some notable antioxidants.

SHISEIDO MAKEUP

FOUNDATION: ✓☺ **$$$ Compact Foundation SPF 15** *($29.50 for powder; $8 for compact)* has an application that's more sheer than Shiseido's Powdery Foundation SPF 14-17, reviewed below, due to a reduced level of talc. The sunscreens are titanium dioxide and zinc oxide, which makes this an effective, gentle option for those with sensitive skin. This pressed-powder foundation has an inordinately light texture that applies smoothly and provides a sheer matte finish. It can be difficult to pick up enough powder to obtain meaningful coverage, so this functions best when applied over a sunscreen or a foundation with sunscreen rated SPF 15 or higher. The shades have improved considerably since last reviewed; among the ten options, only three should be avoided due to their strong pink tone: B20, B40, and B60. The Ochre range is ideal for those with olive skin.

✓ ☺ $$$ **Dual Balancing Foundation SPF 17** *($37.50)* is late to the game, as foundations proclaiming they can balance oily areas while providing moisture to dry spots have been around for years, most notably with Clinique's Superbalanced Makeup and Estee Lauder Equalizer Foundation SPF 10. Shiseido's balancing claims are just as out of whack as those of its predecessors, but the foundation itself exceeds them by offering superior sun protection (featuring in-part titanium dioxide) and a fluid, silky texture that applies like a second skin. Once blended, this sets to a natural matte finish that gives skin an attractive dimensional (rather than flat) quality. It's well-suited for combination skin, but not because it is simultaneously controlling oil and maximizing moisture. You'll net light to medium coverage and the selection of ten shades is promising. The following shades are noticeably pink or peach and best avoided: B40, B60, and I60.

✓ ☺ $$$ **Pureness Matifying Compact Oil-Free SPF 16** *($20 for powder; $8 for compact)* is a slam-dunk recommendation for those with oily to very oily skin looking for an absorbent, matte-finish pressed powder with sun protection. The actives are titanium dioxide and zinc oxide (which are quite absorbent on their own), and the talc-based formula applies well despite feeling too dry. All six shades are recommended.

✓ ☺ $$$ **Stick Foundation SPF 15** *($37.50)* has a wonderfully smooth, light texture and a titanium dioxide sunscreen that blends on with ease, builds from sheer to almost full coverage, and dries to an absorbent powder finish thanks to the amount of clay it contains. It's best for someone with normal to slightly dry or slightly oily skin, since several waxes in it can be problematic for those with breakouts and/or oily skin. Among the shades, avoid B20, which is quite pink, and the noticeably peach B60 and I60. The I00 shade is a beautiful option for someone with very fair skin.

✓ ☺ $$$ **STM Perfect Smoothing Compact Foundation SPF 15** *($30 for powder; $9 for compact)*. Shiseido rarely produces a product with sunscreen that does not provide adequate UVA protection, and they don't disappoint with this pressed-powder foundation and its sole active ingredient of titanium dioxide. The powdery texture is exceptionally silky and leaves skin looking beautifully smooth and polished rather than dry. The satin-matte finish is laced with subtle sparkles that are not distracting for daytime wear. You can get sheer to light coverage that never looks powdery and the formula blends seamlessly. All but one of the shades are stellar, and each goes on more neutral than it looks (which is good, because some of them appear too peachy-gold in the compact). Only #060 may be too gold for some medium skin tones; the rest are highly recommended to those looking for a powder with reliable sunscreen. This foundation is suitable for all skin types except very oily.

✓ ☺ $$$ **Sun Protection Compact Foundation SPF 34 PA+++** *($25.50 for powder; $8 for compact)* is a talc-based pressed-powder foundation that includes an in-part titanium dioxide sunscreen for sufficient UVA protection. It has a smooth texture that's drier than normal, but that's to be expected given the amount of titanium dioxide. What counts beyond sun protection is the natural matte finish this powder leaves while providing sheer to light coverage. All seven shades apply more neutral than they appear in the compact, so don't reject a particular color without trying it first—you may be surprised.

✓☺ **$$$ Sun Protection Liquid Foundation SPF 42 PA+++** *($25.50 for powder; $8 for compact)* deserves much praise not only for offering substantial sun protection via its in-part titanium dioxide sunscreen but also for having a silky, lightweight texture that blends easily. It offers a sheer matte finish but can provide medium to nearly full coverage if needed, all without feeling thick or looking heavy. The silicone-enhanced fluid is ideal for normal to very oily skin and an excellent option for outdoor wear when you're active because it stays in place and is water-resistant. That doesn't mean you can apply it once and sit by the pool or play volleyball all day, but it is one of the few foundations that provide sufficient sun protection and keep looking fresh even through strenuous activities. Seven shades are available, with SP40 and SP50 being a bit too peach for most medium skin tones. The other shades are great options for light and dark (but not very dark) skin.

☺ **$$$ Hydro-Liquid Compact Foundation SPF 17-20** *($28.50 for powder; $10.50 for compact)* isn't liquid at all, but rather a very dry-finish but silky cream-to-powder foundation. The SPF rating varies by shade, but each contains titanium dioxide as the only active ingredient. When carefully blended this can look nearly imperceptible on skin while providing light to medium coverage. Less than perfect blending can result in a heavy appearance because this foundation tends to "grab" over less-than-smooth areas and cannot be easily softened once set. Although 12 shades are available (this is the only Shiseido foundation with colors for dark skin) 5 of them are unacceptably pink or peach. Avoid B20, B40, B60, B80, and I60. The other shades present some attractive options, especially for fair skin.

☺ **$$$ Lifting Foundation SPF 16** *($42.50)* claims to provide "full coverage as beautiful as bare skin," but that's taking it too far (even though it's fun to imagine). With almost 10% titanium dioxide as the active ingredient, this creamy, thick foundation doesn't provide its complete coverage without looking like makeup. It spreads and blends well yet is very concentrated—a tiny dab covers half the face, yet you'll likely need more than that to ensure sufficient sun protection (unless you're applying this foundation over a regular sunscreen). Lifting Foundation SPF 16 has a silky, matte finish that appears somewhat chalky, something that's more apparent with the darker shades. Still, this formula is a huge step forward from the greasy, full-coverage foundations of years past. Among the ten shades, the only poor choices are B60 (very peach) and the slightly peach shades B20 and I40. Lastly, this foundation won't lift the skin—the real reason to consider it is if you need significant coverage and want a foundation with sunscreen.

☺ **$$$ Powdery Foundation SPF 14-17** *($29.50 for powder; $8 for compact)* features titanium dioxide as its sole active ingredient, but the SPF rating varies by shade, which explains why Shiseido listed an SPF range rather than settling on one number. (Note that this is not authorized by FDA or Japanese regulations for sunscreens.) This talc-based, pressed-powder foundation has a dry but silky texture that goes on soft and even, providing seamless light to medium coverage. It can function as your only sunscreen if you apply it liberally, but it works best when dusted over a regular sunscreen or foundation with sunscreen. The shade range is beautifully neutral, but lacks options for dark skin. The only color to avoid is the too-peach B60.

CONCEALER: ☺ **$$$ Concealer** *($20)* is Shiseido's best concealer, but given their other lackluster options that's not necessarily saying much. Still, this liquid concealer has its strong points, including a long-lasting matte finish and a formula that's appropriate for use on blemishes. Because talc is the second ingredient it sets quickly, so blending must be deft. On the plus side, this won't crease and it provides significant coverage. It would be worthy of a Paula's Pick rating if only the four shades were better. If you decide to try this, Light and Dark are the best colors; Light Enhancer is sheer and best used for subtle highlighting.

☺ **$$$ Concealer Stick** *($26.50)* comes in an attractive metal twist-up component and has a creamy texture that glides over skin without being too slippery. It sets to a satin finish and each of the three shades provides considerable coverage, but it has the drawbacks of looking chalky and also being prone to minor creasing. The creasing can be remedied with powder, but the chalky finish keeps this product from earning a higher rating.

☹ **Corrector Pencil** *($17)* is a standard, dry-finish pencil that comes in three average but workable colors. This provides good coverage, but application is an issue, and it looks quite obvious on the skin while also being too stiff to soften.

POWDER: ✓☺ **$$$ Pureness Mattifying Compact Oil-Free SPF 16** *($20 for powder cake; $8 for compact)* is a slam-dunk recommendation for those with oily to very oily skin looking for an absorbent, matte-finish pressed powder with sun protection. The actives are titanium dioxide and zinc oxide (which are quite absorbent on their own), and the talc-based formula applies well, despite feeling too dry. All shades are recommended.

☺ **$$$ Enriched Loose Powder** *($32.50)* has an airy texture whose single shade produces a soft, translucent finish on skin. The look is more satiny than powdery, which makes this best for normal to dry skin. If it weren't so sheer the single shade would be very limiting. By the way, the amount of Shiseido's Advanced Nutrient Factor, said to make this powder moisturizing, is negligible. If this powder did not have such a finely milled texture, it would be a mistake to consider. As it is, if you don't mind the shine for daytime, it's an option.

☺ **$$$ Pressed Powder** *($22.50 for powder; $7.50 for compact)* comes in colors suitable for fair skin and has a talc-based formula that feels smooth but is more powdery than the best options in this category. It's a good option if you have light skin and want a sheer, basic pressed powder, but that's about it.

☺ **$$$ Translucent Loose Powder** *($35)* is a mica- and talc-based loose powder with a gossamer texture and nearly invisible finish on skin. Although this powder appears pure white in the jar, it goes on translucent and is suitable for all skin tones except very dark. Brushed on, it makes skin look beautifully polished and won't interfere with the color of your foundation.

☺ **$$$ Luminizing Color Powder** *($22.50 for powder; $10.50 for compact)* is a talc-based pressed powder that features three colors, one of which is quite shiny, in one powder cake. The color selection ranges from pure white shimmer to glittery bronze, and none of them would help set makeup or reduce shine. These are workable as highlighting powders, but the effect depends on careful application so as not to make your foundation look strange.

BLUSH AND BRONZER: ☺ **$$$ Accentuating Color Stick** *($33)* has a slick, silicone-based texture that is quick to dry out if you don't replace the cap tightly after each use. Think of this as a hybrid cream-to-powder blush that is best applied over moist skin (applying it over powdered skin assures a spotty, streaked look). Each shade goes on almost as bright as it looks, but blending softens the effect and the product sets to a natural matte finish. This works as lip color, too, though it's best paired with a gloss unless you're comfortable with its matte finish.

☺ **$$$ The Makeup Multi-Shade Enhancer** *($26 for powder cake; $10.50 for compact)* is a pressed powder bronzer that is completely average in every way. Designed to be housed in a sold-separately compact, it's composed of five shimmery stripes of graduated colors. When swirled together with a brush, the result is less bronze and more of an iridescent glow, but achieving that look takes work because the powder, though very soft to the touch, does not easily lift onto a brush or adhere well to skin. Two shades are available. The lighter option, Sunset Glow, is a very shiny peach, while Terra-Cotta Glow is more luminous bronze—however, neither shade creates a natural bronzing effect, because real tans don't shimmer!

☺ **$$$ Accentuating Powder Blush** *($29.50)* is a standard pressed-powder blush with the requisite smooth texture and even application. Color deposit is sheer, and each shade has some amount of shine. It's a decent option, though overpriced for what you get. Powder blushes from L'Oreal, Revlon, or Physician's Formula easily best this, in price and in overall performance.

EYESHADOW: ☺ **$$$ Hydro-Powder Eye Shadow** *($24)* has an intriguing water-to-powder texture with enough slip to make it easy to blend over small areas. This sets to a matte (in feel) finish and the shades have an iridescent or metallic flake-free shine, depending on which you choose.

☺ **$$$ Silky Eye Shadow Duos** *($28.50)* must be applied in sheer layers because the formula is pressed so softly that application can be powdery and encourage flaking. If layered, the powder clings well and blends beautifully, with each shade having some degree of shine. Several of the duos are odd or contrasting colors, so unless you're up for a challenge, choose from among the following pairs: S1, S11, S19, or S20.

☹ **Accentuating Color for Eyes** *($21)* may look appealing, but it is completely unremarkable. Each color is intensely shiny and densely filled with chunky particles of mica that definitely reflect light, but also tend to flake all over—bad news for contact lens wearers. In addition, whoever created some of these colors must not realize that bright pink and orange eyeshadows don't accent eyes. Rather, sweeping these particular shades over the lid may make others think that you've been crying all day or have an eye infection. Still, there are always those with avant-garde tastes, where the intensity of the color, not the flaking, is what really matters.

☹ **Silky Eye Shadow Quad** *($36.50)* may look appealing, but it's completely unremarkable. Each color is intensely shiny and densely filled with chunky particles of mica that definitely do reflect light, but also tend to flake all over—bad news for contact lens wearers. In addition, the color combinations are poorly done.

EYE AND BROW SHAPER: ☺ **$$$ The Makeup Accentuating Cream Eyeliner** *($26)* is Shiseido's version of the numerous gel eyeliners offered at cosmetics counters. Their version shares the same formula basics and easy-to-apply traits as the others, yet its finish remains slightly tacky, and that can affect wear time. The included synthetic, angled eyeliner brush is a nice touch, but not enough to propel this above the front-runners in this category (Bobbi Brown, M.A.C., and Stila come to mind).

☺ **$$$ Eyebrow and Eyeliner Compact** *($29.50)* presents a brow powder and powder eyeliner (either may be used wet or dry) in one compact. The brow tones are good for those with brown or black hair only, yet each applies smoothly considering the dry texture, and the color builds well. Oddly, each duo has a slight amount of shine, which doesn't add much to the result (eyebrows aren't supposed to shine). As for the included applicator, it is best tossed in favor of full-size brushes.

☺ **$$$ Fine Eyeliner** *($28)* is another liquid eyeliner with a brush that is only capable of applying a thick line. The color seeps into the brush much like ink in a fountain pen, making it hard to control how much comes out at once, but this can be workable once you adapt to its peculiarities. Watch out for Soft Black, which is really olive green.

☺ **$$$ Translucent Eyebrow Shaper** *($23)* remains one of the most expensive brow gels around, and let me be the first to tell you how indistinguishable this is from the inexpensive version from Cover Girl, which also is less sticky than Shiseido's version.

☹ **Eyebrow Pencil** *($16)* is also below standard, with stiff, dry application and a waxy/tacky finish that's a far cry from the worry-free result of filling in brows with powder. This is disappointing given how attractive the color choice is.

☹ **Eyeliner Pencil** *($16)* is below average due to its creamy texture, which tends to drag over skin, and its smudge-prone finish.

☹ **Eyeliner Pencil Duo** *($21)* is a needs-sharpening dual-sided pencil with a standard eyeliner color on one end and a shiny pastel or vivid tone on the other. Both ends are too creamy and remain so, which invites smearing and fading.

☹ **The Makeup Natural Eyebrow Pencil** *($20)* is an eyebrow pencil that isn't worth considering unless you enjoy exerting much more pressure than you need to with almost every other eyebrow pencil to achieve decent results. The brush on the other end of this needs-sharpening pencil is fine, but it cannot soften this pencil's hard, waxy finish.

LIPSTICK, LIP GLOSS, AND LIPLINER: ✓☺ **$$$ Perfect Rouge Lipstick** *($25)* is truly one of the most elegant lipsticks I have ever reviewed. In stick form this collection of sheer cream lipsticks appears no different from the hundreds of others on the market. But once applied, the silky-smooth texture and beautiful subtle shimmer are gorgeous. This is shimmer done right and it includes a touch of shine. The color selection has expanded to over 20 shades, and ranges from light to dark so there is no doubt you'll find more than one to love. As with any cream lipstick, use of a lipliner is recommended to avoid "feathering" and to extend wear time.

✓☺ **$$$ Perfecting Lipstick** *($22.50)* costs more than a lipstick should, but if you're going to spend this much to paint your lips, it might as well be on a superior product like this. Shiseido has created a modern cream lipstick that moisturizes without feeling greasy and affords a soft gloss or shimmer finish from its brilliant, rich colors. There is not a bad shade in the bunch, which may make it hard to choose, but have fun trying!

☺ **$$$ Lip Gloss** *($21)* makes a wonderfully non-sticky, lightweight finishing touch if you aren't put off by the price. The shade selection sizzles and finishes sheer with sparkles that don't feel grainy.

☺ **$$$ Shimmering Lipstick** *($23.50)* is an emollient, creamy lipstick with a slippery feel that lingers, so count on this making its way into any lines around your mouth. Coverage is moderate while, true to its name, the finish is shimmering.

☺ **$$$ The Makeup Automatic Lip Crayon** *($23)* looks like it needs routine sharpening, but it doesn't. This automatic, retractable creamy lip pencil combines lipstick and gloss in one convenient package. Lightweight yet creamy and slick, this isn't for those prone to lipstick bleeding into lines around the mouth. Others will appreciate the flattering gloss finish and the good stain of each color. Regarding shades, most are bold peaches and pinks.

☺ **$$$ Translucent Gloss Lipstick** *($20)* is a colorless, emollient lip balm that leaves a glossy finish and helps prevent chapping, just like countless other less expensive lip balms, though this one is glossier than most.

☺ **$$$ Lip Liner Pencil** *($16)* is worth considering if you don't mind the price and routine sharpening. It goes on creamy, deposits rich color, and stays in place better than expected given its texture.

☺ **$$$ Sheer Gloss Lipstick** *($22.50)* is accurately named! The color selection is certainly worth a look if you prefer this type of lipstick, though it can feel slightly sticky.

MASCARA: ☺ **$$$ Advanced Volume Mascara** *($22)* promises to thicken lashes for "an intensely dramatic look" and it does that in spades! The trade-off is a heavy application that requires you to comb through with a clean mascara wand for the most attractive results. The reward is long wear without flaking and very dramatic lashes.

☺ **$$$ Distinguish Mascara** *($22)* doesn't distinguish itself from lots of other mascaras that can produce equally impressive length with a hint of fullness. This is a very good mascara, but considering the name and price, upon first use it should give you the impression that it will rise above the rest, and that just doesn't happen.

☺ **$$$ Extra Length Mascara** *($22)* lengthens quickly and without clumps or smearing. You can build some thickness, but this excels primarily at creating long, perfectly defined lashes.

☺ **$$$ Lasting Lift Mascara** *($22)* has a long, thin spiral brush that allows you to reach every lash and extend it for a defined, separated (and, OK, lifted) result. Length is more prominent than thickness, but successive coats add volume.

☹ **$$$ Mascara Base** *($23)* is another clear lash primer meant to boost the application and wear of any mascara. Adding Mascara Base before applying most mascaras produced slightly more length, but no extra thickness. The trade-off was that it's harder to apply mascara evenly over the coating formed on your lashes after you've applied the Base, but, with patience, you can get longer lashes than you can with mascara alone. The difference isn't significant and in the long run, isn't worth the trouble.

FACE AND BODY ILLUMINATING/SHIMMER PRODUCTS: ☺ **$$$ Luminizing Blush Powder** *($45)* wins points for its clever, slim packaging. The cap includes a built-in pressed shimmer powder and the base houses a full, natural-hair powder brush that is concealed with the touch of a button so you can replace the cap without splaying the bristles. Each time you replace the cap, a small amount of powder gets on the tip of the brush, ready for the next application. I wish this weren't so pricey because it is an attractive, convenient way to dust on a sheer layer of shiny powder for special occasions or as evening makeup. The only drawback other than the high price is that the powder doesn't cling to skin as well as it should. If you plan to purchase this product, apply moisturizer or a dry oil spray before powdering so it will cling to your skin more securely.

☹ **$$$ Sheer Enhancer Base SPF 15** *($32)* is a slightly thick liquid base available in two shades: white and a bronze tone that is a bit too coppery for most skin tones. Shiseido maintains that this product "naturally defines facial contours as it minimizes dullness and reflects a translucent brilliance." The slight amount of shimmer in both shades is where the "brilliance" comes into play, but otherwise this isn't a great option for contouring, primarily because it is too sheer and the colors can look strange. The white shade is slightly opaque, and thus provides a bit of camouflage for mild redness or a sallow skin tone. However, the effect is mostly muted once you apply foundation, and you will definitely want to do that because the white shade is not attractive on its own unless you're going for a pasty, pale look. Sheer Enhancer Base has good intentions along with an in-part titanium dioxide sunscreen, but its limitations (and price) should give you pause.

BRUSHES: ☹ **$$$ Shiseido Brushes** *($18-$50)* are supposedly approved by fashion makeup artist Tom Pecheux, and if that's true he must prefer brushes that are mostly too floppy and soft for anything but very sheer application. The only worthwhile brushes in this straightforward collection are the **Concealer** *($20)* and **Eye Shadow Brush Medium** *($24)*, and even they have drawbacks when compared to the options from most other lines.

SPECIALTY PRODUCTS: ☺ **$$$ Brightening Veil SPF 24** *($33.50)* features an all titanium dioxide sunscreen in a silicone and nylon-12 base, so you're assured of a silky finish with some good absorbent properties that those with normal to oily skin will enjoy. Those with breakout-prone skin should avoid this product due to its ceresin (a waxlike substance) content. The single shade is a neutral fair beige tone that can function as a lightweight concealer or can be used as a highlighter. The cream-to-powder texture blends right into the skin, and if the shade is a match for you, it can be used as a stand-alone light-coverage foundation.

☺ **$$$ Matifying Veil SPF 17** *($33.50)* has an in-part titanium dioxide sunscreen and is composed primarily of various silicones, which leave a solid matte finish on the skin. However, this isn't too far removed from the Smoothing Veil below, and each will have the same basic effect on the skin. You may want to sample both before you decide whether one (or both) of these would make a smart addition to your makeup routine. The Matifying version is best for normal to very oily skin and does not contain waxes that may clog pores.

☺ **$$$ Smoothing Veil SPF 16** *($33.50)* is a silicone-based makeup primer with an in-part titanium dioxide sunscreen. This colorless, solid cream leaves a soft, opalescent finish that feels very silky. It's an extra step whose line- and pore-filling benefit won't be all that noticeable, at least not any more than a foundation can provide. For the most part this is just a great way to get sun protection if your favored foundation does not include sunscreen or lacks effective UVA protection. This can be used by all skin types.

☺ **$$$ Eraser Pencil** *($17)* is a wax-based pencil (like almost all other needs-sharpening pencils) that is colorless and designed to remove makeup mistakes, such as those from mascara or eye pencils. You swipe the pencil over the makeup and it wipes off cleanly. This is convenient to have on hand and works quickly, but is not an essential because a bit of foundation, concealer, or a little makeup remover on a cotton swab provides the same results.

SHU UEMURA

SHU UEMURA AT-A-GLANCE

Strengths: Oil-based cleansers for dry to very dry skin; makeup is this line's strong suit; the Pro Concealer provides incredible coverage and comes in a great range of colors; excellent powders, powder blush, and powder eyeshadows; good lipsticks; a brilliant, extremely well-made selection of makeup brushes and all manner of cosmetic applicators.

Weaknesses: Expensive; some sunscreens leave skin vulnerable to UVA damage; no products to manage acne; mediocre toners and moisturizers; irritating masks; for the money, the pencils and mascaras lack even a mild "wow factor"; Lip Fix doesn't fix anything; the Brush Cleaner is inferior to using a gentle shampoo to remove makeup residue and oil from your tools.

For more information about Shu Uemura, owned by L'Oreal, call (888) 748-5678 or visit www.shuuemura-usa.com or www.Beautypedia.com.

SHU UEMURA SKIN CARE

SHU UEMURA DEPSEA PRODUCTS

☺ $$$ **Depsea Moisture Replenishing Lotion** *($30 for 5 ounces)* is a decent moisturizing toner for normal to dry skin. It would be rated higher if it did not contain so many volatile fragrance components.

☹ **Depsea Water** *($24 for 5 ounces)* presents a collection of facial mists, but whether you choose Bergamot, Chamomile, *Hamamelis* (witch hazel), Lavender, Rosemary, Rose, or Sage, each one is nothing more than seawater with potentially irritating fragrance components. The Fragrance-Free version is just water and a preservative. Unbelievable! The company maintains that their seawater, taken from great depths, enriches skin with over 60 minerals. Even if that's true, not all minerals are beneficial for skin and even the good ones are neither a panacea nor even that essential for skin when applied topically in a watered-down mist.

☺ $$$ **Depsea Moisture Replenishing Cream** *($38 for 1 ounce)* contains some wonderfully effective ingredients for dry to very dry skin, including standbys such as mineral oil and petrolatum. Water-binding agents and anti-irritants add to the benefits, which is why it's a shame jar packaging was chosen because it won't keep the handful of antioxidants stable during use.

☺ $$$ **Depsea Moisture Replenishing Emulsion** *($55 for 2.5 ounces)* shares many of the same ingredients as the Depsea Moisture Replenishing Cream above, but with a lighter, lotion-like texture. The omissions are enough to knock this moisturizer down to average status, while the many volatile fragrance components increase the odds of this causing irritation.

☺ $$$ **Depsea Moisture Replenishing Essence** *($60 for 1 ounce)* is a basic serum-type moisturizer for normal to oily skin. It is only worth the cost if you firmly believe that Uemura's seawater is an "empowered" ingredient your skin cannot do without.

SHU UEMURA PHYTO-BLACK LIFT PRODUCTS

☺ $$$ **Phyto-Black Lift Anti-Wrinkle Eye and Lip Contour Cream** *($125 for 1.6 ounces)*. It is nothing short of outrageous that Shu Uemura (a L'Oreal-owned company) charges such an exorbitant price for what amounts to a merely OK moisturizer. It contains a standard roster of emollients and thickening agents along with some effective plant oils, but all of those are standard issue for lots of products that don't come close to this price level. When you consider the jar packaging and that the plant extracts won't stay stable because the container isn't airtight, the price becomes even more ridiculous. The company makes a big deal about the source of their sea water, but after it is purified to the very strict standards used in the cosmetics industry, the sea water is just water. The long and short of it is that this moisturizer is a waste of money. If you want to forgo logic and waste money (not unusual in the cosmetics industry), it is most appropriate for normal to dry skin.

☺ $$$ **Phyto-Black Lift Firming Anti-Wrinkle Cream** *($125 for 1.6 ounces)* is very similar to Shu Uemura's Phyto-Black Lift Anti-Wrinkle Eye and Lip Contour Cream above. As such, the same review applies.

☹ **Phyto-Black Lift Lifting Anti-Wrinkle Essence** *($95 for 1 ounce)*. For nearly $100, you're getting a serum that's mostly water, slip agents, emollient, and alcohol, period. Any well-researched antiwrinkle ingredients are absent in this formula, which makes the price even more insulting. The claims that this product can help reverse signs of aging are baseless, as are its claims of visibly lifting skin. This isn't a "girdle in a bottle," whatever that's supposed to mean!

All the algae, sea water, and plants in the world aren't going to lift skin even one millimeter, and thinking otherwise is literally an invitation to throw your money away.

☹ **Phyto-Black Lift Radiance Boosting Lotion** *($45 for 5 ounces)*. Alcohol is the third ingredient listed in this poorly formulated lightweight moisturizer for normal to oily skin. Alcohol causes free-radical damage as well as irritation and dryness. The Phyto-Black in the product name refers to the form of black tea included, but there is no research showing it has benefit for skin. If it were so special, why doesn't L'Oreal include it in all their products, from Lancome to Vichy? None of the potentially helpful ingredients matter much given that all of them are listed after the alcohol.

☺ **$$$ Phyto-Black Lift Renewing Firming Night Cream** *($150 for 1.6 ounces)* might have been worth the money if it really did firm and stimulate skin while you sleep, but it doesn't. This is a very ordinary moisturizer that will see the effectiveness of its plant oils and extracts compromised due to the jar packaging. Moreover, alcohol appears on the ingredient list before several intriguing ingredients, which isn't good news for skin at any time of day. The price is 100% out of line for what you get, and seawater plus the form of algae Shu Uemura chose have no special benefit when it comes to aging skin. The company makes a big deal about the source of their seawater, but after it is purified to the very strict standards used in the cosmetics industry the seawater is just water. The long and short of it is that this moisturizer is a waste of money.

☹ **Phyto-Black Lift Smoothing Anti-Wrinkle Emulsion** *($125 for 2.5 ounces)*. Nothing about this ultralight moisturizer is antiwrinkle, primarily because alcohol (the kind that causes irritation, dryness, and free-radical damage) is such a prominent ingredient. Given the paltry amount of bells and whistles for the money and the inclusion of several fragrance chemicals known to be irritating, you can only conclude that investing in this moisturizer is a mistake. Those looking to spend in this range for a single skin-care product can check out any of the recommended pricey moisturizers or serums in my Best Products lists on this site.

OTHER SHU UEMURA PRODUCTS

☺ **$$$ Cleansing Beauty Oil Premium A/O** *($32 for 5 ounces)* has the distinction of being the company's best-selling cleanser worldwide, but quite honestly, this mineral oil– and corn oil–based liquid is overwhelmingly standard, and the notion that it is best-selling makes me lament how easily taken in women can be by the cosmetics industry. The oils do a great job of dissolving makeup, and the mild surfactants are water-activated, producing a creamy emulsion that rinses better than plain oil would, but it can still leave a residue. This is an OK option for dry to very dry skin. It does contain several volatile fragrance components.

☺ **$$$ Foaming Cleansing Water** *($28 for 5 ounces)* is a gentle, water-soluble cleansing fluid that is a good option for normal to oily skin. It removes most types of makeup, but doesn't work as well on waterproof or long-wearing formulas as the Cleansing Beauty Oil Premium A/O.

☺ **$$$ High Performance Balancing Cleansing Oil** *($28 for 5 ounces)* is very similar to the Cleansing Beauty Oil Premium A/O above, only with fewer bells and whistles (none of which have much, if any, impact on skin). Otherwise, the same review applies.

☹ **High Performance Balancing Cleansing Oil, Enriched** *($28 for 5 ounces)* is only enriched because the company added some avocado oil, but your skin won't know the difference. The misstep here was including pepper extract, which has no business in a cleanser because it can be very irritating, especially around the eyes and mouth.

☹ **High Performance Balancing Cleansing Oil, Fresh** *($28 for 5 ounces)* creates the illusion of a fresh feeling from the irritating menthol derivative menthoxypropanediol, and is not recommended. Plain mineral oil would work just as well and without hurting skin in the process.

☹ **Ace B-G Reinforcing Emulsion** *($70 for 2.5 ounces)* offers a mixed bag of ingredients for normal to slightly dry skin. The glycerin, silicone, plant oil, and several water-binding agents are all pluses, but the amount of jasmine extract is potentially irritating, and this also contains several volatile fragrance components, including linalool and sensitizing eugenol. For the money, this doesn't translate to a wise investment in the quest for healthier skin.

☺ **$$$ Ace B-G Reinforcing Eye Cream** *($47 for 0.5 ounce)* is an OK, lightweight moisturizer for slightly dry skin, but the amount of jasmine extract makes it a potential problem for use around the eyes. It is unfortunate that the many antioxidants in this product are all present in low amounts. This product cannot minimize dark circles or puffiness as claimed.

☺ **$$$ Ace B-G Signs Preventing Essence** *($60 for 1 ounce)* contains more alcohol than helpful ingredients for skin, and that trumps any benefits possible from the many antioxidants in this nonessential Essence. The jasmine extract in here has no antiaging benefits for skin; it merely adds fragrance.

☺ **$$$ B-G Recharging Night Cream** *($55 for 1 ounce)* has a light yet creamy texture and provides some worthy ingredients to reinforce normal to slightly dry skin's structure, but the jar packaging won't keep the very small amount of antioxidants stable during use.

☺ **$$$ B-G Reinforcing Gel Cream** *($50 for 1 ounce)* is similar to but has a lighter texture than the B-G Recharging Night Cream above, and the same review applies.

☺ **$$$ B-G Reinforcing Booster** *($95 for 4 vials)* is a two-step process involving mixing their Powder with the Depsea Water in this combination system. This is supposed to deliver the maximum dosage of beta-glucan to the inner layers of skin, improving its elasticity and, get this, its immunity. Beta-glucan is a very good antioxidant for skin, but there is no established maximum dosage and the amount Shu Uemura includes barely qualifies as a minimum. The **Powder** is just a blend of sugars and a slip agent with lecithin, cholesterol, and preservatives; the **Depsea Water** is just water. Sure, it is said to come from the sea, but that has no special immunity-boosting benefit for skin. At almost $100 for five days' worth of treatments, this counts as one of the most expensive do-nothing products I have reviewed.

✓ ☺ **$$$ Face Paper** *($12 for 40 sheets)* consists of microscopically thin sheets of tissue paper that have a subtle texture that allows them to be a bit more absorbent than regular blotting papers. I don't think the difference is worth the price—not when you consider that many lines sell the same type of product for less than $6 and you get more sheets per package. Still, these non-powdery papers do the job very well and fit in even the tiniest evening bag.

☺ **$$$ Principe Lip Serum** *($22 for 0.33 ounce)* is a good emollient moisturizing fluid with a small amount of water-binding agents and antioxidant. This is a good option for lips, but the claims that it can exfoliate are completely false.

SHU UEMURA MAKEUP

FOUNDATION: ☺ **$$$ Face Architect Powder Foundation Natural Glow Finish SPF 22** *($45; $32.50 for powder refills)* is a fantastic pressed-powder foundation that contains an in-part titanium dioxide and zinc oxide sunscreen (among other active ingredients). The talc-based texture is exceptionally smooth and the application silky and sheer with a finish that's matte without looking chalky. It is excellent for all skin types except dry, and is best used over a daytime moisturizer or foundation with sunscreen (liberal application of this powder can look too heavy). Almost all of the shades are good and present options for fair to tan skin tones. Consider the slightly pink 364 and slightly peach 554 carefully. This would've earned a Paula's Pick rating if it didn't contain fragrance chemicals that pose a risk of irritation.

☺ **$$$ Face Architect Smoothing Fluid Foundation** *($42)* has a fluid, very light texture that is a pleasure to apply. Blending this liquid foundation takes some time due to the amount of slip, but the sheer, satin-matte finish is worth it. A natural look is attainable, but with that comes the knowledge that more obvious flaws will show through clearly unless you layer this to achieve medium coverage (which takes more foundation than most women want to use). The range of available shades includes many neutral options suitable for fair to dark (but not very dark) skin tones. Those to avoid due to slight overtones of pink, peach, or orange include 345, 355 (may work for some fair skin tones), 554, 734, and 934, which is very peach. For less money, reliable sunscreen, and an equally good selection of shades, check out L'Oreal True Match Super Blendable Makeup at the drugstore (and remember, L'Oreal owns Shu Uemura, so unless you believe the company's Depsea Water is an extraordinary achievement, there's no need to invest in this foundation).

☹ **$$$ Face Architect Remodeling Cream Foundation SPF 10** *($45)* has a great name, which may lead you to think it contains ingredients that can sculpt aging skin into its ideal appearance. Of course, it can't do that. In fact, it does a poor job of even providing basic sun protection because its SPF rating is below SPF 15, the minimum standard set by almost all medical organizations in the world, and it doesn't contain the UVA-protecting ingredients of titanium dioxide, zinc oxide, avobenzone (also known as butyl methoxydibenzoylmethane), Tinosorb, or Mexoryl SX. This jar-packaged foundation has a slightly creamy, smooth texture that blends well and sets to a soft matte finish. Coverage stays in the medium range and the formula is quite fragrant. As usual for Shu Uemura, the shade range is impressive. There are some good choices for fair skin, but no options for dark skin tones. Consider shade 734 carefully due to its slight peach cast. Shade 964 is noticeably yellow, but may work for some Asian skin tones.

CONCEALER: ☹ **$$$ Pro Concealer** *($23)* comes in a broad range of mostly neutral shades. Avoid 5YR Medium, which is too ash no matter how little you apply. This concealer has a heavy finish and is only for those who need full coverage.

☹ **Cover Crayon** *($24)* is a dual-ended pencil concealer with a thick, greasy texture and unappealing colors that look artificial on skin. You've been warned!

POWDER: ✓ ☺ **$$$ Face Powder Matte** *($33)* has a superfine, talc-based texture that creates a polished, not powdered, matte finish from each of the excellent shades. The jar component is equipped with a helpful sifter screen, making this much less messy than the typical loose powder. Although the finish is matte, this is a superior loose powder for all skin types except very dry.

✓ ☺ **$$$ Face Powder Sheer** *($33)* has an airy, sheer feel and an appearance that's amazingly skinlike, making this a prime choice for normal to dry skin. It would be better if there were more than two shades available. The component has the same helpful sifter screen as the Face Powder Matte.

BLUSH AND BRONZER: ✓ ☺ **$$$ Glow On** *($21)* has an enviably silky-smooth application and a soft powder texture that imparts color evenly. The shade selection is extensive, though a few of the colors are too pale or orange to work as blush. Still, this product remains one of the highlights of this Japanese line. The best shades include: M Pink 31C, M Pink 33E, M Pink 31, M Amber 89, M Amber 82, M Amber 85, M Orange 55, and M Peach 44.

☺ **$$$ Bronzing Powder** *($38)* has a dry texture that's non-powdery and applies soft and sheer yet not as evenly as it should. Every shade of this talc-based pressed bronzing powder has shine, and not all of them work convincingly to create bronzed skin; rather, some are better as shiny blush. The shine does cling well but it can still get on clothing, depending on how much you apply.

EYESHADOW: ✓ ☺ **$$$ Pressed Eye Shadow** *($20)* remains a premier powder eyeshadow with a silky feel and a smooth, flake-free application. The palette is huge, and the medium to dark shades (which aren't as dark as they used to be) apply evenly. These are divided into four different finishes: shades labeled **Pearl** have a standard soft-shimmer finish; the **Iridescent** shades have a stronger, more obvious shine than the Pearl; the **Metallic** colors are just that, and include some beautiful options for evening eye makeup; the **Matte** selection is beautiful though not every shade labeled matte is shine-free (still, the shine is really subtle, so these can pass for matte). If you check out one portion of Shu Uemura's makeup, it should be these shadows.

☺ **$$$ Cream Eye Shadow** *($30)* is a silicone- and wax-based cream eyeshadow that goes on smoothly but feels a bit waxy. It has a good amount of slip that eases application yet allows for controlled blending, which is critical for this type of eyeshadow. Most of the shades provide a soft wash of color with moderate shine, though there are a couple of basic matte shades (Sand Brown, Black, and White). Once set, this is minimally prone to creasing and the shine doesn't flake.

EYE AND BROW SHAPER: ✓ ☺ **$$$ Painting Gel Eyeliner** *($24)* differs little from all of the other long-wearing gel formulas available from lines such as Bobbi Brown, L'Oreal, and Paula's Choice. The intense colors go on smoothly and have the look of liquid eyeliner without the inherent drawbacks. The formula sets quickly and lasts all day without fading, smearing, or flaking. Shu Uemura created basic black and brown shades but the rest are Cirque de Soleil-colorful and not recommended unless living the circus life aptly describes you.

☺ **$$$ Liquid Eyeliner** *($33; $15 for refill cartridge)* has a great soft-but-firm brush that allows for one-shot application. The formula dries quickly and wears extraordinarily well (it's actually a bit difficult to remove). Although this is pricey, consider this a must-try if you prefer liquid liner and haven't found one that doesn't smear or fade. Note: This only comes in one shade—black—with a slight iridescent finish.

☺ **$$$ Drawing Pencils** *($19)* need sharpening and all of the colors are infused with glitter, but these pencils apply smoothly, their cream finish remains relatively smudgeproof, and the glitter barely flakes. Not bad, but not exceptional, nor is it preferred to lining the eyes with one of Shu Uemura's Pressed Eye Shadows.

☺ **$$$ Eye Light Pencil White** *($18)* is a dual-ended pencil, with a matte white on one end and a white shimmer on the other. Each end has a creamy but not slippery texture that stays in place surprisingly well. This is workable for highlighting, but keeping it sharpened isn't as convenient as just highlighting with a white or shimmer powder.

☺ **$$$ Eyebrow Manicure, Waterproof** *($25)*. If for some reason you need a waterproof eyebrow mascara, this product offers that benefit, but there is only one color available. That color is black, but it has a subtle, yet visible, metallic green tint that doesn't resemble anyone's real brow color. The effect, for those looking to dramatize brow color and shape, is intense. This really is waterproof yet manages to be non-sticky. The brush is small enough to allow for agile application even on thin brows, and the formula sets quickly. It's just that the metallic green tint is very odd, really limiting this product's appeal.

☹ **Hard Formula Eyebrow Pencil** *($22)* is extremely tricky to use, something the counter staff at Shu Uemura's defend because they have a special sharpening/shaving technique they recommend to get this undeniably hard-textured pencil to work. I can't imagine why anyone would want to go through this trouble given the myriad brow pencils available that pose no downside.

LIPSTICK, LIP GLOSS, AND LIPLINER: ✓ ☺ $$$ **Rouge Unlimited Creme Matte Lipstick** *($23)*. L'Oreal's influence on this Japanese cosmetics brand, which it acquired a few years back, has become more apparent in a few of Shu Uemura's recent product launches, including this Lipstick, which is excellent. These richly pigmented cream lipsticks feel great without being slick or bleeding into lines around the mouth. The finish is semi-matte and it beautifully emphasizes the opacity of the mostly striking colors. Of course, you don't have to spend this much for a quality lipstick, but if you choose to do so and want full coverage and impressive longevity, this won't leave you disappointed.

☺ $$$ **Gloss Unlimited** *($22)* is equipped with an elongated sponge-tip applicator that can be tricky to use if you have small lips. The gloss has a moderately thick texture that feels smooth and balm-like while imparting a soft gloss finish that's minimally sticky. All of the shades contain shimmer and apply more sheer than they look in the package.

☺ $$$ **Rouge Unlimited Lipstick** *($23)* has a smooth, creamy feel and a soft, glossy finish that stays slippery, so this won't last for an "unlimited" amount of time. Still, if you're not prone to lipstick bleeding into lines around the mouth it's worth considering, and the range of 48 shades has something for everyone. As an added bonus, every color goes on exactly the way it looks in the tube, and there are some gorgeous red shades.

☺ $$$ **Drawing Lip Pencil** *($19)* requires routine sharpening so it's not as convenient as automatic lip pencils, but it applies effortlessly and feels comfortably creamy without being prone to smudging. Color-wise, the range favors brown-toned hues and soft pinks, though there are also a few good reds and brighter tones to coordinate with Uemura's vast lipstick palette.

MASCARA: ☺ $$$ **Ultimate Expression Mascara** *($23)* has a slightly curved wand applicator, which I suppose was intended to help application, except that it doesn't. Application tends to be uneven, requiring significant comb-through for presentable results. If you have the patience this mascara demands, you'll get equal parts length and thickness with a dramatic flair. This removes easily with a water-soluble cleanser.

☺ $$$ **Lash Repair** *($22)* won't repair lashes any more than a hair conditioner can repair split ends. This water- and glycerin-based clear gel basically just makes lashes soft and more receptive to curling. It's a lightweight formula that contains several water-binding agents, but it won't strengthen lashes against future damage, at least not any better than wearing regular mascara every day.

☺ $$$ **Mascara Basic** *($27.50)* is a gel-based mascara that supposedly contains the same type of black ink found in Japanese calligraphy pens (which isn't safe for the eye area, so that ends up being a good story and nothing else). This takes lots of effort for minimal payoff and is incredibly difficult to remove because it tends to stain the lashes.

☹ **Precise Volume Mascara Waterproof** *($23)* produces sparse results from its uneven application, leading to merely average length and no thickness. The formula is tenaciously waterproof and more difficult than most to remove, making it a poor contender all around.

BRUSHES: ✓ ☺ $$$ **Shu Uemura Brushes** *($10-$270)*. Shu Uemura's reputation for superior Brushes is well deserved. Few lines offer such an extensive (at times eclectic) assortment of brushes, with all manner of natural hair and synthetic bristles. Although the prices on many of them are out of line, for sheer variety (there are more than 70) this brush collection is hard to beat. The most useful brushes are priced competitively with those from other artistry-driven lines such as M.A.C. and Bobbi Brown. My favorites, due to their shape, density, and overall performance, are the **Synthetic Brush 10** *($35)* and **Synthetic Brush 12** *($40),* both of which are great for eyeshadow application; the **Natural Brush 27** *($60)* for loose powder; **Natural Brush 14H** *($35)* if you have a large eye area to work with; the **Natural Brush 20** *($50)* for blush; the **Natural Brush 10DF** *($45)* for eye contour; and the **Synthetic Brush 6M** *($22)* for lipstick application.

✓ ☺ **$$$ Essential Brush Set & Portable Brush Set** *($164-$275)* are nicely done, but for this amount of money, it's imperative to make sure you'll regularly use every brush that's in these sets!

✓ ☺ **$$$ Kolinsky Brushes** *($45-$270).* If you're feeling indulgent, you won't be disappointed with any of the Kolinsky Brushes—they are luxury redefined! There really are no brushes to avoid, though many are not for everyone due to their differing shapes and cuts.

SPECIALTY PRODUCTS: ☺ **$$$ Base Control** *($22.50)* is a collection of liquid color correctors that mostly omits the standard roster of odd colors; although green is available, it goes on so sheer you can barely tell that the color looks a bit "off." Instead, the collection favors gold, silver, and brown tones that can be skillfully used to highlight or shadow parts of the face. The texture is fluid and silky and application is sheer with a soft matte (in feel) finish. Base Control is best used as a foundation primer or highlighter. It is suitable for all skin types, but it is not for most people's daily makeup routine.

☺ **$$$ Eyelash Curlers** *($19)* are a hot commodity because they're well designed and really work.

☺ **$$$ False Eyelashes** *($16-$50).* Those who want to experiment with false eyelashes will find Shu Uemura tough to beat, and the boutiques have eyelash bars where experts teach you how to tailor the various lashes to suit your needs. Uemura also sells his own Eyelash Adhesive.

☺ **$$$ Makeup Cases** *($35-$700).* Shu Uemura offers expertly designed, durable Makeup Cases; the professional makeup artist and makeup-savvy consumer looking to organize will appreciate these options.

☹ **$$$ UV Under Base SPF 10** *($32 for 2.2 ounces)* is a nearly colorless, airy mousse moisturizer with an in-part titanium dioxide sunscreen. It has a unique texture that is incredibly light, but what a shame the SPF value isn't higher so someone with oily skin could take advantage of this product! As is, you'll need to pair it with a foundation, powder, or regular sunscreen rated SPF 15 or higher.

☹ **Brush Cleaner** *($13 for 4.2 ounces)* is a liquid brush cleanser that contains acetone; the same solvent in many nail-polish removers. It will clean your brushes, but over time it also will break down the hair and make the brush unusable.

SK-II

SK-II AT-A-GLANCE

Strengths: Some well-formulated moisturizers and serums; all of the sunscreens provide sufficient UVA protection.

Weaknesses: Shockingly expensive, especially for the wide assortment of mediocre products; unreliable skin-lightening products; AHA/BHA products that contain an ineffective amount of exfoliant; no products to help manage blemishes; jar packaging.

For more information about SK-II, owned by Procter & Gamble, visit www.sk2.com or www.Beautypedia.com.

Note: Pitera is the cornerstone of the SK-II line and is present in every SK-II product. Pitera is the trade name for *Saccharomycopsis* ferment filtrate (SFF), a form of yeast purportedly unique because of the fermenting and filtering process it goes through before being added to these products. As it turns out, many forms of yeast have anti-inflammatory and antioxidant properties, including SFF (Source: *Journal of Dermatologic Science*, June 2006, pages 249-257). Other than that, all of the information about Pitera comes from papers presented at medical conferences, not from published studies. Presenting papers at medical conferences is not at all the same thing as publishing the results of studies. I frequently present papers and information at medical conferences, and I wouldn't offer that material as proof of anything because it isn't. The standards for presenting a paper at a medical conference are very different from the requirements for publication of study results in most medical journals.

SK-II SKIN CARE PRODUCTS

SK-II SIGNS PRODUCTS

☺ **$$$ Signs Eye Cream** *($105 for 0.5 ounce).* Unless you believe that Pitera (the star ingredient that sets Procter & Gamble-owned SK-II apart from the company's Olay brand) is worth the hefty expense, there is no reason to consider this jar-packaged eye cream over any product from Olay Regenerist, Definity, or Pro-X. A detailed explanation of Pitera is noted above, but basically this is not even remotely a miraculous or even close to a must-have ingredient for skin, and there's not a shred of published, substantiated research that can refute my statement. Signs Eye Cream contains basic emollient ingredients that moisturize dry skin anywhere on the face, helping to improve barrier function, but the jar packaging is a problem for the stability of the teeny amount of beneficial ingredient it does contain. CeraVe Moisturizing Lotion, available at the drugstore for a fraction of the price, is far more elegantly formulated. The bottom line is you don't need to spend anywhere near this offensive amount of money to gain these benefits.

☺ **$$$ Signs Nourishing Cream** *($160 for 1 ounce)* follows the same pattern as other SK-II moisturizers (including eye creams): water, Pitera (listed by its yeast name of *Saccharomycopsis* ferment filtrate), glycerin, thickeners, and niacinamide, the latter the B vitamin that shows up in lots of products, including dozens from Olay (both Olay and SK-II are owned by Procter & Gamble). This moisturizer is supposed to address sagging skin, allowing it to "bounce back beautifully" because it addresses skin's loss of elasticity. It doesn't do that. No skin-care product can do that because once skin starts to sag due to lost elasticity (which occurs from sun damage and gravity, among other factors), cosmetic ingredients can't change that. I know that doesn't stop consumers from thinking that a face-lift-in-a-jar does exist, but it's the truth. At best, this is just a smooth-feeling, ordinary jar-packaged moisturizer that won't keep the teeny amount of beneficial ingredients present stable. There are far better products for a fraction of this price for normal to dry skin.

☺ **$$$ Signs Totality** *($175 for 2.8 ounces).* Aside from the Pitera and the price tag, there is nothing in or about this product that Olay Regenerist's Daily Regenerating Serum can't do far better. Not to mention that Olay's version is in proper packaging designed to keep its ingredients stable, while Signs Totality comes in a jar, making it anything but total.

☺ **$$$ Signs Up-Lifter** *($250 for 1.3 ounces).* Just when you thought you had had enough of Pitera, this product actually contains an even more concentrated version of this strain of yeast, called Pitera 4. It's there along with many of the same ingredients you find in Olay's Regenerist, and that means this is a good, fragrance-free moisturizer for normal to dry skin. I should mention that there are a few extras in Signs Up-Lifter, like *Padina pavonica* extract, from a form of algae that has some antioxidant properties. But as it turns out, a comparison study (my favorite kind) found that a different form of algae had far more potent antioxidant abilities, namely *Caulerpa racemosa* (Source: *Journal of Experimental Marine Biology and Ecology*, July 2005, pages 35-41). This also contains *Crithmum maritimum* extract, another form of algae. There is some research that shows *Crithmum maritimum* has some antioxidant properties, but there is also research showing it can be cytotoxic (toxic to cells) (Source: *Journal of Natural Products*, September 1993, pages 1598-1600). In the greater scheme of things, these extras add up to a whole lot of nothing.

☺ **$$$ Signs Eye Mask** *($105 for 14 pairs).* If I've done my math right, this mask weighs in at almost $400 for 1 ounce of product, making it the most expensive SK-II item. Oddly, you don't even get the "concentrated" amount of Pitera that's present in several other SK-II products. For the money, even if you were a Pitera adherent, this isn't the way to get the stuff on your skin. It has some interesting ingredients, but again, nothing that would make it rank over and above Olay Regenerist or Definity. The few additional plant extracts in here aren't worth the extra expense or time to apply this mask. For example, it contains *Chrysanthellum indicum* extract (from golden chamomile), which has some research showing it reduces irritation and improves the appearance of rosacea. However, the studies didn't compare the extract with other anti-irritant ingredients or protocols, only with a placebo (Source: *Journal of the European Academy of Dermatology & Venereology*, September 2005, page 564).

SK-II WHITENING SOURCE PRODUCTS

☹ **Whitening Source Clear Lotion** *($65 for 5 ounces).* Other than niacinamide and a small amount of ascorbyl glucoside (a form of vitamin C), this toner-like skin-lightening product doesn't contain anything of significance to banish skin discolorations. If you want to see how niacinamide might work on your discolorations, you can purchase any of the serums or lightening products from Olay's Regenerist or Definity lines (Procter & Gamble owns both SK-II and Olay, and Olay has the better products). It's particularly egregious that SK-II includes (and brags about) peppermint extract, which serves only to irritate skin and offers no whitening (though consumers may think the product is working because it tingles). Pitera, the star ingredient found throughout the SK-II line, is front-and-center in this product. The bottom line is that there is no published, substantiated research anywhere proving that it has any benefits for skin, and that includes having any effect on discolorations.

☺ **$$$ Whitening Source Intensive Mask** *($140 for 10 masks).* The repetitiveness of the formulations in the SK-II line is exhausting. Here, as with most of the SK-II products, you get mostly water, Pitera, slip agents, niacinamide, antioxidant, and preservatives. Overall, this mask isn't worth the money or trouble, and it definitely won't affect skin color.

☺ **$$$ Whitening Source Skin Brightener** *($125 for 2.6 ounces).* I should be surprised that a product consisting mostly of silicone, yeast (that's what Pitera is, listed as *Saccharomycopsis* ferment filtrate), slip agent, and preservative has such an inflated price. Sadly, I'm not because this is just one more example of how incredibly out of hand this segment of the cosmetics industry has become. If you were hoping this moisturizer would be the answer for your skin discolorations, think again. The tiny amounts of vitamin C and niacinamide it contains won't make even a freckle sweat, which is to say any lightening you get when using this product is purely coincidental. Any of the products with niacinamide from Olay's Regenerist, Total Effects, or Definity lines would work much better against skin discolorations and at a fraction of the cost (Procter & Gamble owns both Olay and SK-II). This product is really only capable of making skin feel silkier; all of the plant ingredients and antioxidants will deteriorate quickly once you begin using this jar-packaged moisturizer. One more comment to expand on Pitera: A detailed explanation of this ingredient (listed as *Saccharomycopsis* ferment filtrate) is presented in the brand summary for SK-II; suffice it to say it is not a miraculous or even close to a must-have ingredient for skin, and there's not a shred of published, substantiated research to prove otherwise.

OTHER SK-II SKIN CARE PRODUCTS

☺ **$$$ Facial Treatment Cleanser** *($55 for 4 ounces)* is a decent, extremely overpriced, basic, water-soluble, detergent-based cleanser that is an option for normal to oily skin, if only the cost weren't so ludicrous. It does contain Pitera and a few other interesting extras, but in a cleanser they will hardly be on your face before they are rinsed down the drain.

☺ **$$$ Facial Treatment Cleansing Gel** *($55 for 3.5 ounces)* is an extremely standard, mineral oil–based (yes, mineral oil) wipe-off cleanser that, shockingly, comes in a jar! Sticking your fingers into any product is bad news for its stability. This is more reminiscent of a cold cream than anything else, and it's a very expensive cold cream! The only reason to blow $50 on this would be because you actually believed that the Pitera it contains was simply the most important skin-care ingredient ever. It also contains *Crithmum maritimum* extract, from a seaweed commonly known as rock samphire or sea fennel. Some research does show that it has antioxidant properties, but there is also research showing it can be cytotoxic (toxic to cells) (Source: *Journal of Natural Products*, September 1993, pages 1598-1600).

☺ **$$$ Facial Treatment Cleansing Oil** *($55 for 8.4 ounces)* is mostly mineral oil with a few thickening agents, plant extracts, and, of course, Pitera. This is one of the most expensive containers of mineral oil I've ever seen! The few bells and whistles in here aren't nearly enough to make up for the absurd price and the absence of any unique benefit for skin.

☺ **$$$ Facial Treatment Clear Lotion** *($55 for 5 ounces)* is an exceptionally standard toner that is mostly water and Pitera (well, it isn't standard if you think Pitera is the best ingredient ever for skin). There is a tiny, and I mean really tiny, amount of a good water-binding agent, even smaller amounts of salicylic acid, and two alpha hydroxy acids. While the pH is low enough for them to function as exfoliants, the amount of BHA and AHAs is far too low for them to be effective. Spending this much money on what is a basic toner would have to be based only on your faith in Pitera because every other ingredient is easily replaced by better formulations for far less money.

☺ **$$$ Skin Refining Treatment** *($140 for 1.7 ounces)*. I almost fell off my chair when I saw the price of this ordinary salicylic acid (BHA) cream. Other than Pitera—and I have no idea why every product has to have this ingredient—there is no reason to spend this much of your hard-earned money on what amounts to a decent, though basic BHA product. One word of warning: At 2.3, the pH of this product is unusually low, which means there is a high

The Reviews S

potential for irritation. Also, the jar packaging isn't the best. But given that this fragrance-free product contains the teensiest amount of an antioxidant and some aloe water, even that can't really make a difference.

☺ $$$ **Advanced Eye Treatment Film** *($90 for 0.5 ounce)* is mostly Pitera, water, slip agents, preservatives, and comb extract. The comb extract is from hen or rooster combs, which may mislead you into thinking that it is similar to the hyaluronic acid in some dermal fillers such as Restylane. But it isn't—it's not even close. So, aside from the Pitera, this product comes up a big zero; it's actually one of the most contains-nothing products around. This is all about Pitera, and banking on that is not a reliable investment.

☹ **Advanced Protect Essence UV, SPF 15** *($90 for 1 ounce)* is problematic because the cost of any expensive sunscreen means you are unlikely to apply it liberally, which means you won't be getting adequate sunscreen protection. Separate from my concerns about application, this product is not recommended even though it contains an in-part zinc oxide sunscreen. That's because, for unknown reasons, SK-II decided to include the irritating menthol derivative menthyl lactate. Any of Olay's sunscreens with zinc oxide or avobenzone are distinctly preferred to this pricey mistake.

☺ $$$ **De-Wrinkle Essence** *($165 for 0.85 ounce)* is an almost identical copy of Olay Re-generist's Targeted Tone Enhancer, except for the Pitera, of course. The decision about which product to choose seems clear to me, but to be specific, De-Wrinkle is a good, lightweight moisturizer for someone with normal to slightly dry skin. It contains some good antioxidants and a cell-communicating ingredient.

☺ $$$ **Facial Hydrating UV Cream, SPF 15** *($110 for 1.7 ounces)* is almost identical to the Advanced Protect Essence UV, SPF 15 above, but this version omits the irritant menthyl lactate. However, the jar packaging is disappointing. Although that won't affect the SPF, it will affect the teensy amount of vitamin E, as well as the Pitera.

☺ $$$ **Facial Lift Emulsion** *($120 for 3.3 ounces)*. Other than the Pitera (*I'm* getting tired of me saying that), this is a decent, though ordinary, fragrance-free, lightweight moisturizer for normal to dry skin that contains too little of antioxidants and water-binding agents.

☺ $$$ **Facial Treatment Essence** *($145 for 5 ounces)* is supposed to contain "the most concentrated amount of Pitera of all the SK-II skincare products—around 90% pure SK-II Pitera." Indeed, that is all this contains, other than some slip agents, water, and preservatives. What a waste, and what a strange gimmick to thrust on women the world over.

☺ $$$ **Facial Treatment Massage Cream** *($110 for 2.5 ounces)* comes to you in jar packaging that prevents the air-sensitive ingredients from remaining stable. But given that Pitera and a teeny amount of vitamin E are the only ingredients that could be affected, there isn't much to worry about. There is no reason to consider this ordinary water-and-wax basic moisturizer for dry skin.

☺ $$$ **Facial Treatment Repair C** *($150 for 1 ounce)*, despite the name, doesn't contain vitamin C. In fact, all it contains is Pitera, water, slip agents, water-binding agent, and preservatives. The one thing you may be gleaning from this product lineup is that whatever effect Pitera has, P&G must believe it takes a lot of it to provide a benefit. Otherwise, why not just offer one super-Pitera product and call it good, and have this option be something else that is proven to be beneficial for skin?

☺ $$$ **Ultimate Revival Cream** *($330 for 1.7 ounces)* has the distinction of being the second most expensive moisturizer in the SK-II line, and that is saying something when you consider how many moisturizers this line sells and the fact that most of them are in the $100 range. I wonder what the SK-II counter staff tells customers who have been using the "cheaper" moisturizers from this line. I imagine many of those SK-II customers will want to know what makes this "ultimate" cream hundreds of dollars better than the miraculous products they were sold during their last visit. The answer is nothing; it isn't any better or any worse than the ordinary, overpriced moisturizers littering this line. As it turns out, the only miracle is that consumers probably will fall for the claims about this product and buy it thinking they're one up on everyone else struggling to look younger. This is a classic example of expensive absolutely not being better in the world of cosmetics. You might be shocked to discover that the ingredients in this moisturizer are strikingly similar to those in every other moisturizer from SK-II. And you may feel faint (I know I would) if you bought Ultimate Revival Cream only to find out now that texture- and formula-wise it differs little from the moisturizers Olay sells in their Regenerist and Pro-X lines (both Olay and SK-II are owned by Procter & Gamble). The only extra you're getting for your money is the prestige factor SK-II promotes. Too bad a prestigious image doesn't help your skin, and it certainly is not a guarantee of superior antiaging skin care. I really can't stress enough what a waste of time and money this moisturizer is. Yes, it has what it takes to make dry skin feel and look better, and it can improve skin's barrier function to prevent moisture loss, but so can countless other moisturizers whose price tags haven't been catapulted into the stratosphere. SK-II insults even further by packaging this moisturizer in a jar. At this price, that's akin to paying for a 2-karat diamond ring only to find out you bought cubic zirconium (and not even good cubic zirconium). One more comment: Just like almost every SK-II product, this contains an ingredient known as Pitera (*saccharomycopsis* ferment filtrate). A detailed explanation of Pitera is presented in the At-A-Glance section for SK-II; suffice it to say it is not a miraculous or even close to a must-have ingredient for skin, and there's not a shred of published, substantiated research to prove otherwise.

☺ $$$ **Facial Treatment Mask** (*$85 for 6 masks*) is just water, Pitera, slip agents, and preservative. It does contain sodium salicylate, but the pH of the product, combined with the characteristics of this type of salicylate, render it a poor choice for exfoliation.

SK-II MAKEUP

FOUNDATION: ✓ ☺ $$$ **Signs Transform Foundation SPF 20** (*$90 for foundation; $40 for refillable compact*). This impressive, very light, cream-to-powder foundation has a liquid feel on the skin as you apply it and then sets to a solid matte finish. SK-II brags about the pigment technology and radiance-boosting light reflection properties this foundation is supposed to have; well, it does look natural on skin, but it doesn't supersede other well-formulated foundations. This resists creasing into lines and magnifying pores, but its minimally moist finish is ill-suited for those with dry skin unless you apply an emollient moisturizer underneath. The sunscreen is pure titanium dioxide, which is great. Signs Transform Foundation is available in six shades, all of which are recommended and apply and finish more neutral than they appear. The price for this foundation is unusually high, but at least the refill option saves you money if you choose to go with the deluxe compact. This is not an antiaging miracle, not even vaguely, but given the price they had to convince you that this wasn't just foundation you were applying. This deserves praise for its ease of use, sunscreen, and beautiful appearance on skin. This foundation is best for those with normal to oily skin.

☺ **$$$ Air Touch Foundation** (*$165 for starter set; $90 for refills*) is one of the most unusual and absurdly expensive foundations I've ever tested. I was left wondering why anyone would bother with this, and not only because the price is ridiculously out of line for what you get. Air Touch Foundation is said to harness "never-before-seen technology to deliver a precise application that gives an unparalleled result." The "never-before-seen" part must be the large circular component of the packaging; it's roughly the size of a softball, but flatter, and I have to agree that I've never before seen that as a way to get makeup on. There's a silver button in the center that has three settings: on, off, and a teardrop-shaped symbol that you set first to prime the foundation. The priming step supposedly activates the Air Touch Ionizer, a system that's said to give the foundation particles a positive charge while simultaneously preparing to mist a veil of negatively charged ions over skin. Without getting into an in-depth discussion about ions, which are simply atoms that have lost or gained one or more electrons, this Ionizer nonsense is as gimmicky as it gets. Priming this foundation with ionization is not an essential step that allows it to work better than any other foundation, and there's no proof to the contrary, and you won't experience better results, either. Once you turn the dial to "on" this is ready to mist on skin. The mist it produces is ultrafine, and it feels slightly damp as you move the spray around your face to ensure even application and a soft satin finish, but you must be very careful not to spray this into your eye or mouth, that's for sure, or over your hairline. Unless you want very sheer coverage you have to apply quite a bit, which means you'll be buying refills more often than you'd like. Applied normally, holding the device four inches from the face, produces a fine layer of sheer foundation that needs minor blending to smooth things out and produce a uniform soft matte finish. All of the four colors are fine (because they're so sheer) and are suitable for light to medium skin tones. Although Air Touch Foundation is interesting and "never before seen," the results aren't worth the expenditure.

SKINCEUTICALS (SKIN CARE ONLY)

SKINCEUTICALS AT-A-GLANCE

Strengths: Great line to shop if you're looking for well-formulated vitamin C and retinol products; some outstanding sunscreens, and every one provides sufficient UVA protection; one effective AHA product; good self-tanner; several fragrance-free products.

Weaknesses: Mostly problematic cleansers and toners; fruit and sugar extracts trying to substitute for AHA products when the real deal is much better; ineffective BHA products; jar packaging.

For more information about SkinCeuticals, owned by L'Oreal, call (800) 811-1660 or visit www.skinceuticals.com or www.Beautypedia.com.

☺ **$$$ Clarifying Cleanser** (*$29 for 5 ounces*) contains 2% salicylic acid along with the AHAs glycolic and mandelic acids. Although the pH of this cleansing scrub would allow chemical exfoliation, the acids are not in contact with skin long enough for that to occur. This is a good, water-soluble option for normal to oily skin, but keep it away from the eye area.

☹ **Cleansing Cream, for Normal to Dry Skin** (*$29 for 8 ounces*) contains too much sandalwood extract to make this creamy cleanser worth purchasing. The *Phellodendron* extract has anti-inflammatory properties, but they're canceled out by the sandalwood, not to mention the lesser amount of fragrant orange oil also included.

☹ **Foaming Cleanser** *($29 for 5 ounces)* contains several irritating plant extracts, including arnica, ivy, and pellitory, all of which make this otherwise fine water-soluble cleanser not recommended.

☺ **$$$ Gentle Cleanser, for Sensitive Skin** *($29 for 8 ounces)* is a cleansing gel/lotion hybrid that has surprisingly minimal cleansing ability, and the orange oil it contains isn't something that you should apply to sensitive skin. This is an OK option for normal skin when minimal to no makeup needs to be removed.

☺ **$$$ Simply Clean, for Combination or Oily Skin** *($29 for 8 ounces)* does a good job of cleansing and removing makeup for its intended skin types. However, it doesn't deserve a happy face rating due to the problematic plant extracts it includes.

☺ **$$$ Equalizing Toner, for Combination or Oily Skin** *($28 for 8 ounces)* is mostly water, mixed fruit extracts that don't work like AHAs, and aloe, though the amount of witch hazel is potentially irritating, as are the rosemary and thyme extracts.

☹ **Revitalizing Toner, for Normal or Dry Skin** *($28 for 8 ounces)* lists various fruit extracts said to work like AHAs, but they don't. The plants used in this toner are a skin-confusing blend of soothing and irritating, and the fact that it is fragranced with orange oil isn't helpful, either. This really doesn't deserve serious consideration.

☺ **$$$ C + AHA Exfoliating Antioxidant Treatment** *($128 for 1 ounce)* is a good option if you're looking for a stabilized vitamin C serum that contains a blend of 10% AHAs along with an effective though potentially irritating amount of vitamin C in its pure form (ascorbic acid). Vitamin C is not the sole answer for skin and there are less irritating yet still effective AHA products for far less money, but this is an option.

☺ **$$$ A.G.E. Interrupter** *($150 for 1.7 ounces)*. The A.G.E. in this product's name refers to advanced glycation end-products (AGE), which are not good for the body or the skin. AGEs are formed by the body's major fuel source, namely glucose. This simple sugar is essential for energy, but it also binds strongly to proteins (the body's fundamental building blocks), forming abnormal structures—AGEs—that progressively damage tissue elasticity. Once generated, AGEs begin a process that prevents many systems from behaving normally by literally causing tissue to cross-link and become hardened (Source: *Proceedings of the National Academy of Sciences*, March 14, 2000, pages 2809-2813). SkinCeuticals' theory is that by breaking these AGE bonds you can undo or stop the damage they cause. AGEs and free-radical damage may be inextricably linked (Sources: *European Journal of Neuroscience*, December 2001, page 1961; and *Neuroscience Letters*, October 2001, pages 29-32), but none of the studies indicate that there are any substances that can be included in skin-care products to affect this process. Specific to this product, the only ingredient it contains that is known to inhibit the formation of AGEs in skin is one that L'Oreal did the research on. Because L'Oreal owns SkinCeuticals, this research can hardly be considered impartial. Surprisingly, the blueberry extract L'Oreal used in this study (and in this product) did not fare as well as aminoguanidine, another ingredient known to inhibit AGEs (Source: *Experimental Gerontology*, June 2008, pages 584-588). Knowing this, why would you want to purchase this SkinCeuticals product when the parent company's own research shows that what they're including to inhibit AGEs is not as effective as another ingredient that they didn't include? If anything, this product is a big step backwards for SkinCeuticals. It's mostly slip agents, silicones, and wax, plus the questionable AGE-inhibiting blueberry extract, although even if this extract could help, it won't remain potent for long thanks to the jar packaging (not to mention that there's hardly any of it in this product). For $150, you have every right to expect a whole lot more than this no-better-than-average product provides.

☺ **$$$ C E Ferulic Combination Antioxidant Treatment** *($138 for 1 ounce)* is a star product for SkinCeuticals, and it comes complete with all manner of antiaging claims. However, the only ones you can bank on with this product (based on a significant amount of research) are its abilities to reduce free radicals and to defend skin against oxidative stress. It reportedly contains 15% L-ascorbic acid, a form of vitamin C considered an excellent antioxidant and anti-inflammatory agent (Sources: *Experimental Dermatology*, June 2003, pages 237-244; and *Bioelectrochemistry and Bioenergetics*, May 1999, pages 453-461). Because L-ascorbic acid is stable only in low-pH formulations (Source: *Dermatologic Surgery*, February 2001, pages 137-142), the good news is that this product's pH of 3 is low enough to allow this form of vitamin C to be effective. Also present in this water-based antioxidant serum are vitamin E and ferulic acid. Vitamin E, appearing here as alpha tocopherol, also has a well-established reputation as an effective antioxidant (Sources: *Radiation Research*, July 2005, pages 63-72; *Annals of the New York Academy of Sciences*, December 2004, pages 443-447; and *Journal of Investigative Dermatology*, February 2005, pages 304-307). Ferulic acid is relatively new to the skin-care scene, but earlier research suggests that it provides antioxidant and sun-protective benefits to skin while enhancing the stability of topical applications of vitamin E (Sources: *International Journal of Pharmaceutics*, April 10, 2000, pages 39-47; *Anticancer Research*, September-October 1999, pages 3769-3774; *Nutrition and Cancer*, February 1998, pages 81-85; and *Free Radical Biology and Medicine*, October 1992, pages 435-448). As research into this and similar compounds (such as caffeic and ellagic acid) continues, I suspect we will see more antioxidant-based products enhanced with them, which is great news for keeping skin healthy and protecting it from further damage. C E Ferulic Combination Antioxidant Treatment is suitable for all skin types. Its brown glass packaging helps keep its high level of antioxidants stable, although an airless pump applicator would have been better than the dropper tip, because that requires you to remove the cover with each use, exposing the oxygen-sensitive antioxidants to air. That is what keeps this product from earning a Paula's Pick rating. After all, who wants to spend this much on one product only to discover that the efficacy is severely diminished after a period of time?

☹ **Daily Moisture Lightweight Pore-Minimizing Moisturizer, for Normal or Oily Combination Skin** *($55 for 2 ounces)* begins well with its water-based blend of several species of algae and a light moisturizing agent, but all in all, this contains too many potentially problematic plant extracts to make it a slam-dunk for normal to oily skin. Algae extracts cannot make pores smaller, but the cinnamon, ginger, and thyme may make them appear smaller by virtue of the inflammation they cause—yet that's a negative for the long-term health of your skin.

☹ **Emollience Rich, Restorative Moisturizer, for Normal or Dry Skin** *($55 for 2 ounces)* not only features jar packaging that undermines the efficacy of its many antioxidants, but this emollient cream also is bound to cause irritation due to the volatile essential oils it contains.

☹ **$$$ Epidermal Repair** *($68 for 1.33 ounces)* sounds like a serious reparative product, and is recommended for skin compromised by cosmetic corrective procedures or harsh environmental influences. The star ingredients are beta-glucan and *Centella asiatica*, both good anti-irritants and antioxidants. This might be worth the expense if the aforementioned ingredients were front and center, but they're not. In fact, they're barely present. That leaves you with a lightweight, silicone-enhanced moisturizer for normal to dry skin that doesn't have any edge for managing stressed or irritated skin. SkinCeuticals could (and should) have added a lot more to this product to make good on its claims. As is, several other less expensive moisturizers and serums best this formula.

☺ **$$$ Eye Balm Rehabilitative Emollient, for Aging Skin** *($76 for 0.5 ounce)* has a lot going for it, including copious antioxidants and a cell-communicating ingredient, all wrapped up in a lightweight lotion texture for all skin types. What a shame the jar packaging won't keep the state-of-the-art ingredients stable during use.

✓ ☺ **$$$ Eye Cream Firming Treatment** *($55 for 0.67 ounce)* is an excellent, fragrance-free, antioxidant-rich, lightweight moisturizer for slightly dry skin anywhere on the face. It contains a couple of very good water-binding agents and an efficacious plant oil, along with stabilized vitamin C; however, don't expect it to lighten dark circles as claimed.

☺ **$$$ Eye Gel AOX+** *($58 for 0.5 ounce)* is a good water-based moisturizer for slightly dry skin anywhere on the face. It contains impressive amounts of vitamin C, but a fairly inconsequential amount of ferulic acid and sodium hyaluronate. All in all, this is a one-note product and not nearly as elegant as others in this price category or for even less money.

☺ **Eye Renewal Gel Nighttime Line-Minimizing Treatment** *($34 for 1 ounce)* claims to exfoliate delicate skin around the eyes with a 5% hydroxy acid blend, but the fruit and sugarcane extracts are not the same as AHAs, and the lemon extract can be irritating.

☺ **$$$ Face Cream Rehabilitating Cream, for Aging Skin** *($138 for 1.67 ounces)* offers normal to dry skin several rehabilitating ingredients, including good antioxidants and plant oils. However, the ylang-ylang and geranium oils are bad news, and keep this moisturizer from being truly state-of-the-art.

☺ **$$$ Hydrating B5 Gel Moisture Enhancing Gel** *($65 for 1 ounce)* is a simple hydrating mix of a water-binding agent, vitamin B-5 (also known as panthenol), and a preservative. It is suitable for all skin types.

☺ **$$$ Intense Line Defense Potent Nighttime Line-Minimizing Treatment** *($59 for 1 ounce)* is another SkinCeuticals product claiming to exfoliate skin with fruit acids. That's not going to happen, at least not in the same manner and with the same benefits as using a well-formulated AHA or BHA product. Without the reliable exfoliation, you're left with mostly water, an antioxidant, slip agents, and preservatives. Not too intense after all!

☹ **Phloretin CF** *($150 for 1 ounce)*. Dr. Sheldon Pinnell is back with another powerhouse serum, complete with claims on its years of research, patents, and new cosmeceutical buzzwords such as "biodiverse" and "broad-spectrum treatment." Considering the claims and ads for this water-based serum, I am not at all surprised that it has quickly become one of the products readers ask me about most. Aside from the company's exemplary marketing efforts, the product does deserve some discussion in terms of its single unique ingredient, phloretin (because other than that, this is one boring ordinary, potentially skin-damaging product). Phloretin is a white crystalline flavonoid that results from the decomposition or hydrolysis of phlorizin. Naturally, your next question is: What's phlorizin? It's a bitter substance extracted from the root bark of apple trees and from apples, so phloretin does have a natural origin (though what it takes to get phlorizin out of the apple tree to turn it into phloretin is hardly a natural process; you're not going to use phloretin to flavor pie). As for phloretin's value for skin, in vitro and animal research has shown that it has antioxidant ability, can interrupt melanin synthesis to potentially reduce skin discolorations, inhibits the formation of MMP-1 (which breaks down collagen), and also serves as a penetration enhancer, which, as you'll see below, is not a good thing in the case of this product (Sources: *The FEBS Journal*, August 2008, pages 3804-3814; *Phytochemistry*, April 2007, pages 1189-1199; *Biological and Pharmaceutical Bulletin*, April 2006, pages 740-745; *European Journal of Pharmaceutics and Biopharmaceutics*, March 2004, pages 307-312; and *International*

The Reviews S

Journal of Pharmaceutics, April 2003, pages 109-116).Although there are compelling reasons to consider phloretin as another potent, beneficial antioxidant to improve skin's appearance and healthy functioning, in the case of this product it is completely wasted. Why? Because the amount of denatured alcohol in this serum negates any antioxidant benefit of the phloretin. The inclusion of alcohol is extremely disappointing because alcohol causes free-radical damage, cell death, and irritation. That does not help skin in the least and, in fact, makes matters worse. Bottom line: Phloretin may be the antioxidant du jour, but not in this product. Please keep in mind that despite the published research for phloretin and SkinCeuticals claims, it is not the best antioxidant to "attack damage on every level." There are lots of brilliant antioxidants in skin-care products, but there isn't a miracle or magic bullet out there.

☺ $$$ **Phyto Corrective Gel Calming Complexion Gel** *($56 for 1 ounce)* is a water-based serum whose water-binding agents can benefit all skin types, while the *Uva ursi* extract's arbutin content may have a positive impact on skin discolorations. This would be rated higher if not for the thyme extract and the nebulous "herbal fragrance."

☺ $$$ **Renew Overnight Dry Nighttime Skin-Refining Moisturizer, for Normal to Dry Skin** *($55 for 2 ounces)* provides more fruit acids masquerading as AHAs, while jar packaging ruins the effectiveness of the antioxidants in this moisturizer for normal to dry skin. For the money, you're better off investing in a separate AHA product and a stably packaged moisturizer with state-of-the-art ingredients.

☺ $$$ **Renew Overnight Oily Nighttime Skin-Refining Moisturizer, for Normal or Oily Skin** *($55 for 2 ounces)* is a lighter-weight version of the Renew Overnight Dry Nighttime Skin-Refining Moisturizer above, and the same review applies, except that this is indeed better for normal to oily skin.

✓ ☺ $$$ **Retinol 0.5 Refining Night Cream with 0.5% Pure Retinol** *($50 for 1 ounce)* makes many antiaging claims, and because it contains a significant amount of retinol the claims you can bank on are building collagen and stimulating cell regeneration. However, since other ingredients can also do that, or at least assist in the process, it's a bit overly optimistic to hang all your hopes on one specialized ingredient such as retinol. Fortunately, this water- and silicone-based serum does contain many other beneficial ingredients for healthy skin, including ceramides, cholesterol, lecithin, antioxidants, and the anti-irritant bisabolol. The opaque bottle with pump applicator helps maintain the stability of the retinol, which is a prerequisite for products with this ingredient. Retinol 0.5 is suitable for all skin types. Getting back to the claims, SkinCeuticals boasts that this serum will also minimize pore size and correct blemishes. The first claim rests on a subjective judgment. The second claim that retinol is able to correct blemishes is at this point more theoretical than proven. In contrast, tretinoin (the active ingredient in Retin-A) has considerable research supporting its use as a prescription acne treatment. While it's definitely possible that using a retinol serum like this one will result in fewer blemishes, it's not as much of a sure thing as using a tretinoin product. The benefits of retinol versus tretinoin are that retinol has significantly fewer and comparably minor side effects, but the trade-off is reduced efficacy (Source: *Cosmetic Dermatology*, volume 18, issue 1, supplement 1, January 2005, page 19). This product is not recommended for daytime application because it contains photosensitizing St. John's wort.

✓ ☺ $$$ **Retinol 1.0 Maximum Strength Refining Night Cream with 1.0% Pure Retinol** *($48 for 1 ounce)* is similar to the Retinol 0.5 product above, except it contains twice as much retinol. The same basic comments apply (including the one about St. John's wort), but a caution is warranted because using retinol at this level (1%) poses a slight risk of side effects that are similar to, but less pronounced than, those caused by topical tretinoin, including redness, flaking/peeling, and possibly stinging. These effects should be short-term as the skin acclimates to retinol, but if they do not dissipate or if they worsen with continued use, stop using the product; retinol at this level may not be right for your skin.

☺ **$$$ Serum 10 AOX+** *($84 for 1 ounce)* is a water-based serum that contains 10% L-ascorbic acid along with penetration-enhancing ingredients, stabilizers, and a couple of water-binding agents. SkinCeuticals added the antioxidant ferulic acid to their vitamin C serums because research has shown it helps boost efficacy, although the only research on topical application of these antioxidants was done in part by Dr. Pinnell (Source: *Journal of Investigative Dermatology*, October 2005, pages 826-832), so it's not exactly impartial. Still, there is enough research on ferulic acid's antioxidant effects when taken internally to rationalize (and further research) its use in skin-care products.

☺ **$$$ Serum 15 AOX+** *($94 for 1 ounce)* is identical to the Serum 10 AOX+ above, except this version provides 15% L-ascorbic acid. Keep in mind that this amount of vitamin C at the pH that's needed for it to be effective may prove more irritating than beneficial for skin (a fact SkinCeuticals mentions on their Web site and in literature for this product). This is not the type of product you'd want to use nightly with other products such as those with retinol, AHAs, BHA, or topical prescription retinoids because such a combination may send skin into irritation overload, so proceed cautiously to see how your skin reacts.

☺ **$$$ Serum 20 AOX+** *($114 for 1 ounce)* is similar to the Serum 10 AOX+ above, except this pricier version increases the vitamin C content to 20%. Otherwise, the same comments and precautions made for the other two AOX+ serums apply here, too. Interestingly, relatively recent research on formulating vitamin C into skin-care products shows that a thickened microemulsion, not a solution as used here, does a better job of keeping the antioxidants stable (Sources: *Drug Delivery*, April 2007, pages 235-245; and *Pharmaceutical Development and Technology*, November 2006, pages 255-261).

☹ **Skin Firming Cream** *($106 for 1.67 ounces)* lists sandalwood extract as the third ingredient, and also contains fragrant juniper oil, which makes this otherwise good but overpriced moisturizer a problem for all skin types.

☺ **$$$ Hydrating B5 Masque** *($50 for 2.5 ounces)* is an exceptionally boring mask that is absolutely not worth the money. The claims make it seem like the ultimate moisture oasis for dry, parched skin, but it is primarily water, glycerin, pH-adjusting agent, and gel-based thickener. Big deal!

☺ **$$$ Clarifying Clay Masque Deep Pore Cleansing Skin-Refining Masque** *($42 for 2 ounces)* is a standard, but good, clay mask for normal to very oily skin. The fruit and sugar extracts do not exfoliate skin like an AHA product would. This should be thoroughly rinsed from skin because comfrey extract can be irritating if left on skin.

☹ **Phyto + Botanical Gel, for Hyperpigmentation** *($76 for 1 ounce)* lists thyme extract as the second ingredient, which makes this arbutin-enhanced skin-lightening gel a problem for all skin types. Chemical components of thyme have been shown to be irritating for skin (Source: www.naturaldatabase.com).

☺ **$$$ Blemish Control Gel** *($36 for 1 ounce)* puts 1% salicylic acid in a smooth, gel-based formula that does not contain fragrance or needlessly irritating ingredients. What a letdown to realize the pH range of this product (pH 4.8-5.0, as confirmed by the company and our testing) will not permit the salicylic acid to work its magic effectively on blemishes.

✓ ☺ **$$$ Antioxidant Lip Repair Restorative Treatment, for Damaged or Aging Lips** *($34 for 0.3 ounce)* has an interesting texture in an overall emollient formula that provides lips with an impressive selection of antioxidants, water-binding agents, and a peptide, which theoretically has cell-communicating ability. If you're going to spend this much for a lip product, it might as well be loaded with extras like this one is! However, this doesn't contain sunscreen, and so should only be used at night.

SKINCEUTICALS SUN PRODUCTS

☺ **Active UV Defense Sunscreen Cream SPF 15** *($30 for 3.4 ounces)* brings us the Skin-Ceuticals version of a sunscreen with Mexoryl SX (ecamsule) that is nearly identical to those from L'Oreal, Lancome, Kiehl's, and La Roche-Posay. All of them and SkinCeuticals are owned by L'Oreal, the company that holds the patent on the use of Mexoryl SX. Whichever company you choose to purchase from (L'Oreal's Revitalift version costs the least, Lancome's costs the most, and SkinCeuticals' is in the middle), all provide sufficient UVA protection and also contain active ingredients to keep UVB rays from damaging skin. The other similarity is that all of these sunscreens with Mexoryl SX come in lightweight moisturizing bases that are void of any other exciting or state-of-the-art ingredients. I was hoping SkinCeuticals would have at least added some vitamin C or ferulic acid to their contribution, but that's not the case. This is best as a daytime moisturizer for normal to slightly dry or slightly oily skin, and is fragrance-free.

☺ **$$$ Daily Sun Defense SPF 20** *($37 for 3 ounces)* has an in-part zinc oxide sunscreen and does not contain fragrance, but for all of SkinCeuticals talk about antioxidants (particularly vitamin C), it is disappointing that not a single antioxidant shows up in this sunscreen for normal to dry skin not prone to blemishes.

✓ ☺ **$$$ Physical UV Defense SPF 30** *($37 for 3 ounces)* improves on the Daily Sun Defense SPF 20 above by including a couple of antioxidants. This creamy sunscreen contains only titanium dioxide and zinc oxide as its active ingredients, making it an excellent choice for sensitive skin, including those with various forms of dermatitis and rosacea. It is fragrance-free.

✓ ☺ **$$$ Sport UV Defense SPF 45** *($37.50 for 3 ounces)* is a very good, in-part zinc oxide sunscreen for normal to very dry skin not prone to blemishes. The fragrance-free formula contains antioxidant vitamins that have proven to be positive additions to sunscreens.

☺ **$$$ Ultimate UV Defense SPF 30** *($37 for 3 ounces)* is very similar to the Daily Sun Defense SPF 20 above, except that this one contains the higher percentage of active ingredients necessary to attain an SPF 30 rating. Otherwise, the same comments apply.

☺ **$$$ Sans Soleil Moisturizing Sunless Tanner** *($34 for 5 ounces)* is a good self-tanning lotion for normal to dry skin. It combines dihydroxyacetone and the slower-acting erythrulose to turn skin brown, and also includes a tiny amount of antioxidant vitamins. This does contain fragrance.

SMASHBOX (MAKEUP ONLY)

SMASHBOX AT-A-GLANCE

Strengths: A unique Anti-Shine product that is a must-try if you have very oily skin; mostly good foundations with a neutral range of shades; improved powder eyeshadows; the great Photo Finish Lipstick; a lash primer that really makes a difference; well-constructed makeup brushes that cost less than the department-store competition.

Weaknesses: A small, mostly boring assortment of products priced higher than they should be; a couple of products contain irritants that have no benefit for skin; several lackluster makeup categories, including concealer, blush, eye pencils, and brow shaders; the Cream Eyeliner is a mistake if you expect any amount of longevity; several specialty products that should offer more for the money (and the one with sunscreen leaves skin vulnerable to UVA damage).

For more information about Smashbox, call (888) 763-1361 or visit www.smashbox.com or www.Beautypedia.com.

FOUNDATION: ☺ **$$$ Camera Ready Full Coverage Foundation SPF 15** *($38)* is a cream-to-powder foundation that provides almost opaque coverage. It applies creamy but sets to a satin finish that can feel slightly moist. The titanium dioxide sunscreen provides excellent UVA/UVB protection without making skin look chalky. Those with normal to dry skin will find this an excellent option; the formula is too creamy for anyone with combination or oily skin and the waxes are not for anyone with acne-prone skin. Ignore the included too-rough-to-use brush, it's useless. The shade range is limited to options for those with fair to medium skin tones. Watch out for Medium M3 and M4 and for Dark D1, which are too yellow and orange for most to use convincingly. If not for the cumbersome, difficult-to-open compact, this would have rated a Paula's Pick.

☺ **$$$ Conversion Cream to Powder Foundation** *($32)* is a cream-to-powder foundation with a silky-smooth application, yet a somewhat heavy-looking finish. You can achieve medium to full coverage, but the high wax content lends an opacity that tends to camouflage, rather than enhance, skin. Eight shades are available, with the darker colors being particularly good. Watch out for the slightly pink shade 0 and keep in mind that shade 4 is slightly peach. This is best for normal to slightly dry or slightly oily skin that's not prone to blemishes.

☺ **$$$ Function5 Self-Adjusting Powder Foundation** *($36)* is a creamy-feeling pressed-powder foundation made without talc. Smashbox advertises the vitamins in this foundation, and they are present in greater amounts than typically found in makeup. However, the packaging of the product will routinely expose them to light and air, so don't count on this as your sole source of topical antioxidants. Because this powder is pressed lightly, it can be somewhat messy and the application heavier (in terms of the amount picked up on the brush) than with most. The good news is this doesn't look heavy on skin—you'll get sheer to light coverage and a soft matte (in feel) finish with a bit of shine. Among the six shades (all of which go on more neutral than they appear), all but one are recommended; the Fair F1-F2 shade will be too yellow for some pale skin tones. There are no shades for very dark skin.

☺ **$$$ High Definition Healthy F/X Foundation SPF 15** *($38)* is said to be packed with antiaging and firming ingredients that revitalize skin. The in-part titanium dioxide sunscreen deserves most of the credit for antiaging (assuming you apply this daily and liberally), but nothing in this product will revitalize or firm skin. The silky, fluid texture is built around no fewer than six forms of silicone, and they ensure a smooth, even application that meshes well with skin, which is this foundation's strongest point. Blending takes longer than usual but is OK, and this sets to a soft-satin finish appropriate for normal to slightly dry skin (even if it is prone to blemishes). You'll get medium coverage that looks surprisingly skin-like, and this wears quite well. Among the 13 mostly neutral shades, the only ones to consider carefully are Light L3 and Medium M3.

☺ **$$$ Sheer Focus Tinted Moisturizer SPF 15** *($30)* is so sheer that any coverage you get will be accidental! That makes choosing from among the four shades (plus a shimmer shade labeled "Luminous") as easy as figuring out which one comes closest to the depth of your skin tone. The sunscreen includes zinc oxide for sufficient UVA protection, and the fluid, moist texture has good slip so blending is easy. Sheer Focus sets to a satin-matte finish. The vitamins and antiaging peptides Smashbox refers to are barely present—all of them are listed after the preservative—so they don't even come close to qualifying as "packed." Still, this is a good, very sheer tinted moisturizer for normal to dry skin.

☺ $$$ Wet/Dry Foundation ($34) is a talc-based, pressed-powder foundation that is much better used dry than wet. It has a reasonably smooth, slightly dry texture with light to medium coverage and a soft matte finish. There are nine mostly neutral shades that are predominantly best for fair to light skin tones, though Caramel and Cocoa are good, non-ashy shades for lighter African-American skin. The only shade to avoid is Sand, which is too peach for most skin tones.

CONCEALER: ☹ $$$ Camera Ready Full Coverage Concealer ($18) is a creamy, twist-up stick concealer that applies smoothly and blends well, though it remains moist and quickly settles into lines around the eye. Despite the name, this provides full coverage only if you pile it on—and that causes it to crease even more. This is still worth considering if you want a cream concealer and the eight shades are nearly impeccable (shade 1 is too white for just about anyone), but it must be set with powder to minimize the creasing.

☹ $$$ High Definition Concealer ($18) is a water- and silicone-based concealer that has a slightly creamy texture and decent slip for controlled blending. It provides nearly full coverage, but its smooth matte finish has a tendency to look chalky. Another issue is that although it's a squeeze tube, the opening readily dispenses too much product, and putting it back in is a messy endeavor. One more comment: Other than the fact that all of the shades except Medium/Dark are good, this concealer contains angelica root extract, which can cause contact dermatitis.

POWDER: ☹ $$$ Halo Hydrating Perfecting Powder ($59) has a very clever dispenser that's designed to help negate the mess that occurs with many loose powders. The built-in shaver is meant to give you the perfect amount of powder for each use, with no mess. This is a novel approach, but in fact it doesn't end up making Halo any more or less messy than any other loose powder. That's because you will inevitably shave off more powder than you need, and will therefore always have some surplus in the packaging. Dispenser aside, this hugely overpriced powder will do nothing to hydrate skin or help reduce fine lines and wrinkles as Smashbox claims. The first ingredient is mica, a very standard ingredient in many loose powders that provides shine. The "gold" Smashbox brags about in this formulation is nearly last on the ingredient list, a negligible amount at best. Even if it were present at a higher concentration, gold has not been shown anywhere to have benefit for skin, so it's just useless window dressing. If the high price and common formulation don't dissuade you from trying Halo Hydrating Perfecting Powder, also consider the fact that all but the Fair shade tend toward orange, and the included kabuki brush is too small to allow for even application. For considerably less money you can buy better loose powders from several drugstore and department-store lines.

BLUSH AND BRONZER: ✓☺ $$$ Bronze Lights ($28) is one of the best talc-based pressed bronzing powders around. It has a wonderfully smooth texture that makes application nearly foolproof, plus it looks incredibly natural on skin. Even better, both shades (Suntan Matte is preferred, Sunkissed Matte is more peachy than bronze) offer a matte finish! Definitely a consideration if you love bronzing powder but are tired of those with sparkles.

✓ ☺ **$$$ O-Bronze** *($26)* is playing off Smashbox's success with its other O-products, which are hyped as being able to turn a custom color once they are applied to your skin. While the hype is nonsense (these products tend to look the same on almost everyone), O-Bronze Intuitive Cheek Bronzer is a good option for adding a subtle touch of glowing color to your skin. The creamy product dispenses white from the tube, but quickly turns to a sheer bronze tint when blended into the skin. A little goes a long way, so start out with a pea-size amount for your initial application and build from there. O-Bronze comes in only one shade and it favors light to medium skin tones. Those with darker skin will likely find this product is not pigmented enough for their skin tones. This deserves a Paula's Pick rating because of its performance and a formula that's stably packaged to preserve the effectiveness of the antioxidants.

☺ **$$$ Blush Rush** *($24)* is a sheer powder blush whose suede-smooth texture applies beautifully. Each of the shades is infused with some shimmer, but the product application is so sheer that it doesn't pose a problem for daytime wear. Ignore the long-wearing claims because this will wear just as well, but not better than, any other similarly formulated powder blush. The Flush shade is a beautiful pale pink that also works great as a highlighter.

☺ **$$$ Untamed Creamy Cheek Color** *($24)* is a good, traditional cream blush that is easy to apply and leaves a soft, moist finish. Application is enhanced by silicone, but the main ingredient (isopropyl palmitate) makes this best suited for those with dry skin not prone to blemishes.

☹ **$$$ Blush** *($24)* is a very standard, pressed-powder blush whose price tag is uncalled for. It applies nicely (though a bit too softly to register on darker skin tones or to make an impact under studio lights), but many of the colors are very shiny and the shine tends to flake. Whether you want a sheer or more pigmented powder blush, consider options from M.A.C. or Bobbi Brown before this.

☹ **$$$ O-Glow** *($26)*. Remember mood rings? The jewelry that changed color after being in contact with your skin? Smashbox tries to recapture that idea with a silicone-based clear blush they refer to as "intuitive" because "this clear gel reacts with your personal skin chemistry to turn cheeks the exact color you blush, naturally in just seconds!" Sounds like the perfect "natural blush," but the claim is bogus. Yes, this goes on clear and changes color as it blends—but it turns into the same translucent fuchsia hue on everyone. My office staff has a good range of skin tones, from fair to dark. I asked several women to sample this blush and let me know what color it turned on their skin, and did they think it matches how they blush naturally. All of them had the same color response (fuchsia) and none of them claimed to blush this shade (no one does). I admit, it's cool to watch a clear gel turn into a vibrant pink shade as you blend, and this has a smooth powder finish that lasts, but the color itself isn't personalized and the strong color isn't going to work for everyone.

☹ **$$$ Skin Tint** *($28)* is a water-based stick blush that offers a very soft application of translucent color. I previously came down hard on this product because its texture and finish undermine foundation and powder, but it does have a place for those who go foundation-free, have poreless skin, and just want a hint of juicy color to rev up their complexion. Skin Tint is best for normal to dry skin; using this over even slightly oily cheeks will make your skin look too greasy, and applying this over large pores may make your skin look dotted with color.

EYESHADOW: ✓ ☺ **$$$ Waterproof Shadow Liner Duo** *($25)* includes a cream eyeshadow and eyeliner in one compact. Each product has its own compartment, and each compartment is outfitted with a snap-tight closure to prevent it from drying out, which is a nice touch. Both products apply smoothly with rich color payoff and fast dry times. The color pairings are mostly light with dark, with the dark being the obvious choice for use as eyeliner or for creating a sultry eye design. The Smolder duo is glittery and not as sophisticated as the others. This is a very good way to create a long-lasting eye design; you will need an oil- or silicone-based makeup remover handy to take it off!

☺ $$$ **Eye Shadow Trio** *($28)* has the same formula as the Single Eye Shadow and the same comments apply. All three shades in each set have some degree of shine, though many are soft and suitable for daytime wear (assuming you have smooth, unlined eyelids). The most versatile combinations include Shutterspeed, On Stage, Center Stage, and Head Shot.

☺ $$$ **Eyelights Palette** *($34)* presents three creamy-feeling powder eyeshadows in a compact. Each is laden with metallic shine, but they apply amazingly well and offer opaque coverage without flaking. Although not for everyone (and assuredly not for anyone with wrinkles around the eye), this is a dramatic evening eye-makeup option that wears well.

☺ $$$ **Photo Finish Lid Primer** *($20)*. Sold as "an ultra-luxurious lid primer" (I guess when you're offering a superfluous makeup item you need a good adjective to make it sound important), this is merely a peach-tinged liquid concealer that offers slight camouflage and sets quickly to a dry matte finish. The finish has a subtle tackiness to it that doesn't make eyeshadow application easier, but it's not a deal-breaker. The best reason to consider this is if you have oily eyelids and you're not satisfied with the results you get using a regular concealer with a strong matte finish. If that's not your dilemma, this is easy to pass by.

☺ $$$ **Single Eye Shadow** *($16)* has an impressively smooth texture that applies evenly, and only the shiniest shades are mildly prone to flaking (every color has some amount of shine). The only drawback (and for some this may be a plus) is that even the darkest shades tend to go on sheer, so building intensity takes some effort.

☺ $$$ **Untamed Waterproof Shadow Liner Trio** *($29)*. This cleverly packaged product offers three shades of cream eyeshadows (or they may be used as cream eyeliners) in one compact. Each shade has its own compartment, and each compartment has a snap-tight closure to prevent the product from drying out. The silicone-based formula is a cinch to apply and once it sets, the wear time is impressive. All of the colors have shine and go on softer than you'd think. Although they can be used for eyelining, the softness makes them best as cream eyeshadows.

☹ $$$ **Untamed Double-Ended Eye Brightener** *($22)* is a dual-sided pencil that needs routine sharpening. If that doesn't stop you from reading this review … one end of the pencil is a fleshy, pale peach color and the other is a soft gold. Each side has a very smooth, sheer application and soft-shimmer finish that adds a glow and, surprisingly, stays in place beautifully once the formula sets. This would earn a happy face rating if not for the need to routinely sharpen both ends.

EYE AND BROW SHAPER: ☺ $$$ **Jet Set Waterproof Eye Liner** *($22)* is yet another gel eyeliner whose price tag isn't warranted given its blatant, late-to-the-game-yet-with-nothing-new-to-add similarities to several less expensive options. This is waterproof, comes in two classic colors, and wears beautifully. I couldn't fault anyone for using this eyeliner, but I'd be sure to tell them they spent too much money!

☹ $$$ **Brow Tech** *($24)* is described by Smashbox as "the answer to everyone's prayers," but before you reconsider your pleas for world peace or that new car you've always wanted, consider that this is merely a split-pan compact with a shine-infused brow powder that you mix with the other half, which is a clear, thick wax. But no one needs shiny eyebrows, and the wax can look heavy and thick, not a look everyone will appreciate.

☺ **$$$ Brow Tech Wax** *($20)* is available separately and provides twice the amount of product as the regular Brow Tech, just without the powder brow color.

☹ **Cream Eye Liner** *($22)* is an interesting notion that sounds better than it ends up being. In the "pro" column, these do go on very smoothly and intensely. The "cons" include their tendency to fade, smear, and run with the slightest blink or smile, which makes them not worth the effort, especially at this price. For a superior version of this product, consider the silicone-enhanced Gel Eyeliners available from Bobbi Brown, Stila, M.A.C., Trish McEvoy, and Paula's Choice.

☹ **Cream Eye Liner Palette** *($32)* has same review as Cream Eye Liner, above, because this palette provides ten shades (tiny amounts of each), housed in one sleek compact.

LIPSTICK, LIP GLOSS, AND LIPLINER: ✓☺ **$$$ Limitless Long-Wearing Lip Gloss SPF 15** *($21)* is an excellent lip gloss that includes an in-part avobenzone sunscreen. The shade range is pleasing and each shade goes on sheer, leaving a high-gloss finish that feels sticky. The stickiness is a trade-off for the tenacious wear you get from this gloss. It also has minimal slickness so it's a good choice for those who find that gloss barely stays on their lips before they're out the door.

✓☺ **$$$ Reflection High Shine Lip Gloss** *($19)* is an excellent emollient lip gloss. It has a smooth application and highly reflective, dimensional finish that works alone or applied over any shade of lipstick, and it's only minimally sticky.

☺ **$$$ Lip Enhancing Gloss** *($18)* is a standard, moderately sticky but very glossy lip gloss. It is available in three intensities, although applied over an opaque lipstick you won't be able to see much difference. The Sheer Color shades are indeed sheer and come with a brush applicator; The True Color shades offer a bit more color payoff, but have a sponge-tip applicator; the Full Color shades offer the most color and coverage, but are not opaque. These also have a sponge-tip rather than a brush applicator (which is odd, because a brush applicator would deposit more product, which means stronger color).

☺ **$$$ Photo Finish Lipstick with Sila-Silk Technology** *($22)* is a very emollient, almost greasy cream lipstick with an unusual gloss finish that provides a multidimensional, wet-look shine. The shade selection is well edited yet still manages to offer an impressive range, including some great reds and pinks. The Sila-Silk portion is supposed to lend a unique silky feel to this lipstick, but the ingredients that precede it lend a thicker, moist feel rather than creating a sensation of silkiness.

☺ **$$$ Doubletake Lip Color** *($22)* has what it takes, if you want a lip color and lip pencil in one package and don't mind sharpening (which is really inconvenient and unnecessary given the number of twist-up pencils available). The lipliner portion applies sheer and slightly creamy—it's not one that's going to last very long or keep lip color from bleeding into lines around the mouth. The lip color portion is decidedly creamier and applies smoothly. Both ends need routine sharpening, which shortens the lifespan of any pencil and just adds a complication you don't need. As for the pairings, they're mostly muted and nude tones, nothing too shocking or contrived.

☺ **$$$ Lip Brilliance** *($28)* is a three-color lip palette that proclaims "the coverage of a lipstick, the smooth feel of a gloss," and this turns out to be partially true. Although this emollient lipstick/gloss hybrid offers full coverage, the texture is thick and sticky, and for the money this is not preferred to using a standard gloss over a good creamy lipstick.

☺ **Lip Pencil** *($14)* is a standard pencil with a creamy, but firm, texture and a cream finish that's a bit too short-lived, though the colors are versatile.

☺ **$$$ The Nude Lip Liner** *($16)* is a standard, needs-sharpening pencil with a silicone base that helps create a soft, creamy texture that glides on and sets to a slightly tacky, but budge-proof finish. As the name states, the small group of colors are nude/lip-toned shades, each with a brown undertone many will find versatile. The shades correspond to different skin tones from fair to dark, and it's a good way to determine which shade will work best for you. For example, the Dark shade is close to a chocolate brown, and looks much better against a darker skin tone than it does on someone with fair skin. This would earn a happy face rating if not for the need to routinely sharpen.

☺ **$$$ Untamed Lip Gloss** *($18)* has a thick texture and sticky finish that supplies a wet, glossy look and sheer color deposit. As lip glosses go, it's just OK, and this is too expensive to settle for OK.

☹ **O-Gloss** *($22)* is a sheer, sticky gloss that dispenses clear and turns a sheer shade of pink when applied to lips. Hardly an "intuitive" gloss, it turns nearly the same shade on everyone, and not everyone looks great with bubblegum-pink lips. To be honest, there is a slight difference in how the shade reads on lips, depending on the natural color of your lips. On women with darker lips, the colors will be more fuchsia, while women with pink to rosy lips tend to get the bubblegum-pink tone. Despite the novelty, there are several ingredients in this gloss that cause lips to swell and burn (pepper and peppermint oils among them), and as such it is not recommended.

MASCARA: ✓ ☺ **$$$ Bionic Mascara** *($19)* has a silly name and makes even sillier claims (ions do not make eyelashes stronger or longer), but wow: does this mascara deliver dramatic results! With just a few strokes, lashes are thickened, incredibly long, and beautifully defined. The formula is water-resistant (it'll withstand slight tearing or a light mist of rain), but not waterproof (don't swim with this on unless you want raccoon eyes). It removes with a water-soluble cleanser and wears all day without flaking or smearing, which is just more to love about Smashbox's best mascara.

✓ ☺ **$$$ Lash DNA Mascara** *($19)* has a name and claims that are beyond ridiculous. Supposedly, this mascara's "genetic fingerprint" includes a blend of proteins and amino acids that binds to lashes for enhanced strength and damage repair. Whatever happened to mascaras stating they make lashes 300% longer? So now we're into genetics as a means of improving the appearance of lashes?! Let's get real, here! There is no genetic manipulation going on. The ingredient list for this mascara is very standard and it does not include a single amino acid. The amount of protein is insignificant, but protein isn't a must-have for lashes, anyway. This mascara has an impractically large brush that demands dexterity, but rewards the user with long, thick, and perfectly separated lashes. I wish the claims weren't so hokey because this really does provide a fanned-out span of dramatically enhanced lashes—but let's leave the genetic stuff to the scientists, please.

✓ ☺ **$$$ Layer Lash Primer** *($16)* is one of a handful of lash primers that actually do make a difference, even when used with an already outstanding mascara. The effect (especially with the best mascaras) isn't night-and-day, but if you're looking to eke a bit more out of your usual mascara, this product is a decent add-on—and that's a refreshing change of pace! One of the reasons it works where others fail is that its conditioning formula keeps lashes soft and flexible while at the same time allowing a regular mascara to adhere evenly to already pumped-up lashes.

☺ **$$$ That's a Wrap Mascara** *($18)* makes much ado about the "advanced ingredients" and wheat protein it contains to condition and moisturize lashes, but this contains the same roster of ingredients seen in almost every mascara, namely waxes and thickeners. The wheat protein is present in such a tiny amount that your lashes won't notice it's there, but that's OK because several other ingredients do a great job of keeping lashes soft and flexible during wear. Performance-wise, That's a Wrap applies easily, separates lashes well, and lengthens without much thickness. If you prefer mascaras that primarily lengthen without clumping or smudging, this is recommended—but be aware that the same benefit can be had for less money from several drugstore mascaras.

☺ **$$$ Focal Point Lash Building Mascara** *($18)* allows you to gradually build length, but you'll be hard pressed to create thicker lashes, and attempting to do so results in some clumping. Although this is an OK option for making lashes longer, it doesn't compete with the best of what Maybelline New York and L'Oreal have to offer.

☹ **$$$ Limitless Lash** *($22)* is a dual-sided product with one end being a decent lengthening waterproof mascara that isn't as waterproof as it should be and the other being a silicone-based mascara remover applied with a brush. The remover works to dissolve the mascara, but you'll still need to use a regular remover or cleanser to get everything off, and the wand quickly becomes coated with used mascara, which gets kind of gross after a few uses.

FACE AND BODY ILLUMINATING /SHIMMER PRODUCTS: ☺ **$$$ Eye Illusion** *($32)* provides four pastel pressed powders in one large component with dividers between each shade. They have a nice, soft texture that applies evenly and leaves a prismatic shine. It is recommended that you use one or more shades over a medium to deep eyeshadow to change the color and light reflection. It does have an interesting effect for evening wear, assuming you want to make your existing eyeshadow a shinier, pastel shade.

☺ **$$$ Fusion Soft Lights** *($30)* are nearly identical to the regular Soft Lights below, but feature individual strips of color in one unit that can be applied separately or swirled together for a high-shine effect that appears almost glossy (but feels powder dry).

☺ **$$$ Soft Lights** *($28)* is a smooth-textured pressed shimmer powder that blends beautifully and clings better than expected. The shine ranges from subtle (Glow and Hue) to Las Vegas-caliber glitz.

☺ **$$$ Untamed High Lights Cheek Luminizer** *($24)* is a great way for those with dry skin to add a soft, pink shimmer to the cheek area. The product applies easily (be sure to put it on before powdering) and stays moist without looking greasy.

☹ **$$$ Artificial Light Luminizing Lotion** *($30)* has a very silky, fluid feel and produces a shimmer that's softly metallic. It's an OK option for shine, but because this stays moist it is prone to rubbing off and fading. For this amount of money, there should be no drawbacks, and overall this isn't worth considering over better, longer-lasting options from Lorac or Make Up For Ever.

☹ **Hybrid Luminizing 2-in-1 Primer** *($34)* is described by Smashbox as "revolutionary," which is probably one of the most overused words in the cosmetics industry. When have you seen a product advertised as being "commonplace" or "typical"? Answer: never. They're always revolutionary or a similarly grand adjective, even when they're basic or, in some cases, basically useless. What Smashbox claims makes this product so special is that it's a foundation primer and luminizing (read: adds shine) liquid in one product. Big deal! This very fluid, concentrated product is l-o-a-d-e-d with shimmer. So much, in fact, that unless you apply only a tiny amount your face will be shiny enough to find your way out of a dark cave. OK, not quite that shiny, but you get the idea. This feels silky and its lightweight finish makes foundation easier to apply, but so do countless other moisturizers and serums. This primer is recommended only if you crave allover shine and can't get past the notion that a primer is a pre-makeup must.

BRUSHES: **Smashbox Brushes** *($18-$52)* are more realistically priced than those of other artistry-based lines, and there are some expert options to consider, all with snazzy red lacquered handles that visually set them apart from the standard black of other lines. The ones to consider are the ☺ **$$$ #3 Blending,** ☺ **$$$ #12 Angle Brow,** ☺ **$$$ #15 Crease Brush,** ☺ **$$$ #10 Crease Brush,** ☺ **$$$ Face & Body Brush,** and ☺ **$$$ #9 Cream Eye Liner,** the last being one of the better types of this brush around because it's thin enough to use for both upper and lower lash lines and you can make the line as thin or thick as you like using almost any eyeshadow. For those so inclined, Smashbox's synthetic-hair ✓☺ **$$$ #13 Foundation Brush** *($34)* is one of the better brushes of its type available, and the price is comparable to those of most other lines.

SPECIALTY PRODUCTS: ✓☺ **$$$ Anti-Shine** *($27 for 1 ounce)* remains an intriguing product for anyone with very oily skin. It is mostly water and magnesium with a hint of color (a colorless version is also available). Magnesium (as in Phillips' Milk of Magnesia) absorbs oil very well and does not feel as heavy on the skin as clays do. This formula goes on extremely matte and dry and has great staying power; it is definitely worth trying if you have oily to very oily skin, and it works well with a matte-finish foundation. Anti-Shine may be applied under or over foundation to keep oiliness in check.

☺ **$$$ Compact Anti-Shine** *($28)* has the same oil-absorbing, matte-finish goals as the Anti-Shine, except this variation mixes silicone and talc with waxes to keep it in solid form. The wax content reduces the amount of time skin stays shine-free, and also isn't the best to use over blemishes. However, this is a workable option if you need only modest shine control and prefer a portable version.

☺ **$$$ Photo Finish Foundation Primer Light** *($16 for 1 ounce)* may have gotten your attention if you have oily, acne-prone skin because that's Smashbox's target market for this fluid, exceptionally light primer that leaves a silky, refined finish. Although it contains nothing to combat blemishes and has minimal ability to (temporarily) fill in large pores, it does not contain ingredients that aggravate or encourage blemishes, which is a plus. The water-based serum is fragrance-free and contains a tiny amount of vitamin C. It works well under foundation, but if your skin is oily and you're using a matte-finish foundation, this won't provide a significant boost in terms of wear time. It makes application smoother, but that's a tactile sensation rather than a legitimate need (your foundation should go on smoothly if you're using a good one and taking care of your skin). Still, primers have their proponents, and this is one more to consider.

☺ **Brush Cleaner** *($15)* uses primarily water, alcohol, and surfactants to break down built-up makeup and allow it to be rinsed off your brushes. This spray-on product has a low alcohol content, meaning it's mostly water, and that means brushes take some time to dry. I wouldn't choose this method over occasionally shampooing my brushes, toweling them off, and letting them dry overnight, but I suppose some will find this method more convenient.

☺ **$$$ Filter with Dermaxyl Complex** *($28)* has a formula that's similar to the original Photo Finish Foundation Primer reviewed below, but contains the peptide found in the Dermaxyl Complex (a trademark product of Sederma) as well as a high amount of film-forming agent. The product is intended for use around the eyes and lips and is dispensed through an angled-tip applicator. It can temporarily smooth and minimally fill in lines around the eyes, but how long the effect lasts depends on how expressive you are. This doesn't fulfill all its promises, but may be worth testing to see if you like the results—just keep in mind that they are temporary.

☺ **$$$ Lip & Lid Primer** *($24)* is a dual-sided product with both ends approximating creamy concealers. One end is for the eyelid area while the other is for filling in lines on the lips and creating longer-lasting lip color. Although both sides smooth things out and provide coverage, neither takes the place of a regular concealer (and one that's semi-matte to matte for the eyes, because this one stays too creamy). The lip end has minimal "priming" benefit, and can mix with a lipstick for unattractive results.

☺ **$$$ Lip Treatment SPF 15** *($16)* does not contain sufficient UVA protection and so cannot be relied on for sun protection. It is otherwise a standard, castor oil-based lip balm in lipstick form that softens dry lips and adds a glossy shine.

☺ **$$$ Photo Finish Bronzing Foundation Primer** *($38)* is similar to the Photo Finish Foundation Primer below, only with a sheer bronze tint that doesn't leave any shine behind. It's an OK option if you want to try Smashbox's primers and have medium to dark skin.

☹ **$$$ Photo Finish Color Correcting Foundation Primer** *($38)* is a pure silicone-based primer that, like others of its ilk, can make skin feel very silky and appear matte. Such an even canvas can facilitate makeup application, but this Smashbox product offers three strangely tinted shades meant to correct uneven skin tones (such as redness, sallowness, and so on). Thankfully, the peach and lavender shades are so sheer the color change is minimal, meaning that your foundation won't look strange when used with them. However, the green shade has too much color, which gives skin an odd, alien hue that substitutes one problem for another. These are not preferred to Smashbox's other Photo Finish primers.

☺ **$$$ Photo Finish Foundation Primer** *($36 for 1 ounce)* a colorless, silicone-based serum that has little going for it other than being a decent lightweight moisturizer that makes your skin feel smooth, and that can help ensure a semi-matte finish when paired with a matte-finish liquid or powder foundation.

☺ **$$$ Photo Finish Foundation Primer SPF 15 with Dermaxyl Complex** *($17)* does not contain sufficient UVA protection, so the sun protection claims cannot be relied on, and that's never a good sign for an antiaging product. This silicone-based primer does contain several antioxidants, but the translucent glass packaging won't help keep them stable, so that's a loss as well. The Dermaxyl Complex is a trademark of ingredient manufacturer Sederma. The key ingredient is palmitoyl oligopeptide and although this has potentially intriguing benefits for skin, the amount Smashbox includes doesn't measure up to the quantity Sederma recommends for efficacy. That means, at best, that the peptide functions as a water-binding agent, making this Smashbox primer slightly more hydrating than the other Smashbox primers—but the price is unwarranted.

☺ **$$$ Photo Op Under Eye Brightener** *($18)* is a concealer/highlighter combination product applied with a brush. It imparts sheer to light coverage for minor flaws and leaves obvious sparkles on skin (that's the "brightening" part). Smashbox recommends using this with a concealer, which is a good idea if you need more than meager coverage. In photographs, the amount of shine this leaves behind may prove to be too much, and it's definitely overkill for daytime makeup.

☹ **Emulsion Lip Exfoliant** *($18 for 0.75 ounce)* works to exfoliate dead, flaky skin on lips with its blend of plant oil and sugar. However, the inclusion of peppermint oil makes this scrub needlessly irritating. Mixing table sugar with a couple of drops of a nonfragrant plant oil would work too, and without the irritation.

The Reviews S

☹ **O-Plump** *($24)* contains irritating ingredients to create the "plumping" effect you get from this lip gloss, just like almost every other lip plumper on the market. O-Plump's offending irritants are peppermint oil, ginger oil, spearmint extract, wintergreen extract, and capsicum extract. (The latter is what gives hot peppers their heat.) Does that sound like something you want to put on your lips? Nope. This gloss is "intuitive" at only one thing, and that's causing lips to become swollen by virtue of extreme irritation.

SONIA KASHUK

SONIA KASHUK AT-A-GLANCE

Strengths: Affordable and widely available (though exclusive to Target stores nationwide); impressive skin-care products from a makeup-oriented line; very good cleanser; good makeup remover; facial moisturizers with sunscreen provide sufficient UVA protection; the makeup is still the star attraction, with impressive options for foundation, powder, blush, lip color, and especially makeup brushes.

Weaknesses: No AHA or BHA products or options for those with blemishes; jar packaging; lip balm with sunscreen does not contain the right UVA-protecting ingredients; the concealers, eye pencil, and brow shapers are a letdown; the makeup palettes may seem convenient, but several of the included products perform poorly.

For more information about Sonia Kashuk, visit www.soniakashuk.com or www.Beauty-pedia.com.

Note: Sonia Kashuk products are also available at select Bloomingdales locations in New York and California. The company also maintains free-standing stores in New York and New Jersey.

SONIA KASHUK SKIN CARE

✓ ☺ **Cleanse, Tri-Active Cleanser** *($10.99 for 6 ounces)* doesn't really have any toning benefits, but is nevertheless a very good, fragrance-free, water-soluble cleanser for all skin types except very oily. It is adept at removing makeup without leaving skin feeling dry.

✓ ☺ **Remove, Eye Makeup Remover** *($9.99 for 4 ounces)* is a simple, water- and silicone-based makeup remover, but it works beautifully to remove all types of long-wearing makeup and wins extra points for being fragrance-free and including no extraneous ingredients except a tiny amount of coloring agent.

☺ **Wash, Pre-Moistened Towelettes** *($6.99 for 30 towelettes)* contain a gentle, lotion-like formula that works well to remove makeup and leave skin feeling soft. The only objection is the cloying, baby wipe–like fragrance, which lingers on skin. Otherwise, these towelettes are suitable for all skin types except sensitive. As for the claims, these cleansing cloths are so far removed from a "complete regimen" that I don't know what else to say, other than it's pure fantasy to think otherwise.

☺ **Polish, Exfoliant Face Wash** *($12.99 for 4 ounces)* is a cleanser/scrub hybrid that contains diatomaceous earth as the abrasive agent. As a result, this is a grittier scrub that must be used gently. It's best for normal to oily skin.

☺ **Enhance, Firming Eye Cream** *($14.99 for 0.5 ounce)* treats skin to several antioxidants, but they won't hold up for long thanks to jar packaging. This is otherwise a decent emollient moisturizer for dry skin anywhere on the face, and it is fragrance-free.

☺ **Radiant, Tinted Moisturizer SPF 15** *($11.99 for 2 ounces)* remains a lightweight tinted moisturizer with an in-part avobenzone sunscreen. It has a cushiony, moist texture on application, but sets to a soft matte finish with the tiniest hint of shine. You'll achieve soft color and very sheer coverage from each of the three shades, all of them outstanding. This formula is best for normal to dry skin. Those with oily or blemish-prone skin will not appreciate the short-lived matte finish, and the thickeners and waxes aren't the best over breakout-prone areas.

☺ **Replenish, Essential Face Cream SPF 15** *($17.99 for 1.8 ounces)* will provide UVA protection thanks to its in-part avobenzone sunscreen (listed by its chemical name of butyl methoxydibenzoylmethane), but would be a better option for normal to dry skin if it did not use jar packaging. As is, the antioxidant potential will be lost shortly after the product is opened.

☺ **Restore, Intense Moisture Creme** *($17.99 for 1.8 ounces)* is a wonderfully rich moisturizer for dry to very dry skin, but the antioxidant oils and vitamins will be compromised due to jar packaging. This does contain fragrance.

✓ ☺ **Matte, Oil Blotting Papers** *($6.99 for 100 sheets)* are tissue paper–style white blotting papers that work quite well, and they're sized larger than most, which means they aren't the most discreet option to tuck into an evening bag. However, you can mop up more shine with a single sheet, so that may make these more appealing—and the price is right!

☺ **Hydrating Lip Balm SPF 14** *($7.99).* SPF 14 is an odd number to stop at, but it's close enough to the minimum recommendation of SPF 15. However, this isn't a tinted lip balm to turn to if you want broad-spectrum protection because the active ingredients don't provide sufficient UVA protection. This is otherwise a good, sheer lip balm that works well to keep lips conditioned while imparting a glossy sheen that feels slightly sticky.

☹ **Smooth, Lip Balm SPF 15** *($4.99 for 0.1 ounce)* makes lips feel smooth, but leaves them vulnerable to UVA damage because it lacks the UVA-protecting ingredients of titanium dioxide, zinc oxide, avobenzone, Mexoryl SX (ecamsule), or Tinosorb.

SONIA KASHUK MAKEUP

FOUNDATION: ✓ ☺ **Dual Coverage Powder Foundation** *($10.49)* has a very smooth, talc-based texture that applies sheerer than most pressed-powder foundations and looks natural. The soft, dry finish is best for normal to oily skin, and five shades are available. Linen and Sand tend to turn slightly peach, but are workable, while Ivory is suitable for fair skin and Honey for medium to slightly tan skin tones.

☺ **Perfecting Liquid Foundation** *($10.49)* is a very sheer- to light-coverage, dewy finish, liquid foundation for someone with normal to dry skin. It has a great, soft texture thanks to the significant amounts of silicone and mineral oil. Six shades are available, and five are nicely neutral and worth considering by light to medium skin tones. Camel is an OK option that may be too orange for some medium skin tones. Note: The color visible through the bottle does not resemble the product after it has dried on skin, which makes choosing the best shade a bit tricky.

CONCEALER: ☺ **Confidential Concealer with Brightening Pencil** *($6.99)* is a liquid concealer that's so sheer it barely makes a difference if covering dark circles is your goal. It blends well but leaves a shiny finish and is only appropriate for highlighting. The opposite end of this brush-applied concealer is a creamy, retractable pencil that's flesh-toned and loaded with shine. It doesn't so much brighten skin as add sparkles, although they do tend to stay in place.

☺ **Hidden Agenda Concealer Palette** *($9.99)* provides three shades of creamy concealer and one shade of pressed powder in a single compact. The concealer is slightly thick but applies smoothly and covers well. It would be better if it didn't look so heavy with the supplied powder applied over it; a sheerer powder would have worked much better (and the concealer needs to be set with powder to minimize creasing and fading). You'll find only one of the concealer shades is needed, but the range of shades is workable for fair to light/medium skin tones.

☹ **Take Cover Concealing Stick** *($7.99)* is a lipstick-style concealer that offers four shades, but you cannot see the color without breaking the product open, and the shade swatches at the Kashuk display aren't that accurate. Not only does this have an unpleasantly thick texture, it also finishes slightly sticky and creases almost instantly. Getting back to the shades, the only acceptable color is Dusk; the others are too pink, peach, or olive to consider.

POWDER: ✓ ☺ **Bare Minimum Pressed Powder** *($9.99)* comes in three soft, neutral colors best for fair to light skin tones, and it has a sublimely silky texture and seamless application. This is one of those rare talc-based powders that look very skin-like and enhance the complexion rather than dulling it or making skin look too matte and powdery. Well done!

☺ **Barely There Loose Powder** *($8.99)* remains one of the most elegant and gossamer loose powders you'll find in this price range. Its finely milled, silky texture blends beautifully on skin and it comes in three very good colors, best for fair to light skin tones. Two caveats: This contains cornstarch, which can (in theory) be problematic for those with blemishes, and now features a slightly shiny finish, which isn't ideal if you're using powder to temper shine. This powder is best for normal to dry skin.

☺ **Bare Minimum Pressed Bronzer** *($8.99)*. This pressed bronzing powder has a big golden yellow "S" in the middle of it. The "S" is for "Sonia" but when combined with the darker bronzing powder that surrounds it, the result on skin is more golden peach with shimmer than anything resembling a tan. This is an OK option if you want a warm-toned blush, but that's about it.

☺ **Sheer Magic Mineral Face Powder** *($14.99)* offers a **Mineral Concealer**, **Sheer Mineral Powder Foundation**, and **Sheer Mineral Blush** in one cleverly stacked component. The creamy concealer's main ingredient is titanium dioxide, so it goes on opaque and drags a bit during blending. It can easily look too heavy and has a tendency to crease into lines around the eye and magnify large pores. The Sheer Mineral Powder Foundation contains only mica and zinc oxide. The mica provides a silky texture and soft-glow finish while the zinc oxide provides opacity, giving this loose-powder foundation medium coverage. With the exception of the peachy Honey, all of the shades are soft and neutral, and include options for fair skin tones. The Sheer Mineral Blush is almost identical to the Sheer Mineral Powder Foundation, but includes a token amount of gemstones that have no effect on skin. For a loose-powder blush, the pigmentation is stronger than expected, so this is best brushed on lightly. Overall, this earns a neutral face rating due to the concealer's drawbacks and the inherent mess that comes with applying foundation and blush in loose-powder form. The packaging lacks conveniences to minimize this mess, while the openings are too small for many full-sized brushes.

BLUSH AND BRONZER: ✓ ☺ **Beautifying Blush** *($7.99)* is a pressed-powder blush with a super-smooth, non-powdery application and a collection of mostly sheer colors. Building intensity with this blush requires effort, but it's a good option for a hint of color. The matte shades include Nude, Flamingo, Spice, and Pink.

✓ ☺ **Crème Blush** *($9.99)* is best described as cream-to-powder rather than cream. It's initially creamy, but sets to a soft-powder finish that adds an enlivening, non-shimmering glow to cheeks. This is fantastically easy to blend and it lasts longer than a true cream blush. Every shade is beautiful, too!

✓ ☺ **Super Sheer Liquid Tint** *($9.99)* is aptly named! The silky formula imparts super sheer color that gives cheeks a healthy transparent flush. This has a slightly tacky finish, but is much easier to blend than most gel blushes (you get more play time with Kashuk's tint whereas a traditional gel blush sets almost immediately). The shade range is small but impressive, and none go on as dark as the packaging may imply. Fans of gel blush, take note!

☺ **Shimmering Loose Mineral Blush** *($8.99)* is a very sheer, feather-light loose powder blush that leaves a sparkling finish on skin. Definitely more for adding shine than color to cheeks, it is best dusted on to highlight skin for evening makeup. The sparkles are a bit much for casual or professional daytime makeup, though they cling to skin reasonably well.

☺ **Barely There Loose Bronzer** *($8.99)*. This sheer, silky bronzing powder imparts a soft, golden tan glow to skin. The glow comes complete with sparkles, and they have a below average ability to cling to skin. I wouldn't choose this over the less expensive bronzing options from Wet 'n' Wild.

EYESHADOW: ☺ **Enhance Eye Color** *($5.99)* represents Kashuk's single eyeshadows and they have a silky, dry application and sheer color deposit that layers well for more intensity. Most of the shades have a slight shimmer, but there are a few matte colors, too.

☺ **Eye Shadow Duo** *($7.99)* has a slightly different formula than the Enhance Eye Color; it's less dry and slightly creamy, but still applies smoothly and softly. One shade in each duo is shiny (many duos feature two shiny shades), but it's subtle (more subtle than it appears in the compact) and doesn't flake.

☺ **Eye Shadow Palette** *($12.99)* provides six shades of Kashuk's powder eyeshadow along with a sheer cream concealer and dual-sided sponge-tip applicator that should be tossed (Kashuk's eyeshadow brushes are preferred). Each powder shadow applies smoothly but quite sheer. They layer well, so you can achieve more dramatic shaping and shading, and the shades offer both matte and shimmer finishes. The concealer is described as an eyeshadow base, and it has a soft-powder finish that works well to enhance application while evening out minor discoloration on the eyelids. Both sets are great, but Perfectly Neutral is better for shading.

☺ **Eye Shadow Quad** *($9.99)* offers four coordinated eyeshadows in one compact, and the same formula, texture, and application comments mentioned for the Eye Shadow Duo apply here, too. The colors include options for highlighting, contouring, and eyelining, making these practical kits. Most of the sets have at least one shiny shade, but it's low-key and suitable for daytime makeup.

EYE AND BROW SHAPER: ✓ ☺ **Dramatically Defining Long Wearing Gel Liner** *($8.99)* is another excellent long-wearing cream-gel eyeliner to consider, and the price is more than fair for what you get. This applies smoothly and sets to a tenacious, long-wearing finish that resists fading, flaking, and smudging. This type of liner requires an oil- or silicone-based makeup remover. The black and brown shades are excellent; Indigo is best avoided because it is a shocking blue rather than understated navy.

✓ ☺ **Eye Marker** *($5.99)* is a brilliant way to apply liquid eyeliner! This sleek packaging looks like a pen and once uncapped, you'll see the precision felt tip. This is pre-loaded with color, and it makes application a breeze: no skipping, smearing, or flaking. The formula dries lightning fast and stays on until you remove it. Only one shade is available, so good thing it's classic soft black!

☺ **Brow Definer** *($5.99)* is a very standard, but good, brow pencil available in two shades suitable for dark blonde to medium brown brows. Why Kashuk didn't offer more shades is a mystery, but what's here is workable and this has a soft-powder finish. Brow Definer would be rated with a happy face if it didn't require routine sharpening.

☹ **Brow Kit Arch Alert Palette** *($9.99)* includes four shades of creamy, sheer brow wax (for blondes, redheads, and brunettes) and two unbelievably small applicators: a wedge brow brush to apply the wax and a mascara-type wand to groom brows. The wax doesn't do much to enhance brows and the colors are too soft for any real definition, while the tools are difficult to work with when compared to full-size brushes. If you try this you'll most likely only need one shade; why these weren't offered as stand-alone colors (without the nearly useless applicators) is a mystery.

☹ **Eye Definer** *($5.99)* is a substandard pencil that needs routine sharpening, and the oil-based formula tends to fade and smudge without much provocation. Kashuk's powder eyeshadows (in the brown, black, or gray colors) are much better choices for eyelining.

LIPSTICK, LIP GLOSS, AND LIPLINER: ✓ ☺ **Ultra Shine Sheer Lip Gloss** *($8.99)* is a commendable lip gloss with an elegant brush applicator that doesn't splay. It feels emollient without being too slick or greasy, and has a lovely soft-gloss finish that is barely sticky. The shade range presents sheer and juicy hues, and all of them are recommended.

✓ ☺ **Velvety Matte Lip Crayon** *($6.99)* is outstanding, if you prefer a thick pencil for lip color and want an opaque matte finish that feels virtually weightless. The palette of shades is soft and wearable—I can't imagine most women would balk at any of the colors—and all apply with enviable smoothness. For a lipstick in pencil form, the tip stays impressively pointed and isn't prone to becoming smushed down unless you apply with a lot of pressure. The finish is truly matte, and can begin to feel dry, but if you're OK with that then you'll likely love this product.

☺ **Luxury Lip Color** *($7.99)* is a good cross between a gloss and an opaque lipstick. It gives good coverage but has a very slippery, glossy finish. The latest packaging features an improved color swatch that is an accurate representation of how the color will appear on lips. The shades that begin with "Sheer" are indeed softer, more translucent colors.

☺ **Lip Definer** *($5.99)* has a creamy, oil-based formula that's nearly identical to the Eye Definer, but the creaminess is not a problem for the lips, unless lipstick feathering into lines around the mouth is an issue. There aren't many colors available, but they cover the basics and are versatile.

☺ **Velvety Shine Lip Crayon** *($7.99)*. This chunky, sharpening-required lip pencil is essentially a slightly greasy, glossy lipstick. It glides on effortlessly and the colors are soft, but this will easily travel into lines around the mouth. You're better off using Kashuk's Velvety Matte Lip Crayon and topping that with a light layer of lip gloss.

MASCARA: ☺ **Lashify Mascara** *($7.99)* is worth considering if you need a mascara that's better at lengthening than thickening and that wears well without a flake or smear. The packaging now includes a built-in metal lash comb that, while not my personal favorite (plastic combs are safer), works well to add separation to lashes.

☺ **Lashify Mascara with Liner** *($7.99)* is identical to the Lashify Mascara except, instead of the metal lash comb, the opposite end of the component houses an automatic, retractable pencil eyeliner. The creamy-smooth texture glides on but is meant to be smudged (before that happens on its own).

☺ **Lashify Mascara Waterproof** *($7.99)* performs almost as well as the non-waterproof Lashify Mascara, and offers a bit more oomph than many waterproof mascaras (and this one is definitely waterproof). Consider this if you don't want much lash drama, but foresee tears or a rainstorm.

BRUSHES: ✓ ☺ **Sonia Kashuk Brushes** *($7.99-$19.99)* are almost all recommended and a bona fide beauty bargain at these prices. Each brush has an ergonomically designed handle and a polished, futuristic look that's eye-catching. The top choices include **Contoured Large Eye Shadow Brush**, **Contoured Small Eye Shadow Brush**, **Contoured Powder Brush**, and **Contoured/Angled Eye Shadow Brush**, which also works to fill in and define all but very thin brows. Also recommended is the retractable **Travel Blush Brush**, which can also be used to apply powder on the go.

☺ **Synthetic Flat Blusher Brush** *($14.99)* doesn't have the shape or profile of a traditional blush brush (synthetic or natural hair), although it proves to be an interesting departure that produces similar results, as long as you use the flat side of the brush rather than "dotting" blush on with the cut-straight-across brush head. For a synthetic-hair brush, this feels remarkably soft and has superior density, which is ideal for holding and applying powder colors.

Consider the well-designed plastic and rubber ☺ **Dramatic Definition Travel Eyelash Curler** *($9.99)* or the traditional metal-with-rubber-pad **Dramatically Defining Eyelash Curler** *($9.99)* if you're looking to curl your lashes.

SPECIALTY PRODUCTS: ☺ **How to Create the Bronzer Face Cosmetic Palette** *($19.99)* is the best of Kashuk's "How to …" palettes. The combination of eyeshadow, lip, and cheek colors is ideal for creating a balanced bronzed makeup look without any one area being emphasized more than another. The powder blush and powder bronzer work great together, as do the eyeshadows and soft, warm-toned lip colors. This palette is best for light to medium skin tones and comes with helpful application instructions.

☺ **How to Create the Smokey Eye Cosmetic Palette** *($19.99)*. Housed in a sleek cardboard compact are three shades of powder eyeshadow along with complementary colors for lips and cheeks plus a dual-sided applicator that isn't nearly as effective as Sonia Kashuk's brushes (sold separately). The colors in this set can create a smoky eye (and the instructions are a helpful addition) but the overall palette is best for lighter skin tones. This is worth the price if the shades appeal to you.

☺ **How to Organically Look Natural Cosmetic Palette** *($19.99)* is designed for the natural-is-best crowd both for creating a nude, natural look and for anyone interested in certified-organic ingredients. The palette includes powder eyeshadows, blushes, and cream lip colors along with a dispensable applicator. The color balance of this palette is best for fair to light skin tones.

STILA (MAKEUP ONLY)

STILA AT-A-GLANCE

Strengths: Two very good tinted moisturizers, each providing sufficient UVA protection, and one of which is fragrance-free; inexpensive for a department-store/boutique line; the foundations are remarkable in most respects, especially shade selection and texture; excellent concealers; bronzing powder with sunscreen; very good options for blush and eyeshadow; Major Lash Mascara really wows; the Brow Polish and Lip Glaze are standouts; several attractive, versatile shimmer products; great makeup brushes.

Weaknesses: Convertible Eye Color and Kajal Eye Liner; some problematic lip glosses; the lip pencils are average at best.

For more information about Stila, call (866) 415-1332 or visit www.stilacosmetics.com or www.Beautypedia.com.

FOUNDATION: ✓ ☺ **$$$ Illuminating Liquid Foundation** *($38)* is a creamy, mineral oil–based makeup that's very good for dry skin seeking light to medium coverage with a satin-smooth, shimmer finish. The shine is more noticeable than in the Illuminating Powder Foundation below, but with a sheer powder dusted over it this can lend a radiant glow to the skin. All eight shades are soft and neutral whether skin is fair or dark (but not very dark).

✓ ☺ **$$$ Natural Finish Oil-Free Makeup** *($38)* is an outstanding liquid foundation with an exceedingly silky application that blends beautifully and provides light to medium coverage with a satin-matte finish. The formula is oil-free and an excellent choice for normal to oily skin prone to blemishes. Thirteen shades are available, including options for fair to dark skin tones. Within that range, only shades F, H, and L are too peach to consider.

✓ ☺ **$$$ Sheer Color Tinted Moisturizer SPF 15** *($34)* contains an in-part avobenzone sunscreen for sufficient UVA protection and has a lightweight lotion texture that provides a slight hint of coverage and understated, almost see-through, color. All but one of the ten perfectly neutral shades blend well and set to a soft matte finish; the Warm shade is bound to be too peach for its intended skin tone. This tinted moisturizer is ideal for those with normal to slightly dry or slightly oily skin who want something less formal than a regular foundation. Note that although it's a bit pricey, it comes in a 1.7-ounce size, whereas similar options typically offer less product.

☺ **$$$ Sheer Color Tinted Moisturizer SPF 30** *($36)*. Talk about sheer! This tinted moisturizer provides so little coverage you might ask why you bothered—except it does contain a very good in-part zinc oxide sunscreen and has a smooth, moist texture suitable for normal to very dry skin. Formula-wise, the only downside is the inclusion of cinnamon and ginger extracts, both potential irritants. The eight shades are mostly very good, as is typical of all of Stila's complexion-enhancing products. The three lightest shades are nearly interchangeable for those with fair skin, including porcelain skin tones. Only Medium is worth avoiding because of its peachy tint, but this is so sheer it's hardly an issue. This is recommended for its sun protection and moisturization, but not for its coverage. It definitely needs to be set with powder to ensure long wear.

☺ **$$$ Illuminating Powder Foundation SPF 12** *($28)* deserves a happy face rating even though its titanium dioxide–based sunscreen is below the minimum SPF 15. This is recommended with the caveat that it be used over a regular sunscreen or a foundation with sunscreen rated SPF 15 or higher. This talc-based powder foundation is extraordinarily silky and applies seamlessly, offering light, non-powdery coverage and a barely there, slightly shiny finish. The eight shades are terrific and not to be missed if you prefer this type of foundation and don't mind the initially high price.

CONCEALER: ☺ **$$$ Cover-Up Stick** *($20)* is a twist-up stick concealer. Alas, this has a creamy texture that will easily lend itself to creasing under the eye. However, it blends very well and is fine if you need heavier coverage over birthmarks or broken capillaries, and the six colors are uniformly excellent, even if this is not a matte-finish concealer as stated.

☹ **$$$ Perfecting Concealer** *($23)* has a slightly thick, greasy formula that's a step backward when compared to many other modern concealers. You'll get full coverage with an opacity that camouflages redness and dark circles, but it's tricky to blend and is so emollient it will crease into lines no matter how much powder you use for setting. Substantial coverage without the drawbacks of greasiness and persistent creasing is attainable from M.A.C.'s Select Moisturecover, and it costs less, too! If you decide to try Perfecting Concealer, avoid shades H and K, which are too ash and copper for dark skin. The other shades are predominantly neutral and there are some good options for fair skin.

POWDER: ☺ $$$ **Sheer Pressed Powder** *($28)* goes on quite sheer. This talc-based powder doesn't feel the least bit heavy, nor is it too dry or "powdery." It goes on lightly and has a silky matte finish, yet manages to keep excess oil in check without making skin look flat and dull. The palette of shades is a bit odd: Fair is pure white, while Light and Medium are suitable for fair skin tones only. Dark and Deep are best for light to medium skin tones, while Mocha and Cocoa are meant for darker skin or for use as matte bronzing powders. Sorting through the options to find your best match isn't as easy as it should be, but this pressed powder is still recommended for all skin types except blemish-prone. The cornstarch in this product can be a problem for blemishes.

☺ $$$ **Hydrating Finishing Powder** *($32)* is just as it sounds; a powder with water that goes on slightly damp and then dries. This liquid powder has more movement than traditional powders, and can adhere to skin slightly better. I disagree that the water adds hydration though, because water in and of itself isn't going to add or hold moisture to skin (if it did, taking a bath should be all skin needs to be free from dryness and that is absolutely not the case). The main ingredient in here is the very absorbent mineral silica. The texture is nearly weightless and silky, yet, as expected, the silica lends a dry finish. Therefore, this powder with its sole translucent shade (suitable for light to medium skin tones) is best for normal to oily skin.

☺ $$$ **Illuminating Treatment Powder** *($45)* is exclusive to Stila's Web site, but don't let that tempt you to try this liquid loose powder. Yes, it looks cool to see loose powder move around like water yet go on dry (in the case of this product, very dry), but this special effect is simply one more way to formulate powder. Illumination comes from the iridescent gold sheen that this powder leaves behind, along with an uncomfortably dry finish suitable only for oily skin, which is the very skin type that likely doesn't want to add more shine all over. As for treatment benefits, this contains a tiny amount of plant extracts and water-binding agents that you're much better off getting from a moisturizer or serum than from this powder.

BLUSH AND BRONZER: ✓☺ $$$ **Bronzing Tinted Moisturizer SPF 15** *($32)* is a lightweight bronzing lotion that is sheer enough for allover use if desired, but not if your skin is fair to light. Used in key areas of the face for a bronze effect, you'll be impressed with how easily this blends without streaking. The sunscreen includes zinc oxide for sufficient UVA protection, but this is best as an adjunct to another SPF-rated product in your daily routine because if you apply it all over, you will look like you've applied a mask to your skin. The color is a soft, peachy tan with subtle sparkles, and the formula is suitable for normal to oily skin.

✓☺ $$$ **Cheek Color Pan** *($18)* is Stila's pressed-powder blush and it has a silky, almost creamy feel that goes on smoothly and offers a shade range that runs from sheer to deep, so there's something for just about every skin color. Most of the shades are nearly matte, and the shiny ones are readily apparent and best for evening makeup. Interestingly, Sephora stores (where Stila is primarily sold) carry only a handful of the available shades. Check out Stila's Web site for the full selection of colors.

✓☺ $$$ **Stila Sun SPF 15 Bronzing Powder** *($28)* marks the return of Stila's classic pressed bronzing powder, and now it includes an in-part titanium dioxide sunscreen. Although you wouldn't want to use this as your sole source of sun protection unless you're willing to apply it opaquely, it is a fine adjunct to your moisturizer or foundation with sunscreen. This powder has a very smooth texture and sheer application, whose finish leaves a faint trace of shine. Shade 1 is a medium tan with a peachy undertone, while Shade 2 is a darker tan with a more apparent brown tone. Either shade of this talc-based powder is workable for light to medium skin tones. One caution: The amount of cornstarch may make this problematic for those prone to blemishes.

✓ ☺ **$$$ Sun Gel** *($24)* seems pricey at first, but this small tube of bronzing gel is concentrated—a tiny dab is enough to add a translucent bronze glow to the cheeks and temple area, and the shine is kept to a minimum. The single shade available is a fairly convincing tan color, though it can be too orange for fair skin tones. It blends well, but if you're not used to applying gels it will take some practice to ensure smooth, even application. Bronzing gels are best used over bare skin, or carefully applied over sunscreen (give the sunscreen time to be absorbed before dabbing on the gel). This does not blend well over foundation or powder, and is ideally suited for a natural, sun-kissed look.

☺ **$$$ Convertible Color** *($25)* is a find for dry skin. This is basically a sheer, emollient blush that feels more like a lipstick in compact form. This is intended for use on lips and cheeks for a simple, easy, "finger-painted" look. The texture is creamy bordering on greasy (akin to traditional lipstick), and the large color range is exceptional, with a few eye-catching sheer, but bright, hues. The color of each compact is a very good representation of how the shade appears on skin, though of course the product itself is more translucent. The Marigold option is a split pan that offers a sheer bronze and gold tone, the latter being infused with real gold, but that's of no special benefit for your skin.

☹ **Gel Cheek Color** *($16)* has the advantage of being easier to control and blend than liquid cheek tints such as Benefit BeneTint, but this true-gel blush from Stila, while offering three very good translucent colors, leaves a slightly tacky finish. It's an OK option for normal to dry skin, but not preferred to a powder blush.

EYESHADOW: ✓ ☺ **$$$ Eye Shadow Duo** *($20)* has the most sublime powder texture that applies creamy-smooth and has excellent blendability as well as pigmentation. Every shade in each duo has some amount of shine, but it doesn't flake. The only negative is the number of vivid or pastel duos, none of which work well to shape and shade the eye. The best duos include Lilly, Promenade, Dragonfly, Mara Samba, and Vieux Carre.

✓ ☺ **$$$ Eye Shadow Pan** *($18)* has a gorgeous, smooth, suitably dry texture that blends well. Shine rules the roost here, but at least these single eyeshadows apply easily, cling well, and aren't garish. These are meant to be used with any of Stila's refillable compacts.

☺ **$$$ Baked Eye Shadow Trio** *($28)*. If you can get past the domed shape, which makes the lack of dividers between the three colors more apparent and a bit awkward to use, and you want more shiny eyeshadows, then this is an outstanding, beautifully silky trio to consider. The powder-based formula glides over lids and practically blends itself, and its strong shimmer finish doesn't flake. In short, it's an ideal find for those with unwrinkled, smooth eyes looking to really make them sparkle. All of the sets are predominantly warm-toned and are highly recommended—just be sure to use shadow brushes that fit within the borders of each color to avoid turning each trio into a smudgy mess in the container.

☺ **$$$ Eye Shadow Quad** *($38)*. Stila wisely went with its talc-based powder eyeshadow formula for this pair of eyeshadow sets. The quads are well-coordinated, but a bit more tone-on-tone than is useful for many people. Still, each shade applies smoothly and blends well and, for those looking for shine, it's here in varying degrees (from soft shimmer to a strong metallic sheen). This is worth exploring if you find the color groupings to your liking.

☺ **$$$ Smoky Eyes Talking Palette** *($40).* Now here's something I haven't seen before when shopping for makeup, and that's saying something given how much makeup I've seen and tested! This palette of four powder eyeshadows talks to you. OK, it doesn't tell you what career path to follow or what you should wear for your Saturday night date, but with the press of a button you get vocalized step-by-step instructions for using each shade to create perfect smoky eyes. The shadows are laced with shimmer (I guess Stila doesn't care for the matte smoky eyes you see on page after page of fashion magazines) and each has a smooth, dry texture that applies well and builds easily if you desire more intensity. Two shades in each set are dark enough to double as powder eyeliner. Because you won't hear this from the talking palette, I'll tell you: Watch out for the green and blue sets! The Bronzes and The Grays are best.

☹ **$$$ Silky Eye Shadow Wash** *($22)* is a liquid eyeshadow with an angled sponge-tip applicator that comes in one color. The sole shade was inspired by Stila's best-selling eyeshadow shade, Kitten (a pale pink-beige shade with shimmer). In contrast to the eyeshadows, this goes on sheer and imparts noticeable gold sparkles to the eye area. Film-forming agent PVP is the second ingredient, and leaves a slightly tacky finish. Despite this, the initial slip and blending are satisfactory and, for being sheer, it wears better than expected. All told, this nonessential eyeshadow is recommended for Stila devotees only.

☹ **Convertible Eye Color** *($22)* is a dual-ended product that gives you an automatic, retractable eye pencil along with an iridescent-powder eyeshadow dispensed from a sponge tip. The pencil is a breeze to work with but the powder eyeshadow tends to apply unevenly and flake no matter how careful you are. For that reason alone, this product isn't recommended.

☹ **Matte Eye Shadow** *($18)* is Stila's attempt to go matte and jump on the mineral makeup bandwagon with this "mineral-enriched" formula, but ends up a huge letdown. None of the colors are truly matte, despite the fact that they appear that way at first glance, and each is infused with sparkles that tend to flake. Formula-wise, this feels unusually dry and applies unevenly—not good news considering the pigmented shades. Blending is a challenge and wearability is uneven, making this an eyeshadow to ignore. Ironically, it is the minerals in this product (barium sulfate and magnesium carbonate chief among them) that make the texture and application so undesirable.

EYE AND BROW SHAPER: ✓ ☺ **Brow Polish** *($14)* comes in a small container, but the price isn't outrageous for what ends up being a very good brow tint that can do double duty to conceal gray hairs between appointments with your colorist. The dual-sided brush allows for easy application, whether you want soft or more dramatically defined (but not overdone) brows. It dries to a soft, powdery feel and lasts well without flaking or smearing. Two shades are available: Warm for light brown to auburn brows, and Medium for medium to dark brown brows.

☺ **$$$ Glitter Eye Liner** *($18)* is a liquid eyeliner infused with glitter. I can't imagine that this will appeal to most adult women, who are looking to create a sophisticated eye-makeup design, but if the occasional foray into Technicolor glitter is on your beauty list, you could do worse! The brush applies this liner evenly, though it is strictly about glitter, not adding depth and definition like a regular eyeliner would. The formula takes several seconds to set, but once it does, the glitter stays on amazingly well, which is by far the most impressive aspect of this liner.

☺ **$$$ Liquid Eyeliner** *($16)*. Liquid Eyeliner has a very good, firm but flexible brush that applies color evenly and easily (relatively speaking). The dry time is slow and once set the line remains slightly tacky, which can compromise wear. I wouldn't choose this over Stila's Smudge Pots (their version of gel eyeliner), but if you prefer liquid eyeliner, this is an overall impressive one. It's available in black only.

☺ **$$$ Smudge Pots** *($20)* is nearly identical to Bobbi Brown's Long-Wear Gel Eyeliner and M.A.C.'s Fluidline. These types of gel eyeliners are able to stand up to oily eyelids without fading, smearing, or running. Stila mimicked Brown's basic formulation, offering a slightly moist gel-cream eyeliner that sets to a long-wearing matte finish. It is every bit as tenacious as those from Brown and M.A.C., but the application is not as easy because the color intensity does not build as quickly, going on more sheer and requiring you to layer if you want a solid, more dramatic line. How thin or thick a line you create depends entirely on the type of brush you use; a pointed eyeliner brush produces a thin line, while a wedge brush can easily create a thicker line. The only reason to choose Stila's version over similar products is if you're looking more for a sheer application than for a dramatic one. Basic shades of black, brown, and gray are accompanied by wilder hues, including a bright blue and green that are best avoided. The Golden Noir shade includes real gold, but the effect is simply black with gold shimmer.

☺ **$$$ Brow Set** *($18)* offers two slightly shiny brown shades in one pan for defining brows and filling in sparse areas (that's what the lighter shade is intended for). While adding shimmer to brows is just strange, this is an option, though the price is steep for what you get. You can get similar results from a single shade of matte powder eyeshadows.

☹ **Kajal Eye Liner** *($18)* is a rare misstep from Stila, because this is one disappointing, needs-sharpening pencil. It does have a super-soft texture that makes it easy to apply, but it's so creamy (and stays that way) that smearing and fading are inevitable. Yes, you can enhance this pencil's longevity by setting it with a powder eyeshadow, but why not use a pencil (or powder eyeshadow) that lasts well to begin with?

LIPSTICK, LIP GLOSS, AND LIPLINER: ✓☺ **$$$ Pearl Shimmer Gloss** *($22)* is a beautiful brush-on lip gloss in every respect. The slickness and mineral oil base make it the wrong choice for anyone with lines around the mouth, but it has a supremely smooth texture and a completely non-sticky pearlized finish that works with any lip color, from soft pink to beige to deep red.

☺ **$$$ It Gloss** *($18)* is "It" because the company claims it "takes shine to a whole new level." Make no mistake—this brush-on gloss provides not only a wet-look, glossy finish, but also high-wattage shimmer to spare, all without feeling sticky. Still, lots of glosses have these characteristics, and Stila's attempt, nice as it is, is a reinvention of the wheel. The palette of shades is gorgeous, presenting options that range from sheer nudes to vivid wine tones.

☺ **$$$ Mango Crush Lip & Cheek Stain with Shimmer** *($24)*. This lip and cheek stain is housed in a pen-style component outfitted with a synthetic brush applicator. It is much easier to apply to lips than cheeks, but because the formula is a cross between a gel and a cream blush you don't get a very moist finish, so you might end up reaching for lip gloss in addition. Applied to cheeks, this produces a sheer coral-red flush and it blends well.

☺ **$$$ Lip Color** *($17)* is Stila's main lipstick, and it is available in your choice of Creme, Shimmer, or Sheer formulas (thankfully designated on the tester unit so you're not guessing which version you're considering). **Cremes** feel thick and are indeed creamy, though they are greasy enough to slip into lines around the mouth. These provide medium coverage and a good stain. The **Shimmer** formula is smoother and less greasy than the Cremes, and, true to its name, has a shimmer finish. **Sheers** are glossy and fleeting but the soft colors are beautifully appealing.

☺ **$$$ Lip Glaze** *($22)* is a moderately thick, smooth lip gloss with a minimally sticky finish and a glaze-like shine. It's packaged in a click-pen component with a built-in brush applicator and the brush itself is nicely cut to fit the contours of the mouth. Lip Glaze is one of Stila's best-selling products, and numerous shades are available, ranging from translucent with shimmer to glossy reds and berry tones.

☺ **$$$ Lip Polish** *($22)* is a lip gloss in a self-dispensing brush applicator, for more money than this clever packaging is really worth ($22 for lip gloss borders on ridiculous). A few clicks at the base release a flow of gloss onto the lip-brush applicator, and you're on your way to semi-rich color with a soft gloss finish. This is similar to Stila's Lip Glaze but the colors are stronger and the finish less sticky.

☺ **$$$ Long Wear Lip Color** *($18)*. This slim, twist-up lipstick with a rounded tip (rather than angled) goes on slick and stays that way. It feels very light and its staying power comes from the stain effect it has on lips. It's an intriguing way to get lip color that lasts longer than traditional lipstick, but it doesn't take as long as the two-step lip paint/top coat products. Long Wear Lip Color is worth a try if you don't like the lip paint/top coat options, and Stila offers some enticing shades.

☺ **$$$ Silk Shimmer Gloss** *($22)* comes in a single shade inspired by one of Stila's best-selling eyeshadow shades, Kitten (a pale pink-beige shade with shimmer). This silky, lightweight gloss feels great and imparts a sheer beige-pink shimmer, complete with clear crystalline sparkles. The brush applicator is great, and it doesn't splay with repeated use. Despite these positives, this pricey lip gloss is really for devoted Stila fans only because you can find equally impressive lip glosses at the drugstore for one-third the price.

☺ **$$$ Cherry Crush Lip & Cheek Stain** *($24)* is supposed to react to skin's pH and stain your cheeks and lips a customized cherry hue. It works to some extent, but color impact on any skin tone remains a soft, sheer red. This is better for lips than cheeks because on cheeks it feels way too sticky and is difficult to blend. On lips, it functions well as a sheer gloss, though application with the built-in brush can be uneven, so be prepared to be patient. For the money, I wouldn't go for this over the better sheer lip glosses from L'Oreal and Revlon.

☹ **$$$ Hi-Shine Lip Color** *($17)* is an incredibly greasy lipstick with a glossy finish that has minimal staying powder. Most of the colors are quite soft, so this is definitely a lipstick that, while great for dry lips, will need frequent reapplication and can bleed into lines around the mouth.

☹ **$$$ Lip Liner** *($16.50)* needs sharpening, which is inconvenient, but this smooth-textured pencil's slightly dry finish tends to stay put, so the payoff is a long-lasting line that holds up to all but the greasiest lipsticks and glosses. The dozen or so shades consist of mostly nude and neutral tones to complement a variety of lipstick hues.

☹ **$$$ Lip Rouge** *($20)* claims to be a magic marker for the lips. I wouldn't call it indelible, but it has impressive staying power, just not as much as you would expect for the money. Inside a fountain pen–style package, a very pigmented water- and alcohol-based liquid is fed into a brush tip, which is applied to the lips; it then sets into a long-lasting, feels-like-nothing stain. Two cautions: It dries up easily if you don't replace the cap tightly after each use and the hard brush tip makes for less-than-pleasant application.

☺ **$$$ SPF 20 Shine Lip Color** *($22)*. When you consider this lipstick's deficiency—it does not shield lips from the full spectrum of UVA rays—it isn't off to a grand start. Adding to this disappointment is the high price for a creamy lipstick that goes on too sheer and tends to fade quickly. There are plenty of inexpensive lipsticks that outperform this, and some of those also offer broad-spectrum sun protection.

☹ **24kt Gloss** *($22)*. It's nice that this lip gloss is infused with real gold, but with gold prices being what they are, what a waste! Don't worry, however, there's not much gold in here, and keep in mind that gold isn't required to produce the sparkling finish that this gloss provides. More important, pure gold can cause contact dermatitis, so be careful if you use this product—it made my lips burn immediately! More bad news: This gloss feels grainy because of the amount of glitter. The sparkling finish is ultra-shiny, but you can get that from other glosses that don't have the problems this one does.

☹ **Plumping Lip Glaze** *($24)* is Stila's worst lip gloss on several counts. The click-pen dispenser with built-in brush is convenient, but on this version it tends to dial up way too much product (and there's no way to put it back), the gloss itself has an unusually thick, syrupy texture that tends to stick lips together, and the formula contains irritating, menthol-based menthoxypropanediol, an ingredient that plumps lips via irritation, and that's not good news.

MASCARA: ✓ ☺ **$$$ Lash Visor Waterproof Mascara** *($20)*. Lash Visor has been reformulated and has a new brush, and the difference is positive. Most waterproof mascaras are better at lengthening than thickening, but this one excels at the latter—and quickly, too! You'll have to manage minor clumping, but it combs through without much trouble and lashes end up softly fringed. The formula is waterproof and requires a silicone- or oil-based makeup remover.

✓ ☺ **Major Lash Mascara** *($8.50 for 0.18 ounce)* is a major winner if you're looking for an outstanding thickening mascara! It sweeps on with ease, providing almost instant thickness and enough length so that each lash is well defined but not clumpy. This builds well, too, and wears evenly throughout the day.

☺ **$$$ Convertible Mascara** *($22)* is a dual-sided product that includes a long, skinny brush on one end and a fuller (actually, a more standard) brush on the other. Both brushes feature the same acrylate-based mascara formula. The acrylate copolymer forms tiny tubes around each lash, and can be removed with water and slight agitation. Ironically, the formula is water-resistant and lasts all day without smudging, flaking, or smearing. The trick is to be fastidious when removing this, because it's easy for little pieces of the tube to become "stuck" on lashes or the skin around them. The skinny brush side has a wet application with some minor clumps, but produces strong definition and ample length. The thick brush is very similar to the skinny brush, except you can get a bit of thickness. You may want to apply a coat from the thick brush side, then elongate and finish with the skinny brush side.

☺ **$$$ Lash Visor Waterproof Mascara** *($12.50)* makes lashes impressively long while also providing more thickness than most waterproof mascaras. Definitely waterproof, Lash Visor provides good lash separation, doesn't clump, and makes it through the day without a smudge or smear.

☺ **$$$ MAJOR Major Lash Mascara** *($22)* is meant to build on the success and stellar results from Stila's original Major Lash Mascara, which sells for one-third the cost of this. Performance-wise, both "Majors" are nearly equal in that they build thick, long lashes without clumps. However, the brush on MAJOR Major Lash Mascara is enormous, and difficult to maneuver into the inner corner of the eye. No matter how I applied this, I got dots of mascara near my tear duct and also on my eyelid above the outer corner. This was not an issue with the regular Major Lash Mascara, and given that one's convenience and lower price, it remains the better choice (unless you prefer huge mascara brushes and don't mind the extra cost).

☺ **$$$ Multi-Effect Mascara** *($20)* purports to be the ultimate formula that does it all, yet using this tells a different story, and its title is Great Expectations, Depressing Results. This curved-brush mascara is marginally adept at building length with minimal thickness, and leaves lashes slightly curled, if you don't mind a careful application that still creates some clumps and is smear-prone for longer than it should be. Stila dares you to try this; I implore you to consider the superior options from the drugstore, or, for Stila fans, the company's truly impressive Major Lash Mascara.

FACE AND BODY ILLUMINATING/SHIMMER PRODUCTS: ✓☺ **$$$ All Over Shimmer Liquid Luminizer** *($22)* is an improved version of Stila's original All Over Shimmer, which is now only occasionally offered in limited edition products. This widely available version is packaged in a glass bottle and includes a brush applicator. It is more fluid, less slick, and less powdery at dry-down than its predecessor, and is overall a significant improvement. Unlike All Over Shimmer, this stays in place, dries quickly after blending, and looks more natural. Its shimmer is more glow-y than shiny, and the shade selection has been whittled down to four (opalescent white, pale pink, light gold, and peachy bronze), all best for fair to medium skin tones. A little goes a long way, so the price is somewhat justified, not to mention that this product is versatile. This is Stila's best shine-enhancing option.

☺ **$$$ Illuminating Finishing Powder** *($32)* is a talc-based "domed" shimmer powder that's great for adding shine or highlighting areas of the face or body. It sweeps on soft shimmer plus larger flecks of shine, and the latter are prone to flaking. All three shades (Gold, Bronze, and Rose Glow) are accurately named and attractive for most skin tones. This highlighting powder works best for evening or special-occasion makeup.

☺ **$$$ Illuminating Tinted Moisturizer SPF 15** *($32)* has an in-part avobenzone sunscreen to ensure sufficient UVA protection, but unless you're willing to apply this all over the face it is best as an adjunct to another product rated SPF 15 or greater. The one-shade-fits-all concept is fine for most skin tones because this moisturizer imparts more soft radiance than color. The lightweight, luminous finish is attractive and suitable for normal to dry skin, but don't expect any coverage (it's really that sheer).

☺ **$$$ Sun Shimmer Dry Oil** *($26)* is a silicone-based moisturizing body spray that offers a sheer, glowing bronze tint suitable for fair to medium skin tones; it's just too sheer to register on tan to dark skin tones. The fragrant formula (think coconut/floral with tropical fruit) is moisturizing and leaves a sheen wherever you spray it. This works best to complement a self-tan on arms, legs, or décolleté, assuming you're OK with the fragrance. Remember to apply this before sunscreen because it does not offer any sun protection on its own.

☺ **$$$ All Over Glow** *($28)* provides a shimmery pressed-powder blush and coordinating highlighter in one compact. Both have a silky feel and sheer color impact, and the glam, glitter-like shine isn't anyone's definition of subtle. If shiny cheeks are what you're after, this is one (pricey) way to get it.

BRUSHES: Stila Brushes *($15-$50)* mostly have a soft but firm feel and excellent shapes. There are even a few unique dual-sided and retractable options, and almost every brush is available in long- or short-handled versions. Stop by and check these out if you are shopping for brushes, especially the following Paula's Picks: ✓☺ **#26 Perfecting Concealer Brush** *($20)*,

The Reviews S

✓ ☺ **#2 Under Eye Concealer Brush** *($20)*, ✓ ☺ **#9 All Over Blend Brush** *($24)*, ✓ ☺ **#15 Double Sided Brush** *($32)*, ✓ ☺ **#17 Retractable Bronzing Brush** *($26)*, and ✓ ☺ **#20 Eye Enhancer Brush** *($32)*. The synthetic ☺ **$$$ #27 Perfecting Foundation Brush** *($20)* is smaller than most, which means application takes more time.

SPECIALTY PRODUCTS: ☺ **$$$ Hydrating Primer with SPF 15** *($34)*. Labeling this as a primer is only correct in the sense that you would apply this product before foundation. Generally speaking, primers are silicone-based and are designed to add slip to skin to facilitate makeup application. This product is merely a good daytime moisturizer for normal to slightly dry or slightly oily skin. Its in-part avobenzone sunscreen provides sufficient UVA protection and it has a slightly moist finish, which is different from most primers. The texture of this product works well under makeup, but doesn't have the smoothing effect or absorbent quality many other primers possess.

STRIDEX (SKIN CARE ONLY)

STRIDEX AT-A-GLANCE

Strengths: A couple of benzoyl peroxide options that are fragrance- and irritant-free.

Weaknesses: All the pads with salicylic acid contain irritants such as menthol, alcohol, or witch hazel; poor cleansers; no oil-absorbing products; no effective AHA or BHA products.

For more information about Stridex, call (888) 784-2472 or visit www.stridex.com or www.Beautypedia.com.

☹ **Essential Care Triple Action Pads** *($4.29 for 55 pads)* contain menthol, and as such are too irritating for all skin types. Plus, the detergent cleansing agents are not what you want to leave on skin.

☹ **Maximum Strength Triple Action Pads** *($6.49 for 90 pads)* contain menthol and detergent cleansing agents that should not be left on skin.

✓ ☺ **Power Pads** *($6.99 for 28 pads)* are a unique new option to disinfect blemish-prone skin. Featuring an effective concentration of 2.5% benzoyl peroxide and free of irritating ingredients such as alcohol, witch hazel, or peppermint, these larger-than-usual, nonabrasive pads are recommended for all skin types battling acne. These pads contain a mild detergent cleansing agent, so unless your skin is very oily or you have makeup to remove, they will gently cleanse skin while disinfecting, and they do not need to be rinsed. Nice job, Stridex!

☹ **Sensitive Skin Triple Action Pads** *($6.69 for 90 pads)* are advertised as being alcohol-free, and that's great. However, although these pads do not contain alcohol, they are still terrible for sensitive skin because they contain menthol and an essentially ineffective amount of salicylic acid.

☹ **Super Scrub Triple Action Pads** *($3.99 for 55 pads)* are textured pads intended to exfoliate skin, but they're merely a great way to really increase the irritation from the menthol in each pad. In other words, don't bother.

☹ **Dual Solutions Daily Pore Control** *($6.99)* means well, but both products included in this 2-piece anti-acne set have problems that someone with blemish-prone skin doesn't need. The **Cleansing Pads** contain menthol and witch hazel, which are irritating and offer no benefit or help for acne-prone skin. The **Medicated Gel**, despite its 2% salicylic acid content, contains witch hazel and a small amount of alcohol. The alcohol would be tolerable on its own (again, the amount used is small) but the pH above 4 won't permit effective exfoliation to take place, so using the Gel becomes a "why bother?" more than anything else. Together it is just not a solution for anyone's skin.

☺ **Dual Solutions Intensive Acne Repair** *($6.99)* includes one problematic and one recommended product in this 2-piece anti-acne set. The recommended product is the **Medicated Gel**, a lightweight solution that includes 2.5% benzoyl peroxide to disinfect blemish-prone skin. The **Cleansing Pads** present problems for skin due to the menthol they contain. Moreover, the pH of the pads is too high for the 2% salicylic acid to exfoliate, so that ingredient is wasted. The happy face rating pertains to the Medicated Gel only. The Cleansing Pads definitely merit an unhappy face!

STRIVECTIN (SKIN CARE ONLY)

STRIVECTIN AT-A-GLANCE

Strengths: The Eye Cream is worth considering if you don't mind the price.

Weaknesses: Expensive; the original StriVectin-SD product (and every other product sold under this brand name) is absolutely not better than Botox; some of the products contain irritant peppermint oil; the Deep Wrinkle serum is terrible.

For more information about StriVectin, call (800) 621-9553 or visit www.bremennlabs.com or www.Beautypedia.com.

☹ **StriVectin-HS Hydro-Thermal Deep Wrinkle Serum** *($153 for 0.9 ounce)* is a cosmetics rip-off that is a must to avoid. That's not only because it doesn't work as claimed, but because it includes an inaccurate ingredient statement (there's no such ingredient as "Tripeptide"; it should be followed by a number). For over $150, you're getting a water-based serum that temporarily tightens skin because of the amount of sodium polystyrene sulfonate (a film former) and egg white (albumen) it contains. It cannot penetrate to the dermal/epidermal junction and plump deep wrinkles from the bottom up. Wasting money on a few bottles of this would only match the cost for a series of facial peels or Intense Pulsed Light (IPL) treatments, options proven to make a positive difference in skin. (Though even so, neither of these treatments will significantly improve the appearance of deep wrinkles—for that, more invasive procedures are needed.)

☺ **$$$ StriVectin-SD Eye Cream** *($59 for 1.3 ounces)* is a surprisingly good moisturizer for dry skin around the eyes, and the price is better than the original StriVectin-SD. It contains olive-based emollients, nonvolatile plant oils, skin-identical ingredients, and, further down on the list, some very good anti-irritants and antioxidants. Because this is for use around the eyes, manufacturer Klein-Becker wisely omitted the peppermint oil found in the original StriVectin-SD product. Interestingly, the company mentions this on their Web site, stating that "since the original StriVectin-SD formula was designed as a stretch-mark reducer, it contains aromatic agents (such as peppermint) which cause some users' eyes to water when applied to the delicate skin in the orbital eye area...." How thoughtful of them to let us know, though they left out the part about the irritation it can cause skin, and never mind the fact that peppermint oil and other "aromatic compounds" have absolutely no effect on stretch marks! The real question is whether this Eye Cream is the antiaging breakthrough it's made out to be. But it's no surprise the answer is "No!"—though as mentioned above, it is a good moisturizer. Klein-Becker claims the patented pentapeptides in this product are the wrinkle-reducing, dark circle–diminishing wonders, but independent research does not correlate with this claim because there are no independent, peer-reviewed studies analyzing the effects of palmitoyl pentapeptide-3 on wrinkles.

The studies that do exist were paid for by Sederma (now owned by Croda), the ingredient's manufacturer and distributor. Such company-sponsored studies are not a reliable source of information because the company has a vested interest in making sure that whatever tests they conduct show their ingredient performs as intended. Lastly, Sederma's own research mentions that in order to gain maximum benefit from palmitoyl pentapeptide-3, it must be used at a 3% to 5% concentration, yet the amount in StriVectin-SD Eye Cream is unknown, and a look at the ingredient list indicates that it's far less than 3% (Klein-Becker would not reveal the exact percentage when we called). If you still want to know if this ingredient is the miracle the ads claim, Olay Regenerist serums and moisturizers contain the exact same thing, and more of it, for a fraction of this price.

☹ **StiVectin-SD Physicians' Formula SPF 15** *($63 for 2 ounces)* makes a medical association via its name, but this in-part zinc oxide sunscreen is not what the doctor ordered. Not only is it unnecessarily pricey, but—just like the original StriVectin-SD formula — it contains peppermint oil. Further, there is no substantiated research proving that the company's Striadril compound (consisting of glycerin, butylene glycol, peptides, plant extracts, and some good skin-identical ingredients) is the preferred antiaging blend because of its superior stability, tolerability, and effectiveness. The peptides in this complex are beneficial for skin, but whether or not they exert a noticeable effect on wrinkles is undetermined.

☹ **StriVectin-SD Physicians' Formula SPF 30** *($75 for 2 ounces)* is designed to be compared with or used with the original StriVectin product, so Klein-Becker decided to keep the price high while offering it in a smaller container (original StriVectin comes in a 6-ounce tube). Perhaps they did that because the amount of "Striadril Complex" is more prominent in this mineral sunscreen for normal to dry skin. Although this Complex contains peptides and some effective water-binding agents for skin, it isn't an antiwrinkle phenomenon. What I can't understand is why this otherwise gentle sunscreen had to contain peppermint oil. That won't help anyone's skin, and completely eliminates the possibility of recommending this for those with sensitive skin (and a penchant for spending way more than they need to on a sunscreen). Oddly, the directions call for you to apply this sunscreen twice per day if you're using it on wrinkled skin—which means you'll be replacing this every month if you're using it properly (meaning a liberal application each time). Unless you're outdoors for several hours, are perspiring heavily, or swimming, you don't need to apply sunscreen twice daily—it certainly isn't needed at night! The company mentions that the formula is concentrated so that only a small amount is needed per application—but that's dangerous advice for a sunscreen.

☺ **$$$ StriVectin Facial Anti-Oxidant** *($109 for 3.5 ounces)*. Given the ongoing, somewhat confounding success of the original StriVectin-SD, the company decided to launch another product with the same exaggerated, unproven claims as the original. Capitalizing on brand name recognition is good business. The claim is that the antioxidant blend in the product returns the skin-cell renewal rate of a 67-year-old woman back to that of a woman of 29. Of course, that is preposterous, and of course there is no published or peer-reviewed research to support the claim, nor are the details of how the company came to this conclusion available. Given their sketchy background, troubles with the FDA, and legal issues, I'm not the least bit surprised there is no supporting evidence for their turn-back-the-clock claims. Several of the antioxidants StriVectin included in this product show up in hundreds of other products, though I suppose the company would argue that their "synergistic blend" is unique and therefore exerts a stronger benefit. But affecting the renewal rate of skin cells as drastically as claimed is like saying a diet high in antioxidants is going to help your organs go from age 67 to 29. This is not youth restored in a tube any more than the original StriVectin could replace Botox in any way, shape, or form. While the claims for this product are insulting and a mockery, the blend of antioxidants, water-binding agents, and lightweight emollients can help normal to dry skin look and feel better. I'd argue that you don't have to spend nearly this much to get an antioxidant-rich moisturizer in stable packaging, but as long as you don't expect the fantasy claims of this product to come true and don't mind the expense, it is one more moisturizer with antioxidants to consider. (However, encouraging the continued questionable business practices of Klein Becker is something I ask consumers to reconsider.)

☺ $$$ **StriVectin Neck Cream** *($90 for 1.4 ounces)*. The folks behind StriVectin want you to believe this product can get rid of sagging skin on your chin and neck. Why not? They have nothing to lose and women love too-good-to-be-true promises so StriVectin can laugh themselves silly all the way to the bank. "Turkey neck"—you know what it looks like and you know when that description applies to the skin on your neck. StriVectin claims to have the solution for this sign of aging, claiming that this cream can lift, shape, and refine sagging skin, which it cannot do—but more on that in a moment. The appearance of turkey neck on adults occurs when the platysma muscle (which consists of two broad strands of muscles on both sides of the neck) loosens as a result of time and repeated movements. A neck lift corrects this drooping appearance by surgically shortening the platysma muscles or reattaching them to their original position. In some cases, Botox injections can improve the appearance of sagging muscles on the neck, but in advanced cases cosmetic surgery is the only way to eliminate the dreaded turkey neck. But, can a cream do that, or even come close? Absolutely not! There are some absorbent and tightening ingredients in this jar-packaged moisturizer for normal to dry skin, but the tightening effect is temporary and incapable of shoring up loose skin that results from drooping muscles. StriVectin Neck Cream contains a small amount of a form of antiseptic resorcinol, and it may prove irritating.

☹ **StriVectin-SD** *($135 for 6 ounces)*. So is StriVectin better than Botox? The short answer is no—and that means no way, and no how. It isn't even better than the daily use of an effective sunscreen! StriVectin is merely a moisturizer with some good emollients and antioxidants, though the addition of peppermint oil is extremely suspect—the tingle is probably meant to lead women to believe that the product is doing something to their skin. It is doing something: causing irritation without a benefit. Botox prevents the use of facial muscles, and that instantaneously smooths out the skin. StriVectin-SD won't alter the wrinkling on any part of your face, not in the long term, and not in the short term. An impressive study supports this conclusion. Researchers recruited 77 women who were divided into five groups. One group received Botox injections, one used a placebo product, and the other groups applied either StriVectin-SD, Hydroderm, or DDF Wrinkle Relax. Only the group that received Botox injections reported satisfaction with the results; wrinkle depth measurement parameters established for this study proved Botox produced the best results. And StriVectin-SD? It was deemed NOT better than Botox. Actually, three test subjects using StriVectin-SD had to drop out due to "adverse reactions," likely from the peppermint oil in the product (Source: *Dermatologic Surgery*, February 2006, pages 184-197).

☹ **StriVectin-WF, Instant Deep Wrinkle Filler** *($59 for 0.78 ounce)*. In the category of wrinkle-filling products, most are thicker, spackle-like products that rely on a sophisticated blend of silicones and silicone polymers to smooth and temporarily fill in superficial lines and wrinkles. They tend to work reasonably well, but are short-lived and certainly no substitute for cosmetic corrective procedures such as Botox and dermal fillers. This wrinkle-filling contribution from StriVectin doesn't follow formulary suit and as such is no competition for the superior options from lines like Estee Lauder, Good Skin, and Cosmedicine. All you're getting with this overpriced product is a blend of water, glycerin, thickening gum, and some plant extracts. The gum does a poor job of filling in wrinkles and lends a tacky finish anywhere it is placed. It's nice that there are some antioxidants in this wrinkle filler, but the inclusion of comfrey extract (listed by its Latin name *Symphytum officinale*) is cause for concern due to its toxic constituents. Please refer to my *Cosmetic Ingredient Dictionary* at www.Beautypedia.com for more information about comfrey. Reading the detailed claims for this product may sway you, but buyer beware!

TRISH MCEVOY

TRISH MCEVOY AT-A-GLANCE

Strengths: Mostly good cleansers; a well-formulated serum; a good absorbent gel for oily skin; the makeup is the crown jewel of this line, with many superb options, particularly the powders, bronzers, eyeshadows, brow gel, Glaze Lip Color, High-Volume Mascara, and Shimmer Pressed Powder; McEvoy's makeup brushes and makeup planners are practically peerless.

Weaknesses: Expensive; average moisturizers; sunscreens don't provide sufficient UVA protection; no effective AHA or BHA products; jar packaging; the foundations don't have that extra something that raises the bar (yet they should for what they cost); the concealers either crease endlessly or are difficult to work with; disappointing eyeliner options.

For more information about Trish McEvoy, call (800) 431-4306 or visit www.trishmcevoy.com or www.Beautypedia.com.

Note: I must extend a special thank you and acknowledge how unbelievably helpful Trish McEvoy and her team were while my team and I worked on this book. No cosmetics company we've ever contacted (and I've been writing the *Don't Go...* books since 1991) has provided as much helpful material and product as Trish McEvoy. No matter what we asked for or how many follow-up questions we posed, McEvoy's team was prompt, professional, and most importantly, exceedingly helpful. I have had the pleasure of speaking with some of McEvoy's artists at cosmetics counters across the United States, and their makeup application skills and product knowledge are typically excellent. I extend my deepest thanks and gratitude toward everyone at Trish McEvoy for their impeccable service and generosity.

TRISH MCEVOY SKIN CARE

TRISH MCEVOY BEAUTY BOOSTER PRODUCTS

☺ $$$ **Beauty Booster Cream** *($85 for 1.7 ounces)* has a light, silky texture suitable for normal to slightly dry skin, but overall is a bland formula whose antioxidants (olive oil and vitamin E) will be rendered ineffective due to jar packaging. This also contains potentially irritating fragrant components, and is way too expensive for what you (don't) get. Regarding the jar packaging, the company informed me that this product will be available in a tube by the time this book goes to press (late 2009).

☺ $$$ **Beauty Booster Serum** *($125 for 1 ounce)* ends up being a much smarter, though still exorbitantly overpriced, choice compared to the Beauty Booster Cream above. It contains mostly water, acetyl hexapeptide-3, slip agents, another peptide, soothing antioxidant plant extracts, and preservatives. This could have been a much more exciting, well-rounded formula. There is still no substantiated research to support the frequently made claim that acetyl hexapeptide-3 works like Botox by affecting facial muscle contractions; to McEvoy's credit, she does not make such a claim, whereas most companies that sell products containing acetyl hexapeptide-3 do. Considering that peptides have merit as water-binding agents and, theoretically, as cell-communicating ingredients, this serum contains a good amount of them and is an option for all skin types. It's just not as multifaceted as it could have been, owing to the minimal amount of antioxidants or ingredients that mimic the structure of skin, and overall that makes the price even more out of line.

☹ **Beauty Booster SPF 15 Anti-Fatigue Cream Enriched Primer and Mask** *($85 for 1.8 ounces)* isn't a beauty booster, it's a beauty blunder! It is inexcusable that this product lacks the UVA-protecting ingredients of titanium dioxide, zinc oxide, avobenzone (also called butyl methoxydibenzoylmethane), Tinosorb, or Mexoryl SX. As for the base formula, although it has a cushiony, creamy texture that can make for a lush-feeling moisturizing mask, you're not getting much for your money. The instant lift and extended foundation wear claims are completely off base, too. If those were accurate, then even plain Lubriderm would be an antiaging, makeup-enhancing moisturizer!

TRISH MCEVOY EVEN SKIN PRODUCTS

☺ **$$$ Even Skin Glycolic Wash** *($42 for 6.5 ounces)* is a good, though absurdly overpriced, standard, water-soluble cleanser for normal to oily skin, but the "scientifically proven AHA blend," which is chiefly glycolic acid, won't exfoliate skin to even out discolorations because it is rinsed down the drain before it has a chance to work. The pH is low enough for the glycolic acid to function as an exfoliant, but you'd have to leave this on skin longer than what's reasonable for a cleanser. This does contain lavender extract for fragrance.

☺ **$$$ Even Skin Beta Hydroxy Pads** *($65 for 40 pads)* list witch hazel extract as the second ingredient, which makes these pads needlessly irritating. Luckily the witch hazel is countered by some potent anti-irritants and soothing plant extracts, though the lavender isn't a welcome addition. Most disappointing are the tiny amount of salicylic acid and the pH of 5. That means the only exfoliation you'll get is from the act of massaging the pad over your skin, sort of like using a washcloth (except using a washcloth is gentler and more cost-effective).

☹ **$$$ Even Skin Vitamin C Cream** *($68 for 1 ounce)* makes normal to dry skin feel amazingly smooth because of its blend of silky silicones and emollient petrolatum. Vitamin C is on board along with a couple of other very good antioxidants, but the choice of jar packaging, while attractive, won't keep these key ingredients stable during use. In better packaging, this would be an excellent way to experience a moisturizer with vitamin C. Speaking of better packaging, the company informed me that this moisturizer will be switching to a tube in late 2009. As this book goes to press, it is still being sold in a jar. In the tube, this earns a happy face rating.

OTHER TRISH MCEVOY SKIN CARE PRODUCTS

☺ **$$$ Gentle Cleansing Lotion** *($58 for 6.8 ounces)* is a good, fragrance-free, water-rinsable cleansing lotion that's a good choice for someone with normal to dry skin. It does not contain detergent cleansing agents, but the emollients and oils it contains work well to remove makeup. Similar, less expensive options are available from Dove and Neutrogena, which is good to know, since the price of this cleanser is needlessly high for what you get.

☺ **$$$ Gentle Cleansing Wash** *($58 for 6.5 ounces)* is a fairly gentle, water-soluble gel cleanser for normal to oily or slightly dry skin. The small amounts of balm mint, lavender, and lemongrass extract are unpleasant additions, but should not pose a problem unless you get it in your eyes. In case you're wondering if this cleanser is really worth its brow-raising price—no, it is not. This ordinary formulation doesn't warrant even half the price tag. However, for those with money to burn and an affinity for all things McEvoy, it performs well and does remove makeup.

☺ **$$$ Gentle Eye Makeup Remover** *($24 for 4 ounces)* is a good, but exceptionally standard, water-based fluid makeup remover. It is fragrance- and colorant-free, but is easily replaced by other less expensive options.

☹ **$$$ Dry Skin Normalizer** *($60 for 2 ounces)* isn't a poor choice for those needing a fragrance-free moisturizer to remedy dry skin, but for the money, the formula is surprisingly dated and, well ... boring. It contains mostly water, thickeners, emollient, several more thickeners, film-forming agent, paraffin, slip agents, tiny amounts of water-binding agents, silicone, plant oil, a dusting of antioxidants, and preservatives. McEvoy and her team missed an opportunity to offer a state-of-the-art product worthy of its premium price.

☹ **$$$ Intense Eye Treatment** *($48 for 0.5 ounce)* bills itself as a unique formula, but it is a very standard mix of water, aloe, thickeners, and film-forming agents along with minuscule amounts of antioxidants and water-binding agents. It's an OK moisturizer for slightly dry skin around the eyes or elsewhere, but better formulas abound. This contains lavender extract for fragrance.

☹ **$$$ Line Refiner** *($36 for 0.15 ounce)* provides a small amount of a fragrance-free emollient moisturizer for dry skin, packaged in a portable component. It's just water with lots of thickening agents, some silicone, and wax. That works, but your skin deserves more.

☹ **Luxe Moisture Balm SPF 15** *($28 for 0.28 ounce)* lacks the UVA-protecting ingredients of titanium dioxide, zinc oxide, avobenzone, Mexoryl SX (ecamsule), or Tinosorb, and is not recommended. What a shame, because this has a beautifully smooth balm texture.

☹ **Protective Shield Moisturizer SPF 15** *($40 for 2 ounces)* lacks the UVA-protecting ingredients of titanium dioxide, zinc oxide, avobenzone, Mexoryl SX (ecamsule), or Tinosorb, and is not recommended. Shame on McEvoy (and her dermatologist husband Dr. Sherman) for not taking the opportunity to address the issue of UVA protection!

☺ **$$$ Protective Shield SPF 15 Tinted Moisturizer** *($40)* has an in-part avobenzone sunscreen and a creamy but lightweight texture that slips over skin and provides very sheer coverage. This is best regarded as a sunscreen that adds a hint of color to skin; it won't camouflage redness or other minor flaws. Still, it's definitely worth considering for those with normal to dry skin, and the range of five shades is mostly neutral. Porcelain is an outstanding option for those with very fair skin.

TRISH MCEVOY MAKEUP

TRISH MCEVOY EVEN SKIN PRODUCTS

FOUNDATION: ✓ ☺ **$$$ Even Skin Foundation** *($55)* has a liquidy smooth, silicone-enriched texture and flawless application that looks wonderfully smooth and natural on the skin. It offers a satin finish and sheer to light coverage, and is best for those with normal to dry skin who want a foundation that is moist but lightweight. Eight shades are available, and most are outstanding. Shade 1 is ideal for those with very fair skin, while Shades 2, 3, and 4 rival

Stila's best neutral tones. The only slight misstep is Shade 5, which is a bit too peachy. Shade 8 works for dark (but not very dark) skin tones. Note: this fluid foundation requires vigorous shaking before each use.

☹ **$$$ Even Skin Portable Foundation** *($52)* is a silicone-based cream-to-powder makeup packaged in a sleek black compact complete with black velvet bag. Don't let the trappings of attractive packaging fool you, because overall this is a needlessly expensive foundation that doesn't measure up to several superior options from competing lines. A major shortcoming is McEvoy's choice to launch only four shades. All of them are worthwhile, but only if you have fair to light skin. Whatever the reason for this limitation, it doesn't change the fact that this has a slick texture that can be tricky to blend (until you get the hang of it) and that sets to a satin-matte finish. Coverage is sheer to light, but take care to smooth out any dry areas, because this will "grab" them, an unattractive drawback common to most cream-to-powder foundations. Even Skin Portable Foundation is best for normal to oily skin.

CONCEALER: ☹ **$$$ Even Skin Extra Coverage Concealer** *($28)* is a dual-sided concealer with a thick, almost immovable texture that is tricky to blend. This is still thick enough so that trying to make it look natural on skin is a time-consuming task, not to mention that blending the two shades together to attain a perfect match isn't particularly easy. If you're up for the challenge and need significant coverage, the best of the three duos is Beige. The Porcelain Duo is slightly pink, and the Honey Duo is too orange to look convincing on its intended range of skin tones.

POWDER: ✓☺ **$$$ Even Skin Finishing Powder** *($30)* has a texture that would make a feather feel heavy, and it leaves a gorgeous sheer finish and a hint of shine. The formula is talc-based, blends imperceptibly, and comes in three beautiful colors. My only complaint is the tiny amount of product you get for the money, though the component is sleek enough to fit in any makeup bag (and maybe that was the point).

SPECIALTY PRODUCTS: ☹ **$$$ Even Skin Face Primer** *($32)* is a substandard primer whose cream-gel texture belies its basic formula of water, thickeners, and preservative. It's an OK lightweight moisturizer for normal to slightly dry skin, but doesn't make good on its claim of keeping your foundation looking "just applied" all day. A cream-gel moisturizer with silicone (there are countless options available) works much better under foundation, and doesn't pose the risk of irritation this product does (because it contains lavender).

OTHER TRISH MCEVOY MAKEUP PRODUCTS

FOUNDATION: ✓☺ **$$$ Correct & Brighten Loose Mineral Powder SPF 15** *($35)*. Apparently, this loose powder mineral makeup was added to McEvoy's line after her dermatologist husband's patients begged to take this post-procedure powder home due to its perceived effect on their skin. From my perspective, regardless of how this came to be, it's one of the best mineral makeups with sunscreen to consider. The sole active ingredient is zinc oxide, which is great. I don't know how they did it, but given that 25% of this formula is zinc oxide it's surprising that this doesn't look opaque or heavy on skin. It has a sumptuous, silky texture that blends with an ease few mineral makeups (at least those with zinc oxide) do. You get a soft, matte (in feel) finish with a subtle radiant glow (without sparkles, another nice touch). Unlike some mineral makeup that go on opaque and thus provide significant coverage, this has a sheer, soft-focus effect that won't hide major discolorations or blemishes easily. It layers well for added coverage, but that increases the odds that this will look too powdery and dry. The formula contains some

The Reviews T

anti-irritants, too, and is fragrance-free. It is best for normal to slightly oily skin, and would make a wonderful finishing powder to use over your foundation with sunscreen. This mineral foundation is definitely suitable for those with rosacea. All four shades are excellent and best for light to medium skin tones.

✓ ☺ **$$$ Mineral Powder Foundation SPF 15** *($35)* is a talc-free, silicone-based, pressed-powder foundation that provides sun protection with titanium dioxide and zinc oxide (these mineral actives are what create this product's powder texture). The thick but smooth texture doesn't pick up easily on a brush or sponge, but perhaps that was the intent, because applying too much product results in a flat, opaque appearance. Applying this with a brush, as an adjunct to your regular sunscreen or foundation with sunscreen, works best. Doing so imparts a natural matte finish and sheer yet even coverage. Five of the six shades are terrific; avoid Naked, which is noticeably peach unless you apply it very sheer. This fragrance-free powder foundation with sunscreen is excellent for sensitive, rosacea-affected skin.

☺ **$$$ Treatment Foundation SPF 15** *($75)*. There is no rational reason for this foundation to cost double what competing lines charge. Don't get me wrong, Treatment Foundation is very good, but the price isn't justified. You're getting a fluid, silky liquid foundation whose sunscreen is in-part titanium dioxide. It feels moist, takes its time to set to a soft-satin finish suitable for normal to dry skin, and provides medium coverage. The finish doesn't mesh with skin as well as liquid foundations rated a Paula's Pick, but it comes close. If you're willing to spend more money than you need to, this is worth considering. There are nine shades available, and most are very good. Light Beige is slightly peach for many fair skin tones, while Golden Beige is noticeably peachy gold and not recommended. Caramel has limited appeal for medium to tan skin tones, but is worth testing. As for the treatment benefits, this foundation contains some antioxidants and a peptide, but not in amounts prodigious enough to make it a reason to splurge, and the frosted glass bottle packaging is unlikely to keep them stable. Still, such ingredients are a thoughtful addition to a foundation.

CONCEALER: ☺ **$$$ Flawless Concealer** *($36)* is a liquid-to-powder concealer that's packaged in a click-pen component with a built-in synthetic brush applicator. It has a smooth, even application and provides impressive coverage, plus the brush aids rather than hinders application, allowing you to reach along the lash line and into tiny corners. The strong matte finish looks a bit powdery and doesn't provide moisture, so this isn't a great concealer if you have pronounced lines around the eye. The only significant drawback is that half of the four shades are noticeably peach to orange. Shades 4 and 5 are not recommended, but shades 1 and 3 are suitable for fair to light skin tones. The formula for this concealer makes it a good choice for use over blemishes.

☺ **$$$ Brightening Line Minimizing Concealer** *($21)* is a thick, slightly creamy concealer that blends well but not as well as several other concealers with a cream texture. You'll get nearly opaque coverage and a powdery (talc is the second ingredient) matte finish that tends to exaggerate rather than minimize lines. Using concealer—any concealer—over wrinkles will make them look more apparent than if you were bare-faced. Makeup tends to make wrinkles "pop," which is why a "less is more" approach and lighter-textured products tend to work better if your skin is showing "signs of aging" (which is really about sun damage). A heavier concealer like this that contains so much talc is best used away from wrinkles, although this does work quite well to mask redness and skin discolorations. Among the five shades, most of which are commendable, avoid the very peach Honey.

BLUSH AND BRONZER: ✓ ☺ **$$$ Dual Resort Bronzer** *($32)* provides an equal amount of soft copper and golden bronze pressed powders in one compact. Texture and application are exceptionally silky, and although each shade is shiny the effect is more glow than glitter, and it clings well. Both shades work best on fair to light skin tones.

✓ ☺ **$$$ Matte Bronzer** *($28)* doesn't have a true matte finish, but it's close enough to count given the prevailing, here-to-stay shimmer trend (and shimmer done right can be quite attractive). Just like the Dual Resort Bronzer above, this has an amazing silky-smooth feel and applies evenly, allowing you to gradually build color. The sole shade is realistic if you're trying to fake a tan because it is brown-based with a slight red cast.

☺ **$$$ All Over Face Color** *($28)* is another pressed bronzing powder that provides one to four colors in one pan, depending on which option you choose (and various options are rotated in seasonally). The talc-based texture is smooth and dry, and applies fairly well, depositing a strong shimmer finish that for some shades borders on metallic. Pigmentation is greater than usual, so this tends to work best on medium to tan skin tones.

☺ **$$$ Blush** *($20)* is sold as individual powder tablets and it's up to you to decide on a compact or planner page for its placement (the makeup planners are reviewed below). The finely pressed powder feels silky and applies well, depositing more color than you expect. The shade selection presents a good balance of warm and cool tones, and all have some amount of shine.

☺ **$$$ Liquid Face Color** *($32)* is a liquid blush housed in a click-pen component outfitted with a built-in synthetic brush applicator. Once dispensed through the brush, this thin-textured cream is easy to blend, providing a translucent wash of soft, warm pink color imbued with a none-too-subtle amount of gold sparkles. Basically a cross between a cream and gel blush, Liquid Face Color (only available in one shade) is a workable option for those looking to try blush in a different form. This is best for those with normal to slightly dry skin and fair to medium skin tones.

EYESHADOW: ✓ ☺ **$$$ Deluxe Eye Shadow** *($20)* costs more but provides a greater amount of product. These larger powder tablets have a sumptuous texture and seamless application that make them a pleasure to work with. There are only two shades, which is definitely a shortcoming, but I expect the company will launch more in the future.

✓ ☺ **$$$ Eye Definer/Eye Liner** *($16)* is McEvoy's collection of dark powder eyeshadows designed for lining the eyes or creating more dramatic shading (such as for the classic smoky eye). Each has a smooth, dry texture that should be applied in sheer layers to avoid flaking. Application is stellar and pigmentation is excellent, so with patience you can get beautiful results. Every shade is recommended, including those that look obviously blue and purple (because they go on less bright than they look and actually pass for good variations on black). Some of the shades have a sparkling shine, and these are less desirable because the sparkles are quite flyaway so the effect doesn't last.

✓ ☺ **$$$ Glaze Eye Shadow** *($16)* has a non-powdery, beautifully smooth texture and seamless application that begins sheer but builds well. Each shade has great cling, and all are shiny, but the effect is a low-key satin sheen. The Glaze shades have a light to medium pigmentation and blend superbly.

☺ **$$$ Eye Base Essentials** *($24)* is similar to a liquid concealer and is meant to prep the eyelid area prior to eyeshadow application. It applies evenly and leaves a silky, soft matte finish, but doesn't provide as much camouflage as a traditional concealer. It is waterproof, as claimed,

The Reviews T

and is worth considering if you find that using concealer or foundation as an eyeshadow base doesn't work for you. The Malibu and Sheer Gold shades have a sheer metallic sheen.

☺ **$$$ Matte Eye Shadow** *($16)* is only available in one shade, a classic heather/taupe. The texture and application are sublime, but this isn't true matte: it is laced with sheer sparkles that cling reasonably well.

EYE AND BROW SHAPER: ✓ ☺ **$$$ Brow Gel** *($20)* is different from most brow gels because it keeps hairs in place without feeling the least bit tacky, stiff, or sticky. There is only one clear color, so it works only for those who are just trying to keep their brows in place, not trying to create more definition or fullness. If you're going to spend more than you need to for brow gel, this should be the one you buy.

✓ ☺ **$$$ Precision Brow Shaper** *($26)* is a very good twist-up, retractable brow pencil that includes a "spoolie" brow brush on the other end to soften the effect or just groom wayward brows. Although the pencil has a slightly stiff texture, it goes on smoothly with gentle pressure, its fine point allowing you to sketch between brows for a natural effect. Both shades of this pencil (one for dark blonde, one for brunette brows) have a soft powder finish that resists smudging and smearing. If you're keen on shopping for brow pencils at the department store, this is a great pencil to consider; without a doubt, it allows for precise application.

☺ **$$$ Classic Eye Pencil** *($20)* is classic in the sense that it's one more creamy pencil that needs routine sharpening and it comes with a pointed smudger to soften the line. The plus with this option is that, for all its creaminess, it is relatively impervious to smudging.

☺ **$$$ Eye Definer Pencil** *($28)* is a thick, chunky pencil that needs routine sharpening, but that's its only con. If the sharpening doesn't bother you, this is a beautiful way to add depth and shimmering dimension to your lash line. The pencil glides on readily and sets to a minimally creamy finish that's relatively impervious to smearing. Best applied and then softened for a smoky, diffused look, the shimmer finish is best for younger, unwrinkled eyes. This would earn a happy face rating if not for the sharpening requirement.

☹ **Eye Brightener** *($22)* is a standard, chunky pencil that needs sharpening. It glides on but remains greasy enough to smudge, so its brightening effect, while attractive, won't last. You can achieve the same effect with McEvoy's longer-lasting Glaze Eye Shadow.

LIPSTICK, LIP GLOSS, AND LIPLINER: ✓ ☺ **$$$ Beauty Booster SPF 15 Lip Gloss** *($25)*. Yes, the colors and appearance of this tube lip gloss are essentially McEvoy's attempt to mimic Lancôme's popular Juicy Tubes Ultra Shiny Lip Gloss—but this goes further by providing a smoother texture, minimally sticky finish, and an in-part avobenzone sunscreen! This is one of the few lip glosses with reliable broad-spectrum sun protection, which makes it even more beautiful! If there's a color you like, you may find it worth the splurge. Note: this contains a tiny amount of peppermint oil but it does not make lips tingle or burn, so the amount is essentially inconsequential.

✓ ☺ **$$$ Lip Gloss** *($22)* comes with either a sponge-tip or brush applicator, depending on the shade you choose. The emollient formula has been improved and it now feels decadently smooth and luscious while providing a glossy sheen with only a hint of stickiness. Well done!

☹ **Be Prepared Pink Lip Kit** *($28)*. Housed in a small, squat double-decker mirrored compact are eight shades of lip gloss. Each shade provides a tiny amount of product that must be applied with a brush (well, unless you want to use your fingers, which isn't all that sanitary). You get sheer to translucent glossy color that feels emollient and is minimally sticky. This is rated with an unhappy face for two reasons: several shades of the gloss in this compact contain the potent irritants camphor and menthol, and many of them list active sunscreen ingredients but no SPF rating, not to mention the actives do not supply sufficient UVA protection.

☺ **$$$ Cream Lip Color** *($22)* provides nearly full coverage, and comes in only two shades. More greasy than creamy, this moves easily into lines around the mouth, but if that's not an issue there is no reason to not consider this lipstick, assuming you like one of the shades.

☺ **$$$ Glaze Lip Color** *($22)* took a step backward and went from being an excellent creamy lipstick to a slightly greasy sheer lipstick whose shades now have a glittery sheen rather than their former subdued pearlized finish. This is still a good lipstick, it just isn't as distinctive as it used to be.

☺ **$$$ Fast-Track Lips** *($38)* is a sleek, dual-sided pen that houses an automatic, retractable lip pencil on one end and a slim lipstick on the other. Although certainly not ground-breaking, it's a clever, convenient way to tote your lipliner and lipstick. The lip pencil is easy to apply and stays in place well, while the lipstick is creamy and relatively smooth, with little movement once it sets. This isn't for fans of very creamy, emollient, or glossy lipsticks, but the lipliner and lip color combination is workable and may be something you want to splurge on.

☺ **$$$ Sheer Lip Color** *($22)* has an emollient texture and a very glossy finish that's not as sheer as most. The shade selection favors pink and pastel shades. Sheer London is the collection's most versatile color.

☹ **$$$ SPF 15 Lip Color** *($22)* comes in two bright but sheer colors and has a smooth texture and soft glossy sheen. This is a letdown in terms of broad-spectrum sun protection because the active ingredients (octinoxate and oxybenzone) do not provide enough UVA protection.

☹ **$$$ Essential Pencil** *($22)* is a thick, needs-sharpening pencil that feels slick and slightly greasy while leaving a glossy finish and sheer color. It's an OK option, but pricey for what you get.

☹ **$$$ Lip Liner** *($20)* comes in a nice assortment of rich colors, and one end of the pencil has a lip brush. It's a nice touch, but this is too creamy if you're concerned about keeping lipstick in place. If not, and if you don't mind sharpening, it's worth a look.

MASCARA: ✓ ☺ **$$$ High Volume Waterproof Mascara** *($28)* takes some effort to prove its worth, but the reward is long, lush, and perfectly separated lashes without a clump in sight. The formula is waterproof, and one of the better waterproof mascaras from department-store lines.

☺ **$$$ High-Volume Mascara** *($28)* deposits a lot of mascara on lashes, but does so with minimal clumping, and lets you quickly create long, thick lashes. The water-soluble formula removes easily and wears with a slight tendency to flake, but it doesn't smear.

☺ **$$$ Lash Curling Mascara** *($28)* doesn't curl lashes any more than a lot of other mascaras, but it excels at lengthening, though it does take some time to dry (which gives you time to comb out minor clumping). All of McEvoy's mascaras tend to go on wetter than most, but with practice this becomes less objectionable.

☹ **$$$ Lash Builder** *($20)* is a pre-mascara product meant to enhance the performance of any mascara. This ends up being just a standard mascara formulation minus the pigment. It makes a slight difference in terms of making lashes longer, but it also makes mascara application less smooth. Lash Builder helps make an average mascara better, but why are you using an average mascara in the first place?

FACE AND BODY ILLUMINATING/SHIMMER PRODUCTS: ✓ ☺ **$$$ Shimmer Pressed Powder** *($32)* is wonderful. It has a superior smooth texture that blends very well and provides a soft shine that's wearable day or night. All three shades are attractive and the shine doesn't flake. It's an altogether outstanding choice.

☺ **$$$ Luminizer Pen** *($38)*. McEvoy is big on packaging liquid items in click-pen components with built-in brush applicators, and here's another one to consider. This very sheer liquid works well to create subtle highlights anywhere on the face. It is best used to brighten the under-eye area after applying concealer or to highlight the top of the cheekbones. Yves Saint Laurent, Sephora, Lorac, and Maybelline offer more versatile versions of this product; McEvoy only offers one shade and the effect can be so soft you may wonder why you bothered. Definitely one of those items that's best for McEvoy devotees.

BRUSHES: ✓☺ **$$$ Trish McEvoy Brushes** *($14-$90)* can be considered one-stop shopping for those whose budget extends this far. Trish McEvoy has a well-earned reputation for producing some of the softest, most exquisitely shaped makeup brushes anywhere and, aside from the steep price tag that accompanies many of them, you won't be disappointed with their performance and longevity. There isn't a bad brush in the bunch, though of course some of them will be superfluous based on your needs and preferences. In any event, the brushes, which fit in any size of McEvoy's excellent Makeup Planners, are aces when it comes to shape, feel, and, most importantly, performance.

The ☺ **Eyelash Curler** *($18)* is standard fare, but it is well-made and used properly does its job of curling lashes before you apply mascara.

☺ **$$$ Portable Beauty Brush Set Simplicity** *($65)* is a tiny brush set housed in a cute, well-made zippered case. The case includes a pouch that holds all four brushes plus another pouch for additional items such as lipstick or lip gloss. Each of the brushes is, in typical McEvoy fashion, well made and wonderfully soft. The lip, eyeshadow, and eyeliner brush are great but the **Pocketable Blush Brush** is too small for quick, convenient powder blush application. It works in a pinch, but for what this set costs, the blush brush should've been better. Still, it's worth a peek if you're a fan of McEvoy's brushes and want a mini, purse-size set.

☹ **$$$ The Ball Sponge Makeup Applicator** *($16)*. I admit the concept of this foundation sponge is different and certainly intriguing. It's a perfectly round sponge designed to fit the contours of the face for an enhanced foundation application. It works well, but requires more careful blending (and re-blending) than a conventional flat or wedge-shaped sponge. The biggest frustration is that there isn't much surface area to hold on to, and the round shape ensures you get excess foundation on your fingers as you apply, not to mention the ball will roll if you set it down, leaving a streak of foundation in its wake. This is only recommended if you have a lot of patience and for whatever reason are dissatisfied with conventional makeup sponges.

☺ **$$$ Brush Bath** *($20)* is a gentle, detergent-based shampoo for your brushes. Its formula is basically the same as a standard shampoo that does not contain conditioning agents. In other words, this works great to cleanse your brushes, but so would a regular shampoo such as Neutrogena Anti-Residue or Suave Clarifying, both of which cost less than $5.

☺ **$$$ Makeup Brush Cleaner** *($20)* is a good, spray-on brush cleanser that omits fast-drying solvents like alcohol in favor of water and gentle detergent cleansing agents. It dissolves makeup from brushes without damaging the hair, but with the drawback that the brush cannot be used again immediately. This is a fine option for occasional brush cleansing when you have time to let your brushes dry between uses.

SPECIALTY PRODUCTS: ✓☺ **$$$ Makeup Planners** *($58-$425)* resemble a luxury day planner and remain the most distinguishing element of McEvoy's line. A two-ring binder inside an elegant zippered bag holds covered plastic "pages" that can be filled (and refilled) with the colors of your choice. The color tablets affix to the magnetized pages and each page comes with a clear plastic cover. It's pricey, but the bags are handsomely made and exceedingly convenient, especially if you're loyal to Trish McEvoy's color line. You can assemble all the products you need for a complete makeup application, from foundation to lip color, and there are interior pockets and pouches that can hold several brushes or miscellaneous items that won't fit on the pages. The wide price range refers to the material the planners are made from (some are exquisite dyed leather) and how much room each has. This is assuredly a not-to-be-missed item if you're at all interested in McEvoy's makeup collection. Plastic "pages" for the Planners range from $18 to $20 each.

✓ ☺ **$$$ Ultimate Beauty Organizer** *($85)* is basically a soft beauty briefcase that houses McEvoy's famous Makeup Planner (the Classic Black Mini version) plus removable pouches and clear, sturdy plastic storage compartments. This is beauty product packing done right, and is definitely worth a look if you're a McEvoy fan. The craftsmanship is evident, which makes the price easier to understand.

✓ ☺ **$$$ Refillable Double Decker Compacts** *($15-$25 depending on size)* are beautifully made compacts designed to hold various McEvoy makeup products. These are sturdy enough to last for years, and each features a built-in mirror. These compacts are a wise consideration if you don't want to go the Makeup Planner route.

☺ **$$$ Beauty To Go Refillable Pen** *($25)*. If you're a fan of applying foundation with a brush and want an on-the-go option, this is worth a look. The bottom of this thick, pen-like component houses a small plastic tube that can be filled with the liquid foundation (or other liquid makeup) product of your choice. Once the plastic tube is snapped back into the base, you depress a button on the bottom and the liquid is fed onto a synthetic brush applicator. The brush works well, though it is smaller than a traditional foundation brush. Still, as mentioned it's worth a look if you want a portable way to apply liquid foundation.

☺ **$$$ Correct & Brighten Pen** *($38)* appears to be McEvoy's attempt to compete with Yves Saint Laurent's Touche Eclat Radiant Touch or the lesser-known but very good Ideal Light Brush-On Illuminator from Estee Lauder. Housed in a chunky click-pen applicator with a built-in brush is a silky-smooth liquid highlighter. It provides a soft matte (in feel) finish with a soft-glow shine to help reflect light away from shadowed areas. Shade 1 is great, while Shade 2 is too peach for most light to medium skin tones. Overall this compares favorably with its predecessors, but could have surpassed them by offering a larger shade range, a slimmer component, and a lower price. As is, I encourage you to consider Lauder's products first if the concept of a highlighter (rather than a concealer, which provides more coverage) appeals to you. For even less money and the benefit of a liquid concealer too, consider Maybelline New York Instant Age Rewind Double Face Perfector.

☺ **$$$ Finish Line** *($22)* is an alcohol-free, water-based fluid meant to turn any powder eyeshadow into a long-lasting liquid liner. It applies smoothly, dries quickly, and deepens the color payoff of an eyeshadow, making many medium tones suitable for lining. The waterproof claim is accurate, but it's worth noting that even minimal rubbing of your eyes while it's wet causes the product to break down. This is an OK option if you're a fan of eyelining with powders and want to experiment for a different, more intense effect.

☺ **$$$ Beauty Emergency Card** *($28)* is a sleek compact the size of a credit card and almost as thin. Housed inside are two shades of eyeshadow, two powder eyeliners that double if you need darker eyeshadows, a cream concealer, two sheer lip colors and one creamy lip color. It's not everything a person would need to thwart the number of beauty emergencies that may befall them, but if the colors appeal to you, this works great as an extremely portable eye and lip palette. Two of the four powder eye colors are noticeably shiny and the concealer will only work for certain light to medium skin tones, plus it tends to crease unless generously set with powder. The sheer lip colors are not recommended because they contain the irritants camphor and menthol, plus each lists active ingredients that don't provide sufficient UVA protection, not to mention the lack of an SPF rating. All told, this is a pricey convenience with limited appeal.

☺ **$$$ Flawless Lip** *($22)* is a clear, silicone-based pre-lipstick base designed to keep lipstick anchored firmly on the lips. It works marginally well, but still can't keep most of McEvoy's lipsticks from their forward march into lines around the mouth. A better version of this product for less money is The Body Shop's Lip Line Fixer.

☺ **$$$ Instant Pick Me Up** *($38)* is a sheer cream-to-powder makeup that comes in one light, flesh-toned shade. Sold as a portable complexion perfector, it is meant to be used alone or over makeup throughout the day, as touch-ups are needed. The slightly greasy texture can undo a carefully applied foundation and powder, but this does set to a soft matte finish (if you can figure out how to get it on evenly). Still, using it over makeup holds no advantage over touching up with oil-blotting papers and pressed powder, a combination of which, depending on the line you shop, can cost much less than this single, potentially makeup-disrupting product. I suspected this wouldn't last long in McEvoy's line, because it sounds a lot better than what reality reveals when you begin using it, but it seems I was wrong since it's still around.

URBAN DECAY (MAKEUP ONLY)

URBAN DECAY AT-A-GLANCE

Strengths: Workable options in almost every category; excellent powder blush; bonanza for anyone who wants lots of shiny eyeshadows; several super-smooth lip glosses; makeup brushes.

Weaknesses: Average to poor eye and brow pencils; limited foundation shades; disappointing lash primer/waterproofing product; irritating makeup remover and lip plumper.

For more information about Urban Decay, call (800) 784-URBAN or visit www.urbandecay.com or www.Beautypedia.com.

MAKEUP REMOVERS: ☹ **Clean & Sober Makeup Remover** *($18 for 3.4 ounces)* begins as a standard, detergent-based liquid makeup remover, but isn't worth considering over many others (price notwithstanding) because it contains potentially irritating plant extracts and volatile fragrance components that should not be used near the eyes.

FOUNDATION: ☺ **$$$ Surreal Skin Cream to Powder Foundation** *($34)* is described as an ultralightweight formula, and it is. The texture is practically weightless and very silky and application is easy. As you blend, this quickly goes from a creamy glide to a soft-powder finish that leaves a bit of a sheen. The drawback is that unless you blend it impeccably and touch it up during the day it settles into lines and large pores. That drawback applies to many cream-to-powder foundations, so Urban Decay is hardly alone. The nonaqueous formula comes in eight neutral shades, with options for light to tan skin tones. One more comment: If you decide to try this, toss the mini foundation brush that's included because using it produces a streaky, striped result. You can blend it away, but results are faster and more natural-looking using a sponge.

☺ **$$$ Surreal Skin Liquid Makeup** *($26)* comes in a bottle that looks like it could also house a genie (someone tell Christina Aguilera!), but all that's dispensed is a silky, fluid foundation that blends easily and provides medium coverage. This would have earned a Paula's Pick rating if it looked a bit more natural on skin. As is, the strong matte finish, while great for oily to very oily skin, tends to call attention to itself unless blending is meticulous. If that doesn't deter you (and it's not a deal-breaker) four of the five shades are beautifully neutral; Supernatural has a slight orange cast that won't work for most medium skin tones.

☺ $$$ **Surreal Skin Mineral Makeup** *($29)* marks Urban Decay's attempt to bring their brand of street credibility to the overhyped category of mineral makeup. This loose-powder foundation is packaged in a jar with a sponge affixed to the cap. Once opened, the powder is shaken onto the sponge, where it poofs out and allows you to blend it over your skin. The formula is based on mica and bismuth oxychloride (the same as most mineral foundations and powders), and this product shares the same traits typical for this category of makeup, meaning it offers shine, reliable coverage, and a dry finish that can become uncomfortably dry during the day depending on your skin type. Urban Decay's version has a decidedly light texture, and most of the shades are attractive, but you have to accept a slight sparkling effect and the drawbacks of mineral makeup to really enjoy this product. Mineral makeup is not a good choice if you have any degree of dry skin because the ingredients absorb oil (and your moisturizer), making dry skin drier. For someone with very oily skin the makeup typically separates on your skin and pools into pores, which is as unbecoming as it sounds. Getting back to the colors, there are some enticing options for dark (but not very dark) skin tones, but consider Fortune carefully due to its slight orange cast. Fantasy is too copper for most dark skin tones.

CONCEALER: ☺ $$$ **Surreal Skin Creamy Concealer** *($16)* is a liquid concealer with a slightly runny consistency that makes blending tricky and provides coverage that is more sheer than what most people who use concealer want. Still, the two shades (reserved for those with fair to light skin) are good, and this is an OK option if you want sheer coverage and a satin-matte finish. The formula is appropriate for use over blemishes, but don't expect much in the way of camouflage.

☹ $$$ **24/7 Concealer** *($17)* has a blendable, slightly silky texture that provides substantial coverage without looking too thick or feeling greasy, if you don't mind routinely sharpening this creamy pencil. It is slightly prone to creasing into lines around the eye, but tends to stay put once it's set, so fading isn't an issue. All four shades are very good, but are limited for use by those with fair to medium skin tones. The thickeners and wax-like ingredients in this concealer make it not well-suited for use on acne; a liquid concealer is better and there are plenty of options that provide significant coverage (such as Estee Lauder Double Wear or Shiseido The Makeup Concealer).

POWDER: ☺ $$$ **Surreal Skin Universal Mineral Powder** *($29)* is a silky-textured loose powder that comes in one translucent yellow shade that's nearly imperceptible on lighter skin tones, but that can be apparent on darker skin tones. You'll get hints of sparkles from the mineral pigments in this powder, and coverage is very sheer, making this best as a finishing powder that adds shine to skin.

☹ $$$ **De-Slick Mattifying Powder** *($29)*. One-shade-fits-all powders rarely work for everyone, and that's the case with this pale whitish-blue option. The talc-based formula contains a high amount of absorbent calcium carbonate, so it does a good job of absorbing excess oil to keep skin matte. The texture is smooth yet dry, plus it is difficult to pick up enough powder on your brush to sufficiently temper shine. All told, this doesn't replace any of the less expensive pressed powders for oily skin that I recommend from Maybelline New York, Revlon, or Sonia Kashuk.

The Reviews U

BLUSH AND BRONZER: ✓ ☺ **$$$ Afterglow Blush** *($17)* claims to go beyond blushing to make you glow, and it does that thanks to each shade's pearlescent finish. This creamy-feeling powder blush is excellent, with moderately pigmented shades that go on with more intensity than you may expect. Although each shade has shine that's best for evening glamour, the effect is indeed more of a glow than a sparkle-fest, and it doesn't flake.

☺ **$$$ Baked Bronzing Powder** *($24)* is a talc-based pressed bronzing powder that goes on smoothly and has a sheer, dry finish. The shades would be more convincing without shine, but if a shiny tan effect is what you want, it clings well.

EYESHADOW: ☺ **$$$ Deluxe Eyeshadow** *($18)* has deluxe packaging but formula-wise is quite similar to Urban Decay's regular Eye Shadow, save for an application that's a touch smoother due to the silicone content. The small selection of shades favors strong metallic colors, few of which make for an effective eye design unless you're doing eye makeup for shock value. Still, these apply and blend well and the shine stays put, so they're a consideration.

☺ **$$$ Eye Shadow** *($16)* features a rainbow of unusual, sometimes shocking colors sold as singles. Most of them have a superior smooth texture that applies and blends wonderfully. Every shade has some degree of shine, but the good news is that except for the colors with glitter (easily identified), the shine clings well. The almost garish shades that you should consider very carefully are Gash, Acid Rain, Mildew, Vert, Shattered, Goddess, Asphyxia, Stalker, and Last Call.

☺ **$$$ Eyeshadow Primer Potion** *($17)* promises to make eyeshadows last longer while keeping them from creasing, and it works. In addition, it facilitates a smoother application and makes blending even easier. The problem is you can get the same results from a good matte-finish concealer that's silicone-based like this one. Because most of today's best concealers follow this format, a product like this, though it works, seems superfluous (unless you don't use a silicone-based type of concealer).

☺ **$$$ Eyeshadow Primer Potion, Sin** *($17)*. Just like Urban Decay's original Eyeshadow Primer Potion above, this sparkling champagne–colored version would be a welcome addition for anyone who does not mind shimmer and doesn't already use a silicone-based foundation or concealer, which would work similarly to this primer, producing the same shadow-enhancing effect, only with shine added to the application. Urban Decay's Sin version allows eyeshadow to set and intensify quickly with minimal creasing. It naturally complements shiny and iridescent shadows nicely, but the primer's shimmer does pose a problem for darker-hued matte shadows, though it worked surprisingly well with lighter matte shades. Contrary to its marketing, avoid wearing Sin alone, or at least test it first to be sure the appearance is what you're after; it isn't the best application for everyone, that's for sure.

☺ **$$$ Book of Shadows** *($45)* is a playful palette of eyeshadows that bursts open with whimsical (though completely unnecessary) pop-up decorations before you even get to the 16 tiny, individual colors buried beneath. Eight of the shades are supposed to be Urban Decay's top sellers; the other eight are exclusive to this palette, along with a mini-sized Eyeshadow Primer Potion. The shadows' staying power and depth of color is quite reliant on the silicone-based primer, so it's a good thing it's included in the kit, because without it the shadows, while silky, resist setting and appear dull, especially the new charcoal-gray shade Perversion. While the primer is essential for the shadows' longevity, it also makes blending impossible, so either way there are substantial drawbacks. The colors are all somewhat shimmery (this is Urban Decay after all) and the obvious shades that no one should ever wear are unattractively close to being pink or green. However, new shades Gridlock, Scandal, and Shakedown offer rich, neutral pigments if shimmer is your thing. Don't even bother with the teeny-tiny brushes that are included, unless you plan on giving your old Barbie doll a makeover.

☺ $$$ **Get Baked Eyeshadow Palette** *($28)* is a practical-sized palette that contains more misses than hits, making Urban Decay's Get Baked hardly worth the price tag. Granted, the eyeshadow's texture is smooth, and when used with the champagne-colored Eyeshadow Potion Primer Potion, Sin included in the palette, it sets to rich colors that flatter the underlying shimmer rather than overemphasize it. It has a rich bronze color that is a clear standout, but you need to be very cautious of Flipside, a radioactive-glowing, sparkly teal. Included is a decent-size Glide-On Eye Pencil in deep brown called Bourbon, but it is just too creamy to work with the shimmery shadows, or even to keep up with them for that matter, as smudging is nothing short of inevitable.

☺ $$$ **Loose Pigments** *($20)* are shiny, pigment-dense loose powders packaged in containers with a wand that includes a pointed sponge-tip applicator. As you can imagine, this is tricky to apply without making a mess, but those up for the task will find this an intriguing way to add strong color and shine to the eye area. Based on method of application, Loose Pigments works best for smoky-eye designs or for highlighting small areas. Be sure to have an eyeshadow brush or two at the ready to soften hard edges.

☹ **Cream Eyeshadow** *($17)* boasts gel-based silicone technology, which allows this cream-based eyeshadow to set to a vibrant, film-like waterproof finish. So the good news is that once this product dries, it likely won't budge until you apply makeup remover, though even then a few stubborn sparkles might remain because every single color is absolutely teeming with glitter. The bad news, however, is that it's a complete mess to apply using the doe-foot wand applicator. If that weren't drawback enough, the product also thickens up in the tube so easily I can't see how anyone could use it for more than several applications before having to throw it away. Even with a sponge or brush, the product's consistency is downright goopy, making it a difficult product to blend evenly; and the pigmentation is so deep, there's little room for error. Between the glitter, the applicator, and the goop factor, this is an eyeshadow you're better off skipping.

EYE AND BROW SHAPER: ☺ $$$ **Liquid Eye Liner** *($18)* has a long, thin brush that's relatively easy to use, and this liquid liner deposits rich color along the entire lash line. Although it wears well once it sets, the dry time is slower than average, which can lead to slight smearing, especially if you blink a lot.

☺ $$$ **Smoke Out Eye Pencil** *($14)* needs sharpening, so it doesn't earn higher than a neutral face rating. However, if you don't mind sharpening, this is definitely a pencil to check out! It has a smooth texture that glides on and a powder finish that won't smudge or smear once set. The shade selection favors the trendy and odd, but Smoke is a reliable choice that's almost a basic black.

☹ **24/7 Glide-On Eye Pencil** *($16)* does glide on, but this needs-sharpening pencil has a soft tip that's prone to breaking off and a finish that is creamy enough to smudge. It doesn't last all night and isn't the best fit for anyone's "on-the-go" lifestyle, and the colors are mostly clownish.

☹ **Brow Beater** *($14)* is a dual-sided, needs-sharpening pencil that includes a brow pencil on one end and a clear wax for grooming on the other. The brow color portion is thick and tricky to apply, while the wax portion is noticeably sticky.

☹ **Heavy Metal Glitter Liner** *($18)* is a liquid eyeliner that's basically large flecks of colored glitter suspended in a clear fluid. This much shine has its place for those so inclined, but not when the application is as uneven as this, not to mention the slow dry time.

☹ **Ink for Eyes** *($22)* is Urban Decay's contribution to the growing number of gel/cream eyeliners. Unlike their competitors, they opted for a formula that begins creamy and stays creamy (emollient isopropyl palmitate is the first ingredient). Application is smooth, but each color goes on surprisingly sheer and layering will cause it to "chunk up" right along your lash line. As you might imagine, the finish is prone to smearing and the colors fade in short order. Add to this the mostly garish colors and this is most assuredly an eyeliner to avoid.

LIPSTICK AND LIP GLOSS: ✓ ☺ **$$$ Ultraglide Lip Gloss** *($17)* is one of the best lip glosses around if you prize a smooth application, an ultra-glossy finish, and a non-sticky texture that's neither too thin nor too thick. The shade selection is pleasingly versatile and, dare I say, more mainstream than what Urban Decay usually offers.

☺ **$$$ Blow Lip Plumper** *($17)* is said to use a high-tech formula to inflate lips to injection-worthy proportions. It doesn't do that in the least, and, as far as I can tell, lacks ingredients capable of causing lips to swell in any manner. It is otherwise a thin-textured, nearly clear lip gloss whose shiny finish can create the illusion of larger lips, though I'll stress again it's not even close to the results possible from lip injections.

☺ **$$$ Lip Envy** *($17)* is a slightly thick, water-based lip stain. The doe-foot wand helps with precise application, which is critical with a product like this because mistakes aren't easily wiped away. The two sheer shades (each looks quite dark before applying) are both attractive.

☺ **$$$ Lip Primer Potion SPF 15** *($20)* is a colorless lipstick meant to "lay a silky foundation for your favorite lipstick or gloss." It has a silky, thick texture that feels waxy, but it's these wax ingredients that help fill lip lines for a smoother appearance. It leaves a moist yet non-glossy finish that's compatible with most standard lipsticks and glosses. The main letdown is that the sunscreen does not provide sufficient UVA protection. Well, that and the fact that using Lip Primer Potion to stop lipstick from bleeding into lines around the mouth doesn't work that well.

☺ **$$$ Lipstick** *($22)* is a very good cream lipstick whose best qualities are undermined by the fact that almost all of the shades are infused with glitter. What a way to make an elegant lipstick look silly rather than beautiful. Glittery lipsticks can be fun on occasion, but you can find such options at the drugstore for a lot less money. By the way, Gash, one of the few non-glittery shades, remains a riveting red that's sure to attract attention.

☺ **$$$ 24/7 Glide-On Lip Pencil** *($16)* is a lip pencil with a silicone-based formula. The result is an application that glides over lips without being too slick and a long-wearing finish that feels slightly tacky, although the tackiness is barely noticeable when paired with lipstick. This requires routine sharpening, hence, no happy face rating.

☺ **$$$ Pocket Rocket Lip Gloss** *($19)* includes packaging with images of good-looking men you can "strip" by tilting the container from side to side. The provocative package is also supposed to come laced with man-attracting pheromones, which you can (according to the company) emit simply by rubbing the flattened tube; that's really gimmicky, but if you're a teen or twenty-something it would be hard not to giggle the entire time you were testing it at the counter, and probably buying it as well. It's that kind of silly product. As for the product itself, it's pretty standard lip gloss fare: slightly sticky with a tendency to bleed, and a wand brush applicator that easily splays. The iridescent colors—Doug, Jesse, and Julio (that's right, the colors are named after the different hunks adorning the packaging)—are chock-full of sparkle, but the creams and sheers go on quite nicely, with day-glo pink James being the only cream shade with clearly limited appeal. Also worth noting is the unpleasantly strong dessert-y fragrance, which lingers far longer than the gloss does.

☺ **$$$ XXX Shine Lip Gloss** *($16)* has a texture that's syrupy and sticky. The sheer colors last thanks to this gloss' clingy nature, but the peppermint flavor can be irritating and that isn't good for lips.

MASCARA: ☺ **$$$ Skyscraper Multi-Benefit Mascara** *($22)* is positioned as a replacement of Urban Decay's original Skyscraper Mascara. I praised the original formula for its lengthening prowess and its ability to keep lashes soft and attractively fringed. This update performs almost identically, except you get a bit of thickness. Clumping is completely absent, and this separates lashes easily. The shape of the rubber-bristle brush makes it easy to reach every lash, though those with small eyes may find it a bit cumbersome.

☺ **$$$ Eyelash Primer Potion** *($17)*. The main reason to consider this lash primer (which, like most lash primers goes on white and adds bulk to lashes) is that it helps clump-prone mascaras go on better, but that isn't a great reason. It would be better to just not use a clump-prone mascara in the first place. Used with a mascara that doesn't clump, Eyelash Primer Potion makes no difference compared to simply brushing on another coat of mascara.

☹ **$$$ Big Fatty Mascara** *($20)* purports to thicken and lengthen lashes, and its gigantic brush achieves that, though not to the same impressive extent as mascaras with smaller brushes and more variegated bristles. You may think that a big brush equals big results, but that's not the case here, nor has it been with any other enlarged mascara brush I've ever tried, with one exception: Dior's Mascara Diorshow. If you're curious to see how a large mascara brush will work for you, try Dior's version instead of this average mascara from Urban Decay.

☹ **$$$ Big Fatty Waterproof** *($20)* is aptly named because it boasts a huge brush with long, dense bristles. While it does adequately thicken and elongate lashes, the huge brush poses serious logistical problems too big to ignore—problems only made worse by the mascara's tenacious waterproofing. Available only in black (called Gotham), when wet, the mascara's color intensifies beautifully; however, because the big, fat brush is hard to control, it is quite likely a lot of the mascara will end up on your lids, and then it doesn't budge or run until doused with cleanser. So, while it certainly lives up to its waterproof claim, the gigantic brush and quick-setting color is a hazard to any other makeup on or around the eye. For more fool-proof waterproof options consider those from Dior or Maybelline.

☹ **Big Fatty Colored Mascara** *($17)* is Urban Decay's multicolored version of their Big Fatty Mascara, above, and it suffers the fate of many an *über*-hip brightly hued mascara—it just doesn't perform well. The number of coats required to get the color to actually appear on the average dark lash causes clumping, crumbling, and an overall mess. The brush is as large and unwieldy as its name implies, which doesn't help matters unless you like your lids to match your lashes. Once dried, lashes are caked stiff, and the color appears almost chalky. Available in five shades, from burgundy red to teal blue, Big Fatty Colored Mascara will force you to sacrifice everything a mascara should do well for the novelty of bright color.

☹ **Lingerie & Galoshes for Lashes** *($17)* seems like a clever idea: it's a dual-ended product featuring a waterproofing solution on one end and a lash primer on the other. The waterproofing side is designed to be used over a non-waterproof mascara, the idea being that it will make your favorite mascara resistant to tears and water-based activities. Sounds great until you try it—the product doesn't apply easily over lashes and it's not completely waterproof. In fact, mild splashing of the eye area caused smearing and streaking. Adding to this disappointment is that the waterproofing sealer is difficult to remove. The primer's results aren't that great either, but the overall effect is neutral (nearing do-nothing) and it doesn't impede mascara application. All told, there are too many negatives to give this product anything but an unhappy face rating.

FACE AND BODY ILLUMINATING/SHIMMER PRODUCTS: ☺ **$$$ Heavy Metal Glitter Eye Gel** *($18)* is glitter to the max, but if that's the look you're after for a night of clubbing or a Halloween costume, this is excellent. A clear, clingy gel suspends brilliantly shiny particles of glitter, allowing you to apply it with a brush or a fingertip. It takes a moment to set, but the reward is long wear with negligible flaking.

☺ **$$$ Baked Body Glow** *($25)* looks like a large roll-on deodorant, but is a sheer, peachy bronze tint for the body. The thick texture must be warmed on the hand or it doesn't glide over skin well, while the result feels a bit too thick and waxy to make it worth considering over numerous bronzing gels, lotions, or self-tanning products—and this one will come off on clothes.

☺ **$$$ Cocktail Collection—Flavored Body Powder** *($30)* features various sets of cocktail-flavored products, including Piña Colada and Cosmopolitan. This collection features Flavored Body Powder, which has a huge synthetic brush attached to a jar of sparkling powder that clings unevenly but does add head-to-toe gleam. This product is also available in food flavors (such as Marshmallow), which are packaged in cardboard jars and include powder puffs. You'll find that either Powder (food or cocktail flavored) lasts longer if you apply the Body Balm ($25) first, which adds a low-key but still sexy sheen of its own.

☺ **$$$ Flavored Body Powder** *($26)*. I can think of other retail establishments where this product should be sold, but there it was, sitting in Sephora, waiting to be dusted on someone's skin and then be kissed, or licked, off—they're flavored and scented to smell like food. The loose powder provides a strong shimmer finish, but wearing it becomes increasingly bothersome because it makes skin feel sticky, especially if you apply it near areas where you perspire.

☹ **Midnight Cowboy Shimmer Body Lotion** *($28)* is a very standard body lotion imbued with a metallic shimmer. Although the shiny finish clings well, application can be tricky; it's way too easy to go from subtle glow to blinding shimmer in a flash. There's also the fact that this product contains the preservative methylisothiazolinone, which is not recommended for use in leave-on products due to its high risk of causing a sensitized reaction (Sources: *Contact Dermatitis*, November 2001, pages 257-264; and *European Journal of Dermatology*, March 1999, pages 144-160). Overall, this falls short as a shine product and is only a little better than boring as a body moisturizer.

☹ **Santa Tanita Body Bronzer** *($28)*. The packaging and name are the most enticing things about this dud of a body bronzer. Housed in a pressurized metal container and dispensed as a mousse, the foam falls flat and liquefies almost instantly. It is difficult to control, tending to be messy and drippy, and the initial color you get is a sickly looking yellowish brown. This contains the slow-acting self-tanning ingredient erythrulose, so the aforementioned cosmetic tint gives way to a sheer tan color that lasts a few days; however, lots of self-tanners contain this ingredient, and without the mess and unattractive cosmetic tint of this bronzer.

BRUSHES: ✓ ☺ **$$$ Big Buddha Brush** *($36)*. Using a religious icon in a name seems inappropriate, but names aside, this synthetic-hair brush with a squat handle is a brilliant way to apply powder to a large area of skin at once. The brush hair is wonderfully soft and dense, yet flexible enough to enable a sheer dusting of, say, shimmer powder, from the neck down.

If you need a brush like this and don't mind the absence of an elongated handle, this is well worth checking out.

✓☺ **$$$ Big Buddha Brush Set** *($138)* includes all of Urban Decay's well-made brushes in a zippered bag. A brush roll with holders for each tool would be better, but all things considered, this set ends up being functionally proficient and a good value.

☺ **$$$ Good Karma Brushes** *($15-$36)* are all expertly crafted synthetic brushes, making them a distinct highlight and value of this line. Each one has merit depending on your needs and preferences, but generally speaking the standouts are the **Powder Brush** *($35)*, **Shadow Brush** *($18)*, **Blender Brush** *($24)*, and the **Brow Brush** *($15)*, which is also suitable for applying powder eyeliner.

SPECIALTY PRODUCTS: ☺ **$$$ Complexion Primer Potion—Brightening** *($30)* is a good primer that's essentially a lightweight gel-textured fluid that has some beneficial ingredients. It smooths on easily and makes skin feel silky, while leaving a slightly tacky finish that dissipates once makeup is applied. The formula goes above and beyond most primers by offering skin a plentiful range of antioxidants, water-binding agents, and cell-communicating ingredients, and it's also fragrance-free. This product is suitable for all skin types, but best for oily skin.

☺ **$$$ Complexion Primer Potion—Pore Perfecting** *($30)*. Although Urban Decay got creative (to your skin's benefit) with their Complexion Primer Potion—Brightening, the formulary bells and whistles don't sound as loudly here. This slightly thick, silicone-based primer goes on slightly white and leaves a faint white cast. I suppose you could consider that a brightening effect, but it's basically canceled once you apply foundation over it. This primer's silky texture can slightly fill in large pores, but not to the extent that you'll look air-brushed to poreless perfection. It feels light and is compatible with oily skin. The only extra of note is a tiny amount of olive oil, but this is still an interesting primer to consider if you want to add such a product to your routine. It isn't essential, but some consumers really want to try a primer.

☺ **$$$ Eyeshadow Transforming Potion** *($18)* is said to transform eyeshadow into a liquid eye color. This water-based solution is housed in a dual-sided component that provides a synthetic brush meant for drawing wide lines and another for drawing thin, precise lines. Both work well and deepen powder eyeshadow colors, though this requires successive layers because initially the solution causes the color to go on sheer. Once set it wears reasonably well, but it's neither budge-proof nor completely waterproof. The thicker brush tends to dispense too much of the liquid, so be sure to remove some of it before using with a powder eyeshadow.

VIVITÉ (SKIN CARE ONLY)

VIVITÉ AT-A-GLANCE

Strengths: Fragrance-free; good selection of pH-correct AHA products with effective amounts of glycolic acid; good water-soluble cleansers.

Weaknesses: Expensive; the sole sunscreen option does not provide sufficient UVA protection; using the company's recommended routine will result in AHA overload; jar packaging won't keep ingredients stable.

For more information about Vivité, owned by Allergan, call (877) 345-5372 or visit www.viviteskincare.com or www.Beautypedia.com.

☺ **$$$ Daily Facial Cleanser** *($27 for 6 ounces)* is an incredibly pricey water-soluble cleanser that supposedly contains 12% glycolic compound. In any amount, AHAs in a cleanser aren't going to do your skin much good because of their brief contact with skin. Cleansers are designed to be rinsed shortly after application (you don't want to keep them on for longer than needed because you don't want the cleansing agents to disturb skin), so any benefit from the AHA is rinsed down the drain. AHAs also are a problem in cleansers because they can be irritating when used around the eyes. There are far better and far less expensive cleansers to consider than this one.

☺ **$$$ Exfoliating Facial Cleanser** *($39 for 6.76 ounces)* is a standard water-soluble cleanser that contains 15% glycolic acid. It can be irritating, especially if used around the eyes, and the glycolic acid won't exfoliate skin due to its brief contact with it; you don't want to leave a cleanser on skin long enough for the AHA to work because the cleansing agents can disturb skin and cause irritation. Vivité recommends using this two to three times per week, but there is nothing special about this product indicating that you need to ration it to a few times a week; because of the potential problems, you shouldn't even use it that much.

✓ ☺ **$$$ Replenish Hydrating Facial Cleanser** *($27 for 2 ounces)* is similar to my Paula's Choice Moisture Boost One Step Cleanser for Normal to Dry Skin (which is flattering), but Vivité's price is outrageous for such a tiny amount of cleanser. This does have a milky texture that slips over skin and removes makeup efficiently. This cleanser doesn't contain AHA, but that's just fine, because AHAs are best used in products meant to stay on skin; they should not be used in a rinse-off product because there is the potential that it can be splashed into the eyes.

☺ **$$$ Daily Antioxidant Facial Serum** *($109 for 1 ounce)* is a very good, though needlessly expensive, serum with 15% glycolic acid, and it is formulated at a pH of 3.8 so it is an effective exfoliant. However, the amount of AHA is more than what the FDA considers safe for long-term daily use; the FDA recommends a 10% maximum concentration. Routinely applying 15% or greater of AHAs in an acidic base (pH of 3 to 4, which allows AHAs to be effective) to skin may result in pronounced stinging, redness, and irritation. Continued irritation to the skin can cause negative results, just the opposite of what you want.

There has always been a trade-off with using well-formulated AHA products: some irritation (though many formulas contain anti-irritants to counter the problem) versus lots of benefits. You always want to tip the scale in favor of the benefits (smoother skin with a plumped, less lined appearance), while incurring minimal risk, and for most people that's entirely possible by using a pH-correct AHA product containing 5% to 10% glycolic acid. Using higher concentrations can be overkill—and there just isn't any research to support the safety of using such high concentrations daily on a long-term basis.

The Cosmetic Ingredient Review Board (a cosmetics industry–based group) assessed the available data on the effectiveness and safety of glycolic acid, and concluded that AHAs are safe as used, provided that the concentration of glycolic acid does not exceed 10% in a pH of 3.5. Higher concentrations were deemed safe if used "in products designed for brief, discontinuous use followed by thorough rinsing from skin, when applied by trained professionals, and when application is accompanied by directions for the daily use of sun protection." The FDA concurs with this assessment, but goes further, stressing the importance of sun protection while using any AHA product (Sources: *2007 CIR Compendium*, 2007, pages 117-120; and www.fda.gov). The high concentration of AHA in this Facial Serum is what keeps it from earning a Paula's Pick rating. It is worth considering if the expense doesn't bother you (though it should, because MD Formulations offers a 15% concentration AHA product for far less) and you plan to use it, say, once per week as a "booster" to your lower-strength but still effective AHA product.

☹ **Daily Facial Moisturizer with SPF 30** *($49 for 1.7 ounces)* lacks the UVA-protecting ingredients of titanium dioxide, zinc oxide, avobenzone (also known as butyl methoxydibenzoylmethane), Tinosorb, or Mexoryl SX and is not recommended. If you're looking to combine daily sun protection with an AHA moisturizer (though that combination is not particularly helpful for skin), look no further than the excellent options from NeoStrata.

☺ **$$$ Night Renewal Facial Cream** *($79 for 2 ounces)*. This overly expensive AHA moisturizer contains 20% glycolic acid. It is formulated at a pH of 3.8 so it is an effective exfoliant, but the concentration of AHA is higher than what the FDA considers safe for long-term daily use; the FDA recommends 10% as a maximum concentration. Routinely applying 20% AHAs in an effective acidic base (pH of 3 to 4, which allows AHAs to be effective) may result in pronounced stinging, redness, and irritation. Such irritation to the skin, if continued, can cause negative results, just the opposite of what you want. Using higher concentrations can be overkill—and there just isn't any research to support the safety of using such high concentrations daily on a long-term basis.

☺ **$$$ Replenish Hydrating Cream** *($50 for 2 ounces)* is one of the only Vivité products not containing AHAs. It's a good moisturizer for normal to dry skin due to its texture and elegant but lightweight cream feel, but it's disappointing that this intriguing formula is packaged in a jar. That means the antioxidants and other helpful ingredients, which deteriorate when exposed to air, won't remain potent once this product is opened. Also a letdown is that most of the intriguing ingredients are listed after the preservative. At this price, they should have more prominence.

☺ **$$$ Revitalizing Eye Cream** *($69 for 0.5 ounce)* is an intriguing eye cream that contains 10% glycolic acid formulated at a pH of 3.8. Although it will exfoliate and improve skin texture anywhere on the face or body, it's disappointing that jar packaging was chosen because it will render the delicate antioxidants and peptides ineffective once you open it. For a product that prices out to $138 per ounce, that's a significant waste! There are much less expensive ways to apply glycolic acid safely around the eyes, but always take care to not use AHAs too close to your eyes (and never apply AHA products to the eyelid), and 10% is probably far more than the area can tolerate, so proceed with caution.

✓ ☺ **$$$ Vibrance Therapy** *($119 for 1 ounce)* is yet another AHA product from Vivité that contains a potent amount of glycolic acid (15%) at an effective pH of 3.8. This water-based serum comes with claims that it can "brighten" skin, and it does contain a smattering of plant extracts with limited in vitro research demonstrating their ability to fade skin discolorations, along with retinol and some good antioxidants. The main reason to consider this product is its exfoliating ability, though the other ingredients are also quite helpful.

In addition to the steep price tag, 15% glycolic acid can be a problem for skin if used every day. Please refer to the review of Daily Antioxidant Facial Serum above for an explanation as to why daily use of high percentage AHA products can be a problem.

Despite the concerns over AHA content, if you're going to spend money on one Vivité product, make it this fragrance-free one. The key is to make sure you use it only once or twice a week; on the other days use a well-formulated 5% to 8% concentration AHA product.

☺ **$$$ Defining Lip Plumper** *($45 for 0.12 ounce)* is a very standard lip moisturizer that doesn't make good on its claims of increasing lip volume and fullness. Moist lips look fuller than dry, chapped lips, but that's something any lip moisturizer can provide, including several at the drugstore that wouldn't dare charge this much for such an ordinary formula. If your doctor is suggesting this product over lip injections, consider getting a second opinion!

WET 'N' WILD (MAKEUP ONLY)

WET 'N' WILD AT-A-GLANCE

Strengths: Inexpensive; good tinted moisturizer with sunscreen; one of the best bronzing powders at any price; great powder blush; mostly good eyeshadow and lipstick options; one superior lip gloss; a few great liquid shimmer options.

Weaknesses: Unimpressive concealers; large assortment of average to poor eyelining products; the mascaras do little to impress; some lip products suffer from the inclusion of irritants; the makeup brushes.

For more information about Wet 'n' Wild, visit www.wnwbeauty.com or www.Beautypedia.com.

WET 'N' WILD NATURAL WEAR PRODUCTS

POWDER: ☺ **Natural Wear 100% Natural Pressed Powder** *($4.99)* is a mica- and cornstarch-based pressed powder that comes close to being 100% natural, but unless you can show me a glyceryl caprylate plant, I'll stick with my statement. This powder has a silky texture that feels slightly creamy yet leaves skin with a dry-looking powdered finish best for oily skin. Among the four shades are good options for fair to light skin tones (shade 821A is great for fair skin), but there are no options for medium to tan skin tones. Interestingly, considering this product's formula and comparing it with several other pressed powders reveals that they're fairly close to being "100% natural," too.

BRONZER: ✓ ☺ **Natural Wear Bronzer** *($4.99)* is a very smooth, creamy-feeling pressed bronzing powder that looks great on skin if you don't mind its shiny finish. It applies evenly and lends a soft, rosy tan flush to cheeks. In terms of natural ingredients, this cornstarch-based formula has several, including some oils that make it ill-advised for those with oily or blemish-prone skin. For the money and a good formula, this is well worth checking out if you don't mind (or are after) its very shiny finish.

LIPSTICK: ☹ **Natural Wear Lip Shimmer** *($1.99)* contains peppermint oil and several irritating plant extracts that make it impossible to recommend this sheer lipstick. Those ingredients are definitely natural, but it's further proof that natural ingredients aren't automatically better for your skin (or lips).

WET 'N' WILD ULTIMATE MINERALS PRODUCTS

FOUNDATION: ☺ **Ultimate Minerals Powder Foundation** *($4.99)* isn't the ultimate in terms of mineral or powder-based makeup, but for the money, this competes better than you'd think with similar loose-powder makeup from bareMinerals and Jane Iredale, among other mineral-centric cosmetic lines. The mica-based formula has a nearly weightless, surprisingly silky texture that meshes well with skin and provides light to medium coverage. The mica (which is definitely a mineral) also lends noticeable shine to this foundation, but unlike the sparkles you get from many mineral makeups, this is a diffused glow. You don't get any sun protection, nor does this keep shine at bay like several other mineral makeups. All four shades are good (and best for light to medium skin), making this an inexpensive way to discover if mineral makeup is for you or not.

BLUSH AND BRONZER: ☺ **Ultimate Minerals Loose Blush** *($3.99)*. I can't fathom why someone would want to use powder blush in loose rather than pressed form (there is no advantage and it just makes application a bit more tricky), but this product is indeed loose. The main mineral in this blush is mica, a pigment ingredient that's standard in hundreds of makeup products, so this is hardly the "ultimate" in mineral makeup (but that's just a marketing detail). I have to hand it to Wet 'n' Wild for packaging this loose-powder blush to minimize mess. The sifter has a cap that you can close between uses and the dispenser holes are few and small so it's easier to control how much powder comes out at once. Application with a brush is surprisingly smooth, sheer, and even. Cheeks are blushed with soft color and a moderately shiny (but not sparkling) finish. The small shade range is best for fair to light skin tones.

☺ **Ultimate Minerals Bronzer** *($3.99)* contains the same mineral pigments that show up in thousands of loose-powder makeup products, so it's not the "ultimate" for fans of mineral makeup. The packaging is smart because the container includes a special closure for the sifter, which minimizes mess, and the smaller holes in the sifter make controlled dispensing easier. Just like Wet 'n' Wild's Ultimate Minerals Loose Blush above, application with a brush is smooth, sheer, and even. The bronze effect is best described as a peachy tan color with moderate shimmer. This is best for light to medium skin tones.

EYESHADOW: ☹ **Ultimate Minerals Loose Eyeshadow** *($3.99)*. I think loose eyeshadow is a messy waste of time—why bother with it when there are so many good pressed-powder (or cream-to-powder) eyeshadows? Possibly this type of eyeshadow has its fans, because it never goes away completely. Wet 'n' Wild's version is an OK option. The biggest compliment I can give is that it's not as messy as you'd think. Application with the rounded sponge-tip applicator is somewhat uneven and sheer enough that you'll need to layer to build intensity. The sparkling shine of each shade clings decently, but expect some flaking. If you're keen to try this, avoid the bright purple Amethyst shade.

OTHER WET 'N' WILD PRODUCTS

FOUNDATION: ☺ **Ultimate Sheer Tinted Moisturizer SPF 15** *($3.99)* wins instant points for using titanium dioxide as the sole broad-spectrum active sun-protecting ingredient. It has a slightly fluid, thin texture that blends decently and sets to a nearly matte finish suitable for normal to slightly oily skin. True to its name, coverage is sheer and definitely more akin to a tint than a true foundation. All four colors are excellent and there are options for light to tan skin.

CONCEALER: ☹ **Cover All Liquid Concealer** *($2.99)* has a creamy-smooth texture, but although it provides good coverage it's not a "cover all" solution. This is too emollient for use over blemishes, but is an OK option for under-eye use or concealing minor redness. Among the four shades, Medium, Light, and Beige are strongly pink and should be avoided. Fair is recommended for that respective skin tone.

☹ **Cover All Stick** *($1.99)* is a lipstick-style cream concealer that's very greasy, easily creases under the eye, and offers shades that look nothing like real skin.

POWDER: ☺ **Ultimate Touch Pressed Powder with Puff** *($2.99)* comes with the cheapest puff imaginable, but that's OK because powder looks best when applied with a brush. This talc-based powder has a smooth, dry texture and silky matte finish. Four shades are available, and only Warm Beige is a dud due to its peachy tone. This pressed powder is best for normal to oily skin.

BLUSH AND BRONZER: ✓ ☺ **Silk Finish Blush** *($2.99)* For the money, this small collection of powder blushes is among the best at the drugstore. If only the shade selection were more extensive! Heather Silk and Mellow Wine are matte, while Pearlescent Pink has shine. All apply smoothly, and have more pigment than you'd expect, so they really last.

✓ ☺ **Bronzer Ultimate Bronzing Powder** *($2.99)* remains one of Wet 'n' Wild's star products, and for good reason: this inexpensive pressed bronzing powder is one of the best around in terms of smooth application, good intensity, and believable colors. The Light/Medium and Medium/Dark shades are matte, while the others have shine, so you can take your pick (but I suggest saving the shiny ones for evening makeup).

☺ **Silk Finish Three of a Kind Blush** *($4.99)* presents three coordinated shades of blush and highlighter in one compact. There is a divider between the shades, a feature that many expensive lines overlook. Regardless of whether you use one or all of the shades, the result is sheer color with a shimmer finish. The highlighting shade doesn't provide the most flattering results, but is an OK option if you prefer powders to liquids. This applies well, but the pigment level limits their appeal to those with fair to light skin.

EYESHADOW: ☺ **Eye Expressions Eye Shadow/Illuminator** *($3.99)* combines four cream eyeshadows and the MegaGlo Face Illuminator in one compact. The sheer cream eyeshadows apply and blend well, setting to a soft powder finish that doesn't slip or crease, making these a step above the norm. The eyeshadows and Illuminator are shiny, but the shine on the eyeshadows is softer. This is definitely worth a try if you find a color combination you like.

☺ **MegaEyes Cream Eyeshadow** *($1.99)* isn't creamy so much as gel-like. The water- and glycerin-based formula has good initial slip, allowing for blending over the entire eye area. Spot application is tricky and not this product's forte. The effect is sheer color with intense shine, and flaking is scant once the product has set. These don't crease either, making them a workable alternative to powder eyeshadows if you can handle this much shine. Avoid Blue Heaven and Envy, both of which are too clownish.

☺ **MegaEyes Eye Shadow** *($2.99)* is sold as trios and at just $1 per shade deserves mention as a bona fide beauty steal. The creamy-feeling powder texture applies smoothly but sheer, and layered application is recommended to avoid slight flaking. Doing so enhances blending, and every trio has one shade that's dark enough to serve as eyeliner (and these may be applied wet). All of the trios are shiny, which means they're not for wrinkled eyes, but if that doesn't include you these are recommended.

☺ **MegaEyes Shadow Pot** *($1.99)* has a smooth texture and sheer application that make this powder eyeshadow easy to work with and blend. You won't be able to add much depth and there are no shades that are dark enough to serve as eyeliner. All of the shades have some amount of shine; those with visible shiny particles tend to flake while the others do not.

☺ **Ultimate Expressions Eyeshadow Palette** *($4.99)* provides eight powder eyeshadows in one sturdy compact that includes a built-in pop-out mirror. The set of four shades in the middle is what's needed for shaping, shading, and eyelining; the shades on the periphery are best for highlighting. These shadows have a smooth, minimally flaky texture that applies evenly although they tend to rub off easily, so aren't the best if your goal is long-lasting eye makeup. The darker shades have good pigmentation while the light to medium shades go on sheer, imparting more shine than color (all eight shades have shine).

EYE AND BROW SHAPER: ☺ **H2O Proof Liquid Eyeliner** *($3.99)* has a good, firm brush that lays down a continuous line of color and a formula that not only dries quickly but also is tenaciously waterproof. A minor issue is that the color saturation isn't as intense as it could be. This requires layering if you want more definition (and for most of the colors, you will). That's not a deal-breaker, but it's enough to keep this liquid eyeliner from earning a higher rating.

☺ **Perfect Pair Eye Wand** *($3.99)* combines a retractable, shiny eye pencil and creamy eyeshadow in one dual-sided pen component. Both ends work well, with the pencil being preferred for its powder finish. The eyeshadow is very shiny and tends to crease slightly, but this won't be a problem if you use it only to highlight the brow bone.

☹ **H2O Proof Blending Eye Pencils** *($1.99)* need sharpening, but for the money that's not such a bad deal. These pencils apply easily and most of the shades have a metallic or sparkle-infused finish, so this is not the epitome of understated makeup. True to the name, the long-wearing, surprisingly smudge-resistant finish is waterproof. In fact, it takes effort to remove this pencil! How come Wet 'n' Wild can do this for less than $2 and Chanel can't get it right for $25? As you may have guessed, this pencil would be rated higher were it not for the need to routinely sharpen it.

☺ **MegaLiner Liquid Eyeliner** *($2.99)* dries quickly and doesn't flake, chip, or smear once it has set, but this loses points because its long, thin, somewhat flimsy brush makes drawing an even line unusually tricky. If you're adept at handling this type of brush you may want to consider this—but avoid the green, blue, and purple shades unless it's Halloween.

☺ **Purse Size Twin Eye or Lipliner Pencils** *($1.99)* are standard pencils that need sharpening and are indeed small enough to fit in even a tiny purse or evening bag. These have a different, better formula than the Wet 'n' Wild Eyeliner Pencils below. Although they're still creamy, they have better staying powder and are an OK option for a smoky-eye design.

☺ **I-Shimmer Retractable Eye Pencil** *($1.99)* is a very good automatic, retractable eye pencil that suffers from its color choices (only a teal and a blue shade are offered) as well as the fact that the mirror-like shimmer particles tend to flake (but the color remains). What a shame, because this glides on easily and sets to a long-wearing finish.

☹ **Ultimate Brow Color & Set** *($2.99)* is a dual-sided product featuring a creamy brow pencil (that needs sharpening) on one end and a sheer, tinted brow gel on the other. The pencil applies smoothly but suffers from some fading, while the brow gel feels slightly tacky (though it does the trick as far as keeping unruly brows in place). The concept is good, but the execution is not as flawless as it could have been.

☹ **Eyeliner Pencils** *($0.99)* need sharpening, but even if that doesn't bother you, these extra long pencils are way too creamy and stay that way, which just invites smudging and smearing. I suppose this is one of those cosmetic instances where you get what you pay for.

☹ **Brow Pencils** *($0.99)* are almost as creamy as the Wet 'n' Wild Eyeliner Pencils, and tend to ball up and get matted in brow hairs, necessitating more work than filling in and defining the brows should take.

☹ **Idol Eyes Retractable Eye Pencil** *($1.99)* is, without question, one of the worst eye pencils on the market. Yes, it doesn't need sharpening and is retractable, but it tends to drag over skin, deposits color unevenly, and smears with little provocation, plus it is exceedingly difficult to remove. This is a must to avoid.

LIPSTICK, LIP GLOSS, AND LIPLINER: ✓☺ **Wild Shine Lip Lacquer** *($2.99)*. Naming this a lip lacquer is inaccurate because it is really a lightweight cream lipstick—albeit a smooth-textured one that gives some department-store cream lipsticks a run for their money. Application is smooth, coverage and color intensity are moderate, and this sets to a soft cream finish that doesn't readily move into lines around the mouth or require frequent touch-ups. The soft shimmer shades are most attractive, and for the price, you may want to try a few! One more plus: this lipstick is fragrance-free!

☺ **3-of-a-Kind Twist-Up Sticks for Lips, Eyes, and Cheeks** *($3.99)* has a smooth, slightly slick texture that glides over skin and imparts translucent color and a natural, minimally moist finish. Only one shade (#728) is suitable for use as eyeshadow (though using it as such invites some creasing); the others are best for sheer blush. Applied to lips, the lack of emollients is disappointing, as is the fleeting nature of the sheer colors.

☺ **Diamond Brilliance Moisturizing Lip Sheen** *($2.99)* should get an audition from anyone who likes a fairly tenacious lip gloss that imparts sheer color and a blatantly glossy finish. This wand-applicator gloss competes favorably with much more expensive options, and doesn't suffer from a cloying fragrance or artificial fruit- or dessert-like flavors. The majority of colors pair well with any lipstick shade, too, though you must be able to tolerate a slightly sticky finish.

☺ **Glassy Gloss Lip Gel** *($2.99)* is a very good, sheer lip gloss packaged in a tube. It has a slightly runny texture so careful dispensing is needed (especially if the gloss has been kept in a warm environment) but feels lush, smooth, and is not sticky or overly slick. The shades are sheer enough to work with a wide range of lipstick colors. This lip gloss does contain fragrance.

☺ **Jumbo Juicy Lip Balm** *($2.99)* is a chunky lip balm whose candy-bright colors may catch your eye. But color isn't what this smooth, slightly glossy lip balm is all about. Every shade applies translucent, but imparts a fruity flavor. Although this will take care of dry lips, the flavor may encourage lip-licking, and that's not a good way to stop dryness.

☺ **Lip Impressions** *($3.99)* comes in a compact with a generous-size mirror and a chintzy dual-sided lip brush. The product comprises four shades of the Wild Shine Lip Lacquer and one shade of the MegaGlo Face Illuminator reviewed below. It's a fine option if you don't mind applying lip color with a brush and find most of the shades appealing.

☺ **MegaColors Lipstick** *($1.99)* is a traditional cream lipstick that has a lighter feel and less color saturation than most. The finish is creamy with a hint of gloss and the color selection is large enough to offer all the basics and some trendier colors, too.

☺ **MegaLast Long-Lasting Lipcolor** *($3.99)* is Wet 'n' Wild's me-too Lipfinity product, and includes the same two steps (color coat followed by a glossy top coat). The color portion goes on a bit unevenly, requiring more blending before it sets. It's ready for the top coat after a couple of minutes, and even when completely dry, the top coat removes a bit of color (superior options from M.A.C. and Estee Lauder don't do this). Still, this isn't a terrible option for the money, and you'll find that, for the most part, the color wears well and the gloss coat doesn't require frequent touch-ups. This does come off on cups and light kisses, so don't consider it transfer-resistant.

☺ **MegaSlicks Lip Color Retractable Pencil** *($2.99)* looks deceiving because you'd swear it was a pencil that needed to be sharpened. Look closer and it's a cleverly designed automatic pencil whose tip can be wound up or down. This thick pencil has a slightly dry application and semi-matte finish with nearly opaque colors. It wears longer than traditional lipsticks, but you may need to add some gloss for comfort.

☺ **MegaSlicks Lip Gloss** *($1.99)* is a good basic lip gloss that feels slightly thick, isn't too slick, and is slightly sticky. All of the sheer shades have soft to moderate shimmer and are applied with a sponge-tip wand. Note: This lip gloss has a strong fragrance.

☺ **Perfect Pair Lip Wand** *($3.99)* combines a retractable, shimmer-finish lip pencil with a slim, sheer lipstick in one dual-sided unit. The pencil is standard fare in terms of application and wear (it's too creamy to last the day) and the lipstick feels light, provides moderate coverage, and imparts a frosted shimmer. This has more appeal to teens than adults, but for those who use lipliner and lipstick and like strong shimmer, it is convenient.

☺ **Precious Metals Lipstick** *($1.99)* has a lightweight, somewhat slick texture and a strong metallic finish. This actually feels more elegant than the price suggests and is worth exploring if this type of finish appeals to you. One caution: The mica particles in this lipstick tend to cling to the lips as the color wears away, creating a whitish shimmer without color.

☺ **Silk Finish Lipstick** *($1.29)* is Wet 'n' Wild's most opaque lipstick, but also its greasiest. The wide shade selection has a nice stain, helping to keep the color around longer, but this is also greasy enough to immediately bleed into any lines around the mouth. If that's not an issue for you and you want full-coverage color, the price is tough to beat!

☺ **Creme Lipliner Pencil** *($0.99)* is a standard, needs-sharpening pencil that's neither too creamy nor too dry, though the finish is slightly tacky. A few of the colors are excellent versatile shades that you really should check out if you can tolerate the sharpening aspect.

☺ **MegaMixers** *($1.99)* are teen-themed pot lip glosses inappropriately colored and flavored to resemble popular cocktails, such as margaritas and daiquiris (which is not ethical marketing to a young audience). Despite the shades looking bold, each goes on extremely sheer. The product feels more like a light-textured lip balm than a gloss, while the flavors smack of artificiality and have a pervasive, sweet fragrance. Whether you're a teen or an adult, there are better inexpensive glosses available from Cover Girl.

☹ **MegaPlump Plumping Lip Gloss** *($3.99)* burns on application and may make you think you've smeared potpourri on your lips given the pervasive cinnamon scent. Two forms of pure cinnamon oil are part of the formula, and although they plump lips, each does so by causing irritation. Most lip-plumping products take the irritation route to inflating the mouth, but few do so with such strong irritants.

☹ **MegaBrilliance Lip Gloss** *($1.99)* is a lightweight, minimally sticky lip gloss loaded with large flecks of glitter. As you might guess, the glitter feels grainy (almost scratchy) shortly after application, and the effect is far from sophisticated or glamorous.

☹ **Speed Gloss Energizing Lip Shine** *($3.99)* owes the energizing part of this gloss to irritating peppermint oil. What a disappointment, because this gloss and its collection of shimmer-infused shades has a lot going for it, including a smooth texture, non-sticky finish, good pigmentation, and attractive shine.

MASCARA: ☺ **H2O Proof Waterproof Mascara** *($2.99)* sells at a price that makes me wish it was a great recommendation, but mascaras have never been one of Wet 'n' Wild's strong suits. This version produces negligible to very modest length and barely any thickness, but it does apply evenly without clumping or smearing, and it is waterproof. If you're OK with an average mascara (perhaps because you already have long, thick lashes or you just want minimal definition), this is an ordinary, but unquestionably affordable, option.

☺ **Lash Intense Mascara** *($4.99)* brings to market yet another rubber-bristle brush option. This version is unique because one side is a brush for applying the mascara and the other a comb that you use to comb through and separate lashes once the mascara is applied. This could've been handy, were it not for the following problems. First, the newfangled brush causes the mascara to clump easily and does little to either lengthen or thicken lashes. Second, the teeth on the comb side are too short to adequately and easily comb through and separate lashes. You need to use a separate spooly or eyelash comb to break up the clumping. For a few dollars more, there are many better options at the drugstore that create long, thick, separated lashes without the trouble of going through a second step to comb through the glop. Rimmel, L'Oréal, Jane, and Maybelline offer excellent, reasonably priced options.

☺ **MegaLash Lengthening Mascara** *($1.99)* is a reasonably good lengthening mascara if you want something that creates a soft, natural lash look. Performance plateaus quickly, so applying successive coats doesn't produce more dramatic results, but the formula doesn't clump or smear.

☺ **MegaLength Double Action Mascara** *($3.99)* is a two-step product that includes a lash primer and regular mascara. Although the primer does make a slight difference in lash thickness and volume, the mascara portion is lackluster and no match for similar products from L'Oreal (Double Extend), Revlon (Lash Fantasy), or a variety of options from Maybelline.

☺ **MegaPlump Mascara** *($3.99)* has a name that makes you think of thick lashes, perhaps? Well, that's what I was hoping would happen with this, but not even successive coats provided any lengthening or thickening. The only thing plump about it is the tube. It wears well, removes easily, and is an OK option if you want minimally enhanced lashes.

☺ **MegaProtein Mascara** *($2.99)* contains a tiny, not "mega" amount of soy protein, and protein in and of itself isn't the fast track to gorgeous lashes. This mascara, like most of those from Wet 'n' Wild, does little to impress. Its main accomplishment is average length; you cannot build bigger, longer lashes with this no matter how long you try.

☺ **MegaWink Lash Curling Mascara** *($2.99)* is an OK mascara for a really natural look without a hint of thickness. You'll get soft, separated lashes without clumps and a minimal curled effect.

☹ **MegaVolume Thickening Mascara** *($2.99)* is a nearly do-nothing mascara that is seriously misnamed.

FACE AND BODY ILLUMINATING/SHIMMER PRODUCTS: ✓ ☺ **MegaGlo Face Illuminator** *($2.99)* adds an illuminated gleam to skin thanks to its smooth texture and emollient formula that is suitable only for dry to very dry skin. This has a distinctive moist finish, but tends to stay in place quite well because it doesn't remain slippery once blended. Blushing is best as a highlighter, Toasty is great for a bronze effect, and Rosy is good for a shiny blush.

☺ **MegaPump Bronzer** *($3.99)* has the same formula as the MegaPump Shimmer below, but produces a sheer bronze tint with a golden shimmer overtone. The shine level is more intense than that of the MegaPump Shimmer, and looks best on medium to tan skin.

☺ **MegaPump Shimmer** *($3.99)* is a lightweight shimmer lotion with a smooth texture and opalescent finish on skin. The shimmer effect is subtle but can look more intense depending on the room lighting.

☺ **MegaPump Glitter Gel** *($3.99)* is a clear, water- and alcohol-based gel laced with multi-colored glitter particles. The gel base allows the glitter to cling to skin decently, but don't expect this to last all night without some fallout.

☹ **MegaShimmer Illuminating Powder Brush** *($3.99)* houses sheer, shiny color in a cylindrical unit that includes a respectable built-in powder brush. Simply turning the component upside down and shaking it releases powder onto the brush. Application is fine, but cling is poor. Within no time the shiny effect is diminished and the shiny particles are all over everything. Not good.

☹ **MegaShimmer Shimmer Dust** *($2.99)* is a loose shimmer powder that has an unappealingly dry, slightly grainy texture. It imparts subtle to glittery shine depending on the shade, but none of them cling well and they feel terrible on skin when used over large areas (such as the décolletage).

☹ **MegaSparkle Loose Confetti** *($2.99)* is loose glitter that has a dimensional, multicolored effect that can be striking in most lighting. The unhappy face rating is because this product has absolutely no ability to cling to skin, meaning the effect is short-lived and glitter gets all over the place.

BRUSHES: ☹ **Brush Kit** *($1.99)* is a too-tiny kit that gives new meaning to the phrase "Why bother?" and the brushes are all the throwaway variety.

☺ **Plush Brush** *($1.99)* is about as plush as a dry loofah. Unless your budget is incredibly tight, this isn't worth the savings.

SPECIALTY PRODUCTS: ☺ **Travel Size Eyelash Curler** *($1.99)* is a decent option for a portable, functional eyelash curler, and its plastic and rubber parts tend to be gentler on lashes than those made of metal.

YVES SAINT LAURENT

YVES SAINT LAURENT AT-A-GLANCE

Strengths: Every sunscreen includes avobenzone for sufficient UVA protection; some moisturizers with elegant textures; good makeup removers and toners; good lip balm; one superior pressed-powder and eyeshadow formula; Radiant Touch is a favorite for good reason; Variations Blush is a great way to experiment with cheek color; two fantastic mascaras; very good liquid highlighter.

Weaknesses: Expensive; a few sunscreens sport SPF ratings below the benchmark SPF 15; no AHA or BHA products; no products to manage acne or combat skin discolorations; mostly mundane moisturizers and serums; pervasive use of jar packaging; antiwrinkle claims that epitomize ridiculous, yet cost hundreds of dollars; mostly average foundations, sometimes due to SPF rating below the benchmark SPF 15; eyeshadow quads; mostly average lipstick and gloss options.

For more information about Yves Saint Laurent, call (212) 715-7339 or visit www.ysl.com or www.Beautypedia.com.

YVES SAINT LAURENT SKIN CARE

YVES SAINT LAURENT AGE EXPERT PRODUCTS

☺ **$$$ Age Expert Age Defying Crème SPF 15** *($88 for 1 ounce)* makes some far-fetched turn-back-the-clock claims, all hinged on what they refer to as "The cosmetic alternative to DHEA, Age Expert contains Ganoderic Fraction—an exclusive active ingredient with a structure similar to the famous hormone of youthfulness, capable of reactivating the vital functions of the epidermis." DHEA is the abbreviated name for dehydroepiandrosterone, a male hormone produced in the adrenal glands that contributes to bone density, muscle mass, and skin tone. Its popularity as an oral supplement comes from its reputation for increasing strength, boosting the immune system, enhancing memory and concentration, reducing depression, preventing weight gain, and heightening libido function. What does any of that have to do with skin? Aside from the suggested association between DHEA and male hormone levels, and hormone levels having an effect on skin, there is no research showing that DHEA has any impact on aging skin when applied topically, though it can penetrate into the skin (Source: *Drug Delivery*,

September/October 2005, pages 275-280; and *Clinics in Geriatric Medicine*, November 2001, pages 661-672). Besides, it isn't the male hormones that improve the texture and appearance of female skin. The feel and suppleness of a woman's skin are affected by the levels of estrogen and progesterone production (male hormones give men's skin its characteristic appearance). Even more ludicrous, after YSL carries on about this ingredient, it actually doesn't show up in this product (DHEA does appear in other skin-care products). Rather YSL uses a bogus alternative that has nothing to do with DHEA, adding up to a lot of bluster with little substance. "Ganoderic Fraction" is a fancy term for the ingredient this product does contain, which is the extract of *Ganoderma lucidum*, a mushroom. There is definitely research showing that, when eaten, this fungus can have many potential benefits as an antioxidant and anti-inflammatory, and for liver and blood-pressure support. However, there is no research showing that it has miraculous benefit when applied topically to skin in teeny amounts (which is all this product contains), or even in huge amounts. About all this moisturizer for normal to slightly dry skin has to offer is broad-spectrum sun protection (with avobenzone for UVA screening). All of the intriguing ingredients are listed well after the preservatives, and jar packaging won't keep most of them stable once you open it.

☺ $$$ **Age Expert Yeux Age Defying Eye Creme** (*$68 for 0.5 ounce*) contains mostly thickeners, film-forming agents, slip agents, and plant oil. It's an OK moisturizer for dry skin anywhere on the face, but it cannot reduce puffiness or darkness under the eye. If anything, the arnica and cypress can be irritating, though the amount used is likely not cause for concern.

☺ $$$ **Age Expert Nuit Age Defying Night Creme** (*$88 for 1 ounce*) is an emollient blend of mostly water, thickener, film-forming agent, Vaseline, silicone, and more thickeners. It contains a very small amount of water-binding agents and the few antioxidants won't remain stable once this jar-packaged product is opened. Do not expect "ultimate restorative action."

YVES SAINT LAURENT CONTOUR EXPERT PRODUCTS

☹ $$$ **Contour Expert Yeux Lifting and Anti-Puffiness Eye Care** (*$63 for 0.5 ounce*) has a very light texture, and wheat germ extract has water-binding properties for skin. However, several ingredients in this "care" product are cause for concern, including alcohol, tansy, bitter-orange, and cypress. All of the other truly beneficial ingredients appear after these problematic ones, making this option a risky proposition.

☹ **Contour Expert Intensive Lifting and Reshaping Serum** (*$86 for 1 ounce*) promises to restore volume and contour to aging skin, but it absolutely cannot do that. No skin-care product can make sunken features plump and full again, nor can a jawline be redefined. That type of improvement is possible only via cosmetic medical procedures. This serum is primarily water and gum-based thickeners, which have a slight plasticizing effect on skin as they dry. The amount of tansy extract (*Tanacetum vulgare*) is cause for concern because this plant can cause severe contact dermatitis (Source: www.naturaldatabase.com). That alone is reason enough to avoid this product.

☺ $$$ **Contour Expert Reshaping and Lifting Creme SPF 10** (*$88 for 1.6 ounces*) contains less tansy extract than the Contour Expert Intensive Lifting and Reshaping Serum above, but still disappoints because of its low SPF rating (though the sunscreen includes avobenzone for UVA protection) and jar packaging. It's an average option for normal to slightly dry skin and does not stand a ghost of a chance of restoring lost facial contours.

YVES SAINT LAURENT HYDRA FEEL PRODUCTS

☺ **$$$ Hydra Feel Comfort Hydrating Water Crème** *($62 for 1.6 ounces)* has some good emollient ingredients for dry to very dry skin, including macadamia nut oil. However, there's more fragrance here than antioxidants, and what few antioxidants are present won't last long once this jar-packaged moisturizer is opened.

☺ **$$$ Hydra Feel Eye Radiant Hydrating Eye Gel** *($44 for 0.5 ounce)* is said to be enriched with "Baby Skin Complex," so the intent is clear; it is intended to evoke the image of youthful skin all the way back to birth. Regardless of your age, not a single ingredient in this lightweight, banal gel moisturizer is going to take your skin back that far, or even back a few minutes in time. Although suitable for normal to slightly dry skin anywhere on the face, this contains few impressive ingredients for the money, and most of the plant extracts have limited to no research concerning their effectiveness for skin of any age.

☹ **Hydra Feel Fresh Hydrating Water Gel** *($62 for 1.6 ounces)* lists alcohol as the second ingredient, and as such is too drying and irritating for all skin types. The amount of alcohol will also make the acrylate-based film-forming agent (think hairspray-type ingredients) that follows it irritating, and will trigger oil production in the pore lining.

☹ **Hydra Feel Soft Hydrating Water Lotion SPF 15** *($62 for 1.6 ounces)* provides sufficient UVA protection with its in-part avobenzone sunscreen, but the second ingredient is alcohol and that makes this nonhydrating product too irritating for all skin types. The alcohol will also trigger oil production in the pore lining.

☺ **$$$ Hydra Feel Gentle Rehydrating Masque** *($48 for 2.5 ounces)* is a simple but silky blend of water with silicones, slip agents, and a tiny amount of the emollient squalane. It's a good mask for normal to dry skin, but doesn't "rehydrate" better than dozens of other moisturizers, many of which offer skin a balanced blend of what YSL includes, plus antioxidants and skin-identical ingredients. Sadly, this mask contains more fragrance than anything unique (or worthy of this product's price) for skin.

YVES SAINT LAURENT LISSE EXPERT PRODUCTS

☹ **$$$ Lisse Expert Esthetic Line Eraser Kit** *($225)* is composed of a **Peeling Masque**, said to provide a "spectacular cosmetic resurfacing effect," and a **Wrinkle Filler Pen** that supplies a dose of topical hyaluronic acid to plump lines. The Pen is also said to stimulate the skin's own synthesis of hyaluronic acid so it will become plumped from within too, further reducing wrinkles and expression lines. When you're charging a price that approaches the cost of genuine cosmetic corrective procedures, you'd better have a good story. In this case, you can skim the cover and skip to the last page because nothing in this product will resurface skin or plump lines to the same extent as professionally administered treatments. The Masque contains about 5% glycolic acid and has a pH low enough to exfoliate skin. It is formulated in a simple base of water and slip agents to enhance penetration of the AHA. The tiny amounts of water-binding and soothing agents are inconsequential compared with the amount of fragrance in this product. The Wrinkle Filler Pen contains so little hyaluronic acid (used in its salt form, sodium hyaluronate, which is considerably less expensive and less effective than pure hyaluronic acid) that it's barely worth mentioning, particularly since it's minimally capable of exerting any sort of benefit on skin. The product dispensed from this pen is mostly water, film-forming agent, alcohol, and gum-based thickener. The film-forming agent works to temporarily smooth lines, while the alcohol just makes every cell dry and dull. Using a well-formulated AHA product from another line (almost all cost less than YSL's version) will work far better for skin, and then if you want to see if a "filler"-type product works, consider those from Avon, Estee Lauder, or Good Skin. They won't make a "Gee, I don't need an injection after all" difference either, but at least they contain far more state-of-the-art ingredients than this version and cost far less!

☺ $$$ **Lisse Expert Advanced Eye and Lip Intensive Anti-Wrinkle Care** *($63 for 0.25 ounce)* is a dual-sided pen: one end dispenses a water- and silicone-based lotion and the other is meant to be used as a massage tool to make the product work better on lines and wrinkles. It is mostly water, silicone, silicone polymer, and salt. You may get some superficial line filling owing to the texture of the silicones, but the effect is short-lived and it's certainly no substitute for what injectable dermal fillers can do.

☺ $$$ **Lisse Expert Advanced Intensive Anti-Wrinkle Crème** *($83 for 1.6 ounces)* is so ordinary it beautifully drives home the point that fashion designers trying to do skin care may have aesthetically pleasing packaging, while the "fabric" of their formulas is much less impressive; they're just hoping to coast by on image alone. If you must have YSL skin care, this is appropriate for normal to dry skin.

☺ $$$ **Lisse Expert Advanced Intensive Anti-Wrinkle Serum** *($93 for 1 ounce)* is an incredibly basic, overpriced, water- and silicone-based serum for all skin types. The styrene film-forming agent can make skin appear smoother and feel slightly taut, but this won't make skin "just like new" any more than wearing Groucho Marx glasses with a mustache is a brilliant disguise.

☹ **Lisse Expert Esthetic Gel-Patch** *($115 for 0.5 ounce)* is one of the biggest wastes of time and money to ever hit cosmetic counters. Reading the claims for this product might just convince you it's a downright cheap alternative to a face-lift, what with all its talk of signaling the skin's self-repair process and of the diffusion of ingredients precisely where wrinkles need it most. However, the formula tells the true story, and in this case the claims are classic fiction. These supposedly targeted "ultra-technical" patches are mostly water, alcohol, gum-based thickener, and more alcohol. They're very irritating and offer absolutely no hope to anyone concerned about aging skin. At best, the irritants, if left on skin overnight, will cause low-grade inflammation that temporarily makes wrinkled areas look less pronounced. But the long-term cost of assaulting your skin with such irritants (and an accompanying dusting of potentially beneficial ingredients) isn't worth one-quarter of what YSL is charging.

YVES SAINT LAURENT TEMPS MAJEUR PRODUCTS

☺ $$$ **Temps Majeur Lotion** *($90 for 6.6 ounces)* is a good, alcohol-free toner for normal to dry skin. It contains some good water-binding agents, skin-smoothing silicone, and nonvolatile plant extracts, but for the money it's still fairly ordinary and not worth it.

☺ $$$ **Temps Majeur Crème** *($330 for 1.6 ounces)* has an elegantly silky texture and contains ingredients that help normal to slightly dry or slightly oily skin feel and look better, but the antioxidant activity of the mushroom extract will be lost once this ultra-pricey jar-packaged product is opened. This is prestigious in name only; for the money, it should be loaded with a range of state-of-the-art ingredients.

☺ $$$ **Temps Majeur Elixir De Nuit** *($462 for 0.7 ounce)* is positioned as an amazing elixir whose potency comes from the "treasures of traditional Chinese remedies," an odd association given YSL's haute couture French image. Rest assured: No culture's ancient remedies are the solution for youthful skin. After all, think of how much was unknown about skin hundreds of years ago! This tiny bottle contains mostly safflower oil, a triglyceride, and *Crambe abyssinica* seed oil. The latter's oil content is a source of erucic acid, which is used to manufacture plastic and lighting implements. It is also considered one of the cheaper oils available, which doesn't make the price of this mostly worthless product any more convincing (Source: www.ibiblio.org/pfaf/cgi-bin/arr_html?Crambe+abyssinica&CAN=LATIND). *Crambe abyssinica* oil contains a fatty acid that can help dry skin, but it isn't nearly as multifaceted as several other oils are for skin, including olive, evening primrose, and flax seed. This serum-like product is an option for dry skin, but the price is nothing less than ludicrous, and the Chinese remedy claim is just plain hokey.

☺ **$$$ Temps Majeur Eye Contour** *($126 for 0.5 ounce)* is a good emollient moisturizer for dry skin anywhere on the face. What a shame that the jar packaging won't keep the mushroom extract stable once this product is being used. The mineral pigments create a soft shine effect on skin, and can slightly "brighten" shadowed areas (though a concealer works much better, and if you want shine, you can dust some shimmer powder on top).

☹ **$$$ Temps Majeur Fluide Intensive Skin Supplement SPF 12** *($330 for 1.7 ounces)* makes me want to scream, mostly because there are people out there who will be swayed by the outrageous price of this product, figuring that anything that costs this much for so little must be youth concentrated in a bottle. Believe me, it isn't! The actual claims for the product aren't all that enticing, basically stating repeatedly that your skin will be really soft if you use this product. Other than including avobenzone for UVA protection, this YSL daytime moisturizer has barely anything going for it. Speaking of sunscreen, any antiwrinkle product should have an SPF rating of at least 15, and this comes up short. Plus, we know that liberal application is a must to achieve the listed level of protection. But how liberal do you think you're going to be with a sunscreen that costs this much? For those who have already invested in this product, I wish I could say the base formula contained something interesting or significant for skin. Instead, the ordinary nature of this formula (and the amount of fragrance relative to the amount of state-of-the-art ingredients) is shocking. Mushroom extract, which is the basis for YSL's Temps Majeur products, is almost the last ingredient listed. What a waste of money and guarantee of dashed hopes with this injudicious product!

☹ **$$$ Temps Majeur Serum** *($336 for 1.6 ounces)* is only worth the price if you believe mushroom stem extract is the fountain of youth. Most species of mushroom have antioxidant capability and various other attributes that can be helpful for skin. But none of these benefits is in line with what YSL claims this serum can do, and the few other potentially intriguing ingredients are barely present. By the way, the gum base of this serum can lend a slightly sticky finish. All told, I wouldn't choose this over serums from Olay, Neutrogena, Clinique, Estee Lauder, or even Clarins.

☹ **$$$ Temps Majeur Ultra Riche Crème** *($330 for 1.6 ounces)* is a suitable moisturizer for dry to very dry skin, but the workhorse ingredients in this product are found in hundreds of other moisturizers with much more realistic prices. You're not getting anything substantial for your substantial investment; if anything, it's quite a letdown to know that the jar packaging won't keep the efficacious antioxidants in this product stable during use.

☹ **$$$ Temps Majeur Masque** *($158 for 1.6 ounces)* is mostly water and film-forming agent with some thickeners. How this average concoction is supposed to offer skin an "intense burst of energy" is a good question. At best, normal to dry skin will look and feel smoother.

OTHER YVES SAINT LAURENT SKIN CARE PRODUCTS

☺ **$$$ Freshness Rinse-Off Foaming Crème** *($38.50 for 5 ounces)* is a very standard, glycerin-rich, water-soluble cleanser that produces copious foam. The foaming action has no effect as far as cleansing, but many consumers prefer this type of cleanser; so here's another one to consider. The amount of potassium hydroxide is potentially drying, and makes this cleanser preferred for those with oily to very oily skin. I don't know why Yves Saint Laurent is touting the species of tree bark they put in this cleanser; it is barely present and it has no effect on skin anyway—so what's the big deal? And the price is due to the brand not the quality of this product!

☺ **$$$ Pureness Cleansing Satiny Oil** *($38.50 for 6.7 ounces)* is a mineral oil–based fluid cleanser that also contains several nonfragrant plant oils. When mixed with water, the water phase of the cleanser emulsifies with the oils to form a milky liquid that cleanses skin and removes makeup quickly. This is a good option for dry to very dry skin not prone to blemishes, but would be even better without the fragrance (which makes this potentially risky to use for removing eye makeup). Oh and the price, completely unjustified and you could do better and cheaper from a range of product lines.

☹ **Pureness Rinse-Off Instant Foam** *($38.50 for 5 ounces)* begins as a very good, though still standard, foaming gel cleanser for normal to oily skin. However, the inclusion of menthol (which does not detoxify skin) makes it too irritating and not preferred over several gentle cleansing gels, most of which cost a lot less than this.

☺ **$$$ Softness Cleansing Silky Balm** *($38.50 for 5 ounces)* is a very emollient, creamy cleanser for dry to very dry skin. It requires a washcloth for complete removal, and removes all types of makeup. You're not getting anything special for your money (other than the cachet that comes with a fashion designer's name, a point your skin could care less about), but if your skin type fits the bill, this is an indulgent option.

☺ **$$$ Softness Rinse-Off Foaming Water** *($38.50 for 6.7 ounces)* is a very standard but good water-soluble cleanser for all skin types except dry or sensitive (due to the amount of fragrance it contains). It rinses completely and removes all but waterproof makeup easily. This doesn't bring your skin to a state of radiant purity any better than any other water-soluble cleanser, but I guess such descriptions help seduce consumers into spending more than they need to for cleansed skin!

☺ **$$$ 3-in-1 Cleansing Water** *($38.50 for 6.7 ounces)* is a good, fairly gentle liquid makeup remover for all skin types except very oily. It is not the best for use around the eyes because it contains fragrance and citrus peel extract.

☺ **$$$ Freshness Cleansing Milky Veil** *($37 for 6.7 ounces)* is accurately described as a milky gel, and it becomes a fluid when mixed with water. Its formula is similar to those of most dual-phase eye makeup removers, and it certainly works swiftly to remove makeup. In addition to the price, however, another drawback is the large amount of fragrance, which can be a problem, especially if you intend to use it around your eyes. Overall, it's an OK option for all skin types, but you certainly don't need to spend this much to remove makeup.

☺ **$$$ Instant Eye Make-Up Remover** *($30 for 3.4 ounces)* is a standard, dual-phase eye-makeup remover that works very well to remove all types of makeup. It is fragrance-free and suitable for all skin types, and contains soothing plant extracts. The tiny amount of panthenol this contains will not help make eyelashes stronger.

☺ **$$$ Gommage Natural Action Exfoliator** *($44 for 2.5 ounces)* is sold as an exfoliant that does not contain abrasive particles, instead relying on sugars and oils to remove dead skin cells. Although it is admittedly interesting to watch this gel turn oily and then milky when mixed with water and applied to skin, the tiny amount of sugar won't dissolve a single dead skin cell—though your skin will be smoother and softer after using this due to the moisturizing agents it contains.

☺ **$$$ Baume Nourrissant, Moisturizing Lip and Nail Balm** *($25 for 0.5 ounce)* is a standard emollient lip balm that is way overpriced for what you get. However, if you fall for the designer trappings of YSL, at least this product will take good care of dry lips and nails.

☹ **$$$ Gloss Repulpant Shiny Lip Plumper SPF 10** *($25)* includes avobenzone for UVA protection, but would be better if the SPF rating were 15 instead of 10. Although this does not list any of the usual suspect plumping ingredients (read: lip irritants), the minty sensation is there, which isn't great for routine application. Despite that and a lack of wow-inducing plumping results, this sheer lip gloss wears well and imparts sheer, juicy color. This would get a happy face rating if the sunscreen were rated SPF 15.

YVES SAINT LAURENT MAKEUP

FOUNDATION: ☺ **$$$ Perfect Touch Radiant Brush Foundation** *($55)* comes in a unique component that features a built-in synthetic foundation brush. Carefully squeezing the tube pushes a silky liquid foundation onto the brush, allowing you to paint it on. The foundation begins slightly thick but blends very well, providing sheer to light coverage and a luminous finish suitable for normal to dry skin. YSL offers 15 shades, and just over half are remarkably neutral. The following shades are too peach, orange, or copper for most skin tones: #6, #8, #10, #12, #13, and #14. The brush applicator is workable if you prefer this method of applying foundation, though it blends just as well using your fingertips or a makeup sponge.

☺ **$$$ Matt Touch Foundation SPF 10** *($50)* had great potential to be an outstanding oil-absorbing foundation with a long-lasting matte finish for very oily skin. The main problem is the lack of sufficient UVA protection and an SPF rating too low for adequate daytime protection (at least if you're concerned with following sunscreen guidelines from almost every major dermatologic association). The silicone-based texture dispenses from its tube nearly as thick as toothpaste; however, the texture quickly softens as it warms on your skin, and leaves it feeling incredibly silky with a powdery finish. It feels nearly weightless, but the finish will grossly exaggerate even a slight hint of dry skin or flaking. There are 12 shades, which is more than most of YSL's other foundations offer. All blend out softer and more neutral than they first appear, but there are definitely some colors to avoid, including #3, #10, and #11. Shade #6 is slightly peach, but may work for some medium skin tones. I wish all the elements were in place to make this a slam-dunk recommendation for very oily, acne-prone skin. As is, this unique foundation has enough drawbacks for it to not deserve better than a neutral face rating.

☺ **$$$ Teint Compact Hydra Feel SPF 10** *($55)* features an in-part avobenzone sunscreen, yet the SPF rating is frustratingly short of the recommended minimum for daytime protection. This is otherwise an innovative cream-to-powder makeup packaged in an elegant compact complete with a very good sponge applicator. The semi-solid cake doesn't allow you to pick up product as easily as many cream-to-powders, but it smooths onto skin easily and blends to an ultralight satin finish while providing light to medium coverage. It is best for normal to dry skin looking for a radiant yet natural finish. With the exception of shade #6, all of the colors are impeccable and include options for fair to tan skin tones.

☺ **$$$ Teint Eclat de Soie Radiance Smoothing Foundation SPF 8** *($54)* has an SPF rating that's too low for daytime wear, though it is titanium dioxide–based. This liquid foundation has a fluid, silky texture and a very smooth application that sets to a soft, radiant finish. What a shame the sunscreen rating isn't higher! If you decide to pair this with a product rated SPF 15 or greater, it is best for normal to dry skin, and only two of the eight shades (#1 and #3) are a problematic shade of peach.

☺ **$$$ Teint Majeur Luxurious Foundation SPF 18** *($99)* has an enviable, beautifully silky texture and a gorgeous skin-like finish while providing medium coverage. What a shame that the price is so out of line and that the sunscreen lacks the UVA-protecting ingredients of avobenzone, titanium dioxide, zinc oxide, Mexoryl SX, or Tinosorb. Without this key element, there is no way this otherwise terrific foundation (even the shade range is impressively neutral) can work "antiaging miracles" for anyone's skin.

☺ **$$$ Teint Mat Purete Transfer-Resistant Fluid Foundation SPF 15** *($51)* does not contain the UVA-protecting ingredients of titanium dioxide, zinc oxide, avobenzone, Mexoryl SX (ecamsule), or Tinosorb, and should not be relied on for daily sun protection. That's unfortunate, because this is an otherwise excellent foundation for normal to oily or combination skin. The slightly thick consistency becomes silky and fluid during blending, quickly setting to a dimensional (rather than flat or masklike) matte finish. It provides light to medium coverage and offers good staying power, too. Among the eight shades, #1, #2, and #3 are slightly peach, but may work for some light skin tones. The other shades are flawless.

☺ **$$$ Teint Singulier Sheer Powder Creme Veil** *($47)* has a slippery texture that dries to a satin-matte finish, providing sheer coverage that would work for someone with normal to dry skin. Most of the four shades are off-color and tend toward pinks and peaches, but this is so sheer it doesn't really matter. Contrary to the vastly inflated claims, this does not "perfectly shape the face" in any way, nor is it capable of concealing blemishes.

CONCEALER: ☹ **Anti-Cernes Multi-Action Concealer** *($34)*. It takes a lot of chutzpah to charge so much for such a greasy, heavy-looking concealer that creases in no time. If for some reason you prefer this type of product, there are significantly less expensive versions available at the drugstore.

POWDER: ✓ ☺ **$$$ Poudre Compact Eclat et Matite Matt & Radiant Pressed Powder** *($45.50)* is a buttery-smooth, talc-based pressed powder that melds with skin to create a very natural nonpowdery finish. This is an outstanding pressed-powder option for those with normal to dry skin (those with oily skin or oily areas may find this not absorbent enough). All six shades are neutral and matte.

☺ **$$$ Poudre de Soleil SPF 10** *($48)* is a pressed bronzing powder with a beautifully silky texture and a low-wattage shine finish that doesn't flake. The sunscreen is titanium dioxide, and because this product would be used as an adjunct to a regular sunscreen or foundation with sunscreen, it deserves a happy face rating. There are three shades, with the best being Golden Sun 2. Light Sun 1 is almost too sheer to show even a slight tanned appearance, but may work for very fair skin tones. This applies smoothly and evenly and is definitely a bronzing powder worth considering if your budget is generous.

☺ **$$$ Poudre Sur Mesure Semi-Loose Powder** *($58)* comes in a cake form, but the container shaves off the top layer when you twist it, creating a loose powder. It's less messy than conventional loose powder, but this clever convenience doesn't come cheap. The talc- and aluminum starch-based formula goes on sheer and has a dry finish suitable for normal to very oily skin. Each of the five colors has a bit of shine, so this is not for those who want to use powder to keep shine at bay.

BLUSH: ☺ $$$ **Variations Blush** *($44)* features four quilted strips of tone-on-tone colors, which is where the "variations" part of the name comes into play (for example, you get subtle variations on pinks or berry tones). All of the shades in each compact have shine and are incredibly silky, while also being strongly pigmented (which is a plus for dark skin tones). Despite the intensity, this applies smoothly and offers a luminous rather than sparkling finish. Compacts 6 and 11 are great for bronzing or contouring.

☹ $$$ **Touche Blush** *($42)* is a loose-powder blush whose base component comes with an attached cheek-size sponge for on-the-spot application. The concept is intriguing but the execution tends to place blush-colored powder all over your face instead of just on your cheek area, though you can temper this somewhat if you're extra careful about application. Still, applying blush should be easier than this. Four shades are available (additional, limited-edition shades are often seen in seasonal collections), and although all are sheer and workable, each is infused with large particles of sparkle that tend to go everywhere. If the sparkles don't bother you and you're in the mood for a novel way to apply powder blush, you may want to give this an audition if you happen upon a YSL counter.

EYESHADOW: ✓ ☺ $$$ **Ombre Solo Double Effect** *($28.50)* presents two tone-on-tone powder eyeshadows in one sleek compact. This is YSL's silkiest eyeshadow formula, and it applies superbly, builds intensity well, and doesn't flake. All of the duos are shiny, but most are not distractingly so (#5 and #6 are the least shiny).

☺ $$$ **Ombres Duolumieres Eye Shadow Duo** *($41)* are worth considering (price notwithstanding) if you want lots of shine and strong colors. The pairings are much more workable than they used to be, with predominantly brown and gray tones ideal for shadowing and shaping.

☹ $$$ **Frozen Eye Shadow** *($28.50)* is a loose-powder eyeshadow packaged in a small, vial-type bottle that includes a sponge-tip wand applicator. Each of the colors lays down an intense, opaque shine and must be blended quickly because the consistency causes them to set quickly and then become immovable. The good news is that this shadow lasts and lasts; the bad news is it's tricky to get such strong, shiny colors blended well. This is one to test at the counter and see if you like the application and the result.

☹ $$$ **Ombre Solo Mono Eyeshadow** *($28.50)* consists of pressed-powder eyeshadows with a silky but dry texture that hinders application a bit and leads to some flaking. The shade selection favors strong shine. If the flaking weren't an issue the shine would be tolerable, but at this price an eyeshadow should be nearly perfect in every way.

☹ **Ombres Quadralumieres Eye Shadow Quartet** *($54)* is no match for the powder eye-shadows from haute couture fashion competitor Dior, and the prices of the two lines are nearly identical. These YSL quads suffer from a dry texture that makes blending difficult (though they do have some smoothness) and especially from terribly contrasting colors that are for fantasy, not real-world, makeup.

EYE AND BROW SHAPER: ☺ $$$ **Eyeliner Moiré Liquid Eyeliner** *($32)* is a liquid liner with a thin, tapered brush that applies evenly, allowing you to lay down a solid line with one swift stroke. All of the colors (except black) are metallic and the formula takes longer than it should to dry, but if you can endure that, it stays on marvelously well.

☺ $$$ **Dessin du Regard Haute Tenue Long-Lasting Eye Pencil** *($28)* would have earned a happy face rating were it not for the required sharpening. It's an above-average pencil whose performance bests many standard pencils due to its smooth application, suitable range of shades, and smudge-proof finish.

☺ **$$$ Eyebrow Enhancer Duo** *($29)* combines a brow gel and brow color in one dual-sided product. The sheer brow color is applied with a sponge-tip applicator, which is odd but workable if you are really careful, while the brow gel is applied with a regular mascara-like brush. It's an OK option for slightly darkening and grooming brows, but combining the products can feel heavy and give brows a wet look that may or may not be to your liking.

☺ **$$$ Eyebrow Pencil** *($27)* costs a mint and needs routine sharpening, but it's a good, non-greasy eyebrow pencil that won't smudge. It finishes and remains slightly tacky, but that's less of an issue if you apply this softly. Among the standard shades, #4 is puzzlingly shiny.

☺ **$$$ Eyeliner Noir** *($32)* is an average liquid eyeliner with an out-of-line price tag. Application can be tricky because the brush is a bit too long and flimsy, dry time is slow, and it tends to smear if you blink while waiting for it to set.

LIPSTICK, LIP GLOSS, AND LIPLINER: ✓ ☺ **$$$ Gloss Pur Pure Lip Gloss** *($29)* is a brush-on lip gloss that has a decadent, slightly syrupy texture that glides over lips and provides a luscious glossy finish. The colors look quite dark and imposing in the container, but each goes on sheer and may work alone or over lipstick. The ingredient statement lists butyl methoxydibenzoylmethane (aka avobenzone), but it's not listed as active and so you cannot rely on it for UVA protection. Although pricey, this is an undeniably enticing lip gloss with a smooth, non-sticky finish.

✓ ☺ **$$$ Touche Brilliance Sparkling Touch for Lips** *($30)* is a fantastic lip gloss that is packaged just like YSL's Touche Eclat Radiant Touch highlighter, meaning the gloss is dispensed onto a synthetic brush applicator. The texture is superb and the finish is a gleaming shine that's not the least bit sticky. As for the colors, they're an enticing mix of sheer, bright, and bold metallic.

☺ **$$$ Baume d'Ete Tinted Lip Balm SPF 10** *($23)* has an in-part avobenzone sunscreen and although SPF 10 isn't ideal, it's better than no lip sunscreen at all. This sheer, slightly viscous gloss comes in a tube and has a sticky (but not intolerably so) feel that makes it rather tenacious. It's a good option if you don't mind needlessly splurging on lip gloss.

☺ **$$$ Fard a Levres Rouge Pur Pure Lipstick SPF 8** *($29)* offers mostly bright shades (including many warm reds and oranges) in a fairly greasy lipstick formula that goes on opaque and has a glossy finish. These are richly pigmented, which is nice, but the glossiness allows them to easily bleed and feather into lines around the mouth. The sunscreen is all titanium dioxide, and although SPF 8 isn't the benchmark to strive for, when it comes to lipsticks, it's better than nothing.

☺ **$$$ Rouge Vibration Magnetic Glow Comfortable Lipstick** *($29)* is a modern, sophisticated lipstick with a highbrow price. It is indeed comfortable and the slim-line case houses a smooth, lightweight cream lipstick that offers medium opacity and a slight stain complete with a high-shine finish.

☺ **$$$ Dessin des Levres Lip Liner** *($26)* is a very good standard pencil that feels slightly creamy going on, but ends up having a drier than usual finish, which helps keep it in place. The color range has been toned down and now favors browns, mauves, and reds—so there are clearly some missing links between this and Saint Laurent's lipstick palette.

☺ **$$$ Golden Gloss Shimmering Lip Gloss** *($28)* gets its shimmer from particles of glitter, and although the multidimensional effect is striking, the glitter tends to feel slightly grainy as the emollience of the gloss wears away. It's not a bad lip gloss, but for the money it should stay smooth and soft longer.

☺ **$$$ Lisse Gloss Smoothing Lip Gloss** *($27)* is your everyday wand gloss that features sheer, unquestionably glossy colors with a tacky feel. It's an OK option, but if you're all about YSL this isn't preferred to their Touche Brilliance Sparkling Touch for Lips or a dozen options from the drugstore.

☺ **$$$ Rouge Pur Shine Sheer Lipstick SPF 15** *($29)* does not contain the UVA-protecting ingredients of titanium dioxide, zinc oxide, avobenzone, Mexoryl SX, or Tinosorb, so it is not recommended as a reliable lipstick with sunscreen. It is otherwise a slick, shimmer-infused lipstick that feels very light and features some gorgeous soft colors. Its neutral face rating is for not including sufficient UVA protection.

☺ **$$$ Rouge Volupte Lipstick** *($34)* has beautiful packaging and some rich colors that leave a lasting stain on lips. Unfortunately, this expensive lipstick is also one of the greasiest lipsticks around. This will travel into lines around the mouth before you can say "I like this color!" and it has a slick, glossy finish that's more prone to movement than any lipstick I've seen in recent memory.

MASCARA: ✓☺ **$$$ Everlong Mascara Lengthening Mascara** *($28.50)* isn't quite as impressive as the YSL mascara above, but is still worthy of its rating. The short, dense bristles allow you to build prodigious length and enough thickness to satisfy, all with only minor clumps that are easily combed through. This also leaves lashes softly curled, and wears without a smear or flake.

✓☺ **$$$ Volume Effet Faux Cils Luxurious Mascara for a False Lash Effect** *($28.50)* doesn't quite measure up to the effect obtainable from false eyelashes, but it ranks as YSL's best mascara. That's because it builds beautifully and thickens well without clumps. The result is lashes that are dramatic without being over the top, and all with a soft, fringed curl. This mascara also comes off completely with a water-soluble cleanser.

☺ **$$$ Everlong Mascara Waterproof Lengthening Mascara** *($28.50)* produces extra-long, perfectly separated lashes with just a few strokes, if you can get used to this mascara's extra-large, barrel-shaped brush (and don't mind the expense), It isn't much for building noticeable thickness, but its claim to fame is length, and it definitely delivers that! It is waterproof yet keeps lashes soft and requires an oil- or silicone-based makeup remover at the end of the day.

☺ **$$$ Mascara Volume Infini Curl Volumizing Mascara for Infinite Curl** *($28.50)* has a heavy, wet application that leads to smearing if you're not extremely careful, and the effect may not be worth it, depending on your preferences (and budget). This mascara quickly lengthens and uplifts lashes, leading to a sweeping, dramatic effect that begs for shameless flirting. Have a clean mascara wand or lash brush handy because you may need to comb through some minor clumps.

☹ **$$$ Mascara Aquaresistant Mascara Waterproof** *($27.50)* is expertly waterproof, even if lashes get completely soaked. Yet that's about the only exciting aspect of this otherwise ordinary mascara. Lashes get somewhat longer and there are no clumps, but for the money there are much more impressive waterproof mascaras at the drugstore.

FACE ILLUMINATING PRODUCTS: ✓☺ **$$$ Teint Parfait Complexion Enhancer** *($42)* is sold as a sheer highlighter for allover use on the face, and is ideal for this purpose. The easy-to-blend lotion texture imparts a sheer, slight shimmer finish that works under or over foundation. It sets to a matte (in feel) finish and is suitable for all skin types, particularly those with dull complexions. Shade #1 is a pale lilac that may be OK for very fair skin, but test it first; shade #6 has a peachy cast that should also be considered carefully. The four remaining shades are attractive and versatile, and the shimmer stays put.

BRUSHES: ☺ **$$$ Yves Saint Laurent Brushes** *($29.50-$55)* are a small, workable collection of brushes that are better than they used to be, though in terms of overall quality and performance, they still lag behind most other lines (many that charge less for similar brushes), including M.A.C., Stila, Trish McEvoy, and Laura Mercier.

The ☹ **$$$ Powder Brush** *($55)* while very soft, is the weakest (but still worthy) option because it's not dense enough to apply more than a sheer dusting of powder. The other brushes are all worth considering and are readily available for testing at the counter.

SPECIALTY PRODUCTS: ☺ **$$$ Matt Touch** *($42)* has a luxuriously silky, weightless texture that works to slightly fill in pores and make skin feel supremely smooth. Of course this also facilitates foundation application, just as most serums and moisturizers with this kind of texture do. Its oil-control abilities aren't as good as those of similar options from Clinique and Smashbox, but if you happen to come across it and want to try a sample under your makeup, go for it.

☺ **$$$ Touche Eclat Radiant Touch** *($40)* is far and away the most popular YSL makeup item and one that is routinely featured in fashion magazine "best of beauty" lists. It's the original brush-on highlighter, cleverly packaged in a pen-style component with a built-in synthetic brush. Although not much for concealing (the coverage isn't too substantial), it functions well as a highlighter or to add a subtle radiance to shadowy areas, particularly under the eyes. It is light enough to layer over a regular concealer (which you'll need if dark circles are apparent), and the best of the four shades are #1 and #2. Shade #3 is slightly peach but likely too sheer to matter, while #4 has an orange cast that limits its appeal. As an option, and I mean a really impressive option, try Maybelline's Instant Age Rewind Double Face Perfector, which works perfectly and for far less money.

ZIA NATURAL (SKIN CARE ONLY)

ZIA NATURAL AT-A-GLANCE

Strengths: The company provides complete product ingredient lists on their Web site.

Weaknesses: Several products contain one or more irritating ingredients that have no established benefit for skin; several of the sunscreens do not provide sufficient UVA protection; no reliable AHA, BHA, or anti-acne products.

For more information about Zia, call (800) 334-7546 or visit www.zianatural.com or www. Beautypedia.com.

ZIA NATURAL SKIN BASICS PRODUCTS

☹ **$$$ Skin Basics Fresh Cleansing Gel, for Normal Skin** *($17.95 for 8.3 ounces)* is indeed a basic water-soluble cleanser whose main cleansing agent isn't going to remove makeup very well. It's an OK option for those with normal to slightly dry skin, but would be better without the fragrant plant oil. Oh, and the sea algae, even if it could have a benefit, would be rinsed down the drain before it could have any impact on skin.

☺ **Skin Basics Moisturizing Cleanser, for Dry Skin** *($17.95 for 8.3 ounces)*. Those with normal to dry skin who prefer a lotion cleanser without detergent cleansing agents may want to consider this product. With the exception of fragrant ylang-ylang oil (not the best for use around the eyes), this moisture-rich cleanser leaves skin feeling smooth, and it does remove makeup, though a washcloth is advised to avoid leaving a residue.

☹ **Skin Basics Sea Tonic Aloe Toner, for Oily Skin** *($14.95 for 6.7 ounces)* comes up short as far as including a blend of helpful ingredients for skin, and smells more like eau de cologne than anything else. It is not recommended for any skin type because it contains irritating fragrant oils, including cypress and ylang-ylang. Leaving those on your skin isn't smart, because neither has any established benefit that makes the irritation worth the risk.

☹ **Skin Basics Sea Tonic Rosewater & Aloe Toner, for Normal/Dry Skin** *($14.95 for 6.7 ounces)* is closer to eau de cologne than good skin care. The rosewater-based formula is fragrant, and this is intensified by the rose and ylang-ylang oils. Despite claims to the contrary, rose flower oil contains components that can be irritating to skin (Sources: *Journal of Separation Science*, February 2008, pages 262-267; and *Planta*, July 2004, pages 468-478). This isn't basic for any skin type.

☹ **$$$ Skin Basics Bamboo Exfoliant** *($24.95 for 6.7 ounces)* is a topical scrub that exfoliates with ground-up pieces of bamboo, which are gentler than apricot pits or walnut shells, but overall not preferred to other scrub particles (from jojoba beads to polyethylene beads) that can be used in skin-care products, or even a plain washcloth. Although this can be a good scrub for normal to dry skin not prone to blemishes, the inclusion of irritating lemon peel and ylang-ylang oils isn't ideal.

☹ **Skin Basics Daily Moisture Screen SPF 15, for All Skin Types** *($20.95 for 1.6 ounces).* Sun protection is an integral part of any sensible skin-care routine, but this sunscreen leaves skin vulnerable to UVA damage because it lacks the UVA-protecting ingredients of titanium dioxide, zinc oxide, avobenzone, Tinosorb, or Mexoryl SX. It is absolutely not recommended.

☹ **Skin Basics Essential Eye Gel, for All Skin Types** *($23.95 for 0.5 ounce)* is a lightweight, fragrant gel moisturizer that contains a frustrating, skin-confusing blend of beneficial and irritating ingredients. The helpful ingredients are found in many other moisturizers, which makes this option not worth considering, because why subject your skin to needless irritating ingredients if there are better alternatives?

☺ **Skin Basics Everyday Moisturizer, for Normal Skin** *($20.95 for 1.6 ounces)* is a good moisturizer for its labeled skin type, but is probably best for dry to very dry skin. The soybean oil (a main ingredient) is a reliable source of antioxidants and emolliency, while water-binding agents and other emollients are abundant. A greater array of antioxidants and a cell-communicating ingredient or two would've elevated this to Paula's Pick status. Surprisingly, though thankfully, it does not contain fragrance or fragrant plant extracts like most every other Zia product.

☹ **Skin Basics Herbal Moisture Gel, for Oily Skin** *($26.95 for 1.6 ounces)* is a rosewater-based gel moisturizer that contains too many problematic plant extracts along with irritating fragrant oils of tangerine and sandalwood. None of these are beneficial for oily skin (or any type of skin for that matter), and it is not recommended.

☹ **Skin Basics Nourishing Creme** *($36.95 for 1 ounce)* contains nothing nourishing or basic in this fairly standard moisturizer packaged in a jar container, which allows the plant extracts to be exposed to air and therefore diminishes their potency. Although this moisturizer contains some beneficial ingredients for dry skin, it also contains several irritating ingredients, including lavender, lemon peel, and geranium oils. Considering the state-of-the-art moisturizers that are available elsewhere, there is no reason to choose this one.

ZIA NATURAL ULTIMATE PRODUCTS

☹ **Ultimate Cleansing Mousse** *($21.95 for 4 ounces)*. Given the irritating citrus oils, I wouldn't consider this an ultimate cleanser any more than I would consider the telegraph a modern way to communicate. A standard water-soluble foaming cleanser is at its core, the irritants make it a problem for all skin types, and the price tag is irritating as well.

☺ **$$$ Ultimate Deep Pore Cleanser** *($25.95 for 4 ounces)* is not advised if you're looking to thoroughly clean your pores of oil and cellular debris. It does not contain any cleansing agents, and the emollient thickeners pose a risk of clogging pores rather than cleansing them. The fragrant oils aren't helpful, but at least their presence is minimal. You'll get a mild abrasive action from the jojoba beads, but considering the aforementioned drawbacks, your pores would be much happier with a water-soluble cleanser and a washcloth!

☹ **Ultimate Exfoliant** *($29.95 for 2 ounces)*. Zia tries to convince you that this product is a natural source of AHAs, and to some extent that's true—technically, lemon and lime are alpha hydroxy acids due to their citric acid component, but there is no research showing they can effectively exfoliate skin. On the other hand, there is extensive research showing how glycolic and lactic acids can exfoliate. The papaya base of this product also is an issue, not just because the enzymes are unstable, but because the papain enzyme in papaya can be irritating to skin, especially for anyone allergic to latex (Source: www.naturaldatabase.com).

☺ **$$$ Ultimate Toning Mist, for Normal/Dry Skin** *($21.95 for 4 ounces)* would come close to being the ultimate toning mist for its intended skin type if it did not contain cell-damaging lavender oil and irritating rosewood oil. Also present is DMAE (dimethylaminoethanol), which has controversial research detailing its helpfulness, but also has potential problems when applied to skin (for details please see the entry for DMAE in our *Cosmetic Ingredient Dictionary* at www. Beautypedia.com). This is not the ultimate solution for smoothing wrinkles or firming skin.

☹ **Ultimate Toning Mist, for Normal/Oily Skin** *($21.95 for 4 ounces)*. Given that irritating witch hazel is part of the botanical infusion (plant tea), along with the controversial ingredient DMAE (dimethylaminoethanol—see our *Cosmetic Ingredient Dictionary* at www. Beautypedia.com for details) and irritating citrus oils, this is far from the ultimate toning mist for any skin type.

☺ **Ultimate Age-Defying Solar Care Face SPF 30, Oil-Free** *($17.95 for 1.8 ounces)* has an in-part avobenzone sunscreen that will provide broad-spectrum protection and has a base formula that's suitable for normal to dry skin, but the inclusion of balsam peru (a common skin sensitizer) is cause for concern. The amount of balsam is tiny, but it keeps this sunscreen from earning a happy face rating.

☹ **Ultimate "C" Serum** *($39.95 for 0.5 ounce)* is a water-based, antioxidant-loaded serum that comes close in many respects to being the ultimate, but it contains grapefruit oil. Topical application of grapefruit oil can cause contact dermatitis and/or a phototoxic reaction when skin is exposed to sunlight (Source: www.naturaldatabase.com). Oddly, Zia recommends applying this to sunburned skin! Ouch!

☹ **Ultimate Day Renewal** *($40.95 for 1 ounce)* is Zia's answer to a "works-like-Botox" product because it contains acetyl hexapeptide-3, a peptide whose manufacturer claims it has a Botox-like effect, but, of course, there is no substantiated proof. Remember, even Botox itself has no effect on expression lines when applied topically rather than injected into the muscles that control the formation of these lines. Unfortunately, this serum is not recommended, not only because it doesn't work as claimed, but also because it contains several irritating essential (fragrant) oils.

☹ **$$$ Ultimate Eye Creme** *($35.95 for 0.5 ounce)* is loaded with several beneficial ingredients, but it's hard to get past the fact that it is formulated in a base of irritating witch hazel and fragrant rose water. Another detriment is that the jar packaging will allow the antioxidants in this product to degrade. With some slight formulary adjustments and better packaging, this could have been one of the ultimate eye creams for dry to very dry skin.

☹ **Ultimate Moisture** *($39.95 for 1.5 ounces)*. Perhaps this is Zia's "most popular moisturizer" because of its name (it certainly is boastful); however, the product itself has three major weaknesses: jar packaging, which won't keep the many antioxidants and vitamins it contains stable during use; lavender and grapefruit oils, which won't do your skin any favors (though they contribute to this product's natural scent, so maybe that's the draw); and the main floral extract (chrysanthemum), which contains camphor and other irritating fragrant components that serve only to inflame rather than soothe your skin.

☹ **Ultimate Night Renewal** *($40.95 for 1 ounce)* is just a standard emollient moisturizer whose antioxidant capacity will be lessened due to the unfortunate choice of jar packaging. That's a shame, because this contains several notable antioxidants. It also contains the controversial ingredient DMAE (dimethylaminoethanol), though the small amount is likely not cause for concern. The essential oils may please your nose, but they're trouble for your skin, and hardly what you should expect to find in any skin-care product labeled "ultimate."

☹ **Ultimate Oil-Free Moisture** *($33.95 for 2 ounces)*. I could elaborate on why the skin-firming claims for this product are completely bogus and how the botanical extracts in here have no possibility to fight the "signs" of aging or any other signs, besides improving dry skin (and it isn't oil-free in the least because it contains "essential oils"). Instead, I'll just cut to the chase and state that this below-average moisturizer is not recommended because it contains irritating, sensitizing citrus oils, which is a shame because otherwise it would have rated a happy face.

☹ **Ultimate Age Defying Mask** *($29.95 for 3 ounces)*. Although this moisturizing mask has some redeeming qualities, it has a rather unpleasant texture that makes your skin feel a bit sticky, but the bigger issue is the irritating fragrant oils, including rosemary and red mandarin. For the money, the moisturizing masks from Estee Lauder or Aveda are much better for dry to very dry skin.

☺ **Ultimate Age-Defying Solar Care Sunless Tanner** *($17.95 for 4 ounces)* is a standard self-tanning lotion for normal to dry skin. It contains the same ingredient (dihydroxyacetone) found in almost every self-tanner being sold. The negative feature of this product is the inclusion of the known skin sensitizer balsam peru. The small amount isn't likely cause for concern, but why risk irritation at all when there are so many excellent self-tanners that work without the chance of irritating skin?

OTHER ZIA PRODUCTS

☹ **Skin Balancing Tonic** *($27.95 for 3.3 ounces)* contains enough witch hazel water (which is mostly alcohol, not water) to cause dryness and irritation, while the fragrant oils (including eucalyptus) are incapable of balancing skin, although they can cause irritation. The price is insulting for a product that's truly a burn for skin.

☹ **Natural Microdermabrasion Scrub** *($39.95 for 2.5 ounces)* is an incredibly abrasive scrub because it contains pumice, but it also contains several fragrant oils in amounts significant enough to be very irritating. The company claims their magnesium oxide crystals are safer than the aluminum oxide crystals used in traditional microdermabrasion treatments, but there is no proof of that. In fact, the warnings and precautions for both ingredients are equal, and both can exfoliate skin in crystalline form (Source: *Handbook of Cosmetic and Personal Care Additives*, Second Edition, Synapse Information Resources, 2002).

☺ **Citrus Night Time Reversal, for Normal to Dry Skin** *($29.95 for 1.67 ounces)*. How this product is supposed to exfoliate skin is anyone's guess because it doesn't contain any ingredients that can accomplish that. It's merely an emollient moisturizer for normal to dry skin. The acid it contains, which is the result of the sugar cane, buttermilk, and citrus, doesn't work in the same manner as AHAs such as glycolic and lactic acids, and none of them can help make pores look smaller. If anything, the oil in this moisturizer-masquerading-as-an-AHA-product will potentially clog pores or make your skin look greasier, and that can definitely make pores look larger.

☺ **$$$ Deep Moisture Repair Serum** *($36.95 for 0.5 ounce)* has the ability to make normal to slightly dry skin look and feel better. It contains skin-beneficial ingredients—cell-communicating ingredients, water-binding agents, and plant extracts—but also a tiny amount of irritating grapefruit peel oil and a base of fragrant rose water. The latter two additions keep this product from earning a happy face rating, but it is certainly recommended over several other serums and moisturizers from Zia.

☺ **$$$ Moisture Infusion Serum with CoQ10** *($42.95 for 0.5 ounce)*. If you store this nonaqueous serum away from light, it is a very good, simply formulated option for dry to very dry skin. The olive oil base is helpful for dry skin, while the vitamin E and ubiquinone (coenzyme Q10) provide an antioxidant punch. Although not as well-rounded as many other antioxidant serums, and pricey for what you get, it may be worth a try. The fragrance-free formula and the absence of plant irritants make it a contender for those with dry, sensitive skin.

☹ **Seaweed Lift Serum, for All Skin Types** *($36.95 for 0.5 ounce)* is not recommended, whether your skin needs lifting or not (though no serum or moisturizer can lift skin anywhere), because this water-based serum contains irritating lavender, rosewood, geranium, and orange oils along with an unidentified essential oil blend for fragrance. Talk about getting away from what skin really needs to thrive!

☺ **15 Minute Face Lift** *($20.95)* has a name that promises results in 15 minutes; however, a more accurate description would be to say that the results last for 15 minutes or less. The **15 Minute Face Lift Powder** that you're directed to mix with the **Sea Tonic Rosewater & Aloe Toner** is mostly cornstarch and egg white (albumen) with a tiny amount of soothing agents. The Toner is really eau de cologne and not skin care in the least. The floral rose water content along with the other fragrant irritants, despite the few beneficial ingredients, makes this a product to avoid. You are supposed to mix the Powder with the Toner. As expected, no actual lifting takes place. Rather, as the cornstarch and egg white dry, they make your skin feel temporarily tighter. The effect won't last for long, especially if you move your face even a little, and nothing in here has any effect on facial muscles. Thinking otherwise is akin to sitting on your couch and watching an exercise video rather than getting up and following along. Overall, the only thing this kit will lift is money from your pocketbook. Products like this have come and gone over the years (I can't tell you how many I've reviewed) and all of them are a waste of money, and not one of them has put a plastic surgeon out of business!

☹ **Apple Refining Mask** *($24.95 for 1.2 ounces)* contains lots of natural ingredients in this fruity mask, which makes this a prime example of why natural isn't always a slam dunk solution for your skin. The lemon juice is exceedingly irritating, as is the grapefruit oil, and not a single ingredient in this mask will benefit clogged skin. If anything, this amount of food-based ingredients can serve as a source of fuel for the bacteria that trigger blemishes.

☹ **French Clay Purifying Mask** *($24.95 for 1 ounce)*. What could've been an effective, gentle clay mask for oily skin is negated by the inclusion of irritating peppermint, tangerine, and sage oils. These "pure essential oils" do not balance skin or control bacteria, at least not the kind of bacteria that promotes acne, and the irritation they cause results in skin damage, which is not purifying in the least. This mask is not recommended.

☺ **$$$ Fresh Papaya Enzyme Mask, for All Skin Types** *($24.95 for 1.67 ounces)*. Enzymes from papaya or other fruits are not reliable exfoliants for skin, especially not in a cosmetic product that is "cooked" and preserved (enzymes are highly unstable in the presence of heat). It's a good thing this mask is oil- and wax-rich, because those ingredients help shield your skin from the potential irritation from the papaya, not to mention the problems presented by tangerine peel oil. The claim about this mask removing pore blockages is absolutely false—since when did oil and wax become able to do that? This gimmicky mask is an OK option for normal skin, but it certainly doesn't do much to make it worth the price.

☹ **Pumpkin Exfoliating Mask** *($24.95 for 1 ounce)* smells good enough to eat, but this pumpkin-based mask contains plenty of ingredients that are not the least bit good for your skin, such as sweet orange and frankincense oils along with a potentially irritating amount of pineapple juice. A well-formulated AHA or BHA product would be a much better, less irritating way to exfoliate skin and clear pores.

☹ **Super Moisturizing Mask** *($19.95 for 3.3 ounces)*. The shea butter, honey, and cucumber that serve as the main selling points for this moisturizing mask are not going to have much impact on dry skin, primarily because none of them are included in amounts deserving of top billing. Remember, a line with a "natural" angle isn't going to sell products if they call out synthetic ingredients, like glyceryl stearate, so the shea butter and honey win. Although this mask has the potential to make dry skin look and feel better, it contains a range of fragrant plant oils whose detrimental effects on skin make this a mask to avoid.

The Reviews Z

The Best Products Summary

MAKE YOUR LIST, BUT CHECK IT TWICE

Well, here we are—the best of the best—the category-by-category lists of products that really impressed me as I was compiling this book. All of the products included in the lists below either met or exceeded the criteria established for their respective categories. As such, all of these products deserve strong consideration, based on your skin type, skin condition, personal preferences, and cosmetics budget. (Speaking of budget, price was not a factor in determining whether or not a product was included in the lists below.)

First of all, if you turned directly to this chapter, figuring that you'd just cut to the chase and start shopping, let me forewarn you that this approach can backfire. Although the streamlined lists below are indeed helpful, you should also read the full review of any product you're considering. In addition, there may be other favorably reviewed options that will work perfectly well for you, although they may not appear on the lists below. Why not? Because just like in the seventh edition of this book, I decided to include only the products rated as Paula's Picks. The result, in most cases, is that the lists are shorter than ever (in some cases, only one or two products are listed). These shorter lists are in response to frequent requests from my readers and from the media to provide succinct lists of the best of the best—neither group likes too many choices, which I understand completely. To make these shorter lists even easier to navigate, you'll find that the majority of categories are divided according to location as well as to skin type and, in the case of makeup, also according to texture. Of course, the location (drugstore or department/specialty store) gives you an immediate indication of the price tier. Interestingly, the lists in some categories include several department-store options that many consumers would consider expensive, while the list of inexpensive products from the drugstore is comparably short. I did not do this intentionally to spotlight the expensive products or department-store brands; rather, it is simply how the reviews turned out as I read through the book one last time to select the products to include on the best-of-the-best lists.

As comprehensive as this book is, as it goes to press there are new products being created and launched, and there is ongoing publication and release of new research unveiling the promise of ingredients that may have increased benefits or risks for skin. To keep you up to date on the latest products and corresponding ingredient research and to make it easy for you to find the best skin-care and makeup products available, you can turn to my subscription-based Web site, www.Beautypedia.com. Beautypedia includes all of the reviews in this book, and is updated regularly with new reviews, revisions to existing reviews (e.g., when a product is discontinued), and hundreds of complete-line reviews which, for reasons of space and timing, are not included in this book. Beautypedia has been a big success and I continue to look for ways to improve the user experience on this dynamic site. In addition to Beautypedia, I will continue to offer my free online Beauty Bulletin (sign up at www.cosmeticscop.com). These two resources provide more extensive in-depth explanations and clarifications about specific topics than I can possibly provide in this book. Beautypedia.com and the Beauty Bulletin also allow me to provide far more detail about a product's claims and its ingredients. In this book, for almost all products, the goal is to bring more general information together all in one place, giving consumers enough comparative information to find out what works best for them among all the products with great, reliable formulations.

HOW TO AVOID STAYING CONFUSED

You have heard me say it before: Do not automatically buy a company's group of products just because it is recommended for your skin type. Most cosmetics companies recommend skin-care routines for specific skin types. As helpful as this may seem (and at times it *can* be helpful), it often ends up being a waste of money and may even be problematic for your skin. I strongly suggest that you ignore their categories and the corresponding product names. A person with dry skin who automatically follows a cosmetics company's recommendations could end up using too many products that are too emollient or too heavy, which can cause skin cells to build up and result in dull, rough-feeling skin. Loading up dry skin with too many heavy products can also cause breakouts (particularly whiteheads). Conversely, someone with oily skin may be sold products that contain strong irritants, which cause skin to become dry, irritated, red, and flaky, while still leaving you with oily skin. Indeed, someone with oily skin using irritating products will likely experience increased oil production in the pore lining. In other words, the products designed to help oily skin actually make it worse. More often than not, those with blemish-prone skin often end up purchasing products that are ineffective for acne. Please make sure you consider each product individually for its quality and its value to your skin, rather than selecting it based on its placement within a series of products, its promotional ads or brochures, its celebrity or fashion magazine endorsements, or the sales pitches you hear.

Product names are meant to be seductive, not factual. Please keep in mind that a cosmetics company's name for a product does not always correspond with my recommendations. Just because a product label says it "gets rid of wrinkles" or is "good for sensitive skin" or "is a firming and nourishing serum" doesn't mean the formulation itself supports that label or claim. The same is true for eye, chest, or throat creams; despite what the cosmetics industry wants you to believe, these products can be used anywhere on the face, and what counts is what skin type they are good for and whether or not the product contains beneficial ingredients. **There is absolutely nothing about any eye cream reviewed in this book that is unique for use in that area.** What is most shocking is that eye creams have formulations very similar to those of facial moisturizers; the main differences are that usually the product comes in a smaller container (i.e., you get less product) and you usually pay more under the guise that the eye cream is "specially formulated." Of even greater concern is that many specialty eye and face products don't contain sunscreen. So, if you were being diligent about using a sunscreen on your face, but were applying only a designated eye or throat product that didn't contain sunscreen, you would be allowing the sun to harm to the skin in those areas.

In addition, you will find many selections in the following lists of recommended products with names that sound like they should be in the dry-skin group, but that I have included in the oily-skin group, and vice versa. That's because ultimately what counts is how the product is formulated, not what the companies want you to believe about the product.

Remember, putting together the best routine for your skin type and your makeup needs is the overall goal.

The sequence of applying products for a particular skin-care regimen for a wide range of skin types is posted on my Web site, www.cosmeticscop.com and discussed in detail in my book *The Original Beauty Bible*, 3rd Edition. As a general rule, the following sequence is a safe, step-by-step guideline, depending on the products that your skin needs: cleanser; scrub; eye-makeup remover (if needed); toner; AHA or BHA product, topical disinfectant (only for blemish-prone skin); topical retinoid (note that with the exception of Differin [adapalene], retinoids cannot be used with benzoyl peroxide), azelaic acid, MetroGel, MetroLotion, MetroCream, or Noritate (one of the latter five if you have been diagnosed with rosacea); serum, skin-lightening product (only if discolorations are an issue); and during the day sunscreen and at night a moisturizer. Sunscreen is always the last item you apply during the day because you must never dilute a sunscreen.

BEST CLEANSERS (INCLUDING CLEANSING CLOTHS)

All of the cleansers listed below were chosen for their exceptional formulation, which, in most cases, means that fragrance and fragrant plant extracts have been excluded and that the cleanser is gentle yet effective for removing surface dirt, oil, perspiration, and makeup without making skin feel dry or tight. Those with normal to slightly dry, combination, or very oily skin should use a water soluble cleanser; those with normal to very dry skin can use a water soluble cleanser or, if preferred, a cleansing lotion.

Every cleanser on these lists is free of harsh, irritating, or sensitizing ingredients. I never recommend bar soap because the ingredients that keep the bar soap in a bar form can clog pores, and the cleansing agents in them are almost always drying. Emollient wipe-off cleansers may be the only types of cleansers that don't cause dry, sensitive skin to become drier; therefore I recommend them for that skin type, although in most cases such products were not rated Paula's Picks because they are inherently difficult to rinse (and you should never remove a cleanser with tissues—talk about outdated!).

You will notice that I do not specify a group of "medicated" or "anti-acne" cleansers supposedly designed for very oily or blemish-prone skin. This is for two reasons. First, cleansers identified as being good for those skin types generally contain ingredients that are too harsh or irritating, and that is not helpful for any skin type. Cleansing must be gentle and thorough, not harsh and drying. Second, cleansers for blemish-prone skin often contain topical disinfectants such as benzoyl peroxide or the exfoliant (and mild antibacterial agent) salicylic acid, but in a cleanser, these ingredients are rinsed down the drain before they have a chance to affect your blemished skin for the better.

BEST CLEANSERS FOR *ALL SKIN TYPES EXCEPT VERY DRY, AT THE DRUGSTORE: Alpha Hydrox Foaming Face Wash ($7.49 for 6 ounces) and Face Wash ($5.99 for 6 ounces); **Dove** Cool Moisture Facial Cleansing Cloths ($6.49 for 30 cloths) and Cool Moisture Foaming Facial Cleanser ($6.49 for 6.76 ounces); **Eucerin** Aquaphor Gentle Wash for Baby ($5.99 for 8 ounces), Gentle Hydrating Cleanser ($6.99 for 8 ounces) and Redness

Relief Soothing Cleanser ($8.99 for 6.8 ounces); **Marcelle** Gentle Foaming Wash ($13.50 for 6.2 ounces) and Hydra-C ComplexE Gentle Self-Foaming Cleanser ($13.50 for 5.5 ounces); **Neutrogena** Make-Up Remover Cleansing Towelettes ($8.99 for 25 towelettes) and One Step Gentle Cleanser ($7.49 for 5.2 ounces); **Olay** Foaming Face Wash, for Sensitive Skin ($4.49 for 6.78 ounces) and Gentle Foaming Face Wash, for Sensitive Skin ($5.99 for 7 ounces); **Sonia Kashuk** Cleanse, Tri-Active Cleanser ($10.99 for 6 ounces); **Zia Natural** HydraClean Face Wash ($9.95 for 5 ounces).

All of the cleansers on the list above are either recommended for all skin types or are equally suited to normal to oily or normal to dry skin.

BEST CLEANSERS FOR *ALL SKIN TYPES EXCEPT VERY DRY, AT THE DE-PARTMENT/SPECIALTY STORE: Clinique Liquid Facial Soap Mild Formula ($15 for 6.7 ounces); **DHC** Make Off Sheet ($7.50 for 50 sheets); **Dior** Self-Foaming Cleanser ($29 for 5 ounces); **Isomers** Foaming Facial Cleanser ($20 for 4.06 ounces); **Jan Marini** Bioglycolic Bioclean Cleanser ($29 for 8 ounces); **Kiehl's** Ultra Facial Cleanser, for All Skin Types ($17.50 for 5 ounces); **L'Occitane** Ultra Comforting Cleansing Milk ($22 for 6.7 ounces); **M.A.C.** Wipes ($17 for 45 sheets); **Mary Kay** Facial Cleansing Cloths ($15 for 30 cloths); **Patricia Wexler M.D.** Dual Action Foaming Cleanser ($16 for 5.1 ounces); **Paula's Choice** CLEAR Normalizing Cleanser Pore Clarifying Gel for All Skin Types ($10.95 for 6 ounces); Hydralight One Step Face Cleanser, for Normal to Oily/Combination Skin ($15.95 for 8 ounces) and Skin Balancing Cleanser, for Normal to Oily/Combination Skin ($15.95 for 8 ounces); **The Body Shop** Aloe Calming Facial Cleanser, for Sensitive Skin ($14 for 6.75 ounces).

All of the cleansers on the list above are either recommended for all skin types or are equally suited to normal to oily or normal to dry skin.

BEST CLEANSERS FOR NORMAL TO OILY/COMBINATION OR BLEMISH-PRONE SKIN, AT THE DRUGSTORE: Boots Expert Anti-Blemish Cleansing Foam ($5.29 for 5 ounces) and No7 Beautifully Balanced Purifying Cleanser, for Oily/Combination Skin ($7.99 for 6.6 ounces); **Clean & Clear** Daily Pore Cleanser, Oil-Free ($5.49 for 5.5 ounces) and Foaming Facial Cleanser, Sensitive Skin ($5.49 for 8 ounces); **Marcelle** Gentle Foaming Wash ($13.50 for 6.2 ounces); **Neutrogena** Fresh Foaming Cleanser ($6.59 for 6.7 ounces) and Make-Up Remover Cleansing Towelettes ($8.99 for 25 towelettes); **RoC Canada** Dema-quillage Actif Foaming Facial Wash ($16 for 150 ml) and Enydrial Anti-Drying Cleansing Gel ($16 for 200 ml).

BEST CLEANSERS FOR NORMAL TO OILY/COMBINATION OR BLEMISH-PRONE SKIN, AT THE DEPARTMENT/SPECIALTY STORE: Good Skin Perfect Balance Gel Cleanser ($12.50 for 6.7 ounces); **Laura Mercier** Oil-Free Gel Cleanser ($35 for 8 ounces); **Mary Kay** Deep Cleanser Formula 3 ($12 for 6.5 ounces); **Paula's Choice** CLEAR Normalizing Cleanser Pore Clarifying Gel, for All Skin Types ($10.95 for 6 ounces); Hydralight One Step Face Cleanser, for Normal to Oily/Combination Skin ($15.95 for 8 ounces) and Skin Balancing Cleanser, for Normal to Oily/Combination Skin ($15.95 for 8 ounces); **The Body Shop** Aloe Calming Facial Cleanser, for Sensitive Skin ($14 for 6.75 ounces) and Aloe Gentle Facial Wash, for Sensitive Skin ($16 for 4.2 ounces).

BEST CLEANSERS FOR NORMAL TO DRY OR VERY DRY SKIN, AT THE DRUG-STORE: Boots Expert Sensitive Cleansing & Toning Wipes ($4.49 for 30 wipes), Expert Sensitive Gentle Cleansing Lotion ($4.49 for 6.7 ounces), Expert Sensitive Gentle Cleansing Wash ($4.49 for 6.7 ounces), No7 Soft & Soothed Gentle Cleanser, for Normal/Dry Skin ($7.99 for 6.6 ounces) and Time Dimensions Conditioning Cleansing Cream ($8.99 for 6.7

ounces); **CeraVe** Hydrating Cleanser ($11.99 for 12 ounces); **Cetaphil** Gentle Skin Cleanser ($7.99 for 8 ounces); **Marcelle** New•Age Comforting Foaming Cleanser ($14.25 for 5.8 ounces); **Neutrogena** Extra Gentle Cleanser ($7.99 for 6.7 ounces) and Make-Up Remover Cleansing Towelettes ($8.99 for 25 towelettes); **Olay** Daily Facials Skin Soothing Cleansing Cloths, for Sensitive Skin ($5.99 for 30 cloths).

BEST CLEANSERS FOR NORMAL TO DRY OR VERY DRY SKIN, AT THE DE-PARTMENT/SPECIALTY STORE: **Clinique** Comforting Cream Cleanser ($18.50 for 5 ounces), Liquid Facial Soap Extra Mild ($15 for 6.7 ounces), Redness Solutions Soothing Cleanser ($20.50 for 5 ounces), Take The Day Off Cleansing Balm ($27 for 3.8 ounces) and Take The Day Off Cleansing Milk ($25 for 6.7 ounces); **DHC** Cleansing Milk ($24 for 6.7 ounces) and Soft Touch Cleansing Oil ($14 for 5 ounces); **Estee Lauder** Verite LightLotion Cleanser ($23.50 for 6.7 ounces); **Good Skin** All Calm Creamy Cleanser ($15 for 6.7 ounces) and Soft Skin Creamy Cleanser ($12.50 for 6.7 ounces); **Kiehl's** Ultra Moisturizing Cleansing Cream ($14.50 for 8 ounces); **La Roche-Posay** Toleriane Dermo-Cleanser ($19.50 for 6.76 ounces) and Toleriane Purifying Foaming Cream ($21 for 4.22 ounces); **Laura Mercier** Foaming One-Step Cleanser ($35 for 5 ounces) and One-Step Cleanser ($35 for 8 ounces); **MD Formulations** Facial Cleanser, Sensitive Skin Formula ($32 for 8.3 ounces); **Nu Skin** Creamy Cleansing Lotion, for Normal to Dry Skin ($17.10 for 5 ounces); **Paula's Choice** CLEAR Normalizing Cleanser Pore Clarifying Gel, for All Skin Types ($10.95 for 6 ounces); Moisture Boost One Step Face Cleanser, for Normal to Dry Skin ($15.95 for 8 ounces) and Skin Recovery Cleanser, for Normal to Very Dry Skin ($15.95 for 8 ounces); **Physicians Formula** Gentle Cleansing Lotion, for Normal to Dry Skin ($7.25 for 8 ounces); **The Body Shop** Aloe Calming Facial Cleanser, for Sensitive Skin ($14 for 6.75 ounces) and Aloe Gentle Facial Wash, for Sensitive Skin ($16 for 4.2 ounces); **Vivite** Replenish Hydrating Facial Cleanser ($27 for 2 ounces).

BEST TONERS

There are far more similarities than differences among toners. Almost without exception, the majority of toners either are boring concoctions of water and glycerin or contain irritating ingredients such as alcohol, witch hazel, overly fragrant plants, and menthol. The small selection of toners below are only those with truly state-of-the-art formulations. The companies that make these products endeavored to create toners that go beyond just softening skin and/or removing the last traces of makeup. Recognizing that a well-formulated toner can be an integral part of one's skin-care routine, the options below supply skin with antioxidants, skin-identical substances, anti-irritants, and/or cell-communicating ingredients—all essential elements for creating and maintaining healthy, radiant skin.

Note: As this book goes to print there are no drugstore toners rated as Paula's Pick. If this changes in the future, those toners will be reviewed on my Beautypedia Web site.

Second Note: Some toners appear on both lists below. In those cases, the toner in question is suitable for all skin types.

BEST TONERS FOR NORMAL TO OILY/COMBINATION SKIN, AT THE DE-PARTMENT/SPECIALTY STORE: **Estee Lauder** Re-Nutriv Intensive Softening Lotion ($40 for 8.4 ounces); **Paula's Choice** Healthy Skin Refreshing Toner, for Normal to Oily/Combination Skin ($15.95 for 6 ounces) and Skin Balancing Toner, for Normal to Oily/Combination Skin ($15.95 for 6 ounces); **Jane Iredale** Pom Mist ($17.50 for 2 ounces); **MD**

Formulations Moisture Defense Antioxidant Spray ($28 for 8.3 ounces); **Nu Skin** NaPCA Moisture Mist ($10.93 for 8.4 ounces).

BEST TONERS FOR NORMAL TO VERY DRY SKIN, AT THE DEPARTMENT/ SPECIALTY STORE: BeautiControl Skinlogics Platinum Plus Relaxing Tonic ($22.50 for 6.7 ounces); **Estee Lauder** Re-Nutriv Intensive Softening Lotion ($40 for 8.4 ounces); **Jane Iredale** Pom Mist ($17.50 for 2 ounces); **M.A.C.** Lightful Active Softening Lotion; **MD Formulations** Moisture Defense Antioxidant Spray ($28 for 8.3 ounces); **Nu Skin** NaPCA Moisture Mist ($10.93 for 8.4 ounces); **Paula's Choice** Moisture Boost Hydrating Toner, for Normal to Dry Skin ($15.95 for 6 ounces) and Skin Recovery Toner, for Normal to Very Dry Skin ($15.95 for 6 ounces).

BEST SCRUBS

Exfoliating the skin (i.e., getting rid of unwanted, dead, or built-up layers of sun-damaged skin cells and improving skin-cell turnover) is beneficial for almost all skin types, especially for those with sun-damaged skin or a tendency toward breakouts or clogged pores; however, even those with dry skin can benefit for many reasons. Despite the fact that most beauty experts, as well as dermatologists and plastic surgeons, agree that exfoliating the skin is a wonderful way to take care of both oily and dry skin, the method of exfoliating remains a point of contention. Today's assortment of scrubs is, almost without exception, far removed from the 1980s versions that abraded skin with walnut shells, almond pits, and other harsh additives; irritation, dryness, and redness were typical problems for people who used such scrubs. In some respects, that irritation (or at least the potential for it) came back to the forefront in a number of scrubs claiming to be microdermabrasion-in-a-jar. Although these scrubs often contain the same aluminum oxide crystals that are used in professional microdermabrasion treatments, their use at home is not equivalent to a real microdermabrasion session. However, as it turns out, professionally administered microdermabrasion is not all that great either, at least not if your goal is to stave off wrinkles and encourage collagen production to a noticeable degree. I would encourage anyone considering microdermabrasion to keep their expectations low; greater benefits can be obtained from a series of Intense Pulsed Light (IPL) treatments in conjunction with an exfoliation routine done at home.

Although there are some very good scrubs available, I encourage you to consider using a well-formulated AHA or BHA product instead because the benefits of the latter products far outweigh those that you can get from a topical scrub, and they will provide greater visible results all around. I acknowledge that many people like to use scrubs, and that's why I chose the ones below. Those reviewed as best for normal to oily skin are typically gel-based and rinse completely; those reviewed as best for normal to dry skin provide an exfoliating benefit while also cushioning skin with emollients or other moisturizing ingredients. In addition, none of the scrubs below contain common irritants such as menthol, and most are fragrance-free.

Note: Fans of topical scrubs should consider instead just using a washcloth with their normal cleanser. I can almost guarantee you'll get equal results and with less potential for irritation (depending on how zealously you use a scrub); plus, you won't have to add another product to your skin-care routine.

BEST SCRUBS FOR NORMAL TO OILY/COMBINATION SKIN, AT THE DRUG-STORE AND DEPARTMENT/SPECIALTY STORE: Boots Expert Sensitive Gentle Smoothing Scrub ($5.49 for 3.3 ounces); **Good Skin** Polished Skin Gentle Exfoliator ($14 for 3.4 ounces); **Marcelle** Hydra-C ComplexE Facial Exfoliating Gel ($13.50 for 3.4 ounces); **Neutrogena** Fresh Foaming Scrub ($5.99 for 4.2 ounces); **Olay** Definity Pore Redefining Scrub ($10.49 for 5 ounces).

BEST SCRUBS FOR NORMAL TO DRY SKIN, AT THE DRUGSTORE AND DE-PARTMENT/SPECIALTY STORE: Boots Expert Sensitive Gentle Smoothing Scrub ($5.49 for 3.3 ounces); **Kiehl's** Ultra Moisturizing Buffing Cream with Scrub Particles ($14.50 for 4 ounces); **Marcelle** Hydra-C ComplexE Facial Exfoliating Gel ($13.50 for 3.4 ounces); **Neutrogena** Pore Refining Cleanser ($7.99 for 6.7 ounces); **RoC Canada** Demaquillage Actif Gentle Exfoliating Cream ($16 for 40 ml).

BEST MAKEUP REMOVERS

The makeup removers below are all fragrance-free and do not contain ingredients known to be irritating when used around the eyes. Whether you choose a detergent- or silicone-based product, all of the options below work quickly and efficiently with minimal effort. Keep in mind that a cotton swab soaked in makeup remover works great for taking off stubborn eyeliner or waterproof mascara at lash roots, and is easier to control than a cotton pad.

BEST MAKEUP REMOVERS THAT USE GENTLE DETERGENT CLEANSING AGENTS FOR ALL SKIN TYPES, AT THE DRUGSTORE OR DEPARTMENT/SPE-CIALTY STORE: BeautiControl Skinlogics Lash and Lid Bath ($9.75 for 4 ounces); **DHC** Eye Make-Up Remover ($11 for 3.7 ounces); **gloMinerals** gloEye Make Up Remover ($14 for 4 ounces); **La Roche-Posay** Rosaliac Gelee Micellar Make-Up Removal Gel ($23.50 for 6.76 ounces); **Marcelle** Soothing Eye Makeup Remover Gel ($11.50 for 3.5 ounces).

BEST MAKEUP REMOVERS THAT USE SILICONE FOR ALL SKIN TYPES, AT THE DRUGSTORE: L'Oreal Paris Clean Artiste Waterproof & Long Wearing Eye Makeup Remover ($6.99 for 4 ounces); **Neutrogena** Oil-Free Eye Makeup Remover ($7.99 for 5.5 ounces); **Sonia Kashuk** Remove, Eye Makeup Remover ($9.99 for 4 ounces).

BEST MAKEUP REMOVERS THAT USE SILICONE FOR ALL SKIN TYPES, AT THE DEPARTMENT/SPECIALTY STORE: Bobbi Brown Instant Long-Wear Makeup Remover ($22 for 3.4 ounces); **Clinique** Take The Day Off Makeup Remover for Lids, Lashes & Lips ($17.50 for 4.2 ounces); **Dior** Duo-Phase Eye Make-Up Remover ($26 for 4.2 ounces); **Elizabeth Arden** All Gone Eye and Lip Makeup Remover ($16 for 3.4 ounces); **Laura Mercier** Waterproof Eye Makeup Remover ($20 for 4 ounces); **M.A.C.** Wipes ($17 for 45 sheets); **Mary Kay** Oil-Free Eye Makeup Remover ($14 for 3.75 ounces); **Paula's Choice** Gentle Touch Makeup Remover ($12.95 for 4 ounces); **Sephora** FACE Waterproof Eye Makeup Remover ($10 for 4.22 ounces).

BEST LOTION-STYLE MAKEUP REMOVERS THAT WORK BEST FOR DRY TO VERY DRY SKIN, AT THE DRUGSTORE: Physicians Formula Eye Makeup Remover Lotion, for Normal to Dry Skin ($4.75 for 2 ounces).

BEST LOTION-STYLE MAKEUP REMOVERS THAT WORK BEST FOR DRY TO VERY DRY SKIN, AT THE DEPARTMENT/SPECIALTY STORE: The Body Shop Camomile Waterproof Eye Make-Up Remover ($14.50 for 3.3 ounces).

Note: There are limited options in this category because so few lotion-style makeup removers do their job without leaving a greasy residue that ideally should be removed. Several lotion-style makeup removers received a happy face rating, and are worth considering in addition to those above if you prefer this type of product.

BEST TOPICAL DISINFECTANTS (BENZOYL PEROXIDE)

For someone who struggles with blemishes, a topical disinfectant is a fundamental way to effectively treat this condition. One of the primary causes of blemishes is the presence of a bacterium, and killing this bacterium can be of great help to many of those suffering with varying degrees of acne. Benzoyl peroxide is considered the most effective topical disinfectant for the treatment of blemishes. Generally, benzoyl peroxide products come in concentrations of 2.5%, 5%, and 10%, and as a general rule, it's best to start with a lower concentration to see if that works for you. If not, you can then try the next higher concentration. If you find that the higher concentrations don't work, then it may be time for you to consult a dermatologist or health care provider for a prescription topical disinfectant and/or for other topical acne treatments (e.g., Retin-A, Avita, Tazorac, or generic versions of these [active ingredient tretinoin, and, in the case of Tazorac, tazarotene]).

All of the products on this list categorized as "benzoyl peroxide" are Paula's Picks because they contain appropriate concentrations of this active ingredient with no other irritating or harsh additives. Surprisingly, most of the benzoyl peroxide products available from drugstores contain the maximum amount (10%) of benzoyl peroxide. Although this can be effective, this high concentration also increases the chance of side effects, while likely not providing a significantly greater anti-acne benefit relative to that of the lower concentrations.

As a general rule for all forms of breakouts (including blackheads), BHA is preferred over AHA because BHA is better at cutting through the oil inside the pore (Source: *Cosmetic Dermatology*, October 2001, pages 65-72). Penetrating the pore is necessary to exfoliate the pore lining. However, some people (including those allergic to aspirin) can't use BHA, so an AHA is the next option to consider. If that describes you, please refer to the list of Best Alpha Hydroxy Acid Products below.

BEST TOPICAL DISINFECTANTS FOR BLEMISH-PRONE SKIN, AT THE DRUGSTORE: Clean & Clear Persa-Gel 10, Maximum Strength ($5.89 for 1 ounce); **Clearasil** StayClear Tinted Acne Treatment Cream ($6.29 for 1 ounce) and StayClear Vanishing Acne Treatment Cream ($6.29 for 1 ounce); **Oxy** Oxy Spot Treatment ($5.49 for 0.65 ounce); **Stridex** Power Pads ($6.99 for 28 pads).

BEST TOPICAL DISINFECTANTS FOR BLEMISH-PRONE SKIN, AT THE DEPARTMENT/SPECIALTY STORE: Clinique Acne Solutions Emergency Gel Lotion ($13.50 for 0.5 ounce); **Mary Kay** Acne Treatment Gel ($7 for 1 ounce); **Paula's Choice** CLEAR Acne Fighting Treatment 2.5% Benzoyl Peroxide, for All Skin Types ($16.95 for 2.25 ounces) and CLEAR Extra Strength Acne Fighting Treatment 5% Benzoyl Peroxide, for All Skin Types ($17.95 for 2.25 ounces); **ProActiv Solution** Repairing Lotion ($21.75 for 2 ounces); **Serious Skin Care** Clearz-It Acne Medication ($17.50 for 2 ounces).

BEST AHA & BHA PRODUCTS

Alpha hydroxy acids (AHA, such as glycolic acid and lactic acid) and beta hydroxy acid (BHA, which is salicylic acid) work by exfoliating the skin chemically instead of mechanically via abrasion. For many reasons, these can be less irritating and can create results that are more even and smoother than scrubs, which is why facial scrubs have become less and less a part of most daily skin-care routines (though they do have their proponents). There is also research showing that AHAs and BHA can improve skin thickness and cell turnover, increase collagen content, reduce skin discolorations, and improve pore function (i.e., by reducing the number of clogged pores and breakouts). Similar impressive research simply does not exist for scrubs.

The goal with chemical exfoliants is to use one effective AHA (between 5% and 10% concentration) or one BHA (1% to 2% concentration) product, and only as needed—which may be twice a day, once a day, or once every other day, depending on your skin type and its response. The AHA and BHA products recommended below not only have formulations with the appropriate concentrations but also have a pH between 3 and 4, which is critical if those ingredients are to be effective as exfoliants. Just like in the seventh edition of this book, AHA and BHA products rated as Paula's Picks not only meet the basic formulary requirements that allow exfoliation to occur, but also do so without added fragrance or needlessly irritating ingredients. In addition, all of the AHA and BHA options below contain beneficial ingredients such as water-binding agents, antioxidants, and/or anti-irritants. You will find AHA (but no BHA) products reviewed throughout this book with a happy face rating (although not necessarily a Paula's Pick), and these are options if your singular goal is exfoliation. However, the choices below are preferred.

AHAs are best for those with normal to dry skin, and BHA is best for those with normal to oily or blemish-prone skin. This is because AHAs cannot penetrate oil and, therefore, cannot get into the pore lining. BHA can penetrate oil and, therefore, can get into the pore where it can improve and repair pore function while dissolving blockages of dead skin cells and oil that contribute to blackheads and acne. Whichever you choose, always monitor your skin's response, and remember, irritation is never the goal.

Note: Although no AHA products at the drugstore received a Paula's Pick rating, most of those from the inexpensive Alpha Hydrox line were rated with a happy face and are definitely worth considering.

BEST ALPHA HYDROXY ACID PRODUCTS FOR NORMAL TO OILY/COMBINATION SKIN, AT THE DEPARTMENT/SPECIALTY STORE: MD Formulations Vit-A-Plus Night Recovery ($50 for 1 ounce, *contains both AHA and BHA*); **Murad** Night Reform Glycolic Treatment ($66 for 1 ounce); **Paula's Choice** Skin Revealing Body Lotion with 10% Alpha Hydroxy Acid, for All Skin Types ($19.95 for 8 ounces); **Vivite** Vibrance Therapy ($119 for 1 ounce).

BEST ALPHA HYDROXY ACID PRODUCTS FOR NORMAL TO DRY SKIN, AT THE DEPARTMENT/SPECIALTY STORE: DHC Renewing AHA Cream ($39 for 1.5 ounces); **MD Formulations** Moisture Defense Antioxidant Lotion ($50 for 1 ounce), and Vit-A-Plus Illuminating Serum ($65 for 1 ounce); **NeoStrata** Brightening Bionic Eye Cream ($42 for 0.5 ounce), Daytime Protection Cream SPF 15, PHA 10 ($33 for 1.75 ounces), Exuviance Professional Rejuvenating Complex ($45 for 1 ounce) and Renewal Cream, PHA 12 ($43 for 1.05 ounces); **Paula's Choice** 8% Alpha Hydroxy Acid Gel, for All Skin Types ($18.95 for 4 ounces); **Peter Thomas Roth** Glycolic Acid 10% Moisturizer ($45 for 2 ounces); **Vivite** Vibrance Therapy ($119 for 1 ounce).

BEST BETA HYDROXY ACID PRODUCTS FOR NORMAL TO OILY/COMBINATION SKIN, AT THE DRUGSTORE: Neutrogena Oil-Free Acne Stress Control 3-In-1 Hydrating Acne Treatment ($7.99 for 2 ounces).

BEST BETA HYDROXY ACID PRODUCTS FOR NORMAL TO OILY/COMBINATION SKIN, AT THE DEPARTMENT/SPECIALTY STORE: Clinique Skin Conditioning

Treatment ($65 for 1 ounce); **Nu Skin** Clear Action Acne Medication Night Treatment ($38 for 1 ounce); **Paula's Choice** 1% Beta Hydroxy Acid Gel, for All Skin Types ($18.95 for 4 ounces), 1% Beta Hydroxy Acid Lotion, for All Skin Types ($18.95 for 4ounces), 2% Beta Hydroxy Acid Gel, for All Skin Types ($18.95 for 4 ounces), 2% Beta Hydroxy Acid Liquid, for All Skin Types ($18.95 for 4 ounces), 2% Beta Hydroxy Acid Lotion, for All Skin Types ($18.95 for 4 ounces), CLEAR Extra Strength Targeted Acne Relief Toner with 2% Salicylic Acid, All Skin Types ($18.95 for 4 ounces) and CLEAR Targeted Acne Relief Toner with 2% Salicylic Acid, All Skin Types ($18.95 for 4 ounces).

BEST BETA HYDROXY ACID PRODUCTS FOR NORMAL TO DRY SKIN, AT THE DRUGSTORE: Neutrogena Oil-Free Acne Stress Control 3-In-1 Hydrating Acne Treatment ($7.99 for 2 ounces).

BEST BETA HYDROXY ACID PRODUCTS FOR NORMAL TO DRY SKIN, AT THE DEPARTMENT/SPECIALTY STORE: Clinique Skin Conditioning Treatment ($65 for 1 ounce); **Estee Lauder** Fruition Extra Multi-Action Complex ($73 for 1.7 ounces); **Jan Marini** Factor-A Plus Mask ($81 for 2 ounces); **Nu Skin** Clear Action Acne Medication Night Treatment ($38 for 1 ounce*)*; **Paula's Choice** 1% Beta Hydroxy Acid Gel, for All Skin Types ($18.95 for 4ounces), 1% Beta Hydroxy Acid Lotion, for All Skin Types ($18.95 for 4 ounces), 2% Beta Hydroxy Acid Gel, for All Skin Types ($18.95 for 4 ounces), 2% Beta Hydroxy Acid Liquid, for All Skin Types ($18.95 for 4 ounces), 2% Beta Hydroxy Acid Lotion, for All Skin Types ($18.95 for 4 ounces), CLEAR Extra Strength Targeted Acne Relief Toner with 2% Salicylic Acid, All Skin Types ($18.95 for 4 ounces) and CLEAR Targeted Acne Relief Toner with 2% Salicylic Acid, All Skin Types ($18.95 for 4 ounces); **ProActiv Solution** Clarifying Night Cream ($28.75 for 1 ounce).

BEST MOISTURIZERS (INCLUDING EYE CREAMS)

I have written extensively about ingredients that have substantiated research proving they are necessary (if not integral) to creating a truly state-of-the-art moisturizer. Regardless of your skin type (more on that below) or texture preference, all of the moisturizers listed below meet that goal of substantiated research brilliantly. What remains offensive, however, is that most of the moisturizer formulations don't warrant their outlandish claims, ridiculous prices, or your belief that you've finally found the fountain of youth. None of the options below will "eliminate wrinkles," "lift sagging skin," "restore youthful contours," or "make you look years younger." What each will do, to some degree, is restore a healthy barrier (essential for allowing skin to repair itself and generate new collagen), reduce inflammation, help prevent (not completely eliminate) free-radical damage, restore vital elements needed to maintain healthy skin, and create a feeling of smoothness and softness that most will find aesthetically pleasing. A well-formulated moisturizer can do many wonderful things for your skin—provided you keep your expectations realistic. No moisturizer or eye cream is a comparable alternative to cosmetic surgery or cosmetic corrective procedures.

Moisturizers for oily skin are difficult to evaluate. As a rule, if oily skin is not being irritated or assaulted with harsh skin-care products, it does not need a moisturizer. Lotions and creams in general can be problematic for oily skin; even gels and serum-type moisturizers can feel heavy on oily skin. For this reason, I rate moisturizers, regardless of their designation as gels, lotions, antiwrinkle, anti-aging, or otherwise, on the basis of their value for normal to dry or dry to slightly dry or slightly oily skin. As a result, there are no strongly recommended moisturizers for oily skin. Even when a product is labeled as being for someone with oily or combination skin, it is meant to be used only over dry areas, not over oily areas. Those with oily to very oily skin can provide the beneficial ingredients all skin types need via well-formulated toners or serums, which have much lighter textures that those with oily skin will find agreeable.

If you are not using harsh or irritating skin-care products and are not undergoing potentially irritating procedures such as microdermabrasion or facial peels, but still have dry, red patches of skin in areas that are oily, it can be indicative of a skin disorder such as rosacea, dermatitis, psoriasis, or seborrhea. That does not require a moisturizer, but rather a change in how you are taking care of your skin, or an appointment with a dermatologist for a medical diagnosis. If you have oily skin but also have dry areas (and you are certain you have no skin disorders, you are not using irritating skin-care products, and you are not subjecting yourself to irritating non-invasive procedures), consider using the moisturizers reviewed as best for slightly dry or dry skin, but use them only over dry areas, not all over.

Packaging is a big deal for state-of-the-art moisturizers, and I'm not talking about visual appeal (though this entices many a consumer and fashion magazine editor). Rather, I am referring to the need for opaque, non-jar packaging that demonstrates the manufacturer has made efforts to ensure the continuing potency of the bells and whistles, particularly antioxidants, after you start using the product. Almost without exception, antioxidants are prone to degradation when repeatedly exposed to light and air (the manner in which they work to protect our skin bears this out). It is thus very disappointing to report that hundreds of the moisturizers reviewed in this book did not make the lists below and were not rated a Paula's Pick solely because of clear or jar packaging. The Lauder companies are the biggest offenders in this regard. Although their packaging for moisturizers has improved in some respects, they still package the majority of their outstanding moisturizer formulations in jars. Also, using a product that repeatedly requires you to dip your fingers into a jar isn't the most hygienic way to take care of your skin.

The eye creams below are all recommended because they contain an outstanding assortment of beneficial ingredients for skin anywhere on the face. Essentially, these are moisturizer formulas designated as eye-area products, though they contain nothing that is specific or better for skin around the eyes compared to the best facial moisturizers available. You're definitely not getting as much for your money with these products versus moisturizers, but there's no denying that many consumers are convinced they need a separate product to treat skin around the eyes. For those so inclined, the eye creams below are brilliant options. However, keep in mind that you only need a separate eye moisturizer if the skin in this area is drier than on the rest of your face.

Please refer to each moisturizer's individual review for an assessment of claims and information on formulary specifics, such as whether or not it is fragrance-free (many on the lists below are) and, in some cases, comparisons with less expensive options.

BEST LIGHTWEIGHT MOISTURIZERS FOR NORMAL TO SLIGHTLY DRY, OILY, OR COMBINATION SKIN, AT THE DRUGSTORE: Boots Expert Sensitive Light Moisturizing Lotion ($5.99 for 6.7 ounces); **CeraVe** Moisturizing Lotion ($12.99 for 12 ounces).

BEST LIGHTWEIGHT MOISTURIZERS FOR NORMAL TO SLIGHTLY DRY, OILY, OR COMBINATION SKIN, AT THE DEPARTMENT/SPECIALTY STORE: BeautiControl Cell Block-C P.M. Cell Protection ($36.50 for 1 ounce); **Clinique** Super Rescue

Antioxidant Night Moisturizer, for Combination Oily to Oily Skin ($42.50 for 1.7 ounces); **Clinique** Turnaround Concentrate Visible Skin Renewer ($37.50 for 1 ounce); **Dermalogica** AGE Smart Map-15 Regenerator ($85 for 0.3 ounce); **Good Skin** All Calm Moisture Lotion ($24.50 for 1.7 ounces); **MD Formulations** Critical Care Calming Gel ($39 for 1 ounce) and Moisture Defense Antioxidant Hydrating Gel ($45 for 1 ounce); **Paula's Choice** HydraLight Moisture-Infusing Lotion, for Normal to Oily/Combination Skin ($18.95 for 2 ounces) and Skin Balancing Moisture Gel, for Normal to Oily/Combination Skin ($18.95 for 2 ounces).

BEST MOISTURIZERS FOR NORMAL TO DRY SKIN, AT THE DRUGSTORE: **Boots** Expert Sensitive Hydrating Moisturizer ($4.99 for 1.6 ounces) and Expert Sensitive Restoring Night Treatment ($6.99 for 1.69 ounces); **CeraVe** *Moisturizing Cream ($14.99 for 16 ounces).

Note: This product is packaged in a jar but does not contain light- or air-sensitive ingredients.

BEST MOISTURIZERS FOR NORMAL TO DRY SKIN, AT THE DEPARTMENT/ SPECIALTY STORE: Clinique Super Rescue Antioxidant Night Moisturizer, for Dry Combination Skin ($42.50 for 1.7 ounces); **Dermalogica** AGE Smart Map-15 Regenerator ($85 for 0.3 ounce); **Dr. Denese New York** 15 Day SkinScience Booster Program ($74.76 for 1.05 ounces) and Triple Strength Wrinkle Smoother ($54 for 2 ounces); **Estee Lauder** Nutritious Vita-Mineral Moisture Lotion ($36 for 1.7 ounces); **Good Skin** All Bright Moisture Cream ($24.50 for 1.7 ounces); **M.A.C.** Strobe Cream ($29.50 for 1.7 ounces); **Mary Kay** Time-Wise Targeted-Action Line Reducer ($40 for 0.13 ounce); **MD Formulations** Critical Care Calming Gel ($39 for 1 ounce) and Moisture Defense Antioxidant Hydrating Gel ($45 for 1 ounce); **MD Skincare by Dr. Dennis Gross** Hydra-Pure Oil-Free Moisture ($78 for 1 ounce); **NeoStrata** Bionic Eye Cream, PHA 4 ($50 for 0.5 ounce); **Paula's Choice** RESIST Barrier Repair Moisturizer, Skin Remodeling Complex ($22.95 for 1.7 ounces) and Moisture Boost Hydrating Treatment Cream, for Normal to Dry Skin ($18.95 for 2 ounces); **Peter Thomas Roth** Moisturizing Multi-Tasking After Shave Balm ($24 for 3.4 ounces).

BEST MOISTURIZERS FOR DRY TO VERY DRY SKIN, AT THE DRUGSTORE: **Neutrogena** Oil-Free Moisture, for Sensitive Skin ($12.99 for 4 ounces); **Olay** Total Effects 7-In-1 Anti-Aging Moisturizer, Mature Skin Therapy ($19.38 for 1.7 ounces).

BEST MOISTURIZERS FOR DRY TO VERY DRY SKIN, AT THE DEPARTMENT/ SPECIALTY STORE: Caudalie Paris Vinosource Riche Anti-Wrinkle Ultra Nourishing Cream ($50 for 1.3 ounces); **Clinique** Recovery Week Complex ($65 for 1 ounce) and Super Rescue Antioxidant Night Moisturizer, for Very Dry to Dry Skin ($42.50 for 1.7 ounces); **Dermalogica** AGE Smart Map-15 Regenerator ($85 for 0.3 ounce); **DHC** Wrinkle Filler ($27 for 0.52 ounce); **Dr. Denese New York** 15 Day SkinScience Booster Program ($74.76 for 1.05 ounces); **Paula's Choice** RESIST Barrier Repair Moisturizer, Skin Remodeling Complex ($22.95 for 1.7 ounces) and Skin Recovery Moisturizer, for Normal to Very Dry Skin ($18.95 for 2 ounces).

BEST EYE MOISTURIZERS FOR NORMAL TO DRY SKIN, AT THE DRUG-STORE: Olay Pro-X Eye Restoration Complex ($47 for 0.5 ounce), Regenerist Eye Lifting Serum ($18.99 for 0.5 ounce) and Regenerist Touch of Concealer Eye Regenerating Cream ($21.99 for 0.5 ounce).

BEST EYE MOISTURIZERS FOR NORMAL TO DRY SKIN, AT THE DEPART-MENT/SPECIALTY STORE: Aveda Tourmaline Charged Eye Creme ($32 for 0.5 ounce); **BeautiControl** Regeneration Tight, Firm & Fill Eye Firming Serum ($42.50 for 0.46 ounce);

Borghese Fluido Protettivo Advanced Spa Lift for Eyes ($46.50 for 1 ounce); **DDF - Doctor's Dermatologic Formula** Advanced Eye Firming Concentrate ($88 for 0.5 ounce) and Nourishing Eye Cream ($48 for 0.5 ounce); **Elizabeth Arden** Prevage Eye Anti-Aging Moisturizing Treatment ($98 for 0.5 ounce); **Estee Lauder** Idealist Refinishing Eye Serum ($48 for 0.5 ounce) and Verite Special EyeCare ($37.50 for 0.5 ounce); **Kinerase** Pro+ Therapy Ultra Rich Eye Repair ($88 for 0.5 ounce); **MD Skincare by Dr. Dennis Gross** Continuous Eye Hydration Advanced Technology ($45 for 0.5 ounce); **NeoStrata** Bionic Eye Cream, PH4 ($50 for 0.5 ounce); **Nu Skin** Tru Face IdealEyes Eye Refining Cream ($43.70 for 0.5 ounce); **Paula's Choice** Moisture Boost Hydrating Treatment Cream, for Normal to Dry Skin ($18.95 for 2 ounces), RESIST Barrier Repair Moisturizer, Skin Remodeling Complex ($22.95 for 1.7 ounces), and Skin Recovery Moisturizer, for Normal to Very Dry Skin ($18.95 for 2 ounces); **Shiseido** Bio-Performance Super Eye Contour Cream ($55 for 0.53 ounce); **SkinCeuticals** Eye Cream Firming Treatment ($55 for 0.67 ounce).

BEST EYE MOISTURIZERS FOR NORMAL TO OILY/COMBINATION SKIN, AT THE DRUGSTORE: Olay Pro-X Eye Restoration Complex ($47 for 0.5 ounce), and Regenerist Touch of Concealer Eye Regenerating Cream ($21.99 for 0.5 ounce).

BEST EYE MOISTURIZERS FOR NORMAL TO OILY/COMBINATION SKIN, AT THE DEPARTMENT/SPECIALTY STORE: BeautiControl Regeneration Tight, Firm & Fill Eye Firming Serum ($42.50 for 0.46 ounce); **Paula's Choice** HydraLight Moisture-Infusing Lotion, for Normal to Oily/Combination Skin ($18.95 for 2 ounces) and Skin Balancing Moisture Gel, for Normal to Oily/Combination Skin ($18.95 for 2 ounces).

BEST RETINOL PRODUCTS

Because many of you have written me asking about moisturizers and serums with retinol, and because this vitamin A ingredient has more than proven its worth for all skin types, I have also included lists of the best moisturizers with efficacious amounts of retinol. All of these products are packaged to ensure that the retinol remains stable during use, which is absolutely essential for this light- and air-sensitive ingredient. Whether you choose a moisturizer or serum with retinol comes down to preference and skin type (those with dry skin should go with a moisturizer that contains retinol). It is fine to combine any retinol product with an AHA or BHA product. However, because retinol can cause mild flakiness and sensitivity for some people, pay attention to how your skin responds. If you notice undesirable side effects, decrease frequency of use or or apply the retinol product in the evening and exfoliant as part of your daytime routine.

BEST MOISTURIZERS CONTAINING RETINOL, AT THE DRUGSTORE: Alpha Hydrox Retinol Night ResQ ($14.99 for 1.05 ounces); **Neutrogena** Healthy Skin Anti-Wrinkle Cream, Night ($13.99 for 1.4 ounces); **Olay** Pro-X Deep Wrinkle Treatment ($47 for 1 ounce); **RoC** Multi-Correxion Night Treatment ($24.99 for 1 ounce); **RoC Canada** Retin-OL Correxion Intensive Nourishing Anti-Wrinkle Care, for Dry Skin ($44 for 30 ml), Retin-OL Multi-Correxion Multi-Corrective Anti-Ageing Moisturiser, Day/Night ($42 for 30 ml) and Retin-OL Multi-Correxion Multi-Corrective Eye Cream ($32 for 15 ml).

BEST MOISTURIZERS CONTAINING RETINOL, AT THE DEPARTMENT/SPE-CIALTY STORE: DDF - Doctor's Dermatologic Formula Retinol Energizing Moisturizer ($88 for 1.7 ounces); **Paula's Choice** RESIST Barrier Repair Moisturizer, Skin Remodeling Complex ($22.95 for 1.7 ounces) **Remergent** Advanced Retinol Therapy 1% Retinol + L-Ergothioneine ($56 for 1 ounce); **Serious Skin Care** A-Stick, Vitamin A Moisturizer Stick ($8 for 0.17 ounce).

BEST SERUMS CONTAINING RETINOL, AT THE DEPARTMENT/SPECIALTY STORE: BeautiControl Regeneration Overnight Retinol Recovery Eye Capsules ($39.50 for 30 capsules) and Regeneration Overnight Retinol Recovery Serum ($45 for 1 ounce); **Dr. Denese New York** HydroShield Eye Serum ($44 for 0.5 ounce), HydroShield Neck Serum ($44.50 for 1 ounce) and Neck Saver Serum ($34 for 1 ounce); **Estee Lauder** Re-Nutriv Intensive Lifting Serum ($180 for 1 ounce); **Jan Marini** Factor-A Eyes for Dark Circles ($78 for 60 capsules); **MD Skincare by Dr. Dennis Gross** Hydra-Pure Antioxidant Firming Serum ($95 for 1 ounce) and Hydra-Pure Radiance Renewal Serum ($95 for 1 ounce); **Paula's Choice** Skin Balancing Super Antioxidant Mattifying Concentrate, for Normal to Very Oily Skin ($24.95 for 1 ounce) and Skin Recovery Super Antioxidant Concentrate, for Normal to Very Dry Skin ($24.95 for 1 ounce); **Peter Thomas Roth** Retinol Fusion PM ($65 for 1 ounce); **philosophy** eye believe ($30 for 0.5 ounce); **Serious Skin Care** A-Force XR, Retinol Serum ($15.75 for 1 ounce); **SkinCeuticals** Retinol 0.5 Refining Night Cream with 0.5% Pure Retinol ($50 for 1 ounce) and Retinol 1.0 Maximum Strength Refining Night Cream with 1.0% Pure Retinol ($48 for 1 ounce).

BEST SERUMS

Serums have made great strides in terms of their sophisticated formulas. Most of these ingredients have substantiated research proving their benefit for skin of all ages. And many serums have a texture that is suitable for oily or breakout-prone skin. As such, serums can be a brilliant way for those with this skin type and/or condition to obtain the benefits of antioxidants and cell-communicating ingredients, including retinol (serums containing an impressive amount of retinol in stable packaging are listed separately).

You will notice that the longer list of serums is on the expensive side. I wish this weren't the case, but it is. There are two reasons. One is that most cosmetics companies position serums as specialty or targeted products, almost always with an anti-aging angle. Therefore, as the perceived (or the claimed) benefits increase, so does the price. Second, and the more real-world reason for the high prices, is that it is expensive to create serums (most are nonaqueous, and water is the least expensive yet most pervasive skin-care ingredient around) that contain the level and range of state-of-the-art ingredients noted in the products below. The cost of several of the ingredients in these serums is, on a pound-for-pound basis, staggering when compared to the cost of ubiquitous ingredients such as triglycerides, glycerin, or mineral oil. Although most of the best serums are costly, at least you know you're getting an intelligently formulated product whose ingredients have a proven track record of improving skin's health and appearance. Just as with the best moisturizers, please refer to each serum's individual review for an assessment of the claims and information on formulary specifics, such as whether or not it is fragrance-free and, in some cases, comparisons with less expensive options.

BEST SERUMS FOR ALL SKIN TYPES EXCEPT VERY OILY SKIN, AT THE DRUGSTORE: Boots Expert Sensitive Hydrating Serum ($7.49 for 1.6 ounces); **Olay** Regenerist Daily Regenerating Serum ($19.49 for 1.7 ounces) and **Olay** Regenerist Daily Regenerating Serum, Fragrance-Free ($19.49 for 1.7 ounces).

BEST SERUMS FOR ALL SKIN TYPES EXCEPT VERY OILY, AT THE DEPARTMENT/SPECIALTY STORE: BeautiControl Regeneration Platinum Plus Face Serum ($65 for 1 ounce); **Bobbi Brown** Intensive Skin Supplement ($65 for 1 ounce); **Clinique** CX Antioxidant Rescue Serum ($135 for 1 ounce); **DDF - Doctor's Dermatologic Formula**

Mesojection Healthy Cell Serum ($84 for 1 ounce) and Wrinkle Resist Plus Pore Minimizer Moisturizing Serum ($85 for 1.7 ounces); **Elizabeth Arden** Ceramide Advanced Time Complex Capsules Intensive Treatment for Face and Throat ($65 for 60 capsules) and Ceramide Gold Ultra Restorative Capsules ($68 for 0.95 ounce); **Estee Lauder** Advanced Night Repair Concentrate Recovery Boosting Treatment ($85 for 1 ounce), Nutritious Vita-Mineral Radiance Serum ($40 for 1 ounce), Perfectionist [CP+] Wrinkle Lifting Serum ($80 for 1.7 ounces), Re-Nutriv Ultimate Lifting Serum ($200 for 1 ounce); **Good Skin** All Firm Rebuilding Serum ($26 for 1 ounce) and Tri-Aktiline Instant Deep Wrinkle Filler ($39.50 for 1 ounce); **Isomers** Absolutes Anti Redness Serum ($29.99 for 1 ounce); **MD Skincare by Dr. Dennis Gross** Hydra-Pure Redness Soothing Serum ($85 for 1 ounce) and Hydra-Pure Vitamin C Serum ($95 for 1 ounce); **Nu Skin** 180º Night Complex ($66.50 for 1 ounce) and Celltrex CoQ10 Complete ($48.45 for 0.5 ounce); **Patricia Wexler M.D.** Advanced No-Injection Wrinkle Smoother ($29.50 for 0.5 ounce); **Paula's Choice** RESIST Super Antioxidant Concentrate Serum, for All Skin Types ($24.95 for 1 ounce) and Skin Recovery Super Antioxidant Concentrate, for Normal to Very Dry Skin ($24.95 for 1 ounce).

BEST ULTRALIGHT OR MATTIFYING SERUMS FOR VERY OILY SKIN, AT THE DEPARTMENT/SPECIALTY STORE: Bobbi Brown Intensive Skin Supplement ($65 for 1 ounce); **Clinique** CX Antioxidant Rescue Serum ($135 for 1 ounce), Pore Minimizer Instant Perfector ($17.50 for 0.5 ounce) and Repairwear Deep Wrinkle Concentrate for Face and Eyes ($55 for 1 ounce); **DDF - Doctor's Dermatologic Formula** C3 Plus Serum ($68 for 0.5 ounce); **Estee Lauder** Perfectionist [CP+] Wrinkle Lifting Serum ($80 for 1.7 ounces); **Good Skin** All Firm Rebuilding Serum ($26 for 1 ounce); **MD Skincare by Dr. Dennis Gross** Hydra-Pure Radiance Renewal Serum ($95 for 1 ounce), Hydra-Pure Redness Soothing Serum ($85 for 1 ounce) and Hydra-Pure Vitamin C Serum ($95 for 1 ounce); **Nu Skin** Celltrex CoQ10 Complete ($48.45 for 0.5 ounce); **Patricia Wexler M.D.** Advanced No-Injection Wrinkle Smoother ($29.50 for 0.5 ounce); **Paula's Choice** Skin Balancing Super Antioxidant Mattifying Concentrate, for Normal to Very Oily Skin ($24.95 for 1 ounce); **Smashbox** Anti-Shine ($27 for 1 ounce).

BEST DAYTIME MOISTURIZERS WITH SUNSCREEN (SPF 15 OR GREATER, INCLUDING EYE CREAMS)

Many, if not most, of the changes that take place on our skin over the years, such as wrinkles, skin discolorations, loss of elasticity, texture problems, and dryness, are the result of sun damage from exposure to the sun without appropriate or adequate sun protection. Sunscreens are essential for skin care day in and day out, 365 days a year. If applied correctly (meaning liberally and reapplied as often as needed), they are the only true antiwrinkle product. They can also potentially help prevent some forms of skin cancer and are an absolute must if you have already been treated for any type of skin cancer (or have a family history of it). If you are not using a sunscreen of some kind (lotion, cream, gel, serum, or foundation with sunscreen) with SPF 15 or greater and that contains the UVA-protecting ingredients of avobenzone, zinc oxide, titanium dioxide, Mexoryl SX, or, outside the United States, Tinosorb, then you are doing nothing of value for the long-term health of your skin. Really, all of the antiwrinkle, firming, anti-aging, or rejuvenating products in the world are completely and totally useless if you are not protecting your skin from the sun every day. It is of vital importance to the health of your skin to include a well-formulated sunscreen in your daily skin-care routine. Arguably, the most unethical thing the cosmetics industry does is sell women a plethora of antiwrinkle products that more often than not do not include reliable sun protection.

I am pleased that in the last few years many cosmetics chemists have created lightweight sunscreens whose texture and typically smooth matte finish are just what someone struggling with oily skin or oily areas needs. Still, for the face, someone with oily skin may prefer to use a foundation with sunscreen rated SPF 15 or greater, and apply a well-formulated sunscreen from the neck down. This is one area of skin care that is becoming less difficult for someone with oily skin, but it still takes experimentation to figure out what product with sunscreen works best for you. Those dealing with breakout-prone skin should consider sunscreens reviewed as best for normal to slightly dry or oily/combination skin. Keep in mind that despite non-comedogenic or non-acnegenic claims made on labels, no sunscreen is guaranteed to be problem-free for someone struggling with acne.

All of the following sunscreens were rated Paula's Picks for two important reasons. First, each has an SPF 15 or greater and includes avobenzone, titanium dioxide, zinc oxide, Mexoryl SX, or Tinosorb (the latter approved for use outside the United States) as one or more of the active ingredients (if these are listed someplace else on the ingredient list, it does not count toward reliable sun protection). Avobenzone may be listed on an ingredient label by its chemical name, butyl methoxydibenzoylmethane, and Mexoryl SX may be listed as ecamsule. Second, every sunscreen on the lists below contains a range of antioxidants and also includes other skin-beneficial ingredients such as those that mimic healthy skin's structural components. Antioxidants have proven to be an incredibly helpful addition to sunscreens because they not only boost the efficacy of the active ingredients, but also help offset free-radical damage from sun exposure. Selecting a daytime moisturizer with sunscreen or "regular" sunscreen without antioxidants isn't giving your skin much of a fighting chance against the cascade of damage that sun exposure can cause (and that can be dramatically minimized with diligent, liberal application and, when needed, reapplication, of a sunscreen rated SPF 15 or greater).

BEST DAYTIME MOISTURIZERS WITH SUNSCREEN FOR NORMAL TO SLIGHTLY DRY OR OILY/COMBINATION SKIN, AT THE DRUGSTORE: Neutrogena Ageless Intensives Tone Correcting Moisture SPF 30 ($19.99 for 1 ounce) and Healthy Skin Visibly Even Daily SPF 15 Moisturizer ($13.09 for 1.7 ounces); **Olay** Complete Ageless Skin Renewing UV Lotion SPF 20 ($24.99 for 2.5 ounces), Regenerist Advanced Anti-Aging DNA Superstructure UV Cream SPF 25 ($29.99 for 1.7 ounces), Regenerist UV Defense Regenerating Lotion SPF 15 ($19.99 for 2 ounces), and Regenerist UV Defense Regenerating Lotion SPF 50 ($29.99 for 1.7 ounces); **RoC Canada** Retin-OL + Day SPF 30 ($48.99 for 30 ml).

BEST DAYTIME MOISTURIZERS WITH SUNSCREEN FOR NORMAL TO SLIGHTLY DRY OR OILY/COMBINATION SKIN, AT THE DEPARTMENT/SPECIALTY STORE: Avon Ageless Results Renewing Day Cream SPF 15 ($15 for 1.7 ounces), Anew Advanced All-in-One Max SPF 15 Lotion ($16.50 for 1.7 ounces), and Anew Alternative Photo-Radiance Treatment SPF 15 ($25 for 1 ounce); **Avon Mark** For Goodness Face Antioxidant Skin Moisturizing Lotion SPF 30 ($15 for 1.7 ounces); **BeautiControl** Cell Block-C New Cell Protection SPF 20 ($30.50 for 1 ounce); **Borghese** Crema Straordinaria Da Giornio SPF 25 ($66 for 1.7 ounces); **Clinique** City Block Sheer Oil-Free Daily Face Protector SPF 25 ($17.50 for 1.4 ounces), Redness Solutions Daily Protective Base SPF 15 ($17.50 for 1.53 ounces), Sun SPF 30 Face Cream ($17.50 for 1.7 ounces), and Sun SPF 50 Face Cream ($17.50 for 1.7 ounces); **DDF – Doctor's Dermatologic Formula** Daily Organic SPF 15 ($36 for 1.7

ounces), Daily Protective Moisturizer SPF 15 ($40 for 1.7 ounces), and Protect and Correct UV Moisturizer SPF 15 ($60 for 1.7 ounces); **Dr. Denese New York** SPF 30 Defense Day Cream ($34 for 1.5 ounces) and SPF 30 Neck Defense Day Cream UVA/UVB ($32.25 for 2 ounces); **Elizabeth Arden** Extreme Conditioning Cream ($38.50 for 1.7 ounces); **Estee Lauder** DayWear Plus Multi Protection Anti-Oxidant Lotion SPF 15, for Oily Skin ($38.50 for 1.7 ounces); **Good Skin** All Bright Moisturizing Sunscreen SPF 30 ($12 for 1.7 ounces), All Calm Gentle Sunscreen SPF 25 ($12 for 1.7 ounces), and Clean Skin Oil-Free Lotion SPF 15 ($16 for 1.7 ounces); **Jan Marini Skin Research, Inc.** Bioglycolic Facial Lotion SPF 15 ($52 for 2 ounces); **M.A.C.** Studio Moisture Fix SPF 15 ($29.50 for 1.7 ounces); **Mary Kay** TimeWise Day Solution Sunscreen SPF 25 ($36 for 1 ounce); **MD Formulations** Moisture Defense Antioxidant Moisturizer SPF 20 ($36 for 1.7 ounces); **NeoStrata** Oil Free Lotion SPF 15, PHA 4 ($30 for 1.75 ounces); **Paula's Choice** Skin Balancing Daily Mattifying Lotion with SPF 15 and Antioxidants, for Normal to Combination Skin ($20.95 for 2 ounces) and Skin Recovery Daily Moisturizing Lotion with SPF 15 and Antioxidants ($20.95 for 2 ounces).

BEST DAYTIME MOISTURIZERS WITH SUNSCREEN FOR NORMAL TO DRY OR VERY DRY SKIN, AT THE DRUGSTORE: Neutrogena Healthy Skin Visibly Even Daily SPF 15 Moisturizer ($13.09); **Olay** Regenerist Advanced Anti-Aging DNA Superstructure UV Cream SPF 25 ($29.99 for 1.7 ounces), Regenerist UV Defense Regenerating Lotion SPF 15 ($19.99), and Regenerist UV Defense Regenerating Lotion SPF 50 ($29.99).

BEST DAYTIME MOISTURIZERS WITH SUNSCREEN FOR NORMAL TO DRY OR VERY DRY SKIN, AT THE DEPARTMENT/SPECIALTY STORE: Avon Anew Alternative Photo-radiance Treatment SPF 15 ($25 for 1 ounce); **BeautiControl** Cell Block-C New Cell Protection SPF 20 ($30.50 for 1 ounce); **Borghese** Crema Straordinaria Da Giornio SPF 25 ($66 for 1.7 ounces); **Clinique** City Block Sheer Oil-Free Daily Face Protector SPF 25 ($17.50 for 1.4 ounces), Sun SPF 30 Face Cream ($17.50 for 1.7 ounces), and Sun SPF 50 Face Cream ($17.50 for 1.7 ounces); **DDF – Doctor's Dermatologic Formula** Daily Organic SPF 15 ($36 for 1.7 ounces), Daily Protective Moisturizer SPF 15 ($40 for 1.7 ounces), and Protect and Correct UV Moisturizer SPF 15 ($60 for 1.7 ounces); **Dr. Denese New York** SPF 30 Neck Defense Day Cream UVA/UVB ($32.25 for 2 ounces); **Elizabeth Arden** Extreme Conditioning Cream ($38.50 for 1.7 ounces); **Estee Lauder** Resilience Lift Extreme Ultra Firming Lotion SPF 15, for Normal/Combination Skin ($70 for 1.7 ounces) and Time Zone Line & Wrinkle Reducing Moisturizer SPF 15 - Normal/Combination Lotion ($58 for 1.7 ounces); **Good Skin** All Bright Moisturizing Sunscreen SPF 30 ($12 for 1.7 ounces) and All Calm Gentle Sunscreen SPF 25 ($12 for 1.7 ounces); **Jan Marini Skin Research, Inc.** Bioglycolic Facial Lotion SPF 15 ($52 for 2 ounces); **Mary Kay** TimeWise Day Solution Sunscreen SPF 25 ($36 for 1 ounce); **MD Formulations** Moisture Defense Antioxidant Moisturizer SPF 20 ($36 for 1.7 ounces); **NeoStrata** Oil Free Lotion SPF 15, PHA 4 ($30 for 1.75 ounces); **Paula's Choice** Skin Recovery Daily Moisturizing Lotion with SPF 15 and Antioxidants ($20.95 for 2 ounces).

BEST EYE MOISTURIZERS WITH SUNSCREEN, AT THE DRUGSTORE: Zia Natural Dual Protection Eye Cream SPF 15 ($14.95 for 1 ounce).

BEST "MINERAL" DAYTIME MOISTURIZERS WITH SUNSCREEN WHOSE ONLY ACTIVES ARE TITANIUM DIOXIDE AND/OR ZINC OXIDE, WHICH ARE BEST FOR NORMAL TO DRY OR SENSITIVE SKIN, AT THE DEPARTMENT/ SPECIALTY STORE: BeautiControl Cell Block-C New Cell Protection SPF 20 ($30.50

for 1 ounce); **Clinique** City Block Sheer Oil-Free Daily Face Protector SPF 25 ($17.50 for 1.4 ounces) and Redness Solutions Daily Protective Base SPF 15 ($17.50 for 1.35 ounces); **DDF – Doctor's Dermatologic Formula** Daily Organic SPF 15 ($36 for 1.7 ounces); **Good Skin** All Calm Gentle Sunscreen SPF 25 ($12 for 1.7 ounces); **Jan Marini Skin Research, Inc.** Bioglycolic Facial Lotion SPF 15 ($52 for 2 ounces); **Paula's Choice** Skin Recovery Daily Moisturizing Lotion with SPF 15 and Antioxidants ($20.95 for 2 ounces).

Best All-Purpose Sunscreens

BEST SUNSCREENS FOR NORMAL TO SLIGHTLY DRY OR OILY/COMBINA-TION SKIN, AT THE DRUGSTORE: Banana Boat Kids Tear-Free SPF 30 Continuous Lotion Spray ($9.99 for 6 ounces); **Neutrogena** Age Shield Face Sunblock SPF 55 ($10.99 for 4 ounces), Age Shield Sunblock SPF 30 ($10.69 for 4 ounces), Age Shield Sunblock SPF 45 ($10.69 for 4 ounces), Ultra Sheer Dry-Touch Sunblock SPF 30 ($10.69 for 3 ounces), and Ultra Sheer Dry-Touch Sunblock SPF 45 ($10.69) for 3 ounces; **Physicians Formula** Sun Shield For Faces Extra Sensitive Skin SPF 25 ($8.95 for 4 ounces).

BEST SUNSCREENS FOR NORMAL TO SLIGHTLY DRY OR OILY/COMBINA-TION SKIN, AT THE DEPARTMENT/SPECIALTY STORE: Clinique Sun SPF 15 Face/Body Cream ($20 for 5 ounces), Sun SPF 30 Body Cream ($20 for 5 ounces), and Sun SPF 50 Body Cream ($20 for 5 ounces); **DDF – Doctor's Dermatologic Formula** Matte-Finish Photo-Age Protection SPF 30 ($32 for 4 ounces) and Moisturizing Photo-Age Protection SPF 30 ($32 for 4 ounces); **Mary Kay** SPF 30 Sunscreen ($14 for 4 ounces); **MD Skincare by Dr. Dennis Gross** Powerful Sun Protection SPF 30 Sunscreen Lotion ($42 for 5 ounces), Powerful Sun Protection SPF 30 Sunscreen Packettes ($42 for 60 packettes), and Powerful Sun Protection SPF 45 Sunscreen Cream ($42 for 4.2 ounces); **Paula's Choice** Essential Non-Greasy Sunscreen SPF 15, for Normal to Oily/Combination Skin ($14.95 for 5 ounces), Extra Care Moisturizing Sunscreen SPF 30+ for Normal to Dry Skin ($14.95 for 5 ounces), Extra Care Non-Greasy Sunscreen SPF 45 ($14.95 for 5 ounces), Pure Mineral Sunscreen SPF 15, for Normal to Very Dry Skin ($15.95 for 6 ounces), and Ultra Light Weightless Finish SPF 30 Sunscreen Spray, for All Skin Types ($15.95 for 4 ounces); **Peter Thomas Roth** Oil-Free Sunblock SPF 30 ($26 for 4.2 ounces), Uber-Dry Sunscreen Cream SPF 30 ($26 for 4.2 ounces), and Ultra-Lite Oil-Free Sunblock SPF 30 ($26 for 4.2 ounces); **SkinCeuticals** Physical UV Defense SPF 30 ($37 for 3 ounces) and Sport UV Defense SPF 45 ($37.50 for 3 ounces).

BEST SUNSCREENS FOR NORMAL TO DRY OR VERY DRY SKIN, AT THE DRUGSTORE: Neutrogena Age Shield Face Sunblock SPF 55 ($10.99 for 4 ounces).

BEST SUNSCREENS FOR NORMAL TO DRY OR VERY DRY SKIN, AT THE DEPARTMENT/SPECIALTY STORE: Clinique Sun SPF15 Face/Body Cream ($20 for 5 ounces), Sun SPF 30 Body Cream ($20 for 5 ounces) and Sun SPF 50 Body Cream ($20 for 5 ounces); **DDF – Doctor's Dermatologic Formula** Moisturizing Photo-Age Protection SPF 30 ($32 for 4 ounces); **fresh** Sunshield Face and Body SPF 30 ($48 for 5.1 ounces); **MD Skincare by Dr. Dennis Gross** Powerful Sun Protection SPF 30 Sunscreen Lotion ($42 for 5 ounces), Powerful Sun Protection SPF 30 Sunscreen Packettes ($42 for 60 packettes), and Powerful Sun Protection SPF 45 Sunscreen Cream ($42 for 4.2 ounces); **NuSkin** Sunright Body Block SPF 15 ($15.20 for 3.4 ounces) and Sunright Body Block SPF 30 ($15.20 for 3.4 ounces); **Paula's Choice** Extra Care Moisturizing Sunscreen SPF 30+ for Normal to Dry Skin ($14.95 for 5 ounces), Extra Care Non-Greasy Sunscreen SPF 45 ($14.95 for 5 ounces), Pure

Mineral Sunscreen SPF 15, for Normal to Very Dry Skin ($15.95 for 6 ounces), and Ultra Light Weightless Finish SPF 30 Sunscreen Spray, for All Skin Types ($15.95 for 4 ounces); **SkinCeuticals** Physical UV Defense SPF 30 ($37 for 3 ounces) and Sport UV Defense SPF 45 ($37.50 for 3 ounces).

BEST "MINERAL" SUNSCREENS WHOSE ONLY ACTIVES ARE TITANIUM DIOXIDE AND/OR ZINC OXIDE, WHICH ARE BEST FOR NORMAL TO DRY OR SENSITIVE SKIN, AT THE DEPARTMENT/SPECIALTY STORE: Paula's Choice Pure Mineral Sunscreen SPF 15, for Normal to Very Dry Skin ($15.95 for 6 ounces); **Physicians Formula** Sun Shield for Faces Extra Sensitive Skin SPF 25 ($8.95 for 4 ounces); **SkinCeuticals** Physical UV Defense SPF 30 ($37 for 3 ounces).

BEST SELF-TANNERS

By and large, almost all self-tanners will work as indicated, because 99% of them contain the same "active" ingredient, dihydroxyacetone (DHA). DHA reacts with amino acids found in the top layers of skin to create a shade of brown; the effect takes place within two to six hours, and color depth can be built with every reapplication. DHA has a long history of safe use, but it is critical to keep in mind that the "tan" you get from DHA does not provide any sun protection. If you decide to use a self-tanner, be sure you continue to protect exposed skin every day with a well-formulated sunscreen rated SPF 15 or greater and that contains the UVA-protecting ingredients of avobenzone, titanium dioxide, zinc oxide, Mexoryl SX (ecamsule), or Tinosorb.

Self-tanners with sunscreen tend to be a problem if used as your sole source of sun protection. The reason is that ideally, a self-tanner should be applied sparingly while a sunscreen requires liberal application. If you apply a self-tanner with sunscreen liberally, you risk a blotchy or too-dark result. Conversely, applying a self-tanner with sunscreen sparingly will not get you to the level of protection stated on the label, and that puts your skin at risk for damage.

If all self-tanners are similar, how did I decide which ones to rate as Paula's Picks? Good question! Although I have no doubt you will have success with any self-tanner rated with a happy face (for best results, be sure to follow the application instructions exactly), the handful of options below are the self-tanners that, for the most part, are also state-of-the-art moisturizers or gels that just happen to turn skin a beautiful shade of tan. I'd recommend starting with any of the options below before others because what each contains will prove helpful for skin (especially normal to dry skin) while imparting a sunless tan, which is the only kind I (and any dermatologist informed on the dangers of tanning in the sun) recommend.

BEST SELF-TANNERS FOR ALL SKIN TYPES, AT THE DEPARTMENT/SPECIALTY STORE: Clinique Self Sun Body Daily Moisturizer, Light-Medium ($20 for 5 ounces) and Self Sun Body Daily Moisturizer, Medium-Deep ($20 for 5 ounces); **Dr. Denese New York** Glow Younger Clear Self-Tanner for Face and Body ($32 for 6 ounces); **Estee Lauder** Body Performance Naturally Radiant Moisturizer ($35 for 6.7 ounces); **Paula's Choice** Almost the Real Thing Self-Tanning Gel, for All Skin Types ($12.95 for 5 ounces).

BEST FACIAL MASKS

Although I am rarely a woman of few words, I'm not one to get too excited about facial masks. First, as you will see from the limited options below, there are not many exciting, interesting, or particularly helpful facial masks. Many facial masks for normal to oily skin contain clay as their main ingredient, along with some thickening agents, and although that can be a benefit because it absorbs oil, the improvement is short-lived, not long-term. Other masks contain clay as well, but also include water-binding agents and plant oils, and that can make them better for normal to combination or slightly dry skin. Masks for normal to dry skin are often just moisturizers and nothing more, and don't necessarily warrant the extra time it takes to apply them. They aren't bad for skin, they just aren't a necessary step.

There are also masks that contain a plasticizing agent that you subsequently pull or peel off your skin. These do impart a temporary soft feeling to the skin because what you're doing is pulling off a layer of skin, but that is hardly beneficial or lasting (and I did not rate this type of mask favorably).

Facial masks can be a pampering, relaxing interval for women, but for good skin care, what you do daily is vastly more important than what you do once a week or once a month. The Paula's Picks in this category are the masks that either have a unique, beneficial twist (such as a clay mask that absorbs excess oil and imparts soothing agents without stripping skin) or, as is the case for every facial mask for normal to dry or very dry skin, feature outstanding formulas that supply skin with helpful ingredients (and can double as a nighttime moisturizer if you have dry skin). Any of the moisturizing masks for normal to very dry skin will work even better if left on overnight, and there are no ingredients in the masks listed below that are harmful or irritating if left on skin longer than the directions indicate.

Note: There were no facial masks from the drugstore that received a Paula's Pick rating, though some did receive a happy face rating and are worth considering.

BEST MASKS FOR NORMAL TO OILY/COMBINATION AND/OR BLEMISH-PRONE SKIN, AT THE DEPARTMENT/SPECIALTY STORE: Jan Marini Factor-A Plus Mask ($81 for 2 ounces); **Nu Skin** Epoch Glacial Marine Mud ($24.70 for 7 ounces); **Paula's Choice** Skin Balancing Carbon Mask, for Normal to Oily/Combination Skin ($14.95 for 4 ounces).

BEST MASKS FOR NORMAL TO DRY OR VERY DRY SKIN, AT THE DEPART-MENT/SPECIALTY STORE: Aveda Tourmaline Charged Radiance Masque ($29 for 4.2 ounces); **Caudalie Paris** Vinoperfect Radiance Revealing Mask ($42 for 1.3 ounces); **Estee Lauder** Resilience Lift Extreme Ultra Firming Mask ($40 for 2.5 ounces); **Paula's Choice** Skin Recovery Hydrating Treatment Mask, for Normal to Very Dry Skin ($14.95 for 4 ounces); **Peter Thomas Roth** Mega Rich Intensive Anti-Aging Cellular Moisture Masque ($60 for 3.4 ounces).

BEST SKIN-LIGHTENING PRODUCTS

The products listed below either contain the time-proven, safe skin-lightening agent hydroquinone or they contain ingredients related to it, such as arbutin or other agents that research (however limited) has shown hold some promise for lightening sun- or hormone-induced brown skin discolorations. Some of these skin-lightening products also contain an AHA or BHA at the correct pH for exfoliation to occur. The synergistic combination of hydroquinone and a chemical exfoliant not only allows the hydroquinone to work better but also helps remove layers of uneven, sun-damaged skin (and those with BHA can help keep breakouts and blackheads at bay).

Hydroquinone has become a controversial ingredient, despite considerable research demonstrating its safety when properly formulated (meaning following over-the-counter guidelines rather than adulterating products with compounds that can cause skin problems). For detailed information about this "gold standard" skin-lightening agent, please refer to the *Cosmetic Ingredient Dictionary* on www.Beautypedia.com. Over-the-counter hydroquinone products are available in strengths of 1% to 2%; higher concentrations are available from dermatologists and plastic surgeons (e.g., Tri-Luma). Keep in mind that no skin-lightening product will work if you don't use an effective sunscreen daily. Also, if you're using any over-the-counter product with hydroquinone and you haven't noticed any skin-lightening results after three months of daily use (plus daily use of a well-formulated sunscreen rated SPF 15 or greater), you should discontinue use. If this occurs, it is very likely that, for whatever reason, over-the-counter strengths of hydroquinone are not going to be effective for you.

BEST SKIN-LIGHTENING PRODUCTS THAT CONTAIN HYDROQUINONE, AT THE DRUGSTORE: Alpha Hydrox Spot Light Targeted Skin Lightener ($9.99 for 0.85 ounce).

BEST SKIN-LIGHTENING PRODUCTS THAT CONTAIN HYDROQUINONE, AT THE DEPARTMENT/SPECIALTY STORE: Paula's Choice RESIST Clearly Remarkable Skin Lightening Gel, for All Skin Types ($18.95 for 2 ounces) and RESIST Remarkable Skin Lightening Lotion, for All Skin Types ($18.95 for 2 ounces); **ProActiv Solution** Skin Lightening Lotion ($21.75 for 1 ounce).

BEST SKIN-LIGHTENING PRODUCTS THAT DO NOT CONTAIN HYDRO-QUINONE, AT THE DEPARTMENT/SPECIALTY STORE: BeautiControl Cell Block-C Intensive Brightening Elixir ($26 for 1 ounce) and Skinlogics Platinum Plus Brightening Day Creme ($26 for 3.5 ounces); **Dermalogica** AGE Smart Map-15 Regenerator ($85 for 0.3 ounce) and ChromaWhite TRx Extreme C ($85 for 0.3 ounce); **Mary Kay** TimeWise Even Complexion Essence ($35 for 1 ounce); **MD Skincare by Dr. Dennis Gross** Hydra-Pure Radiance Renewal Serum ($95 for 1 ounce); **philosophy** a pigment of your imagination SPF 18 ($30 for 2 ounces).

BEST OIL-ABSORBING PAPERS

This is another category for which it was difficult to pick the top options due to the basic and similar nature of the products in this category. The ones that made the cut did so because they had a nifty convenience feature, were noticeably more absorbent than the competition, or proved to be a very cost-effective option. Keep in mind that the many oil-absorbing papers reviewed in this book and on Beautypedia.com are options as well, though those with added oil, powders, or clays tend to be more troublesome than oil-absorbing papers without these ingredients. The reason they're troublesome is because they tend to leave an uneven deposit of clay and/or powder on skin, necessitating further touch-ups.

BEST OIL-ABSORBING PAPERS FOR NORMAL TO VERY OILY SKIN (ALL RETAIL LOCATIONS): e.l.f. Shine Eraser ($1 for 50 sheets); **Paula's Choice** Oil-Blotting Papers ($6.95 for 100 sheets); **Sephora** Natural Matte Blotting Papers ($8 for 100 sheets); **Shu Uemura** Face Paper ($12 for 40 sheets); **Sonia Kashuk** Matte, Oil Blotting Papers ($6.99 for 100 sheets).

BEST LIP PRODUCTS (INCLUDING LIP EXFOLIATORS)

Lips are certainly a focal point of the face, and an area that should not be ignored when it comes to sun protection and moisturizing. All of the products below are excellent options to remove dry, flaky skin from chapped lips, protect lips from daily sun exposure, or provide broad-spectrum sun protection. Unless you apply an opaque lipstick every day, it is important to use a lip balm or lipstick with sunscreen rated SPF 15 or greater (recommended lipsticks with sunscreen appear in the "Best Lipsticks" below). Taking the time to protect your skin from sun exposure should always include your delicate, sun-vulnerable lips, too.

BEST LIP BALMS WITH SUNSCREEN (SPF 15 OR GREATER), AT THE DRUG-STORE: Banana Boat Sport Performance Lip Balm SPF 50 ($2.99 for 0.02 ounce); **RoC Canada** Minesol High Protection Lipstick SPF 20 ($10 for 3 grams).

BEST LIP BALMS WITH SUNSCREEN (SPF 15 OR GREATER), AT THE DEPART-MENT/SPECIALTY STORE: BeautiControl Skinlogics Lip Balm SPF 20 ($10.50 for 0.6 ounce); **Jane Iredale** Lip Drink SPF 15 ($11.60 for 0.18 ounce); **Mary Kay** Lip Protector Sunscreen SPF 15 ($7.50 for 0.16 ounce); **MD Skincare by Dr. Dennis Gross** Powerful Sun Protection SPF 25 Lip Balm ($18 for 0.25 ounce); **Paula's Choice** Moisturizing Lipscreen SPF 15 ($8.95 for 0.16 ounce); **Shiseido** Sun Protection Lip Treatment SPF 36 PA++ ($20 for 0.14 ounce).

BEST LIP BALMS WITHOUT SUNSCREEN, AT THE DRUGSTORE: Boots Organic Face Lip Balm ($6.99 for 0.33 ounce).

BEST LIP BALMS WITHOUT SUNSCREEN, AT THE DEPARTMENT/SPECIALTY STORE: BeautiControl Lip Apeel ($19.50 for a two-piece set), **BeautiControl** Platinum Regeneration Age Defying Lip Treatment ($23.50 for 0.09 ounce); **Benefit** Lipscription ($32 for a two-piece set); **Estee Lauder** Nutritious Vita-Mineral Lip Treatment ($22 for 0.5 ounce); **La Roche-Posay** Ceralip Lip Repair Cream ($13.50 for 0.5 ounce); **M.A.C.** Lip Conditioner ($12.50 for 0.5 ounce); **Paula's Choice** Lip Recovery Balm ($7.95 for 0.19 ounce); **philosophy** kiss me clear tube ($12 for 0.5 ounce); **SkinCeuticals** Antioxidant Lip Repair Restorative Treatment, for Damaged or Aging Lips ($34 or 0.3 ounce); **The Body Shop** Cocoa Butter Lip Care Stick ($8 for 0.15 ounce) and Hemp Lip Protector ($8 for 0.15 ounce).

BEST MANUAL LIP EXFOLIATORS, AT THE DEPARTMENT/SPECIALTY STORE: BeautiControl Lip Apeel ($19.50 for a two-piece set); **Benefit** Lipscription ($32 for a two-piece set); **Isomers** Lip Exfoliating Balm ($8 for 0.17 ounce).

BEST PRODUCTS FOR SENSITIVE SKIN

The following lists of products are recommended for those with truly sensitive or rosacea-afflicted skin based on one primary criterion: they do not contain ingredients known to be irritating or especially problematic for sensitive skin or rosacea. That means none of these products contain fragrance of any kind, including essential oils and none of them feature inordinately long ingredient lists (which decreases the odds that your skin will suffer a negative reaction). Please be aware that even with careful consideration and adherence to usage guidelines, we cannot guarantee that these products will not cause problems for your sensitive or rosacea-prone skin. No product or product line can make this guarantee (at least not honestly) because of the many variables that can conspire to cause your skin to have a sensitized reaction. Rosacea, in particular, is a disorder that may cause a person's skin to flare with minimal provocation, or from even the most benign cosmetic ingredients, climate changes, hormonal fluctuation, and stress.

The goal of this list is to make it easier for persons with sensitive or rosacea-prone skin to find products that may work for them without making matters worse. Please know that managing rosacea requires the care and supervision of a physician, along with careful use of skin-care products and avoidance of external triggers that worsen this condition. If you experience a lingering reaction to any skin-care product, including those from the list below, discontinue use and consult your physician for advice.

Note: Unlike the other products that comprise the various "Best" lists, not all of the products below received a Paula's Pick rating. This was typically due to packaging concerns, but that doesn't change the fact that the formula itself is suitable for sensitive or rosacea-prone skin.

Second note: Beyond foundations, there are no other listings for best makeup products for those with sensitive or rosacea-prone skin. That's because, generally speaking, makeup tends to contain far fewer potential irritants and typically omits fragrance. Another reason is that some persons with sensitive skin react to various pigments in makeup. In those cases, careful avoidance is mandatory. Otherwise, please refer to the main Best Products list for a selection of the top-rated concealers, powders, blush, eyeshadow, mascara, and so on.

CLEANSERS: Boots Expert Anti-Blemish Cleansing Foam ($5.29 for 5 ounces), Expert Sensitive Cleansing & Toning Wipes ($4.49 for 30 wipes), Expert Sensitive Cleansing Lotion ($4.49 for 6.7 ounces), and Expert Sensitive Gentle Cleansing Wash ($4.49 for 6.7 ounces); **CereVe** Hydrating Cleanser ($11.99 for 12 ounces); **Cetaphil** Gentle Skin Cleanser ($7.99 for 8 ounces); **Clinique** Comforting Cream Cleanser ($18.50 for 5 ounces), Liquid Facial Soap Extra Mild ($15 for 6.7 ounces), Redness Solutions Soothing Cleanser ($20.50 for 5 ounces), Take The Day Off Cleansing Balm ($27 for 3.8 ounces), and Take The Day Off Cleansing Milk ($25 for 6.7 ounces); **DHC** Cleansing Milk ($24 for 6.7 ounces); **Estee Lauder** Verite LightLotion Cleanser ($23.50 for 6.7 ounces); **Eucerin** Aquaphor Gentle Wash for Baby ($5.99 for 8 ounces), Gentle Hydrating Cleanser ($6.99 for 8 ounces) and Redness Relief Soothing Cleanser ($8.99 for 6.8 ounces); **Good Skin** All Calm Creamy Cleanser ($15 for 6.7 ounces); **Kiehl's** Ultra Moisturizing Cleansing Cream ($14.50 for 8 ounces); **Neutrogena** Extra Gentle Cleanser ($7.99 for 6.7 ounces); **L'Occitane** Ultra Comforting Cleansing Milk ($22 for 6.7 ounces); **La Roche-Posay** Toleriane Dermo-Cleanser ($19.50 for 6.76 ounces); **Olay** Daily Facials Skin Soothing Cleansing Cloths, for Sensitive Skin ($5.99 for 30 Cloths), Foaming Face Wash, for Sensitive Skin ($4.49 for 6.78 ounces), and Gentle Foaming Face Wash, for Sensitive Skin ($5.99 for 7 ounces); **Paula's Choice** Hydralight One Step Face Cleanser, for Normal to Oily/Combination Skin ($15.95 for 8 ounces), Moisture Boost One Step Face Cleanser, for Normal to Dry Skin ($15.95 for 8 ounces), and Skin Recovery Cleanser, for Normal to Very Dry Skin ($15.95 for 8 ounces); **Physicians Formula** Gentle Cleansing Lotion, for Normal to Dry Skin ($7.25 for 8 ounces); **The Body Shop** Aloe Calming Facial Cleanser, for Sensitive Skin ($14 for 6.75 ounces) and Aloe Gentle Facial Wash, for Sensitive Skin ($16 for 4.2 ounces).

EYE MAKEUP REMOVERS: Bobbi Brown Instant Long Wear Makeup Remover ($22 for 3.4 ounces); **Clinique** Take The Day Off Makeup Remover for Lids, Lashes & Lips ($17.50 for 4.2 ounces); **DHC** Eye Make-Up Remover ($11 for 3.7 ounces); **La Roche-Posay** Rosaliac Gelee Micellar Make-Up Removal Gel ($23.50 for 6.76 ounces); **Neutrogena** Oil-Free Eye Makeup Remover ($7.99 for 5.5 ounces); **Paula's Choice** Gentle Touch Makeup Remover ($12.95 for 4 ounces).

TONERS: Paula's Choice Moisture Boost Hydrating Toner, for Normal to Dry Skin ($15.95 for 6 ounces) and Skin Recovery Toner, for Normal to Very Dry Skin ($15.95 for 6 ounces).

SCRUBS: Boots Expert Sensitive Gentle Smoothing Scrub ($5.49 for 3.3 ounces); **RoC Canada** Demaquillage Actif Gentle Exfoliating Cream ($16 for 40 ml).

BHA: Paula's Choice 1% Beta Hydroxy Acid Gel, for All Skin Types ($18.95 for 4 ounces) and 1% Beta Hydroxy Acid Lotion, for All Skin Types ($18.95 for 4 ounces).

MOISTURIZERS WITHOUT SUNSCREEN: Boots Expert Sensitive Hydrating Moisturizer ($4.99 for 1.6 ounces), Expert Sensitive Light Moisturizing Lotion ($5.99 for 6.7 ounces), and Expert Sensitive Restoring Night Treatment ($6.99 for 1.69 ounces); **CereVe** Moisturizing Cream ($14.99 for 16 ounces); **Clinique** Recovery Week Complex ($65 for 1 ounce), Super Rescue Antioxidant Night Moisturizer, for Combination Oily to Oily Skin ($42.50 for 1.7 ounces), Super Rescue Antioxidant Night Moisturizer, for Dry to Combination Skin ($42.50 for 1.7 ounces), and Super Rescue Antioxidant Night Moisturizer, for Dry to Very Dry Skin ($42.50 for 1.7 ounces); **DHC** Wrinkle Filler ($27 for 0.52 ounce); **Good Skin** All Calm Moisture Lotion ($24.50 for 1.7 ounces); **MD Formulations** Moisture Defense Antioxidant Hydrating Gel ($45 for 1 ounce); **Neutrogena** Oil-Free Moisture, for Sensitive Skin ($12.99 for 4 ounces); **Paula's Choice** HydraLight Moisture-Infusing Lotion, for Normal to Oily/Combination Skin ($18.95 for 2 ounces), Moisture Boost Hydrating Treatment Cream, for Normal to Dry Skin ($18.95 for 2 ounces), Skin Balancing Moisture Gel, For Normal to Oily/Combination Skin ($18.95 for 2 ounces), RESIST Barrier Repair Moisturizer Skin Remodeling Complex ($22.95 for 1.7 ounces), and Skin Recovery Moisturizer, for Normal to Very Dry Skin ($18.95 for 2 ounces).

MOISTURIZERS WITH SUNSCREEN: BeautiControl Cell Block C New Cell Protection SPF 20 ($30.50 for 1 ounce); **Clinique** City Block Sheer Oil-Free Daily Face Protector SPF 25 ($17.50 for 1.4 ounces) and Redness Solutions Protective Base SPF 15 ($17.50 for 1.35 ounces); **DDF Doctor's Dermatologic Formula** Daily Organic SPF 15 ($36 for 1.7 ounces); **Good Skin** All Calm Gentle Sunscreen SPF 25 ($12 for 1.7 ounces); **Paula's Choice** Skin Recovery Daily Moisturizing Lotion with SPF 15 and Antioxidants ($20.95).

EYE MOISTURIZERS: Estee Lauder Verite Special EyeCare ($37.50 for 0.5 ounce); **Paula's Choice** Moisture Boost Hydrating Treatment Cream, for Normal to Dry Skin ($18.95 for 2 ounces), Skin Balancing Moisture Gel, For Normal to Oily/Combination Skin ($18.95 for 2 ounces), RESIST Barrier Repair Moisturizer Skin Remodeling Complex ($22.95 for 1.7 ounces), and Skin Recovery Moisturizer, for Normal to Very Dry Skin ($18.95 for 2 ounces).

SERUMS: Boots Expert Sensitive Hydrating Serum ($7.49 for 1.6 ounces); **DDF - Doctor's Dermatologic Formula** C3 Plus Serum ($68 for 0.5 ounce); **Elizabeth Arden** Ceramide Gold Ultra Restorative Capsules ($68 for 0.95 ounce); **Isomers** Absolutes Anti Redness Serum ($29.99 for 1 ounce); **Paula's Choice** RESIST Super Antioxidant Concentrate Serum, for All Skin Types ($24.95 for 1 ounce).

TINTED MOISTURIZERS: Clinique Almost Makeup SPF 15 ($20.50); **Laura Geller** Barely There Tinted Moisturizer SPF 20 ($30); **Paula's Choice** Barely There Sheer Matte Tint SPF 20 ($14.95).

FACIAL MASKS: Paula's Choice Skin Balancing Carbon Mask, for Normal to Oily/Combination Skin ($14.95 for 4 ounces) and Skin Recovery Hydrating Treatment Mask, for Normal to Very Dry Skin ($14.95 for 4 ounces).

ALL-PURPOSE SUNSCREENS: Neutrogena Pure & Free Baby Sunblock Stick SPF 60+ with PureScreen ($8.99 for 0.47 ounce); **Paula's Choice** Pure Mineral Sunscreen SPF 15, for Normal to Very Dry Skin ($15.95 for 6 ounces); **Physician's Formula** Sun Shield for

Faces Extra Sensitive Skin SPF 25 (0.95 for 4 ounces); **SkinCeuticals** Physical UV Defense SPF 30 ($37 for 3 ounces).

SPECIALTY PRODUCTS: Paula's Choice Skin Relief Treatment, for All Skin Types ($15.95 for 4 ounces).

FOUNDATION WITH SUNSCREEN: Clinique Dewy Smooth Anti-Aging Makeup SPF 15 ($22.50) and Repairwear Anti-Aging Makeup SPF 15 ($28.50); **Cover Girl** CG Smoothers AquaSmooth Makeup SPF 15 ($9.99); **Jane Iredale** Amazing Base Loose Minerals SPF 20 ($42) and PurePressed Base Mineral Foundation SPF 20 ($49.50); **Paula's Choice** All Bases Covered Foundation SPF 15 ($14.95); **Shiseido** Compact Foundation SPF 15 ($29.50); **Trish McEvoy** Mineral Powder Foundation SPF 15 ($35).

FOUNDATION WITHOUT SUNSCREEN: Lorac Natural Performance Foundation ($35).

BEST FOUNDATIONS WITH SUNSCREEN

Choosing the right foundation color is not only time-consuming, but also exceedingly frustrating. The only way to discover your ideal match is to apply the foundation on your facial skin, perhaps two different colors on either side of your face, and then to check it in daylight. If the color isn't an exact match, you have to go back in and try again. Another hurdle is to find a foundation with a pleasing texture, one that feels soft and silky, but doesn't streak, cake, or look thick, and that takes experimentation, too. Determining how much coverage you want is another factor, and then there's what type of foundation (liquids or creams or stick formulas). Now tell me that isn't a challenge!

Financially, if you can splurge on only one cosmetic product, foundation is it. This is the one category where spending a little bit more is the best option, not because expensive means better, but because it's just way too risky to buy a foundation you can't try on first, either with a tester at the cosmetics counter or with samples you can take home or, in some cases, order online. Still, many mass-market outlets and drugstores have very good hassle-free return policies for used makeup, and it's wise to inquire about that before purchasing makeup in these environments (note: all of them require you to keep your receipt as proof of purchase). Do not keep a foundation that ends up being the wrong color—return it and keep trying until you get it right.

Remember that most cream-to-powder foundations or stick foundations are best for those with normal to slightly dry or slightly oily skin because the ingredients that keep these types of foundations in their cream or stick form can be problematic for oily or blemish-prone skin, and the often-powdery finish isn't flattering on dry skin.

I cannot emphasize enough how much foundation has improved over the last few years. Companies such as Estee Lauder, Lancome, L'Oreal, Revlon, and more continue to raise the bar, which only means better foundations for consumers. The foundations on the list below, whether cream, liquid, cream-to-powder, or powder all have exemplary, class-leading textures, beautiful finishes, reliable coverage, and a selection of neutral shades that match real skin tones (rather than masking skin with an odd shade of pink, rose, or peach). If you have stayed away from foundation because of a previous misstep or negative experience, there has never been a safer time to try it again; the right one can make a huge difference in the appearance of your skin. And if you have oily to very oily skin, choosing a foundation with sunscreen is a great idea because it will help keep excess shine in check while eliminating the need for you to apply two products (when it comes to very oily skin, fewer products is better).

Note: Several foundations with sunscreen reviewed would have earned a Paula's Pick rating had their SPF value been higher. Because it is widely accepted that SPF 15 is the minimum amount of daytime protection needed, I made the decision (with occasional exceptions) to not give foundations with sunscreen below SPF 15 a rating above a neutral face. However, if you are willing to pair such a foundation with another product rated SPF 15 or greater, then you may in fact want to consider those foundations as well. This is one more reason why, depending on your needs and preferences, shopping from the Best Products list alone may not be the best approach.

BEST FOUNDATIONS WITH SUNSCREEN (SPF 15 OR GREATER) FOR VERY OILY SKIN, AT THE DRUGSTORE:

LIQUID: Boots No7 Stay Perfect Foundation SPF 15 ($13.99); **L'Oreal Paris** True Match Super Blendable Makeup SPF 17 ($10.95); **Revlon** ColorStay Active Light Makeup SPF 25 ($12.99).

BEST FOUNDATIONS WITH SUNSCREEN (SPF 15 OR GREATER) FOR VERY OILY SKIN, AT THE DEPARTMENT/SPECIALTY STORE:

LIQUID: Clarins Truly Matte Foundation SPF 15 ($37.50); **Shiseido** Sun Protection Liquid Foundation SPF 42 PA+++ ($33.50).

PRESSED POWDER: Clinique Almost Powder Makeup SPF 15 ($22.50); **Shiseido** Compact Foundation SPF 15 ($29.50).

BEST FOUNDATIONS WITH SUNSCREEN (SPF 15 OR GREATER) FOR NORMAL TO OILY/COMBINATION SKIN, AT THE DRUGSTORE:

LIQUID: Almay Nearly Naked Liquid Makeup SPF 15 ($12.99), Smart Shade Smart Balance Skin Balancing Makeup SPF 15 ($11.99), and TLC Truly Lasting Color 16 Hour Makeup SPF 15 ($12.99); **Boots** No7 Stay Perfect Foundation SPF 15 ($13.99); **L'Oreal Paris** Flawless Liquid Makeup SPF 15 ($13) and True Match Super Blendable Makeup SPF 17 ($10.95); **Revlon,** Beyond Natural Skin Matching Makeup SPF 15 ($13.99) and ColorStay Active Light Makeup SPF 25 ($12.99).

CREAM-TO-POWDER: Cover Girl CG Smoothers AquaSmooth Makeup SPF 15 ($9.99); **Revlon** New Complexion One Step Compact Makeup SPF 15 ($12.99).

BEST FOUNDATIONS WITH SUNSCREEN (SPF 15 OR GREATER) FOR NORMAL TO OILY/COMBINATION SKIN, AT THE DEPARTMENT/SPECIALTY STORE:

LIQUID: Chanel Mat Lumiere Long Lasting Soft Matte Makeup SPF 15 ($54); **Clarins** Truly Matte Foundation ($37.50); **Cle de Peau Beaute** Refining Fluid Foundation SPF 24 ($118); **Clinique** Even Better Makeup ($24.50); **M.A.C.** Studio Sculpt SPF 15 Foundation ($28); **Paula's Choice** Best Face Forward Foundation SPF 15 ($14.95); **Shiseido** Dual Balancing Foundation SPF 17 ($37.50) and Sun Protection Liquid Foundation SPF 42 PA+++ ($33.50).

PRESSED POWDER: Clinique Almost Powder Makeup SPF 15 ($22.50); **Dior** Dior-Skin Forever Compact Flawless & Moist Extreme Wear Makeup SPF 25 ($42); **Estee Lauder** Nutritious Vita-Mineral Loose Powder Makeup SPF 15 ($33.50); **Shiseido** Compact Foundation SPF 15 ($29.50), STM Perfect Smoothing Compact Foundation SPF 15 ($30) and Sun Protection Compact Foundation SPF 34 PA+++ ($25.50).

CREAM-TO-POWDER: Clinique Superbalanced Compact Makeup SPF 20 ($28); **Dior** DiorSkin Compact SPF 20 ($41); **SK-II** Signs Transform Foundation SPF 20 ($90); **The Body Shop** Flawless Skin Protecting Foundation SPF 25 ($25).

BEST FOUNDATIONS WITH SUNSCREEN (SPF 15 OR GREATER) FOR NORMAL TO DRY SKIN, AT THE DRUGSTORE:

LIQUID: Almay TLC Truly Lasting Color 16 Hour Makeup SPF 15 ($12.99); **L'Oreal Paris** H.I.P. Flawless Liquid Makeup SPF 15; **Revlon** Age Defying Makeup With Botafirm SPF 15 ($13.99) and ColorStay Makeup with Softflex, for Normal to Dry Skin SPF 15 ($12.99).

CREAM-TO-POWDER: Maybelline New York Instant Age Rewind Custom Face Perfector Cream Compact Foundation SPF 18 ($7.99); **Revlon** New Complexion One Step Compact Makeup SPF 15 ($12.99).

BEST FOUNDATIONS WITH SUNSCREEN (SPF 15 OR GREATER) FOR NORMAL TO DRY SKIN, AT THE DEPARTMENT/SPECIALTY STORE:

LIQUID: Chanel Mat Lumiere Long Lasting Soft Matte SPF15 ($54); **Cle de Peau Beaute** Refining Fluid Foundation SPF 24 ($118); **Clinique** Dewy Smooth Anti-Aging Makeup SPF 15 ($22.50) and Repairwear Anti-Aging Makeup SPF 15 ($28.50); **Lancome** Absolue BX Makeup Absolute Replenishing Radiant Makeup SPF 18 ($57); **M.A.C.** Select SPF 15 Moistureblend ($29) and Studio Sculpt SPF 15 Foundation ($28); **Paula's Choice** All Bases Covered Foundation SPF 15 ($14.95); **Shiseido** Dual Balancing Foundation SPF 17 ($37.50).

PRESSED POWDER: Clinique Almost Powder Makeup SPF 15 ($22.50); **Dior** DiorSkin Forever Compact Flawless & Moist Extreme Wear Makeup SPF 25 ($42); **Shiseido** Compact Foundation SPF15 ($29.50), STM Perfect Smoothing Compact Foundation SPF 15 ($30) and Sun Protection Compact Foundation SPF 34 PA+++ ($25.50).

CREAM-TO-POWDER AND/OR STICK: Clinique City Stick SPF 15 ($22); **Dior** DiorSkin Compact SPF 20 ($41); **Estee Lauder** Resilience Lift Extreme Ultra Firming Crème Compact Makeup SPF 15 ($34.50); **M.A.C.** Studio Stick Foundation SPF 15 ($29); **Shiseido** Stick Foundation SPF 15 ($37.50).

BEST FOUNDATIONS WITH SUNSCREEN (SPF 15 OR GREATER) FOR DRY TO VERY DRY SKIN, AT THE DRUGSTORE:

LIQUID: Almay TLC Truly Lasting Color 16 Hour Makeup SPF 15 ($12.99); **L'Oreal Paris** HIP Flawless Liquid Makeup SPF 15 ($13); **Revlon** ColorStay Makeup with Softflex for Normal to Dry Skin SPF 15 ($12.99).

BEST FOUNDATIONS WITH SUNSCREEN (SPF 15 OR GREATER) FOR DRY TO VERY DRY SKIN, AT THE DEPARTMENT/SPECIALTY STORE:

LIQUID: Lancome Absolue BX Makeup Absolute Replenishing Radiant Makeup SPF 18 ($57); **M.A.C.** Select SPF 15 Moistureblend ($29).

CREAM-TO-POWDER: Giorgio Armani Designer Shaping Cream Foundation SPF 20 ($65).

BEST SHEER FOUNDATIONS/TINTED MOISTURIZERS WITH SUNSCREEN (SPF 15 OR GREATER) FOR ALL SKIN TYPES EXCEPT VERY OILY, AT THE DRUGSTORE: Boots No7 Soft & Sheer Tinted Moisturizer SPF 15 ($20.50); **Neutrogena** Healthy Skin Enhancer SPF 20 ($11.99) and Healthy Skin Glow Sheers SPF 30 ($12.79); **Olay** Regenerist Touch of Foundation UV Defense Regenerating Moisturizer SPF 15 ($19.99).

BEST SHEER FOUNDATIONS/TINTED MOISTURIZERS WITH SUNSCREEN (SPF 15 OR GREATER) FOR ALL SKIN TYPES EXCEPT VERY OILY, AT THE DEPARTMENT/SPECIALTY STORE: Aveda Inner Light Tinted Moisturizer SPF 15 ($26); **Bobbi Brown** SPF 15 Tinted Moisturizer ($40); **Clinique** Almost Makeup SPF 15 ($20.50); **Estee Lauder** DayWear Plus Multi Protection Anti-Oxidant Moisturizer Sheer Tint Release Formula SPF 15, for All Skin Types ($38.50) and DayWear Plus Multi Protection Tinted Moisturizer SPF 15 ($35); **Laura Geller** Barely There Tinted Moisturizer SPF 20 ($30); **Laura**

Mercier Illuminating Tinted Moisturizer SPF 20 ($42); **Paula's Choice** Barely There Sheer Matte Tint SPF 20 ($14.95); **Stila** Sheer Color Tinted Moisturizer SPF 15 ($34).

BEST FOUNDATIONS WITHOUT SUNSCREEN

BEST FOUNDATIONS *WITHOUT* SUNSCREEN FOR VERY OILY SKIN, AT THE DRUGSTORE:

LIQUID: **Almay** Clear Complexion Liquid Makeup ($12.49).

CREAM-TO-POWDER AND/OR STICK: **Boots** No7 Intelligent Balance Mousse Foundation ($13.99); **Marcelle** Satin Matte Mousse Make-Up ($16.95).

BEST FOUNDATIONS *WITHOUT* SUNSCREEN FOR VERY OILY SKIN, AT THE DEPARTMENT/SPECIALTY STORE:

LIQUID: **Clinique** Perfectly Real Makeup ($22.50) and Superfit Makeup Oil-Free Long Wear ($20.50); **Lancome** Teint Idole Ultra Enduringly Divine & Comfortable Makeup ($40); **Make Up For Ever** HD Invisible Cover Foundation ($40), Mat Velvet + Mattifying Foundation ($34); **Stila** Natural Finish Oil-Free Makeup ($38).

PRESSED POWDER: **Lorac** Oil-Free Wet/Dry Powder Makeup ($36); **Make Up For Ever** Duo Mat Powder Foundation ($32) and Powder Foundation ($40).

CREAM-TO-POWDER AND/OR STICK: **Avon** Beyond Color Line Softening Mousse Foundation ($12); **Clarins** Express Compact Foundation Wet/Dry ($37).

BEST FOUNDATIONS *WITHOUT* SUNSCREEN FOR NORMAL TO OILY/ COMBINATION SKIN, AT THE DRUGSTORE:

LIQUID: **Almay** Clear Complexion Liquid Makeup ($12.49); **Cover Girl** TruBlend Liquid Makeup ($9.39); **Maybelline New York** Dream Liquid Mousse Airbrush Finish ($8.79); **Sally Hansen Natural Beauty Inspired by Carmindy** Your Skin Makeup ($12.99).

PRESSED POWDER: **Sonia Kashuk** Dual Coverage Powder Foundation ($10.49).

CREAM-TO-POWDER: **Boots** No7 Intelligent Balance Mousse Foundation ($13.99); Cover Girl TruBlend Whipped Foundation ($9.60); **Marcelle** Satin Matte Mousse Make-Up ($16.95).

BEST FOUNDATIONS *WITHOUT* SUNSCREEN FOR NORMAL TO OILY/COM-BINATION SKIN, AT THE DEPARTMENT/SPECIALTY STORE:

LIQUID: **Clinique** Perfectly Real Makeup ($22.50) and Superfit Makeup Oil-Free Long Wear ($20.50); **Giorgio Armani** Luminous Silk Foundation ($58); Good Skin All Firm Makeup ($16); **Lancome** Teint Idole Ultra Enduringly Divine & Comfortable Makeup ($40); **Laura Mercier** Silk Crème Foundation ($42); **Lorac** Natural Performance Foundation ($35); **Make Up For Ever** HD Invisible Cover Foundation ($40), Mat Velvet + Mattifying Foundation ($34); **Stila** Natural Finish Oil-Free Makeup ($38).

PRESSED POWDER: **Clinique** Perfectly Real Compact Makeup ($22.50); **Laura Mercier** Foundation Powder; **Lorac** Oil-Free Wet/Dry Powder Makeup ($36); **M.A.C.** Studio Fix Powder Plus Foundation ($26); **Make Up For Ever** Duo Mat Powder Foundation ($32) and Powder Foundation ($40); **Sephora** Mattifying Compact Foundation ($20); **The Body Shop** All in One Face Base ($20).

CREAM-TO-POWDER: **Avon** Beyond Color Line Softening Mousse Foundation ($12); **Clarins** Express Compact Foundation Wet/Dry ($37).

BEST FOUNDATIONS *WITHOUT* SUNSCREEN FOR NORMAL TO DRY SKIN, AT THE DRUGSTORE:

LIQUID: Maybelline New York Dream Liquid Mousse Airbrush Finish ($8.79).

CREAM-TO-POWDER: Cover Girl TruBlend Whipped Foundation ($9.60).

BEST FOUNDATIONS *WITHOUT* SUNSCREEN FOR NORMAL TO DRY SKIN, AT THE DEPARTMENT/SPECIALTY STORE:

LIQUID: Clarins Extra Firming Foundation ($42); **Giorgio Armani** Luminous Silk Foundation ($58); **Good Skin** All Firm Makeup ($16); **Laura Mercier** Moisturizing Foundation ($42); **Lorac** Natural Performance Foundation ($35); **Stila** Illuminating Liquid Foundation ($38); **Trish McEvoy** Even Skin Foundation ($55).

PRESSED POWDER: Avon Mark Powder Buff Natural Skin Foundation ($8); **Clinique** Perfectly Real Compact Makeup ($22.50); **Lancome** Dual Finish Fragrance Free Versatile Powder Makeup ($35.50) and Dual Finish Versatile Powder Makeup ($35.50); **Lorac** Oil-Free Wet/Dry Powder Makeup ($36); **M.A.C.** Studio Fix Powder Plus Foundation ($26); **Make Up For Ever** Powder Foundation ($40); **The Body Shop** All in One Face Base ($20).

CREAM-TO-POWDER: Bobbi Brown Moisturizing Cream Compact Foundation ($40) and Oil-Free Even Finish Compact Foundation ($40); **Clarins** Express Compact Foundation Wet/Dry ($37).

BEST LIQUID FOUNDATIONS *WITHOUT* SUNSCREEN FOR DRY TO VERY DRY SKIN, AT THE DEPARTMENT/SPECIALTY STORE:

LIQUID: Clinique Perfectly Real Makeup ($22.50); **Stila** Illuminating Liquid Foundation ($38).

CREAM-TO-POWDER: Bobbi Brown Moisturizing Cream Compact Foundation ($40); **Clarins** Express Compact Foundation Wet/Dry ($37).

BEST FOUNDATIONS WITH MAXIMUM COVERAGE, REGARDLESS OF SKIN TYPE, WITH AND WITHOUT SUNSCREEN, AT ALL STORES: BeautiControl Secret AGEnt Undercover Makeup ($15); **Cle de Peau Beaute** Teint Naturel Cream Foundation ($110); **Estee Lauder** Maximum Cover Camouflage Makeup for Face & Body SPF 15; **Exuviance by Neostrata** CoverBlend Concealing Treatment Makeup SPF 20 ($22..50); **M.A.C.** Pro Full Coverage Foundation ($28); **Smashbox** Camera Ready Full Coverage Foundation SPF 15 ($38).

BEST FOUNDATION PRIMERS

Foundation primers truly aren't essential yet many women have been led to believe that skipping this step is absolutely ruinous to a beautiful makeup application. The fact is, most of us are already priming our skin for makeup by virtue of following a food skin-care routine beforehand. You don't need a special product labeled "primer" before applying foundation, and there is nothing in foundation that skin needs to be protected from. The primers on the list below are included not only because their formulas surpass standard primers but because my readers continue to ask me for my favorites in this group. Although all of the recommendations below are great, you can achieve similar results applying a state-of-the-art serum or lightweight moisturizer instead. You definitely don't need a well-formulated moisturizer, serum *and* primer. That's definitely going overboard and can cause your makeup to not last as long—just the opposite of what primers are said to do.

BEST FOUNDATION PRIMERS, AT THE DRUGSTORE: Revlon Age Defying Instant Firming Face Primer for Dry Skin ($13.99) and Age Defying Instant Firming Face Primer for Normal/Combination Skin ($13.99).

BEST FOUNDATION PRIMERS, AT THE DEPARTMENT/SPECIALTY STORE: **Clarins** Instant Light Complexion Perfector ($32); **Giorgio Armani** Light Master Primer ($55); **M.A.C.** Prep + Prime Line Filler ($19.50).

BEST CONCEALERS

Although there are lots of good concealers available in all price ranges, the options below represent the elite, whether you prefer a liquid formula (generally best for normal to oily skin or for use on blemishes) or cream formula (generally best for normal to dry skin not prone to blemishes or for under-eye use). Each concealer below has a beautiful texture, provides moderate to significant coverage without looking thick or cakey, and has an impressive wear time with minimal to no risk of creasing into lines around the eye. I have no doubt you will be pleased with almost any concealer on this list, but please refer to each individual review for details before making your final decision.

I do not recommend color-correcting concealers because they rarely (if ever) look convincing in natural light, and they often substitute one visible discoloration for another.

BEST LIQUID CONCEALERS, AT THE DRUGSTORE: L'Oreal Paris True Match Concealer ($8.95) and Visible Lift Line-Minimizing & Tone-Enhancing Under Eye Concealer SPF 20 ($8.99); **Maybelline New York** Instant Age Rewind Double Face Perfector ($7.09).

BEST LIQUID CONCEALERS, AT THE DEPARTMENT/SPECIALTY STORE: Benefit Lyin' Eyes ($18); **Cargo** One Base Concealer + Foundation in One ($24); **Chanel** Correcteur Perfection Long Lasting Concealer ($40); **Dior** DiorSkin Sculpt Lifting Smoothing Concealer ($30); **Elizabeth Arden** Flawless Finish Concealer ($16); **Lancome** Maquicomplet Eclat Eye Brightening Concealer ($27.50); **Origins** Quick, Hide! Easy Blend Concealer ($14.50).

BEST CREAM, CREAM-TO-POWDER, AND STICK CONCEALERS, AT THE DEPARTMENT/SPECIALTY STORE: Cle de Peau Beaute Concealer ($70); **Clinique** All About Eyes Concealer ($15.50); **Flirt** Pretty Easy Quick Cover ($10); **M.A.C.** Select Cover-Up ($15.50); **Make Up For Ever** Full Cover Concealer ($30); **Mary Kay** Concealer ($10); **Paula's Choice** Soft Cream Concealer ($9.95).

BEST POWDERS

Quite honestly (well, I'm always honest in my reviews, but it deserves mention here), it is getting more and more difficult to find a bad loose or pressed powder. For the most part, all of them have an appreciable degree of silkiness and do their jobs of setting makeup, absorbing excess oil, and helping made-up skin look finished. The powders below are those whose qualities surpass the norm, set new benchmarks, and perform beautifully, with most setting to a finish that resembles a second skin (albeit a better looking one). Those who find the lists below too limiting should know that any powder rated with a happy face is also worth considering (but, for various reasons, isn't in the same league as the powders below). Depending on your preferences and expectations, the powder field is mostly wide open (and the shade options for women of color continue to improve; ashy powders are few and far between these days unless you're shopping for a mineral powder).

Expense does not distinguish powders one from the other; there are equally beautiful options at the drugstore as there are at the department store. For example, L'Oreal and Lancome (owned by L'Oreal) each have equally impressive loose powders for normal to dry skin. Lancome's has more elegant packaging, but that doesn't affect the outcome on your face.

A separate category of pressed powders are those that contain sunscreen with an SPF 15 and the mineral-based UVA-protecting ingredients of titanium dioxide or zinc oxide. These are excellent options as a way to touch up makeup and add sunscreen protection over your foundation to be sure you have all-day coverage. Because of their thicker texture, these can also double as powder foundation, though they are best used over a regular sunscreen or over a foundation with sunscreen to ensure sun protection.

Note: The recommendations for skin type in each powder review are more interchangeable than you might expect. Choosing a powder truly has more to do with your preference (what kind of finish you like), how much of the product you use, and what kind of foundation you wear. However, powders reviewed as best for dry skin typically have a satiny (as opposed to dry matte) finish, which is a more attractive choice for women with dry skin who use powder. Conversely, powders recommended for normal to oily skin have a drier, noticeably matte finish (though none of the matte-finish powders below make skin look flat or dull).

BEST LOOSE POWDERS FOR NORMAL TO OILY/COMBINATION OR VERY OILY SKIN, AT THE DRUGSTORE: Almay Nearly Naked Loose Powder ($12.49); **Boots** No7 Perfect Light Loose Powder ($11.99) and No7 Perfect Light Portable Loose Powder ($12.99).

BEST LOOSE POWDERS FOR NORMAL TO OILY/COMBINATION OR VERY OILY SKIN, AT THE DEPARTMENT/SPECIALTY STORE: Avon Mark Powder-matic Go Anywhere Loose Powder ($8); **Bobbi Brown** Sheer Finish Loose Powder ($34); **Chanel** Poudre Universelle Libre Natural Finish Loose Powder ($52); **DHC** Q10 Face Powder ($17); **Laura Mercier** Loose Setting Powder ($34); **M.A.C.** Prep + Prime Transparent Finishing Powder ($21) and Select Sheer Loose Powder ($21); **Make Up For Ever** Super Matte Loose Powder ($24); **Shiseido** Translucent Loose Powder ($35); **Shu Uemura** Face Powder Matte ($33); **Trish McEvoy** Even Skin Finishing Powder ($30).

BEST LOOSE POWDERS FOR NORMAL TO DRY SKIN, AT THE DRUGSTORE: Almay Nearly Naked Loose Powder ($12.49); **L'Oreal Paris** Translucide Naturally Luminous Powder ($10.59); **Marcelle** Face Powder ($13.50); **Physicians Formula** Loose-to-Go Multi-Colored Loose Powder ($11.95).

BEST LOOSE POWDERS FOR NORMAL TO DRY SKIN, AT THE DEPARTMENT/ SPECIALTY STORE: Avon Ideal Shade Loose Powder ($9); **Avon Mark** Powder-matic Go Anywhere Loose Powder ($8); **Bobbi Brown** Sheer Finish Loose Powder ($34); **Chanel** Poudre Universelle Libre Natural Finish Loose Powder ($52); **Clarins** Loose Powder ($35); **Clinique** Blended Face Powder & Brush ($19); **DHC** Q10 Face Powder ($17); **Giorgio Armani** Micro-fil Loose Powder ($48); **Good Skin** Totally Natural Loose Powder ($16); **La Mer** The Powder ($65); **Lancome** Absolue Powder Radiant Smoothing Powder ($52); **Laura Mercier** Loose Setting Powder ($34); **M.A.C.** Prep + Prime Transparent Finishing Powder ($21) and Select Sheer Loose Powder ($21); **Make Up For Ever** Super Matte Loose Powder ($24); **Shiseido** Translucent Loose Powder ($35); **Shu Uemura** Face Powder Matte ($33) and Face Powder Sheer ($33); **Trish McEvoy** Even Skin Finishing Powder ($30).

BEST PRESSED POWDERS FOR NORMAL TO OILY/COMBINATION OR VERY OILY SKIN, AT THE DRUGSTORE: Cover Girl Advanced Radiance Age-Defying Pressed Powder ($8.05) and TruBlend Pressed Powder ($7.99); **L'Oreal** True Match Super Blendable Powder; **Maybelline New York** Dream Matte Face Powder ($6.49); **Revlon** ColorStay Pressed Powder ($9.99); **Sonia Kashuk** Bare Minimum Pressed Powder ($9.99)

BEST PRESSED POWDERS FOR NORMAL TO OILY/COMBINATION OR VERY OILY SKIN, AT THE DEPARTMENT/SPECIALTY STORE: Avon Ideal Shade Pressed Powder ($9); **Avon Mark** Matte-Nificent Oil-Absorbing Facial Powder ($8); **Bobbi Brown** Sheer Finish Pressed Powder ($34); **Estee Lauder** AeroMatte Ultralucent Pressed Powder ($26); **Giorgio Armani** Luminous Silk Powder ($44); **Korres Natural** Multivitamin Compact Powder ($28); **Lancome** Color Ideal Pressed Powder Precise Match Skin Perfecting Pressed Powder ($33); **Laura Mercier** Pressed Setting Powder ($30); **Lorac** Translucent Touch Up Powder ($32); **M.A.C.** Select Sheer Pressed Powder ($21); **Paula's Choice** Healthy Finish Pressed Powder SPF 15 ($14.95).

BEST PRESSED POWDERS FOR NORMAL TO DRY SKIN, AT THE DRUGSTORE: Almay Line Smoothing Pressed Powder ($13.99); **Cover Girl** Advanced Radiance Age-Defying Pressed Powder ($8.05) and TruBlend Pressed Powder ($7.99); **L'Oreal** True Match Super Blendable Powder; **Sally Hansen Natural Beauty Inspired by Carmindy** Luminous Matte Pressed Powder ($11.99); **Sonia Kashuk** Bare Minimum Pressed Powder ($9.99).

BEST PRESSED POWDERS FOR NORMAL TO DRY SKIN, AT THE DEPART-MENT/SPECIALTY STORE: Bobbi Brown Sheer Finish Pressed Powder ($34); **Cle de Peau Beaute** Luminizing Relief Powder ($45); **Estee Lauder** AeroMatte Ultralucent Pressed Powder ($26); **Korres Natural** Rice and Olive Oil Compact Powder ($28) and Wild Rose Compact Powder ($28); **Lancome** Color Ideal Pressed Powder Precise Match Skin Perfecting Pressed Powder ($33); **Laura Mercier** Pressed Setting Powder ($30); **Lorac** Translucent Touch Up Powder ($32); **M.A.C.** Select Sheer Pressed Powder ($21); **Mary Kay** Sheer Mineral Pressed Powder ($16); **The Body Shop** Pressed Face Powder ($18.50); **Yves Saint Laurent** Poudre Compact Eclat et Matite Matt & Radiant Pressed Powder ($45.50).

BEST PRESSED POWDERS WITH SUNSCREEN FOR ALL SKIN TYPES, AT THE DEPARTMENT/SPECIALTY STORE: Avon Anew Beauty Age-Transforming Pressed Powder SPF 15 ($12); **Paula's Choice** Healthy Finish Pressed Powder SPF 15 ($14.95); **Shiseido** Pureness Mattifying Compact Oil-Free SPF 16 ($20).

BEST BRONZING POWDERS, GELS, AND LIQUIDS

The short lists below represent what I found to be the top-performing bronzing products, whether you prefer powder (the predominant form) or a gel-type product. Each bronzing product not only is easy to apply and blend, but also produces a convincing, real-tan color and is suitable for a range of skin tones. Those looking for a bronzing powder or liquid with noticeable shine should refer to the list of Best "Face/Body Illuminating/Shimmer Products" below. The bronzing powders on this list have a matte or semi-matte finish, which is far more natural (at least for daytime) than trying to create a fake tan that glistens.

BEST PRESSED BRONZING POWDERS, AT THE DRUGSTORE: Rimmel Natural Bronzer ($5.49); **Sally Hansen Natural Beauty Inspired by Carmindy** Sun Glow Powder Bronzer ($12.99); **Wet `n` Wild** Bronzer Ultimate Bronzing Powder ($2.99) and Natural Wear Bronzer ($4.99).

BEST PRESSED BRONZING POWDERS, AT THE DEPARTMENT/SPECIALTY STORE: Avon True Color Bronzer ($10); **Clarins** Sun Face Palette SPF 20 ($35); **Dior** Bronze Harmonie de Blush ($42) and Dior Bronze Matte Sunshine SPF 20 ($40); **fresh** Marbella Gold and Tunisian Bronze Face Lusters ($45); **M.A.C.** Bronzing Powder ($21); **Stila** Sun SPF 15 Bronzing Powder ($28); **Trish McEvoy** Dual Resort Bronzer ($32) and Matte Bronzer ($28).

BEST BRONZING GELS, AT THE DEPARTMENT/SPECIALTY STORE: Bobbi Brown All Over Bronzing Gel SPF 15 ($28); **Cargo** Multi-Mix Bronzer ($28); **Giorgio Armani** Bronze Mania Skin Tint ($55); **Stila** Sun Gel ($24).

BEST BRONZING CREAMS AND LIQUIDS, AT THE DRUGSTORE: Maybelline New York Dream Mousse Bronzer ($5.99).

BEST BRONZING CREAMS AND LIQUIDS, AT THE DEPARTMENT/SPECIALTY STORE: Benefit Glamazon ($26); **Giorgio Armani** Body Tints Bronzer ($75) and Bronze Mania Summer Foundation; **gloMinerals** gloSheer Tint Base Bronzing Gel ($30); **Lorac** TANtalizer Body Bronzing Luminizer ($30); **Smashbox** Bronze Lights ($28) and O-Bronze ($26); **Stila** Bronzing Tinted Moisturizer ($32).

BEST BLUSHES

Today's best powder blushes have silky-smooth textures, apply evenly, don't fade, and come in a range of pigment density (so you can create either a dramatic or soft appearance with little effort). For the most part, blush is probably one of the easiest cosmetics to get right because it is nearly impossible to buy a bad blush. Not that there aren't some real losers out there, but there are far more winners. The problem with blush is usually in application, and that is where good brushes come into play. Using the proper brush is essential for getting blush to go on correctly. With very few exceptions, you should just discard the mini-brushes that come packaged with a powder blush in favor of an elegant, professional-size blush brush.

Powder blush is by far the most popular form of this makeup staple, but for variety's sake many lines offer cream, cream-to-powder, and liquid or gel blushes. Those that proved particularly impressive (or easier than usual to work with) earned my top rating and are on the lists below. Because most blushes in all forms have some degree of shine (clearly, many women must want shiny cheeks), I did not take a matte finish into consideration as strongly as I have in the past. There are some terrific matte blushes on the lists below, but, for the most part, what passes for matte today still has a hint of shine. Any noticeably shiny blush on the lists below was included because the shine does not flake or interfere with a smooth application. Please refer to each blush's individual review for comments on its finish (matte, almost matte, or level of shine).

Note: The cream blushes on the lists below are recommended only for dry to very dry skin that is not prone to blemishes.

BEST POWDER BLUSHES, AT THE DRUGSTORE: L'Oreal Feel Naturale Light Softening Blush ($11.99) and True Match Super-Blendable Blush ($10.95); **Sonia Kashuk** Beautifying Blush ($7.99); **Wet `n` Wild** Silk Finish Blush ($2.99).

BEST POWDER BLUSHES, AT THE DEPARTMENT/SPECIALTY STORE: American Beauty Blush Perfect Cheek Color ($15.50) and Beloved Rose Powder Blush ($18); **Avon Mark** Good Glowing Mosaic Blush ($7); **Cargo** Blu-Ray Blush/Highlighter ($24); **Clarins** Powder Blush Compact ($29.50); **Dior** DiorBlush ($38); **DHC** Face Color Perfect Pro Cheek ($9); **fresh** Here Comes the Sun Face Palette ($45); **Good Skin** Naturally Cheeky Powder Blush ($15); **Korres Natural** Blush ($22); **Laura Mercier** Second Skin Cheek Colour ($24); **Lorac** Blush ($19); **Make Up For Ever** Sculpting Blush Powder Blush ($24); **NARS** Blush ($25); **Shu Uemura** Glow On ($21); **Stila** Cheek Color Pan ($18); **Urban Decay** Afterglow Blush ($17).

BEST CREAM-TO-POWDER OR STICK BLUSHES, AT THE DRUGSTORE: Maybelline New York Dream Mousse Blush ($5.99); **Revlon** Cream Blush ($9.79); **Sonia Kashuk** Crème Blush ($9.99).

BEST CREAM-TO-POWDER OR STICK BLUSHES, AT THE DEPARTMENT/ SPECIALTY STORE: Avon Mark Just Pinched Instant Blush Tint ($6); **Clarins** Multi-Blush ($28.50); **Clinique** Blushwear Cream Stick ($18.50); **Dior** Pro Cheeks Ultra-Radiant Blush ($30); **Estee Lauder** Signature Satin Crème Blush ($26); **Lancome** Color Design Blush Sensational Effects Cream Blush, Smooth Hold ($27); **Sheer Cover** Mousse Blush ($24.95); **Laura Geller** Tint Hint ($23); **Lorac** Sheer Wash ($20).

BEST LIQUID OR GEL BLUSHES, AT THE DRUGSTORE: Sonia Kashuk Super Sheer Liquid Tint ($9.99).

BEST LIQUID OR GEL BLUSHES, AT THE DEPARTMENT/SPECIALTY STORE: Benefit BeneTint ($28); **NARS** Color Wash ($25).

BEST TRADITIONAL CREAM BLUSHES, AT THE DEPARTMENT/SPECIALTY STORE: Avon Mark Just Pinched Instant Blush Tint ($6); **Bobbi Brown** Pot Rouge for Lips and Cheeks ($22); **Laura Geller** Cheek Sweeps ($17); **Laura Mercier** Creme Cheek Colour ($22).

BEST EYESHADOWS

In much the same way loose and pressed powders continue to improve for the better, so do eyeshadows. Those listed below have enviable silky textures, apply seamlessly, blend and build well, and have staying power. You can shop the cosmetics counters in both the drugstores and the department stores and find wonderful textures and colors, although when it comes to variety of matte shades, the scales remain tipped in favor of the department stores (primarily in the makeup artist–driven lines such as M.A.C., Stila, and Bobbi Brown). Those of you who love eyeshadow with some shine will find these options almost limitless, regardless of where you shop. The good news is that today's best shiny eyeshadows add more glow than glitter to your eyes, and the shine clings much better than in the past (though there are still plenty of shiny eyeshadows that flake, none of which are on the lists below). Eyeshadows on this list include singles, duos, trios, and quads. Please keep in mind that purchasing multiple eyeshadows as part of a set only makes sense if you'll really use the color combinations provided (and in many cases, you won't want to, at least not if you want to create a classic, understated eye design).

BEST POWDER EYESHADOWS (INCLUDING SINGLES, DUOS, TRIOS and QUADS), AT THE DRUGSTORE: Marcelle Wet & Dry Eyeshadow Quad ($13.95); **NYX Cosmetics** Eyeshadow ($4.99); **Physicians Formula** Bright Collection Shimmery Quads Eye Shadow ($6.75), Matte Collection Quad Eye Shadow ($6.75), and Shimmer Strips Custom Eye Enhancing Shadow & Liner ($10.95).

BEST POWDER EYESHADOWS (INCLUDING SINGLES, DUOS, TRIOS and QUADS), AT THE DEPARTMENT/SPECIALTY STORE: Cargo Essential Eyeshadow Palette ($32); **Clarins** Single Eye Colour ($20); **Clinique** Colour Surge Eye Shadow Duo ($17.50), Colour Surge Eye Shadow Quad ($25), Colour Surge Eye Shadow Soft Shimmer ($14) and Colour Surge Eye Shadow Stay Matte ($14); **Dior** 1-Colour Eyeshadow ($24.50), 2-Colour Eyeshadow ($35), and 5-Colour Eyeshadow Compact ($54); **DHC** Eye Shadow Moon ($6) and Eye Shadow Perfect Pro ($21); **Elizabeth Arden** Color Intrigue Eyeshadow ($15) and Color Intrigue Eyeshadow Duo ($24.50); **Estee Lauder** Pure Color Eye Shadow ($17.50); **Jane Iredale** Duo Eye Shadows ($27); **Giorgio Armani** Maestro Eye Shadow Quads ($58); **Korres Natural** Eyeshadow ($16); **Lancome** Ombre Absolue Duo Radiant Smoothing Eye Shadow Duo 6 Hour Hold ($35); **Laura Mercier** Eye Colour Trio ($38), Luster Eye Colour ($22), and Matte Eye Colour ($22); **M.A.C.** Eye Shadows, Veluxe ($14.50) and Matte

Eye Shadow ($14.50); **Sephora** Colorful Mono Eyeshadow ($12); **Shu Uemura** Pressed Eye Shadow ($20); **Stila** Eye Shadow Duo ($20) and Eye Shadow Pan ($18); **Trish McEvoy** Deluxe Eye Shadow ($20), Eye Definer/Eye Liner ($16), and Glaze Eye Shadow ($16); **Urban Decay** Matte Eyeshadow ($16); **Yves Saint Laurent** Ombre Solo Double Effect ($28.50).

BEST CREAM-TO-POWDER, STICK, GEL, LIQUID, AND CREAM EYESHAD-OWS, AT THE DRUGSTORE: **L'Oreal Paris H.I.P. Makeup** Cream Shadow Paint ($12), **Revlon** Illuminance Creme Eyeshadow ($6.50).

BEST CREAM-TO-POWDER, STICK, GEL, LIQUID, AND CREAM EYESHAD-OWS, AT THE DEPARTMENT/SPECIALTY STORE: **Bobbi Brown** Long-Wear Cream Shadow ($22); **M.A.C.** Paint Pot ($16.50).

BEST EYE AND BROW SHAPERS

There are numerous options to line eyes and define the brows, depending on your mood, makeup style, and the amount of time you have to apply such products.

I am still a fan of lining eyes with a matte-powder eyeshadow, used wet or dry (with wet application producing a more intense effect). However, I have abandoned my powder eyeshadow in favor of the various gel-type eyeliners available. The ones below apply easily; allow me to create any kind of line I'd like (depending on the brush I use); and last all day without smearing, flaking, or fading. In some respects, these are similar to liquid eyeliners, but they tend to dry faster and are easier to apply, plus the effect is softer, and they last longer. There are, however, some incredible liquid eyeliners to consider if that is your preference.

When it comes to eye and brow pencils, those rated as standard tend to have more similarities than differences. I did not rate any pencil that needed routine sharpening a Paula's Pick because there are enough excellent automatic (no sharpening required) pencils available; I just can't understand why anyone would bother with the other kind, though this is still the dominant version both at drugstores and department stores. The eye and brow pencils on the lists below have quick, smooth applications and a long-wearing finish. The eye pencils tend to be creamier but don't smear, while the brow pencils have a drier texture and powder-like finish (much better for brows than wax-laden, greasy brow pencils).

Several companies sell tinted eyebrow gels as a way to fill, groom, and define the brow. There are also a few companies that make a clear brow gel that isn't much different from using hairspray on a toothbrush and brushing it through the brow. For the most part, the natural-colored brow gels are great, and I strongly recommend them as another way to make eyebrows look fuller but not artificial. If you can learn how to use the eyebrow "mascaras," they are a great alternative (or adjunct) to brow pencils. The brow gels listed below are those that keep brows groomed while not feeling sticky or making brow hairs feel stiff or look obviously coated.

BEST LIQUID, CAKE, OR GEL EYELINERS, AT THE DRUGSTORE: **Almay** Liquid Eyeliner ($7.49); **L'Oreal Paris** Lineur Intense Felt Tip Liquid Eyeliner ($8.29) and Voluminous Eyeliner ($7.49); **L'Oreal Paris H.I.P. Makeup** Color Truth Cream Eyeliner ($12); **Maybelline New York** Line Stiletto Ultimate Precision Liquid Eyeliner ($6.99); **Physicians Formula** Eye Definer Felt-Tip Eye Marker ($6.95); **Revlon** ColorStay Liquid Eye Pen ($8.99) and ColorStay Liquid Liner ($7.49); **Sonia Kashuk** Dramatically Defining Long Wearing Gel Liner ($8.99) and Eye Marker ($5.99).

BEST LIQUID, CAKE, OR GEL EYELINERS, AT THE DEPARTMENT/SPECIALTY STORE: **Avon** Perfectly Portable Liquid Eye Liner ($4.99); **BeautiControl** Liquid Eye Liner

($9.50); **Bobbi Brown** Long-Wear Gel Eyeliner ($21); **Cargo** Liquid Liner ($22); **Clinique** Brush-On Cream Liner ($14.50); **Estee Lauder** Double Wear Zero-Smudge Liquid Eyeliner ($19.50); **Lancome** Artliner Precision Point EyeLiner ($28); **Lorac** Front of the Line PRO ($22) and Front of the Line Waterproof Eyeliner ($20); **M.A.C.** Fluidline ($15) and Penultimate Eyeliner ($16.50); **Paula's Choice** Constant Color Gel Eyeliner ($12.95); **Sephora** Long Lasting Metallic Eyeliner ($10); **Smashbox** Waterproof Shadow Liner Duo ($25); **Shu Uemura** Painting Gel Eyeliner ($24); **The Body Shop** Liquid Eyeliner ($13.50); **Trish McEvoy** Eye Definer/Eye Liner ($16).

BEST AUTOMATIC EYE PENCILS, AT THE DRUGSTORE: **Cover Girl** Outlast Smoothwear All-Day Eyeliner ($6.99); **Maybelline New York** Expertwear Defining Liner ($5.79), Line Stylist Eyeliner ($5.79), and Unstoppable Smudge-Proof Waterproof Eyeliner ($7.29); **Rimmel** Exaggerate Full Colour Eye Definer ($6.29).

BEST AUTOMATIC EYE PENCILS, AT THE DEPARTMENT/SPECIALTY STORE: **DHC** Eyeliner Perfect Pro Pencil ($7); **M.A.C.** Technakohl Liner ($14.50); **Trish McEvoy** Precision Brow Shaper ($26).

BEST AUTOMATIC EYEBROW PENCILS, AT THE DRUGSTORE: **Maybelline New York** Define-A-Brow Eyebrow Pencil ($5.49); **Physicians Formula** Brow Definer Automatic Brow Pencil ($5.95).

BEST AUTOMATIC EYEBROW PENCILS, AT THE DEPARTMENT/SPECIALTY STORE: **M.A.C.** Eye Brow Pencils ($14.50); **Origins** Fill in the Blanks Eyebrow Enhancer ($15).

BEST EYEBROW GELS, WAXES, AND BROW TINTS, AT THE DRUGSTORE: **e.l.f.** Wet Gloss Lash & Brow Clear Mascara ($1).

BEST EYEBROW GELS, WAXES, AND BROW TINTS, AT THE DEPARTMENT/SPECIALTY STORE: **Bobbi Brown** Natural Brow Shaper ($19); **Dior** DiorShow Brow Fixing Gel ($17); **Jane Iredale** PureBrow Colours ($16); **Laura Geller** Eyebrow Tint & Tamer ($21.50); **Paula's Choice Brow/Hair Tint** ($9.95); **Sephora** Arch It Brow Kit ($35); **Stila** Brow Polish ($14); **Trish McEvoy** Brow Gel ($20).

BEST LIPSTICKS

How does one decide what constitutes a "best" lipstick? Given the number of lipsticks available and women's wide range of preferences for this essential cosmetic (some like sheer with a glossy finish, others want moderate coverage with a satin finish, or semi-matte textures with shimmer, and on and on and on…). The top picks listed below include all of that and more, with the widest range of choice being the cream lipsticks. Cream lipsticks are middle-of-the-road options that balance what most women want from a lipstick (comfort, moisture, and long-wearing color) with what they don't like but are willing to tolerate (slippery feel, routine touch-ups, and lipstick coming off on coffee cups and significant others). The cream lipsticks rated Paula's Picks have remarkably smooth yet non-greasy textures that provide lots of moisture without slip-sliding all over your mouth. The color range for each was taken into consideration as well, and almost without exception (such as the case with a couple of matte-finish options), the shade range includes soft pink, rose, and nude tones along with deeper reds, burgundies, and plum tones. That being said, it must be noted that the numerous lipsticks rated with a happy face are also worth considering. It all depends on your preferences; that's why it was so difficult to narrow down the list of the best options in this category. Despite the struggle, I feel confident that after all of the lipsticks I tested at counters (not on my lips, nor did I show a bias for lipsticks whose colors looked great on me), those listed below are exemplary in their category and worthy of must-see status.

BEST MATTE OR SEMI-MATTE LIPSTICKS, AT THE DRUGSTORE: Revlon Matte Lipstick ($7.99); **Sonia Kashuk** Velvety Matte Lip Crayon ($6.99).

BEST MATTE OR SEMI-MATTE LIPSTICKS, AT THE DEPARTMENT/SPECIALTY STORE: Clinique Long Last Soft Matte Lipstick ($14); **Estee Lauder** Double Wear Stay-in-Place Lipstick ($22); **M.A.C.** Lipsticks, Mattes ($14); **NARS** Semi-Mattes ($24); **Shu Uemura** Rouge Unlimited Creme Matte Lipstick ($23).

BEST CREAM LIPSTICKS, AT THE DRUGSTORE: Cover Girl Queen Collection Vibrant Hue Color ($6.29); **L'Oreal Paris H.I.P. Makeup** Intensely Moisturizing Lipcolor ($10); **Maybelline New York** Color Sensational Lipcolor ($7.19); **Revlon** Super Lustrous Lipstick ($7.99); **Rimmel** Lasting Finish Intense Wear Lipstick ($5.19) and Lasting Finish Lipstick ($4.99); **Wet `n` Wild** Wild Shine Lip Lacquer ($2.99).

BEST CREAM LIPSTICKS, AT THE DEPARTMENT/SPECIALTY STORE: Clarins Joli Rouge ($23.50); **Clinique** Long Last Soft Shine Lipstick ($14); **DHC** Lip Color Perfect Pro Creme ($20); **Elizabeth Arden** Ceramide Plump Perfect Lipstick ($21.50) and Color Intrigue Lipstick ($19.50); **Estee Lauder** Signature Hydra Lustre Lipstick ($19.50); **Giorgio Armani** Armanisilk Lipstick ($25); **gloMinerals** gloLip Stick ($16.50); **Lancome** Color Design Sensational Effects Lipcolor Smooth Hold ($22); **Laura Geller** Creme Couture Soft Touch Matte Lipstick ($15.50); **Laura Mercier** Lip Velvet ($22); **M.A.C.** Lipsticks, Amplified Cremes ($14) and Lipsticks, Satins ($14); **Mary Kay** Creme Lipstick ($13); **Shiseido** Perfect Rouge Lipstick ($25) and Perfecting Lipstick ($22.50).

BEST SHEER LIPSTICKS, AT THE DRUGSTORE: Boots No7 Sheer Temptation Lipstick ($9.99).

BEST SHEER LIPSTICKS, AT THE DEPARTMENT/SPECIALTY STORE: Avon Glazewear Diamonds Lipstick ($8).

BEST LIPSTICKS WITH SUNSCREEN RATED SPF 15 OR GREATER, AT THE DRUGSTORE: Neutrogena MoistureShine Lipstick with SPF 20 ($9.49).

BEST LIPSTICKS WITH SUNSCREEN RATED SPF 15 OR GREATER, AT THE DEPARTMENT/SPECIALTY STORE: Chanel Aqualumiere Sheer Colour Lipshine SPF 15 ($28.50); **Clinique** High Impact Lipstick SPF 15 ($14); **Paula's Choice** Sheer Cream Lipstick SPF 15 ($10.95).

Note: Although there are very few lipsticks that meet the requirements for being outstanding products that included broad-spectrum sun protection, those listed above are highly recommended. Each includes at least one of the critical UVA-protecting active ingredients to shield lips while providing beautiful color.

BEST LIP PAINTS/STAINS AND LONG-WEARING LIPCOLOR

BEST LIP PAINTS/STAINS LONG-WEARING LIPCOLOR, AT THE DRUGSTORE: Cover Girl Outlast All-Day Lipcolor ($9.99) and Outlast Smoothwear All-Day Lipcolor ($10.30); **Maybelline New York** Superstay Lipcolor ($9.19); **Rimmel** Lasting Finish Kiss & Stay Lipgloss ($7.99).

BEST LIP PAINTS/STAINS LONG-WEARING LIPCOLOR, AT THE DEPARTMENT/SPECIALTY STORE: American Beauty Super Plush 10-Hour Lipcolor ($16.50);

Estee Lauder Double Wear Stay-in-Place Lip Duo ($24); **Lorac** Co-Stars ($19); **M.A.C.** Pro Longwear Lipcolour ($20) and Pro Longwear Lustre Lipcolour ($21).

BEST LIP GLOSSES

Lip gloss is an incredibly popular item for women of all ages. Regardless of where I went or what line I was looking at, if there was one makeup item that made women positively glee-ful, it was lip gloss. I don't know whether it's the low-commitment sheer colors or the glossy finish reminiscent of youth and sex appeal (ads for lip gloss have become quite racy of late, and it's often associated with lingerie). Sephora can be a veritable madhouse of women trying on lip glosses, further testament to the popularity of this type of lip makeup. The lip glosses below feature sheer and opaque options. Sheer lip glosses may be worn alone or over a lipstick; opaque or nearly opaque lip glosses (also known as liquid lipsticks) may be worn alone or over a bold lipstick for added depth and color impact. Each option comes in a gorgeous range of shades and does not have a sticky, gooey, or syrup-like finish. Of course, spending a lot on lip gloss isn't the best idea because it is fleeting, but for those so inclined, there are some great expensive options, too.

BEST SHEER (COLOR) LIP GLOSSES, AT THE DRUGSTORE: Boots Botanics Lip Gloss ($7.99); **Burt's Bees** Super Shiny Lip Gloss ($7); **Cover Girl Queen Collection** Lip Gloss ($5.49); **L'Oreal Paris** Colour Riche Lip Gloss ($5.49) and Bare Naturale Gentle Lip Conditioner ($9.95); **L'Oreal Paris** H.I.P. Makeup Jelly Balm ($9); **Marcelle** Vita-Lip Plumping Gloss ($10.95); **Neutrogena** MoistureShine Gloss ($7.65); **Revlon** Beyond Natural Cream Lip Gloss ($7.99); **Sonia Kashuk** Ultra Shine Sheer Lip Gloss ($8.99).

BEST SHEER (COLOR) LIP GLOSSES, AT THE DEPARTMENT/SPECIALTY STORE: Avon Hollywood Lights Lip Gloss ($7.99); **Cargo** Classic Lip Gloss ($22), High Intensity Gloss ($22), and Lip Gloss Quad ($16.80); **Chanel** Aqualumiere Gloss High-Shine Sheer Concentrate ($27); **Clarins** Colour Quench Lip Balm ($20); **Clinique** Superbalm Moisturizing Gloss ($13.50) and Vitamin C Smoothie Antioxidant Lip Colour ($17.50); **Giorgio Armani** Lip Shimmer ($26); **M.A.C.** Cremesheen Glass ($18) and Lipgelee ($14); **Make Up For Ever** Fascinating Lip Gloss ($18) and Super Lip Gloss ($16); **philosophy** kiss me red tube ($14); **Smashbox** Reflection High Shine Lip Gloss ($19); **Trish McEvoy** Lip Gloss ($22); **Yves Saint Laurent** Touche Brilliance Sparkling Touch for Lips ($30).

BEST PIGMENTED/OPAQUE LIP GLOSSES, AT THE DRUGSTORE: L'Oreal Paris Glam Shine Dazzling Plumping Lipcolour ($8.99); **L'Oreal Paris** H.I.P. Makeup Shine Struck Liquid Lipcolor ($12); **Maybelline New York** Color Sensational Lip Gloss ($6.19); **Rimmel** Vinyl Lip ($5.79).

BEST PIGMENTED/OPAQUE LIP GLOSSES, AT THE DEPARTMENT/SPECIALTY STORE: Avon Glazewear Liquid Lip Color/Glazewear Metallics Lip Gloss ($6); **BeautiCon-trol** Lip Gloss ($14); **Cargo** Lip Gloss Duo ($14); **Clarins** Colour Quench Lip Balm ($20); **Dior** Creme de Gloss ($25.50); **Giorgio Armani** Midnight Lip Shimmer ($26); **gloMinerals** gloLiquid Lips ($14.75; **Korres Natural** Cherry Full Color Gloss ($16); **Laura Geller** Lip Shiner ($16); **Laura Mercier** Liquid Crystal Lip Glace ($22); **Make Up For Ever** Liquid Lip Color ($20); **NYX Cosmetics** Goddess of the Night Lip Gloss with Mega Shine ($4.99); **Trish McEvoy** Lip Gloss ($22); **Urban Decay** Ultraglide Lip Gloss ($17); **Yves Saint Laurent** Gloss Pur Pure Lip Gloss ($29) and Touche Brilliance Sparkling Touch for Lips ($30).

BEST LIP GLOSSES WITH SUNSCREEN RATED SPF 15 OR GREATER, AT THE DRUGSTORE: e.l.f. Super Glossy Lip Shine SPF 15 ($1).

BEST LIP GLOSSES WITH SUNSCREEN RATED SPF 15 OR GREATER, AT THE DEPARTMENT/SPECIALTY STORE: Aveda Lip Tint SPF 15 ($12); **Mark Kay** Tinted Lip Balm with Sunscreen SPF 15 ($13); **Smashbox** Limitless Long-Wearing Lip Gloss SPF 15; **Trish McEvoy** Beauty Booster SPF 15 Lip Gloss ($25).

BEST LIP PENCILS

Automatic lip pencils (i.e., do *not* need-sharpening) are the only ones that earned a Paula's Pick rating. If you don't mind routinely sharpening pencils, there are some good ones to consider outside of the short lists presented here. Otherwise, the pencils below come in a superb range of shades, glide on easily, and have a long-wearing finish that doesn't fade easily.

BEST AUTOMATIC LIP PENCILS, AT THE DRUGSTORE: Almay Ideal Lipliner Pencil ($7.49); **L'Oreal Paris** Infallible Never Fail Lipliner ($8.99); **Revlon** ColorStay Lip Liner ($7.99).

BEST AUTOMATIC LIP PENCILS, AT THE DEPARTMENT/SPECIALTY STORE: Clarins Retractable Lip Definer ($22.50); **Clinique** Quickliner for Lips ($14); **Dior** RougeLiner Automatic Lip Liner ($25); **Lancome** Le Crayon Lip Contour ($22); **Origins** Automagically Lip Lining Pencil ($14.50); **Paula's Choice** Long-Lasting Anti-Feather Lipliner, Clear ($7.95); **The Body Shop** Lip Line Fixer ($11).

BEST MASCARAS

I must hand it to the cosmetics chemists involved in formulating mascaras, because the wealth of superior choices is expanding almost monthly! I should also mention the wide variety of mascara brushes that are available, from a thin comb with serrated edges to a tightly packed full row of nylon bristles, each providing different effects and each deserving of experimentation to see if you prefer the results from one type of brush over another. Performance of any mascara comes down to the perfect marriage of brush and formula, with packaging components (such as the wiper) coming in a close second. The rest is preference-related depending on the lash look you want. I am ecstatic to report there are excellent mascaras in all price ranges, and obviously it is not logical to buy the most expensive mascara when reasonably priced ones are equally good. Given that this is one product you can't readily test at the counters, try a few of the inexpensive ones listed below and see if that isn't the most sensible and beautiful decision.

Because the mascaras listed below are only those rated Paula's Pick, you'll find that each has its own "wow factor"; that is, they offer impressive results quickly and go the distance when it comes to superior application and wear. Although there are plenty of formidable options here, you should also know that any mascara rated with a happy face in this book is worth considering, again, depending on your preferences.

BEST MASCARAS, AT THE DRUGSTORE: Almay Intense i-Color Mascara Volumizing Lash Color ($7.49), One Coat Nourishing Mascara Lengthening ($7.01), and One Coat Nourishing Mascara Triple Effect ($8.19); **Cover Girl** Lash Blast Mascara ($8.69); **e.l.f.** Wet Gloss Lash & Brow Clear Mascara ($1); **L'Oreal Paris** Double Extend Lash Extender & Magnifier Mascara ($10.49), Lash Architect 3-D Dramatic Mascara ($8.29), Lash Architect 3-D Dramatic Mascara, Curved Brush ($8.29), Voluminous Full Definition Volume Building Mascara ($6.99), and Voluminous Naturale Natural-Looking Volume & Definition Mascara

($6.99); **L'Oreal Paris** H.I.P. Makeup High Drama Volumizing Mascara ($10); **Maybelline New York** Define-a-Lash Volume Mascara ($6.29), Full 'n Soft Mascara ($6.59), Intense XXL Volume + Length Microfiber Mascara ($6.79), Lash Discovery Mascara ($6.59), Sky High Curves Extreme Length and Curl Mascara ($6.49), The Colossal Volum' Express Colossal Mascara ($5.99), Volum' Express Mascara 3X ($6.69), Volum' Express Mascara 3X, Curved Brush ($6.69), Volum' Express Turbo Boost Mascara 7X ($7.79), XXL Curl Power Volume + Length Microfiber Mascara ($6.79), XXL Extensions XX-Treme Length Microfiber Mascara ($7.59), and XXL Volume + Length Microfiber Mascara ($7.59); **NYX Cosmetics** Doll Eye Mascara Longlash ($10.99) and Doll Eye Mascara Volume ($10.99); **Revlon** 3D Extreme Mascara ($13.99) and Fabulash Mascara ($6.99); **Rimmel** Eye Magnifier Exact Definition Clean Definition Lengthening Mascara ($6.99), Eye Magnifier Eye Opening Mascara ($6.99), Lash Maxxx 3X Lash Multiplying Effect Mascara ($7.49), Volume Flash Instant Thickening Mascara ($7.49), and Volume Flash Mousse Air-Whipped Volumizing Mascara ($6.99).

　　BEST MASCARAS, AT THE DEPARTMENT/SPECIALTY STORE: Avon Mark Comb Out Lash Lifting Mascara ($6); **BeautiControl** SpectacuLash Mascara ($10) and Spectacu-Lash Thickening Primer and Maximum Length Mascara ($18.50); **Chanel** Exceptionnel De Chanel Intense Volume and Curl Mascara ($30); **Clarins** Pure Curl Mascara ($24) and Pure Volume Mascara ($23.50); **Clinique** High Impact Mascara ($14) and Lash Doubling Mascara ($14); **DHC** Mascara Perfect Pro Double Protection ($17.50); **Dior** Diorshow Iconic Mascara ($27); **Elizabeth Arden** Ceramide Lash Extending Treatment Mascara ($20); **Estee Lauder** Double Wear Zero-Smudge Lengthening Mascara ($19.50) and Sumptuous Bold Volume Lifting Mascara ($19.50); **Giorgio Armani** Soft Lash Mascara ($26); **Kiehl's** Marvelous Mineral Mascara ($16.50); **Korres** Abyssinia Oil Volumising/Strengthening Mascara ($20); **Lancome** Definicils High Definition Mascara ($24), Fatale Exceptional Volume Sculpting 3D Comb Mascara ($23), and L'Extreme Instant Extensions Lengthening Mascara ($24); **Laura Geller** Creamy Mascara ($15.50); **Laura Mercier** Thickening and Building Mascara ($20); **Lorac** Visual Effects Curling, Separating, and Lengthening Mascara ($19.50); **M.A.C.** Pro Lash Mascara ($12) and Zoom Lash Mascara ($12); **Make Up For Ever** Lengthening Mascara ($19); **Paula's Choice** Great Big Lashes Mascara ($9.95) and Lush Mascara ($9.95); **Sephora** Atomic Volume Mascara ($16), Lash Plumper ($16), and Lengthening Mascara ($10); **Smashbox** Bionic Mascara ($19) and Lash DNA Mascara ($19); **Stila** Major Lash Mascara ($8.50); **Yves Saint Laurent** Everlong Mascara Lengthening Mascara ($28.50) and Volume Effet Faux Cils Luxurious Mascara for a False Lash Effect ($28.50).

　　BEST WATERPROOF MASCARAS, AT THE DRUGSTORE: Almay One Coat Nourishing Mascara Triple Effect Waterproof ($7.99); **Maybelline New York** Define-A-Lash Volume Waterproof Mascara ($6.99), Define-A-Lash Waterproof Lengthening Mascara ($6.29), Lash Discovery Waterproof Mascara ($5.99), Sky High Curves Extreme Length and Curl Mascara Waterproof ($6.49), and The Colossal Volum' Express Waterproof Mascara ($6.99); **Revlon** Beyond Natural Defining Mascara Waterproof ($7.99).

　　BEST WATERPROOF MASCARAS, AT THE DEPARTMENT/SPECIALTY STORE: American Beauty Perfectly Waterproof Mascara ($12); **Bobbi Brown** No Smudge Mascara ($22); **Chanel** Inimitable Waterproof Mascara ($30); **Clarins** Wonder Waterproof Mascara ($23.50); **Dior** DiorShow Waterproof Mascara ($24); **Lancome** Definicils Waterproof High Definition Mascara ($24); **Make Up For Ever** Lengthening Waterproof Mascara ($20); **Stila** Lash Visor Waterproof Mascara ($20); **Trish McEvoy** High Volume Waterproof Mascara ($28).

BEST MASCARA PRIMER, AT THE DEPARTMENT/SPECIALTY STORE: Smashbox Layer Lash Primer ($16).

BEST FACE AND BODY ILLUMINATING/SHIMMER PRODUCTS

Given that most cosmetics lines offer at least a few shine-enhancing options, it made sense for this growing, seemingly here-to-stay group of products to have its own category of Paula's Picks. The options below favor liquid shimmer products because they not only tend to be the most versatile but also tend to have the most flattering finishes and shine that clings well to skin. These products are recommended for evening or special-occasion makeup (except weddings if you're the bride; shimmer and shine tend to register as greasy, glossy skin in photographs).

BEST LIQUID, CREAM, CREAM-TO-POWDER, OR GEL SHIMMER PRODUCTS, AT THE DRUGSTORE: Wet 'n' Wild MegaGlo Face Illuminator ($2.99).

BEST LIQUID, CREAM, CREAM-TO-POWDER, OR GEL SHIMMER PRODUCTS, AT THE DEPARTMENT/SPECIALTY STORE: Avon Mark All Lit Up Face Brightening Wand ($8) and Get Bright Hook Up Highlighter ($6); **Chanel** Brillance Pur Sheer Brilliance ($45) and Eclat Lumiere Highlighter Face Pen ($40); **Dior** DiorSkin Shimmer Star ($43); **Giorgio Armani** Fluid Sheer ($58); **Lorac** Oil Free Luminizer ($28) and TANtalizer Body Bronzing Luminizer ($30); **Stila** All Over Shimmer Liquid Luminizer ($22).

BEST PRESSED POWDER WITH SHIMMER, AT THE DEPARTMENT/SPECIALTY STORE: Benefit 10 ($28); **Cle de Peau Beaute** Luminizing Relief Powder ($45); **Clinique** Fresh Bloom Allover Colour ($29.50); **DHC** Face Color Perfect Pro Highlighter ($9); **Lancome** Color Ideal Illuminateur Sheer Highlighting Pressed Powder ($31); **Laura Mercier** Shimmer Bloc ($38); **Lorac** Perfectly Lit Oil-Free Luminizing Powder ($32); **Trish McEvoy** Shimmer Pressed Powder ($32); **Yves Saint Laurent** Teint Parfait Complexion Enhancer ($42).

BEST MINERAL MAKEUP

Mineral Makeup is a hot trend these days, and it doesn't seem to be going away anytime soon. Clearly, many women enjoy this type of makeup, though it definitely has its limitations and isn't nearly as awe-inspiring as companies selling it want you to believe. A detailed summary of mineral makeup can be found on my Web site, www.Beautypedia.com. Nonsubscribers can access this summary for free; simply go to the Master Brand List page and, from the alphabetical list of brands, click on Mineral Makeup. Although I am not a big fan of mineral makeup, the products below are truly impressive and a great place to start if this type of makeup appeals to you.

Note: All of the SPF-rated mineral makeup products below provide sufficient UVA protection. The powders can be an excellent adjunct to your daytime moisturizer or liquid foundation with sunscreen.

BEST MINERAL FOUNDATIONS, AT THE DRUGSTORE: Cover Girl TruBlend Minerals Pressed Mineral Foundation ($9.39); **Neutrogena** Mineral Sheers Powder Foundation SPF 20 ($12.99); **Revlon** ColorStay Mineral Mousse Makeup SPF 20 ($13.99).

BEST MINERAL FOUNDATIONS, AT THE DEPARTMENT/SPECIALTY STORE: Cover FX Powder FX Mineral Powder Foundation ($32); **Estee Lauder** Nutritious Vita-Mineral Loose Powder Makeup SPF 15 ($33.50); **Jane Iredale** Amazing Base Loose Minerals SPF 20 ($42) and PurePressed Base Mineral Foundation SPF 20 ($49.50); **Laura Mercier** Mineral

Powder SPF 15 ($35); **Mary Kay** Mineral Powder Foundation ($18); **Trish McEvoy** Mineral Powder Foundation SPF 15 ($35).

BEST MINERAL POWDERS, AT THE DRUGSTORE: **e.l.f.** Mineral Glow ($8); **L'Oreal Paris** Bare Naturale Soft-Focus Mineral Finish ($15.25); **Physicians Formula** Mineral Wear Talc-Free Mineral Face Powder ($12.95).

BEST MINERAL POWDERS, AT THE DEPARTMENT/SPECIALTY STORE: Jane **Iredale** Amazing Matte Loose Powder ($31); **Lancome** Ageless Minerale Perfecting and Setting Mineral Powder with White Sapphire Complex ($36); **M.A.C.** Mineralize Skinfinish ($26.50); **Trish McEvoy** Correct & Brighten Loose Mineral Powder SPF 15 ($35).

BEST MINERAL BLUSHES, AT THE DRUGSTORE: **L'Oreal Paris** Bare Naturale Gentle Mineral Blush ($15.25).

BEST MINERAL BLUSHES, AT THE DEPARTMENT/SPECIALTY STORE: **BeautiControl** BC Color Mineral Blush ($16); **Jane Iredale** PurePressed Blush ($26).

BEST MINERAL EYESHADOWS, AT THE DEPARTMENT/SPECIALTY STORE: **Jane Iredale** PurePressed Eye Shadows ($17.50); **Mary Kay** Mineral Eye Color ($6.50).

BEST MINERAL LIPSTICKS, AT THE DRUGSTORE: **e.l.f.** Mineral Lip Gloss ($3) and Mineral Lipstick ($5).

BEST MAKEUP BRUSHES

Professional-size brushes are available in all price ranges. Keep in mind that the density, shape, and cut of the brush is more important than the source of the bristles. Although many cosmetics companies love to brag about the type and grade of animal hair used for their brushes, remember, you are not buying a mink coat. Hair softness, brush shape, and firmness (which affect application) are what matters the most, no matter the source. A few companies offer synthetic brushes that are often exquisite replications of natural-hair brushes that must be felt to be believed. These synthetic hair brushes are perfectly worthwhile options, and an easy solution for anyone conflicted about using animal-hair brushes for applying makeup. Please note that not every single brush in the lines listed below is rated a Paula's Pick. For comments on individual brushes and individual Paula's Pick brushes, please refer to the respective cosmetics company's review elsewhere in this book. A brush collection that rates a Paula's Pick represents a superior combination of performance, craftsmanship, and value.

BEST MAKEUP BRUSHES (INCLUDING INDIVIDUAL BRUSHES AND BRUSH SETS), AT THE DRUGSTORE: **e.l.f. Studio** Brushes ($3-$30); **L'Oreal Paris** All Purpose Shadow Brush ($7.89); **Sonia Kashuk** Brushes ($7.99-$21.99).

BEST MAKEUP BRUSHES (INCLUDING INDIVIDUAL BRUSHES AND BRUSH SETS), AT THE DEPARTMENT/SPECIALTY STORE: **Aveda** Flax Sticks ($12-$34); **Chanel** Brushes ($27-$52); **Elizabeth Arden** Face Powder Brush ($28); **Jane Iredale** Brushes ($10.50-$48.50); **Lancome** Ageless Minerale Mineral Powder Foundation Brush ($36); **M.A.C.** Brushes ($11-$125); **Make Up For Ever** Brushes ($13-$65); **NARS** Brushes ($21-$75); **Origins** Brushes ($16-$33.50); **Paula's Choice** Brushes ($9.95-$38.95); **Sephora** Brushes ($5-$58); **Shu Uemura** Brushes ($10-$270); **Smashbox** #13 Foundation Brush ($34); **Stila** Brushes ($15-$50); **Trish McEvoy** Brushes ($14-$90); **Urban Decay** Big Buddha Brush and Big Buddha Brush Set ($36-$138).

BEST SPECIALTY PRODUCTS

Following is a list of miscellaneous products that have interesting effects, are available by prescription only (yet definitely worth considering if their pharmacologic action applies to your needs), or have an intriguing premise that just doesn't fit squarely into the above categories. For details about these products, please refer to the individual reviews in this book.

BEST SPECIALTY PRODUCTS, ALL TYPES, ALL RETAIL LOCATIONS: Eucerin Aquaphor Baby Healing Ointment ($6.99 for 3 ounces); **Clinique** Redness Solutions Urgent Relief Cream ($30 for 1 ounce); **La Prairie** Cellular Lip Line Plumper ($85 for 0.08 ounce); **M.A.C.** Prep + Prime Line Filler ($19.50 for 0.5 ounce) and Prep + Prime Lip ($14.50); **Mary Kay** TimeWise Age-Fighting Lip Primer ($22); **Paula's Choice** Cuticle & Nail Treatment ($10.95 for 0.06 ounce) and Skin Relief Treatment, for All Skin Types ($15.95 for 4 ounces); **Peter Thomas Roth** Lashes to Die For ($125 for 0.2 ounce); **Trish McEvoy** Makeup Planners, Beauty Organizers, and Refillable Compacts ($15-$425); **Urban Decay** Complexion Primer Potion—Brightening ($30).

LINES WHOSE PRODUCTS DID NOT EARN A SINGLE PAULA'S PICK

Although none of the companies listed below has a single product that was rated a Paula's Pick, several of them do offer good options that may be worth considering depending on your needs and preferences. Please do not let these companies' inclusion on this list dissuade you from reading reviews of their products. As a consumer, the final choice about what to purchase and use is up to you. Lines indicated with an asterisk are flagged because it is especially disappointing that, given the cumber of products available, not a single product received a Paula's Pick rating.

Ahava, *Arbonne, *Aubrey Organics, Biore, Coppertone, *Darphin Paris, *Decleor, *Dr. Brandt, Garnier Nutritioniste, *Jurlique International, *Lush, Nivea, Noxzema.

CHAPTER SEVEN

Cosmetic Ingredient Dictionary Online

You can access my comprehensive *Cosmetic Ingredient Dictionary* FREE online in the Learn section of my Web site at www.Cosmeticscop.com or under the Free Reviews & Information section on my Web site at www.Beautypedia.com. This unique, online resource is a great way to find information for over 3,500 cosmetic ingredients ranging from specific antioxidants, anti-wrinkle ingredients, anti-acne ingredients, hundreds of plant extracts, vitamins, minerals, cleansing agents, preservatives, and on and on.

The conclusions reached for all of the skin-care product reviews in this book are based around the product's formulation and what the published scientific research and literature shows to be true about those ingredients. All the details for almost every ingredient can be found in our online *Cosmetic Ingredient Dictionary*. Use this dictionary to gain an understanding of the significance of an ingredient in terms of its claims and its potential (if any) for irritation. You can then use this information to make comparisons among products before you make a purchase. My team and I routinely update this dictionary with new terms and changes to existing terms as new research is published. I hope it helps you demystify the exaggerated and overhyped claims you've been bombarded with by the cosmetics industry.